THERAPY
IN SLEEP
MEDICINE

THERAPY IN SLEEP MEDICINE

Teri J. Barkoukis, MD
Director, Sleep Medicine Fellowship
Professor of Medicine
Division of Pulmonary, Critical Care, Sleep Medicine, and Allergy
Department of Internal Medicine
University of Nebraska Medical Center
Omaha, Nebraska

Jean K. Matheson, MD
Associate Professor of Neurology
Harvard Medical School
Division Chief, Sleep Medicine
Department of Neurology
Beth Israel Deaconess Medical Center
Boston, Massachusetts

Richard Ferber, MD
Associate Professor of Neurology
Harvard Medical School
Director, Center for Pediatric Sleep Disorders
Children's Hospital Boston
Boston, Massachusetts

Karl Doghramji, MD
Professor of Psychiatry and Human Behavior, Neurology, and Medicine
Medical Director, Jefferson Sleep Disorders Center
Thomas Jefferson University
Philadelphia, Pennsylvania

ELSEVIER
SAUNDERS

ELSEVIER
SAUNDERS

1600 John F. Kennedy Blvd.
Ste 1800
Philadelphia, PA 19103-2899

Notice

Knowledge and best practice in this field are constantly changing. As new research and experience broaden our understanding, changes in research methods, professional practices, or medical treatment may become necessary.

Practitioners and researchers must always rely on their own experience and knowledge in evaluating and using any information, methods, compounds, or experiments described herein. In using such information or methods they should be mindful of their own safety and the safety of others, including parties for whom they have a professional responsibility.

With respect to any drug or pharmaceutical products identified, readers are advised to check the most current information provided (i) on procedures featured or (ii) by the manufacturer of each product to be administered, to verify the recommended dose or formula, the method and duration of administration, and contraindications. It is the responsibility of practitioners, relying on their own experience and knowledge of their patients, to make diagnoses, to determine dosages and the best treatment for each individual patient, and to take all appropriate safety precautions.

To the fullest extent of the law, neither the Publisher nor the authors, contributors, or editors, assume any liability for any injury and/or damage to persons or property as a matter of products liability, negligence or otherwise, or from any use or operation of any methods, products, instructions, or ideas contained in the material herein.

Library of Congress Cataloging-in-Publication Data

Therapy in sleep medicine / Teri J. Barkoukis ... [et al.]; pharmacology editor, Jeffrey L. Blumer; section editors, Steven W. Lockley, Carlos H. Schenck.
     p. ; cm.
Includes bibliographical references and index.
ISBN 978-1-4377-1703-7 (hardcover : alk. paper) 1. Sleep disorders—Treatment. I. Barkoukis, Teri J.
[DNLM: 1. Sleep Disorders—therapy. WL 108]
     RC547.T44 2012
     616.8'49806—dc23

2011025305

Associate Acquisitions Editor: Julie Goolsby
Senior Developmental Editor: Ann Ruzycka Anderson
Publishing Services Manager: Patricia Tannian
Senior Project Manager: Sharon Corell
Design Direction: Ellen Zanolle

Printed in the United States of America

Last digit is the print number: 9   8   7   6   5   4   3   2   1

Jeffrey Blumer, PhD, MD
Pharmacology Editor

Steven W. Lockley, PhD
Section 8 Editor
CIRCADIAN RHYTHM DISORDERS

Carlos H. Schenck, MD
Section 10 Editor
PARASOMNIAS IN ADULTS

CONTRIBUTORS

Imran Ahmed, MD
Assistant Professor of Neurology
Director of the Sleep Medicine Fellowship
Albert Einstein College of Medicine
Associate Director, Sleep-Wake Disorders Center
Montefiore Medical Center
Bronx, New York, USA

Donna L. Arand, PhD
Research Associate Professor
Department of Neurology
Wright State University School of Medicine
Dayton, Ohio, USA

Elda Arrigoni, PhD
Assistant Professor
Department of Neurology
Harvard Medical School
Beth Israel Deaconess Medical Center
Assistant Professor
Division of Sleep Medicine
Harvard Medical School
Boston, Massachusetts, USA

Hrayr Attarian, MD
Associate Professor
Department of Neurology
Northwestern University
Chicago, Illinois, USA

Laura K. Barger, PhD
Instructor in Medicine
Division of Sleep Medicine
Harvard Medical School
Associate Physiologist
Department of Medicine
Division of Sleep Medicine
Brigham and Women's Hospital
Boston, Massachusetts, USA

Teri J. Barkoukis, MD
Director, Sleep Medicine Fellowship
Professor of Medicine
Division of Pulmonary, Critical Care, Sleep Medicine,
    and Allergy
Department of Internal Medicine
University of Nebraska Medical Center
Omaha, Nebraska, USA

Kendra Becker, MD, MPH
Sleep Medicine Physician
Department of Sleep Medicine
Kaiser Permanente, Fontana Medical Center
Fontana, California, USA

Kathleen L. Benson, PhD
Research Associate
Department of Psychiatry
Harvard Medical School
Boston, Massachusetts, USA
Research Associate
Brain Imaging Center
McLean Hospital
Belmont, Massachusetts, USA

Matt T. Bianchi, MD, PhD, MMSc
Instructor
Harvard Medical School
Assistant in Neurology
Department of Neurology, Sleep Division
Massachusetts General Hospital
Boston, Massachusetts, USA

Michel M. Billiard, MD
Honorary Professor of Neurology
School of Medicine
Montpellier, France

Sabin R. Bista, MD, MBBS, FAASM
Assistant Professor
Department of Internal Medicine
Division of Pulmonary, Critical Care, Sleep Medicine
    and Allergy
University of Nebraska Medical Center
Nebraska Medical Center
Omaha, Nebraska, USA

Jeffrey Blumer, PhD, MD
Chair, Department of Pediatrics
The University of Toledo
Toledo, Ohio, USA

Michael H. Bonnet, PhD
Professor
Department of Medicine
Wright State University Boonshoft School of Medicine
Dayton, Ohio, USA
Clinical Director
Department of Sleep Disorders
Kettering Medical Center
Kettering, Ohio, USA

George Brainard, PhD
Professor
Department of Neurology
Thomas Jefferson University
Philadelphia, Pennsylvania, USA

Brenda Byrne, PhD
Clinical Assistant Professor
Department of Neurology
Jefferson Medical College
Thomas Jefferson University
Psychologist
Margolis Berman Byrne Health Psychology PC
Philadelphia, Pennsylvania, USA

Rosalind D. Cartwright, PhD, FAASM
Professor Emerita
Neurological Sciences Graduate Division
Rush University Medical Center
Chicago, Illinois, USA

Sudhansu Chokroverty, MD, FRCP
Professor
Department of Neuroscience
Seton Hall University
South Orange, New Jersey, USA
Professor and Co-Chair of Neurology
New Jersey Neuroscience Institute at JFK Medical Center
Edison, New Jersey, USA
Clinical Professor
Department of Neurology
Robert Wood Johnson Medical School
New Brunswick, New Jersey, USA

Daniel A. Cohen, MD, MMSc
Director, Cognitive and Behavioral Neurology
Sentara Neurology Specialists
Sentara Norfolk General Hospital
Norfolk, Virginia, USA

Nancy A. Collop, MD
Professor of Medicine
Director, Emory Sleep Center
Emory University
Atlanta, Georgia, USA

Leopoldo P. Correa, BDS, MS
Assistant Professor
Head, Dental Sleep Medicine
Craniofacial Pain Center
Tufts University School of Dental Medicine
Boston, Massachusetts, USA

Bernadette M. Cortese, PhD
Assistant Professor
Department of Psychiatry and Behavioral Sciences
Medical University of South Carolina
Charleston, South Carolina, USA

Valerie McLaughlin Crabtree, PhD
Director of Clinical Services and Training
Department of Psychology
St. Jude Children's Research Hospital
Memphis, Tennessee, USA

Norma G. Cuellar, RN, DSN, FAAN
Professor
Department of Nursing
University of Alabama
Tuscaloosa, Alabama, USA

Jamie A. Cvengros, PhD, CBSM
Laboratory Director, Sleep Disorders Center
Rush University Medical Center
Assistant Professor of Behavioral Sciences
Rush Medical College
Chicago, Illinois, USA

Nicholas A. DeMartinis, MD
Assistant Clinical Professor
Department of Psychiatry
University of Connecticut Health Center
Farmington, Connecticut, USA
Neuroscience Research Unit
Pfizer Worldwide Research & Development
Groton, Connecticut, USA

Jennifer L. DeWolfe, DO
Assistant Professor of Neurology
Director, UAB Neurology Sleep Services
Epilepsy Division
University of Alabama at Birmingham
Director, BVAMC Sleep Center
Birmingham, Alabama, USA

Christina Diederichs, BA
Sleep Disorders and Research Center
Henry Ford Hospital
Detroit, Michigan, USA

Paul Dieffenbach, MD
Resident Physician
Department of Medicine
Section of General Medicine
Yale University School of Medicine
New Haven, Connecticut, USA

Ehren R. Dodson, PhD
Adjunct Professor
Behavioral Sciences Department
St. Louis Community College
St. Louis, Missouri, USA
Volunteer
Sleep Medicine and Research Center
St. Luke's Hospital
Chesterfield, Missouri, USA

Karl Doghramji, MD
Professor of Psychiatry and Human Behavior, Neurology, and Medicine
Medical Director, Jefferson Sleep Disorders Center
Thomas Jefferson University
Philadelphia, Pennsylvania, USA

Charmane I. Eastman, PhD
Professor
Behavioral Sciences Department
Director
Biological Rhythms Research Laboratory
Rush University Medical Center
Chicago, Illinois, USA

Colin A. Espie, PhD, MAppSci, CPsychol, FBPsS, FCS
Professor of Clinical Psychology
Director
University of Glasgow Sleep Centre
Sackler Institute of Psychobiological Research and Institute
    of Neuroscience & Psychology
College of Medical, Veterinary and Life Sciences
University of Glasgow
Scotland, United Kingdom

Richard Ferber, MD
Associate Professor of Neurology
Harvard Medical School
Director, Center for Pediatric Sleep Disorders
Children's Hospital Boston
Boston, Massachusetts, USA

Michael Friedman, MD, FACS
Professor and Chairman
Section of Sleep Surgery
Rush University Medical Center
Professor and Chairman
Section of Otolaryngology
Advocate Illinois Masonic Medical Center
Medical Director
Advanced Center for Specialty Care
Chicago, Illinois, USA

Suzanne Ftouni, BSc (Hons)
School of Psychology and Psychiatry
Monash University
Melbourne, Victoria, Australia

Patrick M. Fuller, PhD
Assistant Professor
Department of Neurology
Division of Sleep Medicine
Harvard Medical School
Assistant Professor
Department of Neurology
Beth Israel Deaconess Medical Center
Boston, Massachusetts, USA

Hlynur Georgsson, MD
Research Fellow
Department of Neurology and Sleep Medicine
Sunnybrook Health Sciences Centre
University of Toronto
Toronto, Ontario, Canada

Nalaka S. Gooneratne, MD, MSc
Assistant Professor
Divisions of Geriatric Medicine and Sleep Medicine
University of Pennsylvania School of Medicine
Attending Physician
Divisions of Geriatric Medicine and Sleep Medicine
Hospital of the University of Pennsylvania
Associate Director
Clinical and Translational Research Center
Institute for Translational Medicine and Therapeutics
University of Pennsylvania
Philadelphia, Pennsylvania, USA

Madeleine M. Grigg-Damberger, MD
Professor of Neurology
Medical Director, Pediatric Sleep Medicine Services
Associate Director of the Clinical Neurophysiology
    Laboratory
University of New Mexico School of Medicine
University of New Mexico
Albuquerque, New Mexico, USA

Constance Guille, MD
Assistant Professor
Department of Psychiatry and Behavioral Science
Medical University of South Carolina
Charleston, South Carolina, USA

Alex D. Hakim, MD
Sleep Medicine Fellow
Pulmonary and Critical Care Fellow
Departments of Pulmonary and Critical Care Medicine
Cedars-Sinai
Los Angeles, California, USA

Philip A. Hanna, MD
Associate Professor of Neurology
Neurology Residency Program Director
New Jersey Neuroscience Institute at JFK Medical Center
Edison, New Jersey, USA
Seton Hall University School of Health and Medical Sciences
Neurological Director for the Huntington's Disease Unit
JFK Hartwyck at Cedar Brook
Plainfield, New Jersey, USA

Susan M. Harding, MD
Professor of Medicine
Medical Director
UAB Sleep/Wake Disorders Center
Department of Medicine
Division of Pulmonary, Allergy and Critical Care Medicine
University of Alabama at Birmingham
Birmingham, Alabama, USA

David G. Harper, PhD
Assistant Professor of Psychology
Department of Psychiatry
Harvard Medical School
Associate Psychologist
Department of Psychiatry
McLean Hospital
Belmont, Massachusetts, USA

Peter J. Hauri, PhD
Professor Emeritus
Department of Psychiatry and Psychology
Mayo Medical School
Consultant Emeritus
Department of Sleep Medicine
Mayo Clinic
Rochester, Minnesota, USA

Max Hirshkowitz, PhD
Tenured Associate Professor
Department of Medicine and Menninger
Department of Psychiatry
Baylor College of Medicine
Director
Sleep Disorders and Research Center
Michael E. DeBakey Veterans Affairs Medical Center
Houston, Texas, USA

Michael J. Howell, MD
Assistant Professor
Department of Neurology
University of Minnesota
Director, Parasomnia Program
Sleep Disorders Center
University of Minnesota Medical Center
Minneapolis, Minnesota, USA

Thomas D. Hurwitz, MD
Department of Psychiatry/Sleep Medicine
Minneapolis Veterans Affairs Medical Center
Assistant Professor
University of Minnesota Medical School
Minneapolis, Minnesota, USA

Anna Ivanenko, MD, PhD
Associate Professor of Clinical Psychiatry and Behavioral
    Sciences
Feinberg School of Medicine Northwestern University
Associate Professor of Clinical Psychiatry and Behavioral
    Sciences
Division of Child and Adolescent Psychiatry
Children's Memorial Hospital
Chicago, Illinois, USA
Pediatric Sleep Medicine Director
Department of Neuroscience
Central DuPage Hospital
Winfield, Illinois, USA
Pediatric Sleep Medicine Director
Chicago Sleep Group
Elk Grove Village, Illinois, USA

Kyle P. Johnson, MD
Associate Professor
Departments of Psychiatry and Pediatrics
Oregon Health & Science University
Portland, Oregon, USA

Adrienne Juarascio, MS
Doctoral Candidate
Department of Psychology
Drexel University
Philadelphia, Pennsylvania, USA

Naveen Kanathur, MD
Division of Sleep Medicine
Department of Medicine
National Jewish Health
Denver, Colorado, USA

Eliot S. Katz, MD
Assistant Professor in Pediatrics
Harvard University School of Medicine
Department of Respiratory Diseases
Children's Hospital, Boston
Boston, Massachusetts, USA

Abigail L. Kay, MD, MA
Assistant Professor
Department of Psychiatry and Human Behavior
Medical Director, Narcotic Addiction Rehabilitation
    Program
Department of Psychiatry and Human Behavior
Division of Substance Abuse
Thomas Jefferson University Hospital
Philadelphia, Pennsylvania, USA

Suresh Kotagal, MD
Professor
Department of Neurology
Consultant
Division of Child Neurology and the Center for Sleep
    Medicine
Mayo Clinic
Rochester, Minnesota, USA

James M. Krueger, PhD
Regents Professor
Program in Neuroscience
Sleep and Performance Research Center
WWAMI Medical Education Program
Washington State University
Spokane, Washington, USA

Andrew D. Krystal, MD, MS
Director, Insomnia and Sleep Research Program
Professor of Psychiatry and Behavioral Sciences
Duke University School of Medicine
Durham, North Carolina, USA

Brett R. Kuhn, PhD, CBSM
Associate Professor, Pediatrics and Psychology
Department of Psychology
Munroe-Meyer Institute for Genetics and Rehabilitation
University of Nebraska Medical Center
Director, Behavioral Sleep Medicine Services
Children's Sleep Disorders Center
Children's Hospital & Medical Center
Omaha, Nebraska, USA

Simon D. Kyle, PhD
University of Glasgow Sleep Centre
Sackler Institute of Psychobiological Research and Institute
  of Neuroscience & Psychology
College of Medical, Veterinary and Life Sciences
University of Glasgow
Scotland, United Kingdom

Gert Jan Lammers, MD, PhD
Associate Professor
Department of Neurology and Clinical Neurophysiology
Leiden University Medical Center
Leiden, Netherlands

Teofilo L. Lee-Chiong, MD
Professor of Medicine
Chief, Division of Sleep Medicine
Department of Medicine
National Jewish Health
Professor of Medicine
School of Medicine
University of Colorado Denver
Denver, Colorado, USA

Christopher W. Leesman, DO
Research Fellow
Advanced Center for Specialty Care
Chicago, Illinois, USA

Michael R. Littner, MD, FCCP
Emeritus Professor of Medicine
David Geffen School of Medicine at University of California,
  Los Angeles
Los Angeles, California, USA
Volunteer Faculty
Department of Medicine/Pulmonary, Critical Care and Sleep
VA Greater Los Angeles Healthcare System
Sepulveda, California, USA

Steven W. Lockley, PhD
Assistant Professor of Medicine
Division of Sleep Medicine
Harvard Medical School
Associate Neuroscientist
Department of Medicine
Division of Sleep Medicine
Brigham and Women's Hospital
Boston, Massachusetts, USA
Honorary Associate Professor in Sleep Medicine
Clinical Sciences Research Institute
Warwick Medical School
Coventry, United Kingdom
Adjunct Associate Professor
School of Psychology and Psychiatry
Monash University
Melbourne, Australia
Research Associate Woolcock Institute of Medical Research
Sydney, Australia

Liudmila Lysenko, MD
Sleep Medicine Chief Fellow
JFK Medical Center
Edison, New Jersey, USA

Mark W. Mahowald, MD
Minnesota Regional Sleep Disorders Center
Hennepin County Medical Center
Minneapolis, Minnesota, USA

Beth Ann Malow, MD, MS
Professor of Neurology and Pediatrics
Director, Sleep Disorders Division
Vanderbilt University
Director, Vanderbilt Sleep Disorders Center
Nashville, Tennessee, USA

Jennifer L. Martin, PhD
Adjunct Assistant Professor
Department of Medicine
University of California, Los Angeles
Research Health Scientist/Psychologist
Geriatric Research, Education and Clinical Center
VA Greater Los Angeles Healthcare System
Los Angeles, California, USA

Jean K. Matheson, MD
Associate Professor of Neurology
Harvard Medical School
Division Chief, Sleep Medicine
Department of Neurology
Beth Israel Deaconess Medical Center
Boston, Massachusetts, USA

Noshir R. Mehta, BDS, DMD, MDS, MS
Professor and Chair General Dentistry
Director, Craniofacial Pain, Headache and Sleep Center
Associate Dean International Collaborations
Tufts University School of Dental Medicine
Boston, Massachusetts, USA

Murray A. Mittleman, MD, DrPH
Associate Professor of Medicine and Epidemiology
Harvard Schools of Medicine and Public Health
Director, Cardiovascular Epidemiology Research Unit
Beth Israel Deaconess Medical Center
Boston, Massachusetts, USA

Babak Mokhlesi, MD, MSc
Associate Professor of Medicine
Section of Pulmonary and Critical Care
Director, Sleep Disorders Center and Sleep Fellowship
  Program
University of Chicago
Chicago, Illinois, USA

Harvey Moldofsky, MD, Dip.Psych, FRCPC
Professor Emeritus
Faculty of Medicine
Department of Psychiatry
University of Toronto
Honorary Staff
Department of Psychiatry
Toronto Western Hospital
University Health Network
Consultant
Department of Psychiatry
Centre for Addiction and Mental Health
President and Medical Director
Sleep Disorders Clinics
Centre for Sleep and Chronobiology
Toronto, Ontario, Canada

Brian J. Murray, MD, FRCPC D, ABSM
Associate Professor
Department of Neurology and Sleep Medicine
Sunnybrook Health Sciences Centre
University of Toronto
Toronto, Ontario, Canada

David N. Neubauer, MD
Associate Professor
Department of Psychiatry
Johns Hopkins University School of Medicine
Associate Director
Johns Hopkins Sleep Disorders Center
Baltimore, Maryland, USA

Seiji Nishino, MD, PhD
Professor
Department of Sleep and Circadian Neurobiology Laboratory
Stanford University School of Medicine
Palo Alto, California, USA

Sushmita Pamidi, MD, FRCPC
Division of Respiratory Medicine
McGill University Health Centre
Montreal, Quebec, Canada

Rafael Pelayo, MD
Associate Professor
Stanford Sleep Medicine Center
Stanford University School of Medicine
Associate Professor
Department of Psychiatry
Stanford University Medical Center
Redwood City, Canada

Barbara A. Phillips, MD, MSPH, FCCP
Professor
Division of Pulmonary, Critical Care and Sleep Medicine
Department of Internal Medicine
University of Kentucky College of Medicine
Director, Sleep Disorders Center
Good Samaritan University of Kentucky Hospital
Lexington, Kentucky, USA

Grace W. Pien, MD, MS
Assistant Professor of Medicine
Divisions of Sleep Medicine and Pulmonary & Critical Care
Department of Medicine
University of Pennsylvania School of Medicine
Philadelphia, Pennsylvania, USA

Charles Poon, MD
Pulmonary and Critical Care Fellow
Department of Medicine
University of California, Davis
Davis, California, USA
Pulmonary and Critical Care Fellow
Department of Internal Medicine
University of California Davis Medical Center
Sacramento, California, USA

Tanya Pulver, MD
Research Fellow
Advanced Center for Specialty Care
Chicago, Illinois, USA

Stuart F. Quan, MD
Professor of Medicine
Division of Sleep Medicine
Harvard Medical School
Boston, Massachusetts, USA
Professor Emeritus of Medicine
Arizona Respiratory Center
University of Arizona College of Medicine
Tucson, Arizona, USA

Shantha M.W. Rajaratnam, PhD, LLB(Hons)
Associate Professor
School of Psychology and Psychiatry
Monash University
Clayton, Victoria, Australia
Lecturer in Medicine
Division of Sleep Medicine
Brigham and Women's Hospital
Harvard Medical School
Boston, Massachusetts, USA

Winfried J. Randerath, MD
Department of Pneumology
Institute of Pneumology at the University of Witten/
    Herdecke
Department of Pneumology
Bethanien Hospital
Solingen, North Rhine-Westphalia, Germany

Victoria L. Revell, BSc (Hons), PhD
Faculty of Health and Medical Sciences
University of Surrey
Guildford, Surrey, United Kingdom

Brandy M. Roane, MS, LPA, PLMHP
Pediatric Intern
Department of Psychology
Munroe-Meyer Institute for Genetics and Rehabilitation
University of Nebraska Medical Center
Omaha, Nebraska, USA

Timothy A. Roehrs, PhD
Henry Ford Hospital
Sleep Disorders and Research Center
Department of Psychiatry and Behavioral Neurosciences
Wayne State University, School of Medicine
Detroit, Michigan, USA

Carol L. Rosen, MD
Professor
Department of Pediatrics
Case Western Reserve University School of Medicine
Medical Director, Pediatric Sleep Center
Department of Pediatrics
Division of Pulmonology, Allergy and Immunology, and
    Sleep Medicine
Rainbow Babies and Children's Hospital
University Hospitals-Case Medical Center
Cleveland, Ohio, USA

Gerald Rosen, MD
Associate Professor
Department of Pediatrics
University of Minnesota School of Medicine
Minneapolis, Minnesota, USA
Director
Department of Pediatric Sleep Medicine
Children's Hospital of Minnesota
St. Paul, Minnesota, USA
Minnesota Regional Sleep Disorders Center
Hennepin County Medical Center
Minneapolis, Minneapolis, USA

Thomas Roth, PhD
Henry Ford Hospital
Sleep Disorders and Research Center
Department of Psychiatry and Behavioral Neurosciences
Wayne State University, School of Medicine
Detroit, Michigan, USA

David B. Rye, MD, PhD
Professor of Neurology
Emory University School of Medicine & Program in Sleep
Atlanta, Georgia, USA

Noriaki Sakai, DVM, PhD
Visiting Scholar
Department of Sleep and Circadian Neurobiology Laboratory
Stanford University School of Medicine
Palo Alto, California, USA

Carlos H. Schenck, MD
Professor
Department of Psychiatry
University of Minnesota Medical School
Senior Staff Physician
Department of Psychiatry
Minnesota Regional Sleep Disorders Center
Hennepin County Medical Center
Minneapolis, Minnesota, USA

Paula K. Schweitzer, PhD
Director of Research
Sleep Medicine and Research Center
St. Luke's Hospital
Chesterfield, Missouri, USA

Steven J. Scrivani, DDS, DMedSc
Professor
Craniofacial Pain, Headache and Sleep Center
Tufts University School of Dental Medicine
Adjunct
Department of Public Health and Community Medicine
Pain Research, Education and Policy Program
Tufts University School of Medicine
Boston, Massachusetts, USA

Ronald Serota, MD
Assistant Professor
Department of Psychiatry and Human Behavior
Medical Director, Maternal Addiction Treatment Education
    and Research Program
Department of Psychiatry and Human Behavior
Division of Substance Abuse
Thomas Jefferson University Hospital
Philadelphia, Pennsylvania, USA

Rajinder Singh, DO
Fellow in Clinical Neurophysiology
Department of Neurology
Loyola University Chicago
Stritch School of Medicine
Maywood, Illinois, USA

Tracey L. Sletten, BSc (Hons), PhD
School of Psychology and Psychiatry
Monash University
Melbourne, Victoria, Australia

Krystal R. Stober, PsyD
Clinical Instructor
Department of Psychiatry and Human Behavior
Coordinator of Treatment and Training Services
Division of Substance Abuse Programs
Thomas Jefferson University
Philadelphia, Pennsylvania, USA

Shannon S. Sullivan, MD
Assistant Professor
Division of Sleep Medicine
Department of Psychiatry and Behavioral Sciences
Stanford University School of Medicine
Stanford, California, USA
Clinical Assistant Professor
Stanford Sleep Medicine Center
Stanford University Medical Center
Redwood City, California, USA

Michael O. Summers, MD
Director, Nebraska Medical Center Sleep Disorders Center
Assistant Professor of Medicine
Division of Pulmonary, Critical Care, Sleep Medicine,
    and Allergy
Nebraska Medical Center
Omaha, Nebraska, USA

Elizabeth R. Super, MD
Assistant Professor
Department of Pediatrics
Oregon Health and Sciences University
Portland, Oregon, USA

Celeste Thirlwell, MD, FRCPC
Director Sleep/Wake Health Maintenance Program
Sleep Disorders Clinics
Centre for Sleep and Chronobiology
Toronto, Ontario, Canada

Michael J. Thorpy, MD
Director, Sleep-Wake Disorders Center
Montefiore Medical Center
Professor of Neurology
Albert Einstein College of Medicine
Bronx, New York, USA

Lynn Marie Trotti, MD, MS
Assistant Professor of Neurology
Emory University School of Medicine & Program in Sleep
Atlanta, Georgia, USA

Makoto Uchiyama, MD, PhD
Department of Psychiatry
Nihon University School of Medicine
Itabashi-ku, Tokyo, Japan

Thomas W. Uhde, MD
Professor and Chair
Department of Psychiatry and Behavioral Sciences
Medical University of South Carolina
Charleston, South Carolina, USA

Richard L. Verrier, PhD, FACC
Associate Professor of Medicine
Harvard Medical School
Beth Israel Deaconess Medical Center
Harvard-Thorndike Electrophysiology Institute
Boston, Massachusetts, USA

Alvin G. Wee, DDS, MS, MPH
Associate Professor and Director of Maxillofacial
    Prosthodontics
Department of Prosthodontics
Creighton University School of Dentistry
Staff Maxillofacial Prosthodontist
Department of Surgery
VA Nebraska-Western Iowa Health Care System
Affiliate Member
Cancer Prevention and Control Program
University of Nebraska Medical Center Eppley Cancer Center
Omaha, Nebraska, USA

Stephen P. Weinstein, PhD
Professor
Director, Division of Substance Abuse Programs
Psychologist
Department of Psychiatry and Human Behavior
Thomas Jefferson University
Philadelphia, Pennsylvania, USA

Andrew Winokur, MD, PhD
Professor and Dr. Manfred J. Sakel Distinguished
Chair in Psychiatry
University of Connecticut Health Center
Farmington, Connecticut, USA

James K. Wyatt, PhD, DABSM, CBSM
Director, Sleep Disorders Center
Rush University Medical Center
Associate Professor of Behavioral Sciences
Rush Medical College
Chicago, Illinois, USA

H. Klar Yaggi, MD, MPH
Associate Professor of Medicine
Department of Internal Medicine
Pulmonary, Critical Care, Sleep Section
Yale University School of Medicine
New Haven, Connecticut, USA
VA Connecticut Clinical Epidemiology Research Center
West Haven, Connecticut, USA

Mark R. Zielinski, PhD
Research Assistant Professor
Program in Neuroscience
Sleep and Performance Research Center
WWAMI Medical Education Program
Washington State University
Spokane, Washington, USA

PREFACE

The field of sleep medicine has experienced an explosion of publications over the past few decades. The reader may then wonder, "Why another sleep medicine textbook?" *Therapy in Sleep Medicine* is the first compendium of current, state-of-the-art knowledge in the field of sleep medicine applicable specifically to the management and treatment of sleep disorders. It is unique therefore in that its focus is on treatment rather than the disease process itself.

Although we exercised the greatest of care to present the most recent advances in therapies, we remind our readers that scientific discovery is ongoing. Already, since the publication of this textbook, certain guidelines and standards for treatment may have changed. Every effort has been made to ensure that our treatment recommendations are evidence based and consistent with professional guidelines to the extent that current knowledge permits.

In clinical practice, drugs may be used for indications and at doses that are not covered by the package label (i.e., off-label). Therefore we advise readers to consult the peer-reviewed literature as well as the label to obtain the most up-to-date information regarding recommended doses, safety profiles, indications, and other guidelines. Detailed information on any medication can be found through use of the FDA search engine at: http://www.accessdata.fda.gov/scripts/cder/drugsatfda/index.cfm.

Also, new safety alerts first appear on the FDA website at: http://www.fda.gov/Safety/Recalls/default.htm.

It is our sincere hope that you will enjoy the wealth of information presented here to help you manage patients with sleep disorders. We are excited to be able to put a therapeutic manual into your hands to improve both the lives and sleep of your patients. We hope that you will find this book useful to you in your practice, and we welcome readers' suggestions for improvements for future editions.

Editors:

Teri J. Barkoukis

Jean K. Matheson

Richard Ferber

Karl Doghramji

Jeffrey L. Blumer

ACKNOWLEDGMENTS

The goal of this textbook is to provide state-of-the-art information on the treatment of sleep disorders. It spans the entire field of sleep medicine. Therefore its completion involved considerable effort on the part of many to whom we owe our gratitude.

First of all, we extend our thanks to all the chapter contributors who so carefully and critically reviewed the relevant and available information to provide up-to-date guidelines to the readers of this work. This was not an easy task because new information is published daily, and consensus among experts is lacking in many areas. We also gratefully acknowledge the work of our section editors, Dr. Carlos Schenck, editor for the section on adult parasomnias, and Dr. Steven Lockley, editor for the section on circadian rhythm disorders. They provided special levels of expertise and knowledge that helped guide chapter content in these important areas.

Secondly, we extend our deepest appreciation to Dr. Jeffrey Blumer, pharmacology editor for this entire volume. Dr. Blumer reviewed each of the chapters for accuracy regarding drug indication and usage guidelines. Accuracy in such a textbook on therapy is of particular importance and required enormous effort, far more then he likely anticipated when he accepted the task.

We also thank Elsevier staff members, many of whom worked with us from conception to completion. Specifically, we wish to acknowledge the efforts of Adrianne Brigido, who was with us from the outset and whose guidance in formulating the overall plan was invaluable; Dolores Meloni, who offered guidance during the implementation of this work; Julie Goolsby, who joined in to provide important guidance that helped us finish this text; and Ann Ruzycka Anderson, who stood by our side throughout this project, tackling manuscripts, permissions, and illustrations with exceptional skill. We also thank the book designers and other members of the production staff for their skillful finishing touches to this textbook on therapy in sleep medicine.

Finally, we wish to thank the many members of our respective families and friends without whose loving support this work would not have been possible.

Teri J. Barkoukis

Jean K. Matheson

Richard Ferber

Karl Doghramji

A NOTE ON NOMENCLATURE

In 1968 a committee of sleep researchers, led by Drs. Alan Rechtschaffen and Anthony Kales, published the first standard guidelines for the recording and scoring of sleep stages. This document, *A Manual of Standardized Terminology, Techniques and Scoring System for Sleep Stages of Human Subjects* (typically referred to as the *Rechtschaffen and Kales manual* or the *R&K manual*), was the international gold standard until 2007 when the American Academy of Sleep Medicine (AASM) developed a new set of guidelines.[1,2] These revisions evolved from concerns that the R&K manual: 1) allowed for significant variability in the visual interpretation of sleep stages, and 2) was developed with reference to young healthy adults and therefore was not always applicable to variations seen with disease and aging.[3] The new manual is based on an extensive review of the literature and sets forth guidelines for both adult and pediatric studies. Its guidelines encompass digital recording and analysis, reporting parameters, and visual scoring of sleep stages. Definitions are provided for the scoring of arousals, cardiac and respiratory events, and sleep-related movements.

The major changes introduced by the AASM manual were: 1) the recommendation of three (frontal, central, and occipital) rather than two EEG derivations, 2) the merging of stages 3 and 4 into one stage (N3), 3) the abolition of "movement time," and 4) the simplification of some context rules. From a terminological standpoint, the most readily apparent changes are that R&K NREM stages S1, S2, S3, and S4 are now referred to as N1, N2, and N3—with R&K slow wave sleep (SWS) stages S3 and S4 merged into a single stage N3—and stage REM is now referred to as stage R.

The references within this textbook are based on studies that utilized either the older R&K manual or the newer AASM manual guidelines. Rather than apply a uniform nomenclature throughout the textbook, the editors made the decision to adhere to the original nomenclature utilized by referenced studies in order to maintain the accuracy of the original observations and conclusions. Therefore the reader will find both terminologies throughout the text.

1. Rechtschaffen A, Kales A. A Manual of Standardized Terminology, Techniques and Scoring System for Sleep Stages of Human Subject. Washington, D.C.: US Government Printing Office, National Institute of Health Publication, 1968.
2. Iber C, Ancoli-Israel S, Chesson A, Quan SF, eds. The AASM Manual for the Scoring of Sleep and Associated Events: Rules, Terminology, and Technical Specification, 1st ed. Westchester, IL: American Academy of Sleep Medicine, 2007.
3. Danker-Hopfe H, Kunz D, Gruber G, et al. Interrater reliability between scorers from eight European sleep laboratories in subjects with different sleep disorders. *J Sleep Res* 2004;13:63-9.

CONTENTS

SECTION 1
Introduction to Sleep Medicine

Chapter 1   History of Sleep in Society, Sleep Science, and Sleep Medicine, 3
STUART F. QUAN

Chapter 2   Approach to the Patient with a Sleep Disorder, 10
MICHAEL J. THORPY / IMRAN AHMED

Chapter 3   Introduction to Sleep Medicine Diagnostics in Adults, 28
MAX HIRSHKOWITZ

SECTION 2
Background to Sleep Medicine Therapeutics

Chapter 4   An Overview of Sleep, 43
ELDA ARRIGONI / PATRICK M. FULLER

Chapter 5   Essentials of Sleep Neuropharmacology, 62
MATT T. BIANCHI

SECTION 3
Pharmacology Principles

Chapter 6   Stimulant Pharmacology, 85
NORIAKI SAKAI / SEIJI NISHINO

Chapter 7   Pharmacology of Benzodiazepine Receptor Agonist Hypnotics, 99
TIMOTHY A. ROEHRS / CHRISTINA DIEDERICHS / THOMAS ROTH

Chapter 8   Pharmacology of Psychotropic Drugs, 109
NICHOLAS A. DeMARTINIS / ANDREW WINOKUR

Chapter 9   Alternative Therapeutics for Sleep Disorders, 126
ADRIENNE JURASCIO / NORMA G. CUELLAR / NALAKA S. GOONERATNE

SECTION 4
Insomnias

Chapter 10   Overview of Insomnia, 143
MICHAEL H. BONNET / DONNA L. ARAND

Chapter 11   Sleep/Wake Lifestyle Modifications, 151
PETER J. HAURI

Chapter 12   Cognitive Behavioral and Psychological Therapies for Chronic Insomnia, 161
COLIN A. ESPIE / SIMON D. KYLE

Chapter 13   Pharmacotherapeutic Approach to Insomnia in Adults, 172
DAVID N. NEUBAUER

Chapter 14   The Role of Psychology in Sleep Disorders and in Their Treatment, 181
ROSALIND D. CARTWRIGHT

SECTION 5
Sleep-Related Breathing Disorders

Chapter 15   Behavioral and Medical Interventions in Sleep-Related Breathing Disorders, 195
SABIN R. BISTA / MICHAEL O. SUMMERS

Chapter 16   Positive Airway Pressure Therapy for Obstructive Sleep Apnea, 206
NAVEEN KANATHUR / MAX HIRSHKOWITZ / TEOFILO L. LEE-CHIONG

Chapter 17   Surgical Therapy for Obstructive Sleep Apnea/Hypopnea Syndrome, 218
MICHAEL FRIEDMAN / CHRISTOPHER W. LEESMAN / TANYA PULVER

Chapter 18   Oral Appliances in Snoring and Sleep Apnea Syndrome, 230
ALVIN G. WEE

Chapter 19   Central and Mixed Sleep-Related Breathing Disorders, 243
WINFRIED J. RANDERATH

Chapter 20   Nocturnal Ventilation in Chronic Hypercapnic Respiratory Diseases, 254
SUSHMITA PAMIDI / BABAK MOKHLESI

Chapter 21   Sleep-Related Disorders in Chronic Pulmonary Disease, 270
ALEX D. HAKIM / MICHAEL R. LITTNER

SECTION 6
Central Hypersomnolence

Chapter 22   Narcolepsy, 289
GERT JAN LAMMERS

Chapter 23   Non-Narcoleptic Hypersomnias of Central Origin, 297
MICHAEL M. BILLIARD

xvii

SECTION 7
Movement Disorders Affecting Sleep

Chapter 24   Restless Legs Syndrome and Periodic Limb
Movement Disorders, 307
DAVID B. RYE / LYNNE MARIE TROTTI

Chapter 25   Sleep-Related Bruxism, 324
NOSHIR R. MEHTA / STEVEN J. SCRIVANI / LEOPOLDO P. CORREA /
JEAN K. MATHESON

Chapter 26   Sleep Disorders in Parkinson's Disease and
Parkinsonian Syndromes, 330
HLYNUR GEORGSSON / BRIAN J. MURRAY

Chapter 27   Sleep Disruption from Movement Disorders, 345
LIUDMILA LYSENKO / PHILIP A. HANNA /
SUDHANSU CHOKROVERTY

SECTION 8
Circadian Rhythm Disorders

Chapter 28   Overview of the Circadian Timekeeping System
and Diagnostic Tools for Circadian Rhythm Sleep
Disorders, 363
STEVEN W. LOCKLEY

Chapter 29   Shift Work Disorder, 378
SUZANNE FTOUNI / TRACEY L. SLETTEN / LAURA K. BARGER /
STEVEN W. LOCKLEY / SHANTHA M.W. RAJARATNAM

Chapter 30   Jet Lag and Its Prevention, 390
VICTORIA L. REVELL / CHARMANE I. EASTMAN

Chapter 31   Delayed and Advanced Sleep Phase Disorders, 402
JAMES K. WYATT / JAMIE A. CVENGROS

Chapter 32   Other Circadian Rhythm Disorders, 411
STEVEN W. LOCKLEY / DANIEL A. COHEN / DAVID G. HARPER /
MAKOTO UCHIYAMA

SECTION 9
Therapy in Pediatric Sleep-Related Disorders

Chapter 33   Sleep Apnea in Children, 427
CAROL L. ROSEN

Chapter 34   Disorders of Central Respiratory Control During
Sleep in Children, 434
ELIOT S. KATZ

Chapter 35   Pediatric Insomnia and Behavioral
Interventions, 448
BRETT R. KUHN / BRANDY M. ROANE

Chapter 36   Sleep Pharmacotherapeutics for Pediatric
Insomnia, 457
ELIZABETH R. SUPER / KYLE P. JOHNSON

Chapter 37   Circadian Rhythm Disorders in Children, 465
GERALD ROSEN

Chapter 38   Parasomnias, Periodic Limb Movements, and
Restless Legs in Children, 475
SURESH KOTAGAL

Chapter 39   Narcolepsy in Children, 485
SHANNON S. SULLIVAN / RAFAEL PELAYO

Chapter 40   Sleep and Sleep Problems in Children with
Neurologic Disorders, 493
MADELEINE M. GRIGG-DAMBERGER

Chapter 41   Sleep and Sleep Problems in Children with Medical
Disorders, 519
MADELEINE M. GRIGG-DAMBERGER

Chapter 42   Sleep and Sleep Problems in Children with
Psychiatric Disorders, 539
ANNA IVANENKO / VALERIE McLAUGHLIN CRABTREE

SECTION 10
Parasomnias in Adults

Chapter 43   REM Sleep Parasomnias in Adults, 549
CARLOS H. SCHENCK / MARK W. MAHOWALD

Chapter 44   NREM Sleep Parasomnias in Adults, 559
MICHAEL J. HOWELL / CARLOS H. SCHENCK

Chapter 45   Other Parasomnias in Adults, 573
CARLOS H. SCHENCK / THOMAS D. HURWITZ

SECTION 11
Sleep-Related Medical Disorders

Chapter 46   Sleep-Related Cardiac Disorders, 585
RICHARD L. VERRIER / MURRAY A. MITTLEMAN

Chapter 47   Sleep, Chronic Pain, and Fatigue in Rheumatic
Disorders, 595
CELESTE THIRLWELL / HARVEY MOLDOFSKY

Chapter 48   Inflammation and Sleep, 607
MARK R. ZIELINSKI / JAMES M. KRUEGER

Chapter 49   Sleep-Related Gastroesophageal Reflux Disease, 617
SUSAN M. HARDING

SECTION 12
Neurologic Disorders and Sleep

Chapter 50   Approach to Sleep-Related Seizure Identification
and Management, 629
JENNIFER L. DeWOLFE / BETH ANN MALOW

Chapter 51   Sleep-Disordered Breathing and Cerebrovascular
Disease, 647
H. KLAR YAGGI / PAUL DIEFFENBACH

Chapter 52   Sleep Disorders Associated with Dementia, 656
DANIEL A. COHEN

Chapter 53   Sleep Disturbances and Disorders and Their
Treatment in Multiple Sclerosis, 666
RAJINDER SINGH / HRAYR ATTARIAN

SECTION 13
Therapy of Sleep Disturbances Associated with Psychiatric Disorders

Chapter 54   Sleep in Mood Disorders, 675
ANDREW D. KRYSTAL

Chapter 55   Sleep in Anxiety Disorders, 682
CONSTANCE GUILLE / BERNADETTE M. CORTESE /
THOMAS W. UHDE

Chapter 56   Seasonal Affective Disorder, 695
BRENDA BYRNE / GEORGE BRAINARD

Chapter 57   Schizophrenia and Its Associated Sleep Disorders, 705
KATHLEEN L. BENSON

SECTION 14
Special Situations and the Future

Chapter 58   Sleep in Women, 717
GRACE W. PIEN / BARBARA A. PHILLIPS / NANCY A. COLLOP

Chapter 59   Sleep Disorders in Geriatric Patients, 735
KENDRA BECKER / CHARLES POON / JENNIFER L. MARTIN

Chapter 60   Drug Abuse, Dependency, and Withdrawal, 749
ABIGAIL L. KAY / KRYSTAL R. STOBER / RONALD SEROTA /
STEPHEN P. WEINSTEIN

Appendix   Effects of Drugs on Sleep, 761
PAULA K. SCHWEITZER / EHREN R. DODSON

SECTION 1

Introduction to Sleep Medicine

History of Sleep in Society, Sleep Science, and Sleep Medicine

Chapter 1

STUART F. QUAN

The mystery of sleep has been the topic of writings by philosophers, literary writers, religious leaders, and scientists since the beginning of recorded history. However, only in the last century has the seemingly impenetrable cloak surrounding the unconscious state ubiquitously known as "sleep" become more transparent. As in many scientific disciplines, there have been exponential advances in basic and clinical sleep science in recent years with the advent of molecular and genetic tools, as well as the ability to obtain large amounts of detailed information from studies of large populations. There is every reason to anticipate that these rapid advances will continue. Nonetheless, often the best perspective for the future is framed in the context of past events and accomplishments. There have been several reviews of the history of sleep and sleep medicine from different perspectives.[1-5] However, the intent of this chapter is to highlight important events in the development of sleep science and sleep medicine as a scientific discipline and a medical specialty with an update on more recent developments.

SLEEP IN EARLY CIVILIZATION

The Greeks and Romans personified sleep through their deities, Hypnos and Somus, respectively. Moreover, references to sleep can be found in ancient writings. In his epic, *The Odyssey*, the Greek poet Homer wrote in 800 BC, "In his first sleep, call up your hardiest cheer," referring to the segmented sleep pattern commonly practiced at that time. This consisted of two separate periods of waking and sleeping during a 24-hour day.[6] The ancient physician Hippocrates was probably the first to comment on the importance of sleep in relation to health. In section 2 of *Aphorisms*,[7] he writes, "Both sleep and insomnolency, when immoderate, are bad," an observation that is still true today. The ancient Greek philosopher Aristotle wrote an entire treatise entitled *On Sleep and Sleeplessness* in approximately 350 BC.[8] In this essay, Aristotle proposes that "waking and sleep appertain to the same part of an animal, inasmuch as they are opposites, and sleep is evidently a privation of waking." Thus, even in ancient civilizations, it was obvious that sleep and wake are inextricably linked. In his review of historic accounts of obstructive sleep apnea (OSA) syndrome, Kryger notes several ancient accounts of the condition.[9] One of the most compelling is the description of Dionysius, the tyrant of Heracleia in Pontus during the reign of Alexander the Great about 360 BC. It has been written that Dionysius was corpulent, short of breath, and subject to fits of choking. In addition, his physicians prescribed that fine needles be thrust into his abdomen whenever he fell asleep, presumptively to awaken him when he became apneic.

Other ancient civilizations also gave some thought to the purpose of sleep.[6] The Rishis of India contain writings pertaining to waking consciousness and dreaming.[6] In ancient Egypt, temple priests engaged in a form of hypnosis and dream interpretation.[6] References to sleep are found in early Chinese writings as well.[6]

During more recent years, perhaps some of the most notable descriptions of sleep were provided by William Shakespeare (1564-1616). In *Hamlet* appears the well-known phrase "To sleep, perchance to dream...."[10] In *Henry IV*, Shakespeare provides descriptions of what appear to be OSA and Cheyne-Stokes breathing.[6] A few centuries later, another famous literary figure, Dickens, also wrote about OSA in *The Posthumous Papers of the Pickwick Club*. In this 1836 novel,[11] Dickens describes "Joe the Fat Boy," who is depicted as obese, sleepy, and a chronic snorer. As a result of these writings, the "Pickwickian Syndrome" was originally used by Burwell to describe patients with OSA in 1956.[12] Historians believe that Napoleon Bonaparte had the disorder as well. It is well known that he was short and obese, had a thick neck, and took daytime naps.[6] One wonders if the course of history may have been different had Napoleon not been afflicted with the condition. Could, for example, Napoleon have defeated Wellington at Waterloo?

The past few decades have provided numerous examples of the role of sleep disorders in determining the course of history. In the 1950s, then Secretary of State John Foster Dulles failed to negotiate a treaty with Egypt for the United States to build the Aswan Dam because of sleep deprivation from jet lag. Dulles had participated in key meetings with Egyptian leaders immediately after arriving in Egypt from the United States. He later attributed his poor performance to jet lag.[13] More recently, sleep deprivation has been cited as contributing factors to the Challenger and the Exxon Valdez disasters.[13]

A number of events in history have shaped modern day culture with respect to sleep and wakefulness.[6] In 1807, gas lighting was introduced in the city of London, thus enabling city-dwellers to more safely engage in activities normally only performed during daytime.[6] This was quickly replaced in 1879 by the incandescent light bulb, which was invented by Thomas Edison.[6] This discovery opened up the possibility of being active during all hours of the day and night. This factor, combined with the ability to perform work-related activities from virtually anywhere in the world via computers and the Internet, have fostered the notion of a 24-hour society, which dismisses the importance of time spent asleep.

EARLY SCIENTIFIC OBSERVATIONS RELATED TO SLEEP

Although physicians, scientists, and philosophers have made numerous scientific observations and hypotheses related to sleep and biologic rhythms for centuries, it was not until the invention of the electroencephalogram (EEG) that electrophysiologic correlates of sleep and wakefulness could be gathered. The ability to record brain electrical activity was first described by Caton in 1875.[14] This subsequently led to the development of the EEG by Berger in 1929.[15] The first descriptions of what today is known as non-REM (NREM) sleep were made by Loomis and co-workers in 1937.[16] In their writings, they proposed that sleep be divided into five stages, A through E, ranging from the normal waking rhythm (A) to deep sleep and a predominance of delta waves (E). Drowsiness to light sleep occurred in stage B, and spindle activity was described in stages C and D. Nathaniel Kleitman, often called the father of modern sleep research, and his graduate student, Eugene Aserinsky, were the first to describe rapid eye movement (REM) sleep in 1953.[17] Sleep was then reclassified into stages 1 though 4 of NREM and a fifth stage of REM. Subsequently in 1957, the recurring pattern of NREM and REM sleep was observed in the first human all-night sleep recordings by William Dement, who was working with Nathaniel Kleitman as a medical student at the time.[18,19] The international community soon made important contributions to the physiologic study of sleep, as noted by Michel Jouvet's observation that REM sleep was associated with the suppression of skeletal muscle activity.[20]

Armed with the ability to make electrophysiologic recordings of sleep, sleep research in the decade of the 1960s began to accelerate. However, the seminal observations of Loomis and Kleitman[16-18] did not provide a basis for the standardization of how sleep was to be reported or recorded. It was not until 1967 that such standardization was provided, when a group of investigators led by Alan Rechtschaffen and Anthony Kales developed and published a standard sleep recording and scoring system.[21] This system was used by sleep researchers and clinicians without modification until the introduction of a revised version in 2005.

SLEEP MEDICINE AND SLEEP SCIENCE IN THE MODERN ERA

Despite the report of the Pickwickian Syndrome in 1956,[12] sleep medicine remained a rather obscure field until Gastaut and colleagues in 1965 described the presence of obstructive apneic episodes occurring in "Pickwickian" patients.[22] After this report, the practice of sleep medicine, as well as scientific discoveries related to sleep science and circadian biology, accelerated.

In 1971, Konopka and Benzer identified the first circadian clock gene in *Drosophila* and named it *per*.[23] Shortly thereafter, in 1972, the suprachiasmatic nucleus (SCN), a cluster of about 50,000 neurons located in the hypothalamus, was discovered as the site of the body's internal circadian pacemaker.[24,25] Also in 1972, the French spelunker, Michel Siffre, spent 6 months in a cave without external time cues such as light or clocks. His biologic clock became "free-running," stabilizing with a period of approximately 25 hours.[6] Years later, Charles Czeisler and his colleagues demonstrated that the actual human

free-running period was about 24.2 hours.[26] Over the course of the 2 decades spanning 1980 to 2000, important contributions in the field of circadian biology included the introduction of the two process model of sleep regulation, in which the homeostatic sleep drive and a circadian alertness system interact to produce our daily periods of sleep and wakefulness; the discovery that melatonin is important in the regulation of the internal circadian clock and that its secretion is suppressed by light; and that transplantation of the SCN into animals whose SCN had been previously ablated resulted in the restoration of circadian rhythmicity.[6] In the first decade of the 21st century, scientific advances have continued. Circadian clock genes in humans were identified and an inherited mutation in one of them was linked to familial advanced sleep phase syndrome.[27] In addition, a light-sensitive pigment called "melanopsin" was found in retinal ganglion cells to provide light-dark signaling via the retinal retinohypothalamic tract to the SCN.[28]

During the past 20 to 30 years, there have been a number of advances in our understanding of the central mechanisms governing the production of sleep.[6] In 1996, Saper and colleagues identified the ventrolateral preoptic (VLPO) area of the hypothalamus as an area that controls sleep and wakefulness.[29] They described a "sleep switch". When this "switch" is in the "on" position, VLPO neurons are active and wakefulness-promoting pathways are silenced, resulting in sleep; when set in the "off" position, the VLPO area is inactive and wakefulness-promoting areas are active, resulting in wakefulness. Adenosine, which accumulates with sleep deprivation, was demonstrated to induce sleep.[6] This finding provided a mechanism to explain how adenosine antagonists such as caffeine may promote wakefulness. Finally, a number of scientists investigated the interactions of sleep and wakefulness states on metabolic function, temperature regulation, behavioral processes such as learning and memory, and a variety of organ systems.[6]

Clinical research into sleep disorders during the past 20 years has flourished. Drug development studies have paved the way for the development of new pharmacologic compounds to treat insomnia, restless legs syndrome, and narcolepsy, among others. Two milestone clinical studies are also of significance. In 1995, the Sleep Heart Health Study was initiated by the National Institutes of Health (NIH) to investigate whether OSA is a risk factor for cardiovascular disease.[30] It was the first longitudinal cohort study with a primary sleep outcome. Recently published findings from this study demonstrate that OSA is an independent risk factor primarily in men for coronary heart disease, stroke, and increased all-cause mortality rate.[31-33] In addition, in 2003, the NIH sponsored the Apnea Positive Pressure Long-term Efficacy Study (APPLES).[34] APPLES was the first large multicentered randomized controlled clinical trial to be sponsored by the NIH in the area of sleep disorders. It was designed to determine whether continuous positive airway pressure (CPAP) is effective in improving neurocognitive performance in patients with OSA. Analyses of the results of APPLES are currently ongoing.

Although nocturnal polysomnography quickly became the core research and clinical tool for the assessment of sleep and sleep disorders, an objective method for the assessment of daytime sleepiness was not available until 1978 when William Dement and Mary Carskadon described a technique that formed the basis of the multiple sleep latency test, which measures the time it takes a person to fall asleep in a series of daytime naps.[35] It is still used today for research and clinical assessments of daytime sleepiness.

In the past 20 to 30 years, there have been a number of historic highlights related to the pathogenesis and treatment of sleep disorders. In 1972, tracheostomy was introduced as the first definitive treatment for OSA.[36] However, in 1981, Colin Sullivan's description of the application of nasal CPAP revolutionized the treatment of this condition.[37] To this day, CPAP is the primary treatment for OSA. In 1999 and 2000, a deficiency of hypocretin was discovered to be the cause of narcolepsy in animals, and the cause of the disorder in most humans, raising the possibility of replacement therapy sometime in the future and providing additional insights into the role of neurotransmitters in controlling sleep and wakefulness.[38,39] Iron deficiency was discovered to be a core finding in many cases of restless legs syndrome (RLS). In addition, large-scale genetic linkage studies have identified loci on several genes in association with RLS.[40,41] In 2007, the American Academy of Sleep Medicine published the first revision of sleep scoring rules since the original Rechtshaffen and Kales manual and extended their applicability by constructing rules for scoring sleep-disordered breathing, leg movements, cardiac rhythms, digital recording, and pediatric studies.[42]

ORGANIZED SLEEP MEDICINE

The history of organized sleep medicine has been described in detail elsewhere.[2,4] This section provides an updated summary of this area, focusing on the United States.

Sleep Research Society

The wealth of information that emerged from EEG studies of the sleeping brain brought researchers together in informal scientific meetings in the 1960s. Eventually, this group formally organized and became the Association for the Psychophysiological Study of Sleep (first APSS), elected officers, and held annual meetings, which featured formal presentations and published abstracts. With the growth of sleep science to encompass areas other than psychology and physiology, the scientific base of the first APSS broadened, and the society evolved into today's Sleep Research Society (SRS). The first APSS began as an organization of basic sleep researchers and focused on the presentation and advancement of sleep science. Its successor, the SRS, has grown to a membership of greater than 1200 and still has fostering sleep science as its core mission, but with the development of clinical sleep medicine and the recognition that sleep and circadian biology are integral to the function of many systems, SRS members are not only scientists with backgrounds in psychology, and physiology, but also those who specialize in endocrinology, neural sciences, pharmacology, chronobiology, pulmonology, epidemiology, clinical sleep research, and many other fields.

Evolution of Clinical Sleep Professional Societies

The first clinical sleep program ever to be established focused on treating a single sleep disorder, namely narcolepsy. It was established in 1964 by William Dement at Stanford University. Unfortunately[2] it was not financially viable and closed rather quickly. Nonetheless, it was the precursor of a more

enduring initiative, which began in 1970, for a comprehensive sleep clinic at Stanford University. This clinic is still in existence today. Subsequently, several other academic centers started comprehensive sleep evaluation units. Under William Dement's leadership, five centers (Stanford University, the University of Cincinnati, Ohio State University, Baylor College in Houston, and Montefiore Medical Center in New York City) organized in 1975 to form the Association of Sleep Disorders Centers (ASDC). William Dement was elected as the first president and served in this capacity for the next 12 years. The ASDC expanded rapidly, fueled by the growing body of clinical knowledge in sleep disorders and by the recognition that many of these disorders could be effectively treated. Nonetheless, it became apparent that an organization whose basis for membership was "sleep disorders centers" did not meet the professional needs of individual practitioners. This led to the formation of a companion entity, the Clinical Sleep Society, in 1984. However, it was soon realized that two separate clinical organizations, one representing centers and the other individuals, was not efficient. Thus, in 1987, the two entities merged to form the American Sleep Disorders Association (ASDA). The ASDA quickly became recognized as the organization representing the emerging clinical discipline of sleep medicine within the structure of organized medicine in the United States. The ASDA was granted membership in the House of Delegates of the American Medical Association, and became the specialty's representative in interactions with local, state, and federal government agencies. In 1999, under the presidency of Stuart Quan, concerns were raised that the organization's name may lend itself to misidentification as a patient support or advocacy group. This led to a change in name to the American Academy of Sleep Medicine (AASM). Today, the AASM comprises more than 8400 sleep medicine clinicians, researchers, and polysomnographic (PSG) technologists, as well as more than 1200 sleep disorders center members. Its activities include representation of the specialty of sleep medicine to governmental agencies, legislative bodies, and other branches of organized medicine; organization of educational initiatives for its members and the general public; promoting and sponsoring research-related basic sleep mechanisms and clinical sleep medicine; developing accreditation standards for sleep disorders centers; developing standards of practice for sleep medicine; and the publication of the *Journal of Clinical Sleep Medicine*.

The AASM and the SRS, representing the fields of sleep medicine and sleep research, respectively, have overlapping interests. In fact, a number of individuals are members of both organizations. Despite the unsuccessful attempt under then AASM President David White in 1998 to merge the organizations, it remains likely that they will remain distinct entities for the foreseeable future given their separate albeit somewhat overlapping membership and missions.

Associated Professional Sleep Societies

In 1986, the ASDC, SRS, and the Association of Polysomnographic Technologists (APT) formed a federation, which they named the Association of Professional Sleep Societies (second APSS). Its purpose was to operate and plan annual meetings of relevance for sleep researchers and clinicians, and to publish the scientific journal *SLEEP*. By coincidence, the acronym, APSS, is the same as that of the former Association for the Psychophysiological Study of Sleep (first APSS). The APT later left the federation. Subsequently, the federation's name changed to the Associated Professional Sleep Societies, maintaining the same acronym. The second APSS continues to organize the annual "sleep" meeting and to publish the journal *SLEEP*.

World Federation of Sleep Research and Sleep Medicine Societies

Worldwide, sleep research and clinical sleep medicine have emerged as important scientific and clinical disciplines. This growth has led to national and regional organizations of sleep researchers and clinicians. These professional sleep organizations conduct periodic scientific meetings and publish their own scientific journals. In 1988, the SRS, Federation of Latin American Sleep Societies, Asian Sleep Research Society, Canadian Sleep Society, European Sleep Research Society, and the Australasian Sleep Society formed the World Federation of Sleep Research Societies (WFSR). The AASM joined the WFSR in 2003 and the name changed to the World Federation of Sleep Research and Sleep Medicine Societies (WFSRSM). The mission of the WFSRSM is multifaceted: (1) facilitate international collaborations and cooperation among professional sleep societies around the world; (2) promote sleep health as a worldwide public health priority; (3) disseminate globally professional information on sleep medicine and sleep science; (4) foster awareness of the importance of sleep research and the impact of sleep disorders; (5) sponsor international congresses on state-of-the-art developments in sleep medicine and sleep research; and (6) support international training in clinical sleep medicine and sleep research.[43] The WFSRSM organizes a worldwide conference every 4 years and holds a smaller interim conference between the larger meetings.

World Association of Sleep Medicine

Stimulated by the perceived need for a worldwide organization of individual sleep medicine practitioners and researchers, Sudhansu Chokroverty led the effort to form the World Association of Sleep Medicine (WASM) in 2003. As written on their website, "The goal of the World Association of Sleep Medicine (WASM) is to advance knowledge about sleep and sleep disorders among health care personnel and among the public worldwide. WASM was founded to improve sleep health worldwide and to encourage prevention and treatment of sleep disorders." The WASM holds a conference every 4 years.[44]

American Association of Sleep Technologists

Following the emergence of polysomnography and widespread acceptance of it as a valid diagnostic test, the Association of Polysomnographic Technologists (APT) was formed in 1978 to serve the professional needs of polysomnographic technologists. The APT joined the ASDA and the SRS in 1986 to form the second APSS but separated from the APSS several years later. Nevertheless, the APT continues to hold its annual meetings simultaneously with those of the APSS. In 2007, the APT changed its name to the American Association of Sleep Technologists to reflect the broader responsibilities of its members and to enhance recognition of the organization by other entities.

American Academy of Dental Sleep Medicine

In 1991, a small group of dentists who were interested in the use of oral appliances to treat OSA organized the Sleep Disorders Dental Society. The purpose of the society is to foster and disseminate knowledge related to the use of oral appliances and surgery for the treatment of OSA. Over ensuing years, the society grew in membership and its name changed to the American Academy of Dental Sleep Medicine. The AADSM now has more than 1800 members and has held annual meetings in conjunction with the APSS since 1991.

CLINICAL TRAINING IN SLEEP MEDICINE IN THE UNITED STATES

Until the late 1980s, formal training in clinical sleep medicine did not exist. Clinical expertise was acquired through "on the job training" with supervision by those with more experience or by informal, nonstandardized training. In 1989, the ASDA, through its Fellowship Training Committee, defined standards for clinical training and later established a process for the accreditation of fellowship training programs for physicians. Fellowships were to be 1 year long and were to include training in all aspects of sleep medicine. However, it was argued that those who came from a pulmonary medicine background needed little additional training in the care and treatment of patients with sleep-disordered breathing. Therefore, a second type of fellowship was created for physicians specializing in pulmonary medicine and required only 6 months of training in nonpulmonary aspects of sleep medicine in recognition of prior training related to sleep-disordered breathing during the pulmonary fellowship. In these latter fellowships, training in sleep medicine occurred within a 3-year pulmonary/critical care medicine fellowship.

In 2002, as part of its efforts to have sleep medicine certification recognized by the American Board of Medical Specialties, the AASM board of directors successfully completed an application to the Accreditation Council for Graduate Medical Education (ACGME), which resulted in the latter organization's assuming the responsibility of providing accreditation for training programs in sleep medicine. This program led to the development of a set of common training requirements by a committee that included representatives of ACGME, impacted specialties (adult pulmonary, neurology, pediatrics, and psychiatry), and the AASM.* These requirements were approved in 2004, and subsequently served as the basis for the accreditation of 1-year sleep medicine fellowships beginning in 2005. Simultaneously, the AASM ended its accreditation program. The ACGME considers sleep medicine to be a dependent subspecialty. Therefore, all programs must fall under the sponsorship of one of the "parent" specialties, which currently are internal medicine, pediatrics, psychiatry, neurology, and otolaryngology. Initially, each fellowship program was evaluated for accreditation by the Residency Review Committee of the parent specialty. This review revealed variability in the interpretation of the common standards. Consequently, in

---

*The initial Sleep Medicine Training Requirement Development Committee consisted of Michael Sateia, Stuart Quan, Angeline Lazarus, Jasper R. Daube, Andrew Chesson, Daniel Glaze, David Nahrwold, Gail A. McGuinness, Carol B. Lindsley, Karl Doghramji, and John Heffner. Later participants were Aaron Sher and Eric Olson.

2010 the ACGME decided that all sleep medicine fellowship programs, irrespective of parent specialty, would be evaluated for accreditation by the Internal Medicine Residency Review Committee. There are now 72 ACGME accredited sleep medicine fellowships nationwide with 179 fellowship positions open to individuals who have complete ACGME accredited residencies in internal medicine, pediatrics, neurology, psychiatry, otolaryngology, anesthesiology, and family medicine.

The history of clinical training for doctoral level nonphysician clinicians, most of whom are psychologists specializing in behavioral interventions in the treatment of patients with sleep disorders, has followed a course similar to that of physicians. Edward Stepanski spearheaded an initiative between 2001 and 2003, which produced guidelines for training in behavioral sleep medicine in the context of clinical psychology programs. However, as yet there are relatively few training programs in this field.

Originally, training for polysomnographic technologists was informal and consisted primarily of "on the job training" with most technologists entering the field with either little relevant experience, or previous training in EEG or respiratory therapy. In 2003, the Commission on Accreditation of Allied Health Education Programs recognized polysomnographic technology. This recognition led to development and accreditation of 2-year training programs in community colleges, a process that is now overseen by the Committee on Accreditation of Education for Polysomnographic Technologists. In addition, the AASM has established the Accredited Sleep Technology Education Program, or A-STEP, which is a curriculum used by AASM-accredited centers to train polysomnographic technologists.

BOARD CERTIFICATION IN SLEEP MEDICINE

American Board of Sleep Medicine

The need for certification and recognition of competence in polysomnography and sleep medicine was recognized quickly after the formation of the ASDC. The first examination in polysomnography was administered in 1978, and participation grew steadily under the direction of Helmut Schmidt. It eventually became a two-part examination: Part 1 consisted of multiple choice questions and Part 2, which was available for those who passed Part 1, consisted of handwritten interpretations of polysomnograms. Initially, it was administered by the ASDC and its successor, the ASDA. However, in 1980, the ASDA separately incorporated the American Board of Sleep Medicine (ABSM) for the purpose of administering the examination. The examination was open to both physicians and those with PhD degrees. Ultimately, 3445 individuals became diplomates of the ABSM. In 2006, the ABSM ceased administering these examinations, as that task was handed to the ABMS. However, it continues to administer the certification examination in behavioral sleep medicine and to maintain the records of those whom it previously certified.

American Board of Medical Specialties

ABSM Presidents Wolfgang Schmidt-Nowara and Barbara Phillips led overtures over the course of many years supporting the ABMS's acquisition of the sleep medicine certification process. However, these efforts were unsuccessful until the ACGME, prompted by the efforts of Marvin Dunn, accepted the AASM's application for accreditation of sleep medicine training. Shortly thereafter, five-member boards of the ABMS, internal medicine, pediatrics, psychiatry, neurology, otolaryngology, and family medicine agreed to certify physicians as sleep medicine specialists after successful completion of common training requirements and a common examination. The American Board of Anesthesiology became a co-sponsoring board in 2011. The examination was first administered under the administrative auspices of the American Board of Internal Medicine in 2007 and is offered every other year.[45]

NONPHYSICIAN CERTIFICATION

From its inception, the ABSM examination allowed for certification by doctoral-trained nonphysicians, usually individuals with a PhD in clinical psychology. However, when physician certification became the purview of the ABMS, this pathway was no longer available. Therefore, in order to recognize the special role of PhD-trained individuals in the delivery of behavioral interventions to treat sleep disorders, the AASM, under the leadership of Edward Stepanski, began offering certification in behavioral sleep medicine in 2003. In 2008, administration of the examination was transferred to the ABSM.

Recognizing the need to establish a certification examination to for polysomnographic technologists, the APT established a committee to develop an examination that eventually became the American Board of Registered Polysomnographic Technologists. It subsequently changed its name to the Board of Registered Polysomnographic Technologists (BRPT). Originally, the BRPT operated under the auspices of the APT, but it became an independent entity in 2000. More recently, an alternative examination was developed and is now being offered by the National Board for Respiratory Care for respiratory therapists who perform sleep testing. However, it is unclear whether this new examination will gain acceptance by the sleep medicine community and by regulatory agencies. Certification by the BRPT is required for polysomnographic technologist licensure in most cases and is gaining importance as more states require licensing for these professionals.

ACCREDITATION OF SLEEP DISORDERS CENTERS

Accreditation of sleep disorders centers began shortly after the inauguration of the ASDC in 1975. Accreditation by the ASDC, and subsequently by its successors, the ASDA and the AASM, implied that programs met professional standards for the diagnosis and treatment of the gamut of sleep disorders. Accreditation standards have evolved in response to changes in the practice of sleep medicine over time. Many health insurance companies now require AASM accreditation status for reimbursement for services performed in sleep disorders centers. Although the AASM is the most widely recognized accreditation body, boasting over 1200 accredited facilities, other organizations also accredit sleep diagnostic facilities.

NATIONAL CENTER FOR SLEEP DISORDERS RESEARCH

Led by the efforts of William Dement and Senator Mark Hatfield, the National Center for Sleep Disorders Research (NCSDR) was established within the National Institutes of Health (NIH) by an act of the United States Congress in 1993.[4] The NCSDR is housed with the National Heart, Lung and Blood Institute. Although it does not directly fund sleep research, it develops a national sleep research plan that is updated periodically, and serves to coordinate and stimulate sleep research within all of the constituent institutes within the NIH. It also assists in the dissemination of sleep educational materials to the general public.

OTHER ORGANIZATIONS

The emergence of sleep medicine as a recognized clinical discipline spawned the creation of several disease-specific patient support and advocacy groups, including the American Sleep Apnea Association, the Restless Legs Syndrome Foundation, Kleine-Levin Syndrome Foundation, and the Narcolepsy Network. These organizations provide patient educational material, engage in patient advocacy activities, organize meetings, and fund small research projects.

In addition to patient support and advocacy groups, there are several sleep-focused tax-exempt foundations. The ASDA formed the National Sleep Foundation in 1990. It advocates for research and education related to sleep disorders. The most notable activity of the NSF is its annual Sleep in America Poll in which a sample of Americans is surveyed regarding sleep habits and symptoms. In addition, the NSF provides patient educational materials and funds sleep research fellowships and grants. The American Sleep Medicine Foundation and the Sleep Research Society Foundations are the charitable 501c(3) affiliates of the American Academy of Sleep Medicine and the Sleep Research Society, respectively. Through various fund-raising activities, both of these organizations fund research or provide fellowships for research training.

FINAL THOUGHTS

Sleep occupies one third of people's lives. Nevertheless, sleep science and sleep medicine have only recently been established as scientific and medical disciplines. Advances in knowledge and treatment have been accelerating and have resulted in improvements in the quality of life of the human populace. The magnitude of the accomplishments of this field in such a short period of time give many sleep medicine researchers and clinicians greater courage to continue advancing knowledge in this field to better serve all patients.

REFERENCES

1. Deak M, Epstein LJ. History of polysomnography. *Sleep Med Clin*. 2009;4(3):313-321.
2. Dement WC. History of sleep medicine. *Sleep Med Clin*. 2008;3(2):147-156.
3. Kirsch D. There and back again: A current history of sleep medicine. *Chest*. 2011 Apr;139(4):939-946.
4. Shepard Jr JW, Buysse DJ, Chesson Jr AL, et al. History of the development of sleep medicine in the United States. *J Clin Sleep Med*. 2005;1(1):61-82.
5. Thorpy MJ. The history of sleep and man. In: Pollack CP, Thorpy MJ, Yager J, eds. *The Encyclopedia of Sleep and Sleep Disorders (Facts on File Library of Health and Living)*. Chicago, IL: American Library Association; 2009:ix.
6. Shea SA. *Healthy Sleep*. 2008: Available at http://healthysleep.med.harvard.edu/interactive/timeline.
7. Adams CD. *The Genuine Works of Hippocrates*. 1868: Available at http://www.chlt.org/sandbox/dh/Adams/page.49.a.php.
8. Aristotle. *On Sleep and Sleeplessness*. 350 BC. Available at http://www.scribd.com/doc/9321/Aristotle-On-Sleep-Sleeplessness.
9. Kryger MH. Sleep apnea. From the needles of Dionysius to continuous positive airway pressure. *Arch Intern Med*. 1983;143(12):2301-2303.
10. Shakespeare W. Hamlet. 1599: Available at http://shakespeare.mit.edu. ezproxy1.library.arizona.edu/hamlet/full.html.
11. Dickens C. *The Posthumous Papers of the Pickwick Club*. 1836: Available at http://dickens.thefreelibrary.com/The-Posthumous-Papers-Of-The-Pickwick-Club.
12. Bickelmann AG, Burwell CS, Robin ED, et al. Extreme obesity associated with alveolar hypoventilation; a Pickwickian syndrome. *Am J Med*. 1956;21(5):811-818.
13. *How much is sleep deprivation costing you?* 2004: Available at http://health.ninemsn.com.au/azindex/689685/how-much-is-sleep-deprivation-costing-you.
14. Caton R. The electric currents of the brain as reported at the Forty-Third Annual Meeting of the British Medical Association. *Br Med J*. 1875;2(765):278.
15. Berger H. Über das Elektroenkephalogramm des Menschen. *Arch Psychiatr Nervenkr*. 1929;97(1):6-26.
16. Loomis AL, Harvey EN, Hobart GA. Cerebral states during sleep as studied by human brain potentials. *J Exp Psychol*. 1937;21(2):127-144.
17. Aserinsky E, Kleitman N. Regularly occurring periods of eye motility, and concomitant phenomena, during sleep. *Science*. 1953;118(3062):273-274.
18. Dement W, Kleitman N. Cyclic variations in EEG during sleep and their relation to eye movements, body motility, and dreaming. *Electroencephalogr Clin Neurophysiol*. 1957;9(4):673-690.
19. Dement WC. Knocking on Kleitman's door: The view from 50 years later. *Sleep Med Rev*. 2003;7(4):289-292.
20. Jouvet M, Michel F, Courjon J. Sur un stade d'activite electrique cerebrale rapide au cours dusommeil physiologique. *C R Seances Soc Biol Fil*. 1959;153(3):1024-1028.
21. Rechtschaffen A, Kales A. *A Manual of Standardized Terminology, Techniques and Scoring System for Sleep Stages of Human Subject*. Washington, DC: U.S. Government Printing Office, National Institute of Health Publication; 1968.
22. Gastaut H, Tassinari CA, Duron B. Polygraphic study of diurnal and nocturnal (hypnic and respiratory) episodal manifestations of Pickwick syndrome. *Rev Neurol (Paris)*. 1965;112(6):568-579.
23. Konopka RJ, Benzer S. Clock mutants of *Drosophila melanogaster*. *Proc Natl Acad Sci U S A*. 1971;68(9):2112-2116.
24. Moore RY, Eichler VB. Loss of a circadian adrenal corticosterone rhythm following suprachiasmatic lesions in the rat. *Brain Res*. 1972;42(1):201-206.
25. Stephan FK, Zucker I. Circadian rhythms in drinking behavior and locomotor activity of rats are eliminated by hypothalamic lesions. *Proc Natl Acad Sci U S A*. 1972;69(6):1583-1586.
26. Klein T, Martens H, Dijk DJ, et al. Circadian sleep regulation in the absence of light perception: Chronic non-24-hour circadian rhythm sleep disorder in a blind man with a regular 24-hour sleep-wake schedule. *Sleep*. 1993;16(4):333-343.
27. Toh KL, Jones CR, He Y, Eide EJ, Hinz WA, et al. An hPer2 phosphorylation site mutation in familial advanced sleep phase syndrome. *Science*. 2001;291(5506):1040-1043.
28. Gooley JJ, Lu J, Chou TC, et al. Melanopsin in cells of origin of the retinohypothalamic tract. *Nat Neurosci*. 2001;4(12):1165.
29. Sherin JE, Shiromani PJ, McCarley RW, et al. Activation of ventrolateral preoptic neurons during sleep. *Science*. 1996;271(5246):216-219.
30. Quan SF, Howard BV, Iber C, et al. The sleep heart health study: design, rationale, and methods. *Sleep*. 1997;20(12):1077-1085.
31. Gottlieb DJ, Yenokyan G, Newman AB, et al. Prospective study of obstructive sleep apnea and incident coronary heart disease and heart failure: the sleep heart health study. *Circulation*. 2010;122(4):352-360:(Epub 2010, July 12).
32. Punjabi NM, Caffo BS, Goodwin JL, et al. Sleep-disordered breathing and mortality: a prospective cohort study. *PLoS Med*. 2009;6(8):e1000132:(Epub 2009, Aug 18).
33. Redline S, Yenokyan G, Gottlieb DJ, et al. Obstructive sleep apnea-hypopnea and incident stroke: the sleep heart health study. *Am J Respir Crit Care Med*. 2010;182(2):269-277:(Epub 2010, Mar 25).
34. Kushida CA, Nichols DA, Quan SF, et al. The Apnea Positive Pressure Long-term Efficacy Study (APPLES): Rationale, design, methods, and procedures. *J Clin Sleep Med*. 2006;2(3):288-300.
35. Richardson GS, Carskadon MA, Flagg W, et al. Excessive daytime sleepiness in man: multiple sleep latency measurement in narcoleptic and control subjects. *Electroencephalogr Clin Neurophysiol*. 1978;45(5):621-627.

36. Coccagna G, Mantovani M, Brignani F, et al. Tracheostomy in hypersomnia with periodic breathing. *Bull Physiopathol Respir (Nancy)*. 1972;8(5):1217-1227.

37. Sullivan CE, Issa FG, Berthon-Jones M, et al. Reversal of obstructive sleep apnoea by continuous positive airway pressure applied through the nares. *Lancet*. 1981;1(8225):862-865.

38. Chemelli RM, Willie JT, Sinton CM, et al. Narcolepsy in orexin knockout mice: molecular genetics of sleep regulation. *Cell*. 1999;98(4):437-451.

39. Nishino S, Ripley B, Overeem S, et al. Hypocretin (orexin) deficiency in human narcolepsy. *Lancet*. 2000;355(9197):39-40.

40. Stefansson H, Rye DB, Hicks A, et al. A genetic risk factor for periodic limb movements in sleep. *N Engl J Med*. 2007;357(7):639-647.

41. Winkelmann J, Schormair B, Lichtner P, et al. Genome-wide association study of restless legs syndrome identifies common variants in three genomic regions. *Nat Genet*. 2007;39(8):1000-1006.

42. Iber C, Ancoli-Israel S, Chesson A, et al. *The AASM Manual for the Scoring of Sleep and Associated Events: Rules. Terminology and Technical Specifications*. 1st ed. Westchester, IL: American Academy of Sleep Medicine; 2007, 57.

43. *The World Federation of Sleep Research & Sleep Medicine Societies*. Available at http://www.wfsrsms.org/mission.aspx.

44. World Association of Sleep Medicine. Available at http://www.friglobalevents.com/wasmonline/.

45. Quan SF, Berry RB, Buysse D, et al. Development and results of the first ABMS subspecialty certification examination in sleep medicine. *J Clin Sleep Med*. 2008;4(5):505-508.

Chapter 2

Approach to the Patient with a Sleep Disorder

MICHAEL J. THORPY / IMRAN AHMED

PREVALENCE

Complaints relating to sleep and wakefulness are ubiquitous in the general population. Approximately 10% of adults experience insomnia that occurs every night for 2 weeks or more[1] and 30% experience sleep disturbance for a few nights every month. Excessive daytime sleepiness occurring at least 3 days per week has been reported in between 4% and 21% of the population, and severe excessive daytime sleepiness is reported at 5%.[2] Parasomnia behaviors, which are undesirable physical events or experiences that occur during entry into sleep, within sleep, or during arousals from sleep, occur in approximately 90% of the population during their lifetimes, with 12% experiencing five or more parasomnias.[3]

Nevertheless, the majority of people with sleep complaints do not present for treatment. For example, only 6% of people with sleep disturbance seek a physician specifically to address their sleep problem, and over 70% of those with insomnia have never discussed the sleep problem with a physician; the majority resort to over-the-counter medications or self-remedies in order to alleviate the sleep disturbance.[4] Furthermore, about 28% of patients with insomnia have an associated mental disorder that would require management.[5]

CONSEQUENCES

Sleep disorders are associated with significant morbidity and mortality rates. Insomnia, for example, is associated with the future development of depressive and anxiety disorders.[6] Obstructive sleep apnea syndrome (OSA) predisposes to cardiovascular and cerebrovascular disorders and to sudden death during sleep.[7] Because daytime sleepiness can lead to impaired functional ability during the daytime there is the possibility of sleepiness causing motor vehicle or industrial accidents.[8] Several major catastrophic events that have affected society have been ascribed to disturbances of the sleep-wake cycle in the individuals responsible. The Exxon Valdez ship accident in Alaska which led to a major environmental oil disaster, the Challenger space shuttle accident, and the Chernobyl nuclear power station accident are all are examples of major industrial accidents that were in part caused because of human errors as a result of an inadequate sleep-wake pattern.[8]

CLASSIFICATION OF SLEEP DISORDERS

Publication of the International Classification of Sleep Disorders (ICSD) resulted in a unified approach to the classification of over 80 sleep disorders, and greatly enhanced clinical research on patients with sleep-related complaints.

The current classification schema represents the second edition, which was published in 2005, and its structure is based on both symptomatic presentation and underlying pathophysiology (Box 2-1).[9]

CARDINAL SYMPTOMS OF SLEEP DISORDERS

When a patient presents to a physician with a sleep-related complaint, further clarification may be necessary to understand whether the complaint is one of insomnia, excessive daytime sleepiness, or a parasomnia. Once the chief complaint has been identified, a systematic exploration should attempt to identify the nature and severity of the complaint, and the specific sleep disorders that underlie the chief complaint. The rest of this chapter will outline guidelines for this process, yet Box 2-2 lists key questions that can expedite this additional evaluation in routine clinical settings. Nevertheless, a detailed sleep history, coupled with a medical, psychiatric, social, and family history; appropriate questionnaires; and a physical examination are all important in creating a differential diagnosis (Box 2-3).

Presentation

Patients present with one of three major categories of symptoms. The first is insomnia, which may include any combination of difficulty in falling asleep, staying asleep, not sleeping long enough, or feeling unrested upon awakening. The second category is excessive sleepiness or fatigue, which may manifest as cognitive impairment such as difficulty in concentrating, memory or coordination difficulties, tiredness or lack of energy, or sleepiness that may be pervasive and associated with naps or falling asleep at inappropriate times. The third category consists of abnormal events that occur during sleep that can be sensory or motor in nature.

Underlying Factors

The factors motivating the expression of the main complaint and for the clinical presentation must be clearly understood. For example, a complaint of snoring may be an indication of significant marital stress; patients who snore loudly may have moved out of the bedroom to prevent the snoring from disturbing the bed partner. A complaint of insomnia may reflect a concern about potential loss of employment because of poor work efficiency. Patients may have been referred by a physician, or may have been asked to present for treatment by a family member, acquaintance, or work colleague. In addition, the patient may report having no symptoms but the referring

BOX 2-1 *ICSD-2 Sleep Disorder Categories and Individual Sleep Disorders*

Insomnias	ICD-9-CM	ICD-10-CM
Adjustment insomnia (acute insomnia)	307.41	F51.02
Psychophysiological insomnia	307.42	F51.04
Paradoxical insomnia (formerly sleep state misperception)	307.42	F51.03
Idiopathic insomnia	307.42	F51.01
Insomnia due to mental disorder	307.42	F51.05
Inadequate sleep hygiene	V69.4	Z72.821
Behavioral insomnia of childhood	307.42	—
Sleep-onset association type	—	Z73.810
Limit-setting sleep type	—	Z73.811
Combined type	—	Z73.812
Insomnia due to drug or substance	292.85	G47.02
Insomnia due to medical condition (code also the associated medical condition)	327.01	G47.01
Insomnia not due to a substance or known physiological condition, unspecified	780.52	F51.09
Physiological (organic) insomnia, unspecified; (organic insomnia, NOS)	327.00	G47.09
Sleep-Related Breathing Disorders		
Central sleep apnea syndromes		
Primary central sleep apnea	327.21	G47.31
Central sleep apnea due to cheyne stokes breathing pattern	768.04	R06.3
Central sleep apnea due to high altitude periodic breathing	327.22	G47.32
Central sleep apnea due to a medical condition, not cheyne stokes	327.27	G47.31
Central sleep apnea due to a drug or substance	327.29	F10-19
Primary sleep apnea of infancy	770.81	P28.3
Obstructive sleep apnea syndromes		
Obstructive sleep apnea, adult	327.23	G47.33
Obstructive sleep apnea, pediatric	327.23	G47.33
Sleep-related hypoventilation/hypoxemic syndromes		
Sleep-related nonobstructive alveolar hypoventilation, idiopathic	327.24	G47.34
Congenital central alveolar hypoventilation syndrome	327.25	G47.35
Sleep-related hypoventilation/hypoxemia due to a medical condition		
Sleep-related hypoventilation/hypoxemia due to pulmonary parenchymal or vascular pathology	327.26	G47.36
Sleep-related hypoventilation/hypoxemia due to lower airways obstruction	327.26	G47.36
Sleep-related hypoventilation/hypoxemia due to neuromuscular or chest wall disorders	327.26	G47.36
Other sleep-related breathing disorder		
Sleep apnea/sleep-related breathing disorder, unspecified	320.20	G47.30
Hypersomnias of Central Origin		
Narcolepsy with cataplexy	347.01	G47.411
Narcolepsy without cataplexy	347.00	G47.419
Narcolepsy due to medical condition	347.10	G47.421
Narcolepsy, unspecified	347.00	G47.43
Recurrent hypersomnia	780.54	G47.13
Kleine-levin syndrome	327.13	G47.13
Menstrual related hypersomnia	327.13	G47.13
Idiopathic hypersomnia with long sleep time	327.11	G47.11
Idiopathic hypersomnia without long sleep time	327.12	G47.12
Behaviorally induced insufficient sleep syndrome	307.44	F51.12
Hypersomnia due to medical condition	327.14	G47.14
Hypersomnia due to drug or substance	292.85	G47.14
Hypersomnia not due to a substance or known physiological condition	327.15	F51.1
Physiological (organic) hypersomnia, unspecified (organic hypersomnia, NOS)	327.10	G47.10
Circadian Rhythm Sleep Disorders		
Circadian rhythm sleep disorder, delayed sleep phase type	327.31	G47.21
Circadian rhythm sleep disorder, advanced sleep phase type	327.32	G47.22
Circadian rhythm sleep disorder, irregular sleep-wake type	327.33	G47.23
Circadian rhythm sleep disorder, free-running (nonentrained) type	327.34	G47.24
Circadian rhythm sleep disorder, jet lag type	327.35	G47.25
Circadian rhythm sleep disorder, shift work type	327.36	G47.26
Circadian rhythm sleep disorders due to medical condition	327.37	G47.27
Other circadian rhythm sleep disorder	327.39	G47.29
Other circadian rhythm sleep disorder due to drug or substance	292.85	G47.27

Continued

BOX 2-1 *ICSD-2 Sleep Disorder Categories and Individual Sleep Disorders—cont'd*

	ICD-9-CM	ICD-10-CM
Parasomnias		
Disorders of arousal (from non-REM sleep)		
Confusional arousals	327.41	G47.51
Sleepwalking	307.46	F51.3
Sleep terrors	307.46	F51.4
Parasomnias usually associated with REM sleep		
REM sleep behavior disorder (including parasomnia overlap disorder and status dissociatus)	327.42	G47.52
Recurrent isolated sleep paralysis	327.43	G47.53
Nightmare disorder	307.47	F51.5
Sleep related dissociative disorders	300.15	F44.9
Sleep enuresis	788.36	N39.44
Sleep related groaning (catathrenia)	327.49	G47.59
Exploding head syndrome	327.49	G47.59
Sleep-related hallucinations	368.16	R29.81
Sleep-related eating disorder	327.49	G47.59
Parasomnia, unspecified	227.40	G47.50
Parasomnia due to a drug or substance	292.85	G47.54
Parasomnia due to a medical condition	327.44	G47.54
Sleep-Related Movement Disorders		
Restless legs syndrome (including sleep-related growing pains)	333.49	G25.81
Periodic limb movement sleep disorder	327.51	G47.61
Sleep-related leg cramps	327.52	G47.62
Sleep-related bruxism	327.53	G47.63
Sleep-related rhythmic movement disorder	327.59	G47.69
Sleep-related movement disorder, unspecified	327.59	G47.90
Sleep-related movement disorder due to drug or substance	327.59	G47.67
Sleep-related movement disorder due to medical condition	327.59	G47.67
Isolated Symptoms, Apparently Normal Variants, and Unresolved Issues		
Long sleeper	307.49	R29.81
Short sleeper	307.49	R29.81
Snoring	786.09	R06.83
Sleep talking	307.49	R29.81
Sleep starts (hypnic jerks)	307.47	R25.8
Benign sleep myoclonus of infancy	781.01	R25.8
Hypnagogic foot tremor and alternating leg muscle activation during sleep	781.01	R25.8
Propriospinal myoclonus at sleep onset	781.01	R25.8
Excessive fragmentary myoclonus	781.01	R25.8
Other Sleep Disorders		
Other physiological (organic) sleep disorder	327.8	G47.8
Other sleep disorder not due to a known substance or physiological condition	327.8	G47.9
Environmental sleep disorder	307.48	F51.8
APPENDIX A:		
Sleep Disorders Associated with Conditions Classifiable Elsewhere		
Fatal familial insomnia	046.8	A81.8
Fibromyalgia	729.1	M79.7
Sleep related epilepsy	345	G40.5
Sleep related headaches	784.0	R51
Sleep related gastroesophageal reflux disease	530.1	K21.9
Sleep related coronary artery ischemia	411.8	I25.6
Sleep related abnormal swallowing, choking, and laryngospasm	787.2	R13.1
APPENDIX B:		
Other Psychiatric/Behavioral Disorders Frequently Encountered in the Differential Diagnosis of Sleep Disorders		
Mood disorders	—	—
Anxiety disorders	—	—
Somatoform disorders	—	—
Schizophrenia and other psychotic disorders	—	—
Disorders usually first diagnosed in infancy, childhood, or adolescence	—	—
Personality disorders	—	—

From *ICD-9, International Classification of Diseases,* Ninth Revision; *ICD-10, International Classification of Diseases,* Tenth Revision; *ICSD-2, International Classification of Sleep Disorders,* 2nd ed. Courtesy of the American Academy of Sleep Medicine, Westchester, IL, 2005.

- What time do you go to bed and get up on weekdays and weekends?
- Do you have difficulty falling asleep, staying asleep, or awakening in the morning?
- Do you feel rested after a night's sleep?
- Do you have discomfort of your legs or jerking at night?
- Do you snore, gasp, choke, or stop breathing during sleep?
- Do you have any abnormal behavior during the night?
- Do you doze easily or feel sleepy in quiet or monotonous situations?
- Do you take naps?

BOX 2-3 *Differential Diagnosis for the Major Sleep Complaints*

Insomnia
- Insomnia disorders (e.g., psychophysiological insomnia, paradoxical insomnia, inadequate sleep hygiene)
- Sleep-related breathing disorders (e.g., obstructive sleep apnea syndrome, central sleep apnea syndrome)
- Circadian rhythm disorders (e.g., advanced sleep phase syndrome, delayed sleep phase syndrome, shift work disorder)
- Sleep-related movement disorders (e.g., restless legs syndrome, periodic limb movement disorder)
- Isolated symptoms, apparently normal variants and unresolved issues (e.g., sleep starts)
- Medical disorders (e.g., sleep-related gastroesophageal reflux, sleep-related headaches)
- Psychiatric disorders (e.g., anxiety disorders, mood disorders)

Excessive Sleepiness
- Hypersomnias of central origin (e.g., narcolepsy, idiopathic hypersomnia, recurrent hypersomnia)
- Sleep related breathing disorders (e.g., obstructive sleep apnea syndrome)
- Circadian rhythm sleep disorders (e.g., delayed sleep phase syndrome, shift work disorder)
- Sleep related movement disorders (e.g., periodic limb movement disorder)
- Medical disorders (e.g., sleep-related epilepsy)
- Psychiatric disorders (e.g., mood disorders)

Abnormal Events During Sleep
- Parasomnias (e.g., arousal disorders, REM parasomnias, other)
- Sleep-related movement disorders (e.g., restless legs syndrome, periodic limb movement disorders, bruxism, rhythmic movement disorder)
- Sleep-related breathing disorders (e.g., obstructive sleep apnea syndromes, central sleep apnea syndromes)
- Isolated symptoms, apparently normal variants and unresolved issues (e.g., sleep starts, propriomyoclonus at sleep onset)
- Medical disorders (e.g., sleep-related epilepsy, sleep-related gastroesophageal reflux)
- Psychiatric disorders (e.g., post-traumatic stress disorder, nocturnal panic disorder, conversion disorder, Munchausen syndrome by proxy, malingering)

physician may suspect a sleep disorder such as the existence of OSA in the context of obesity, hypertension, or unexplained pulmonary hypertension. Therefore, understanding how the chief complaint affects the patient's relationship and exploring the circumstances surrounding the referral will ensure that the main concern is addressed by the evaluation.

HISTORY OF THE CHIEF COMPLAINT

Insomnia

Sleep-Wake Features and Schedule

Patients with insomnia complain of either difficulty in falling asleep at night, frequent awakenings during the night, early morning awakening, or feeling unrested after sleeping all night. The complaint of disturbed nighttime sleep is usually associated with some impairment of function during the daytime, for example, tiredness or fatigue but not usually excessive sleepiness (defined later in this chapter). Typically, patients with psychophysiologic insomnia are unable to nap during the daytime.[9] The difficulty in sleeping is a 24-hour problem; falling asleep is impaired at night and during the daytime. However, occasionally, patients with psychophysiologic insomnia experience a transient tendency to fall asleep when sedentary and relaxed, in the early evening.

Patients with psychophysiologic insomnia tend to worry throughout the day about the prospect of not sleeping well during the ensuing night. As nighttime approaches, this concern can intensify and, unlike other patients with insomnia who retire early due to tiredness and fatigue, they delay going to bed at night until very sleepy. In addition, patients with insomnia often stay in bed longer in the morning following a night of poor sleep in an attempt to make up for lost sleep. As a result, the timing of their sleep period can become erratic and spread out over a larger portion of the 24-hour day[10] as they spend, for example, anywhere from 8 PM to 8 AM in bed. Any sleep that occurs, therefore, occurs within a 12-hour window and at irregular times. The patient's bedtimes, times to fall asleep, times of awakening, and final wake times are, therefore, very important aspects of the sleep-wake history.

Daytime Symptoms

Typically, insomnia patients complain about tiredness, fatigue, irritability, and mood changes during the daytime and are unable to carry on their usual activities such as housework or activities related to their occupation without a great increase in effort. They also complain of memory, concentration, and attention problems as well as headaches or feelings of abnormal fuzziness or grogginess that may occur intermittently or continuously throughout the day.[9]

Daytime Habits and Behaviors. For a detailed review of daytime habits and behaviors, their effects on sleep and wakefulness, and supporting references, readers are referred to Chapter 11.

The assessment of daytime and evening behaviors is important because they can affect sleep quality. Examples of influencial factors include exercise frequency and timing, and degree of exposure to bright light. Bright light exposure and daytime activity can strengthen circadian rhythms that ultimately improve sleep quality. Bright light exposure is particularly important in immobile or elderly patients, who may spend the majority of the day inside a poorly lit room. Ensuring an adequate amount of inside light exposure during the daytime and an appropriate amount of darkness during the sleep period is important, especially with institutionalized patients. Exposure to dim light, such as that of a computer screen, within a few hours of bedtime can also prolong sleep onset.

Physical activity during the day promotes good sleep at night and inactivity during the daytime may be counterproductive to good sleep. Active exercise close to bedtime may increase stimulation, thereby making sleep onset more difficult.

Caffeine intake can have a negative effect on sleep because its psychostimulant effects can produce psychological activation, preventing sleep onset, and its effects can persist into the sleep period, resulting in fragmented sleep. The effects of caffeine on sleep are highly variable and subject to individual differences in absorption, time of consumption, dosage, and length of consumption, among others. Nevertheless, even one cup of a caffeine-containing drink in the morning can have adverse effects in vulnerable patients.[11] Alcohol is a sedative and can enhance sleep onset, yet it can also have deleterious effects on sleep owing to its rapid metabolism and an ensuing rebound effect, which, in turn, can lead to awakenings in the second half of the night. Large meals, excessive fluid intake, smoking, stimulating foods, and emotionally and physically stimulating activities close to bedtime can all be counterproductive.

Napping. There is a significant negative correlation between total sleep time at night and the mean sleep latency on the following day in primary insomnia patients.[12] Therefore, the inability to sleep at night is related to the same inability during the course of the day in insomnia. This phenomenon is likely due to hyperarousal, a central feature of primary insomnia. Therefore, primary insomnia patients who report little sleep at night also report the inability to nap, despite attempts to do so, to resolve unrelenting daytime fatigue. In contrast, some patients with psychophysiologic insomnia doze momentarily, or nap unintentionally when in a relaxed situation.[9] Napping is common in the elderly and it has been shown that those who nap in the daytime and evening have better quality sleep than those who do not nap,[13] suggesting that nappers have a lower level of hyperarousal or that they suffer from another, co-morbid, sleep disorder. Excessive and regular napping in conjunction with the complaint of insomnia also suggests the presence of co-morbid sleep disorders such as insufficient nocturnal sleep, circadian rhythm disorders, and OSA, among others.

Psychological and Psychiatric Effects

Approximately 30% of patients with chronic insomnia have either a mood or an anxiety disorder; however, most patients with insomnia have some depressive or anxiety features even though they do not meet specific criteria for an Axis I psychiatric diagnosis.[14] Therefore, it is important to ask about hallmark symptoms of depression, such as reduced appetite, tearfulness, depressive affect, and suicidal ideation, and ideally use a questionnaire such as the patient health questionnaire (PHQ9)[15] (Fig. 2-1). If a patient is suspected of having an anxiety disorder, the Generalized Anxiety Disorder Assessment questionnaire, the GAD-7 can be helpful[16] (Fig. 2-2). Alternative questionnaires that can be used include the Beck Depression Inventory Second Edition (BDI-II), a 21-item self-report

instrument intended to assess the existence and severity of symptoms of depression, and the State-Trait Anxiety Inventory (STAI), which differentiates between the temporary condition of state anxiety and the long-standing quality of trait anxiety.[17,18]

Abnormal expectations about sleep can underlie the patient's complaint regarding insomnia.[19] Patients may feel that they need more than 8 hours to adequately function during the daytime or that a small amount of loss of sleep will impair their functional ability during the daytime. Cognitive behavior therapy (CBT) can help eliminate some of these misattributions about sleep.

Circadian Rhythm Sleep Disorders

Complaints of insomnia, coupled with daytime sleepiness can indicate the possibility of circadian rhythm sleep disorders as a cause of these complaints.[9] An evaluation of bedtimes and wake times during the work week and on weekends and days off work can assist in establishing these disorders. The elderly with the complaint of early morning awakening should be particularly evaluated for advanced sleep phase syndrome (ASP), and young adults with the complaint of sleep onset difficulties should be evaluated for delayed sleep phase syndrome (DSP). Shift workers have bedtimes that are not in conformity with social norms and which usually change significantly on days off and with change in shift schedules. A sleep log or diary to show the daily sleep pattern is most important in these evaluations. A 2-week actigraphic evaluation of the sleep pattern can provide further, objective, information.[20]

Excessive Daytime Sleepiness

Excessive Daytime Sleepiness versus Fatigue

Patients who complain of excessive daytime sleepiness (EDS) may use vague terms such as "tired," "fatigued," and "no energy," among others; strictly speaking, however, EDS is defined as the inability to stay awake and alert during the major waking episode of the day, resulting in unintended lapses into drowsiness or sleep.[9] Fatigue, on the other hand, is a physical or psychological feeling of tiredness and occurs with various disorders such as multiple sclerosis and depression. Unlike EDS, it is not associated with an exaggerated physiologic drive for sleep; therefore, fatigued individuals do not fall asleep inappropriately in situations that promote inactivity, such as relaxing in front of a television, sitting and reading quietly, or attending a lecture or a social event with the lights dimmed. Fatigue is promoted by exercise, such as jogging several miles, yet the same situation would not necessarily result in an exaggerated tendency to fall asleep. This distinction between fatigue and EDS is important because EDS indicates problems with sleep at night and specific sleep disorders, whereas fatigue indicates an underlying medical or psychological problem that is not necessarily associated with specific sleep disruption.[21] Fatigue and EDS can coexist in disorders such as multiple sclerosis and Parkinson's disease.[22,23]

Consequences of Excessive Daytime Sleepiness

Because EDS is not always subjectively recognized, questions regarding the predisposition for falling asleep in everyday situations are more revealing.[24,25] These situations include

---

PATIENT HEALTH QUESTIONNAIRE (PHQ-9)—Depression Scale

Patient Name _____ Date _____

Read each item carefully, and circle your response.	Not at all	Several days	More than half the days	Nearly every day
1. Over the last 2 weeks, how often have you been bothered by any of the following problems?				
a. Little interest or pleasure in doing things				
b. Feeling down, depressed, or hopeless				
c. Trouble falling asleep or staying asleep, or sleeping too much				
d. Feeling tired or having little energy				
e. Poor appetite or overeating				
f. Feeling bad about yourself, feeling that you are a failure, or feeling that you have let yourself or your family down				
g. Trouble concentrating on things such as reading the newspaper or watching television				
h. Moving or speaking so slowly that other people could have noticed or being so fidgety or restless that you have been moving around a lot more than usual				
i. Thinking that you would be better off dead or that you want to hurt yourself in some way				
2. If you checked off any problem on this questionnaire so far, how difficult have these problems made it for you to do your work, take care of things at home, or get along with other people?	Not difficult at all	Somewhat difficult	Very difficult	Extremely difficult

How to score PHQ-9
Scoring Method for Diagnosis

Major Depressive Syndrome is suggested if:
• Of the nine items, five or more are circled as at least "More than half the days"
• Either item 1a or 1b is positive, that is, at least "More than half the days"
Minor Depressive Syndrome is suggested if:
• Of the nine items, b, c, or d is circled as at least "More than half the days"
• Either item 1a or 1b is positive, that is, at least "More than half the days"

Scoring Method for Planning and Monitoring Treatment

Question One:
• To score the first question, tally each response by the number value of each response:
Not at all = 0
Several days = 1
More than half the days = 2
Nearly every day = 3
• Add the numbers together to total the score
• Interpret the score by using the guide listed below:

Score	**Action**
≤4	The score suggests the patient may not need depression treatment.
≥5-14	Physician uses clinical judgment about treatment, based on patient's duration of symptoms and functional impairment
≥15	Warrants treatment for depression, using antidepressant, psychotherapy, and/or a combination of treatment

Question Two:
In question two the patient's responses can be one of four: Not difficult at all, Somewhat difficult, Very difficult, Extremely difficult. The last two responses suggest that the patient's functionality is impaired. After treatment begins, the functional status is again measured to see if the patient is improving.

Figure 2-1 Patient Health Questionnaire (PHQ-9) — Depression Scale. (Courtesy of Pfizer, Inc.)

sedentary ones, such as watching television, using a computer, and reading, and more active settings, such as driving. A tendency to doze off when waiting at red traffic lights, or when in stop-and-go traffic, can cause the patient's foot to slip off the brake and may result in damage to the vehicle in front, and implies a high level of EDS that warrants heightened attention. More severe accidents and deaths can result from falling asleep when traveling at higher speeds. The occurrence of sleepiness while driving is a medical emergency; all patients need to be thoroughly evaluated to determine the cause, and appropriate

THE GENERALIZED ANXIETY DISORDER ASSESSMENT (GAD-7)				
	Not at all sure	Several days	Over half the days	Nearly every day
Over the last 2 weeks, how often have you been bothered by the following problems?				
Feeling nervous, anxious, or on edge	0	1	2	3
Not being able to stop or control worrying	0	1	2	3
Worrying too much about different things	0	1	2	3
Trouble relaxing	0	1	2	3
Being so restless that it's hard to sit still	0	1	2	3
Becoming easily annoyed or irritable	0	1	2	3
Feeling afraid as if something awful might happen	0	1	2	3
Add the score for each column Total Score (*add your column scores*)				
If you checked off any problems, how difficult have these problems made it for you to do your work, take care of things at home, or get along with other people? Not difficult at all_____ Somewhat difficult_____ Very difficult_____ Extremely difficult_____				

Scoring: Add the results for question number one through seven to get a total score. If you score 10 or above you might want to consider one or more of the following: discuss your symptoms with your doctor, contact a local mental health care provider or contact my office for further assessment and possible treatment. Although these questions serve as a useful guide, only an appropriate licensed health professional can make the diagnosis of Generalized Anxiety Disorder.

Figure 2-2 The Generalized Anxiety Disorder Assessment (GAD-7). (Data from Spitzer RL, Kroenke K, Williams JB, Lowe B. A Brief Measure for Assessing Generalized Anxiety Disorder: The GAD-7. *Arch Intern Med.* 2006;166[10]:1092-1097.)

treatment should be instituted.[26,27] Excessive sleepiness can also result in chronic cognitive changes, resulting in poor educational and work performance and in an increased risk of accidents at work or in the home. EDS in narcolepsy patients has been associated with impairments in occupational performance, promotion, earning capacity, fear of or actual job loss, and increased disability insurance, as well as work and home accidents. In addition, there are negative effects on education, recreation, and personality related to the disease.[27] EDS may also be associated with depressed affect, although patients may not meet diagnostic criteria for major depression.[9]

Napping

Patients with a complaint of EDS tend to nap excessively during the day. After the nap, the patient may awaken feeling refreshed or still feeling sleepy. Awakening feeling refreshed is a classic description in narcolepsy, whereas awakening unrefreshed is more typical of disorders of disrupted nighttime sleep such as OSA or idiopathic hypersomnia (IH).[9,26] Nap duration greater than 1 hour has an 87% sensitivity and specificity in distinguishing IH from narcolepsy.[28]

Sleep Patterns

Excessive sleepiness limited to the morning hours and associated with sleep onset insomnia, introduces the possibility of delayed sleep phase disorder, whereas EDS limited to the evening hours, especially when associated with early morning awakening, suggests the possibility of advanced sleep phase disorder.[9] Intermittent sleep episodes throughout the 24-hour day suggests an irregular sleep-wake rhythm. A sleep log or diary or an actigraphic evaluation can demonstrate the daily sleep pattern and help establish the diagnosis.

Time Spent in Bed

Short bedtimes can produce EDS. Behaviorally induced insufficient sleep syndrome occurs when an individual persistently fails to obtain the amount of sleep required to maintain normal levels of alertness and wakefulness.[9] Persistent work or leisure activities prior to bedtime, an ultrashort sleep latency, and the use of alarms to awaken in the morning can point to such a difficulty.

Excessive time in bed can be associated with an insomnia disorder, but nocturnal sleep exceeding 10 hours in duration that is accompanied by daily naps can indicate the presence of IH with long sleep time or may indicate a long sleeper if there are no EDS complaints.[9] Nevertheless, actigraphic studies with patients with a presumed diagnosis of IH with long sleep time have indicated that some overestimate sleep duration and actually meet diagnostic criteria for IH with short sleep duration.[29]

Depressed patients with psychomotor retardation typically spend an excessive amount of time in bed both night and day. In turn, prolonged time in bed during the daytime can predispose to napping and result in a reduced quality and quantity of nocturnal sleep.[30]

Abnormal Events During Sleep

Patients may report unusual sensations or motor activity during sleep; they range from unexpected gastrointestinal, respiratory, or cardiac events to violent activity with vocalization to the level of screaming or shouting. Accordingly, when taking a history the clinician needs to consider in the differential diagnosis the diagnostic categories of parasomnias, sleep-related breathing disorders, sleep-related movement disorders, isolated symptoms, apparently normal variants and unresolved issues, sleep disorders classifiable elsewhere, and other psychiatric and behavioral disorders.

Parasomnias

Parasomnias are undesirable physical events or experiences that occur during entry into sleep, within sleep, or during arousals from sleep.[9] Parasomnias comprise abnormal sleep-related movements, behaviors, emotions, perceptions, dreaming, and autonomic nervous system functioning, which includes disorders such as nightmares, sleepwalking, or REM sleep behavior disorder (RBD). They often involve complex, seemingly purposeful and goal-directed behaviors, which are acted outside the conscious awareness of the individual. Most of the parasomnias are defined by their specific behavioral features. Therefore, the characteristics of the disturbance should be carefully noted. As these events may not reach the patient's awareness, reports by bed partners or family members are usually revealing. The age of the patient, the time of occurrence of the event during the night, the presence of dreaming, and the physical features of the condition all help with diagnosis.

Episodes of confusion with mumbling or few spoken words, or nonpurposeful movements such as sitting up in bed, reaching out, or holding something may reflect a confusional arousal. More elaborate activities such as walking during sleep, falling out of bed, or shouting or screaming at night may reflect disorders such as sleepwalking, sleep terrors, or RBD. The time of night that the activities occur can suggest the sleep stage, as sleepwalking and sleep terrors occur in slow wave sleep, which typically occurs in the first third of the night, whereas nightmares and RBD occur in REM sleep, which is more typical in the latter third of the night. Prolonged expiratory groaning during sleep, particularly during the second half of the night, may indicate catathrenia.[9]

Nightmares may not be overly frightening, but simply may evoke a dysphoric emotion such as sadness or anger and can result in insomnia resulting from the fear of going to bed or falling back to sleep and re-experiencing the nightmares. Age often helps in the differential diagnosis, as some disorders such as sleep terrors and sleepwalking are more common in children and young adults, whereas RBD is more common in the elderly. Some activities may be violent. Violent behaviors are reported in nearly 2% of the general population over the age of 15 and are more prevalent in those under the age of 35.[31] Abnormal sexual ("sexsomnia") and violent activity during sleep can pose the risk of harm to self and others and can enhance legal liability.

Sleep-Related Breathing Disorders

Typical symptoms of OSA include snoring, gasping or choking, cessation of breathing during sleep, dry or painful mouth upon awakening, and hyperhidrosis, among others, yet snoring can be the only symptom.[9] Disturbed sleep can be present, whose only manifestation may be bed covers that are unexplicably disheveled. Central sleep apnea syndrome and sleep-related hypoventilation feature symptoms of shallow or absent breathing during sleep that is not accompanied by snoring, at times followed by a hyperventilation phase that follows the apnea episode. In all of these disorders, patients are typically unaware of these symptoms; therefore, to elicit them it is helpful to interview a bed partner or family member. Knowing the patient's sleep position may be helpful, for sleeping on the back may be associated with higher OSA severity.

Sleep-Related Movement Disorders

These disorders are characterized by relatively simple, usually stereotyped, movements that disturb sleep, or monophasic movements such as muscle cramps.[9] The most common disorders that produce subjective symptoms are restless legs syndrome (RLS) and sleep-related leg cramps. The patient either reports discomfort or pain that occurs before sleep onset, or causes awakenings during the night. Periodic limb movement disorder may be experienced by the patient as a jerking movement of the legs, or more rarely the arms. However, it is often asymptomatic and therefore a report from a bed partner of repetitive episodes of leg jerking activity that occur at intervals of 20 to 40 seconds throughout the night may suggest this diagnosis. There can be many other "mimics" for RLS and periodic limb movement disorder such as neuropathies, arthritis, or skin conditions.[32]

Sleep-related movement disorder is a rhythmic movement activity that occurs prior to sleep onset or during sleep that involves large muscle groups. The body may be rocked backward and forward or from side to side and can be associated with physical injury. More common in infants or young children, however, it can persist into adulthood.

Sustained jaw clenching or a series of repetitive muscle contractions, termed rhythmic masticatory muscle activity (RMMA), that occur during sleep may indicate sleep-related bruxism.[9]

Other Sleep Disorders

Abnormal sleep behaviors during the night including restlessness, frequent urination, excessive sweating, gastroesophageal reflux, other abnormal movement activity, and vocalization during sleep should be determined. Episodic and sudden abnormal events, awakening with tongue biting, or urinary incontinence may be signs of a seizure disorder.[33] The clinical features considered in differentiating parasomnias from nocturnal frontal lobe epilepsy (NFLE) episodes include the quality and nature of the behaviors, the progression of the episode, and the nature of the offset. Parasomnias are more likely to have sobbing and "normal" arousal behaviors (such as scratching and face rubbing) and they vary in intensity, with increasing interaction as the event progresses. NFLE episodes more frequently have dystonic posturing and limb or axial automatisms and tend to be brief with limited environmental interaction. Parasomnia motor behaviors taper off, making it difficult to clearly delineate the end of an episode, whereas the offset of events is usually distinct in NFLE and followed by full wakefulness. However, a detailed history from an observer, or ideally a video recording, may be essential in determining the exact nature of these abnormal events.[9]

Episodes of chest pain or acute shortness of breath during sleep may indicate cardiac disease, such as congestive heart failure, ischemic heart disease, and cardiac arrhythmias; breathing disturbances such as COPD and OSA; gastroesophageal reflux; or panic disorder.[9]

MEDICAL, PSYCHIATRIC, SOCIAL, AND FAMILY HISTORY

These aspects of history taking are essential components of any standard clinical evaluation and should, therefore, be included in the routine evaluation of all sleep-related complaints.

Medical and Psychiatric History

In addition to current and past medical and psychiatric disorders and their treatments, the sleep-specific history should elicit greater detail in the area of cardiovascular, nasopharyngeal, neurologic, and psychiatric symptoms. A history of hypertension, heart failure, ischemic heart disease, leg edema, palpitations, or cerebrovascular problems should be inquired about. Many sleep disorders, such as OSA, are sensitive to changes in body habitus; therefore, information on the height, weight, weight change, and any attempts at weight reduction over the prior 5 years should be noted. Sleep-disordered breathing can also be suggested by chronic upper airway obstruction, symptoms of which include obligatory mouth breathing, rhinitis, postnasal drip, and other symptoms of chronic sinusitis, all of which can cause frequent visits to an otolaryngologist or upper airway surgical treatments such as tonsilloadenoidectomy.

A neurologic history should include any change in cognitive functioning such as concentration, focus, and memory. Any prior history of head trauma or central nervous system vascular events or infections may be particularly relevant.

A history of, or symptoms associated with, metabolic and endocrine disturbances such as hypo- or hyperthyroidism and renal and hepatic disease should be inquired about, as these areas are associated with sleep-related complaints.[34] Constipation, loss of smell, and mood disturbances can represent premotor symptoms of Parkinson's disease and early manifestations of RBD.[35] Mood disorders such as major depression and bipolar disorder, and anxiety disorders such as generalized anxiety disorder and panic disorder, are common psychiatric diagnoses that are co-morbid with insomnia.

Childhood and Family History

Family history is relevant in insomnia. There is a familial vulnerability to insomnia, possibly owing, at least in part, to genetic factors; a higher concordance of sleep difficulties has been noted in monozygotic as compared to dizygotic twins.[9] The childhood and family history is particularly relevant in the parasomnias because, as noted earlier, age of onset can be an important clue as to the type of parasomnia. Both ASP and DSP can have an autosomal dominant mode of inheritance and a positive family history may be present in 40% of those with DSP. DSP can be associated with polymorphisms in several factors including the circadian clock gene hPer3, and some families with ASP have a mutation of the hPer2 gene.[9] Other familial disorders include OSA, narcolepsy, and RLS.[9]

Medication and Substances

Medications and substances can have an adverse effect on sleep at night or cause impaired alertness during the daytime. The effects of these medications on sleep and wakefulness are noted in corresponding chapters in this text.

Social and Occupational History

The social history should include family and extended relationships; interpersonal strife can precipitate disturbed sleep and can lead to excessive times spent in bed to avoid family members. Financial and occupational stressors can also contribute to disturbed sleep. The patient's physical activity, light exposure, and a history of drugs, alcohol, excessive caffeine, or smoking is also relevant. For a detailed review of these effects, readers are directed to Chapter 11. Individuals in certain occupations such as commercial drivers, train operators, pilots, and physicians are predisposed to shift work sleep disorder, which features the complaints of insomnia and EDS.[9]

PHYSICAL EXAMINATION

Blood pressure, pulse, body habitus, height, weight, body mass index (BMI), neck circumference, and distribution of body fat (abdominal, neck, etc.) are recorded. A high BMI is associated with OSA.[9] The upper airway should be evaluated for thyromegaly, pharyngeal narrowing, enlarged tonsillar tissue, a large tongue, a low-lying soft palate, and an enlarged and edematous uvula, all potential indicators of OSA.[9]

The Mallampati score, which is based on the inspection of the upper airway, is a sensitive predictor of OSA.[36] The patient is instructed to open the mouth as wide as possible while protruding the tongue as far as possible. There are four classes:

Class I: the soft palate and entire uvula are visible
Class II: the soft palate, hard palate, and upper portion of the uvula are visible
Class III: the soft palate, hard palate, and base of the uvula are visible
Class IV: only the hard palate is visible

For every 1-point increase in the score, the odds of having OSA increase more than twofold. Although this procedure may be useful for nonsleep specialists, in a sleep clinic population the Mallampati class does not significantly modify the likelihood of severe OSA or absence of OSA and is therefore of limited value[37] in that setting.

When appropriate, especially if surgery is being contemplated, the patient should be referred to an otolaryngologist or pulmonologist for endoscopic evaluation of the upper airway to determine if a more specific obstruction is present in the posterior nasopharynx or hypopharynx.

The neurologic examination should include focal neurologic sensory and motor deficits; the latter can indicate the presence of seizures, strokes, or other structural lesions of cortical, subcortical, or brainstem regions. Strategically located lesions in these regions predispose patients to sleep disruption or the development of RBD.[9] The examination should also assess for signs of parkinsonism or Parkinson's disease (bradykinesia, tremor, cogwheel rigidity, postural instability). Evidence of a focal neurologic lesion might also contribute to understanding the etiology of a patient's central sleep apnea.[9] Olfactory dysfunction testing with Sniffin' Sticks, pen-like odor dispensing devices, may confirm hyposmia in patients with RBD or narcolepsy.[38,39] The evaluation of the motor and sensory function of the extremities can indicate neuropathy or a radiculopathy, both of which may present with symptoms mimicking RLS.[32] Poor distal pulses or pedal edema suggest a vascular cause of leg symptoms (e.g., vascular claudication) that is also occasionally confused with RLS.

MENTAL STATUS EXAMINATION

Appearance, attitude, behavior and psychomotor activity, speech (rate, amount, tone, impairments), mood/affect, perception (hallucinations, illusions, depersonalization, derealization), thought process (loose associations, tangential thinking, circumstantiality, blocking, perseveration, echolalia, flight of ideas), thought content (delusions, obsessions, suicidal/homicidal thoughts), judgment, and insight help understand the psychiatric functioning of a patient.

Cognitive function, such as memory and orientation to time, place, and person, should be assessed. The mini-mental status examination (MMSE), a 30-point questionnaire that takes just 10 minutes to complete, can detect dementia, yet it lacks sensitivity and may miss mild cognitive impairment.[40] Neuropsychological testing focusing on conceptualization, motor programming, or inhibitory control may be more sensitive and diagnostically useful than the MMSE.[41]

The Frontal Assessment Battery (FAB) is an evaluation of mental status that can be helpful in patients complaining of cognitive difficulties associated with tiredness, fatigue, or excessive sleepiness.[42] The designed battery consists of six subtests exploring the following: conceptualization, mental flexibility, motor programming, sensitivity to interference, inhibitory control, and environmental autonomy. It takes approximately 10 minutes to administer.

PRIOR MEDICAL REPORTS

These reports can help establish the nature of past and current illnesses as many sleep disorders are chronic in duration. Therefore, patients with these disorders can present for a second opinion or for continued care. Prior sleep medicine evaluations, including polysomnographic study results, and associated treatments are, therefore, of importance.

QUESTIONNAIRES AND INVENTORIES

The comprehensive evaluation of the patient with a sleep disorder includes not only the sleep, medical, and psychiatric history, and the physical examination, but typically includes administration of one or more questionnaires (Box 2-4).

A comprehensive sleep questionnaire such as the Montefiore Sleep Questionnaire (Fig. 2-3) completed by the patient prior to the office consultation may be helpful in expediting the history-taking process.

The Berlin Questionnaire (BQ) is an explorative tool of 13 questions designed to identify patients with OSA. The questions are targeted toward key symptoms of snoring, apneas, daytime sleepiness, hypertension, and excessive weight.[43]

The STOP-BANG questionnaire is a brief questionnaire that is also used as a screening tool for OSA[44] but may be less useful for sleep specialists who need to perform a more in-depth sleep evaluation.

The Insomnia Severity Index (ISI) is a reliable and valid instrument to quantify perceived insomnia severity[45] (Fig. 2-4). The ISI is a clinically useful tool for patients

---

BOX 2-4 *Assessment of the Patient with a Sleep Disorder*

- Clinical interview
  - Direct observation
  - Frequency, nature, and impact of the sleep disorder
  - Perspective of spouse, family member, bed partner
  - Thorough medical, psychiatric, medication, family, and psychosocial history
- Physical examination
- Questionnaires
  - Insomnia Severity Index
  - Epworth Sleepiness Scale (ESS)
  - Karolinska Sleepiness Scale (KSS)/VAS
  - Sleep diary
  - PHQ-9, GAD-7
- Sleep-wake studies
  - Videopolysomnography (PSG)
  - Multiple Sleep Latency Test (MSLT)
  - Maintenance of Wakefulness Test (MWT)
  - Psychomotor Vigilance Test (PVT)
  - Actigraphy
- Additional studies
  - Blood tests (e.g., chemistry, endocrine, immune)
  - Cerebrospinal fluid analysis (hypocretin)
  - Fiberoptic endoscopy, cephalometric x-ray studies
  - Neuroimaging
  - Electromyogram (EMG) and nerve conduction velocity (NCV) studies
  - Electroencephalogram (EEG)
  - Neuropsychological/performance testing

---

with insomnia but is more often used in research studies of insomnia.

Epworth Sleepiness Scale (ESS) is a valuable instrument for determining the presence of daytime sleepiness over 2 weeks[46] (Fig. 2-5). The patient scores the likelihood of dozing in eight common everyday situations on a rating scale of 0 to 3, leading to a maximum score of 24. Patients with a score of 10 or higher are considered to have significant daytime sleepiness, and those who score over 15 have severe daytime sleepiness.

Karolinska Sleepiness Scale (KSS) is a simple scale that assesses sleepiness at a particular point in time[47] (Box 2-5). It is a variation of a previously used scale called the *Stanford Sleepiness Scale,* and consists of statements whereby the patient assesses himself on a 10-point scale as very alert through very sleepy and ranks an alertness level. An alternative to the KSS is a visual analog scale (VAS) with a 10-cm line that has very alert at one end and very sleepy at the other, and the patient marks an appropriate point along the line.

The Pittsburgh Sleep Quality Index (PSQI) is a self-rated questionnaire that assesses sleep quality and disturbances over a 1-month time interval.[48] Nineteen individual items generate seven "component" scores: subjective sleep quality, sleep latency, sleep duration, habitual sleep efficiency, sleep disturbances, use of sleeping medication, and daytime dysfunction. The sum of the scores for these seven components yields one global score.

Name: _____ Date: _____

Age: _____ Occupation: _____

Marital Status: _____

Do not write in
this column

MONTEFIORE SLEEP QUESTIONNAIRE

Instructions: Please complete this questionnaire and return it to the clinician who interviews you at the time of your initial evaluation. Your responses will give your doctors an overview to your sleep problems, therefore helping to give you the best services possible in an efficient manner. *It is important that you fully answer these questions to the best of your ability.* You will notice that most of the questions are "yes/no" with some requiring you to fill in the blank. The questionnaire should take approximately 20 minutes to complete.

If you have additional questions before your initial appointment, please contact our staff at xxx-xxx-xxxx. We look forward to being able to evaluate your problem and to provide you with therapeutic advice.

NATURE OF SLEEP-WAKE PATTERN

Why are you seeking treatment at this time?

☐ Excessive daytime sleepiness   ☐ Snoring   ☐ Difficulty staying asleep
☐ Disruptive behaviors during sleep   ☐ Difficulty falling asleep   ☐ Other

How does this problem affect you? _____

CURRENT SLEEP-WAKE SCHEDULE

What time do you usually: turn out the bedroom light on **workdays?** _____ AM / PM
wake up on **workdays?** _____ AM / PM
turn out the bedroom light on **weekends?** _____ AM / PM
wake up on **weekends?** _____ AM / PM

On *average*, how long after going to bed do you fall asleep? _____ minutes
How long after finally awakening do you get out of bed? _____ minutes
How many times do you usually awaken during the night? _____ times
What is the *average* length of time of your awakenings? _____ minutes
What do you do during these arousals (check one or more)? ☐ Go to bathroom
Other: _____   ☐ Lie in bed
_____   ☐ Eat/drink
_____   ☐ Get out of bed

Do you awaken earlier than you'd like and have trouble returning to sleep? ☐ Yes ☐ No
On average, how much sleep in total do you think you get per night? _____ hrs _____ min
Do you follow a regular, nightly routine every night before getting into bed? ☐ Yes ☐ No
If yes, what do you do? _____

SNORING/BREATHING WHILE ASLEEP

Do you snore loudly or have been told you snore loudly? ☐ Yes ☐ No
Do you ever awaken choking, gasping, or gulping for air? ☐ Yes ☐ No
Has anyone said that you have trouble breathing or stop breathing while asleep? ☐ Yes ☐ No
Do you often awaken with a dry mouth or sore throat? ☐ Yes ☐ No
Do you ever awaken with headaches? ☐ Yes ☐ No
Do you use the bathroom frequently at night? ☐ Yes ☐ No
Do you experience heartburn or acid indigestion at night? ☐ Yes ☐ No
Have you ever received any treatment for sleep apnea? ☐ Yes ☐ No
Have you had your tonsils and/or adenoids removed? ☐ Yes ☐ No

DAYTIME FUNCTIONING

Do you feel sleepy, sluggish or fatigued most mornings? ☐ Yes ☐ No
Do you usually feel fatigued and/or sleepy during the day? ☐ Yes ☐ No
Do you notice problems with attention, concentration or memory during the day? ☐ Yes ☐ No
Do you tend to fall asleep in inactive situations? ☐ Yes ☐ No
Have you fallen asleep while driving or while stopped at a traffic light? ☐ Yes ☐ No
Have you had a motor vehicle accident due to sleepiness or fatigue? ☐ Yes ☐ No
Do you usually nap during the day? ☐ Yes ☐ No
If yes, how long do you usually nap? _____ minutes
What time of day do you usually nap (morning, afternoon, evening)? _____
How many naps do you usually take per day? _____
How many naps do you take per week? _____
Has your weight changed recently? ☐ Yes ☐ No
If so, how: _____

Figure 2-3 The Montefiore Sleep Questionnaire.

	Do not write in this column

WORK HOURS

If you work, what are your usual work hours?... _____ to _____
Do you work shifts (evenings, nights, rotating shifts)? .... ☐Yes ☐No
Do you work multiple jobs? .... ☐Yes ☐No

SLEEP ENVIRONMENT

Is there any aspect of your sleep environment that seems to contribute to your sleep
problem (e.g., light, temperature, humidity, bed comfort, etc.)? .... ☐Yes ☐No
     If yes, explain: _____
Do you sleep with anyone else in the same room or same bed?...................... ☐Yes ☐No
     If yes, are you bothered by your bed partner's snoring or movements
     during sleep?... ☐Yes ☐No
     If yes, do you sleep in the same room or bed with your children?............. ☐Yes ☐No
Do you sleep in the same bed with a pet?... ☐Yes ☐No
Do you usually eat or drink liquid before getting into bed or while in bed?........ ☐Yes ☐No
Do you tend to watch the clock while in bed?.. ☐Yes ☐No
Have you tried any relaxation exercises to help you sleep or while in bed?....... ☐Yes ☐No
Do you do any of the following while in bed? (Check all that apply.) .... ☐Read
                ☐Watch TV
                ☐Eat/Drink
                ☐Use Computer

MOVEMENTS WHILE ASLEEP

Do you have painful or unusual feelings in your legs that make it difficult to fall asleep? ☐Yes ☐No
Do you ever experience twitching or jerking of your legs while asleep?.................. ☐Yes ☐No

OTHER SLEEP SYMPTOMS

Upon falling asleep or waking up, have you ever had the experience of seeing things
or hearing things that weren't really there?.. ☐Yes ☐No
When falling asleep or waking up, have you ever been unable to move your arms or
legs even though you tried?.. ☐Yes ☐No
Have you ever experienced sudden muscle weakness while awake that was brought
on my an intense emotion?... ☐Yes ☐No
Do you start dreaming right after you fall asleep? .... ☐Yes ☐No

OTHER SLEEP DISTURBANCES

Do you recall dreaming? [ ] rarely [ ] occasionally [ ] often [ ] very often
Do you sleepwalk (or have you or have you ever)?... ☐Yes ☐No
Do you have recurrent/frequent nightmares? .... ☐Yes ☐No
Do you injure yourself/others while asleep or have you fallen out of bed? .... ☐Yes ☐No
Do you eat while asleep?.. ☐Yes ☐No
Do you wet the bed while asleep? .... ☐Yes ☐No
Do you ever scream loudly at night?.. ☐Yes ☐No
Do you talk during your sleep? .... ☐Yes ☐No

LIFESTYLE FACTORS

Do you have caffeine (e.g., soda, coffee, chocolate, tea) within 6 hours of bedtime? .... ☐Yes ☐No
Do you use caffeine to help you stay awake? .... ☐Yes ☐No
Do you use alcohol to help you fall asleep? .... ☐Yes ☐No
Do you smoke? .... ☐Yes ☐No
     If yes, how many cigarettes, cigars, pipes do you smoke per day? .... _____
     Do you smoke just before bed or during the night? .... ☐Yes ☐No
Do you use any illicit drugs (e.g., marijuana, heroin, crack, cocaine)? .... ☐Yes ☐No
Do you use any illicit drugs to help you fall asleep? .... ☐Yes ☐No
Do you eat a large meal two hours before bedtime?....................................... ☐Yes ☐No

MEDICATION USE

Please list all prescription and over-the-counter medications that you currently use.

Medication Name	Dose	Reason Used	Used to Treat a Sleep Problem?	Prescribing Doctor
			Yes / No	
			Yes / No	
			Yes / No	
			Yes / No	
			Yes / No	
			Yes / No	
			Yes / No	
			Yes / No	

Do you have any medication allergies? If so, list:

Figure 2-3, cont'd.

MEDICAL/PSYCHIATRIC HISTORY

What is your height?.. _____ ft _____ in
What is your current weight?.. _____ pounds
What was your weight one year ago?... _____ pounds
Have you ever had surgery?... ☐Yes ☐No
    If yes, what:_____

            _____
            _____

Have you ever been treated for any psychiatric problems?....................... ☐Yes ☐No
    If yes, what:_____
Are you currently being treated by a psychologist/psychiatrist?............... ☐Yes ☐No
    If so, whom?_____

Have you had any of the following medical problems? (Please check any that apply.)

☐ Stroke	☐ Heart attack	☐ Hypothyroidism
☐ Glaucoma	☐ Hypertension	☐ Hyperthyroidism
☐ Cataracts	☐ Irregular heartbeat	☐ Seasonal allergies
☐ Deviated nasal septum	☐ Headache	☐ Environmental allergies
☐ Chronic congestion	☐ Seizure	☐ Head injury
☐ Broken nose	☐ Nerve damage	☐ Ulcers/gastrointestinal problems
☐ Broken jaw	☐ GERD	☐ Kidney/renal disease
☐ COPD	☐ Overweight	☐ Cancer
☐ Asthma	☐ Diabetes	☐ Other: _____

FAMILY AND SOCIAL HISTORY

Please give the following family information:

            Age   Illnesses
Mother: _____   _____
Father: _____   _____

Number of brothers/sisters:_____ Number of children:_____
Does anyone in your family have any sleep problems?............................... ☐Yes ☐No
    If so, who and what:_____
Has anyone in your family ever been treated for any serious medical problems?......... ☐Yes ☐No
    If yes, what:_____
Has anyone in your family ever been treated for any psychiatric problems? .... ☐Yes ☐No
    If yes, what:_____

Do not write in this column

Figure 2-3, cont'd.

INSOMNIA PROBLEM	None	Mild	Moderate	Severe	Very
1. Difficulty falling asleep	0	1	2	3	4
2. Difficulty staying asleep	0	1	2	3	4
3. Problems waking up too early	0	1	2	3	4

	Very Satisfied	Satisfied	Moderately Satisfied	Dissatisfied	Very Dissatisfied
4. How SATISFIED/DISSATISFIED are you with your CURRENT sleep	0	1	2	3	4
5. How NOTICEABLE to others do you think your sleep problems are in terms of impairing the quality of your work?	0	1	2	3	4
6. How WORRIED/DISTRESSED are you about your current sleep problem?	0	1	2	3	4
7. To what extent do you consider your sleep problem to INTERFERE with your daily functioning (e.g., daytime fatigue, mood, ability to function at work/daily chores, concentration)	0	1	2	3	4

Add the scores for all seven items = _____ your total score

Total score categories:
0–7 = No clinically significant insomnia
8–14 = Subthreshold insomnia
15–21 = Clinical insomnia (moderate severity)
22–28 = Clinical insomnia (severe)

Figure 2-4 The Insomnia Severity Index. (Data from Bastien CH, Vallières A, Morin CM. Validation of the Insomnia Severity Index as an outcome measure for insomnia research. *Sleep Med.* 2001;2[4]:297-307.)

Indicate your chance of falling asleep under the following situations:

    0 = no chance of dozing
    1 = slight chance of dozing
    2 = moderate chance of dozing
    3 = high chance of dozing

Situation

	Chance of Dozing
1. Sitting and reading	___
2. Watching television	___
3. Sitting inactive in a public place (e.g., a theater or meeting)	___
4. As a passenger in a car for an hour without a break	___
5. Lying down to rest in the afternoon when circumstances permit	___
6. Sitting and talking to someone	___
7. Sitting quietly after a lunch without alcohol	___
8. In a car, while stopped for a few minutes in traffic	___

Abnormal > 10, Severe Sleepiness > 15

Figure 2-5 The Epworth Sleepiness Scale. (Data from Johns MW. A new method for measuring daytime sleepiness: The Epworth Sleepiness Scale. *Sleep*. 1991;14[6]:540-545.)

BOX 2-5 *Karolinska Sleepiness Scale (KSS)*

On a scale of 1 through 10, indicate how sleepy you are feeling:

    1 = extremely alert
    2 = very alert
    3 = alert
    4 = rather alert
    5 = neither alert nor sleepy
    6 = some signs of sleepiness
    7 = sleepy, but no effort to keep awake
    8 = sleepy, some effort to keep awake
    9 = very sleepy, great effort to keep awake, fighting sleep
    10 = extremely sleepy, can't keep awake

From Akerstedt T. Subjective and objective sleepiness in the active individual. *Int J Neurosci.* 1990;52:29-37.

Ullanlinna Narcolepsy Scale (UNS) is a simple questionnaire used to measure the symptoms of the narcoleptic syndrome.[49] The 11-item scale (range 0-44) assesses the two main features of the narcoleptic syndrome, the abnormal sleeping tendency and cataplexy. The UNS sum score reliably distinguishes patients with the narcoleptic syndrome from patients with sleep apnea, multiple sclerosis, and epilepsy. The mean score in patients with the narcoleptic syndrome is approximately 27.

The sleep log or sleep diary documents, over a period of approximately 2 weeks, the time of sleep onset and wake time, awakenings during the night, and daytime naps. The clinician can readily see the circadian sleep pattern, the number and frequency of awakenings, and number and duration of naps. The sleep log can also record other events, such as abnormal events and medication intake.

The Dysfunctional Beliefs and Attitudes Sleep Scale (DBAS) is a useful patient-reported measure that helps identify particular, salient, irrational, and often affect-laden thoughts that intrude prior to sleep onset, such as misconceptions and misattributions, or amplifications of the consequences of insomnia; unrealistic sleep expectations; diminished perceptions of control; and faulty beliefs about sleep-promoting practices.[50] It consists of 16 analog-scaled items that evaluate the role of sleep-related beliefs and attitudes in insomnia and can be used to monitor change in cognitive variables.

Other sleep-related questionnaires include the Horne and Ostberg Questionnaire (HOQ), which evaluates morningness-eveningness to determine an individual's chronotype to determine whether someone is a "morning person" or an "evening person."[51] The Parkinson's Disease Sleep Scale (PDSS) is a simple bedside instrument for evaluation of sleep disturbances in Parkinson's disease.[52] Several RLS scales have been developed, and include: (1) the International RLS Severity Rating (IRLS) scale that helps determine RLS severity (used mainly in research studies[53]) and (2) the Cambridge-Hopkins RLS questionnaire (CH-RLSq) that is useful in distinguishing RLS from disorders that mimic RLS.[54] The Augmentation Severity Rating Scale (ASRS) is useful in determining symptom augmentation in patients on dopaminergic medications for RLS.[55] The Frontal Lobe Epilepsy and Parasomnias (FLEP) scale is a brief, validated clinical questionnaire that is useful in distinguishing nocturnal frontal lobe epilepsy from parasomnias on the basis of the historical information.[56]

INVESTIGATIONS

Nocturnal Polysomnography

Polysomnographic recordings (see Chapter 3 for greater detail) are performed according to the recommended criteria of the American Academy of Sleep Medicine.[57] Video monitoring with an extended EEG montage documents abnormal events that occur during sleep to differentiate between a parasomnia and an epileptic disorder.[58] Polysomnography is most useful for the diagnosis of sleep-related breathing disorders, narcolepsy, periodic limb movement disorder, and RBD. If a sleep-related breathing disorder is confirmed, the patient may need to return for a second night of polysomnography to determine if positive airway pressure (PAP) is an effective treatment modality. On the other hand, many other sleep disorders do not require polysomnography for diagnosis, including psycho-physiologic insomnia, RLS, and circadian rhythm disorders.[59]

Multiple Sleep Latency Testing

The Multiple Sleep Latency Test (MSLT) (see Chapter 3 for greater detail) establishes the severity of sleepiness and is useful for the diagnosis of narcolepsy and IH.[60] It can detect sleepiness in a patient who might otherwise deny sleepiness, such as an older individual who may insist on driving a motor vehicle despite pleas to the contrary by family members who may have observed severe daytime sleepiness. This objective measure of sleepiness may demonstrate to the patient that potentially dangerous sleepiness is present and the need for behavioral change or other treatment.

Maintenance of Wakefulness Testing

The Maintenance of Wakefulness Test (MWT) (see Chapter 3 for more detail), a variation of the MSLT, assesses the ability of the patient to remain awake on daytime nap opportunities and is most useful in determining the effects of treatment on daytime sleepiness.[60,61] A patient on alerting medications during the daytime or a patient who has been treated by means of nasal PAP may undergo an MWT to demonstrate the ability to remain awake when desired. It has also been used to determine the propensity to fall asleep during daytime activities, particularly those that are work-related.

Psychomotor Vigilance Test

The psychomotor vigilance test (PVT) measures a patient's concentration; although not typically used in clinical practice, research studies of sleepiness often employ this performance test to assess the behavioral consequences of excessive sleepiness. The PVT measures the patient's ability to sustain attention by using reaction time to successive stimuli to measure deficits in attention and performance.[62] In a study comparing two versions of the PVT on 21 patients, both versions demonstrated an increase in reaction time with increasing hours of wakefulness.[63]

Actigraphy

Actigraphy (see Chapter 3 for more detail) is a wristwatch-like monitor that detects rest and activity that approximately equates with the sleep-wake cycle It is useful to record the pattern of sleep over at least 1 or 2 weeks, and is most useful for patients with prolonged sleep episodes or patients with circadian rhythm sleep disorders.[64]

Ancillary Tests

Additional investigations may be required, depending upon the presumed diagnosis.

Upper Airway Investigations

Fibreoptic endoscopy of the upper airway, preferably during sleep (sleep endoscopy), in the OSA patient assesses nasopharyngeal obstruction, such as enlarged turbinates, small choanae, enlarged adenoids or tonsils, or a prolapsing epiglottis, to demonstrate obstruction that cannot be visualized by an oral

visual examination.[65] Cephalometric radiographs for a patient who has micrognathia or retrognathia, will demonstrate the abnormal jaw position and can be helpful if mandibular surgery or an oral appliance is contemplated.[66,67] Computed tomography (CT) or magnetic resonance imaging (MRI) studies of the upper airway may be helpful, although there is not enough evidence that these techniques are superior to the routine clinical assessment.[68]

Blood and Urine Tests

Routine hematologic testing and blood chemistry analysis should be performed at or prior to the sleep evaluation to help exclude an underlying medical cause of symptoms, especially in patients who complain of insomnia, fatigue, or excessive sleepiness. Specific blood testing should be predicated upon the underlying disorder under investigation. Patients with daytime sleepiness or with OSA do not require routine thyroid testing, as the likelihood of a positive return is low.[69] Patients who have features suggestive of RLS should be tested for serum ferritin level and iron levels.[70] A serum ferritin level of less than 50 µg/L, indicates a need for iron replacement therapy. Low vitamin D levels might be associated with hypersomnia.[71] Salivary melatonin levels during dim light exposure (dim light melatonin onset [DLMO]) are useful for determining a patient's circadian phase if circadian rhythm disorders such as ASP or DSP are suspected.[72] Urine drug screening for illicit drug use may be helpful, particularly in adolescents or young adults with unexplained daytime sleepiness, as eveningness and EDS are associated with an increase in risky behaviors in adolescents.[60,73]

Genetic Testing

A positive HLA DQB1*0602 test increases the likelihood of narcolepsy in patients who exhibit features suggestive of narcolepsy but with a negative MSLT result.[74] Ninety-eight percent of patients with narcolepsy and cataplexy and hypocretin-1 deficiency are positive for HLA DQB1*0602; however, 26% of the general population is also positive for HLA DQB1*0602. Therefore, a negative HLA DQB1*0602 does not exclude the diagnosis of narcolepsy. HLA DQB1*0602 positivity also predicts interindividual differences in physiologic sleep, sleepiness, and fatigue after sleep deprivation.[75]

In unexplained EDS where myotonic dystrophy (MD) might be considered, genetic testing for cytosine-thymine-guanine (CTG) trinucleotide repeat in the gene *DMPK* can help substantiate the diagnosis of type 1 (MD1).[76] In infants with congenital alveolar hypoventilation syndrome testing for a mutation in the *PHOX2B* gene can confirm the diagnosis.[77]

Lumbar Puncture

A cerebrospinal (CSF) hypocretin level of 110 pg/mL or less is consistent with a diagnosis of narcolepsy with cataplexy[9] and is rarely noted in narcolepsy without cataplexy. This test is most useful in patients who have established cataplexy but who have also demonstrated a normal MSLT result, and those who cannot undergo an MSLT, or whose MSLT is not interpretable or is inconclusive.[74] However, CSF hypocretin level can be reduced in hypersomnias because of other neurologic disorders such as traumatic brain injury, Parkinson's disease, Prader-Willi syndrome, and Guillain-Barré syndrome.[74]

Electromyography and Nerve Conduction Velocity Tests

Electromyography (EMG) and nerve conduction velocity (NCV) studies should be performed if it is suspected that a neuropathy or radiculopathy might be mimicking RLS.[32]

Electroencephalography

Electroencephalography (EEG) may be required to evaluate a possible seizure disorder. A full montage EEG is capable of detecting epileptic features better than polysomnography and should be performed in any patient suspected of having a seizure disorder. Continuous in-hospital or ambulatory EEG monitoring may be helpful in the evaluation of episodic epileptic disorders. Frontal lobe epilepsy, which commonly manifests itself during sleep, can be diagnosed by the clinical features, such as stereotypy but may have no EEG manifestations on polysomnography or on continuous EEG monitoring.[78] An intracranial EEG study, sometimes coupled with functional magnetic resonance imaging (fMRI) may be necessary to localize a seizure source for possible epilepsy surgery.[79]

Neuroimaging

Neuroimaging, such as CT scan or MRI, should be performed in a patient with IH if there is clinical suspicion of an underlying brain lesion.[9] In addition, neuroimaging might show brainstem pathologic changes in RBD[80] and cerebrovascular disease or brainstem disorders, such as Chiari malformations, in unexplained central sleep apnea syndrome.[81] Newer functional neuroimaging techniques such as positron emission tomography (PET), single photon emission computed tomography (SPECT), and fMRI can be helpful in demonstrating cerebral dysfunction in neurologic patients with sleep disorders.[82]

FOLLOW-UP AND REEVALUATION

It is not unusual for more than one sleep disorder to be present in a particular patient. Narcolepsy is a diagnosis that can be missed when it is co-morbid with another cause of EDS, and it can even be misdiagnosed as an insomnia disorder because one if its features is disturbed nocturnal sleep. In a study of narcolepsy patients, 25% had a concomitant diagnosis of OSA, and in 30% of those with narcolepsy and OSA the narcolepsy diagnosis was delayed because it was initially missed by the clinician.[83] Active follow-up is essential to ensure the presenting symptoms have resolved and to consider alternative diagnoses in patients whose symptoms have not resolved.

Follow-Up Evaluation

The appropriate follow-up interval is clearly dependent on the disorder under treatment and the patient. In case of excessive sleepiness or insomnia an interval of follow-up of approximately 2 weeks is appropriate after starting therapy. At the follow-up, a sleep log or diary may be useful. Repeat ESS questionnaires are helpful at every follow-up visit, no matter what the underlying sleep diagnosis. Behavioral therapy may require frequent interval visits to adjust behavioral recommendations and repeat questionnaire evaluations, such as the ISI or DBAS, during and at the end of treatment.

If PAP therapy has been instituted, the patient's follow-up evaluation should be scheduled no less than 4 weeks later to determine effectiveness of treatment and compliance and, if necessary, to consider the need for a change of mask or the addition of a humidifier. Then, if the patient is doing well, follow-up visits at 3 months, 6 months, and then yearly are appropriate.

Polysomnographic Reevaluation

Once a patient has had confirmatory sleep studies for narcolepsy these studies do not need to be repeated unless there is a major change in the patient's status. However, patients with IH should have repeat polysomnographic studies performed after 1 year to determine the patient's current status or if there has been a change to narcolepsy.

Patients on PAP treatment need reevaluation if their treatment becomes ineffective, there is a major weight change, or their symptoms of sleepiness do not resolve and a question of narcolepsy is raised. If continuous PAP (CPAP) tolerance or effectiveness is an issue, then patients may need reevaluation with PAP treatment other than CPAP, such as bilevel PAP, or adaptive servoventilation (ASV) if there is a prominent central apneic component.

If the ability to drive or operate dangerous equipment is an issue, then reevaluation by means of the MWT may be required to demonstrate the ability to keep awake.

CONCLUSION

Once a clinical history has been taken and appropriate investigations, which often include polysomnography, have been performed, the physician is in a good position to understand the nature and treatment direction for most sleep disorders. It may be necessary to refer the patient to a consultant specialist, such as a psychiatrist, otolaryngologist, or cardiologist, if an underlying psychiatric, otolargyngologic, or cardiac illness is suspected. Other consultations may be requested as appropriate.

With recent advances in sleep medicine every sleep disorder can be helped if the physician takes an accurate history, performs the appropriate investigative tests, formulates a differential diagnosis, and develops an effective treatment plan.

REFERENCES

1. Ohayon MM, Roth T. What are the contributing factors for insomnia in the general population? *J Psychosom Res.* 2001;51(6):745-755.
2. Ohayon MM. From wakefulness to excessive sleepiness: What we know and still need to know. *Sleep Med Rev.* 2008;12(2):129-141.
3. Bjorvatn B, Grønli J, Pallesen S. Prevalence of different parasomnias in the general population. *Sleep Med.* 2010;11:1031-1034.
4. The Gallup Organization for the National Sleep Foundation. Sleep in America. Princeton, NJ: National Sleep Foundation; 1995.
5. Ohayon MM, Roth T. Place of chronic insomnia in the course of depressive and anxiety disorders. *J Psychiatr Res.* 2003;37(1):9-15.
6. Breslau N, Roth T, Rosenthal L, et al. Sleep disturbance and psychiatric disorders: A longitudinal epidemiological study of young adults. *Biol Psychiatry.* 1996;39(6):411-418.
7. Calvin AD, Somers VK. Obstructive sleep apnea and cardiovascular disease. *Curr Opin Cardiol.* 2009;24(6):516-520.
8. Mitler M, Carskadon MA, Czeisler CA, et al. Catastrophes, sleep, and public policy: Consensus report. *Sleep.* 1988;11:100-109.
9. ICSD-2. *International Classification of Sleep Disorders.* 2nd ed. Westchester, IL: American Academy of Sleep Medicine; 2005.

10. Spielman AJ, Saskin P, Thorpy MJ. Treatment of chronic insomnia by restriction of time in bed. *Sleep*. 1987;10(1):45-56.
11. Tiffin P, Ashton H, Marsh R, et al. Pharmacokinetic and pharmacodynamic responses to caffeine in poor and normal sleepers. *Psychopharmacology (Berl)*. 1995;121(4):494-502.
12. Stepanski E, Zorick F, Roehrs T, et al. Daytime alertness in patients with chronic insomnia compared with asymptomatic control subjects. *Sleep*. 1988;11:54-60.
13. Dautovich ND, McCrae CS, Rowe M. Subjective and objective napping and sleep in older adults: Are evening naps "bad" for nighttime sleep? *J Am Geriatr Soc*. 2008;56(9):1681-1686:Epub 2008 Aug 5.
14. Ford DE, Kamerow DB. Epidemiologic study of sleep disturbances and psychiatric disorders. An opportunity for prevention? *JAMA*. 1989;262(11):1479-1484.
15. Kroenke K, Spitzer RL. The PHQ-9: A new depression and diagnostic severity measure. *Psychiatr Ann*. 2002;32:509-521.
16. Spitzer RL, Kroenke K, Williams JB, Lowe B. A brief measure for assessing generalized anxiety disorder: The GAD-7. *Arch Intern Med*. 2006;166(10):1092-1097.
17. Beck AT, Ward CH, Mendelson M, Mock J, Erbaugh J. An inventory for measuring depression. *Arch Gen Psychiatry*. 1961;4:561-571.
18. Spielberger CD, Gorsuch RL, Lushene R. *STAI Manual*. Palo Alto, CA: Consulting Psychologists Press; 1970.
19. Chesson Jr A, Hartse K, Anderson WM, et al. Practice parameters for the evaluation of chronic insomnia. An American Academy of Sleep Medicine report. Standards of Practice Committee of the American Academy of Sleep Medicine. *Sleep*. 2000;23(2):237-241.
20. Sack RL, Auckley D, Auger RR, et al. Circadian rhythm sleep disorders: Part I, basic principles, shift work and jet lag disorders. An American Academy of Sleep Medicine review. *Sleep*. 2007;30(11):1460-1483.
21. Neu D, Linkowski P, le Bon O. Clinical complaints of daytime sleepiness and fatigue: How to distinguish and treat them, especially when they become 'excessive' or 'chronic'? *Acta Neurol Belg*. 2010;110(1):15-25.
22. Merkelbach S, Schulz H, Kölmel HW, Gora G, Klingelhöfer J, et al. Fatigue, sleepiness, and physical activity in patients with multiple sclerosis. *J Neurol*. 2011;258:74-79:Epub 2010 Aug 18.
23. Chaudhuri KR. Nocturnal symptom complex in PD and its management. *Neurology*. 2003;61(6) (Suppl 3):S17-S23.
24. Pigeon WR, Sateia MJ, Ferguson RJ. Distinguishing between excessive daytime sleepiness and fatigue: Toward improved detection and treatment. *J Psychosom Res*. 2003;54(1):61-69.
25. Merino-Andreu M, Arnulf I, Konofal E, et al. Unawareness of naps in Parkinson's disease and in disorders with excessive daytime sleepiness. *Neurology*. 2003;60(9):1553-1554.
26. Thorpy M. Current concepts in the etiology, diagnosis and treatment of narcolepsy. *Sleep Med*. 2001;2(1):5-17.
27. Broughton R, Ghanem Q, Hishikawa Y, et al. Life effects of narcolepsy in 180 patients from North America, Asia and Europe compared to matched controls. *Can J Neurol Sci*. 1981;8(4):299-304.
28. Anderson KN, Pilsworth S, Sharples LD, et al. Idiopathic hypersomnia: A study of 77 cases. *Sleep*. 2007;30:1274-1281.
29. Ali M, Auger RR, Slocumb NL, Morganthaler TI. Idiopathic hypersomnia: Clinical features and response to treatment. *J Clin Sleep Med*. 2009:562-568.
30. Ohayon MM, Caulet M, Philip P, et al. How sleep and mental disorders are related to complaints of daytime sleepiness. *Arch Intern Med*. 1997;157(22):2645-2652.
31. Ohayon MM, Schenck CH. Violent behavior during sleep: Prevalence, comorbidity and consequences. *Sleep Med*. 2010;11(9):941-946.
32. Hening WA, Allen RP, Washburn M, et al. The four diagnostic criteria for restless legs syndrome are unable to exclude confounding conditions ("mimics"). *Sleep Med*. 2009;10(9):976-981:Epub 2009 Jan 29.
33. Mahowald MW, Schenck CH. Diagnosis and management of parasomnias. *Clin Cornerstone*. 2000;2(5):48-57.
34. Katz DA, McHorney CA. Clinical correlates of insomnia in patients with chronic illness. *Arch Intern Med*. 1998;158(10):1099-1107.
35. Tolosa E, Compta Y, Gaig C. The premotor phase of Parkinson's disease. *Parkinsonism Relat Disord*. 2007;13(Suppl):S2-S7:Epub 2007 Jul 27.
36. Nuckton TJ, Glidden DV, Browner WS, Claman DM. Physical examination: Mallampati score as an independent predictor of obstructive sleep apnea. *Sleep*. 2006;29(7):903-908.
37. Hukins C. Mallampati class is not useful in the clinical assessment of sleep clinic patients. *J Clin Sleep Med*. 2010;6(6):545-549.
38. Buskova J, Klaschka J, Sonka K, Nevsimalova S. Olfactory dysfunction in narcolepsy with and without cataplexy. *Sleep Med*. 2010;11(6):558-561:Epub 2010 May 23.
39. Fantini ML, Postuma RB, Montplaisir J, Ferini-Strambi L. Olfactory deficit in idiopathic rapid eye movements sleep behavior disorder. *Brain Res Bull*. 2006;70(4-6):386-390:Epub 2006 Aug 7.
40. Shiroky JS, Schipper HM, Bergman H, Chertkow H. Can you have dementia with an MMSE score of 30? *Am J Alzheimers Dis Other Demen*. 2007;22(5):406-415.
41. Rami L, Bosch B, Valls-Pedret C, et al. Discriminatory validity and association of the mini-mental test (MMSE) and the memory alteration test (MAT) with a neuropsychological battery in patients with amnestic mild cognitive impairment and Alzheimer's disease. *Rev Neurol*. 2009;49(4):169-174.
42. Dubois B, Slachevsky A, Litvan I, Pillon B, The FAB. a Frontal Assessment Battery at bedside. *Neurology*. 2000;55(11):1621-1626.
43. Netzer NC, Stoohs RA, Netzer CM, et al. Using the Berlin Questionnaire to identify patients at risk for the sleep apnea syndrome. *Ann Intern Med*. 1999;131(7):485-491.
44. Chung F, Elsaid H. Screening for obstructive sleep apnea before surgery: Why is it important? *Curr Opin Anaesthesiol*. 2009;22(3):405-411.
45. Bastien CH, Vallières A, Morin CM. Validation of the Insomnia Severity Index as an outcome measure for insomnia research. *Sleep Med*. 2001;2(4):297-307.
46. Johns MW. A new method for measuring daytime sleepiness: The Epworth sleepiness scale. *Sleep*. 1991;14(6):540-545.
47. Akerstedt T. Subjective and objective sleepiness in the active individual. *Int J Neurosci*. 1990;52:29-37.
48. Buysse DJ, Reynolds 3rd CF, Monk TH, et al. The Pittsburgh Sleep Quality Index: A new instrument for psychiatric practice and research. *Psychiatry Res*. 1989;28(2):193-213.
49. Hublin C, Kaprio J, Partinen M, et al. The Ullanlinna Narcolepsy Scale: Validation of a measure of symptoms in the narcoleptic syndrome. *J Sleep Res*. 1994;3(1):52-59.
50. Morin CM, Vallières A, Ivers H. Dysfunctional beliefs and attitudes about sleep (DBAS): Validation of a brief version (DBAS-16). *Sleep*. 2007;30(11):1547-1554.
51. Horne JA, Ostberg O. A self-assessment questionnaire to determine morningness-eveningness in human circadian rhythms. *Int J Chronobiol*. 1976;4(2):97-110.
52. Chaudhuri KR, Pal S, DiMarco A, et al. The Parkinson's disease sleep scale: A new instrument for assessing sleep and nocturnal disability in Parkinson's disease. *J Neurol Neurosurg Psychiatry*. 2002;73(6):629-635.
53. Abetz L, Arbuckle R, Allen RP, et al. The reliability, validity and responsiveness of the International Restless Legs Syndrome Study Group rating scale and subscales in a clinical-trial setting. *Sleep Med*. 2006;7(4):340-349:Epub 2006 May 19.
54. Allen RP, Burchell BJ, MacDonald B, et al. Validation of the self-completed Cambridge-Hopkins questionnaire (CH-RLSq) for ascertainment of restless legs syndrome (RLS) in a population survey. *Sleep Med*. 2009;10(10):1097-1100:Epub 2009 Feb 4.
55. García-Borreguero D, Kohnen R, Högl B, et al. Validation of the Augmentation Severity Rating Scale (ASRS): A multicentric, prospective study with levodopa on restless legs syndrome. *Sleep Med*. 2007;8(5):455-463:Epub 2007 May 31.
56. Derry C, Duncan J, Berkovic S. Paroxysmal motor disorders of sleep: The clinical spectrum and differentiation from epilepsy. *Epilepsia*. 2008;49:2125-2129.
57. The AASM. *Manual for the Scoring of Sleep and Associated Events*. Westchester, IL: American Academy of Sleep Medicine; 2007.
58. Aldrich M, Jahnke B. Diagnostic value of video-EEG polysomnography. *Neurology*. 1991;41:1060-1066.
59. Littner M, Hirshkowitz M, Kramer M, et al. Practice parameters for using polysomnography to evaluate insomnia: An update. *Sleep*. 2003;26(6):754-760.
60. Standards of Practice Committee of the American Academy of Sleep Medicine. Practice parameters for clinical use of the multiple sleep latency test and the maintenance of wakefulness test. *Sleep*. 2005;28(1):113-121.
61. Mitler MM, Gujavarty KS, Browman CP. Maintenance of wakefulness test: A polysomnographic technique for evaluating treatment efficacy in patients with excessive somnolence. *Electroencephalogr Clin Neurophysiol*. 1982;53:658.
62. Stoohs RA, Philip P, Andries D, et al. Reaction time performance in upper airway resistance syndrome versus obstructive sleep apnea syndrome. *Sleep Med*. 2009;10(9):1000-1004.
63. Lamond N, Jay SM, Dorrian J, et al. The sensitivity of a palm-based psychomotor vigilance task to sleep loss. *Behav Res Methods*. 2008;40(1):347-352.

64. Morgenthaler TI, Lee-Chiong T, Alessi C, et al. Standards of Practice Committee of the American Academy of Sleep Medicine. Practice parameters for the clinical evaluation and treatment of circadian rhythm sleep disorders. An American Academy of Sleep Medicine report. *Sleep.* 2007;30(11):1445-1459.

65. den Herder C, van Tinteren H, de Vries N. Sleep endoscopy versus modified Mallampati score in sleep apnea and snoring. *Laryngoscope.* 2005;115(4):735-739.

66. Olszewska E, Sieskiewicz A, Rozycki J, et al. A comparison of cephalometric analysis using radiographs and craniofacial computed tomography in patients with obstructive sleep apnea syndrome: Preliminary report. *Eur Arch Otorhinolaryngol.* 2009;266(4):535-542:Epub 2008 Oct 28.

67. Liu Y, Lowe AA, Fleetham JA, Park YC. Cephalometric and physiologic predictors of the efficacy of an adjustable oral appliance for treating obstructive sleep apnea. *Am J Orthod Dentofacial Orthop.* 2001;120(6):639-647.

68. Stuck BA, Maurer JT. Airway evaluation in obstructive sleep apnea. *Sleep Med Rev.* 2008;12(6):411-436:Epub 2007 Nov 28.

69. Mickelson SA, Lian T, Rosenthal L. Thyroid testing and thyroid hormone replacement in patients with sleep disordered breathing. *Ear Nose Throat J.* 1999;78(10):768-771:774–775.

70. Kryger MH, Otake K, Foerster J. Low body stores of iron and restless legs syndrome: A correctable cause of insomnia in adolescents and teenagers. *Sleep Med.* 2002;3(2):127-132.

71. McCarty DE. Resolution of hypersomnia following identification and treatment of vitamin D deficiency. *J Clin Sleep Med.* 2010;6(6):605-608.

72. Rahman SA, Kayumov L, Tchmoutina EA, Shapiro CM. Clinical efficacy of dim light melatonin onset testing in diagnosing delayed sleep phase syndrome. *Sleep Med.* 2009;10(5):549-555:Epub 2008 Aug 23.

73. Gau SS, Shang CY, Merikangas KR, et al. Association between morningness-eveningness and behavioral/emotional problems among adolescents. *J Biol Rhythms.* 2007;22(3):268-274.

74. Bourgin P, Zeitzer JM, Mignot E. CSF hypocretin-1 assessment in sleep and neurological disorders. *Lancet Neurol.* 2008;7(7):649-662.

75. Goel N, Banks S, Mignot E, Dinges DF. DQB1*0602 predicts interindividual differences in physiologic sleep, sleepiness, and fatigue. *Neurology.* 2010;75(17):1509-1519.

76. Turner C, Hilton-Jones D. The myotonic dystrophies: Diagnosis and management. *J Neurol Neurosurg Psychiatry.* 2010;81(4):358-367:Epub 2010 Feb 22.

77. Weese-Mayer DE, Rand CM, Berry-Kravis EM, et al. Congenital central hypoventilation syndrome from past to future: Model for translational and transitional autonomic medicine. *Pediatr Pulmonol.* 2009;44(6):521-535.

78. Foldvary-Schaefer N, De Ocampo J, Mascha E, et al. Accuracy of seizure detection using abbreviated EEG during polysomnography. *J Clin Neurophysiol.* 2006;23(1):68-71.

79. Vulliemoz S, Carmichael DW, Rosenkranz K, et al. Simultaneous intracranial EEG and fMRI of interictal epileptic discharges in humans. *Neuroimage.* 2011;54(1):182-190:Epub 2010 Aug 11.

80. Culebras A, Moore JT. Magnetic resonance findings in REM sleep behavior disorder. *Neurology.* 1989;39(11):1519-1523.

81. Gosalakkal JA. Sleep-disordered breathing in Chiari malformation type 1. *Pediatr Neurol.* 2008;39(3):207-208.

82. Desseilles M, Dang-Vu T, Schabus M, et al. Neuroimaging insights into the pathophysiology of sleep disorders. *Sleep.* 2008;31(6):777-794.

83. Sansa G, Iranzo A, Santamaria J. Obstructive sleep apnea in narcolepsy. *Sleep Med.* 2010;11(1):93-95:Epub 2009 Aug 20.

Chapter 3

Introduction to Sleep Medicine Diagnostics in Adults

MAX HIRSHKOWITZ

OVERVIEW

This chapter reviews laboratory and nonlaboratory procedures used to diagnose or confirm diagnosis of important sleep disorders. These procedures, in some cases, also guide therapeutic intervention. The procedures reviewed here include attended polysomnography, multiple sleep latency testing, maintenance of wakefulness testing, suggested immobilization test, actigraphy, and home sleep testing. The current American Academy of Sleep Medicine (AASM) standards of practice guidelines concerning these procedures are summarized. This chapter also provides clinical information concerning indications for testing, technical details about procedures, and guidance for interpreting test results. To a large degree the field of sleep medicine evolved from laboratory polysomnography developed originally for the psychophysiologic study of sleep. This endeavor, lent its name (the Association for the Psychophysiological Study of Sleep later changed to the Associated Professional Sleep Societies) and initials (APSS) to the original scientific society established to foster communication in the field. Although sleep medicine clearly developed into an independent clinical specialty, the laboratory procedures remain at its heart. Only recently have home sleep testing and actigraphy made a similar transition from research methodology to recognized clinical practice, and this progression may represent the next horizon in sleep medicine.

BRIEF DESCRIPTIONS OF PROCEDURES

Laboratory Procedures

Attended laboratory clinical polysomnography[1,2] (often referred to as a *sleep study*) involves recording brain activity, eye movements, muscle tone, breathing, leg movements, and heart rhythm during sleep. The resulting *polysomnogram* may take the form of a baseline diagnostic study, a positive airway pressure titration, or a split-night diagnostic-titration study. Polysomnography is primarily used to diagnose sleep-related breathing disorders and to determine the positive airway pressure level needed to support ventilation in afflicted patients. Attended laboratory polysomnography, synchronized with video recording, is also used to diagnose an array of other sleep disorders and to differentiate parasomnias from sleep-related seizure disorders.

The *multiple sleep latency test*[3] is a procedure primarily used to diagnose or confirm narcolepsy. It also provides an objective measure of physiologic sleepiness. It follows overnight attended laboratory polysomnography and involves four or five nap opportunities (the number depending upon outcomes). These nap opportunities, scheduled at 2-hour intervals throughout the day, begin approximately 2 hours after initial arising from the major sleep period. During each test session, the patient lies down in bed while polysomnographic parameters are recorded. The patient is instructed to try to fall asleep.

Maintenance of wakefulness testing follows similar procedures to those used in the multiple sleep latency test; however, patients are instructed to "resist falling asleep" and to "try to remain awake." The test is used to objectively index an individual's manifest sleepiness. Four test sessions, scheduled at 2-hour intervals begin approximately 2 or 3 hours after awakening from the previous major sleep period. During each test session, the patient reclines (remaining semi-upright) while electroencephalographic, electro-oculographic, and submentalis electromyographic parameters needed to differentiate sleep from wakefulness are recorded.

Suggested immobilization test[4] can help confirm restless legs syndrome. At 90 minutes before bedtime, the patient semi-reclines in bed with legs outstretched and eyes open. Patients are instructed not to fall asleep and not to move during this single, 1-hour test session. Concurrent electroencephalographic, electro-oculographic, and electromyographic (from submentalis and both right and left anterior tibialis) recordings are made.

Home Testing Procedures

Actigraphy[5] records movement using accelerometers and semiconductor memory mounted in a wristwatch-like device. The actigraph provides information about an individual's rest and activity levels during a period ranging from several days to weeks. These data help document a person's sleep-wake schedule and pattern. Many actigraphs also incorporate a photosensor to record concurrent environmental light and darkness.

Home sleep testing[6-8] refers to a variety of procedures used principally to diagnose sleep-related breathing disorders in symptomatic patients. The most common device configuration consists of a cardiopulmonary recorder with oximetry. Other devices range from pulse volume tonometry coupled with oximetry to essentially full polysomnography adapted for unattended recording. As the name suggests, patients undergoing this procedure usually sleep at home; however, home sleep testing devices are also used in hospitals for in-patient bedside monitoring.

BASELINE DIAGNOSTIC POLYSOMNOGRAPHY

Indications

Approved clinical indications for polysomnography include sleep-disordered breathing diagnosis, positive airway pressure titration, narcolepsy diagnosis (when followed by a multiple sleep latency test), and parasomnia/seizure-disorder assessment. Routine use of laboratory polysomnography to evaluate insomnia is not recommended. However, it can be appropriate when the insomnia is resistant to treatment because occult pathophysiologic conditions may exist.

Procedures

Clinical laboratory polysomnography evolved from a research methodology and became the foundation of modern sleep medicine. This procedure provides a psychophysiologic portrait of the sleeper. Current technique includes electroencephalogram (EEG) activity, eye movement detection (electro-oculogram, EOG), and skeletal muscle tone measures (electromyogram [EMG] from submentalis). These measures unveil sleep state, awakenings from sleep, brief central nervous system arousals, and aberrant brain discharges. Polysomnography also includes measurements of airflow, respiratory effort, oxyhemoglobin level, and heart rhythm to reveal cardiopulmonary functioning. Finally, leg muscle activity and concurrent video monitoring help expose unexpected, abnormal, and inappropriate movements during sleep. Table 3-1 provides specific details concerning the recording montage used for routine clinical sleep studies.

Electroencephalogram, Electro-Oculogram, and Electromyogram

Current polysomnographic technique involves continuously recording of frontal (F), central (C), and occipital (O) EEG throughout an entire major sleep period (usually overnight). Monopolar derivations from F4, C4, and O2, referenced to contralateral mastoid (M), serve as primary data. Homologous left-sided EEGs serve as backup in case primary signals become eroded or compromised during the many hours of recording. The AASM guidelines also permit use of an alternate recording montage that substitutes midline bipolar recordings from frontal and occipital derivations. EOG recordings derive from electrodes placed near the eyes' right and left outer canthi, each referenced to a neutral site (usually the mastoid) and recorded on separate channels. One eye electrode should be placed 1 cm above and the other 1 cm below the outer canthus. Thus, lateral eye movements produce robust out-of-phase EOG activity as the eye's positive corneal potential moves toward one electrode and away from the other. This characteristic out-of-phase signature allows easy differentiation of eye movements from frontal EEG activity (presenting as in-phase activity at the same electrodes). Some appreciation of vertical eye movements is afforded by placing one electrode slightly above and the other slightly below each eye's horizontal plane. For clinicians wishing to better visualize vertical eye movements, an optional

TABLE 3-1

Polysomnography Recording Montage

Channels (with Abbreviations)	Activity	Purpose
Frontal, central, and occipital EEGs (F3-M1, F4-M2, C3-A2, C4-M1, O1-M2, O2-M1)	Brain activity	To classify sleep stages, to help recognize sleep onset, and identify CNS arousals
Left and right electro-oculograms on separate channels (LOC-M1 and ROC-M1)	Eye movements	To classify sleep stages and help recognize sleep onset
Submentalis (chin) electromyogram	Skeletal muscle tone	To classify sleep stages and identify CNS arousals during REM sleep
Single-channel electrocardiogram	Heart rhythm	To screen for arrhythmias
Nasal-oral thermistors and nasal pressure transducer	Airflow	To identify sleep apnea, hypopnea, and respiratory effort–related arousal events
Esophageal pressure, chest wall, and abdominal movement and/or intercostal electromyogram	Respiratory effort	To differentiate central from obstructive SRBD events
Pulse oximetry set to an averaging time of ≤3 sec	Oxygenation	To identify oxyhemoglobin desaturations and score hypopnea events
Left and right anterior tibialis electromyograms	Leg movements	To identify activity associated with restless legs syndrome and periodic limb movement disorder

C, central EEG placement; *CNS*, central nervous system; *EEG*, electroencephalogram; *F*, frontal EEG placement; *LOC*, left outer canthus; *M*, mastoid; *O*, occipital EEG placement; *REM*, rapid eye movement; *ROC*, right outer canthus; *SRBD*, sleep-related breathing disorder.

recording montage (with right and left eye outer canthi electrodes both placed 1 cm below the horizontal plane and referenced to the middle of the forehead) is permitted. Submentalis EMG activity derives from an electrode pair placed 1 cm above (on the horizontal midline) and the other placed 2 cm below the mandible's inferior edge (2 cm to the right of midline). A backup electrode is placed 2 cm to the left of midline.

In patients exhibiting unusual sleep behaviors or those suspected of possible nocturnal seizure activity, polysomnographic recordings include additional EEG derivations. Appropriate recording montages are described in texts devoted to this topic.[9,10] Sleep deprivation has long been known to provoke epileptiform activity in susceptible individuals. Therefore, in an attempt to provoke what is often an irregularly occurring or even rare event, laboratories may request a patient to curtail sleep by several hours on the night before polysomnography. In the past when polysomnograms were recorded using ink pen tracings made on chart drive moving paper, channels and temporal resolution had to be selected "on the fly" from available electrode inputs and discrete paper speeds. By contrast, modern digital polysomnographic equipment makes it relatively easy to select preprogrammed montages to enhance abnormal activity localization and visualization. Recordings can be rescaled in the temporal domain at will. Additionally, some recording systems allow re-referencing signals to any other recorded channel.

Cardiopulmonary Measures

During the past 2 to 3 decades, the vast majority of all polysomnographic procedures serve to diagnose or optimize treatment for sleep-related breathing disorders. Before the AASM Manual was published, no officially endorsed clinical procedure existed to guide recording and scoring technique for sleep-related cardiopulmonary activity. The de facto standard derived from Sharon Keenan's chapter in Guilleminault's *Indications and Techniques*.[11] With some revision, the basic principles remain unchanged.

Required measures include airflow, respiratory effort, oxyhemoglobin saturation, sleep disturbance (derived from EEG recordings described previously), and a single channel electrocardiogram. For adult patients, current AASM approved clinical technique requires the five data channels: (1) a thermal sensor placed at the nose and mouth, (2) a nasal pressure transducer, (3) an esophageal manometer, chest/abdominal inductance plethysmograph, or intercostal EMG (to detect respiratory effort changes), (4) a pulse oximeter (with a maximum 3-second signal averaging time), and (5) a single modified electrocardiographic lead II placed on the torso aligned parallel to the right shoulder and the left hip. It should be noted that end-tidal CO_2 measurement can be useful for assessing hypoventilation but is not currently part of the AASM standard for adults.

Sometimes during diagnostic polysomnography, sleep-disordered breathing becomes readily apparent early during recording. If a patient meets treatment criteria for positive airway pressure therapy during the first 2 hours, the baseline recording montage can be switched to one more appropriate for titration, and treatment commences. However, once the patient is wearing a mask or nasal pillow interface, airflow sensor recording (nasal-oral thermistors and nasal pressure transducers) becomes problematic. A flow signal from the positive pressure device is substituted for the channels removed. Additionally, a signal or marker indicating pressure level is added to assist the sleep specialist in determining optimal therapeutic setting (details concerning titration procedure and interpretation are presented elsewhere in this book).

Detecting and Measuring Movement

Discovery of periodic leg movements during sleep prompted clinicians to routinely record leg EMG activity during polysomnography. Pioneering work by Richard Coleman with methodology described in Guilleminault's *Indications and Techniques* became the unofficial guideline.[12] The approach was endorsed (with minor revision) by the AASM taskforce publication[13] and re-endorsed with some refinements in the *AASM Manual*. Standard clinical polysomnographic technique currently recommends using a pair of surface electrodes placed longitudinally at homologous sites on the belly of each leg's anterior tibialis muscle (approximately 2-3 cm apart). Preferably, right and left leg EMGs are recorded separately on different channels. The anterior tibialis EMG recordings can also assist in detecting hypnagogic foot tremor and excessive fragmentary myoclonus.

Other unexpected, abnormal, or inappropriate movements during sleep may require additional recording channels (for example, EMG from arms for upper extremity movements or jaw for bruxism). Also, concurrent video monitoring provides crucial information about movements characterizing sleep walking, rapid eye movement (REM) sleep behavior disorder (and its variants), rhythmic movement disorder, and movements accompanying seizures.

Interpretation

Brain Activity

Sleep Macroarchitecture. From the very beginning, the sheer volume of data collected during a sleep study necessitated creation of schema to summarized results. Thus, sleep staging was invented (Fig. 3-1). All sleep staging systems attempt to group recorded segments of EEG activity within a designated time domain (epoch) according to similarities. (NOTE: Current practice uses a 30-second epoch.) In this manner, a simple categorical name replaces a myriad of complex variations that in turn makes it easier (nay, possible) to characterize the general architecture of sleep and wakefulness. However, the purpose of grouping according to similarities is ultimately to accentuate categorical differences. We will begin with the most rudimentary differentiation: wakefulness versus sleep.

Differentiating sleep and wakefulness sounds simple and is straightforward in most individuals. However, in some people recognizing sleep onset can be quite difficult. EEG differentiation between sleep and wakefulness dates back to Berger's initial discovery of brain waves activity in humans.[14] During eyes-closed, relaxed wakefulness, a 7- to 14-cycle per second (cps) waveform dominates the EEG. This rhythm (named *alpha* by Berger himself) disappears at sleep onset. So what is the problem? Some individuals have little or no alpha activity. In fact, Loomis and colleagues,[15] who performed the first continuous all-night sleep studies in humans, found it so difficult to score sleep-wake transition in such individuals that they discarded those recordings from their analysis. As clinicians, we do not have that luxury, and determining the exact moment of sleep onset can be a challenge. However, improved recording equipment, standard use of occipital EEG derivations (that accentuate the alpha rhythm), and better knowledge of alternate sleep markers have improved this technique.

Nonetheless, differentiating sleep and wakefulness immediately allows characterization of sleep initiation, integrity, and continuity. The amount of time it takes to fall asleep (latency to sleep onset) affords the measure "sleep latency." We can consider simple *sleep latency* as the time to reach any epoch categorized as sleep or a more complex *latency to persistent sleep* as the elapsed time to reach 10 minutes of continuous uninterrupted sleep (a measure considered more sensitive and commonly used in insomnia treatment trials).[16] Once an individual falls asleep, *sleep efficiency* (time spent asleep, i.e., *total sleep time*, as a percentage of *time in bed*) can index sleep's general integrity. The time from first falling asleep to the final awakening represents the *total sleep period* and sleep continuity measures within this period include the *number of awakenings* and the duration of *wake after sleep onset*.

Within epochs classified as sleep, differentiation next proceeds according to general EEG background activity and specific waveforms (Fig. 3-2). The relatively low voltage, mixed frequency background activity seen when the alpha rhythm disappeared becomes increasingly punctuated by large, somewhat sharp waves. These waves stand out from the background

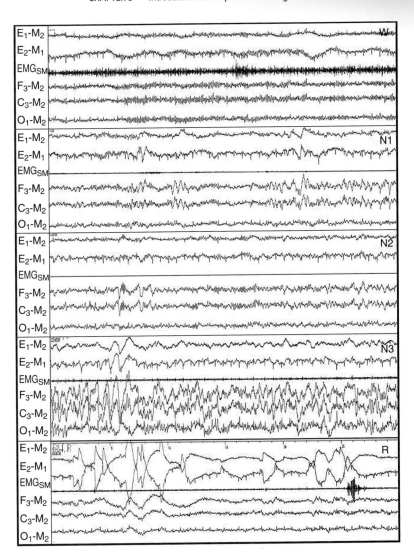

Figure 3-1 Sleep stages. These five panels illustrate eye movement, submentalis electromyographic parameters, and electroencephalographic activity correlated with wakefulness *(W)* and sleep stages *N1, N2, N3,* and *R* (rapid eye movement) sleep in the normal young adult. Electrode placement notation: E_1, outer cantus of left eye; E_2, outer cantus of right eye; EMG_{SM}, submentalis electromyogram; F_3, left frontal; C_3, left central; O_1, left occipital; M_2, right mastoid.

and may be either unidirectional or biphasic. Concurrently, short bursts of 12- to 16-cps waves (that form a spindle-shaped envelope) superimpose on the background. Finally, in most people (especially healthy, young subjects) the background activity begins transforming into higher voltage, slow waves. When the amplitude exceeds 75 microvolts and the frequency drops below 2 cps the wave is officially designated as a *slow wave*. The categorical designation for an epoch containing large, somewhat sharp, biphasic waves (*K complexes*) or spindle-shaped bursts (*sleep spindles*) is N2 unless there are 6 (or more) seconds of *slow waves*, which would make it N3. By contrast, an epoch with low-voltage, mixed-frequency background EEG devoid of *K complexes* and *sleep spindles* and less than 6 seconds of *slow wave* activity can provisionally be considered as stage N1. If, however, rapid eye movements (REMs) are present in the EOG and submentalis EMG level is very low, the epoch is classified as stage R (or REM) sleep.

The amount, sequence, and pattern of sleep stages vary from individual to individual; however, commonalities do exist. In normal young adults, nightly sleep stage pattern is fairly consistent (Fig. 3-3). N1 typically accounts for 5% or less of sleep time, N2 takes up about 50%, N3 occupies 12.5% to 20% (mostly occurring in the first third of the sleep period), and REM sleep encompasses 20% to 25%. REM sleep first

appears approximately 90 minutes after sleep onset (*REM sleep latency*) and reappears every 90 to 100 minutes thereafter (with notable regularity). The initial REM sleep episode duration is short (5-15 minutes) but successive episodes elongate as the night progresses. Consequently, the majority of REM sleep usually occurs in the second half of the sleep period.

Interestingly, some disorders are associated with abnormal REM sleep patterns. For example, sleep in patients with narcolepsy may begin with REM sleep. Increased REM sleep duration occurs in response to REM sleep deprivation caused by curtailing scheduled sleep time or when discontinuing REM-suppressing drugs. It is precisely for this reason that a week of actigraphy monitoring and drug screening is recommended as part of the diagnostic workup for narcolepsy.

Patients with major depressive disorder may also demonstrate shorter than normal *REM sleep latency* (but not the extent seen in narcolepsy). This change may be accompanied by a reverse pattern of REM episode durations (i.e., longer duration episodes at the beginning, rather than the end, of the sleep period), displacement of N3 to after the first occurrence of REM sleep, and overall diminished N3 duration. By contrast, generally reduced REM sleep duration can also result from a wide variety of factors, including stress, pain, discomfort, noise, taking medications with anticholinergic

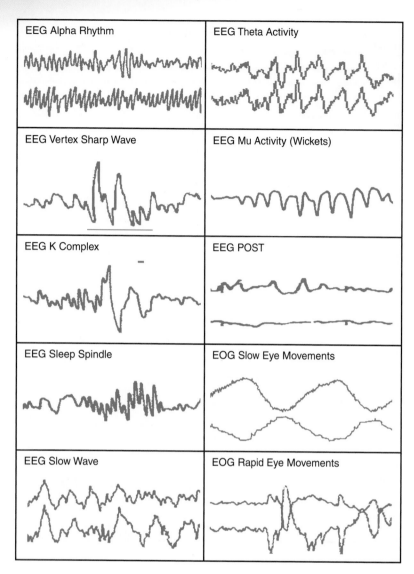

Figure 3-2 Electroencephalographic (EEG) and electro-oculographic (EOG) waveforms. These 10 panels illustrate normal EEG and EOG waveforms commonly observed during sleep. Some of these waveforms represent activity specifically used to classify sleep stages (alpha, vertex sharp waves, K complexes, sleep spindles, slow waves, slow eye movements, and rapid eye movements), and others are less common and not as essential for summarizing nocturnal sleep (mu rhythms, POSTS [positive occipital sharp transients of sleep], and theta rhythms).

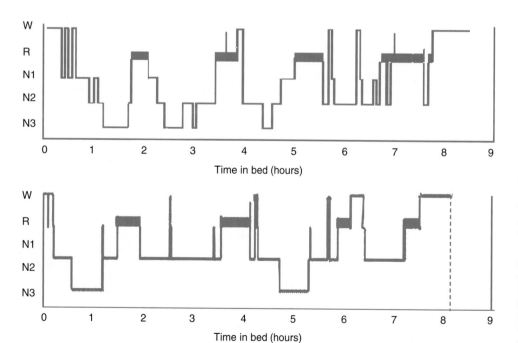

Figure 3-3 Normal sleep histograms. These two sleep histograms were recorded from a normal young adult. The variation in sleep architecture is apparent with the top panel (first night) indicating a longer latency to sleep onset and a prolonged latency to arising (typical when an individual sleeps in the laboratory). The second night *(bottom panel)* was marked by quicker sleep onset and fewer awakenings. *W,* stage wake; *R,* stage REM sleep; *N,* NREM sleep.

properties, ingesting a drug or substance having aminergic agonist properties (e.g., amphetamines), sleep-related breathing disorders, and neurologic disease. REM suppression can also be provoked by something as simple as sleeping in the laboratory for the first time (the so-called *first night effect*).

Over the lifespan, sleep macroarchitecture changes. The adult pattern of having a single major period usually develops by the second decade of life. Although infants enter sleep immediately via "active sleep" (REM sleep) the adult pattern emerges by the end of a year. Total sleep time gradually decreases during childhood with notable decreasing N3 after adolescence, a trend that continues through the lifespan with N3, sometimes disappearing altogether in old age. REM sleep declines spectacularly from birth to adolescence (from 50% to 25%), remains quite stable for the next 4 to 5 decades, and then may decline slightly thereafter. Overall, total sleep time, but not necessarily time in bed, decreases with age; thus, many seniors spend more time in bed but less time sleeping. Decreased *total sleep time*, increased *number of awakenings*, and increased *wake after sleep onset* commonly reflect accumulated pathologic changes that invariably accompany aging. Pain and other pathologic conditions often suppress REM and N3 sleep. Finally, premature N3 sleep decline is a known correlate of certain neurologic and psychiatric disorders, common in the elderly.

Sleep Microarchitecture. *Sleep microarchitecture* refers to the individual waveforms and events that occur during sleep. Some of these events fundamentally define sleep stages (e.g., slow waves); others do not (e.g., EEG theta rhythms). Even though a particular waveform may be somewhat represented, its propensity or amplitude cannot be appreciated from macroarchitectural measures. For example, an epoch of N2 with a single sleep spindle is scored the same as an epoch with 10 sleep spindles, even though the actual tracings look radically different. However, to quantify these differences requires specialized computer analysis or a tremendous amount of time and herculean effort. For years the promise of computed waveform analysis has been dangled in front of clinicians but its practical utility is slow in coming.

The central nervous system (CNS) arousal likely represents the most clinically important (and useful) sleep microarchitectural element (Fig. 3-4). Sleep appears to require continuity in order to optimally achieve its restorative function. Sleep that is fragmented by CNS arousals often leaves the individual tired or drowsy. However, patients with disrupted sleep may complain of insomnia, restless sleep, or awakening unrefreshed. CNS arousals are defined by EEG alpha intrusions into sleep that are too brief to meet criteria as awakening (i.e., less than 15 seconds in a 30-second epoch) but long enough to be visually scored reliably (3 seconds or more).[17] A patient

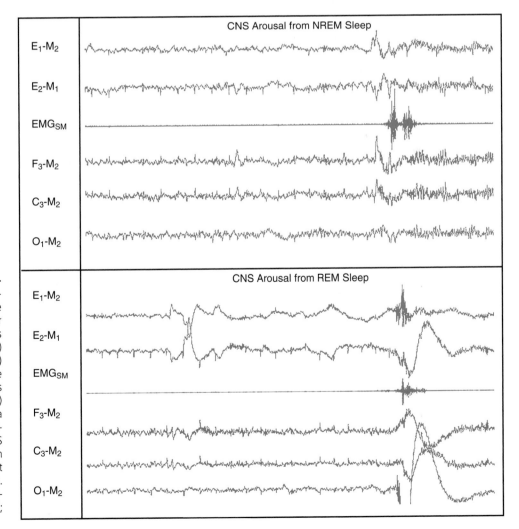

Figure 3-4 Central nervous system (CNS) arousals. Brief awakenings (of insufficient duration to be classified as stage W [wake]) occur during sleep. This figure illustrates CNS arousals from non-REM (NREM) and (rapid eye movement (REM)) sleep. Arousals such as these can be caused by pathophysiologic events (e.g., an episode of sleep apnea) or an environmental factor (e.g., a noise), or they may occur spontaneously. Regardless of origin, the CNS arousal represents a disturbance in the continuity of sleep that may not be captured by sleep stage scoring. *E*, eye; *M*, mastoid; *EMG*, electromyogram; *SM*, submentalis; *F*, frontal; *C*, central; *O*, occipital.

must be asleep in order to score an arousal, and to meet criteria when REM sleep is present, there must be an accompanying increase in submentalis EMG activity. When the EEG alpha activity intrudes into N3 sleep but does not interrupt the ongoing background activity, it is noted as alpha-delta sleep and is not tabulated as an arousal. Nonetheless, alpha-delta sleep is commonly associated with outcomes similar to sleep disturbed by arousals (i.e., unrefreshing sleep and tiredness). CNS arousals can be provoked by a specific pathophysiology (e.g., a sleep-disordered breathing event) or can occur spontaneously (which may just mean that we are not recording, and therefore have not identified, the eliciting event).

The cyclic alternating pattern (CAP) is composed of a burst-quiescent EEG rhythm (Fig. 3-5). The burst portion can incorporate many waveforms, including K complex, slow waves, high-amplitude alpha activity, or a combination of these. When the burst is devoid of alpha activity, it likely represents sleep instability (CAP type I), but as the alpha content increases it begins to resemble periodic arousal (CAP type II has alpha activity composing less than half of its duration but in a type III burst 50% or more of the burst contains EEG alpha activity). In fact, CAP type III burst phases correlate 95% with arousals scored by AASM criteria.[18]

Excessive EEG beta and sleep spindle activity should alert the clinician to possible drug ingestion. Many medications increase spindle activity (e.g., benzodiazepines and γ-aminobutyric acid [GABA$_A$] receptor agonists) and EEG beta activity (e.g., barbiturates and amphetamines). Patients with major depressive disorder reportedly also manifest increased EEG beta activity during sleep. Sharp waves, spikes, and spike and wave patterns are EEG events commonly associated with seizure disorders. However, they occasionally occur unexpectedly during routine sleep evaluations conducted for other purposes. The sleep specialist must be able to recognize these waveforms and have a working knowledge of their associated disorders. Evaluating clinical correlation with abnormal sleep-related behaviors (e.g., tongue biting) is imperative whenever these EEG events are observed. Additionally, spikes and other abnormal EEG waveforms should not be confused with benign but odd-looking phenomena (e.g., wickets [see Fig. 3-2], benign epileptiform transients of sleep, posterior occipital transients of sleep [see Fig. 3-2], and phantoms).

Cardiopulmonary Measures

Most sleep studies performed on any given night are conducted to diagnose or treat sleep-related breathing disorders. It is also now widely recognized that sleep-disordered breathing varies in etiology, presentation (Fig. 3-6), severity, and morbidity.

A sleep-related 10-second (or longer) arrest in ventilation constitutes a *sleep apnea episode*. If provoked by an inspiratory effort pause, it is labeled central. If caused by airway occlusion, it is labeled obstructive. If it is a combination of both central and obstructive elements, it is called mixed. The operational definition of a sleep apnea episode is a *10-second (or longer) 90% drop (or greater) in the nasal/oral airflow channel's peak-to-trough amplitude persisting for at least 90% of the event's duration.* By contrast, a hypopnea is merely a shallow breath (and they occur all the time during wakefulness). In sleep, a hypopnea is considered pathophysiologic because of its consequence. The AASM-recommended operational definition designates *hypopnea as a 10-second (or longer) 30% drop (or greater) in nasal pressure signal amplitude (compared to baseline) persisting for at least 90% of the event's duration and associated with a 4% or greater drop in oxygen saturation.* Thus, a hypopnea is a shallow breath associated with oxyhemoglobin desaturation. When the shallow breath is a consequence of inspiratory airway resistance and the increased effort to breath provokes an arousal, it is labeled a respiratory

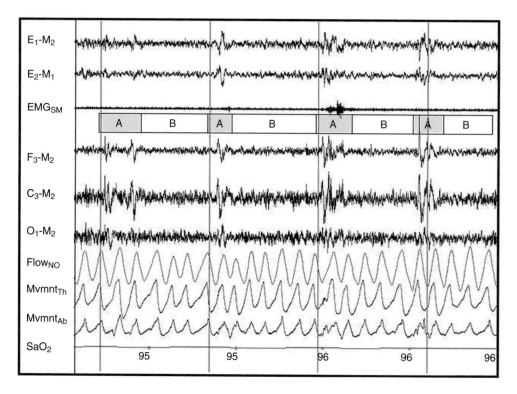

Figure 3-5 Cyclic alternating pattern (CAP). This sequence of sleep-related events is classified as CAP. The burst-quiescence pattern depicted is not caused by any obvious pathophysiology and likely represents unstable sleep. Recording notation: E_1, outer cantus of left eye; E_2, outer cantus of right eye; EMG_{SM}, submentalis electromyogram; F_3, left frontal; C_3, left central; O_1, left occipital; M_2, right mastoid; $Flow_{NO}$, nasal-oral airflow; $Mvmnt_{Th}$, thoracic movment; $Mvmnt_{Ab}$, abdominal movement; Sao_2, oxyhemoglobin saturation.

effort–related arousal (RERA). AASM's operational definition for RERA is *a 10-second (or greater) respiratory effort increase (manifest as "flattening" in the nasal pressure channel) provoking a CNS arousal.* If an event meets criteria for both a hypopnea and a RERA, designation as a hypopnea takes precedent. Nasal pressure signals are used for hypopnea and RERA detection because they are more sensitive to subtle respiratory events than nasal-oral thermistors (if the sleeper is not mouth breathing).

Diagnostic criteria depend on severity, co-morbidity, and presentation. In general, a sleep-related breathing disorder exists when five or more sleep-disordered breathing events (apnea, hypopnea, and RERA) occur per hour of sleep (summarized as the respiratory disturbance index, RDI). It must be noted, however, that Medicare indexes sleep-disordered breathing according to the number of apnea and hypopnea episodes per hour (apnea-hypopnea index, AHI) rather than RDI. If the majority of breathing events are obstructive, obstructive sleep apnea is diagnosed; otherwise the diagnosis is one or another form of central sleep apnea. The specific central apnea diagnosis depends largely on presumed cause and co-morbidities. Patients with significant contributions of both obstructive and central events (particularly if central events emerge during positive airway

pressure titration) are designated as having complex sleep apnea by some clinicians.

According to AASM practice guidelines, positive airway pressure therapy is indicated in nonsleepy patients with RDI greater than or equal to 15 and sleepy patients with RDI of 5 or more during full-night, attended polysomnography. Positive airway pressure therapy is also indicated in nonsleepy patients with AHI at or above 40 and sleepy patients with AHI at or above 20 during a 2-hour (or longer) baseline portion of a split-night polysomnographic study. Medicare guidelines are notably different in that they currently use AHI rather than RDI. Additionally, Medicare uses the lower AHI (five events per hour) when sleepiness, insomnia, hypertension, heart disease, or depression is present.

AASM recommends reporting the following cardiac events: sustained rates of 90 (or more) beats per minute (bpm), or sinus tachycardia; sustained rates below 40 bpm, or bradycardia; 3-second (or greater) pauses, or asystole; and other ectopic beats considered clinically significant. Sleep-related wide complex tachycardia is designated when the rate of three consecutive beats exceed 100 bmp with a 120-msec QRS duration (or greater) and narrow complex tachycardia is designated when similar rates occur but with QRS duration less than 120 msec.

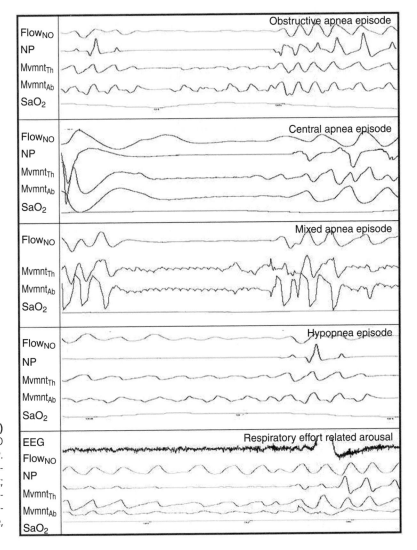

Figure 3-6 Sleep-related breathing disorder (SRBD) events. These five common pathophysiologic types of SRBD events are commonly seen during clinical polysomnography. Recording notation: *EEG,* electroencephalogram; *Flow$_{NO}$,* nasal-oral airflow; *NP,* nasal pressure; *Mvmnt$_{Th}$,* thoracic movment; *Mvmnt$_{Ab}$,* abdominal movement; *Sao$_2$,* oxyhemoglobin saturation. See text for definitions for obstructive apnea episode, central apnea episode, mixed apnea episode, hypopnea episode, and respiratory effort related arousal.

Detecting and Measuring Movement

For periodic leg movements, the "movement" begins when EMG amplitude acutely increases to 8 μV or greater above resting EMG level. The "movement" ends when EMG level returns to within 2 μV of the resting level. The increased level must persist for at least 0.5 second but not more than 5 seconds. A sequence of four or more EMG bursts (with inter-movement interval ranging from 5 to 90 seconds) must occur to call a sequence "periodic." Leg movements can be unilateral or bilateral, or may alternate. Most important, movements may be associated with CNS arousals. Periodic leg movements during wakefulness often occur in patients with restless legs syndrome (Fig. 3-7). Patients with restless legs syndrome may also show other leg EMG patterns during polysomnography.

Rudimentary polysomnographic criteria exist for other sleep-related movement disorders, including hypnagogic foot tremor, excessive fragmentary myoclonus, sleep bruxism, REM sleep behavior disorder, and rhythmic movement disorder. Video and audio recordings made during and synchronized with polysomnographic activity are often critical for interpreting the sleep study findings. Discussion of recording, scoring, and interpreting technique for these other movements is beyond the scope of this chapter (for details see the *AASM Manual*).[1]

MULTIPLE SLEEP LATENCY TEST

Indications

The AASM Standards of Practice Guideline currently endorses using the Multiple Sleep Latency Test (MSLT) to confirm and differentiate narcolepsy from other nonapneic forms of hypersomnia. In the past, some clinicians used MSLT to objectively document sleepiness; however, such use is no longer sanctioned for routine clinical practice. Nonetheless, MSLT unquestionably provides a sensitive objective measure for sleepiness and as such is considered a "standard." Consequently, MSLT is widely used in basic, clinical, and pharmacologic sleep research.

Procedures

The current protocol for MSLT involves providing a series of five nap opportunities (test session) scheduled at 2-hour intervals (measured from start time to start time). In some cases, if REM sleep occurs on two (or more) test sessions, testing

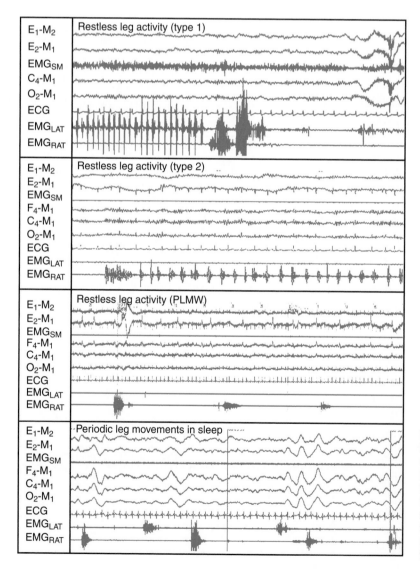

Figure 3-7 Leg movement events. These three types of leg movements may be associated with restless legs syndrome and a sequence of alternating periodic leg movements during sleep. Recording notation: E_1, outer cantus of left eye; E_2, outer cantus of right eye; EMG_{SM}, submentalis electromyogram; F_4, right frontal; C_4, right central; O_2, right occipital; M_1, left mastoid; *ECG*, electrocardiographic rhythm; EMG_{LAT}, electromyogram from left anterior tibialis; EMG_{RAT}, electromyogram from right anterior tibialis; *PLMW*, periodic leg movement during wakefulness.

can be concluded after the forth nap opportunity. Test sessions commence approximately 2 hours (ranging from 1.5 to 3.0 hours) after awakening from the prior major sleep period. It is recommended that a light breakfast be consumed 1 hour, or more before the first test session. Recommended lunch time is immediately after the second test session. The prior major sleep period must include attended, laboratory polysomnographic recording in order to appreciate sleep quantity and quality. This polysomnography must not be a "split-night" diagnostic-titration study. Furthermore, if total sleep time during the prior major sleep period is less than 6 hours, results are compromised.

The patient's sleep habits, sleep-wake schedule, and medication regimen for the past month provides helpful information, and sleep logs for 1 or more weeks before testing are recommended. Stimulants and REM-suppressing medications should be withdrawn for 2 weeks before testing, if possible. Patients should have drug screen samples collected before MSLT commences. Patients must avoid vigorous physical activity, exposure to bright sunlight, and caffeinated beverages before and between MSLT test sessions.

Individuals undergoing an MSLT must not smoke or ingest tobacco (or nicotine in any form) for 30 minutes before each nap opportunity and must abstain from engaging in any stimulating activity 15 minutes before each test session. Patients should use the toilet, if necessary, before each test session, and once they are in bed, they must be allowed time to get comfortable. "Biocalibrations" (i.e., maneuvers performed to check equipment function) should precede each nap opportunity. This calibration includes instructing the patient to relax with eyes open for 30 seconds, look right, look left, repeat twice (some also like patients to look up and down) without moving head, blink five times slowly, and clench teeth. The patient should then be encouraged to get comfortable and is instructed to "Please lie quietly, assume a comfortable position, keep your eyes closed, and try to fall asleep." Lights are then turned off and the test session begins.

During each test session, polysomnograms are recorded using left and right central (C3 and C4) and occipital (O1 and O2) EEG derivations referenced to the contralateral mastoid (M2 and M1, respectively). Left and right eye EOGs, submentalis EMG, and electrocardiogram are also recorded. Sleep rooms must be dark and quiet during testing.

If sleep does not occur, the test session is terminated after 20 minutes. If sleep onset occurs (defined as the first 30-second epoch with 15 seconds, or more, of cumulative sleep), the test session continues for 15 more minutes. For each test session, the beginning and ending time, latency to sleep onset, REM sleep latency from sleep onset (if present), and tabulation of each sleep stage during the nap opportunity are recorded. Individual test sessions in which no sleep occurred receive a latency to sleep onset score of 20 minutes.

Between nap opportunities, patients must get out of bed and should be monitored by sleep center personnel to assure that they do not nap or self-administer caffeine or unapproved medications.

Interpretation

MSLT measures physiologic sleep drive. More important, from a clinical perspective, MSLT also detects abnormal REM sleep tendency. Increased propensity for REM sleep during napping strongly suggests narcolepsy. A short mean sleep latency and REM sleep appearing on 2, or more, MSLT nap opportunities confirm narcolepsy, especially in patients with cataplexy, sleep paralysis, or hypnagogia (or hypnapompia).

Sleep latency in normal adults ranges from 10 to 20 minutes. Traditionally, an MSLT mean sleep latency of 5 minutes, or less, is considered pathologic (particularly for patients with suspected narcolepsy). A clinical MSLT should not be conducted during drug withdrawal (especially from stimulants or REM sleep suppressing medications), while sedating medications are pharmacologically active, or after a night of profoundly disturbed sleep.

MAINTENANCE OF WAKEFULNESS TEST

Indications

Maintenance of Wakefulness Test (MWT) is an indicated procedure to evaluate excessive sleepiness that is severe enough to overpower an individual's ability to remain awake. MWT is commonly used as a supporting metric for establishing "fitness for duty" after a sleep-related accident or therapeutic intervention for a sleep disorder associated with sleepiness. Testing can follow from suspicion or probable cause in individuals in whom lapses into sleep would constitute a hazard to personal or public safety.

Procedures

Individual trial sessions, scheduling, timing, and recording technique for MWT follow much the same protocol as that used for MSLT, with a few key differences. Most important, with respect to the differences, the patient attempts to remain awake rather than allowing him- or herself to fall asleep. Additionally, during test sessions, patients sit reclining on the bed with a bolster pillow (not laying down) in a dimly lit room (0.10-0.13 lux level, not total darkness) for a maximum of 40 (not 20) minutes if they do not fall asleep. A 7.5-watt nightlight located 1 foot from the floor and 3 feet lateral to the patient's head will provide proper illumination. If the patient actually falls asleep, the test session terminates once unequivocal sleep onset is determined (rather than 15 minutes later as on MSLT). Unequivocal sleep is reached at the first occurrence of one epoch of stage N2, N3, or REM; when one epoch of stage N1 is followed by an epoch of stage N2, N3, or REM; or there are three consecutive epochs of N1. Although this termination rule seems rather complicated, it represents a solution to a simple problem: avoiding terminating a test session prematurely.

One principle employed during MWT is to avoid accumulating sleep as part of the testing. To achieve this goal, we awaken patients once they have fallen asleep and terminate the test session. Stage N1 sleep is difficult to score consistently, even in the best circumstances. Interscorer reliability ranges from 60% to 70%. Stage N1 scoring problems derive from the fact that stage N1 lacks defining features and is usually scored in the absence of spindles, slow wave activity, rapid eye movements, or alpha rhythm. Complicating this difficulty is the need to score online while data are being collected. If a stage-defining feature (for example, a sleep spindle) occurs, sleep onset is clear. However, if otherwise featureless low-amplitude, mixed-frequency activity is present the certainty of sleep onset is in doubt. Terminating a test session that later review fails to find sleep onset renders that entire test session useless. Requiring three consecutive epochs of stage N1 sleep (when no other stage is observed) reduces the probability of inadvertent data loss.

Like MSLT, the first MWT session commences approximately 2 hours (ranging from 1.5 to 3.0 hours) after initial awakening from the major sleep period. Unlike MSLT, the patient is not required to undergo polysomnography during the major sleep period before a MWT. The beginning of each of the three subsequent test sessions is scheduled at 2-hour intervals. Subjects are tested under standardized conditions, seated on the bed with a bolster pillow, in their street clothes, and are not allowed to read, watch television, talk on the phone, or listen to the radio during test sessions. During MWT there is no task other than attempting to remain awake. Also, the individual may not remain in bed between test sessions. Individuals are instructed to "attempt to remain awake and not fall asleep."

Recording montage includes brain activity from central and occipital electroencephalographic derivations (C3-M2, C4-M1, O1-M2, and O2-M1 electrode site pairs). Eye movements (from left and right outer canthi), submentalis EMG, and electrocardiogram are recorded. Other channels used for overnight polysomnogram are not recorded because patients are awakened once sleep onset has occurred; therefore, detecting sleep-related pathophysiologic conditions is unnecessary. For each test session, beginning and ending time, latency to sleep onset (first 30-second epoch with 15 seconds or more of cumulative sleep), and occurring sleep stages are recorded. Individual test sessions in which no sleep occurred receive a latency to sleep score of 40 minutes.

Interpretation

MWT assesses an individual's capability to maintain wakefulness in a passive, sedentary, nonstimulating, soporific situation. If the wakefulness system fails, sleepiness becomes manifest. This laboratory test attempts to simulate conditions paralleling circumstances in which sleep onset occurs inadvertently in drowsy individuals. MWT objectively evaluates the ability to remain awake if the individual is actually attempting to do so. If an individual's agenda is to appear sleepy, MWT findings are compromised (because the patient is not trying to resist falling asleep). Therefore, clinicians must consider the patient's motives in terms of both primary and secondary gains, when interpreting test results.

As a test for the ability to remain awake, the principle outcome measure is mean sleep latency across the four MWT test sessions. Individuals whose activity directly affects public safety (e.g., commercial pilots) are characteristically held to a high standard. In such cases a perfect score (mean sleep latency of 40 minutes, i.e., no sleep onset on any trial) may be required. Normative data reveal this outcome in 59% of individuals tested. Normative data also found only 2.5% of individuals fell asleep in less than 8 minutes and this outcome is used to define excessive (abnormal) sleepiness. The significance of mean sleep latencies between 8 and 40 minutes is uncertain. One must also remember that MWT test results do not assure alertness in other environments, at other times, at other circadian phases, when sleep deprived, when taking medication or recreational substances, or after many uninterrupted hours on task. Clinical judgment must ultimately prevail when rendering interpretive decisions.

SUGGESTED IMMOBILIZATION TEST

Indications

The suggested immobilization test (SIT) provides a laboratory procedure to evaluate patients with suspected restless legs syndrome. The procedure is not part of recommended standards of clinical practice at this time; however, researchers needing objective quantitative measures find it useful. A similar procedure called the forced immobilization test has also been described, but SIT is preferred.

Procedures

SIT involves a 1-hour session conducted 1.5 hours before laboratory polysomnography scheduled for a patient's major sleep period. Standard polysomnographic recording technique is used. Patients sit in bed at a 45-degree angle with their eyes open and their legs outstretched in front of them. They are instructed not to move and not to fall asleep. If a patient falls asleep, he or she is awakened after 20 seconds and the test continues.

Recordings include left and right central (C3 and C4) and occipital (O1 and O2) EEG (referenced to contralateral mastoid), left and right eye electrooculograms, and submentalis EMG. SIT recordings also include anterior tibialis EMGs, left and right legs. A pair of longitudinally placed electrodes on the belly of each leg's anterior tibialis muscle (approximately 2-3 cm apart) record activity on separate channels.

Interpretation

All leg movements with durations ranging from 0.5 to 10 seconds are counted if separated by a 4-second interval. Left only, right only, and bilateral (if left and right are within 4 seconds of one another) leg movements are tabulated separately. Total movement indices (number per hour) are calculated. Patients with restless legs syndrome have significantly higher indices than control subjects (76 vs. 27 per hour, respectively) and a greater preponderance in the second half of the test (98 vs. 55 per hour, respectively). Most movements are bilateral, but some patients have only unilateral movements. Receiver-operator characteristic analysis places overall threshold at 40 movements per hour, which provides an 81% sensitivity and 81% specificity.

ACTIGRAPHY

Indications

Like many clinical procedures in sleep medicine, actigraphy began as a research tool and evolved into a clinical procedure as the field of sleep medicine grew. Originally used mainly to assess specific circadian rhythm disorders, actigraphy now enjoys wider application. AASM standards of practice endorse actigraphy for evaluating many circadian rhythm disorders, including advanced sleep phase syndrome, delayed sleep phase syndrome, shift work sleep disorder, jet lag, non-24-hour sleep-wake syndrome, and blindness-related dyssomnia. As an adjunct measure, actigraphy can objectively document the sleep-wake pattern during the week (or longer) leading up to a multiple sleep latency test. The AASM also endorses using actigraphy for estimating total sleep time during cardiopulmonary monitoring when polysomnography is not available.

Other approved actigraphic assessments include evaluations for insomnia (including those with co-morbid depression) and hypersomnia, especially in circumstances problematic for laboratory polysomnography (e.g., nursing home residents), and as a treatment outcome measure for various sleep disorders.

Procedures

Most actigraphs used in sleep medicine resemble a wristwatch. They contain accelerometers, an internal clock, a digital memory device, event markers, and often a photo sensor. Modern actigraphs are lightweight and water resistant. Patients wear the device continuously on their nondominant wrist usually for a week (or more) and they concurrently maintain a "sleep diary." Event marker use varies; however, at a minimum, getting into bed and out of bed should be indicated. For some applications, an actigraph may be worn on an ankle or attached to the body. After the device acquires data for the designated period of time, the patient returns the actigraph and a computer extracts its stored activity information.

Interpretation

Simply stated, the fundamental rationale for actigraphy is that reduced movement occurs during sleep and increased movement occurs during wakefulness. Therefore, by continuously monitoring movement we can gain insight into an individual's rest-activity cycle and circadian rhythm alignment with clock time. Advanced and delayed sleep phase, as well as other circadian rhythm disorders are easily visualized as misalignments between desired bed time, clock time, and active-inactive periods. Insufficient sleep schedule or movements occurring at a time the patient is sleeping or attempting to sleep can be readily determined. In a complementary fashion, chronically low activity levels or sudden inactivity during wake periods can alert clinicians to subwakefulness, hypersomnia, or lapses into sleep. Finally, comparing pre- and posttreatment actigraphic profiles can reveal consolidation, improved timing, lengthening, or increased differentiation of the sleep-wake cycle.

HOME SLEEP TESTING

Indications

Home sleep testing (HST) as an accepted (and reimbursable) diagnostic procedure for sleep apnea represents a relatively recent development in sleep medicine. Central Medicare Services approved HST in 2008 with an indication for evaluating patients with highly probable sleep apnea. Clinical suspicion derives from signs, symptoms, and risk factors, including sleepiness, disruptive snoring, awakening with gasping or choking, witnessed breathing cessations, obesity, hypertension, depression, and heart disease. Patients with symptoms suggesting sleep disorders other than sleep apnea (for example, sleep paralysis, cataplexy, sleepwalking, or dream enactment with injury) should be referred for laboratory evaluation. Unattended studies are also more susceptible to patient tampering and should not be used forensically or in regulatory matters unless adequate validation safeguards are in place. And at the risk of stating the obvious, HST is inappropriate when attendant-related procedures are required (e.g., continuous positive airway pressure titration).

Properly conducted HST can facilitate sleep-disordered breathing recognition. However, successful clinical application depends on (1) proper patient selection, (2) appropriate portable recorder selection and application, (3) accurate interpretation (by a sleep specialist), and (4) readily available sleep laboratory access (to follow up on negative tests or residual problems following treatment). Additionally, in our experience a successful home sleep testing program requires close clinical follow-up at every step along the clinical pathway. Finally, HST provides an option for patients who, for a variety of reasons, cannot be studied in the sleep laboratory.

Procedures

HST involves recording cardiopulmonary data usually packaged as a Holter-type device principally designed for unattended use in the home. AASM devised a classification scheme for home testing devices based on recorded parameters compared to standard laboratory technique (Table 3-2). HST recorders are classified as levels II, III, and IV. Most HST devices fall into the level III category (cardiopulmonary recorders) by acquiring heart rhythm and three or more respiratory channels. Data are stored in memory and subsequently transferred to a computer for review and analysis. Systems with a single (or possibly two) data channels fall into the level IV category (and usually include oximetry).

TABLE 3-2		
Classification of Laboratory and Home Sleep Tests		
Level	**Designation**	**Description**
I	Attended laboratory polysomnography	Conducted in a sleep laboratory
		Includes recordings of EEG, EOG, EMG-SM, airflow, respiratory effort, ECG, Sao_2 , EMG-AT
		Technologist in attendance
II	Unattended polysomnography	Usually conducted in patient's home but sometimes recorded in a hospital bedroom or care unit
		Includes recordings of EEG, EOG, EMG-SM, airflow, respiratory effort, ECG, Sao_2, EMG-AT
		No technologist in attendance
III	Unattended cardiopulmonary recording	Usually conducted in patient's home but sometimes recorded in a hospital bedroom or care unit
		Usually 4 or more channels, including airflow, snoring sounds, respiratory effort, ECG, and/or Sao_2
		No technologist in attendance
IV	Unattended single- or dual-channel recording	Usually conducted in a patient's home but sometimes recorded in a hospital bedroom or care unit
		Usually records 1 or 2 channels, typically ECG and Sao_2
		No technologist in attendance

ECG, electrocardiogram; *EEG,* electroencephalogram; *EMG-AT,* electromyogram–anterior tibialis; *EMG-SM,* electromyogram–submentalis; *EOG,* electro-oculogram; *Sao_2,* oxygen saturation.

HST devices typically include some measure of airflow, respiratory effort, cardiac rhythm, and blood oxygen saturation. Most HST recorded measures derive from those used in standard polysomnography (e.g., temperature transducers or nasal pressure sensors for airflow, diaphragm movement for respiratory effort, finger or ear oximetry for oxyhemoglobin saturation). However, some HST devices use unique measurements (e.g., peripheral arterial tonometry, forehead reflectance oximetry, transformed breathing sounds, accelerometers attached to the legs, and forehead EEG). Some of these novel methods are well validated surrogate measures, and others require further testing.

Interpretation

Some HST devices, in the proper hands, can reliably confirm sleep-related breathing disorders. However, because HST is less sensitive (compared to attended laboratory polysomnography) and more prone to data loss (due to uncorrected technical failures), the results can "rule-in" but not "rule-out" sleep apnea. The clinician reviewing and interpreting HST (who should be an experienced sleep practitioner) must continually keep in mind that it is an abbreviated test that can miss subtle sleep-disordered breathing events. Patients failing to reach unequivocal sleep apnea diagnostic criteria (usually AHI ≥ 15) should either be (a) scheduled for repeat testing (if technical issues rendered the test uninterruptable) or (b) scheduled for attended, laboratory polysomnography.

Medicare qualifies any patient for positive airway pressure therapy when HST finds 15 or more apnea or hypopnea (using the definition requiring a ≥ 4% oxyhemoglobin desaturation) episodes per hour of testing with a 2-hour baseline minimum duration. A lower treatment threshold (AHI ≥ 5) qualifies patients with co-morbid sleepiness, insomnia, hypertension, heart disease, a history of stroke, impaired cognition, or mood disorder. AASM criteria may allow use of the alternate definition for hypopnea for calculating these indices, but the guidelines are not completely clear. Since Medicare criteria can change, the reader is referred to www.cms.gov for further information.

Recommended scoring technique for detecting respiratory events during HST is largely borrowed from polysomnography (and may or may not be completely appropriate). HST clinical interpretation is much more specifically focused (compared to polysomnography) on simply determining if a patient has and needs sleep-disordered breathing treated. In our experience, interpretation depends much more on pattern recognition and subtleties seen when inspecting actual recordings (raw data) rather than summary parameters. Thus, the sleep specialist reading the home sleep test needs greater direct understanding and control over set-up, recording, downloading, and summarization to assure quality. In fact, perhaps the most important judgment is a global assessment of a recording's technical quality and interpretability. All decisions about diagnostic outcome, when to retest, and who to treat are all based on medical judgments relating back to the HST quality control assessment.

Continuously monitored oxygen saturation levels has long been used in patients with significant lung disease to determine the need for possible supplemental oxygen. Sometimes a clear oxyhemoglobin desaturation-resaturation pattern can be observed and this can indicate sleep apnea. Nonetheless, single-channel overnight oximetry is not recommended for diagnosing sleep-related breathing disorders.

SUMMARY

This chapter summarizes the major diagnostic procedures used in sleep medicine practice. The AASM standards concerning these procedures are also reviewed. Sleep specialists must be familiar with the details of these test procedures, their appropriate use, and methods for interpretation of findings. Clinical correlation with signs, symptoms, and co-morbid conditions requires insight into normal sleep mechanisms and the pathophysiologic associations. As refined as these procedures may be, clinical interview and assessment remain paramount.

REFERENCES

1. Iber C, Ancoli-Israel S, Chesson A, Quan SF. *for the American Academy of Sleep Medicine. The AASM Manual for the Scoring of Sleep and Associated Events: Rules, Terminology and Technical Specifications.* 1st ed. Westchester, IL: American Academy of Sleep Medicine; 2007.
2. Standards of Practice Committee of the American Academy of Sleep Medicine. Practice parameters for the indications for polysomnography and related procedures: An update for 2005. *Sleep.* 2005;28:499-521.
3. Standards of Practice Committee of the American Academy of Sleep Medicine. Practice parameters for clinical use of the multiple sleep latency test and the maintenance of wakefulness test. *Sleep.* 2005;28: 113-121.
4. Montplaisir J, Boucher S, Nicolas A, Lesperance P, Gosselin A, et al. Immobilization tests and periodic leg movements in sleep for the diagnosis of restless legs syndrome. *Movement Disord.* 1998;13:324-329.
5. Standards of Practice Committee of the American Academy of Sleep Medicine. Practice parameters for the use of actigraphy in the assessment of sleep and sleep disorders: An update for 2007. *Sleep.* 2007;30:519-529.
6. American Sleep Disorders Association Standards of Practice Committee. Practice parameters for the use of portable recording in the assessment of obstructive sleep apnea. *Sleep.* 1994;14:372-377.
7. Collop NA, Anderson WM, Boehlecke B, Claman D, Goldberg R, et al. Clinical guidelines for the use of unattended portable monitors in the diagnosis of obstructive sleep apnea in adult patients. *J Clin Sleep Med.* 2007;3(7):737-747.
8. Littner M, Hirshkowitz M, Sharafkhaneh A, Goodnight-White S. Nonlaboratory assessment of sleep-related breathing disorders. *Sleep Med Clin.* 2006;1:461-463.
9. Malow B. Neurologic monitoring techniques. In: Kryger MH, Roth T, Dement WC, eds. *Principles and Practice of Sleep Medicine.* St. Louis: Elsevier-Saunders; 2011:1646-1656.
10. Chokroverty S, Montagna P. Sleep and epilepsy. In: Chokroverty S, ed. *Sleep Disorders Medicine.* 3rd ed. Philadelphia: Saunders; 2009:499-529.
11. Bornstein SK. Respiratory monitoring during sleep: Polysomnography. In: Guilleminault C, ed. *Sleeping and Waking Disorders: Indications and Techniques.* Menlo Park, CA: Addison-Wesley; 1982:183-212.
12. Coleman RM. Periodic movements in sleep (nocturnal myoclonus) and restless legs syndrome. In: Guilleminault C, ed. *Sleeping and Waking Disorders: Indications and Techniques.* Menlo Part, CA: Addison-Wesley; 1982:267-295.
13. Bonnet M, Carley D, Guilleminault C, Hirshkowitz M, Keenan S, et al. Recording and scoring leg movements. ASDA Report. *Sleep.* 1993;16: 748-759.
14. Berger H. Uber das elektroenkephalogramm des Menschen. *J Psychol Neurol.* 1930;40:160-179.
15. Loomis AL, Harvey N, Hobart GA. Cerebral states during sleep, as studied by human brain potentials. *J Exp Psychol.* 1937;21:127-144.
16. Roth T, Stubbs D, Walsh JK. Rameleton (TAK-375), A selective MT_1-/MT_2-receptor agonist, reduces latency to persistent sleep in a model of transient insomnia related to a novel sleep environment. *Sleep.* 2005; 28(3):303-307.
17. Bonnet M, Carley D, Carskadon M, Easton P, Guilleminault C, et al. EEG arousals: Scoring rules and examples: ASDA Report. *Sleep.* 1992;15: 173-184.
18. Parrino L, Smerieri A, Rossi M, Terzano MG. Relationship of slow and rapid EEG components of CAP to ASDA arousals in normal sleep. *Sleep.* 2001;24:881-885.

SECTION 2

Background to Sleep Medicine Therapeutics

An Overview of Sleep:
Physiology and Neuroanatomy

Elda Arrigoni / Patrick M. Fuller

One of the first recorded descriptions of alterations in consciousness can be found in the Hindu textbook *Upanishad* (about 1000 BC), which described four states of "vigilance," two of which correspond to the sleeping state: non-rapid eye movement (NREM) sleep and rapid eye movement (REM) sleep. The first true "theory of sleep," however, is credited to Lucretius, who in the 1st century BC hypothesized that sleep was a passive phenomenon and reflected only the cessation of wake. Lucretius's theory became the predecessor to the "deafferentation theory," which persisted for many years and held that sleep is initiated passively when sensory inputs fall below a threshold necessary to maintain cortical arousal. Contemporary models of sleep-wake regulation, which are reviewed herein, reflect a deeper understanding of the neuronal substrates underlying different states of vigilance and, in particular, hold sleep to be an active process requiring the participation of specific sleep-promoting neurons.

The Phenomenology of Sleep

Sleep is a behavioral state characterized by a reduction in motor activity (as measured by the electromyogram, EMG), a decreased sensitivity to stimuli, and stereotypic posture and, unlike other states of altered consciousness, such as coma and anesthesia, is rapidly reversible and self-regulating.[1] The state transition to sleep also involves dramatic changes in the cortical electroencephalogram (EEG; Fig. 4-1). During wakefulness, the cortical EEG typically contains desynchronized high-frequency, low-amplitude waves in the 14- to 30-Hz range that are thought to reflect differences in the timing of processing of cognitive, motor, and perceptual functions. Although the transition from wakefulness to sleep is generally viewed as rapid and relatively complete, humans typically exhibit graded and stereotypic changes in the cortical EEG during this transition period. During the earliest stage of the transition from wake to sleep, commonly referred to as "quiet wakefulness" or "quiet rest," EEG oscillations predominate in the 8- to 13-Hz range and are referred to as *alpha rhythm*. At the onset of NREM sleep, the EEG waves become larger in amplitude, reflecting increased cortical synchrony, and the EEG frequency slows. In humans, NREM sleep has been classically described as being composed of four stages. During stage 1 (N1), conscious awareness of the external environment disappears and the EEG slows further, with oscillations predominating in the 4- to 7-Hz theta range. Stage 2 (N2) is typified by a complete loss of conscious awareness as well as

the appearance of sleep spindles and K-complexes in the EEG. During stages 3 and 4 (now together referred to as stage N3, see later discussion), commonly termed "deep sleep," delta waves appear in the EEG. Delta waves are oscillations that predominate in the 1- to 4-Hz range and are commonly referred to as *slow wave activity* in the EEG. It follows that an increase in the total power, amplitude, and incidence of delta waves in the cortical EEG during NREMS forms the operational definition of increasing sleep intensity. The appearance of delta waves in the EEG is also thought to primarily reflect synchronized oscillations of thalamocortical circuit activity[2] (reviewed later), although the neocortex is also capable of generating intrinsic slow oscillations (primarily 0.5-1.0 Hz, but also 1.0-4.0 Hz). In addition to NRM sleep, humans and other mammals spend part of their lives in the behavioral state of REM sleep (stage R), which is a state characterized by activation of the cortical and hippocampal EEG, rapid eye movements (REMs) (as measured by the electro-oculogram, EOG), profound skeletal muscle atonia, and often dreaming. REM sleep cycles periodically with NREM sleep and produces striking changes in the cortical EEG, including the transition to high-frequency, low-amplitude activity resembling stage N1 sleep and wake in humans. It is important to note that the American Academy of Sleep Medicine (AASM) has recently published an updated set of rules used for the staging of human sleep. In the updated AASM manual the three behavioral states of wake, NREM sleep, and REM sleep are still conceptualized on the basis of the EEG, EOG, and EMG; however, stages 3 and 4 of NREM sleep are now combined into a single stage (N3) that is characterized by epochs consisting of 20% or more slow wave activity of frequency 0.5 to 2 Hz and amplitude greater than 75 μV as measured over the frontal regions.[3]

EEG and Behavioral Arousal

The Brainstem Ascending Reticular Activating System

In order to fully understand the behavioral state of sleep, it is first useful to review the brain substrates necessary for maintaining an arousal cortex (i.e., an activated EEG) and wakeful consciousness. Nearly one century ago and around the time of the First World War, the Viennese neurologist Baron Constantine von Economo (Fig. 4-2) evaluated patients with a viral encephalitis that profoundly affected sleep-wake regulation (i.e., encephalitis lethargica). In these seminal clinico-anatomic studies, von Economo (1930)[4] reported that the preponderance of the lethargica victims slept excessively, some more than 20 hours per day, typically waking only to eat or void. Postmortem brain analysis revealed that these individuals had lesions at the junction of the midbrain and posterior hypothalamus, suggesting to von Economo that this area of the brain contained wake-promoting circuitry. Interestingly, and quite paradoxically (at least at the time), a small percentage of individuals afflicted with encephalitis lethargica became insomniac, often sleeping only a few hours each day. Postmortem analysis revealed that these insomniac individuals had lesions involving not the midbrain-diencephalon junction but, rather, the basal forebrain and anterior hypothalamus, suggesting that this area of the brain likely contained sleep-promoting circuitry. Nearly 20 years later, von Economo's observations in the encephalitis lethargica victims was recapitulated experimentally by Ranson through his demonstration of hypersomnolence in rhesus monkeys sustaining lesions of the posterior hypothalamus.[5] Around this same time, in 1935, Frederic Bremer[6] uncovered evidence of an ascending arousal system necessary for cortical arousal (Fig. 4-3). In his seminal studies, Bremer demonstrated that transection of the brainstem at the pontomescephalic level (i.e., cerveau isole), but not

the spinomedullary junction (i.e., encephale isole), produced coma in cats. Bremer hypothesized that the resulting reduction in "cerebral tone" following the cerveau isole was due to interruption of ascending sensory inputs, lending significant credence to the passive "deafferentation theory" of sleep that prevailed at the time. More than a decade after Bremer's transection experiments, Moruzzi (who was a student of Bremer's) and Magoun[7] demonstrated that electrical stimulation of the rostral pontine reticular formation produced a desynchronized EEG (as electrophysiologic correlate of the conscious state, per earlier mention) and that transections at this same level (i.e., the so-called "intercollicular" transections) caused acute coma. Moruzzi and Magoun interpreted their experimental data as evidence for an active "waking center" in the mesopontine reticular formation, essentially refuting the deafferentation theory of sleep. Moruzzi and Magoun coined the term "ascending reticular activating system" (ARAS) for this brainstem system, and the functional integrity of this system was henceforth considered the sine qua non for cortical arousal and wakeful consciousness. Subsequent studies showed that lesions at the level of the rostral pons, but not in the midpons or more caudally, could cause coma both in animals[8] and in humans.[9,10] Hence the origin of the ascending arousal system must begin in the rostral pons.

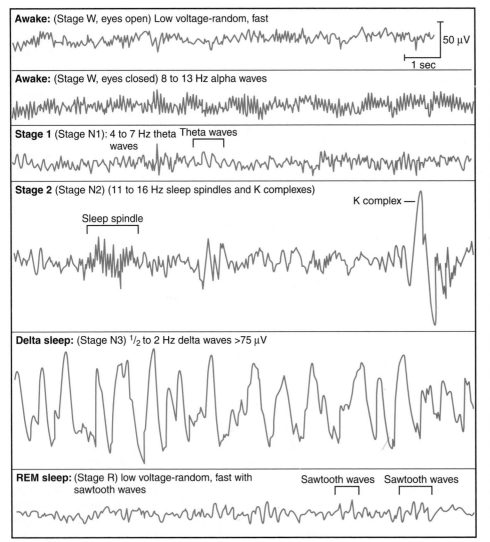

Figure 4-1 The electroencephalogram (EEG) characterizing the waking state contains desynchronized high-frequency, low-*amplitude waves.* The "quiet wake" EEG with the eyes closed contains waves in the 8- to 13-Hz range that are termed *alpha waves.* During stage N1 of NREM sleep the EEG becomes slower and theta waves (4- to 7-Hz, with "sawtooth" appearance) emerge. During stage N2 of NREM sleep both sleep spindles (phasic burst of 11 to 16 Hz) and K-complexes (a well-delineated negative sharp wave followed immediately by a positive component) appear in the EEG. During stages 3 and 4 (now combined into stage N3 in the 2007 *AASM Manual,* see text) of NREM sleep high-amplitude slow waves (also called *delta waves*) in the .5 to 2 Hz range appear. Finally, during REM sleep (stage R) the EEG transitions to a high-frequency, low-amplitude activity that resembles stage N1 of NREM sleep, and conjugate saccades are seen in the electro-oculograph (EOG) *(not shown),* reflecting the rapid eye movements that occur and give this behavioral state its name. NREM sleep, non-rapid eye movement sleep; REM sleep, rapid eye movement sleep. (Redrawn with modification from Amlaner CJ, Buxton OM, eds: The Sleep Research Society Basics of Sleep Guide, Slide Set 7, Section 1 [Caples SM, Lanfranchi PA, Somers VK; Sleep Physiology, Sleep and the Autonomic Nervous System]. Darien, IL: Sleep Research Society, 2007, with permission.)

In the 1970s and 1980s, experiments revealed that, contrary to popular conception, the origin of the ARAS was not a neurochemically and functionally homogeneous collection of neurons in the undifferentiated reticular formation but, rather, comprised specific cell groups using specific neurotransmitters that projected to the cortex via two distinct anatomic branches and "relays"[11-14] (Fig. 4-4, *A*). The dorsal branch of the ARAS consists of cholinergic neurons that project to the forebrain and are found in the pedunculopontine tegmental (PPT) and laterodorsal tegmental (LDT) nuclei of the mesopontine tegmentum.[15] Cholinergic PPT and LDT neurons project to the midline and intralaminar nuclei of the thalamus

and are thought to play a critical role in gating thalamocortical transmission by preventing relay neurons from being hyperpolarized and entering into burst mode, thus clearing the way for thalamocortical sensory transmission (see following discussion for more on thalamus). PPT and LDT neurons fire most rapidly during wakefulness and REM sleep (W/REMS) and most slowly during NREM sleep, suggesting that they participate in cortical activation and EEG desynchronization.[2,16]

The ventral branch of the ARAS, which largely bypasses the thalamus (although not completely, as a small population of axons target the thalamic intralaminar and reticular nuclei), consists of a series of wake-promoting monoaminergic cell groups, also predominately of mesopontine tegmentum origin, that project to the lateral hypothalamus, basal forebrain, and cerebral cortex.[17-20] The monoaminergic systems include the noradrenergic ventrolateral medulla and locus ceruleus, the dopaminergic neurons of the ventrolateral periaqueductal gray matter (just adjacent to the dorsal raphe nucleus [DRN]), the serotoninergic dorsal and median raphe nuclei, and histaminergic neurons in the hypothalamic tuberomammillary nucleus (see Fig. 4-4, *A*). In general, neurons in all of these cell groups fire more during wakefulness than during NREM sleep and show virtually no activity during REM sleep.[17-20] It is important to recognize that while the traditional model of the ARAS has emphasized the critical role of the cholinergic and monoaminergic neurons in cortical activation, cell-body specific lesions in these cell groups have produced limited alterations in wakefulness, at least in rats and cats.[21-25] In fact, even combined lesions including the locus ceruleus (LC), tuberomammillary nucleus (TMN), and basal forebrain cholinergic neurons have had little effect on overall wakefulness and hence the origin of the arousing influence has never been fully explained, and the source has been presumed to be the collective input from all of these structures so that lesions of any one of them will not produce a loss of consciousness. An alternative, and only recently explored, source of arousal-promoting inputs from the rostral pons may be glutamatergic neurons in the parabrachial nucleus and adjacent precoeruleus area, which project to the lateral hypothalamus, basal forebrain, and cerebral

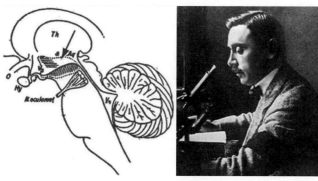

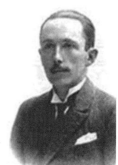

Figure 4-2 An active role for the brain in sleep-wake behavior was first indicated in 1916 when Baron Constantine von Economo performed postmortem brain analysis on victims of a viral encephalitis that profoundly affected sleep-wake regulation (i.e., encephalitis lethargica or von Economo's sleeping sickness). As seen at top, in the original drawing taken from von Economo's clinico-anatomic studies, lesions at the junction of the midbrain and posterior hypothalamus (*diagonal hatching*) produced hypersomnolence. By contrast, lesions of the basal forebrain and anterior hypothalamus (*horizontal hatching*) produced profound insomnia. von Economo also observed that lesions between these two sites (see *arrow*), which included the lateral hypothalamic area, caused narcolepsy. For many years, however, the nature of the circuitry subserving these putative wake/arousal- and sleep-promoting brain regions remained elusive. (From von Economo C: Sleep as a problem of localization. *J Nerv Ment Dis.* 1930;71:249-259.)

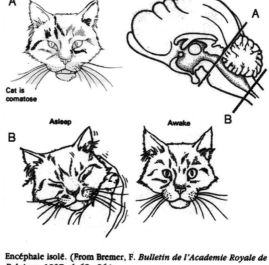

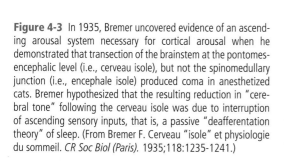

Figure 4-3 In 1935, Bremer uncovered evidence of an ascending arousal system necessary for cortical arousal when he demonstrated that transection of the brainstem at the pontomesencephalic level (i.e., cerveau isole), but not the spinomedullary junction (i.e., encephale isole) produced coma in anesthetized cats. Bremer hypothesized that the resulting reduction in "cerebral tone" following the cerveau isole was due to interruption of ascending sensory inputs, that is, a passive "deafferentation theory" of sleep. (From Bremer F. Cerveau "isole" et physiologie du sommeil. *CR Soc Biol (Paris).* 1935;118:1235-1241.)

Encéphale isolé. (From Bremer, F. *Bulletin de l'Academie Royale de Belgique,* 1937, *4,* 68–86.)

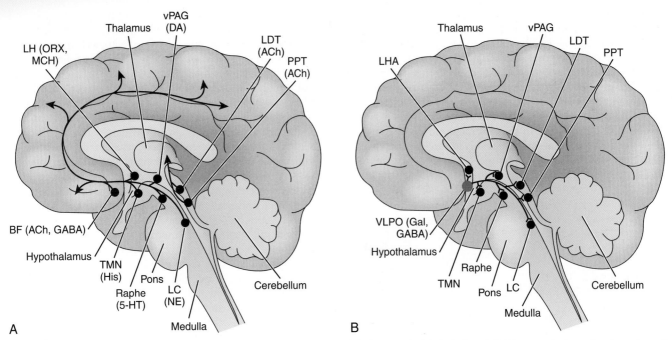

Figure 4-4 A, The ascending arousal system consists of noradrenergic (NE) neurons of the locus ceruleus (LC), cholinergic (ACh) neurons in the pedunculopontine and laterodorsal tegmental (PPT/LDT) nuclei, serotoninergic (5-HT) neurons in the raphe nucleus, dopaminergic (DA) neurons of the ventral periaqueductal gray matter (vPAG), and histaminergic (His) neurons of the tuberomammillary nucleus (TMN). These systems produce cortical arousal via two pathways: a dorsal route through the thalamus and a ventral route through the hypothalamus and basal forebrain (BF). The latter pathway receives contributions from the orexin (ORX) and melanin-concentrating hormone (MCH) neurons of the lateral hypothalamic (LH) area as well as from GABAergic, glutamatergic, or acetylcholine (Ach) neurons of the basal forebrain (BF). **B,** For many years it remained unclear how this arousal system was turned "off" so that sleep could be initiated and maintained. Although work by Nauta (1946) and Bremer (1935) provided support for the concept of sleep-promoting circuitry in the anterior hypothalamus/preoptic area, it was not until the mid-1990s that the identity of this sleep-promoting circuitry was revealed. In these recent investigations, it was demonstrated that the ventrolateral preoptic nucleus (VLPO) contains sleep-active cells, which contain the inhibitory neurotransmitters GABA and galanin (Gal). The VLPO (*blue circle*) projects to all of the main components of the ascending arousal system. Inhibition of the arousal system by the VLPO during sleep is critical for the maintenance and consolidation of sleep. (Modified from Fuller PM, Gooley JJ, Saper CB. Neurobiology of the sleep-wake cycle: Sleep architecture, circadian regulation, and regulatory feedback. *J Biol Rhythms.* 2006;21[6]:482-493.)

cortex.[26-28] Consistent with an important arousal-promoting role, it has recently been reported that cell-specific lesions of the parabrachial-preceruleus complex produce behavioral unresponsiveness and a monotonous sub-1 Hz cortical EEG in the rat.[28] The preceruleus also sends projections to the medial septum, which, in turn, projects to the hippocampus and is presumably important in ascending control of hippocampal function.

The Forebrain Arousal System

In addition to the brainstem arousal-promoting systems, several forebrain neuronal networks are critically involved in supporting EEG and behavioral arousal. In general, these forebrain systems depend upon the brainstem arousal influence, although it is important to recognize that nearly all patients with brainstem lesions eventually recover wake-sleep cycles if they receive sufficient medical support. These observations suggest that after injury to the brainstem arousal system, forebrain cell groups can support cycles of cortical arousal.[10,29] The most caudally located wake-promoting forebrain arousal population is found in the posterior hypothalamus, near the midbrain junction. This brain region includes the aforementioned histaminergic TMN whose neurons represent the sole source of CNS histamine.[20,30] TMN neurons also contain the inhibitory neurotransmitter GABA as well as the μ-opioid peptide endomorphin.[31] Neurons of the TMN project widely across

the neuraxis, and similar to brainstem monoaminergic groups, TMN neurons are most active during waking and mostly quiescent during sleep. The neurotransmitter histamine has potent arousal-promoting properties and, accordingly, histamine antagonists (e.g., antihistamines, which are commonly prescribed to treat allergies) often produce drowsiness. Just rostral to the TMN and in the lateral hypothalamic area are neurons containing the orexin neuropeptides (orexin-A and -B, also called hypocretin-1 and -2). Many of the orexin neurons co-localize glutamate and virtually all contain the neuropeptide dynorphin.[32] The orexin neurons project to the basal forebrain, to the cerebral cortex, and in a reciprocal manner, to components of the brainstem arousal systems, in particular the TMN and LC.[33] Orexin neurons also innervate the intralaminar nuclei of the thalamus, albeit to a lesser degree than the other brain regions described. Orexin neurons are active during wakefulness, firing particularly briskly during behavioral exploration, and increase the firing rates of neurons in the TMN, LC, and DRN.[34] Mice and humans lacking orexin neurons (or orexin receptors) demonstrate narcolepsy-like symptoms,[35-37] including profound behavioral state instability in the form of frequent state transitions and cataplexy (i.e., sudden bilateral loss of skeletal muscle tone without loss of consciousness) (Fig. 4-6). The orexin neurons are also implicated in the regulation of REM sleep. A second population of neurons containing the peptide melanin-concentrating hormone (MCH) is intermingled with the lateral hypothalamic orexin neurons. MCH neurons, which also contain GABA, have very similar projections to the orexin neurons but are mostly active during REM sleep, during which time they are thought to inhibit the ascending monoaminergic systems.[38,39] Interestingly, damage to the posterior lateral hypothalamus in humans and animals can produce much more extreme hypersomnolence than can be explained by loss of just orexin or MCH neurons alone.[5,40,41] It has therefore been suggested that a third population of wake-promoting neurons must exist in the posterior-lateral hypothalamic (PLH) region. Recent anatomic work has revealed the presence of cortically projecting glutatmatergic neurons in this region, suggesting a possible critical role for PLH glutatmatergic neurons in maintaining the waking state.[26,42,43]

The most rostral of the wake-promoting forebrain arousal systems is located in the basal forebrain (BF). The BF corticopetal system is a complex continuum of large, subcortical and highly heterogeneous neurons that intermingle in roughly the same regions and project to sensory and motor areas of the cortex as well as to hippocampal and limbic cortical areas.[44,45] Overall, the magnocellular corticopetal group occupies the medial septal-diagonal band complex, the medial globus pallidus, the magnocellular preoptic nucleus, and the substantia innominata (SI; corticopetal neurons within the SI are also called the nucleus basalis). These neurons receive inputs from many regions of the neuraxis, including inputs from the amygdala, nucleus accumbens, locus ceruleus, raphe nuclei, ventral tegmental area, reticular formation, and in particular, the parabrachial nucleus.[28]

Neurons of the BF serve as the ventral, extrathalamic "relay" from the ARAS to the cortex and are believed to play a critical role in maintaining cortical arousal and wakeful consciousness.[46] The BF neurons comprise intermingled cholinergic, GABAergic, and glutamatergic cells that project directly to cortical pyramidal cells or interneurons.[47] A close relationship between the BF and cortical activity has been long appreciated; for example, direct stimulation of the BF has pronounced activating effects on the cortical EEG, increases cerebral blood flow, and modifies (enhances) the responsiveness to sensory input.[46,48,49] There is also an extensive literature demonstrating that neurons in the BF fire in bursts that are time-locked to EEG waves and that stimulation of the BF can activate the EEG, whereas inhibition of BF firing can slow the EEG.[50,51] Recent work[52] has further established a strong correlation between the *in vivo* discharge properties of specific BF neuronal population and spectral shifts in the cortical EEG (in unanesthetized, head-fixed rats).

While a more complete understanding of the individual roles of the cholinergic, GABAergic, and glutamatergic BF cell groups in EEG and neurobehavioral arousal is the focus of on-going research, recent work has revealed some of the electrophysiologic characteristics of these BF populations. For example, BF cholinergic neurons fire in association with the waking and REM sleep EEG, whereas BF GABAergic and glutamatergic neurons comprise multiple sleep-wake subgroups.[52] About 70% of BF GABAergic neurons fire during wakefulness and REM sleep, whereas 30% are NREM sleep active and discharge at a higher rate during slow wave sleep. Of the three BF neuronal populations, the glutamatergic population appears to be the most heterogeneous population with respect to state-specific activity. For example, some BF glutamatergic neurons are similar to BF cholinergic and

GABAergic neurons insofar as they discharge at a higher rate during waking and REM sleep, whereas other BF glutamatergic neurons fire in association with NREM sleep, and finally, some discharge in positive association with EMG amplitude. Based upon their discharge properties, these latter BF glutamatergic neurons have been suggested to play a unique role in facilitating muscle tone and behavioral arousal via a downstream projection to the posterior hypothalamus (including the orexin neurons) and brainstem.[52]

Historically, the functional integrity of the thalamus has been widely considered to be necessary for generating the EEG correlates of cortical arousal and a wakeful state as well as for "gating" sensory transmission during sleep and wake.[53,54] In fact, thalamic relay nuclei (e.g., the anterior, ventral, and lateral thalamic cell groups; medial and lateral geniculate nuclei; mediodorsal nucleus; and pulvinar) are the most abundant sources of subcortical afferents to the cerebral cortex. The contemporary model of the thalamocortical system holds that thalamocortical (TC) neurons fire in two distinct modes, one in NREM sleep (burst mode) and another in wakefulness and REM sleep (transmission mode). The firing mode is dependent on the input activity of the cholinergic PPT and LDT, which influences the membrane potential of the TC cells. When the membrane potential of the TC neurons is near threshold (as during wake when the PPT and LDT are active), they respond to incoming stimuli by firing single spikes. However, when the TC neurons are hyperpolarized (as during NREM sleep when the PPT and LDT fall silent), a low-threshold calcium channel is de-inactivated. In this state, incoming excitatory postsynaptic potentials now produce calcium spikes that are prolonged and produce a depolarized plateau, from which the neuron fires a series or burst of action potentials. When the TC cell is in burst mode, thalamocortical sensory transmission is inhibited, and oscillatory communication between TC neurons, cortical neurons, and reticular thalamus neurons results in several characteristics of the sleep EEG, namely slow wave activity (0.5-4 Hz) and spindles (Fig. 4-5).

Consistent with the electrophysiologic characteristics of the TC neurons during sleep and wakefulness, early electrical stimulation studies also suggested that the midline and intralaminar thalamic nuclei might constitute a diffuse, "nonspecific" cortical activating system. Surprisingly, however, lesions of the midline and intralaminar nuclei do not prevent cortical activation.[55] Equally remarkable is the finding that near-complete ablation of the thalamus actually produced an increase in wakefulness in cats, and had little if any effect on wakefulness or EEG waveforms in rats, other than to eliminate sleep spindles.[28,56] In addition, lesions of the thalamic relay nuclei in humans usually produce focal neurologic deficits related to the specific cortical regions that they innervate, rather than overall deficits of arousal.[10] These findings suggest that while the thalamus may be important in supplying the content of the waking state, it is difficult to reconcile these observations with the thalamus playing a critical role in regulating overall EEG or behavioral arousal. Rather, these observations strongly argue that activating influences from the brainstem may reach the neocortex via an extrathalamic route.

Finally, one recent study has suggested a potentially important wake-promoting role for the basal ganglia, in particular, the striatum and globus pallidus, in the regulation of sleep-wake behaviors.[57] Given that the basal ganglia are involved in numerous neurobiologic processes that operate on the basis

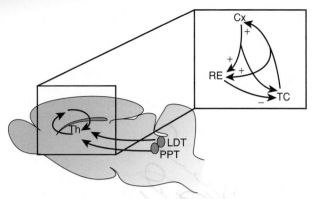

Figure 4-5 During cortical arousal the electroencephalogram (EEG) directly reflects the collective synaptic potentials of inputs largely to pyramidal cells within the neocortex and hippocampus. The thalamocortical system has been widely considered to be a major source of this activity. The overall level of activity in the thalamocortical system, in turn, is thought to be regulated by the ascending arousal system. Today, it is generally accepted that a brainstem cholinergic activating system, located in the pedunculopontine tegmental (PPT) and laterodorsal tegmental (LDT) nuclei (*grey circles*), induces tonic and phasic depolarization effects upon thalamocortical (TC) neurons to produce the low-voltage, mixed-frequency, fast activity of the waking and rapid eye movement (REM) sleep EEG. The PPT and LDT cease firing during non-REM (NREM) sleep, which hyperpolarizes the TC neurons to produce two important effects: (1) sensory transmission through the thalamus to the cortex is blocked; and (2) oscillatory activity between TC neurons, cortical neurons (Cx), and reticular thalamus (RE) neurons (see *inset*) is unmasked to manifest several characteristics of the sleep EEG: slow wave activity (0.5-4 Hz) and spindles. Thus the thalamus (Th) appears to be a critical relay for the ascending arousal system for "gating" sensory transmission to the cortex during sleep and wake. (Modified from Steriade M, McCormick DA, Sejnowski TJ. Thalamocortical oscillations in the sleeping and aroused brain. *Science*. 1993;262:679-685.)

of wakefulness, this finding is perhaps not surprising. At present, however, the specific role of the two efferent basal ganglia pathways (i.e., striatonigral versus striatopallidal) in maintaining wakefulness remains unclear.

Turning off the ARAS: Sleep-Promoting Circuitry

As outlined previously, projections from brainstem cholinergic, monoaminergic, glutamatergic, and histaminergic cell groups and forebrain orexinergic, cholinergic, GABAergic, and glutamatergic neurons act collectively to produce arousal. But what turns off this arousal system to produce sleep? As indicated previously, von Economo inferred the presence of sleep-promoting circuitry in the BF and anterior hypothalamic area based upon postmortem brain analysis of his insomniac patients. Although von Economo's prediction was borne out experimentally by Nauta (1946)[41] and by McGinty and Sterman (1968),[58] who showed a reduction in sleep in rats and cats, respectively, following lesions of the preoptic-BF region, the exact population of sleep-promoting neurons remained unresolved for many years. In 1996, Sherin and colleagues identified a population of neurons in the ventrolateral preoptic nucleus (VLPO) that are sleep-active, contain the inhibitory neurotransmitters GABA and galanin, and are reciprocally connected with the major components of the ARAS[59,60] (see Fig. 4-4, *B*). Consistent with their putative sleep-promoting function, cell-specific lesions of the VLPO produce profound insomnia and sleep fragmentation in rats.

Recent experiments have shown that loss of neurons in the VLPO "cluster" correlated closely with loss of NREM sleep and delta wave power and loss of neurons in the "extended" VLPO correlated with the loss of REM sleep.[61]

A second population of sleep-active neurons is found in the median preoptic nucleus (MnPO), although their ability to cause sleep is less clear. Similar to VLPO neurons, these neurons fire rapidly during NREM sleep and REM sleep and become quiescent during wakefulness.[62] In the MnPO, there are at least three known neuronal groups including GABAergic, glutamatergic, and nitric oxide neurons.[63] Of these MnPO cell groups, the GABAergic population is most tightly linked to sleep control given their sleep-discharge profile and projections to ARAS nodes including the lateral hypothalamic orexin neurons, the DRN neurons, and the LC. Studies using cell-specific lesion techniques or genetic silencing approaches are eagerly awaited because they will greatly inform our understanding of the *in vivo* role of the MnPO neurons in sleep-wake regulation.

Because even large lesions of the VLPO, including those encompassing large portions of the MnPO, do not completely eliminate sleep, it is likely that other sleep-promoting circuitry contributes to the inhibition of the ARAS during sleep. For example, the presence of putative sleep-promoting circuitry in the medullary brainstem has long been suggested.[8] To date, however, the location of these neurons has remained elusive and therefore the status of this cell group has been relegated to that of sleep "lore."

BEHAVIORAL STATE TRANSITIONS

Sleep Switches

The interaction between the VLPO and components of the ARAS (e.g., TMN, LC, DRN) has been demonstrated to be mutually inhibitory, and as such, these pathways function analogously to an electronic "flip-flop" switch/circuit (Fig. 4-7). Within the framework of the flip-flop model, the VLPO represents the "sleep side," whereas the ARAS nodes represent the "arousal side."[13] The flip-flop model further predicts that orexin neurons of the lateral hypothalamus act as a "finger on the switch" to both prevent unwanted transitions into sleep and to stabilize wakefulness. By virtue of the self-reinforcing nature of these switches—that is, when each side is firing, it reduces its own inhibitory feedback—the flip-flop switch is inherently stable in either end state but avoids intermediate states. In short, the flip-flop design ensures stability of behavioral states and facilitates relatively rapid switching between behavioral states. Flip-flop switches also possess, at times, the undesirable property of abruptly undergoing unwanted state transitions. The frequency of unwanted state transitions may increase if one side of the switch is "weakened," as the weakened side becomes less able to inhibit the other side, thereby biasing the switch toward a midpoint where smaller perturbations may trigger a state transition. As an example, it has been suggested that cell loss in the VLPO during aging may weaken the switch, ultimately leading to sleep fragmentation and daytime napping, both of which are frequent complaints in the elderly. Another example is that of narcolepsy, a neurologic disorder associated with the inability to maintain normal wakefulness, and the intrusion of fragments of REM sleep into wakefulness such as atonia, which

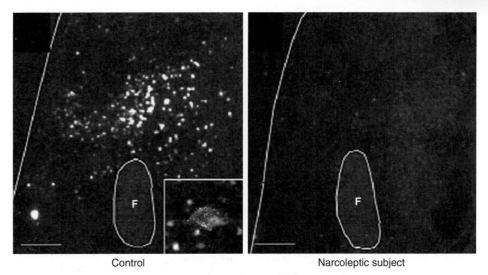

Figure 4-6 Most patients with narcolepsy-cataplexy have low or undetectable levels of orexin in the cerebrospinal fluid. This figure shows that "prepro-orexin" transcripts are detected in the hypothalamus of control subjects but not narcoleptic subjects. *F*, fornix. (Modified from Peyron C, Faraco J, Rogers W, Ripley B, Overeem S, et al. A mutation in a case of early onset narcolepsy and a generalized absence of hypocretin peptides in human narcoleptic brains. *Nat Med.* 2000;6:991-997.)

Control   Narcoleptic subject

manifests as cataplexy.[64] Recent research has established that it is the selective loss of orexin signaling that causes narcolepsy (Fig. 4-6), although both the pathogenic basis of narcolepsy and what actually "triggers" cataplexy in the absence of orexin signaling remain open questions. Whatever the case, narcolepsy is an excellent clinical example of how disruption of one component of the sleep-switch circuitry can destablize behavioral state control.

CIRCUITRY REGULATING REM SLEEP

Aserinksy and Kleitman first described the behavioral state of REM sleep in a seminal report in 1953.[65] As described previously, REM sleep in humans and other mammals cycles periodically with NREM sleep and is characterized by the appearance of fast, desynchronized rhythms in the cortical EEG, rapid eye movements (REM), autonomic activation, and a loss of muscle tone (of the muscles only the extraocular, middle ear, external sphincters, and diaphragm are unaffected). Finally, because the cortical EEG of REM sleep closely resembles that of the waking state,[66] REM sleep has been alternatively termed "paradoxical sleep" or, by some investigators, "active sleep."

The pathways and transmitter systems governing REM sleep regulation have only recently been elaborated. In one of the first published studies on REM sleep mechanisms, Jouvet and Michel (1960)[67] showed that physiologic REM sleep was blocked by systemic administration of the cholinergic antagonist atropine and enhanced by the cholinergic agonist physostigmine, suggesting that acetylcholine promoted REM sleep. Two years later, Jouvet demonstrated that electrical stimulation of the caudal mesencephalic region of the pontine tegmentum produced a desynchronized sleep-like state in cats that was, excepting in duration, indistinguishable from physiologic REM sleep.[68] Interestingly, transections at this same level (i.e., the "pretrigeminal" cat preparation) had previously been shown to result in chronic EEG desynchronization, although this was not linked to REM sleep regulation at the time. Neuropharmacologic experiments over the next 2 decades provided additional support for a "mesopontine cholinergic" hypothesis of REM sleep regulation but also indicated an important role for brainstem monoaminergic neurons (the same cell groups composing the ARAS, see Fig. 4-4 and previous discussion).

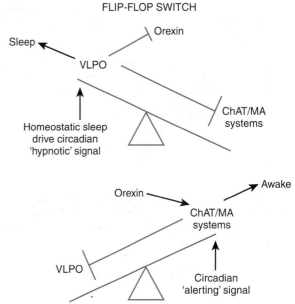

Figure 4-7 Neurons of the ventrolateral preoptic nucleus (VLPO) are sleep active, and loss of VLPO neurons produces profound insomnia and sleep fragmentation. The VLPO sends projections to brainstem cholinergic choline acetyltrans ferase (ChAT) and monoaminergic (MA) systems that compose the ascending arousal system. This interaction between the VLPO and components of the arousal systems is mutually inhibitory, and as such, these pathways function analogously to an electronic flip- flop switch. The lateral hypothalamic orexin neurons are thought to play a stabilizing role for the switch. Circadian and homeostatic processes influence both sides of the switch to produce consolidated bouts of sleep and wake. (Adapted from Fuller PM, Gooley JJ, Saper CB. Neurobiology of the sleep-wake cycle: Sleep architecture, circadian regulation, and regulatory feedback. *J Biol Rhythms.* 2006;21[6]:482-493.)

In 1975, McCarley and Hobson[69] proposed a "reciprocal interaction" model for REMS regulation.[69] This model, which until recently has remained the most widely accepted model of REM sleep regulation, cast the pontine REM sleep circuitry as a population of presumptive cholinergic neurons of the mesopontine tegmentum (which fire most rapidly during REM sleep, hence "REM-on" neurons) and brainstem monoaminergic neurons (which cease firing during REM sleep, hence

"REM-off" neurons) that reciprocally interact to generate the ultradian rhythm of sleep. In the original conception of the model, REM-on cholinergic neurons of the medial pontine reticular formation (i.e., PPT and LDT neurons) are essential for the generation of the tonic and phasic physiologic events of REM sleep (i.e., neocortical EEG activation, atonia and ponto-geniculo-occipital [PGO] waves).[70,71] During waking, the cholinergic REM sleep generator is tonically inhibited by REM-off monoaminergic neurons, but during NREM sleep inhibitory monoaminergic tone gradually wanes and cholinergic excitation waxes until REM sleep is generated. Although this model has been modified several times over the past 30 years, the basis framework of aminergic-cholinergic interplay has remained the same.[72] In general, neuropharmacologic and electrophysiologic experiments have provided strong support for the pontine reciprocal interaction model and the critical role of the PPT-LDT neurons as REM-on cell groups. Importantly, however, this model does not fully explain several other, more recent experimental findings, including (1) limited alterations in REM sleep following selective lesions of brainstem cholinergic and monoaminergic nuclei and (2) limited c-Fos expression in cholinergic PPT and LDT neurons during REM sleep.

Recent work directed at reconciling the apparent incongruities between the widely accepted cholinergic-aminergic model of REM sleep and the aforementioned experimental findings has revealed the presence of REM sleep switching circuitry in the mesopontine tegmentum. In the rat, this circuitry takes the form of putative REM-off neurons located in the ventrolateral periaqueductal gray (vlPAG) and lateral pontine tegmentum (LPT) and putative REM-on neurons located in the sublaterodorsal nucleus (SLD) and the adjacent preceruleus (PC) area. This circuit arrangement also involves mutually inhibitory GABAergic interactions between the vlPAG-LPT REM-off and SLD-PC REM-on neurons, suggesting a flip-flop switch arrangement in which each side (by inhibiting the other) also disinhibits (and thus reinforces) its own firing (Fig. 4-8). Consistent with this flip-flop circuit arrangement, cell-specific lesions of the vlPAG and LPT result in a doubling of REM sleep, including an increase in both the number and duration of bouts of REM sleep. By contrast, cell-specific lesions of the

PC result in loss of hippocampal theta during REM sleep, and cell-specific lesions of SLD, in particular the ventral SLD, result in a phenomenon known as REM sleep without atonia, which manifests as simple and complex motor behaviors during the normally atonic REM sleep.[24] These aberrant motor behaviors seen in animals with lesions of the SLD are highly reminiscent of that observed in human REM sleep behavior disorder (RBD; see Chapter 43) and suggest that the primary tonic control mechanism for producing the atonia of REM sleep involves descending projections from the SLD to the ventral spinal horn.

Yet more recent work has demonstrated that spinally projecting neurons of the SLD are glutamatergic and so, from a clinical perspective, these findings may also provide a framework for understanding the pathophysiology of REM sleep-related disorders, in particular RBD. Human RBD is a parasomnia that typically manifests as "dream enactment" behavior, meaning involuntary nocturnal movements that include kicking, shouting, punching, and leaping during REM sleep.[73] Accumulating evidence also suggests that, importantly, RBD may represent an early pathophysiologic manifestation of evolving Parkinson's disease (PD) and other synucleinopathies, such as Lewy body dementia (LBD), multiple system atrophy (MSA), and pure autonomic failure.[74-76] Consistent with a possible role for the SLD in RBD pathology, in 2007, Mathis and colleagues[77] reported a rare case of RBD in a 30-year-old individual following an encephalitis-induced lesion that was restricted to the dorsal pontine tegmentum (presumably involving the SLD bilaterally). Equally interesting is the recent report of RBD development following a unilateral stroke affecting the right SLD region.[78] On the basis of these findings, others have hypothesized that SLD glutamatergic neurons are gradually damaged as a part of the pathogenesis of RBD. If this were to be the case, it also raises the interesting question of why SLD glutamatergic neurons and glutamatergic neurons in general (e.g., cortical glutamatergic neurons) exhibit and apparent heighten selective vulnerability in the pathogenesis of these neurodegenerative conditions.

As indicated previously, substantial data support an important role for both cholinergic and monoaminergic neurons in REM sleep regulation. First, it has been long known that

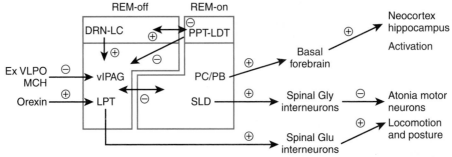

Figure 4-8 In the rapid eye movement (REM) sleep flip-flop switch model, the REM switch consists of two halves: "REM-on" and "REM-off." The REM-off region is identified by the overlap of inputs from the extended VLPO (eVLPO) and orexin neurons. These REM-off neurons in the ventrolateral periaqueductal gray matter (vlPAG) and lateral pontine tegmentum (LPT) have a mutually inhibitory interaction with REM-on GABAergic neurons of the ventral sublaterodorsal nucleus (SLD) and the preceruleus (PC)-parabrachial (PB) nucleus. Although the cholinergic neurons of the pedunculopontine and laterodorsal tegmental nuclei (PPT-LDT) are REM-on and likely inhibit the LPT, these neurons are not directly inhibited by the LPT and are thus external to the switch. This is also true for the dorsal raphe and noradrenergic locus ceruleus (DR-NLC) neurons that can activate the REM-off area but are not inhibited directly by the SLD. Neurons of the SLD produce atonia during REM sleep through direct glutamatergic spinal projections to interneurons that inhibit spinal motor neurons by both glycinergic and GABAergic mechanisms. Glutamatergic inputs from the REM-on PC region (and possibly from the adjacent PB nucleus) to the medial septum and the basal forebrain (BF) appear to play a key role in generating hippocampal and cortical activation during REM sleep. (Modified from Lu J, Sherman D, Devor M, Saper CB. A putative flip-flop switch for control of REM sleep. *Nature.* 2006;441[7093]:589-594.)

carbachol injected in the medial pontine reticular formation (mPRF) produces a REM sleep-like state characterized by EEG desynchronization, REMs, PGO waves, and muscle atonia. Although several sites in the mPRF have been identified at which carbachol elicits REM sleep-like phenomena,[70] there is a general consensus that the most effective place is the region corresponding to the aforementioned SLD[70,71] and, perhaps not surprisingly, REM-on SLD neurons are indeed activated by carbachol.[79] Second, single unit recording in the region of the cholinergic LDT/PPT have identified two subsets of REM sleep-active neurons: neurons that discharge at a high rate during wakefulness and REM sleep (W/REM-on neurons) and neurons that discharge selectively during REM sleep (REM-on neurons).[16,80,81] Taken together, these findings demonstrate that many cholinergic neurons of the LDT/PPT are active during REM sleep and some are active during both waking and REM sleep (W/REM-on). It is, however, the case that these two groups of cholinergic neurons may play different roles in promoting muscle atonia, PGO wave generation, and cortical activation, with W/REM-on neurons more likely involved in control of cortical activation and REM-on neurons more likely involved in the generation of PGO waves and REM sleep-atonia.[71,82] Finally, there is general agreement that muscarinic receptors are involved in promoting REM sleep and the carbachol-induced REM sleep-like state; however, the identification of the muscarinic receptor subtypes (M_2 vs. M_3) remains unresolved.[83-87]

Counterposed with the cholinergic LDT/PPT REMS-on neurons, noradrenergic and serotoninergic neurons of the LC and DRN have long been viewed as REM-off neurons.[17,88-91] The active silencing of the LC and DRN during REM sleep has been attributed to both recurrent inhibition and GABAergic input from REM-on neurons.[71] In addition to natural REM sleep, the silencing of monoaminergic neurons has also been shown to occur during carbachol-induced REM sleep-like state.[70,92] The reduced activity of brainstem monoaminergic neurons has been proposed to play a permissive role in the generation of REM sleep. Specifically, this model predicts that noradrenergic and serotoninergic inputs to the mPRF directly inhibit REM sleep-generating neurons, including the REM sleep-atonia neurons of the SLD and the REM sleep-promoting neurons of the LDT/PPT (cholinergic REM-on). Alternatively, or in combination with the permissive role of reduced monoaminergic activity in the generation of REM sleep, the silencing of brainstem noradrenergic and serotoninergic neurons has been proposed to reduce the excitatory drive to motor neurons, in turn, promoting the muscle atonia characteristic of REM sleep. Conversely, it has been proposed that enhanced brainstem monoaminergic tone (possibly via orexin-mediated activation of the LC and DRN) prevents cataplexy by increasing the activity of motor neurons. Although a reduction in monoaminergic tone appears to be the primary mechanism for the generation of REM sleep-atonia in hypoglossal motor neurons,[93-95] it is generally accepted that the major inhibitory drive to the spinal motor neurons during REM sleep is instead mediated by glycine release,[96] which, in turn, is regulated by descending supraspinal glutamatergic inputs from the SLD neurons.[24]

In summary, significant advances have been made in our understanding of how pontine brain circuits, including specific neurotransmitter systems, regulate REM sleep phenomena. It remains the case, however, that neither the vlPAG-LPT/SLD-PC "flip-flop" model nor the cholinergic-monoaminergic model fully explains, at least in isolation, REM sleep regulation. One possibility is that brainstem aminergic and cholinergic groups are more correctly characterized as REM sleep modulators and not REM sleep generators. For example, the REM-on cholinergic neurons of the PPT-LDT may inhibit the LPT (as cholinergic agonists injected into this region cause REM sleep state), but they themselves are not directly inhibited by the LPT and thus the PPT-LDT is not a part of the "flip-flop" switch, which forms the "core" of the REM sleep pontine circuitry. Alternatively, REM-on PPT-LDT cholinergic neurons may excite REM-on SLD neurons, but again remain external to the switch. Similarly, serotoninergic DRN and noradrenergic LC neurons may inhibit REM-on SLD neurons or activate REM-off circuitry. Nevertheless, like the PPT-LDT, DRN-LC neurons are not inhibited directly by the SLD, and hence are not a part of the mutually inhibitory flip-flop switch. Whatever is the case ultimately, delineating these mechanisms is an important research goal, in particular because doing so may provide insight into how monoamine inhibitors, such as antidepressants, can dramatically suppress REM sleep and, also, prevent cataplexy.

HOMEOSTATIC REGULATION OF SLEEP

Sleep Drive and Adenosine

Although a unified theory of sleep function has remained elusive, the deleterious cognitive and physiologic consequences of sleep deprivation clearly indicate a restorative effect of sleep for the brain and body (Fig. 4-9). The neurobiologic underpinning of sleep need or, alternatively, "sleep drive" is unknown, but has been conceptualized as a homeostatic pressure that builds during the waking period and is dissipated by sleep.[97,98] This homeostatic process, or sleep homeostat, thus represents the need for sleep (i.e., sleep propensity). The nature of what accumulates in the brain during waking to initiate sleep is not entirely clear. At present, the best candidate for a sleep-promoting compound is adenosine (Fig. 4-10), which may accumulate extracellularly as a rundown product of cellular metabolism at least in some parts of the brain.[99,100]

Adenosine is a nucleoside widely distributed throughout the intracellular and the extracellular spaces of the body, and its relative concentration across the cell membrane is maintained by membrane transporters.[101] Intracellular adenosine serves as a precursor for the nucleic acid adenine and adenosine triphosphate (ATP), whereas extracellular adenosine acts as a modulator of cellular activity via the activation of four G protein–coupled receptors (A_1 A_{2A}, A_{2B}, and A_3) (see Chapter 5). Each adenosine receptor subtype has a specific tissue distribution, intracellular signaling pathway, and pharmacologic profile. For example, A_1 and A_3 receptors are inhibitory while A_{2A} and A_{2B} receptors are excitatory. It is interesting to note that while physiologic levels of adenosine can activate the A_1, A_{2A}, and A_3 receptors, the A_{2B} receptor is activated only by supraphysiologic levels of adenosine.

It was first proposed in the early 1990s that adenosine, as a terminal by-product of ATP hydrolysis, might represent a cellular signal for energy demand in the brain.[102,103] Taken together with the established "restorative" effects of sleep, it was further suggested that adenosine might also represent an endogenous homeostatic sleep-promoting factor that accumulates during wakefulness and inhibits wake-active neurons to promote sleep.[99,103,104] Several studies have provided evidence in general support of this theory, including

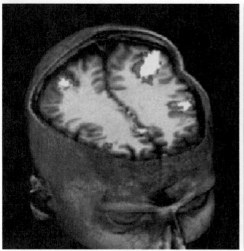

Normal sleep   Sleep deprivation

Figure 4-9 Impaired brain response during an arithmetic working memory task during sleep deprivation. *Left panel*, Brain regions responsive to task demands after a normal night of sleep include the inferior parietal lobes, bilateral dorsolateral prefrontal cortex, and anterior cingulate cortex. *Right panel*, The same regions are significantly less responsive to the same task demands following 35 hours of total sleep deprivation. (Modified from Drummond SPA, Brown GG, Stricker JL, Buxton RB, Wong EC, Gillin JC. Sleep deprivation-induced reduction in cortical functional response to serial subtraction. *Neuroreport.* 1999;10[18]:3745-3748.)

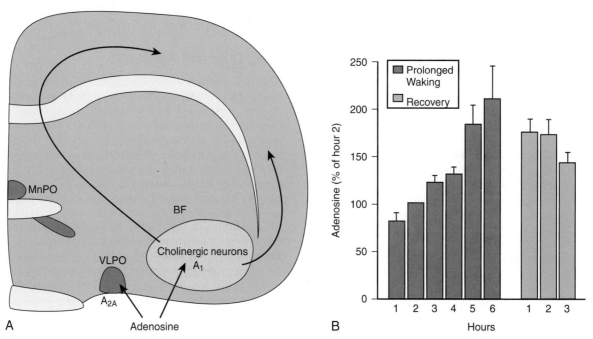

Figure 4-10 A, Even though significant progress has been made in delineating the neuronal circuitry that controls wake and sleep, the cellular determinant of homeostatic sleep drive is unknown, although a putative endogenous somnogen, adenosine (AD), is thought to play a critical role. AD is a naturally occurring purine nucleoside that is hypothesized to accumulate during wake and upon reaching sufficient concentrations, inhibits neural activity in wake-promoting circuitry of the basal forebrain (via A_1 receptors located on BF cholinergic neurons), and likely activates sleep-promoting VLPO neurons (via A_{2A} receptors) located adjacent to the basal forebrain. **B,** Mean basal forebrain extracellular adenosine values by hour during 6 hours of prolonged wakefulness and in the subsequent 3 hours of spontaneous recovery sleep in felines. Microdialysis values in the six animals are normalized relative to the second hour of wakefulness. (**A,** Adapted from Porkka-Heiskanen T, Strecker RE, Thakkar M, Bjorkum AA, Greene RW, McCarley RW. Adenosine: A mediator of the sleep-inducing effects of prolonged wakefulness. *Science.* 1997;276[5316]:1265-1268; **B,** Adapted from Basheer R, Strecker RE, Thakkar MM, McCarley RW. Adenosine and sleep-wake regulation. *Prog Neurobiol.* 2004;73[6]:379-396.)

the following: (1) adenosine accumulates in the extracellular space in response to increased metabolism and increased neuronal activity;[105-107] (2) extracellular adenosine accumulates during spontaneous and prolonged wakefulness when metabolic rate is higher and, importantly, adenosine levels decline during recovery sleep;[108-112] (3) adenosine has hypnogenic effects—when given systemically or centrally adenosine increases sleep time and EEG slow wave activity;[99,100,113,114] and (4) adenosine inhibits all of the primary wake-promoting neurons including lateral hypothalamic orexin neurons, histaminergic neurons of the TMN, noradrenergic neurons of

the LC, and cholinergic neurons of the BF and LDT.[104,115-121] In addition, adenosine may also promote sleep by activating sleep-active neurons of the VLPO.[122-126]

Additional strong support for the role of adenosine as an endogenous sleep-promoting factor comes from the stimulatory action of caffeine (Fig. 4-11), which, among other central effects, acts as a competitive antagonist at adenosine receptors. Caffeine is the most widely used psychoactive drugs and its suppresive effect on sleep is the primary reason for its use. In the Western world the daily consumption of caffeine from all dietary sources (coffee, tea, cocoa beverages, chocolate bars,

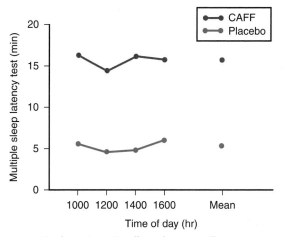

Figure 4-11 This figure shows the effects of 250 mg caffeine in two groups of healthy, but moderately sleepy individuals. The alerting effect of caffeine in these individuals is shown using the standard Multiple Sleep Latency Test (MLST). (Modified from Zwyghuizen-Doorenbos A, Roehrs TA, Lipschutz L, et al. Effects of caffeine on alertness. *Psychopharmacology.* 1990;100:36-39.)

and several soft drinks) yields caffeine blood levels in the low micromolar ranges, which is consistent with caffeine's stimulatory effect being mediated by the blockade of adenosine receptors.[127] The effects of caffeine on sleep are also well documented. In both animal and humans caffeine prolongs sleep latency, reduces slow wave activity, and reduces the buildup of theta activity that occurs after sleep deprivation, suggesting that caffeine interferes with NREM sleep homeostasis.[128] Additional data from studies using adenosine receptor knockout mice indicate that caffeine's arousal effects are mediated by the antagonizing of A_{2A} receptors. In agreement with this result it has been shown that a polymorphism in the A_{2A} receptor gene in humans is associated with the subjective and objective effects of caffeine on sleepiness and sleep, respectively.[129,130] Nevertheless, other studies have suggested that caffeine could act through both A_1 and A_{2A} receptors[127] and therefore the relative role of A_{2A} or A_1 receptors in mediating the wake-promoting effects of caffeine remains a question of debate.

Similar to the debate on the type of adenosine receptor that mediates the caffeine responses, it is still unresolved whether the hypnogenic effects of adenosine are mediated through the A_1 or A_{2A} receptors or both. Based on both their distribution within the CNS and the inhibitory action of A_1 receptors it was assumed that adenosine effects on sleep are primarily mediated by A_1 receptors, and several pharmacologic and electrophysiologic studies have provided support for this hypothesis.[105,131] However, more recent studies from adenosine receptor knockout animals have shown that mice lacking A_1 receptors have normal sleep-wake cycles and normal homeostatic sleep regulation, whereas A_{2A} receptor knockout mice have blunted responses to homeostatic sleep pressure.[130,132,133] Thus, although these findings are intriguing and strongly support the involvement of the A_{2A} receptors in sleep regulation, results from studies employing constitutive knockout mice must be interpreted cautiously owing to the possibility, if not likelihood, of compensatory developmental changes.[125,126,134] In summary, it is conceivable that both A_1 and A_{2A} receptors are involved in promoting sleep and in the control of sleep homeostasis, but their action is also likely to be site specific. To this end, the A_1 receptor may mediate

adenosine responses in brain regions containing wake-active neurons while the A_{2A} responses may be restricted to areas with a high density of sleep-promoting neurons, such as the preoptic area.[105,135,136]

Extracellular levels of adenosine are tightly regulated by the rate of both production and metabolism. There are two primary sources of extracellular adenosine—adenosine released through equilibrative membrane transporters (during high cellular demand) and adenosine formation via hydrolysis of ATP.[107,137] Once in the extracellular space, adenosine is cleared by one of two main mechanisms: either adenosine is taken up by neurons and astrocytes through the equilibrative transporters, or adenosine is metabolized by adenosine deaminase in the extracellular matrix.[107,138] A recent study has shown that 10% of the healthy population carries a polymorphism that lowers adenosine deaminase activity and these individuals have longer NREM sleep bouts and higher cortical slow wave activity, presumably secondary to the elevated extracellular adenosine levels.[128,139] In agreement with this result, manipulations of the adenosine metabolism in animal models that produce elevated extracellular adenosine levels also prolong sleep and increases EEG slow wave activity.[108,116,140-142] Interestingly, ethanol has been shown to produce accumulation of extracellular adenosine by inhibiting adenosine uptake,[143] which may contribute to the impairment of cognitive and motor functions and the drowsiness associated with acute ethanol intake.[144,145] A popular belief is that coffee can offset, in part, the intoxicating effects of alcohol and this may be related to caffeine's ability to antagonize extracellular adenosine.[127,146]

Although the accumulating experimental evidence would suggest that adenosine receptors and the enzymes and transporters that control adenosine levels are promising targets for treating sleep-wake disorders, the ubiquity of adenosine receptors and the consequent wide range of possible side effects makes this possibility a complicated proposition. Differential affinities of selective ligands among species might further complicate preclinical testing in animal models. Thus, although targeting the adenosine system to treat sleep disorders is intriguing, it seems that before this could happen it might require the development of brain-specific drugs.[147] Finally, it is unlikely that adenosine alone can explain the homeostatic drive for sleep, and thus additional homeostatic factors driving sleep remain under investigation (see later discussion under "Humoral Regulation of Sleep").

CIRCADIAN REGULATION OF SLEEP

Timing, Duration, and Consolidation

The circadian system provides temporal organization for virtually all neurobiologic, physiologic, and biochemical processes (Fig. 4-12). The fundamental adaptive advantage of circadian organization is that it permits predictive rather than entirely reactive homeostatic regulation of function.[148] For example, prior to waking, body temperature, plasma cortisol, and sympathetic tone all rise in anticipation of the increased energetic demands of the day. A "master" circadian pacemaker that is located in the hypothalamic suprachiasmatic nuclei (SCN; Fig. 4-13) generates these daily rhythms. SCN neurons themselves are autonomously rhythmic and their rhythmicity is governed by a network of transcriptional/translational/post-translational feedback loops that regulate the

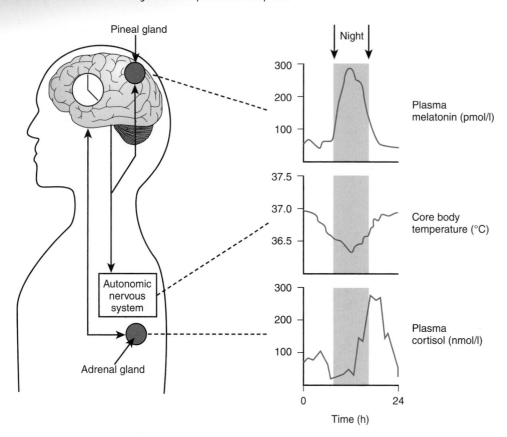

Figure 4-12 The circadian timing system provides temporal organization for virtually all physiologic, neurobiologic, and biochemical processes. Signals from the suprachiasmatic nucleus (SCN) (see Fig. 4-13) are communicated to the periphery via synaptic and humoral mechanisms to generate circadian rhythms. Examples of these rhythms are shown and parameters affected by them include plasma melatonin, body temperature, and plasma cortisol. (Redrawn from Hastings M. The brain, circadian rhythms, and clock genes. *BMJ.* 1998;317[7174]: 1704-1707.)

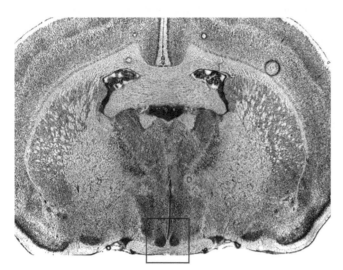

Figure 4-13 The suprachiasmatic nucleus (SCN) is the master biologic clock and is located in the anteroventral hypothalamus just dorsal (hence, "supra") to the optic chiasm and immediately lateral to the third ventricle (the SCNs are the black circular structures contained in the blue box in this coronal section from a rat). The SCN projects to several other hypothalamic nuclei, including the neighboring dorsomedial nucleus and paraventricular nucleus that play important and wide-ranging roles in the regulation of biologic function. (Courtesy of PM Fuller.)

expression of circadian clock genes.[149,150] The so-called "clock genes" are themselves transcription factors that regulate the expression of hundreds, if not thousands of other genes. Neurons of the SCN are synchronized to the daily light-dark cycle primarily by inputs from melanopsin-containing intrinsically photosensitive retinal ganglion cells, although rods and cones also provide input under some circumstances.[151,152] Lesions of the SCN, or disruption of the expression of key clock genes, result in loss of most circadian rhythms.[153-155]

In addition to providing temporal regulation for behavioral states, including sleep-wakefulness, the SCN also plays a significant role in determining the duration, intensity, and propensity of sleep. For example, regulation of the sleep-wake cycles by the SCN is evident because sleep-wake cycles continue on an approximate 24-hour basis even in the absence of environmental cues.[154] In addition, a clear circadian variation in sleep propensity and sleep structure has been demonstrated in humans by uncoupling the rest-activity cycle from the output of the SCN (i.e., so-called "forced desynchrony protocol"). Finally, experimentally placed lesions of the SCN in monkeys and rodents also result in the loss of 24-hour sleep-wake rhythms.[154]

In 1985, Borbely and Tobler[98] proposed a two-process model of sleep regulation in which a homeostatic process (i.e., sleep drive; see earlier discussion) builds during the day and declines exponentially during sleep and interacts with a circadian process that is independent of sleep and waking (Fig. 4-14). At its most fundamental level, this model was an attempt to explain how in humans a consolidated bout of sleep of approximately 8 hours is achieved each night. Further elaborations of the two-process model have been proposed, including an "opponent process" model of sleep-wake regulation that identified a specific role for the SCN in actively facilitating the initiation and maintenance of wakefulness and opposing homeostatic sleep tendency during the day. In other words, the opponent process model predicts a wake-promoting, but not sleep-promoting, role for the SCN in sleep-wake regulation. Human sleep studies have yielded data largely consistent with both the two-process

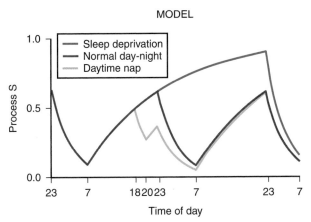

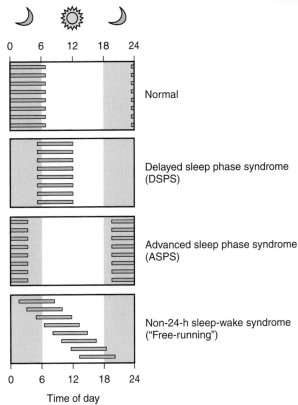

Figure 4-14 The effect on homeostatic sleep drive or "Process S" of a normal day and night *(gray)*, sleep deprivation/wake extension *(dark blue)*, and a daytime nap *(light blue)*. Whenever sleep occurs, Process S is reduced and the rate of dissipation of Process S during sleep follows an exponential decline. (Modified from Borbély AA. A two process model of sleep regulation. *Hum Neurobiol.* 1982; 1[3]:195-204.)

Figure 4-15 Sleep patterns in three of the most common circadian rhythm sleep disorders. Individuals with delayed sleep phase syndrome (DSPS) tend to fall asleep at very late times and have difficulty waking up in the morning. Individual with advanced sleep phase syndrome (ASPS) tend to experience sleepiness in the early evening, which leads to an early time of sleep onset and, also, early rising. Individual with free-running (or so-called non-24-hour sleep-wake syndrome) show a circadian sleep drive that is not entrained to conventional sleep-wake times and so they may sleep during the day and wake during the night. (Modified from Ebisawa T. Circadian rhythms in the CNS and peripheral clock disorders: Human sleep disorders and clock genes. *J Pharmacol Sci.* 2007;103:150-154.)

and opponent process models, in particular that the human sleep-wake cycle is regulated by the interaction of homeostatic and circadian process. More specifically, work by many, but in particular Dijk and Czeisler in 1995,[156] has demonstrated (1) a paradoxical increase in circadian drive for wakefulness during the course of the waking day that opposes the wake-dependent increase in sleep-propensity, resulting in a consolidated bout of wakefulness; and (2) an increase in circadian sleep drive during the course of the night that opposes the decline in homeostatic sleep drive during sleep (i.e., dissipation of the sleep homeostat), resulting in a consolidated bout of sleep.

Circadian sleep disorders can arise due to SCN dysfunction but more often arise when the timing of the individual's endogenous sleep-wake rhythm and exogenous geophysical (e.g., light-dark cycle) and social factors (e.g., night-shift work) are misaligned.[157] For example, while sleep is optimized when the sleep period coincides with the timing of the circadian rhythm of sleep, disruption of this temporal relationship can lead to insomnia or excessive daytime sleepiness. Although circadian rhythm sleep disorders will be discussed in greater detail later in the book (see Section 8), three of the more common circadian rhythm disorders will be introduced here (Fig. 4-15). The first is delayed sleep phase syndrome (DSPS), which is characterized by habitual wake-sleep times that are delayed (i.e., they occur later than desired), often resulting in extreme difficulty in awakening in the morning. By contrast, individuals with advanced sleep phase syndrome (ASPS) experience profound sleepiness in the early evening and wake up earlier than desired. A third circadian rhythm sleep disorder and one that is most common in totally blind individuals is the so-called *free-running* (or nonentrained) type and is characterized by a variable sleep-wake pattern and results in complaints of insomnia or excessive sleepiness.

In light of the demonstrated role for the SCN in governing the timing and consolidation of sleep, it is rather remarkable that the SCN itself has very limited monosynaptic outputs to sleep-regulatory centers such as the VLPO and lateral hypothalamus and none at all to brainstem arousal sites.[158] The densest projection from the SCN terminates dorsally and caudally in the adjacent subparaventricular zone (SPZ). Similar

to the effects of SCN ablation, lesions that include the ventral SPZ abolish behavioral circadian rhythms, including sleep-wake and feeding cycles.[159] By contrast, lesions of the dorsal SPZ have little effect on rhythms of sleep-wake but do eliminate the circadian rhythm of body temperature. Therefore, and taken together, these observations suggest that neurons of the ventral and dorsal SPZ function as obligate relays to maintain circadian rhythms of sleep-wake and temperature, respectively. Similar to the SCN, the SPZ has limited projections to the major components of the sleep-wake regulatory system. The SCN and SPZ do, however, project densely to the dorsomedial hypothalamic nucleus (DMH). Lesions of the DMH also abolish circadian rhythms of sleep-wake, feeding and corticosteroid secretion, but they do not eliminate the rhythm of body temperature. Interestingly, the DMH sends a dense glutamatergic projection to the lateral hypothalamic orexin neurons as well as an intense GABAergic projection to the VLPO, suggesting a primary wake-promoting role for the DMH and a possible substrate for the circadian regulation of sleep-wake cycles.[160] Although these experimental findings suggest that the neurons of the SCN regulate circadian rhythms via multiple and divergent pathways, they also raise the questions of

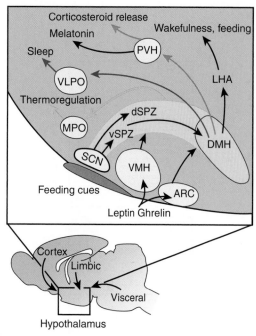

Figure 4-16 Circadian regulation of sleep-wake cycles. The circadian rhythm of sleep-wake is regulated at multiple levels in the hypothalamus. The circadian clock in the SCN sends an indirect projection to the DMH via the SPZ that is critical for the circadian rhythm of sleep-wake. The DMH, in turn, provides rhythmic output to brain regions critical for the regulation of sleep-wake, hormone synthesis and release, and feeding. This multistage regulation of circadian behavior in the hypothalamus allows for the integration of multiple time cues from the environment to shape daily patterns of sleep-wake. (Redrawn from Saper CB, Scammell TE, Lu J. Hypothalamic regulation of sleep. *Nature*. 2005;437:1257-1263.)

why circadian rhythms of behavior and physiology are regulated by a complex multisynaptic pathway rather than a simple, direct projection from the SCN to wake-sleep centers of the brain. The answer may lie within the functional anatomy of the system. Considering that in both nocturnal and diurnal animals the SCN is active (i.e., highest firing rate) during the waking portion of the 24-hour cycle and the VLPO, also irrespective of circadian phenotype, is active during the sleeping portion of the 24-hour cycle, additional (intervening) neural circuitry would be required to organize diurnal and nocturnal programs because the clock inputs and sleep-control systems are identical between the two chronotypes. In consideration of the fact that the timing of environmental pressures such as feeding, food availability, mating opportunities, and predation do not always track with the solar day, having flexibility in circadian organization may be very adaptive.[13,14,161] For example, the series of hypothalamic relays (SCN, SPZ, DMH) could allow for the integration of light entrained circadian cues from the SCN with environmental time cues (e.g., feeding, temperature, social cues) to sculpt patterns of rest-activity and sleep-wake cycles that are optimal for survival (Fig. 4-16).

Melatonin: A Circadian Link to Sleep Consolidation?

Melatonin is a hormone produced by the pineal gland that is suggested to play a role in sleep-wake regulation and whose daily rhythm of production and secretion[162] occurs independent of a light-dark cycle. Melatonin is also thought to play a possible physiologic role as both a potent antioxidant and may exert neuroprotective effects as it relates to aging and neurodegenerative disorders.[163] Circulating melatonin levels are elevated by about 10-fold during the night (in both diurnal and

nocturnal species) relative to the day and so melatonin provides a biologic signal for the subjective night (i.e., quiescent period in diurnal animals and behaviorally active period in nocturnal animals). As an endogenous correlate for the length of the night period (so-called "scotoperiod"), melatonin provides, at least in lower mammals, an important physiologic signal for seasonal behaviors, such as reproduction. In mammals, melatonin production and secretion is under the control of the SCN and this regulation occurs via a rather circuitous retina-SCN-pineal pathway.[148] The SCN sends GABAergic projections to preautonomic neurons of the paraventricular hypothalamus, which in turn send projections to the intermediolateral (IML) cell column of the spinal cord. IML preganglionic cholinergic fibers then project to the superior cervical ganglia, which in turn send noradrenergic sympathetic postganglionic axons along the carotid artery back into the skull to reach the pineal gland. Lesions of this pathway at the level of the upper thoracic or lower cervical spinal cord (tetraplegia, Horner's syndrome) result in a complete loss of production of melatonin and this may explain, in part, the disrupted sleep of patients with tetraplegia (Fig. 4-17).

In humans, exogenously administered melatonin promotes sleep; specifically, melatonin administration during the subjective day promotes early sleep onset and longer sleep duration and daily ingestion of melatonin entrains free-running circadian rhythms in totally blind (i.e., enucleated) individuals.[162,164] In addition, pharmacologic suppression of nocturnal melatonin levels produce an increase in total wake time and a concomitant decrease in NREM sleep and REM sleep.[165] The circadian rhythm of plasma melatonin also has a temporal association with circadian rhythms in EEG activity during sleep in humans, further supporting a direct linkage between melatonin and sleep-wake regulation.[166] Melatonin

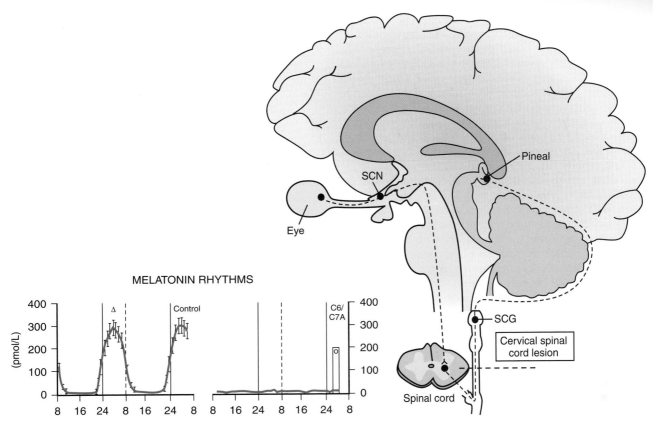

Figure 4-17 The rhythm of melatonin in a normal, healthy individual and in an individual with a cervical spinal cord lesion. Because of the long SCN-pineal projection via the intermediolateral cell column of the spinal cord, high-level spinal injuries completely disrupt both melatonin production and its rhythmic secretion. The absence of a melatonin rhythm in individuals with spinal injuries has been linked to the disrupted sleep patterns of these individuals. *SCG*, superior cervical ganglion; *SCN*, suprachiasmatic nucleus. (Right, redrawn from Ganong WF. *Review of Medical Physiology*. 18th ed. Stamford, CT: Appleton & Lange; 1997:433.)

supplementation has been used clinically for circadian and sleep-wake disorders. In summary, while much remains to be clarified with regard to melatonin's "endogenous role" in sleep-wake regulation, one prevailing thought is that SCN-driven rhythmic release of melatonin feeds back to the SCN to regulate its activity, which in turn contributes to the consolidation of the sleep-wake rhythm.

Other Sleep "Drives"

Arousal state is also invariably influenced by visceral, emotional, and cognitive inputs. Humans and animals alike are often confronted with environmental "stressors" that require rapid and specific alterations in sleep-wake behavior. These so-called "allostatic loads"[167] may, for example, produce a state of hyperarousal by overriding the homeostatic and circadian drives for sleep, thereby enhancing cognitive and physical performance. Although this transient hyperarousal state is clearly adaptive in certain contexts (i.e., presence of a predator or a potential mate), chronic or inappropriate activation of arousal circuitry, such as might occur during psychological stress or depression, is maladaptive. Even though little is known regarding the mechanisms by which allostatic loads influence the regulation of sleep and wake, studies have demonstrated extensive interconnectivity between corticolimbic (prefrontal cortex, infralimbic cortex, bed nucleus of the stria terminalis, ventral subiculum) and components of the sleep-wake system, suggesting at least a potential substrate for

these interactions.[168,169] One recent study has demonstrated that activation of medial prefrontal and amygdaloid circuitry can drive arousal circuitry even when the VLPO is active.[170] Increased activation of these corticolimbic sites has also been demonstrated in human subjects with insomnia.[171]

HUMORAL REGULATION OF SLEEP

Although the concept of sleep induction by "vapors" is an ancient one, the first formal hypothesis that sleep is regulated by humoral factors dates back to 1892 (Rosenbaum).[172] The first experimental evidence linking humoral factors to sleep induction is credited to the independent studies of Ishimori (1909)[173] in Japan and Legendre and PieAron (1913)[174] in France who showed that the cerebrospinal fluid (CSF) of sleep-deprived dogs contained a sleep-promoting factor. The humoral theory of sleep was however rapidly overtaken by the circuit-based theories of sleep proposed by von Economo, Moruzzi and Magoun, and others (see earlier discussion). In the 1960s additional evidence for humoral sleep regulatory factors began to re-emerge from several laboratories, in particular from the laboratory of John Pappenheimer at Harvard Medical School. In a seminal paper published in 1967, Pappenheimer and colleagues[175] showed that the CSF from sleep-deprived goats rapidly increased sleep and decreased locomotor activity in recipient rats. It was later revealed that the sleep-active factor in the CSF (so-called "factor S") was in fact muramyl peptide, a component of bacterial cell walls. Thus, even though muramyl peptide is not an endogenously produced somnogen, the identification of muramyl peptide as the "sleep-promoting factor" suggested a hitherto unrecognized interrelationship between brain sleep and immune function. It was in fact subsequently shown that muramyl peptide induced the synthesis and secretion of the proinflammatory cytokine interleukin 1 (IL-1). Ensuing studies demonstrated that central administration of IL-1 produces increased EEG (slow wave NREM sleep) and behavioral sleep and this is true in all species studied to date including mice, rats, rabbits, sheep, cats, monkeys, and humans.

So, what actually constitutes a "sleep factor"? Krueger and colleagues,[176] who over the past 3 decades have been at the forefront of research in humoral sleep factors, have proposed a list of criteria to be met for a substance to be considered a sleep regulatory factor: (1) when administered, the factor should induce or maintain physiologic sleep, (2) the factor should act on sleep regulatory circuits, (3) the level of the factor should increase with sleep drive, (4) if the factor is inhibited, sleep should be reduced; and (5) the level of the factor should be increased in pathologic states associated with increased sleep. At present, the list of putative humoral factors regulating NREM sleep and meeting these criteria include IL-1, tumor necrosis factor-α (TNF-α), growth hormone releasing hormone (GHRH), prostaglandin D_2 (PGD$_2$), adenosine (discussed earlier), and uridine.[176] For example, and similar to IL-1, TNF-α enhances NREM sleep, inhibition of TNF-α inhibits spontaneous sleep, brain TNF-α levels increase with sleep deprivation, TNF-α is elevated in patients with clinical conditions involving sleep disorders, and finally, a TNF-α variant (G-308A) is associated with sleep apnea.[177] How and why immune signaling molecules such as IL-1 and TNF-α modulate sleep (intensity, duration, and architecture) remain open questions and are currently areas of intense investigation.

SUMMARY

Although a unified teleologic explanation for sleep continues to elude neuroscientists, it is an established fact that sleep is necessary for optimal physiologic, psychological, and cognitive function. As detailed in this chapter, remarkable progress has been made over the past century in understanding the neural circuitry underlying the regulation of sleep-wake states. For example, specific neuronal pathways, transmitters, and receptors have been identified that are now the target of pharmaceutical manipulation for the treatment of sleep-wake disorders. Moreover, recent studies have indicated that sleep and wakefulness are regulated by mutually inhibitory populations of neurons in the hypothalamus and brainstem, which together ensure behavioral state stability and facilitate rapid switching between sleep and wakefulness. Nevertheless, and despite these advances, significant gaps remain in our knowledge. As one example, the signaling pathway(s) that mediate homeostatic sleep drive remain unknown. However, the recent advent of a wide range of technical advances is expected to produce rapid advances in an understanding of the detailed anatomic and molecular circuitry governing sleep-wake regulation. Finally, and from a more "basic science" perspective, the development of new methods and technical approaches will also shed light on some of the most enduring mysteries in systems neuroscience, including "why do we sleep?"

REFERENCES

1. Rechtschaffen A, Kales A, (Eds.) *A Manual of Standardized Terminology, Techniques and Scoring System of Sleep Stages of Human Subjects.* Washington, DC: U.S. Department of Health Education, and Welfare, Public Health Service—NIH/NINDS; 1968.
2. Steriade M, McCormick DA, Sejnowski TJ. Thalamocortical oscillations in the sleeping and aroused brain. *Science.* 1993;262(5134):679-685.
3. Iber C, Ancoli-Israel S, Chesson A, Quan SF. American Academy of Sleep Medicine for the Scoring of Sleep and Associated Events: Rules, Terminology and Technical Specifications. Westchester, IL: American Academy of Sleep Medicine, 2007.
4. von Economo C. Sleep as a problem of localization. *J Nerv Ment Dis.* 1930;71:249-259.
5. Ranson SW. Somnolence caused by hypothalamic lesions in monkeys. *Arch Neurol Psychiatry.* 1939;41:1-23.
6. Bremer F. Cerveau isole et physiologie du sommeil. *C R Soc Biol (Paris).* 1935;118:1235-1242.
7. Moruzzi G, Magoun HW. Brain stem reticular formation and activation of the EEG. *Electroencephalogr Clin Neurophysiol.* 1949;1(4):455-473.
8. Batini C, Moruzzi G, Pelestini M, et al. Effects of complete pontine transections on the sleep-wakefulness rhythm: The midpontine pretrigeminal preparation. *Arch Ital Biol.* 1959;97:1-12.
9. Parvizi J, Damasio AR. Neuroanatomical correlates of brainstem coma. *Brain.* 2003;126(Pt 7):1524-1536.
10. Posner JB, Saper CB, Schiff ND, et al. *Plum and Posner's Diagnosis of Stupor and Coma.* New York: Oxford University Press; 2008:1-37.
11. Jones BE. From waking to sleeping: Neuronal and chemical substrates. *Trends Pharmacol Sci.* 2005;26(11):578-586.
12. Saper CB, Chou TC, Scammell TE. The sleep switch: Hypothalamic control of sleep and wakefulness. *Trends Neurosci.* 2001;24(12):726-731.
13. Saper CB, Scammell TE, Lu J. Hypothalamic regulation of sleep and circadian rhythms. *Nature.* 2005;437(7063):1257-1263.
14. Fuller PM, Gooley JJ, Saper CB. Neurobiology of the sleep-wake cycle: Sleep architecture, circadian regulation, and regulatory feedback. *J Biol Rhythms.* 2006;21(6):482-493.
15. Hallanger AE, Levey AI, Lee HJ, Rye DB, Wainer BH. The origins of cholinergic and other subcortical afferents to the thalamus in the rat. *J Comp Neurol.* 1987;262(1):105-124.
16. el Mansari M, Sakai K, Jouvet M. Unitary characteristics of presumptive cholinergic tegmental neurons during the sleep-waking cycle in freely moving cats. *Exp Brain Res.* 1989;76(3):519-529.
17. Aston-Jones G, FE Bloom M. Activity of norepinephrine-containing locus coeruleus neurons in behaving rats anticipates fluctuations in the sleep-waking cycle. *J Neurosci.* 1981;1(8):876-886.
18. Dahlstrom A, Fuxe K. Localization of monoamines in the lower brain stem. *Experientia.* 1964;20(7):398-399.
19. Lu J, Jhou TC, Saper CB. Identification of wake-active dopaminergic neurons in the ventral periaqueductal gray matter. *J Neurosci.* 2006;26(1):193-202.
20. Panula P, Pirvola U, Auvinen S, Airaksinen MS. Histamine-immunoreactive nerve fibers in the rat brain. *Neuroscience.* 1989;28(3): 585-610.
21. Webster HH, Jones BE. Neurotoxic lesions of the dorsolateral pontomesencephalic tegmentum-cholinergic cell area in the cat. II. Effects upon sleep-waking states. *Brain Res.* 1988;458(2):285-302.
22. Denoyer M, Sallanon M, Buda C, Kitahama K, Jouvet M. Neurotoxic lesion of the mesencephalic reticular formation and/or the posterior hypothalamus does not alter waking in the cat. *Brain Res.* 1991;539(2):287-303.
23. Shouse MN, Siegel JM. Pontine regulation of REM sleep components in cats: Integrity of the pedunculopontine tegmentum (PPT) is important for phasic events but unnecessary for atonia during REM sleep. *Brain Res.* 1992;571(1):50-63.
24. Lu J, Sherman D, Devor M, Saper CB. A putative flip-flop switch for control of REM sleep. *Nature.* 2006;441(7093):589-594.
25. Blanco-Centurion CA, Shiromani A, Winston E, Shiromani PJ. Effects of hypocretin-1 in 192-IgG-saporin-lesioned rats. *Eur J Neurosci.* 2006;24(7):2084-2088.
26. Hur EE, Zaborszky L. Vglut2 afferents to the medial prefrontal and primary somatosensory cortices: A combined retrograde tracing in situ hybridization study [corrected]. *J Comp Neurol.* 2005;483(3):351-373.
27. Saper CB, Loewy AD. Efferent connections of the parabrachial nucleus in the rat. *Brain Res.* 1980;197(2):291-317.
28. Fuller PM, Sherman D, Pedersen NP, Saper CB, Lu J. Reassessment of the structural basis of the ascending arousal system. *J Comp Neurol.* 2010;519:933.

29. Saper CB. Personal communication. Clifford B. Saper, MD, Chairman, Department of Neurology, Harvard Medical School, Boston, MA.

30. Steininger TL, Stevens DR, Haas HL, McGinty D, Szymusiak R. Sleep-waking discharge of neurons in the posterior lateral hypothalamus of the albino rat. *Brain Res.* 1999;840(1-2):138-147.

31. Greco MA. Opioidergic projections to sleep-active neurons in the ventrolateral preoptic nucleus. *Brain Res.* 2008;1245:96-107.

32. Chou TC, Lee CE, Lu J, et al. Orexin (hypocretin) neurons contain dynorphin. *J Neurosci.* 2001;21(19):RC168.

33. Peyron C, Tighe DK, van den Pol AN, et al. Neurons containing hypocretin (orexin) project to multiple neuronal systems. *J Neurosci.* 1998;18(23):9996-10015.

34. Lee MG, Hassani OK, Jones BE. Discharge of identified orexin/hypocretin neurons across the sleep-waking cycle. *J Neurosci.* 2005;25(28):6716-6720.

35. Lin L, Faraco J, Li R, et al. The sleep disorder canine narcolepsy is caused by a mutation in the hypocretin (orexin) receptor 2 gene. *Cell.* 1999;98(3):365-376.

36. Chemelli RM, Willie JT, Simon CM, et al. Narcolepsy in orexin knock-out mice: Molecular genetics of sleep regulation. *Cell.* 1999;98(4):437-451.

37. Thannickal TC, Moore RY, Nienhuis R, et al. Reduced number of hypocretin neurons in human narcolepsy. *Neuron.* 2000;27(3):469-474.

38. Hassani OK, Lee MG, Jones BE. Melanin-concentrating hormone neurons discharge in a reciprocal manner to orexin neurons across the sleep-wake cycle. *Proc Natl Acad Sci U S A.* 2009;106(7):2418-2422.

39. Verret L, Goutagny R, Fort P, et al. A role of melanin-concentrating hormone producing neurons in the central regulation of paradoxical sleep. *BMC Neurosci.* 2003;4:19.

40. Gerashchenko D, Kohls MD, Greco M, et al. Hypocretin-2-saporin lesions of the lateral hypothalamus produce narcoleptic-like sleep behavior in the rat. *J Neurosci.* 2001;21(18):7273-7283.

41. Nauta W. Hypothalamic regulation of sleep in rats. An experimental study. *J Neurophysiol.* 1946;9:285-314.

42. Grove EA. Neural associations of the substantia innominata in the rat: Afferent connections. *J Comp Neurol.* 1988;277(3):315-346.

43. Saper CB. Organization of cerebral cortical afferent systems in the rat. II. Hypothalamocortical projections. *J Comp Neurol.* 1985;237(1):21-46.

44. Zaborszky L, Buhl DL, Pobalashingham S, Bjaalie JG, Nadasdy Z. Three-dimensional chemoarchitecture of the basal forebrain: Spatially specific association of cholinergic and calcium binding protein-containing neurons. *Neuroscience.* 2005;136(3):697-713.

45. Saper CB. Organization of cerebral cortical afferent systems in the rat. II. Magnocellular basal nucleus. *J Comp Neurol.* 1984;222(3):313-342.

46. Jones BE. Activity, modulation and role of basal forebrain cholinergic neurons innervating the cerebral cortex. *Prog Brain Res.* 2004;145:157-169.

47. Manns ID, Mainville L, Jones BE. Evidence for glutamate, in addition to acetylcholine and GABA, neurotransmitter synthesis in basal forebrain neurons projecting to the entorhinal cortex. *Neuroscience.* 2001;107(2):249-263.

48. Dringenberg HC, Vanderwolf CH. Involvement of direct and indirect pathways in electrocorticographic activation. *Neurosci Biobehav Rev.* 1998;22(2):243-257.

49. Sato A, Sato Y, Uchida S. Activation of the intracerebral cholinergic nerve fibers originating in the basal forebrain increases regional cerebral blood flow in the rat's cortex and hippocampus. *Neurosci Lett.* 2004;361(1-3):90-93.

50. Berridge CW, Foote SL. Enhancement of behavioral and electroencephalographic indices of waking following stimulation of noradrenergic beta-receptors within the medial septal region of the basal forebrain. *J Neurosci.* 1996;16(21):6999-7009.

51. Lee MG, Hassani OK, Alonso A, Jones BE. Cholinergic basal forebrain neurons burst with theta during waking and paradoxical sleep. *J Neurosci.* 2005;25(17):4365-4369.

52. Hassani OK, Lee MG, Henny P, Jones BE. Discharge profiles of identified GABAergic in comparison to cholinergic and putative glutamatergic basal forebrain neurons across the sleep-wake cycle. *J Neurosci.* 2009;29(38):11828-11840.

53. Morrison JL, Dempsey EW. A study of thalamo-cortical relations. *Am J Physiol.* 1942;135:281-292.

54. Steriade M. Thalamic origin of sleep spindles: Morison and Bassett (1945). *J Neurophysiol.* 1995;73(3):921-922.

55. Starzl TE, Taylor CW, Magoun HW. Ascending conduction in reticular activating system, with special reference to the diencephalon. *J Neurophysiol.* 1951;14(6):461-477.

56. Villablanca J, Marcus R. Sleep-wakefulness, EEG and behavioral studies of chronic cats without neocortex and striatum: The "diencephalic" cat. *Arch Ital Biol.* 1972;110(3):348-382.

57. Qiu MH, Vetrivelan R, Fuller PM, Lu J. Basal ganglia control of sleep-wake behavior and cortical activation. *Eur J Neurosci.* 2010;31(3):499-507.

58. McGinty DJ, Sterman MB. Sleep suppression after basal forebrain lesions in the cat. *Science.* 1968;160(833):1253-1255.

59. Sherin JE, Shiromani PJ, McCarley RW, Saper CB. Activation of ventrolateral preoptic neurons during sleep. *Science.* 1996;271(5246):216-219.

60. Chou TC, Bjorkum AA, Gaus SE, Lu J, Scammell TE, Saper CB. Afferents to the ventrolateral preoptic nucleus. *J Neurosci.* 2002;22(3):977-990.

61. Lu J, Greco MA, Shiromani P, Saper CB. Effect of lesions of the ventrolateral preoptic nucleus on NREM and REM sleep. *J Neurosci.* 2000;20(10):3830-3842.

62. Suntsova N, Szymusiak R, Alam MN, Guzman-Marin R, McGinty D. Sleep-waking discharge patterns of median preoptic nucleus neurons in rats. *J Physiol.* 2002;543(Pt 2):665-677.

63. Gong H, McGinty D, Guzman-Marin R, et al. Activation of c-Fos in GABAergic neurons in the preoptic area during sleep and in response to sleep deprivation. *J Physiol.* 2004;556(Pt 3):935-946.

64. Peyron C, Faraco J, Rogers W, Ripley B, Overeem S, et al. A mutation in a case of early onset narcolepsy and a generalized absence of hypocretin peptides in human narcoleptic brains. *Nat Med.* 2000;6(9):991-997.

65. Aserinsky E, Kleitman N. Regularly occurring periods of eye motility, and concomitant phenomena, during sleep. *Science.* 1953;118(3062):273-274.

66. Dement W. The occurrence of low voltage, fast, electroencephalogram patterns during behavioral sleep in the cat. *Electroencephalogr Clin Neurophysiol.* 1958;10(2):291-296.

67. Jouvet M, Michel F. [New research on the structures responsible for the "paradoxical phase" of sleep.]. *J Physiol (Paris).* 1960;52:130-131.

68. Jouvet M. [Research on the neural structures and responsible mechanisms in different phases of physiological sleep.] *Arch Ital Biol.* 1962;100:125-206.

69. McCarley RW, Hobson JA. Neuronal excitability modulation over the sleep cycle: A structural and mathematical model. *Science.* 1975;189(4196):58-60.

70. Kubin L. Carbachol models of REM sleep: Recent developments and new directions. *Arch Ital Biol.* 2001;139(1-2):147-168.

71. McCarley RW. Neurobiology of REM and NREM sleep. *Sleep Med.* 2007;8(4):302-330.

72. Pace-Schott EF, Hobson JA. The neurobiology of sleep: Genetics, cellular physiology and subcortical networks. *Nat Rev Neurosci.* 2002;3(8):591-605.

73. Boeve BF, Dickson DW, Olson EJ, et al. Pathophysiology of REM sleep behaviour disorder and relevance to neurodegenerative disease. *Brain.* 2007;130(Pt 11):2770-2788.

74. Braak E, Bohl JR, Muller CM, Rüb U, de Vos RA, Del Tredici K. Stanley Fahn Lecture: The staging procedure for the inclusion body pathology associated with sporadic Parkinson's disease reconsidered. *Mov Disord.* 2005;21:2042-2051.

75. Braak E, Sandmann-Keil D, Rüb U, et al. Alpha-synuclein immunopositive Parkinson's disease-related inclusion bodies in lower brainstem nuclei. *Acta Neuropathol.* 2001;101(3):195-201.

76. Braak H, Rüb U, Sandmann-Keil D, et al. Parkinson's disease: Affection of brain stem nuclei controlling premotor and motor neurons of the somatomotor system. *Acta Neuropathol (Berl).* 2000;99(5):489-495.

77. Mathis J, Hess CW, Bassetti C. Isolated mediotegmental lesion causing narcolepsy and rapid eye movement sleep behavior disorder: A case evidencing a common pathway in narcolepsy and rapid eye movement sleep behavior disorder. *J Neurol Neurosurg Psychiatry.* 2007;78(4):427-429.

78. Xi Z, Luning W. REM sleep behavior disorder in a patient with pontine stroke. *Sleep Med.* 2009;10(1):143-146.

79. Sakai K, Crochet S, Onoe H. Pontine structures and mechanisms involved in the generation of paradoxical (REM) sleep. *Arch Ital Biol.* 2001;139(1-2):93-107.

80. Kayama Y, Ohta M, Jodo E. Firing of "possibly" cholinergic neurons in the rat laterodorsal tegmental nucleus during sleep and wakefulness. *Brain Res.* 1992;569(2):210-220.

81. Thakkar MM, Strecker RE, McCarley RW. Behavioral state control through differential serotonergic inhibition in the mesopontine cholinergic nuclei: A simultaneous unit recording and microdialysis study. *J Neurosci.* 1998;18(14):5490-5497.

82. Jones BE. Paradoxical REM sleep promoting and permitting neuronal networks. *Arch Ital Biol.* 2004;142(4):379-396.

83. Velazquez-Moctezuma J, Gillin JC, Shiromani PJ. Effect of specific M_1, M_2 muscarinic receptor agonists on REM sleep generation. *Brain Res.* 1989;503(1):128-131.

84. Imeri L, Bianchi S, Angeli P, Mancia M. Selective blockade of different brain stem muscarinic receptor subtypes: Effects on the sleep-wake cycle. *Brain Res.* 1994;636(1):68-72.

85. Sakai K, Sastre JP, Salvert D, Touret M, Tohyama M, Jouvet M. Tegmentoreticular projections with special reference to the muscular atonia during paradoxical sleep in the cat: An HRP study. *Brain Res.* 1979;176(2):233-254.

86. Baghdoyan HA, Lydic R. M_2 muscarinic receptor subtype in the feline medial pontine reticular formation modulates the amount of rapid eye movement sleep. *Sleep.* 1999;22(7):835-847.

87. Goutagny R, Comte JC, Salvert D, Gomeza J, Yamada M, Wess J, et al. Paradoxical sleep in mice lacking M_3 and M_2/M_4 muscarinic receptors. *Neuropsychobiology.* 2005;52(3):140-146.

88. Hobson JA, McCarley RW, Wyzinski PW. Sleep cycle oscillation: Reciprocal discharge by two brainstem neuronal groups. *Science.* 1975;189(4196):55-58.

89. McGinty DJ, Harper RM. Dorsal raphe neurons: Depression of firing during sleep in cats. *Brain Res.* 1976;101(3):569-575.

90. Trulson ME, Jacobs BL. Raphe unit activity in freely moving cats: Correlation with level of behavioral arousal. *Brain Res.* 1979;163(1):135-150.

91. Maloney KJ, Mainville L, Jones BE. Differential c-Fos expression in cholinergic, monoaminergic, and GABAergic cell groups of the pontomesencephalic tegmentum after paradoxical sleep deprivation and recovery. *J Neurosci.* 1999;19(8):3057-3072.

92. Woch G, Davies RO, Pack AI, Kubin L, et al. Behaviour of raphe cells projecting to the dorsomedial medulla during carbachol-induced atonia in the cat. *J Physiol.* 1996;490(Pt 3):745-758.

93. Kubin L, Reignier C, Tojima H, et al. Suppression of hypoglossal motoneurons during the carbachol-induced atonia of REM sleep is not caused by fast synaptic inhibition. *Brain Res.* 1993;611(2):300-312.

94. Morrison JL, Sood S, Liu H, et al. Role of inhibitory amino acids in control of hypoglossal motor outflow to genioglossus muscle in naturally sleeping rats. *J Physiol.* 2003;552(Pt 3):975-991.

95. Fenik VB, Davies RO, Kubin L. REM sleep-like atonia of hypoglossal (XII) motoneurons is caused by loss of noradrenergic and serotonergic inputs. *Am J Respir Crit Care Med.* 2005;172(10):1322-1330.

96. Chase MH, Morales FR. The control of motoneurons during sleep. In: Kryger MH, Roth T, Dement WC, eds. *Principles and Practice of Sleep Medicine.* Philadelphia: WB Saunders; 1994:163-175.

97. Achermann P, Borbely AA. Mathematical models of sleep regulation. *Front Biosci.* 2003;8:S683-S693.

98. Borbely AA, Tobler I. Homeostatic and circadian principles in sleep regulation in the rats in brain mechanisms of sleep. In: McGinty D, Drucker-Colin R, Morrison A, Parmeggiani PL, eds. *Brain Mechanisms of Sleep.* New York: Raven Press; 1985:35-44.

99. Radulovacki M, Virus RM, Djuricic-Nedelson M, Green RD. Adenosine analogs and sleep in rats. *J Pharmacol Exp Ther.* 1984;228(2):268-274.

100. Radulovacki M. The pharmacology of the adenosine system. In: Kales A, ed. *The Pharmacology of Sleep.* Berlin: Springer-Verlag; 1995:307-319.

101. Latini S, Pedata F. Adenosine in the central nervous system: Release mechanisms and extracellular concentrations. *J Neurochem.* 2001; 79(3):463-484.

102. Chagoya de Sanchez V, Hernández Múñoz R, Suárez J, et al. Day-night variations of adenosine and its metabolizing enzymes in the brain cortex of the rat—Possible physiological significance for the energetic homeostasis and the sleep-wake cycle. *Brain Res.* 1993;612(1-2):115-121.

103. Benington JH, Heller HC. Restoration of brain energy metabolism as the function of sleep. *Prog Neurobiol.* 1995;45(4):347-360.

104. Rainnie DG, Grunze H, McCarley R, Greene R. Adenosine inhibition of mesopontine cholinergic neurons: Implications for EEG arousal. *Science.* 1994;263(5147):689-692.

105. Basheer R, Strecker RE, Thakkar MM, McCarley RW. Adenosine and sleep-wake regulation. *Prog Neurobiol.* 2004;73(6):379-396.

106. Burnstock G. Physiology and pathophysiology of purinergic neurotransmission. *Physiol Rev.* 2007;87(2):659-797.

107. Dunwiddie TV, Masino SA. The role and regulation of adenosine in the central nervous system. *Annu Rev Neurosci.* 2001;24:31-55.

108. Porkka-Heiskanen T, Strecker RE, Thakkar M, Bjorkum AA, Greene RW, McCarley RW. Adenosine: A mediator of the sleep-inducing effects of prolonged wakefulness. *Science.* 1997;276(5316):1265-1268.

109. Huston JP, Haas HL, Boix F, Pfister M, Decking U, et al. Extracellular adenosine levels in neostriatum and hippocampus during rest and activity periods of rats. *Neuroscience.* 1996;73(1):99-107.

110. Murillo-Rodriguez E, Blanco-Centurion C, Gerashchenko D, et al. The diurnal rhythm of adenosine levels in the basal forebrain of young and old rats. *Neuroscience.* 2004;123(2):361-370.

111. Madsen PL, Schmidt JF, Wildschiodtz G, et al. Cerebral O_2 metabolism and cerebral blood flow in humans during deep and rapid-eye-movement sleep. *J Appl Physiol.* 1991;70(6):2597-2601.

112. Maquet P, Peters JM, Aerts J, et al. Functional neuroanatomy of human slow wave sleep. *J Neurosci.* 1997;17(8):2807-2812.

113. Strecker RE, Thakkar M, Bjorkum AA, et al. Adenosinergic modulation of basal forebrain and preoptic/anterior hypothalamic neuronal activity in the control of behavioral state. *Behav Brain Res.* 2000;115(2):183-204.

114. Steriade M, McCarley RW. *Brain Control of Wakefulness and Sleep.* New York: Kluwer Academic/Plenum; 2005.

115. Liu ZW, Gao XB. Adenosine inhibits activity of hypocretin/orexin neurons by the A_1 receptor in the lateral hypothalamus: A possible sleep-promoting effect. *J Neurophysiol.* 2007;97(1):837-848.

116. Oishi Y, Huang ZL, Fredholm BB, Urade Y, Hayaishi O. Adenosine in the tuberomammillary nucleus inhibits the histaminergic system via A_1 receptors and promotes non-rapid eye movement sleep. *Proc Natl Acad Sci U S A.* 2008;105(50):19992-19997.

117. Pan WJ, Osmanovic SS, Shefner SA. Characterization of the adenosine A_1 receptor-activated potassium current in rat locus ceruleus neurons. *J Pharmacol Exp Ther.* 1995;273(1):537-544.

118. Arrigoni E, Chamberlin NL, Saper CB, McCarley RW. Adenosine inhibits basal forebrain cholinergic and noncholinergic neurons in vitro. *Neuroscience.* 2006;140(2):403-413.

119. Alam MN, Szymusiak R, Gong H, King J, McGinty D. Adenosinergic modulation of rat basal forebrain neurons during sleep and waking: Neuronal recording with microdialysis. *J Physiol.* 1999;521(Pt 3): 679-690.

120. Thakkar MM, Ramesh V, Strecker RE, McCarley RW. Microdialysis perfusion of orexin-A in the basal forebrain increases wakefulness in freely behaving rats. *Arch Ital Biol.* 2001;139(3):313-328.

121. Rai S, Kumar S, Alam MA, et al. A_1 receptor mediated adenosinergic regulation of perifornical-lateral hypothalamic area neurons in freely behaving rats. *Neuroscience.* 2010;167(1):40-48.

122. Chamberlin NL, Arrigoni E, Chou TC, et al. Effects of adenosine on GABAergic synaptic inputs to identified ventrolateral preoptic neurons. *Neuroscience.* 2003;119(4):913-918.

123. Moriarty S, Rainnie D, McCarley R, Greene R. Disinhibition of ventrolateral preoptic area sleep-active neurons by adenosine: A new mechanism for sleep promotion. *Neuroscience.* 2004;123(2):451-457.

124. Gallopin T, Luppi PH, Cauli B, et al. The endogenous somnogen adenosine excites a subset of sleep-promoting neurons via A_{2A} receptors in the ventrolateral preoptic nucleus. *Neuroscience.* 2005;134(4): 1377-1390.

125. Methippara MM, Kumar S, Alam MN, Szymusiak R, McGinty D. Effects on sleep of microdialysis of adenosine A_1 and A_{2a} receptor analogs into the lateral preoptic area of rats. *Am J Physiol Regul Integr Comp Physiol.* 2005;289(6):R1715-R1723.

126. Scammell TE, Gerashchenko DY, Mochizuki T, et al. An adenosine A_{2a} agonist increases sleep and induces Fos in ventrolateral preoptic neurons. *Neuroscience.* 2001;107(4):653-663.

127. Fredholm BB, Battig K, Holmen J, et al. Actions of caffeine in the brain with special reference to factors that contribute to its widespread use. *Pharmacol Rev.* 1999;51(1):83-133.

128. Landolt HP. Sleep homeostasis: A role for adenosine in humans? *Biochem Pharmacol.* 2008;75(11):2070-2079.

129. Retey JV, Adam M, Khatami R, et al. A genetic variation in the adenosine A_{2A} receptor gene (*ADORA2A*) contributes to individual sensitivity to caffeine effects on sleep. *Clin Pharmacol Ther.* 2007;81(5):692-698.

130. Huang ZL, Qu WM, Eguchi N, et al. Adenosine A_{2A}, but not A_1, receptors mediate the arousal effect of caffeine. *Nat Neurosci.* 2005;8(7): 858-859.

131. Stenberg D. Neuroanatomy and neurochemistry of sleep. *Cell Mol Life Sci.* 2007;64(10):1187-1204.

132. Stenberg D, Litonius E, Halldner L, et al. Sleep and its homeostatic regulation in mice lacking the adenosine A_1 receptor. *J Sleep Res.* 2003;12(4):283-290.

133. Ferre S, Diamond I, Goldberg SR, et al. Adenosine A_{2A} receptors in ventral striatum, hypothalamus and nociceptive circuitry implications for drug addiction, sleep and pain. *Prog Neurobiol.* 2007;83(5):332-347.

134. Satoh S, Matsumura H, Hayaishi O. Involvement of adenosine A$_{2A}$ receptor in sleep promotion. *Eur J Pharmacol.* 1998;351(2):155-162.

135. Satoh S, Matsumura H, Hayaishi O. Involvement of adenosine A$_{2A}$ receptor in sleep promotion. *Eur J Pharmacol.* 1998;351:155-162.

136. Huang ZL, Urade Y, Hayaishi O. Prostaglandins and adenosine in the regulation of sleep and wakefulness. *Curr Opin Pharmacol.* 2007;7(1):33-38.

137. Fredholm BB, et al. Structure and function of adenosine receptors and their genes. *Naunyn Schmiedebergs Arch Pharmacol.* 2000;362(4-5):364-374.

138. Fredholm BB, Arslan G, Halldner L, et al. Adenosine and brain function. *Int Rev Neurobiol.* 2005;63:191-270.

139. Retey JV, Adam M, Honegger E, et al. A functional genetic variation of adenosine deaminase affects the duration and intensity of deep sleep in humans. *Proc Natl Acad Sci U S A.* 2005;102(43):15676-15681.

140. Okada T, Mochizuki T, Huang ZL, et al. Dominant localization of adenosine deaminase in leptomeninges and involvement of the enzyme in sleep. *Biochem Biophys Res Commun.* 2003;312(1):29-34.

141. Radulovacki M, Virus RM, Djuricic-Nedelson M, Green RD. Hypnotic effects of deoxycorformycin in rats. *Brain Res.* 1983;271(2):392-395.

142. Radek RJ, Decker MW, Jarvis MF. The adenosine kinase inhibitor ABT-702 augments EEG slow waves in rats. *Brain Res.* 2004;1026(1):74-83.

143. Krauss SW, Ghirnikar RB, Diamond I, Gordon AS. Inhibition of adenosine uptake by ethanol is specific for one class of nucleoside transporters. *Mol Pharmacol.* 1993;44(5):1021-1026.

144. Crews FT, Morrow AL, Criswell H, Breese G. Effects of ethanol on ion channels. *Int Rev Neurobiol.* 1996;39:283-367.

145. Dar MS. Brain adenosinergic modulation of acute ethanol-induced motor impairment. *Alcohol Suppl.* 1993;2:425-429.

146. Fredholm BB, Chen JF, Masino SA, Vaugeois JM. Actions of adenosine at its receptors in the CNS: Insights from knockouts and drugs. *Annu Rev Pharmacol Toxicol.* 2005;45:385-412.

147. Jacobson KA, Gao ZG. Adenosine receptors as therapeutic targets. *Nat Rev Drug Discov.* 2006;5(3):247-264.

148. Moore RY. Neural control of the pineal gland. *Behav Brain Res.* 1996;73(1-2):125-130.

149. Jin X, Shearman LP, Weaver DR, et al. A molecular mechanism regulating rhythmic output from the suprachiasmatic circadian clock. *Cell.* 1999;96(1):57-68.

150. Reppert SM, Weaver DR. Coordination of circadian timing in mammals. *Nature.* 2002;418(6901):935-941.

151. Gooley JJ, Lu J, Chou TC, Scammell TE, Saper CB. Melanopsin in cells of origin of the retinohypothalamic tract. *Nat Neurosci.* 2001;4(12):1165.

152. Hattar S, Liao HW, Takao M, Berson DM, Yau KW. Melanopsin-containing retinal ganglion cells: Architecture, projections, and intrinsic photosensitivity. *Science.* 2002;295(5557):1065-1070.

153. Bunger MK, Wilsbacher LD, Moran SM, et al. Mop3 is an essential component of the master circadian pacemaker in mammals. *Cell.* 2000;103(7):1009-1017.

154. Edgar DM, Dement WC, Fuller CA. Effect of SCN lesions on sleep in squirrel monkeys: Evidence for opponent processes in sleep-wake regulation. *J Neurosci.* 1993;13(3):1065-1079.

155. Moore RY, Eichler VB. Loss of a circadian adrenal corticosterone rhythm following suprachiasmatic lesions in the rat. *Brain Res.* 1972;42(1):201-206.

156. Dijk DJ, Czeisler CA. Contribution of the circadian pacemaker and the sleep homeostat to sleep propensity, sleep structure, electroencephalographic slow waves, and sleep spindle activity in humans. *J Neurosci.* 1995;15(5 Pt 1):3526-3538.

157. Moore-Ede MC, Sulzman FM, Fuller CA. *The clock that times us: Physiology of the circadian timing system.* Cambridge, MA: Harvard University Press; 1982.

158. Watts AG, Swanson LW. Efferent projections of the suprachiasmatic nucleus: II. Studies using retrograde transport of fluorescent dyes and simultaneous peptide immunohistochemistry in the rat. *J Comp Neurol.* 1987;258(2):230-252.

159. Lu J, Zhang YH, Chou TC, et al. Contrasting effects of ibotenate lesions of the paraventricular nucleus and subparaventricular zone on sleep-wake cycle and temperature regulation. *J Neurosci.* 2001;21(13):4864-4874.

160. Chou TC, Scammell TE, Gooley JJ, et al. Critical role of dorsomedial hypothalamic nucleus in a wide range of behavioral circadian rhythms. *J Neurosci.* 2003;23(33):10691-10702.

161. Gooley JJ, Schomer A, Saper CB. The dorsomedial hypothalamic nucleus is critical for the expression of food-entrainable circadian rhythms. *Nat Neurosci.* 2006;9(3):398-407.

162. Lockley SW, Skene DJ, James K, et al. Melatonin administration can entrain the free-running circadian system of blind subjects. *J Endocrinol.* 2000;164(1):R1-6.

163. Wang X. The antiapoptotic activity of melatonin in neurodegenerative diseases. *CNS Neurosci Ther.* 2009;15(4):345-357.

164. Sack RL, Brandes RW, Kendall AR, et al. Entrainment of free-running circadian rhythms by melatonin in blind people. *N Engl J Med.* 2000;343(15):1070-1077.

165. Van Den Heuvel CJ, Reid KJ, Dawson D. Effect of atenolol on nocturnal sleep and temperature in young men: Reversal by pharmacological doses of melatonin. *Physiol Behav.* 1997;61(6):795-802.

166. Dijk DJ, Shanahan TL, Duffy JF, et al. Variation of electroencephalographic activity during non-rapid eye movement and rapid eye movement sleep with phase of circadian melatonin rhythm in humans. *J Physiol.* 1997;505(Pt 3):851-858.

167. McEwen BS. Allostasis and allostatic load: Implications for neuropsychopharmacology. *Neuropsychopharmacology.* 2000;22(2):108-124.

168. Dong HW, Petrovich GD, Watts AG, Swanson LW. Basic organization of projections from the oval and fusiform nuclei of the bed nuclei of the stria terminalis in adult rat brain. *J Comp Neurol.* 2001;436(4):430-455.

169. Aston-Jones G, Cohen JD. Adaptive gain and the role of the locus coeruleus-norepinephrine system in optimal performance. *J Comp Neurol.* 2005;493(1):99-110.

170. Cano G, Mochizuki T, Saper CB. Neural circuitry of stress-induced insomnia in rats. *J Neurosci.* 2008;28(40):10167-10184.

171. Nofzinger EA, Berman S, Fasiczka A, et al. Functional neuroimaging evidence for hyperarousal in insomnia. *Am J Psychiatry.* 2004;161(11):2126-2128.

172. Rosenbaum E. Warum Mussen Wir Schlafen? Eine Neue Theorie des Schlafens. [Why to we need sleep? A new theory of sleep.] Berlin: Hirschwald. 1892.

173. Ishimori K. True cause of sleep: A hypnogenic substance as evidenced in the brain of sleep-deprived animals. *Tokyo Igakkai Zasshi.* 1909;23:429-457.

174. Legendre R, PieAron H. Recherches sur le besoin de commeil consecutif a une veille prolongee. *Z Allgem Physiol.* 1913;14:235-262.

175. Pappenheimer JR, Miller TB, Goodrich CA. Sleep-promoting effects of cerebrospinal fluid from sleep-deprived goats. *Proc Natl Acad Sci U S A.* 1967;58(2):513-517.

176. Krueger JM. The role of cytokines in sleep regulation. *Curr Pharm Des.* 2008;14(32):3408-3416.

177. Imeri L, Opp MR. How (and why) the immune system makes us sleep. *Nat Rev Neurosci.* 2009;10(3):199-210.

Chapter 5

Essentials of Sleep Neuropharmacology

MATT T. BIANCHI

The endogenous substances implicated in sleep-wake state modulation span diverse molecular categories, each with distinct considerations regarding circumstances of release, mechanisms of cellular response, and time-course of target exposure. For example, classical neurotransmitters such as glutamate and γ-aminobutyric acid (GABA) generally involve synaptic vesicle release, brief (milliseconds) exposure of postsynaptic receptors, followed by voltage changes that are short-lived for ionotropic receptors (tens to hundreds of milliseconds) or longer lived for metabotropic receptors (hundreds to thousands of milliseconds). Neuropeptides, such as orexin, also undergo vesicular release, but generally act upon target receptors at the time scale of seconds or longer. Other substances, such as hormones and cytokines, are released, circulate in the blood and cerebrospinal fluid (CSF), and affect sleep-wake states through diverse mechanisms, extending over even longer time scales.

Modulation of sleep-wake control via exogenous compounds involves interactions with the endogenous systems that facilitate sleep or wakefulness. Exogenous agents can be considered to fall into one of three categories: prescription therapeutics aimed at improving sleep-wake symptoms; therapeutics given for other indications that carry side effects impacting sleep or wakefulness; or dietary supplements and natural substances taken to modulate sleep or wakefulness. Although the precise mechanisms of many of these compounds remain the subject of active research, a common strategy is to focus investigations toward their receptor targets in hopes of building a bottom-up understanding within the context of the anatomy and physiology of sleep-wake systems. Information from each perspective informs the other, and indeed top-down and bottom-up approaches are indispensable as we progress toward improved pharmacologic interventions in this domain.

OVERVIEW OF SLEEP-WAKE NEUROCHEMISTRY: THE MAJOR PLAYERS

Extensive basic research has delineated a network of neuro-anatomic and neurochemical components controlling mammalian sleep and wake behavioral states[1-3] (see Chapter 4). The main sleep-promoting nuclei are in the preoptic area (POA), which utilizes the neurotransmitter GABA and the neuropeptide galanin, and the basal forebrain (BF), which is a major player in adenosine-mediated sleepiness. The main wake-promoting regions (and their signals) are the posterior hypothalamus (orexin), the tuberomammillary nucleus (TMN; histamine), the laterodorsal and pedunculopontine

tegmentum (LDT/PPT; acetylcholine), the locus ceruleus (LC; norepinephrine), and the dorsal raphe (DR; serotonin). The basal forebrain cholinergic neurons are important for cortical activation associated with waking as well as REM (rapid eye movement) sleep. The substantia nigra and ventral tegmental area (dopamine) are also implicated in wakefulness. A rich literature spanning pharmacology, physiology, lesion studies, and genetics generally supports these roles.[2-8] Interactions among these nuclei may form "flip-flop" switches, as proposed by Saper and colleagues, in which reciprocal negative interactions occur between wake- and sleep-promoting centers, as well as REM and NREM (non-REM) promoting centers.[9]

HISTORICAL BACKGROUND

The search for endogenous substances involved in sleep regulation began with experiments in which CSF or blood from sleep-deprived animals was transferred to nondeprived animals. This classical approach assumed that the sleepiness caused by sleep deprivation would involve concomitant accumulation of sleep-promoting substance(s). These early experiments demonstrated that CSF and central venous blood contained one or more humoral "somnogens" capable of inducing sleep in the recipient animals. The main components identified by these early experiments were factor S (later identified as muramyl peptide, a bacterial cell wall component), sleep-promoting substance (SPS; later identified as uridine and oxidized glutathione), and the delta sleep–inducing peptide (DSIP), which was isolated from rabbit central venous blood after median thalamic stimulation. Although the search for specific sleep substances has given way to a growing appreciation of the large number of molecular players influencing the sleep-wake system, the pioneering experiments of Pieron, Schendorf, Pappenheimer, and Inoue remain the foundation of modern sleep pharmacology.[6]

The variability in reported effects in the field of sleep pharmacology is a recurrent theme that serves as a reminder of several important points worth considering. For example, human and animal studies of the sleep-wake effects of DSIP have shown variable effects, including no impact on sleep or even insomnia. The ever-growing list of substances (endogenous and exogenous) that modulate sleep, and their interactions with genetic and environmental factors (Fig. 5-1), serve as a cautionary backdrop against which to interpret the experimental findings that support modern theories of drug mechanisms important for sleep-wake regulation. Even the routine quantification of NREM and REM sleep may not capture the dynamics of sleep architecture or its response to perturbation in sleep pharmacology experiments. For example, patients with severe sleep apnea have similar percentages of awake, REM sleep, and NREM sleep stages as normal subjects; however, analyzing sleep stage transition probabilities revealed marked fragmentation of sleep architecture.[10]

Most mechanistic studies contributing to our knowledge of the receptors involved in sleep-wake pharmacology come from nonhuman animal experiments, which are more amenable to genetic and pharmacologic manipulations. Although clinical effects (e.g., those measured by polysomnography) of various drugs on human sleep and wake physiology are well studied, much of the mechanistic receptor work is derived from rodent studies and, to a lesser extent, studies on cats, rabbits, and primates.

OVERVIEW OF RECEPTORS

Membrane receptors respond to neurotransmitters, neuropeptides, and other molecular signals through two main mechanisms: ionotropic or metabotropic (Fig. 5-2). In both types of receptor, multiple subunit proteins (each typically encoded by their own gene) assemble to form the functional receptor complex, which includes extracellular, transmembrane, and intracellular domains. The extracellular domain faces outside the cell and contains the binding site for the appropriate neurotransmitter, neuropeptide, or neurohormone. The transmembrane domain of ionotropic receptors contains the channel pore itself, which opens in response to neurotransmitter binding in the extracellular domain. The transmembrane domain of metabotropic receptors conveys extracellular signals (e.g., neurotransmitter binding) to intracellular signaling cascades (see Fig. 5-3). Thus, both ionotropic and metabotropic receptors can be understood as detectors of extracellular signals (such as neurotransmitters) to facilitate regulation of neuronal activity.

Ionotropic receptors are cell surface proteins that contain an intrinsic ion channel pore formed at the center of the assembled subunit proteins. Ion channels that are activated by extracellular signals such as neurotransmitters are known as *ligand-gated ion channels.* Activation of these ligand-gated ion channels modulates neuronal excitability depending on which types of ions are allowed to pass. Excitatory ligand-gated channels generally are permeable to sodium or calcium ions, which increase neuronal activity by causing membrane depolarization. In contrast, inhibitory ligand-gated channels generally are permeable to chloride, resulting in decreased neuronal activity due to hyperpolarization. The canonical excitatory ligand-gated ion channels mediate depolarization in response to one of the main excitatory neurotransmitters: glutamate, serotonin (5-HT [5-hydroxytryptamine]), or acetylcholine (ACh). The neurotransmitters γ-aminobutyric acid (GABA) and glycine each activate a distinct chloride-permeable channel and are classified as inhibitory, or hyperpolarizing. It is worth mentioning that although transmitters and channels carry the labels of inhibitory or excitatory, their capacity to hyperpolarize or depolarize neurons is not an intrinsic property; rather, the voltage response depends on the local ion gradients. The importance of ionic homeostasis in neuronal excitability is emphasized by the physiologic occurrence of altered chloride gradients that can render GABA-gated ion channels depolarizing. Note that not all ion channels are ligand-gated: numerous voltage-gated ion channels also regulate neuronal excitability, such as the voltage-gated sodium and potassium channels that underlie axonal action potentials. Some ion channels are controlled by intracellular G-protein signals, and this is a critical mechanism of some metabotropic receptor signaling, as will be discussed further in this chapter.

Metabotropic receptors respond to extracellular signals by activating one or more of several well-described intracellular signal transduction pathways.[11] The common theme across these cascades is the role of intracellular signals called

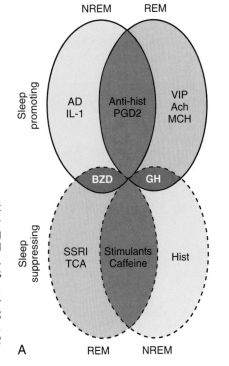

Figure 5-1 Sleep pharmacology considerations. A, The impact of endogenous and exogenous compounds on sleep is typically dichotomized into sleep-promoting *(solid border ovals)* or sleep-suppressing *(dashed border ovals),* which can refer to NREM *(light blue fill)* or REM *(light gray fill)* sleep, or both *(dark gray fill).* For some compounds, opposing effects on REM and NREM are seen *(dark blue fill).* **B,** Factors that may influence the pharmacology of sleep-related substances. *Ach,* acetylcholine; *AD,* adenosine; *Anti-hist,* anti-histamine; *BZD,* benzodiazepine; *GH,* growth hormone; *Hist,* histamine; *IL-1,* interleukin-1; *MCH,* Melanin-concentrating hormone; *PGD2,* prostaglandin D2; *SSRI,* selective serotonin reuptake inhibitor; *TCA,* tricyclic antidepressant; *VIP,* vasoactive intestinal peptide.

Potential influences on sleep-wake pharmacology:
- Age
- Sex
- Species
- Genetic background
- Circadian phase
- Stress
- Temperature
- Delivery route
- Concentration
- Exposure duration
- Brain region
- Neuron type
- Disease state
- Other modulators
- Measurement technique

G proteins, and thus these receptors are known collectively as G protein–coupled receptors (GPCRs). There are several different kinds of G proteins, each of which activates or inhibits a certain intracellular signaling pathway to stimulate or inhibit neuronal activity. Many metabotropic receptors are associated with, or "coupled" to, more than one G protein, enabling a diversity of signaling to targets including enzymes and ion channels.

The details of GPCR signaling are shown in Figure 5-3. As already mentioned, receptor activation by extracellular ligands is conveyed to the intracellular domain, where G proteins reside in a resting state. Upon activation, guanosine triphosphate (GTP) circulating in the intracellular compartment is allowed to bind to the G protein by replacing the diphosphate (guanosine diphosphate, GDP) associated with the resting state. GTP binding initiates the dissociation of the G protein subunits, called α and $\beta\gamma$, from the intracellular domain of the receptor, whereupon they diffuse into the intracellular space to initiate a spectrum of downstream signaling cascades. The major G protein signaling pathway involves the enzyme adenylate cyclase (AC), which catalyzes the formation of cyclic adenosine monophosphate (cAMP), the small molecule that activates protein kinase A (PKA). Depending on the specific G protein subunit involved, this cascade can yield either enhancement ($G_{\alpha s}$) or inhibition ($G_{\alpha i}$) of the AC enzyme. Another G protein signaling pathway involves stimulation of the enzyme phospholipase C (PLC), via specific types of G proteins called $G_{\alpha q}$ and $G_{\alpha 11}$. PLC catalyzes the conversion of phosphatidylinositol-4,5-bisphosphate (PIP$_2$) into diacylglycerol (DAG) and inositol triphosphate (IP$_3$). DAG activates protein kinase C (PKC), while IP$_3$ increases Ca^{2+} concentration via intracellular stores. The intermediate molecule PIP$_2$ may itself serve a signaling role by enhancing K$^+$ channels. The $\beta\gamma$ subunits also play important signaling roles, and are best known for their activation of K$^+$ channels and inhibition of Ca^{2+} channels, both of which reduce neuronal firing.

COMPLEXITY OF RECEPTOR SIGNALING

Because the diversity of known receptors far exceeds that of signaling pathways, there is considerable potential for overlap, and understanding how signaling specificity is achieved is an area of ongoing study (extensively elaborated in the context of serotonin signaling[12]). This diversity is illustrated in Figure 5-4, an overview of signaling classifications and major mechanisms. Table 5-1 also summarizes the types of signaling

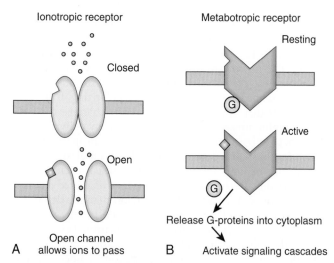

Figure 5-2 Ionotropic and metabotropic receptors. A, An ionotropic, ligand-gated receptor. Binding of ligand *(open square)* triggers opening of the channel gate, allowing ions *(dots)* to flux across the phospholipid bilayer membrane. **B,** A metabotropic receptor, which also responds to extracellular neurotransmitter *(open square)*. In this case, a conformation change in the receptor protein activates intracellular G-protein signaling. Although certain G proteins go on to activate other, downstream, ion channels (see text), the metabotropic receptors do not themselves contain ion channels.

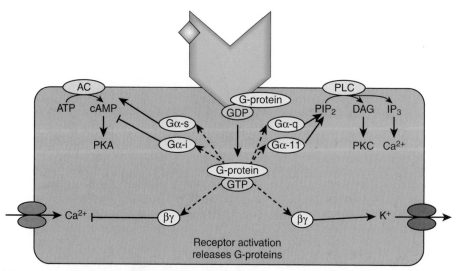

Figure 5-3 Metabotropic receptor signaling through intracellular G proteins. Upon binding of extracellular ligand (such as a neurotransmitter or neurohormone), the metabotropic receptor undergoes a conformational change that allows guanosine diphosphate (GDP) (present at rest) to be replaced by guanosine triphosphate (GTP) (which is circulating in the cytoplasm). This exchange allows the G proteins to dissociate from the receptor and engage in signaling activity. Several types of G proteins are shown, each with a particular signaling pathway (dotted arrows). The Gα-s subunits activate the adenylate cyclase (AC) enzyme to generate cAMP, while the Gα-i subunits inhibit AC. The Gα-q and Gα-11 subunits activate the phospholipase C (PLC) enzyme to generate diacylglycerol (DAG) and inositol triphosphate (IP$_3$). The $\beta\gamma$ subunits activate certain types of K$^+$ and inhibit certain types of Ca^{2+} channels, such that metabotropic receptors may be indirectly coupled to membrane excitability.

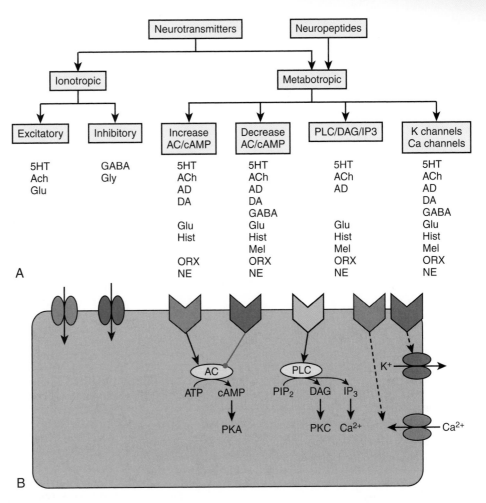

Figure 5-4 Neurotransmitters, neuropeptides, and their primary signaling mechanisms. A, Categories of neurotransmitters (interacting with ionotropic and metabotropic receptors) and neuropeptides/hormones (all of which interact with metabotropic receptors). The receptor mechanisms employed by the major neurotransmitters and orexin are listed. **B,** Signaling mechanisms are vertically aligned to each category, including excitatory *(dark gray)* and inhibitory *(dark blue)* ion channels, and metabotropic receptors that either activate *(dark gray)* or inhibit *(dark blue)* adenylate cyclase (AC), or activate phospholipase C (PLC; *light blue*). *5HT,* 5-hydroxytryptamine; *AC,* adenylate cyclase; *ACh,* acetylcholine; *AD,* adenosine; *ATP,* adenosine triphosphate; *Ca²⁺,* calcium; *cAMP,* cyclic adenosine monophosphate; *DA,* dopamine; *DAG,* diacylglycerol; *GABA,* gamma aminobutyric acid; *Gly,* glycine; *Glu,* gluamate; *Hist,* histamine; *IP₃,* inositol triphosphate; *K⁺,* potassium; *Mel,* melatonin; *ORX,* orexin; *NE,* norepinephrine; *PIP₂,* phosphatidylinositol-4,5-bisphosphate; *PKA,* protein kinase A; *PKC,* protein kinase C.

mechanisms available to the major neurotransmitters. In addition to these classical signaling pathways, certain GPCRs are capable of signal transduction independent of their G protein subunits.[13] As discussed later. Most of the major neurotransmitters interact with multiple receptor subtypes: ionic and metabotropic, located in pre- and postsynaptic compartments, capable of regulating excitability across a spectrum from excitation to inhibition (see Fig. 5-4).

Presynaptic receptors are particularly important regulators of neurotransmitter release, often mediating negative feedback as autoreceptors.[14] Extrasynaptic receptor signaling is an area of growing interest, as classical transmitters (especially GABA and serotonin) and other substances (hormones, lipids, adenosine, cytokines, nitric oxide) are not restricted to synaptic communication. There is also growing interest in compartmentalization of signaling via membrane specializations called *lipid rafts*.[15] Neurotransmitter transporters, a prominent class of targets in CNS pharmacology, also regulate excitability via intrinsic electrical properties.[16] Figure 5-5 summarizes the primary aspects of neurotransmission that may be modulated pharmacologically. Box 5-1 summarizes the basic concepts of receptor pharmacology, including affinity, efficacy, desensitization, agonism, antagonism, and partial agonism.

Chemical transfer of information in the brain is diverse and complex, with each class of receptor containing multiple subtypes, whose particular structure or subunit composition can have dramatic impact on receptor expression, signaling

pathways, and pharmacology. In addition to this combinatorial complexity at the level of individual receptors and their potentially interacting signaling mechanisms, there is increasing evidence for ligand-receptor promiscuity, direct (protein-protein) cross-talk between receptors, and receptor-receptor intermixing at the level of assembly.[17-19] Receptor localization adds to the complexity, as the classical postsynaptic receptors adjacent to the axon terminal awaiting vesicular release are complemented by nonsynaptic receptors that respond to slower fluctuations of generally low concentrations of agonists and modulators. Appreciating this richly complex landscape of receptor signaling mechanisms serves as a background for interpreting the growing field of sleep-wake pharmacology.

NEUROTRANSMITTER SIGNALING

Synthesis pathways for the neurotransmitters are shown in Figure 5-6.

Acetylcholine

Overview

Acetylcholine (ACh) is synthesized from choline via the presynaptic enzyme choline acetyltransferase. Synaptic ACh is cleared through enzymatic breakdown via acetylcholinesterase (AChE), and to a lesser degree by presynaptic uptake transporters. Receptors for ACh include ionotropic and

TABLE 5-1

Neurotransmitter Receptor Signaling Mechanisms

Neurotransmitter	Ionotropic	Metabotropic			
		AC	PLC	K⁺	Ca²⁺
ACETYLCHOLINE					
Nicotinic	•				
M_1			▲		
M_2		▼		▲	▼
M_3			▲		
M_4		▼		▲	▼
M_5			▲		
5-HYDROXYTRYPTAMINE (5-HT, SEROTONIN)					
$5\text{-}HT_1$		▼		▲	▼
$5\text{-}HT_2$			▲		
$5\text{-}HT_3$	•				
$5\text{-}HT_4$		▲			
$5\text{-}HT_5$		▼	▲		
$5\text{-}HT_6$		▲			
$5\text{-}HT_7$		▲			
NOREPINEPHRINE					
α_1			▲	▲	▼
α_2		▼	▲	▲	▼
β_1		▲			
β_2		▲			
β_3		▲			
DOPAMINE					
D_1		▲			
D_2		▼		▲	▼
D_3		▼			
D_4		▼			
D_5		▲	▲		
GLUTAMATE					
NMDA	•				
AMPA	•				
Kainate	•				
$mGluR_1$		▼	▲	▲	
$mGluR_2$		▼			▲
$mGluR_3$		▼			▲
$mGluR_4$		▼			
$mGluR_5$		▼	▲	▲	
$mGluR_6$		▼			
$mGluR_7$		▼			
$mGluR_8$		▼			
GABA					
$GABA_A$	•				
$GABA_B$		▼		▲	▼
ADENOSINE					
A_1			▲	▲	▼
A_{2A}		▲			
A_{2B}		▲	▲		
A_3			▲		
HISTAMINE					
H_1			▲		▲
H_2		▲			
H_3		▼			

The subtypes of each neurotransmitter are shown, along with symbols indicating the types of signaling mediated by each subtype: •, ionotropic receptor; ▲, increases signaling activity; ▼, decreases signaling activity.

AC, adenylate cyclase; *AMPA*, α-amino-3-hydroxy-5-methyl-4-isoxazole proprionate; *GABA*, γ-aminobutyric acid; *NMDA*, N-methyl-D-aspartate; *PLC*, phospholipase C.

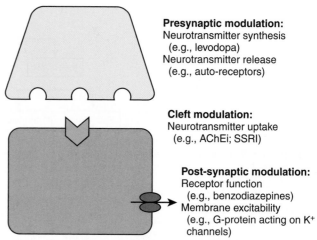

Presynaptic modulation:
Neurotransmitter synthesis (e.g., levodopa)
Neurotransmitter release (e.g., auto-receptors)

Cleft modulation:
Neurotransmitter uptake (e.g., AChEi; SSRI)

Post-synaptic modulation:
Receptor function (e.g., benzodiazepines)
Membrane excitability (e.g., G-protein acting on K⁺ channels)

Figure 5-5 Regulation of synaptic transmission. Summary of the possible sites at which neurotransmission can be regulated. Presynaptic control involves the synthesis and release of neurotransmitter. Drugs such as levo-dopa, a precursor of dopamine, enhances dopaminergic transmission by facilitating dopamine synthesis. Autoreceptors (see Box 5-1) provide feedback about neurotransmitter release back to the presynaptic terminal, which is often a negative feedback point of regulation. Neurotransmitter concentration in the synaptic cleft is another important point of regulation and therapeutic intervention. Antidepressant selective serotonin reuptake inhibitors (SSRIs) block the serotonin transporter, and antidementia cholinesterase inhibitors (AChEi) block the breakdown of acetylcholine, both of which lead to increased neurotransmitter concentration. Postsynaptic regulation is perhaps most diverse, and can range from extracellular modulation of receptors (e.g., benzodiazepine enhancement of $GABA_A$ receptors), intracellular modulation such as phosphorylation, or G protein regulation of other ion channels.

metabotropic types, which are known as *nicotinic* or *muscarinic receptors,* respectively (Fig. 5-7, *A*). The nicotinic channels are expressed in both pre- and postsynaptic locations, where they mediate fast excitatory currents, and thus enhance neurotransmitter release as well as postsynaptic excitability. Neuronal nicotinic acetylcholine (nACh) channels expressed in the brain (and sympathetic neurons peripherally) are structurally related to, but encoded by different genes than, the ACh-gated channels at the neuromuscular junction. Neuronal and muscle ACh channels are structurally related to ion channels gated by GABA, glycine, and serotonin.[20] The muscarinic ACh receptors (mACh), located centrally and peripherally, are GPCRs that include several subtypes,[21] associated with different signaling pathways (see Fig. 5-7, *A*). M_1, M_3, and M_5 subtypes activate the PLC pathway, but M_2 and M_4 subtypes inhibit the AC/cAMP pathway. The M_5 subtype may also inhibit the AC/cAMP pathway. M_2 receptors are the dominant presynaptic type, although M_4 receptors may also be presynaptic; these subtypes serve to inhibit neurotransmitter release. The M_2 and M_4 subtypes also inhibit postsynaptic neuronal excitability by enhancing K⁺ and inhibiting Ca²⁺ channel function. M_2 receptors may be enriched in GABAergic terminals, where inhibiting release causes indirect excitation of downstream target neurons.

Sleep-Wake Regulation

Cholinergic neurons in the basal forebrain (BF) project widely to the cortex, providing activating inputs characteristic of waking and REM sleep physiology, whereas brainstem cholinergic nuclei (LDT/PPT) are important regulators of REM sleep.[3,22] Accordingly, in animals and humans, enhancing

BOX 5-1 *Receptor Pharmacology Terminology*

Ligand-receptor interactions typically are described in terms of affinity and efficacy. **Affinity** typically refers to the dissociation constant obtained from in vitro ligand-binding studies and is interpreted as a measure of "selectivity" among receptor targets or subtypes. The term *efficacy* refers to the signaling activity available to the target receptor. **Agonists** trigger or enhance receptor function, and the modifiers *full* or *partial* reflect the extent to which a receptor can be activated. Although a full agonist usually is defined in terms of the "cognate" ligand (e.g., glutamate at a glutamate receptor), many exceptions exist. **Antagonists** are divided, based on location of binding, into *competitive* (at the agonist site) and *noncompetitive* (at any other site) subtypes. **Inverse agonists** decrease the receptor activity via binding to the agonist binding site; this implies some baseline receptor activity, from which a decrease could be measured. For receptors without constitutive (spontaneous) activity, a competitive antagonist and an inverse agonist would be pharmacologically distinguishable. The term *modulator* may refer to any nonagonist molecule that directly alters receptor function.

Desensitization refers generally to the decrease in receptor response to agonist activation. Multiple mechanisms of desensitization are possible, and they may occur over varied time scales. For some receptors (e.g., synaptic ligand-gated ion channels), desensitization is a conformational change occurring within milliseconds of agonist exposure, with recovery over hundreds to thousands of milliseconds. Longer-scale desensitization often involves internalization, usually requiring extended agonist exposure.

Receptors on the presynaptic terminal often are involved in regulating neurotransmitter release and are called *autoreceptors* if they respond to the same agonist being released at that terminal, or **heteroreceptors** if they respond to any other neurotransmitter, such as that released by another axon terminal. *Autocrine signaling* typically refers to a diffusible signal acting on the same cell (or more broadly, cell type) that released it, whereas **paracrine** refers to effects at nearby cells (or other cell types). Excitatory presynaptic receptors enhance vesicular release, whereas inhibitory presynaptic receptors decrease release. A single neurotransmitter (or drug) may interact with excitatory or inhibitory receptors, at presynaptic or postsynaptic locations, to modulate excitability (Fig. A). Of note, competitive antagonists block agonist-triggered signaling, whereas inverse agonists require spontaneous receptor activity in the absence of agonist.

The pharmacologic modulation of receptor function can be visualized using **concentration-response curves** (CRCs) (Fig. B). Isolated affinity changes yield pure left or right shift of the CRC (for increased [+][a] or decreased [−][c] affinity, respectively). Efficacy changes, by contrast, are manifested as upward or downward shifts in the CRC (for increased [+][b] or decreased [−][d] efficacy, respectively). Inverse agonists [−][e] decrease activity present in the absence of agonist. A single compound may exhibit multiple effects on a receptor, presumably via distinct binding sites; for example, barbiturates affect $GABA_A$ receptors at low concentration as enhancing modulators, at moderate concentration as direct agonists, and at high concentration as noncompetitive antagonists. Of note, in vitro CRCs may appear quite different from CRCs based on drug effects in a behaving organism (often called a *dose-response curve*, reflecting that the concentration encountered by the receptor is not known). Preclinical and early clinical drug studies use methods of **pharmacokinetics**, which refers to drug metabolism, and **pharmacodynamics**, which refers to drug effects on the physiology or behavior of the organism.

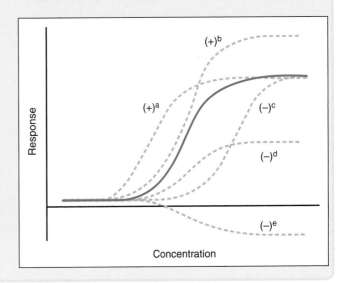

cholinergic transmission, either with agonists or by inhibiting the catabolic cholinesterase enzyme, has been shown to promote REM sleep, whereas anticholinergic compounds decrease REM sleep. Wakefulness has also been shown, in some cases, to be increased by cholinergic substances (e.g., when cholinesterase inhibitors are given during normal waking in humans). Enhancement of REM sleep can be seen with systemic administration, intraventricular delivery, or local injection of cholinergic agents into several brainstem nuclei.[23,24]

Clinical Correlations

Nicotine, the primary exogenous agonist of nACh channels, is rapidly absorbed during smoking, and has a 1- to 2-hour half-life. The complex effects of nicotine include acute vasodilation, chronic reduction in cerebral blood flow, and variable electrical impact on brainstem cholinergic neurons. Nicotine decreases REM sleep in animals and humans, and may also increase objective wakefulness, despite the common clinical report of relaxation.[8,25]

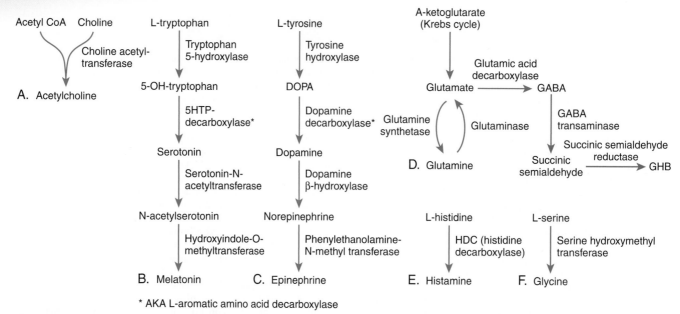

Figure 5-6 **Synthesis pathways for the neurotransmitters. A,** Acetylcholine. **B,** Serotonin and melatonin. **C,** Dopamine, norepinephrine, and epinepnrine. **D,** Glutamate, glutamine, GABA (γ-aminobutyric acid), and GHB (γ-hydroxybutyrate). **E,** Histamine. **F,** Glycine. *5HTP,* 5-Hydroxytryptophan; *CoA,* co-enzyme A; *GABA,* gamma aminobutyric acid; *GHB,* gamma hydroxybutyrate; *OH,* hydroxy.

Serotonin

Overview

Serotonin, or 5-hydroxytryptamine (5-HT), is synthesized from tryptophan, and is itself a substrate for the synthesis of melatonin. 5-HT clearance occurs via reuptake into neurons and via catabolism by monoamine oxidase (MAO), an enzyme in glia and presynaptic terminals involved in the breakdown of several monoamine transmitters (serotonin, dopamine, norepinephrine, epinephrine, melatonin). The reuptake occurs via (mainly presynaptic) membrane proteins known as *transporters,* which shuttle extracellular 5-HT back into the cell for repackaging into vesicles. The serotonin transporter is blocked by new generation antidepressants (selective serotonin reuptake inhibitors [SSRIs] and serotonin-norepinephrine reuptake inhibitors [SNRIs]; Box 5-2). 5-HT activates an ionotropic receptor as well as several metabotropic receptors[12,26] (Fig. 5-7, *B*). The excitatory 5-HT$_3$ channel is structurally similar to GABA$_A$, glycine, and nACh channels. The metabotropic 5-HT receptors exhibit a variety of G protein signaling mechanisms. 5-HT$_1$ receptors inhibit the AC/cAMP pathway, and they are the dominant presynaptic subtype, where they regulate 5-HT release. 5-HT$_1$ receptors also inhibit postsynaptic neuronal excitability by enhancing K$^+$ and decreasing Ca^{2+} channel function. The 5-HT$_2$ and 5-HT$_5$ subtypes mediate postsynaptic activation of the PLC pathway, although the 5-HT$_5$ subtype also inhibits the AC/cAMP pathway. The remaining subtypes, 5-HT$_4$, 5-HT$_6$, and 5-HT$_7$, activate the AC/cAMP pathway and are mainly postsynaptic.

Sleep-Wake Regulation

The brainstem dorsal raphe (DR) nucleus is the main source of ascending serotoninergic projections. Although early studies suggested that 5-HT circuits were sleep-promoting, these projections are now considered wake-promoting.[5] Accordingly,

serotonin transporter blockers, which increase the concentration of serotonin, are generally considered "activating" and may contribute to insomnia. Subtype selective drugs, as well as receptor subtype knockout mice (see Box 5-2), have provided some insight into the potential roles of different 5-HT receptors in sleep-wake regulation.[4,5] However, many inconsistencies remain from the extensive animal literature, and it is difficult to precisely assign sleep-wake functions to the many subtypes. In many cases, the effect of serotoninergic drugs on sleep depended on dose, species, and location of delivery (for microinjection studies).[27-29] Some of the discrepancies relate to the synaptic location of receptors: for example, the inhibitory 5-HT$_{1A}$ receptors are presynaptic in the dorsal raphe (where an agonist would decrease 5-HT signaling), and postsynaptic in most other locations (where an agonist would increase 5-HT signaling). The ionotropic 5-HT$_3$ subtype appears to be wake-promoting, as an agonist increased wake time at the expense of both NREM and REM sleep, whereas an antagonist had the opposite effect.[30]

Clinical Correlations

Antidepressant SSRI and SNRI drugs are the major therapeutic classes acting on serotoninergic transmission. Most of these drugs suppress REM sleep, and may increase leg movements. Certain "atypical" antipsychotic medications are thought to block 5-HT$_{2A}$ receptors (but also have mixed agonist and antagonist actions on other subtypes, which may relate to their REM suppression) in addition to their dopamine receptor antagonism. Aripiprazole, which is distinct from other neuroleptics in that it is a D$_2$ partial agonist, has mixed agonist and antagonist action at a variety of 5-HT subtypes. Agomelatine, a novel antidepressant also with multiple target mechanisms, is thought to antagonize 5-HT$_{2C}$ as well as activate melatonin receptors. The ion channel subtype, 5-HT$_3$, is the target of antiemetic drugs such as ondansetron, which is a 5-HT$_3$ antagonist. The migraine abortive tryptan

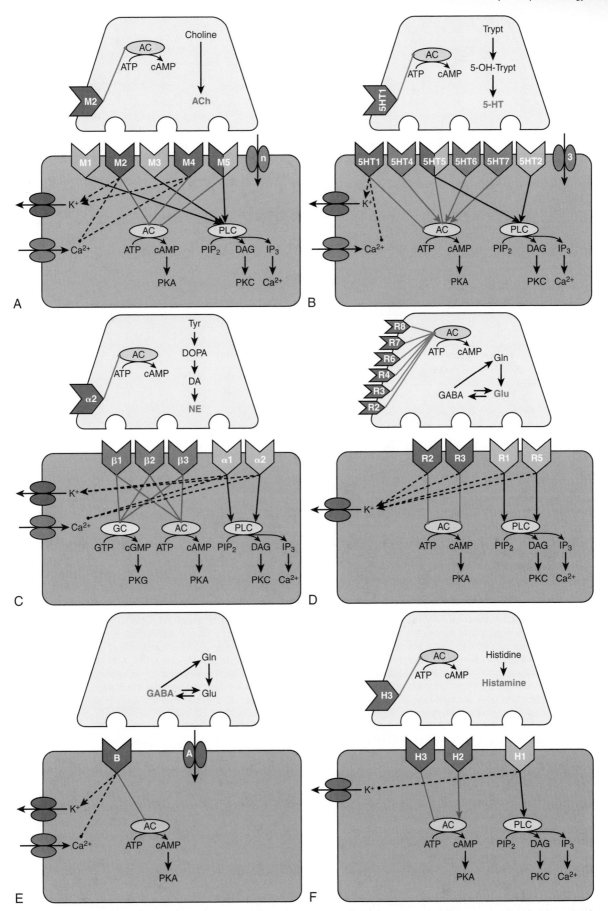

Figure 5-7 Neurotransmitter receptor subtypes. Synaptic transmission is illustrated for **A,** acetylcholine (ACh), **B,** serotonin (5-HT), **C,** norepinephrine (NE), **D,** glutamate, **E,** γ-aminobutyric acid (GABA), and **F,** histamine.

Continued

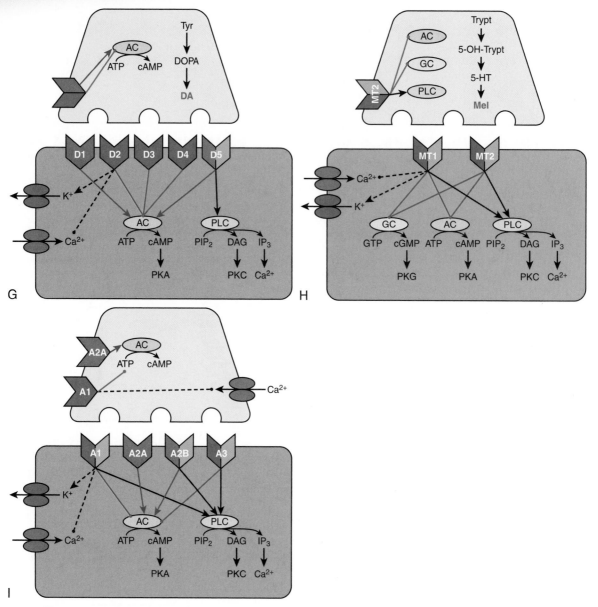

Figure 5-7, cont'd Synaptic transmission is illustrated for **G,** dopamine, **H,** melatonin, and, **I,** adenosine. In each panel, the presynaptic terminal contains the main biosynthesis step(s) and major receptor types that regulate synaptic release, as well as postsynaptic receptor subtypes and coupled mechanisms. Note that melatonin and adenosine do not undergo vesicular synaptic release, but may act as heteroreceptors. Excitatory *(dark gray)* and inhibitory *(dark blue)* ion channels are shown as ovals. Metabotropic receptors may activate *(dark gray)* or inhibit *(dark blue)* adenylate cyclase (AC) or activate phospholipase C (PLC; *light blue*). *5HT*, 5-hydroxytryptamine; *5HT1-7*, 5-hydroxytryptamine receptor 1-7; *A and B (panel E)*, GABA-A and GABA-B receptors; *A1-3*, adenosine receptor 1-3; *AC*, adenylate cyclase; *ACh*, acetylcholine; *α1-2*, alpha adrenergic receptor 1-2; *ATP*, adenosine triphosphate; *β1-3*, beta adrenergic receptor 1-3; *Ca²⁺*, calcium; *cAMP*, cyclic adenosine monophosphate; *cGMP*, cyclic guanosine monophosphate; *D1-5*, dopamine receptor 1-5; *DA*, dopamine; *DAG*, diacylglycerol; *DOPA*, L-3,4-dihydroxyphenylalanine; *GABA*, gamma aminobutyric acid; *GC*, guanylate cyclase; *Gln*, glutamine; *Glu*, gluamate; *Gly*, glycine; *H1-3*, histamine receptor 1-3; *Hist*, histamine; *IP₃*, inositol triphosphate; *K⁺*, potassium; *M1-5*, muscarinic receptor 1-5; *Mel*, melatonin; *MT1-2*, melatonin receptor 1-2; *n*, nicotinic; *ORX*, orexin; *NE*, norepinephrine; *OH*, hydroxy; *PIP₂*, phosphatidylinositol-4, 5-bisphosphate; *PKA*, protein kinase A; *PKC*, protein kinase C; *PKG*, protein kinase G; *R1-8*, glutamate receptor 1-8; *Trypt*, tryptophan; *Tyr*, tyrosine.

medications are antagonists at the 5-HT₁ subtype. Although the hypnotic mechanism of valerian remains uncertain, there is evidence for agonist action at 5-HT₅ₐ receptors.

Norepinephrine

Overview

Norepinephrine (NE) is synthesized from dopamine by dopamine β-hydroxylase (DBH), and synaptic NE is cleared by a presynaptic membrane transporter. The NE transporter (NET) is inhibited by the tricyclic antidepressants (TCAs), and has

variable degree of blockade by SNRI (and even some SSRI) antidepressants. NET belongs to the family of Na/Cl-dependent transporters, which also includes transporters for dopamine (DAT) and for serotonin (SERT; also known as *5-HTT*). These transporters are indirectly energy-dependent because of the Na⁺ ion gradient requirement. In addition to clearance via transporters, NE is broken down by MAO, and catechol-*O*-methyltransferase (COMT). Epinephrine is formed from NE, and is present at low levels in the brain (in contrast to the high epinephrine levels in the adrenal medulla).

NE interacts with a family of adrenergic receptor subtypes, all of which are metabotropic GPCRs (Fig. 5-7, *C*). The

BOX 5-2 *Glossary*

Goldman equation: The membrane potential at any time is dependent on the relative conductance, or permeability, of various ion species. Without membrane ion channels, the neuronal membrane would not be permeable to ions, and no transmembrane voltage gradient could be assessed. At rest, mostly "leak" K^+ channels (but also some Cl^- channels) are active, such that the membrane potential follows the K^+ equilibrium (or Nernst) potential. During an action potential, for example, the opening of large numbers of Na^+ channels, which far outnumber the leak channels, drive the membrane potential transients toward the Na^+ equilibrium potential (>0 mV), causing depolarization.

Ion channel gating: Certain ion channels are activated only upon binding of neurotransmitter (ligand-gated), whereas others are activated upon changes in membrane potential (voltage-gated). Some Ca^{2+} and K^+ channels are modulated by intracellular G protein ($\beta\gamma$ subunit) signaling, representing an indirect step between extracellular transmitter action and downstream ion channel activity. Still other ion channels are active at rest, without requiring ligand or voltage changes (leak channels).

Knockin mice: Genetically altered mice in which a gene has been altered such that its protein product contains a particular mutation. The phenotype resulting from a gene knockin is taken to suggest a role for the specific function of the protein that was disrupted by the introduced mutation (other protein functions may remain intact, offering potential advantages over gene knockouts that abolish all functions). For example, the $GABA_A$ receptor subtypes involved in hypnotic versus anxiolytic effects of benzodiazepines were determined by "knocking in" a single amino acid mutation that blocks benzodiazepine binding onto each subunit, one at a time, and measuring the behavioral responses to benzodiazepine administration.

Knockout mice: Genetically altered mice in which a gene has been disrupted such that its protein product is no longer produced.

The phenotype resulting from a gene knockout is taken to suggest a functional role for that protein or its pathway. For example, a serotonin transporter knockout mouse would be expected to have higher extracellular serotonin levels (owing to inability to transport serotonin into neurons).

Nernst equation: The eponymous name for the equilibrium potential of a given type of ion (e.g., Na^+, K^+, Ca^{2+}, Cl^-). The equilibrium potential depends largely on its transmembrane gradient (concentration outside versus inside the cell). It is the point at which concentration and voltage driving forces are balanced and can be thought of as the "target" voltage when a given type of ion channel opens. In the presence of multiple permeant ions, the Nernst equation for each one is used in the Goldman equation to calculate the overall membrane potential.

Serotonin-norepinephrine reuptake inhibitor (SNRI): SNRIs are a class of new-generation antidepressant agents (e.g., duloxetine, venlafaxine) that act by blocking both the serotonin and norepinephrine transporters.

Selective serotonin reuptake inhibitor (SSRI): SSRIs are a class of antidepressant agents (e.g., fluoxetine) that act by blocking the serotonin transporter, thus increasing the concentration of extracellular serotonin.

Suprachiasmatic nucleus (SCN): small hypothalamic nucleus that serves as a central regulator of circadian rhythms. The SCN receives input from the retina regarding light exposure and has efferent connections to the pineal gland to regulate melatonin synthesis.

Transporter: Neurotransmitter transporters are membrane proteins that shuttle neurotransmitters from the extracellular to the intracellular space, or from the intracellular space into synaptic vesicles. Some transporters also are located on glial cells, such as the excitatory amino acid transporter (EAAT) involved in glutamate clearance.

α_1 receptor mediates postsynaptic activation of PLC. The α_2 receptor is primarily presynaptic, where it inhibits neurotransmitter release via inhibiting the AC/cAMP pathway, activating K^+ channels, and inhibiting Ca^{2+} channels. The postsynaptic β_1 to β_3 subtypes activate the AC/cAMP pathway, and stimulate cGMP production by the enzyme guanylate cyclase (GC).

Sleep-Wake Regulation

Projections of the wake-promoting locus ceruleus (LC) are widely distributed to the forebrain as well as to other brainstem nuclei. Drugs enhancing NE transmission generally have alerting effects, while sedation may occur with antagonists (e.g., beta blockers) especially if they cross the blood-brain barrier. Local injection of NE, or an α_2 agonist, in or near the LC decreases REM sleep, which can be attenuated by concomitant administration of an α_2 antagonist. Similarly, selective α_1 agonists decrease, and α_1 antagonists increase, the amount of REM sleep. Systemic β_1 or β_2 antagonists decrease REM sleep.

Clinical Correlations

The tendency of TCAs to cause sedation despite the increase in NE levels may relate to antihistaminergic, anticholinergic, or other "off-target" effects. Trazodone, for example, is a $5\text{-}HT_{2a}$ antagonist (but has only mild antihistamine activity). Beta blockers (in particular those that penetrate the CNS, propranolol and metoprolol) can decrease REM sleep, as can

the α_2 agonist clonidine. These adrenergic antagonists carry a risk of sedation, but are not commonly used for the purpose of treating insomnia.

Glutamate

Overview

Glutamate is the considered the main excitatory neurotransmitter, although it also has inhibitory receptor subtypes. Glutamate can be synthesized from either GABA (via GABA transaminase) or from glutamine (via glutaminase). Synaptic glutamate is cleared by presynaptic and glial excitatory amino acid transporters (EAAT; see Box 5-2). Glutamate receptors include both ionotropic and metabotropic GPCR receptor classes[31,32] (Fig. 5-7, *D*). The ion channels are further classified into α-amino-3-hydroxy-5-methyl-4-isoxazole proprionate (AMPA), *N*-methyl-D-aspartate (NMDA), and kainate subtypes. All three types are sodium-permeable, while NMDA channels (and some AMPA and kainate isoforms) are also Ca^{2+} permeable. The NMDA channels are unique in two respects: (1) glycine is an obligatory co-agonist with glutamate, and (2) the channel also exhibits voltage-sensitivity—that is, it is both ligand-gated and voltage-gated. This unique voltage sensitivity is an indirect consequence of magnesium ions present in the extracellular space blocking the channel pore; these blocking ions are expelled from the pore during neuronal membrane depolarization. In other words, a neuron must already be active (depolarized) in order for glutamate to effectively open the NMDA channel. Because NMDA channels require concurrent ligand binding and postsynaptic depolarization in order to function, they are known as "coincidence detectors," a critical concept for synaptic (Hebbian) theories of memory formation.

The metabotropic glutamate receptor family includes subtypes 1 to 8. $mGluR_1$ and $mGluR_5$ are postsynaptic GPCRs that stimulate the PLC pathway, and also enhance K^+ channel function. The other subtypes inhibit the AC/cAMP pathway; of these, $mGluR_2$ and $mGluR_3$ are found in postsynaptic locations, and the other subtypes are predominantly presynaptic, where they regulate neurotransmitter release.

Sleep-Wake Regulation

Glutamate is the main transmitter of cortical pyramidal neurons, as well as thalamocortical neurons that ascend from thalamic nuclei to innervate the cortex broadly. As the major excitatory transmitter in the brain, glutamate signaling tends to be wake-promoting, while blockade causes sedation (or in the extreme case, anesthesia, which may share physiologic mechanisms with sleep).[23,33-35] Accordingly, agonists of ionotropic GluRs applied to the BF are wake-promoting, while glutamate channel antagonism is sedating.[36] Inhibiting ionotropic GluRs in the suprachiasmatic nucleus blocks light entrainment in rodents.[37] Kainate delivery to the peri-LC of the cat enhances REM sleep.[38] Systemic delivery of an $mGluR_2/mGluR_3$ agonist was REM suppressing in rats, while an $mGluR_2/mGluR_3$ antagonist actually suppressed both NREM and REM sleep.[39]

Clinical Correlations

Therapeutic modulation of glutamatergic transmission is the subject of active investigation,[40] but therapeutic options related to sleep are not yet available. Riluzole, which has shown some benefit as a glutamate antagonist (and Na^+ channel blocker) for treatment of amyotrophic lateral sclerosis, has been reported to increase both REM and NREM sleep in rats.[41] In addition to the role of NMDA receptors in synaptic plasticity and memory, they are also implicated in glutamate-mediated excitotoxicity. This latter effect may be the basis for the proposed clinical benefits of the NMDA channel antagonists memantine and amantadine in Alzheimer's disease. Glutamate is also involved in the atonia accompanying REM sleep, likely via exciting local glycinergic neurons that inhibit spinal motor neurons.

GABA

Overview

GABA is widely considered the major inhibitory neurotransmitter in the brain. However, it is involved in diverse physiologic processes beyond simple postsynaptic inhibition, including timing of cortical oscillations, and network dynamics in the hippocampus and between the thalamus and cortex.[42,43] GABA is synthesized from glutamate via glutamic acid decarboxylase, and is a precursor for synthesis of γ-hydroxybutyrate (GHB), a formulation of which, sodium oxybate (SXB), is used to treat narcolepsy with cataplexy. Synaptic GABA is cleared via presynaptic membrane transporters. GABA interacts with three families of membrane receptors

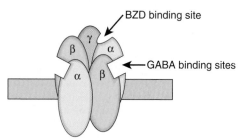

Figure 5-8 The γ-aminobutyric acid class A (GABA_A) receptor: a ligand-gated ion channel. The main type of neuronal GABA_A receptor is a pentameric assembly of α, β, and γ subunits. The channel pore, which is permeable to chloride ions in the open state, is formed by the central interface of the five subunits. The two GABA binding sites are pockets at the interface of the α and β subunits. The single benzodiazepine binding site, in contrast, is formed by a pocket at the interface of the α and γ subunits. Barbiturates and neurosteroids bind to yet another site, distinct from both the GABA site and the benzodiazepine site *(not shown)*. *BZD*, benzodiazepine.

(Fig. 5-7, *E*). The GABA_A receptor is itself a family of ionotropic chloride channels widely expressed in the brain.[44] The predominant type consists of a pentameric complex of two α subunits, two β subunits, and one γ subunit. There are two GABA binding sites, located at the interface between the α and β subunits (Fig. 5-8). The benzodiazepine binding site is located at the interface between the α and the γ subunit. Benzodiazepines are therefore considered "modulators" of the GABA_A receptor, since they bind at a distinct site (not the GABA binding site) and increase the ability of GABA to activate the channel (rather than directly opening the channel). The GABA_C receptor is also a ligand-gated chloride channel, predominantly expressed in the retina. The GABA_B receptors are GPCRs that decrease neuronal excitability by inhibiting the AC/cAMP pathway, activating K^+ channels, and inhibiting Ca^{2+} channels.

GABA_A receptors are important for synaptic signaling, in which vesicular release of GABA activates hyperpolarizing or shunting currents over a rapid time scale of 10 to 100 milliseconds. Extrasynaptic receptors also contribute to neuronal excitability through slower fluctuations and lower GABA concentration thought to occur via spillover from synaptic signaling. GABA_B receptor signaling also occurs via synaptic GABA release, but the downstream effects differ in time scale and mechanism compared to GABA_A. The postsynaptic inhibition occurs on a slower time scale, in the range of 100 to 1000 milliseconds, and is mediated not by chloride but by the βγ G proteins that activate inhibitory K^+ channels.

Sleep-Wake Regulation

Although GABA_A and GABA_B receptors are widely expressed, the most relevant localizations for sleep-wake regulation are the BF, POA, and the thalamus. GABAergic neurons in the POA and BF project to the posterior-lateral hypothalamus, including orexin neurons, as well as to the TMN histaminergic neurons, and to the LC. Thalamic projections also occur, and may play an important role in the hyperpolarization-mediated thalamocortical oscillations characteristic of NREM sleep physiology. GABAergic inhibition has been linked to the decreased firing of LC and DR neurons during REM sleep.

In general, enhancing GABAergic transmission has sedating and sleep-promoting effects,[35] although this depends on anatomic location of drug delivery in animal studies.[45] REM sleep is also regulated by GABA transmission, although the effect also depends on site of drug injection. For example, local delivery of GABA$_A$ antagonists to the rodent LC, dorsolateral pontine tegmentum, or periaqueductal gray, increases REM sleep, although nearby in the PPT, GABA$_A$ antagonists suppressed REM.[38,46,47] GABA$_A$ agonists are sleep-promoting when injected into the TMN,[48] which is expected given the role of histamine as an alerting neurotransmitter system (see later discussion). Although no longer used clinically, synthetic neurosteroids cause sedation/anesthesia; endogenous neurosteroids induce sedation in part via enhancing GABA$_A$ receptor function.[49]

Clinical Correlations

Therapeutic manipulation of GABA$_A$ receptors is dominated by the benzodiazepines, which exhibit a combination of hypnotic, anxiolytic, myorelaxant, and anticonvulsant properties. A series of transgenic (knock-in; see Box 5-2) studies have demonstrated the specific GABA$_A$ subtypes mediating each of these clinical effects.[50,51] The new generation "Z" hypnotics (zolpidem, zaleplon, zopiclone and eszopiclone) bind to the benzodiazepine binding site, but are structurally distinct from classic benzodiazepines, and thus are called "nonbenzodiazepines" based on structural differences rather than binding site preference. Two of these drugs, zolpidem and zaleplon, represent a rational targeting of the GABA$_A$ receptor α_1 subtype that is most important for the hypnotic effects, but offer little in the way of anticonvulsant or anxiolytic properties.

Histamine

Overview

Histamine is synthesized from histidine via decarboxylation, and synaptic histamine is cleared by a presynaptic membrane transporter. All histamine receptors are metabotropic GPCRs (Fig. 5-7, F).[52] The H$_1$ subtype mediates postsynaptic activation of the PLC pathway, and may also increase excitability via K$^+$ channel inhibition. H$_2$ receptors mediate postsynaptic activation of the AC/cAMP pathway, and newer antihistamines (e.g., ranitidine) that interact mainly with this subtype have much lower sedation potential. H$_3$ receptors negatively couple to the AC/cAMP pathway, and are the main presynaptic subtype (although they are also expressed in postsynaptic membranes). The H$_4$ subtype is expressed on mast cells and is involved in degranulation.

Sleep-Wake Regulation

The tuberomammillary nucleus (TMN) of the hypothalamus is the only source of brain histamine, and this wake-promoting center projects widely. In animal studies, histamine is a well-studied wake-promoting substance when delivered to the BF, the preoptic area, the TMN, or intraventricularly.[53,54] Subtype selective agents implicated the excitatory postsynaptic H$_1$ receptor for promoting wakefulness, and H$_1$ antagonists accordingly are sleep-promoting in various animals.[53,55] The H$_2$ subtype is also excitatory and postsynaptic, but systemic antagonists have little effect on sleep. Several studies have shown that antagonists of the presynaptic inhibitory H$_3$ subtype are wake-promoting, while agonists generally cause sedation.[56]

Clinical Correlations

The sedation caused by first-generation antihistamine drugs (e.g., diphenhydramine) is thought to depend on the H$_1$ subtype. The sedation accompanying these nonselective antihistamines is the basis of their over-the-counter use as sleep aids. In human studies, diphenhydramine is reported to have no objective impact on sleep in healthy volunteers, but was sleep-promoting in patients with insomnia.[57,58] Off-target antihistamine blockade may contribute to sedation side effects of certain medications, such as the antidepressants doxepin and mirtazapine.

Dopamine

Overview

Dopamine is synthesized from tyrosine, and is a substrate for NE synthesis. Synaptic dopamine is cleared by the dopamine transporter (DAT), which is a target for drugs such as cocaine, amphetamine, and the antidepressant bupropion; breakdown occurs via MAO and COMT enzymes. All dopamine receptors are metabotropic GPCRs,[59] which are divided into two groups, D$_1$-like and D$_2$-like, based on early pharmacologic characterization (Fig. 5-7, G). D$_1$-like subtypes include D$_1$ and D$_5$, which mediate postsynaptic activation of the AC/cAMP pathway. D$_2$-like subtypes include D$_2$, D$_3$, and D$_4$, which inhibit the AC/cAMP pathway and also decrease excitability via $\beta\gamma$-mediated enhancement of K$^+$ channels and inhibition of Ca^{2+} channels. D$_5$ may also couple to PLC activation, unlike the D$_1$ subtype. Both D$_1$-like and D$_2$-like receptors may be expressed in presynaptic terminals to regulate neurotransmitter release.

Sleep-Wake Regulation

The substantia nigra and the ventral tegmentum are the dopaminergic circuits most implicated for sleep-wake control, although these neurons do not change their firing patterns across arousal state as clearly as the other wake- and sleep-promoting centers.[60] Drugs that enhance dopamine receptor function or increase release of dopamine increase alertness. The amphetamine-related stimulants are an important example of wake-promoting pharmacology that act, in large part, through dopaminergic signaling. Rodent studies show that systemic and intraventricular delivery of D$_1$-like agonists is wake-promoting, and D$_1$-like antagonists are sleep-promoting.[61] D$_2$-like agonists have dose-dependent impact on sleep, with low doses being sedating, and high doses being alerting.

Clinical Correlations

Dopamine antagonists (e.g., neuroleptics) tend to cause sedation, which may be a combination of dopaminergic and other mechanisms. Neuroleptics tend to suppress REM sleep, and although they increase NREM sleep (N2 and, in some cases also N3), they are not generally recommended as hypnotic agents. Notable exceptions to the general idea that dopamine signaling plays an alerting role include the dopamine agonists pramipexole and ropinorole (high affinity D$_2$-D$_4$ receptor agonists), used to treat restless legs syndrome and periodic limb movements of sleep, which can cause sedation.

One potential side effect of dopaminergic stimulant use for daytime sleepiness is nocturnal insomnia, particularly for longer acting agents, or when taken later in the day.

Glycine

Glycine is the major inhibitory signal in the spinal cord, although its receptors are also widely expressed in the brain. Glycine is synthesized from serine, and synaptic glycine is cleared via presynaptic uptake transporters. Structurally similar to the $GABA_A$ receptor, glycine receptors are chloride-permeable channels. The main relevance of glycine receptors in sleep-wake regulation involves the motor atonia of REM sleep. Glycine inhibits anterior horn motor neurons via medullary nuclei that use glutamate to excite local glycinergic neurons in the cord. Although the benzodiapzepine clonazepam is the most studied treatment for RBD (REM sleep behavior disorder), glycine receptors are not a target of this drug, and clonazepam does not restore the normal atonia of REM sleep despite suppressing dream enactment.[62]

NEUROPEPTIDES, NEUROHORMONES, AND OTHER SIGNALING MOLECULES

Neuropeptides and neurohormones subserve a diversity of signaling functions in the brain.[7,63-66] Neuropeptides undergo vesicular release like classical neurotransmitters, but their time course of action is generally on a longer time scale. Hormone-, steroid-, and lipid-based signaling also occurs on a longer and more gradual time scale, but does not involve vesicular release. The interactions among systemic hormones, neurohormones, inflammatory, and cytokine signals are becoming increasingly evident.[67-72] The interaction between these systems and sleep is surely bidirectional, as primary alterations in inflammatory or stress systems can alter sleep (e.g., exogenous steroid therapy, or autoimmune inflammatory disorders), and primary sleep disorders have been linked to altered inflammatory/ stress markers (e.g., sleep apnea and insomnia). However, most of the mechanistic information reviewed in this section derives from animal studies.

Melatonin

Overview

Melatonin is synthesized from serotonin in the pineal gland, circulates into the blood and CSF, and is implicated in sleep, circadian rhythms (see Chapter 28), and many other functions.[73,74] Light exposure inhibits melatonin synthesis in the pineal gland by the following pathway: light is first detected by melanopsin-containing ganglion cells of the retina, and conveyed to the suprachiasmatic nucleus (SCN) by the retinohypothalamic tract, and subsequently to the pineal gland by way of the superior cervical ganglion. Melatonin metabolism is mainly hepatic; a small fraction is secreted in saliva or excreted in urine, which may be measured as a marker of circadian phase.

Sleep-Wake Regulation

Although melatonin is lipophilic and may interact with intracellular/nuclear receptors, the best studied signaling occurs via metabotropic GPCRs, which are enriched in the SCN but are also found in the retina (Fig. 5-7, *H*). The MT_1 and MT_2 subtypes inhibit the AC/cAMP pathway and the GC/cGMP pathway, and stimulate the PLC pathway. Melatonin is also linked to decreased excitability via inhibiting Ca^{2+} channels and enhancing K^+ channels. MT_1 has been implicated in the hypnotic effect of melatonin, which inhibits SCN firing, while the MT_2 receptor has been implicated in the phase shifting effects of melatonin.[73,75]

Clinical Correlations

Although melatonin signals "darkness" in mammals, it is only associated with sleep in diurnal species. Mice, for example, are active in the dark phase despite elevated melatonin levels. Although exogenous melatonin is used for both hypnotic and circadian entrainment reasons, clinical use of melatonin is complicated by nonstandardized preparations, intersubject variability of blood levels, and potentially supraphysiologic concentrations after even small oral doses. Improved sleep metrics may be seen with 0.1 and 0.3 mg doses, which generally lead to physiologic plasma concentrations.[76] Despite the variability in preparation and dose-response dynamics, meta-analysis suggested that melatonin improved objective sleep measures such as latency, efficiency, and total sleep time, although effects were small and possibly influenced by subjects with delayed circadian phase.[77,78] The hypnotic agent ramelteon, which was FDA-approved for insomnia in 2005, is a synthetic agonist at both MT_1 and MT_2 receptors. Placebo-controlled trials have demonstrated improvements in sleep onset latency in a variety of clinical populations.[79] Melatonin, in combination with light therapy and schedule modification, is often utilized clinically to facilitate phase advances in patients suffering from delayed sleep phase syndrome.[80] Exogenous melatonin has been shown to advance the circadian temperature nadir, as well as the endogenous melatonin rhythm.[81]

Adenosine

Overview

Adenosine is generated intracellularly via dephosphorylation of adenosine triphosphate (ATP) associated with energy consumption, and extracellularly by degrading enzymes acting on ATP after synaptic release. Uptake occurs across membranes mainly via nucleoside transporters. Glial cells also play a central role in adenosine signaling and homeostasis in the context of sleep-wake regulation.[82] Adenosine receptors are alternatively known as P_1 receptors, a subset of the large purine receptor family, which also includes P_{2X} (ionotropic) and P_{2Y} (metabotropic) receptors for the purine ATP.[83]

The main adenosine GPCR subtypes expressed in the brain include A_1 and A_{2A}, which are found in neurons as well as glia[84] (Fig. 5-7, *I*). A_1 receptors, which have the highest affinity for adenosine, reduce neuronal excitability by decreasing AC/cAMP activity, and, via $\beta\gamma$ subunits, blocking Ca^{2+} channels and enhancing K^+ channels. The A_1 subtype can be found in pre- and postsynaptic locations, and may also stimulate the PLC pathway in the latter. In contrast, A_{2A} receptors activate AC/cAMP signaling mainly in postsynaptic locations, but may also be presynaptic. The postsynaptic A_{2B} subtype stimulates the PLC pathway as well as the AC/cAMP pathway. The postsynaptic A_{3A} subtype inhibits the AC/cAMP pathway and stimulates the PLC pathway.

Sleep-Wake Regulation

The evidence for adenosine as an endogenous sleep-promoting substance[85] derives from its accumulation during wakefulness, its ability to induce sleep and enhance slow wave EEG activity, and the utility of adenosine receptor antagonists (most notably, caffeine[86]) to enhance alertness. However, the literature contains some inconsistencies. For example, cholinergic BF lesions, which attenuated adenosine build-up during deprivation, failed to alter recovery sleep,[87] suggesting that other mechanisms contribute to homeostatic sleep drive. Nevertheless, animal studies show that systemic, intraventricular, and BF delivery of A_1 receptor agonists is sleep-promoting, while A_1 receptor antagonists are wake-promoting.[88] However, the sleep-wake patterns (NREM sleep and REM sleep) and the response to sleep deprivation, all remain normal (not different from wild-type mice) in mice harboring the A_1 receptor gene knockout,[89,90] suggesting that other receptor subtypes may be involved in the effects of adenosine homeostasis on sleep. Several lines of evidence implicate the A_{2A} subtype as the principle mechanism of adenosine-mediated sleep regulation.[91-94] Of note, a human polymorphism in the adenosine deaminase enzyme, which causes impaired adenosine breakdown, is associated with sleepiness and increased delta sleep.[95]

Clinical Correlations

Caffeine is the major over-the-counter modulator of adenosine transmission. By antagonizing adenosine receptors, caffeine is thought to counteract the homeostatic accumulation of sleep drive that occurs with prolonged wakefulness. Adenosine has also been implicated in diverse processes spanning sleep, seizures, pain, inflammation, trauma, and ischemia, and thus has been an attractive focus for research in mechanisms and pharmacologic treatments of diverse CNS conditions.[96]

Nitric Oxide

Along with carbon monoxide (CO) and hydrogen sulfide (H_2S), nitric oxide (NO) is an endogenous gas involved in neuronal signaling. The lipid-soluble NO molecule is synthesized from L-arginine via the enzyme nitric oxide synthase (NOS), which requires NADPH (reduced form of nicotine adenine dinucleotide phosphate) and produces L-citrulline.[97] NO and both the neuronal form (nNOS) and the inducible form (iNOS) of the NO synthesis enzymes have been implicated in sleep-wake regulation.[85] In particular, brain NO signaling has been linked to increased adenosine levels. NOS is activated by Ca^{2+}/calmodulin, and the resulting NO is thought to function primarily as a retrograde diffusible messenger, stimulating guanylyl cyclase to generate cGMP, which activates protein kinase G, as well as cyclic nucleotide gated membrane channels. NO can also directly modulate proteins via S-nitrosylation of cysteine residues. The variable effects of systemic or CNS delivery of NOS donors or inhibitors is now known to be explained, at least in part, by the demonstration of a circadian variation in the impact of NO signaling on sleep.[98] Mice lacking the neuronal NOS enzyme exhibit decreased REM sleep, whereas those lacking the inducible NOS have increased REM sleep and decreased NREM sleep.[99]

Gamma-Hydroxybutyric Acid

Endogenous GHB is synthesized from GABA, and may weakly activate $GABA_B$ receptors, in addition to binding to its own GPCR.[100] Although it is known for its abuse potential, the sodium salt of GHB, sodium oxybate, is FDA-approved for narcolepsy with cataplexy (see Chapter 22). It causes sedation, improves sleep continuity, and increases slow wave sleep.[101] Although off-label uses include insomnia and fibromyalgia, a recent FDA advisory committee recommended against approval for the latter.

Orexin

Although the peptide orexin (ORX) is best recognized clinically for the pathophysiologic connection to narcolepsy with cataplexy,[102,103] there is a growing list of physiologic functions in which ORX is implicated.[104] ORX receptors stimulate the PLC pathway, and can enhance or inhibit AC/cAMP pathway, as well as couple to K^+ and Ca^{2+} channels to regulate excitability mainly through postsynaptic localization. Disruption of orexin signaling either by gene deletion[105,106] or by transgenic silencing of orexin neurons,[107] causes sleep-wake fragmentation with some increase in REM percentage. Intraventricular delivery of ORX increased wake and decreased REM sleep, which was blocked by systemic administration of an H1 receptor antagonist.[108,109] Wakefulness was stimulated with local injection of ORX to the LC or the TMN as well, although REM was decreased only in the former site.[110] Although these studies implicated histamine as a downstream effector of the wake-promoting action of the ORX system, subsequent work showed that the alerting effect of ORX neuron activation was preserved in knockout mice that lacked histamine.[111]

Stress Axis Hormones

Corticotropin-releasing hormone (CRH) acts via widely expressed GPCRs (including arousal nuclei), which stimulate the AC/cAMP pathway, resulting in increased wakefulness.[112] CRH may modulate sleep-wake systems independent of stress, as rat strains with lower CRH levels spend less time awake at baseline. CRH and downstream ACTH and corticosteroids suppress NREM and REM sleep, possibly via downstream interleukin 1 signaling.

Neuropeptide S

NPS is a wake-promoting peptide with high expression near the LC. NPS receptors are widely expressed throughout the brain.[113] Exogenous NPS increased waking activity at the expense of NREM and REM sleep in mice; anxiolytic effects were also noted.

Galanin

Along with GABA, galanin is expressed in the inhibitory neurons of the sleep-promoting ventrolateral preoptic area (VLPO). GAL_1 receptors are GPCRs that inhibit the AC/cAMP pathway, and GAL_2 receptors stimulate the PLC pathway. Intravenous pulses of galanin enhanced REM sleep in humans.[114] Galanin is also expressed in the spinal cord, and galanin knockout mice have increased sensitivity to pain.

Vasoactive Intestinal Peptide

Vasoactive intestinal peptide (VIP) interacts with a widely expressed GPCR that stimulates AC/cAMP pathway. Similar to the enhanced REM seen in humans given intravenous (IV) VIP, animals show increased REM sleep following systemic, intraventricular, or brainstem VIP delivery; on the other hand, a VIP antagonist is REM suppressing.[115,116]

Cholecystokinin

The CNS form of cholecystokinin, CCK-8, is a truncated but active form of the gut peptide. It is co-expressed in dopamine-containing neurons along with the peptide neurotensin, in thalamic neurons along with neuropeptide Y and VIP, and in the medulla along with substance P. In addition to influences on sleep, it is involved in pain signaling and possibly anxiety. CCK-8 binds to two receptors, CCK-A and CCK-B, which are both GPCRs that activate the PLC pathway. Although signaling in the CCK pathway is largely sleep-promoting in animals, CCK-A antagonists were sleep-promoting in humans, pointing to another example of species differences. Peripheral administration may alter sleep, despite lack of blood-brain barrier penetration, via vagus nerve afferents. Of note, CCK-A deficient rats have normal sleep.[117]

Somatostatin

Although somatostatin (SS) is best known for its release from the hypothalamus to inhibit pituitary GH secretion, this inhibitory neuropeptide is also synthesized and released by neurons elsewhere in the brain.[118] The SS receptors are GPCRs that inhibit the AC/cAMP pathway (SST_1, SST_3, SST_4, SST_5), activate the PLC pathway (SST_2, SST_3, SST_5), and decrease excitation via enhancing K^+ and decreasing Ca^{2+} channel activity (SST_2, SST_4, SST_5). SS exhibits acute wake-promoting activity in humans, likely via feedback inhibition of the sleep-promoting GHRH (see following section).[119] However, animal studies suggest that intraventricular SS enhances REM sleep, while SS depletion, SS antagonists, and anti-SS antibodies all decrease REM sleep. The sleep-promoting effects of SS are attenuated in mice lacking GHRH. Cortistatin, a sleep-promoting peptide expressed primarily in cortical GABAergic interneurons, interacts with SS receptors.[120]

Growth Hormone and Growth Hormone Releasing Hormone

Growth hormone-releasing hormone (GHRH) is expressed in the arcuate nucleus and other hypothalamic regions, and increases the AC/cAMP pathway through its GPCR. GHRH promotes NREM sleep independent of increasing growth hormone (GH) levels, as the effect persisted in rats after hypophysectomy. Administration of a GHRH antagonist or antibodies to GHRH was wake-promoting in animal studies.[121] GH signaling occurs through a receptor tyrosine kinase pathway.[122] Exogenous administration of GH enhances REM sleep in multiple species.[123] In humans, serum GH levels rise with sleep onset, peaking during the first periods of NREM sleep of the night. The surge in GH is delayed, and is larger in magnitude, when humans are sleep-deprived by delaying nocturnal sleep onset. Replacement of GH in deficient patients improves their sleep architecture.[124] There is also evidence that adiposity negatively impacts GH secretion and may contribute through hormonal mechanisms (in addition to increasing apnea risk) to sleep fragmentation.[125]

Melanin-Concentrating Hormone

Melanin-concentrating hormone (MCH) is a REM-promoting peptide expressed in the tuberal hypothalamus.[126] Both MCH receptor subtypes inhibit the AC/cAMP pathway and stimulate the PLC pathway. The pharmacology of this region is interesting, with NE, 5-HT, carbachol, and $GABA_A$ agonist inhibiting MCH neurons (the latter also suppressed REM sleep); in contrast, ORX stimulates these neurons. Decreasing MCH function via an MCH antagonist, or by gene knockout, increased wakefulness and caused fragmentation, with decreases in both REM and NREM sleep.[127] However, in another study MCH knockout mice were hypersomnolent.[128]

Prolactin

Prolactin (PRL) (acting through receptor tyrosine kinase pathway), and its releasing factor (acting via its GPCR), increase REM sleep in several species, including humans, and hypoprolactinemia is associated with decreased REM sleep.[129] Prolactin antibodies suppress REM in animal studies, and block the increased REM seen with VIP administration. Mice lacking PRL, accordingly, showed decreased REM sleep, and failed to increase REM sleep in response to VIP.[130] Although benzodiazepine treatment has been shown to increase PRL during sleep, these drugs nevertheless exhibit REM-suppressing effects.

Arginine Vasopressin

Arginine vasopressin (AVP, antidiuretic hormone) acts at the $AVPR_1$ receptor centrally (to stimulate the PLC pathway), and at the $AVPR_2$ receptor peripherally (to increase the AC/cAMP pathway).[131] Vasopressin promotes NREM sleep while suppressing REM sleep in animal studies, while antibodies against this peptide enhanced REM sleep. Administration in humans appears to selectively increase REM sleep.

Ghrelin and Leptin

Several peptides are implicated in feeding control, including ghrelin, leptin, ORX, NPY, CCK, and MCH. Ghrelin acts through the GH secretagogue receptor, a GPCR that stimulates AC/cAMP and PLC pathways. Ghrelin promotes food intake, whereas leptin mediates satiety. Other satiety mediators, such as insulin and CCK, have sedative actions, even with intraventricular delivery. Chronic partial sleep restriction elevates ghrelin and decreases leptin.[132] Interestingly, sleep-wake stage percentages were intact in ghrelin receptor knockout mice, even during food restriction, although increased fragmentation was noted,[133,134] emphasizing that stage transitions dynamics are a more sensitive measure of architecture than global metrics such as sleep efficiency or stage percentages.[10,135] IV ghrelin delivery in humans increased NREM and decreased REM sleep.[136] Leptin binds to a specific receptor of the cytokine receptor family. Exogenous leptin increased NREM sleep and decreased REM sleep in rats.[137] However, leptin-deficient mice, *ob/ob*, exhibit increased NREM and decreased REM, with overall increased fragmentation as well.[138] In studies of patients with insomnia, or healthy subjects undergoing sleep restriction, elevated ghrelin and decreased leptin levels have been observed.[67,132,139,140] This relationship was proposed to provide a basis for the increased obesity seen in short sleepers or in patients with insomnia.

Neuropeptide Y

Neuropeptide Y (NPY) has diverse functions in the brain, most notably regulation of feeding, likely via arcuate nucleus expression. NPY interacts with six types of receptors, which inhibit the AC/cAMP pathway. Although the Y_1 subtype is mainly postsynaptic, and Y_2 is mainly presynaptic, both inhibit the AC/cAMP pathway and also decrease excitability via βγ subunit activation of K^+ channels.[141] The presynaptic subtype inhibits Ca^{2+} channels. The impact of NPY on sleep appears to be species-specific, with intravenous NPY being sleep-promoting in humans,[142,143] but in rats, intraventricular or hypothalamic delivery of NPY is wake-promoting.[144]

Opiates

The peptide pro-opio-melanocortin (POMC) is expressed in the pituitary and hypothalamus. It undergoes cleavage to form β-endorphin, an endogenous opioid, corticotropin, α-MSH, and the enkephalin peptides. Endogenous and therapeutic opioids act through a family of receptors (δ, μ, κ). Although clinically sedating, opiates in fact cause sleep fragmentation and suppression of REM and NREM3 stages.

Prostaglandins

Prostaglandins (PGs) are a family of fatty acid ecosanoids synthesized from arachidonic acid via cyclooxygenase, an enzyme involved in the synthesis of PGs, prostacyclin, and thromboxane, and the target of anti-inflammatory agents such as ibuprofen. PGs have diverse CNS roles, including sleep-wake regulation.[145] In animal studies, PGD_2 stimulates NREM, and in most cases also REM sleep. Although systemic or intraventricular delivery of PGD_2 is generally sleep-promoting, some studies suggested that the effect is limited to the preoptic area and the subarachnoid space near the BF,[146] where PGD2 may increase local adenosine levels to induce sleepiness. PGD_2-mediated hypnosis is attenuated in mice lacking the PGD_2 receptor.[147] Although inhibition of PGD synthase (which is normally expressed in meninges, choroid, and glia) is wake-promoting,[148] mice overexpressing the PGD synthase enzyme had normal baseline sleep despite increased PGD_2 levels.[149] Consistent with the sleep-promoting role of PGD, cyclooxygenase (COX) inhibitors decrease NREM and sleep efficiency in humans. PGD_1 and PGD_3 had no effect on sleep, but PGE_2 studies were variable: some suggested wake-promoting activity, but others showed that PGE_2 induces sleep. Note that although both PGD_2 and PGE_2 are pyrogenic, the sleep-promoting activity of the former is independent of fever. PGD_2 signaling occurs downstream of the cytokines interleukin 1 (IL-1) and tumor necrosis factor α (TNF-α), both of which are sleep-promoting (see later discussion). Other arachidonic acid derivatives may also play a role in sleep regulation: the lipoxins LXA_4 and LXB_4 have both been shown to increase NREM sleep, as has the leukotriene, LTD_4.

Fatty Acid Amides: Cannabinoids and Oleamide

The fatty acid amide family includes anandamide and oleamide, which are synthesized from membrane phospholipids, and degraded by fatty acid amide hydrolase (FAAH), a process that generates arachidonic acid.[150] Cannabinoids (CBs) are thought to mediate retrograde signaling to modulate presynaptic activity, via CB receptors, which inhibit the AC/cAMP pathway, and may also stimulate the PLC pathway. Anandamide is sleep-promoting, an effect that is blocked by CB1 antagonists, although CB1 antagonism alone is wake-promoting.[145,151] Accordingly, mice lacking the FAAH gene (and thus have increased cannabinoid levels) have enhanced NREM sleep at the expense of wake.[152] 1-Methylhelptyl-gamma-bromoacetate, an endogenous bromide, is a REM sleep-promoting substance that may act through inhibition of FAAH. Oleamide decreased latency, increased NREM sleep and total sleep time, and the hypnotic effects were attenuated in mice lacking the $GABA_A$ receptor β3 subunit.[153]

Immune Signals and Cytokines

Multiple cytokines, known primarily for their roles in inflammation and immune functions, have also been implicated in sleep-wake regulation, and may act within the brain or in the periphery through vagus nerve afferent signaling.[66,154] The interleukin 1 (IL-1) family includes IL-1β, IL-1α, and the IL-1 receptor antagonist (IL-1RA). IL-1 receptors are expressed widely in the brain, utilizing several signaling cascades such as AC/cAMP, adenosine, NO, prostaglandins, and the transcription factor NFκB, among others. IL-1β is one of the best-studied cytokines, exhibiting sleep-promoting activity in animals and humans. Anti-IL-1β antibodies and soluble IL-1RA inhibited NREM sleep. Factors that induce IL-1β are sleep-promoting, such as the bacteria-derived muramyl peptides. Other bacterial components are also somnogens, including lipopolysaccharide (endotoxin) and its derivative, lipid A. The inflammatory cytokines (IL-1, IL-6, TNF-α) are sleep-promoting, while anti-inflammatory cytokines (IL-4, IL-10, and IL-13) tend to be wake-promoting.

Although generally sleep-promoting, the impact of IL-1β on sleep may depend on factors such as location of action, circadian time, and dose. For example, high doses and daytime administration of IL-1β are wake-promoting. Mice lacking IL-1 receptors have slightly decreased baseline NREM sleep and intact REM sleep. The hypnotic effects of exogenous IL-1β are attenuated in these mice, but that of TNF-α remains intact.[155]

TNF-α is a proinflammatory sleep-promoting cytokine that interacts with two primary receptors, expressed in neurons and glia. Intraventricular TNF-α promotes NREM and enhances EEG slow waves in several species. REM sleep is inhibited by TNF-α, mainly at high doses. NREM sleep is increased by factors that increase TNF-α, such as endotoxin, and is decreased by substances that block TNF-α signaling, such as anti-TNF-α antibodies, soluble receptor fragments, or anti-inflammatory cytokines (IL-4, IL-10, IL-13). TNF-α levels are elevated in OSA, and a TNF-α polymorphism is implicated in obesity and OSA in humans.[156]

Other cytokines and peptide signaling factors have been implicated in sleep-wake regulation, but are not as extensively studied. Sleep-promoting effects were observed with interferon-α (IFN-α), IL-6, IL-15, IL-18, nerve growth factor (NGF), brain-derived neurotrophic factor (BDNF), glial-derived neurotrophic factor (GDNF), erythrocyte growth factor (EGF), fibroblast growth factor (FGF), and colony-stimulating factor. Consistent with the hypnotic potential for IFN, mice lacking the IFN receptor have increased waking, and reduced REM sleep,[157] and sleepiness may be seen as a side effect of interferon therapy in humans. However, mice lacking IL-6 had decreased wake time (and increased REM sleep).[158] Wake-promoting effects are seen with transforming growth factor (TGF-β), insulin-like growth factor, and α-melanocyte-stimulating hormone (α-MSH).

Although experimental manipulation of inflammatory mediators and cytokines is more commonly studied in animals, extensive correlation studies have been performed in humans with normal sleep and with sleep disorders.[69,70] For example, serum IL-1 levels peak with sleep onset, and are increased with sleep deprivation.[159] IL-6 also peaks with sleep onset, and the peak is delayed with experimental delayed sleep onset in healthy volunteers.[160]

VOLTAGE-GATED ION CHANNELS AND GAP JUNCTIONS

Chemical signaling mechanisms are complemented by membrane proteins governing so-called "intrinsic" excitability of neurons, because they do not require transmitters or other extracellular signals to operate. These proteins consist mainly of voltage-gated ion channels, but voltage-independent "leak" channels, also regulate membrane excitability. K^+ channels are the dominant channel type shaping the resting membrane potential, and because they are open constantly, without requiring any signal to activate them, they are known as *leak channels.* The membrane potential at any time depends upon which ions are permeable, that is, which ion channels are active (a concept expressed by the Goldman equation, see Box 5-2). At rest, the leak K^+ channels are the main channels open, such that the membrane potential approaches the K^+ equilibrium potential, which is typically around −70 mV (according to the Nernst equation, see Box 5-2). Upon activation of Na^+ or other excitatory channels, the membrane potential is driven to depolarization by outweighing the basal K^+ leak. Some leak channels can be blocked by G proteins, as described above—this action indirectly leads to excitation by permitting the membrane to depolarize (by reducing the contribution of the leak K^+ channels to the membrane potential). Although not "receptors" in the classical sense, many CNS-active drugs modulate these channels either directly (e.g., anticonvulsants) or indirectly (through GPCRs), which may be relevant for therapeutic and side effects of drugs.

Several voltage-gated ion channels have been implicated in sleep regulation, as knockout mice have shown prominent sleep architecture abnormalities.[161-166] For example, mice harboring a restricted thalamic deficiency in T-type Ca^{2+} channels, which underlie thalamocortical burst firing associated with slow wave sleep, demonstrated sleep fragmentation.[161] Gap junctions also regulate excitability by allowing direct electrical coupling between adjacent neurons, and may be important for sleep regulation.[43,167-169]

ALTERNATIVE THERAPIES

The use of over-the-counter remedies related to sleep-wake complaints is common, although individual responses are variable and well-designed clinical studies of these agents are largely lacking. In addition to melatonin and antihistamine preparations, other agents such as valerian and chamomile (both of which may interact with $GABA_A$ receptors; the latter likely via flavonoid components) are used to facilitate sedation.[170] Although many patients may experiment with over-the-counter and alternative medicines, caution should be exercised regarding possible interactions of natural or herbal substances with prescription medications.[171] For example, melatonin should be used with caution in patients anticoagulated with warfarin, as the international normalized ratio (INR) may be elevated by melatonin.

THERAPEUTIC MECHANISMS OF SLEEP-WAKE MODULATION

Several excellent reviews, as well as Section 3 in this book summarize current thinking about the receptor targets that mediate the therapeutic or side effects of various drugs.[172-174] Sedation may occur as a side effect of many drugs used in neurology and psychiatry, and occasionally this feature is used as an advantage if insomnia accompanies the primary indication for the drug. Given their design to decrease neuronal excitability, anticonvulsants carry the potential for sedation by a variety of target mechanisms. Tricyclic antidepressants (TCAs) may induce sedation via antihistamine, anticholinergic, or anti-α-adrenergic mechanisms, which may be a benefit if insomnia accompanies the depression or headaches for which the TCA is prescribed. Certain antidepressants are considered activating, including protriptyline and many of the SSRIs. Many neuroleptics have antihistamine and anti-5-HT$_2$ action in addition to blocking dopamine receptors, which may contribute to sedation. On the other end of the dopamine spectrum, amphetamine-like stimulants and antiparkinsonism medications tend to cause insomnia, with the exception of the dopamine agonists pramipexole and ropinirole. Antihypertensives may also induce sedation, including beta blockers (especially lipophilic propranolol, in contrast to hydrophilic atenolol), and the presynaptic α_2 agonist clonidine. However, individual responses may be quite variable to CNS-active medications, and insomnia can be seen with beta blockers, and sedation can be seen with SSRIs. Nicotine and caffeine are stimulants that act either directly (nACh receptor agonist) or indirectly (adenosine receptor antagonist) to enhance neuronal excitability and thus wakefulness. Cholinesterase inhibitors tend to be activating, decreasing sleep efficiency, and increasing REM sleep, consistent with enhancement of cholinergic signaling. Although clinically not prominent, decreased sleep efficiency can be seen with COX-inhibitors, which may relate to decreased endogenous sleep-promoting prostaglandins.

SUMMARY

The approach to sleep-wake regulation has shifted from the search for one or a few sleep-related substances to a vast spectrum of signaling mechanisms spanning neurotransmitters, neuropeptides, hormones, lipids, and immune signals, many of which exhibit interactions and cross-talk at the level of receptor stimulation and signal transduction pathways. Despite this complexity, improved understanding of the factors contributing to variability in sleep-wake pharmacology may yield greater promise for individualized medicine in the future. Improved mechanistic information at the cellular and receptor level will continue to dovetail with behavioral approaches, such that ever more rational approaches to the clinical neuropharmacology of sleep can be realized.

REFERENCES

1. Saper CB, Scammell TE, Lu J. Hypothalamic regulation of sleep and circadian rhythms. *Nature.* 2005;437(7063):1257-1263.
2. Espana RA, Scammell TE. Sleep neurobiology for the clinician. *Sleep.* 2004;27(4):811-820.
3. Jones BE. From waking to sleeping: Neuronal and chemical substrates. *Trends Pharmacol Sci.* 2005;26(11):578-686.
4. Ursin R. Serotonin and sleep. *Sleep Med Rev.* 2002;6(1):55-69.
5. Monti JM, Jantos H. The roles of dopamine and serotonin, and of their receptors, in regulating sleep and waking. *Prog Brain Res.* 2008;172:625-646.
6. Borbely AA, Tobler I. Endogenous sleep-promoting substances and sleep regulation. *Physiol Rev.* 1989;69(2):605-670.
7. Steiger A. Neurochemical regulation of sleep. *J Psychiatr Res.* 2007;41(7):537-552.
8. Boutrel B, Koob GF. What keeps us awake: The neuropharmacology of stimulants and wakefulness-promoting medications. *Sleep.* 2004;27(6):1181-1194.
9. Fuller PM, Gooley JJ, Saper CB. Neurobiology of the sleep-wake cycle: Sleep architecture, circadian regulation, and regulatory feedback. *J Biol Rhythms.* 2006;21(6):482-493.
10. Swihart BJ, Caffo B, Bandeen-Roche K, Punjabi NM. Characterizing sleep structure using the hypnogram. *J Clin Sleep Med.* 2008;4(4):349-355.
11. Harmar AJ, Hills RA, Rosser EM, Jones M, Buneman OP, et al. IUPHAR-DB: The IUPHAR database of G protein-coupled receptors and ion channels. *Nucleic Acids Res.* 2009;37(database issue):D680-685.
12. Millan MJ, Marin P, Bockaert J, la Cour CM. Signaling at G-protein-coupled serotonin receptors: Recent advances and future research directions. *Trends Pharmacol Sci.* 2008;29(9):454-464.
13. Heuss C, Gerber U. G-protein-independent signaling by G-protein-coupled receptors. *Trends Neurosci.* 2000;23(10):469-475.
14. Engelman HS, MacDermott AB. Presynaptic ionotropic receptors and control of transmitter release. *Nat Rev Neurosci.* 2004;5(2):135-145.
15. Ostrom RS, Insel PA. The evolving role of lipid rafts and caveolae in G protein-coupled receptor signaling: Implications for molecular pharmacology. *Br J Pharmacol.* 2004;143(2):235-245.
16. Richerson GB, Wu Y. Dynamic equilibrium of neurotransmitter transporters: Not just for reuptake anymore. *J Neurophysiol.* 2003;90(3):1363-1374.
17. Fuxe K, Canals M, Torvinen M, Marcellino D, Terasmaa A, et al. Intramembrane receptor-receptor interactions: A novel principle in molecular medicine. *J Neural Transm.* 2007;114(1):49-75.
18. Ben-Shlomo I, Hsueh AJ. Three's company: Two or more unrelated receptors pair with the same ligand. *Mol Endocrinol.* 2005;19(5):1097-1109.
19. Brink CB, Harvey BH, Bodenstein J, Venter DP, Oliver DW. Recent advances in drug action and therapeutics: Relevance of novel concepts in G-protein-coupled receptor and signal transduction pharmacology. *Br J Clin Pharmacol.* 2004;57(4):373-387.
20. Ortells MO, Lunt GG. Evolutionary history of the ligand-gated ion-channel superfamily of receptors. *Trends Neurosci.* 1995;18(3):121-127.
21. Ishii M, Kurachi Y. Muscarinic acetylcholine receptors. *Curr Pharm Des.* 2006;12(28):3573-3581.
22. Vanni-Mercier G, Sakai K, Lin JS, Jouvet M. Mapping of cholinoceptive brainstem structures responsible for the generation of paradoxical sleep in the cat. *Arch Ital Biol.* 1989;127(3):133-164.
23. Van Dort CJ, Baghdoyan HA, Lydic R. Neurochemical modulators of sleep and anesthetic states. *Int Anesthesiol Clin.* 2008;46(3):75-104.
24. Imeri L, Bianchi S, Angeli P, Mancia M. Selective blockade of different brain stem muscarinic receptor subtypes: Effects on the sleep-wake cycle. *Brain Res.* 1994;636(1):68-72.
25. Jaehne A, Loessl B, Barkai Z, Riemann D, Hornyak M. Effects of nicotine on sleep during consumption, withdrawal and replacement therapy. *Sleep Med Rev.* 2009;13(5):363-377.
26. Barnes NM, Sharp T. A review of central 5-HT receptors and their function. *Neuropharmacology.* 1999;38(8):1083-1152.
27. Monti JM, Jantos H. Effects of the 5-HT1A receptor ligands flesinoxan and WAY 100635 given systemically or microinjected into the laterodorsal tegmental nucleus on REM sleep in the rat. *Behav Brain Res.* 2004;151(1-2):159-166.
28. Boutrel B, Franc B, Hen R, Hamon M, Adrien J. Key role of 5-HT1B receptors in the regulation of paradoxical sleep as evidenced in 5-HT1B knock-out mice. *J Neurosci.* 1999;19(8):3204-3212.
29. Monti JM, Jantos H. Effects of the serotonin 5-HT2A/2C receptor agonist DOI and of the selective 5-HT2A or 5-HT2C receptor antagonists EMD 281014 and SB-243213, respectively, on sleep and waking in the rat. *Eur J Pharmacol.* 2006;553(1-3):163-170.
30. Ponzoni A, Monti JM, Jantos H, Altier H, Monti D. Increased waking after intra-accumbens injection of m-chlorophenylbiguanide: prevention with serotonin or dopamine receptor antagonists. *Eur J Pharmacol.* 1995;278(2):111-115.
31. Benarroch EE. Metabotropic glutamate receptors: Synaptic modulators and therapeutic targets for neurologic disease. *Neurology.* 2008;70(12):964-968.
32. Dingledine R, Borges K, Bowie D, Traynelis SF. The glutamate receptor ion channels. *Pharmacol Rev.* 1999;51(1):7-61.
33. Alkire MT, Hudetz AG, Tononi G. Consciousness and anesthesia. *Science.* 2008;322(5903):876-880.
34. Boveroux P, Bonhomme V, Boly M, Vanhaudenhuyse A, Maquet P, Laureys S. Brain function in physiologically, pharmacologically, and pathologically altered states of consciousness. *Int Anesthesiol Clin.* 2008;46(3):131-146.
35. Lydic R, Baghdoyan HA. Sleep, anesthesiology, and the neurobiology of arousal state control. *Anesthesiology.* 2005;103(6):1268-1295.
36. Manfridi A, Brambilla D, Mancia M. Stimulation of NMDA and AMPA receptors in the rat nucleus basalis of Meynert affects sleep. *Am J Physiol.* 1999;277(5 Pt 2):R1488-1492.
37. Ebling FJ. The role of glutamate in the photic regulation of the suprachiasmatic nucleus. *Prog Neurobiol.* 1996;50(2-3):109-132.
38. Boissard R, Gervasoni D, Schmidt MH, Barbagli B, Fort P, Luppi PH. The rat ponto-medullary network responsible for paradoxical sleep onset and maintenance: A combined microinjection and functional neuroanatomical study. *Eur J Neurosci.* 2002;16(10):1959-1973.
39. Feinberg I, Schoepp DD, Hsieh KC, Darchia N, Campbell IG. The metabotropic glutamate (mGLU)2/3 receptor antagonist LY341495 [2S-2-amino-2-(1S,2S-2-carboxycyclopropyl-1-yl)-3-(xanth-9-yl)propanoic acid] stimulates waking and fast electroencephalogram power and blocks the effects of the mGLU2/3 receptor agonist ly379268 [(-)-2-oxa-4-aminobicyclo[3.1.0]hexane-4,6-dicarboxylate] in rats. *J Pharmacol Exp Ther.* 2005;312(2):826-833.
40. Byrnes KR, Loane DJ, Faden AI. Metabotropic glutamate receptors as targets for multipotential treatment of neurological disorders. *Neurotherapeutics.* 2009;6(1):94-107.
41. Stutzmann JM, Lucas M, Blanchard JC, Laduron PM. Riluzole, a glutamate antagonist, enhances slow wave and REM sleep in rats. *Neurosci Lett.* 1988;88(2):195-200.
42. Beenhakker MP, Huguenard JR. Neurons that fire together also conspire together: Is normal sleep circuitry hijacked to generate epilepsy? *Neuron.* 2009;62(5):612-632.
43. Crunelli V, Blethyn KL, Cope DW, Hughes SW, Parri HR, et al. Novel neuronal and astrocytic mechanisms in thalamocortical loop dynamics. *Philos Trans R Soc Lond B Biol Sci.* 2002;357(1428):1675-1693.
44. Mehta AK, Ticku MK. An update on GABAA receptors. *Brain Res Brain Res Rev.* 1999;29(2-3):196-217.
45. Xi MC, Morales FR, Chase MH. Interactions between GABAergic and cholinergic processes in the nucleus pontis oralis: Neuronal mechanisms controlling active (rapid eye movement) sleep and wakefulness. *J Neurosci.* 2004;24(47):10670-10678.
46. Pollock MS, Mistlberger RE. Rapid eye movement sleep induction by microinjection of the GABA-A antagonist bicuculline into the dorsal subcoeruleus area of the rat. *Brain Res.* 2003;962(1-2):68-77.
47. Sastre JP, Buda C, Kitahama K, Jouvet M. Importance of the ventrolateral region of the periaqueductal gray and adjacent tegmentum in the control of paradoxical sleep as studied by muscimol microinjections in the cat. *Neuroscience.* 1996;74(2):415-426.

48. Lin JS, Sakai K, Vanni-Mercier G, Jouvet M. A critical role of the posterior hypothalamus in the mechanisms of wakefulness determined by microinjection of muscimol in freely moving cats. *Brain Res.* 1989;479(2):225-240.
49. Rupprecht R. Neuroactive steroids: Mechanisms of action and neuropsychopharmacological properties. *Psychoneuroendocrinology.* 2003;28(2):139-168.
50. Mohler H. GABA(A) receptor diversity and pharmacology. *Cell Tissue Res.* 2006;326(2):505-516.
51. Bianchi MT. The pharmacology of insomnia: Targeting GABAA receptor function. *Int J Sleep Dis.* 2007;1(3):102-110.
52. Haas HL, Sergeeva OA, Selbach O. Histamine in the nervous system. *Physiol Rev.* 2008;88(3):1183-1241.
53. Lin JS, Hou Y, Sakai K, Jouvet M. Histaminergic descending inputs to the mesopontine tegmentum and their role in the control of cortical activation and wakefulness in the cat. *J Neurosci.* 1996;16(4):1523-1537.
54. Ramesh V, Thakkar MM, Strecker RE, Basheer R, McCarley RW. Wakefulness-inducing effects of histamine in the basal forebrain of freely moving rats. *Behav Brain Res.* 2004;152(2):271-278.
55. Lin JS, Sakai K, Jouvet M. Evidence for histaminergic arousal mechanisms in the hypothalamus of cat. *Neuropharmacology.* 1988;27(2):111-122.
56. Lin JS, Dauvilliers Y, Arnulf I, Bastuji H, Anaclet C, et al. An inverse agonist of the histamine H(3) receptor improves wakefulness in narcolepsy: Studies in orexin-/- mice and patients. *Neurobiol Dis.* 2008;30(1):74-83.
57. Rickels K, Morris RJ, Newman H, Rosenfeld H, Schiller H, Weinstock R. Diphenhydramine in insomniac family practice patients: A double-blind study. *J Clin Pharmacol.* 1983;23(5-6):234-242.
58. Borbely AA, Youmbi-Balderer G. Effect of diphenhydramine on subjective sleep parameters and on motor activity during bedtime. *Int J Clin Pharmacol Ther Toxicol.* 1988;26(8):392-396.
59. Vallone D, Picetti R, Borrelli E. Structure and function of dopamine receptors. *Neurosci Biobehav Rev.* 2000;24(1):125-132.
60. Monti JM, Monti D. The involvement of dopamine in the modulation of sleep and waking. *Sleep Med Rev.* 2007;11(2):113-133.
61. Isaac SO, Berridge CW. Wake-promoting actions of dopamine D1 and D2 receptor stimulation. *J Pharmacol Exp Ther.* 2003;307(1):386-394.
62. Gagnon JF, Postuma RB, Mazza S, Doyon J, Montplaisir J. Rapid-eye-movement sleep behaviour disorder and neurodegenerative diseases. *Lancet Neurol.* 2006;5(5):424-432.
63. Czeisler CA, Klerman EB. Circadian and sleep-dependent regulation of hormone release in humans. *Recent Prog Horm Res.* 1999;54:97-130:discussion 132.
64. Rashid AJ, O'Dowd BF, George SR. Minireview: Diversity and complexity of signaling through peptidergic G protein-coupled receptors. *Endocrinology.* 2004;145(6):2645-2652.
65. Merighi A. Costorage and coexistence of neuropeptides in the mammalian CNS. *Prog Neurobiol.* 2002;66(3):161-190.
66. Obal Jr F, Krueger JM. Biochemical regulation of non-rapid-eye-movement sleep. *Front Biosci.* 2003;8:d520-550.
67. Mullington JM, Haack M, Toth M, Serrador JM, Meier-Ewert HK. Cardiovascular, inflammatory, and metabolic consequences of sleep deprivation. *Prog Cardiovasc Dis.* 2009;51(4):294-302.
68. Ryan S, Taylor CT, McNicholas WT. Systemic inflammation: a key factor in the pathogenesis of cardiovascular complications in obstructive sleep apnoea syndrome? *Postgrad Med J.* 2009;85(1010):693-698.
69. Kapsimalis F, Basta M, Varouchakis G, Gourgoulianis K, Vgontzas A, Kryger M. Cytokines and pathological sleep. *Sleep Med.* 2008;9(6):603-614.
70. Kapsimalis F, Richardson G, Opp MR, Kryger M. Cytokines and normal sleep. *Curr Opin Pulm Med.* 2005;11(6):481-484.
71. Krueger JM, Majde JA, Obal F. Sleep in host defense. *Brain Behav Immun.* 2003;17(Suppl 1):S41-47.
72. Kotronoulas G, Stamatakis A, Stylianopoulou F. Hormones, hormonal agents, and neuropeptides involved in the neuroendocrine regulation of sleep in humans. *Hormones (Athens).* 2009;8(4):232-248.
73. Dubocovich ML, Rivera-Bermudez MA, Gerdin MJ, Masana MI. Molecular pharmacology, regulation and function of mammalian melatonin receptors. *Front Biosci.* 2003;8:d1093-1108.
74. Pandi-Perumal SR, Srinivasan V, Maestroni GJ, Cardinali DP, Poeggeler B, Hardeland R. Melatonin: Nature's most versatile biological signal? *FEBS J.* 2006;273(13):2813-2838.
75. Turek FW, Gillette MU. Melatonin, sleep, and circadian rhythms: Rationale for development of specific melatonin agonists. *Sleep Med.* 2004;5(6):523-532.
76. Buscemi N, Vandermeer B, Pandya R, Hooton N, Tjosvold L, et al. Melatonin for treatment of sleep disorders. *Evidence report technology assessment.* 2004;108:(AHRQ Publication No. 05-E002-2).
77. Buscemi N, Vandermeer B, Hooton N, Pandya R, Tjosvold L, et al. The efficacy and safety of exogenous melatonin for primary sleep disorders. A meta-analysis. *J Gen Intern Med.* 2005;20(12):1151-1158.
78. Brzezinski A, Vangel MG, Wurtman RJ, Norrie G, Zhdanova I, et al. Effects of exogenous melatonin on sleep: A meta-analysis. *Sleep Med Rev.* 2005;9(1):41-50.
79. Doghramji K. Melatonin and its receptors: A new class of sleep-promoting agents. *J Clin Sleep Med.* 2007;3(5 Suppl):S17-23.
80. Arendt J. In what circumstances is melatonin a useful sleep therapy? Consensus statement, WFSRS focus group, Dresden, November 1999. *J Sleep Res.* 2000;9(4):397-398.
81. Rajaratnam SM, Middleton B, Stone BM, Arendt J, Dijk DJ. Melatonin advances the circadian timing of EEG sleep and directly facilitates sleep without altering its duration in extended sleep opportunities in humans. *J Physiol.* 2004;561(Pt 1):339-351.
82. Halassa MM, Florian C, Fellin T, Munoz JR, Lee SY, et al. Astrocytic modulation of sleep homeostasis and cognitive consequences of sleep loss. *Neuron.* 2009;61(2):213-219.
83. Abbracchio MP, Burnstock G, Verkhratsky A, Zimmermann H. Purinergic signalling in the nervous system: An overview. *Trends Neurosci.* 2009;32(1):19-29.
84. Dunwiddie TV, Masino SA. The role and regulation of adenosine in the central nervous system. *Annu Rev Neurosci.* 2001;24:31-55.
85. Basheer R, Strecker RE, Thakkar MM, McCarley RW. Adenosine and sleep-wake regulation. *Prog Neurobiol.* 2004;73(6):379-396.
86. Fredholm BB, Battig K, Holmen J, Nehlig A, Zvartau EE. Actions of caffeine in the brain with special reference to factors that contribute to its widespread use. *Pharmacol Rev.* 1999;51(1):83-133.
87. Blanco-Centurion C, Xu M, Murillo-Rodriguez E, Gerashchenko D, Shiromani AM, et al. Adenosine and sleep homeostasis in the basal forebrain. *J Neurosci.* 2006;26(31):8092-8100.
88. Methippara MM, Kumar S, Alam MN, Szymusiak R, McGinty D. Effects on sleep of microdialysis of adenosine A_1 and A_{2a} receptor analogs into the lateral preoptic area of rats. *Am J Physiol Regul Integr Comp Physiol.* 2005;289(6):R1715-1723.
89. Stenberg D, Litonius E, Halldner L, Johansson B, Fredholm BB, Porkka-Heiskanen T. Sleep and its homeostatic regulation in mice lacking the adenosine A1 receptor. *J Sleep Res.* 2003;12(4):283-290.
90. Bjorness TE, Kelly CL, Gao T, Poffenberger V, Greene RW. Control and function of the homeostatic sleep response by adenosine A1 receptors. *J Neurosci.* 2009;29(5):1267-1276.
91. Coleman CG, Baghdoyan HA, Lydic R. Dialysis delivery of an adenosine A_{2A} agonist into the pontine reticular formation of C57BL/6J mouse increases pontine acetylcholine release and sleep. *J Neurochem.* 2006;96(6):1750-1759.
92. Hong ZY, Huang ZL, Qu WM, Eguchi N, Urade Y, Hayaishi O. An adenosine A receptor agonist induces sleep by increasing GABA release in the tuberomammillary nucleus to inhibit histaminergic systems in rats. *J Neurochem.* 2005;92(6):1542-1549.
93. Urade Y, Eguchi N, Qu WM, Sakata M, Huang ZL, et al. Sleep regulation in adenosine A_{2A} receptor-deficient mice. *Neurology.* 2003;61(11 Suppl 6):S94-96.
94. Scammell TE, Gerashchenko DY, Mochizuki T, McCarthy MT, Estabrooke IV, et al. An adenosine A2a agonist increases sleep and induces Fos in ventrolateral preoptic neurons. *Neuroscience.* 2001;107(4):653-663.
95. Retey JV, Adam M, Honegger E, Khatami R, Luhmann UF, et al. A functional genetic variation of adenosine deaminase affects the duration and intensity of deep sleep in humans. *Proc Natl Acad Sci U S A.* 2005;102(43):15676-15681.
96. Benarroch EE. Adenosine and its receptors: Multiple modulatory functions and potential therapeutic targets for neurologic disease. *Neurology.* 2008;70(3):231-236.
97. Guix FX, Uribesalgo I, Coma M, Munoz FJ. The physiology and pathophysiology of nitric oxide in the brain. *Prog Neurobiol.* 2005;76(2):126-152.
98. Ribeiro AC, Kapas L. Day- and nighttime injection of a nitric oxide synthase inhibitor elicits opposite sleep responses in rats. *Am J Physiol Regul Integr Comp Physiol.* 2005;289(2):R521-R531.
99. Chen L, Majde JA, Krueger JM. Spontaneous sleep in mice with targeted disruptions of neuronal or inducible nitric oxide synthase genes. *Brain Res.* 2003;973(2):214-222.
100. Crunelli V, Emri Z, Leresche N. Unravelling the brain targets of gamma-hydroxybutyric acid. *Curr Opin Pharmacol.* 2006;6(1):44-52.

101. Wong CG, Bottiglieri T, Snead 3rd OC. GABA, gamma-hydroxybutyric acid, and neurological disease. *Ann Neurol.* 2003;54(Suppl 6):S3-12.

102. Chemelli RM, Willie JT, Sinton CM, Elmquist JK, Scammell T, et al. Narcolepsy in orexin knockout mice: Molecular genetics of sleep regulation. *Cell.* 1999;98(4):437-451.

103. Lin L, Faraco J, Li R, Kadotani H, Rogers W, et al. The sleep disorder canine narcolepsy is caused by a mutation in the hypocretin (orexin) receptor 2 gene. *Cell.* 1999;98(3):365-376.

104. Adamantidis A, de Lecea L. The hypocretins as sensors for metabolism and arousal. *J Physiol.* 2009;587(Pt 1):33-40.

105. Mochizuki T, Crocker A, McCormack S, Yanagisawa M, Sakurai T, Scammell TE. Behavioral state instability in orexin knock-out mice. *J Neurosci.* 2004;24(28):6291-6300.

106. Anaclet C, Parmentier R, Ouk K, Guidon G, Buda C, et al. Orexin/hypocretin and histamine: distinct roles in the control of wakefulness demonstrated using knockout mouse models. *J Neurosci.* 2009;29(46):14423-14438.

107. Matsuki T, Nomiyama M, Takahira H, Hirashima N, Kunita S, et al. Selective loss of GABA(B) receptors in orexin-producing neurons results in disrupted sleep/wakefulness architecture. *Proc Natl Acad Sci U S A.* 2009;106(11):4459-4464.

108. Hagan JJ, Leslie RA, Patel S, Evans ML, Wattam TA, et al. Orexin A activates locus coeruleus cell firing and increases arousal in the rat. *Proc Natl Acad Sci U S A.* 1999;96(19):10911-10916.

109. Bourgin P, Huitron-Resendiz S, Spier AD, Fabre V, Morte B, et al. Hypocretin-1 modulates rapid eye movement sleep through activation of locus coeruleus neurons. *J Neurosci.* 2000;20(20):7760-7765.

110. Huang ZL, Qu WM, Li WD, Mochizuki T, Eguchi N, et al. Arousal effect of orexin A depends on activation of the histaminergic system. *Proc Natl Acad Sci U S A.* 2001;98(17):9965-9970.

111. Carter ME, Adamantidis A, Ohtsu H, Deisseroth K, de Lecea L. Sleep homeostasis modulates hypocretin-mediated sleep-to-wake transitions. *J Neurosci.* 2009;29(35):10939-10949.

112. Chang FC, Opp MR. Corticotropin-releasing hormone (CRH) as a regulator of waking. *Neurosci Biobehav Rev.* 2001;25(5):445-453.

113. Xu YL, Reinscheid RK, Huitron-Resendiz S, Clark SD, Wang Z, et al. Neuropeptide S: A neuropeptide promoting arousal and anxiolytic-like effects. *Neuron.* 2004;43(4):487-497.

114. Murck H, Antonijevic IA, Frieboes RM, Maier P, Schier T, Steiger A. Galanin has REM-sleep deprivation-like effects on the sleep EEG in healthy young men. *J Psychiatr Res.* 1999;33(3):225-232.

115. Bourgin P, Lebrand C, Escourrou P, Gaultier C, Franc B, et al. Vasoactive intestinal polypeptide microinjections into the oral pontine tegmentum enhance rapid eye movement sleep in the rat. *Neuroscience.* 1997;77(2):351-360.

116. Mirmiran M, Kruisbrink J, Bos NP, Van der Werf D, Boer GJ. Decrease of rapid-eye-movement sleep in the light by intraventricular application of a VIP-antagonist in the rat. *Brain Res.* 1988;458(1):192-194.

117. Sei M, Sei H, Shima K. Spontaneous activity, sleep, and body temperature in rats lacking the CCK-A receptor. *Physiol Behav.* 1999;68(1-2):25-29.

118. Viollet C, Lepousez G, Loudes C, Videau C, Simon A, Epelbaum J. Somatostatinergic systems in brain: Networks and functions. *Mol Cell Endocrinol.* 2008;286(1-2):75-87.

119. Obal Jr F, Alt J, Taishi P, Gardi J, Krueger JM. Sleep in mice with nonfunctional growth hormone-releasing hormone receptors. *Am J Physiol Regul Integr Comp Physiol.* 2003;284(1):R131-139.

120. de Lecea L. Cortistatin—Functions in the central nervous system. *Mol Cell Endocrinol.* 2008;286(1-2):88-95.

121. Obal Jr F, Payne L, Kapas L, Opp M, Krueger JM. Inhibition of growth hormone-releasing factor suppresses both sleep and growth hormone secretion in the rat. *Brain Res.* 1991;557(1-2):149-153.

122. Nyberg F. Growth hormone in the brain: Characteristics of specific brain targets for the hormone and their functional significance. *Front Neuroendocrinol.* 2000;21(4):330-348.

123. Obal Jr F, Bodosi B, Szilagyi A, Kacsoh B, Krueger JM. Antiserum to growth hormone decreases sleep in the rat. *Neuroendocrinology.* 1997;66(1):9-16.

124. Astrom C. Interaction between sleep and growth hormone. Evaluated by manual polysomnography and automatic power spectrum analysis. *Acta Neurol Scand.* 1995;92(4):281-296.

125. Veldhuis JD, Iranmanesh A. Physiological regulation of the human growth hormone (GH)-insulin-like growth factor type I (IGF-I) axis: Predominant impact of age, obesity, gonadal function, and sleep. *Sleep.* 1996;19(Suppl 10):S221-224.

126. Peyron C, Sapin E, Leger L, Luppi PH, Fort P. Role of the melanin-concentrating hormone neuropeptide in sleep regulation. *Peptides.* 2009;30(11):2052-2059.

127. Willie JT, Sinton CM, Maratos-Flier E, Yanagisawa M. Abnormal response of melanin-concentrating hormone deficient mice to fasting: Hyperactivity and rapid eye movement sleep suppression. *Neuroscience.* 2008;156(4):819-829.

128. Adamantidis A, Salvert D, Goutagny R, Lakaye B, Gervasoni D, et al. Sleep architecture of the melanin-concentrating hormone receptor 1-knockout mice. *Eur J Neurosci.* 2008;27(7):1793-1800.

129. Garcia-Garcia F, Drucker-Colin R. Endogenous and exogenous factors on sleep-wake cycle regulation. *Prog Neurobiol.* 1999;58(4):297-314.

130. Obal Jr F, Garcia-Garcia F, Kacsoh B, Taishi P, Bohnet S, et al. Rapid eye movement sleep is reduced in prolactin-deficient mice. *J Neurosci.* 2005;25(44):10282-10289.

131. Birnbaumer M. Vasopressin receptors. *Trends Endocrinol Metab.* 2000;11(10):406-410.

132. Taheri S, Lin L, Austin D, Young T, Mignot E. Short sleep duration is associated with reduced leptin, elevated ghrelin, and increased body mass index. *PLoS Med.* 2004;1(3):e62.

133. Szentirmai E, Kapas L, Sun Y, Smith RG, Krueger JM. The preproghrelin gene is required for the normal integration of thermoregulation and sleep in mice. *Proc Natl Acad Sci U S A.* 2009;106(33):14069-14074.

134. Szentirmai E, Kapas L, Sun Y, Smith RG, Krueger JM. Spontaneous sleep and homeostatic sleep regulation in ghrelin knockout mice. *Am J Physiol Regul Integr Comp Physiol.* 2007;293(1):R510-517.

135. Bianchi MT, Cash SS, Mietus J, Peng CK, Thomas R. Obstructive sleep apnea alters sleep stage transition dynamics. *PLoS One.* 2010;5(6):e11356.

136. Weikel JC, Wichniak A, Ising M, Brunner H, Friess E, et al. Ghrelin promotes slow-wave sleep in humans. *Am J Physiol Endocrinol Metab.* 2003;284(2):E407-415.

137. Sinton CM, Fitch TE, Gershenfeld HK. The effects of leptin on REM sleep and slow wave delta in rats are reversed by food deprivation. *J Sleep Res.* 1999;8(3):197-203.

138. Laposky AD, Shelton J, Bass J, Dugovic C, Perrino N, Turek FW. Altered sleep regulation in leptin-deficient mice. *Am J Physiol Regul Integr Comp Physiol.* 2006;290(4):R894-903.

139. Spiegel K, Tasali E, Penev P, Van Cauter E. Brief communication: Sleep curtailment in healthy young men is associated with decreased leptin levels, elevated ghrelin levels, and increased hunger and appetite. *Ann Intern Med.* 2004;141(11):846-850.

140. Motivala SJ, Tomiyama AJ, Ziegler M, Khandrika S, Irwin MR. Nocturnal levels of ghrelin and leptin and sleep in chronic insomnia. *Psychoneuroendocrinology.* 2009;34(4):540-545.

141. Benarroch EE. Neuropeptide Y: Its multiple effects in the CNS and potential clinical significance. *Neurology.* 2009;72(11):1016-1020.

142. Antonijevic IA, Murck H, Bohlhalter S, Frieboes RM, Holsboer F, Steiger A. Neuropeptide Y promotes sleep and inhibits ACTH and cortisol release in young men. *Neuropharmacology.* 2000;39(8):1474-1481.

143. Held K, Antonijevic I, Murck H, Kuenzel H, Steiger A, Neuropeptide Y. (NPY) shortens sleep latency but does not suppress ACTH and cortisol in depressed patients and normal controls. *Psychoneuroendocrinology.* 2006;31(1):100-107.

144. Szentirmai E, Krueger JM. Central administration of neuropeptide Y induces wakefulness in rats. *Am J Physiol Regul Integr Comp Physiol.* 2006;291(2):R473-480.

145. Chen C, Bazan NG. Lipid signaling: Sleep, synaptic plasticity, and neuroprotection. *Prostaglandins Other Lipid Mediat.* 2005;77(1-4):65-76.

146. Matsumura H, Nakajima T, Osaka T, Satoh S, Kawase K, et al. Prostaglandin D2-sensitive, sleep-promoting zone defined in the ventral surface of the rostral basal forebrain. *Proc Natl Acad Sci U S A.* 1994;91(25):11998-12002.

147. Mizoguchi A, Eguchi N, Kimura K, Kiyohara Y, Qu WM, et al. Dominant localization of prostaglandin D receptors on arachnoid trabecular cells in mouse basal forebrain and their involvement in the regulation of non-rapid eye movement sleep. *Proc Natl Acad Sci U S A.* 2001;98(20):11674-11679.

148. Qu WM, Huang ZL, Xu XH, Aritake K, Eguchi N, et al. Lipocalin-type prostaglandin D synthase produces prostaglandin D2 involved in regulation of physiological sleep. *Proc Natl Acad Sci U S A.* 2006;103(47):17949-17954.

149. Pinzar E, Kanaoka Y, Inui T, Eguchi N, Urade Y, Hayaishi O. Prostaglandin D synthase gene is involved in the regulation of non-rapid eye movement sleep. *Proc Natl Acad Sci U S A.* 2000;97(9):4903-4907.

150. McKinney MK, Cravatt BF. Structure and function of fatty acid amide hydrolase. *Annu Rev Biochem*. 2005;74:411-432.
151. Koh B, Crews CM. Chemical genetics: A small molecule approach to neurobiology. *Neuron*. 2002;36(4):563-566.
152. Huitron-Resendiz S, Sanchez-Alavez M, Wills DN, Cravatt BF, Henriksen SJ. Characterization of the sleep-wake patterns in mice lacking fatty acid amide hydrolase. *Sleep*. 2004;27(5):857-865.
153. Laposky AD, Homanics GE, Basile A, Mendelson WB. Deletion of the GABA(A) receptor beta 3 subunit eliminates the hypnotic actions of oleamide in mice. *Neuroreport*. 2001;12(18):4143-4147.
154. Moldofsky H. Central nervous system and peripheral immune functions and the sleep-wake system. *J Psychiatry Neurosci*. 1994;19(5):368-374.
155. Fang J, Wang Y, Krueger JM. Effects of interleukin-1 beta on sleep are mediated by the type I receptor. *Am J Physiol*. 1998;274(3 Pt 2):R655-660.
156. Sookoian SC, Gonzalez C, Pirola CJ. Meta-analysis on the G-308A tumor necrosis factor alpha gene variant and phenotypes associated with the metabolic syndrome. *Obes Res*. 2005;13(12):2122-2131.
157. Bohnet SG, Traynor TR, Majde JA, Kacsoh B, Krueger JM. Mice deficient in the interferon type I receptor have reduced REM sleep and altered hypothalamic hypocretin, prolactin and 2',5'-oligoadenylate synthetase expression. *Brain Res*. 2004;1027(1-2):117-125.
158. Morrow JD, Opp MR. Sleep-wake behavior and responses of interleukin-6-deficient mice to sleep deprivation. *Brain Behav Immun*. 2005;19(1):28-39.
159. Uthgenannt D, Schoolmann D, Pietrowsky R, Fehm HL, Born J. Effects of sleep on the production of cytokines in humans. *Psychosom Med*. 1995;57(2):97-104.
160. Redwine L, Hauger RL, Gillin JC, Irwin M. Effects of sleep and sleep deprivation on interleukin-6, growth hormone, cortisol, and melatonin levels in humans. *J Clin Endocrinol Metab*. 2000;85(10):3597-3603.
161. Anderson MP, Mochizuki T, Xie J, Fischler W, Manger JP, et al. Thalamic Cav3.1 T-type Ca^{2+} channel plays a crucial role in stabilizing sleep. *Proc Natl Acad Sci U S A*. 2005;102(5):1743-1748.
162. Beuckmann CT, Sinton CM, Miyamoto N, Ino M, Yanagisawa M. N-type calcium channel alpha1B subunit (Cav2.2) knock-out mice display hyperactivity and vigilance state differences. *J Neurosci*. 2003;23(17):6793-6797.
163. Joho RH, Marks GA, Espinosa F. Kv3 potassium channels control the duration of different arousal states by distinct stochastic and clock-like mechanisms. *Eur J Neurosci*. 2006;23(6):1567-1574.
164. Douglas CL, Vyazovskiy V, Southard T, Chiu SY, Messing A, et al. Sleep in Kcna2 knockout mice. *BMC Biol*. 2007;5:42.
165. Wu MN, Joiner WJ, Dean T, Yue Z, Smith CJ, et al. SLEEPLESS, a Ly-6/neurotoxin family member, regulates the levels, localization and activity of Shaker. *Nat Neurosci*. 2010;13(1):69-75.
166. Pang DS, Robledo CJ, Carr DR, Gent TC, Vyssotski AL, et al. An unexpected role for TASK-3 potassium channels in network oscillations with implications for sleep mechanisms and anesthetic action. *Proc Natl Acad Sci U S A*. 2009;106(41):17546-17551.
167. Beck P, Odle A, Wallace-Huitt T, Skinner RD, Garcia-Rill E. Modafinil increases arousal determined by P13 potential amplitude: An effect blocked by gap junction antagonists. *Sleep*. 2008;31(12):1647-1654.
168. Franco-Perez J, Paz C. Quinine, a selective gap junction blocker, decreases REM sleep in rats. *Pharmacol Biochem Behav*. 2009;94(2):250-254.
169. Garcia-Rill E, Heister DS, Ye M, Charlesworth A, Hayar A. Electrical coupling: novel mechanism for sleep-wake control. *Sleep*. 2007;30(11):1405-1414.
170. Meolie AL, Rosen C, Kristo D, Kohrman M, Gooneratne N, et al. Oral nonprescription treatment for insomnia: an evaluation of products with limited evidence. *J Clin Sleep Med*. 2005;1(2):173-187.
171. Izzo AA, Ernst E. Interactions between herbal medicines and prescribed drugs: An updated systematic review. *Drugs*. 2009;69(13):1777-1798.
172. DeMartinis NA, Winokur A. Effects of psychiatric medications on sleep and sleep disorders. *CNS Neurol Disord Drug Targets*. 2007;6(1):17-29.
173. Brown WD. The effect of medication on sleep. *Respir Care Clin North Am*. 2006;12(1):81-99.
174. Qureshi A, Lee-Chiong Jr T. Medications and their effects on sleep. *Med Clin North Am*. 2004;88(3):751-766.

SECTION 3

Pharmacology Principles

Stimulant Pharmacology

NORIAKI SAKAI / SEIJI NISHINO

Chapter
6

Central nervous system (CNS) stimulant is a loosely defined scientific term despite its wide use. In *Handbook of Sleep Disorders* J.D. Parkes describes CNS stimulation as "an increase in neuronal activity due to enhanced excitability, with a change in the normal balance between excitatory and inhibitory influences. This may result from blockage of inhibition, enhancement of excitation, or both."[1] In this chapter, the generic term "CNS stimulants" will be used for all wake-promoting compounds of potential use in the treatment of excessive daytime sleepiness (EDS), which is a common symptom in patients with sleep disorders and in the general population at large.

CNS stimulants currently used in sleep medicine include amphetamine-like compounds (L- and D-amphetamine and methamphetamine, L- and D-methylphenidate, and pemoline), mazindol, modafinil, some antidepressants with stimulant properties (e.g., bupropion), and caffeine. Though not all are indicated for this use by the U.S. Food and Drug Administration (FDA), CNS stimulants are generally effective in the management of EDS independently of its underlying cause. A list of compounds discussed in this chapter and their FDA indications appear in Table 6-1. However, caution should be paid to their potential for misuse and abuse. The effects of most of these drugs on wakefulness are primarily mediated via an inhibition of dopamine reuptake/transport and in some cases via increased dopamine release. Inhibition of adrenergic uptake also likely has some stimulant effects. Biogenic monoamine transporters (for dopamine [DA], norepinephrine [NE], and serotonin [5-HT]) are located at nerve terminals, and play an important role on terminating transmitter action and maintaining transmitter homeostasis. In the past decade, monoamine transporters have been cloned and their molecular mechanisms have been elucidated. Genetically engineered mice lacking these molecules (knockout mice) have also become available. In parallel with these discoveries, potent and selective ligands for DA, NE, and 5-HT transporters have been developed. The results of pharmacologic studies using these new ligands in canines and knockout mice models suggest the importance of the DA transporter for the mode of action of amphetamines and amphetamine-like compounds (as well as mazindol and bupropion) on wakefulness. Importantly, however, the various stimulants also have differential effects on dopamine storage (via vesicular monoamine transporter [VMAT] inhibition) or release, and in most cases have substantial effects on other monoaminergic systems. The mode of action of modafinil, a more recent compound that rapidly became a first-line treatment for EDS in narcolepsy, is controversial to date, but is increasingly suggested to be primarily mediated by dopamine reuptake inhibition. Other wake-promoting modes include adenosine receptor antagonism, such as those found in caffeine. More recently, novel classes of wake-promoting therapeutics including glutamatergic and histaminergic modulators are being developed and preclinical and clinical evaluations are in progress.

In this chapter, we will review the neurochemical, neurophysiologic, and neuropharmacologic properties of the CNS stimulants most commonly used in sleep medicine. We will also discuss a perspective on future stimulant treatments.

AMPHETAMINES AND AMPHETAMINE-LIKE COMPOUNDS

Historical Perspective and Limitations

Amphetamine was first synthesized by Gordon Alles in 1897, but its stimulant effects were not recognized until 1929. Amphetamine increases energy, elevates mood, prevents fatigue, increases vigilance and prevents sleep, stimulates respiration, and causes electrical and behavioral arousal from natural- or drug-induced sleep. It was rapidly shown to be a safer and cheaper alternative to ephedrine, recently banned, as a stimulant. In World War II, amphetamine was massively supplied to paratroopers and commandos to induce alertness and reduce fatigue.

Narcolepsy was probably the first condition for which amphetamine was used clinically. It revolutionized therapy for the condition, although it was not curative. The piperazine derivative of amphetamine, methylphenidate, was introduced by Yoss and Daly in 1959.[2]

The use of amphetamine in treating parkinsonism dates back to 1937, when it was initially used to alleviate the muscular rigidity of postencephalitic parkinsonism. By 1968, its use in the treatment of this condition was largely suspended thanks to the availability of more effective dopaminergic agents. Until the risks of amphetamine dependence and abuse became recognized, amphetamine had been widely used in the treatment of obesity. It had also been prescribed in the treatment of sedative abuse and alcoholism to offset sleepiness and lethargy.

Bradley and Bowen (1941) first reported the effectiveness of amphetamine to modify antisocial behavior (withdrawn or lethargic) in children.[3] A paradoxic calming effect was also noted in some children and aggressive adults. Most notably, hyperactive children tended to move less, and to be calmer and not as quarrelsome after treatment with amphetamine. In 1958, methylphenidate was introduced to treat hyperactivity

TABLE 6-1

Pharmacologic Compounds Commonly Used for Excessive Daytime Sleepiness (EDS)

Stimulant Compound	Usual Daily Dose*	Half-life (hr)	FDA Indications	Side Effects/Notes
AMPHETAMINE/AMPHETAMINE-LIKE CNS STIMULANTS				
D-Amphetamine sulfate (II)	5-60 mg (15, 100 mg)	16-30	Narcolepsy, ADHD	Irritability, mood changes, headaches, excessive sweating, palpitations, tremors, insomnia
Methamphetamine HCl† (II)	5-60 mg (15, 80 mg)	9-15	ADHD, exogenous obesity	Same as for D-amphetamine May have greater central over peripheral effects than for D-amphetamine
Methylphenidate HCl (II)	10-60 mg (30, 100 mg)	~3	Narcolepsy, ADHD	Same as for amphetamines; better therapeutic index than for D-amphetamine, with less reduction of appetite or increase in blood pressure Short duration of action
Pemoline (IV)	20-115 mg (37.5, 150 mg)	11-13	ADHD	Less sympathomimetic effect, milder stimulant, slower onset of action Occasionally produces liver toxicity and has been withdrawn from the U.S. market
DOPAMINE-NOREPINEPHRINE UPTAKE INHIBITOR				
Mazindol (IV)	2-6 mg (NA)	10-13	Exogenous obesity	Weaker CNS-stimulant effects, anorexia, dry mouth, irritability, headaches, gastrointestinal symptoms Less potential for abuse
OTHER AGENTS FOR TREATMENT OF EDS				
Modafinil‡ (IV)	200-400 mg (NA)	9-14	Narcolepsy, OSAS, SWSD	No peripheral sympathomimetic action; headaches, nausea Less potential for abuse
Armodafinil (IV)	150-250 mg (NA)	10-15	Narcolepsy, OSAS, SWSD	Similar to those for modafinil
MAO INHIBITORS WITH ALERTING EFFECT				
Selegiline	5-40 mg (NA)	2	Parkinson's disease	Low abuse potential Partial (10-40%) interconversion to amphetamine
XANTHINE DERIVATIVE				

Caffeine§	100-200 mg (NA)	3-7	Multiple purpose	Weak stimulant effect; 100 mg of caffeine roughly equivalent to 1 cup of coffee
				    Generally recognized as safe
				    Palpitations, hypertension

All listed compounds are DEA-scheduled compounds, except for selegiline and caffeine, and the DEA schedule is given in *parentheses*.

*Dosages are those recommended by the American Academy of Sleep Medicine (formerly the American Sleep Disorders Association) Usual starting dose and maximal dose recommended in the treatment of narcolepsy are given in *parentheses*.

†Methamphetamine is reported to have more central effects and may predispose to amphetamine psychosis. The widespread misuse of methamphetamine has led to severe legal restriction on its manufacture, sale, and prescription in many countries. L-Amphetamine (dose range, 20-60 mg) is not available in the United States but probably has no advantage over D-amphetamine in the treatment of narcolepsy (it may even be a slightly weaker stimulant).

‡The half-life of the *S*-enatiomer is short at 3 to 4 hours, so the half-life of racemic modafinil mostly reflects the half-life of armodafinil (*R*-enantiomer).

§Caffeine can be purchased without a prescription in the form of tablets (NoDoz, 100 mg caffeine; Vivarin, 200 mg caffeine) and is used by many patients with narcolepsy before their diagnosis.

ADHD, attention deficit hyperactivity disorder; *CNS*, central nervous system; *DEA*, U.S. Drug Enforcement Administration; *FDA*, U.S. Food and Drug Administration; *MAO*, monoamine oxidase; *NA*, not applicable; *OSAS*, obesity sleep apnea syndrome; *SWSD*, shift work sleep disorder.

Source: Practice parameters for the use of stimulants in the treatment of narcolepsy. Standards of Practice Committee of the American Sleep Disorders Association. Sleep 1994;17:348-351.

in children.[4] These observations preceded reports on the effects of amphetamine and methylphenidate in children who are hyperkinetic, a disorder which is now referred to *as attention deficit hyperactivity disorder (ADHD)*.

Although no controlled trials have been done, many case series suggest the effectiveness of stimulants in some cases of treatment-resistant depression. Part of the beneficial effects of amphetamine on depression may be due a reduction of fatigue and apathy, rather than a genuine antidepressant effect. Combined therapy with stimulants, monoamine oxidase inhibitors (MAOIs), and tricyclic antidepressants is generally not advised because of significant hypertension or hyperthermia

noted in certain cases. Amphetamines are often prescribed in combination with low (anticataplectic) doses of tricyclic agents in narcolepsy-cataplexy patients.

From a historical perspective, indications for amphetamine stimulants have been considerably limited over the years to primarily narcolepsy, ADHD, and intractable depression. The rationale for this change has been the realization of the risk of abuse and dependence with these compounds. The introduction of other effective therapies for these conditions (e.g., modafinil for narcolepsy, atomoxetine for ADHD) has also led to narrower indications. In addition, many new formulations and isomer-specific preparations have been recently

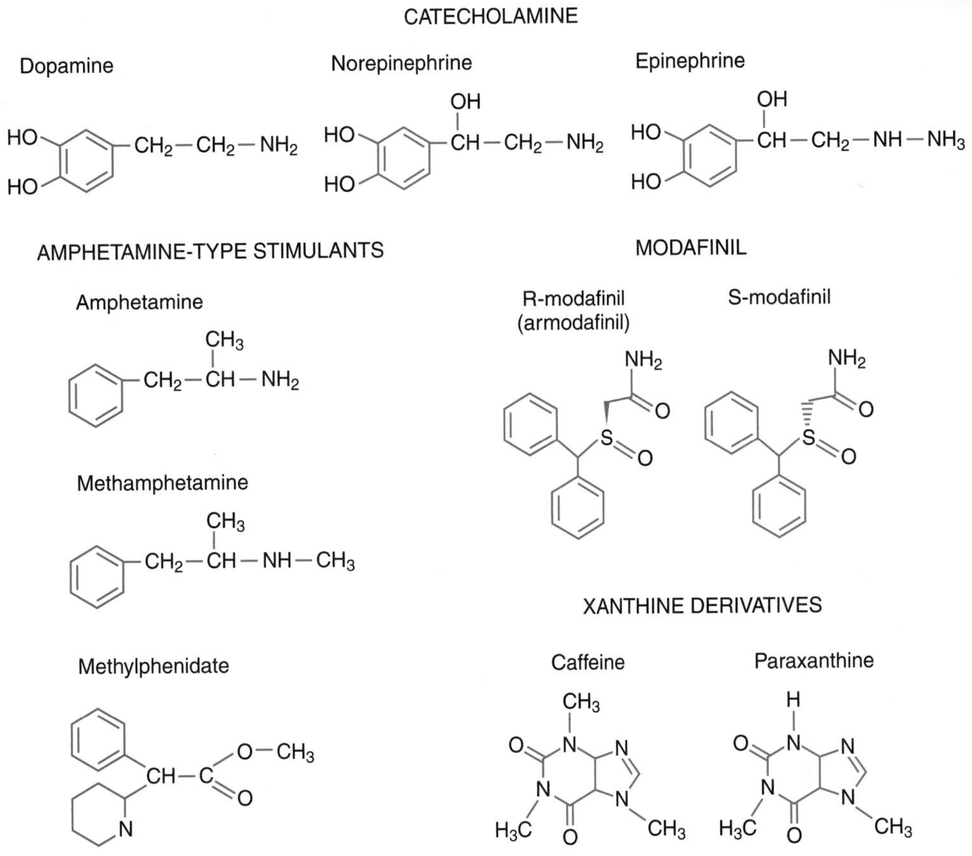

Figure 6-1 Chemical structures of amphetamine-like stimulants, modafinil, armodafinil, and xanthine derivatives, as compared to catecholamine.

developed and are increasingly used, mostly for the treatment of ADHD.

Structure-Activity Relationships and Major Chemical Entities

Amphetamine has a simple chemical structure resembling endogenous catecholamines (Fig. 6-1). This backbone forms the template for a wide variety of pharmacologically active substances. Although amphetamine possesses strong central stimulant effects, minor structural modifications can result in a broad spectrum of effects, including nasal decongestion, anorexia, vasoconstriction, antidepressant effects, and hallucinogenic properties.

The structure of amphetamine can be divided into three components: (1) a terminal amine, (2) an aromatic nucleus, and (3) an isopropyl side chain. Substitution at the amine group is the most common alteration. Methamphetamine, which is characterized by an additional methyl group attached to the amine (a secondary substituted amine), is more potent than amphetamine, probably because of increased CNS penetration. Substitution on the aromatic nucleus generally produces less potent, if not entirely inactive, stimulants.[5] Substitution of two or more methoxy groups plus addition of ethyl, methyl, or bromine groups on the aromatic nucleus creates hallucinogens of various potencies. The drug Ecstasy (MDMA [methylenedioxymethamphetamine]) is built on a methamphetamine backbone, with a dimethoxy ring extending from the aromatic group. If a similar compound is synthesized with a primary amine (without the methyl group), then it creates a drug known as Love

(MDA [methylenedioxyamphetamine]). An intact isopropyl side chain appeared to be needed to maintain stimulant efficacy. For example, changing the propyl to an ethyl side chain creates phenylethylamine, an endogenous neuroamine. The compound has mood- and energy-enhancing properties but is less potent and has a much shorter half-life than amphetamine.

The pharmacologic effects of most amphetamine derivatives are isomer-specific. These differential effects occur both at the pharmacokinetic level (absorption, distribution, metabolism, elimination) and the pharmacodynamic level (actual pharmacologic effects). In electroencephalographic (EEG) studies, D-amphetamine is four times more potent than L-amphetamine in inducing wakefulness.[6] However, not all effects are stereospecific. For example, both enantiomers are equipotent at suppressing REM sleep in humans and rats and at producing amphetamine psychosis.

Amphetamine-like compounds, such as methylphenidate, pemoline, and fencamfamin are structurally similar to amphetamines; all compounds include a benzene core with an ethylamine group side chain (see Fig. 6-1). Both methylphenidate and pemoline were commonly used for the treatment of EDS in narcolepsy, but pemoline has been withdrawn from the market in several countries because of liver toxicity (Table 6-1). The most common form of methylphenidate commercially available is a racemic mixture of both a D- and L-enantiomer. In this preparation, the D-methylphenidate mainly contributes to its clinical effects, especially after oral administration, while L-methylphenidate undergoes a significant first-pass effect. A single isomer form of D-methylphenidate (Focalin) is also available.

Amphetamines are highly lipophilic molecules that are well absorbed by the gastrointestinal tract. Peak levels in plasma are achieved approximately 2 hours after oral administration, with rapid tissue distribution and brain penetration. Protein binding is highly variable, with an average volume of distribution (V_D) of 5 L/kg. Amphetamines are inactivated by both hepatic metabolism and renal excretion. Amphetamine can be metabolized in the liver by either aromatic or aliphatic hydroxylation, yielding biologically active metabolites parahydroxyamphetamine or norephedrine, respectively. Thirty-three percent of the oral dose is excreted unchanged in the urine. Urinary excretion of amphetamine and many amphetamine-like stimulants is greatly influenced by urinary pH. At urinary pH 5.0, the elimination half-life of amphetamine is short (~5 hours), but at pH 7.3 it increases to 21 hours. Sodium bicarbonate will delay excretion of amphetamine and prolong its clinical effects, whereas ammonium chloride will shorten amphetamine action (and can possibly induce toxicity).

Methylphenidate is almost totally and rapidly absorbed after oral administration. Methylphenidate has low protein binding (15%) and is short acting; effects last approximately 4 hours, with a half-life of 3 hours. The primary pathway of clearance is through the urine, in which 90% is excreted.

Molecular Targets of Amphetamine Action

The molecular targets mediating amphetamine-like stimulant effects are complex and vary depending on the specific analog/isomer used and on the dose administered. Amphetamine per se increases catecholamine (DA and NE) release and inhibits reuptake from presynaptic terminals. This results in increase in catecholamine concentrations in the synaptic cleft and enhances postsynaptic stimulation. The presynaptic modulations by amphetamines are mediated by specific catecholamine transporters[7] (Fig. 6-2). The responsible molecules, the DA transporter (DAT) and the NE transporter (NET), have now been cloned and characterized. Amphetamine derivatives are known to inhibit the uptake and enhance the release of DA, NE, or both, by interacting with the DAT and the NET. These transporters normally move DA and NE from the outside to the inside of the cell. This process is sodium-dependent; sodium and chloride bind to the DA/NE transporter to immobilize it at the extracellular surface and to alter the conformation of the DA/NE binding site so that it facilitates substrate binding. Substrate binding allows movement of the carrier to the intracellular surface of the neuronal membrane, driven by sodium concentration gradients. Interestingly, in the presence of some drugs such as amphetamine, the direction of transport appears to be reversed (see Fig. 6-2). DA and NE are thus moved from the inside of the cell to the outside through a mechanism called *exchange diffusion,* which occurs at low doses (1-5 mg/kg) of amphetamine. This mechanism, rather than a simple inhibition of monoamine reuptake, is involved in the enhancement of extracellular catecholamine release by amphetamine. It explains why amphetamine is in particular more potent than expected based on its relatively low binding affinity for DAT and NET.[8,9] A recent in vitro experiment has shown that amphetamine transport causes an inward sodium current. As intracellular sodium ions become more available, a DAT-mediated reverse transport of DA occurs, following DA release through the DAT transporter.

At higher dose, other effects are involved. Increased serotonin (5-HT) release is also observed. Moderate to high doses of amphetamine (>5 mg/kg) also interact with the vesicular monoamine transporter 2 (VMAT2).[7] The vesicularization of the monoamines (DA, NE, serotonin, and histamine) in the nerve terminal is dependent on VMAT2; VMAT2 regulates the size of the vesicular and cytosolic DA pools. Amphetamine is highly lipophilic and easily enters nerve terminals by diffusing across plasma membranes. Once inside, amphetamine depletes vesicular monoamine stores by several mechanisms. First, it binds directly, albeit with low affinity, to VMAT2 thereby inhibiting vesicular uptake. Second, amphetamine, a weak base, diffuses across the vesicular membrane in its uncharged (lipophilic) form and accumulates in the granules in its charged form (because of the lower pH of the synaptic vesicle interior). As vesicular amphetamine concentration increases, the buffering capacity of the catecholamine-containing vesicle is lost. As a result, the vesicular pH gradient diminishes, followed by the decrease of vesicular monoamine uptake. All these mechanisms lead to a diffusion of the native monoamines out of the vesicles into the cytoplasm along a concentration gradient. Amphetamine can therefore be considered as a physiologic VMAT2 antagonist that releases the vesicular DA/NE loaded by VMAT2 into the cytoplasm. High doses of amphetamine also inhibit MAO activity. These mechanisms, as well as the reverse transport and the blocking of reuptake of DA/NE, all lead to an increase in NE and DA synaptic concentrations,[7] and these are independent of the phasic activity of the neurons.

Various amphetamine derivatives have slightly different effects on all these systems. For example, methylphenidate also binds to the NET and DAT and enhances catecholamine release. It has, however, less effect on the granular storage via VMAT than native amphetamine. Similarly, D-amphetamine has proportionally more releasing effect on the DA than the NE system compared to L-amphetamine. MDMA (Ecstasy) has more effect on 5-HT release than on catecholamine release. Of note, other medications acting on monoaminergic systems (e.g., bupropion or mazindol, see later discussion) tend to exert their actions by simply blocking the reuptake mechanism.

It is well established that MDMA shows the serotoninergic neurotoxicity in both humans and animals. Similarly, amphetamine derivatives with strong effects on monoamine release have neurotoxic effects on DA systems at high dose in animal studies, especially in the context of repeated administration mimicking drug abuse.

Presynaptic Modulation of the Dopaminergic System: EEG Arousal Effects

Although amphetamine-like compounds are well known to stimulate catecholaminergic transmission, the exact mechanism by which they promote EEG arousal is still uncertain. A canine model of the sleep disorder narcolepsy has been used to explore its mechanism. Canine narcolepsy is a naturally occurring animal model of the human disorder.[8] Similar to human patients, narcoleptic dogs are excessively sleepy (i.e., short sleep latency), have fragmented sleep patterns, and display cataplexy.[7]

Using narcoleptic and control Dobermans, the effects of ligands specific for the DA (GBR12909, bupropion, and

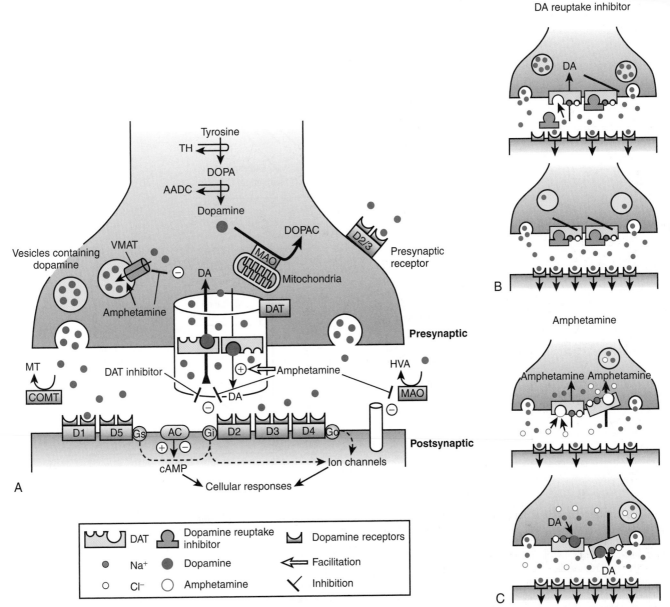

Figure 6-2 **Schematic representations of dopaminergic terminal neurotransmission in relation to mode of action of dopamine reuptake inhibitors and amphetamine. Effects of dopamine reuptake inhibitors and amphetamines at the dopaminergic nerve terminal. A,** DA transporter (DAT) is one of the most important molecules that regulate dopaminergic neurotransmission and the favorite molecular target of several CNS stimulants. i, Amphetamine interacts with the DAT carrier to facilitate DA release from the cytoplasm through an exchange diffusion mechanism (see part C). At higher intracellular concentrations, ii, amphetamine also disrupts vesicular storage of DA and, iii, inhibits monoamine oxidase (MAO). Both these actions increase cytoplasmic DA concentrations. iv, Amphetamine also inhibits DA uptake by virtue of its binding to and transport by the DAT. These mechanisms all lead to an increase in DA synaptic concentrations, and these are independent on the phasic activity of the neurons. Increased synaptic concentration of DA stimulates postsynaptic DA receptors (D_1 type [1, 5] and D_2 type [2, 3, 5] receptors). **B,** Sodium and chloride bind to the DAT to immobilize it at the extracellular surface. This binding alters the conformation of the DA binding site on the DAT to facilitate substrate (i.e., DA) binding. DAT reuptake inhibitors bind to DAT competitively and inhibit DA-DAT bindings, followed by the increase of DA concentrations in the synaptic cleft. **C,** Amphetamine, in competition with extracellular DA, binds to the transporter. Substrate binding allows the movement of the carrier to the intracellular surface of the neuronal membrane, driven by the sodium and amphetamine concentration gradients. Amphetamine dissociates from the transporter, making the binding site available to cytoplasmic DA. DA binding to the transporter enables the movement of the transporter to the extracellular surface of the neuronal membrane, as driven by the favorable DA concentration gradient. Thus, it results in a reversal of the flow of DA uptake. DA dissociates from the transporter, making the transporter available for amphetamine, and thus another cycle. *AADC,* aromatic acid decarboxylase; *AC,* adenylyl cyclase; *cAMP,* cyclic adenosine monophosphate; *CNS,* central nervous system; *COMT,* catechol-*O*-methyltransferase; D_1-D_5, dopamine receptors 1 through 5; *DA,* dopamine; *DAT,* dopamine transporter; *DOPA,* 3,4-dihydroxyphenylalanine; *DOPAC,* dihydroxyphenylacetic acid; *Gi, Go,* and *Gs,* protein subunits; *HVA,* homovanillic acid; *MAO,* monoamine oxidase; *TH,* tyrosine hydroxylase; *VMAT,* vesicular monoamine transporter.

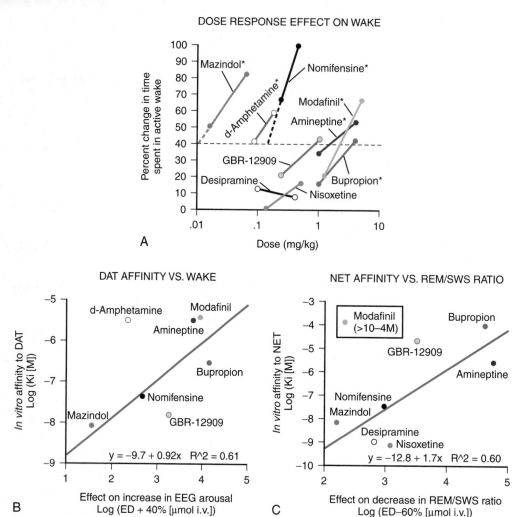

Figure 6-3 **Effects of various dopamine (DA) and norepinephrine (NE) uptake inhibitors and amphetamine-like stimulants on the electroenceph-alographic (EEG) arousal of narcoleptic dogs and correlation between in vivo EEG arousal effects or REM sleep and in vitro DA or NE transporter binding affinities. A,** The effects of various compounds on daytime sleepiness were studied using 4-hour daytime polygraphic recordings (10:00-14:00) in four to five narcoleptic animals. Two doses were studied for each compound. All DA uptake inhibitors and central nervous system (CNS) stimulants dose-dependently increased EEG arousal and reduced slow wave sleep (SWS) in comparison to vehicle treatment. In contrast, nisoxetine and desipramine, two potent NE uptake inhibitors, had no significant effect on EEG arousal at doses that completely suppressed cataplexy. Compounds with both adrenergic and dopaminergic effects (nomifensine, mazindol, D-amphetamine) were active on both EEG arousal and cataplexy. The effects of the two doses performed for each stimulant were used to approximate a dose-response curve; the drug dose that increased the time spent in wakefulness by 40% above baseline (vehicle session) was estimated for each compound. The order of potency of the compounds obtained was mazindol > (amphetamine) > nomifensine > GBR 12,909 > amineptine > modafinil > bupropion. **B,** In vitro DA transporter (DAT) binding was performed using [³H]-WIN 35,428 onto canine caudate membranes. Affinity for the various DA uptake inhibitors tested varied widely between 6.5 nM and 3.3 mM. In addition, it was also found that both amphetamine and modafinil have low but significant affinity (same range as amineptine) for the DAT. A significant correlation between in vivo and in vitro effects was observed for all 5 DA uptake inhibitors and modafinil. Amphetamine, which had potent EEG arousal effects, has a relatively low DAT binding affinity, suggesting that other mechanisms, most probably monoamine releasing effects or monoamine oxidase inhibition, are also involved. In contrast, there was no significant correlation between in vivo EEG arousal effects and in vitro NE transporter binding affinities for DA and NE uptake inhibitors. These results suggest that presynaptic enhancement of DA transmission is the key pharmacologic property mediating the EEG arousal effects of most wake-promoting CNS stimulants. **C,** In vitro NE transporter (NET) binding was performed using [³H]-nisoxetine. A significant correlation between in vivo potencies on the REM/SWS and in vitro affinity to the NET suggests that presynaptic modulation of NE transmission is important for the pharmacologic control of REM sleep. This may explain why most monoamine uptake inhibitors and monoamine-oxidase inhibitors strongly reduce REM sleep in humans and experimental animals.

amineptine), NE (nisoxetine and desipramine), or both the DA and NE (mazindol and nomifensine) transporters, as well as amphetamine and a nonamphetamine stimulant modafinil, were studied to dissect wake-promoting mechanisms.[9] The results indicate that prototypical DA uptake inhibitors such as GBR12909 and bupropion dose-dependently increased EEG arousal in narcoleptic dogs, while nisoxetine and desipramine, two potent NE uptake inhibitors, had no effect on EEG arousal at doses that almost completely suppressed REM sleep and

cataplexy (Fig. 6-3).[9] Furthermore, the EEG arousal potency of various DA uptake inhibitors correlated tightly with in vitro DA transporter binding affinities, and a reduction in REM sleep correlated with in vitro NET binding affinities (see Fig. 6-3),[9] suggesting that DA uptake inhibition is critical for the EEG arousal effects of these compounds.

D-Amphetamine has a relatively low DA transporter binding affinity but potently (i.e., need for a low mg/kg dose) promotes alertness (see Fig. 6-3). It is also generally considered

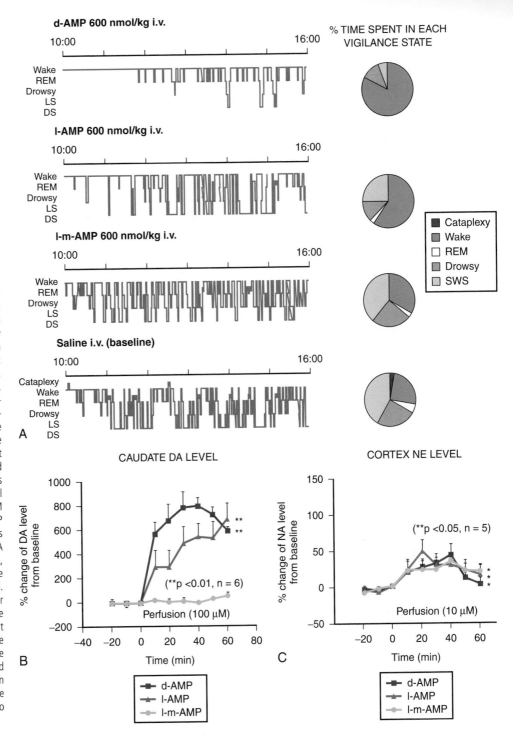

Figure 6-4 Effect of amphetamine derivatives on sleep parameters during 6-hour electroencephalographic (EEG) recordings. Typical effects of amphetamine derivatives on sleep architecture in a narcoleptic dog (600 nmol/kg IV). Local perfusion of amphetamine derivatives: effects on caudate dopamine (DA) and cortex norepinephrine (NE) levels. **A,** Representative hypnograms with and without drug treatment are shown. Recordings lasted for 6 hours, beginning at approximately 10 AM. Vigilance states are shown in the following order from top to bottom: cataplexy, wake, REM sleep, drowsy, light sleep (LS), and deep sleep (DS). The amount of time spent in each vigilance stage (expressed as % of recording time) is shown on the right side of each hypnogram. D-amphetamine (D-AMP) was found to be more potent than L-amphetamine (L-AMP), and L-methamphetamine (L-m-AMP) was found to be the least potent, while all isomers equipotently reduced REM sleep. **B,** Local perfusion of D-AMP (100 µM) raised DA levels eight times above baseline. L-AMP also increased DA levels up to seven times above baseline, but this level was obtained only at the end of the 60-minute perfusion period. L-m-AMP did not change DA levels under these conditions. **C,** In contrast, all three amphetamine isomers had equipotent enhancements on NE release. These results suggest that the potency of these derivatives on EEG arousal correlated well with measurements of DA efflux in the caudate of narcoleptic dogs, while effects on NE release may be related to REM suppressant effects.

more efficacious (i.e., can produce more alertness with high dose) than pure DAT reuptake inhibitors in promoting wakefulness. The DA releasing effects of amphetamine are likely to explain the unusually high potency and efficacy of amphetamine in promoting EEG arousal.

In vitro studies have demonstrated that the potency and selectivity for enhancing release or inhibiting uptake of DA and NE vary between amphetamine analogs and isomers.[10] Amphetamine derivatives thus offer a unique opportunity to study the pharmacologic control of alertness in vivo. To dissect wake-promoting effects of amphetamine, the effects of various amphetamine analogs (D-amphetamine, L-amphetamine, and

L-methamphetamine) on EEG arousal and in vivo effects on brain extracellular DA levels were compared using narcoleptic dogs.[11] In canine narcolepsy, D-amphetamine is 3 times more potent than L-amphetamine, and 12 times more potent than L-methamphetamine in increasing wakefulness and reducing slow wave sleep (Fig. 6-4).[11]

Microdialysis experiments in the same narcoleptic dogs suggest that wake-promoting effects of amphetamine derivatives correlate well with their effects on dopamine efflux (i.e., intracellular concentration, a net effect of dopamine release and dopamine uptake block). The local perfusion of D-amphetamine raised DA levels nine times above baseline (see Fig. 6-4).[11]

L-Amphetamine also increased DA levels by up to seven times, but maximum DA level was only obtained at the end of the 60-minute perfusion period. L-Methamphetamine did not change DA levels under these conditions. NE was also measured in the frontal cortex during perfusion of amphetamine analogs. Although all compounds increased NE efflux, no significant difference in potency was detected among the three analogs.

The fact that the potency of amphetamine derivatives on EEG arousal correlates with effects on DA efflux in the caudate of narcoleptic dogs further confirms that the enhancement of DA transmission by presynaptic modulation mediates the wake-promoting effects of amphetamine analogs. This result is also consistent with data obtained with DA transporter blockers (see Fig. 6-3). Considering the fact that other amphetamine-like stimulants, such as methylphenidate and pemoline, also inhibit DA uptake and enhance release of DA, presynaptic enhancement of DA transmission is likely to be the key pharmacologic property mediating wake-promotion for all amphetamines and amphetamine-like stimulants. In contrast, there is little evidence that enhancing adrenergic transmission is wake promoting in animal studies.

The role of the DA system in sleep regulation was further assessed using mice, which genetically lacked the DAT gene. Consistent with a role of DA in the regulation of wakefulness, these animals have reduced NREM sleep time and increased wakefulness consolidation (independently from locomotor effects).[12] The most striking finding was that DAT knockout mice were completely unresponsive to the wake-promoting effects of methamphetamine, GBR12909, and modafinil. These results further confirm the critical role of DAT in mediating the wake-promoting effects of amphetamines and modafinil (see Figs. 6-3 and 6-4)[12] (see also modafinil discussion). Interestingly, DAT knockout animals were also found to be more sensitive to caffeine,[12] suggesting functional interactions between adenosinergic and DA systems in the control of sleep and wakefulness.

Anatomic Targets Mediating Dopaminergic Effects on Wakefulness

Anatomic studies have demonstrated two major subdivisions of the ascending DA projections from mesencephalic DA nuclei (ventral tegmental area [VTA, A10], substantia nigra [SN, A9], and retrorubral nucleus [A8]): One is the mesostriatal system, which originates in the SN (and in part from the VTA) and retrorubral nucleus and terminates in the dorsal striatum (principally the caudate and putamen).[13] The other is the mesolimbocortical DA system, which consists of the mesocortical and mesolimbic DA systems. The mesocortical system originates in the VTA and the medial SN and terminates in the limbic cortex (medial prefrontal, anterior cingulate, and entorhinal cortices). Interestingly, DA reuptake is of physiologic importance for the elimination of DA in cortical hemispheres, limbic forebrain, and striatum, but not in midbrain DA neurons.[14] It is thus possible that amphetamine, modafinil, and DA uptake inhibitors induce wakefulness acting on DA terminals of the cortical hemispheres, limbic forebrain, and striatum. Local perfusion experiments of DA compounds in rats and canine narcolepsy have suggested that the VTA, but not the SN, is critically involved in EEG arousal regulation.[15] DA terminals of the mesolimbocortical DA system may thus be

important in mediating wakefulness after DA-related CNS stimulant administration. The involvement of other, less studied dopaminergic cell groups, such those located in the hypothalamus or in the ventral periaqueductal gray (recently suggested to be wake active[16]), is also possible and would be worthy of further exploration.

Dopamine agonists and L-dopa (dopamine precursor) drugs typically used in the therapy of Parkinson's disease are generally not strongly wake-promoting in clinical practice, but rather mildly sedative. It has been explained by the primary presynaptic effect of these compounds at low dose, an effect that may in fact reduce DA transmission in some projection areas.[17]

Uses

Amphetamine and methylphenidate are primarily indicated for narcolepsy and ADHD. Other therapeutic uses are controversial, because of their abuse potential. This potential also imparts to them a schedule II classification under the Controlled Substances Act of 1970. Moreover, certain states (e.g., Wisconsin) have passed even more restrictive legislation limiting the access and the use of these substances.[18] The use of these compounds is highly regulated by federal policy and in some states requires triplicate prescription and monthly renewal.

Side Effects and Toxicity

Amphetamine releases not only DA but also NE. NE indirectly stimulates α- and β-adrenergic receptors, a profile common to all indirectly acting sympathomimetic compounds. This results in significant cardiovascular effects.[19] α-Adrenergic stimulation produces vasoconstriction, thereby increasing both systolic and diastolic blood pressure. Heart rate may slightly slow down in reflex at low dose, but with large doses, tachycardia and cardiac arrhythmias may occur. Cardiac output is not modulated by therapeutic doses, and cerebral blood flow is unchanged. In general, smooth muscles respond to amphetamine as they do to other sympathomimetic drugs. There is a contractile effect on the urinary bladder sphincter.[19] Pain and difficulty in micturition may occur. Methamphetamine (and to a lesser extent amphetamine) can be neurotoxic at high dose. In dopaminergic neurons, the neurotoxicity is mediated by the formation of peroxynitrite.[20]

Common side effects occurring during long-term treatment in narcolepsy include irritability, headache, bad temper, and profuse sweating (reported by over one third of subjects). Less common side effects include anorexia, gastric discomfort, nausea, talkativeness, insomnia, orofacial dyskinesia, nervousness, palpitations, muscle jerking, chorea, and tremor. Psychiatric symptoms such as delusions or hallucinations may also occur, but are rather rare in narcoleptic patients who receive amphetamine.

The side effect profile of methylphenidate is similar to that of amphetamine and includes nervousness, insomnia, and anorexia, as well as dose-related systemic effects such as increased heart rate and blood pressure. Methylphenidate overdose may lead to seizures, dysrhythmias, or hyperthermia. For common side effects of CNS stimulant drugs for EDS, refer to Table 6-1.

Abuse and Misuse of Amphetamine Stimulants

Methamphetamine, amphetamine, and methylphenidate all have clear street value for abusers. Whereas reinforcement occurs in the early stages of drug use, tolerance is common during long-term administration. Appetite-suppressing effects are also common. Interestingly, anecdotal data suggest that psychostimulant abuse in narcoleptic subjects is extremely rare,[21,22] a finding also supported by some animal data.[23] Nevertheless, there is a negative stigma associated with the administration of amphetamine-like compounds in patients with narcolepsy. The mechanisms underlying abuse of amphetamine-like stimulants are complex but have been shown to primarily involve stimulation of the VTA-DA systems.[24] Downstream changes in adrenergic and serotoninergic systems, particularly via α_{1b}-adrenergic and 5-HT$_{2a}$ receptor, may also be important.[25,26]

Drug-Drug Interactions

Drug-drug interactions with amphetamine and methylphenidate are generally pharmacodynamic/neurochemical in nature.[27] Small percentages of amphetamine and methylphenidate are metabolized by cytochrome P-450 (CYP) 2D6. Theoretically, drugs that are competitively metabolized by CYP2D6 or that inhibit CYP2D6 can increase plasma levels of amphetamine. This action is, however, rarely a significant problem with therapeutic doses. Tricyclic drugs competitively inhibit the metabolism of amphetamine and amphetamine-like stimulants and enhance their behavioral effects. The combination of amphetamine with tricyclics could theoretically increase blood pressure (because of the combined effects of NE reuptake and release), but in practice amphetamine 10 to 16 mg (and methylphenidate 10-60 mg, mazindol 2-12 mg), have been safely given with imipramine and clomipramine 10 to 100 mg to treat narcolepsy-cataplexy.[19] The dosage of amphetamine required to control narcolepsy may be reduced by a third by the simultaneous use of tricyclic drugs. MAO-A inhibitors (e.g., nialamide, pargyline, and tranylcypromine) inhibit the metabolism of amphetamine by liver, and greatly potentiate the behavioral effects of amphetamine. Co-administration of MAO inhibitors and amphetamine derivatives is contraindicated. In contrast to tricyclic drugs and MAO-A inhibitors, haloperidol, reserpine, and atropine have no effect on amphetamine hydroxylation in the animal liver, although they may reduce the central effects of amphetamine.[28] Chlorpromazine, trifluoperazine, perfenazine and thioproperazine increase the half-life of amphetamine in the brain, but inhibit central behavioral effects, such as stereotypical behavior in animals and euphoria in humans.[28] Hypnotic drugs will prevent many behavioral effects of amphetamines, although chlordiazepoxide and diazepam increase amphetamine tissue levels.[28]

Modafinil and Armodafinil

Structure and Pharmacokinetics

Racemic modafinil (2-[diphenylmethylsulfinyl]acetamide, Fig. 6-1) was first developed in France and has been available in Europe since 1986. Modafinil was first approved in 1998 in the United States for the treatment of narcolepsy. More recently, it has been approved for shift-work sleep disorder (SWSD) and for residual sleepiness in treated patients with the obstructive sleep apnea syndrome (OSAS).

Modafinil is rapidly absorbed but slowly cleared. It is approximately 60% bound to plasma proteins and a V_D of 0.8 L/kg, suggesting that the compound is readily able to penetrate into tissues. Its half-life is 9 to 14 hours. Up to 60% of modafinil is converted into inactive metabolites, modafinil acid and modafinil sulfone. Metabolism primarily occurs via CYP3A4/CYP3A5, but the compound has also been reported to induce CYP2C19 in vitro.[29] Modafinil is currently available as a racemic mixture of two active isomers and as an *R*-isomer only preparation (Armodafinil). The *R*-enantiomer of modafinil has a half-life of 10 to 15 hours, which is longer than that of the *S*-enantiomer (3-4 hours).[30]

Uses

Modafinil is one of the few compounds that have been specifically developed for the treatment of narcolepsy. Early clinical trials in France and Canada showed that 100 to 300 mg modafinil is effective in improving EDS in narcolepsy and hypersomnia without interfering with nocturnal sleep, but that it has limited efficacy on cataplexy and other symptoms of abnormal REM sleep.[31-33] Pharmacologic experiments in canine narcolepsy also demonstrated that modafinil has no effects on cataplexy, but it significantly increases time spent in wakefulness.[34] A double-blind trial of 283 narcoleptic subjects in 18 centers in the United States revealed that 200 mg and 400 mg of modafinil significantly reduced EDS and improved patients' overall clinical condition.[35]

Armodafinil was approved by the FDA in June 2007 for the treatment of excessive sleepiness in association with narcolepsy, effectively treated obstructive sleep apnea syndrome, and shift work sleep disorder (i.e. for the same indications as those of racemic modafinil).[30] At steady state, armodafinil produces higher plasma drug concentrations late in the day than modafinil when compared on a milligram-to-milligram basis. In addition, a preliminary study with healthy volunteers who were administered armodafinil during the course of their usual night noted that armodafinil improved the ability to sustain wakefulness for a longer time throughout the night.[36,37] Nevertheless, direct comparisons between modafinil and armodafinil still need to be performed to demonstrate differences in efficacy across time in clinical populations.

Besides the FDA-approved indications for modafinil and armodafinil, several preliminary reports have suggested that modafinil may also be effective for the treatment of ADHD, fatigue in multiple sclerosis, and EDS in myotonic dystrophy.[38,39]

Side Effects

Modafinil is well tolerated. The most frequent side effects reported are headache and nausea.[38] In addition, modafinil should be used at lower doses in hepatic dysfunction because of its hepatic metabolism. Caution is needed in patients with severe renal insufficiency because of substantial increases in levels of modafinil acid, although dosage recommendations in such patients cannot be made.[39] Modafinil also has a number of potential drug interactions. The most substantive interactions observed in clinical studies were with ethinylestradiol and triazolam, apparently through induction of CYP3A4, primarily in the gastrointestinal system. For this reason, it is recommended that women taking low estrogen contraception use alternative or concomitant methods of contraception during the use of modafinil, and for 1 month after its discontinuation.[40] Interestingly, modafinil has been shown to be well tolerated, and to have additive effects on alertness, when administered with sodium oxybate in narcolepsy.[41] Rare cases of serious rash, including Stevens-Johnson syndrome, requiring hospitalization and discontinuation of treatment have been reported in adults and children in association with the use of modafinil.[40] Therefore, modafinil should be discontinued at the first sign of rash, unless the rash is clearly not drug-related. Other rare side effects include multiorgan hypersensitivity and angioedema.

Several factors make modafinil an attractive alternative to amphetamine-like stimulants. First, clinical studies have shown no significant changes in mean heart rate or systolic and diastolic blood pressure in patients receiving modafinil, although the requirement for antihypertensive medication was slightly greater in patients receiving modafinil compared to placebo.[40] In addition, clinical studies have shown small, but consistent, increases in average values for mean systolic and diastolic blood pressure and average pulse rate in patients receiving armodafinil, and a slightly greater proportion of patients on armodafinil required new or increased use of antihypertensive medications.[42] Therefore, increased monitoring of blood pressure may be appropriate in patients on these compounds. Second, data obtained to date suggest that dependence is limited in humans with this compound,[31,43] although a recent animal study suggests cocaine-like discriminative stimulus and reinforcing effects of modafinil in rats and monkeys. Modafinil is not "liked" by cocaine or stimulant abusers, and does not have a high street value. Third, modafinil has minimal effects on the neuroendocrine system. In a study of healthy volunteers who were sleep-deprived for 36 hours, those who received modafinil did not differ from those who did not with respect to cortisol, melatonin, and growth hormone levels.[44] Fourth, clinical experience suggests that the pharmacologic profiles of modafinil might be qualitatively different from those observed with amphetamine.[31] In general, patients feel less irritable and less agitated with modafinil than with amphetamines[31] and do not experience severe rebound hypersomnolence (seen in patients treated with amphetamine) after modafinil is eliminated. This differential profile is substantiated by animal experiments.[34,45] This profile contrasts with the intense recovery sleep observed after amphetamine-induced wakefulness.[46] The safety profile of modafinil is likely the basis for the fact that it has replaced amphetamine-like stimulants as a first-line treatment for EDS in narcolepsy.[35]

Mechanism of Action

The mechanism of action of modafinil/armodafinil is the subject of controversy, although, in our opinion, it is, as in the case of other stimulants, most likely related to DAT inhibition. Because there are a limited number of studies addressing the mode of action of armodafinil, this section will mostly discusses the actions of the racemic modafinil mixture. Modafinil/armodafinil has not been shown to bind to or inhibit receptors or enzymes for most known neurotransmitters, with

the exception of the DAT protein.[9,47] In vitro, modafinil/armodafinil binds to the DAT and inhibits dopamine reuptake.[9,30,47] These binding inhibitory effects have been shown to be associated with increased extracellular DA levels in the striatum of rats and dogs, suggesting functional effects. Finally, most important, modafinil's effects on alertness are entirely abolished in mice without the DAT protein,[12] and in animals lacking D_1 and D_2 receptors.[48] Given these similarities in mechanism to other DAT inhibitors, it is puzzling that modafinil has a low potential for abuse.

Clinical observations provide strong evidence that modafinil is not primarily an adrenergic compound. Amphetamine and adrenergic reuptake blockers cause dilation of the pupils by increasing NE signaling, but modafinil has no effect on pupil size. Heart rate and blood pressure changes have been modest (see the section of "Side effects"); in contrast, adrenergic reuptake blockers are well known to slightly increase blood pressure and heart rate. These clinical observations suggest that at usual clinical doses, modafinil may not increase adrenergic signaling in humans.

Interestingly, Madras and associates[49] recently reported, in a study involving rhesus monkeys undergoing positron emission tomography (PET) imaging, that modafinil intravenous (IV) occupied striatal DAT sites (5 mg/kg: 35%; 8 mg/kg: 54%). In the thalamus, modafinil occupied NET sites (5 mg/kg: 16%; 8 mg/kg: 44%). The authors also showed that modafinil inhibited [³H] dopamine (IC50 6.4 M) transport 5 times and 80 times more potently than [³H] norepinephrine (IC50 35.6 M) and [³H] serotonin (IC50 500 M) transport, respectively, in cell lines that expressed the human DAT, NET, and serotonin transporter. These data provide compelling evidence that modafinil occupies the DAT in the living brains of rhesus monkeys, consistent with the DAT hypothesis, but suggest that modafinil may also act on NET depending on drug dose, brain structure, and other physiologic conditions. Furthermore, a recent human PET study in 10 healthy humans with [¹¹C] cocaine (DAT radioligand) and [¹¹C] raclopride (D_2/D_3 radioligand sensitive to changes in endogenous dopamine) also demonstrated that modafinil (200 mg and 400 mg given orally) decreased [¹¹C] cocaine binding potential in caudate (53.8%, $P < 0.001$), putamen (47.2%, $P < 0.001$), and nucleus accumbens (39.3%, $P = 0.001$),[50] the results being consistent with the DAT hypothesis. In addition, modafinil also reduced [¹¹C] raclopride binding potential in caudate (6.1%, $P = 0.02$), putamen (6.7%, $P = 0.002$), and nucleus accumbens (19.4%, $P = 0.02$), suggesting the increases in extracellular dopamine were caused by DAT blockades.[50] The authors also pointed out the potential for abuse potency of modafinil because drugs that increase dopamine in the nucleus accumbens have this potency.

MAZINDOL

Mazindol is a schedule IV controlled drug and is rarely used in the United States. At 2 to 8 mg daily, mazindol produces central stimulation, a reduction in appetite, and an increase in alertness, but has little or no effect on mood or the cardiovascular system.[51] Mazindol is effective for the treatment of both EDS and cataplexy in humans[52] and in canine narcolepsy, possibly due to its blocking properties of DA and NE reuptake.[9] This compound has a high affinity for the DA and NE transporters,[9] yet interestingly this compounds has a low abuse potential. Problematically, however, mazindol often causes significant side effects including anorexia, gastrointestinal discomfort, insomnia, nervousness, dry mouth, nausea, constipation, urinary retention, and occasionally angioneurotic edema, vomiting, and tremor.

BUPROPION

Bupropion is not scheduled by the DEA. Although the selectivity for the dopamine transporter is not absolute, bupropion blocks DA uptake. Bupropion shows a weak inhibition of NE reuptake and very limited serotoninergic effects. Although not indicated for these uses, bupropion may be useful for the treatment of EDS associated with narcolepsy at 100 mg given three times per day.[9,53] It may be especially useful in cases associated with atypical depression.[53] Risk of convulsion increases dose-dependently (0.1% at 100-300 mg, and 0.4% at 400 mg).

SELEGILINE

Selegiline (L-desprenyl) is a methamphetamine derivative and a potent, irreversible, MAO-B selective inhibitor primarily used for the treatment of Parkinson's disease.[54,55] Because it is often considered as a simple MAO-B inhibitor, it is worth mentioning that selegiline is an amphetamine precursor. This compound is metabolized into L-amphetamine (20-60% in urine) and L-methamphetamine (9-30% in urine).[55]

In the canine model of narcolepsy, selegiline (2 mg/kg oral administration) was demonstrated to be an effective anticataplectic agent, but this effect was found to be mediated by its amphetamine metabolites rather than via MAO-B inhibition.[56] Several trials in human narcolepsy have demonstrated a good therapeutic efficacy of selegiline on both sleepiness and cataplexy with relatively few side effects.[57,58] Ten mg of selegiline daily has no effect on the symptoms of narcolepsy, but 20 to 30 mg improves alertness and mood, and reduces cataplexy, showing an effect comparable to D-amphetamine at the same dose. Selegiline may be an interesting alternative to the use of more classical stimulants, as its potential for abuse has been reported to be very low.

ATOMOXETINE AND REBOXETINE

Atomoxetine and reboxetine (in Europe) are selective adrenergic reuptake inhibitors. Both compounds were developed as antidepressants, but atomoxetine is now mainly used in the therapy of ADHD.[59] Although these compounds are not stimulants per se, they are slightly wake-promoting[60,61] and reduce REM sleep. These compounds can be helpful in some cases of narcolepsy and idiopathic hypersomnia. Atomoxetine needs twice daily administration due to its short half-life. Reboxetine was shown to reduce mean sleep latency in narcoleptic patients.[61] These compounds, however, increase heart rate and blood pressure. Sexual side effects are also common, but there is no risk of abuse.

CAFFEINE

Caffeine is probably the most popular and widely consumed CNS stimulant in the world. Tea, cola drinks, chocolate, and cocoa all contain significant amounts of caffeine. An average cup of coffee contains 50 to 150 mg of caffeine. Caffeine can also be available over the counter (OTC) (NoDoz, 100 mg caffeine; Vivarin, 200 mg caffeine), and is commonly used by narcoleptic patients prior to diagnosis.

Taken orally, caffeine is rapidly absorbed. The half-life of caffeine is 3.5 to 5 hours. The behavioral effects of caffeine include increased mental alertness, a faster and clearer flow of thought, wakefulness, and restlessness.[62] Fatigue is reduced and sleep onset delayed. The physical effects of caffeine include palpitations, hypertension, increased gastric acid secretion, and increased urine output.[62] Heavy consumption (12 or more cups of coffee a day, or 1.5 g of caffeine) causes caffeine intoxication, evidenced by agitation, anxiety, tremors, rapid breathing, and insomnia.[62]

Adenosine has been proposed to be a sleep-promoting substance both accumulating in the brain during prolonged wakefulness[63] and possessing neuronal inhibitory effects. In animals, sleep can be induced after administration of adenosine A_1 receptors (A_{1R}) or A_{2A} receptors (A_{2AR}) agonist. The mechanism of action of caffeine on wakefulness involves nonspecific adenosine receptor antagonism. In particular, Huang and colleagues[64] recently reported that wake-promotion effects of caffeine is abolished in A_{2AR} knockout mice, while the effects were not altered in A_{1R} knockout mice, suggesting a primary effect of caffeine through the A_{2AR}, at least in this species.

Caffeine is metabolized into three active metabolites, paraxanthine, theobromine, and theophylline. We recently demonstrated that paraxanthine significantly promoted wakefulness and proportionally reduced NREM and REM sleep in both control and narcoleptic mice.[56] The wake-promoting potency of paraxanthine (100 mg/kg orally) is greater than that of the parent compound, caffeine (92.8 mg/kg orally), and comparable to that of modafinil (200 mg/kg orally). High doses of caffeine and modafinil induced hypothermia and reduced locomotor activity, but paraxanthine did not. In addition, behavioral tests revealed that the compound possessed lesser anxiogenic effects than caffeine. Although further evaluation in humans should be needed, paraxanthine may be a better wake-promoting agent for normal individuals as well as for patients suffering hypersomnia associated with neurodegenerative diseases.

FUTURE STIMULANT TREATMENTS

Hypocretin-Based Therapies

Hypocretin deficiency is a main cause of human narcolepsy. Intracerebroventricular injections of hypocretin strongly promote wakefulness in dogs, mice, and rats. Animal experiments using ligand-deficient narcoleptic dogs show that very high systemic doses are required for hypocretin to penetrate the CNS, and that only a short-lasting therapeutic effect is observed after intravenous administration of hypocretin. Stable and centrally active hypocretin analogs (possibly nonpeptidic synthetic hypocretin ligands) after peripheral administration will need to be developed.[65,66] Studies have also noted a normalization of the sleep-wake patterns and behavioral arrest episodes (equivalent to cataplexy and REM sleep onset) in hypocretin-deficient mice following the central administration of hypocretin-1.[67] Hypocretin may, therefore, one day prove to be effective in the treatment of both EDS (i.e., fragmented sleep-wake pattern) and cataplexy. Such studies also open the door to the possibility of cell transplantation-based and gene-based therapies.

To address whether hypocretin receptor function is intact after long-term hypocretin deficiency, Mishima and associates[68] recently studied hypocretin receptor gene expressions of ligand-deficient narcolepsy in mice, dogs, and humans. A substantial decline (by 50-71%) in the expression of hypocretin receptor genes was observed in ligand-deficient humans and dogs. Similar murine studies suggested that this decline is progressive over age. Importantly, however, about 50% of baseline expression was still observed in old ligand-deficient narcoleptic human subjects. Further, because narcoleptic Dobermans heterozygous for the hypocretin receptor 2 mutation (with 50% receptor levels and normal levels of hypocretin) are asymptomatic, it is likely that an adequate ligand supplementation will prevent narcolepsy in hypocretin-deficient patients even if receptors are partially nonfunctional.

Histaminergic H₃ Antagonists

Histamine has long been implicated in the control of vigilance, as H_1 antagonists are strongly sedative. The excitatory effects of hypocretins on the histaminergic system via hypocretin receptor 2 are likely to be important in mediating the wake-promoting properties of hypocretin.[69] In fact, brain histamine levels are reduced in narcoleptic dogs.[70] Reduction of histamine levels is also observed in human narcolepsy and other hypersomnias of central origin.[71,72] Although centrally injected histamine or histaminergic H_1 agonists promote wakefulness, the systemic administration of these compounds induces various unacceptable side effects via peripheral H_1 receptor stimulation. In contrast, the histaminergic H_3 receptors are regarded as inhibitory autoreceptors and are enriched in the CNS. H_3 antagonists enhance wakefulness in normal rats and cats[73] and in narcoleptic mice models.[74] Histaminergic H_3 antagonists might be a useful as wake-promoting compounds for the treatment of EDS or as cognitive enhancers and are being studied by several pharmaceutical companies.[75]

Thyrotropin-Releasing Hormone

Another possible avenue of treatment, though one that currently enjoys less interest by pharmaceutical companies, is the use of thyrotropin-releasing hormone (TRH) direct or indirect agonists. TRH itself is a small peptide, which penetrates the blood-brain barrier at very high doses. Small molecules with agonistic properties and increased blood-brain barrier penetration have been developed (i.e., CG3703, CG3509, or TA0910), thanks, in part, to the small nature of the starting peptide.[76] TRH (at the high dose of several mg/kg) and TRH agonists increase alertness, have been shown to be wake-promoting and anticataplectic in the narcoleptic canine model,[77,78] and have excitatory effects on motor neurons. Initial studies demonstrated that TRH enhances DA and NE neurotransmission and that these properties may partially contribute to the wake-promoting and anticataplectic effects of TRH. Interestingly, recent studies have suggested that TRH may promote wakefulness by directly interacting with the thalamocortical network; TRH itself and TRH type 2 receptors are abundant in the reticular thalamic nucleus. Local application of TRH in the thalamus abolishes spindle wave activity,[79] and in the slice preparations, TRH depolarized thalamocortical and reticular/perigenuculate neurons by inhibition of leak K^+ conductance.[79]

Locomotor activation by TRH injected in the lateral hypothalamus induced locomotor activation in mice, but this effect was attenuated in hypocretin knockout mice, suggesting that the stimulant effects of TRH are partially mediated by stimulation of hypocretin neurons.[80] TRH also excites the histaminergic tuberomammillary nucleus.[81] Considering that TRH provokes arousal from hibernation,[82] TRH may be a potentially important wake-promoting system, although further studies are needed to disclose the roles of TRH in sleep-wake regulation.

Glutamatergic Compounds

Glutamatergic transmission is the major excitatory transmission of the mammalian brain and is increasingly believed to play a role in the generation of sleep homeostasis through changes in cortical synaptic plasticity.[83] Not surprisingly, therefore, compounds that are allosteric modulators of glutamatergic transmission, the ampakines, are being developed as wake-promoting compounds, and may have counteracting effects on sleep deprivation.[84] Similarly, GluR subtype specific compounds are likely to regulate sleep based on available knockout data and pharmacologic experiments.[85,86]

SUMMARY

Amphetamine-like stimulants have been used in the treatment of narcolepsy and various other conditions for decades, yet only recently has the mode of action of these drugs on vigilance been characterized. In almost all cases, the effects on vigilance were found to be mediated via effects on the DA transporter, DAT, leading to the widely accepted notion that the wake-promoting effects of these agents cannot be disentangled from their abuse potential. Importantly, however, the various medications available have differential effects and potency on the DA transporter and on monoamine storage and release. The various available stimulants are more or less selective for dopamine versus other amines. Although much work remains to be done in this area, it appears more and more likely that other properties (e.g., the ability to release DA rather than simply block reuptake), plus the combined effects on other monoamines (such as serotonin), may be important to explain abuse potential. Differential binding properties on the DAT transporter itself may also be involved, together with drug potency and compound solubility. The lack of solubility of some low potency compounds may, for example, result in an inability to administer the drug via snorting or intravenously. Finally, lower abuse potential for these compounds has long been suspected in narcolepsy-cataplexy patients, either because of the biochemical hypocretin abnormality, or because of the social aspects of treating narcolepsy as a disease.

The mode of action of modafinil remains controversial and probably involves dopaminergic rather than nondopaminergic effects. Whatever its mode of action is, the compound is generally found to be safer and to have a lower abuse potential than amphetamine stimulants. Its favorable side effect profile has led to an increasing use outside the narcolepsy indication, most recently in the context of shift work disorder and residual sleepiness in treated sleep apnea patients. This recent success exemplifies the need for developing novel wake-promoting compounds with low abuse potential. A need for treating daytime sleepiness extends well beyond the relatively rare indication of narcolepsy-cataplexy.

REFERENCES

1. Thorpy MJ, ed. *Handbook of Sleep Disorders, Central nervous system stimulant drugs,* 1st ed, 1990:755-778

2. Yoss RE, Daly DD. Treatment of narcolepsy with ritalin. *Neurology.* 1959;9:171-173.

3. Bradley C, Bowen M. Amphetamine (benzedrine) therapy of children's behavior disorders. *Am J Orthospychiatry.* 1941;11:92-103.

4. Anders TF, Ciaranello RD. Pharmacologic treatment of minimal brain dysfunction syndrome. In: Barchas JD, Berger PA, Ciaranello RD, eds. *Psychopharmacology: From Theory to Practice.* New York: Oxford University Press; 1977:425-435.

5. Glennon RA. Psychoactive phaenylisopropylamines. In: Meltzer HY, ed. *Psychopharmacology: The Third Generation of Progress.* New York: Raven; 1987:1627.

6. Hartmann A, Cravens J. Sleep: Effect of *d-* and *l-*amphetamine in man and rat. *Psychopharmacology.* 1976;50:171-175.

7. Kuczenski R, Segal DS. Neurochemistry of amphetamine. In: Cho AK, Segel DS, eds. *Psychopharmacology, Toxicology and Abuse.* San Diego: Academic Press; 1994:81-113.

8. Nishino S, Mignot E. Pharmacological aspects of human and canine narcolepsy. *Prog Neurobiol.* 1997;52(1):27-78.

9. Nishino S, Mao J, Sampathkumaran R, Shelton J, Mignot E. Increased dopaminergic transmission mediates the wake-promoting effects of CNS stimulants. *Sleep Res Online.* 1998;1:49-61. Available at http://www.sro.org/1998/Nishino/49/.

10. Kuczenski R, Segal DS, Cho A, Melega W. Hippocampus norepinephrine, caudate dopamine and serotonin and behavioral responses to the stereoisomers of amphetamine and methamphetamine. *J Neurosci.* 1995;15:1308-1317.

11. Kanbayashi T, Nishino S, Honda K, Shelton J, Dement WC, Mignot E. Differential effects of D-and L-amphetamine isomers on dopaminergic trasmission: Implication for the control of alertness in canine narcolepsy. *Sleep Res.* 1997;26:383.

12. Wisor JP, Nishino S, Sora I, Uhl GH, Mignot E, Edgar DM. Dopaminergic role in stimulant-induced wakefulness. *J Neurosci.* 2001;21(5):1787-1794.

13. Björklund A, Lindvall O. Dopamine-containing systems in the CNS. In: Björklund A, Hökfelt T, eds. *Handbook of Chemical Neuroanatomy, Vol 2, Classical Transmitter in the CNS, Part I.* Amsterdam: Elsevier; 1984:55-121.

14. Nissbrandt N, Engberg G, Pileblad E. The effects of GBR 12909, a dopamine re-uptake inhibitor, on monoaminergic neurotransmission in rat striatum, limbic forebrain, cortical hemispheres and substantia nigra. *Naunyn-Schmiedeberg's Arch Pharmacol.* 1991;344:16-28.

15. Honda K, Riehl J, Mignot E, Nishino S. Dopamine D3 agonists into the substantia nigra aggravate cataplexy but do not modify sleep. *Neuro Report.* 1999;10(17):3717-3724.

16. Lu J, Jhou TC, Saper CB. Identification of wake-active dopaminergic neurons in the ventral periaqueductal gray matter. *J Neurosci.* 2006;26(1):193-202.

17. Monti JM, Monti D. The involvement of dopamine in the modulation of sleep and waking. *Sleep Med Rev.* 2007;11(2):113-133.

18. Piscopo A, ed. *The impact of prescription drug diversion control systems on medical practice and patient care.* Bethesda, MD: National Institute on Drug Abuse Technical Review Meeting; 1991.

19. Nishino S, Mignot E. CNS stimulants in sleep medicine: Basic mechanisms and pharmacology. In: Kryger MH, Roth T, Dement WC, eds. *Principles and Practice of Sleep Medicine.* 4th ed. Philadelphia: Elsevier Saunders; 2005:468-498.

20. Virmani A, Gaetani F, Imam S, Binienda Z, Ali S. The protective role of L-carnitine against neurotoxicity evoked by drug of abuse, methamphetamine, could be related to mitochondrial dysfunction. *Ann N Y Acad Sci.* 2002;965:225-232.

21. Guilleminault C, Carskadon M, Dement WC. On the treatment of rapid eye movement narcolepsy. *Arch Neurol.* 1974;30:90-93.

22. Parkes JD, Baraitser M, Marsden CD, Asselman P. Natural history, symptoms and treatment of the narcoleptic syndrome. *Acta Neurol Scand.* 1975;52:337-353.

23. de Lecea L, Jones BE, Boutrel B, Borgland SL, Nishino S, et al. Addiction and arousal: Alternative roles of hypothalamic peptides. *J Neurosci.* 2006;26(41):10372-10375.

24. Koob GF, Nestler EJ. The neurobiology of drug addiction. *J Neuropsychiatry Clin Neurosci.* 1997;9(3):482-497.

25. Drouin C, Darracq L, Trovero F, Blanc G, Glowinski J, et al. Alpha-1b-adrenergic receptors control locomotor and rewarding effects of psychostimulants and opiates. *J Neurosci.* 2002;22(7):2873-2884.

26. Salomon L, Lanteri C, Godeheu G, Blanc G, Gingrich J, Tassin JP. Paradoxical constitutive behavioral sensitization to amphetamine in mice lacking 5-HT2A receptors. *Psychopharmacology (Berl).* 2007;194(1):11-20.

27. Markowitz JS, Patrick KS. Pharmacokinetic and pharmacodynamic drug interactions in the treatment of attention-deficit hyperactivity disorder. *Clin Pharmacokinet.* 2001;40(10):753-772.

28. Parkes JD. Central nervous system stimulant drugs. In: Thorpy M, ed. *Handbook of Sleep Disorders.* New York: Marcel Dekker; 1990:755-778.

29. Robertson P, DeCory HH, Madan A, Parkinson A. In vitro inhibition and induction of human hepatic cytochrome P450 enzymes by modafinil. *Drug Metab Dispos.* 2000;28(6):664-671.

30. Nishino S, Okuro M. Armodafinil for excessive daytime sleepiness. *Drugs Today (Barc).* 2008;44(6):395-414.

31. Bastuji H, Jouvet M. Successful treatment of idiopathic hypersomnia and narcolepsy with modafinil. *Prog Neuropsychopharmacol Biol Psychiat.* 1988;12:695-700.

32. Besset A, Tafti M, Villemine E, Billiard M. Effect du modafinil (300 mg) sur le sommeil, la somnolence et la vigilance du narcoleptique. *Neurophysiol Clin.* 1993;23:47-60.

33. Boivin DB, Montplaisir J, Petit D, Lambert C, Lubin S. Effect of modafinil on symptomatology of human narcolepsy. *Clin Neuropharmacol.* 1993; 16:46-53.

34. Shelton J, Nishino S, Vaught J, Dement WC, Mignot E. Comparative effects of modafinil and amphetamine on daytime sleepiness and cataplexy of narcoleptic dogs. *Sleep.* 1995;18:817-826.

35. Randomized trial of modafinil for the treatment of pathological somnolence in narcolepsy. U.S. Modafinil in Narcolepsy Multicenter Study Group. *Ann Neurol.* 1998;43(1):88-97.

36. Dinges DF, Arora S, Darwish M, Niebler GE. Pharmacodynamic effects on alertness of single doses of armodafinil in healthy subjects during a nocturnal period of acute sleep loss. *Curr Med Res Opin.* 2006;22(1):159-167.

37. Darwish M, Kirby M, Hellriegel ET. Comparison of steady-state plasma concentrations of armodafinil and modafinil late in the day following morning administration: Post hoc analysis of two randomized, double-blind, placebo-controlled, multiple-dose studies in healthy male subjects. *Clin Drug Investig.* 2009;29(9):601-612.

38. Fry J, group TMs, eds. *A new alternative in the pharmacologic management of somnolence: A phase III study of modafinil in narcolepsy.* Miami, FL: American Neurology Association Meeting; 1996.

39. Kumar R. Approved and investigational uses of modafinil: An evidence-based review. *Drugs.* 2008;68(13):1803-1839.

40. *Modafinil prescribing information from Cephalon (accessed October 2010).* Available at http://www.provigil.com/media/PDFs/prescribing_info.pdf.

41. Black J, Houghton WC. Sodium oxybate improves excessive daytime sleepiness in narcolepsy. *Sleep.* 2006;29(7):939-946.

42. *Armodafinil prescribing information from Cephalon (accessed October 2010).* Available at http://www.nuvigil.com/media/Full_Prescribing_Information.pdf.

43. LaGarde D, ed. *Sustained/continuous operations subgroup of the department of defense human factors engineering technical group: Program summary and abstracts from the 9th semiannual meeting, March 1990.* Pensacola, FL: Naval Aerospace Medical Research Laboratory; 1990.

44. Brun J, Chamba G, Khalfallah Y, Girard P, Boissy I, et al. Effect of modafinil on plasma melatonin, cortisol and growth hormone rhythms, rectal temperature and performance in healthy subjects during a 36 h sleep deprivation. *J Sleep Res.* 1998;7(2):105-114.

45. Edgar DM, Seidel WF, Contreras P, Vaught JL, Dement WC. Modafinil promotes EEG wake without intensifying motor activity in the rat. *Can J Physiol Pharmacol.* 1994;72:362.

46. Edgar DM, Seidel WF. Modafinil induces wakefulness without intensifying motor activity or subsequent rebound hypersomnolence in the rat. *J Pharmacol Exp Ther.* 1997;283(2):757-769.

47. Mignot E, Nishino S, Guilleminault C, Dement WC. Modafinil binds to the dopamine uptake carrier site with low affinity. *Sleep.* 1994;17:436-437.

48. Qu WM, Huang ZL, Xu XH, Matsumoto N, Urade Y. Dopaminergic D1 and D2 receptors are essential for the arousal effect of modafinil. *J Neurosci.* 2008;28(34):8462-8469.

49. Madras BK, Xie Z, Lin Z, Jassen A, Panas H, et al. Modafinil occupies dopamine and norepinephrine transporters in vivo and modulates the transporters and trace amine activity in vitro. *J Pharmacol Exp Ther.* 2006;319(2):561-569.

50. Volkow ND, Fowler JS, Logan J, Alexoff D, Zhu W, et al. Effects of modafinil on dopamine and dopamine transporters in the male human brain: Clinical implications. *JAMA*. 2009;301(11):1148-1154.

51. Parkes JD, Schachter M. Mazindol in the treatment of narcolepsy. *Acta Neurol Scand*. 1979;60:250-254.

52. Iijima S, Sugita Y, Teshima Y, Hishikawa Y. Therapeutic effects of mazindol on narcolepsy. *Sleep*. 1986;9(1):265-268.

53. Rye DB, Dihenia B, Bliwise DL. Reversal of atypical depression, sleepiness, and REM-sleep propensity in narcolepsy with bupropion. *Depress Anxiety*. 1998;7(2):92-95.

54. Golbe LI. Deprenyl as symptomatic therapy in Parkinson's disease. *Clin Neuropharmacol*. 1988;11:387-400.

55. Reynolds GP, Elsworth JD, Blau K, Sandler M, Lees AJ, Stern GM. Deprenyl is metabolized to methamphetamine and amphetamine in man. *Br J Clin Pharmacol*. 1978;6(6):542-544.

56. Nishino S, Arrigoni J, Kanbayashi T, Dement WC, Mignot E. Comparative effects of MAO-A and MAO-B selective inhibitors on canine cataplexy. *Sleep Res*. 1996;25:315.

57. Hublin C, Partinen M, Heinonen EH, Puukka P, Salmi T. Selegiline in the treatment of narcolepsy. *Neurology*. 1994;44(11):2095-2101.

58. Mayer G, Meier E, Hephata K. Selegiline hydrochloride in narcolepsy: A double-blind placebo-controlled study. *Clin Neuropharmacol*. 1995;18(4):306-319.

59. Findling RL. Evolution of the treatment of attention-deficit/hyperactivity disorder in children: A review. *Clin Ther*. 2008;30(5):942-957.

60. Bart Sangal R, Sangal JM, Thorp K. Atomoxetine improves sleepiness and global severity of illness but not the respiratory disturbance index in mild to moderate obstructive sleep apnea with sleepiness. *Sleep Med*. 2008;9(5):506-510.

61. Larrosa O, de la Llave Y, Bario S, Granizo JJ, Garcia-Borreguero D. Stimulant and anticataplectic effects of reboxetine in patients with narcolepsy: A pilot study. *Sleep*. 2001;24(3):282-285.

62. Rall TR. Central nervous system stimulants. In: Gilman AG, Goodman LS, Rall TW, Murad F, eds. *The Pharmacological Basis of Therapeutics*. 7th ed. New York: Pergamon Press; 1985:345-382.

63. Porkka-Heiskanen T, Strecker RE, Thakkar M, Bjorkum AA, Greene RW, McCarley RW. Adenosine: A mediator of the sleep-inducing effects of prolonged wakefulness. *Science*. 1997;276(5316):1265-1268.

64. Huang ZL, Qu WM, Eguchi N, Chen JF, Schwarzschild MA, et al. Adenosine A2A, but not A1, receptors mediate the arousal effect of caffeine. *Nat Neurosci*. 2005;8(7):858-859.

65. Fujiki N, Ripley B, Yoshida Y, Mignot E, Nishino S. Effects of IV and ICV hypocretin-1 (orexin A) in hypocretin receptor-2 gene mutated narcoleptic dogs and IV hypocretin-1 replacement therapy in a hypocretin ligand deficient narcoleptic dog. *Sleep*. 2003;6(8):953-959.

66. Schatzberg SJ, Barrett J, Cutter Kl, Ling L, Mignot E. Case study: Effect of hypocretin replacement therapy in a 3-year-old Weimaraner with narcolepsy. *J Vet Intern Med*. 2004;18(4):586-588.

67. Mieda M, Willie JT, Hara J, Sinton CM, Sakurai T, Yanagisawa M. Orexin peptides prevent cataplexy and improve wakefulness in an orexin neuron-ablated model of narcolepsy in mice. *Proc Natl Acad Sci U S A*. 2004;101(13):4649-4654.

68. Mishima K, Fujiki N, Yoshida Y, Sakurai T, Honda M, et al. Hypocretin receptor expression in canine and murine narcolepsy models and in hypocretin-ligand deficient human narcolepsy. *Sleep*. 2008;31(8):1119-1126.

69. Huang ZL, Qu WM, Li WD, Mochizuki T, Eguchi N, et al. Arousal effect of orexin A depends on activation of the histaminergic system. *Proc Natl Acad Sci U S A*. 2001;98(17):9965-9970.

70. Nishino S, Fujiki N, Ripley B, Sakurai E, Kato M, et al. Decreased brain histamine contents in hypocretin/orexin receptor-2 mutated narcoleptic dogs. *Neurosci Lett*. 2001;313(3):125-128.

71. Kanbayashi T, Kodama T, Kondo H, Satoh S, Inoue Y, et al. CSF histamine contents in narcolepsy, idiopathic hypersomnia and obstructive sleep apnea syndrome. *Sleep*. 2009;32(2):181-187.

72. Nishino S, Sakurai E, Nevsimalova S, Yoshida Y, Watanabe T, et al. Decreased CSF histamine in narcolepsy with and without low CSF hypocretin-1 in comparison to healthy controls. *Sleep*. 2009;32(2):175-180.

73. Lin JS, Sakai K, Vanni-Mercier G, Arrang JM, Garbarg M, et al. Involvement of histaminergic neurons in arousal mechanisms demonstrated with H3-receptor ligands in the cat. *Brain Res*. 1990;523(2):325-330.

74. Shiba T, Fujiki N, Wisor J, Edgar D, Sakurai T, Nishino S. Wake promoting effects of thioperamide, a histamine H3 antagonist in orexin/ataxin-3 narcoleptic mice. *Sleep*. 2004;27(suppl):A241-A242.

75. Parmentier R, Anaclet C, Guhennec C, Brousseau E, Bricout D, et al. The brain H3-receptor as a novel therapeutic target for vigilance and sleep-wake disorders. *Biochem Pharmacol*. 2007;73(8):1157-1171.

76. Sharif NA, To ZP, Whiting RL. Analogs of thyrotropin-releasing hormone (TRH): Receptor affinities in brain, spinal cords, and pituitaries of different species. *Neurochem Res*. 1991;16:95-103.

77. Riehl J, Honda K, Kwan M, Hong J, Mignot E, Nishino S. Chronic oral administration of CG-3703, a thyrotropin releasing hormone analog, increases wake and decreases cataplexy in canine narcolepsy. *Neuropsychopharmacology*. 2000;23(1):34-45.

78. Nishino S, Arrigoni J, Shelton J, Kanbayashi T, Tafti A, et al. Effects of thyrotropin-releasing hormone and its analogs on daytime sleepiness and cataplexy in canine narcolepsy. *J Neurosci*. 1997;17:6401-6408.

79. Broberger C, McCormick DA. Excitatory effects of thyrotropin-releasing hormone in the thalamus. *J Neurosci*. 2005;25(7):1664-1673.

80. Hara J, Gerashchenko D, Wisor JP, Sakurai T, Xie X, Kilduff TS. Thyrotropin-releasing hormone increases behavioral arousal through modulation of hypocretin/orexin neurons. *J Neurosci*. 2009;29(12):3705-3714.

81. Parmentier R, Kolbaev S, Klyuch BP, Vandael D, Lin JS, et al. Excitation of histaminergic tuberomamillary neurons by thyrotropin-releasing hormone. *J Neurosci*. 2009;29(14):4471-4483.

82. Stanton TL, Winokur A, Beckman AL. Seasonal variation in thyrotropin-releasing hormone (TRH) content of different brain regions and the pineal in the mammalian hibernator, *Citellus lateralis*. *Regul Pept*. 1982;3(2):135-144.

83. Tononi G, Cirelli C. Sleep function and synaptic homeostasis. *Sleep Med Rev*. 2006;10(1):49-62.

84. Porrino LJ, Daunais JB, Rogers GA, Hampson RE, Deadwyler SA. Facilitation of task performance and removal of the effects of sleep deprivation by an ampakine (CX717) in nonhuman primates. *PLoS Biol*. 2005;3(9):E299.

85. Joo DT, Xiong Z, MacDonald JF, Jia Z, Roder J, et al. Blockade of glutamate receptors and barbiturate anesthesia: Increased sensitivity to pentobarbital-induced anesthesia despite reduced inhibition of AMPA receptors in GluR2 null mutant mice. *Anesthesiology*. 1999;91(5):1329-1341.

86. Steenland HW, Kim SS, Zhuo M. GluR3 subunit regulates sleep, breathing and seizure generation. *Eur J Neurosci*. 2008;27(5):1166-1173.

Pharmacology of Benzodiazepine Receptor Agonist Hypnotics

TIMOTHY A. ROEHRS / CHRISTINA DIEDERICHS / THOMAS ROTH

Most of the drugs currently indicated for the treatment of insomnia in the United States are the benzodiazepine receptor agonists (BZRAs), which are recommended as first-line pharmacologic therapy for insominia.[1,2] The name of this group of drugs is derived from their recognized mechanism of action involving the occupation of benzodiazepine receptors on the γ-aminobutyric acid (GABA), type A receptor complex, resulting in the opening of chloride ion channels and facilitation of GABA inhibition. Some of these drugs have a benzodiazepine chemical structure (e.g., estazolam, flurazepam, quazepam, temazepam, triazolam) and others do not (e.g., zaleplon, zolpidem, eszopiclone). Other BZRAs that are not indicated by the Food and Drug Administration (FDA) as hypnotics are often used as hypnotics on an off-label basis. Typically, these BZRAs are indicated for anxiety. They share the same mechanism of action, but have longer durations of action, optimized for daytime anxiolytic effects. For example, when hypnotic prescription patterns in a large managed-care population were assessed over an 18-month period, 7% of patients were receiving one or more hypnotic prescriptions: 55% were for anxiolytics (e.g., alprazolam, clonazepam, and lorazepam), 25% for antidepressants, and 20% for hypnotics. [3]

This chapter reviews the mechanisms of action, pharmacokinetics, efficacy, and safety of BZRAs used to treat insomnia, both hypnotics and anxiolytics. A thorough understanding of the basic pharmacology of this group of drugs will inform the clinician regarding the potential effectiveness and the side effect profile of these drugs when used to treat insomnia. Generally, both the efficacy and safety of these drugs can be related to their mechanism of action and pharmacokinetics.

GABA AND THE CONTROL OF SLEEP AND WAKE

GABA is the major inhibitory neurotransmitter in the brain and is thought to have a major role in the control of sleep and wakefulness. Briefly, GABAergic neurons in the ascending reticular activating system, the anterior hypothalamus-preoptic area, and the basal forebrain are thought to play a critical role in the control of the processes governing sleep.[4,5] Within the reticular activating system GABAergic interneurons inhibit excitatory glutamatergic and cholinergic neurons and neurons of the thalamic reticular nucleus, which contain GABA, inhibit thalamic relay neurons that transmit afferent input to the cortex. These inhibitory postsynaptic potentials underlie the spindling and slow wave activity seen on cortical electroencephalographs (EEGs) during sleep. Projections from the ventrolateral preoptic nucleus, which contain GABA, inhibit the major ascending excitatory systems including cholinergic neurons of the pedunculopontine and laterodorsal tegmental nuclei, histaminergic neurons of the tuberomammillary nucleus, serotoninergic neurons of the dorsal raphe nucleus, and noradrenergic neurons of the locus ceruleus.

GABA acts at three receptor subtypes: $GABA_A$, $GABA_B$, and $GABA_C$.[6] The $GABA_A$ receptor is linked to chloride ion channels on the postsynaptic membrane and GABA occupation produces membrane hyperpolarization through fast inhibitory postsynaptic potentials (IPSPs). Barbiturates, benzodiazepines, and alcohol all act at the $GABA_A$ receptor. The $GABA_B$ receptor activates the second messenger system to alter both potassium and calcium ion channels, and GABA occupation at this receptor produces slow IPSPs. The muscle relaxant drug baclofen acts at $GABA_B$ receptors, and γ-hydroxybutyrate and its sodium salt, sodium oxybate, are thought to act weakly at this receptor. $GABA_C$ receptors, primarily found in the retina, comprise another class of ion channel gating receptors, but these have not been extensively explored for their therapeutic potential.

THE GABA$_A$ RECEPTOR COMPLEX

The $GABA_A$ receptor is a pentameric protein that forms the postsynaptic chloride channel and is composed of a number of classes of subunits including α_1 to α_6, β_1 to β_3, γ_1 to γ_3, δ, ε, θ, and π.[7] Usually the receptor contains an α, β, and γ subunit and the BZ site lies between the α and γ subunit (Fig. 7-1).[8] BZ occupation at this recognition site on the $GABA_A$ receptor complex acts allosterically to facilitate channel opening and chloride conduction. Thus, in the absence of GABA occupation at the receptor, the chloride channel is not opened. However, BZ agonist binding results in the opening of the chloride ion channel and the enhancement of flow of negatively charged chloride ions into the neuron, resulting in a change in the postsynaptic membrane potential. The neuron is thus rendered less likely to achieve an action potential. Through a number of genetic studies using knock-in mice and medicinal chemical studies assessing behavior in rats the functional significance of the α subunits have been identified (Table 7-1).[7] The sedative and amnestic activities of BZRAs are mediated through α_1 subunits and anxiolytic activity through α_2 and α_3 subunits.[7] The α_1 subunit also has some anticonvulsant activity and the α_2 and α_3 subunits have some mylorelaxant activity. However, studies of such differential receptor subtype activities in human subjects are limited.

The differential brain distribution of α subtypes is further supportive of the behavioral specificity of the distinct

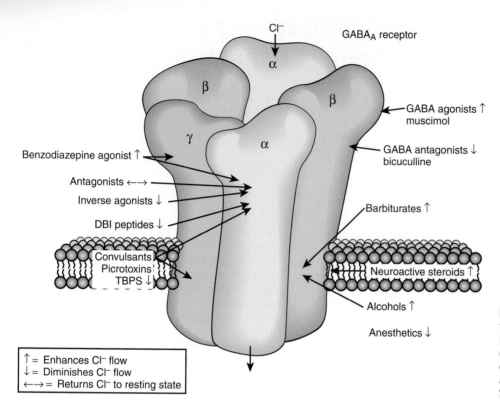

Figure 7-1 **GABA$_A$ receptor.** (Redrawn from Mendelson WB. Hypnotic medications: Mechanisms of action and pharmacologic effects. In: Kryger MH, Roth T, Dement WC, eds. *Principles and Practice of Sleep Medicine.* 4th ed. Philadelphia: Elsevier Saunders; 2005:446.)

GABA$_A$ receptor

GABA agonists ↑ muscimol

GABA antagonists ↓ bicuculline

Barbiturates ↑

Neuroactive steroids ↑

Alcohols ↑

Anesthetics ↓

Benzodiazepine agonist ↑

Antagonists ←→

Inverse agonists ↓

DBI peptides ↓

Convulsants
Picrotoxins
TBPS ↓

↑ = Enhances Cl⁻ flow
↓ = Diminishes Cl⁻ flow
←→ = Returns Cl⁻ to resting state

TABLE 7-1

GABA$_A$ Receptor Subtypes Based on Alpha Subunit

Alpha Subunit	Percentage of CNS GABA$_A$ Receptors	Known Action Mediated
α_1	60	Sedation, amnesia, partial anticonvulsant
α_2	15-20	Anxiolytic, myorelaxation
α_3	10-15	Myorelaxation (only at high doses)
α_4	<5	Insensitive to BZRAs
α_5	<5	Partial myorelaxation
α_6	<5	Insensitive to BZRAs

BZRAs, benzodiazepine receptor agonists; *CNS,* central nervous system; *GABA$_A$,* γ-aminobutyric acid class A.
Data from Rudolph U, Mohler H. GABA-based therapeutic approaches: GABA$_A$ receptor subtype functions. *Curr Opin Pharmacol.* 2006;6:18-23.

pharmacologic effects associated with a receptor subtype.[9] For example, the α_1 is distributed in the hippocampus where learning and memory are controlled. The α_1 is also distributed in the cortex and thalamus where receptor activation leads to inhibition of sensory input and results in a sedative effect.

PHARMACOKINETICS OF THE BENZODIAZEPINE RECEPTOR AGONISTS

All the BZRAs, with a hypnotic indication, reach peak plasma concentrations rapidly at approximately 60 to 90 minutes after oral ingestion. The hypnotic BZRAs were chosen for development as hypnotics due to their relatively rapid onset of effect. That is not the case for some of the nonhypnotic

BZRAs. For example, clonazepam and oxazepam reach peak plasma concentration more slowly, that is, over 1 to 4 hours. A rapid onset of effect is clearly of particular importance for insomniacs with sleep onset problems. To that end, currently, there are two additional preparations of zolpidem: sublingual and transmucosal.[10] Although the sublingual preparation has been FDA approved, it is still new to physicians and patients, as well as the field of sleep research. Sublingual zolpidem has been shown to decrease latency to persistent sleep with little or no side effects.[11,12]

The half-lives of the hypnotic BZRAs vary from ultrashort (1 hour), to short (2-5 hours), to intermediate (5-12 hours), and long (>12 hours) (Table 7-2).[13] The ultrashort half-life drug, zaleplon, has an indication for sleep onset only and is not likely to improve sleep maintenance insomnia. Some intermediate half-life drugs may have next-morning residual effects as the sedative activity of the drug extends to the waking hours. Long-acting drugs will clearly produce residual effects (see "Safety of the Benzodiazepine Receptor Agonists" for discussion of residual effects). It is important to note that the half-life does not increase in extended-release forms of zolpidem. The nonhypnotic BZRAs generally have longer half-lives as they were chosen for development to provide anxiolytic activity throughout the day and consequently will have daytime sedative effects. For the patient with insomnia coupled with anxiety disorders these longer acting drugs could be appropriate. Tolerance to the sedative effects of benzodiazepines is considered to be rapid, although tolerance to the anxiolytic effects is limited and develops more slowly, making the topic of tolerance part of a much more complex issue.[14] (See discussion of tolerance and dose escalation under "Dependence Liability" for additional information.)

Typically the BZRAs are metabolized in the liver through the cytochrome P-450 system by the CYP3A4 enzyme. Some of

TABLE 7-2

FDA-Approved Hypnotics Benzodiazepine Receptor Agonists

Drug	Dose (mg)	Half-Life ($t_{1/2}$) (hr)	Active Metabolite	Metabolism
Estazolam	1, 2	8-24	N	Oxidation
Flurazepam	15, 30	48-120	Y	Oxidation
Quazepam	7.5, 15	48-120	Y	Oxidation
Temazepam	7.5, 15, 22.5, 30	8-20	N	Conjugation
Triazolam	0.125, 0.25	2-4	N	Oxidation
Eszopiclone	1, 2, 3	5-7	N	Oxidation
Zaleplon	5, 10	~1.0	N	Oxidation
Zolpidem	5, 10	1.5-2.4	N	Oxidation
Zolpidem ER	6.25, 12.5	2.8-2.9	N	Oxidation
Zolidem Oral Spray	5, 10	1.7-8.4	N	Oxidation
Zolpidem Sublingual	5, 10	1.6-6.7	N	Oxidation

Data from Walsh JK, Roehrs T, Roth T. Pharmacologic treatment of primary insomnia. In: Kryger MH, Roth T, Dement WC, eds. Principles and Practice of Sleep Medicine. 4th ed. Philadelphia: Elsevier Saunders; 2005:751; Clinical Pharmacology [database online]. Tampa, FL: Gold Standard, Inc.; 2010. Available at http://www.clinicalpharmacology.com (accessed April 2010).

the drugs are metabolized to active compounds and others to inactive metabolites that are readily excreted (see Table 7-2). Those with active metabolites that have long half-lives can be expected to produce continued sedative effects during the daytime, and when administered nightly, plasma levels will increase. Quazepam and flurazepam are examples of drugs with active metabolites. Some of the BZRAs are not metabolized by the CYP3A4 enzyme (e.g., temazepam, lorazepam, and oxazepam), but rather by direct conjugation with glucuronic acid to inactive metabolites. This characteristic reduces the likelihood of drug-drug interactions and other side effects, an especially useful feature in patients with compromised liver function and in older adults.[15]

Drugs that either induce or inhibit the CYP3A4 enzyme have the potential to produce drug-drug interactions with the BZRAs (Box 7-1). Alcohol is known to induce liver enzymes and the consequence for any of the BZRAs is a potentially reduced hypnotic efficacy, especially in heavy alcohol drinkers. Other enzyme inducers include ethotoin, phenytoin (or fosphenytoin), barbituates, bosentan, rifamycins (e.g., rifampin, rifabutin, oxcarbazepine, and rifapentine), nevirapine, and troglitazone.[15]

CYP3A4 inhibitors that may reduce metabolism of BZRAs and hence produce greater or longer duration hypnotic effects include amiodarone, clarithromycin, cyclosporine, dalfopristin, quinupristin, delavirdine, diltiazem, efavirenz (inducer or inhibitor), erythromycin, ergotamine, fluoxetine, paroxetine, fluvoxamine, imatinib, STI-571, mifepristone, RU-486, nicardipine, probenecid, nifedipine, ranolazine, troleandomycin, verapamil, and zafirlukast, which inhibit oxidative metabolism. Antifungal agents also inhibit liver enzymes including fluconazole, itraconazole, ketoconazole, intravenous miconazole, and voriconazole. In addition, some of the antiretroviral protease inhibitors inhibit the CYP34A enzymes, and others can induce these enzymes.[15]

Pharmacodynamic drug-drug interactions are also possible. Additive effects with other sedating drugs can be anticipated, including antihistamines, antipsychotics (e.g., clozapine, molindone, olanzapine, pimozide, quetiapine, or risperidone), anticonvulsants, antiparkinsonian drugs (e.g., entacapone, pramipexole, ropinirole, and tolcapone), chloral hydrate, cannabinoids (e.g., dronabinol, THC), ethanol, general anesthetics, nabilone, opiate agonists, mixed opiate agonist/antagonists (e.g., buprenorphine, butorphanol, nalbuphine, pentazocine), phenothiazines, pregabalin, tramadol, and tricyclic antidepressants, which can potentiate the CNS effects (i.e., increased sedation or respiratory depression) of either agent.[15]

Caffeine-containing products including medications (i.e., theophylline) and dietary supplements such as guarana, kava kava, and beverages (e.g., coffee, green tea, other teas, or colas)

BOX 7-1 *Agents That May Interact with Hypnotics**

Alcohol
Anticonvulsants
Anitfungal agents
Antihistamines
Anitconvulsant drugs
Antipsychotics
Antiretroviral protease inhibitors
Barbiturates
Benzodiazepines
Caffeine and certtain beverages (e.g., tea, green tea)
Cannabinoids
Cytochrome P-450 (CYP) 3A4 inhibitors not listed
Ephedrine and pseudoephedrine
General anesthetics
Medications for hypertension (e.g., bosentan) and other cardiovascular conditions (e.g., ranolazine)
Opiate and mixed opiate agonists
Oral contraceptives
Other drugs with sedating effects
Other hypnotics
Rifamycins
Some supplements (e.g., kava kava, St. John's wort, guarana)
Tricyclic antidepressants

*This should not be considered an exhaustive list; each patient's drug history should be reviewed carefully.
   Data from Clinical Pharmacology [database online]. Tampa, FL: Gold Standard, Inc.; 2010. Available at http://www.clinicalpharmacology.com (accessed April 2010).

may also pharmacodynamically antagonize the sedative effects of the BZRAs. Obviously, any of the psychomotor stimulant medications will produce pharamacodynamic antagonism of BZRA effects. Sometimes overlooked is the fact that various over-the-counter preparations contain ephedrine or pseudoephedrine, both having robust stimulatory effects.[15] It is important to note that not all of these interactions have been clinically demonstrated, nor are they of equal clinical importance. Many factors contribute to interactions in addition to different levels of effect. Practitioners and patients should be mindful of potential interactions ranging from current medications, supplements, and even some foods or beverages. (See www.clinicalpharmacology.com[15] for a complete listing of potential drug-drug interactions.)

HYPNOTIC EFFICACY OF THE BENZODIAZEPINE RECEPTOR AGONISTS

Benzodiazepine Receptor Agonists with a Hypnotic Indication

Assessments of hypnotic efficacy involve polysomnographic (PSG) or patient estimates of the induction or maintenance of sleep, or both. Sleep latency (whether PSG or self-report) is the standard sleep induction variable, and number of awakenings and minutes of wake after sleep onset (WASO) is the common sleep maintenance measure. Total sleep time and sleep efficiency reflect both the sleep induction and sleep maintenance properties of a given drug. The qualitative measures of efficacy that are also used include morning ratings of sleep quality, sleep depth, or global impression ratings of insomnia severity or therapeutic improvement by either an investigator or the patient. The monitoring of motor activity with a wrist-worn sensor (actigraphy) has also been used to evaluate hypnotic efficacy. A new dry electrode system that is worn as a headband (Zeo), as well as other ambulatory EEG systems, which yield estimates of total sleep time, rapid eye movement (REM) time, and non-REM (NREM) time, have not been evaluated as of yet, but may show potential for the future.

Many studies have documented the hypnotic efficacy of BZRAs using patient reports or PSG outcomes, or both.[1,2] Generally, the PSG and subjective data regarding hypnotic efficacy parallel each other across doses with subjective sleep latency reported as being longer and sleep time shorter than PSG results.[16] A meta-analysis in 1997 concluded that the benzodiazepines and zolpidem produce reliable improvements in sleep in persons with chronic insomnia, although the median duration of the studies included was only one week.[17] Other meta-analyses largely concur regarding short-term efficacy. However, the utility of these meta-analyses to assist the clinician is fairly low, because they combine data from multiple drugs with widely different pharmacokinetics. Additionally, two or more doses of a drug may be included in a given analysis. It is much more instructive to examine the strengths and weaknesses of individual drugs at any given dose as opposed to generalizing across all BZRAs at multiple doses. Clearly, higher doses are likely to produce greater efficacy, but at what cost in terms of side effects? Here, similarities among BZRAs will be discussed in terms of their risks and benefits, and important differences among drugs will be emphasized.

All of the BZRA hypnotics reduce sleep latency and most increase total sleep time. The exception is zaleplon, which does not reliably increase total sleep time. The reduction of sleep latency is attributable to a rapid onset of hypnotic effects. Specific sleep maintenance variables, distinct from total sleep time, have not commonly been emphasized until recently. Investigations assessing number of awakenings and WASO typically find that the longer the drug's duration of action (i.e., a longer half-life or higher dose will increase duration of action), the more likely it is that the drug will show efficacy on these measures.

Previous to the recent National Institutes of Health (NIH) consensus conference the indications for all FDA-approved hypnotics included limitations on duration of use (typically 2-4 weeks). It was generally assumed that tolerance developed with chronic use beyond 2 to 4 weeks.[1] However, more than 30 years ago, Oswald and colleagues[18] reported that lormetazepam and nitrazepam, two BZRAs, retained their effect during 24 weeks of use, based on patient reports of their hypnotic effects. More recently, in rigorous PSG studies the nonbenzodiazepine BZRAs, zolpidem 10 mg and zaleplon 10 mg, were shown to retain their efficacy for 5 weeks of nightly use.[19,20] Recent landmark studies of several hundred patients with primary insomnia in each study reported continued hypnotic efficacy of eszopiclone for 6 to 12 months of nightly use, although only the first 6 months were controlled.[21,22] In these studies, self-reported sleep latency, WASO, and sleep time were improved with 3 mg as compared to placebo at each monthly time point.

Given concerns for tolerance development in chronic use, the efficacy of non-nightly use of zolpidem 10 mg has been investigated for up to 12 weeks.[23,24] Additionally, improved sleep was sustained in a study conducted over a 24-week period.[25] In these studies, ratings of sleep latency, total sleep time, number of awakenings, and sleep quality were all improved on nights when zolpidem was taken, as compared with placebo. Investigators used global ratings that considered both medication nights and nonmedication nights, which indicated reduced insomnia severity with zolpidem. Total sleep time data on nights when a pill (either zolpidem or placebo) was taken immediately after a zolpidem night indicated no evidence of rebound insomnia (see "Safety of the Benzodiazepine Receptor Agonists" for further discussion of rebound insomnia).[23] In a study of the safety and efficacy of ramelton, a non-BZRA hypnotic that acts by occupation of melatonin receptors, latency to persistent sleep was reduced over a 6-month period with no next-morning residual effects or rebound insomnia.[26] Ramelton is the first melatonin-receptor agonist approved in the United States for the treatment of insomnia, and additional long-term studies are needed.

Effects on Sleep Staging

BZRAs are known to reduce stage 3-4 sleep, albeit mildly. For example, estazolam 2 mg in 35-year-old insomniacs reduced stage 3-4 from 4% to 1%.[27] Temazepam 15 mg and 30 mg reduced stage 3-4 sleep from 8% to 5% in 38-year-old insomniacs.[28] In elderly insomniacs (60-85 years), triazolam 0.125 mg had no effect on sleep stages; stage 1 was 22% and stage 3-4 was 5% on both placebo and active drug.[29] In each of the studies, however, total sleep time was increased, which in part explains the reduction in percentage of stage 3-4 in the one study. Interestingly, despite the reduction in stage 3-4 in the one study, self-reported sleep quality was improved. Additionally, in the study of elderly insomniacs in which no sleep stage changes were observed, the improved sleep time in that study was associated with an improvement in daytime alertness as measured by the multiple sleep latency test (MSLT). As these contrasting results show, it is important to be cautious in interpreting the significance of stage 3-4 changes and the biology associated with them. In humans, for example, stage 3-4 sleep is associated with the highest arousal threshold[30] and the BZRAs have been shown to increase arousal threshold, but reduce stage 3-4 sleep.

The nonbenzodiazepine RAs do not appear to consistently alter stage 3-4 sleep.[31] In one study of healthy 21- to 35-year-old normal subjects over a dose range of 2.5 to 20 mg, zolpidem did not affect stage 3-4.[16] In young insomniacs, zopiclone 5 to 15 mg only reduced stage 3-4 (9% to 4%) at the higher doses.[32] Eszopiclone 0, 1, 2, 3, and 3.5 mg also did not reduce stage 3-4 sleep relative to the 10% of the placebo group.[33] In all these studies the BZRA being assessed improved total sleep time or efficiency using self-reports of sleep quality.

To the extent that stage 1 sleep is elevated (>10%) in the insomnia population being studied, both benzodiazepine and nonbenzodiazepine RAs have been shown to reduce the percentage of stage 1 sleep, which is thought to reflect the consolidation of sleep. For example, in the same study cited previously, zopiclone 5 to 15 mg reduced stage 1 from 12% to 8%.[32] Both estazolam and temazepam have been shown to reduce stage 1 as well, from 11% and 16% to 9%.[27,28] At clinical doses, all BZRAs do not suppress REM sleep. In the zolpidem study cited previously, only the high dose (20 mg) of zolpidem, or twice the clinical dose, reduced REM sleep,[16] and in the zopiclone study REM sleep was reduced from 20% to 18%, again only at twice the clinical dose.[32]

Benzodiazepine Receptor Agonists Not Indicated as Hypnotics

Benzodiazepines, with an anxiolytic indication, have similar effects on sleep architecture and sleep efficiency, depending on the dose. Unfortunately, there are few reports of data describing the dose range for hypnotic efficacy of anxiolytics used as hypnotics, as well as the safe dose range for such effects. However, as noted in the introduction, medications other than those with indications for insomnia are utilized to treat insomnia. In a large managed-care system alprazolam was the most frequently prescribed medication for sleep, and together with other anxiolytics, accounted for 55% of all prescriptions over an 18-month period.[3]

A study comparing alprazolam 1 mg to placebo in healthy normal men found alprazolam significantly increased total sleep time and stage 2 sleep, while decreasing slow wave sleep,[34] as is often found with other hypnotic benzodiazepines. In addition, subjective assessments of sleep latency and the perceived quality of sleep were improved. However, alprazolam was also found to significantly increase REM latency and reduce the duration of REM sleep. A sleep EEG study was performed in a study of alprazolam in patients with major depressive disorder and showed decreased REM.[35] Drug administration was increased weekly from 4 mg/day to a maximum of 9 mg/day, at the physician's discretion over a 6-week period. Both mean time in bed

and total sleep time increased significantly over the 6-week period. The subjects also experienced an increase in minutes and percentage of stage 2 sleep, but again a decrease in minutes and percentage of REM was reported.

In a 1972 study, lorazepam 2 mg was assessed for its effects on sleep.[36] Nine normal subjects were studied over eight to nine nights. With the BZRA both REM and wake stages were reduced. In a study of 11 normal men, lorazepam 4 mg significantly decreased REM, whereas triazolam 0.5 mg did not.[37] Both drugs were also found to decrease stage 1, and increase stage 2, while not affecting stage 3-4.

Clonazepam 1 to 2 mg was administered over a 2-week period to six patients with combat-related posttraumatic stress disorder and sleep disturbances. The results showed no effect of clonazepam on their sleep disturbance. However, this may be due to the small sample size and the type of patient population being studied.[38] A study from 1991 found clonazepam 0.5 mg to be very effective in six insomniac subjects.[39] Total wake time was reduced and sleep efficiency was increased, while the number of awakenings was reduced after only 1 week of administration. Patients experienced an increase in stage 2 sleep but did not experience a significant change in REM sleep. Subjectively study participants rated their overall sleep more positively with clonazepam.

Although the dose range for efficacy in insomnia without REM sleep suppression is established for most of the BZRAs with a hypnotic indication, that is not the case for the BZRAs without a hypnotic indication. Although they are generally associated with improvement in both objective and subjective assessments of sleep, most studies utilizing these agents have revealed a suppression of REM sleep time. Furthermore, it is difficult to assess the relation of hypnotic effects to REM suppressive effects because these studies, unlike the hypnotic BZRA studies, did not include subjects diagnosed with any of the accepted diagnostic criteria for insomnia.

Benzodiazepine Receptor Agonists and Daytime Function

According to the *Diagnostic and Statistical Manual of Mental Disorders-IV-TR*[40] and the International Classification of Sleep Disorders revised, *Diagnostic and Coding Manual*,[41] diagnostic criteria for insomnia typically include some form of subjective daytime impairment or distress caused by the sleep disturbance. Theoretically, it should be possible to demonstrate an insomnia-related performance impairment that is then followed by a subsequent attenuation of the impairment with improved sleep. Elimination or improvement of the daytime impairment in primary insomnia patients should be concurrent to the improvement of sleep.

The demonstration of improvement in daytime function has, however, eluded investigators until the recent past, owing, in large part, to the finding that patients with primary insomnia do not demonstrate expected findings in terms of daytime sleepiness/alertness and other measures of daytime function on standard tests. Rather than showing greater daytime sleepiness, as might be expected given their disturbed and insufficient sleep, as well as reports of daytime tiredness, patients with insomnia have greater daytime alertness as reflected by longer daytime sleep latencies on the MSLT than age-matched normal subjects.[42,43] Metabolic rate, heart rate variability, body temperature, and cortisol levels also suggest a trait of hyperarousal in patients with insomnia, which is hypothesized to lead to their disrupted sleep and high MSLT sleep latencies.[43,44] Previous failures to explain this phenomenon may be due to the short duration of studies and the use of insensitive variables. Recently, however, a 6-month eszopiclone study of patients with primary insomnia demonstrated improvement in patient reports of daytime alertness, ability to function during the daytime, and physical sense of well-being in the eszopiclone group compared to the placebo group.[45] In another study, eszopiclone 3 mg relative to placebo enhanced quality of life and reduced work limitations over 6 months of treatment, improvements that were associated with a concurrent reduction of insomnia severity.[46]

The pattern of hyperarousal that is seen in primary insomnia is not evident in all types of insomnia. For example, patients with insomnia co-morbid with periodic limb movement disorder[47] or co-morbid with rheumatoid arthritis have been shown to have lower than optimal MSLT sleep latencies, which, in turn, improved significantly after six nights of treatment with triazolam.[48] A study of older adult patients showed increased daytime alertness on the MSLT resulting from increased sleep time with triazolam treatment.[49] However, these are isolated studies and research assessing the nature of the daytime impairment with a common set of metrics in insomnia populations is needed.

SAFETY OF THE BENZODIAZEPINE RECEPTOR AGONISTS

In general, BZRAs are well tolerated with few significant safety concerns. Adverse reactions recorded in clinical trials or in clinical practice are infrequent, are most commonly rated as mild, and are related to their primary pharmacologic activity, sedation. For inpatient use in a large academic hospital, the median rate of adverse events, across all hypnotics, was found to be about 1 in every 10,000 doses.[50] This assessment was derived from spontaneous reports recorded in patients' medical records. Although specific data on the frequency of abuse of hypnotic medications is not available, a study in Switzerland in the early 1980s indicated that abuse of all benzodiazepines, not limited to those used as hypnotics, occurred at the rate of only 2 per 10,000 prescriptions.[51] Specific safety issues for hypnotics are discussed in the following sections.

Amnestic Effects

One side effect, in part, related to the sedative effects of hypnotics is anterograde amnesia, memory failure for information presented after consumption of the drug. It is also associated with other hypnotics, including all the BZRAs, alcohol, and barbiturates. The extent of amnesia is related to the drug's plasma concentration at the time items for recall are presented, to the time since the drug was ingested, and to the dose ingested.[52,53] Furthermore, maintaining wakefulness for 10 to 15 minutes after presentation of memory material, rather than allowing a drug-induced rapid return to sleep, attenuates the amnesia.[54] Amnesia would be anticipated given the GABA$_A$ receptor subtype specificity of effects (see Table 7-1) and the brain distribution for the α1 receptor, as discussed earlier.

Residual Effects

Other side effects associated with BZRAs are also mediated by their primary pharmacologic activity, sedation.[55] Residual sedation, which is merely a prolongation of the hypnotic effect of the drug after sleep, results in adverse reactions such as drowsy feelings, sleepiness, and impairment in psychomotor performance. The likelihood of residual sedation is primarily determined by two factors: the elimination rate and the dose of the drug.[56] Many studies have shown differences in residual effects between short- and long-acting drugs and between different doses of the same drug using MSLT and performance assessments.

Falls and Cognitive Effects

Falls and cognitive impairment are of particular concern in the elderly, who also represent a significant proportion of hypnotic medication users.[56] Age-related physiologic changes cause changes in the pharmacokinetics and pharmacodynamics of certain drugs. This effect can cause differences in drug absorption, first-pass metabolism and bioavailability, drug distribution, as well as drug clearance.[57] Also, due to the increased prevalence of medical and neurologic disorders in older adults, the common use of concomitant medications (e.g., particularly other drugs with CNS activity; see the drug-drug interaction discussion earlier in the chapter), and the changes in drug pharmacokinetics that occur with aging, the therapeutic index for hypnotics in older adults is probably narrower than for younger adults.

Drugs that are primarily metabolized by conjugation are safer for patients who are older and for those with liver disease (see Table 7-2). In these two categories of patients, the pharmacokinetics of oxidatively metabolized drugs are altered, resulting in an increased area under the plasma concentration curve. This alteration is a consequence of increasing the peak plasma concentration for some drugs (e.g., triazolam) and of extending the duration of significant plasma levels for others (e.g., flurazepam) (Fig. 7-2). For most, hypnotic use of the lower recommended dose, especially when treating older patients, will diminish the likelihood of adverse events.[56]

Studies have demonstrated an increased risk of falls for institutionalized older adults taking BZRAs and other psychotropic medications. Results of early studies of community-dwelling older adults were inconsistent,[58-60] but recent large-scale studies suggest an elevated risk of injurious falls for seven categories of medications.[61] After controlling for co-morbid illness, the elevated risk was only significant for antidepressants (selective serotonin reuptake inhibitors and tricyclic antidepressants), anticonvulsants, and benzodiazepines. Data from another study showed that the risk for fractures was elevated for those taking narcotics and antidepressants, but was not affected by use of benzodiazepines and anticonvulsants.[62] Previous studies had indicated that long-acting sedative drugs increase the risk for falls more than short-acting drugs,[56] but recent studies have not shown the same distinction.[63] Most importantly a variety of CNS-active medications statistically increased fall rates in older adults, antidepressants often being associated with the highest rates.[64,65]

To our knowledge, the risk of falls in insomniacs taking exclusively hypnotics for insomnia, in comparison to those taking no medication, has yet to be evaluated. Furthermore,

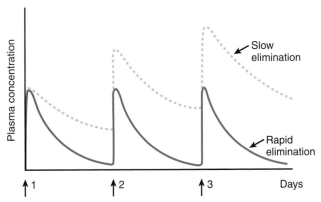

Figure 7-2 Plasma concentration. (Redrawn from Mendelson WB. Hypnotic medications: Mechanisms of action and pharmacologic effects. In: Kryger MH, Roth T, Dement WC, eds. *Principles and Practice of Sleep Medicine.* 4th ed. Philadelphia: Elsevier Saunders; 2005:448.)

studies have not differentiated among BZRAs to determine if receptor selectively affects fall risk, which would be expected if the degree of mylorelaxation impacts falls. Poor sleep, however, has been identified as a risk factor for falls in older adults. Reported sleep problems, but not psychotropic medication use, was an independent risk factor for falls in a large sample of community-dwelling adults aged 64 to 99 years.[66] Clearly, further studies are needed to determine the independent fall risk for sleep disturbance and the drugs used to treat the sleep disturbance.

Reports have claimed long-term BZRA use is associated with cognitive decline in older adults. [67] However, this is not a universal finding.[68] Additionally, these studies do not allow a firm conclusion regarding causality, since their designs were predominantly cross-sectional and retrospective, making it impossible to isolate the effects of various factors such as the aging process, co-morbid conditions, and other drugs. Cognitive changes that have been identified have been subtle,[69] and their clinical significance has been questioned.[70] Despite these areas of uncertainty, the possibility of cognitive impairment should be borne in mind by clinicians when treating the elderly with hypnotic agents and other psychotropic agents.

An elevated mortality risk has been associated with use of medications for sleep, yet the reasons for these findings remain unclear.[71,72] A number of factors limit the conclusions that can be drawn from these studies. The medications responsible for the elevated mortality risk are not constant from study to study, and in most cases the drug name or class is not known. Data from one study were collected in 1959 to 1960,[71] when barbiturates were the most commonly used hypnotics; for the second study data were collected in 1982,[72] when benzodiazepines were the most commonly used hypnotics. The studies grouped findings for prescription and nonprescription drugs, and relied on respondents' reports to identify medications taken for sleep, without regard for whether they were indicated as hypnotics or whether prescribing physicians actually intended them to be used for insomnia. In contrast, in another study in which the identities of the drugs were known, sedative-hypnotics were not associated with an increased mortality risk. Rather, "other drugs," typically analgesics, often utilized on an off-label basis for sleep, were associated with a higher mortality risk.[73] Clearly, prospective studies are needed to clarify whether hypnotic medications increase mortality risk.

Discontinuation Effects

The major discontinuation effect most frequently attributed to BZRAs is rebound insomnia. Typically, sleep is worsened, relative to the patient's baseline, for one to two nights after discontinuation. Rebound insomnia can occur following short-term use and does not increase in severity following 1 to 12 nights of repeated use.[74] There was no evidence of rebound insomnia following 6 months of treatment with zolpidem extended release 12.5 mg,[25] and after 6 months of treatment with eszopiclone 3 mg.[45] Rebound insomnia is more likely to occur following the administration of doses that are high and beyond clinical range, and following the administration of short- and intermediate-acting BZRAs.[74] Therefore, it can usually be avoided by using the lowest effective dose. It is unlikely to occur with long-acting drugs because of the inherent gradual tapering of plasma concentrations over a few nights.

One must differentiate rebound insomnia from recrudescence and from a withdrawal syndrome. Recrudescence, a return of the original symptom at its original severity, typically does not disappear with time as does rebound insomnia. Rebound insomnia is the exacerbation of an existing sleep disturbance that lasts for one to two nights. Rebound insomnia does not increase the likelihood of continued hypnotic use as shown in laboratory studies of hypnotic self-administration.[53] Patient expectancies can also play a role in the experience of rebound insomnia. Discontinuing placebo pills, that is, stopping pill-taking per se, has been found to produce a mild sleep disturbance.[75] Withdrawal syndrome refers to the emergence of a new cluster of symptoms (not present prior to treatment), which lasts several days to weeks, rather than the one or two nights characteristic of rebound, and is associated with higher doses and longer durations of use.

Dependence Liability

Drug abuse consists of two components, physical dependence and behavioral dependence.[40] Physical dependence is evident in the expression of a withdrawal syndrome when the drug is discontinued or an antagonist is administered. However, physical dependence does not necessarily indicate drug abuse or dependence. Physical dependence may be a component of behavioral dependence, but it is not a sufficient condition for it. Behavioral dependence is characterized by a recurring pattern of compulsive drug-seeking behavior and consumption, despite aversive psychosocial, legal, and medical consequences.[40]

Concerns regarding dependence on hypnotic medication are common despite minimal evidence to support them. Epidemiologic data indicate that the majority of patients (74%) use hypnotics for 2 weeks or less.[76,77] Only 14% of individuals use hypnotics nightly on a chronic basis (i.e., for months or years), but with rare dose escalation, at a rate of 8%.[78] Given the low likelihood of dose escalation or nontherapeutic use of the medication (i.e., in the absence of insomnia, or during the daytime), it is unlikely that a nightly pattern of use reflects dependence (i.e., physiologic or behavioral). Although there are some reports of physical dependence at therapeutic doses in long-term daytime use of BZRAs, there is a lack of data to support this claim for hypnotics. Studies of drug self-administration during the day, which assess the reinforcing effects of these drugs, provide further evidence that they have a low behavioral dependence liability.[79] Additional studies, specifically of the behavioral dependence liability of BZRAs used as hypnotics, have found similar results.[75,80] In double-blind, self-administration studies in insomniacs, when given an opportunity to take multiple capsules before sleep (0.125 mg triazolam or 5 mg zolpidem) dose escalation did not occur after prior short-term or long-term nightly hypnotic use.[80,81] In addition, daytime use of hypnotics (0.125 or 0.25 mg triazolam) by insomniacs (self-administration opportunities at 9 AM) was infrequent.[82] Those few insomniac patients who did take hypnotic medication during the daytime showed significant physiologic hyperarousal as seen on a MSLT.[82]

The self-administration of hypnotics in insomniac patients can be described as therapy-seeking behavior, in that it does not lead to short-term dose escalation, it infrequently generalizes to daytime use (i.e., it does not occur outside the therapeutic context), and the rate of self-administration varies as a function of the severity of the sleep problem. In fact, in a 2002 study of hypnotic self-administration by insomniacs, rate of self-administration was a function of the degree of sleep disturbance during the preceding night.[83]

The potential relation between BZRA receptor subtype affinity and dependence liability is also of research interest. To the degree that anxiolytic and mylorelaxant properties may be associated with the abuse liability of BZRAs, it is plausible to hypothesize that more selective BZRAs (i.e., those with low affinity for receptors with α_2 subunits) may have less dependence liability. Unfortunately, as yet, the hypothesis has not been tested and thus data are not yet available to support or refute this hypothesis.

Amnestic Parasomnia Episodes

Parasomnia-like activity in association with BZRA hypnotics use has been reported in public media.[84] These include "global amnesia," somnambulism, sleep driving, complex behaviors in sleep, and sleep-related eating disorder. Deriving conclusions from such reports is problematic, as they are published in venues that are not peer-reviewed, are usually not independently documented, and are thus subject to confirmation bias. It is possible, therefore, that they overrepresent the real risk.

Case reports of parasomnia-like behaviors in association with BZRA use have also appeared in the scientific-medical, peer-reviewed literature.[56] Here, too, caution is advised in interpreting the data. Although case reports do provide some information about contributing factors, they are not placebo-controlled and the relative contribution of the medication itself to these behaviors is, therefore, unknown. Additionally, the relative risk of BZRA-associated parasomnia events is unknown because the rate of exposure, as assessed by the number of prescriptions written and doses consumed (the "denominator problem") is not known. The appearance of media reports and medical publications in such controversial areas may also artificially increase the frequency at which patients report the same side effect.[85] Yet, the FDA has taken these concerns seriously enough to recommend that manufacturers insert language regarding precautions for parasomnias in the drug labeling of this class of compounds.

As noted earlier, transient global amnesia has been reported in association with the use of triazolam by otherwise healthy individuals experiencing sleep disturbance.[86] The memory loss for the autobiographical events transpired over an 8- to 12-hour period after administration of the medication. In the case reports, prior stress and sleep deprivation may have combined to produce the amnesia. Supraclinical doses and alcohol ingestion are also likely contributory factors. It is unlikely that this phenomenon is unique to triazolam, as similar kinds of amnesia are produced by the intravenous administration of other benzodiazepines.[87]

Somnambulism has been reported with zolpidem and zaleplon.[88,89] These episodes of somnambulism have occurred with two to three times the clinical doses of the drug, in individuals with a prior history of somnambulism, and in individuals with prior traumatic head injury. Zolpidem-associated somnambulism has also been reported in combination with antidepressant treatment.[90] Somnambulism is believed to be associated with partial arousals from sleep, which alcohol and sleep deprivation also exacerbate. Not surprisingly both alcohol and sleep deprivation exacerbate somnambulism.

Finally, there are case reports of sleep-related eating associated with psychotropic medications, including BZRAs.[91-93] There is a dispute as to whether sleep-related eating disorder represents a partial arousal from sleep with altered levels of consciousness or a psychiatric disorder of nocturnal eating with awareness and recall.[94,95] Zolpidem was reported to exacerbate sleep-related eating disorder and in several cases induce it de novo.[95] In some of these cases, doses greater than 10 mg zolpidem were being used and in other cases there was use of sedating antidepressants. Sleep-related eating disorder has also been reported with triazolam.[96,97]

A common thread runs through these reports—excessive sleep drive and hypnotic activity. Excessive sleep drive (e.g., very rapid sleep onset, MSLT less than 2 minutes[98]), can occur as a result of high doses, or even clinical doses utilized in vulnerable individuals (i.e., a history of various sleep disorders or brain injury), clinical or high doses combined with prior sleep deprivation due to stress or illness, or clinical or high doses combined with the prior consumption of alcohol or other CNS drugs with sedative effects. Sleep deprivation produces increased slow wave sleep during ensuing nights of sleep.[99] In turn, abrupt arousals from slow wave sleep following sleep deprivation can result in automatic behavior, complex motor activity with little memory and consciousness.[86] Sleep deprivation is known to induce somnambulism in individuals with a previous history of somnambulism.[100] Together the data raise the possibility that parasomnia reports associated with BZRAs are the result of excessive hypnotic/sedative activity in vulnerable individuals. These findings emphasize the need to ensure that patients utilizing hypnotic agents use proper sleep hygiene practices and avoid alcohol and other unnecessary sedatives and that proper dosages are utilized. Patients should also be carefully screened for co-morbid medical and psychiatric disorders and histories of parasomnia.

SUMMARY

The BZRAs act at the BZ site on the $GABA_A$ receptor complex to inhibit the major excitatory transmitter systems in the brain. Those drugs with a hypnotic indication generally have a rapid onset of effect, but differing half-lives. In numerous studies, hypnotic BZRAs have been shown to increase sleep time by producing a rapid sleep induction and, depending on pharmacokinetics, by maintaining sleep. They remain effective in chronic use and show little discontinuation effects and abuse liability when used at clinical doses. The other major side effects are generally related to their primary effect, sedation. Anxiolytic BZRAs, while often used as hypnotics, may be less desirable choices as the dose ranges for efficacy and safety in primary insomnia are unknown.

REFERENCES

1. National Institute of Health. State of the Science Conference: Manifestation and management of chronic insomnia in adults, June 13-15, 2005. *Sleep.* 2005;28(1):1049-1057.
2. American Psychiatric Association Task Force on Benzodiazepines Dependency. *Benzodiazepine Dependence, Toxicity, and Abuse.* Washington, DC: American Psychiatric Association; 1990.
3. Roehrs T, Roth T. "Hypnotic" prescription patterns in a large managed-care population. *Sleep Med.* 2004;5:463-466.
4. Jones BE. Basic mechanisms of sleep-wake states. In: Kryger MH, Roth T, Dement WC, eds. *Principles and Practice of Sleep Medicine.* 4th ed. Philadelphia: Elsevier Saunders; 2005:136-153.
5. Saper CB, Chou TC, Scammell TE. The sleep switch: Hypothalamic control of sleep and wakefulness. *Trends Neurosci.* 2001;24:726-731.
6. Foster AC, Kemp JA. Glutamate- and GABA-base CNS therapeutics. *Curr Opin Pharmacol.* 2006;6:7-17.
7. Rudolph U, Mohler H. GABA-based therapeutic approaches: GABA$_A$ receptor subtype functions. *Curr Opin Pharmacol.* 2006;6:18-23.
8. Mendelson WB. Hypnotic medications: Mechanisms of action and pharmacologic effects. In: Kryger MH, Roth T, Dement WC, eds. *Principles and Practice of Sleep Medicine.* 4th ed. Philadelphia: Elsevier Saunders; 2005:444-451.
9. Da Settimo F, Taliani S, Trincavelli ML, et al. GABA/Bz receptor subtypes as targets for selective drugs. *Curr Med Chem.* 2007;14:2680-2701.
10. Nuelbauer DN. The latest insomnia medications: What's old is new. *Prim Psychiatry.* 2010;17:28-30.
11. Roth T, Mayleben D, Corser BC, et al. Daytime pharmacodynamic and pharmacokinetic evaluation of low-dose sublingual transmucosal zolpidem hemitartrate. *Hum Psychopharmacol Clin Exp.* 2008;23:13-20.
12. Roth T, Hull SG, Lankford A, et al. Low-dose sublingual zolpidem tartrate is associated with dose-related improvement in sleep onset and duration in insomnia characterized by middle-of-the-night (MOTN) awakenings. *Sleep.* 2008;31(9):1277-1284.
13. Walsh JK, Roehrs T, Roth T. Pharmacologic treatment of primary insomnia. In: Kryger MH, Roth T, Dement WC, eds. *Principles and Practice of Sleep Medicine.* 4th ed. Philadelphia: Elsevier Saunders; 2005:749-760.
14. Busto U, Sellers EM. Pharmacologic aspects of benzodiazepine tolerance and dependence. *J Subs Abuse Treat.* 1991;8:29-33.
15. Clinical Pharmacology [database online]. Tampa, FL: Gold Standard, Inc; 2010. Available at http://www.clinicalpharmacology.com (accessed April 2010).
16. Merlotti L, Roehrs T, Koshorek G, et al. The dose effects of zolpidem on the sleep of healthy normals. *J Clin Psychopharmacol.* 1989;1:9-14.
17. Nowell PD, Mazumdar S, Buysse DJ, et al. Benzodiazepines and zolpidem for chronic insomnia: A meta-analysis of treatment efficacy. *JAMA.* 1997;278:2170-2177.
18. Oswald I, French C, Adam K, et al. Benzodiazepine hypnotics remain effective for 24 weeks. *Br Med J (Clin Res Ed).* 1982;284:860-863.
19. Scharf MB, Roth T, Vogel GW, et al. A multicenter, placebo-controlled study evaluating zolpidem in the treatment of chronic insomnia. *J Clin Psychiatry.* 1994;55:192-199.
20. Walsh JK, Vogel GW, Scharf M, et al. A five week, polysomnographic assessment of zaleplon 10 mg for the treatment of primary insomnia. *Sleep Med.* 2000;1:41-49.
21. McCall WV, Erman M, Krystal AD, et al. A polysomnography study of eszopilone in elderly patients with insomnia. *Current Medical Research and Opinion.* 2006;22(9):1633-1642.
22. Roth T, Walsh JK, Krystal A, et al. An evaluation of the efficacy and safety of eszopiclone over 12 months in patients with chronic primary insomnia. *Sleep Med.* 2005;6:487-495.
23. Walsh JK, Roth T, Randazzo AC, et al. Eight weeks of non-nightly use of zolpidem for primary insomnia. *Sleep.* 2000;23:1087-1096.
24. Perlis M, McCall WV, Krystal, et al. Long-term, non-nightly administration of zolpidem in the treatment of patients with primary insomnia. *J Clin Psychiatry.* 2004;65:1128-1137.
25. Krystal AD, Erman M, Zammit GK, et al. Long-term efficacy and safety of zolpidem extended-release 12.5 mg, administered 3 to 7 per week for 24 weeks, in patients with chronic primary insomnia: A 6-month, randomized, double-blind, placebo-controlled, parallel-group, multicenter study. *Sleep.* 2008;31:79-90.
26. Mayer G, Wang-Weigand S, Roth-Schechter B, et al. Efficacy and safety of 6-month nightly ramelteon administration in adults with chronic primary insomnia. *Sleep.* 2009;32(3):351-360.
27. Lamphere J, Roehrs T, Zorick F, et al. Chronic hypnotic efficacy of estazolam. *Drugs Exp Clin Res.* 1986;12:687-692.
28. Roehrs T, Vogel G, Vogel F, et al. Dose effects of temazepam tablets on sleep. *Drugs Exp Clin Res.* 1986;12:693-699.
29. Roehrs T, Zorick F, Wittig R, Roth T. Efficacy of reduced triazolam dose in elderly insomniacs. *Neurobiol Aging.* 1985;6:293-296.
30. Roehrs T, Merlotti L, Rosenthal L, Roth T. Benzodiazepine associated reversal of the effects of experimental sleep fragmentation. *Hum Psychopharmacol.* 1993;8:351-356.
31. Walsh J, Roehrs T, Decerck AC. Polysomnographc studies of the effects of zolpidem in patients with insomnia. In: Freeman H, Puech AJ, Roth T, eds. *Zolpidem: An update of Its Pharmacological Properties and Therapuutic Place in Management of Insomnia.* Paris: Elsevier; 1996:129-139.
32. Lamphere JK, Roehrs TA, Zorick F, et al. The dose effects of zopiclone. *Hum Psychopharm.* 1989;4:41-46.
33. Rosenberg R, Caron J, Roth T, Amato D. An assessment of the efficacy and safety of eszopiclone in the treatment of transient insomnia in healthy adults. *Sleep Med.* 2005;6:15-22.
34. Hindmarch I, Dawson J, Stanley N. A double-blind study in healthy volunteers to assess the effects on sleep of pregabalin compared with alprazolam and placebo. *Sleep.* 2005;28:187-193.
35. Hubain PP, Castro P, Mesters P, et al. Alprazolam and amitriptyline in the treatment of major depressive disorder: A double-blind clinical and sleep EEG study. *J Affect Disord.* 1990;18:67-73.
36. Globus GG, Phoebus EC, Fishbein W, et al. The effect of lorazepam on sleep. *J Clin Psychopharmacol.* 1972;12:331-336.
37. Roth T, Hartse KM, Saab PG, et al. The effects of flurazepam, lorazepam, and triazolam on sleep and memory. *Psychopharmacology.* 1980;70:231-237.
38. Cates ME, Bishop MH, Davis LL, et al. Clonazepam for treatment of sleep disturbances associated with combat-related posttraumatic stress disorder. *Psychiatry.* 2004;38:1395-1399.
39. Kales A, Manfredi R, Vgontzaz AN, et al. Clonazepam: Sleep laboratory study of efficacy and withdrawal. *J Clin Psychopharmacol.* 1991;11:189-193.
40. American Psychiatric Association. *Diagnostic and Statistical Manual of Mental Disorders.* 4th ed. Washington, DC: American Psychiatric Publishing; 2000.
41. American Academy of Sleep Medicine. *International Classification of Sleep Disorders: Diagnostic and Coding Manual, rev.* Chicago: American Academy of Sleep Medicine; 2001.
42. Stepanski E, Zorick FJ, Roehrs TA, et al. Daytime alertness in patients with chronic insomnia compared with asymptomatic control subjects. *Sleep.* 1988;18:39-46.
43. Bonnet MH, Arand DL. 24-Hour metabolic rate in insomniacs and normal sleepers. *Sleep.* 1995;18:581-588.
44. Bonnet MH, Arand DL. Heart rate variability in insomniacs and matched normal sleepers. *Psychosom Med.* 1998;60:610-615.
45. Krystal AD, Walsh JK, Laska E, et al. Sustained efficacy of eszopiclone over 6 months of nightly treatment: Results of a randomized, double-blind, placebo-controlled study in adults with chronic insomnia. *Sleep.* 2003;26:793-799.
46. Walsh JK, Krsytal AD, Amato DA, et al. Nightly treatment of primary insomnia with eszopiclone for six months: Effects on sleep, quality of life, and work limitations. *Sleep.* 2007;30:959-968.
47. Doghramji K, Browman CP, Gaddy JR, et al. Triazolam diminishes daytime sleepiness and sleep fragmentation in patients with periodic leg movements in sleep. *J Clin Psychopharmacol.* 1991;11:284-290.
48. Walsh JK, Muehlbach MJ, Lauter SA, et al. Effects of triazolam on sleep, daytime sleepiness, and morning stiffness in patients with rheumatoid arthritis. *J Rheumatol.* 1996;23:245-252.
49. Roehrs T, Zorick F, Wittig R, et al. Efficacy of reduced triazolam dose in elderly insomniacs. *Neurobiol Aging.* 1985;6:293-296.
50. Mendelson WB, Thompson C. Frank T. Adverse reactions to sedative/hypnotics: Three years' experience. *Sleep.* 1996;19:702-706.
51. Ladewig D. Abuse of benzodiazepines in western European society: Incidence and prevalence, motives, drug acquisition. *Pharmacopsychiatria.* 1983;16:103-106.

52. Roth T, Roehrs TA, Stepanski EJ, et al. Hypnotics and behavior. *Am J Med*. 1990;8:435-465.
53. Greenblatt D, Harmatz JS, Shapiro L, et al. Sensitivity to triazolam in elderly. *N Engl J Med*. 1991;324:1691-1698.
54. Roehrs T, Zorick F, Sicklesteel J, et al. Effects of hypnotics on memory. *J Clin Psychopharmacol*. 1983;3:310-313.
55. Roth T, Roehrs T. Issues in the use of benzodiazepine therapy. *J Clin Psychiatry*. 1992;53:S14-S18.
56. Roehrs T, Roth T. Safety of insomnia pharmacotherapy. *Sleep Med Clin*. 2006;1:399-407.
57. Mangoni AA, Jackson SHD. Age-related changes in pharmacokinetics and pharmacodynamics: Basic principles and practical applications. *BR J Clin Pharmacol*. 2003;57(1):6-14.
58. Cambell AJ, Borrie MJ, Spears GF. Risk factors for falls in a community based prospective study of people 70 years and older. *J Gerontol*. 1989;44:M112-M117.
59. Tinetti ME, Speechley M, Ginter SF. Risk factors for falls among elderly persons living in the community. *N Engl J Med*. 1988;319:1701-1707.
60. Nevitt MC, Cummings SR, Kidd S, et al. Risk factors for recurrent non-syncopal falls: A prospective study. *JAMA*. 1989;261:2663-2668.
61. Kelly KD, Pickett W, Yiannakoulias N, et al. Medication use and falls in community-dwelling older persons. *Age Aging*. 2003;32:503-509.
62. Ensrud KE, Blackwell TL, MAngione CM, et al. Central nervous system active medications and risk for fractures in older women. *Arch Intern Med*. 2003;163:949-957.
63. Ensrud KE, Blackwell TI, Mangione CM, et al. Central nervous system-active medications and risk for falls in older women. *J Am Geriatr Soc*. 2002;50:1629-1637.
64. Kallin K, Lundin-Olson L, Jensen J, et al. Predisposing and precipitating factors for falls among older people in residential care. *Pub Health*. 2002;116:263-271.
65. Thapa PB, Gideon P, Cost TW, et al. Antidepressants and the risk of falls among nursing home residents. *N Eng J Med*. 1998;339:875-882.
66. Brassington GS, King AC, Bliwise DL. Sleep problems as a risk factor for falls in a sample of community-dwelling adults aged 64-99 years. *J Am Geriatr Soc*. 2000;48:1234-1240.
67. Paterniti S, Dufouil C, Alperovitch A. Long-term benzodiazepine use and cognitive decline in the elderly: The epidemiology of vascular aging study. *J Clin Psychopharmacol*. 2002;22:285-293.
68. Allard J, Artero S, Ritchie K. Consumption of psychotropic medication in the elderly: A re-evaluation of its effect on cognitive performance. *Int J Geriatr Psychiatry*. 2003;18:874-878.
69. Curran HV, Collins R, Flectcher S, et al. Older adults and withdrawal from benzodiazepine hypnotics in general practice: Effects on cognitive function, sleep, mood and quality of life. *Psychol Med*. 2003;33:1223-1237.
70. McAndrews MP, Weiss RI, Sandor P, et al. Cognitive effects of long-term benzodiazepine use in older adults. *Hum Psychopharmacol*. 2003;18:51-57.
71. Kripke DF, Simons RN, Garfinkel L, et al. Short and long sleep and sleeping pills: Is increased mortality associated? *Arch Gen Psychiatry*. 1979;36:103-116.
72. Kripke DF, Klauber MR, Wingard DL, et al. Mortality hazard associated with prescription hypnotics. *Biol Psychiatry*. 1998;43:687-693.
73. Rumble R, Morgan K. Hypnotics, sleep, and mortality in elderly people. *J Am Geriatr Soc*. 1992;40:787-791.
74. Roehrs T, Vogel G, Roth T. Rebound insomnia: Its determinants and significance. *Am J Med*. 1990;88:S39-S42.
75. Roehrs T, Merlotti L, Zorick F, et al. Rebound insomnia and hypnotic self administration. *Psychopharmacology*. 1992;107:480-484.
76. Melliginer GD, Balter MB, Uhlenhuth EH. Insomnia and its treatment. *Arch Gen Psychiatry*. 1985;42:225-232.
77. Roehrs T, Hollebeck E, Drake C, et al. Substance use for insomnia in Metropolitan Detroit. *J Psychosom Res*. 2002;53:571-576.
78. Balter MB, Uhlenhuth EH. New epidemiologic findings about insomnia and its treatment. *J Clin Psychiatry*. 1992;53(12):34-39.
79. Griffith RR, Roache JD. Abuse liability of benzodiazepines: A review of human studies evaluating subjective and/or reinforcing effects. In: Smith DE, Wesson DR, eds. *The Benzodiazepines: Current Standards for Medical Practice*. Ingman, MA: MTP Press; 1985:209-225.
80. Roehrs T, Pedrosi B, Rosentha L, et al. Hypnotic self administration and dose escalation. *Psychopharmacology*. 1996;127:150-154.
81. Roehrs TA, Randall S, Harris E, et al. Twelve months of nightly zolpidem does not lead to dose escalation: A prospective placebo controlled study. *Sleep*. 2010;34(2). (in press)
82. Roehrs T, Bonahoom A, Pedrosi B, et al. Disturbed sleep predicts hypnotic self administration. *Sleep Med*. 2002;3:61-66.
83. Roehrs T, Boanahoom A, Pedrosi B, et al. Nighttime versus daytime hypnotic self-administration. *Psychopharmacology*. 2002;161:137-142.
84. The Associated Press. 2007. *FDA says pills can cause "sleep-driving." The Washington Post*. Available at http://www.washigntonpost.com/wp-dyn/content/article/2007/03/14 AR2007031401027.html.
85. Barsky AJ, Saintfort R, Rogers MP, et al. Nonspecific medication side effects and the nocebo phenomenon. *JAMA*. 2002;287(5):622-627.
86. Morris HH, Estes ML. Traveler's amnesia: Transient global amnesia secondary to triazolam. *JAMA*. 1987;258:945-946.
87. George KA, Dundee JW. Relative amnesic actions of diazepam, flunitrazepam and lorazepam in man. *Br J Clin Pharmacol*. 1977;4:45-50.
88. Yang W, Dollear M, Muthukrishnan SR. One rare side effect of zolpidem – sleepwalking: A case report. *Arch Phys Med Rehabil*. 2005;86:1265-1266.
89. Liskow B, Pikalov A. Zaleplon overdose associated with sleepwalking and complex behavior. *J Am Acad Child Adoles Psychiatry*. 2004;43:927-928.
90. Lange CL. Medication-associated somnambulism. *J Am Acad Child Adoles Psychiatry*. 2005;44:211-212.
91. Paquet V, Strul J, Servais L, et al. Sleep-related eating disorder induced by olanzapine. *J Clin Psychiat*. 2002;63:7.
92. Lu ML, Shen WW. Sleep-related eating disorder induced by risperidone. *J Clin Psychiatry*. 2004;65:273-274.
93. Morgenthaler TI, Silber MH. Amnestic sleep-related eating disorder associated with zolpidem. *Sleep Med*. 2002;3:323-327.
94. Schenk CH, Mahowald MW. Review of nocturnal sleep-related eating disorders. *Int J Eat Disord*. 1994;15:343-356.
95. Vetrugno R, Manconi M, Strembi LF, et al. Nocturnal eating: Sleep related eating disorder or nocturnal eating syndrome? A videopolysomnographic study. *Sleep*. 2006;29:876-877.
96. Menkes DB. Triazolam-induced nocturnal bingeing with amnesia. *Aust N Z J Psychiatry*. 1992;26:320-321.
97. Lauerma H. Nocturnal wandering caused by restless legs and short-acting benzodiazepines. *Acta Psychiatr Scand*. 1991;83:492-493.
98. Roehrs T, Carskadon MA, Dement WC, et al. Daytime sleepiness and alertness. In: Kryger MH, Roth T, Dement WC, eds. *Principles and Practice of Sleep Medicine*. 4th ed. Philadelphia: Elsevier Saunders; 2005:39-50.
99. Bonnet MH. Acute sleep deprivation. In: Kryger MH, Roth T, Dement WC, eds. *Principles and Practice of Sleep Medicine*. 4th ed. Philadelphia: Elsevier Saunders; 2005:51-66.
100. Zandra A, Pilon M, Montplaisir J. Polysomnographic diagnosis of sleepwalking: Effects of sleep deprivation. *Ann Neurol*. 2008;63:513-519.

Pharmacology of Psychotropic Drugs

Chapter 8

NICHOLAS A. DeMARTINIS / ANDREW WINOKUR

The focus of this chapter on psychotropic pharmacology brings together an emphasis on drugs used in the treatment of major psychiatric disorders with a consideration of the effects of psychotropic drugs on sleep physiology and sleep architecture. Historically, clinicians have long recognized that alternations in sleep patterns represented common and core manifestations of major psychiatric disorders. Hippocrates (460-357 BC) described melancholia (a term from antiquity to describe severe depression, literally referring to "black bile") as a state of "aversion to food, despondency, sleeplessness, irritability and restlessness."[1] Ancient Greek clinicians recognized that insomnia represents a core feature of severe depression. Similarly, for patients who presented with what is now referred to as "mixed state" bipolar disorder, with a simultaneous presentation of mania and depression, the Greek clinician Soranus, in the first century BC, noted the expected presence of "continual wakefulness and fluctuating states of anger and merriment, and sometimes of sadness and futility."[1] In a landmark epidemiologic study of the relationship of sleep disturbances and psychiatric disorders, Ford and Kamerow[2] started with data on 7954 respondents from a community sample who were questioned at baseline and 1 year later for follow-up evaluation. Over 10% of the sample reported symptoms of insomnia at baseline, and an additional 3.2% of the baseline sample reported symptoms of hypersomnia. Forty percent of the subjects presenting with insomnia and 46.5% of the subjects initially describing symptoms of hypersomnia were found to have a psychiatric disorder at follow-up evaluation, as compared to a prevalence of 16.4% in the subjects who reported no sleep complaints at baseline evaluation. Patients with an initial presentation of sleep disturbance were particularly likely to present with depression or anxiety disorder diagnoses at the 1 year follow-up evaluation, thus further reinforcing the importance of interrelationships between sleep and psychiatric disorders. Additionally, sleep problems have been noted to be highly prevalent in patients with schizophrenia.[3,4] Finally, in an overview on the clinical features of psychiatric disorders, Yager and Gitlin[5] comment: "Insomnia is a common, often chronic symptom or sign of many different psychiatric disorders and conditions including substance abuse, depressive disorder, generalized anxiety disorder, panic attacks, manic episodes (in which the diminished sleep does not always provoke a complaint), and acute schizophrenia." Thus, a complex and often bidirectional relationship between sleep disturbance and psychiatric disorder has increasingly been recognized in recent years.

With the advent of the "psychopharmacologic revolution" starting in the early 1950s, the importance of pharmacologic treatment interventions for the management of major psychiatric disorders has become an increasingly important and frequently employed component of treatment for a broad array of psychiatric disorders. Virtually all of the psychotropic drugs utilized in contemporary treatment algorithms in psychiatric practice have been found to exert prominent effects on a broad array of neurotransmitters and neuroreceptors.[6] Notably, the majority of neurotransmitter systems modulated by these psychotropic drugs have been implicated in the regulation of sleep and arousal as well as in the regulation of transitions between the major sleep states. Thus, the importance of considering effects of psychotropic drugs on sleep and arousal is based on both clinical empirical experience with respect to their effects on sleep and wakefulness and also on the emerging neurobiologic mechanisms demonstrated to be relevant to effects of psychopharmacologic agents on sleep and circadian rhythms.

This chapter discusses selected topics related to the antidepressant drugs, antipsychotic agents, antiepileptics, drugs used to treat anxiety disorders, and antihistaminic agents. Each section starts with a brief review of basic and clinical pharmacology of relevance to the therapeutic agents under consideration. Next follows a review of studies examining effects of the drugs in this category on sleep architecture based on polysomnographic studies, where available. We then discuss practical clinical approaches to the use of the respective classes of psychotropic drugs in the management of sleep disorders. Finally, we provide a discussion of pertinent pharmacologic features of relevance to the sleep clinician in using these agents for therapeutic application, particularly with reference to managing symptoms of sleep disorders.

Characteristics of selected psychotropic medications are given in Table 8-1.

ANTIDEPRESSANTS

Critical Points

- Antidepressants have a broad range of effects on sleep, sleep physiology, and sleep disorders ranging from beneficial to detrimental, even among individuals with the same medication.
- These effects are mediated by a broad range of pharmacologic mechanisms, sometimes including multiple mechanisms within the same drug.

TABLE 8-1

Selected Psychotropic Medication Characteristics

Medication/Class	Indication(s)	Dosing	Side Effects	Precautions	Drug Interactions
TRICYCLIC ANTIDEPRESSANTS					
Amitriptyline, imipramine, doxepin	Depression	10–50 mg qhs	Dry mouth, constipation, urinary retention, sedation, weight gain	Suicidal thoughts, suicide, worsening of depression. *Contraindications*: cardiac conduction abnormalities, recent cardiac events, narrow-angle glaucoma	Drugs that significantly inhibit CYP2D6 (e.g., quinidine, fluoxetine, paroxetine, amiodarone)
Trazodone	Depression	25–100 mg qhs for insomnia, 200–600 mg for depression	Constipation, diarrhea, loss of appetite, nausea, vomiting, weight gain, dizziness, priapism	Suicidal thoughts, suicide, worsening of depression	Triazolam, sibutramine
Mirtazepine	Depression	7.5–45 mg qhs	Somnolence, increased appetite, constipation, diarrhea, vomiting, weight gain	Suicidal thoughts, suicide, worsening of depression	
SSRIS					
Paroxetine, fluoxetine, sertraline, escitalopram, citalopram	Depression, anxiety disorders	Paroxetine: 10–50 mg qhs Fluoxetine: 20–80 mg qam Sertraline: 50–200 mg qd Escitalopram: 5–20 mg qd Citalopram: 20–60 mg qd	Somnolence (greater with paroxetine), insomnia, nausea, diarrhea, dyspepsia, loss of appetite, asthenia, decreased libido, sexual dysfunction, headache, weight gain	Suicidal thoughts, suicide, worsening of depression. Discontinuation syndrome. Paroxetine: pregnancy category D	Paroxetine, fluoxetine: CYP2D6 inhibitor: use caution in combination with drugs metabolized by CYP2D6
SNRIS					
Venlafaxine, duloxetine	Depression, anxiety disorders	Venlafaxine: 37.5–225 mg qd Duloxetine: 30–90 mg qam	Insomnia, nausea, dyspepsia, sweating, constipation or diarrhea, decreased libido, sexual dysfunction, headache, weight gain, increased blood pressure, sedation, dysuria	Suicidal thoughts, suicide, worsening of depression. Discontinuation syndrome	Use caution in combination with drugs that are CYP2D6 inhibitors
ANTIPSYCHOTICS					
Risperidone	Schizophrenia, bipolar disorder	0.25–6 mg	Dizziness, drowsiness, fatigue, nausea, constipation, runny nose, increased appetite, weight gain, nervousness, acne, dry skin, difficulty concentrating, decreased sexual ability/desire or difficulty sleeping, dystonia. *Infrequent*: hyperglycemia/diabetes, tardive dyskinesia, neuroleptic malignant syndrome	Increased risk for cerebrovascular events and increased risk of death in elderly patients treated for dementia-related psychosis	Use caution in combination with drugs that are CYP2D6 inhibitors

Drug	Indication	Dosage	Side Effects	Warnings	Interactions
Quetiapine	Schizophrenia, bipolar disorder	50-800 mg	Constipation, drowsiness, dizziness, dry mouth, headache, stomach pain/upset, fatigue, weight gain, hyperlipidemia, *Infrequent:* hyperglycemia/diabetes, movement disorders, neuroleptic malignant syndrome	Increased risk for cerebrovascular events and increased risk of death in elderly patients treated for dementia-related psychosis	May add to hypotensive effects of antihypertensives
Olanzapine	Schizophrenia, bipolar disorder	5-20 mg	Constipation, drowsiness, dizziness, dry mouth, stomach pain/upset, fatigue, weight gain, hyperlipidemia, hyperglycemia *Infrequent:* tardive dyskinesia, neuroleptic malignant syndrome	Increased risk for cerebrovascular events and increased risk of death in elderly patients treated for dementia-related psychosis	
ANTICONVULSANTS					
Tiagabine	Adjunctive treatment of partial seizures	32-56 mg/day, bid-qid dosing	Dizziness, headache, sleepiness, inability to concentrate, tremor	Risk of suicidal thoughts and behavior Seizure in patients without epilepsy	
Gabapentin	Postherpetic neuralgia, epilepsy	900 to 1800 mg/day, tid dosing	Drowsiness, dizziness, unsteadiness, fatigue, vision changes, weight gain, nausea, dry mouth, constipation	Risk of suicidal thoughts and behavior Dose adjustment for compromized renal function	
Pregabalin	Fibromyalgia, neuropathic pain associated with diabetic peripheral neuropathy, postherpetic neuralgia, adjunctive therapy for adult patients with partial-onset seizures	150-600 mg/day, bid or tid dosing	Dizziness, somnolence, dry mouth, peripherial edema, blurred vision, weight gain and difficulty with concentration/attention	Risk of suicidal thoughts and behavior	
ANTIHISTAMINES					
Diphenhydramine	Seasonal allergies, allergic reactions	Diphenhydramine: 12.5-50 mg qhs Hydroxyzine: 25-100 mg qhs	Drowsiness, dizziness, headache, constipation, stomach upset, blurred vision, irritability, decreased coordination, dry mouth, confusion	Increased risk for psychomotor adverse events in the elderly	Additive effects with other anticholinergic medications

SNRIs, serotonin–norepinephrine reuptake inhibitors; *SSRIs,* selective serotonin reuptake inhibitors.

- Knowledge of these impacts on sleep and sleep physiology can assist clinicians in managing sleep-related adverse effects and leveraging beneficial effects in the management of conditions for which they are approved, and in selective management of sleep disorders when existing approved treatments are ineffective or poorly tolerated.

Basic and Clinical Pharmacology

All of the first-generation tricyclic antidepressant compounds (TCAs) and the majority of the second-generation antidepressant drugs, including the selective serotonin reuptake inhibitors (SSRIs), the serotonin-norepinephrine reuptake inhibitors (SNRIs), and the dopamine and norepinephrine reuptake inhibitor bupropion, are speculated to produce their antidepressant effects by maintaining released monoamine neurotransmitters in the synaptic space for a longer period, enhancing the effect on the postsynaptic receptor. Only the monoamine oxidase inhibitors (MAOIs) nefazodone and mirtazapine appear to exert mood-elevating effects via a mechanism that does not primarily involve reuptake site inhibition for a monoamine transporter. In the case of the MAOIs, potent, irreversible inhibition of intracellular MAO leads to an increase in the concentration of the monoamines norepinephrine (NE), serotonin (5-HT), and dopamine (DA) in the presynaptic neuron. Subsequent firing of an action potential results in an increased amount of monoamine neurotransmitter substances being released into the synaptic space, thereby leading to increased activation of postsynaptic neurons. In the case of nefazodone, the primary mechanism of action of relevance to its antidepressant efficacy appears to involve rather weak inhibition of the 5-HT uptake site presynaptically coupled with potent inhibition of postsynaptic 5-HT$_2$ receptors. The presumptive mechanism of action of mirtazapine is even more complex. Mirtazapine is an α_2-adrenergic receptor antagonist, which leads to enhanced release of NE from the presynaptic neuron. Subsequent to the enhanced release of NE, an action of released NE on postsynaptic neurons results in increased stimulation of the release of 5-HT. Mirtazapine also exerts potent blockade of postsynaptic 5-HT$_2$ and 5-HT$_3$ receptors, and inhibition of histamine H$_1$ receptors. Notably, the blockade of 5-HT$_2$ receptors and the H$_1$ receptor are relevant to the effects of mirtazapine on sleep.

The TCAs have been demonstrated to produce a variety of pharmacologic effects apart from the monoamine reuptake site inhibition, which may be of high relevance to the broad array of side effects associated with these compounds.[7,8] Blockade of histamine H$_1$ receptors by TCAs, an effect that is clearly more prominent with some TCAs than others, has been linked to the liability for producing increased appetite, weight gain, and daytime somnolence.

Of the SSRIs, paroxetine is characterized by exerting prominent inhibitory effects on muscarinic cholinergic receptors and histamine H$_1$ receptors. These effects are thought to be relevant to its profile of being somewhat sedating and also being associated with an enhanced degree of weight gain liability among the SSRIs. Finally, as noted previously mirtazapine has a broad pharmacologic profile with one of its prominent effects being potent inhibition of the histamine H$_1$ receptor. The clinical implications of this pharmacologic effect include enhancement of nocturnal sleep, daytime somnolence, and weight gain liability.

Effects on Sleep Architecture and Physiology

Progress in studying neurobiologic mechanisms related to the regulation of sleep and wakefulness have identified the role of numerous neuroactive substances.[6] Among the most extensively implicated neurotransmitters have been several of the monoamine neurotransmitters: 5-HT, NE, and acetylcholine (ACh). The reciprocal inhibition hypothesis of rapid eye movement (REM) sleep regulation of Hobson and McCarley invokes a key role for ACh in triggering the onset of REM sleep via effects on specialized REM-on neurons and roles for both NE and 5-HT in terminating a REM sleep episode via effects exerted on REM-off neurons.[9,10] In light of the well-established pharmacologic effects of virtually all antidepressant drugs on these monoamine neurotransmitter systems that have been implicated in sleep-wake regulation and in REM sleep regulation in recent years, numerous studies carried out in recent years employing polysomnographic (PSG) techniques have produced information delineating effects of various antidepressant drugs on both sleep continuity measures (i.e., maintenance of sleep versus production of sleep disruption and increased wakefulness) and on various aspects of sleep architecture[11] (Table 8-2).

Tricyclic Antidepressants

From a clinical perspective, it was quickly recognized that some of the available TCAs exerted pronounced sedating effects, and clinicians soon chose to administer the sedating TCAs, such as amitriptyline, doxepin, and clomipramine to their patients with major depressive disorder (MDD) who demonstrated prominent associated insomnia symptoms.[11] In contrast, a subset of TCAs (e.g., desipramine and protriptyline) were characterized as having limited sedating effects and were actually rather activating. The sedating TCAs demonstrated more prominent modulatory effects on 5-HT activity, exerted prominent histamine H$_1$ receptor blockade and produced pronounced muscarinic cholinergic blocking effects.[8] In contrast, the more activating TCAs exerted prominent effects in enhancing NE activity.

TABLE 8-2

Antidepressant Medication Impact on Sleep Physiology

Medication/Class	Sleep-Related Pharmacology	Effects on Sleep Architecture
SSRI	5-HT reuptake inhibition	REM suppression, increased REM latency
SNRI	5-HT, NE reuptake inhibition	REM suppression, increased REM latency
Trazodone/nefazodone	5-HT$_2$ antagonism	Decreased sleep latency, increased SWS
Mirtazapine	5-HT$_2$ antagonism, H$_1$ antagonism	Decreased sleep latency, increased SWS
Tricyclic antidepressants	5-HT, NE reuptake inhibition, H$_1$ antagonism	Decreased sleep latency, REM suppression, increased REM latency

H$_1$, histamine H$_1$ receptor; *5-HT*, 5-hydroxytryptamine; *NE*, norepinephrine; *REM*, rapid eye movement (sleep); *SSRI*, selective serotonin reuptake inhibitor; *SWS*, slow wave sleep.

The use of PSG laboratory techniques has produced reports cataloging the effects of various TCAs on sleep EEG parameters. In general, effects reported on the basis of PSG analyses supported the clinical observations. Thus, TCAs such as amitriptyline and doxepin, which demonstrate a sedating effect clinically, were found to shorten sleep onset latency (SOL) and increase sleep continuity measures such as total sleep time (TST) and reduced wake time after sleep onset (WASO).[11,12] Additionally, these studies found that activating TCAs such as desipramine and protriptyline tended to prolong sleep latency, shorten TST, and increase WASO and number of awakenings during the night. An additional effect of the various TCAs on sleep architecture, across the spectrum of sedating, neutral, and activating TCAs, involved the suppression of REM sleep.[13] The one TCA that represented an exception to the REM suppressant profile of the TCA class was trimipramine.[11,14] The pharmacologic profiles of the TCAs as potent enhancers of the activity of NE, 5-HT, or both had a logical connection to the potent REM suppression observed across this class of agents in light of the identified role of both NE and 5-HT in terminating REM sleep.[9,10]

Monoamine Oxidase Inhibitors

The most widely employed MAOIs in the United States have been phenelzine and tranylcypramine. Phenelzine may be rather sedating for some patients, whereas tranylcypramine, which has pharmacologic similarities to stimulant drugs, is noted to be more activating and may be associated with producing insomnia in some patients. Based on PSG studies, tranylcypramine can produce an increase in SOL and reduction in TST and sleep continuity measures.[6,15,16] Additionally, both of the commonly used MAOIs have been noted to produce very prominent suppression of REM sleep. Moreover, termination of treatment with MAOIs can be associated with REM rebound if a patient is studied in the sleep laboratory shortly after an MAOI has been discontinued. Clinically, patients who discontinue the use of an MAOI may report having more frequent and possibly more intense dreams and nightmares.

Trazodone and Nefazodone

Trazodone and nefazodone demonstrate unique pharmacologic profiles characterized by weak presynaptic uptake inhibition of 5-HT, accompanied by antagonism of 5-HT$_2$ receptors.[7] They also exert minimal muscarinic cholinergic blocking effects.[8] When trazodone was initially introduced as an antidepressant drug, it was typically prescribed in a dosage range of 300 to 600 mg per day in divided doses and was associated with the production of pronounced daytime somnolence. In recent years, trazodone has become infrequently used as an antidepressant because of the high liability for sedating effects, but has now become routinely used off-label to treat symptoms of insomnia, particularly in the context of treating patients with depression plus insomnia who are being treated with an antidepressant drug. In PSG studies, trazodone has been reported to increase TST, and in some, but not all, studies to increase slow wave sleep as well.[11,17] Inconsistent reports have appeared with respect to the potential for trazodone to suppress REM sleep. Clinically, nefazodone can be associated with reports of somnolence in some patients being treated for MDD. In a large PSG study in which patients with MDD plus insomnia complaints were randomized to treatment with fluoxetine or nefazodone, nefazodone was associated with a higher sleep continuity measures than fluoxetine, and nefazodone demonstrated a lack of suppression of REM sleep parameters with respect to fluoxetine.[18-20]

Selective Serotonin Reuptake Inhibitors

In 1988, fluoxetine was the first of the six marketed SSRIs to be approved by the Food and Drug Administration (FDA) in the United States. From the initial clinical trial experience with fluoxetine, it was clear that prominent effects on sleep were readily apparent, as evidenced by a self-reported incidence of insomnia up to 20% of depressed patients in early trials.[11,19] Another common adverse effect reported in patients being treated with fluoxetine was daytime somnolence.[21] This variability of effect of fluoxetine on sleep symptoms might be related to the important and diverse roles exerted by 5-HT in the regulation of both sleep and wakefulness. Reports on adverse effects of all of the other SSRIs have replicated the original findings with fluoxetine with respect to the occurrence of both insomnia and daytime somnolence in a subset of patients being treated with these agents for MDD.

Early PSG studies found fluoxetine to be associated with a prolongation of SOL and a disruption of sleep continuity, a constellation of findings referred to in one report as a "lightening effect on sleep."[19,20,22] In addition to effects on sleep continuity, all studies to date have reported that fluoxetine produces pronounced suppression of REM.[12,23] Additional sleep-related findings include an increase in limb movements during sleep and a report of increased non-REM eye movements.[24-26] Although the other SSRIs have been studied less extensively than fluoxetine, the consensus has been to replicate the findings reported for fluoxetine, suggesting that these effects on sleep physiology represent a class effect.

Serotonin-Norepinephrine Reuptake Inhibitors

Three SNRIs are currently on the market in the United States for the treatment of major depressive disorder, including venlafaxine, duloxetine, and desvenlafaxine. Few PSG studies have been reported involving the SNRIs, with the available literature mainly involving venlafaxine. Clinically, the SNRIs have been reported to be associated with self-reported side effects of both insomnia and daytime somnolence. A limited number of studies utilizing PSG techniques have reported on effects exerted by venlafaxine and by duloxetine on sleep physiology in normal subjects and in patients with MDD.[27-30] No sleep studies have been reported for desvenlafaxine. The most prominent effect seen in studies with both desvenlafaxine and duloxetine, including studies conducted in normal control subjects and studies carried out with patients diagnosed with MDD, has been a suppression of REM sleep, reflected by a delay in the time of the first REM onset and a reduction in overall REM sleep time. In studies involving administration of venlafaxine to normal subjects and to patients with MDD, increases in WASO were reported, indicating a disruption of sleep continuity. In the study with venlafaxine administered to normal control subjects, an increase in periodic limb movements of sleep (PLMS) was also reported.[28] In a study involving administration of the SNRI duloxetine to patients, a significant increase in stage III sleep was reported, along with suppression of REM sleep.[30]

Bupropion

Bupropion demonstrates a unique mechanism of action among the currently available antidepressants characterized by presynaptic uptake inhibition of DA and NE.[7] Bupropion is notable for lacking any pharmacologic modulatory effects on 5-HT. Clinically, bupropion has been noted to be associated with reports of insomnia in some patients with MDD. In laboratory studies involving PSG analysis, the most striking finding has been a shortening of the time to initial REM onset and an overall increase in total REM sleep time throughout the night, a finding that stands in sharp contract to effects reported for the majority of antidepressant drugs, most of which produce prominent REM suppression.[31,32]

Mirtazapine

Some of the pharmacologic effects associated with mirtazapine administration, including inhibition of histamine H_1 and 5-HT$_2$ receptors, would suggest the potential to exert potent effects on sleep maintenance.[7] In clinical trial studies, a subset of patients with MDD who were treated with mirtazapine reported symptoms of daytime somnolence. In PSG studies, patients with MDD on mirtazapine showed a shortening of SOL and a significant increase in TST and sleep efficiency. Additionally, administration of mirtazapine appears to be associated with little or no suppression of REM sleep.[33,34]

Clinical Evidence for Efficacy in Sleep Disorders

Although there is only one example to date of an antidepressant drug being formally approved for the treatment of a sleep disorder or a sleep-related symptom, a number of antidepressant drugs are used off-label because of their effects on sleep symptoms. Examples to be discussed in this section include the use of antidepressant drugs to treat insomnia, fibromyalgia, and cataplexy in narcoleptic patients.

The Use of Antidepressant Drugs in the Treatment of Insomnia

Dating back to the early years of antidepressant drug use, clinicians observed that a subset of TCAs (e.g., amitriptyline, doxepin, clomipramine) were somewhat to markedly sedating. When these antidepressant agents were studied in the sleep laboratory, a shortening of SOL or an improvement in TST, associated with a decrease in the number of awakenings and in WASO, was typically observed.[7,11] Clinicians found that adding a sedating TCA, in particular amitriptyline or doxepin, in a relatively low dose (e.g., 25-50 mg at bedtime) to a primary second-generation antidepressant drug such as an SSRI, SNRI, or bupropion led to improvement in symptoms of insomnia associated with depression. The perceived success of this empirical clinical strategy has led to the use of the sedating TCAs for the treatment of insomnia in individuals who do not have a coexisting depressive or anxiety disorder.

Doxepin has been examined in studies enrolling subjects with primary insomnia. At doses of 1, 3, or 6 mg at bedtime (doses far below established antidepressant efficacy), doxepin has been reported to shorten SOL and to improve indices of sleep maintenance. Notably, when administered in this dose range, doxepin is characterized pharmacologically by exerting virtually exclusively potent histamine H_1 receptor antagonism,

an effect associated with enhancement of sleep in preclinical studies.[35,36] Stahl has noted a greater-than-2 orders of magnitude potency difference between doxepin's histamine H_1 receptor blocking potency and its potency in blocking the monoamine reuptake transporters.[37]

In March 2010 the FDA approved a low-dose preparation of doxepin (3 mg or 6 mg) for use in the treatment of chronic or transient insomnia characterized by difficulty with sleep maintenance. Unlike the majority of drug products that have been approved by the FDA for an insomnia indication, the low-dose doxepin formulation is not scheduled and has not been reported to be associated with problems with tolerance, withdrawal, amnesia, or complex behaviors. The most commonly reported side effect with the 3 mg or 6 mg doxepin formulation was drowsiness.[38,39]

Among the second-generation antidepressants, trazodone is widely employed in modest dose ranges, such as 50 to 100 mg at bedtime, to treat insomnia symptoms in a broad array of patients, including patients with psychiatric disorders associated with insomnia and in patients with insomnia who have no coexisting psychiatric diagnosis. In a study enrolling subjects with a diagnosis of primary insomnia, trazodone (50 mg, h.s.) produced improvements in SOL, TST and WASO compared to subjects randomized to placebo after 1 week.[40] However, after 2 weeks, the subjects treated with trazodone did not differ significantly from the subjects randomized to placebo on the various sleep parameters examined. The SSRI paroxetine, administered at an average dose of 20 mg over a 6-week period, was evaluated in an open-label study in patients with primary insomnia. Paroxetine produced improvement in subjective variables of sleep disturbance, but did not produce significant improvement in objective PSG variables.[41] Mirtazapine has been noted to be prominently sedating in some patients being treated for depression, presumably based on its pharmacologic profile, as noted previously. In a study enrolling subjects with MDD plus insomnia, patients randomized to mirtazapine demonstrated a significant shortening of SOL and a significant increase in TST compared to patients randomized to fluoxetine.[34]

The Use of Antidepressant Drugs in the Treatment of Fibromyalgia

Fibromyalgia is a disorder characterized by diffuse, widespread pain, fatigue, depression, and sleep disturbance.[42,43] PSG studies involving patients with fibromyalgia have documented a finding that is characteristic, though not specific, for patients with this disorder, namely, the intrusion of alpha wave activity into slow wave sleep—a finding referred to as *alpha-delta sleep*. Antidepressant drugs that exert a spectrum of pharmacologic effects characterized by modulation of NE and 5-HT neurotransmission have been reported to exert beneficial effects for symptoms of fibromyalgia, particularly characterized by improvement in pain symptoms, but also frequently associated with improvements in fatigue symptoms, depression, and self-reported sleep disturbance.[43]

The Use of Antidepressant Drugs in the Treatment of Cataplexy in Patients with Narcolepsy

Cataplexy, a symptom characterized by sudden loss of muscle tone that is typically triggered by intense emotion, is a prominent manifestation of narcolepsy. Various symptoms of narcolepsy have been speculated to represent components of REM sleep intruding into wakefulness.[44] Because of the potency of the majority of antidepressant drugs in suppressing REM sleep, a number of antidepressant drugs have been employed to manage cataplectic attacks in patients with narcolepsy. This treatment option has become particularly important in recent years because modafinil, one of the current first-line treatments for symptoms for excessive sleepiness and sleep attacks in narcoleptic patients, does not have established efficacy to alleviate cataplectic symptoms. Thus, co-administration of modafinil to manage daytime sleepiness and sleep attacks, with a REM-suppressing antidepressant drug, to prevent or reduce cataplectic episodes, represents a commonly employed treatment strategy. Although the stimulant drugs, such as dextroamphetamine or methylphenidate, do exert some potency with respect to suppressing cataplectic attacks, patients with narcolepsy may not achieve sufficient relief from symptoms of cataplexy with a stimulant drug as monotherapy and may require the addition of a REM-suppressing antidepressant agent in order to achieve sufficient control of their symptoms of cataplexy.[45] Typically, a more activating antidepressant drug is employed for this purpose, such as the TCA desipramine or protriptyline as well as an SSRI, such as fluoxetine. All of the antidepressants listed here are characterized by being potent REM-suppressing agents, and this combination of a potentially activating profile plus robust REM suppression appears to be particularly beneficial for the purpose of treating symptoms of cataplexy in patients with narcolepsy.

Clinical Management: Initiation, Maintenance, Precautions, and Abuse Potential

As noted earlier, the use of antidepressant drugs for treatment of sleep disturbances has been "off-label," but recently the low-dose doxepin formulation has been approved by the FDA for the treatment of insomnia, and duloxetine has received FDA approval for the treatment of fibromyalgia. A general principle with respect to the use of antidepressant drugs to treat insomnia has been to scale down the dose from the typical range associated with antidepressant efficacy. In light of the long half-life for most antidepressant drugs, clinical management should strive to minimize next-day sedating effects associated with these compounds while providing beneficial effects on SOL and sleep maintenance parameters. Some antidepressant drugs have active metabolites that demonstrate longer half-lives than the parent compound.[46] An example is fluoxetine, which has an active metabolite, desmethylfluoxetine, that has a distinctly longer half-life than is the case for fluoxetine. Because it can produce disruptive effects on sleep continuity, attention must be paid to the potential contribution of its active metabolite with respect to problems with sustained sleep disruption.

Some antidepressant drugs can produce inhibitory effects on various cytochrome P-450 (CYP) hepatic enzymes. Notable examples of this phenomenon include fluoxetine and paroxetine, both of which act as potent inhibitors of the CYP2D6 enzyme.[46] A clinically relevant circumstance related to this enzyme inhibition can ensue from the combined administration of fluoxetine as an antidepressant agent and trazodone to manage symptoms of insomnia. Trazodone's active metabolite m-chlorophenylpiperazine (mCPP) acts as an agonist at

$5-HT_2$ receptors.[47] As a consequence, mCPP can produce insomnia. mCPP is metabolized by CYP2D6. When fluoxetine is administered as an antidepressant drug along with trazodone, inhibition of CYP2D6 by fluoxetine can lead to the accumulation of larger amounts of mCPP, potentially producing greater disruption of sleep maintenance.

There is a notable lack of data from controlled studies regarding the sustained efficacy of antidepressants with respect to SOL and TST in long-term maintenance therapy. As noted earlier, in a study examining effects of trazodone administration in patients with primary insomnia, statistically significant improvements were documented at the end of week 1 of treatment with trazodone as compared to placebo, but no significant advantage for trazodone was observed at the end of week 2.[48] From a clinical perspective, many patients who are placed on an antidepressant drug such as amitriptyline, doxepin, trazodone, or mirtazapine appear to experience improvement in symptoms of insomnia and to report an improved quality of sleep over a prolonged period of time. However, since systematic controlled studies are lacking, decisions about the duration of treatment with an antidepressant drug for insomnia complaints must be made strictly on the basis of clinical assessment and judgment.

Discontinuation of treatment with an antidepressant drug, particularly if the termination of treatment involves an abrupt discontinuation, can be associated with the development of discontinuation/withdrawal reactions, which may involve both physical symptoms, such as shakiness, dizziness, diaphoresis, and nausea, and well as emotional symptoms including an abrupt increase in anxiety and depression.[49] Discontinuation syndromes associated with the termination of therapy were initially described with respect to cessation of treatment with TCAs, and the mechanism underlying this reaction was initially attributed to the anticholinergic effects associated with many of the TCAs. More recently, such reactions have also been reported for many of the second-generation antidepressant drugs with the exception of fluoxetine, whose long half-life appears to provide a built-in safeguard against discontinuation reactions. Based on clinical experience, termination of treatment with venlafaxine and with paroxetine may be associated with a particularly high likelihood of discontinuation reactions as well as with more prominent and severe symptoms of withdrawal. Overall, termination of treatment with an antidepressant drug should virtually always involve a gradual taper of the dose attained for maintenance therapy. Patients should be advised at the start of treatment to take their medication on a regular basis and to avoid inadvertent discontinuation of treatment.

Some patients started on an antidepressant drug, whether it has been prescribed as an antidepressant treatment or off-label to treat symptoms of insomnia, may report a change in their experience of dreaming, which is most frequently characterized by more frequent, disturbing, or more intense dreaming activity.[50] Although these effects may appear surprising in a class of drugs that typically produces prominent REM suppression, it is possible that initial REM suppression can cause subsequent REM rebound, as the effects of the drug dissipate during the course of the day. With termination of antidepressant drug treatment, patients may again report an increase in dreaming activity, more intense dreams, and disturbing dreams. In this case, the explanation for the alteration in the experience of dreaming activity is likely to be explained on the basis of "REM rebound," a phenomenon that predictably occurs with the removal of a drug that had been producing potent, sustained REM suppression.

ANTIPSYCHOTICS

Critical Points

- Antipsychotic medications, particularly the second-generation or atypical antipsychotics, have sleep-promoting effects demonstrated through clinical studies and examination of their effects on sleep physiology.
- Clinicians can utilize knowledge of these effects and differences within this class to target specific sleep-related symptoms in the management of illnesses for which they are approved.
- Use of these medications for sleep symptoms and conditions for which they have not been fully evaluated should be approached with caution, and only in the context of careful balancing of their known risks versus potential benefits in subjects who demonstrated nonresponse or poor tolerability with standard treatments.

Basic and Clinical Pharamcology

The antipsychotic drugs are conventionally grouped into two categories: the typical antipsychotic drugs and the atypical (or second-generation) antipsychotic drugs. Several categories of typical antipsychotic drugs have been described on the basis of chemical structure, including the phenothiazines (e.g., chlorpromazine), the thioxanthines (e.g., thiothixene), and the butyrophenones (e.g., haloperidol). From a pharmacologic perspective, all of the typical antipsychotic drugs demonstrate potent inhibition of DA D_2 receptors, and minimal receptor blocking effects at DA D_1 receptors, leading to the characterization of typical antipsychotic drugs as demonstrating a very high ratio of $D_2:D_1$ blockade.[51,52]

Even though a great deal of attention with respect to the typical antipsychotic drugs has been directed to their inhibitory effects on various DA receptors, it should be emphasized that these agents exert a broad spectrum of pharmacologic effects, including inhibition of 5-HT$_{2A}$ and 5-HT$_{2C}$ receptors, muscarinic cholingeric receptors, α_1-adrenergic receptors and histamine H_1 receptors.[7,53] Several of the pharmacologic effects produced, to varying degrees, by different antipsychotic drugs are likely to produce prominent effects on sleep physiology and on the subjective sense of sleepiness. The potential effects of these receptors on sleep and wakefulness have been described earlier. The atypical antipsychotics, exemplified by the first drug from this class, clozapine, differ from the typical antipsychotics in their much more potent inhibition of 5-HT$_2$ receptors, particularly relative to their inhibition of DA D_2 receptors. Clozapine also exhibits a lower occupancy of the DA D_2 receptor at therapeutic concentrations (in the range of 60%) as compared to an occupancy rate of 80% or higher for the typical antipsychotic drugs, and it exerts more prominent inhibition of the DA D_1 receptor site, so the ratio of DA D_2 to DA D_1 blockade is much more balanced for clozapine than is the case for the typical antipsychotic drugs.[7,53] Since the initial marketing of clozapine in the United States in 1990, seven additional drugs have been marketed in this country, initially for the treatment of schizophrenia, and are also referred to as

atypical antipsychotic agents: risperidone (1993), olanzapine (1994), quetiapine (1997), ziprasidone (2000), aripiprazole (2002), asenapine (2009), and iloperidone (2009). In general, these agents demonstrate a more balanced ratio of DA D_2:DA D_1 blockade, and also show prominent receptor blockade for 5-HT$_{2A}$ and 5-HT$_{2C}$ receptors to varying degrees. Aripiprazole has a novel mechanism in that it is a DA D_2 partial agonist.[54,55] As is the case with clozapine, the other atypical antipsychotic agents demonstrate a broad but variable range of effects on other receptors sites that may be most relevant to their respective adverse event profiles, such as muscaranic cholinergic, α_1-adrenergic and histamine H_1 receptors.

The primary clinical application for the typical antipsychotic drugs has been in the treatment of schizophrenia, where they are effective in reducing or eliminating positive symptoms such as hallucinations, delusions, paranoid ideation, and excited, disorganized behaviors. They have, however, proved much less effective with respect to negative symptoms such as poverty of speech and thought, amotivation, and social withdrawal and isolation.[4,37,56] These agents have also been shown to be clinically useful in the management of positive psychotic symptoms related to other causes, including substance-induced psychoses, manic excitation, and psychotic depression.

Blockade of DA D_2 receptors by the typical antipsychotics is linked to their most common group of adverse events: the production of extrapyramidal side effects acutely, and tardive dyskinesia with more long-term treatment.[7] Another common adverse effect associated with the typical antipsychotic drugs involves an increase in prolactin levels, which can lead to problems such as gynecomastia in men and galactorrhea and amenorrhea in female subjects. Because DA plays a key role in inhibiting the secretion of prolactin, the potent effect of the typical antipsychotic drugs in blocking DA D_2 receptors provides a clear mechanism to explain this adverse effect as well.

Effects on Sleep Architecture and Sleep Physiology

Although a moderate number of studies have examined effects of typical and atypical antipsychotic drugs on sleep architecture employing PSG techniques, these studies have been limited by a number of methodologic shortcomings.[3,56,57] Among these methodologic limitations have been the inclusion of a rather small number of patients in most studies, enrollment of rather variable clinical populations of schizophrenic patients in most studies, marked differences in terms of the presence of potentially confounded concomitant medications and variable intervals since discontinuing treatment with antipsychotic agents, and different durations of treatment across the various studies. Despite these methodologic shortcomings, some observations have been reported that represent generally consistent findings across these array of studies involving typical and atypical antipsychotic drugs with respect to effects on sleep architecture, as is described here (Table 8-3).

Cumulative findings obtained in seven studies examining effects of typical antipsychotic drugs including haloperidol, thiothixene, flupenthixol, and assorted other typical antipsychotic agents by PSG techniques have been reviewed in Winokur and Kamath.[56] In general, these drugs increase TST and sleep efficiency, shorten SOL, and decrease WASO.

TABLE 8-3

Antipsychotic Medication Impact on Sleep Physiology

Medication	Sleep-Related Pharmacology	Effects on Sleep Architecture
Typical antipsychotic	D_2 antagonism, H_1 antagonism, anticholinergic	↑ TST ↑ Sleep efficiency ↓ SOL ↓ WASO ↔ SWS ↑ REM latency
Atypical antipsychotic	D2 antagonism, 5-HT$_2$ antagonism, H_1 antagonism	↑ TST ↑ Sleep efficiency ↓ SOL ↓ WASO ↑ SWS

D_2, dopamine D_2 receptor; H_1, histamine H_1 receptor; *5-HT*, 5-hydroxytryptamine; *NE*, norepinephrine; *REM*, rapid eye movement [sleep]; *SOL*, sleep onset latency; *SWS*, slow wave sleep; *TST*, total sleep time; *WASO*, wake after sleep onset.

SWS was not significantly altered across these various studies, and REM latency tended to increase.

Studies of effects of atypical antipsychotic drugs on sleep architecture assessed by PSG techniques are particularly pertinent to contemporary clinical practice in light of the fact that the atypical antipsychotic agents represent the predominant modality currently being prescribed in the United States. Clozapine, the original and prototypical atypical antipsychotic agent, has been reported to reduce SOL while increasing TST and sleep efficiency in schizophrenic patients.[4,56] In one study involving administration of clozapine to patients with treatment-refractory bipolar disorder, subjects were reported to manifest an average time of going to bed that was 55 minutes earlier than they reported at baseline assessment, perhaps as a reflection of the rather prominent sedating effects associated with clozapine.[58]

Risperidone demonstrates minimal affinity for muscarinic cholinergic and histamine H_1 receptors.[53] In studies examining effects of risperidone on sleep in schizophrenic patients compared to patients randomized to treatment with the typical antipsychotic drug haloperidol, risperidone was associated with an increase in sleep maintenance parameters and a decrease in number of awakenings.[56,59,60] In a study that employed haloperidol as a comparator agent, administration of risperidone was associated with an increase in SWS.[61] Additionally, a study involving administration of risperidone to healthy control subjects reported a reduction in REM sleep time.[62] Paliperidone extended release (ER) is the 9-hydroxy metabolite of risperidone, and has a similar pharmacologic profile. Probably the most extensive PSG study involving an atypical antipsychotic drug was carried out with paliperidone ER in a group of patients with schizophrenia who were stable at the time of enrollment in terms of schizophrenia symptomatology but who reported prominent symptoms of insomnia.[63] Enrolled patients were carefully screened with regard to being drug free for at least a 2-week period prior to baseline PSG assessment, a feature that differentiated this study from most other studies examining effects of other antipsychotic drugs in schizophrenic populations. Additional methodologic rigor associated with the paliperidone ER sleep study that distinguished it from other comparable studies in the field included

careful attention to the sleep-wake schedule of study participants, restriction of daytime napping, and strict limitations with respect to caffeine consumption and smoking. A total of 36 patients with schizophrenia completed the baseline assessments, 2-week treatment interval, and end of study two-night repeat PSG assessment on paliperidone ER or placebo. The results obtained included significant improvements in TST, sleep efficiency, stage 2 sleep, and REM sleep time and decreases in SOL, WASO, number of awakenings, and stage 1 sleep.

Olanzapine has a structural similarity to clozapine, and has also been noted to produce prominent inhibition of muscarinic cholinergic receptors and of histamine H_1 receptors. PSG sleep studies with olanzapine in schizophrenic patients have produced reports documenting significant decreases in wake time and light stage 1 sleep and significant increases in TST, stage 2 sleep, and SWS.[28,62] In studies with normal volunteer subjects, administration of olanzapine was reported to increase TST, sleep efficiency (SE), and SWS and to decrease SOL, WASO, and REM total sleep time.[64] In the majority of studies in which effects of olanzapine on sleep physiology have been evaluated, significant increases in SWS have been observed, an effect that is generally linked to its potency in blocking 5-HT$_2$ receptors.[4,56]

Quetiapine is notable, from a pharmacologic perspective, for exerting only moderate DA D_2 receptor blockade and 5-HT$_{2a}$ receptor blockade.[7] It demonstrates potent blockade of α_2-adrenergic receptors, which is probably related to its potential to produce orthostatic hypotension, and moderate antagonism at both histamine H_1 receptors and at muscarinic cholinergic receptors. In early clinical trial studies with quetiapine, prominent daytime somnolence was noted, with rates of 18% to 34% of patients reporting symptoms of daytime somnolence based on data cited in the package insert for quetiapine. The most extensive PSG sleep study with quetiapine involved a study with healthy male volunteer subjects.[65] Administration of quetiapine was reported to produce increases in TST, sleep efficiency, and stage 2 sleep and decreases in SOL and WASO. In a non-PSG-based study examining subjective sleep reports of sleep symptoms in patients with post-traumatic stress disorder (PTSD), improvement in the Pittsburgh Sleep Quality Index global sleep score was noticed with administration of relatively low doses of quetiapine, along with improvements in subjective reports of sleep quality, SOL, and TST and reductions in episodes of terror and acting out of dreams.[66]

Ziprasidone has been reported to produce potent blockade of DA D_2 receptors and 5-HT$_2$ receptors.[7] It exerts low to moderate inhibition of muscarinic cholinergic receptors, α_1-adrenergic receptors and histamine H_1 receptors. Other pharmacologically defining features of ziprasidone, among the atypical antipsychotic drugs, include agonist effects at the 5-HT$_{1a}$ receptor and relatively potent blockade of the 5-HT and the NE presynaptic transporters.[4] Only a single PSG sleep study has been reported with ziprasidone to date, in healthy male volunteer subjects.[65] Administration of ziprasidone in this study produced increases in TST, sleep efficiency, stage 2 sleep, and REM latency and decreases in SWS, WASO, stage 1 sleep, number of awakenings, and percentage of REM sleep time. Ziprasidone also produced prominent suppression of REM sleep, an effect not typically seen in studies involving atypical antipsychotic agents; PSG studies have been performed with the majority of antidepressant drugs that share its monoamine reuptake inhibition effects.

Notably, there appears to be a lack on information regarding effects of several of the more recently marketed atypical antipsychotic drugs, with no reported PSG studies being available, to our knowledge, for aripiprazole, asenapine, or iloperidone. Additionally, as noted previously, data are lacking with regard to sleep studies conducted in patients with schizophrenia, the original clinical indication leading to FDA approval with respect to quetiapine or ziprasidone. Therefore, even though all of the atypical antipsychotic drugs demonstrate a range of pharmacologic effects suggestive of the possibility that they may exert prominent effects on various aspects of sleep architecture, rather limited data are currently available on this class of therapeutic agents, and PSG sleep study data are currently available from studies conducted in schizophrenic patients for only five of the eight currently marketed, atypical antipsychotic drugs.

Clinical Evidence for Efficacy in Sleep Disorders

The antipsychotic drugs' effects on sleep may be mediated through 5-HT_2 receptors, which offer the promise of increasing SWS, and through histamine H_1 inhibitory effects, which might contribute to a shortening of SOL and an improvement in TST and sleep efficiency. However, broad pharmacologic profiles of the antipsychotic drugs convey substantial risk for unwanted adverse effects that might significantly limit their therapeutic potential with respect to the treatment of sleep disorders. In particular, the typical antipsychotic drugs are associated with a significant risk of producing extrapyramidal motor symptoms (EPS), whereas a number of the atypical antipsychotic agents can produce significant weight gain and increased risk for metabolic syndrome, as well as the potential for causing excessive daytime somnolence in some cases.[7] Strategies for managing these risks and developing agents that have the potential to be more useful in the treatment of sleep disorders include: (1) developing drugs with more selective pharmacologic profiles, as exemplified by some selective 5-HT_2 receptor antagonists that have recently been evaluated in phase III clinical trials for the treatment of insomnia, or (2) scaling down the doses of antipsychotic agents substantially in order to find a dose range that utilizes pharmacologic effects of these drugs that have the potential to facilitate sleep while minimizing the risk associated with other pharmacologic effects that are minimally expressed with administration in low dose ranges.[6] For example, clinical experience indicates that quetiapine is being utilized quite frequently in low dose ranges to manage severe insomnia problems in patients who fail to respond to more traditional hypnotic agents that act through effects on the benzodiazepine-GABA (γ-aminobutyric acid) macromolecular complex. When administered in this fashion, the predominant pharmacologic effect exerted by quetiapine relates to its potent histamine H_1 inhibitory effects. However, it is necessary to balance the sleep-promoting effects of quetiapine, administered in dose ranges of 25 to 100 mg at bedtime, with the potential that some patients may still experience excessive daytime somnolence, and others may experience problems with weight gain or glucose intolerance. Although the incidence of EPS with quetiapine in clinical populations has been observed to be low, and although the low doses used

for insomnia may further minimize this risk, the potential for occurrence of these adverse effects cannot be excluded.

Quetiapine also has some clinical reports suggesting utility in the treatment of sleep problems associated with PTSD. In a retrospective study of Vietnam War veterans with PTSD who reported prominent sleep problems, administration of quetiapine was reported to produce improvement in subjective reports of sleep disturbance in 62% of patients and improvement in 25% of patients reporting problems with disturbing nightmares.[67] The possible benefit of quetiapine in PTSD awaits more systematic research in the context of randomized controlled studies, preferably utilizing PSG monitoring. In an open label pilot study recruiting patients with primary insomnia, quetiapine 25 mg at bedtime produced improvements in subjective sleep quality and increases in TST and SE at both 2 and 6 weeks of treatment, but it did not bring about a shortening of SOL.[68] Clearly, further studies are needed to fully evaluate the potential efficacy as well as the adverse event profile of a low dose regimen of quetiapine in patients with primary insomnia.

Clinical Management: Initiation, Maintenance, Precautions, and Abuse Potential

Some antipsychotic drugs are quite sedating, and administration of these agents in the evening might help address symptoms of insomnia. Examples of more notable sedating antipsychotic drugs include chlorpromazine, thioridazine, and thiothixene among the typical antipsychotic drugs, and clozapine, olanzapine, and quetiapine among the atypical antipsychotic agents.[56] However, a number of the antipsychotic drugs may be of less benefit to address problems with SOL due to their relatively long time to achieve a maximum concentration in plasma (e.g., T_{max} values of approximately 5 hours after ingestion for olanzapine and ziprasidone).[4] In contrast, quetiapine demonstrates a T_{max} value of 1 hour, perhaps partially explaining its notable popularity among the atypical antipsychotic agents for treating problems related to sleep difficulties.

Antipsychotic drugs also differ substantially with respect to their half-lives. For example, quetiapine demonstrates a relatively short half-life on the order of 7 hours (although a sustained release form of quetiapine has recently been marketed[46]), which suggests the potential for it to be capable of being administered in the evening with minimal daytime somnolence. Other antipsychotic drugs are associated with considerably longer half-lives. For example, olanzapine, with a reported half-life of 30 hours, particularly when administered on a repeated basis, would be expected to have a significant liability for producing daytime somnolence.

In addition to the potential for EPS, weight gain, and metabolic syndrome, antipsychotic agents (especially risperidone) may cause or exacerbate periodic limb movements in sleep (PLMS) and restless legs syndrome (RLS).[4] Weight gain associated with many of the atypical antipsychotic drugs, in particular clozapine, olanzapine, and quetiapine, may lead to the development of obstructive sleep apnea syndrome. Thus, in consideration of the potential to utilize the antipsychotic drugs for their potential sleep-enhancing effects, consideration needs to be given to the risk-benefit ratio for this drug class, especially in light of the fact that many of the standard hypnotic compounds used to treat insomnia complaints demonstrate favorable adverse event profiles.

ANTIEPILEPTICS

Critical Points

- The most promising potential beneficial effect on sleep of the antiepileptic drugs discussed in this section is an increase in the percentage of slow wave sleep and a decrease in awakenings.
- Clinicians can utilize knowledge of these effects to target specific sleep-related symptoms in the management of illnesses for which they are indicated.
- Use of these medications for sleep symptoms and conditions for which they have not been fully evaluated should be approached with caution; clinicians considering such use should carefully consider the known risks of this group of medications and judiciously balance those risks against potential benefits in making individual decisions on patient management.

Basic and Clinical Pharmacology

Antiepileptics modulate neuronal excitability via a broad set of pharmacologic actions that affect glutamate and GABA neurotransmitter systems through direct and indirect effects. They have been observed to exert widely varying effects on sleep architecture, daytime somnolence, and the sleep-wake cycle in the epilepsy population,[69,70] although findings of disturbed sleep and alterations in sleep architecture and physiology in the epilepsy population itself[71] complicate interpretation of these findings. The first-generation antiepileptics are associated with excessive daytime somnolence and other adverse effects that have limited exploration of their use for primary sleep disorders.[72]

Effects on Sleep Architecture and Sleep Physiology

The development of newer-generation antiepileptics with improved tolerability profiles has facilitated the evaluation of a number of additional clinical uses in clinical trials, including studies examining treatment of insomnia. To date, the most studied antiepileptics in clinical sleep physiology and sleep disorder treatment are tiagabine, gabapentin, and pregabalin, although none of these medications has received regulatory approval for management of primary sleep disorders. In keeping with the general goals of this chapter, the remainder of this section will focus on data available for gabapentin, pregabalin, and tiagabine in terms of potential utility for sleep disorders among all of the older and newer generation antiepileptic drugs that are currently marketed. Tiagabine inhibits neuronal and glial reuptake of GABA, increasing synaptic concentrations of GABA, which in turn prolong inhibitory postsynaptic potentials at $GABA_A$ receptors, in addition to effects on presynaptic $GABA_B$ receptors. Tiagabine may enhance inhibition by increasing $GABA_A$ receptor-mediated tonic inhibition, by increasing synaptic $GABA_A$ receptor-mediated currents, and by increasing activation of $GABA_B$ heteroreceptors.[73] Tiagabine can, however, also have some proepileptic effects, such as desensitization of $GABA_A$ receptors. Gabapentin and pregabalin modulate neuronal calcium flux through actions on the $\alpha_2\delta$ subunit of voltage-gated calcium channels, and have been found to increase synaptic GABA concentrations and GABA

turnover.[74] The latter effects appear most likely to mediate their impact on sleep, although there may be indirect effects of their modulation of calcium flux through downstream modulation of monoamine neurotransmitters relevant to sleep physiology including glutamate, substance P, and norepinephrine.[73]

Tiagabine has been demonstrated in healthy volunteers to increase slow wave sleep and decrease WASO[75,76] and to reverse the impact of sleep restriction on sustained attention measures.[77] In healthy elderly subjects, a placebo-controlled study found that both 4 mg and 8 mg tiagabine decreased WASO, and increased the duration of SWS, but only the 4-mg dose increased TST and only the 8-mg dose improved a sleep-continuity index.[78] A multiple-dose (4, 8, 12, 16 mg), randomized, placebo-controlled crossover trial of tiagabine in primary insomnia patients found dose-dependent increases in SWS and decreases in WASO; tests of alertness and psychomotor performance were unaffected up to and including the 8-mg dose.[76] A similar study in 207 elderly adults with primary insomnia found significant increases in slow wave sleep with 4, 6, and 8 mg tiagabine, and significantly decreased awakenings at 6 and 8 mg.[77] The 8-mg dose was poorly tolerated, however, and was associated with reduced alertness as measured by the Digital Symbol Substitution Test.

The effect of gabapentin on sleep and sleep physiology has been investigated in healthy volunteers and in patient populations. In a single-dose placebo-controlled study of sleep disruption caused by alcohol in healthy control subjects, gabapentin doses of 300 mg and 600 mg were found to decrease awakenings, increase sleep efficiency, and decrease stage 1 sleep compared to placebo.[79] The 600-mg dose was associated with increased SWS, decreased arousals, and decreased REM sleep. In an open-label study in healthy volunteers with an external control group, gabapentin was titrated to 600 mg three times daily over a 7-day period and then continued for a 7- to 10-day stable dosing period; treatment was associated with significant increases in SWS, with no effect on other PSG variables.[80] Although it is being utilized clinically on an empirical basis,[81] gabapentin has not been examined in controlled trials in primary insomnia. Gabapentin has, though, been studied in the treatment of symptoms of insomnia in alcohol dependence, in RLS and in menopausal women experiencing hot flashes. A clinic-based, unblinded comparison of gabapentin versus trazodone treatment of insomnia in 55 alcoholic outpatients demonstrated improvement in self-reported sleep scores similar to that with trazodone with less morning tiredness in the gabapentin group.[82] A double-blind crossover study of the use of gabapentin in 24 RLS patients using polysomnography found significant improvement in TST, sleep efficiency, and SWS compared to placebo treatment at a mean daily dose of 1855 mg.[83] In a 12-week study examining treatment of 59 postmenopausal women with hot flashes, subjects who were randomized to receive gabapentin, escalating to 300 mg three times daily had significantly greater improvement in a subjective measure of sleep quality (the Pittsburgh Sleep Quality Index) than placebo-treated subjects.[84]

The effects of pregabalin on sleep have been evaluated in studies in healthy volunteers and in clinical populations. A randomized, blinded, crossover trial evaluated the effect of pregabalin on sleep physiology in healthy subjects compared with alprazolam and placebo.[85] Subjects received pregabalin 150 mg, alprazolam 1 mg, or placebo given three times per day over 3-day treatment periods with 7-day washouts in between periods. Treatment with pregabalin was associated with increased SWS, increased stage 4 sleep, reduction in SOL, reduced REM duration, and decreased number of awakenings compared to placebo. Treatment with alprazolam produced modest, but significant, reduction in SOL compared with placebo, but significantly reduced SWS, increased REM latency, and reduced REM duration. Pregabalin 300 mg per day in a small ($N = 15$) 4-week, double-blind, placebo-controlled study in epilepsy patients was found to decrease awakenings and improve subjective measures of sleep disturbance and sleep quality.[86] Pregabalin's effect on sleep parameters in 370 patients with postherpetic neuralgia was assessed with the Medical Outcomes Study (MOS) sleep questionnaire[87]; improvement in pain measures was accompanied by significant improvements in the "sleep-disturbance" and "sleep-adequacy" factors of the MOS sleep scale by week 1 of treatment. An analysis of two studies involving a total of 1493 subjects with fibromyalgia found that treatment with pregabalin significantly improved MOS sleep disturbance, quantity of sleep, and sleep problems index scores relative to placebo.[88] Although pregabalin has not been approved for marketing for generalized anxiety disorder (GAD) in the United States, a study of six double-blind placebo-controlled trials in GAD examined the impact of pregabalin on GAD patients with high levels of insomnia.[89] Treatment with pregabalin in a range of 300 mg to 600 mg per day resulted in significant improvement in insomnia scores over 4 to 6 weeks of treatment, which was comparable to the improvement seen with benzodiazepine comparators (alprazolam or lorazepam).

The postmarketing observation of seizures in patients without epilepsy being treated with tiagabine has limited the extension of its use into other clinical populations. The clinical empirical use of gabapentin for insomnia is not supported by controlled data in primary insomnia, although its effects on sleep in treatment of RLS are consistent with improvements in sleep parameters observed in healthy controls, and it has shown some efficacy in insomnia associated with alcohol dependence. Both gabapentin and pregabalin, which share a common mechanism of action, increase slow wave sleep and decrease WASO and arousals in healthy volunteers, but their use in treatment of primary insomnia has not been evaluated in large-scale safety and efficacy trials. Treatment with pregabalin has been associated with improved sleep quality and decreased awakenings in clinical populations for which it is approved, including postherpetic neuralgia and fibromyalgia.

Clinical Management: Initiation, Maintenance, Precautions, and Abuse Potential

While evidence is accumulating to demonstrate that a number of antiepileptic medications may have beneficial effects on sleep in healthy subjects and clinical populations, including the primary indications of epilepsy, neuropathic pain, and fibromyalgia, it is important to note and assess key risks associated with their use when extending the results of relatively small studies to other clinical populations that have not been evaluated in standard large-scale Phase 3 clinical trials. For example, postmarketing reports have shown that tiagabine use has been associated with new onset seizures and status epilepticus in patients without epilepsy, possibly related to dosage, although seizures have been reported in patients taking

TABLE 8-4

Antiepileptic Medication Impact on Sleep Physiology

Medication	Sleep-Related Pharmacology	Effect(s) on Sleep Architecture
Tiagabine	GABA reuptake inhibitor	↑ SWS ↓ WASO
Gabapentin	$\alpha_2\delta$ voltage-gated calcium channel antagonist	↑ SWS
Pregabalin	$\alpha_2\delta$ voltage-gated calcium channel antagonist	↑ SWS ↓ SOL

GABA, γ-aminobutyric acid; *SOL*, sleep onset latency; *SWS*, slow wave sleep; *WASO*, wake after sleep onset.

daily doses of tiagabine as low as 4 mg per day. Another key risk to assess relates to the December 2008, FDA press release announcing a warning that antiepileptic drugs (AEDs) can increase the risk of suicidal thoughts or behavior in patients taking these drugs for any indication.[90] The warning stated that patients treated with any AED for any indication should be monitored for the emergence or worsening of depression, suicidal thoughts or behavior, and any unusual changes in mood or behavior. It should be noted that of the medications discussed in this section, pregabalin is listed on DEA Schedule V,[91] indicating that abuse of pregabalin may lead to limited physical dependence or psychological dependence relative to the drugs or other substances on Schedule I through IV. Case reports[92,93] and epidemiologic evidence[94] support this finding as well; thus, caution should be used with patients that are at risk for abuse or dependence.

The most promising beneficial effect of the antiepileptic drugs discussed in this section is an increase in the percentage of slow wave sleep and a decrease in awakenings, although decreased sleep latency has also been observed (Table 8-4). Thus, when considering options for treatment within their respective indications, selection of tiagabine, gabapentin, or pregabalin may be preferred over alternative treatments that have not demonstrated similar effects on sleep for patients who have prominent complaints of insomnia. Each of these medications is typically administered in divided doses, so an additional consideration would include adjusting the proportion of the total daily dose that is administered at bedtime to optimize the impact on insomnia symptoms as long as that approach would not be expected to adversely impact control of symptoms of the primary diagnosis.

Clinicians considering the use of antiepileptic drugs off-label for treatment of insomnia should carefully review their known risks and ensure that medications currently approved for treatment of insomnia have been utilized and found ineffective or poorly tolerated. In addition, the clinician should ensure appropriate informed consent by discussing and documenting risks and potential benefits associated with their use in the individual patient under consideration. Prudent clinical practice would suggest targeting the lower end of the known dose range associated with observed effects on sleep and insomnia in clinical trials, and performing ongoing assessment of potential risks associated with their use in addition to confirming that the balance of risks and benefits supports continuing treatment. As noted with the literature on use of antidepressants for sleep disorders, there is a lack of available studies evaluating efficacy and safety of antiepileptic drugs in long-term treatment of sleep disorders; as a result, the clinician should engage in careful evaluation of clinical benefits and risks if maintenance or chronic treatment is considered.

ANTIHISTAMINES

Critical Points

- Even though their use as over-the-counter treatments for insomnia is widespread, evidence for efficacy of the antihistamines (H_1 antagonists) in the treatment of insomnia is limited. Although short-term treatment studies show modest efficacy for mild to moderate insomnia, there is a lack of long-term data on the safety and maintenance of efficacy for these compounds.
- Use of antihistamines for mild to moderate insomnia in adults appears to have a reasonable balance of risk and benefit, but clinicians should monitor patients for daytime somnolence and cognitive effects.
- Use of antihistamines in the elderly and pediatric populations should be approached with greater caution given findings of increased risk for cognitive impairment in the elderly, and potential for daytime somnolence and cognitive effects in children

Basic and Clinical Pharmacology

Histamine is a neurotransmitter known to promote wakefulness and vigilance. The brain histamine system innervates the tuberomammillary nucleus of the hypothalamus, and projects diffusely to various regions of the cerebral cortex where it interacts with histamine H_1 receptors. Histaminergic neurons are highly active during waking and attention and less active or inactive during sleep. Activation of H_1 receptors promotes wakefulness, and histaminergic neurons have been found to be silent or exhibit very low activity during sleep.[95] The classical antihistamines are histamine H_1 receptor antagonists that were initially developed for treatment of seasonal allergies and allergic reactions. Preclinical studies demonstrate sedating effects of H_1 receptor antagonism,[96] and a common adverse event noted during development and clinical use of these antihistamines was sedation.[97,98] The available sedating antihistamines also have clinically relevant anticholinergic effects.[99]

Effects on Sleep Architecture and Sleep Physiology

There are few studies available examining the impact of H_1 antagonists on sleep physiology by polysomnography. The H_1 antagonist chlorpheniramine was examined in a single-dose three-way crossover study with placebo and fenofexadine, a poorly CNS-penetrant H_1 antagonist, in healthy Japanese subjects that included polysomnography and psychomotor assessments.[100] This study found a significant increase in SOL with 6 mg chlorpheniramine compared to placebo, rather than a decrease as might be expected. Chlorpheniramine was associated with an increase in REM latency and suppression of REM sleep compared to placebo. Assessments on the day after administration of chlorpheniramine found decreased latency to daytime sleep and decrements in psychomotor performance on tests of attention, vigilance, and working memory

compared to placebo treatment. A three-way crossover study examining sedation and psychomotor effects of daytime-administered diphenhydramine 50 mg three times a day compared to loratidine 10 mg daily and placebo in healthy male subjects found no difference in nocturnal polysomnography parameters between the three treatments, including SOL, TST, WASO, or sleep stage percentages.[98]

A number of studies that utilized PSG endpoints to evaluate daytime somnolence with H_1 antagonist treatment in healthy subjects have demonstrated decreased latency to sleep, as assessed by the multiple sleep latency test (MSLT), and decreased performance on psychomotor testing with diphenhydramine 50 mg[101-103] and hydroxyzine 20 to 25 mg[104,105] compared to placebo. A study of clinical tolerance to daytime somnolence with H_1 antagonists was conducted in 15 healthy male subjects using a double-blind placebo-controlled crossover design.[106] This study examined the effect of 4 days of treatment with diphenhydramine 50 mg twice a day and placebo with a 2-week washout period between treatments. Actigraphy was used to measure TST at night, and daytime somnolence was assessed using MSLT and the Stanford Sleepiness Scale. Daytime psychomotor performance was assessed using a battery of measures that included the divided attention task. This analysis revealed significantly decreased latency to sleep and increased subjective sleepiness on day 1 of treatment with diphenhydramine, which did not differ from the placebo condition by day 4 of treatment. Similarly, diphenhydramine was associated with decrements in performance on the divided attention task on day 1 compared to placebo, but this finding was also no longer present by day 4 of treatment. The physiologic basis for next day residual sedation was illuminated by a positron emission tomography (PET) H_1 receptor occupancy assessment in a double-blind, placebo-controlled crossover study of eight healthy male subjects.[107] Assessment of H_1 receptor occupancy approximately 13 hours after an evening dose of 50 mg diphenhydramine revealed 45% receptor occupancy, with a trend finding for increased sedation with diphenhydramine on the Stanford Sleepiness Scale compared to placebo.

Clinical Evidence for Efficacy in Sleep Disorders

Despite the widespread use of H_1 antagonists as over-the-counter treatments for insomnia,[108] there are few controlled studies examining the efficacy of these agents in treatment of insomnia.[109] A study of 111 family practice patients with mild to moderate insomnia was conducted using a double-blind crossover design with 1 week of treatment with 50 mg of diphenhydramine and placebo.[110] Efficacy assessments included a sleep diary and subjective measures of morning restfulness and patient satisfaction. This study found decreased latency to sleep onset, increased TST, decreased WASO, and subjective improvement of sleep quality with diphenhydramine that was significantly greater than that found with placebo. Diphenhydramine was also associated with significant improvement in subjective morning restfulness and was significantly more preferred by patients compared to placebo. The effect of 2 weeks of treatment with 50 mg diphenhydramine was compared to 4 weeks of treatment with an herbal preparation of valerian and hops in a placebo-controlled, parallel group study in 184 subjects with mild insomnia.[111] Efficacy endpoints included subjective sleep diaries, PSG evaluation, clinical ratings, and a quality-of-life measure. Diphenhydramine treatment was associated with a significantly greater increase in sleep efficiency compared to placebo, with a trend for increased TST. Subjective ratings of insomnia severity were also improved with diphenhydramine compared to placebo. No significant differences were found between diphenhydramine and placebo on slow wave sleep, REM sleep, or sleep continuity variables.

The efficacy of diphenhydramine 50 mg has also been assessed in comparison to temazepam 15 mg and placebo in two crossover studies in elderly patients with insomnia. An outpatient study in 25 elderly patients with primary insomnia utilized 2-week treatment periods with a minimum 2-week washout; efficacy was assessed using subjective sleep diaries, and next-day psychomotor effects were assessed by the digit symbol substitution test (DSST), the manual tracking test (MTT), and a free recall assessment of memory.[112] Although temazepam was associated with improvement compared to placebo for sleep quality, TST, number of awakenings, and SOL, only the number of awakenings were improved compared to placebo for diphenhydramine. Neither temazepam nor diphenhydramine demonstrated significant differences from placebo on the DSST, MTT, or the free recall assessment of memory. Dry mouth and lightheadedness were more common with diphenhydramine than placebo or temazepam, and imbalance and anxiety were more common with temazepam than diphenhydramine or placebo. One subject experienced a fall during temazepam treatment. A second study in 17 elderly nursing home patients used 5-day treatment periods with a 3-day washout and identical medication doses to the previous study.[113] Efficacy endpoints included observer sleep diaries and subjective morning sleep questionnaires, and next-day effects were assessed using a set of psychomotor and cognitive assessments. Treatment with diphenhydramine was associated with reduction in subjective SOL and increased sleep duration on observer assessments compared to placebo, as well as decreased performance on psychomotor and cognitive assessments and increased rates of daytime somnolence compared to placebo.

Pediatric use of diphenhydramine (1 mg/kg) for children with a variety of sleep disorders was examined in a 2-week, double-blind, placebo-controlled crossover study using parent completed sleep diary endpoints.[114] Fifty subjects between 2 and 12 years of age participated in the study; significant improvements in SOL and frequency of awakenings were observed with diphenhydramine compared to placebo, with a trend for improvement in sleep duration.

The efficacy of diphenhydramine in a mixed group of patients with psychiatric disorders in inpatient and outpatient settings was examined in a double-blind, placebo-controlled study with a clinical assessment as the efficacy endpoint.[115] Doses of diphenhydramine examined in the study included 12.5, 25, and 50 mg over a 2-week treatment period. The proportion of subjects with at least minimal improvement was significantly greater for the overall diphenhydramine treatment group versus placebo. The absence of previous medication treatment for insomnia was a predictor of treatment response to diphenhydramine in the study.

Adverse events associated with the use of H₁ antagonists in clinical surveillance studies include somnolence, grogginess, dizziness, dry mouth, fatigue, and weakness in a general hospital setting, and delirium and cognitive impairment in hospitalized elderly patients.[116,117]

Clinical Management: Initiation, Maintenance, Precautions, and Abuse Potential

Although the use of H_1 antagonists as over-the-counter and prescribed treatments for insomnia is widespread and well precedented clinically, there are few controlled studies evaluating the efficacy and safety of these medications for treatment of sleep disorders or comparative data relative to other treatment options for insomnia. The available controlled studies demonstrate modest efficacy for mild to moderate insomnia with short-term treatment, but long-term studies examining the durability of treatment effects and safety are lacking. Study findings suggest that the sedating effect of H_1 antagonists during daytime tolerates relatively rapidly,[106] but it is unclear whether this applies to their effects on nighttime sleep with longer-term treatment. Dizziness and daytime hangover effects, including somnolence and impairment of psychomotor performance, are the most common adverse events noted in clinical trials and clinical practice. Elderly patients may exhibit higher rates of confusion and other cognitive impairment, likely due to the combination of sedation adverse events and the anticholinergic activity present in the H_1 antagonists prescribed for insomnia. Thus, the use of H_1 antagonists for treatment of insomnia in the elderly should be approached with caution with close monitoring for psychomotor impairment adverse events. These risks should be balanced against the well-characterized risks for psychomotor adverse events with other treatment options such as the benzodiazepines and nonbenzodiazepine hypnotics, however, when selecting a treatment option for insomnia in the elderly. The very limited efficacy data in pediatric populations suggest modest efficacy for sleep disorders in children, but this potential benefit should also be carefully weighed against the risk for psychomotor effects that have been well characterized in acute administration studies in children.[118]

Although there is some preclinical evidence for potential abuse liability of antihistamines,[119] clinical abuse liability studies have demonstrated this risk only with supratherapeutic doses that also cause undesirable effects,[120] and clinical surveys have found relatively low risk in comparison to other hypnotic medications.[121]

SUMMARY

The impact of antidepressants, antipsychotics, antiepileptic, and antihistaminergic drugs on sleep has been observed and documented from the earliest days of their discovery and initial clinical use. These effects can be beneficial, mitigating the negative impact of sleep-related symptoms on quality of life and functioning, or contribute to tolerability problems and deficits in functioning, depending on the specific drug characteristics and the substantial individual variation in the response to these medications. Knowledge of the specific pharmacologic mechanisms mediating these effects has been steadily accumulating through preclinical experiments that permit detailed investigations into their many specific impacts on the highly conserved systems regulating sleep and wakefulness in mammals. The effects of these medications on sleep parameters and clinical symptoms have been demonstrated in studies of their effects on sleep and sleep physiology in healthy volunteers, and from the results of treatment studies in patient populations. This accumulating knowledge may be utilized by clinicians in the selection of treatments to address sleep-related symptoms for their approved disease indications, in the management of sleep-related adverse effects, and in carefully considered use for sleep symptoms that are poorly tolerated or refractory to conventional treatments. Finally, investigations of the mechanisms of action on sleep physiology for these drug classes as well as basic and clinical studies of the pathophysiology of sleep disorders are identifying new targets for developing more effective and better tolerated treatments for sleep disorders.

REFERENCES

1. Akiskal HS, Bourgeois ML, Angst J, et al. Re-evaluating the prevalence of and diagnostic composition within the broad clinical spectrum of bipolar disorders. *J Affective Dis.* 2000;59(Suppl 1):S5-S30.
2. Ford DE, Kamerow DB. Epidemiologic study of sleep disturbances and psychiatric disorders: An opportunity for prevention? *JAMA.* 1989;262(11):1479-1484.
3. Monti JM, Monti D. Sleep disturbance in schizophrenia. *Int Rev Psychiatry.* 2005;17(4):247-253.
4. Krystal AD, Goforth HW, Roth T. Effects of antipsychotic medications on sleep in schizophrenia. *Int Clin Psychopharmacol.* 2008;23(3):150-160.
5. Yager J, Gitlin MJ. Clinical manifestations of psychiatric disorders. In: Sadock BJ, Sadock VA, eds. *Kaplan & Sadock's Comprehensive Textbook of Psychiatry.* Philadelphia: Lippincott Williams & Wilkins; 2005:987-988.
6. DeMartinis NA, Winokur A. Effects of psychiatric medications on sleep and sleep disorders. *CNS Neurol Disord Drug Targets.* 2007;6(1):17-29.
7. Stahl SM. *Stahl's Essential Psychopharmacology.* 3rd ed. New York: Cambridge University Press; 2008.
8. Richelson E. Synaptic effects of antidepressants. *J Clin Psychopharmacol.* 1996;16(3 Suppl 2):1S-7S:discussion 7S-9S.
9. Hobson JA. Sleep mechanisms and pathophysiology: Some clinical implications of the reciprocal interaction hypothesis of sleep cycle control. *Psychosom Med.* 1983;45(2):123-140.
10. McCarley RW, Hobson JA. Neuronal excitability modulation over the sleep cycle: A structural and mathematical model. *Science.* 1975;189(4196):58-60.
11. Winokur A, Gary KA, Rodner S, Rae-Red C, Fernando AT, et al. Depression, sleep physiology, and antidepressant drugs. *Depress Anxiety.* 2001;14(1):19-28.
12. Wilson S, Argyropoulos S. Antidepressants and sleep: A qualitative review of the literature. *Drugs.* 2005;65(7):927-947.
13. Vogel GW, Buffenstein A, Minter K, Hennessey A. Drug effects on REM sleep and on endogenous depression. *Neurosci Biobehav Rev.* 1990;14(1):49-63.
14. Wolf R, Dykierek P, Gattaz WF, Maras A, Kohnen R, et al. Differential effects of trimipramine and fluoxetine on sleep in geriatric depression. *Pharmacopsychiatry.* 2001;34(2):60-65.
15. Wyatt RJ, Fram DH, Kupfer DJ, Snyder F. Total prolonged drug-induced REM sleep suppression in anxious-depressed patients. *Arch Gen Psychiatry.* 1971;24(2):145-155.
16. Kupfer DJ, Bowers Jr MB. REM sleep and central monoamine oxidase inhibition. *Psychopharmacologia.* 1972;27(3):183-190.
17. Mendelson WB. A review of the evidence for the efficacy and safety of trazodone in insomnia. *J Clin Psychiatry.* 2005;66(4):469-476.
18. Gillin JC, Rapaport M, Erman MK, Winokur A, Albala BJ. A comparison of nefazodone and fluoxetine on mood and on objective, subjective, and clinician-rated measures of sleep in depressed patients: A double-blind, 8-week clinical trial. *J Clin Psychiatry.* 1997;58(5):185-192.
19. Armitage R, Yonkers K, Cole D, Rush AJ. A multicenter, double-blind comparison of the effects of nefazodone and fluoxetine on sleep architecture and quality of sleep in depressed outpatients. *J Clin Psychopharmacol.* 1997;17(3):161-168.
20. Rush AJ, Armitage R, Gillin JC, Yonkers KA, Winokur A, et al. Comparative effects of nefazodone and fluoxetine on sleep in outpatients with major depressive disorder. *Biol Psychiatry.* 1998;44(1):3-14.
21. Beasley Jr CM, Sayler ME, Weiss AM, Potzin JH. Fluoxetine: Activating and sedating effects at multiple fixed doses. *J Clin Psychopharmacol.* 1992;12(5):328-333.
22. Oberndorfer S, Saletu-Zyhlarz G, Saletu B. Effects of selective serotonin reuptake inhibitors on objective and subjective sleep quality. *Neuropsychobiology.* 2000;42(2):69-81.
23. Vogal G, Cohen J, Mullis D, Kensler T, Kaplita S. Nefazodone and REM sleep: How do antidepressant drugs decrease REM sleep? *Sleep.* 1998;21(1):70-77.
24. Keck Jr PE, Hudson JI, Dorsey CM, Campbell PI. Effect of fluoxetine on sleep. *Biol Psychiatry.* 1991;29(6):618-619.
25. Schenck CH, Mahowald MW, Kim SW, et al. Prominent eye movements during NREM sleep and REM sleep behavior disorder associated with fluoxetine treatment of depression and obsessive-compulsive disorder. *Sleep.* 1992;15(3):226-235.
26. Dorsey CM, Lukas SE, Cunningham SL. Fluoxetine-induced sleep disturbance in depressed patients. *Neuropsychopharmacology.* 1996;14(6):437-442.
27. Luthringer R, Toussaint M, Schaltenbrand N, et al. A double-blind, placebo-controlled evaluation of the effects of orally administered venlafaxine on sleep in inpatients with major depression. *Psychopharmacol Bull.* 1996;32(4):637-646.
28. Salin-Pascual RJ, Herrera-Estrella M, Galicia-Polo L, Laurrabaquio MR. Olanzapine acute administration in schizophrenic patients increases delta sleep and sleep efficiency. *Biol Psychiatry.* 1999;46(1):141-143.
29. Chalon S, Pereira A, Lainey E, et al. Comparative effects of duloxetine and desipramine on sleep EEG in healthy subjects. *Psychopharmacology (Berl).* 2005;177(4):357-365.
30. Kluge M, Schussler P, Steiger A. Duloxetine increases stage 3 sleep and suppresses rapid eye movement (REM) sleep in patients with major depression. *Eur Neuropsychopharmacol.* 2007;17(8):527-531.
31. Nofzinger EA, Reynolds CF 3rd, Thase ME, et al. REM sleep enhancement by bupropion in depressed men. *Am J Psychiatry.* 1995;152(2):274-246.
32. Ott GE, Rao U, Lin KM, et al. Effect of treatment with bupropion on EEG sleep: Relationship to antidepressant response. *Int J Neuropsychopharmacol.* 2004;7(3):275-281.
33. Winokur A, Sateia MJ, Hayes JB, et al. Acute effects of mirtazapine on sleep continuity and sleep architecture in depressed patients: A pilot study. *Biol Psychiatry.* 2000;48(1):75-78.
34. Winokur A, DeMartinis III NA, McNally DOP, et al. Comparative effects of mirtazapine and fluoxetine on sleep physiology measures in patients with major depression and insomnia. *J Clin Psychiatry.* 2003;64(10):1224-1229.
35. Cusack B, Nelson A, Richelson E. Binding of antidepressants to human brain receptors: Focus on newer generation compounds. *Psychopharmacology (Berl).* 1994;114(4):559-565.
36. Tatsumi M, Groshan K, Blakely RD, Richelson E. Pharmacological profile of antidepressants and related compounds at human monoamine transporters. *Eur J Pharmacol.* 1997;340(2-3):249-258.
37. Stahl SM. Selective histamine H1 antagonism: Novel hypnotic and pharmacologic actions challenge classical notions of antihistamines. *CNS Spectr.* 2008;13(12):1027-1038.
38. Roth T, Rogowski R, Hull S, et al. Efficacy and safety of doxepin 1 mg, 3 mg, and 6 mg in adults with primary insomnia. *Sleep.* 2007;30(11):1555-1561.
39. Singh H, Becker PM. Novel therapeutic usage of low-dose doxepin hydrochloride. *Expert Opin Investig Drugs.* 2007;16(8):1295-1305.
40. Walsh JK, Erman M, Erwin CW, et al. Subjective hypnotic efficacy of trazodone and zolpidem in DSMIII-R primary insomnia. *Hum Psychopharmacol Clin Exp.* 1998;13(3):191-198.
41. Nowell PD, Reynolds III CF, Buysse DJ, et al. Paroxetine in the treatment of primary insomnia: preliminary clinical and electroencephalogram sleep data. *J Clin Psychiatry.* 1999;60(2):89-95.
42. Arnold LM, Keck Jr PE, Welge JA. Antidepressant treatment of fibromyalgia. A meta-analysis and review. *Psychosomatics.* 2000;41(2):104-113.
43. Lawson K. Pharmacological treatments of fibromyalgia: Do complex conditions need complex therapies? *Drug Discov Today.* 2008; 13(7-8):333-340.
44. DeMartinis NA, Kamath J, Winokur A. New approaches for the treatment of sleep disorders. *Adv Pharmacol.* 2009;57:187-235.
45. Morgenthaler TI, Kapur VK, Brown T, et al. Practice parameters for the treatment of narcolepsy and other hypersomnias of central origin. *Sleep.* 2007;30(12):1705-1711.
46. Stahl SM. *Essential Psychopharmacology: The Prescriber's Guide.* Cambridge, UK: Cambridge University Press; 2005.

47. Stahl SM. Mechanism of action of trazodone: A multifunctional drug. *CNS Spectr.* 2009;14(10):536-546.

48. Walsh JK, Erman M, Erwin CW, et al. Subjective hypnotic efficacy of trazodone and zolpidem in DSMIII-R primary insomnia. *Hum Psychopharmacol Clin Exp.* 1998;13(3):191-198.

49. Warner CH, Bobo W, Warner C, et al. Antidepressant discontinuation syndrome. *Am Fam Physician.* 2006;74(3):449-456.

50. Parish JM. Violent dreaming and antidepressant drugs: Or how paroxetine made me dream that I was fighting Saddam Hussein. *J Clin Sleep Med.* 2007;3(5):529-531.

51. Creese I, Burt DR, Snyder SH. Dopamine receptor binding predicts clinical and pharmacological potencies of antischizophrenic drugs. *Science.* 1976;192(4238):481-483.

52. Farde L, Nordström AL, Wiesel FA, et al. Positron emission tomographic analysis of central D1 and D2 dopamine receptor occupancy in patients treated with classical neuroleptics and clozapine. Relation to extrapyramidal side effects. *Arch Gen Psychiatry.* 1992;49(7):538-544.

53. Richelson E. Receptor pharmacology of neuroleptics: Relation to clinical effects. *J Clin Psychiatry.* 1999;60(Suppl 10):5-14.

54. Reynolds GP. Receptor mechanisms in the treatment of schizophrenia. *J Psychopharmacol.* 2004;18(3):340-345.

55. Burris KD, Molski TF, Xu C, et al. Aripiprazole, a novel antipsychotic, is a high-affinity partial agonist at human dopamine D2 receptors. *J Pharmacol Exp Ther.* 2002;302(1):381-389.

56. Winokur A, Kamath J. The effect of typical and atypical antipsychotic drugs on sleep of schizophrenic patients. In: Monti J, Pandi-Perumal SR, Jacobs BL, Nutt D, eds. *Serotonin and Sleep: Molecular, Functional and Clinical Aspects.* Basel: Birkhauser-Verlag; 2008.

57. Monti JM, Monti D. Sleep in schizophrenia patients and the effects of antipsychotic drugs. *Sleep Med Rev.* 2004;8(2):133-148.

58. Armitage R, Cole D, Suppes T, Ozcan ME. Effects of clozapine on sleep in bipolar and schizoaffective disorders. *Prog Neuropsychopharmacol Biol Psychiatry.* 2004;28(7):1065-1070.

59. Dursun SM, Patel JK, Burke JG, Reveley MA. Effects of typical antipsychotic drugs and risperidone on the quality of sleep in patients with schizophrenia: A pilot study. *J Psychiatry Neurosci.* 1999;24(4):333-337.

60. Haffmans PMJ, Oolders JM, Hoencamp E, Arends JB. The effect of risperidone versus haloperidol on sleep patterns of schizophrenic patients—Results of a double-blind, randomised pilot trial. *Eur Neuropsycbopharmacol.* 2001;11(Suppl 3):S260.

61. Yamashita H, Morinobu S, Yamawaki S, et al. Effect of risperidone on sleep in schizophrenia: A comparison with haloperidol. *Psychiatry Res.* 2002;109(2):137-142.

62. Sharpley AL, Bhagwagar Z, Hafizi S, et al. Risperidone augmentation decreases rapid eye movement sleep and decreases wake in treatment-resistant depressed patients. *J Clin Psychiatry.* 2003;64(2):192-196.

63. Luthringer R, Staner L, Noel N, et al. A double-blind, placebo-controlled, randomized study evaluating the effect of paliperidone extended-release tablets on sleep architecture in patients with schizophrenia. *Int Clin Psychopharmacol.* 2007;22(5):299-308.

64. Sharpley AL, Vassallo CM, Cowen PJ. Olanzapine increases slow-wave sleep: Evidence for blockade of central 5-HT(2C) receptors in vivo. *Biol Psychiatry.* 2000;47(5):468-470.

65. Cohrs S, Meier A, Neumann AC, et al. Improved sleep continuity and increased slow wave sleep and REM latency during ziprasidone treatment: A randomized, controlled, crossover trial of 12 healthy male subjects. *J Clin Psychiatry.* 2005;66(8):989-996.

66. Robert S, Hamner MB, Kose S, et al. Quetiapine improves sleep disturbances in combat veterans with PTSD: sleep data from a prospective, open-label study. *J Clin Psychopharmacol.* 2005;25(4):387-388.

67. Sokolski KN, Denson TF, Lee RT, Reist C. Quetiapine for treatment of refractory symptoms of combat-related post-traumatic stress disorder. *Mil Med.* 2003;168(6):486-489.

68. Cohrs S, Rodenbeck A, Guan Z, et al. Sleep-promoting properties of quetiapine in healthy subjects. *Psychopharmacology (Berl).* 2004;174(3):421-429.

69. Geurkink EA, Sheth RD, Gidal BE, Hermann BP. Effects of anticonvulsant medication on EEG sleep architecture. *Epilepsy Behav.* 2000;1(6):378-383.

70. Placidi F, Scalise A, Marciani MG, et al. Effect of antiepileptic drugs on sleep. *Clin Neurophysiol.* 2000;111(Suppl 2):S115-S119.

71. Shouse MN, da Silva AM, Sammaritano M. Circadian rhythm, sleep, and epilepsy. *J Clin Neurophysiol.* 1996;13(1):32-50.

72. Bazil CW. Epilepsy and sleep disturbance. *Epilepsy Behav.* 2003; 4(Suppl 2):S39-S45.

73. Angehagen M, Ben-Menachem E, Rönnbäck L, Hansson E. Novel mechanisms of action of three antiepileptic drugs, vigabatrin, tiagabine, and topiramate. *Neurochem Res.* 2003;28(2):333-340.

74. Czapinski P, Blaszczyk B, Czuczwar SJ. Mechanisms of action of antiepileptic drugs. *Curr Top Med Chem.* 2005;5(1):3-14.

75. Mathias S, Wetter TC, Steiger A, Lancel M. The GABA uptake inhibitor tiagabine promotes slow wave sleep in normal elderly subjects. *Neurobiol Aging.* 2001;22(2):247-253.

76. Walsh JK, Zammit G, Schweitzer PK, Ondrasik J, Roth T. Tiagabine enhances slow wave sleep and sleep maintenance in primary insomnia. *Sleep Med.* 2006;7(2):155-161.

77. Walsh JK, Randazzo AC, Stone K. Tiagabine is associated with sustained attention during sleep restriction: Evidence for the value of slow-wave sleep enhancement? *Sleep.* 2006;29(4):433-443.

78. Roth T, Wright Jr KP, Walsh J. Effect of tiagabine on sleep in elderly subjects with primary insomnia: A randomized, double-blind, placebo-controlled study. *Sleep.* 2006;29(3):335-341.

79. Bazil CW, Battista J, Basner RC. Gabapentin improves sleep in the presence of alcohol. *J Clin Sleep Med.* 2005;1(3):284-287.

80. Foldvary-Schaefer N, De Leon Sanchez I, Karafa M, et al. Gabapentin increases slow-wave sleep in normal adults. *Epilepsia.* 2002;43(12):1493-1497.

81. Winkelman J, Pies R. Current patterns and future directions in the treatment of insomnia. *Ann Clin Psychiatry.* 2005;17(1):31-40.

82. Karam-Hage M, Brower KJ. Open pilot study of gabapentin versus trazodone to treat insomnia in alcoholic outpatients. *Psychiatry Clin Neurosci.* 2003;57(5):542-544.

83. Garcia-Borreguero D, Larrosa O, de la Llave Y, et al. Treatment of restless legs syndrome with gabapentin: A double-blind, cross-over study. *Neurology.* 2002;59(10):1573-1579.

84. Yurcheshen ME, Guttuso T Jr, McDermott M, et al. Effects of gabapentin on sleep in menopausal women with hot flashes as measured by a Pittsburgh Sleep Quality Index factor scoring model. *J Womens Health (Larchmt).* 2009;18(9):1355-1360.

85. Hindmarch I, Dawson J, Stanley N. A double-blind study in healthy volunteers to assess the effects on sleep of pregabalin compared with alprazolam and placebo. *Sleep.* 2005;28(2):187-193.

86. de Haas S, Otte A, de Weerd A, et al. Exploratory polysomnographic evaluation of pregabalin on sleep disturbance in patients with epilepsy. *J Clin Sleep Med.* 2007;3(5):473-478.

87. Sabatowski R, Gálvez R, Cherry DA, et al. Pregabalin reduces pain and improves sleep and mood disturbances in patients with post-herpetic neuralgia: Results of a randomised, placebo-controlled clinical trial. *Pain.* 2004;109(1-2):26-35.

88. Russell LJ, Crofford LJ, Leon T, et al. The effects of pregabalin on sleep disturbance symptoms among individuals with fibromyalgia syndrome. *Sleep Med.* 2009;10(6):604-610.

89. Montgomery SA, Herman BK, Schweizer E, Mandel FS. The efficacy of pregabalin and benzodiazepines in generalized anxiety disorder presenting with high levels of insomnia. *Int Clin Psychopharmacol.* 2009;24(4):214-222.

90. Information for Healthcare Professionals. *Suicidal Behavior and Ideation and Antiepileptic Drugs.* Available at http://www.fda.gov/Drugs/DrugSafety/PostmarketDrugSafetyInformationforPatientsandProviders/ucm100192.htm; 2008:12/16/2008 (cited November 30, 2010); Postmarket Drug Safety Information for Patients and Providers.

91. Schedules of Controlled Substances. Placement of Pregabalin into Schedule V. Drug Scheduling Actions. Available at http://www.deadiversion.usdoj.gov/fed_regs/rules/2005/fr0728.htm; 2005:(cited October 20, 2010).

92. Grosshans M, Mutschler J, Hermann D, et al. Pregabalin abuse, dependence, and withdrawal: A case report. *Am J Psychiatry.* 2010;167(7):869.

93. Filipetto FA, Zipp CP, Coren JS. Potential for pregabalin abuse or diversion after past drug-seeking behavior. *J Am Osteopath Assoc.* 2010;110(10):605-607.

94. Schwan S, Sundström A, Stjernberg E, et al. A signal for an abuse liability for pregabalin—Results from the Swedish spontaneous adverse drug reaction reporting system. *Eur J Clin Pharmacol.* 2010;66(9):947-953.

95. Haas H, Panula P. The role of histamine and the tuberomamillary nucleus in the nervous system. *Nat Rev Neurosci.* 2003;4(2):121-130.

96. Mignot E, Taheri S, Nishino S. Sleeping with the hypothalamus: Emerging therapeutic targets for sleep disorders. *Nat Neurosci.* 2002;5(Suppl):1071-1075.

97. Tashiro M, Mochizuki H, Iwabuchi K, et al. Roles of histamine in regulation of arousal and cognition: Functional neuroimaging of histamine H1 receptors in human brain. *Life Sci.* 2002;72(4-5):409-414.

98. Roth T, Roehrs T, Koshorek G, et al. Sedative effects of antihistamines. *J Allergy Clin Immunol.* 1987;80(1):94-98.

99. Orzechowski RF, Currie DS, Valancius DA. Comparative anticholinergic activities of 10 histamine H1 receptor antagonists in two functional models. *Eur J Pharmacol.* 2005;506(3):257-264.

100. Boyle J, Eriksson M, Stanley N, et al. Allergy medication in Japanese volunteers: Treatment effect of single doses on nocturnal sleep architecture and next day residual effects. *Curr Med Res Opin.* 2006;22(7):1343-1351.

101. Roehrs T, Claiborue D, Knox M, Roth T. Effects of ethanol, diphenhydramine, and triazolam after a nap. *Neuropsychopharmacology.* 1993;9(3):239-245.

102. Roehrs T, Zwyghuizen-Doorenbos A, Roth T. Sedative effects and plasma concentrations following single doses of triazolam, diphenhydramine, ethanol and placebo. *Sleep.* 1993;16(4):301-305.

103. Schweitzer PK, Muehlbach MJ, Walsh JK. Sleepiness and performance during three-day administration of cetirizine or diphenhydramine. *J Allergy Clin Immunol.* 1994;94(4):716-724.

104. Seidel WF, Cohen S, Bliwise NG, Dement WC. Direct measurement of daytime sleepiness after administration of cetirizine and hydroxyzine with a standardized electroencephalographic assessment. *J Allergy Clin Immunol.* 1990;86(6 Pt 2):1029-1033.

105. Seidel WF, Cohen S, Bliwise NG, Dement WC. Cetirizine effects on objective measures of daytime sleepiness and performance. *Ann Allergy.* 1987;59(6 Pt 2):58-62.

106. Richardson GS, Roehrs TA, Rosenthal L, et al. Tolerance to daytime sedative effects of H1 antihistamines. *J Clin Psychopharmacol.* 2002;22(5):511-515.

107. Zhang D, Tashiro M, Shibuya K, et al. Next-day residual sedative effect after nighttime administration of an over-the-counter antihistamine sleep aid, diphenhydramine, measured by positron emission tomography. *J Clin Psychopharmacol.* 2010;30(6):694-701.

108. Walsh JK. Drugs used to treat insomnia in 2002: Regulatory-based rather than evidence-based medicine. *Sleep.* 2004;27(8):1441-1442.

109. Krystal AD. A compendium of placebo-controlled trials of the risks/benefits of pharmacological treatments for insomnia: The empirical basis for U.S. clinical practice. *Sleep Med Rev.* 2009;13(4):265-274.

110. Rickels K, Morris RJ, Newman H, et al. Diphenhydramine in insomniac family practice patients: A double-blind study. *J Clin Pharmacol.* 1983;23(5-6):234-242.

111. Morin CM, Koetter U, Bastien C, et al. Valerian-hops combination and diphenhydramine for treating insomnia: A randomized placebo-controlled clinical trial. *Sleep.* 2005;28(11):1465-1471.

112. Glass JR, Sproule BA, Herrmann N, Busto UE. Effects of 2-week treatment with temazepam and diphenhydramine in elderly insomniacs: A randomized, placebo-controlled trial. *J Clin Psychopharmacol.* 2008;28(2):182-188.

113. Meuleman JR, Nelson RC, Clark Jr RL. Evaluation of temazepam and diphenhydramine as hypnotics in a nursing-home population. *Drug Intell Clin Pharm.* 1987;21(9):716-720.

114. Russo RM, Gururaj VJ, Allen JE. The effectiveness of diphenhydramine HCI in pediatric sleep disorders. *J Clin Pharmacol.* 1976;16(5-6):284-288.

115. Kudo Y, Kurihara M. Clinical evaluation of diphenhydramine hydrochloride for the treatment of insomnia in psychiatric patients: A double-blind study. *J Clin Pharmacol.* 1990;30(11):1041-1048.

116. Shapiro S, Slone D, Lewis GP, Jick H. Clinical effects of hypnotics. II. An epidemiologic study. *JAMA.* 1969;209(13):2016-2020.

117. Agostini JV, Leo-Summers LS, Inouye SK. Cognitive and other adverse effects of diphenhydramine use in hospitalized older patients. *Arch Intern Med.* 2001;161(17):2091-2207.

118. Del Cuvillo A, Sastre J, Montoro J, et al. Use of antihistamines in pediatrics. *J Investig Allergol Clin Immunol.* 2007;17(Suppl 2):28-40.

119. Halpert AG, Olmstead MC, Beninger RJ. Mechanisms and abuse liability of the anti-histamine dimenhydrinate. *Neurosci Biobehav Rev.* 2002;26(1):61-67.

120. Mumford GK, Silverman K, Griffiths RR. Reinforcing, subjective, and performance effects of lorazepam and diphenhydramine in humans. *Exp Clin Psychopharmacol.* 1996;4(4):421-430.

121. Jaffe JH, Bloor R, Crome I, et al. A postmarketing study of relative abuse liability of hypnotic sedative drugs. *Addiction.* 2004;99(2):165-173.

Chapter 9

Alternative Therapeutics for Sleep Disorders

ADRIENNE JUARASCIO / NORMA G. CUELLAR / NALAKA S. GOONERATNE

The National Center for Complementary and Alternative Medicine (NCCAM) defines complementary and alternative medicine (CAM) as a large group of medical and health care systems, practices, and products that are not typically considered to be a part of conventional medicine.[1] Although complementary medicine and alternative medicine are typically linked together, they refer to differing uses. *Complementary medicine* describes medicine and health care practices that are "used together with conventional medicine," whereas *alternative medicine* refers to medicine and health care practices that are "used in place of conventional medicine."[1] It is also possible for a medicine or medical practice that was once designated as CAM to become part of more mainstream medical treatment as more evidence-based research is collected on that type of CAM and it becomes more widely accepted. CAM therapy is often used with patients whose illness is not well treated by current conventional medical treatments.[1] For example, insomnia remains difficult to treat even with more conventional sleeping medicine.[2]

CAM therapies represent a large collection of products and practices, with current estimates putting the total number of CAM therapies well above several hundred.[1] NCCAM uses a classification method to group CAM therapies into five distinct categories:

1. Biologic compounds that are typically found in nature (e.g., herbal products)
2. Mind-body medicine, which relies on the belief that systems of thought affect bodily functioning (e.g., meditation, tai chi, yoga, biofeedback)
3. Manipulative and body-based practices, which involve the movement of specific body parts (e.g., massage-based therapies)
4. Energy medicine, which uses energy fields (e.g., bioelectromagnetic therapies)
5. Alternative medical systems, which rely on theories and beliefs that have developed apart from conventional medical practices (e.g., acupuncture, ayurvedic medicine, homeopathy)

These domains are not clear cut, as some treatments may overlap them.

In the United States, the use of CAM as a form of medical treatment is rising. For example, between 1990 and 1997, the proportion of American citizens who reported using at least one type of CAM treatment for any health condition rose from 33.8% to 42.1%.[3] In particular, this survey also suggested increased usage for all types of CAM for the treatment of insomnia, with figures increasing from 20.4% (in 1990) to 26.4% (in 1997).[3] In addition, a recent telephone survey of 1559 older adults conducted by the American Association of Retired Persons (AARP) and the NCCAM found that 54% of persons aged 65 or older had used at least one type of CAM therapy or practice.[4] Among a sample of patients with insomnia, 18.5% reported using a CAM-based therapy to treat their sleep disorder, whereas only 11.8% reported using a conventional medicinal product, demonstrating that for some disorders, CAM may be more popular than conventional medicine.[3] This preference may be due to the ease of obtaining many types of CAM therapy, especially biologic compounds, which can be purchased over the counter. Therefore, it may be easier for some to use CAM substances than to see their doctor for a prescription. CAM products are also often considered particularly safe and free of side effects because they are available over the counter and can be taken without doctor supervision. This availability, too, may explain their popularity. However, CAM products are not necessarily safe, as will be discussed further in this chapter.

Several factors can be used to determine which adults are more likely to use CAM therapy; individuals of a higher income bracket, those with more years of college education,[4] and younger adults are more likely to use CAM, whereas older adults are more likely to use a prescribed medicine.[5] More health-conscious individuals and those who engage in healthier lifestyle behaviors are more likely to use CAM medicine than a prescribed medicine.[5] Lastly, depression and anxiety seem to be higher among those who use prescribed medication rather then CAM therapies.[5] The results of a Canadian survey on the prevalence of CAM use are shown in Figure 9-1.

Pearson and associates, in their analysis of the National Health Interview Survey (NHIS) dataset, noted that 4.5% of adults used some form of CAM for their insomnia or trouble sleeping in the past year (Fig. 9-2).[6] In comparison, other sedative-hypnotic prescription drugs are used by approximately 5% to 10% of adults with insomnia.[7] Biologically based therapies and mind-body therapies were most commonly used (64.8% and 39.1% of adult CAM users, respectively).[6] Patients with restless legs syndrome (RLS) also commonly use CAM therapy.[8] Previous research has indicated that 65% reported using CAM, with the average use being approximately 2.5 types of biologically based CAM therapies and 0.9 non–biologically based CAM therapies.[8]

Patients typically obtain information regarding CAM therapies from sources other than their health care providers. A survey of older adults indicated that their primary source of CAM information was from family or friends (22%), publications (14%), or radio/TV/Internet (20%).[4] CAM users discussed CAM with their physicians in 31% of cases, yet only 12% viewed their physician as their primary source of information about CAM.[4] These data suggest that physicians are largely unaware of their patients' CAM usage. This finding is of concern, because it jeopardizes the process of providing education to patients regarding CAM and potential medical interactions; 75% of those who take an herbal or dietary product during their lifetime also take one or more prescription medications concurrently.[4]

There is a limited body of evidence-based research on CAM therapy. CAM therapies, especially those that are biologically based, are generally regulated by the Dietary Supplemental

and Education Act of 1994, whose guidelines differ from those of the U.S. Food and Drug Administration (FDA) for prescription medications. Accordingly, these biologic agents do not need to undergo the same degree of scrutiny for purity, safety, and efficacy. This relaxed regulation allows potential inconsistency between medical compounds with identical names across research groups. Therefore, the specific ingredients or the dosages used in such products may vary widely across research studies. This can, in turn, lead to difficulty in the interpretation of research data from different centers on similar CAM products. Readers are urged to keep these considerations in mind when interpreting the results of the studies listed in this chapter (Fig. 9-3).

This chapter will present a summary of research on CAM treatments for sleep disturbances in adults. Although the chapter will focus on treatments for insomnia, which is the most studied sleep disorder, we will also briefly discuss treatments for other disorders, such as fibromyalgia, when evidence-based studies are available.

BIOLOGIC COMPOUNDS

Biologic compounds for the treatment of insomnia appear in Figure 9-4.

Melatonin

Melatonin, a hormone produced by the pineal gland (*N*-acetyl-5-methoxytryptamine), is believed to be an important factor in the regulation of the sleep-wake cycle through

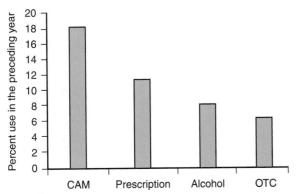

Figure 9-1 Prevalence of complementary and alternative medicine (CAM) use. Results of postal survey of 997 Canadians (of 5991 people initially contacted, 2001 agreed to initial telephone interview, 1473 agreed to postal survey, 997 responded). *OTC*, Over-the-counter medication. (Data from Sanchez-Ortuno MM, Belanger L, Ivers H, et al. The use of natural products for sleep: A common practice? *Sleep Med.* 2009;10(9):982-987.)

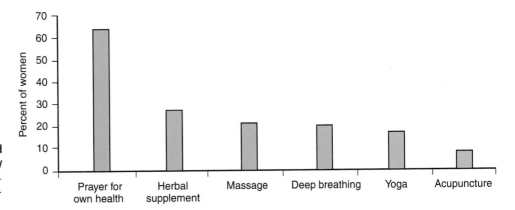

Figure 9-2 Complementary and alternative medicine (CAM) use by females. (Data from *http://mchb.hrsa.gov/whusa09/hsu/pages/302cam.html.*)

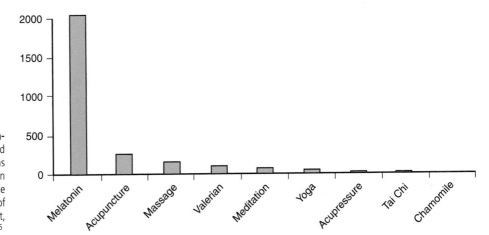

Figure 9-3 Complementary and alternative medicine (CAM) research. Pubmed search for articles that include the terms "sleep" and the treatment modality listed in the figure. No published studies on chamomile are available despite the fact that it is one of the most commonly used CAM biologic agent, according to Sanchez-Ortuno and associates.[5]

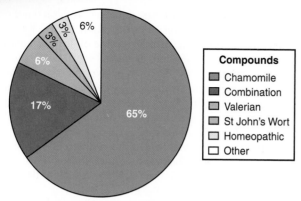

Figure 9-4 Complementary and alternative medicine (CAM) biologic compounds for treatment of insomnia. (Data from Sanchez-Ortuno MM, Belanger L, Ivers H, et al: The use of natural products for sleep: A common practice? *Sleep Med.* 2009;10(9):982-987.)

Summary of Key Melatonin Research Studies

Authors*	Study Population	Findings
Smits et al., 2003[182]	Children with sleep-onset insomnia	Reduced sleep latency, improved QoL
Van der Heijden et al., 2007[183]	Children with ADHD	Improved sleep, but no effect on cognition or QoL
Hoebert et al., 2009[63]	Children with ADHD—follow-up study to 2007 study by Van der Heijden et al.	Improved sleep onset latency, no significant side effects at an average 3.7 years of follow-up
Baskett et al., 2003[31]	Older adults with insomnia	No significant effect (actigraphy)
Garfinkel et al., 1995[184]	Older adults with insomnia	Improved sleep efficiency (actigraph)
Hughes et al., 1998[36]	Older adults with insomnia	No significant effect (polysomnography)
Singer et al., 2003[32]	Alzheimer's disease patients with sleep disturbances	No significant effect (actigraph)
Sack et al., 2000[41]	Blind patients with circadian phase abnormalities	Significant circadian phase entrainment noted
Riemersma-van der Lek et al., 2008[33]	Nursing home patients (irrespective of existing sleep disorders)	Improved sleep latency and sleep duration, but worsened mood; recommended that melatonin be used with light therapy.
Luthringer et al., 2009[35]	Patients 55 years or older with primary insomnia	Improvement in sleep onset latency (9 min) and sleep quality

*Studies in this table are listed in the references at the end of the chapter and are cited in the chapter text where appropriate.
ADHD, attention deficit hyperactivity disorder; QoL, quality of life.

its circadian rhythm effects.[9,10] In particular, melatonin can cause direct inhibition of the suprachiasmatic nucleus via a feedback loop.[11-13] Melatonin can also induce sleep when injected into other brain areas, such as the medial preoptic area.[13] Because of these physiologic effects, melatonin is believed to prepare the body for sleep readiness; its release may cause drowsiness and may induce sleep.[14]

Melatonin may also have a link to age-related insomnia because melatonin levels tend to decrease with age, such that older adults may have markedly decreased levels of melatonin at night compared to younger patients.[15-17] It is hypothesized that this age-related decrease in melatonin levels may be due to a decline in pinealocytes,[18] neuronal degeneration of the suprachiasmatic nucleus,[19] or the effects of co-morbid conditions/medications. A variety of medicines, such as beta blockers and primary conditions (e.g., chronic pain, myocardial interactions, ischemic stroke), are associated with decreased melatonin levels.[20-22] Several studies have sought to examine whether melatonin decrement might mediate insomnia, but the results have been mixed.[19,23-27] Several key melatonin research studies are summarized in Table 9-1.

Insomnia

Studies into the efficacy of exogenous melatonin for the treatment of insomnia has generally used dosages ranging from 0.1 mg to 0.3 mg (which results in physiologic melatonin levels) to 5 mg to 10 mg (pharmacologic melatonin levels). A few early studies revealed modest benefit, but the results were not consistent.[28,29] For example, although one study demonstrated improvement in sleep onset latency,[30] other studies indicated that melatonin did not significantly alter sleep onset latency.[31] One of the largest studies to date that employed an objective measure, wrist activity monitors, involved 157 older adults with Alzheimer's disease and randomized them into three groups: placebo, melatonin 2.5 mg sustained release, and melatonin 10 mg.[32] It should be noted that actigraphy is not regarded as a definitive means for the assessment of hypnotic response. This study found that there was no objectively or subjectively measured difference in sleep onset latency between the three groups of Alzheimer disease patients. However, caregivers did report an improvement in sleep quality (as measured by the Sleep Disorders Inventory) for those using the 2.5 mg sustained release formula compared

to placebo or the 10-mg immediate release formula.[32] Another major study in older adults that used wrist activity monitors observed an 8.2-minute reduction in sleep onset latency and increased sleep duration of 27 minutes over a 15-month (average) follow-up period.[33]

Research studies using polysomnography have also demonstrated mixed results, with some studies showing a benefit[30,34,35] and others not showing a benefit[36,37] in various sleep parameters. In an attempt to synthesize these conflicting results, a meta-analysis of melatonin therapy for sleep was conducted.[38] The results of this meta-analysis indicated the following key findings (values presented are weighted mean differences):

1. Melatonin decreased sleep onset latency significantly in people with delayed sleep phase syndrome (38.8 minutes improvement; 95% CI: 50.3 minutes, 27.3 minutes)
2. A small but statistically significant reduction in sleep onset latency in patients with primary insomnia (4.3 minutes improvement; 95% CI: 8.4 minutes, 0.1 minute)
3. Reduction in sleep onset latency in patients older than 65 years was slightly larger but was not statistically significant (7.8 minutes improvement; 95% CI: 17.4 minutes, −1.7 minutes)

4. Melatonin had larger effects on sleep onset latency in children than in adults (in children sleep onset latency was reduced by 17.0 minutes; 95% CI: 33.5 minutes, 0.5 minute)
5. Melatonin induced a small but statistically significant increase in sleep efficiency in secondary sleep disorders (1.9% improvement; 95% CI: 0.5%, 3.3%).[38]

There were no changes in other measures, such as sleep efficiency in primary insomnia, or wakefulness after sleep onset (any form of insomnia). This led the authors to conclude that the main effects of melatonin on sleep were circadian, not sedative. Of note, these weighted mean difference estimates combined data across a variety of measures (polysomnography, sleep diary, actigraphy) to calculate estimates. The authors attempted to determine if there were differences in the weighted mean differences across measurement methodologies, but there were too few studies in each group to make this determination.

Prolonged-release formulations of melatonin have also been developed. In Europe, Neurim Pharmaceuticals has received approval from the European Medicines Association to market prolonged-release melatonin 2 mg (Circadin) for the short-term treatment of primary insomnia in patients aged older than 55 years.[39] The European Medicines Association review included a pooled analysis that concluded that approximately 32% of patients in the prolonged-release melatonin arm, relative to approximately 19% in the placebo arm, experienced improvement on a combined endpoint defined as sleep quality and behavior following wakefulness (as measured by the quality of sleep items and behavior following wakefulness items on the Leeds Sleep Evaluation Questionnaire); a statistically significant difference but with a small effect size. Polysomnographic data presented in the review showed a small, but statistically significant 9-minute reduction in sleep latency, but no other significant changes in sleep efficiency or other metrics.

One potential area of future investigation is the role of baseline melatonin levels in modulating response to exogenous melatonin. For example, one study found no overall benefit of melatonin therapy, but did note that the most prominent improvement occurred in patients who had only a short duration of endogenous melatonin secretion.[36] Another study noted only an improvement in sleep onset latency for those with low endogenous melatonin levels.[40] These results suggest that the mixed results with melatonin may be due to differential response rates across subgroups of participants. Future research is needed to determine who benefits from melatonin and how best to use this product to treat insomnia.

Circadian Rhythm Disorders

As noted earlier,[38] the Agency for Healthcare Research and Quality (AHRQ) meta-analysis of melatonin therapy identified delayed sleep phase disorder as an area in which melatonin had clinically significant effects. Melatonin may also be beneficial in blind patients, who have free-running circadian rhythms, starting at a 10-mg dose.[41] Several studies have also shown a role for melatonin to ameliorate jet lag in doses of up to 5 mg.[42]

Pediatric Patients

Doses used in pediatric patients range from 0.5 mg to 7.5 mg.[43] Most studies have involved patients with attention deficit disorder[44] and autism[45] and have observed a benign side effect profile. Although the available studies are limited because of small sample size, most have shown improvements in sleep onset latency or total sleep time.[44] A recent meta-analysis in pediatric patients with intellectual disability concluded that melatonin improved sleep onset latency by 34 minutes and total sleep time by 50 minutes.[46] Additional larger studies with longer duration are needed to confirm these findings.

Side Effect and Safety Profile

Overall, exogenous melatonin is associated with a relatively benign side effect profile. Melatonin is well tolerated in the dose range of 0.1 mg to 10 mg.[47-49] Higher doses of melatonin have also been associated with daytime side effects such as reduced alertness, headache, dizziness, and irritability.[50] Melatonin is less likely to lead to dependence and abuse, as occurs with other sedative-hypnotics, because it does not cause euphoria and does not act primarily on γ-aminobutyric acid (GABA) receptors.[51]

A relatively large body of data, derived from efficacy studies or from dedicated safety studies utilizing structured side effect inventories, is available regarding the safety profile of melatonin compared to other types of CAM therapies. Two major reviews have summarized existing clinical trial safety data. The first review was conducted by the Institute of Medicine/National Academies.[52] This report revealed a small increase in blood pressure in patients taking calcium channel blockers. On the other hand, in patients who are not on calcium channel blockers, exogenous melatonin has been demonstrated to result in a mild reduction in blood pressure when a physiologic dose is used (systolic blood pressure -3.77 ± 1.7 mm Hg, $P = 0.0423$; diastolic blood pressure -3.63 ± 1.3 mm Hg, $P = 0.0153$; and mean blood pressure -3.71 ± 1.3 mm Hg, $P = .013$).[53] A second large review of melatonin, published by the AHRQ, determined that melatonin appeared to be a safe substance.[38] The European Medicines Agency also concluded that melatonin was generally safe and noted that there were no safety concerns in hypertensive patients treated for 4 weeks. However, the European Medicines Agency did not recommend the use of melatonin in patients with autoimmune disorders or with severe hepatic or renal disease or pregnant/breastfeeding patients owing to a paucity of safety data in these patient groups.[39]

One concern with any sedative agent is the risk of daytime sleepiness. For melatonin, the sedative effects can persist up to 7 hours after ingestion.[54,55] The sedative effects may be more prominent when melatonin is ingested during the daytime because the melatonin receptors on the suprachiasmatic nucleus are down-regulated at night.[56] Other important daytime consequences include the risk of dysphoria or depression: Riemersma-van der Lek and associates noted in their long-term study (average 15 months, maximum of 3.5 years) of melatonin 2.5 mg in group-care facilities that there were higher levels of withdrawn behavior and negative affect in the melatonin arm and that in the melatonin with bright light arm, these findings were not present, leading the authors to conclude that melatonin should be given with bright light therapy.[33]

Some studies have indicated a proinflammatory role for those with autoimmune arthritis,[57,58] but other studies have indicated that melatonin may actually protect against the development of autoimmune disorders.[59] Melatonin may cause an increase in the apnea-hypopnea index (AHI) in patients with obstructive sleep apnea syndrome (OSA). One study documented mild to moderate increases in the AHI in

OSA patients taking melatonin.[60] Follicle-stimulating hormone (FSH), luteotropic hormone (LH), and thyroid hormones may be affected by melatonin; however, melatonin has not been found to have significant clinical effects in older adults at the doses usually used for managing insomnia.[61,62] Melatonin's sex hormone effects in children are not well studied, which is an important consideration in light of the higher drug concentrations that may result when a given (adult) dose of melatonin (3 mg or 10 mg) is given to a child.[43] One study with an average 3.7-year follow-up did not identify any significant abnormalities in sexual development in children.[63] Other side effects include headache and pruritus, which have occurred in less than 10% of subjects.[64] One potential limitation of using exogenous melatonin is its potential for impact on endogenous melatonin levels. Research has suggested that in individuals with bipolar disorder, the use of melatonin for an extended period of time (10 mg for 3 months) may lead to suppression of endogenous melatonin and result in an unentrained or free running sleep-wake cycle following the withdrawal from exogenous melatonin.[65]

Conclusions

The current body of clinical trials literature on melatonin suggests that it has clinically significant effects for circadian rhythm disorders, such as delayed sleep phase disorder. For other conditions, such as primary or co-morbid insomnia, the effects of melatonin are smaller and in some cases clinically/statistically nonsignificant. At doses ranging from 0.3 mg to 10 mg, melatonin is relatively well tolerated. Specific areas of concern are sex-hormone suppression and depression. Inadequate data are available regarding safety in patients with autoimmune disorders, those with severe renal or hepatic disease, and those who are pregnant/breastfeeding.

Valerian

Valerian has been used for centuries as a sleep aid and anxiolytic, and remains one of the most widely used nonprescription medications for its hypnotic and sedative properties.[66] It is prepared from the roots of the flowering plant *Valeriana officinalis*. In the 2002 National Health Interview Survey of 31,044 interviews, 5.9% of the population used valerian for insomnia.[3]

Over 250 species of valerian are used for medicinal purposes worldwide (Box 9-1).[67-69] Valerian contains over 150 substances, many known to be physiologically active such as the volatile oils and their sesquiterpenes (e.g., valerenic acid and derivatives), iridoids and their monoterpenes (e.g., valepotriates), other alkaloids, and amino acids. The composition varies not only with species, subspecies, and variety but also with the age of the plant, its growing conditions, and the type and age of the extract.[69]

The most unstable components of valerian are the valepotriates (mainly valtrate and isovaltrate) present as 0.05% to 0.67% of the root content. Valepotriates rapidly decompose with moisture and form their degradation products, the baldrinals. These in turn react to form polymers with possible mutagenic effects in vitro. Fortunately, valepotriates are so unstable that they are usually not present in most commercial supplements.

Although many physiologically active substances have been identified in valerian, its mechanism of action on the central nervous system has yet to be clarified.[70] The effects on sleep may involve multiple compounds.[70,71] Potential mechanisms of action include agonist activity at the GABA recognition site, which also mediates the effects of barbiturates and benzodiazepine agents, or at the adenosine and serotonin receptors. Table 9-2 provides descriptions of the possible mechanisms of action for valerian.

Insomnia

Valerian is widely used to treat insomnia and anxiety. Valerian has received approval for use as a sleep aid by regulatory authorities in several countries including Germany.[69] However, studies into the use of valerian have significant methodologic shortcomings. Long-term studies are lacking,[72-74] and many studies examining the effects of valerian use subjective sleep parameters and lack objective parameters such as actigraphy and polysomnography. A variety of valerian preparations

---

BOX 9-1 *Some Species of Family Valerianaceae**

Valeriana officinalis (America and Northern Europe)
Valeriana wallichii (India)
Valeriana jatamansji (India)
Valeriana edulis (Mexico)
Valeriana fauriei (Japan)
Valeriana hardwickii (China)
Valeriana dioica (Britain)
Valeriana pyrenaica (Pyrenees)
Valeriana pyrolaefolia (Himalayas)

*Approximately 250 species exist.

TABLE 9-2

Possible Mechanisms of Action of Valerian

Neurotransmitter	Mechanisms
GABA[77,160-172]	Has been shown to increase activity at GABA receptors which are involved in regulating normal sleep associated with GABA$_A$ receptor chloride channel
	May inhibit GABA uptake and induce the release of [^{3}H]-GABA
	May increase levels of GABA which may contribute to the hypnotic effect resulting in improvement in non-REM sleep
Adenosine[77,165,167,173-179]	May serve as an agonist at human adenosine receptor sites
	Exhibits partial agonist activity at the A$_1$ adenosine receptor subtype
Serotonin[160,167,180,181]	Valerenic acid is the most active component at the G protein–coupled receptor 5-HT$_{5A}$
	Neurobiologic mechanisms have been attributed to activity at the A$_1$ adenosine receptor, the 5-HT$_{5A}$ serotonin receptor, and potentiation of GABAergic transmission (increased release and/or decreased reuptake)

GABA, γ-aminobutyric acid; *5-HT$_{5A}$*, 5-hydroxytryptamine receptor 5A; *REM*, rapid eye movement.

are utilized, making it difficult to compare results across studies. Sample sizes are small, limiting the ability to generalize study results.

Animal studies have shown a depressant effect of valerian on the central nervous system as well as antioxidative and vasorelaxant activities.[70,75-80] In human studies, valerian is associated with a reduction in rapid eye movement (REM) sleep during the first part of the night but an increase during the latter stages of sleep, minimizing natural sleep stage composition. These studies also suggest at least a subjective benefit in sleep quality, night awakenings, and possibly sleep onset latency in health volunteers and those with insomnia.[66-68,81-91] Clinical trials suggest that with repeated administration, valerian produces sleep-inducing effects without altering sleep architecture at modest doses.[66-68,81-91] Doses generally range from 400 mg to 900 mg of valerian taken before bedtime. It is not known whether higher doses may be more effective because of a paucity of safety and efficacy data at higher doses.

Restless Legs Syndrome

Few studies have examined the use of valerian specifically for RLS. Valerian's potential beneficial role in this disorder may be related to its effect on the GABA receptor complex. In a randomized clinical trial, 37 participants with RLS[92] received either 800 mg of valerian or a placebo. There were no differences between placebo and valerian arms on Pittsburgh Sleep Quality Index, Epworth Sleepiness Scale (ESS), and International RLS Symptom Severity Scale assessments, in part because both groups reported improvement in RLS symptom severity and sleep. In a nested analysis comparing subjects in the valerian arm ($n = 17$) who had RLS with daytime sleepiness (ESS score >10) versus those who had RLS without daytime sleepiness (ESS score <10), significant improvements were found in RLS symptom severity ($p = 0.02$) in the former group, suggesting that valerian may have a more prominent effect in those with RLS and daytime sleepiness.

Side Effect and Safety Profile

Safety issues revolve around the predictable and idiosyncratic reactions to valerian and interactions with other agents, as well as those effects attributable to products whose contents are not well defined or do not contain a substantial amount of valerian. Safety data are difficult to interpret, however, as few studies have been specifically designed to investigate safety issues. Adverse events are not significantly different between valerian and placebo, yet, as noted previously, these studies were not specifically designed to evaluate these effects. It should also be noted that hops has been used in conjunction with valerian in some studies included here for safety discussion; the clinical efficacy of hops for sleep disorders is discussed in a later section in this chapter. Generally, the use of valerian root is considered safe for periods of 4 to 6 weeks in the relief of insomnia, at daily doses not exceeding 400 mg to 900 mg of an extract. Side effects include urticaria, restlessness, agitation, nervousness, headache/migraine attack, gastrointestinal complaint, vivid dreams, daytime drowsiness, heavy sleep, and depression with no adverse effects noted during the washout period of valerian.[67,87,88,92] However, there is a case report of a patient developing benzodiazepine-like withdrawal symptoms after abrupt cessation of valerian; in

this particular case, the patient had been taking 0.5 g to 2 g of valerian several times a day.[93]

Concerns exist about the use of valerian and subsequent hepatotoxicity.[71] In rats, doses three times that recommended for human use showed an increase in the rate of bile flow and an increase in serum alkaline phosphatase.[94] Although few reports of hepatotoxicity in valerian users exist, caution should be taken in any person with liver failure, cirrhosis, or alcoholism when using any herb or natural product.

Pharmacodynamic interactions with sedative agents including the barbiturates can be expected. The biggest concern is related to sedative medications whose actions may be potentiated when used with valerian. Although no human studies have confirmed this, animal studies have shown that valepotriates enhance the effects of barbiturates, prolonging sleep time in mice.[95] Therefore, caution must be used if valerian and sedative medicines are used together.

Conclusions

Although widely used to treat insomnia and anxiety, the data on the use of valerian for sleep are hampered by weak study design, small sample sizes, and lack of objective measures of sleep. Studies on valerian are also limited by the lack of purity in many valerian products, variations in potency across compounds, and uncertainty regarding which ingredients possess the soporific properties of the compound. Valerian has been shown to have sleep-inducing effects in some studies. Studies suggest at least a subjective benefit in sleep quality and possibly sleep onset latency in healthy volunteers and those with insomnia and RLS. The long-term efficacy of valerian is unknown, and its effects on subgroups warrants further research.

Hydroxytryptophan

5-Hydroxytryptophan (5-HTP) is a naturally occurring amino acid and is a precursor to the neurotransmitter serotonin.[96] It is currently sold in the United States as a sleep aid, although it is also used as a CAM therapy for depression and as an appetite suppressant.[97]

Insomnia

Several small studies have indicated some improvement in subjective and objective sleep quality following administration of 5-HTP.[96] For example, one study that used a 200-mg dose demonstrated an increase in REM sleep.[98] Despite the initial evidence suggesting it might be a useful treatment for insomnia, research studies have been small in number and have shared methodologic limitations. Additional work replicating these findings would allow for greater certainty in 5-HTP's effectiveness.

Side Effect and Safety Profile

Initial dosage for treating insomnia is usually 100 mg to 300 mg before bed. Case studies have indicated that higher dosages are associated with vivid nightmares during sleep. Additional reported side effects include nausea and headaches. There is direct and indirect evidence for potential heart valve damage or disease in rare cases,[99] acute serotonin syndrome if combined with selective serotonin reuptake inhibitors (SSRIs) or monoamine oxidase inhibitors (MAOIs),[100] and vomiting and nausea when combined with carbidopa.[101] Because 5-HTP has not been thoroughly studied in clinical settings, potential side effects and interactions with other drugs are not well known.

Chamomile

Chamomile, or *Matricaria recutita,* is one of the most widely used types of CAM therapy for promoting sleep and treating insomnia.[102] The active ingredients in chamomile are chamazulene, apigenin, and bisabolol.[103] The sedative effects of chamomile may be due to a benzodiazepine-like compound in the flower head. Although chamomile tea has a popular reputation as a relaxing tea that facilitates sleep, there are no randomized clinical studies supporting its use.[5] Some animal trials suggest that it is efficacious as a mild sedative and anxiolytic.[97]

Side Effect and Safety Profile

Chamomile is part of the Compositae family; thus, patients hypersensitive to the Asteraceae/Compositae family, which includes ragweed, chrysanthemums, marigolds, daisies, and other herbs, should be alert for allergy symptoms.[97] When ingested in the form of a highly concentrated tea, it has also been shown to induce vomiting. It is also possible that chamomile might interact with anticoagulant and antiplatelet drugs as well as any drug with sedative properties such as benzodiazepine. Chamomile may inhibit cytochrome P-450.[97] Therefore, patients who are taking other drugs metabolized by the enzyme system should used caution when ingesting chamomile products.

St. John's Wort

St. John's wort is a flowering herb used orally as a treatment for a sleep disturbances and insomnia.[104] Most preparations with this herb also include a large variety of other substances including naphthodianthrones (hypericin, pseudohypericin, isohypericin), flavonoids (kaempferol, hyperoside, quercetin), phloroglucinols (hyperforin, adhyperforin), tannins, procyanidins, essential oils, amino acids, and other components.[97] This highlights the fact that most compounds of St. John's wort may have multiple mechanisms of action, and the quantity of the herb among preparations may vary dramatically. It also makes it difficult to know which properties may be affecting sleep behavior. The main active ingredients are thought to be hyperforin and hypericin, although other ingredients have been shown to be bioactive as well. Recent work has suggested that hyperforin may be the most active ingredient, and that it functions by inhibiting reuptake of serotonin, norepinephrine, dopamine, GABA, and L-glutamate.[105] Many commercial products are standardized as to the hypericin content, which was previously considered to be the only active ingredient.

Insomnia

Most studies that have investigated St. John's wort in a clinical context were for the treatment of depression, not insomnia. Few published scientific studies of St. John's wort for insomnia not associated with depression were found. One double-blind placebo-controlled study investigated the effects of St. John's wort on health subjects free of mood or sleep disturbances. Polysomnography was used as the main objective measure.[106] The dose of 0.9 mg was found to significantly increase REM

sleep onset latency when compared to placebo. However, a second study that used 10 subjects and a slightly higher dose of St. John's wort (1.8 mg) did not find any difference in REM latency compared to placebo. Among older adults, a randomized placebo-controlled study found an increase in slow wave activity among 10 of 11 subjects when taking St John's wort, but statistical significance was not reported owing to small sample size.[107] The constituents and method of extraction varied from study to study, hampering the generalization of results. Overall, although there are currently some data indicating that St. John's wort might improve sleep onset latency and total sleep time, the results have been mixed. Given the small sample size, use of healthy adults without insomnia, and the heterogeneous nature of the St. John's wort used across studies, little can be concluded about the efficacy of this CAM therapy for insomnia.

Side Effect and Safety Profile

In an observational study of 3250 patients using a commercially available preparation of St. John's wort, gastrointestinal symptoms, allergic reactions, tiredness, anxiety, and confusion were most often reported.[97,108] Photosensitivity and phototoxicity have been reported. St. John's wort also has potentially severe drug interactions. St. John's wort has been demonstrated to induce cytochrome P-450 (CYP), including isoenzyme CYP3A4.[108] Because many drugs are metabolized by CYP3A4, drug interactions would be common. However, the compound that is responsible for CYP3A4 induction, hyperforin, is not standardized among commercial products. The most significant interactions potentially involve patients with cardiovascular disease, human immunodeficiency virus (HIV), cancer, and depression because levels of the following medications may be decreased: antiretroviral medications for HIV, calcium channel blockers, digoxin, cyclosporin, and certain chemotherapeutic agents (e.g., irinotecan).[108-110] Other important effects include the risk of unwanted pregnancies in women on oral anticontraceptives.[110] Individuals taking SSRIs are warned not to take St. John's wort because it increases the risk of serotonin syndrome.[111]

Hops

Hops, or humulus lupulus, is most widely known for its use as a bittering agent in beer. It also has a long-standing history as a CAM treatment for insomnia.[112] Its potential use as a CAM treatment was discovered when hop harvesters reported feeling sleepy after they harvested the flowers. Hops primarily acts as a treatment for restlessness, irritability, anxiety, tension, and disordered sleep.[112] Currently, hops is available in over-the-counter supplements, but the dosage and any additional ingredients in the supplement can vary dramatically.

The active ingredient in hops is currently not known. Hops consists of over 100 different compounds, making the exact compound responsible for its sedative effects difficult to determine.[113] Research has indicated that at least one of these compounds does seem to exert sedative effects in animals. In humans, a combined treatment of valerian and hops did demonstrate small improvement in subjective sleep onset latency (but no significant changes in objective measures).[84] Most of the randomized controlled studies using hops have investigated hops in combination with other compounds as part of a brand name formulation. Therefore, it is difficult to determine how effective this compound alone may be in promoting sleep.

Side Effect and Safety Profile

Hops may cause a hypersensitivity reaction, such as dermatitis, and some individuals are allergic to this product.[50] Hops should be used with caution by patients taking another central nervous system depressant or an antipsychotic, as this could potentially interact with the sedative effects of this medication.[50]

ALTERNATIVE MEDICAL SYSTEMS

Traditional Chinese Medicine: Acupuncture

Acupuncture refers to the process of inserting and removing small filiform needles into various places in the body.[114] These anatomic locations are referred to as meridians and are pathways for vital energy, or qi. Historically, acupuncture has been a common Eastern medical practice, but recently it has become more widely used as a type of CAM therapy in the United States. There is evidence to suggest that acupuncture may be a beneficial treatment for insomnia and fibromyalgia. One limitation of the available literature is that there are several possible acupuncture meridians that could be used in the treatment of sleep disorders, with research studies often using different meridians.

Insomnia

Acupuncture was shown to be as effective as standard medical treatments for improving total sleep duration in studies directly comparing both acupuncture and sedative-hypnotics, and appeared to improve sleep duration when combined with the sedative-hypnotics based on one meta-analysis, but further trials have been recommended.[115] Another meta-analysis of acupuncture therapy for insomnia indicated that acupuncture was an effective treatment for insomnia, but that many of the studies included were poorly designed, lacked sophisticated controls, or used small samples of subjects.[116] In addition, the results tended to focus primarily on a short data collection period, with little to no information about long-term benefits. A meta-analysis that only used randomized controlled trials found that only seven studies met criteria for inclusion,[117] indicating that additional research is needed. Acupuncture has also been examined as a treatment for sleep disruption due to other conditions, including insomnia following stroke[118] and after menopausal symptoms.[119,120] Other sleep disorders that have been treated with acupuncture include OSA. A study comparing acupuncture to sham acupuncture and a second control arm noted a reduction in the AHI from 19.9 events per hour to 10.1 events per hour in the acupuncture arm compared to no change or worsening in the sham acupuncture and control arm over a 12-week period.[121]

Although the available evidence seems to indicate that acupuncture may be a beneficial CAM therapy for insomnia, there are several limitations to the current data. First, few studies had sufficient methodologic rigor and a large enough sample size to be conclusive. More work is needed to determine if the initial findings hold up over time and with repeated measurement. Lastly, it is important to consider that acupuncture

refers to a broad range of procedures, and that the current body of research contains a heterogeneous sampling of the types of acupuncture used in practice. Future research is needed to determine which types and meridian targets may be the most beneficial.

Fibromyalgia

Acupuncture has also shown evidence of improving sleep quality and reducing sleep disturbances among this patient population.[122,123] Although acupuncture has demonstrated some benefit in clinical trials in several different studies,[124] two meta-analyses demonstrated variable and inconsistent findings.[125,126] The meta-analyses indicate that although acupuncture seems to reduce the pain associated with fibromyalgia, it may have little direct benefit on sleep quality.

Side Effect and Safety Profile

Due to the invasive nature of acupuncture treatments, it is important to ensure that it is performed safely. Current research does indicate that acupuncture is safe when administered by well-trained practitioners using sterile needles, with rare (<3%) side effects including hemorrhage, dizziness, and paresthesias.[127]

Traditional Chinese Medicine: Acupressure

Acupressure involves stimulation of meridians on the body using finger pressing movements. Several randomized trials have been conducted with acupressure, some of which have used sham treatment arms to provide a more comparable placebo arm.[128,129] Several of these studies have involved patient populations drawn from institutionalized settings[128,130] or specific patient groups, such as renal failure patients.[129] A recent meta-analysis concluded that acupressure demonstrated a benefit on subjective sleep quality relative to placebo, but that further research was needed.[115]

Acupressure can also be applied directly to the ear as auricular therapy using magnets, pressure, or seeds.[131,132] One randomized, single-blind, placebo-controlled study with wrist-activity monitoring in insomnia patients noted improvements in sleep time[133] that were sustained over 6 months.[134] Acupressure reviews generally suggest that it is beneficial, but that there is a need for further large trials to confirm the initial findings and that various means of administering acupressure may not be equivalent.[131,132]

Ayurvedic Medicine

Ayurveda is a system of traditional medicine that is native to the Indian subcontinent. It focuses on a combined use of herbs, massage, yoga, and other therapies to treat a variety of illnesses. There is currently a limited body of research on ayurveda as a treatment for insomnia. One study demonstrated that among 25 healthy volunteers suffering from insomnia, a traditional ayurvedic supplement formulated for insomnia was associated with a small but significant reduction in sleep latency compared to placebo.[135] An additional study with a large sample size (69 participants, 23 receiving ayurvedic therapies) found that ayurveda demonstrated no significant change in sleep latency when compared to a wait-list control group.[136] Additional research is needed that better clarifies what exactly is included in the ayurvedic compounds and with larger samples and more rigorous methodology.

Side Effect and Safety Profile

In some traditional ayurveda treatments, toxic metals, herbs, and minerals are used. A 2004 study found toxic heavy metals such as lead, mercury, and arsenic in 20% of ayurvedic preparations that were made in South Asia and sold in the Boston area.[137] In addition, a study in 2008 demonstrated that about 20% of remedies, and 40% of a specific type of remedy known as *rasa shastra medicine,* that were purchased online contained lead, mercury, or arsenic despite the fact that 75% of the sites claimed adhering to good manufacturing practices.[138] The presence of toxic heavy metals is due to the belief that these metals can be rendered safe and can aid in the cure of some illnesses. Given these safety concerns and the lack of evidence supporting the efficacy of this treatment, the use of ayurvedic supplements for treating insomnia requires further research.

Mind-Body Treatments

Meditation

Meditation refers to a holistic discipline wherein the person who is meditating attempts to move the mind beyond reflexive "thinking" into a deeper state of relaxation or awareness.[139] Although there are many types of meditation, the one that is most commonly used as a CAM therapy for insomnia is mindfulness meditation.[139-143] This refers to a state of complete nonjudgmental awareness of one's thoughts, without trying to control or alter the thought content in any way. Meditation has shown some benefit as a treatment for insomnia in several preliminary studies.[139,141,144]

When mindfulness training was combined with cognitive behavioral therapy for insomnia, results indicated an improvement in total wake time and sleep efficiency as well as statistically significant reductions in presleep arousal and sleep effort;[145] this study, however, lacked a control arm and further research is needed. Mindfulness-based stress reduction (MBSR) is another standardized intervention that has demonstrated some efficacy for insomnia. Currently there is some evidence that MBSR participants experience a decrease in sleep-interfering cognitive processes such as worry and anxiety.[139,140] In addition to stress reduction, there may also be differences in slow wave sleep as a result of meditation.[146] However, Winbush and colleagues conducted a systematic review of the effects of MBSR as a treatment for sleep disturbances and were unable to make any distinct conclusions. This result was largely due to methodologic limitations in the literature that precluded conclusions about the efficacy of this treatment approach.[147] Overall, it seems that although mindfulness meditation may reduce presleep arousal and potentially help treat insomnia, additional research is necessary. Mindfulness meditation is considered a safe procedure with no known side effects.

Yoga

Yoga is a mind-body approach wherein body movements, breathing exercises, and meditation are integrated into a single multidimensional practice.[148] Yoga as a type of CAM therapy typically involves the use of physical postures, relaxation techniques, voluntarily regulated breathing, and information on the yoga philosophy. Yoga has been demonstrated to improve sleep quality and sleep latency in a small number of studies.[136,149] For example, after 6 months of practicing yoga, participants reported an improved sleep latency, an increase in the total number of hours slept, and a subjective feeling of being more rested in the morning.[136] Individuals who have been practicing yoga for at least 3 years report a better sleep quality than control subjects.[149] One reason that yoga may help treat insomnia is that it could combat the cognitive and physiologic arousal often associated with chronic insomnia. Subjects with insomnia who participated in an 8-week yoga intervention demonstrated improvements in sleep diary sleep efficiency, total sleep time, total wake time, sleep onset latency, and wake time after sleep onset.[150] However, this was an uncontrolled study, limiting the utility of these findings. Overall, yoga appears to be a possibly efficacious type of CAM therapy for the treatment of insomnia, largely owing to reductions in presleep arousal. However, the studies to date have been small and lack methodologic rigor, preventing more firm conclusions.

Side Effect and Safety Profile

Yoga is considered a safe procedure with limited side effects when practiced correctly. Older adults, those who are inactive, and those new to yoga should take care to gradually increase difficulty of postures to prevent muscle strain. When practicing yoga it is important to stretch adequately and warm up muscles prior to engaging in positions. Yoga injuries can occur when positions are done incorrectly.

Tai Chi

Tai chi is an internal Chinese martial art often practiced for health reasons. It involves the use of deliberate slow movements using the leverage of the joints, and is believed to open circulation in the body.[151] Focusing the mind solely on the movements of the form purportedly helps to bring about a state of mental calm and clarity. It essentially is a combination of a low to moderate intensity exercise with meditation. Tai chi has shown some benefit as a type of CAM therapy for insomnia. For example, older adults with moderate sleep complaints who were trained in a 6-month tai chi program reported a better quality of sleep and less daytime sleepiness.[151] A shorter 4-month program was also found to be effective, with older adult subjects reporting greater sleep quality, sleep efficiency, and sleep duration.[152] These two trials were relatively large and had adequate control procedures, suggesting that tai chi may be a beneficial type of CAM therapy for insomnia. However, the results were entirely based on self-report, and future research using objective measures of sleep are needed. In addition, both studies focused on an older adult population with moderate sleep difficulties. Additional research is needed on younger adults and on those with full threshold insomnia.

Side Effect and Safety Profile

Like yoga, tai chi is considered a safe procedure with limited side effects when practiced correctly. Musculoskeletal soreness may occur when patients are first starting tai chi.

MANIPULATION TREATMENTS

Massage

Massage therapy is the practice of soft tissue manipulation through the use of pressure.[153] It is considered to be a natural way of promoting relaxation through the activation of the parasympathetic nervous system. Massage is considered a safe procedure when performed by a massage therapist with proper training.

Insomnia

As a CAM therapy for insomnia massage has received only a minimal amount of research. One study reported that among a group of critically ill patients, massage resulted in improvements in self-reported sleep quality and had a trend toward a significant improvement in polysolmnographic sleep efficiency ($p = 0.06$) when compared to a group receiving relaxation exercises.[154] There is a paucity of research examining whether massage could improve insomnia in an otherwise healthy patient population. Future research is needed to establish whether this could be an effective CAM treatment.

Fibromyalgia

There is relatively little research on CAM treatments for this disorder; however, in one study of patients with fibromyalgia, massage was found to significantly improve sleep quality.[155] These improvements were associated with changes in substance P levels as well, suggesting a biologic mechanism of action.[155]

Balneotherapy

Balneotherapy is a type of hydrotherapy. It involves using water or bathing to treat illness, such as a warm bath in the evening, or baths taken in water with altered mineral content. It is commonly used for sleep problems by the general public.[156]

Insomnia

Warm baths may exert a beneficial effect on sleep by temporarily increasing core body temperature, with the subsequent decline in core body temperature after the bath promoting sleep. Despite its common use, few studies have examined the role of balneotherapy for insomnia. Several have suggested a beneficial effect of warm bath balneotherapy.[157] For therapy to be effective, it should be performed in the evening, with at least 20 to 30 minutes between the end of the bath and bedtime to allow for initiation of core body temperature cooling. Balneotherapy can also be used on the extremities or in water with elevated mineral content, but the available literature is extremely sparse and no evidence-based recommendations can be made at this time.

Fibromyalgia

A meta-analysis of balneotherapy demonstrated that it is an effective treatment for fibromyalgia, and consistently improves sleep quality for this population.[158] One study comparing balneotherapy to pool-based exercise noted an improvement in both groups.[159] Balneotherapy alone may thus be a viable option for patients unable to perform pool exercises.

CONCLUSION

This chapter presented research on commonly used CAM therapies for sleep disorders in adults. The largest body of available research involves biologic compounds such as melatonin and valerian. The evidence suggests that the melatonin is effective in treating circadian sleep disorders. The role of melatonin and valerian for insomnia is less well established. Other biologic compounds have demonstrated mixed results, with many concerns arising from variations in extraction and formulation of these compounds. Other types of CAM therapy have also showed some promise for the treatment of insomnia, with tai chi, yoga, and acupuncture demonstrating some positive findings. For fibromyalgia, massage and balneotherapy may be beneficial. However, most of the research using nonbiologic treatments has methodologic limitations. Additional research using more rigorous study designs, objective measures of sleep, and larger samples are needed for most types of CAM therapy to establish their efficacy and safety. Overall, most of the CAM therapies are reasonably safe and have a favorable side effect profile. There are some exceptions though, with certain biologic compounds causing drug interactions and treatments like ayurveda often being processed with heavy metal toxins. Therefore, patients should be advised to discuss CAM therapies under consideration with their physicians for an evaluation of potential side effects and interactions with standard medications. The studies reviewed in this chapter indicate that certain types of CAM therapy could have a role in the treatment of sleep disorders.

REFERENCES

1. National Center for Complementary and Alternative Medicine. *What Is CAM?* NCCAM Publication No. D347, 2007.
2. Richardson GS. Managing insomnia in the primary care setting: Raising the issues. *Sleep.* 2000;23(Suppl 1):S9-S12:discussion S13–S5.
3. Bliwise DL, Ansari FP. Insomnia associated with valerian and melatonin usage in the 2002 National Health Interview Survey. *Sleep.* 2007;30(7):881-884.
4. American Association of Retired Persons and National Center for Complementary and Alternative Medicine. *Complementary and Alternative Medicine: What People 50 and Over Are Using and Discussing with Their Physicians.* Washington, DC: AARP; 2007:26.
5. Sanchez-Ortuno MM, Belanger L, Ivers H, et al. The use of natural products for sleep: A common practice? *Sleep Med.* 2009;10(9):982-987.
6. Pearson NJ, Johnson LL, Nahin RL. Insomnia, trouble sleeping, and complementary and alternative medicine: Analysis of the 2002 national health interview survey data. *Arch Intern Med.* 2006;166(16):1775-1782.
7. Hatoum HT, Kania CM, Kong SX, et al. Prevalence of insomnia: A survey of the enrollees at five managed care organizations. *Am J Manag Care.* 1998;4(1):79-86.
8. Cuellar N, Galper DI, Taylor AG, et al. Restless legs syndrome. *J Altern Complement Med.* 2004;10(3):422-423.
9. Akerstedt T, Froberg JE, Friberg Y, et al. Melatonin excretion, body temperature and subjective arousal during 64 hours of sleep deprivation. *Psychoneuroendocrinology.* 1979;4(3):219-225.
10. Brzezinksi A. Melatonin in humans. *N Engl J Med.* 1997;336(3):186.
11. Dubocovitch M. Melatonin receptors: Are there multiple subtypes? *Trends Pharmacol Sci.* 1995;16:50-56.
12. Liu C, Weaver DR, Jin X, et al. Molecular dissection of two distinct actions of melatonin on the suprachiasmatic circadian clock. *Neuron.* 1997;19(1):91-102.
13. Mendelson WB. Melatonin microinjection into the medial preoptic area increases sleep in the rat. *Life Sci.* 2002;71(17):2067-2070.
14. Zhdanova IV. Melatonin as a hypnotic: Pro. *Sleep Med Rev.* 2005;9(1):51-65.
15. Touitou Y, Fevre M, Lagoguey M, et al. Age- and mental health-related circadian rhythms of plasma levels of melatonin, prolactin, luteinizing hormone and follicle-stimulating hormone in man. *J Endocrinol.* 1981;91(3):467-475.

16. Zhou JN, Liu RY, Van Heerikhuize J, et al. Alterations in the circadian rhythm of salivary melatonin begin during middle-age. *J Pineal Res.* 2003;34(1):11-16.

17. Sharma M, Palacios-Bois J, Schwartz G, et al. Circadian rhythms of melatonin and cortisol in aging. *Biol Psychiatry.* 1989;25(3):305-319.

18. Humbert W, Pevet P. Calcium content and concretions of pineal glands of young and old rats. A scanning and x-ray microanalytical study. *Cell Tissue Res.* 1991;263(3):593-596.

19. Kripke DF, Elliot JA, Youngstedt SD, et al. Melatonin: Marvel or marker? *Ann Med.* 1998;30(1):81-87.

20. Almay BG, von Knorring L, Wetterberg L. Melatonin in serum and urine in patients with idiopathic pain syndromes. *Psychiatry Res.* 1987;22(3):179-191.

21. Brugger P, Marktl W, Herold M. Impaired nocturnal secretion of melatonin in coronary heart disease. *Lancet.* 1995;345(8962):1408.

22. Fiorina P, Lattuada G, Silvestrini C, et al. Disruption of nocturnal melatonin rhythm and immunological involvement in ischaemic stroke patients. *Scand J Immunol.* 1999;50(2):228-231.

23. Lushington K, Dawson D, Kennaway DJ, et al. The relationship between 6-sulphatoxymelatonin and polysomnographic sleep in good sleeping controls and wake maintenance insomniacs, aged 55-80 years. *J Sleep Res.* 1999;8(1):57-64.

24. Riemann D, Klein T, Rodenbeck A, et al. Nocturnal cortisol and melatonin secretion in primary insomnia. *Psychiatry Res.* 2002;113(1-2):17-27.

25. Hajak G, Rodenbeck A, Staedt J, et al. Nocturnal plasma melatonin levels in patients suffering from chronic primary insomnia. *J Pineal Res.* 1995;19(3):116-122.

26. Youngstedt SD, Kripke DF, Elliott JA, et al. Circadian abnormalities in older adults. *J Pineal Res.* 2001;31(3):264-272.

27. Baskett JJ, Wood PC, Broad JB, et al. Melatonin in older people with age-related sleep maintenance problems: A comparison with age matched normal sleepers. *Sleep.* 2001;24(4):418-424.

28. Garfinkel D, Laudon M, Nof D, et al. Improvement of sleep quality in elderly people by controlled-release melatonin. *Lancet.* 1995; 346(8974):541-544.

29. Jean-Louis G, von Gizycki H, Zizi F. Melatonin effects on sleep, mood, and cognition in elderly with mild cognitive impairment. *J Pineal Res.* 1998;25(3):177-183.

30. Monti JM, Alvarino D, Cardinali D, et al. Polysomnographic study of the effect of melatonin on sleep in elderly patients with chronic primary insomnia. *Arch Gerontol Geriatr.* 1999;28:85-98.

31. Baskett JJ, Broad JB, Wood PC, et al. Does melatonin improve sleep in older people? A randomised crossover trial. *Age Ageing.* 2003;32(2):164-170.

32. Singer C, Tractenberg RE, Kaye J, et al. A multicenter, placebo-controlled trial of melatonin for sleep disturbance in Alzheimer's disease. *Sleep.* 2003;26(7):893-901.

33. Riemersma-van der Lek RF, Swaab DF, Twisk J, et al. Effect of bright light and melatonin on cognitive and noncognitive function in elderly residents of group care facilities: A randomized controlled trial. *JAMA.* 2008;299(22):2642-2655.

34. Zhdanova IV, Wurtman RJ, Regan MM, et al. Melatonin treatment for age-related insomnia. *J Clin Endocrinol Metab.* 2001;86(10):4727-4730.

35. Luthringer R, Muzet M, Zisapel N, et al. The effect of prolonged-release melatonin on sleep measures and psychomotor performance in elderly patients with insomnia. *Int Clin Psychopharmacol.* 2009;24(5):239-249.

36. Hughes RJ, Sack N, Lewy AJ. The role of melatonin and circadian phase in age-related sleep-maintenance insomnia: Assessment in a clinical trial of melatonin replacement. *Sleep.* 1998;21(1):52-68.

37. Dawson D, Rogers NL, van den Heuvel CJ, et al. Effect of sustained nocturnal transbuccal melatonin administration on sleep and temperature in elderly insomniacs. *J Biol Rhythms.* 1998;13(6):532-538.

38. Buscemi N, Vandermeer B, Pandya R, et al. Melatonin for Treatment of Sleep Disorders. Agency for Healthcare Research and Quality. Prepared by the University of Alberta Evidence-based Practice Center, under Contract No. 290-02-0023. Rockville, MD. 2004:310.

39. European Medicines Agency. *Assessment Report for Circadin: Procedure No. EMEA/H/C/695.* London, England: European Medicine Agency; 2007:52.

40. Haimov I, Lavie P, Laudon M, et al. Melatonin replacement therapy of elderly insomniacs. *Sleep.* 1995;18(7):598-603.

41. Sack RL, Brandes RW, Kendall AR, et al. Entrainment of free-running circadian rhythms by melatonin in blind people. *N Engl J Med.* 2000; 343(15):1070-1077.

42. Herxheimer A, Petrie KJ. Melatonin for the prevention and treatment of jet lag. *Cochrane Database Syst Rev.* 2002(2):CD001520.

43. Shamseer L, Vohra S. Complementary, holistic, and integrative medicine: Melatonin. *Pediatr Rev.* 2009;30(6):223-228.

44. Bendz LM, Scates AC. Melatonin treatment for insomnia in pediatric patients with attention-deficit/hyperactivity disorder. *Ann Pharmacother.* 2010;44(1):185-191.

45. Wirojanan J, Jacquemont S, Diaz R, et al. The efficacy of melatonin for sleep problems in children with autism, fragile X syndrome, or autism and fragile X syndrome. *J Clin Sleep Med.* 2009;5(2):145-150.

46. Braam W, MG. Smits R, Didden R, et al. Exogenous melatonin for sleep problems in individuals with intellectual disability: A meta-analysis. *Dev Med Child Neurol.* 2009;51(5):340-349.

47. Siegrist C, Benedetti C, Orlando A, et al. Lack of changes in serum prolactin, FSH, TSH, and estradiol after melatonin treatment in doses that improve sleep and reduce benzodiazepine consumption in sleep-disturbed, middle-aged, and elderly patients. *J Pineal Res.* 2001;30(1):34-42.

48. Seabra ML, Bignotto M, Pinto Jr LR, et al. Randomized, double-blind clinical trial, controlled with placebo, of the toxicology of chronic melatonin treatment. *J Pineal Res.* 2000;29(4):193-200.

49. Buscemi N, Vandermeer B, Hooton N, et al. The efficacy and safety of exogenous melatonin for primary sleep disorders. A meta-analysis. *J Gen Intern Med.* 2005;20(12):1151-1158.

50. Gardiner PK, Kemper KJ. Insomnia: Herbal and dietary alternatives to counting sheep. *Contemp Pediatr.* 2002;19(2):69-75.

51. Dawson D, van den Heuvel CJ. Integrating the actions of melatonin on human physiology. *Ann Med.* 1998;30(1):95-102.

52. National Academies Committee on the Framework for Evaluating the Safety of Dietary Supplements. Prototype Monograph on Melatonin. *Dietary Supplements: A Framework for Evaluation Safety.* Washington, DC: The National Academies Press; 2004:D1-D71.

53. Sewerynek E. Melatonin and the cardiovascular system. *Neuroendocrinol Lett.* 2002;23(Suppl 1):79-83.

54. Rogers NL, Phan O, Kennaway DJ, et al. Effect of daytime oral melatonin administration on neurobehavioral performance in humans. *J Pineal Res.* 1998;25(1):47-53.

55. Kamei Y, Hayakawa T, Urata J, et al. Melatonin treatment for circadian rhythm sleep disorders. *Psychiatry Clin Neurosci.* 2000;54(3):381-382.

56. Wyatt JK, Dijk DJ, Ritz-de Cecco A, et al. Sleep-facilitating effect of exogenous melatonin in healthy young men and women is circadian-phase dependent. *Sleep.* 2006;29(5):609-618.

57. Hansson I, Holmdahl R, Mattsson R. Constant darkness enhances autoimmunity to type II collagen and exaggerates development of collagen-induced arthritis in DBA/1 mice. *J Neuroimmunol.* 1990;27(1):79-84.

58. Maestroni GJ, Sulli A, Pizzorni C, et al. Melatonin in rheumatoid arthritis: Synovial macrophages show melatonin receptors. *Ann N Y Acad Sci.* 2002;966:271-275.

59. Bilici D, Akpinar E, Kiziltunc A. Protective effect of melatonin in carageenan-induced acute local inflammation. *Pharmacol Res.* 2002;46(2):133-139.

60. Maksoud A, Moore CA, Harshkowitz M. The effect of melatonin administration on patients with sleep apnea. *Sleep Res.* 1997;26:114.

61. Olde Rikkert MG, Rigaud AS. Melatonin in elderly patients with insomnia. A systematic review. *Z Gerontol Geriatr.* 2001;34(6):491-497.

62. Bellipanni G, Bianchi P, Pierpaoli W, et al. Effects of melatonin in perimenopausal and menopausal women: A randomized and placebo controlled study. *Exp Gerontol.* 2001;36(2):297-310.

63. Hoebert M, van der Heijden KB, van Geijlswijk IM, et al. Long-term follow-up of melatonin treatment in children with ADHD and chronic sleep onset insomnia. *J Pineal Res.* 2009;47(1):1-7.

64. Attele AS, Xie JT, Yuan CS. Treatment of insomnia: An alternative approach. *Altern Med Rev.* 2000;5(3):249-259.

65. Leibenluft E, Feldman-Naim S, Turner EH, et al. Effects of exogenous melatonin administration and withdrawal in five patients with rapid-cycling bipolar disorder. *J Clin Psychiatry.* 1997;58(9):383-388.

66. Balderer G, Borbely AA. Effect of valerian on human sleep. *Psychopharmacology.* 1985;87(4):406-409.

67. Donath F, Quispe S, Diefenbach K, et al. Critical evaluation of the effect of valerian extract on sleep structure and sleep quality. *Pharmacopsychiatry.* 2000;33(2):47-53.

68. Glass JR, Sproule BA, Herrmann N, et al. Acute pharmacological effects of temazepam, diphenhydramine, and valerian in healthy elderly subjects. *J Clin Psychopharmacol.* 2003;23(3):260-268.

69. Houghton PJ. The scientific basis for the reputed activity of valerian. *J Pharm Pharmacol.* 1999;51(5):505-512.

70. Piccinelli AL, Arana S, Caceres A, et al. New lignans from the roots of *Valeriana prionophylla* with antioxidative and vasorelaxant activities. *J Nat Prod.* 2004;67(7):1135-1140.

71. Lefebvre T, Foster BC, Drouin CE, et al. In vitro activity of commercial valerian root extracts against human cytochrome P450 3A4. *J Pharm Pharmaceut Sci.* 2004;7(2):265-273.

72. Stevinson C, Ernst E. Valerian for insomnia: A systematic review of randomized clinical trials. *Sleep Med.* 2000;1(2):91-99.

73. Taibi DM, Landis CA, Petry H, et al. A systematic review of valerian as a sleep aid: Safe but not effective. *Sleep Med Rev.* 2007;11(3):209-230.

74. Bent S, Padula A, Moore D, et al. Valerian for sleep: A systematic review and meta-analysis. *Am J Med.* 2006;119(12):1005-1012.

75. Shinomiya K, Fujimura K, Kim Y, et al. Effects of valerian extract on the sleep-wake cycle in sleep-disturbed rats. *Acta Med Okayama.* 2005;59(3):89-92.

76. Ugalde M, Reza V, Gonzalez-Trujano ME, et al. Isobolographic analysis of the sedative interaction between six central nervous system depressant drugs and *Valeriana edulis* hydroalcoholic extract in mice. *J Pharm Pharmacol.* 2005;57(5):631-639.

77. Fields AM, Richards TA, Felton JA, et al. Analysis of responses to valerian root extract in the feline pulmonary vascular bed. *J Altern Complement Med.* 2003;9(6):909-918.

78. Hazelhoff B, Malingre TM, Meijer DK. Antispasmodic effects of valeriana compounds: An in-vivo and in-vitro study on the guinea-pig ileum. *Arch Int Pharmacodyn Ther.* 1982;257(2):274-287.

79. Tokunaga S, Takeda Y, Niimoto T, et al. Effect of valerian extract preparation (BIM) on the sleep-wake cycle in rats. *Biol Pharmaceut Bull.* 2007;30(2):363-366.

80. Dimpfel W, Brattstrom A, Koetter U. Central action of a fixed valerian-hops extract combination (Ze 91019) in freely moving rats. *Eur J Med Res.* 2006;11(11):496-500.

81. Leathwood PD, Chauffard F, Heck E, et al. Aqueous extract of valerian root (*Valeriana officinalis* L.) improves sleep quality in man. *Pharmacol Biochem Behav.* 1982;17(1):65-71.

82. Lindahl O, Lindwall L. Double blind study of a valerian preparation. *Pharmacol Biochem Behav.* 1989;32(4):1065-1066.

83. Schulz H, Stolz C, Muller J. The effect of valerian extract on sleep polygraphy in poor sleepers: A pilot study. *Pharmacopsychiatry.* 1994;27(4):147-151.

84. Morin CM, Koetter U, Bastien C, et al. Valerian-hops combination and diphenhydramine for treating insomnia: A randomized placebo-controlled clinical trial. *Sleep.* 2005;28(11):1465-1471.

85. Poyares DR, Guilleminault C, Ohayon MM, et al. Can valerian improve the sleep of insomniacs after benzodiazepine withdrawal? *Prog Neuropsychopharmacol Biol Psychiatry.* 2002;26(3):539-545.

86. Andreatini R, Sartori VA, Seabra ML, et al. Effect of valepotriates (valerian extract) in generalized anxiety disorder: A randomized placebo-controlled pilot study. *Phytother Res.* 2002;16(7):650-654.

87. Wheatley D. Stress-induced insomnia treated with kava and valerian: Singly and in combination. *Hum Psychopharmacol.* 2001;16(4):353-356.

88. Coxeter PD, Schluter PJ, Eastwood HL, et al. Valerian does not appear to reduce symptoms for patients with chronic insomnia in general practice using a series of randomised n-of-1 trials [see comment]. *Complementary Ther Med.* 2003;11(4):215-222.

89. Jacobs BP, Bent S, Tice JA, et al. An internet-based randomized, placebo-controlled trial of kava and valerian for anxiety and insomnia. *Medicine.* 2005;84(4):197-207.

90. Dimpfel W, Suter A. Sleep improving effects of a single dose administration of a valerian/hops fluid extract—A double blind, randomized, placebo-controlled sleep-EEG study in a parallel design using electrohypnograms. *Eur J Med Res.* 2008;13(5):200-204.

91. Koetter U, Schrader E, Kaufeler R, et al. A randomized, double blind, placebo-controlled, prospective clinical study to demonstrate clinical efficacy of a fixed valerian hops extract combination (Ze 91019) in patients suffering from non-organic sleep disorder. *Phytother Res.* 2007;21(9):847-851.

92. Cuellar NG, Ratcliffe SJ. Does valerian improve sleepiness and symptom severity in people with restless legs syndrome? *Altern Ther Health Med.* 2009;15(2):22-28.

93. Garges HP, Varia I, Doraiswamy PM. Cardiac complications and delirium associated with valerian root withdrawal [letter]. *JAMA.* 1998;280(18):1566-1567.

94. Vo LT, Chan D, King RG. Investigation of the effects of peppermint oil and valerian on rat liver and cultured human liver cells. *Clin Exper Pharmacol Physiol.* 2003;30(10):799-804.

95. Hendriks H, Bos R, Woerdenbag HJ, et al. Central nervous depressant activity of valerenic acid in the mouse. *Planta Med.* 1985(1):28-31.

96. Birdsall TC. 5-Hydroxytryptophan: A clinically-effective serotonin precursor. *Altern Med Rev.* 1998;3(4):271-280.

97. Meolie AL, Rosen C, Kristo D, et al. Oral nonprescription treatment for insomnia: An evaluation of products with limited evidence. *J Clin Sleep Med.* 2005;1(2):173-187.

98. Wyatt RJ, Zarcone V, Engelman K, et al. Effects of 5-hydroxytryptophan on the sleep of normal human subjects. *Electroencephalogr Clin Neurophysiol.* 1971;30(6):505-509.

99. Gustafsson B, Tømmerås K, Nordrum I, et al. Long-term serotonin administration induces heart valve disease in rats. *Circulation.* 2005;111(12):1517-1522.

100. Izumi T, Iwamoto N, Kitaichi Y, et al. Effects of co-administration of a selective serotonin reuptake inhibitor and monoamine oxidase inhibitors on 5-HT-related behavior in rats. *Eur J Pharmacol.* 2006;532(3):258-264.

101. Jacobs GE, Kamerling IM, de Kam ML, et al. Enhanced tolerability of the 5-hydroxytryptophane challenge test combined with granisetron. *J Psychopharmacol.* 2010;24(1):65-72.

102. Wheatley D. Medicinal plants for insomnia: A review of their pharmacology, efficacy and tolerability. *J Psychopharmacol.* 2005;19(4):414-421.

103. Cauffield JS, Forbes HJ. Dietary supplements used in the treatment of depression, anxiety, and sleep disorders. *Lippincotts Prim Care Pract.* 1999;3(3):290-304.

104. Barnes J, Anderson LA, Phillipson JD. St John's wort (*Hypericum perforatum* L.): A review of its chemistry, pharmacology and clinical properties. *J Pharm Pharmacol.* 2001;53(5):583-600.

105. Zanoli P. Role of hyperforin in the pharmacological activities of St. John's wort. *CNS Drug Rev.* 2004;10(3):203-218.

106. Sharpley AL, McGavin CL, Whale R, et al. Antidepressant-like effect of *Hypericum perforatum* (St. John's wort) on the sleep polysomnogram. *Psychopharmacology (Berl).* 1998;139(3):286-287.

107. Schulz H, Jobert M. Effects of hypericum extract on the sleep EEG in older volunteers. *J Geriatr Psychiatry Neurol.* 1994;7(Suppl 1):S39-43.

108. Woelk H, Burkard G, Grunwald J. Benefits and risks of the hypericum extract LI 160: Drug monitoring study with 3250 patients. *J Geriatr Psychiatry Neurol.* 1994;7(Suppl 1):S34-38.

109. Di YM, Li CG, Xue CC, et al. Clinical drugs that interact with St. John's wort and implication in drug development. *Curr Pharm Des.* 2008;14(17):1723-1742.

110. Borrelli F, Izzo AA. Herb-drug interactions with St. John's wort (*Hypericum perforatum*): An update on clinical observations. *AAPS J.* 2009;11(4):710-727.

111. Gordon J. SSRIs and St. John's wort: Possible toxicity? *Am Fam Physician.* 1998;57:950-953.

112. Zanoli P, Zavatti M. Pharmacognostic and pharmacological profile of *Humulus lupulus* L. *J Ethnopharmacol.* 2008;116(3):383-396.

113. Schiller H, Forster A, Vonhoff C, et al. Sedating effects of *Humulus lupulus* L. extracts. *Phytomedicine.* 2006;13(8):535-541.

114. Huang W, Kutner N, Bliwise DL. A systematic review of the effects of acupuncture in treating insomnia. *Sleep Med Rev.* 2009;13(1):73-104.

115. Cao H, Pan X, Li H, et al. Acupuncture for treatment of insomnia: A systematic review of randomized controlled trials. *J Altern Complement Med.* 2009;15(11):1171-1186.

116. Sok SR, Erlen JA, Kim KB. Effects of acupuncture therapy on insomnia. *J Adv Nurs.* 2003;44(4):375-384.

117. Cheuk D, Yeung W, Chung K, et al. Acupuncture for insomnia. *Cochrane Syst Rev.* 2007;3:CD005472.

118. Kim YS, Lee SH, Jung WS, et al. Intradermal acupuncture on shen-men and nei-kuan acupoints in patients with insomnia after stroke. *Am J Chin Med.* 2004;32(5):771-778.

119. Huang MI, Nir Y, Chen B, et al. A randomized controlled pilot study of acupuncture for postmenopausal hot flashes: Effect on nocturnal hot flashes and sleep quality. *Fertil Steril.* 2006;86(3):700-710.

120. Carpenter JS, Neal JG. Other complementary and alternative medicine modalities: Acupuncture, magnets, reflexology, and homeopathy. *Am J Med.* 2005;118(Suppl 12B):109-117.

121. Freire AO, Sugai GC, Chrispin FS, et al. Treatment of moderate obstructive sleep apnea syndrome with acupuncture: A randomised, placebo-controlled pilot trial. *Sleep Med.* 2007;8(1):43-50.

122. Rooks DS. Fibromyalgia treatment update. *Curr Opin Rheumatol.* 2007;19(2):111-117.

123. Holdcraft LC, Assefi N, Buchwald D. Complementary and alternative medicine in fibromyalgia and related syndromes. *Best Pract Res Clin Rheumatol.* 2003;17(4):667-683.

124. Targino RA, Imamura M, Kaziyama HH, et al. A randomized controlled trial of acupuncture added to usual treatment for fibromyalgia. *J Rehabil Med.* 2008;40(7):582-588.

125. Langhorst J, Klose P, Musial F, et al. Efficacy of acupuncture in fibromyalgia syndrome—A systematic review with a meta-analysis of controlled clinical trials. *Rheumatology.* 2010;49(7):1421.

126. Martin-Sanchez E, Torralba E, Diaz-Dominguez E, et al. Efficacy of acupuncture for the treatment of fibromyalgia: Systematic review and meta-analysis of randomized trials. *Open Rheumatol J.* 2009;3:25-29.

127. Ernst G, Strzyz H, Hagmeister H. Incidence of adverse effects during acupuncture therapy—A multicentre survey. *Complement Ther Med.* 2003;11(2):93-97.

128. Chen ML, Lin LC, Wu SC, et al. The effectiveness of acupressure in improving the quality of sleep of institutionalized residents. *J Gerontol A Biol Sci Med Sci.* 1999;54(8):M389-394.

129. Tsay SL, Chen ML. Acupressure and quality of sleep in patients with end-stage renal disease—A randomized controlled trial. *Int J Nurs Stud.* 2003;40(1):1-7.

130. Yang MH, Wu SC, Lin JG, et al. The efficacy of acupressure for decreasing agitated behaviour in dementia: A pilot study. *J Clin Nurs.* 2007;16(2):308-315.

131. Lee MS, Shin BC, Suen LK, et al. Auricular acupuncture for insomnia: A systematic review. *Int J Clin Pract.* 2008;62(11):1744-1752.

132. Chen HY, Shi Y, Ng CS, et al. Auricular acupuncture treatment for insomnia: A systematic review. *J Altern Complement Med.* 2007;13(6):669-676.

133. Suen LK, Wong TK, Leung AW. Effectiveness of auricular therapy on sleep promotion in the elderly. *Am J Chin Med.* 2002;30(4):429-449.

134. Suen LK, Wong TK, Leung AW, et al. The long-term effects of auricular therapy using magnetic pearls on elderly with insomnia. *Complement Ther Med.* 2003;11(2):85-92.

135. Farag NH, Mills PJ. A randomised-controlled trial of the effects of a traditional herbal supplement on sleep onset insomnia. *Complement Ther Med.* 2003;11(4):223-225.

136. Manjunath NK, Telles S. Influence of yoga and ayurveda on self-rated sleep in a geriatric population. *Indian J Med Res.* 2005;121(5):683-690.

137. Saper RB, Kales SN, Paquin J, et al. Heavy metal content of ayurvedic herbal medicine products. *JAMA.* 2004;292(23):2868-2873.

138. Saper RB, Phillips RS, Sehgal A, et al. Lead, mercury, and arsenic in US- and Indian-manufactured ayurvedic medicines sold via the Internet. *JAMA.* 2008;300(8):915-923.

139. Carlson LE, Garland SN. Impact of mindfulness-based stress reduction (MBSR) on sleep, mood, stress and fatigue symptoms in cancer outpatients. *Int J Behav Med.* 2005;12(4):278-285.

140. Carlson LE, Speca M, Patel KD, et al. Mindfulness-based stress reduction in relation to quality of life, mood, symptoms of stress and levels of cortisol, dehydroepiandrosterone sulfate (DHEAS) and melatonin in breast and prostate cancer outpatients. *Psychoneuroendocrinology.* 2004;29(4):448-474.

141. Cuellar NG. Mindfulness meditation for veterans—Implications for occupational health providers. *AAOHN J.* 2008;56(8):357-363.

142. Heidenreich T, Tuin I, Pflug B, et al. Mindfulness-based cognitive therapy for persistent insomnia: A pilot study. *Psychother Psychosom.* 2006;75(3):188-189.

143. Gross CR, Kreitzer MJ, Russas V, et al. Mindfulness meditation to reduce symptoms after organ transplant: A pilot study. *Adv Mind Body Med.* 2004;20(2):20-29.

144. Gardner-Nix J, Backman S, Barbati J, et al. Evaluating distance education of a mindfulness-based meditation programme for chronic pain management. *J Telemed Telecare.* 2008;14(2):88-92.

145. Ong JC, Shapiro SL, Manber R. Combining mindfulness meditation with cognitive-behavior therapy for insomnia: A treatment-development study. *Behav Ther.* 2008;39(2):171-182.

146. Mason LI, Alexander CN, Travis FT, et al. Electrophysiological correlates of higher states of consciousness during sleep in long-term practitioners of the Transcendental Meditation program. *Sleep.* 1997;20(2):102-110.

147. Winbush NY, Gross CR, Kreitzer MJ. The effects of mindfulness-based stress reduction on sleep disturbance: A systematic review. *Explore (NY).* 2007;3(6):585-591.

148. Cohen L, Warneke C, Fouladi RT, et al. Psychological adjustment and sleep quality in a randomized trial of the effects of a Tibetan yoga intervention in patients with lymphoma. *Cancer.* 2004;100(10):2253-2260.

149. Vera FM, Manzaneque JM, Maldonado EF, et al. Subjective sleep quality and hormonal modulation in long-term yoga practitioners. *Biol Psychol.* 2009;81(3):164-168.

150. Khalsa SB. Treatment of chronic insomnia with yoga: A preliminary study with sleep-wake diaries. *Appl Psychophysiol Biofeedback.* 2004;29(4):269-278.

151. Li F, Fisher KJ, Harmer P, et al. Tai chi and self-rated quality of sleep and daytime sleepiness in older adults: A randomized controlled trial. *J Am Geriatr Soc.* 2004;52(6):892-900.

152. Irwin MR, Olmstead R, Motivala SJ. Improving sleep quality in older adults with moderate sleep complaints: A randomized controlled trial of tai chi chih. *Sleep.* 2008;31(7):1001-1008.

153. Gauthier DM. The healing potential of back massage. *Online J Knowl Synth Nurs.* 1999;6:5.

154. Richards KC. Effect of a back massage and relaxation intervention on sleep in critically ill patients. *Am J Crit Care.* 1998;7(4):288-299.

155. Field T, Diego M, Cullen C, et al. Fibromyalgia pain and substance p decrease and sleep improves after massage therapy. *J Clin Rheumatol.* 2002;8(2):72-76.

156. Aritake-Okada S, Kaneita Y, Uchiyama M, et al. Non-pharmacological self-management of sleep among the Japanese general population. *J Clin Sleep Med.* 2009;5(5):464-469.

157. Liao WC. Effects of passive body heating on body temperature and sleep regulation in the elderly: A systematic review. *Int J Nurs Stud.* 2002;39(8):803-810.

158. Baranowsky J, Klose P, Musial F, et al. Qualitative systemic review of randomized controlled trials on complementary and alternative medicine treatments in fibromyalgia. *Rheumatol Int.* 2009;30(1):1-21.

159. Altan L, Bingol U, Aykac M, et al. Investigation of the effects of pool-based exercise on fibromyalgia syndrome. *Rheumatol Int.* 2004;24(5):272-277.

160. Dietz BM, Mahady GB, Pauli GF, et al. Valerian extract and valerenic acid are partial agonists of the 5-HT5a receptor in vitro. *Brain Res Mol Brain Res.* 2005;138(2):191-197.

161. Santos MS, Ferreira F, Cunha AP, et al. An aqueous extract of valerian influences the transport of GABA in synaptosomes. *Planta Med.* 1994;60(3):278-279.

162. Santos MS, Ferreira F, Cunha AP, et al. Synaptosomal GABA release as influenced by valerian root extract—Involvement of the GABA carrier. *Arch Int Pharmacodyn Ther.* 1994;327(2):220-231.

163. Santos MS, Ferreira F, Faro C, et al. The amount of GABA present in aqueous extracts of valerian is sufficient to account for [^{3}H]GABA release in synaptosomes. *Planta Med.* 1994;60(5):475-476.

164. Ortiz JG, Nieves-Natal J, Chavez P. Effects of Valeriana officinalis extracts on [^{3}H]flunitrazepam binding, synaptosomal [^{3}H]GABA uptake, and hippocampal [^{3}H]GABA release. *Neurochem Res.* 1999;24(11):1373-1378.

165. Schumacher B, Scholle S, Holzl J, et al. Lignans isolated from valerian: Identification and characterization of a new olivil derivative with partial agonistic activity at A(1) adenosine receptors. *J Nat Prod.* 2002;65(10):1479-1485.

166. De Feo V, Faro C. Pharmacological effects of extracts from *Valeriana adscendens* Trel. II. Effects on GABA uptake and amino acids. *Phytother Res.* 2003;17(6):661-664.

167. Abourashed EA, Koetter U, Brattstrom A. In vitro binding experiments with a valerian, hops and their fixed combination extract (Ze91019) to selected central nervous system receptors. *Phytomedicine.* 2004;11(7-8):633-638.

168. Dunaev VV, Trzhetsinskii SD, Tishkin VS, et al. [Biological activity of the sum of the valepotriates isolated from *Valeriana alliariifolia*]. *Farmakol Toksikol.* 1987;50(6):33-37.

169. Khom S, Baburin I, Timin E, et al. Valerenic acid potentiates and inhibits GABA(A) receptors: Molecular mechanism and subunit specificity. *Neuropharmacology.* 2007;53(1):178-187.

170. Malva JO, Santos S, Macedo T. Neuroprotective properties of *Valeriana officinalis* extracts. *Neurotox Res.* 2004;6(2):131-140.

171. Trauner G, Khom S, Baburin I, et al. Modulation of GABA$_A$ receptors by valerian extracts is related to the content of valerenic acid. *Planta Med.* 2008;74(1):19-24.

172. Neuhaus W, Trauner G, Gruber D, et al. Transport of a GABA$_A$ receptor modulator and its derivatives from *Valeriana officinalis* L. s. l. across an in vitro cell culture model of the blood-brain barrier. *Planta Med.* 2008;74(11):1338-1344.

173. Svensson M, Malm C, Tonkonogi M, et al. Effect of Q_{10} supplementation on tissue Q_{10} levels and adenine nucleotide catabolism during high-intensity exercise. *Int J Sport Nutr.* 1999;9(2):166-180.

174. Retey JV, Adam M, Honegger E, et al. A functional genetic variation of adenosine deaminase affects the duration and intensity of deep sleep in humans. *Proc Natl Acad Sci U S A.* 2005;102(43):15676-15681.

175. Vissiennon Z, Sichardt K, Koetter U, et al. Valerian extract Ze 911 inhibits postsynaptic potentials by activation of adenosine A_1 receptors in rat cortical neurons. *Planta Med.* 2006;72(7):579-583.

176. Schellenberg R, Sauer S, Abourashed EA, et al. The fixed combination of valerian and hops (Ze91019) acts via a central adenosine mechanism. *Planta Med.* 2004;70(7):594-597.

177. Muller CE, B Schumacher EA, Brattstrom A, et al. Interactions of valerian extracts and a fixed valerian-hop extract combination with adenosine receptors. *Life Sci.* 2002;71(16):1939-1949.

178. Ikeda M, Ikeda-Sagara M, Okada T, et al. Brain oxidation is an initial process in sleep induction. *Neuroscience.* 2005;130(4):1029-1040.

179. Lacher SK, Mayer R, Sichardt K, et al. Interaction of valerian extracts of different polarity with adenosine receptors: Identification of isovaltrate as an inverse agonist at A1 receptors. *Biochem Pharmacol.* 2007;73(2):248-258.

180. Giedke H. On the role of serotonin in sleep regulation and depression. A commentary on "neurobiological bases for the relation between sleep and depression" (J. Adrien) [comment]. *Sleep Med Rev.* 2003;7(1):101-102:author reply 103–105.

181. Stiasny-Kolster K, Moller JC, Zschocke J, et al. Normal dopaminergic and serotonergic metabolites in cerebrospinal fluid and blood of restless legs syndrome patients. *Mov Dis.* 2004;19(2):192-196.

182. Smits MG, van Stel HF, van der Heijden K, et al. Melatonin improves health status and sleep in children with idiopathic chronic sleep-onset insomnia: a randomized placebo-controlled trial. *J Am Acad Child Adolesc Psychiatry.* 2003;42(11):1286-1293.

183. Smits EJ, Van Someren, et al. Effect of melatonin on sleep, behavior, and cognition in ADHD and chronic sleep-onset insomnia. *J Am Acad Child Adolesc Psychiatry.* 2007;46(2):233-241.

184. Garfinkel D, Laudon M, Nof D, et al. Improvement of sleep quality in elderly people by controlled-release melatonin. *Lancet.* 1995;346(8974):541-544.

SECTION 4

Insomnias

Overview of Insomnia:
DIAGNOSTIC AND THERAPEUTIC APPROACH

Chapter 10

MICHAEL H. BONNET / DONNA L. ARAND

DEFINITION

Insomnia is defined as a complaint of difficulty initiating sleep (sleep onset insomnia), difficulty maintaining sleep (sleep maintenance insomnia), or waking up too early without being able to return to sleep. Patients may also complain of nonrestorative or poor quality sleep. These difficulties occur despite an adequate opportunity to sleep and must be associated with a daytime impairment.[1] The degree of subjective sleep disturbance may vary from 30 minutes or more to fall asleep or a total sleep time of 6 hours or less to complete inability to sleep for several nights. This sleep disturbance occurs on three or more nights per week. The *International Classification of Sleep Disorders,* Second Edition (ICSD-2) from the American Academy of Sleep Medicine[1] lists nine types of daytime impairment associated with the poor sleep that can be considered sufficient to diagnose insomnia, and these symptoms are listed in Box 10-1.

Insomnia differs from sleep deprivation, where the opportunity for sleep is decreased, resulting in a reduction of sleep, which then returns to normal when a sufficient time for sleep becomes available. In addition, each person has an individual sleep need so that some people only need to sleep for a short time, say 6 hours, to feel awake and refreshed. People who have a short sleep requirement without evidence of daytime impairment or daytime feelings of fatigue or malaise are called *short sleepers* and are not given a diagnosis of insomnia.

BOX 10-1 *Types of Daytime Impairment Associated with a Diagnosis of Insomnia*

- Fatigue/malaise
- Attention, concentration, or memory impairment
- Social/vocational dysfunction or poor school performance
- Mood disturbance/irritability
- Daytime sleepiness
- Motivation/energy/initiative reduction
- Proneness for errors/accidents at work or while driving
- Tension headaches or gastrointestinal symptoms in response to poor sleep
- Concerns or worries about sleep

From International Classification of Sleep Disorders: *Diagnostic and Coding Manual,* 2nd ed. Westchester, IL: American Academy of Sleep Medicine; 2005.

PREVALENCE

Insomnia is the most common sleep disorder and one of the most common medical complaints with 69% of primary care patients reporting at least occasional insomnia.[2] Unfortunately, almost 70% of patients with insomnia do not spontaneously discuss their sleep problem with their physician.[3] Population estimates vary based upon the specific definition of insomnia used, but poor sleep is typically reported in about 30% of the population, and chronic insomnia with residual daytime deficits as described earlier has been reported in about 10% of respondents.[4-6]

The prevalence of insomnia increases with age. In elderly populations, only about 12% of respondents reported normal sleep and 57% had a chronic insomnia complaint.[7] Adult women report insomnia about 50% more often than men.[4] There is also a higher prevalence of insomnia in persons of lower socioeconomic status, the unemployed, and divorced, widowed, or separated individuals.[6]

ASSOCIATED IMPAIRMENTS

The diagnosis of insomnia requires that patients report a carryover of dysphoria into their daily life. Insomnia patients commonly report increased fatigue, sleepiness, confusion, tension/anxiety, and depression compared to control subjects.[8] This dysphoria starts to pervade other areas of life so that patients with insomnia also have significantly decreased quality of life.

Quality of Life

A standard measure of quality of life, the Medical Outcomes Study Short Form (SF-36) has shown that patients with insomnia report significant problems in both medical (including pain) and emotional aspects of life, and the level of discomfort is of a similar magnitude to that seen in patients with other significant and chronic medical conditions such as congestive heart failure and depression.[9] Quality of life (QoL) can also be measured by looking at promotions, sick time, or other employment metrics. For example, insomnia patients have been shown to be less likely to receive promotions, to have more errors and accidents, to have more absenteeism from work, and to have more health care consequences in general.[8,10] Poor work performance and other health issues imply that patients with insomnia will require intervention and will therefore have increased costs to society, and these costs have been estimated both individually and globally.[11,12]

Performance

Insomnia patients are almost universally concerned that their poor sleep has direct negative consequences on their performance of daily tasks and consistently report subjective performance deficits.[13] However, insomnia patients tend to overestimate both the magnitude of their sleep deficits compared with objective measures and the magnitude of the performance deficit when compared with objectively measured performance. Numerous studies have examined psychomotor performance in insomnia patients matched with control subjects. The only consistent problem found in the insomnia patients was a decrement in balance, although about 20% of measures involving memory were also significantly decreased in insomnia patients.[8] However, these decrements could be due to elevated central nervous system arousal in patients (see discussion under "Physiologic Effects") rather than to sleep loss.

Physiologic Effects

Chronic primary insomnia appears to be related to physiologic activation. A majority of studies have found large effects (effect size greater than or equal to 0.8) for increased physiologic activation as measured by cardiac, metabolic, hormone, and high-frequency EEG measures.[8] Recent studies have shown increased activity during sleep in hypothalamic areas and reduced hippocampal volume in insomnia patients compared with control subjects.[14,15]

Association with Other Medical Problems

As primary insomnia is associated with sympathetic nervous system activation,[16] patients with chronic insomnia would be expected to have an increased risk of hypertension[17] and cardiac disease including heart attack,[18] and many studies have reported these associations. One recent laboratory sleep study has shown that patients with primary insomnia without sleep-related breathing disorders had significantly higher diastolic blood pressure than control subjects both at night and during the day, with significantly higher systolic blood pressure at night.[19] A risk assessment study that also measured and controlled breathing disorders during sleep[20] showed that patients with primary insomnia and short sleep times (compared with normal sleepers having short sleep times) were at increased risk for the development of hypertension.

Treatment Response

In the last few years, research protocols have become more sensitive to daytime deficits and have begun to measure them in addition to changes in sleep as treatment outcomes. For example, three studies with eszopiclone (2 mg and 3 mg) in patients with primary and co-morbid insomnia compared with parallel placebo groups have shown significant increases in daytime alertness, physical well-being, and ability to function at the end of treatment.[21-23] Zolpidem extended release 12.5 mg taken as needed for 6 months has also been shown to produce decreased morning sleepiness and improved ability to concentrate.[24] In one study in which the SF-36 was administered after 6 months of treatment with eszopiclone 3 mg, quality of life scores for the vitality, social functioning and mental health scales improved to be both significantly greater than the placebo control group and at or above the U.S. population norms.[25] One recent study used the Work Limitations Questionnaire[26] to assess time demands, physical demands, mental demands, output demands, and work productivity loss in primary insomnia patients given eszopiclone 3 mg or placebo in a double-blind design for 6 months. Patients receiving medication were significantly improved compared to placebo on all scales for the 1- to 6-month average score. Scores at the end of the study were in the range of normal scores on all of the scales except time demands, but there was large variability. In another study using the same questionnaire,[27] patients given zolpidem extended release 12.5 mg versus placebo in a double-blind study for 12 weeks showed significant improvement on the time demands and output demands scales at the end of the study.

CLASSIFICATION AND DIFFERENTIAL DIAGNOSIS

Many classification schemes have been proposed for insomnia. The DSM-IV simply classifies insomnia as primary or as related to another medical condition (or more recently referred to as *co-morbid insomnia*).[28] The ICSD-2, from the American Academy of Sleep Medicine,[1] contains 11 sub-classifications for insomnia that are grouped into five summary categories (Box 10-2). This grouping includes acute or situation-specific insomnia, insomnia that is associated with learned behaviors, insomnia co-morbid with other medical disorders, insomnia judged as a primary problem, and paradoxical insomnia.

Acute (Adjustment) Insomnia

Most individuals have had a poor night of sleep at some time in their life. Environmental stimuli, including almost any change to habitual sleeping times, surroundings, or sleep preparatory routine can have a negative impact on sleep. Acute stress, pain, or other discomfort can reduce sleep quality. Acute insomnia is triggered by a specific onset event and has a time course of less than 3 months.[1] However, as with chronic insomnia, acute insomnia is reported more frequently in females than males and more frequently in older adults.[1] A partial list of

---

BOX 10-2 *Subclassifications of Insomnia*

- Acute (adjustment) insomnia—lasts for 3 months or less and typically is related to transient stress or adjustment
- Inappropriate behavioral conditioning
  - Learned (psychophysiologic) insomnia
  - Inadequate sleep hygiene
  - Behavioral insomnia of childhood (sleep-incompatible behaviors)
- Insomnia related to medical issues (co-morbid)
  - Mental disorders
  - Medical condition
  - Drug or substance use/abuse/withdrawal
- Primary (idiopathic) insomnia (adults and children)
- Paradoxical insomnia (insomnia complaint not verified by electroencephalographic recordings)

potential events that might produce acute insomnia can be found in Box 10-3.

It was thought for many years that insomnia was usually a situational problem or would resolve upon successful treatment of another condition; it is now known that 80% or more of patients with an insomnia problem continue to report insomnia 2 or more years later.[29,30] The remaining insomnia categories are therefore presumed to be associated with a chronic insomnia problem in which the term "chronic" is typically defined as lasting for more than 1 month. Some of the common behavioral and medical associates of insomnia are presented in Box 10-4.

Inappropriate Behavioral Conditioning

Insomnia may develop in response to stressful life experiences. In a model proposed by Spielman and associates,[31] insomnia begins with a stressful event. If the patient then responds in an inappropriate manner by spending more time in bed, using alcohol, starting to have irregular sleep habits, or engaging in other sleep inappropriate behavior, poor sleep continues after the acute stress has passed, and this problem results in chronic insomnia. These patients may begin to worry about their inability to fall asleep or the consequences of poor sleep, which, in turn, further exacerbates the problem. The ICSD-2 lists five symptoms to help identify patients with conditioned sleep difficulty,[1] and they are presented in Box 10-5.

Insomnia may also develop from inadequate sleep hygiene practices. These behaviors include detrimental diet choices such as caffeine or alcohol, especially if consumed in close proximity to bedtime, irregular sleep or waking times associated with shift work or college class schedules, and increased activity in the evening, among others. Common elements that can be associated with inadequate sleep hygiene are listed in Box 10-6. Readers are referred to Chapter 12 of this text for a more detailed discussion of sleep hygiene impairments.

Insomnia can also develop when specific objects or behaviors (teddy bear, bottle, television) become conditionally associated with relaxation and sleep onset and then become unavailable. In children, such a disorder can also be associated with setting limits (the child falls asleep rapidly if consistently

---

BOX 10-3 *Potential Causes of Acute (Adjustment) Insomnia*

- Changes in bedroom (bed, furnishings, light, temperature, occupants)
- Changes in type or level of background noise
- Stressful life events such as arguments, loss of a loved one, divorce, loss of employment, or work or school demands
- Illnesses (particularly any illness or injury resulting in pain or discomfort)
- Use of or withdrawal from caffeine, nicotine, or alcohol, or foods or other substances containing caffeine, nicotine, or alcohol
- Ingestion of medications that have contain stimulants (theophylline, beta blockers, corticosteroids, thyroxine, bronchodilators) or withdrawal from central nervous system depressant medications
- Changes in time or work shift

BOX 10-4 *Selected Disorders in the Differential Diagnosis for Insomnia*

Behaviorally conditioned
- Elevated mental arousal or somatic tension at bedtime (psychophysiologic insomnia)
- Poor sleep hygiene
- Limit setting disorder (children)

Mental disorders
- Major depression and other mood disorders
- Anxiety disorders
- Post-traumatic stress disorder

Medical conditions
- Pulmonary disease
  - Chronic obstructive pulmonary disease
  - Bronchial asthma including nocturnal asthma
- Musculoskeletal disease
  - Arthritis
  - Chronic pain
  - Fibromyalgia and other rheumatic disorders
- Heart disease
  - Congestive heart failure
  - Ischemic heart disease
  - Nocturnal angina
- Hypertension
- Neurologic disease
  - Neurodegenerative disease: Alzheimer's disease, Parkinson's disease
  - Neuromuscular disorders, including painful peripheral neuropathies
  - Cerebral hemispheric and brainstem strokes
  - Brain tumors
  - Traumatic brain injury causing post-traumatic insomnia
  - Headache syndromes: migraine, cluster, hypnic headaches; exploding head syndromes
  - Fatal familial insomnia, a rare prion disease
- Gastrointestinal (gastroesopheageal reflux)
- Urinary (nocturia)
- Diabetes
- Lyme disease
- Acquired immunodeficiency syndrome (AIDS)
- Chronic fatigue syndrome
- Menopause
- Systemic cancer
- Dermatologic disorders (itching)

Substance use/abuse/withdrawal (stimulants, sedatives, alcohol, caffeine, nicotine)

Medications
- Central nervous system stimulants
- Bronchodilators
- Antidepressants
- Beta antagonists
- Corticosteroids

Other sleep disorders
- Sleep-disordered breathing
- Restless legs syndrome
- Periodic limb movement disorder
- Circadian rhythm disorders

Primary insomnia

Paradoxical insomnia

put in bed by the parent, but will not go to sleep without such intervention). As many as 10% to 30% of children may have some component of this behavior/sleep association at some point.[1]

Insomnia Related to Medical Issues

Based upon the most recent National Institute of Health (NIH) Insomnia State-of-the-Science Conference, insomnia that interacts with other medical issues including psychiatric disorders such as depression and substance abuse, cardiopulmonary disorders, and musculoskeletal pain disorders[32] should be referred to as "co-morbid." The *co-morbid* term indicates that insomnia may be a separate problem that could increase severity or limit treatment efficacy in other medical conditions and that treatment of insomnia might also result in improved treatment for the other medical problem.

Mental Disorders

As many as 44% of chronic insomnia cases are associated with mental disorders.[6] Insomnia is a separate diagnosis when the insomnia complaint is predominant or severe enough to warrant independent attention[1] and may be treated independently of the underlying disorder. Disorders for which insomnia is a common and significant problem include mood disorders such as major depression, dysthymic disorder, bipolar disorder,

or cyclothymic disorder; or anxiety disorders such as panic disorder, post-traumatic stress disorder, or generalized anxiety.

Insomnia precedes and predicts the development of a number of psychiatric illnesses including major depression, anxiety disorders, and substance abuse disorders.[33,34] One large epidemiologic study found that individuals with insomnia at baseline were 34 times more likely to develop a new psychiatric disorder (particularly major depression) within 1 year compared to individuals without insomnia, and insomnia remained predictive for depression for many years[34] in a sample of medical students.

The diagnosis of depression based upon Diagnostic and Statistical Manual of Mental Disorders 4th Edition Revised (DSM4R) requires a patient to display either depressed mood or anhedonia, and four of eight other symptoms. Three of the eight symptoms are insomnia or hypersomnia, fatigue or loss of energy during the day, and trouble thinking or concentrating during the day (elements also associated with insomnia). The inclusion of insomnia items in diagnostic inventories for major depression may be one of the factors responsible for the observations that insomnia is reported by 80% of depressed patients,[35] and that resolution of insomnia predicts positive treatment response (insomnia scores decrease with the relief of depression). This does not rule out the possibility, however, that there may be causal connections between insomnia reduction and relief from depression. Early morning awakening is a hallmark symptom of depression, but adolescents and young adults with depression may report difficulty initiating sleep instead.

Insomnia is reported in about 80% of patients with an anxiety disorder. Insomnia is also a hallmark symptom of generalized anxiety disorder; the diagnosis of generalized anxiety disorder based upon DSM4R requires a patient to display anxiety and three of six other symptoms, which are insomnia, fatigue, restlessness, difficulty concentrating, irritability, and muscle tension. In turn, these symptoms can also be associated with an insomnia disorder. Therefore, there is considerable overlap between these two disorders. Insomnia predicts the development of generalized anxiety disorder[33] in some cases. However, while patients more frequently report the onset of insomnia prior to the development of a depressive episode than during or following the depressive episode, insomnia more typically occurs concurrently (about 38% of the time) with the appearance of an anxiety disorder[36] or following the appearance of anxiety (about 44% of the time). Most patients (70-91%) with post-traumatic stress disorder have difficulty falling or staying asleep, and this is frequently associated with nightmares and fear of falling asleep or returning to sleep.[37]

Medical Conditions

Insomnia is a common complaint in many medical disorders that produce discomfort or pain, and about 11% of insomnia cases have been specifically associated with medical conditions or medications.[6] However, patients with a diagnosis insomnia have an increased prevalence of medical problems in general (not always directly related to the insomnia). In one study, 86% reported other medical problems compared with 48% of correspondents who did not have insomnia.[38] Conversely, patients with any other medical problem were also more likely to report insomnia (38% of patients with other medical problems reported insomnia while only 8% without other medical problem had insomnia).[38] Table 10-1 summarizes reported

TABLE 10-1

Prevalence of Medical Problems in Patients Who Have Insomnia and Insomnia Complaints in Patients Who Have Medical Problems

	Prevalence			
	Patients with Insomnia		Patients with Medical Diagnosis	
Medical Problem	**+ Diagnosis**	**− Diagnosis**	**+ Insomnia**	**− Insomnia**
Pulmonary	60%*	21%	25%*	6%
Pain	49%*	17%	50%*	18%
Heart disease	44%*	23%	22%*	10%
Hypertension	44%*	19%	43%*	19%
Neurologic	67%*	24%	7%*	1%
Gastrointestinal	55%*	20%	34%*	9%
Urinary	42%*	23%	20%*	10%
Cancer	41%*	25%	9%	4%
Diabetes	47%	24%	13%	5%

*Significant differences $p < 0.05$.
Columns 2 and 3 compare patients with a complaint of insomnia who had the diagnosis listed in the left column (+ Diagnosis) and control subjects who did not have that diagnosis (− Diagnosis). The last two columns show the prevalence of the medical problem in the left column in patients with insomnia (+ Insomnia) compared with control subjects without insomnia (− Insomnia).
From Taylor DJ, Mallory LJ, Lichstein KL, et al. Comorbidity of chronic insomnia with medical problems. *Sleep.* 2007;30(2):213-218.

prevalence differences by specific category of medical complaint. Significant prevalence differences, adjusted for depression, anxiety, and other sleep disorder symptoms, as assessed by screening questionnaire scores, can be seen in Table 10-1. Of interest is that more than 50% of patients with insomnia also had self-reported neurologic, respiratory, and gastrointestinal disorders compared with control values of about 22%. The right column of Table 10-1 shows prevalence rates for several medical problems in patients with insomnia and control subjects. Because some medical problems are more common than others, the important differences in the table are seen in the comparison of prevalence of a disorder with and without the insomnia complaint. For example, the table shows a low percentage of control subjects with neurologic problems (1%). Patients with insomnia were seven times more likely to have neurologic problems (7%), and this may reflect the high prevalence of sleep complaints associated with dementia[39] or Parkinson's disease.[40] Disease rates associated with insomnia were also much higher for gastrointestinal conditions (34% vs. 9%), respiratory disorders (25% vs. 6%), pain disorders, and hypertension. Elevated insomnia prevalence in these medical disorders probably reflects nocturnal discomfort associated with gastrosophageal reflux, dyspnea,[41] or pain. Sympathetic arousal may be implicated in both insomnia and hypertension.[20]

Substance Use, Abuse, and Withdrawal

Insomnia is common in patients at risk for substance abuse, in active abusers, and during withdrawal states. For example, one survey found that 13% of a representative community-based sample of 2181 Detroit residents had used alcohol in the last year to help to fall asleep.[42] The prevalence of alcohol abuse/dependence was about twice as high in patients with a history of insomnia,[34] and patients with insomnia were more than twice as likely to develop alcohol abuse in the next year.[43] During withdrawal from alcohol, 60% to 91% of patients report insomnia as a continuing problem.[44] The relapse rate was twice as high (60%) in patients with a prior history of insomnia, and insomnia was the major predictor of relapse.[45]

Medications

Medications that may cause insomnia include stimulants, anorectics, beta antagonists, calcium channel blockers, corticosteroids, and antidepressants.[46] It is well known that stimulants such as caffeine used in the evening produce insomnia. However, respiratory stimulants such as theophylline taken in the evening can also cause insomnia. Appetite-suppressing medications can produce insomnia by virtue of their central stimulant properties. Beta antagonists such as propranolol, metoprolol, and pindolol may produce sleep onset insomnia or increased awakenings and dreams. Tricyclic antidepressants are normally considered sedating, but some, such as protriptyline, may produce insomnia. Monoamine oxidase inhibitors produced insomnia in up to 67% of patients in some studies.[46] Selective serotonin reuptake inhibitors, such as fluoxetine, produced insomnia in 5% to 35% of depressed patients.[46] Norepinephrine and dopamine reuptake inhibitors, such as bupropion, have been associated with insomnia in 5% to 19% of patients.[46] Selective serotonin and norepinephrine reuptake inhibitors, such as venlafaxine, were related to insomnia in 4% to 18% of patients.[46] Corticosteroids, such as prednisone and cortisol, produce increased wakefulness during the night.[46] Prednisone produced insomnia in 50% to 71% of patients.[46]

Other Sleep Disorders

Patients with obstructive sleep apnea syndrome (OSA) have pauses in respiration during sleep that are associated with brief arousals when they resume respiration. Although patients infrequently remember respiration related arousals, they may report poor sleep, frequent awakenings, nocturia, or daytime deficits. It has been reported that 50% to 55% of patients undergoing evaluation for OSA report insomnia symptoms.[40,47] In one study, 29% of older insomnia patients were found to have OSA, as defined by and apnea/hypopnea index greater than 15.[48] Therefore, the sleep history of insomnia patients, especially older individuals, needs to include evaluation for snoring and other signs of OSA, and patients who are treated for OSA may need further evaluation to identify residual poor sleep, which may, in turn, require independent management.

Because restless legs syndrome (RLS) is a complaint of discomfort in the extremities that is of maximal intensity in the evening or when the patient is at rest, it is commonly associated with insomnia. The temporal placement, discomfort, and movement response of restless legs all contribute to sleep onset insomnia. One estimate suggests that 85% of patients with RLS have difficulty falling asleep.[49] However, patients are also likely to awaken frequently during the night from the paresthesias.

Patients with periodic limb movement disorder (PLMD) have movements as frequently as every 15 to 40 seconds during sleep.[49] These movements may be accompanied by partial arousals that can cause sleep fragmentation and sleep maintenance insomnia. It is estimated that 80% to 90% of patients with RLS also have at least five periodic limb movements per hour during sleep.[1]

Insomnia is a major component of the diagnostic criteria for all of the circadian rhythm sleep disorders listed in the ICSD-2.[1] Because all circadian rhythm disorders involve violation of underlying sleep/wake rhythms, all can produce either difficulty falling asleep or poor sleep maintenance. Insomnia secondary to circadian rhythm disorders is often acute (as in "jet lag") but may also be periodic, as in shift work disorder, or chronic, as seen in patients with delayed or advanced sleep phase disorders. Suspicion that an insomnia complaint may be secondary to circadian rhythm factors is typically assessed by having the patient complete sleep logs for a week or longer to allow the clinician to asses the pattern of sleep times and wake times.

Primary Insomnia

Insomnia that is not associated with any other identifiable medical, psychiatric, or sleep disorders is classified as primary insomnia. These patients account for about 15% of all insomnia patients seen in sleep disorders centers.[1,6] Patients with primary insomnia are characterized by heightened physiologic activation, as indexed by cardiac,[16] metabolic,[14] hormone,[50] and EEG measures.[51] Patients with primary insomnia commonly find it difficult to relax and may complain of muscle tension or recurring thoughts as they are trying to fall asleep. If these patients focus on their inability to relax and start to worry, the anxiety produces additional activation and the problem intensifies. The great majority of research on insomnia (and reported here) has been performed with patients having primary insomnia.

Studies have shown that, when individuals with normal sleep patterns are subjected to a mildly stressful situation such as sleeping in a sleep laboratory for the first time or caffeine administration in the evening, some continue to have normal sleep while others have insomnia. Further, one study showed that the same individuals who had poor sleep in response to the first night in the hospital also had poor sleep after their bedtime was advanced or after they were given caffeine, and this suggested that poor sleep was a general response to many stressors.[52] These individuals with situational insomnia were found to have faster heart rates and increased sympathetic activation,[52] which implies the existence of a physiologic predisposition to the development of insomnia. Such a predisposition

is supported by several studies that have shown a strong genetic influence in insomnia.[53-55] About 73% of primary insomnia patients have a family history of insomnia.[54,56] One twin study showed a heritability estimate of 57% for insomnia (as contrasted with 73% for obesity and 38% for sleepiness),[53] and evidence of association with specific genotypes is beginning to appear.[57] Such data suggest that a genetic predisposition to elevated physiologic activation associated with stress can produce insomnia. Individuals with greater predisposition to activation or individuals developing additional sympathetic activation associated with normal aging, for example, could account for many cases of primary insomnia.

If primary insomnia is seen as a physiologic problem, it implies that it should be possible to develop an animal model. In a recent experiment in which rats were exposed to an acute stress, it was found that the animals displayed both long sleep latency and reduced sleep time in addition to continuing activation in limbic, arousal, and autonomic systems along with elevated high-frequency electroencephalographic (EEG) activity (human marker for insomnia).[58] The investigators described the findings as continuing activation of arousal centers during sleep.[58] When lesions were made in the areas of the limbic or arousal system previously activated by stress, sleep was normal without elevated high-frequency EEG activation after exposure to the stress. These data also suggest that insomnia may be a problem of inappropriate activation and imply that treatment could be directed to decrease arousal.

Paradoxical Insomnia

Patients who complain of insomnia but who are found to have normal sleep latency and total sleep time scores during polysomnography despite a subjective impression of insomnia are given the diagnosis of paradoxical insomnia. Paradoxical insomnia cannot be differentiated from primary insomnia without a polysomnogram for comparative purposes. Patients with paradoxical insomnia have been shown to have increased whole body metabolic rate and high-frequency EEG activity during sleep,[59,60] and this suggests that their subjective overestimation and daytime dysphoria could be related to increased physiologic activation during sleep that is not indexed by sleep stage measures.

ELEMENTS OF A SLEEP HISTORY FOR PATIENTS WITH INSOMNIA

A sleep history should begin with a careful description of the sleep pattern with emphasis on items that seem problematic to the patient. It is useful to identify a typical bedtime, sleep latency, number and length of awakenings during the night, wake time, impression of sleep quality and level of daytime alertness, placement and length of daytime naps, and indication of whether these naps were planned or spontaneous. It is also useful to know if the pattern described applies every night or if sleep habits differ on the weekend or, in the case of insomnia, if there are better and worse nights and what factors might be related. Daytime consequences (see Box 10-1) should be noted. The clinician should note the duration and the frequency of the insomnia problem and should note any precipitating and perpetuating factors. For example, are there easily identifiable causes (see Box 10-3) or evidence of poor sleep hygiene (see Box 10-6) that can be addressed rapidly and perhaps without need for specialized referral or treatment? Is there evidence that learned behaviors play a major role (see Box 10-5) and that referral for behavioral therapy may be an option?

After consideration of sleep habits, it is appropriate to determine if other sleep disorders (OSA, RLS, PLMD, circadian rhythm disorders) may underlie the insomnia complaint. Finally, a more general medical history to include review of other medical and psychiatric problems, medications used, laboratory findings (thyroid hormones, blood sugar level), legal and illegal substances used, and the possible interaction of these problems and treatments with the insomnia problem (see Box 10-4) should be gathered. Considerations for interaction include avoiding use of stimulating medications or substances near bedtime or sedating medications or substances during the day; timing of other medications (diuretics, pain medication, inhalers) to provide maximum benefit with minimal disturbance during the sleep period; and determining if other medical problems are inadequately treated and whether sleep might improve if the other medical problems were treated in a different manner.

INTRODUCTION TO THERAPEUTICS

The discussion of insomnia provides the rationale for the common treatment strategies to be discussed at length in the chapters to follow. It is clear that insomnia is a common problem that is frequently encountered in association with many other medical problems. Historically, clinicians were advised to treat the "underlying" psychiatric or medical problem with the expectation that the "secondary" insomnia problem would no longer be a significant issue. However, such assumptions have been challenged by numerous studies, including data showing that more than 40% of major depressive patients who respond to treatment with an antidepressant still report poor sleep.[61] In addition an NIH review in 2005 emphasized that insomnia that coexists with other disorders may be viewed as an independent entity, and can interact with these disorders in a bidirectional manner.[32] Such observations raise the intriguing possibility that the direct treatment of insomnia may improve both sleep and the associated disorder, although data supporting such an understanding are by no means definitive in nature,[62,63] and further research is needed in this area.

Historical treatments for insomnia were based on improving sophistication in the use of sedative hypnotics. More recently, cognitive behavioral therapy has been used increasingly to avoid some of the side effects associated with medications. As insomnia is a combination of physiology and behavioral adjustments to that physiology, both approaches have merit, and behavioral and pharmacologic therapies have also been combined in some settings. Finally, it is hoped that a more complete knowledge of the neurophysiology of insomnia will lead to new treatments based on limiting or reversing arousal.

REFERENCES

1. *International Classification of Sleep Disorders: Diagnostic and Coding Manual.* 2nd ed. Westchester, IL: American Academy of Sleep Medicine; 2005.
2. Schochat T, Umphress J, Israel AG, et al. Insomnia in primary care patients. *Sleep.* 1999;22(Suppl 2):S359-365.
3. Ancoli-Israel S, Roth T. Characteristics of insomnia in the United States: Results of the 1991 National Sleep Foundation Survey. I. *Sleep.* 1999;22(Suppl 2):S347-353.
4. Mellinger GD, Balter MB, Uhlenhuth EH. Insomnia and its treatment: Prevalence and correlates. *Arch Gen Psychiat.* 1985;42:225-232.
5. Johnson EO. Epidemiology of insomnia: From adolescence to old age. In: Roth T, ed. *Sleep Medicine Clinics: Insomnia.* Philadelphia: Elsevier; 2006:305-317.
6. Ohayon MM. Epidemiology of insomnia: What we know and what we still need to learn. *Sleep Med Rev.* 2002;6(2):97-111.
7. Foley DJ, Monjan AA, Brown SL, et al. Sleep complaints among elderly persons: An epidemiologic study of three communities. *Sleep.* 1995;18(6):425-432.
8. Bonnet MH, Arand DL. Consequences of insomnia. *Sleep Med Clin.* 2006;1:351-358.
9. Katz D, McHorney C. The relationship between insomnia and health-related quality of life in patients with chronic illness. *J Fam Pract.* 2002;51:229-235.
10. Leger D, Massuel MA, Metlaine A. Professional correlates of insomnia. *Sleep.* 2006;29(2):171-178.
11. Ozminkowski RJ, Wang S, Walsh JK. The direct and indirect costs of untreated insomnia in adults in the United States. *Sleep.* 2007;30:263-273.
12. Walsh JK, Engelhardt CL. The direct economic costs of insomnia in the United States for 1995. *Sleep.* 1999;22(Suppl 2):S386-393.
13. Vignola A, Lamoureux C, Bastien CH, et al. Effects of chronic insomnia and use of benzodiazepines on daytime performance in older adults. *J Gerontol B Psychol Sci Soc Sci.* 2000;55(1):P54-62.
14. Nofzinger EA, Buysse DJ, Germain A, et al. Functional neuroimaging evidence for hyperarousal in insomnia. *Am J Psychiatry.* 2004;161(11):2126-2128.
15. Riemann D, Voderholzer U, Spiegelhalder K, et al. Chronic insomnia and MRI-measured hippocampal volumes: A pilot study. *Sleep.* 2007;30:955-958.
16. Bonnet MH, Arand DL. Heart rate variability in insomniacs and matched normal sleepers. *Psychosom Med.* 1998;60:610-615.
17. Suka M, Yoshida K, Sugimori H. Persistent insomnia is a predictor of hypertension in Japanese male workers. *J Occup Health.* 2003;45:344-350.
18. Bonnet MH, Arand DL. Cardiovascular implications of poor sleep. *Sleep Med Clin.* 2007;2:529-538.
19. Lanfranchi PA, Pennestri M, Fradette L, et al. Nighttime blood pressure in normotensive subjects with chronic insomnia: implications for cardiovascular risk. *Vasc Health Risk Manag.* 2009;32:760-766.
20. Vgontzas AN, Liao D, Bixler EO, et al. Insomnia with objective short sleep duration is associated with a high risk for hypertension. *Sleep.* 2009;32:491-497.
21. Scharf M, Erman M, Rosenberg R, et al. A 2-week efficacy and safety study of eszopiclone in elderly patients with primary insomnia. *Sleep.* 2005;28(6):720-727.
22. Soares CN, Joffe H, Rubens R, et al. Eszopiclone in patients with insomnia during perimenopause and early postmenopause: A randomized controlled trial. *Obstet Gynecol.* 2006;108(6):1402-1410.
23. Krystal AD, Walsh JK, Laska E, et al. Sustained efficacy of eszopiclone over 6 months of nightly treatment: Results of a randomized, double-blind, placebo-controlled study in adults with chronic insomnia. *Sleep.* 2003;26(7):793-799.
24. Krystal AD, Erman M, Zammit GK, et al. Long-term efficacy and safety of zolpidem extended-release 12.5 mg, administered 3 to 7 nights per week for 24 weeks, in patients with chronic primary insomnia: A 6-month, randomized, double-blind, placebo-controlled, parallel-group, multicenter study. *Sleep.* 2008;31(1):79-90.
25. Walsh JK, Krystal AD, Amato DA, et al. Nightly treatment of primary insomnia with eszopiclone for six months: Effect on sleep, quality of life, and work limitations. *Sleep.* 2007;30:959-968.
26. Lerner D, Amick BC, Rogers WH, et al. The Work Limitations Questionnaire. *Med Care.* 2001;39:72-85.
27. Erman M, Guiraud A, Joish VN, et al. Zolpidem extended-release 12.5 mg associated with improvements in work performance in a 6-month randomized, placebo-controlled trial. *Sleep.* 2008;31(10):1371-1378.
28. American Psychiatric Association. *DSM-IV: Diagnostic and Statistical Manual of Mental Disorders.* 4th ed. Washington, DC: American Psychiatric Press; 1994.
29. Johnson EO, Roth T, Schultz L, et al. Epidemiology of DSM-IV insomnia in adolescence: Lifetime prevalence, chronicity, and an emergent gender difference. *Pediatrics.* 2006;117(2):e247-256.
30. Katz DA, McHorney CA. Clinical correlates of insomnia in patients with chronic illness. *Arch Intern Med.* 1998;158(10):1099-1107.
31. Spielman AJ, Caruso L, Glovinsky P. A behavioral perspective on insomnia treatment. *Psychiatr Clin North Am.* 1987;10(4):541-553.

32. National Institutes of Health State-of-the-Science Conference Statement on Manifestations and Management of Chronic Insomnia in Adults. *Sleep.* 2005;28:1049-1057.

33. Breslau N, Roth T, Resenthal L, et al. Sleep disturbance and psychiatric disorders: A longitudinal epidemiological study of young adults. *Biol Psychiatry.* 1996;39:411-418.

34. Ford DE, Kamerow DB. Epidemiologic study of sleep disturbances and psychiatric disorders an opportunity for prevention. *JAMA.* 1989;262:1479-1484.

35. Krystal AD. Psychiatric comorbidity: the case for treating insomnia. *Sleep Med Clin.* 2006;1:359-365.

36. Ohayon MM, Roth T. Place of chronic insomnia in the course of depressive and anxiety disorders. *J Psychiatr Res.* 2003;37(1):9-15.

37. Maher M, Reqo S, Asnis G. Sleep disturbances in patients with posttraumatic stress disorder: Epidemiology, impact and approaches to management. *CNS Drugs.* 2006;20:567-590.

38. Taylor DJ, Mallory LJ, Lichstein KL, et al. Comorbidity of chronic insomnia with medical problems. *Sleep.* 2007;30(2):213-218.

39. Moran M, Lynch CA, Walsh C, et al. Sleep disturbance in mild to moderate Alzheimer's disease. *Sleep Med.* 2005;6(4):347-352.

40. Banno K, Kryger MH. Comorbid insomnia. *Sleep Med Clin.* 2006;1:367-374.

41. George CF, Bayliff CD. Management of insomnia in patients with chronic obstructive pulmonary disease. *Drugs.* 2003;63:379-387.

42. Johnson EO, Roehrs T, Roth T, et al. Epidemiology of alcohol and medication as aids to sleep in early adulthood. *Sleep.* 1998;21(2):178-186.

43. Weissman MM, Greenwald S, Nino-Murcia G, et al. The morbidity of insomnia uncomplicated by psychiatric disorders. *Gen Hosp Psychiatry.* 1997;19(4):245-250.

44. Arnedt JT, Conroy DA, Brower KJ. Treatment options for sleep disturbances during alcohol recovery. *J Add Dis.* 2007;26:41-54.

45. Brower KJ. Insomnia, alcoholism and relapse. *Sleep Med Rev.* 2003;7(6):523-539.

46. Schweitzer PK. Drugs that disturb sleep and wakefulness. In: Kryger M, Roth T, Dement WC, eds. *Principles and Practice of Sleep Medicine.* New York: WB Saunders; 2005:499-518.

47. Krell SB, Kapur VK. Insomnia complaints in patients evaluated for obstructive sleep apnea. *Sleep Breath.* 2005;9:104-110.

48. Gooneratne NS, Gehrman PR, Nkwuo JE, et al. Consequences of comorbid insomnia symptoms and sleep-related breathing disorder in elderly subjects. *Arch Intern Med.* 2006;166(16):1732-1738.

49. Allen RP, Picchietti D, Hening WA, et al. Restless legs syndrome: Diagnostic criteria, special considerations, and epidemiology. A report from the restless legs syndrome diagnosis and epidemiology workshop at the National Institutes of Health. *Sleep Med.* 2003;4(2):101-119.

50. Vgontzas AN, Bixler EO, Lin H, et al. Chronic insomnia is associated with nyctohemeral activation of the hypothalamic-pituitary axis: Clinical implications. *J Clin Endocrinol Metab.* 2001;86:3787-3794.

51. Perlis ML, Smith MT, Andrews PJ, et al. Beta/gamma EEG activity in patients with primary and secondary insomnia and good sleeper controls. *Sleep.* 2001;24(1):110-117.

52. Bonnet MH, Arand DL. Situational insomnia: Consistency, predictors, and outcomes. *Sleep.* 2003;26:1029-1036.

53. Watson NF, Goldberg J, Arguelles L, et al. Genetic and environmental influences on insomnia, daytime sleepiess, and obesity in twins. *Sleep.* 2006;29:645-649.

54. Heath AC, Kendler KS, Eaves LJ, et al. Evidence for genetic influences on sleep disturbance and sleep pattern in twins. *Sleep.* 1990;13:318-335.

55. Beaulieu-Bonneau S, LeBlanc M, Merette C, et al. Family history of insomnia in a population-based sample. *Sleep.* 2007;30(12):1739-1745.

56. Dauvilliers Y, Morin C, Cervena K, et al. Family studies in insomnia. *J Psychosom Res.* 2005;58:271-278.

57. Delisle TT, Werch CE, Wong AH, et al. Relationship between frequency and intensity of physical activity and health behaviors of adolescents. *J Sch Health.* 2010;80(3):134-140.

58. Cano G, Mochizuki T, Saper CB. Neural circuitry of stress-induced insomnia in rats. *J Neurosci.* 2008;28(40):10167-10184.

59. Bonnet MH, Arand DL. Physiological activation in patients with sleep state misperception. *Psychosom Med.* 1997;59:533-540.

60. Krystal Ad Edinger JD, Wohlgemuth WK, et al. Non-REM sleep EEG frequency spectral correlates of sleep complaints in primary insomnia subtypes. *Sleep.* 2002;25:630-640.

61. Nierenberg A, Keefe B, Leslie V, et al. Residual symptoms in depressed patients who respond acutely to fluoxetine. *J Clin Psychiatry.* 1999;60(4):221-225.

62. Fava M, McCall WV, Krystal A, et al. Eszopiclone co-administered with fluoxetine in patients with insomnia coexisting with major depressive disorder. *Biol Psychiatry.* 2006;59:1052-1060.

63. Fava M, Asnis GM, Shrivastava R, et al. Zolpidem extended-release improves sleep and next-day symptoms in comorbid insomnia and generalized anxiety disorder. *J Clin Psychopharmacol.* 2009;29(3):222-230.

Sleep/Wake Lifestyle Modifications:
SLEEP HYGIENE

PETER J. HAURI

Chapter 11

The hurry and excitement of modern life is quite correctly held to be responsible for much of the insomnia of which we hear, and most of the articles and letters are full of good advice to live more quietly and of platitudes concerning the harmfulness of rush and worry. The pity of it is that so many people are unable to follow this good advice and are obliged to lead a life of anxiety and high tension.

Hence the search for some sovereign panacea that will cure the evil. Many are the remedies suggested: hot baths, cold baths, hot drinks, cold drinks, long walks (some say on bare foot) before retiring to rest, and so forth. Some recommend the well-known plan of steady and monotonous counting, while others advise the more difficult feat of thinking about nothing. There can, however, be no doubt that different remedies suit different cases. …We would advise what the sufferer finds to be most soothing to his temperament. Some will find this in a long walk, while others will only be excited by the undue exercise; some may find a hot bath, others a cold bath beneficial; some are lulled by tobacco, others by novel reading; others still by a glass of grog. To be read off to sleep by a gentle voice is, perhaps, the pleasantest way of all…. Others have apparently adopted more heroic measures if we may judge from their letters. We give a quotation from one of these: Soap your head with the ordinary yellow soap; rub it into the roots of the hair until your head is just lather all over, tie it up in a napkin, go to bed, and wash it out in the morning. Do this for a fortnight. Take no tea after 6 P.M. I did this and have never been troubled with sleeplessness since.

The British Medical Journal, **Sleeplessness, Sept. 29, 1894, p 719.**
As related by Dr. MICHAEL PERLIS, University of Rochester, NY

What can we do consciously to improve our sleep? How can we change our behaviors, our environment, and other factors to make us sleep better? Answers to these questions have been sought throughout the ages (see the preceding quote from 1894), but they have acquired more "authority" now, ever since sleep has become an object of intense scientific study during the past half century.

The author's first list considering behaviors and activities to improve sleep, published in 1977,[1] was called "Sleep Hygiene." The more descriptive title "Sleep/Wake Lifestyle Modifications" is preferred for this chapter, but over the past 30 years the shorter title "Sleep Hygiene" seems to have established itself in the literature. The two terms will be used interchangeably here.

Sleep hygiene advice is different from practicing cognitive behavior therapy for insomnia (CBT-I), which generally involves a learning or conditioning process to improve sleep and that takes time (now occasionally as little as only 2 hours).[2] Examples of CBT-I are learning how to relax more deeply and learning how to reassociate the bedroom stimuli with sleep rather than with wakefulness. Sleep hygiene, by contrast, involves simple, direct advice on what to do, such as "hide the bedroom clock" or "exercise in the late afternoon." Of course, while such advice does sound straightforward, it is not always easy to comply with. Consider the simple sleep hygiene rule to "avoid alcohol, especially in the evening." It is a simple rule, but for some patients quite difficult to follow.

This chapter is subdivided into four sections:
1. Rules of sleep hygiene
2. Evidence that sleep hygiene therapy is effective in the treatment of insomnia
3. Evidence and controversies concerning individual sleep hygiene rules
4. Application of sleep hygiene instructions

WHAT ARE THE RULES OF SLEEP HYGIENE

In their review of sleep hygiene, Stepansky and Wyatt[3] found that no two published lists of sleep hygiene rules are the same. Searching for a common core of sleep hygiene advice, Stepansky and Wyatt then compared seven published sets of such rules: Hauri's original 1977 rules,[1] Hauri's 1992 updated list of the rules,[4] the diagnostic criteria of the International Classification of Sleep Disorders used to define a diagnosis of "insomnia associated with poor sleep hygiene,"[5] Schoicket, Bertelson, and Lacks' 1988 list,[6] Hauri's list of 1993,[7] Guilleminault and associates' list of 1995,[8] and Friedman and associates' list from 2000.[9] The review here will follow Stepanski and Wyatt's[3] methodology but update and streamline the data input by dropping two of Hauri's lists[1,7] to avoid duplication and dropping the list of Guilleminault and associates[8] (because it is not uniquely concerned with sleep hygiene and only contains four rules), but adding the sleep hygiene list published by Perlis in 2009.[10] The summary of this updated review is presented in Table 11-1.

To get the results reported in Table 11-1, the original sleep hygiene rules of some authors occasionally had to be paraphrased. For example, the term "exercise" (rule 9) includes authors who only want to keep or increase exercise as well as those who want to assign exercise to a specific time of day (usually late afternoon). Also, the advice to "avoid sleeping pills" was eliminated from Table 11-1. Although probably cogent as a sleep hygiene rule in the 1970s and 1980s, the issue

151

TABLE 11-1

Sleep Hygiene Rules Across Five Publications

Study Factor/Rule	No. of Studies that Agree	Schoicket et al, (1988)[6]	Hauri (1993)[7]	ICSD Definition of Sleep Hygiene (1997)[5]	Friedman et al (2000)[9]	Perlis et al (2005)[10]
Number of recommendations		8	8	11	12	15
A. REVIEW OF THE SLEEP ENVIRONMENT						
1. Eliminate bedroom noise*	4	X		X	X	X
2. Regulate bedroom temperature	3			X	X	X
3. Make bedroom comfortable	3	X		X		X
4. Use the bed only for sleep	2			X	X	
5. Eliminate bedroom clock	2		X			X
B. RULES ABOUT BEDTIMES AND WAKE TIMES						
6. Curtail or eliminate napping*	4	X	X	X		X
7. Decrease time in bed	3		X	X		X
8. Keep regular sleep times	2			X		X
C. EVENING ACTIVITIES THAT HELP SLEEP						
9. Exercise*	5	X	X	X	X	X
10. Relaxing activities before sleep	2	X		X		
11. Make a worry list	2				X	X
12. Hot baths	1				X	
D. INTAKE BEFORE BEDTIME						
13. Limit or avoid caffeine*	5	X	X	X	X	X
14. Avoid alcohol, esp. during evening*	5	X	X	X	X	X
15. Eat a light snack before bedtime*	4	X	X		X	X
16. Decrease or avoid smoking	2				X	X
17. Limit all liquids before bedtime	2				X	X
E. ATTITUDES DURING THE NIGHT						
18. Avoid trying hard to sleep	2		X			X
19. Leave the bed when unable to sleep	1				X	

*Sleep hygiene rules described by at least four of the five publications.

of sleeping pills has become much more complex with the advent of apparently non–habit-forming hypnotics. Readers are referred to Chapter 7 (Pharmacology of Benzodiazepine Receptor Agonist Hypnotics) in this book for a more detailed discussion on this topic.

Of the 19 rules of sleep hygiene that are identified in Table 11-1, only three of them are mentioned in all five publications, and only three more are mentioned in four of the five publications. An asterisk (*) has been placed next to the six most frequently quoted rules to emphasize them. Half the rules in Table 11-1 are only mentioned in one or two lists. Obviously, as Stepansky and Wyatt[3] have already observed, *no generally agreed upon set of sleep hygiene rules has emerged*, although some rules are more widely accepted than others.

Conceptually, the 19 sleep hygiene rules listed in Table 11-1 can be clustered into five subgroups:
- Review of the sleep environment
- Rules about bedtimes and wake-up times
- Evening activities conducive to sleep
- Intake before bedtime
- Attitudes during the night

For the rest of this chapter, the 19 sleep hygiene rules are presented in the sequence shown in Table 11-1. These sleep hygiene rules are introduced much like the clinician would when talking with an insomnia patient. Later, in the third part of this chapter, some of the scientific bases for each of these

rules will be reviewed, as well as some of the controversies about them.

Review of the Sleep Environment

1. *Eliminate bedroom noise:* Occasional loud noises disturb sleep, and one apparently cannot habituate to them. Sound insulating the bedroom helps, as does sound screening (e.g., with a constantly running fan or with a white noise machine).
2. *Regulate bedroom temperature:* Extremes in room temperature (both too hot and too cold) disturb sleep. Most people prefer the bedroom temperature to be somewhat lower than the daytime house temperature, but there are wide individual differences. You need to find your own comfort zone. For example, some like it cool but with heavy blankets, others like it warmer but with fewer blankets.
3. *Make the bedroom comfortable:* What makes for comfort in the bedroom depends, to a large extent, on individual preferences. For example, some like it very, very, quiet, others not so much; some sleep better with open windows; some like soft mattresses, while others sleep better on a harder surface. Sleep clinicians seem to believe that the bedroom should be free of electronics such as TV, videogames, and access to the Internet, especially for children and adolescents. Unless there

are mitigating factors such as phobias, almost all sleep clinicians advise a dark bedroom because light, even when filtered through closed eyelids, can have modulating effects on the sleep/wake rhythm.

4. *Use the bed only for sleep (and sex):* Clearly, sleep is not helped if the bedroom is used as a secondary office, with computers and cell phones reachable from bed and active during the night. Most sleep clinicians expressly forbid any other activity in bed except sleeping and sex. However, others allow activities, such as watching TV and listening to music (see rule 18).

5. *Eliminate the bedroom clock:* Insomniacs who find themselves watching the clock and, in turn, becoming increasingly frustrated and panicking by the realization that time is slipping away while they remain awake may benefit from eliminating all bedroom clocks or other objects that might provide information regarding the time. For many poor sleepers, this is an extremely difficult but very powerful rule.

Rules About Bedtimes and Wake Times

6. **Curtail or eliminate napping:* Sleep requirements vary from person to person, but each day we need about the same amount of sleep per 24 hours. If we use up much of that time for napping during the day, we are likely to sleep less and less soundly during the night.

7. *Decrease time spent in bed:* Longer times in bed lead to more shallow and fragmented sleep. In contrast, cutting down on time spent in bed leads to deeper and more continuous sleep. Poor sleepers should cut down their time in bed to slightly less than the amount of time that they used to spend in bed before the development of insomnia. This advice to insomniacs to decrease time in bed is opposite to the advice typically given to many good sleepers who habitually curtail their bedtime much too short, leading to daytime sleepiness.

8. *Keep regular bedtimes:* It seems intuitive that going to bed at irregular times can disturb the circadian cycle, while regular bed and arousal times reinforce this 24-hour rhythm, thereby facilitating sleep. A regular arousal time, somewhat earlier than desired, is important for those who have difficulties falling asleep and for the young, because these groups commonly struggle with a delayed sleep pattern. On the other hand, for the elderly, a slight delay in bedtime may be desirable to overcome the tendency for an advanced sleep pattern.

Evening Activities Conducive to Sleep

9. **Exercise:* Physically fit people usually sleep better than unfit ones, although there are many exceptions. The effects of exercise during one day on subsequent sleep depend on the intensity and timing of the exercise. Moderate exercise during the morning usually has little effect on that night's sleep. In contrast, exercise too close to bedtime may be activating and delay sleep, although this is not true for everyone. Usually, it is recommended that a person with sleep problems exercise aerobically at least three times per week, starting to exercise between 4 and 6 hours before bedtime.

10. *Engage in relaxing activities before going to bed:* Most of us take a few hours to unwind before going to bed. Working intensely up to bedtime seems counterproductive. Unwinding in the evening may be even more important for poor sleepers who usually are more activated biologically than are good sleepers.

11. *Make a worry list:* Some complain that they cannot "turn off" their minds and that their thoughts race when they are trying to sleep. It is advisable for such patients to set aside about 20 minutes early in the evening to focus on their worries and concerns, which may be responsible for keeping them awake. They might make a list of all issues that are of concern to them and then think carefully about each of those concerns, with the goal of identifying an action (even if small) that they might be able to take *tomorrow* to address each issue. For example, financial problems might be addressed by an appointment with a counselor, relationship problems might need speaking tomorrow with a friend or therapist. Yet other concerns may, realistically, have few solutions other than offering support. Patients facing such concerns might be instructed: "If you are distressed, for example, regarding the health of a hospitalized friend, you might decide to give him a supportive telephone call, or drop him a note, or find out more about his illness to clarify whether your concerns are realistic. Once you have faced each of your concerns, write down (next to that worry on your list) the decisions you have made to address it, so that you can implement them tomorrow." The objective in all this is to consciously and squarely deal with each worry, looking for something that one might change tomorrow, even if small. This process often leads to the cessation of the mind's "racing" at night.

12. *Hot bath:* Hot baths help relaxation, especially if taken 1 to 2 hours before bedtime. After increasing core body temperature artificially, either by exercise or by hot baths, a rebound cooling effect ensues, and seems to promote falling asleep.

Intake Before Bedtime

13. **Limit or avoid caffeine:* Caffeine is used commonly to promote wakefulness, but it can also disturb sleep. Therefore, most clinicians recommend limiting the intake of beverages containing caffeine to 1 cup in the morning to help in waking up, and others recommend the avoidance of such beverages altogether. Indeed, some patients with insomnia are more sensitive to the effects of caffeine and other stimulating substances than are good sleepers and need to stay away from all stimulating substances including chocolate, tea, and some medications and supplements.

Occasionally, patients claim that they sleep better when they go to bed immediately after drinking a caffeine-containing beverage. These patients may habitually drink large amounts of caffeine-containing beverages and may be in a state of caffeine withdrawal at bedtime. The withdrawal process itself can interfere with sleep initiation, and the ingestion of caffeine mitigates this.

14. **Avoid alcohol, especially during the evening hours:* Alcohol is a relaxant and may help tense persons fall

asleep more readily. Self-medicating with alcohol is quite common in poor sleepers. However, alcohol, even if consumed as early as 6 hours before bedtime, can lead to unrefreshing, shallow, and disturbed sleep with long awakenings after falling asleep. Furthermore, excessive and chronic use of alcohol may disturb sleep for up to 12 months or longer after a return to sobriety. Therefore, alcohol is a poor sleep aid.

15. *Eat a light snack before bedtime:* Hunger disturbs sleep. Therefore, many advocate a light snack prior to bedtime. Some specifically suggest foods that contain L-tryptophan, a sleep-promoting substance that is found in poultry, milk, and other foods; however, there are exceptions. For example, patients with gastroesophageal reflux disease should not eat just before going to bed.

16. *Decrease or avoid smoking:* Nicotine is a stimulant. Heavy smoking is associated with disturbed sleep in most cases.

17. *Limit all liquids before bedtime:* Those who suffer from frequent bathroom calls during the night may benefit from decreasing liquid intake before bedtime; however, excessive thirst can also interfere with sleep.

Attitudes During the Night

18. *Avoid trying too hard to sleep:* "Trying" hard to fall asleep may actually lead to greater frustration and greater difficulty in falling asleep. It is not surprising, therefore, that many insomnia sufferers fall asleep easily when watching TV or reading in the living room, as these activities have a relaxing effect by virtue of diminishing stimulating physical activity and keeping the mind focused on thoughts other than the challenge of falling asleep. Sleep cannot be forced; it must be passively allowed. Although reading and watching TV in bed are contrary to sleep hygiene rule 4, some patients who are anxious about falling asleep find reading themselves to sleep or watching some TV in bed to be quite helpful.

19. *Leave the bed when unable to sleep:* Lying in bed awake can result in augmenting sleeplessness, frustration, and anger, thereby further delaying sleep onset. Therefore, patients who are unable to fall asleep readily may benefit from getting out of bed and doing something comfortable and relaxing elsewhere. They should return to bed when they feel sleepy and more relaxed.

EVIDENCE THAT SLEEP HYGIENE THERAPY IS EFFECTIVE IN THE TREATMENT OF INSOMNIA

In 1993, Buysse and colleagues[11] performed a study to address the question of how diagnostic formulations affected treatment recommendations for chronic insomniacs. A total of 216 patients from five different sites were interviewed by two clinicians each (one clinician in each pair was a sleep specialist). The clinicians could suggest more than one sleep therapy for each case. Buysse and co-workers found that sleep hygiene treatment was the most often recommended therapy for almost all chronic insomniac patients.

On the other hand, two task forces appointed by the American Academy of Sleep Medicine (AASM), the first in 1999 and the second in 2006, reviewed the accumulated scientific evidence concerning many psychological treatments for insomnia.[12,13] Both task forces found insufficient evidence to recommend sleep hygiene as a stand-alone treatment! Other reviewers have since agreed with those AASM findings.[14] Therefore, more than 60 years after the 1894 *British Medical Journal* quotation made at the beginning of this chapter, many of us now realize that much of what was proposed as proper sleep hygiene in earlier years is not built on solid evidence. One is, therefore, confronted with an apparent paradox: sleep hygiene advice is the most frequently suggested therapy for chronic insomnia, but it is not recommended as a stand-alone treatment for insomnia.

One explanation for this paradox is that the evidence may be flawed. In almost all studies in which sleep hygiene advice was compared with a type of CBT-I, sleep hygiene was found to be less effective than CBT-I. This was true even when sleep hygiene advice was compared with only 2 hours of CBT-I.[2] However, in almost all of these studies, sleep hygiene was used as the "active placebo," and was compared with the researcher's own form of CBT-I.[15,16] It is possible, therefore, that sleep hygiene was presented with less enthusiasm or with less knowledge than the active CBT-I treatment.

Another possible explanation for this paradox is the possibility that sleep hygiene practices in insomniacs may not differ substantially from those of good sleepers. Comparing more than 250 insomniacs with matched control subjects, Jefferson and associates[17] did, indeed, note that their insomnia patients engaged in some poor sleep hygiene habits; they smoked more often close to bedtime, drank more alcohol, took more naps per week, and slept longer on days not worked. However, Jefferson and associates found no differences between good and poor sleepers in caffeine intake and in the total time spent in bed. That is, both groups practiced similar sleep hygiene habits in those areas. Others have found *low or no correlations* between sleep quality and the sleep hygiene practices of good and poor sleepers.[18,19] Paradoxical findings have even been reported: Cheek and associates[20] found that middle-aged poor-sleeping women varied less in their bedtimes than well-sleeping women, and that they drank less coffee and less alcohol (that is, they showed better sleep hygiene than those who slept well).

There is also some evidence that insomnia patients may respond differently to some sleep hygiene rules than do good sleepers. Yang and associates[21] found that among good sleepers, almost all aspects of sleep hygiene correlated with the quality of their sleep, but among insomniacs, only activities that caused presleep arousal correlated with sleep quality. The violation of other sleep hygiene rules by insomniacs had no effect on their sleep in that study!

Despite these reports, there is considerable anecdotal evidence suggesting that individualized sleep hygiene discussions can be enormously useful in specific cases. An anecdote from the author's experience is that of a 56-year-old businessman who had traveled well over 2000 miles just to get advice for his severe insomnia. A year after consultation, he sent a letter that said, in part, "…I am sleeping quite well now, cured by one sentence you uttered during our two-hour-long discussion: 'Get rid of all bedroom clocks!' It was amazing how that worked for me!"

Nevertheless, the bulk of research supports the overall conclusion of both AASM task forces[12,13]: *There is little evidence that sleep hygiene may be effective as a stand-alone treatment for most insomniacs.* Therefore, it should rarely be used as a stand-alone treatment! Rather, the review of sleep hygiene principles is recommended as an integral part of an overall insomnia treatment plan that includes CBT-I, therapeutic maneuvers to diminish daytime distress and anxiety, and the use of hypnotics, among others. Unfortunately, studies into the relative contribution of sleep hygiene advice to this overall treatment "package" have yet to be conducted. Studies are also warranted to determine if certain insomnia subtypes show differential responses to sleep hygiene interventions.

EVIDENCE AND CONTROVERSIES CONCERNING INDIVIDUAL SLEEP HYGIENE RULES

Given the frequent use of sleep hygiene advice by sleep clinicians, one would expect that this area would be well researched. On the contrary! As will be noted later in this section, except for certain rules such as exercise or regular bedtimes, sleep hygiene recommendations are highly underrepresented in the overall realm of sleep research. And the little research available is almost exclusively based on subjective reports; studies involving polysomnography or other "objective" tests are almost nonexistent.

The following list reviews the research evidence and controversies surrounding each sleep hygiene rule included in Table 11-1.

1. **Eliminate bedroom noise:* There are significant individual differences in the threshold for the noise level that is necessary to cause an awakening. As early as 1966, Rechtschaffen and associates[22] found that some healthy young sleepers awakened to a 15-dBA noise (approximately equivalent to a mere whisper), while others needed 100 dBA to wake up from the same stage of sleep (approximately equivalent to the loudness in a night club). Research also indicates that a consistent volume of background noise is less arousing to sleepers than irregular bursts of loud noise. LaVere and associates[23] studied the effects of nine simulated aircraft overflights per night on the laboratory sleep of good sleepers and found that, on average, sleepers awakened for about 5 minutes after each simulated overflight, even though in the morning, most sleepers could not remember a single overflight noise or a single awakening. More importantly, daytime performance declined after each "flyover" night.[24] Globus and colleagues[25] performed home polysomnography on two groups of Los Angeles residents. The first group had lived for at least 6 years near the airport, and the other group had lived far away from it for the same period of time. Although those near the airport believed that they had totally adapted to the aircraft noise, their sleep recording showed that almost each low-flying aircraft aroused them. Those near the airport still slept about 45 minutes less and had significantly less delta (deep) sleep than those who lived in quieter neighborhoods, even after 6 years of "adaptation."

What is the remedy? Sound proofing (e.g., by special windows) helps, as do earplugs.[26] Sound screening is also effective, such as by running a fan or a "white noise machine" throughout the night.

Not all irregular sound is arousing. Studying older community-dwelling men, Lai and Good[27] found that playing soothing music throughout the night improved their sleep as well as their daytime functioning.

2. *Regulate bedroom temperature:* Excessively hot temperatures (above 75° F)[28] and excessively cold environments (below 41° F) have been shown to disturb sleep,[29] but little research has been performed on environmental temperatures between 41° F and 75° F. Within reason, the temperature conducive to sleep seems to be an individual factor.

3. *Make the bedroom comfortable:* Sleeping on a wooden board causes more body movements and lighter sleep than sleeping on a softer surface.[30] Except for this extreme, the quality of a mattress seems to have little or no effect on sleep.[31] Couples sleeping on the same mattress show less deep sleep and less REM sleep than when sleeping apart.[32] Children who have a television set in their bedroom, who play electronic games in bed, and who surf the Internet at night fall asleep as much as an hour later than children who do not. They also sleep later on weekends, and are more tired throughout each day.[33]

4. *Use the bed only for sleep (and sex):* Environmental stimuli have a profound effect on our behavior. We start to feel hungry when we see food, and the 10 PM news triggers sleepiness in many. Insomniacs often lie in bed agitated and frustrated because they cannot fall asleep. Bootzin[34] speculated that over time these bedroom stimuli might then trigger conditioned arousal and frustration in insomniacs (while in good sleepers, they usually trigger an expectation of relaxation and falling asleep easily). To treat this maladaptive conditioning in insomniacs, Bootzin developed the following stimulus-control rules:
   1. Go to bed only when sleepy.
   2. Use the bed only for sleeping; do not read, watch TV, or eat in bed.
   3. If you cannot fall asleep easily, get out of bed, and return to it only when you feel you might now fall asleep more easily.
   4. Repeat step 3 as often as necessary throughout the night.
   5. Get up at the same time each morning, regardless of how much sleep you got during the night.
   6. Do not nap during the day.

Taking these six rules together, Bootzin's technique is one of the most powerful and effective CBT-I therapies and is abundantly documented by excellent research.[35] However, there is no evidence that individual components of this technique can be used effectively as stand-alone sleep hygiene rules. Indeed, using individual components may even be counterproductive. For example, when patients are instructed only that they cannot read or watch TV in bed, but are not given the full set of Bootzin's rules, they often lie in bed for hours, becoming increasingly frustrated and tense. This strengthens the maladaptive association between the bedroom stimuli and arousal, which is exactly the opposite of the therapeutic goal.

Insomniacs often report that they fall asleep easily when watching television or reading in the living room, but become aroused upon going to bed. In addition to the previously mentioned tendency of insomniacs to associate bedroom stimuli with frustration, falling asleep when reading or watching TV may also result from the fact that doing so keeps the body in a quiet and relaxed position, and keeps the mind focused away from frustrating attempts to fall asleep. Support for the habit of reading or TV in bed is derived from Gallup polls, which indicate that about one third of all U.S. adults read themselves to sleep or fall asleep watching television in bed. Watching television has also been associated with falling asleep more easily on multiple sleep latency testing (MSLT).[36] Nevertheless, there is considerable controversy regarding this recommendation, focused mainly on the success of Bootzin's rules when used as a whole. Clinicians may, therefore, first advise the use of the bed only for sleeping, but if that does not help, they may suggest a trial of reading or watching TV in bed.

5. *Eliminate the bedroom clock:* There is no formal research on this rule. Rather, during a research study on sleeping pills, whose subjects were insomniacs who slept poorly in the laboratory, it was noted that that more than 75% of otherwise well-qualified candidates slept too well in the laboratory to qualify for the study. During a subsequent interview, these insomniacs said that the laboratory bedroom was "very far removed from reality;" and they noted that they were totally unaware of the course of time during their night in the laboratory. After a small clock was introduced into each of the laboratory bedrooms, only 3 of the next 20 possible candidates for the study had to be rejected for sleeping too well in the laboratory!

6. **Curtail or eliminate napping:* The effects of napping have been extensively studied, although most of this work involves normal sleepers. In 2003, Takahashi 3 reviewed this area in depth. He reported that when one is sleep-deprived, a short daytime nap improves subsequent alertness and performance.[38] Also, the usefulness of naps depends on their length and on their timing.[39,40] Short naps, lasting less than 30 minutes, are recommended, because they improve wakefulness and performance for at least 2 hours (after a short period of sleep inertia) without affecting sleep during the subsequent night.[38] Longer naps (90 minutes or more) usually disturb sleep on the following night.[41] Naps coinciding with the midday dip in circadian alertness seem to be most beneficial for improved performance after the nap.[42] Thus, napping might be recommended for those who do not obtain sufficient amounts of nocturnal sleep, and for the elderly, who often cannot sleep well at night. Obviously, this rule of no daytime naps is not pertinent for many insomniacs who have found that they cannot possibly fall asleep during the day due to hyperarousal.[43]

In a population of elderly patients who sleep poorly, Ancoli-Israel and Martin[44] did not find a consistent relationship between daytime napping and sleep quality during the subsequent night. They concluded that the question of whether napping is beneficial, neutral, or detrimental has not yet been established. Similarly, Dautovich and associates,[45] studying 60- to 89-year-old good and poor sleepers, noted that napping was not associated with impaired subsequent sleep in their sample and that the uniform recommendation to restrict or eliminate napping may not meet the needs of all older individuals.

It is true that frequent napping in the elderly is associated with increased illness and morbidity rates.[46-48] However, the frequent naps in these patients may be a marker of some existing underlying disorder, rather than its cause. On the positive side, Newman and colleagues[49] reported that a 20-minute nap, four times per week or more, improved cardiovascular status of patients with cardiovascular disease and Asada and colleagues[50] found that three or more 30-minute naps per week *decreased* the risk of Alzheimer's disease. Thus, the categorical "do not nap!" sleep hygiene rule may also be inappropriate in many medically ill poor sleepers.

Factors to consider prior to making a recommendation on naps include the length and timing of naps, whether they are the result of prior sleep deprivation, whether the insomniac is actually able to nap during the day, health status, and individual differences. Some can "power nap" and feel more alert afterward, whereas others feel "wiped out" for the rest of the day after a nap.

7. *Decrease time spent in bed:* As individuals develop insomnia, they tend to stay in bed longer in an effort to recapture some of their lost sleep. However, longer times in bed result in more shallow and fragmented sleep.[51] Conversely, shorter times in bed result in deeper and more continuous sleep.[52] These findings are the basis for Spielman's sleep restriction therapy[53] for insomniacs. The question of whether the simple admonition to decrease time in bed is useful as a stand-alone rule has not been studied.

8. *Keep regular bedtimes:* The research in this area is confusing. Brown and associates[54] found that variable sleep schedules were indeed associated with poor sleep. Also, Manber and associates[55] report that college students who modified their bedtime schedule so that it was regular and included a minimum of 7 hours per night experienced an improvement in their daytime alertness and well-being. However, when Bonnet and Alter[56] imposed a drastically more regular sleep/wake regimen on irregularly sleeping college students for 5 weeks, not much effect was found on sleep quality, daytime performance, or mood. Possibly, it might have been the 7-hour minimum bedtime that was imposed in the Manber study, not the regularized sleep schedule, that led to the improved waking performance.

Of course, the variability of sleep and wake times affects the circadian rhythm, which will be discussed in Chapters 28 to 32 of this book.

9. *Exercise:* Ramakrishnan and Scheid[57] claim that exercise improves sleep as effectively as benzodiazepines. Studies in healthy people show that those who exercise regularly generally do sleep better than unfit people, although there are exceptions.[58-60] In one study, when poor sleepers increased their general fitness over about 4 months, they rated themselves as falling asleep faster, sleeping longer, and sleeping more deeply.[61] Cardiac patients suffering from insomnia also rated their sleep as improved after exercise.[62] Gerber and associates[63] speculate that merely being physically fit may produce

a self-perception of health that then influences one's perception of sleep in a positive direction, and vice-versa.

The effects of acute exercise on subsequent sleep are more complex. Exercise early in the morning and exercise just before sleep either have little effect on sleep during the following night[64,65] or impair sleep,[36] but exercise 4 to 6 hours before bedtime seems to improve sleep.[66]

Horne and Staff[67] reported that the effects of exercise on sleep are mediated by elevated core body temperature. Horne and Reid[68] showed that passively heating the body through a hot bath (41° C) from 2:30 PM to 5:30 PM) and then going to bed around 10:30 PM had beneficial effects on sleep that were similar to those of exercise (decreased time to fall asleep, longer time in delta [deep] sleep). Edinger and associates[69] found that high levels of body heating just before bedtime caused sleep to *deteriorate* (e.g., more awakenings from sleep) in both fit and unfit people. It seems that sleep is improved not by the high core temperature itself, but by the rebound decrease in core temperature that occurs naturally after heating. Therefore, morning exercise may have no effect on sleep because the rebound cooling would have already dissipated by nightfall, whereas exercise just prior to bedtime may impair sleep by causing body temperature to rise during the sleep period.

10. *Relaxing activities before bedtime:* Most of us take a few hours to unwind before going to bed, and this may be even more important for insomniacs who are typically hyperaroused.[70] Poor sleepers who remain active, working with computers and doing household chores up to bedtime, risk not being able to fall asleep easily. One report published in 1966 showed that intense studying right up to bedtime delays sleep onset even in good young sleepers.[65]

11. *Make a worry list:* In one study, writing down worries and concerns helped poor sleepers fall asleep more easily.[71] A number of behavioral approaches have been developed to assist patients in controlling their worries and anxieties. The author developed the one described in this chapter in cooperation with Dr. J. G. Lindsley from Sleep Well in Lexington, Massachusetts. Many patients say that it works well for them, but to date there has been no research on it.

12. *Hot baths:* The discussion of rule 9 (exercise) explains at least part of the beneficial effects of hot baths on sleep, but it may be that the relaxation achieved by hot water also plays a significant role.

13. **Limit or avoid caffeine:* Coffee significantly disturbs sleep,[72,73] especially in those who are vulnerable to stress.[74] This is true even in those who do not subjectively experience a caffeine effect.[75] There is some evidence of habituation; the chronic daily use of up to seven cups of coffee seemed to have no effect on sleep in a middle-aged working population.[76] Bonnet and Arand[77] found that the effects of 400 mg of caffeine on good sleepers were quite variable; some sleepers demonstrated no effect on sleep, yet sleep in others was quite disturbed. Also, some insomniacs seem to be more sensitive to the effects of caffeine than good sleepers.[78] Most sleep clinicians now suggest only one cup of coffee in the morning, and no coffee intake from lunch onward. Occasionally, patients claim that they sleep better after a cup of coffee. As noted earlier, this may represent the positive effect of caffeine on a state of chronic caffeine withdrawal in those who consume large quantities of caffeine-containing beverages.[79]

14. **Avoid alcohol, especially during the evening:* Alcohol is a relaxant; it may help tense insomniacs fall asleep more easily.[80] Self-medication with alcohol is common in insomnia patients.[81] However, alcohol, even if consumed as early as 6 hours before bedtime, leads to a significant fragmentation of subsequent sleep.[82] Also, the excessive and chronic use of alcohol disturbs sleep for up to 12 months after sobriety.[83]

15. **Eat a light snack before bedtime:* Food deprivation and weight loss are associated with shorter and more fragmented sleep, whereas gaining weight is associated with longer and less interrupted sleep. This has been demonstrated for both animals and humans.[84] Insomnia is a common symptom in anorexia nervosa,[85] and when such patients gain weight, their sleep improves.

Although the association between caloric intake and sleep is not absolute, chronic insomniacs and those awakening too early might try a bedtime snack. Southwell and associates[86] have demonstrated that milk improves sleep, as does "Horlicks," the Scottish milk-cereal drink that was investigated by Brezinova and Oswald.[87]

16. *Decrease or avoid smoking:* Nicotine is a stimulant. It causes difficulties falling asleep and sleep fragmentation during the night, as well as excessive daytime sleepiness.[88] Withdrawal from heavy smoking improved sleep almost immediately, despite the daytime distress associated with smoking cessation. In one study of heavy smokers who stopped smoking, a gradual improvement in sleep continued over the next 12 months.[89]

17. *Limit all liquids before bedtime:* This may be especially important if one suffers from urinary frequency during the night. However, Brown and associates[54] found that going to bed thirsty also contributes to poor sleep.

18. *Avoid trying hard to sleep:* The harder one tries to sleep, the more awake and frustrated one typically gets.[90] The goal of rule 18 is to keep one's mind off the challenge of trying to sleep. Some accomplish this by using imagery at sleep onset or by rethinking positive experiences they have had in the past; others do so by trying to find names starting with a certain letter or by counting backward in sevens from 1000. Also, paradoxical intention can be effective; trying to stay awake in bed all night leads to sleep much more easily than trying desperately to sleep.[91]

19. *Leave the bed when unable to sleep:* This is one of the highly successful stimulus control rules mentioned when discussing rule 4. However, as a stand-alone sleep hygiene rule, it has not been researched. Although it makes intuitive sense not to remain in bed when the lack of sleep aggravates the patient, without the other rules of stimulus-control therapy, one worries that the patient will remain out of bed for too long and then sleep very late into the morning.

In summary, this review of the sleep hygiene rules suggests that they are not a set of absolute edicts to be followed blindly, but a set of suggestions that need to be explored with each patient. It seems interesting that adequate research into some of these rules (e.g., napping, exercise) has led to much more nuanced suggestions, as contrasted with the absolute commands often given in the name of sleep hygiene.

APPLICATION OF SLEEP HYGIENE INSTRUCTIONS

Sleep hygiene rules can be broadly and uniformly disseminated to many individuals in a large population or selectively applied to fit the specific needs of an individual patient. For example, Strom and asociates[92] made available sleep hygiene rules through the medium of the internet and reported improvement in the sleep of those who followed their rules. Morin and asociates[93] utilized a somewhat more selective approach by providing a group of insomniacs with brochures containing sleep hygiene instructions. One brochure was provided each week, over the course of 6 weeks. The authors reported improvement in a number of sleep measures in the group of insomniacs. The most selective application of sleep hygiene education is employed by the sleep clinician, who tailors treatment by choosing a specific set of instructions for an individual patient.[94]

While the broad application of sleep hygiene rules is clearly effective for groups of insomniacs and has the advantage of being less labor-intensive, it does not produce beneficial results in each and every individual in the group, because each rule does not apply to every patient. Not all insomniacs are alike.[95,96] In fact, it is likely that many of the insomniacs who later seek the assistance of sleep clinicians are those who have failed this global approach. In such patients, the clinician is best served by performing a detailed evaluation of the patient's complaint and, prior to utilizing sleep hygiene recommendations, considering whether alternative treatments, such as CBT-I and pharmacotherapy, may be better suited for the patient's needs. If sleep hygiene rules appear to be the optimal choice, the clinician should devise an individualized treatment plan that takes into consideration a variety of clinical factors such as the nature of the insomnia complaint, the patient's sleep patterns, comorbidities, and the nature of, and response to, prior treatments. As a general rule, sleep hygiene recommendations that have previously failed should not be re-applied. However, if they appear to be optimal for the patient's specific needs, they may prove to be effective if modified to better fit the patient's personality. Following their application, if the patient's condition does not improve sufficiently, the rules that are being utilized can be modified, or even abandoned, and different rules can be introduced. Optimally, the combination of rules and their application should be tailored to the patient's individual needs.

CONCLUSION

A review of current sleep hygiene rules shows a remarkable lack of consistency among the authors who have written these rules and an even more remarkable paucity of research into most of them. Additionally, there is no empirical evidence that sleep hygiene alone can significantly alleviate insomnia. Nevertheless, sleep hygiene modifications may be an important ingredient in enhancing the success of other treatment approaches for insomnia. The areas touched by sleep hygiene seem important in helping patients improve their sleep.

Clinically, an individual approach to sleep/wake lifestyle modifications is recommended, learning first what a patient has already tried, then enlisting him as "co-scientist" in the attempt to solve the puzzle of why he sleeps so poorly, and finally in implementing sleep hygiene modifications that are individually tailored for that patient's insomnia.

REFERENCES

1. Hauri P. *Current Concepts: The Sleep Disorders.* Kalamazoo: The Upjohn Company; 1977.
2. Edinger JD, Sampson WS. A primary care "friendly" cognitive behavioral insomnia therapy. *Sleep.* 2003;26(2):177-182.
3. Stepanski EJ, Wyatt JK. Use of sleep hygiene in the treatment of insomnia. *Sleep Med Rev.* 2003;7(3):215-225.
4. Hauri P. Sleep hygiene, relaxation therapy, and cognitive interventions. In: Hauri PJ, ed. *Case Studies in Insomnia.* New York: Plenum; 1992: 65-84.
5. American Sleep Disorders Association. *The International Classification of Sleep Disorders, Revised: Diagnostic and Coding Manual.* Rochester, MN: American Sleep Disorders Association; 1997.
6. Schoicket S, Bertelson A, Lacks P. Is sleep hygiene a sufficient treatment for sleep-maintenance insomnia? *Behav Ther.* 1988;19:183-190.
7. Hauri P. Consulting about insomnia: A method and some preliminary data. *Sleep.* 1993;16:344-350.
8. Guilleminault C, Clark A, Black J, Labanowski M, Pelayo R, Claman D. Nondrug treatment trials in psychophysiologic insomnia. *Arch Intern Med.* 1995;155:838-844.
9. Friedman L, Benson K, Noda A, Zarcone V, Wicks D, et al. An actigraphic comparison of sleep restriction and sleep hygiene treatments for insomnia in older adults. *J Geriatr Psychiatry Neurol.* 2000;13:17-27.
10. Perlis ML, Jugquist C, Smith MT, Posner D. *Cognitive behavioral treatment of insomnia: A session-by-session guide.* New York: Springer Science + Business Media; 2005:18.
11. Buysse DJ, Reynolds CF III, Kupfer DJ, Thorpy MJ, Bixler E, et al. Effects of diagnosis on treatment recommendations in chronic insomnia—A report from the APA/NIMH DSM-IV Field Trial. *Sleep.* 1997;20(7): 542-552.
12. Chesson Jr AL, Anderson WM, Littner M, Davila D, Hartse K, et al. Practice parameters for the nonpharmacologic treatment of chronic insomnia. An American Academy of Sleep Medicine report. Standards of Practice Committee of the American Academy of Sleep Medicine. *Sleep.* 1999;22(8):1128-1133.
13. Morgenthaler T, Kramer M, Alessi C, Friedman L, Boehlecke B, et al. Practice parameters for the psychological and behavioral treatment of insomnia: An update. An American Academy of Sleep Medicine report. *Sleep.* 2006;29(11):1415-1419.
14. McCurry SM, Logsdon RG, Teri L, Vitiello MV. Evidence-based psychological treatments for insomnia in older adults. *Psychol Aging.* 2007;22(1):18-27.
15. Morin C, Hauri P, Espie C, Spielman A, Buysse D, Bootzin R. Nonpharmacologic treatment of chronic insomnia. An American Academy of Sleep Medicine review. *Sleep.* 1999;22:1134-1156.
16. Rybarczyk B, Lopez M, Benson R, Alsten C, Stepanski E. Efficacy of two behavioral treatment programs for comorbid geriatric insomnia. *Psychol Aging.* 2002;17:288.
17. Jefferson CD, Drake CL, Scofield HM, Myers E, McClure T, et al. Sleep hygiene practices in a population-based sample of insomniacs. *Sleep.* 2005;28(5):611-615.
18. Cheek RE, Shaver JL, Lentz MJ. Lifestyle practices and nocturnal sleep in midlife women with and without insomnia. *Biol Res Nurs.* 2004;6(1):46-58.
19. van der Heijden KB, Smits MG, Gunning WB. Sleep hygiene and actigraphically evaluated sleep characteristics in children with ADHD and chronic sleep onset insomnia. *J Sleep Res.* 2006;15(1):55-62.
20. Cheek RE, Shaver JL, Lentz MJ. Variations in sleep hygiene practices of women with and without insomnia. *Res Nurs Health.* 2004;27(4):225-236.
21. Yang CM, Lin SC, Hsu SC, Cheng CP. Maladaptive sleep hygiene practices in good sleepers and patients with insomnia. *J Health Psychol.* 2010;15(1):147-155.
22. Rechtschaffen A, Hauri P, Zeitlin M. Auditory awakening thresholds in REM and NREM sleep stages. *Percept Mot Skills.* 1966;22:927-942.
23. LaVere TE, Bartus RT, Hart FD. Electroencephalographic and behavioral effects of nocturnally occurring jet aircraft sounds. *Aerospace Med.* 1972;43:384-389.

24. Ettema JH, Zielhuis RLI. Health effects of exposure to noise, particularly aircraft noise. *Int Arch Occup Environ Health.* 1977;40:163-164.
25. Globus G, Friedmann J, Cohen H, et al. The effects of aircraft noise on sleep electrophysiology as recorded in the home. In: Ward WD, ed. *Proceedings of the International Congress on Noise as a Public Health Problem.* Washington, DC: U.S. Environmental Protection Agency; 1974:414-418.
26. Otto E. In: Koella WP, Levin P, eds. *Sleep. First European Congress on Sleep Research, Basel. Physiological analysis of sleep disturbances induced by noise and increased room temperature.* 1973. Basel: S. Karger; 1972:414-418.
27. Lai HL, Good M. Music improves sleep quality in older adults. *J Adv Nurs.* 2005;49(3):234-244.
28. Otto E, Kramer H, Bräuer D. Einfluss erhöhter Raumlufttemperatur auf Herzschlagfrequenz, Bewegungshäufigkeit, Rectaltemperatur und Electroencephalogramm schlafender Menschen. *Int Arch Arbeitsmed.* 1971;28:189-202.
29. Angus RG, Pearce DG, Buguet AGC, et al. Vigilance performance of men sleeping under arctic conditions. *Aviat Space Environ Med.* 1979;50(4):692-696.
30. Kinkel HJ, Maxion H. Schlafphysiologische Untersuchungen zur Beurteilung verschiedener Matratzen. *Int Zeit Angewand Physiol.* 1970;28:247-262.
31. Coenen A, Kolff M, Hofman W. Sleep quality and body motility of healthy subjects sleeping on two types of mattresses. In: Sleep-Wake. Research in the Netherlands. Annual Proceedings of the NSWO. *Entschede.* 2009:57-60.
32. Monroe LJ. Transient changes in EEG sleep patterns of married good sleepers: The effects of altering sleeping arrangement. *Psychophysiology.* 1969;6:330-337.
33. van den Bulck J. Television viewing, computer game playing, and internet use and self-reported time to bed and time out of bed in secondary-school children. *Sleep.* 2004;27(1):101-104.
34. Bootzin RR, Nicassio PN. Behavioral treatments for insomnia. In: Hersen M, Eisler R, Miller P, eds. *Progress in Behavior Modification.* New York: Academic Press; 1978.
35. Morin C, Hauri P, Espie C, Spielman A, Buysse D, Bootzin R. Nonpharmacologic treatment of chronic insomnia. An American Academy of Sleep Medicine review. *Sleep.* 1999;22:1134-1156.
36. Bonnet MH, Arand DL. Sleepiness as measured by modified multiple sleep latency testing varies as a function of preceding activity. *Sleep.* 1998;21:477-483.
37. Takahashi M. The role of prescribed napping in sleep medicine. *Sleep Med Rev.* 2003;7(3):227-235.
38. Tietzel AJ, Lack LC. The short-term benefits of brief and long naps following nocturnal sleep restriction. *Sleep.* 2001;24:293-300.
39. Hayashi M, Ito S, Hori T. The effects of a 20-min nap at noon on sleepiness, performance and EEG activity. *Int J Psychophysiol.* 1999;32:173-180.
40. Hayashi M, Watanabe M, Hori T. The effects of a 20 min nap in the mid-afternoon on mood, performance and EEG activity. *Clin Neurophysiol.* 1999;110:272-279.
41. Monk TH, Buysse DJ, Carrier J, et al. Effects of afternoon "siesta" naps on sleep, alertness, performance, and circadian rhythms in the elderly. *Sleep.* 2001;24:680-687.
42. Strogatz SH, Kronauer RE, Czeisler CA. Circadian pacemaker interferes with sleep onset at specific times each day: Role in insomnia. *Am J Physiol Ther.* 1987;253:R172-R178.
43. Bonnet MH, Arand DL. 24-hour metabolic rate in insomniacs and matched normal sleepers. *Sleep.* 1995;18(7):581-588.
44. Ancoli-Israel S, Martin JL. Insomnia and daytime napping in older adults. *J Clin Sleep Med.* 2006;2(3):333-342.
45. Dautovich ND, McCrae CS, Rowe M. Subjective and objective napping and sleep in older adults: Are evening naps "bad" for nighttime sleep? *J Am Geriatr Soc.* 2008;56(9):1681-1686.
46. Campos H, Siles X. Siesta and the risk of coronary heart disease: Results from a population-based, case-control study in Costa Rica. *Int J Epidemiol.* 2000;29:429-437.
47. Bursztyn M, Ginsberg G, Hammerman-Rozenberg R, et al. The siesta in the elderly: Risk factor for mortality? *Arch Intern Med.* 1999;159:1582-1586.
48. Hays JC, Blazer DG, Foley DJ. Risk of napping: excessive daytime sleepiness and mortality in an older community population. *J Am Geriatr Soc.* 1996;44:693-698.
49. Newman AB, Spiekerman CF, Enright P, et al. Daytime sleepiness predicts mortality and cardiovascular disease in older adults. The Cardiovascular Health Study Research Group. *J Am Geriatr Soc.* 2000;48:115-123.
50. Asada T, Motonaga T, Yamagata Z, et al. Associations between retrospectively recalled napping behavior and later development of Alzheimer's disease: association with APOE genotypes. *Sleep.* 2000;23:629-634.
51. Hartmann E. Sleep requirement: Long sleepers, short sleepers, variable sleepers, and insomniacs. *Psychosomatics.* 1973;14:95-103.
52. Benoit O, Foret J, Bouard G. The time course of slow wave sleep and REM sleep in habitual long and short sleepers: Effect of prior wakefulness. *Hum Neurobiol.* 1983;2:91-96.
53. Spielman AJ, Saskin P, Thorpy MJ. Treatment of chronic insomnia by restriction of time in bed. *Sleep.* 1987;10:45-56.
54. Brown FC, Buboltz Jr WC, Soper B. Relationship of sleep hygiene awareness, sleep hygiene practices, and sleep quality in university students. *Behav Med.* 2002;28(1):33-38.
55. Manber R, Bootzin R, Acebo C, Carskadon M. The effects of regularizing sleep-wake schedules on daytime sleepiness. *Sleep.* 1996;19:432-441.
56. Bonnet MH, Alter J. Effects of irregular versus regular sleep schedules on performance, mood and body temperature. *Biol Psychol.* 1982;14(3-4):287-296.
57. Ramakrishnan K, Scheid DC. Treatment options for insomnia. *Am Fam Physician.* 2007;76(4):517-526.
58. Kubitz KA, Landers DM, Petruzzello SJ, Han M. The effects of acute and chronic exercise on sleep. A meta-analytic review. *Sports Med.* 1996;21:277-291.
59. O'Connor PJ, Youngstedt SD. Influence of exercise on human sleep. In: Holloszy JO, ed. *Exercise and Sport Sciences Review.* 23rd ed. Baltimore: Williams & Wilkins; 1995:105-134.
60. Nojomi M, Ghalhe Bandi MF, Kaffashi S. Sleep pattern in medical students and residents. *Arch Iran Med.* 2009;12(6):542-549.
61. King AC, Oman RF, Brassington GS, Bliwise DL, Haskell WL. Moderate-intensity exercise and self-rated quality of sleep in older adults. A randomized controlled trial. *JAMA.* 1997;277(1):32-37.
62. Paparrigopoulos T, Tzavara C, Theleritis C, Soldatos C, Tountas Y. Physical activity may promote sleep in cardiac patients suffering from insomnia. *Int J Cardiol.* 2010;143(2):209-211.
63. Gerber M, Brand S, Holsboer-Trachsler E, Pühse U. Fitness and exercise as correlates of sleep complaints—Is it all in our minds? *Med Sci Sports Exer.* 2010;42(5):893-901.
64. Hauri P. Effects of evening activity on early night sleep. *Psychophysiology.* 1968;4:267-277.
65. Hauri P. The influence of evening activity on the onset of sleep. *Psychophysiology.* 1969;5:426-430.
66. Youngstedt SD, O'Connor PJ, Dishman RK. The effects of acute exercise on sleep: A quantitative synthesis. *Sleep.* 1997;20:203-214.
67. Horne JA, Staff LH. Exercise and sleep: Body heating effects. *Sleep.* 1983;6:36-46.
68. Horne JA, Reid AJ. Night-time sleep EEG changes following body heating in a warm bath. *Electroencephalogr Clin Neurophysiol.* 1985;60:154-157.
69. Edinger JD, Morey MC, Sullivan RJ, Higginbotham MB, Marsh GR, et al. Aerobic fitness, acute exercise and sleep in older men. *Sleep.* 1993;16(4):351-359.
70. Bonnet MHG, Arand DL. 24-hour metabolic rate in insomniacs and matched normal sleepers. *Sleep.* 1995;18(7):581-588.
71. Harvey AG, Farrell C. The efficacy of a Pennebaker-like writing intervention for poor sleepers. *Behav Sleep Med.* 2003;1(2):115-124.
72. Karacan I, Thornby JI, Anch AM, Booth GH, Williams RL, Salis PJ. Dose-related sleep disturbances induced by coffee and caffeine. *Clin Pharmacol Ther.* 1976;20(6):682-689.
73. Nicholson AN, Stone BM. Heterocyclic amphetamine derivatives and caffeine on sleep in man. *Br J Clin Pharmacol.* 1980;9:195-203.
74. Drake CL, Jefferson C, Roehrs T, Roth T. Stress-related sleep disturbance and polysomnographic response to caffeine. *Sleep Med.* 2006;7(7):567-572:[Epub 2006 Sept 22.].
75. Landolt HP, Werth E, Borbely AA, Dijk DJ. Caffeine intake (200 mg) in the morning affects human sleep and EEG power spectra at night. *Brain Res.* 1995;675:67-74.
76. Sanchez-Ortuno M, Moore N, Taillard J, Valtat C, Leger D, et al. Sleep duration and caffeine consumption in a French middle-aged working population. *Sleep Med.* 2005;6(3):247-251.
77. Bonnet MH, Arand DL. Situational insomnia: Consistency, predictors, and outcomes. *Sleep.* 2003;26:1029-1036.
78. Tiffin P, Ashton H, Marsh R, Kamali F. Pharmacokinetic and pharmacodynamic responses to caffeine in poor and normal sleepers. *Psychopharmacology (Berl).* 1995;121(4):494-502.
79. Silverman K, Evans SM, Strain EC, Griffiths RR. Withdrawal syndrome after the double-blind cessation of caffeine consumption. *N Engl J Med.* 1992;327(16):1109-1113.

80. Roehrs T, Zwyghuizen-Doorenbos A, Roth T. Sedative effects and plasma concentrations following single dose of triazolam, diphenhydramine, ethanol and placebo. *Sleep.* 1993;16:301-305.

81. Ancoli-Israel S, Roth T. Characteristics of insomnia in the United States: Results of the 1991 National Sleep Foundation Survey. I. *Sleep.* 1999;22:S347-S353.

82. Landolt HP, Roth C, Dijk DJ, Borbely AA. Late-afternoon ethanol intake affects nocturnal sleep and the sleep EEG in middle-aged men. *J Clin Psychopharmacol.* 1996;16:428-436.

83. Brower K, Aldrich M, Robinson E, Zucker R, Greden JF. Insomnia, self-medication, and relapse to alcoholism. *Am J Psychiatry.* 2001;158:399-404.

84. Jacobs BL, McGinty DJ. Effects of food deprivation on sleep and wakefulness in the rat. *Exp Neurol.* 1971;30:212-222.

85. Lacey JH, Crisp AH, Kalucy RS, et al. Weight gain and the sleeping electroencephalogram: Study of 10 patients with anorexia nervosa. *Br Med J.* 1975;4:556-558.

86. Southwell PR, Evans CR, Hunt JN. Effect of a hot milk drink on movements during sleep. *Br Med J.* 1972;2:429-431.

87. Brezinova V, Oswald I. Sleep after a bedtime beverage. *Br Med J.* 1972;2:431-433.

88. Wetter DW, Young TB. The relation between cigarette smoking and sleep disturbance. *Prevent Med.* 1994;23:328-334.

89. Soldatos CR, Kales JD, Scharf MB, Bixler EO, Kales A. Cigarette smoking associated with sleep difficulty. *Science.* 1988;207:551-553.

90. Kohn L, Espie CA. Sensitivity and specificity of measures of the insomnia experience: A comparative study of psychophysiologic insomnia, insomnia associated with mental disorder and good sleep. *Sleep.* 2005;28:104-112.

91. Ladouceur R, Gros-Louis Y. Paradoxical intention vs. stimulus control in the treatment of severe insomnia. *J Behav Ther Exp Psychiatry.* 1986;17:267-269.

92. Ström L, Pettersson R, Andersson G. Internet-based treatment for insomnia: A controlled evaluation. *J Consult Clin Psychol.* 2004;72:113-120.

93. Chambers MJ, Keller B. Alert insomniacs: Are they really sleep deprived? *Clin Psychol Rev.* 1993;13(7):649-666.

94. Bilsbury CD, Rajda M. What's wrong with sleep hygiene? *Sleep Med.* 2004;5(5):513.

95. Karacan I, Williams RL, Littell RC, Salis PJ. Insomniacs: Unpredictable and idiosyncratic sleepers. In: Koella WP, Levin P, eds. *Sleep: Physiology, Biochemistry, Psychology, Clinical Implications.* Basel: S. Karger; 1973:120-132.

96. Morin CM, Beaulieu-Bonneau S, LeBlanc M, Savard J. Self-help treatment for insomnia: A randomized controlled trial. *Sleep.* 2005;28(10):1319-1327.

Cognitive Behavioral and Psychological Therapies for Chronic Insomnia

COLIN A. ESPIE / SIMON D. KYLE

Chronic insomnia is a prevalent complaint of sleep disturbance that impairs daytime functioning and degrades overall quality of life (QoL). A large number of individuals with chronic sleep disturbance fail to seek treatment; and those who do are typically prescribed hypnotic medications. There are, however, a number of alternative, effective nonpharmacologic therapies that can improve sleep in those with persistent insomnia. These therapies are based on cognitive and behavioral principles, and have a strong evidence base for effectively ameliorating core insomnia symptoms. This chapter begins by outlining contemporary models of insomnia, particularly those that emphasize cognitive and behavioral abnormalities as relevant to the initiation and maintenance of the insomnia disorder. Cognitive behavioral therapies (CBTs) are next described, placing direct focus on implementation in clinical practice. Finally, the evidence base for CBT effectiveness is reviewed and developing research strands considered.

INSOMNIA: DEFINING FEATURES

The core symptoms of insomnia, specified in major disease and sleep disorder classification manuals,[1-4] correspond to difficulties with initiating and maintaining sleep, or nonrestorative sleep (poor quality sleep). To achieve disorder "status," sleep disturbance must not be simply a function of restricted sleep opportunity (curtailment), or environmental perturbation (e.g., noise, bed partner snoring). Importantly, the diagnosis of insomnia disorder is made only when impairment in daytime functioning is present and is linked (attributionally) to nighttime sleep difficulties. Indeed it is often these daytime impairments that motivate patients to seek treatment for their sleep disturbance.[5] Daytime impairments may be measured with reference to isolated symptoms, such as fatigue and concentration,[1,4] but also to more global dysfunction and quality of life impairment, for example, in areas of social and occupational functioning.[2,6]

CONTEMPORARY MODELS OF INSOMNIA

Over the years, several "single factor" as well as multifactorial models have been put forward to account for the cause and maintenance of chronic insomnia. These "single factor" accounts have tended to focus on specific, focused abnormalities, which have some degree of support in the existing literature, and include stimulus dyscontrol and instrumental conditioning,[7] altered sleep homeostasis,[8] alterations in the circadian parameters involved in the timing of sleep,[9] and physiologic hyperarousal preventing the de-aroused state necessary

for sleep.[10,11] Although these "models" are well formulated, it is likely that multicomponent perspectives are required to capture the heterogeneity of insomnia symptoms, associated subtypes, and insomnia development/trajectory. Although it is beyond the scope of this brief chapter to describe each multicomponent model in detail, it is worth outlining some of the main accounts, which are inclusive and encompassing with regard to associated characteristics of insomnia disorder, and place emphasis on cognitive and behavioral factors.

The Predisposing, Precipitating, Perpetuating Model: A General Framework

The main framework for most working models of insomnia was set out in 1987 by Spielman and associates[12] in the form of the predisposing, precipitating, perpetuating (3P) model (Fig. 12-1).[13] This stress-diathesis conceptualization outlines how chronic insomnia may develop over time; proposing, as a first step, that acute sleep disturbance occurs as a consequence of both predisposing (e.g., altered neurotransmission, trait arousal, genetic susceptibility, ruminative personality) and precipitating factors (life stressors such as occupational stress, emotional and health problems). *Perpetuating factors* refer to maladaptive sleep practices, which interact with experienced insomnia symptoms and are aimed at coping with the consequences of poor sleep during the day (e.g., drinking coffee to improve alertness), or directly trying to increase the probability of "achieving" sleep (e.g., extending time in bed). After the precipitant resolves, most individuals will return to the default mode of sleep automaticity, but in those with a predisposition for sleep disturbance, combined with the continued practice of maladaptive perpetuating behaviors, sleep disturbance may become chronic.

Thus, a main assumption of this model is that sleep disturbance may, over time, become dislocated from the precipitating trigger.[14] Such a framework is intuitively appealing because it suggests that treatment should target, specifically, perpetuating factors involved in the maintenance of insomnia. Indeed, this is exactly what cognitive behavioral therapy for insomnia (CBT-I) attempts to do, with an emphasis on correcting maladaptive coping strategies, behaviors, and sleep-related dysfunctional beliefs and attitudes.[15]

Neurocognitive Model

Perlis and colleagues[16] extend this behavioral perspective, acknowledging that acute insomnia is initially precipitated by life stress, is similarly maintained by maladaptive coping

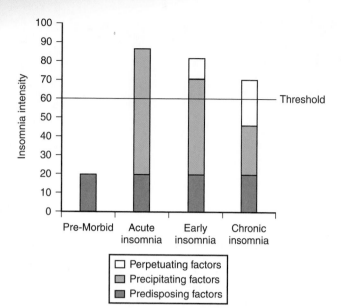

Figure 12-1 Factors contributing to the development of insomnia, according to the 3P framework. (Redrawn, with permission, from Spielman AJ, Glovinsky PB: The varied nature of insomnia. In: Hauri P, ed. *Case Studies in Insomnia.* New York: Plenum Press; 1991:1-15.)

strategies (e.g., extending time in bed), but that, importantly, the associated wakefulness becomes classically conditioned in terms of arousal (somatic, cognitive, and cortical). It is argued that increased cortical arousal (as measured by fast rhythms in the Electroencephalogram (EEG)[17]) at sleep onset, during sleep, and middle of the night awakenings, subsequently disrupts sleep initiation and maintenance through enhanced sensory/information processing and attenuated mesograde amnesia. These altered cognitive parameters may subsequently help explain sleep-state misperception. A later addition to this model also includes the possibility that sleep-related objects (bed, pillow, etc.) become conditioned stimuli for cortical arousal and hence contribute to the perpetuation of continued sleep disturbance.[18]

Cognitive Model

Harvey[19] describes a (maintenance) model of insomnia that focuses primarily on dysfunctional cognitive processes, based upon a large body of work from the anxiety disorders literature. Because it is arguably the first model to give equal attention to both daytime and nighttime factors, it is worth outlining some of its main features. Harvey argues that individuals with insomnia tend to excessively worry about sleep and "catastrophize" about the consequences of not getting adequate sleep (in relation to impact on health and daytime functioning). Ensuing negatively toned cognitive activity, typically about sleep but also other (negatively valenced) life issues, coupled with the application of maladaptive safety behaviors, results in elevated autonomic arousal and emotional distress. As a consequence of this heightened stress state, individuals with insomnia tend to monitor for sleep-related threat cues (internal and external) to confirm that they have not slept and that functioning is adversely affected. Preexisting dysfunctional beliefs exacerbate the situation. Otherwise innocuous cues are subsequently misinterpreted as evidence for sleep and daytime deficits, "tricking" the individual into overestimating

both the level of sleep and daytime impairment. This serves to cause further worry and concern about not sleeping, which may, through feedback mechanisms, increase anxiety and cognitive load, leading to the enhanced possibility of a "real" deficit occurring in both sleep and daytime functioning. The main assumption of this model is that cognitive processes have a causal role in the maintenance of an insomnia state.

Psychobiologic Inhibition/Attention-Intention-Effort Model

Espie[20] and Espie and colleagues[21] take a starting point of normal sleep for their model of insomnia. They acknowledge that normal sleep is governed by two oscillatory processes—a self-sustained oscillating circadian rhythm and an "hourglass" sleep homeostat—rendering the (adaptive) sleep process automatic, involuntary and, hence, not under direct control. Acute stressful life events can however create both physiologic and psychological "over-arousal," which interacts negatively with normal sleep-wake regulation, leading to acute sleep disturbance. For most individuals, the "plasticity" of the sleep system accommodates such transient disruptions, without any lasting chronic modifications. However, it is argued that the development of acute to chronic insomnia, where the defining feature is a fundamental difficulty in inhibiting wakefulness, is precipitated by three related cognitive processes.[21] Attending to sleep-related stimuli, explicitly intending to sleep, and applying voluntary effort to the sleep onset process all represent an attempt to control sleep, an otherwise automatic process. These attempts have the opposite effect: preventing de-arousal by failure to reach a level of inhibitory sufficiency. Factors relevant to this resultant "sleep effort syndrome"[22] include enhanced sleep-preoccupation, affect dysregulation, sleep-incompatible conditioning, dysfunctional beliefs and expectations about sleep, and enhanced focus on the consequences of poor sleep.

PSYCHOLOGICAL MANAGEMENT OF INSOMNIA: A FOCUS ON COGNITIVE BEHAVIORAL PRINCIPLES

It is important to note, first, that the majority of individuals with insomnia do not actually seek treatment for their sleep difficulties; with approximately only 10% to 40% consulting a health professional specifically for insomnia symptoms.[5,23] Although only a small amount of work has been carried out to understand why this is the case, it appears likely that the following play a role: (1) perception of sleep as not being viewed important by the medical profession,[6,24] (2) poor understanding and recognition of sleep disturbances by health care providers,[6] and (3) limited public knowledge of available treatments.[25] For those with chronic insomnia who do seek treatment in primary care, the outcome tends to be long-term prescription of sleep-promoting hypnotics. It is important to note, however, that this is not evidence-based practice: there are no convincing data to suggest that long-term treatment with hypnotics successfully resolves persistent insomnia beyond the termination of active treatment.[26,27] Furthermore, when presented with a list of possible treatments, insomnia patients show preference for nonpharmacologic interventions.[28,29]

Given that maladaptive behaviors and cognitive processes are thought to underlie the maintenance of insomnia, it is

TABLE 12-1

Cognitive and Behavioural Treatments Endorsed by the American Academy of Sleep Medicine (AASM[32]) and Level of Endorsement

Therapy	Level of AASM endorsement	
	Standard (high degree of clinical certainty)	Guideline (moderate degree of clinical certainty)
Siemulus control	x	-
Sleep restriction	-	x
Relaxation training	x	-
Biofeedback	-	x
Paradoxical intention	-	x
CBT with or without relaxation therapy	x	-
Multicomponent therapy (without cognitive-based techniques)	-	x

BOX 12-1 *Key Components of Stimulus Control Therapy*

A Go to bed only when sleepy.
B The bed should only be used for the purposes of sleeping. That is, all other activities, including reading, watching TV, and eating, are prohibited. The only exception to this rule relates to sexual activity.
C If you do not fall asleep within approximately 15 minutes, get up out of bed, exit the bedroom and relocate to another room. Only when feeling sufficiently sleepy again should you return to bed. This process should be repeated as many times as necessary and for sleep re-initiation during middle of the night awakenings.
D Set an alarm clock for a consistent rising time each morning.
E Refrain from daytime napping.

intuitive that therapy targets these factors directly.[30] Cognitive behavioral therapy for insomnia (CBT-I) is an evidence-based treatment modality, containing a number of supported techniques to improve sleep. Practice parameters set out by the American Academy of Sleep Medicine (AASM) recommend and endorse the following single component therapies: stimulus control therapy, sleep restriction therapy, paradoxical intention therapy, progressive muscular relaxation, and biofeedback[31,32] (Table 12-1 shows the level of AASM endorsement for each component). In addition, two multicomponent CBT approaches are also supported. Indeed, most outcome research has focused on multicomponent, multisession CBT interventions, which typically contain a combination of behavioral components (e.g., sleep restriction therapy, stimulus control therapy, muscle relaxation) and cognitive-based techniques (e.g., challenging dysfunctional beliefs about sleep, paradoxical intention to reduce applied sleep effort). Key components are outlined in the following sections, with particular emphasis on practice points to guide effective implementation.

Stimulus Control Treatment

The principle underlying stimulus control treatment is that it increases the bedroom's cueing potential for successful sleep.[7] For good sleepers, the pre-bedtime period and the stimulus environment trigger positive associations of sleepiness and sleep. For the poor sleeper, however, the bedroom triggers associations with restlessness and lengthy nighttime wakening via a stimulus-response relationship, thereby continuing to promote wakefulness and arousal. The concept is similar to phobic conditions in which a conditioned stimulus precipitates an anxiety response. Treatment involves three main elements (Box 12-1 provides a detailed summary). First, all potentially sleep-incompatible stimuli are removed from the bedroom environment. Reading and watching television, for example, are confined to living rooms. Second, sleeping is excluded from living areas and from the daytime period (no napping), and wakefulness is excluded from the bedroom.

Finally, the individual is instructed to "get up and go to another room if not asleep within 15 to 20 minutes" (known simply as "the quarter of an hour rule"). The patient should return to the bedroom only when he begins to feel sleepy. This process should also be repeated for middle of the night awakenings. Conceptually, stimulus control is a reconditioning treatment that enforces discrimination between daytime (waking) and nighttime (sleeping) environments.

Sleep Restriction Therapy

Sleep restriction confines sleep to the length of time the person is likely to sleep.[33] This practice may be equivalent to promoting "core sleep" at the expense of "optional sleep." Sleep restriction primarily aims to improve sleep efficiency. Because sleep efficiency is the ratio of time asleep to time in bed, it can be improved either by increasing the numerator (time spent asleep) or by reducing the denominator (time spent in bed). People with insomnia generally seek the former (typically by extending time in bed), but this may not be necessary, either biologically or psychologically.

Sleep restriction first involves recording nightly sleep parameters in a sleep diary and calculating average nightly sleep duration (Box 12-2 provides a detailed summary of sleep restriction guidelines). The aim, then, is to obtain this average each night. This goal is achieved by setting rising time as an "anchor" each day and delaying going to bed until a "threshold time," which permits this designated amount of sleep. Thus, the sleep period is reduced and sleep efficiency is likely to increase. The permitted "sleep window" can then be titrated week by week in 15-minute increments in response to sleep efficiency improvements. Specifically, if sleep efficiency for the week is 90% or greater, then the sleep window is typically increased by 15 minutes; if sleep efficiency is less than 85%, then the sleep window is decreased by a further 15 minutes; and if values fall between 85% and 89% then no change is made to the schedule. The minimum possible sleep window duration is usually set at 5 hours, to limit the potential for inducing excessive sleepiness and other daytime impairments. Clinically, patients often report feeling sleepier during the day than prior to treatment initiation, and although this is a desired consequence of sleep restriction therapy, patients should be warned not to take risks driving or operating heavy machinery if feeling excessively sleepy.

This "resetting" of the sleep pattern may have a number of parallel therapeutic effects, influencing factors thought to be critical in the pathophysiology of insomnia. For example, standardizing bed and rising times may help to realign circadian parameters important in modulating the timing and maintenance of the sleep period. Restricting sleep opportunity can also acutely induce a mild sleep deprivation state, which, through increased sleep pressure, may help to overcome a malfunctioning sleep homeostat or excessive arousal.[8] Potentiating the correct functioning of these two oscillatory processes subsequently leads to reduced sleep latencies and wake time during the night, ultimately leading to improvements in sleep efficiency.

Paradoxical Intention

Paradoxical intention (PI) is useful for those patients with an intense preoccupation about sleep, sleep loss, and its consequences. The guiding rationale is that because sleep is essentially an involuntary physiologic process, attempts to place it under voluntary control are likely to make matters worse. The paradoxical instruction is to allow sleep to occur naturally through passively attempting to remain quietly wakeful, rather than attempting to fall asleep. PI is thought to work by reducing performance anxiety (the poor sleeper's inability to produce the criterion performance for good sleep) and by reducing associated sleep worry and sleep preoccupation.

A useful way of preparing the patient prior to PI implementation is to get the patient to consider "*How does a good sleeper do it*?" It must be a difficult thing to be a good sleeper, or so people with insomnia might think. They usually have spent months, more likely years, trying to find a solution to their problem, to find a key that will unlock their sleep. But here there is a special secret. Good sleepers are good sleepers precisely because what they do is second nature to them. They just do not really think about it, nor do they "do" anything in particular. The purpose of the *How does a good sleeper do it*? exercise is to communicate that good sleepers are not students of sleep. Their perspective simply supports sleep coming automatically and naturally—nothing more, nothing less. If the insomnia patient wants to become a good sleeper, one of the biggest challenges will be to develop the mindset of the good sleeper, who is relatively "care-less" about sleep.

So what advice would PI therapy specifically offer for sleep-related behavior? Box 12-3 describes two methods for implementing PI therapy in bed.

Method 1 is a "giving up trying" method,[35] and parts of it come close to the notion of acceptance and mindfulness. This method has been referred to as turning the tables.[36] The use of humor is powerful in helping people to take a different perspective. It helps to reduce to dust the edifices of our exaggerated conclusions and emotions. Specifically, patients are encouraged to ask, "What is the worst that can happen?" And rather than just challenging the true likelihood of all their wild imaginings (as one would do in cognitive restructuring), the therapist should try going with the flow, rather than against it, by posing less resistance.

Method 1 may not appeal to all patients, but this more light-hearted approach could help to reduce anxiety and effort around sleep. Patients using this approach often talk about developing a completely different attitude. Indeed, the idea of accepting situations, rather than fighting them all the time, has its roots in a number of ancient philosophies and religions.

BOX 12-2 *Sleep Restriction Therapy Guidelines*

1. Patient instructed to record a sleep diary for 2 weeks to obtain average nightly sleep duration (e.g., 5 hours 45 minutes [rounded to nearest 15 minute interval]). This acts as the designated sleep window.
2. Therapist, in collaboration with patient, sets a morning "rising time" (e.g., 7 AM)
3. A "threshold time" is then calculated by subtracting average nightly sleep duration from the specified morning rising time (e.g., 7 AM–5 hours 45 minutes = threshold time 1:15 AM).
4. Participants are instructed not to enter bed prior to their designated "threshold time" and to exit bed on, or prior to, set "rising time".
5. Follow this prescribed schedule every night, including weekends.
6. Weekly modifications to the sleep window are based on sleep efficiency values (total time asleep/total time in bed x 100):
   - If sleep efficiency > 90% increase sleep window by 15 minutes
   - If sleep efficiency < 85% decrease sleep window by 15 minutes

---

BOX 12-3 *Two Methods for Implementing Paradoxical Intention Instructions*

Method 1: Turn the Tables	Method 2: Try to Stay Awake
1 Take every opportunity to be carefree about your insomnia	1 Lie comfortably in your bed with the lights off, but keep your eyes open.
2 Relish opportunities to get out of bed whenever you can.	2 Give up any effort to fall asleep.
3 Try to imagine as many catastrophes as you can that will happen, just because you are awake at night. See them as exaggerated and absurd.	3 Give up any concern about still being awake.
4 Be prepared to accept you have insomnia. Even tell others about it.	4 When your eyelids feel like they want to close, say to yourself gently "Just stay awake for another couple of minutes, I'll fall asleep naturally when I'm ready".
5 Think of wakefulness as an opportunity, not a disaster. Use the time when you are up, to do something useful or something you enjoy.	5 Do not purposefully make yourself stay awake; but if you can shift the focus off attempting to fall asleep, you will find that sleep comes naturally.

From Espie CA. *Overcoming Insomnia and Sleep Problems: A Self-Help Guide Using Cognitive Behavioral Techniques.* This edition first published by Robinson, an imprint of Constable & Robinson Ltd., London, 2006.

Acceptance leads to a problem having a less dominating position and influence. Where sleep is concerned a more mellow perspective is an adaptive outlook, and one that can lead to improved sleep.

Method 2 is more explicitly paradoxical; the patient is (paradoxically) encouraging the symptoms that they don't want to have to keep going. The goal becomes that of staying awake, instead of getting to sleep. By deciding to stay awake, the patient is completely giving up trying to sleep. When that happens, there is a strong possibility that the patient will find himself falling asleep, in spite of efforts to remain awake. It can be enormously reassuring for the patient to be overtaken by sleep. These patients often say things like, "*I don't know what happened last night. I was trying to stay awake just a few minutes longer, and the next thing I knew it was morning.*" At this point patients begin to realize that they can be normal sleepers.

In the Method 2 approach, people should go to bed at a normal time when they feel sleepy and put the lights off, but their explicit intention is to remain awake rather than to fall asleep, and therefore, they are instructed to keep their eyes open and to make no effort whatsoever to sleep. This is a passive approach rather than an active one, in the sense that they should not deliberately try to keep themselves aroused. They are not given explicit direction to think about something stimulating, to move their arms and legs, or stay physically active to remain awake; rather, they are to resist the tendency for their eyelids to close by reopening them and keeping them open, and encouraging themselves to remain awake until sleep comes naturally. They should follow the same instructions if they waken during the night and do not quickly return to sleep. Like the good sleeper, sleep should be allowed to come to them.

Relaxation and Biofeedback

There is a wide range of relaxation methods, including progressive relaxation, imagery training, biofeedback, meditation, hypnosis, and autogenic training, but little evidence to indicate the superiority of any one approach. Biofeedback and progressive relaxation techniques, however, have the most solid evidence base for individual component use.[31,32]

Relaxation should ultimately be viewed as a skill that requires training and practice, and, of course, patience.[37] In Glasgow, the authors tend to combine aspects of muscle tension release, breathing control, and imagery to create a progressive relaxation program. The context in which relaxation is carried out is essential to the process. Patients are instructed to "wind down" prior to going to bed, ceasing stimulating activities 1 to 2 hours before retiring for sleep. Once in bed, the patient is guided through a series of exercises, directed at making them aware of muscle tension increase and release, as well as the impact of breathing exercises in promoting relaxation (see pp. 57-58 in Morin and Espie[37] for a transcription of a relaxation CD the authors use with our patients).

Relaxation techniques traditionally target somatic arousal, but there are no adequate data that relaxation has its effect through autonomic change. Consequently, and at the cognitive level, these techniques may act through distraction and the promotion of mastery and self-efficacy. During relaxation, the mind focuses upon alternative themes such as visualized images or physiologic responses. Thus, relaxation may be effective for thought processes that are anxiety-based or that flit from topic to topic.

Biofeedback refers to a broad category of techniques that involve the monitoring of participants' physiologic signals, typically through an electronic/computerized interface. An example might be the real-time viewing of the sensorimotor rhythm (SMR), an indicator of reduced attention to sensory input and decreased motor output, which is captured from scalp electrodes placed over the sensorimotor cortex. Based on the notion of instrumental conditioning, patients, over successive trials, learn to modulate the displayed physiologic parameter. This modulation is often achieved through relaxation techniques. A handful of studies by Hauri and colleagues[38,39] demonstrated biofeedback to be effective in improving core insomnia symptoms, but issues concerning expense, resources, and expertise continue to limit its application in the day-to-day management of insomnia. Interestingly, there have been recent renewed efforts into the evaluation of bio/neurofeedback as viable treatment options for insomnia.[40,41] In addition, neural conditioning, using real-time functional magnetic resonance image-derived reward feedback, is currently under exploratory investigation for therapeutic application,[42] which may have important implications for the treatment of neurologic and psychiatric disorders.

Cognitive Approaches

Within multicomponent CBT-I there is usually a session dedicated to challenging misattributions about insomnia and its consequences, as well as other faulty beliefs that are presumed to maintain wakefulness.[37,43] Dysfunctional sleep-related attitudes and beliefs are generally accepted to be a central feature of insomnia, and can be measured with the dysfunctional belief and attitudes about sleep scale (Fig. 12-2[44]). For example, Morin and associates[45] found that people with insomnia endorsed more dysfunctional beliefs about sleep compared to control subjects, a finding replicated many times since.[46,47] The primary mechanism by which dysfunctional beliefs affect sleep is thought to be through the relationship between attitudes and sleep-incompatible behaviors. An individual who believes that he needs 8 hours of sleep is more likely to reduce his sleep efficiency by attempting to obtain sleep during the day, lying in bed when not asleep, or going to bed earlier—all of which are sleep-incompatible behaviors and are likely to exacerbate the problem.

Dysfunctional beliefs may be particularly pertinent for older adults, whose sleep patterns can change as a function of normal aging. Specifically, changes in the timing of the circadian rhythm, as well as structural changes in sleep architecture, can render the belief "*...that 8 hours of consolidated sleep is essential for normal functioning...*" even more unrealistic.[48] Thus, the dissonance between this expectation and perceived reality becomes greater and more anxiety provoking, ultimately exerting even more negative impact on perceptions of sleep quality and subsequent functioning.

Once key dysfunctional beliefs have been elicited, through therapist questioning and questionnaire completion, their validity should be examined in a systematic fashion. This approach involves guiding the patient to appreciate that her thoughts and beliefs represent just one perspective, and that many other interpretations exist, in other words, reinforcing the notion that there is no absolute truth. A number of general strategies can then be used in collaboration with the therapist

---

DYSFUNCTIONAL BELIEFS AND ATTITUDES ABOUT SLEEP

Several statements reflecting people's beliefs and attitudes about sleep are listed below. Please indicate to what extent you personally agree or disagree with each statement. There is no right or wrong answer. For each statement, circle the number that corresponds to your own **personal belief**. Please respond to all items even though some may not apply directly to your own situation.

Example: If I sleep too much, I don't perform as well the next day.

| 0 | 1 | 2 | 3 | 4 | 5 | 6 | (7) | 8 | 9 | 10 |

STRONGLY
DISAGREE   STRONGLY
                                                                          AGREE

1. I need 8 hours of sleep to feel refreshed and function well during the day.

| 0 | 1 | 2 | 3 | 4 | 5 | 6 | 7 | 8 | 9 | 10 |

STRONGLY
DISAGREE   STRONGLY
                                                                          AGREE

2. When I don't get proper amount of sleep on a given night, I need to catch up the next day by napping or the next night by sleeping longer.

| 0 | 1 | 2 | 3 | 4 | 5 | 6 | 7 | 8 | 9 | 10 |

STRONGLY
DISAGREE   STRONGLY
                                                                          AGREE

3. I am concerned that chronic insomnia may have serious consequences for my physical health.

| 0 | 1 | 2 | 3 | 4 | 5 | 6 | 7 | 8 | 9 | 10 |

STRONGLY
DISAGREE   STRONGLY
                                                                          AGREE

4. I am worried that I may lose control over my ability to sleep.

| 0 | 1 | 2 | 3 | 4 | 5 | 6 | 7 | 8 | 9 | 10 |

STRONGLY
DISAGREE   STRONGLY
                                                                          AGREE

5. I know that a poor night's sleep will interfere with my daily activities the next day.

| 0 | 1 | 2 | 3 | 4 | 5 | 6 | 7 | 8 | 9 | 10 |

STRONGLY
DISAGREE   STRONGLY
                                                                          AGREE

6. In order to be alert and function well during the day, I believe I would be better off taking a sleeping pill than having a poor night's sleep.

| 0 | 1 | 2 | 3 | 4 | 5 | 6 | 7 | 8 | 9 | 10 |

STRONGLY
DISAGREE   STRONGLY
                                                                          AGREE

Figure 12-2 Dysfunctional beliefs and attitudes about sleep scale (DBAS-16). (Redrawn, with permission, from Morin CM, Vallieres A, Ivers H. Dysfunctional beliefs and attitudes about sleep (DBAS): Validation of a brief version (DBAS-16). *Sleep.* 2007;30:1547-1554.)

to help "restructure" these beliefs and attitudes about sleep. Box 12-4, adapted from Morin and Espie,[37] provides a list of key strategic areas to be investigated in the therapist-patient interaction, and their desired route of impact.

Cognitive Control

The main complaint of the great majority of insomnia patients relates to an "overactive mind" or the experience of a "racing mind" during both sleep onset and middle of the night awakenings. Cognitive control procedures help to try and remove cognitive activity from the bedroom.[49] In this sense, these procedures are an extension of stimulus control therapy, recognizing that thoughts and worries are incompatible with the de-aroused state necessary for sleep onset. Indeed, in Glasgow, the authors often introduce cognitive control procedures in combination with "sleep scheduling," which includes both sleep restriction and stimulus control therapy (see Morin and Espie[37]). Box 12-5 details an instructional set the authors use with our patients to help address potentially worrisome thoughts long before the sleep onset period.

7. When I feel irritable, depressed, or anxious during the day, it is mostly because I did not sleep well the night before.

0	1	2	3	4	5	6	7	8	9	10

STRONGLY DISAGREE .... STRONGLY AGREE

8. When I sleep poorly on one night, I know it will disturb my sleep schedule for the whole week.

0	1	2	3	4	5	6	7	8	9	10

STRONGLY DISAGREE .... STRONGLY AGREE

9. Without an adequate night's sleep, I can hardly function the next day.

0	1	2	3	4	5	6	7	8	9	10

STRONGLY DISAGREE .... STRONGLY AGREE

10. I can't ever predict whether I'll have a good or poor night's sleep.

0	1	2	3	4	5	6	7	8	9	10

STRONGLY DISAGREE .... STRONGLY AGREE

11. I have little ability to manage the negative consequences of disturbed sleep.

0	1	2	3	4	5	6	7	8	9	10

STRONGLY DISAGREE .... STRONGLY AGREE

12. When I feel tired, have no energy, or just seem not to function well during the day, it is generally because I did not sleep well the night before.

0	1	2	3	4	5	6	7	8	9	10

STRONGLY DISAGREE .... STRONGLY AGREE

13. I believe insomnia is essentially the result of a chemical imbalance.

0	1	2	3	4	5	6	7	8	9	10

STRONGLY DISAGREE .... STRONGLY AGREE

14. I feel insomnia is ruining my ability to enjoy life and prevents me from doing what I want.

0	1	2	3	4	5	6	7	8	9	10

STRONGLY DISAGREE .... STRONGLY AGREE

15. Medication is probably the only solution to sleeplessness.

0	1	2	3	4	5	6	7	8	9	10

STRONGLY DISAGREE .... STRONGLY AGREE

16. I avoid or cancel obligations (social, family) after a poor night's sleep.

0	1	2	3	4	5	6	7	8	9	10

STRONGLY DISAGREE .... STRONGLY AGREE

Figure 12-2, cont'd.

CBT as an Integrated Psychological Therapy

It is important to note that there is thought to be considerable synergy between the elements of the CBT approach. This is part of the reason that CBT is a psychotherapy method, and not merely a collection of strategies. Some examples may help to illustrate.

In stimulus control therapy, patients are encouraged not to read in bed but to protect the bedroom environment exclusively for sleep and sexual activity. They often say that they

---

BOX 12-4 *Cognitive Strategies for Changing Beliefs and Attitudes about Sleep*

1	Keep expectations realistic	For example, understanding individual sleep needs and the "8-hour fallacy" to help reduce performance anxiety/feelings of inadequacy.
2	Revise attributions about causes of insomnia	For example, consider a more multidimensional account of insomnia instead of focusing on one factor (e.g., "chemical imbalance"). Emphasis should be placed on those factors that the patient can exert direct influence over (e.g., napping, time in bed) to move away from perceived helplessness.
3	Sleeplessness does not account for all daytime impairments	Guide the patient to challenge the notion that poor sleep uniquely explains daytime dysfunction and to consider other sources of impairment (e.g., relationships, work).
4	Do not catastrophise after a poor night's sleep	Assess for exaggerations of the impact of insomnia, and guide patient to put in perspective their concerns (e.g., "What is the worst that can happen if you don't sleep tonight?"). Reinforce the notion that insomnia is, on the whole, not dangerous.
5	Do not place too much emphasis on sleep	Encourage patient to shift the focus away from sleep as the centre of existence. Discuss safety behaviors and the impact of these behaviors (e.g., avoiding social activities). Reduce feelings of being a helpless victim.
6	Develop tolerance to effects of sleep loss	Encourage patient to continue with normal, daily routine/activities after poor sleep. Prescribe a behavioral experiment in which patient engages in a pleasurable activity after a poor night of sleep to directly challenge and disprove the belief that sleeplessness impairs enjoyment of all daily activities.
7	Never try to sleep	Explain to patient that sleep is an automatic process that cannot be intiated by willful effort. Consider asking patient to try and stay awake (paradoxical intention) in order to reduce associated performance anxiety.

Adapted from Morin CM, Espie CA. *Insomnia: A Clinical Guide to Assessment and Treatment.* 2003. Kluwer Academic/Plenum Publishers.

BOX 12-5 *Cognitive Control Instructions for Patients to Help "Put the Day to Rest"*

PUTTING THE DAY TO REST

1   Set aside 20 minutes in the early evening, the same time every night if possible (say around 7 PM).
2   Sit down somewhere you are not going to be disturbed.
3   All you need is a notebook, your diary, and a pen.
4   Think of what has happened during the day, how events have gone, and how you feel about the kind of day it has been.
5   Write down some of the main points. Put them to rest by committing them to paper. Write down what you feel good about and also what has troubled you.
6   Write down anything you feel you need to do on a "to do" list with steps that you can take to tie up any loose ends or unfinished business.
7   Now think about tomorrow and what is coming up. Consider things that you are looking forward to as well as things that may cause you worry.
8   Write down your schedule in your diary , or check it if it is already there.
9   Write down anything you are unsure about and make a note in your diary of a time in the morning when you are going to find out about that.
10 Try to use your 20 minutes to leave you feeling more in control. "Close the book on the day".
11 When it comes to bedtime, remind yourself that you have already dealt with all these things if they come into your mind.
12 If new thoughts come up in bed, note them down on a piece of paper at your beside to be dealt with the following morning.

From Espie CA. *Overcoming Insomnia and Sleep Problems: A Self-Help Guide Using Cognitive Behavioral Techniques.* This edition first published by Robinson, an imprint of Constable & Robinson Ltd., London, 2006.

---

know many people who read in bed who are good sleepers, and so may not understand the instruction, and may not be motivated to apply it. Certainly, a rationale can be given, in terms of operant and classical conditioning theory, that serves to explain how these are differing conditioned relationships. However, by considering the synergy across the CBT approach it can also be clarified that there may be differences in personal intention in each case associated with the habit of reading. Whereas the intention of the good sleeper is normally to remain awake *in order to read* (and is unable to do so), the intention of the person with insomnia is normally to use book reading as a hypnotic aid *in order to fall asleep*. The good sleeper ultimately is frustrated in this goal, being overtaken by the homeostatic pressure for sleep, and has to put the book down, whereas poor sleepers are ultimately frustrated in their goal, not yet being asleep, and are overtaken by a vicious circle of mental and somatic arousal, which is a *pressure for wakefulness*. This example, therefore, reveals not only the cognitive behavioral interactions in CBT, but also demonstrates how CBT is best applied as a psychobiologic therapy.

Another example could be drawn from sleep restriction therapy, which is typically seen as a behavioral strategy. Yet, it too may be psychobiologic, having cognitive and biologic effects. Reducing the sleep window involves staying up late and getting up early, according to a preplanned, personally tailored protocol. Not only does that approach take decision processing out of the equation, it also, inevitably, leads to a series of what strict cognitive therapists would call "behavioral experiments"—tests that might disprove a dysfunctional mental hypothesis. What happens, if people follow the instruction, is that they fall asleep quickly (without trying to), that they find it problematic to remain awake leading up to bedtime (when they have to), and that they remain sleepy at rising time (when they do not expect to do so). However, it is the biologic imperative that permits sleep restriction to be effective, and homeostatic drive and personal sleep requirement guides the titration process in subsequent weeks.

A final example can be drawn from the emerging therapy area being applied to primary insomnia, and this is mindfulness-based therapy.[50] This so-called "third wave" psychological therapy is seen as going beyond a cognitive approach, which emphasizes (re-)evaluative strategies, to a more acceptance-based model that does not attempt to correct belief and attitude systems. In part, acceptance is seen as a therapeutic goal and outcome that enables the person to move on. However, in the context of existing *behavioral* strategies for insomnia, this may not be particularly novel. The quarter of an hour rule within stimulus control, for example, involves accepting that you are not asleep, not trying to fix that in any way but rather "giving up" trying to sleep and getting out of bed. This could be seen as a similar philosophical position to take in relation to wakeful experiences in bed. Explicitly paradoxical approaches also involve acceptance at some level, or at least adopting an entirely new relationship to this personal problem.

CBT-I: The Evidence Base

CBT-I has a large and extensive evidence base (spanning over 20 years) in treating insomnia as a primary disorder, and mounting evidence for the successful improvement of insomnia symptoms in the context of coexisting conditions.[26,51,52] Two reviews carried out by the American Academy of Sleep Medicine (AASM) taskforce revealed that CBT-I improves sleep parameters in approximately 70% of insomnia patients.[51,53] These clinical benefits reflect moderate to large effects for the following parameters: sleep onset latency (SOL), wake time after sleep onset (WASO), sleep efficiency (SE), number of awakenings (NAWK), and subjective sleep quality.[26] Effectiveness studies in primary care settings similarly report strong CBT-I effects, including those in which patients are already on prescription hypnotics.[43,54] Studies have also demonstrated maintenance of sleep improvements long after active treatment—indeed, up to 2 years follow-up.[55,56] Maintenance of gains is important given the persistent and chronic nature of insomnia,[57] explaining why CBT is the treatment of choice for the management of chronic insomnia. This was appropriately summarized in 2005 by the recent National Institutes of Health (NIH) state-of-the-science conference statement[27]:

"…[CBT] has been found to be as effective as prescription medications are for brief treatment of chronic insomnia. Moreover, there are indications that the beneficial effects of CBT, in contrast to those produced by medications, may last well beyond the termination of active treatment." (p.1052)

Direct comparisons between CBT and pharmacotherapy reinforce this conclusion: treatment gains are similar during the acute treatment phase, but medicated individuals tend to regress after treatment cessation, compared with CBT-treated individuals who maintain, or improve on, established gains.[55,58,59] CBT-I has been demonstrated to be effective with middle-aged and older adults,[60] and demographic and insomnia severity factors do not appear to moderate CBT-I response.[61] A growing body of work also suggests that improving sleep through CBT-I strategies may also positively impact the course of co-morbid conditions. For example, effectively improving insomnia in depressed patients was also found to

enhance the antidepressant response of escitalopram relative to a control group.[62] Finally, mounting data suggest that CBT-I can lead to improvements in daytime functioning and quality of life variables, providing evidence for successful treatment of the "whole patient," beyond simply nighttime symptoms.[43,63-65]

Despite strong evidential support and demonstrations of cost-effectiveness,[66] access to CBT-I remains limited. Thus, as *Espie*[67] notes:

"The challenge for CBT is no longer to prove its credentials, but to punch its weight. For at least a decade, CBT should have been a contender as the treatment of first choice for insomnia. In reality, however, it has had very little impact on the high volume of insomnia patient care. Indeed, it has amounted to little more than a patchy cottage industry." (p.1549)

Solutions to making CBT-I more available are currently being formulated and tested and include innovative health care models,[67] telephone consultations,[68] condensed brief CBT-I interventions,[69,70] bibliotherapy,[71] DVD and television broadcasts,[72] and Internet programs.[73,74] This work has important implications for how CBT research and evidence can be translated into everyday clinical practice.

Recent Developments in Cognitive and Behavioral Therapeutics

Two recent developments in the psychological management of insomnia warrant attention. The first relates to a novel intervention called intensive sleep retraining (ISR).[75,76] ISR is an in-laboratory behavioral conditioning treatment involving 50 30-minute sleep onset trials, beginning in the evening, approximately 2 hours before habitual bedtime. Within each trial the participant attempts sleep onset, and when the person enters *sleep* (defined as a 50% reduction in baseline alpha power in three consecutive epochs), the experimenter verbally intervenes to reintroduce wakefulness. This process ultimately induces significant sleep deprivation in patients, over time, resulting in a reduction in sleep onset latencies with increasing trials.

ISR rationale is based on the stimulus control model; attempting to recondition the bed, bedroom environment, and associated sleep onset factors, as reliable and discriminative stimuli for cueing sleep initiation (as opposed to arousal and wakefulness). It is presumed to work via a similar route as both sleep restriction therapy and stimulus control; harnessing sleep pressure as a psychobiologic reconditioning agent. It is clear to see, also, that ISR may have powerful cognitive effects on patients, particularly those who have nightly difficulties with sleep initiation. This may relate, for example, to the direct challenge of the long-held belief that *"I don't have the capacity to fall asleep like a normal sleeper,"* that is, in a rapid involuntary manner. The realization that sleep onset can occur very quickly and, indeed, several times in a row, may serve to challenge such conclusions and reinstate perceptions of "sleep ability."

It should be kept in mind that ISR is still early in development and future data, particularly from randomized controlled trials, are required to further evaluate efficacy and durability of response. One uncontrolled trial was recently published,[75] demonstrating promising results in terms of improvements in subjective SOL, WASO, total sleep time (TST), and SE.

Actigraphy data also revealed significant improvements in WASO and SE. Both subjective and objective sleep parameters remained improved at the 2-month follow-up assessment.

Another novel development in the field relates to the creation of an intervention based entirely on cognitive principles. As noted previously, cognitive therapies are typically delivered and evaluated within multicomponent CBT-I. Cognitive therapies have taken various forms, ranging from sleep education and low-level cognitive interventions to in-depth cognitive restructuring and paradoxical intention. These components are typically delivered alongside stimulus control and sleep restriction, making it difficult to understand and assess their individual contribution.

One recent paper described the development and implementation of a stand-alone cognitive therapy intervention.[77] Based on Harvey's[19] cognitive model, and using a mainly Socratic questioning approach, this therapy involved three phases (case formulation, personalized experiments with guided discovery, and planning for continued success while preventing relapse). The therapeutic aim was to reverse the five main cognitive processes thought to maintain insomnia: (1) worry and rumination, (2) attentional bias and monitoring for sleep-related threat, (3) unhelpful beliefs about sleep, (4) the use of safety behaviors that maintain unhelpful beliefs, and (5) misperception of sleep and daytime deficits.[78,79]

Data from 19 individuals with primary insomnia, followed up at 3, 6, and 12 months after intervention, revealed strong and sustained improvements in global insomnia severity, subjective SOL, WASO, and TST. Of note, strong effects were also found for daytime functioning, in addition to standard assessments of depression and anxiety. These results are promising because this "pure" cognitive intervention gives equal attention to both daytime and nighttime processes, providing a truly 24-hour interventional perspective. Clearly, formal assessment within the context of randomized controlled trials is required to further evaluate efficacy, as well as cost-effectiveness in terms of being a feasible alternative to CBT-I.

SUMMARY

CBT-I has a strong and comprehensive evidence base for effectively treating insomnia. Not only are CBT-I approaches effective, but they are durable, and tend to be favored by patients relative to pharmacologic options. Important work still remains to determine how CBT-I can be implemented in a cost-effective manner and to the widest number of poor sleepers possible. The development of novel cognitive and behavioral therapeutic techniques may further extend and enhance the psychological management of chronic insomnia.

REFERENCES

1. American Academy of Sleep Medicine. *ICSD-2: International Classification of Sleep Disorders: Diagnostic and Coding Manual.* 2nd ed. Westchester, IL: American Academy of Sleep Medicine; 2005.
2. American Psychiatric Association. *DSM-IV: Diagnostic and Statistical Manual of Mental Disorders.* 4th ed. Washington, DC: American Psychiatric Press; 1994.
3. World Health Organization. *The ICD-10 Classification of Mental and Behavioural Disorders. Clinical Descriptions and Diagnostic Guidelines.* Geneva: World Health Organization; 1992.
4. Edinger JD, Bonnet MH, Bootzin RR, Doghramji K, Dorsey CM, et al. Derivation of research diagnostic criteria for insomnia: Report of an American Academy of Sleep Medicine workgroup. *Sleep.* 2004;27:1567-1596.
5. Morin CM, LeBlanc M, Daley JP, Merette C. Epidemiology of insomnia: Prevalence, self-help treatments, consultations, and determinants of help-seeking behaviors. *Sleep Med.* 2006;7:123-130.
6. Kyle SD, Espie CA, Morgan K. "...Not just a minor thing, it is something major, which stops you from functioning daily": Quality of life and daytime functioning in insomnia. *Behav Sleep Med.* 2010;8:123-140.
7. Bootzin RR. Stimulus control treatment for insomnia. *Proceedings of the 80th American Psychological Society Annual Convention,* Washington. 1972:395-396.
8. Pigeon WR, Perlis ML. Sleep homeostasis in primary insomnia. *Sleep Med Rev.* 2006;10:247-254.
9. Lack LC, Wright HR. Treating chronobiological components of chronic insomnia. *Sleep Med.* 2007;8:637-644.
10. Bonnet MH, Arand DL. Hyperarousal and insomnia. *Sleep Med Rev.* 1997;1:97-108.
11. Richardson GS. Human physiological models of insomnia. *Sleep Med.* 2007;8:S9-14.
12. Spielman A, Caruso L, Glovinsky P. A behavioral perspective on insomnia treatment. *Psychiatr Clin North Am.* 1987;10:541-553.
13. Spielman AJ, Glovinsky PB. The varied nature of insomnia. In: Hauri P, ed. *Case Studies in Insomnia.* New York: Plenum Press; 1991:1-15.
14. Ebben MR, Spielman AJ. Non-pharmacological treatment for insomnia. *J Behav Med.* 2009;32:244-254.
15. Espie CA, Kyle SD. Primary insomnia: An overview of practical management using cognitive behavioural techniques. *Sleep Med Clin.* 2009;4:559-569.
16. Perlis ML, Giles DE, Mendelson WB, Bootzin RR, Wyatt JK. Psychophysiological insomnia: The behavioral model and a neurocognitive perspective. *J Sleep Res.* 1997;6:179-188.
17. Perlis ML, Smith MT, Andrews PJ, Orff H, Giles DE. Beta/gamma EEG activity in patients with primary and secondary insomnia and good sleeper controls. *Sleep.* 2001;24:110-117.
18. Perlis M, Shaw P, Cano G, Espie C. Models of insomnia. In: Kryger MH, Roth T, Dement W, eds. Principles and Practices of Sleep Medicine, 5th ed. 2010, Saunders.
19. Harvey AG. A cognitive model of insomnia. *Behav Res Ther.* 2002;40:869-893.
20. Espie CA. Insomnia: Conceptual issues in the development, persistence, and treatment of sleep disorders in adults. *Annu Rev Psychol.* 2002;52:215-243.
21. Espie CA, Broomfield NM, MacMahon KM, Macphee LM, Taylor LM. The attention-intention-effort pathway in the development of psychophysiological insomnia: A theoretical review. *Sleep Med Rev.* 2006;10:215-245.
22. Espie CA. Understanding insomnia through cognitive modelling. *Sleep Med.* 2007;8:S3-8.
23. Bartlett DJ, Marshall NS, Williams A, Grunstein RR. Predictors of primary medical care consultation for sleep disorders. *Sleep Med.* 2008;9:857-864.
24. Stinson K, Tang NKY, Harvey AG. Barriers to treatment seeking in primary insomnia in the United Kingdom: A cross-sectional perspective. *Sleep.* 2006;29:1643-1646.
25. Ancoli-Israel S, Roth T. Characteristics of insomnia in the United States: Results of the 1991 National Sleep Foundation Survey. I. *Sleep.* 1999;22:S347-353.
26. Riemann D, Perlis ML. The treatments of chronic insomnia: A review of benzodiazepine receptor agonists and psychological and behavioral therapies. *Sleep Med Rev.* 2009;13:205-214.
27. National Institutes of Health (NIH) state-of-the-science conference statement on manifestations and management of chronic insomnia in adults. *Sleep.* June 13-15, 2005;(28):1049-1057.
28. Vincent N, Lewycky S. Logging on for better sleep: RCT of the effectiveness of online treatment for insomnia. *Sleep.* 2009;32:807-815.
29. Morin CM, Gaulier B, Barry T, Kowatch RA. Patients' acceptance of psychological and pharmacological therapies in insomna. *Sleep.* 1992;15:302-305.
30. Edinger JD, Means MK. Cognitive-behavioral therapy for primary insomnia. *Clin Psychol Rev.* 2005;25:539-558.
31. Chesson AL, Anderson WM, Littner M, Davila D, Hartse K, et al. Practice parameters for the nonpharmacologic treatment of chronic insomnia. *Sleep.* 1999;22:1128-1133.
32. Morgenthaler T, Kramer M, Alessi C, Friedman L, Boehlecke B, et al. Practice parameters for the psychological and behavioral treatment of insomnia: An update. An American Academy of Sleep Medicine Report. *Sleep.* 2006;29:1415-1419.
33. Spielman AJ, Saskin P, Thorpy MJ. Treatment of chronic insomnia by restriction of time in bed. *Sleep.* 1987;10:45-56.

34. Espie CA. Overcoming Insomnia CA. *Sleep Problems: A Self-Help Guide Using Cognitive Behavioral Techniques*. London: Constable & Robinson; 2006.
35. Fogle DO, Dyall JA. Paradoxical giving up and the reduction of sleep performance anxiety in chronic insomniacs. *Psychother Theory Res Pract*. 1983;20:21-30.
36. Espie CA, Lindsay WR. Paradoxical intention in the treatment of chronic insomnia: Six case studies illustrating variability in therapeutic response. *Behav Res Ther*. 1985;23(6):703-709.
37. Morin CM, Espie CA. *Insomnia: A Clinical Guide to Assessment and Treatment*. New York: Kluwer Academic/Plenum; 2003.
38. Hauri P. Treating psychophysiologic insomnia with biofeedback. *Arch Gen Psych*. 1981;38:752-758.
39. Hauri PJ, Percy L, Hellekson C, Hartmann E, Russ D. The treatment of psychophysiologic insomnia with biofeedback: A replication study. *Biofeedback Self Regul*. 1982;7:223-235.
40. Hoedlmoser K, Pecherstorfer T, Gruber G, Anderer P, Klimesch W, Schabus M. A nonpharmacological alternative for the treatment of insomnia. Instrumental Conditioning of Brain Oscillations. 23rd Annual Meeting of the Associated Professional Sleep Societies (APSS), June 6-11, 2009, Seattle, WA. *Sleep*. 2009;32:A251-252.
41. Cortoos A, DeValck E, Arns M, Breteler MH, Cluydts R. An exploratory study on the effects of tele-neurofeedback and tele-biofeedback on objective and subjective sleep in patients with primary insomnia. *Appl Psychophysiol Biofeedback*. 2010;35:125-134.
42. Bray S, Shimjo S, O'Doherty JP. Direct instrumental conditioning of neural activity using functional magnetic resonance image-derived reward feedback. *J Neurosci*. 2007;27:7498-7507.
43. Espie CA, MacMahon KM, Kelly H, Broomfield NM, Douglas NJ, et al. Randomized clinical effectiveness trial of nurse-administered small-group cognitive behaviour therapy for persistent insomnia in general practice. *Sleep*. 2007;30:574-584.
44. Morin CM, Vallieres A, Ivers H. Dysfunctional beliefs and attitudes about sleep (DBAS): Validation of a brief version (DBAS-16). *Sleep*. 2007;30:1547-1554.
45. Morin CM, Stone J, Trinkle D, Mercer J, Remseberg S. Dysfunctional beliefs and attitudes about sleep among older adults with and without insomnia complaints. *Psychol Aging*. 1993;8:463-467.
46. Carney CE, Edinger JD. Identifying critical beliefs about sleep in primary insomnia. *Sleep*. 2006;29:342-350.
47. Carney CE, Edinger JD, Morin CM, Manber R, Rybarczyk B, et al. Examining maladaptive beliefs about sleep across insomnia patient groups. *J Psychosom Res*. 2010;68:57-65.
48. Lichstein KL, Fischer SM. Insomnia. In: Hersen M, Bellack AS, eds. *Handbook of Clinical Behavior Therapy with Adults*. New York: Plenum Press; 1985:319-352.
49. Espie CA, Lindsay WR. Cognitive strategies for the management of severe sleep-maintenance insomnia: A preliminary investigation. *Behav Psychother*. 1987;15:388-395.
50. Ong JC, Shapiro SL, Manber R. Combining mindfulness meditation with cognitive-behavior therapy for insomnia: A treatment-development study. *Behav Ther*. 2008;39(2):171-182.
51. Morin CM, Bootzin RR, Buysse DJ, Edinger JD, Espie CA, Lichstein KL. Psychological and behavioural treatment of insomnia update of the recent evidence (1998-2004). *Sleep*. 2006;29:1398-1414.
52. Edinger JD, Olsen MK, Stechuchak KM, Means K, Lineberger MD, et al. Cognitive behavioral therapy for patients with primary insomnia or insomnia associated predominantly with mixed psychiatric disorders: A randomized clinical trial. *Sleep*. 2009;32:499-510.
53. Morin CM, Hauri PJ, Espie CA, Spielman AJ, Buysse DJ, Bootzin RR. Nonpharmacological treatment of chronic insomnia. An American Academy of Sleep Medicine Review. *Sleep*. 1999;15:1134-1156.
54. Morgan K, Dixon S, Mathers N, Thompson J, Tomeny M. Psychological treatment for insomnia in the management of long-term hypnotic drug use: A pragmatic randomised controlled trial. *Br J Gen Pract*. 2003;53:923-928.
55. Morin CM, Colecchi C, Stone J, Sood R, Brink D. Behavioral and pharmacological therapies for late-life insomnia: A randomized controlled trial. *JAMA*. 1999;281:991-999.
56. Espie CA, Lindsay WR, Brooks N, Hood EM, Turvey T. A controlled comparative investigation of psychological treatments for chronic sleep-onset insomnia. *Behav Res Ther*. 1989;27:79-88.
57. Morin CM, Belanger L, LeBlanc M, Ivers H, Savard J, et al. The natural history of insomnia: A population-based 3-year longitudinal study. *Arch Intern Med*. 2009;169:447-453.
58. Jacobs GD, Pace-Schott EF, Stickgold R, Otto MW. Cognitive behavior therapy and pharmacotherapy: A randomized controlled trial and direct comparison. *Arch Intern Med*. 2004;164:1888-1896.
59. Sivertsen B, Omvik S, Pallesen S, Bjorvatn B, Havik OE, et al. Cognitive behavioral therapy vs. zopiclone for treatment of chronic primary insomnia in older adults. A randomized controlled trial. *JAMA*. 2006;295:2851-2858.
60. Irwin MR, Cole JC, Nicassio PM. Comparative meta-analysis of behavioral interventions for insomnia and their efficacy in middle-aged adults and in older adults 55+ years of age. *Health Psychol*. 2006;25:3-14.
61. Espie CA, Inglis SJ, Harvey L. Predicting clinically significant response to cognitive behavior therapy for chronic insomnia in general medical practice: Analysis of outcome data at 12 months post treatment. *J Consult Clin Psychol*. 2001;69:58-66.
62. Manber R, Edinger JD, Gress JL, San Pedro-Salcedo MG, Kuo TF, Kalista T. Cognitive behavioral therapy for insomnia enhances depression outcome in patients with comorbid major depressive disorder and insomnia. *Sleep*. 2008;31:489-495.
63. Dixon S, Morgan K, Mathers N, Thompson J, Tomeny M. Impact of cognitive behavior therapy on health-related quality of life among adult hypnotic users with chronic insomnia. *Behav Sleep Med*. 2006;4:71-84.
64. Kyle SD, Morgan K, Espie CA. Insomnia and health-related quality of life. *Sleep Med Rev*. 2010;14:69-82.
65. Krystal AD. Treating the health, quality of life, and functional impairments in insomnia. *J Clin Sleep Med*. 2007;3:63-72.
66. Morgan K, Dixon S, Mathers N, Thompson J, Tomeny M. Psychological treatment for insomnia in the regulation of long-term hypnotic drug use. *Health Tech Assess*. 2004;8:1-68.
67. Espie CA. "Stepped care": A health technology solution for delivering cognitive behavioral therapy as a first line insomnia treatment. *Sleep*. 2009;32:1549-1558.
68. Bastien CH, Morin CM, Ouellet M, Blais FC, Bouchard S. Cognitive-behavior therapy for insomnia: Comparison of individual therapy, group therapy, and telephone consultations. *J Consult Clin Psychol*. 2004;72:653-659.
69. Edinger JD, Sampson WS. A primary care "friendly" cognitive behavioral therapy. *Sleep*. 2003;26:177-182.
70. Germain A, Moul DE, Franzen PL, Miewald JM, Reynolds CF, et al. Effects of a brief behavioural treatment for late-life insomnia: preliminary findings. *J Clin Sleep Med*. 2007;2:407-408.
71. Mimeault V, Morin CM. Self-help treatment for insomnia: Bibliotherapy with and without professional guidance. *J Consult Clin Psychol*. 1999;67:511-519.
72. Van Straten A, Cuijpers P, Smit F, Spermon M, Verbeek I. Self-help treatment for insomnia through television and book: A randomized trial. *Patient Educ Couns*. 2009;74:29-34.
73. Ritterband LM, Thorndike FP, Gonder-Frederick LA, Magee JC, Bailey ET, et al. Efficacy of an internet-based behavioral intervention for adults with insomnia. *Arch Gen Psychiatry*. 2009;66:692-698.
74. Vincent N, Lionberg C. Treatment preference and patient satisfaction in chronic insomnia. *Sleep*. 2001;15:411-417.
75. Harris J, Lack L, Wright H, Gradisar M, Brooks A. Intensive sleep retraining treatment for chronic primary insomnia: A preliminary investigation. *J Sleep Res*. 2007;16:276-284.
76. Lack LC, Baraniec M. Intensive sleep onset training for sleep onset insomnia. *Sleep*. 2002;25:A478.
77. Harvey AG, Sharpley AL, Ree MJ, Stinson K, Clark DM. An open trial of cognitive therapy for chronic insomnia. *Behav Res Ther*. 2007;45:2491-2501.
78. Harvey AG, Tang NKY, Browning L. Cognitive approaches to insomnia. *Clin Psychol Rev*. 2005;25:593-611.
79. Kaplan KA, Talbot LS, Harvey AG. Cognitive mechanisms in chronic insomnia: processes and prospects. *Sleep Med Clin*. 2009;4:541-548.

Chapter 13

Pharmacotherapeutic Approach to Insomnia in Adults

DAVID N. NEUBAUER

Chronic insomnia is a common clinical condition that often represents a management challenge. Both physiologic and psychologic processes contribute to the regulation of the normal sleep-wake cycle, and a very diverse range of factors may represent vulnerabilities, triggers, and perpetuating influences on the symptoms of insomnia.[1] Further, the relative influence of these factors typically shifts over time.[2] Advice for improving sleep is abundant in popular health literature, numerous products are marketed as sleep aids, and selected medications are approved by the U.S. Food and Drug Administration (FDA) with formal indications for treating insomnia. Standard therapeutic approaches include cognitive behavioral therapy for insomnia (CBT-I) and pharmacotherapy, primarily with the FDA-approved insomnia medications. However, effective insomnia treatment may be complicated by the under-recognition of the disorder by patients and providers, misconceptions regarding insomnia causes and therapies, the frequent presence of co-morbid conditions, and limited access to medications and trained therapists.

Historically, many different types of sedating substances have been used to promote sleep. For millennia people have used fermented beverages and opium-related compounds specifically for their sleep-inducing characteristics. Several hundred years ago laudanum, an opium and alcohol concoction, first was used as a remedy for insomnia and it became a mainstay of treatment for centuries. In the mid-19th century, paraldehyde and chloral hydrate became available, followed in the early to mid-20th century by various barbiturates and related compounds. With the 1960s popularity of chlordiazepoxide and diazepam came other benzodiazepine-structured compounds specifically marketed as hypnotics beginning in the 1970s. These benzodiazepine receptor agonist hypnotics rapidly became the primary pharmacologic treatments for insomnia due to their improved risk-benefit ratio in comparison with most previous insomnia medications. The 1990s saw the development of a new generation of benzodiazepine receptor agonists sharing fundamental pharmacodynamic properties but not containing the classic benzodiazepine structure. These nonbenzodiazepine hypnotics soon became popular choices for prescribers. The only other types of medications approved by the FDA for the treatment of insomnia have been a selective melatonin receptor agonist (ramelteon) and a low-dose formulation of a histamine H_1-receptor antagonist antidepressant (doxepin). In general terms, the evolution of compounds recommended for treating insomnia has represented improvements in their safety profiles. Many of the historical compounds effectively promoted sleep, yet shared serious safety problems and occasional dire consequences.

The assortment of substances that people currently ingest with the intention of enhancing their sleep can be categorized into four groups. First are the medications assessed for efficacy and safety in people with insomnia and approved by the FDA for the treatment of insomnia. Second are FDA-approved medications that are not specifically indicated for the treatment of insomnia, but which may have sedating properties that promote sleep. The third group constitutes the FDA-regulated over-the-counter (OTC) sleep aids, all of which contain antihistamines as the active ingredients. The final category is made up of the diverse unregulated compounds marketed as dietary supplements and homeopathic preparations, and those employed as folk remedies. Mention also should be made of the frequent and misguided use of alcoholic beverages in the attempt to enhance sleep. This chapter will focus primarily on the pharmacologic treatment of chronic insomnia with the medications indicated for that purpose by the FDA. Issues related to the use of the other categories of compounds will be reviewed briefly, as these approaches are discussed in greater detail elsewhere in this volume. This chapter also will address prescribing guidelines, investigational compounds being evaluated as possible insomnia treatments, and key future research questions.

The unregulated pharmacologic approaches often are considered in the realm of complementary and alternative medicine, and may be available as formulations of single compounds, as with melatonin and L-tryptophan, or as plant extracts or other preparations including numerous individual molecules, as with valerian formulations.[3] These products may be synthetic or derived from plant roots, stems, flowers, buds, or leaves.[4] Often multiple herbal ingredients and possibly various vitamins and minerals are combined in a consumer product. In addition to *Valeriana officinalis*, plant-derived remedies for insomnia may come from such species commonly known as *kava kava, passionflower, skullcap, chamomile,* and *hops*. Generally these plant-derived products have not been well studied with regard to efficacy or safety in people with insomnia. The few efficacy studies typically have not demonstrated significant sleep-related benefits relative to placebo use. Melatonin, in contrast, has been studied extensively. Meta-analyses of melatonin as a treatment for insomnia have demonstrated limited benefit in the treatment of insomnia; however, there is stronger support of its value in populations with circadian rhythm disorders or in the treatment of jet lag.[5]

One potential problem with the unregulated substances is a lack of consistency in concentration and purity. Readers are referred to Chapter 10 of this text for a more detailed discussion of complementary and alternative treatments for sleep disorders.

Antihistamines are available as OTC sleep aids and by prescription at higher doses. Pharmacodynamically they are central histamine H_1-receptor antagonists. Histamine is a key wake-promoting hypothalamic neurotransmitter and the reduction of histaminic activity has a sedating effect.[6] The OTC sleep aids contain either diphenhydramine or doxylamine either alone or combined with analgesics. These antihistamines are relatively long acting and may be associated with next-morning grogginess. In addition to antihistamine effects, they exhibit postsynaptic muscarinic antagonism and therefore can produce anticholinergic effects, such as confusion, delirium, dry mouth, constipation, urinary retention, and exacerbation of narrow angle glaucoma.[7] The risk of anticholinergic effects is greater in elderly individuals and in people concomitantly taking other medications with anticholinergic activity. An additional concern with the continued use of antihistamine sleep aids is the potential development of tolerance to the sedating effects.[8] Although marketed as sleep aids, these compounds are not specifically indicated for the treatment of insomnia.

Available prescription medications that are not indicated for the treatment for insomnia, but which commonly are recommended for this purpose most typically are antidepressants, antipsychotics, and anticonvulsants.[9] Combinations of antagonist effects on histamine, acetylcholine, serotonin, and norepinephrine neurotransmitter systems likely contribute to their sedating properties.[10] Antidepressants most frequently prescribed for insomnia include trazodone, doxepin, amitriptyline, and mirtazapine. Quetiapine is the antipsychotic medication most often prescribed for insomnia. Gabapentin and pregabalin are anticonvulsants sometimes recommended for insomnia. Although these medications prescribed on an off-label basis for the treatment of insomnia may be beneficial for sleep onset and maintenance, and in some cases may enhance slow-wave sleep, they typically have not been well studied for their efficacy and safety in populations of insomnia patients. It is important to recognize that the risk-benefit ratio may be very different for insomnia patients compared with the psychiatric conditions for which most of these medications are indicated.[7,11,12]

FDA-Approved Insomnia Medications

At present, all of the medications approved by the Federal Drug Administration (FDA) for the treatment of insomnia are either benzodiazepine receptor agonist (BZRA) hypnotics, a selective melatonin receptor agonist, or a histamine H_1-antagonist antidepressant. Compounds recently investigated as possible insomnia treatments, including some currently being reviewed by the FDA, are discussed later in this chapter. The FDA-approved insomnia medications all have been evaluated for their safety profiles and have demonstrated efficacy in at least one type of sleep disturbance associated with insomnia. Randomized, placebo-controlled clinical trials for these medications have been performed with populations of healthy individuals and insomnia subjects, and generally have included both objective sleep laboratory and subjective

assessments. All of the medications have been assessed with short-term efficacy trials lasting a few weeks, although the drugs approved in recent years have also been evaluated with longer term placebo-controlled studies of up to 6 months duration and open-label safety assessments up to 1 year. The exceptions are the alternate delivery formulations of previously approved medications for which the FDA has not required new efficacy trials. Tables 13-1, 13-2, and 13-3 respectively list all of the FDA-approved benzodiazepine, nonbenzodiazepine, and two miscellaneous mechanism of action insomnia medications with their generic and common brand names, available doses, approximate elimination half-lives, indications, common side effects, pregnancy category, U.S. Drug Enforcement Agency (DEA) schedule, and the year first approved.

The medications discussed in this section have certain individual and shared potential safety concerns that are highlighted in the approved prescribing information for each drug. The FDA additionally has required that all medications approved for the treatment of insomnia include the same safety warning language regarding two issues. One relates to rare cases of severe anaphylactic and anaphylactoid reactions. It is recommended that patients exhibiting these symptoms not be rechallenged with the same medication. The other concern relates to the possibility of abnormal thinking and behavioral changes, which may include complex behaviors associated with amnesia, such as driving, preparing and eating food, making phone calls, or having sex while not fully awake. The warning suggests discontinuation of the medication if a patient exhibits any complex sleep behavior. Label warnings for insomnia medications also note the possibility of people feeling drowsy the morning following medication use and the recommendation not to drive or do other potentially dangerous activities until feeling fully awake.

Benzodiazepine Receptor Agonist Hypnotics

The general class of BZRA hypnotics has been the mainstay of insomnia pharmacotherapy since the early 1970s.[12] The BZRA hypnotics include the older benzodiazepines, incorporating the characteristic seven-member diazepine ring linked with a benzene ring, and the more recent nonbenzodiazepine compounds with alternate structures but exhibiting similar pharmacodynamic activity. The earlier hypnotics in this class tended to have long elimination half-lives; however, the more recent trend has been toward the development of short- to intermediate-acting compounds that minimize the potential for residual daytime effects. For several decades only immediate-release tablet or capsule formulations of BZRA hypnotics were available, but recently pharmacokinetic modifications have allowed extended-release and alternate delivery formulations that have been approved by the FDA. The onset and duration of action of hypnotics also may be influenced by the individual compound pharmacokinetic and pharmacodynamic features. The DEA categorizes all of the BZRA hypnotics as Schedule IV controlled substances, suggesting an abuse potential that is relatively low. Clinical trials of the BZRA hypnotics have not demonstrated the presence of tolerance to the sleep-promoting effects, but they may be associated with rebound insomnia during the first few days following abrupt discontinuation. These hypnotic medications generally are well tolerated, with the more common adverse events reported in clinical trials being headache, dizziness, nausea, somnolence, and fatigue.[13]

TABLE 13-1

Benzodiazepine Receptor Agonist Hypnotics: Benzodiazepines

Generic Name	Brand Name	Available Doses (mg)	Elimination Half-life (hr)	Indications	Most Common Side Effects	DEA Class	Pregnancy Category	Initial FDA Approval
BENZODIAZEPINE IMMEDIATE RELEASE								
Flurazepam	Dalmane	15, 30	48-120	Treatment of insomnia characterized by difficulty in falling asleep, frequent nocturnal awakenings, and/or early morning awakening	Dizziness, drowsiness, lightheadedness, staggering, loss of coordination, falling	IV	X	1970
Temazepam	Restoril	7.5, 15, 22.5, 30	8-20	Short-term treatment of insomnia	Drowsiness, dizziness, lightheadedness, difficulty with coordination	IV	X	1981
Triazolam	Halcion	0.125, 0.25	2-4	Short-term treatment of insomnia	Drowsiness, headache, dizziness, lightheadedness, "pins and needles" feelings on the skin, difficulty with coordination	IV	X	1982
Quazepam	Doral	7.5, 15	48-120	Treatment of insomnia characterized by difficulty in falling asleep, frequent nocturnal awakenings, and/or early morning awakenings	Drowsiness, headache	IV	X	1985
Estazolam	ProSom	1, 2	8-24	Short-term management of insomnia characterized by difficulty in falling asleep, frequent nocturnal awakenings, and/or early morning awakenings; administered at bedtime improved sleep induction and sleep maintenance	Somnolence, hypokinesia, dizziness, abnormal coordination	IV	X	1990

DEA, U.S. Drug Enforcement Administration; *FDA,* U.S. Food and Drug Administration.[33-37]

The BZRA hypnotics are positive allosteric modulators of γ-aminobutyric acid (GABA) responses at the GABA$_A$ receptor complex, which is a pentameric transmembrane structure with a central ligand-gated chloride channel.[14] GABA is the most widespread inhibitory central nervous system (CNS) neurotransmitter. GABA agonist activity allows an influx of negative chloride ions that promotes hyperpolarization. BZRA compounds interact with an allosteric benzodiazepine recognition site that typically is at the interface of α and γ GABA$_A$ receptor glycoprotein subunits. With an agonist present at the benzodiazepine recognition site, there is a conformational change that allows a greater number of chloride ions to enter the cell in response to GABA molecules leading to an enhancement of the typical inhibitory effect. The widespread CNS distribution of GABA$_A$ receptors may contribute to the sedating effect, although targeted GABAergic action within the hypothalamic ventrolateral preoptic nucleus likely plays a key role in promoting sleep.[10]

The pharmacokinetic properties of the BZRA hypnotics vary considerably. All are rapidly absorbed and should be beneficial for sleep onset. The elimination half-lives determine the duration of the sedating effect in promoting sleep during the nighttime, but also the potential for undesired next-day residual sedation and cognitive impairment. It is notable that the elimination half-lives among the BZRA hypnotics range from about 1 hour to as long as several days.[12] Additional pharmacokinetic and pharmacodynamic characteristics also may influence the onset and duration of action of these medications.

Benzodiazepine Hypnotics

The benzodiazepine hypnotics, all approved by the FDA between 1970 and 1990, are flurazepam, temazepam, triazolam, quazepam, and estazolam. All are available only in immediate-release capsule or tablet formulations. Estazolam, flurazepam, and quazepam have active metabolites. The elimination half-lives and corresponding duration of potential sedating effects range from the moderately short-acting triazolam to the long-acting flurazepam and quezepam. A meta-analysis demonstrated that the most commonly reported adverse events were headache, dizziness, nausea, and fatigue.[13]

Nonbenzodiazepine Hypnotics

The nonbenzodiazepine BZRA hypnotics became available in the United States beginning in the 1990s. The basic compounds available in the United States are zolpidem, zaleplon, and eszopiclone. Zopiclone is widely used in many other countries. Initially all were approved only as immediate-release tablets, but more recently extended-release and alternate delivery formulations of zolpidem have been approved. The latter include

TABLE 13-2

Benzodiazepine Receptor Agonist Hypnotics: Nonbenzodiazepines

Generic Name	Brand Name	Available Doses (mg)	Elimination Half-life (hr)	Indications	Most Common Side Effects	DEA Class	Pregnancy Category	Initial FDA Approval
NONBENZODIAZEPINE IMMEDIATE RELEASE								
Zolpidem	Ambien	5, 10	1.5-2.4	Short-term treatment of insomnia characterized by difficulties with sleep initiation	Drowsiness, dizziness, diarrhea, "drugged" feeling	IV	C	1992
Zaleplon	Sonata	5, 10	1	Short-term treatment of insomnia; has been shown to decrease the time to sleep onset	Drowsiness, lightheadedness, dizziness, "pins and needles" feeling on the skin, difficulty with coordination	IV	C	1999
Eszopiclone	Lunesta	1, 2, 3	5-7	Treatment of insomnia; administered at bedtime decreased sleep latency and improved sleep maintenance	Unpleasant taste in mouth, dry mouth, drowsiness, dizziness, headache, symptoms of the common cold	IV	C	2004
NONBENZODIAZEPINE EXTENDED RELEASE								
Zolpidem ER	Ambien CR	6.25, 12.5	2.8-2.9	Treatment of insomnia characterized by difficulties with sleep onset and/or sleep maintenance (as measured by wake time after sleep onset)	Headache, sleepiness, dizziness	IV	C	2005
NONBENZODIAZEPINE ALTERNATE DELIVERY								
Zolpidem Oral spray	Zolpi-Mist	5, 10	~2.5	Short-term treatment of insomnia characterized by difficulties with sleep initiation	Drowsiness, dizziness, diarrhea, "drugged" feeling	IV	C	2008
Zolpidem Sublingual	Edluar	5, 10	~2.5	Short-term treatment of insomnia characterized by difficulties with sleep initiation	Drowsiness, dizziness, diarrhea, "drugged" feeling	IV	C	2008

DEA, U.S. Drug Enforcement Administration; *FDA,* U.S. Food and Drug Administration.[38-43]

TABLE 13-3

Miscellaneous FDA-Approved Insomnia Medications

Generic Name	Brand Name	Available Dose(s) (mg)	Elimination Half-life (hr)	Indications	Most Common Side Effects	DEA Class	Pregnancy Category	Initial FDA Approval
Ramelteon	Rozerem	8	1-2.6	Treatment of insomnia characterized by difficulty with sleep onset	Drowsiness, tiredness, dizziness	None	C	2005
Doxepin	Silenor	3, 6	15.3	Treatment of insomnia characterized by difficulties with sleep maintenance	Somnolence/sedation, nausea, upper respiratory tract infection	None	C	2010

DEA, U.S. Drug Enforcement Administration; *FDA,* U.S. Food and Drug Administration.

sublingual dissolvable and oral spray formulations. The elimination half-lives and duration of action of the nonbenzodiazepine BZRA hypnotics range from the short-acting zaleplon to the moderately short-acting zolpidem and intermediate duration eszopiclone (Table 13-4). It has been suggested that improved tolerability of the nonbenzodiazepine BZRA hypnotics compared with the benzodiazepines might result from their $GABA_A$ subunit subtype selectivity profiles (although this connection has yet to be made in humans) and from their generally shorter half-lives.[15] It also has been argued that this newer generation of hypnotics has decreased potential for pharmacokinetic drug-drug interactions due to having multiple hepatic metabolic pathways.[16] The same meta-analysis reviewing the benzodiazepine hypnotics demonstrated that the most commonly reported adverse events for the nonbenzodiazepines were headache, dizziness, nausea, and somnolence.[13]

Selective Melatonin Receptor Agonist

Although several compounds with the pharmacodynamic properties of melatonin receptor agonists have been investigated for possible insomnia and circadian rhythm disorder

---

TABLE 13-4

Characteristics of Nonbenzodiazepine Hypnotics

Drug Characteristic	Zaleplon	Zolpidem Immediate-Release	Zolpidem Sublingual	Zolpidem Oral Spray	Zolpidem Extended-Release	Eszopiclone
Approved doses (mg)	5, 10, 20	5, 10	5, 10	5, 10	6.25, 12.5	1, 2, 3
T_{max} (hours)	1	1.6	1.4	0.9	1.5	1
Sleep onset latency	↓	↓	↓	↓	↓	↓
Wake after sleep onset	—	—	—	—	↓	↓
Total sleep time	↑ (20 mg)	↑	↑	↑	↑	↑

↓, decrease; ↑, increase.

indications, at the time of this writing ramelteon is the only medication of this type that has been approved by the FDA. The indication is for the treatment of insomnia characterized by difficulty with sleep onset and there is no implied limitation on the duration for which it may be used. The compound is a single (*S*)-enantiomer of a tricyclic indan derivative that is a selective agonist for the MT_1 and MT_2 melatonin receptor subtypes without significant interactions with other key neurotransmitter systems. Clinical trials employing both objective sleep laboratory and subjective assessments have established its efficacy in populations of adults and older adults.[17] Owing to the lack of any abuse potential, it is considered nonscheduled by the DEA.

Ramelteon is a nonsedating medication that is believed to promote sleep onset by attenuating the evening circadian arousal signal that normally helps to sustain wakefulness. Melatonin MT_1 agonists decrease the firing rate of selected neurons in the suprachiasmatic nucleus while MT_2 agonists influence the timing of the circadian system that strongly influences the phase of the sleep-wake cycle. The compound is readily absorbed and has an elimination half-life of approximately 2.6 hours, and it has one active metabolite with a half-life under 5 hours and sharing similar pharmacodynamic properties at a reduced potency.[18]

Ramelteon is manufactured as a single 8 mg strength tablet that represents the recommended dose for adults, older adults, and patients with mild-to-moderate chronic obstructive pulmonary disease (COPD), sleep apnea, and hepatic impairment.[19] Because ramelteon is metabolized largely through the hepatic cytochrome P-450 (CYP) 1A2 isozyme, it should not be used concomitantly with fluvoxamine, which is a potent inhibitor of the enzyme. The label suggests that it may be taken approximately 30 minutes prior to bedtime and that patients should avoid activities after taking the medication. Ramelteon is well tolerated, with the most common adverse events in clinical trials being drowsiness, tiredness, and dizziness.[19] It is not associated with discontinuation effects when patients stop taking the medication.

Patients with difficulty falling asleep or remaining asleep during the early portion of the night may benefit from the use of ramelteon. Although placebo-controlled sleep laboratory studies demonstrated improvements in sleep onset the first night when using ramelteon, patients may not experience the maximum benefits with the medication for several days or weeks. Patients should be educated about the medication characteristics, including the lack of sedation and gradual improvement in sleep.

Selective Histamine H_1-Receptor Antagonist

Doxepin has been among the sedating antidepressants that for many years have been prescribed on an off-label basis specifically for the treatment of insomnia. Doxepin originally was approved by the FDA for the treatment of depression in 1969. Although typically prescribed in antidepressant doses from 75 mg to 300 mg, it has been available in pill formulations ranging from 10 mg to 150 mg. The rationale for using doxepin to treat insomnia rests with the compound's very high selectivity for an antihistaminic effect, thereby minimizing undesired side effects from other receptor interactions at low doses. In recent years, 1-, 3-, and 6-mg doses of doxepin have been investigated for the treatment of insomnia in randomized, placebo-controlled studies with insomnia subjects. These low doses were found to be well tolerated and they promoted both subjective and objective improvements in sleep throughout the night.[20,21] The most prominent effects were on sleep maintenance with benefits persisting to the last hour of the night.

In 2010, the FDA approved 3 mg and 6 mg doxepin tablets for the treatment of insomnia characterized by difficulties with sleep maintenance.[22] The prescribing guidelines recommend the 6-mg dose for adults and the 3-mg dose initially for elderly insomnia patients. The total daily dose should not exceed 6 mg. The indication does not suggest any limitation on the duration of use. It should be taken within 30 minutes of bedtime. Due to the potential effect of food causing an absorption delay, it should not be taken within 3 hours of a meal. Somnolence/sedation and nausea were reported at rates 2% or higher in subjects taking low-dose doxepin relative to subjects in placebo groups. The contraindications are hypersensitivity to the ingredients, co-administration with monoamine oxidase inhibitors, and the presence of untreated narrow angle glaucoma or severe urinary retention. The prescribing information for these low-dose doxepin formulations does not contain the black-box suicidality warning present at the higher doxepin antidepressant doses. At these low doses, doxepin is classed as pregnancy category C. Because of an absence of abuse potential, the DEA considers doxepin to be a nonscheduled medicine.

PRESCRIBING GUIDELINES

Decisions regarding pharmacotherapy for insomnia patients should be in the context of a broad treatment plan developed following a comprehensive evaluation that has included a detailed history, review of systems, and physical examination.[9] Typically the recommendations for the use of medications to improve sleep are made along with educational plans incorporating sleep hygiene guidelines and possibly one or more components of established psychological and behavioral therapies for insomnia. The use of medications for insomnia should be monitored over time for efficacy and possible side effects and adverse events. Having patients maintain sleep logs or diaries can be very useful in assessing the efficacy of all treatment modalities. Special attention should be given to outcomes related to the initial chief complaints, which may have related primarily to daytime symptoms. Sleep logs and diaries may offer a subjective reflection of how long patients take to fall asleep, the number of times they awaken, how long they sleep, the quality of their sleep, how they feel the following day, and whether they nap. Patients can note whether they used a medication or other therapeutic activity to promote sleep on individual nights. The daily monitoring of sleep is useful because it helps avoid the tendency for some patients at their follow-up visits to suggest that their worst nights are typical of most of their nights. These logs or diaries can provide a broad temporal perspective that can aid in decision making about the continued use or changes in specific therapies. Patient evaluations may be supplement by actigraphy and polysomnography with selected patients. Polysomnographic studies are especially valuable in identifying possible sleep-related breathing disorders or movement disorders during sleep. Although sleep laboratory studies may be performed during the initial evaluation of patients having risk factors for these disorders, polysomnographic testing also may be useful for chronic insomnia patients who do not benefit from standard treatments in order to determine whether the presence of these disorders might be contributing to their sleep disturbance. Sleep laboratory testing also would provide evidence regarding those patients that might be diagnosed with paradoxical insomnia. Actigraphic monitoring over a period of 1 or more weeks can provide valuable supplementary evidence regarding a patient's sleep-wake schedule and an estimation of how much and when the person is sleeping.

Important considerations regarding the possible use of medications for insomnia include the patient's specific sleep-related and daytime symptoms; co-morbid conditions, including any medical, psychiatric, and sleep disorders; concomitant medications with special attention to possible effects on sleep and potential interactions with insomnia medications; past experiences with sleep-promoting medications; lifestyle routines, including typical work and sleep schedules; substance use habits, including caffeine, alcohol, and other abused substances; age; and reproductive status with a consideration of medication pregnancy categories. Elderly individuals and people with debilitating medical conditions generally require lower doses of medications prescribed for the treatment of insomnia. Potential sedating properties and other possible adverse effects should be reviewed carefully; especially when patients already are taking medications that might exacerbate these effects. Special attention should be given to hepatic impairment that might contribute to excessive medication blood levels and the need recommend a low dose. Costs and treatment availability may also be important factors. Some insomnia medications are available in lower-cost generic formulations, and some brand-name products may have higher insurance copay amounts. Pharmacy benefit plans may limit the number of insomnia medications and require prior authorization before they can be dispensed.

Although specific recommendations must be customized for individual patients, typically it is more appropriate to begin treatment with a short to intermediate acting BZRA hypnotic, ramelteon, or low-dose doxepin, as these medications have been reviewed for safety and efficacy and have been approved by the FDA for the treatment of insomnia. Also, these medications are less likely to promote daytime sedation and other residual effects that may be associated with several of the benzodiazepine hypnotics. If this approach is not successful, it may be followed by a trial with another one of the above-mentioned medications. In the context of co-morbid mood or anxiety disorders, the use of a sedating antidepressant may be beneficial, perhaps in combination with one of the approved insomnia medications. Sedating anticonvulsant (mood stabilizer) or antipsychotic medications may be useful in patients with appropriate co-morbid conditions. Based upon current safety and efficacy evidence, there is little reason to recommend unregulated dietary supplements, antihistamines, and older sedating medications with greater safety concerns, such as barbiturates and chloral hydrate.[9] In all cases, specific treatment goals related to medication use should be developed and reviewed with patients. Further, patients should be educated about their specific medications, including instructions regarding the timing and strength of the doses, and potential side effects and interactions.

Although the clinical trials evaluating the efficacy and safety of the FDA-approved insomnia medications have been performed almost exclusively with primary insomnia subjects, a large percentage of real-world insomnia patients have one or more co-morbid conditions that may affect their insomnia symptoms as well as decisions regarding pharmacologic approaches. For example, patients being treated for depressive and anxiety disorders often are prescribed antidepressants, which may be associated with either sleep-promoting or sleep-disturbing effects, depending on the class of medication. The use of a single medication, such as a sedating antidepressant, for the treatment of depression or anxiety, as well as to enhance sleep is appealing for its simplicity. Although this strategy sometimes may be effective, often the antidepressant sedating effects become an undesired daytime side effect, particularly when a standard antidepressant dose is prescribed. In recent decades selective serotonin reuptake inhibitor (SSRI) antidepressants have been the preferred medications in treating anxiety and depressive disorders; however, these medications are more likely to have neutral or negative effects on sleep. Advantages to prescribing separate medications for the insomnia and psychiatric disorders include the possibility of drawing from a wider range of medications and the ability to change medication selections and dosages independently according to the clinical circumstances. For example, a depressed patient with marked insomnia symptoms might be started on both an SSRI or related antidepressant and a hypnotic. The hypnotic may provide rapid relief of the insomnia, could help protect against a potential sleep-disturbing side effect of the antidepressant, and could be discontinued when no longer necessary while the use of the antidepressant is maintained. Analogous strategies may be relevant for insomnia patients with co-morbid pain syndromes, such as fibromyalgia.

The BZRA hypnotics and low-dose doxepin all are available in at least two dosage strengths, and ramelteon comes in a single dose. The lower BZRA doses are most appropriate for elderly patients and individuals with significant debilitating medical co-morbidities. Hepatic impairment generally warrants cautious use with low dosages. Rarely is it necessary to recommend doses beyond the instructions in the approved label for each medication. None of the insomnia treatment medications are approved for the treatment of children. During pregnancy there should be a greater emphasis on nonpharmacologic approaches and medications should be recommended more conservatively. The benzodiazepine hypnotics are pregnancy category X, while all other FDA-approved insomnia medications are category C. A more conservative use of BZRA hypnotics also is recommended with patients having histories of substance abuse. Ramelteon or doxepin may be more appropriate for these patients, depending upon their specific insomnia symptoms. Ramelteon has been evaluated in populations of patients with mild to moderate obstructive sleep apnea and in others with mild to moderate COPD with results showing no worsening of the apnea or oxygen desaturations.[23,24] The frequency and duration of insomnia medication use should be individualized for each patient, and the recommendations may change over time depending upon the patient's symptoms. The frequency options include nightly, intermittent (e.g., a few nights per week) and as-needed use. Often patients begin with nightly use for several days or weeks and then transition to intermittent or occasional as-needed use; however, some individuals benefit from extended periods of nightly use. A common scenario is a patient with insomnia in the context of a particular stressor who is able to sleep better with an insomnia medication that can be used less frequently over time. Insomnia patients complaining of significant sleep difficulty on a nightly basis typically require nightly medication use initially whereas those with occasional sleep problems may benefit from as-needed use.

The selection of an insomnia medication should include a consideration of the pharmacokinetic properties and label indications. Patients with exclusive sleep onset difficulty may do well with a short-acting BZRA hypnotic or ramelteon, and those with sleep maintenance insomnia may do best with an intermediate-acting hypnotic or low-dose doxepin. Medication adjustments may be necessary for patients who seem to be rapid or slow medication metabolizers. Presently no insomnia medications have been granted indications for middle-of-the-night dosing for when patients awaken and have difficulty returning to sleep, although short-acting hypnotics sometimes are recommended cautiously for this purpose. Clinical trials currently are underway with alternate delivery hypnotic formulations to support a future middle-of-the-night indication. If the sedating effects of a medication extend into the daytime, a decreased dose or shorter-acting medication may be more appropriate. If the medication duration of action is too short, an upward dose adjustment or switching to a longer duration may be helpful.

The BZRA hypnotics should be taken by patients at or very shortly before their bedtimes. These medications all may be associated with amnesia and ataxia at peak serum levels. There may be increased risk of undesired effects when patients take their sleep medications well before their bedtime with the hope that they will fall instantly upon getting into bed. Patients certainly should be advised not to drive or perform other hazardous activities after taking a hypnotic. None of the insomnia medications should be combined with alcohol. Generally the insomnia medications are absorbed more rapidly and demonstrate improved efficacy when taken on an empty stomach. A recent high-fat meal is likely to slow absorption considerably.

Until recently, all of the BZRA hypnotics were approved by the FDA with indications for the short-term treatment of insomnia. Among these hypnotics are the five benzodiazepines and the nonbenzodiazepines zaleplon and zolpidem. The recent sublingual and oral spray zolpidem formulations also have the same short-term indications as the original immediate-release zolpidem. Longer-term clinical trials, extended clinical experience with hypnotics, and pharmacodynamic considerations have led to changes in FDA indications. Several of the insomnia treatment medications approved in recent years (e.g., eszopiclone, ramelteon, zolpidem extended-release) demonstrated continued efficacy and safety in long-term, placebo-controlled clinical trials of at least 6 months. The approvals of eszopiclone in 2004, zolpidem extended-release and ramelteon in 2005, and low-dose doxepin in 2010 had indications with no implied limitations for the duration of use of the medications, suggesting that they may be used as long as medically necessary. Nevertheless, when patients are prescribed chronic use of hypnotics they should be monitored on a regular basis regarding continued efficacy and side effects, and whether a dose reduction, discontinuation, or switch to a less frequent dosing schedule would be appropriate.

Abundant evidence has demonstrated the short- and long-term efficacy and the durability of CBT-I. Generally the short-term benefits of pharmacotherapeutic approaches and CBT-I have been found to be comparable.[25] One recent study by Morin and colleagues[26] evaluated the 6-week acute treatment efficacy of CBT-I therapy in groups of chronic insomnia patients with and without concomitant pharmacotherapy (zolpidem). This was followed by a 6-month maintenance treatment phase in which the CBT-I alone group continued with monthly CBT-I sessions and the patients receiving the combined acute treatment were divided into CBT-I alone or CBT-I with intermittent hypnotic maintenance groups. CBT-I with the addition of the hypnotic resulted in added benefits for the patients during the acute phase of treatment; however, the best long-term benefit was found in the group in which the hypnotic had been discontinued during the long-term phase.[26]

INVESTIGATIONAL COMPOUNDS

In recent years a rich assortment of compounds has been evaluated as possible pharmacologic agents for the treatment of insomnia. Some are variations on medications that currently are available; others represent novel approaches based upon emerging neurophysiologic evidence regarding the regulation of sleep and waking.

Benzodiazepine Receptor Agonists

As noted previously, the majority of medications approved for the treatment of insomnia are BZRA hypnotics, with the most recently marketed being alternate delivery formulations of zolpidem. Studies currently are underway to support regulatory approval of zolpidem and zaleplon with different formulations, at different doses, or with new indications. In addition to the current oral spray and sublingual tablet, studies have evaluated inhalation and nasal spray drug deliveries for this class of hypnotics. At present, no insomnia medications are approved with indications for middle-of-the-night (MOTN) dosing, although this therapeutic strategy sometimes now is employed with short half-life hypnotics. Several new BZRA formulations have been investigated for MOTN use. Approval for MOTN dosing would require appropriate efficacy studies as well as sufficient safety data to assure a very low risk of next-morning impairment.

The nonbenzodiazepine BZRA hypnotics all have some degree of GABA$_A$ receptor subunit subtype selectivity relative to the benzodiazepine compounds.[14] All have greater affinity for GABA$_A$ receptors containing the α_1 subunit subtype and eszopiclone additionally has high affinity for the α_3 subtype. New investigational molecules have incorporated partial agonist activity, α_3 preferential binding, or a combination of these characteristics.

Melatonin Receptor Agonists

Although ramelteon remains the only FDA-approved melatonin receptor agonist, several other compounds with this pharmacodynamic activity have been investigated for the treatment of insomnia and circadian rhythm disorders.[27] A serotonin 5-HT$_{2C}$ antagonist with melatonin receptor agonist action (agomelatine) has been investigated as an antidepressant. Because agomelatine shares with ramelteon the pharmacodynamic property of melatonin agonist activity, it may also be effective for insomnia.

Serotonin 5-HT$_{2A}$ Receptor Antagonists

Antagonist activity at the serotonin 5-HT$_{2A}$ receptor is a pharmacodynamic action of a variety of antidepressants (e.g., trazodone) and antipsychotics (e.g., quetiapine) that sometimes are recommended to promote sleep and sometimes are prescribed for insomnia on an off-label basis. Generally these medications have other pharmacologic properties that make them less appropriate as insomnia medications due to the side effect profiles. However, several novel compounds with 5-HT$_{2A}$ receptor antagonism have been investigated as possible insomnia treatments. Variations have included 5-HT$_{2A}$ inverse agonists, a molecule with combined 5-HT$_{2A}$ and histamine H$_1$ antagonism, and a tetracyclic with 5-HT$_{2A}$, H$_1$, and α_2 receptor effects.

Histamine H$_1$ Receptor Antagonists

Medications that modulate brain histamine activity may be used in the future for the treatment of insomnia. Because histamine is a wake-promoting neurotransmitter, there is logic in the attempt to promote sleep with a central histamine antagonist. There is ample experience with the sedating effects of available antihistamines. However, the current OTC antihistamine sleep aids are not ideal for the treatment of chronic insomnia. A more selective and shorter acting H$_1$ antagonist might have a more desirable risk-benefit ratio. Another possibility might be a compound with agonist activity at the presynaptic H$_3$ autoreceptor that theoretically could promote sleep through a reduction in histamine-related stimulation.[28]

Orexin Antagonists

The two orexin (also termed hypocretin) neuropeptides and their key roles in stabilizing wakefulness were discovered in the late 1990s.[6] The recognition that excessively sleepy narcolepsy patients had very low orexin activity led to the idea that reducing orexin activity might benefit excessively aroused insomnia patients by allowing them to achieve enhanced sleep.[29] Several compounds that function as antagonists at one or both of the orexin receptors have been evaluated as possible insomnia treatments and at least two compounds have undergone phase 3 clinical trials.[30]

Miscellaneous Compounds

Among the additional pharmacodynamic approaches that have been considered as possible insomnia treatments have been calcium channel modulators, neurokinin-1 receptor antagonists, 5-HT$_{1A}$ agonists, and 5-HT$_6$ antagonists, corticotropin-releasing hormone antagonists, and adenosine enhancers.[31]

FUTURE RESEARCH QUESTIONS

In spite of the efficacy and safety clinical trials that have been performed with the FDA-approved insomnia medications, many issues regarding the pharmacotherapy of insomnia have not been adequately investigated.[25,32] The medication studies mostly have been acute trials lasting only a few weeks. Only the most recently approved new compounds have been evaluated in long-term studies. Although placebo-controlled clinical trials have been done with all of the approved medications, there have been few comparative studies among different compounds. Further, the populations studied have been subject to multiple inclusion and exclusion criteria and do not necessarily represent typical patients treated in clinical practice. Therefore, longer term clinical research with populations representing different age groups and patients with co-morbid conditions would be useful to help guide patient care. Further, very little research has evaluated the safety and efficacy of the antidepressants and antipsychotics commonly prescribed for the treatment of insomnia. Investigations also should better elaborate how pharmacotherapy and CBT can best be combined.

Beyond the simple efficacy studies with sleep parameter outcomes, there is a great need for research into the effectiveness of the pharmacotherapy of insomnia. Greater evidence is necessary regarding how treating the sleep disturbance of insomnia improves the daytime functioning and quality of life of patients. The potential beneficial effects of insomnia pharmacotherapy on health care utilization, absenteeism, and work productivity, and future health risks all should be explored in longitudinal studies. Finally, the safety implications of long-term medication treatment of insomnia should be more fully delineated.

CONCLUSION

There have been major advances in the pharmacotherapy of chronic insomnia with significant innovations in pharmacodynamics with new compounds and in pharmacokinetics with new medication formulations. The FDA-approved insomnia medications all have been evaluated for efficacy and safety, and have specific indications and labeling regarding their recommended use. Currently the approved insomnia medications include several BZRA hypnotics in varying formulations and a selective melatonin receptor agonist, although novel mechanism of action compounds are being investigated as possible future insomnia treatments. New drug development has been guided by breakthroughs in the neuroscience of sleep-wake cycle regulation. Future research should better characterize the effectiveness and changes in future health risks associated with insomnia treatment.

REFERENCES

1. Buysse DJ. Chronic insomnia. *Am J Psychiatry*. 2008;165(6):678-686.
2. Ebben MR, Spielman AJ. Non-pharmacological treatments for insomnia. *J Behav Med*. 2009;32(3):244-254.
3. AASM position statement: Treating insomnia with herbal supplements. *American Academy of Sleep Medicine*. 2006:Available from http://www.aasmnet.org/Articles.aspx?id=254.
4. Wheatley D. Medicinal plants for insomnia: A review of their pharmacology, efficacy and tolerability. *J Psychopharmacol*. 2005;19(4):414-421.
5. Buscemi N, Vandermeer B, Hooton N, et al. The efficacy and safety of exogenous melatonin for primary sleep disorders. A meta-analysis. *J Gen Intern Med*. 2005;20(12):1151-1158.
6. Saper CB, Chou TC, Scammell TE. The sleep switch: Hypothalamic control of sleep and wakefulness. *Trends Neurosci*. 2001;24(12):726-731.
7. National Institutes of Health. National Institutes of Health state of the science conference statement on manifestations and management of chronic insomnia in adults, June 13-15, 2005. *Sleep*. 2005;28(9):1049-1057.
8. Richardson GS, Roehrs TA, Rosenthal L, Koshorek G, Roth T. Tolerance to daytime sedative effects of H_1 antihistamines. *J Clin Psychopharmacol*. 2002;22(5):511-515.
9. Schutte-Rodin S, Broch L, Buysse D, Dorsey C, Sateia M. Clinical guidelines for the evaluation and management of chronic insomnia in adults. *J Clin Sleep Med*. 2008;4(5):487-504.
10. Fuller PM, Gooley JJ, Saper CB. Neurobiology of the sleep-wake cycle: Sleep architecture, circadian regulation, and regulatory feedback. *J Biol Rhythms*. 2006;21(6):482-493.
11. Roehrs T, Roth T. 'Hypnotic' prescription patterns in a large managed-care population. *Sleep Med*. 2004;5(5):463-466.
12. Walsh JK, Roehrs T, Roth T. Pharmacologic treatment of primary insomnia. In: Kryger MH, Roth T, Dement WC, eds. *Principles and Practice of Sleep Medicine*. Philadelphia, PA: Elsevier; 2005:749-760.
13. Buscemi N, Vandermeer B, Friesen C, et al. The efficacy and safety of drug treatments for chronic insomnia in adults: A meta-analysis of RCTs. *J Gen Intern Med*. 2007;22(9):1335-1350.
14. Bateson AN. Further potential of the GABA receptor in the treatment of insomnia. *Sleep Med*. 2006;7(Suppl 1):S3-9.
15. Rudolph U, Mohler H. GABA-based therapeutic approaches: $GABA_A$ receptor subtype functions. *Curr Opin Pharmacol*. 2006;6(1):18-23.
16. Hesse LM, von Moltke LL, Greenblatt DJ. Clinically important drug interactions with zopiclone, zolpidem and zaleplon. *CNS Drugs*. 2003;17(7):513-532.
17. Neubauer DN. A review of ramelteon in the treatment of sleep disorders. *Neuropsychiatr Dis Treat*. 2008;4(1):69-79.
18. Kato K, Hirai K, Nishiyama K, et al. Neurochemical properties of ramelteon (TAK-375), a selective MT_1/MT_2 receptor agonist. *Neuropharmacology*. 2005;48(2):301-310.
19. Takeda Pharmaceuticals North America. *Rozerem prescribing information*. 2005.
20. Roth T, Rogowski R, Hull S, et al. Efficacy and safety of doxepin 1 mg, 3 mg, and 6 mg in adults with primary insomnia. *Sleep*. 2007;30(11):1555-1561.
21. Lankford A, Segal S, Borders J, et al. Efficacy and safety of doxepin 6 mg in a 4-week outpatient trial of elderly adults with primary insomnia. *Sleep*. 2008;31(suppl):A256.
22. Somaxon Pharmaceuticals. I. Silenor prescribing information. 2010.
23. Kryger M, Wang-Weigand S, Roth T. Safety of ramelteon in individuals with mild to moderate obstructive sleep apnea. *Sleep Breath*. 2007;11(3):159-164.
24. Kryger M, Roth T, Wang-Weigand S, Zhang J. The effects of ramelteon on respiration during sleep in subjects with moderate to severe chronic obstructive pulmonary disease. *Sleep Breath*. 2009;13(1):79-84.
25. Riemann D, Perlis ML. The treatments of chronic insomnia: A review of benzodiazepine receptor agonists and psychological and behavioral therapies. *Sleep Med Rev*. 2009;13(3):205-214.
26. Morin CM, Vallieres A, Guay B, et al. Cognitive behavioral therapy, singly and combined with medication, for persistent insomnia: A randomized controlled trial. *JAMA*. 2009;301(19):2005-2015.
27. Hardeland R. New approaches in the management of insomnia: Weighing the advantages of prolonged-release melatonin and synthetic melatoninergic agonists. *Neuropsychiatr Dis Treat*. 2009;5:341-354.
28. Parmentier R, Anaclet C, Guhennec C, et al. The brain H_3-receptor as a novel therapeutic target for vigilance and sleep-wake disorders. *Biochem Pharmacol*. 2007;73(8):1157-1171.
29. Nishino S. The hypocretin/orexin receptor: Therapeutic prospective in sleep disorders. *Expert Opin Investig Drugs*. 2007;16(11):1785-1797.
30. Brisbare-Roch C, Dingemanse J, Koberstein R, et al. Promotion of sleep by targeting the orexin system in rats, dogs and humans. *Nat Med*. 2007;13(2):150-155.
31. Neubauer DN. Insomnia: Recent advances in pharmacological management. *Drug Benefit Trends*. 2009;21(10):266-271.
32. Krystal AD. A compendium of placebo-controlled trials of the risks/benefits of pharmacological treatments for insomnia: The empirical basis for U.S. clinical practice. *Sleep Med Rev*. 2009;13(4):265-274.
33. West-Ward Pharmaceutical Corp. Dalmane prescribing information. 2009.
34. Mylan Pharmaceuticals Inc. Restoril prescribing information. 2010.
35. Roxane Laboratories Inc. Halcion prescribing information. 2009.
36. Questor Pharmaceuticals Inc. Doral prescribing information. 2010.
37. Abbott Laboratories. ProSom prescribing information. 2006.
38. Sanofi-Aventis. Ambien prescribing information. 2009.
39. King Pharmaceuticals, Inc. Sonata prescribing information. 2006.
40. Sepracor, Inc. Lunesta prescribing information. 2009.
41. Sanofi-Aventis. Ambien CR prescribing information. 2009.
42. Meda Pharmaceuticals. Edluar prescribing information. 2009.
43. NovaDel Pharma, Inc. ZolpiMist prescribing information. 2008.

The Role of Psychology in Sleep Disorders and in Their Treatment

Chapter 14

ROSALIND D. CARTWRIGHT

A Short History

It is well known that the history of sleep medicine dates from the mid-1950s with the discovery of rapid eye movement (REM) sleep. This finding was originally hailed as an exciting breakthrough largely because of the close association of REM with the presence of dreaming: an unconscious mental activity with hallucinatory characteristics. The fact that this stage of sleep was easily and reliably identifiable in laboratory studies, and was also predictably regular in appearance and present in all normal humans, meant that dreams were now open to systematic study as never before possible. The importance of this study was based on the belief that dreams held the key to the causes of mental disorders, and the fact that the most prominent treatment method, psychoanalysis, rested on bringing the meaning of dreams into waking consciousness.[1]

However, by the time the discovery of REM sleep was published, treatment of the mental disorders based on dream interpretation had begun to be challenged. It was too slow, too expensive, and not verified by empirical research. The premise that it was necessary to retrieve the unremembered early childhood past and to expose underlying conflict was being replaced by more direct treatment methods: new pharmacologic agents and shorter psychotherapies designed to target present unhealthy behaviors. Two psychological treatments emerged at that time: cognitive behavior therapy (CBT)[2] and psychodynamic psychotherapy (PPT).[3] These methods had sharply defined differences: CBT aimed to change patients' dysfunctional thinking and PPT to bring unrealistic emotion-based behaviors under rational control. Both were focused on the "here and now" rather than on the distant past.

Meanwhile the investigation of normal sleep proceeded rapidly and with it came the recognition that sleep is subject to a number of new disorders. Whether these problems were primarily physiologic in nature, neurologic, psychological, or some combination, treatments needed to be developed for their control. Thus the standardized protocol for all-night, laboratory-based diagnostic studies was developed, the polysomnogram (PSG). From these studies the length and quality of sleep could be calculated as well as the percentages of time in the various stages of non-REM (NREM) and REM sleep. The aim was to study patients' sleep by objective measures to determine how long and how continuously they slept and whether there were objective indicators of disruption. Dream reports were not part of this single-night diagnostic test because such evaluation would require additional awakenings over and above those natural to the sleeper.

Dream studies did continue as research investigations. Reports were collected by interrupting each REM sleep episode in different demographic groups, as well as control awakenings from NREM sleep on an alternate night to compare the reports to those from REM. This work formed the basis for understanding the mental life, the psychology of sleep, between various groups and within individuals' reports by sleep stages and by early and late times of the night.[4,5] These studies proved that the mind is continuously active throughout sleep and that the reports differed in kind by arousal level (Table 14-1).

These findings resulted in a shift in perspective, from seeing sleep as an empty time of nonconsciousness to a state of continuing mental activity. A lively debate arose over whether all this mental life served some psychological function or was only random noise.

Among the various proposed answers to the question "Why do we dream?," the most popular was the "activation synthesis" model of Hobson and McCarley.[6] These authors argued that dreams have no inherent meaning or function. Their thesis was that the images recalled after waking from REM sleep are the result of stimulation of random brain activation from the pontogeniculo-occipital (PGO) spikes to which the sleeper adds some meaning from associations to these images as they awaken. The dream story, according to this theory, is constructed after the fact by the waking brain.

An alternative to this answer was the "tonic phasic" hypothesis of dream construction proposed by Molinari and Foulkes.[7] Here the characteristics of REM sleep were employed to account for how dreams are formed. The episodic (phasic) REMs, the conjugate movements (single or series of bursts) of the eyes, are the observable indication that one or more images are being experienced, and the pause between them (the tonic component), of continuing awake-looking electroencephalogram (EEG), along with profound loss of muscle tone, is responsible for adding meaning to the images activated from memory. Dream meaning in this model is inherent in each REM episode—the product of the sensory images and the narrative connecting thoughts. This model has had mixed support from research.[8]

There are now two contemporary hypotheses concerning the function of dreaming, both of which have been tested and supported by a good deal of recent research: (1) the mood regulatory hypothesis[9,10] and (2) memory consolidation.[11,12]

181

TABLE 14-1

Psychological Experience in High and Low Arousal Levels in Waking and in Sleep

| State | Arousal Level | |
	High	Low
Waking	Organized thoughts	Loose images
Sleep	Organized images	Loose thoughts

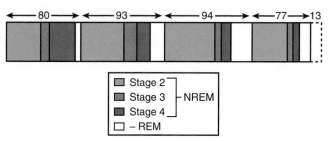

Figure 14-1 This illustrates that waking too early, after 344 minutes of sleep (5.75 hours), would cut off at least 13 minutes of expected REM if the 90-minute cycling were continued. (Adapted from Feinberg I: Effect of age on human sleep patterns. In Kales A, ed. *Sleep: Physiology and Pathology.* Philadelphia: Lippincott; 1969.)

They are not opposing proposals, as they could be combined in one more general theory of dreams. The mood regulation hypothesis states that the content of the reported dreams is related to unresolved waking emotional concerns of the dreamer and that the emotional tone of these concerns changes within the night toward a reduction of negative and increase of positive emotional tone from the first to last dream. This shift of mood within a night is responsible for an improvement in mood as reported and tested next morning. Tests of this model have compared healthy control subjects to matched sample subjects who are clinically depressed. These studies have demonstrated that the change within sleep in expressed mood is predictive of remission from mood disorders.[13,14]

The memory consolidation hypothesis predicts that efforts to learn new materials or skills prior to sleep will be followed by improved performance the next day, if sleep is experienced between the presleep and postsleep tests of the amount learned. This work has been conducted using both neutral and emotionally toned stimuli and has demonstrated that both the early NREM sleep and the following REM cooperate to preserve new learning in long-term memory better than equal amounts of wake time.[15] Also, materials that evoke emotional feelings are better recalled than neutral stimuli[16,17] and sleep deprivation interferes with this process.[18,19]

Research testing of these two hypotheses has supported that sleep plays an important role in the psychological functions of learning, memory, and mood regulation. This has revitalized the interest in testing the negative impact of sleep disorders, especially those interfering with the timing and amount of REM, on waking psychological health. New treatments to control the symptoms of sleep disorders now need to test not only their effectiveness in improving sleep but also the consequent psychological functioning in waking.

REM AND DREAM CORRELATES OF SLEEP DISORDERS

On the basis of the 60 years of research into the sleeping mind of well-functioning humans in comparison to those complaining of sleep or dream disorders, we now know the expected amount of REM sleep and the characteristics of dream reports in normal sleepers, and when these features are not normal, we also know what these alterations indicate regarding the possible need for treatment intervention. The emphasis on the importance of REM sleep to normal functioning so dominated the early research that only studies of the last decade have widened the perspective to recognize that disturbances of any sleep stages have the potential for negative effects on waking mood and behavior. Now, finally,

major theorists state all three states—waking, sleep, and dreaming—are intimately interconnected in maintaining psychological health.[20]

The normal proportion of time in REM sleep to total sleep time remains at a stable 20% to 25%, from adolescence until old age, providing that the amount of total sleep remains relatively constant when calculated to include naps. If the amount of time asleep is reduced (e.g., from 8 hours to 6 hours) the proportion of time in REM sleep will be more severely reduced than will the proportion in NREM sleep. This is due to the normal increase in the proportion of REM to NREM in the second half of the night. This means if sleep time is reduced, either voluntarily, or due to some inability to sleep as much as usual, the first hours of the night will always be higher in proportion of NREM to REM and the second half of the night will have a disproportionate loss of REM sleep that typically dominates the end of the night (Fig. 14-1).

Of what consequence is that loss? This question was raised in the earliest experimental work, which sought to learn the function of dreaming by suppressing REM sleep.[21] From this work we learned several lessons. First, REM is difficult to suppress—it has an insistence demonstrated by an increasing number of attempts to enter this stage during nights it is being aborted and an increasing proportion of REM above baseline for a few nights following the lifting of this restriction (REM rebound). The second finding is that loss of REM was followed by increased anxiety, and the third is that the brain has many ways to work around any loss (the plasticity of the brain). With REM loss some people adapt by dreaming in other stages of sleep and then do not show the expected increase in REM percentage when allowed uninterrupted sleep.[22] REM sleep, then, is the brain state most compatible with the experience of dreaming; when the brain is in high arousal and sensory input from the outside is restricted,[23] and when dreaming is defined by four characteristics:

1. A dream consists of hallucinated sensory images (most of which are visual but may also be of other perceptions such as of dogs barking, rain falling, and music playing) occurring during sleep.
2. These images are linked in a story-like narrative structure (although some claim that the linkage may be added as we awaken).
3. This dream story often contains an emotional component.
4. There is an accompanying loss of reality testing (acceptance of these events as if actually taking place even when they are improbable). For example, "I was delighted to find a money tree growing in my backyard."

TABLE 14-2

Some REM and Dream Abnormalities and Their Possible Diagnostic Implications

Abnormal REM	Criterion	Potential Cause(s)	Dream Abnormality
Early REM	<65 min	Narcolepsy Major depression	Poor dream recall Flat affect
Late REM	≥3 hr	NREM Parasomnia	?
REM interruptions	Short awakenings	RBD PTSD	Dream enactment Nightmares
REM % low	<15%	Medication effect	Short dreams
REM % high	>35%	Medication discontinued	Long elaborate dreams

NREM, non-REM; *PTSD,* post-traumatic stress disorder; *RBD,* REM behavior disorder, *REM,* rapid eye movement.

The reports retrieved from NREM sleep, on the other hand, are typically of a different nature. Rather than sensory perceptions:

1. NREM reports are most often of fragmentary thoughts.
2. The sleeper is aware that these are not actual events but are taking place in the mind.

These two types of cognition normally alternate throughout the night when sleep is normal in quantity and quality, long enough to sustain 20% of time in REM and with few disruptions in its overall continuity.

The warning signs in the diagnostic testing of sleep in relation to the hypothetical functions of REM and dreaming are shown in Table 14-2.

The sleep study may either confirm a preliminary diagnosis, or more often will reveal a sleep disorder needing to be addressed with a treatment plan.

THE ROLE OF PSYCHOLOGY IN SELECTED SLEEP AND DREAM DISORDERS

Insomnia

The most prevalent of the sleep complaints, insomnia, has been examined to find if there are personality types who are more vulnerable to this disorder. The common culprit in many studies is described as presleep cognitive arousal, in plain language "worrying."[24] Further, good sleepers feel they are in control of their bedtime thinking before they fall asleep; insomniacs report they are not.

Although there have been some controversial findings in studies of personality traits contributing to insomnia, "perfectionism" and "physiologic arousal" are the two most frequently noted. Those with excessively high expectations of themselves are more likely to "worry." An early study showed that those with self-reported sleep-onset insomnia, when awakened in the laboratory 5 minutes after the onset of established stage 2 sleep, report that they are certain they are still awake and having continued anxious and worry-related thoughts. This report was not found in the control subjects who slept well.[25] This finding suggests that treatment of sleep onset insomnia should address control of presleep obsessive worrying in order to reduce the chance that this will persist into sleep and have a disrupting effect on its continuity.

The importance of this approach as a treatment imperative followed the landmark epidemiologic study of insomnia by Ford and Kamerow.[26] Nearly 8000 participants were interviewed about their sleep, their psychiatric history, and their current mental health status on two occasions, 1 year apart. Those who reported chronic insomnia at both interviews were found on the second visit to have developed a new psychiatric diagnosis: Anxiety disorders or major depression were now found at a significantly higher rate than in those whose insomnia had resolved by the second interview or who were good sleepers at both testing points. On the basis of this surprising finding the authors called for a prevention effort to be mounted. If insomnia were treated promptly, they argued, psychiatric consequences may well be avoided. Since then, there has been much debate about the cause-and-effect order of these two—does insomnia predate the psychiatric disorder or is the emerging psychiatric disorder the primary cause of insomnia?

Given that all sleep disorders show some disruption of smooth cycling between NREM and REM sleep it is not surprising that those with chronically reduced amounts and quality of sleep will have measurable negative effects on the consolidation into memory of recent learning. This is especially problematic for those whose treatment program includes new learning directed to changing their presleep worrying behavior.

Very few studies have looked into the content of dreams in patients with an insomnia diagnosis. One such study by Ermann (published in German) is quoted in a recent review article by Schredl.[27] The main finding for the REM collected dreams of insomnia patients was they had more negative self-descriptions. This was confirmed in another study when the dreams were collected only in the morning following a night of PSG laboratory testing. This study also found more health-related dream themes and fewer positive emotions in insomnia patients than in healthy control subjects. Neither study tested the effects of these more negative dreams on the morning mood. If dreams in normal sleepers are an important intervening variable between an anxious presleep mood and an improved postsleep emotional state, what are the characteristics of dreams that contribute to bringing about this mood regulation effect?

A study of the dream reports of healthy sleepers[28] tested their mood before and after sleep using the Profile of Mood States (POMS) test.[29] Improvement in morning mood was related to the same three characteristics that had been established to predict remission from untreated depression:[13,14] (1) The dream stories included a highly disturbing concern of the sleeper documented on a presleep test; (2) the dreams also include directly expressed emotion; and (3) the dream story includes elements from older memories, such as a setting in a previous home or school or the characters are younger than their present ages. Thus, *what* is dreamed, not just the amount of REM time or frequency of the eye movements, contributes to sleep-related mood regulation in healthy humans. These three dream characteristics suggest that dreams that appear to contribute to the regulation of negative emotion do so by continuing in sleep mental consideration of some waking concern along with the emotion attached to it, and that this activates a network of older memories related to that concern, which then appear as dream images. When all of the three to five dreams of a night are recorded in order, they display a shift in the emotion from being predominantly negative in the first half of the night to being positive in the second half of the night. This fails to happen when sleep is too short to complete this typical shift (see Fig. 14-1) or when repeated interruptions interfere with this dream sequence.

Insomnia Treatment

Current research supports Morin's model of chronic insomnia as the product of reciprocal interactions among four major variables: dysfunctional thinking, maladaptive habits, a high arousal level, and their waking consequences.[30] This type is the most vicious of the vicious circle models of insomnia (Fig. 14-2).

Treatments designed to break into this cycle are roughly grouped as psychotherapy, behavioral treatments, pharmacologic treatments, and combinations of these. For the purposes of this chapter the focus will be on a treatment designed to improve both sleep and dreams by controlling those behaviors that delay sleep onset and interfere with overnight mood regulation. This short treatment program is made up of two components; the first is to prepare for sleep by reducing the presleep physiologic and psychological levels of arousal in order to shorten sleep onset time. The second trains the patient to shift the emotional tone of dreams from negative to those with more positive emotions.

Controlling Worrying. To address the presleep obsessive worrying, it is important to separate this behavior from bedtime. The patient is instructed:

1. Do the "worrying" well before getting into bed, in the late afternoon or early evening instead.
2. Spend 20 to 30 minutes writing a worry diary listing items of concern in one column.
3. Opposite each worry write a practical plan to resolve or make progress on handling that issue.
4. If one or more items are not solvable now, note that it is out of your hands at this time.
5. Close the book and recognize that you have organized your thinking about these issues and can now relax; you have completed your worrying for the day.

Reducing Physiologic Arousal. The next step is to reduce the level of physiologic arousal. This may be done by systematic muscle relaxation techniques and deep breathing or by taking a very hot bath 2 hours before a set bedtime.[31]

The hot baths also can reduce muscle tension, but the primary aim is to reduce the core body temperature, which in good sleepers drops at sleep onset and remains low until shortly before waking. Poor sleepers have a higher core temperature before sleep which remains high throughout the night. This makes sleep lighter and more easily disrupted.

1. Soak for 20 minute in very hot water. This both relaxes tense muscles and raises the core temperature. Adding bath oil to the surface of the water will help keep the temperature hot and moisturize the skin to prevent dryness.
2. Following the bath do quietly relaxing activities for the next hour and a half, such as viewing a movie or reading, but avoid horror movies, family arguments, or checkbook balancing. During this interval the core body temperature will begin automatically to regulate downward. This drop in temperature induces a sensation of drowsiness.
3. Going to bed then assures a shortened sleep onset time.
4. Repeat this routine every night for 2 weeks. Keep a log of sleep onset time and awake times.

Changing Dream Scenarios. Techniques for improving dream content include two methods. The first method employs practice in the waking state, called Imaging Rehearsal Therapy; this will be discussed later in this chapter. The second method makes changes directly in sleep and is referred to as the RISC method.[32] In the RISC method, patients are instructed that dreams are their own creation and therefore can be changed by them as well. Patients must, thereafter, remind themselves at bedtime to watch out for bad dreams. The method to bring about change has four steps:

1. *Recognize* when you are having a dream that has some negative feeling aspect, one that makes you feel anxious, frightened, helpless, or guilty, by becoming aware while you are dreaming that the plot is not going well.
2. *Identify* what it is about the dream that makes you feel uncomfortable, specifically the negative characteristics of the dream plot.
3. *Stop* the bad dream from continuing even by remembering that you can always force your eyes to open and so assert your control.
4. *Change* the dream emotion from negative to positive before going back to sleep by visualizing an opposite scene. This positive image should then be recalled on

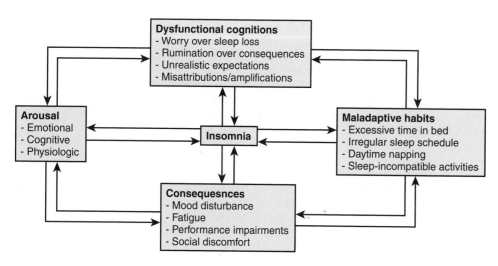

Figure 14-2 Morin's model of chronic insomnia as a vicious circle: chronic insomnia is the product of reciprocal interactions among four major variables: dysfunctional thinking, maladaptive habits, a high arousal level, and their waking consequences. (Adapted from Morin CM: *Insomnia: Psychological Assessment and Management.* New York: Guilford Press; 1993:57.)

awaking. Practicing recall of this positive image makes it easier to initiate changes in a dream without awakening.

This treatment targets dreams in which the dreamer feels helpless, weak, alone, sick, or frightened and trains the dreamer to imagine a scenario with the opposite quality. This method is best begun following a night in the sleep laboratory with REM collections recorded and transcribed for the therapist and patient to use in the first treatment session. In this hour the patient and therapist work together to identify the repeated negative aspects to be changed. The patient is then instructed to remember to change any negative dream experience to the opposite and to keep a home dream diary of recalled dreams on awakening for use in the next sessions. The RISC is typically a short-term therapy of 5 to 10 weekly sessions. Any step can be repeated as necessary. The hot baths, for example, can be resumed if the patient is again having a delayed onset of sleep.

Mood Disorders

One of the characteristic polysomnographic findings in patients suffering a mood disorder is a reduced latency to the first REM episode of the night, typically less than 65 minutes. This early REM has proved to be a robust marker also present in the first-degree relatives of depressed patients who have never suffered a depressive episode.[33] Thus, there is a strong evidence of a genetic component to this disorder, which is supported by the persistence of the reduced REM onset into periods of remission.[13] There is also a correlation between the measured severity of the depression symptoms and the shortness of the time to the first REM.

A negative correlation is also found between the severity of the depression and the degree of recall of dreams. This poor recall is a characteristic finding even when REM awakenings are made to elicit recall and these dream reports are most often short and flat in affect. One of the first brain imaging findings of psychiatric patients suggested an explanation for this result. Nofzinger and associates[34] reported depressed patients differed from control subjects in having more activation in the prefrontal brain areas during REM sleep than did healthy control subjects. The limbic system showed more activation in REM than in waking in both depressed and healthy control subjects. This finding supports the view that dreams have an emotional component, but the high activity in the prefrontal area in the scans of depressed patients was interpreted as being responsible for dampening their recall and lessening the emotion in the dreams.

When the severity of the depression is in the mild to moderate range, there is sufficient access to dream recall to use for training in the control of dreamed emotion as part of a treatment program. Beck and Ward[35] had noted that masochism is a discriminating characteristic of the dreams depressed patients reported when asked to recall a dream during an intake interview. This was in contrast to the dreams recalled by all of the other psychiatric patients being evaluated whose diagnosis was not depression.[35] In this way the dreams of the depressed resemble those of insomnia patients who were noted to have negative self-descriptions in comparison to the dreams of good sleepers. This persistently negative self-image of the insomnia patient, if not challenged and changed, may be what leads to the onset of major depression.

Another abnormality in the REM sleep of depressed patients is the frequency and density of REMs. These have been reported to be both abnormally frequent and to occur in extended bursts without the usual tonic periods between them. On the basis of the "tonic-phasic" hypothesis of dream formation, the too dense REMs would not provide the conditions necessary for developing a memorable dream story. There would not be the time between the images for the linkages to be formed from older associations.

Treatment of Mood Disorders

The consensus following extensive federally funded research is that when a mood disorder is severely disabling, the best course is to treat with a combination of antidepressant medication and psychotherapy. Just which drugs at what dosage will be most successful for any one case is still a matter of trial and error. There are many choices and often several may be tried before the one giving the best response is found. There are also several psychotherapy programs that have been tested for their efficacy in patients with mood disorders. Interpersonal therapy (IPT),[36] CBT,[2] and PPT[3] have all been shown to be helpful in reversing symptoms in a shorter time frame when coupled with a medication than when medication is the only intervention.

When the depression symptoms are mild to moderate, approximately 60% of patients receiving no formal treatment will experience a remission within 6 months to a year.[14,37,38] The study of depression following a marital breakup identified a group of variables predictive of who would be likely to go into remission without treatment. This ability to predict remission in the absence of treatment has been replicated in a second study.

The strongest predictor of remission from an untreated depression was found in the first night of laboratory dream collection. Those whose dreams showed a change from predominantly negative to predominantly positive dreams across the night were more likely to be in remission 1 year later, but those whose dreams became more negative at the end of the night remained depressed.[14] This pattern is in line with the finding that depressed persons have their lowest mood of the day first thing in the morning.[39] A second study over a shorter time period confirmed and expanded on the findings of the first study. Testing the depression mood scores before sleep and in the following morning, those who were in remission after 5 months showed a consistent trend to decrease their negative mood overnight and to hold that gain during the day and then to have a further sleep-related mood regulation the following night. Those remaining depressed showed a waxing and waning change of mood pattern; they had a small improvement in depressed mood overnight but failed to maintain their better mood during the day. An explanation for this difference appears to be that those who fail to remit without treatment have a stronger biologic basis for the depression and a poverty of dream construction within the nights. These patients are the depressed individuals who will need an active treatment intervention.

In research settings, patients who present with difficulty sleeping who are suspected of having a mood disorder on the basis of a previous history of episodes or additional symptoms, such as loss of appetite, a low interest in sex, or withdrawal from social activities, should be scheduled for two PSGs, one for the clinical screening and the second during a REM/dream collection night. If patients have poor recall of dreams with an increase of those with negative emotion at the end of the night, they should be referred for an active treatment program. Those who have good dream recall with an across the night pattern of mood regulation in their dream reports can be followed with a supportive program to assure the disorder does not become more severe. This would be a cost-effective approach to treatment based on research data.

Nightmares and Post-Traumatic Stress Disorders

Nightmares are defined as awakenings, most often from late night REM sleep, caused by strongly frightening dreams with vivid recall. Nightmares are common in young children and are rarely brought to a clinician as a primary complaint. The frequency of nightmares decreases as children begin to develop more waking coping skills. By middle adolescence there begins to be a difference in frequency by gender. Females report more nightmares than males by the age of 15 and this margin continues as a significant gender difference. Females actually show an increase in nightmare frequency between the ages of 10 to 19, but males do not. Psychiatric patients also have a high frequency of disturbing nightmares as adults.[40] Along with the implication that nightmares are more common in those who are more vulnerable to being emotionally overwhelmed, there is evidence of a genetic basis from twin studies. Some medications are also known to increase the frequency of nightmares, as is the withdrawal from alcohol. Neuroleptics, beta blockers, antidepressants, and benzodiazepine hypnotics all have been implicated in nightmare experiences.

Recent research on personality types has shown that a test designed by Hartmann[41] to measure the thickness or thinness of the boundaries of the mind finds those with thin boundaries, defined as those who have difficulty separating reality from fantasy, are more nightmare prone. This group includes artistically creative persons and those who are schizotypal.

Recently there has been an increasing effort to subclassify nightmares as idiopathic, recurrent, or symptomatic of post-traumatic stress disorder (PTSD). Not all those with troublesome nightmares meet the criteria of PTSD as this is just one of several symptoms that define the disorder. The PTSD patient also has *flashbacks* of the trauma that intrude into waking, *numbing* (a reduced responsiveness and avoidance of reminders of the trauma), and *hypervigilance* (watching out for trouble and an exaggerated response to sudden noises), but the repetitive nightmares are the most troublesome symptom. Certainly the PTSD diagnosis has become a focus of attention, as the veterans of our current wars in Iraq and Afghanistan return home. Although the estimated prevalence of this disorder is not firmly established, as few as 50% and as many as 70% of veterans have been said to show PTSD symptoms.[42] Of course, there are traumas other than those of war that have been followed by PTSD diagnoses. Accidents, rape, natural disasters, and terrorist attacks are some of these traumas. This prevalence has prompted a good deal of work to find effective treatments.

Treatment of Nightmares

The rush to be of help to the large number of military personnel led to a number of false starts. One of these was due to a failure to understand this as a unique disorder requiring careful diagnostic studies to differentiate it from a clinical depression, alcohol or drug abuse, and a lifelong history of nightmares. Often the first response, an antidepressant medication, was rarely successful unless there was evidence that a major depression was also present. Only recently have placebo-controlled studies shown that one drug, prazosin, is a promising treatment for post-traumatic nightmares.[43] This treatment does have a downside: nightmares have been found to return when this drug is discontinued.

The behavioral treatments have, in general, been more successful. There have been many variations and combinations of the principles and methods applied, often in samples too small to be able to show a significant effect, and with only subjective (self-report) criteria measures. This has left therapists somewhat at sea about what treatment to employ. A recent review found only 12 studies that met the minimal criteria of being randomized controlled studies of patients with no concurrent pharmacologic treatment, no current alcohol or drug abuse, and no major psychosis, and were not a single case study.[44]

The treatments reviewed varied in length from a single session to 6 weekly sessions and the follow-up ranged from 2 weeks to 18 months. The type of intervention also varied from daytime imagery rehearsal therapy (IRT), the treatment type most frequently used in controlled studies, to recording the nightmare and replaying it while practicing progressive muscle relaxation and deep breathing, to changing the nightmare directly in sleep (like the RISC method described previously). The criterion measure is typically the weekly or monthly frequency of nightmares as reported by the patient in a morning dream log. Other experimental treatments are hypnosis and eye movement desensitization and reprocessing (EMDR).[45] EMDR has less empirical support. The classical insight-oriented psychotherapy was found to be most appropriate for idiopathic nightmares, and not for PTSD patients. In fact, it was determined to be detrimental for those traumatized during the 9/11 attack on the Twin Towers who were better off moving ahead rather than reliving the experience.[46] Also exposure therapy, found to be helpful for those with phobias, is specifically discouraged for nightmare sufferers in the IRT protocol.

The method for carrying out the IRT program is outlined in detail by Krakow and Zadra[47] as a group program consisting of four 2-hour weekly treatment sessions with home practice in between. There are four components:

1. The first session is educational, aimed at relating nightmares to insomnia by pointing out how patients learn to avoid sleep (delaying bedtime), have fears of returning to sleep after a nightmare awakening, and use sleep-inducing substances, all of which they need to recognize interfere with good sleep.
2. The second component involves training patients in imaging while awake, specifically to practice having pleasant images for 5 to 20 minutes every day. Patients are encouraged to select pleasant experiences from their own life for this training to make it easy to elicit positive images under their conscious control.
3. The group next discusses how their identity has been affected by seeing themselves as being a nightmare sufferer and that they now must change to see themselves as a former sufferer just as a previous smoker can become a proud former smoker. This leads to the fourth and last session.

4. In this session, direct change of the disturbing nightmare is finally addressed. Once they have practiced calling up pleasant images, not the threatening nightmare, they are instructed to change the nightmare in any way they like.

Some of the IRT studies have selected a single type of patient (those whose nightmares followed a sexual attack); others included mixed groups of PTSD patients, lifelong nightmare sufferers, and victims of traumas who do not meet PTSD diagnostic criteria. Although the results of this model of treatment look promising, the studies have utilized small numbers of subjects and have relied on self-report measures. In view of the large number of potential patients just within the military, this is an area in which additional careful research should be encouraged.

NREM Parasomnias: Sleepwalking and Sleep Terrors

NREM parasomnias have not been a traditional focus for the clinical practice of sleep medicine, as these disorders were historically considered to be benign in children and rare in adults. Also they were episodic in frequency, and many believed they did not show distinctive markers in the standard PSG. This has changed recently owing to the publicity surrounding an increasing number of court cases for murder, sexual assault, and other episodes of criminal behaviors, such as breaking and entering and alcohol-related driving accidents, in which a plea of not guilty has been entered, and the defense claims the act was committed while the defendant was in a nonconscious state of a sleep disorder. Sleepwalking, which occurs with no memory or motivation for the incident, has drawn controversy regarding its validity but has also brought patients not yet in trouble with the law to ask for treatment to control their parasomnia episodes. As these disorders are covered in detail in other chapters of this book, this chapter will focus on the psychology of these disorders.

The more precise spectral analysis scoring method reveals that those with a sleepwalking history have abnormally low delta wave activity (not seen in the standard delta percent scoring) in the first sleep cycle in comparison to nonsleepwalking control subjects.[48-50] This may explain the proclivity of these patients to exhibit arousals during the first hour of sleep and their vulnerability to a variety of strange behaviors in the mixed sleep/wake state: sleep eating, fighting, and sexual activities that are performed without conscious awareness at the time or memory after waking.[20] This finding also suggests treatment possibilities; for example, clonazepam, the treatment of choice, may reduce delta sleep and frequency of arousals in the first hour, making for an uninterrupted transition from NREM to REM sleep.

The low delta activity is not by itself responsible for a NREM parasomnia episode, or these episodes would occur nightly rather than intermittently; there must be an additional immediate trigger. The one most often cited is sleep deprivation, especially when this is a consequence of a prolonged unresolved emotional response to some stressful event. An accumulated loss of sleep is typically followed by a "rebound," in this case, a longer period of delta sleep in the first hour of the night. An additional precipitant is an alerting stimulus during delta sleep, such as an external noise or internal event like a full bladder or obstructed respiration.[51,52] This stimulus sets up a push for more deep sleep and a pull for arousal, resulting in an abnormal behavioral state of partial sleep and partial waking.

Among the substances that can trigger a NREM parasomnia, alcohol is most often noted but caffeine and many antipsychotic medications as well as lithium and amitriptyline have been noted in many publications. Recently the newer sleep medicines zolpidem and eszopiclone have been required by the Food and Drig Administration (FDA) in the United States to carry warning labels citing a side effect of sleepwalking.

Case studies of the personality particular to the aggressive sleepwalker suggest there is no clear pattern of traits associated with this disorder, most likely because the number of cases is small. Frequently these cases are described as engaging in "uncharacteristic" behavior.[53] It is instructive to note the types of behaviors that are taking place. These acts appear to be motivated by the common basic survival drives: attacking the enemy, consuming food, procreating, exploring new territory, and protecting loved ones. These behaviors demonstrate that primitive drives appear to be active in deep sleep in an unsocialized form when the brain areas related to higher cognitive control (frontoparietal cortices) are less active than they are in waking and when the protective motor dampening effect of sleep is genetically impaired. If not for the frequent arousals from delta sleep that delay the onset of REM, the sleeper would most likely proceed into dreaming where these drives would be expressed in dream scenarios and down-regulated through being associated to older memories.

Treatment of NREM Parasomnias

Clonazepam, though not FDA approved for NREM parasomnias, has been successfully utilized to treat them. However, the psychological characteristics of aggression, inappropriate sexual behavior, eating of noxious foods, and wandering into danger suggest a psychological treatment may be a useful alternative. Hypnosis has been successfully employed to control these episodes,[54,55] with just one training session. The patient learns to exert self-control to sleep peacefully throughout the night or if aroused, to awaken fully once the foot touches the floor. As is true with treatments of other sleep disorders, a combination of the drug plus some psychotherapy is often used with a phasing out of the medication once control is established. Case studies have also shown that psychotherapy aimed to develop better methods of handling unresolved emotional issues reduces these episodes in adults.

Until very recently the understanding of the psychological basis for the dysfunctional behaviors in NREM parasomnia events has been limited by the patient's own lack of recall and the difficulty of observing them in a standard sleep study. However, in a new protocol, published by Pilon and associates,[56] consisting of two PSG studies with 25 hours of sleep deprivation between the two and the use of auditory tones with increasing volume to initiate an arousal during the second (recovery) sleep test, sleepwalking behavior has been documented to take place in 100% of patients with a history of this disorder and only awakenings into full consciousness in control subjects. Once this protocol has been accepted for establishing the diagnosis, the REM periods that follow could be interrupted to sample the ongoing mental activity in comparison to matched control subjects. This would be very useful for therapists of those patients referred for a more traditional psychotherapy.

PSYCHOTHERAPY TREATMENTS FOR SLEEP DISORDERS

The first step in treating any sleep disorder patient referred for psychotherapy is a good history of both the patient's sleep troubles and those of the immediate family, and the patient's psychiatric history. Next is a detailed inquiry into the current sleep problem, its frequency, severity, the degree to which it affects daily living, and what steps have already been tried to overcome the problem. All of this background will help the clinician decide the motivation of the patient to undertake a treatment program and the willingness to change this behavior. If a clinical sleep study has not been done, it should be ordered. If it has been done recently, a new study may still be ordered if the diagnosis is unclear or is needed to confirm a preliminary diagnosis and rule out any additional diagnosis. Because some treatments target dysfunctional dreams, an initial assessment may include a second laboratory night devoted to collecting REM reports.

Psychodynamic Treatments

Freud's original goal of psychoanalytic treatment is still the aim of many contemporary psychotherapists practicing PPT. This therapy is designed to bring the patient's ongoing unconscious cognitions, which have a negative effect on waking behavior choices, under the control of the more rational conscious mind. This method has been shortened and organized into a standardized manual.[57] It still has the aim of making patients aware, in the safety of the treatment session, of their misunderstandings and misperceptions and the long-lasting emotional consequences of these that undermine their current health and happiness. This is accomplished, with the therapist's help, by uncovering the connection between the sleep symptoms and dreams to the present problems, through the patient's associations to the sleep disorder and dream images. These illuminate the emotional memory networks involved in perpetuating these misperceptions of their self-concept and the deleterious effects of these assumptions.

Leaving aside the critiques of Freud's theory, there are practical problems connected with its implementation as a treatment for troubled sleepers. Many have difficulty recalling their dreams and it takes patience and some training to stimulate their recall. Whether dreams are self-reported in a home dream diary or are collected in the laboratory, the one most commonly recalled is the last one, even if all REM periods have been interrupted and a verbal report recorded each time. The last dream is most memorable by being the one closest to the morning awakening and is the longest, with the most complex structure, the most emotional punch, and the most bizarre elements and usually includes the highest number of dream characters. Thus, it may not be representative of the three or four others but is likely to be the richest one for therapeutic understanding. Still, the difficulty of recalling dreams still needs to be addressed.

In one study,[58] the sleep laboratory was used for just that purpose: to prepare patients to be productive in outpatient psychotherapy who were identified at intake as alexithymic or not being "psychologically minded." The aim was to test whether a training program to increase the recall and understanding of their dreams would reduce the early dropout rate

of such patients and increase their ability to engage in therapeutic work in the first 10 treatment hours. Three groups of 12 patients each were involved. Two groups spent four nights a week for 2 weeks in the sleep laboratory: group 1 had four nights of REM interruptions to collect their dream reports, and group 2 was a matched group that had four nights of NREM awakenings with collection of their reports. Both groups had practice in remembering and discussing these awakenings the next morning. All were asked: "What do you remember from last night?" "Do you see any way in which these reports relate to each other?" and "Do you see any way in which these relate to anything happening in your life now?" Group 3 (the control group) had no preparation training but went directly into therapy. Those with dream access training had a markedly lower dropout rate of 31%. The dropout rate of group 3 (the controls) was 62%. The training program clearly helped patients remain in treatment. But did the training help patients who stayed learn how to make use of therapy to understand themselves and make positive changes in their behavior? The first 10 treatment sessions were recorded. Transcripts of the first and tenth hours were given in pairs to be judged by raters who did not know which was the first and which the tenth hour or which of the interviews were from patients who had been trained and which were not. The ratings showed training in dream recall helped patients identify an emotional issue and to express it with feeling, a necessary condition for "talk" therapy.

The study aimed to test whether patients identified as having little ability to identify and talk about an emotional issue would learn from practicing understanding their dreams how to attend to their own inner thoughts and feelings and so better understand themselves in treatment. Other patients, such as those with a history of nightmares or a PTSD diagnosis, have no difficulty recalling their disturbing dreams—quite the opposite. These patients are less appropriate candidates for insight-oriented psychotherapy. In fact, the post 9/11 studies show this type of mental health intervention did more harm than good in prolonging the vivid memories and disturbed affect.[46] Other treatments have been developed for trauma victims in which the emphasis is not on understanding their disturbing dreams but in reshaping or suppressing the associated fear by recalling them while practicing relaxation techniques to reduce their arousal levels.[47]

Summary of Psychological Treatments for Sleep Disorders

Today there are two trends in the marketplace of psychological treatments. On one hand, there has been a proliferation of named brands with unknown differences between them (rather like toothpastes). An opposite trend comes from the pressure for evidence-based treatments and has led to spelling out the essential elements in treatment manuals so that they can be used for formalizing training in specific treatment techniques. This approach allows testing to determine which of the components correlate with overall efficacy of the whole package as compared to no treatment or to other treatment models. The two major brands, CBT[2] and the revised PPT[57] have been the subject of many studies of their effectiveness. A recent article[59] reviews these studies and offers some important conclusions that apply to treating sleep disorder patients whose sleep difficulty is part of a generalized anxiety disorder (GAD) or major mood disorder (MMD). The main symptom in GAD is chronic, pervasive, uncontrollable worry, which is also common to the diagnosis of insomnia and MMD.

The comparison of effectiveness of CBT and PPT involves measuring the therapists' adherence to the manual for each treatment and the relation of that to the outcome of the treatment. These studies have consistently reported the same surprising results. Therapists whose behavior conforms to the psychodynamic model as measured in the transcripts have more successful outcomes, whether the treatment offered was called *PPT* or *CBT*, and those who behave according to the CBT manual in their interactions in the treatment hours have little or no relation to the outcome. To clarify just what this means specifically, randomly selected transcripts of outpatient treatment hours were judged on three variables: the quality of the *therapeutic alliance*; how the therapist addresses the patients' *cognitive distortions*; and the level of *experiencing*, that is, the patient's dawning awareness of previously implicit feelings and meanings. In this study the degree to which the treatment focused on the patient-therapist relationship, *the working alliance*, and worked on deepening the *experiencing level* predicted patient improvement on all outcome measures; while the therapists' adherence to the cognitive treatment by working on the patients' *cognitive distortions* predicted poorer outcome in the sample of depressed patients. Success of CBT depended on *how* the therapist carried out the aim of working to correct the patients' cognitive distortions. If this were performed in a dogmatic, rigid manner—a misinterpretation of the good to be derived from delivering treatment "by the book"—it actually defeated that purpose.

The bottom line from these studies is that treatments that use the interaction between therapist and patient in the hour as a sample of the patient's actual behavior to be modified and understood, and pursue this by encouraging deeper levels of the patient's self-understanding, are more likely to have a successful outcome. These two are what have been called the "active ingredients" of all psychotherapies, regardless of brand name.

The Reason to Focus on Dreams

When any psychotherapy is being considered as the treatment choice for a sleep disorder patient, a sleep study with REM collections is useful for the therapist by providing data of a different order than the patient is typically able to verbalize initially about themselves. If a full laboratory collection is not available, a home dream diary can substitute for examining the patient's ongoing concerns and repeating themes they may not be aware of and can serve as a vehicle for deepening their self-understanding. How to work with dreams in short-term treatment has been outlined in two recent books. The Hill method[60] emphasizes a principle that applies to CBT as well: therapists should avoid offering their own interpretation but act as a prompting guide: "How did you feel at that point?" and "Did it remind you of anything?" The RISC method,[32] discussed earlier, works to identify the organizing concepts, called *dream dimensions*, each of which has a paired opposite aspect for defining the self and others, such as warm-cold, smart-dumb, trustworthy-dangerous. These are the keys to understanding the way the patient habitually organizes his or her experience. Once identified, these concepts are used to explore ways in which negative self-references can be replaced by the more positive descriptors.

In a recent review of CBT and PPT,[61] the authors point out that the criteria of effective psychotherapy need to go beyond relief of initial symptoms to include growth in positive indicators such as empathy for others, resolution of past painful experiences, contentment in life's activities, and satisfaction in pursuing long-term goals. These may be apparent in dreams before they are evident in the treatment sessions. The investigation of these more subtle changes as a product of psychotherapeutic treatments and determining which patients can best benefit from this treatment await further studies.

SUMMARY

If there is one point that stands out from this review of the current state of the psychological causation and treatments for sleep disorders, it is that sleep disorders occur in an interactive mind/body system. With this as the basic unit of concern, the division between the psychology of sleep and that of waking is arbitrary and better understood as an interactive continuum. The psychological traits and the more immediate states of the waking patient influence the psychological functioning both during and following sleep. What is on the mind before sleep has both cognitive content and an emotional weight. When this is an unresolved issue with a disturbing negative affect, a worry for example, it is likely to be continued into NREM sleep. The strength of the emotional value influences the nature of the ensuing sleep. That memory continues to be active until REM sleep where it stimulates associated memories from long-term networks stored as condensed images. This interaction of NREM thoughts and REM dreams repeats three or four times within a night. The late night dreams display more generalized remote memory components. The degree to which this results in some resolution of the negative emotional component depends on the integrity of the sleep and the content of the memories available from past experiences. When sleep is disrupted by awakenings, this process is also disrupted. When the older memories associated to the present concern are as negative in tone as the current concern, the following waking emotional state will not be changed by morning. Targeted psychotherapy can be focused here. If the memories associated are very strong, they may awaken the sleeper in a nightmare, which may prevent the completion of the mood regulation process and require remedial treatment.

For most people, the progression from dream to dream proceeds with more faded negative affect[62,63] followed by a reduction in the negative mood next morning. The healthy mood regulatory function of dreams is part of the reason why good sleep is followed by good psychological functioning. This is seen in better retention of new learning, better decisions, and a more positive outlook. It also contributes to the ability to "spontaneously" remit from mild or moderate MMD over time and to profit from various short-term psychological treatments with similar "active ingredients"—the provision of a nonjudgmental, emotionally supportive relationship within which the patient is safe to explore what the CBT model calls "distorted thinking" and PPT describes as "unconscious defenses against unacceptable negative wishes." When a dream transcript alerts the sleep clinician that the regulatory process is not occurring, an active intervention is needed. How the patient-therapist relationship is conducted differs in the two psychological manuals. If the therapist behaves in ways that frees the patient from disabling fears so that the patient is no longer limited by irrational interpretations of self and others, the patient will not only experience symptom relief but an expanding sense of confidence for the future.

Psychotherapy is not the only treatment for sleep disorders with a strong psychological basis. However, it has been underutilized in spite of being proved effective for GAD and MMD patients, who often present to sleep clinics with "I'm having trouble sleeping." Many sleep clinicians are unfamiliar with the various nonmedication options. The access to REM sleep reports in these cases is a tremendous asset to both patient and therapist. This need can be met by adding a request for the technician to ask at the end of a diagnostic study "What was going on in your mind just before I called you?" This inquiry would provide valuable additional information at no additional cost. If this were standard procedure, and patients were instructed before sleep to expect this, a large database could easily be collected for future understanding and treatment of some of the sleep disorders discussed here.

REFERENCES

1. Freud S. The psychology of the dream processes. In: Freud S, ed. *The Interpretation of Dreams*. New York: Basic Books; 1955:509-610.
2. Beck A. *Cognitive therapy and the emotional disorders*. New York: Penguin Books; 1979:233–262.
3. Luborsky L. *Principles of psychoanalytic psychotherapy: A manual for supportive-expressive treatment*. New York: Basic Books; 1984.
4. Monroe L, Rechtschaffen A, Foulkes D, et al. Discriminability of REM and NREM reports. *J Abnorm Psychol*. 1965;2:456-460.
5. Foulkes D. Dream reports from different stages of sleep. *J Abnorm Soc Psychol*. 1962;65:14-28.
6. Hobson JA, McCarley R. The brain as a dream-state generator: An activation-synthesis hypothesis of the dream process. *Am J Psychiatry*. 1977;134:1335-1348.
7. Molinari S, Foulkes D. Tonic and phasic events during sleep: Psychological correlates and implications. *Percept Motor Skills*. 1969;29:343-368.
8. Pivik T. Tonic states and phasic events in relation to sleep mentation. In: Ellman S, Antrobus J, eds. *The Mind in Sleep: Psychology and Psychophysiology*. 2nd ed. New York: John Wiley; 1991:214-247.
9. Kramer M. The selective mood regulatory function of dreaming: An update and revision. In: Moffitt A, Kramer M, Hoffman, eds. *The Functions of Dreaming*. Albany: State University of New York Press; 1993:139-195.
10. Cartwright R. Dreaming as a Mood Regulation System. In: Kryger M, Roth T, Dement W, eds. *Principles and Practice of Sleep Medicine*. 4th ed. Philadelphia: Elsevier Saunders; 2005:565-572.
11. Walker M, Stickgold R. Sleep dependent learning and memory consolidation. *Neuron*. 2004;44:121-133.
12. Rasch B, Born J. Reactivation and consolidation of memory during sleep. *Curr Direct Psychol Sci*. 2008;17:188-192.
13. Cartwright R, Young M, Mercer P, et al. The role of REM sleep and dream variables in the prediction of remission from depression. *Psychiatry Res*. 1998;80:249-255.
14. Cartwright R, Baehr E, Kirkby J, et al. REM sleep reduction mood regulation and remission from untreated depression. *Psychiatry Res*. 2003;121:159-167.
15. Wagner U, Gais S, Born J. Emotional memory formation is enhanced across sleep intervals with high amounts of rapid eye movement sleep. *Learning Memory*. 2001;8:112-119.
16. Wagner U, Hallschmid M, Rasch B, et al. Brief sleep after learning keeps emotional memories alive for years. *Biol Psychiatry*. 2006;60:788-790.
17. Payne J, Stickgold R, Swanberg K, et al. Sleep preferentially enhances memory for emotional components of scenes. *Psychol Sci*. 2008;19:781-788.
18. Yoo S-S, Hu P, Gujar N, et al. A deficit in the ability to form new human memories without sleep. *Nat Neurosci*. 2007;10:385-392.

19. Lara-Carrasco J, Nielsen T, Salomonova E, et al. Over-night emotional adaptation to negative stimuli is altered by REM sleep deprivation and is correlated with intervening dream emotions. *J Sleep Res*. 2009;18:178-187.
20. Cartwright R. *The Twenty-four Hour Mind: The Role of Sleep and Dreaming in Our Emotional Lives*. New York: Oxford University Press; 2010.
21. Dement W. The effect of dream deprivation. *Science*. 1960;131:255-264.
22. Cartwright R, Monroe L, Palmer C. Individual differences in response to REM deprivation. *Arch Gen Psychiatry*. 1967;16:297-303.
23. Antrobus J. Dreaming: Cortical activation and perceptual thresholds. *J Mind Behav*. 1986;7:193-212.
24. Van de Laar M, Verbeek I, Pevernagle D, et al. The role of personality traits in insomnia. *Sleep Med Rev*. 2010;14:61-68.
25. Borkevec T, Lane T, Van Oot P. Phenomenology of sleep among insomniacs and good sleepers: Wakefulness experience when cortically asleep. *J Abnorm Psychol*. 1981;90:607-609.
26. Ford D, Kamerow D. Epidemiologic study of sleep disturbances and psychiatric disorders: An opportunity for prevention. *JAMA*. 1989;262:1479-1484.
27. Schredl M. Dreams in patients with sleep disorders. *Sleep Med Rev*. 2009;13:215-221.
28. Cartwright R, Luten A, Young M, et al. Role of REM sleep and dream affect in overnight mood regulation: A study of normals. *Psychiatry Res*. 1998;81:1-8.
29. McNair D, Lorr M, Droppleman L. *Profile of mood states*. San Diego: Educational and Testing Service; 1981.
30. Morin C. *Insomnia: Psychological Assessment and Management*. New York: Guilford Press; 1993.
31. Horne J, Shackell B. Slow wave sleep elevations after body heating: Proximity to sleep and effects of aspirin. *Sleep*. 1987;10:383-392.
32. Cartwright R, Lamberg L. *Crisis Dreaming: Using Your Dreams to Solve Your Problems*. New York: ASJA Press; 2000:32–51.
33. Giles D, Roffwarg H, Rush AJ. REM latency concordance in depressed family members. *Biol Psychiatry*. 1987;22:910-914.
34. Nofzinger E, Buysse D, Germain A. Increased activation of anterior paralimbic and executive cortex from waking to rapid eye movement sleep in depression. *Arch Gen Psychiatry*. 2004;61:695-702.
35. Beck A, Ward C. Dreams of depressed patients: Characteristic themes in manifest dreams. *Arch Gen Psychiatry*. 1961;5:462-467.
36. Klerman G, Weissman M, Rounsaville B, et al. *Interpersonal Psychotherapy of Depression*. New York: Basic Books; 1984.
37. Clayton P, Halikas J, Maurice W. The depression of widowhood. *Br J Psychiatry*. 1972;120:71-77.
38. Cartwright R, Agargun M, Kirkby J, et al. The relation of dreams to waking concerns. *Psychiatry Res*. 2006;141:261-270.
39. Hamilton M. Development of a rating scale for primary depressive illness. *Br J Soc Clin Psychol*. 1967;6:278-296.
40. Nielsen T, Zadra A. Nightmares and other common dream disturbances. In: Kryger M, Roth T, Dement W, eds. *Principles and Practice of Sleep Medicine*. 4th ed. Philadelphia: Elsevier Saunders; 2005:926-935.
41. Hartmann E. *Boundaries in the Mind: A New Psychology of Personality*. New York: Basic Books; 1991.
42. Spoormaker V, Montgomery P. Disturbed sleep in post-traumatic stress disorder: Secondary symptom or core feature? *Sleep Med Rev*. 2008;12:169-184.
43. Raskind M, Peskind E, Hoff D. A parallel group placebo controlled study of prazosin for trauma nightmares and sleep disturbance in combat veterans with post-traumatic stress disorder. *Biol Psychiatry*. 2007;8:928-934.
44. Lancee J, Spoormaker V, Krakow B, et al. A systematic review of cognitive-behavioral treatment for nightmares: Toward a well-established treatment. *J Clin Sleep Med*. 2008;4:475-480.
45. Shapiro F. Efficacy of eye movement desensitization procedure in treatment of traumatic memories. *J Traum Stress*. 1989;2:199-223.
46. Seeley K. *Therapy After Terror: 9/11, Psychotherapists, and Mental Health*. New York: Cambridge University Press; 2008: [Previously published as: Imagery rehearsal therapy. *Behav Sleep Med*. 2006;4:45-70.].
47. Karkow B, Zadra A. Clinical management of chronic nightmares: Imagery rehearsal therapy. *Behav Sleep Med*. 2006;4:45-70.
48. Espa E, Ondze B, Deglise P, et al. Sleep architecture, slow-wave activity, and sleep spindles in adult patients with sleepwalking and sleep terrors. *Clin Neurophysiol*. 2000;111:929-939.
49. Gaudreau H, Jonas S, Zadra A, et al. Dynamics of slow-wave activity during NREM sleep of sleepwalkers and control subjects. *Sleep*. 2000;23:1-6.

50. Guilleminault C, Poyares D, Abat F, et al. Sleep and wakefulness in somnambulism: A spectral analysis study. *J Psychosom Res.* 2001;51:411-416.

51. Broughton R. Sleep disorders: Disorders of arousal? *Science.* 1968;159:1070-1078.

52. Nofzinger E, Wettstein R. Homoscidal behavior and sleep apnea: A case report and a medicolegal discussion. *Sleep.* 1995;18:776-782.

53. Bonkalo A. Impulsive acts and confusional states during incomplete arousal from sleep: Criminal and forensic implications. *Psychiatr Q.* 1974;48:400-408.

54. Hurwitz T, Mahowald M, Schenck C, et al. A retrospective outcome study and review of hypnosis of treatment of adults with sleepwalking and sleep terror. *J Nerv Ment Dis.* 1991;179:228-233.

55. Hauri P, Silber M, Boeve B. The treatment of parasomnias with hypnosis: A five-year follow-up study. *J Clin Sleep Med.* 2007;3:369-373.

56. Pilon M, Montplaisier J, Zadra A. Precipitating factors in somnambulism: Impact of sleep deprivation and forced arousals. *Neurology.* 2008;70:2284-2290.

57. Crits-Christoph P, Wolf-Palacio D, Ficher M, et al. Brief supportive-expressive psychodynamic therapy for generalized anxiety disorder. In: Barber J, Crits-Christoph P, eds. *Dynamic Therapies for Psychiatric Disorders (Axis I).* New York: Basic Books; 1995:43-88.

58. Cartwright R, Tipton L, Wicklund J. Focusing on dreams: A preparation program for psychotherapy. *Arch Gen Psychiatry.* 1980;37:275-277.

59. Shedler J. The efficacy of psychodynamic psychotherapy. *Am Psychol.* 2010;65:98-109.

60. Hill C. *Dream Work in Therapy: Facilating Exploration, Insight and Action.* Washington, DC: American Psychological Association; 2004.

61. Leichsenring F, Salzer S, Jaeger U, et al. Short-term psychodynamic psychotherapy and cognitive-behavioral; therapy in generalized anxiety disorder: A randomized, controlled trial. *Am J Psychiatry.* 2009;8:875-881.

62. Ritchie T, Skowronski J. Perceived change in the affect associated with the fading affect bias and its moderators. *Dreaming.* 2008;18:27-43.

63. Walker M, van der Helm E. Overnight therapy? The role of sleep in emotional brain processing. *Psych Bull.* 2009;135:731-748.

SECTION 5

Sleep-Related Breathing Disorders

Behavioral and Medical Interventions in Sleep-Related Breathing Disorders

Chapter 15

SABIN R. BISTA / MICHAEL O. SUMMERS

Behavioral interventions (e.g., weight loss and lifestyle modifications) and pharmacologic interventions that have been utilized to treat obstructive sleep apnea (OSA) and its consequences will be discussed in this chapter. Weight loss can either cure or decrease the overall severity of sleep apnea, especially in obese patients without obvious anatomic abnormalities. Likewise, central nervous system (CNS) depressants (e.g., alcohol, narcotics, and sedative/hypnotics) may trigger apneas or worsen snoring and are best avoided. If sleeping in a primarily supine position triggers a sleep-related breathing disorder, then limiting sleep to alternative positions may suffice as a remedy in some patients, or may at least help in alleviating overall severity. Positive airway pressure (PAP) therapy indeed is the treatment of choice; however, some patients simply cannot tolerate it. It then becomes imperative to explore other treatment modalities such as oral appliances, upper airway (UA) surgeries, and medications. Pharmacologic agents provide a novel approach to treat sleep apnea, but studies have shown that improvement in an apnea-hypopnea index (AHI) is not efficacious enough to recommend as a primary therapy for treatment of sleep apnea. Protriptyline has been used with mixed results in patients who have sleep apnea primarily evident in rapid eye movement (REM) stage of sleep. Some patients continue to complain of excessive daytime sleepiness despite optimal treatment and adequate sleep opportunity. A wake-promoting agent such as modafinil has been used successfully in such patients to increase daytime alertness.

BEHAVIORAL INTERVENTIONS

Certain behavioral factors may increase the risk of developing or further worsening sleep-related breathing disorders. Consequently, interventions to modify such factors are helpful adjuncts in managing such patients. The decision to apply one or more behavioral interventions is made for individual patients as indicated.

Weight Loss

The role of weight loss in alleviating OSA is well studied and can be accomplished medically or surgically. Obesity is a strong risk factor for OSA and the prevalence correlates with increasing body mass index (BMI).[1,2] Obesity leads to fat deposition inside and around the pharyngeal airway, which can cause narrowing of the UA and alteration of function with consequent mass loading and increased collapsibility.[3-5] Weight loss causes a decrease in adipose tissue volume, an increase in UA cross-sectional area, and reduced collapsibility,

thereby improving critical collapsing pressure (Pcrit), with consequent reduction of apneas and hypopneas.[4,6] The Sleep Heart Health Study demonstrated that the overall respiratory disturbance index (RDI) improved or worsened with changes in weight and this association was stronger with men than women (Fig. 15-1).[7] Another longitudinal study also showed that relative to a stable weight, a 10% weight loss would predict a 26% decrease in the AHI.[8]

Interventional studies examining effects of weight loss on OSA have employed strict dietary caloric restriction ranging from a very low calorie diet (VLCD), 600 to 800 kcal per day,[9,10] to a low calorie diet (LCD), 1000 to 1500 kcal per day,[11] both of which have positive outcomes on weight reduction and improvement in AHI. In the recent VLCD study, with every 5-kg weight reduction from initial baseline weight, there was a reduction in AHI by 2.[9] This benefit was seen after 3 months and maintained for up to 1 year with strict adherence (Fig. 15-2). In this group all patients had mild OSA (5-15 events per hour); the average weight loss was 10.7 kg,[9] and OSA was cured in some individuals. The LCD study enrolled obese patients with mild to moderate OSA and the reported outcome suggested that the improvement in AHI may be greater in patients with worse initial OSA despite the fact that all patients remained in the obesity range after intervention.[11]

Smith and colleagues[12] randomized severe sleep apnea patients with at least 35% more weight than ideal to control and weight loss groups. The weight loss group had been asked to lose 0.45 to 0.9 kg per week but no specific diet or behavioral interventions were prescribed. When at least 5% weight loss from baseline was achieved, which took about 5 months, the AHI had improved in both non-REM (NREM; baseline 55 ± 7.5 to 29.2 ± 7.1) and REM sleep (baseline 57.0 ± 3.2 to 37.6 ± 5.7).

Exercise helps with weight reduction and may independently influence OSA severity. A retrospective analysis of data from the Sleep Heart Health Study suggests that vigorous physical activity of at least 3 hours per week may be an adjunct modality of treatment but a prospective trial is lacking to confirm this association.[13]

Different strategies, including counseling, have been designed to assist with weight reduction in sleep apnea patients. Weight loss counseling can be very challenging; however, some behavioral approaches have shown benefits, including counseling in a nurse-managed outpatient program,[14] cognitive-behavioral programs,[15] and programs with guidance to increase the intake of vegetables and fruit.[16]

Orlistat is a well-established antiobesity medication,[17] but its use in sleep apnea patients has not been studied. Only two antiobesity drugs have been studied in patients with OSA: fenfluramine and sibutramine. Although fenfluramine did help decrease AHI in obese patients,[18] the side effect of valvular regurgitation from its use[19] led to its withdrawal from the U.S. market. There are conflicting data regarding the efficacy of sibutramine. One study utilizing a pharmacologic approach with closely monitored sibutramine-assisted weight loss showed modest benefit,[20] especially in obese patients with moderate to severe OSA, without an increase in blood pressure. A more recent Canadian study compared sibutramine-assisted weight loss head-to-head with continuous PAP (CPAP) as a means of treating obese OSA patients. These patients had controlled hypertension and type 2 diabetes mellitus. At the 1-year follow-up, a mean decrement of 2 kg/m^2 in BMI was seen in the sibutramine group, whereas BMI remained the same in the CPAP group. Despite weight loss, sibutramine did not improve sleep-disordered breathing, whereas CPAP therapy improved all respiratory variables. There were no increments in blood pressure or arrhythmias.[21] Sibutramine is a centrally acting monoamine reuptake inhibitor. Because it causes small increases in blood pressure and pulse rate, it was deemed not suitable for use in patients with uncontrolled hypertension, preexisting cardiovascular disease, or tachycardia.[22] Sibutramine was voluntarily pulled off the market in October 2010, at the request of the Food and Drug Administration (FDA), based on data from the Sibutramine Cardiovascular Outcomes (SCOUT)[23] trial* that showed risk outweighing benefit. The difference in mean percent change in body weight between medicine and placebo was around 2.5%, but there was 16% increase in risk of major cardiovascular adverse events.

With nonsurgical treatment modalities, weight reaccumulation would occur should the strategies be discontinued. The weight loss obtained is below 10% at baseline.[24] Unlike nonsurgical treatment, surgical procedures cause typical weight loss of 35% to 40% and appear to be the most durable, with surgical effect lasting up to 15 years.[25] Surgery is an option for patients with severe obesity, and in whom other methods of treatment have failed. However, recurrence of sleep apnea without concomitant increase in weight has been reported in some patients after 7 to 8 years of follow-up.[26] This recurrence seems to be true for nonsurgery weight loss management as well.[27]

Bariatric weight loss surgery studies as applied to OSA have been mostly gastric restriction rather than malabsorptive procedures such as Roux-en-Y gastric bypass (RYGB) and gastric banding. Whereas gastric banding is predominantly restrictive, RYGB is actually a hybrid procedure with both restrictive and limited malabsorption components. There are four prospective studies to date, two for each surgical modality utilized in markedly obese patients (average BMI > 50) followed for at least 1 year after surgery. These data demonstrate that although there is significant improvement in BMI and AHI after weight loss, the residual mean BMI is still elevated above 30 and the OSA remains residual in many patients[28-31] (Table 15-1). In a 1-year follow-up study of 24 consecutive patients with baseline AHI 47.9 ± 33.8 who underwent gastric banding procedure, the authors noted that only 1 patient had complete resolution of OSA (AHI < 5) while the remaining 23 patients still had persistent OSA (AHI > 5); and 71% continued to have AHI greater than 14. The baseline Epworth Sleepiness Scale (ESS) score had been 16.1 ± 4.5, but 13 patients (54%) continued to have ESS greater than 10.[28] Likewise, in the study of 101 obese patients with baseline RDI 51 ± 4 who underwent RYGB surgery,

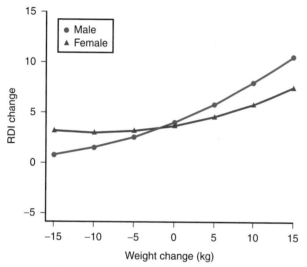

Figure 15-1 Change in respiratory disturbance index (RDI) by change in weight. Note that the relationship is not linear; RDI increased more with weight gain than it decreased with weight loss. (Reproduced with permission Newman AB, Foster G, Givelber R, et al. Progression and regression of sleep-disordered breathing with changes in weight. *Arch Intern Med* 2005;165(20):2411. Copyright ©2005 American Medical Association. All rights reserved.)

*Readers are advised to access www.fda.gov/safety/medwatch for details

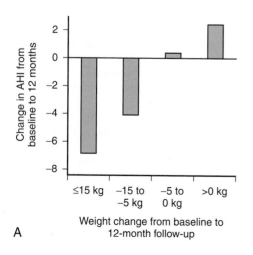

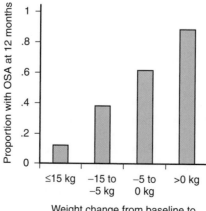

Figure 15-2 A, Changes in apnea-hypopnea index (AHI) in relation to changes in body weight. **B,** The proportion of patients (expressed as a percentage) with obstructive sleep apnea (OSA) in relation to the weight change categories. (Reproduced with permission from Tuomilehto HP, Seppä JM, Partinen MM, et al. Lifestyle Intervention with weight reduction: First line treatment in mild OSA. *Am J Respir Crit Care Med* 2009;179(4):324.)

TABLE 15-1

Bariatric Weight Loss Surgery: Summary of Four Prospective Studies

Study	N	Type of Surgery	Preoperative		Postoperative	
			BMI*	AHI	BMI	AHI
Dixon et al, 2005[29]	25	LAGB	52.7 (9.5)	61.6 (31.9)	37.2 (7.2)	13.4 (13.0)
Lettieri et al, 2008[28]	24	Gastric banding	51.0 (10.4)	47.9 (33.8)	32.1 (5.5)	24.5 (18.1)
Haines et al, 2007[31]	101	Roux-en-Y	56.0 (1.0)	51.0 (4.0)	38.0 (1.0)	15.0 (2.0)
Fritscher et al, 2007[30]	12	Roux-en-Y	51.5 (10.1)	46.5 (33-140)	34.1 (8.1)	16 (0.9-87)

*BMI expressed as kg/m². Values are means, with standard deviation in parentheses, except for AHI in Fritscher study, for which values are medians, with range in parentheses.
BMI, body mass index; *AHI*, apnea-hypopnea index; *OSA*, obstructive sleep apnea; *LAGB*, laparoscopic adjustable gastric band placement; *PSG*, polysomnogram.

Haines and associates[31] noted that, after a median follow-up of 11 months, the RDI, though improved, had been residual at 15 ± 2. The ESS score, however, had improved significantly from baseline 10 ± 1 to 6 ± 1 at 3 months, and to 4 ± 1 at 2 years. With the drop in AHI, therapeutic CPAP level requirement did improve[28] and with the drop in BMI, oxygen saturation also improved.[30] The studies, however, noted that many patients had stopped using CPAP after surgery. The treating clinician should be cognizant that these improvements do not necessarily mean OSA is cured, and patients should be counseled about this before pursuing surgery. The level of CPAP that is required to overcome OSA decreases considerably when patients are undergoing weight loss.[28,32] There is no evidence that one surgical modality is superior to the other regarding AHI. For this reason repeat overnight polysomnography (PSG) should be done after significant weight loss is obtained to assess for any residual sleep apnea. The optimal timing for this repeat PSG is not clear but preferably should be done once the weight loss trend plateaus. Autotitrating CPAP can be considered in the meantime to obtain the new pressure requirement.[32] Bariatric surgery and any weight loss measures alike should be an adjunct in the treatment of OSA and not the sole treatment.

There is a growing body of evidence to support preoperative screening and management of OSA in patients who are pursuing bariatric surgery. OSA is often missed during clinical evaluation and remains underdiagnosed in patients undergoing bariatric surgery.[33] One study employed a prediction model in this high-risk group, but it did not correctly predict OSA.[34] The prevalence of OSA is high and ranges from 77% to 84% in bariatric centers that have utilized routine preoperative screening.[34,35] Mandatory OSA screening and optimal treatment before surgery may substantially reduce a respiratory related intensive care unit (ICU) stay after surgery.[35] Anastomotic leak is a potentially lethal complication of RYGB surgery. OSA was found to be an independent risk factor for such a leak in a multivariate analysis involving 3073 patients.[36] Some case reports raised a concern that PAP therapy in the postoperative period might lead to leak secondary to bowel distention.[37] However, prospective series with larger numbers of patients have shown no correlation between CPAP and bilevel PAP (BiPAP) use and the incidence of leaks.[31,38]

CPAP use per se may also alter BMI as reported by two retrospective studies showing conflicting results. Whereas short-term weight loss of 4.5 kg was seen after 6 months in compliant CPAP users, as defined by use of more than 4 hours nightly on a habitual basis, in one study,[39] no significant decrease in BMI was seen in the CPAP-treated group when followed after 1 year

in another study. Interestingly, an increase in BMI was noted in women and nonobese patients.[40] Good prospective studies are required to conclude any such association and are currently lacking. As there is a beneficial effect of even marginal weight loss on the severity and the likelihood of developing OSA, all patients with sleep apnea should be counseled about lifestyle intervention, including weight loss. The National Heart, Lung and Blood Institute in cooperation with North American Association for the Study of Obesity has published a guideline for clinicians to identify, evaluate, and treat overweight and obese adults. (Fig. 15-3 and Table 15-2).

Positional Therapy

Sleeping supine can be a risk factor for pharyngeal airway narrowing. Gravity alone can pull the bulk of the tongue muscle and soft palate to fall posteriorly, thereby narrowing the upper airway diameter. This supine influence on increase in collapsibility can lead to worsening of sleep apnea severity.[41,42] Patients whose OSA severity is substantially greater in the supine position than in the lateral recumbent position are said to have positional sleep apnea.[43] Thus, as compared to the supine position, lower CPAP will be needed in the lateral position.[41] Even though there is improvement in the overall severity in the lateral position, clinically important AHI in a high range may still persist, especially in very obese patients.[44]

Positional therapy simply consists of strategies that prevent subjects from sleeping on their backs. The tennis ball technique, elevated head and trunk sleep posture, posture alarm, and specially designed pillows are examples of such strategies. The tennis ball technique uses a tennis ball either fastened to a chest belt or placed inside a pocket sewn into a sleeping garment in the middle of the back. The rationale is that pressure from the ball when lying on one's back would force the subject to roll to the side. Over time, the subject becomes trained to sleep in the lateral position. A tennis ball technique in a study involving 12 patients with positional OSA showed reduction of supine sleep time from 79% to 12%, and mean AHI decreased from 46.5 ± 19.9 to 17.5 ± 19.4.[45] Another study utilized a soft ball for positional treatment and was compared to CPAP in a randomized crossover trial of 13 men with mild-moderate OSA. Whereas CPAP therapy was more effective than positional treatment to reduce events, the mean difference in the reduction of overall AHI was only 6. Positional therapy alone reduced events by AHI of 8. There was no difference, however, in sleep architecture, cognitive performance tests, mood scales, and quality of life measures.[46] The optimal duration of utilizing this technique in order to get trained in sleeping

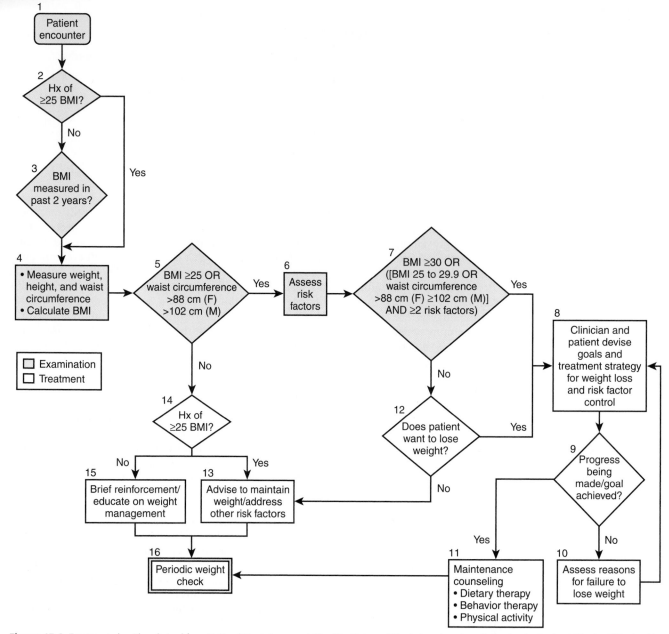

Figure 15-3 Treatment algorithm derived from National Heart, Lung, and Blood Institute and North American Association for the Study of Obesity. This algorithm applies only to assessment of obesity and not to the overall evaluation of other conditions. (From *The Practical Guide: Identification, Evaluation, and Treatment of Overweight and Obesity in Adults.* Bethesda, MD: National Institute of Health; 2000. NIH Publication No. 00-4084.)

lateral without need for physical reminder is not clear. Long-term follow-up studies based on mail-in questionnaires have nonetheless been done for the tennis ball technique. Whereas the 6-month compliance was only 38%,[45] it further declined to less than 10% at 2.5 years after the initial prescription.[47] The main reason for noncompliance was that the technique was uncomfortable.[45,47] Of those 62% who were noncompliant at 6 months, 24% reported having learned to avoid supine sleep and 38% quit using the technique within a few months because they did not learn to do so.

Studies on cervical pillows that intend to improve neck and body positioning have shown some efficacy. One such pillow is a custom-fit design to promote neck extension, thereby increasing upper airway caliber. It demonstrates effectiveness

in mild to moderate OSA,[48] with overall AHI decreasing by 4, but not in severe OSA.[49] Another studied pillow is a triangular pillow with an inclined surface and space to place one's arm under the head designed to help sleep on one's side. The sleeping position allows the mandible to fall gently forward due to gravity and helps maintain UA patency. A nonrandomized study of 22 adults with OSA and an average RDI of 17 demonstrated a decrease to less than 5 while using the pillow, along with reducing snoring and improving oxyhemoglobin saturation.[50] However, these studies have looked at OSA in general and not exclusively positional OSA.

Sleeping in an elevated posture can affect UA collapsibility. Pcrit is more negative, indicating less collapsibility, in an elevated posture of 30 degrees to horizontal as compared to

TABLE 15-2

Treatment Selection Guidelines for Overweight and Obese Adults

Treatment	BMI Category				
	25-26.9	27-29.9	30-34.9	35-39.9	≥40
Diet, physical activity, and behavioral therapy	Two or more risk factors or co-morbid illnesses	Two or more risk factors or co-morbid illnesses	+	+	+
Pharmacotherapy		Two or more risk factors or co-morbid illnesses	+	+	+
Surgery				Two or more risk factors or co-morbid illnesses	

BMI expressed as kg/m². + indicates the use of recommended treatment regardless of co-morbidity. Pharmacotherapy should be considered only if weight loss of 1 lb per week is not achieved despite 6 months of combined lifestyle interventions. Weight loss surgery should be considered if other nonsurgical attempts have failed. The co-morbid illnesses and risk factors to look for are atherosclerotic diseases including coronary heart disease (CHD), type 2 diabetes mellitus, sleep apnea, smoking, hypertension, high LDL cholesterol, low HDL cholesterol, impaired fasting glucose, family history of premature CHD, age 45 years or older for male patients and age 55 or older for female patients.

BMI, body mass index; *HDL,* high-density lipoprotein; *LDL,* low-density lipoprotein.

Adapted from *The Practical Guide: Identification, Evaluation, and Treatment of Overweight and Obesity in Adults. NHLBI, North American Association for the Study of Obesity.* 2000; NIH publication number 00-4084, table 3.

supine and lateral positions.[51] Another study with sitting at a 60-degree angle showed a significant decrease in AHI from 48.9 ± 5.4 to 19.6 ± 6.9, and the more obese subjects tended to have a better response.[52] Shoulder-head elevation pillow (SHEP) is designed to help sleep in the upright position. A crossover randomized study compared a SHEP with CPAP in 14 adult male patients with mild to severe OSA. With SHEP, the mean AHI decreased from 27 ± 12 to 21 ± 17. Seven patients (50%) continued to have AHI greater than 16. The mean AHI with CPAP was 5 ± 3.[53]

Positional therapy can be utilized as a primary therapy in selected patients as well as an adjunct to CPAP in treating OSA. However, because positional therapy does not always normalize AHI, correction of OSA after implementing any such therapy may require confirmation with an appropriate test.[54] Patients with mild to moderate positional OSA are more likely to benefit from positional therapy than with severe OSA.

Sleep Hygiene, Alcohol, and Smoking Cessation

Practicing good sleep hygiene is a part of the treatment of all sleep disorders, including OSA. Sleep fragmentation increases upper airway collapsibility.[55] Similarly, sleep deprivation diminishes genioglossus muscle activity[56] and attenuates ventilatory chemosensitivity because both hypoxic and hypercapnic ventilatory responses are decreased.[57] OSA is known to trigger sleep fragmentation and thus could exacerbate sleep apnea. Hence, an adequate sleep opportunity must be ensured simultaneous with treating OSA, thereby preventing the vicious circle.

Alcohol is known to affect one's sleep hygiene and adversely affect OSA. Acute alcohol consumption adversely affects UA stability. Animal studies have shown a dose-dependent reduction of respiratory motor activity of hypoglossal and laryngeal nerves with increasing alcohol intake.[58,59] Reduced genioglossus electromyographic activity has also been seen in humans.[60] This reduced activity combined with increased inspiratory resistance[61,62] and increased inspiratory effort[62] could collapse the UA. Alcohol is well documented to trigger or worsen snoring,[63] precipitate apneas in snorers,[61] and increase the frequency and duration of apneas

in patients with OSA.[63-66] The effect seems to be most pronounced during the first 1 to 2 hours after bedtime alcohol consumption.[61,63] Of note, most of these studies have used 45% to 50% ethanol by volume in the range of 0.5 to 2 mL/kg. Moderate alcohol consumption even 6 hours before bedtime can disturb sleep consolidation[67] and potentially exacerbate OSA. It becomes intuitive that patients with OSA who use CPAP will require higher therapeutic pressure levels on the nights after ethanol consumption. However, the literature on such impact is inconsistent. The CPAP level required to eliminate snoring in asymptomatic snorers who ingest alcohol is increased.[61] However, acute moderate alcohol ingestion of 1.5 to 2.0 mL/kg of 40% to 50% alcohol by volume does not increase the therapeutic CPAP level requirement in existing OSA, irrespective of whether autoset-CPAP[68] or manual titration is done.[64] Two population-based studies suggested that long-term habitual alcohol consumption increased the risk for sleep-disordered breathing.[69,70] This risk association was seen with male drinkers only, and the increased risk thereof was for mild OSA only. Female drinkers and nondrinkers (those who never drank) did not have increased risk. Therefore, merely advising patients with OSA to avoid bedtime alcohol may not be enough. They should be encouraged to generally reduce alcohol consumption at any time of day or abstain completely.

The prevalence of smoking is higher in OSA patients. A recent study indicates that 35% of patients with OSA are smokers; whereas 18% of the population without OSA does not smoke.[71] Current smokers have a two- to threefold greater odds ratio for snoring and are 2.5 to 4.4 times more likely to have sleep-disordered breathing than nonsmokers. Heavy smoking (> two packs/day) presents the greatest risk for sleep disturbances.[71,72] Former smokers are not at increased risk compared to current smokers; and therefore, counseling for smoking cessation should be a part of treatment and prevention of OSA.

Sedatives and Hypnotics

Patients with underlying OSA could be prescribed benzodiazepines and nonbenzodiazepine hypnotics and sedatives. The effects of such medications on UA stability and breathing during sleep need to be assessed for optimal management and will be discussed in this section.

Benzodiazepines are CNS depressants and may affect the ventilation control during sleep by blunting the hypoxic and hypercapnic arousal responses.[74] Use of these agents in patients with underlying chronic obstructive pulmonary or cardiac disease may cause worsening of sleep-disordered breathing.[75] Temazepam is a fairly commonly used sedative-hypnotic benzodiazepine. A study done in elderly insomnia patients with mild OSA did not show an increase in AHI at doses ranging from 15 to 30 mg.[76] Alternatively, flurazepam, another benzodiazepine hypnotic, not only worsens OSA[77,78] but also increases frequency and duration of apneas in otherwise asymptomatic subjects.[79]

Newer nonbenzodiazepine hypnotics are more commonly used now. A higher 20-mg zolpidem dose worsens OSA similar to flurazepam,[78] but with a 10-mg dose, there is a nonsignificant increase in AHI in patients with OSA[80] or snorers without OSA.[81] Eszopiclone does not worsen AHI at the usual dose of 3 mg.[82,83] Both zolpidem and eszopiclone may actually improve quality of CPAP titration by allowing the patient to sleep better.[80,83] Zaleplon does not worsen AHI in patients with OSA on CPAP therapy.[84] These studies were done in mild to moderate OSA patients and the results may not be applicable in severe OSA. Benzodiazepines are best avoided if feasible, and if necessary, nonbenzodiazepine hypnotics could be used in selected patients.

Opioids

Sleep-disordered breathing may develop in chronic opioid users and can be obstructive, central, or a combination of both.[85-89] The central sleep apnea that develops is not of a Cheyne-Stokes pattern, but is rather atypical and a part of ataxic breathing.[85,87] CPAP alone may not be enough, and may worsen central apneic events. BiPAP with added breathing rate may be useful in such cases.[90] There are conflicting results on efficacy of adaptive servoventilation (ASV)[91,92] because residual ataxic breathing might continue.[92] Any OSA patient on opioids should be monitored for possible worsening of the underlying sleep-related breathing disorder along with evaluation for oxygen desaturation in wakefulness[86] and in NREM sleep.[85,88] Sleep-disordered breathing events and oxygen saturation do not seem to worsen in REM sleep.[85] The current evidence for resolution of sleep-related breathing disorder after opioid withdrawal is only anecdotal.[93] Additional oxygen supplementation may be required to correct hypoxemia.

PHARMACOLOGIC INTERVENTIONS

The most consistently effective treatment for OSA remains some form of PAP therapy. Despite this, PAP's success is dependent on patient compliance and tolerance. Certain subsets of patients, despite extensive attempts, cannot tolerate any sort of PAP device. Because of this, one area of research in evaluating novel treatments for OSA is exploration of the use of pharmacotherapeutics. In 2006, the American Academy of Sleep Medicine released a position paper on the use of medical therapy in the treatment of obstructive sleep apnea, with a subsequent review by the Medical Therapy for Obstructive Sleep Apnea Task Force.[54,73] In this section are brief overviews of some of the medications that have been evaluated in the treatment of OSA.

Serotoninergic Agents

Serotonin (5-hydroxytryptamine, 5-HT) is a monoamine neurotransmitter that functions as a signaling molecule in the body. In the brain, it is primarily produced by the raphe nuclei. There are a total of seven known families of serotonin receptors, six of which are G protein–coupled receptors. The only known exception to this is the 5-HT$_3$ receptor, which belongs to the ligand-gated cation superfamily of receptors.[94] Within these families of serotonin receptors, a number of specific subtypes have been further characterized (Table 15-3).

The difficulty with the serotoninergic system is that activation of some of the subtypes result in inhibition of UA dilator muscles and ventilatory drive, while activation of other subtypes may result in excitation of these same motor neurons and drive.[95] To further complicate the matter, certain data suggest that intermittent hypoxia (as a model for sleep apnea oxygenation patterns) alters the responsiveness of UA nerves to serotonin.[96] As a result, some serotoninergic agents may be beneficial while others may worsen sleep apnea, and within these groups of patients may be subsets of patients who could have different responses to these medications based on their oxygenation patterns and hypoxic exposure. Research on this exceptionally complex system in ongoing, but the details are beyond the scope of this text.

Studies have looked at paroxetine and fluoxetine as a possible treatment for OSA.[97-99] These studies have shown little or no significant effect on either AHI or subjective sleepiness.

Tricyclic antidepressants (TCAs) are known to decrease REM sleep, which is the stage of sleep typically associated with the most severe obstructive sleep apneic episodes. Recently, mirtazapine (a TCA) has been proposed as a

---

TABLE 15-3

Serotonin Receptors and Subtypes

Family	Number of Subtypes	Type	Mechanism of Action	Potential
5-HT$_1$	5	G protein–coupled	Decreases cellular levels of cAMP	Inhibitory
5-HT$_2$	3	G protein–coupled	Increases cellular levels of IP$_3$ and DAG	Excitatory
5-HT$_3$	1	Ligand-gated ion channel	Depolarizing plasma membrane	Excitatory
5-HT$_4$	1	G protein–coupled	Increases cellular levels of cAMP	Excitatory
5-HT$_5$	1	G protein–coupled	Decreases cellular levels of cAMP	Inhibitory
5-HT$_6$	1	G protein–coupled	Increases cellular levels of cAMP	Excitatory
5-HT$_7$	1	G protein–coupled	Increases cellular levels of cAMP	Excitatory

cAMP, cyclic adenosine monophosphate; *DAG*, diacylglycerol; *5-HT$_1$ to 5-HT$_7$*, 5-hydroxytryptamine (serotonin) receptors 1 to 7; *IP$_3$*, inositol 1,4,5-triphosphate.

possible treatment for OSA.[73] Since this proposal, there have been two studies that have specifically looked at the effects of mirtazapine on OSA.[100,101] Both of these studies were randomized control trials. One of the studies showed a halving of the AHI,[101] but the other showed no significant effect on the AHI.[100] Both studies came to the conclusion that mirtazapine is not recommended for treatment of OSA. This conclusion primarily revolves around the fact that a significant portion of patients on mirtazapine report unacceptable levels of somnolence. In addition, significant weight gain, which could worsen underlying OSA, was reported in subjects while on the medication.

REM Sleep Suppressant Therapy

Certain known populations of patients with OSA experience almost exclusively REM-related events. As such, it makes sense that, in these patients, finding a medication that suppresses REM sleep may result in an improved AHI.

Protriptyline is a TCA that has both serotoninergic and noradrenergic reuptake inhibition, in addition to anticholinergic effects. Although as a rule, TCAs are known to suppress REM sleep, their effects on REM suppression are not consistent or clear. There have been multiple randomized, double-blind, placebo-controlled trials looking at the effects of protriptyline on sleep apnea.[99,102-106] The results of the studies have varied, and although many of them showed a subjective decrease in reported sleepiness and objective decrease in AHI, the decrease in AHI was not sufficient to justify the use of protriptyline as a primary therapy for the treatment of OSA.

Ventilatory Stimulants

The methylxanthine drugs (e.g., aminophylline) have been studied because of their known ventilatory stimulant effects (felt primarily due to their adenosine receptor antagonistic effects). There have been a handful of studies looking specifically at the use of aminophylline and its effectiveness on OSA, the most recent of which was more than 10 years ago.[107-110] These studies have all shown relatively insignificant to no improvement in obstructive events. In addition, aminophylline resulted in a significant decrease in sleep efficiency and total sleep time in all the studies performed. These findings, coupled with the significant potential for cardiac toxicity, including intractable ventricular arrhythmias,[111-113] with aminophylline, preclude any recommendation of aminophylline as a treatment option in OSA.

Other studies have looked at opioid antagonists, doxapram, and nicotine in the treatment of OSA.[114-117] Although some of these have shown a mild reduction in AHI,[114] it is a negligible, inconsistent decrease, and the side effects and lack of practicality (doxapram, for example, is IV only) in using some of these medications preclude recommending them for treatment of OSA.

Oxygen Therapy

Oxygen supplementation has consistently been shown to decrease the severity of hypoxic events in patients with OSA.[118-121] One study has shown a reduction in severity of obstructive breathing events with administration of supplemental oxygen.[119] Also of significance is the patient's subjective sense of decreased sleepiness with the use of supplemental oxygen. It is important to note, however, that treatment with supplemental oxygen often does not result in decrease of obstructive breathing events to normal levels, and as such, oxygen therapy does not treat OSA. Rather, it decreases the severity of hypoxia, resulting in improved mean oxyhemoglobin saturation for the sleep period.

Several studies have looked at some of the potential problems associated with the use of supplemental oxygen when used to treat OSA.[122-124] Specifically, there were concerns that although administration of supplemental oxygen decreased the severity of the hypoxia, the durations of the apneas could be prolonged. The study by Martin and colleagues[124] showed that one of the eight subjects did have a prolonged apneic time with administration of supplemental oxygen, one patient had no change in their apnea duration, and the other six patients had a significant decrease in their apnea durations. Kearley and associates[122] looked at the frequency and duration of oxygen desaturations and sleep-disordered breathing during sleep in patients with known chronic obstructive lung disease. They found that oxygen therapy, as would be expected, decreased the frequency of desaturations per hour. Interestingly, they also found that there was no difference between room air versus oxygen in either number of episodes or duration of sleep-related breathing events. They concluded that "in most patients with stable chronic obstructive lung disease, administration of oxygen at 2 liters per minute improved oxygenation, prolongs sleep, but does not adversely affect sleep disordered breathing."

Nasal Insufflation Therapy

In 2007, McGinley and associates[125] looked at the possibility of treating OSA with high-flow (up to 20 L/minute) nasal insufflation with air via a nasal cannula. Though the number of subjects who completed the study was small,[11] the study did seem to suggest that this might be a viable option in the correctly chosen patient population. Subjects had AHIs ranging from 5 to 58. As would be expected, the less severe the sleep apnea, the closer to normal were the AHIs they were able to achieve.

Wake-Promoting Agents in Obstructive Sleep Apnea

There is a subset of patients with OSA that, despite adequate total sleep time and good PAP compliance, still have persistent subjective sleepiness. It has been shown that up to 22% of patients who use CPAP for at least 6 hours per night still report excessive sleepiness.[126] In addition, 52% also had objective evidence, as measured by multiple sleep latency test (MSLT), of physiologic sleepiness.[126]

Weaver and colleagues[127] conducted a study in which they pooled data from two randomized, placebo-controlled trials looking at the effects of modafinil in 480 patients with residual sleepiness. They concluded that "in patients with OSA and residual excessive sleepiness despite regular CPAP use, modafinil treatment was associated with improvements in patients' functional outcomes, including activity, productivity, intimacy, and vigilance and in their ability to engage in a broad array of everyday activities, as confirmed through analysis of data pooled from studies lasting up to 12 weeks."[127]

TABLE 15-4

Modafinil versus Armodafinil*

Drug Characteristic	Modafinil	Armodafinil
Half-life	12-15 hours	12-15 hours
Starting dose	100 mg qd	50-150 mg qd
Maximum dose	200 mg bid	250 mg qd
Metabolism	Hepatic	Hepatic
Common side effects	Headache, insomnia, nausea	Headache, insomnia, nausea
Cmax	2-4 hours	2-4 hours
Pregnancy category	C	C
Available pill dosages	100 mg, 200 mg	50 mg, 150 mg, 250 mg

*Both medications have been shown to decrease the effectiveness of oral contraceptives, so an alternative method of birth control is recommended for female patients taking this medication.
Cmax, peak serum concentration of a drug.

Armodafinil has been recently introduced to the market as a wake-promoting agent. This drug is FDA approved for use in patients with persistent sleepiness despite adequate total sleep time and good CPAP compliance.[128] Armodafinil is the *R*-isomer of modafinil. Its primary benefit over modafinil seems to be related to its higher bioavailability (as measured by AUC, area under the curve) (69% greater than modafinil) and Cmax (37% higher than modafinil) resulting in, typically, once daily dosing as opposed to the more common twice daily dosing needed with modafinil (Table 15-4).

Nasal Patency Medical Therapy

Studies have looked at the effectiveness of treating patients with nasal corticosteroids as possible pharmacologic monotherapy in patients with OSA.[129,130] In one study, patients were randomized to the use of fluticasone nasal spray or placebo.[130] The study found that there was a significant decrease in AHI, but not to a level that would be considered normal (AHI reduced to 12 from 20).

Another study looked at the effect of nasal inhaled corticosteroids plus positional therapy on treatment of OSA.[129] The study results showed that a decrease in AHI occurred only when both positional therapy and the nasal corticosteroid were used. The nasal corticosteroid as monotherapy did not result in a significant decrease in obstructive breathing events.

As a result of these two studies, it is recommended that patients with nasal congestion may benefit from nasal corticosteroids, but this therapy alone would likely not result in adequate treatment of OSA.

A recent study by Larrain and associates[131] looked at the effects of a combination of pseudoephedrine and domperidone in treatment of OSA. Domperidone is not approved for use in the United States, but has been prescribed for its prokinetic properties in other countries.[132] Larrain and associates[133] had previously shown that this combination of medications was effective in reducing or eliminating snoring and the question was posed as to whether this combination might also treat OSA. The study was a retrospective case series, and no polysomnography (PSG) data was obtained. They did, however, collect overnight oximetry information as well as subjective sleepiness as measured by ESS. Snoring and observed apneas disappeared in most patients, and improvement in subjective sleepiness was noted (mean ESS score of 14.1 down to 4.2). There was also a statistically significant decrease in oxygen desaturation index (ODI; a mean baseline of 41.5 down to 25.9).

Although these limited data are encouraging, and represent some of the most recent attempts at finding effective and consistent pharmacotherapy to treat OSA, future studies with PSG using a randomized, placebo-controlled trial could prove beneficial.

REFERENCES

1. Young T, Palta M, Dempsey J, et al. The occurrence of sleep-disordered breathing among middle-aged adults. *N Engl J Med.* 1993;328(17):1230-1235.
2. Young T, Peppard PE, Gottlieb DJ. Epidemiology of obstructive sleep apnea: A population health perspective. *Am J Respir Crit Care Med.* 2002;165(9):1217-1239.
3. Kairaitis K, Howitt L, Wheatley JR, et al. Mass loading of the upper airway extraluminal tissue space in rabbits: Effects on tissue pressure and pharyngeal airway lumen geometry. *J Appl Physiol.* 2009;106(3):887-892.
4. Shelton KE, Woodson H, Kay S, et al. Pharyngeal fat in obstructive sleep apnea. *Am Rev Respir Dis.* 1993;148(2):462-466.
5. Ryan CF, Love LL. Mechanical properties of the velopharynx in obese patients with obstructive sleep apnea. *Am J Respir Crit Care Med.* 1996;154(3 Pt 1):806-812.
6. Schwartz AR, Gold AR, Schubert N, et al. Effect of weight loss on upper airway collapsibility in obstructive sleep apnea. *Am Rev Respir Dis.* 1991;144(3 Pt 1):494-498.
7. Newman AB, Foster G, Givelber R, et al. Progression and regression of sleep-disordered breathing with changes in weight: The Sleep Heart Health Study. *Arch Intern Med.* 2005;165(20):2408-2413.
8. Peppard PE, Young T, Palta M, et al. Longitudinal study of moderate weight change and sleep-disordered breathing. *JAMA.* 2000;284(23):3015-3021.
9. Tuomilehto HP, Seppä JM, Partinen MM, et al. Lifestyle intervention with weight reduction: First-line treatment in mild obstructive sleep apnea. *Am J Respir Crit Care Med.* 2009;179(4):320-327.
10. Kansanen M, Vanninen E, Tuunainen A, et al. The effect of a very low-calorie diet-induced weight loss on the severity of obstructive sleep apnoea and autonomic nervous function in obese patients with obstructive sleep apnoea syndrome. *Clin Physiol.* 1998;18(4):377-385.
11. Hernandez TL, Ballard RD, Weil KM, et al. Effects of maintained weight loss on sleep dynamics and neck morphology in severely obese adults. *Obesity (Silver Spring).* 2009;17(1):84-91.
12. Smith PL, Gold AR, Meyers DA, et al. Weight loss in mildly to moderately obese patients with obstructive sleep apnea. *Ann Intern Med.* 1985;103(6):850-855.
13. Quan SF, O'Connor GT, Quan JS, et al. Association of physical activity with sleep-disordered breathing. *Sleep Breath.* 2007;11(3):149-157.
14. Lojander J, Mustajoki P, Ronka S, et al. A nurse-managed weight reduction programme for obstructive sleep apnoea syndrome. *J Intern Med.* 1998;244(3):251-255.
15. Kajaste S, Brander PE, Telakivi T, et al. A cognitive-behavioral weight reduction program in the treatment of obstructive sleep apnea syndrome with or without initial nasal CPAP: A randomized study. *Sleep Med.* 2004;5(2):125-131.
16. Svendsen M, Blomhoff R, Holme I, et al. The effect of an increased intake of vegetables and fruit on weight loss, blood pressure and antioxidant defense in subjects with sleep related breathing disorders. *Eur J Clin Nutr.* 2007;61(11):1301-1311.
17. Sjostrom L, Rissanen A, Andersen T, et al. Randomised placebo-controlled trial of orlistat for weight loss and prevention of weight regain in obese patients. European Multicentre Orlistat Study Group. *Lancet.* 1998;352(9123):167-172.
18. Strobel RJ, Rosen RC. Obesity and weight loss in obstructive sleep apnea: A critical review. *Sleep.* 1996;19(2):104-115.
19. Dahl CF, Allen MR, Urie PM, et al. Valvular regurgitation and surgery associated with fenfluramine use: An analysis of 5743 individuals. *BMC Med.* 2008;6:34.
20. Yee BJ, Phillips CL, Banerjee D, et al. The effect of sibutramine-assisted weight loss in men with obstructive sleep apnea. *Int J Obes (Lond).* 2007;31(1):161-168.

21. Ferland A, Poirier P, Series F. Sibutramine versus continuous positive airway pressure in obese obstructive sleep apnoea patients. *Eur Respir J.* 2009;34:694-701.

22. Padwal RS, Majumdar SR. Drug treatments for obesity: Orlistat, sibutramine, and rimonabant. *Lancet.* 2007;369(9555):71-77.

23. Torp-Pedersen C, Caterson I, Coutinho W, et al. Cardiovascular responses to weight management and sibutramine in high-risk subjects: An analysis from the SCOUT trial. *Eur Heart J.* 2007;28(23):2915-2923.

24. Bray GA. Lifestyle and pharmacological approaches to weight loss: Efficacy and safety. *J Clin Endocrinol Metab.* 2008;93(11):81-88.

25. Cummings DE, Overduin J, Foster-Schubert KE. Gastric bypass for obesity: Mechanisms of weight loss and diabetes resolution. *J Clin Endocrinol Metab.* 2004;89(6):2608-2615.

26. Pillar G, Peled R, Lavie P. Recurrence of sleep apnea without concomitant weight increase 7.5 years after weight reduction surgery. *Chest.* 1994;106(6):1702-1704.

27. Sampol G, Munoz X, Sagales MT, et al. Long-term efficacy of dietary weight loss in sleep apnoea/hypopnoea syndrome. *Eur Respir J.* 1998;12(5):1156-1159.

28. Lettieri CJ, Eliasson AH, Greenburg DL. Persistence of obstructive sleep apnea after surgical weight loss. *J Clin Sleep Med.* 2008;4(4):333-338.

29. Dixon JB, Schachter LM, O'Brien PE. Polysomnography before and after weight loss in obese patients with severe sleep apnea. *Int J Obes (Lond).* 2005;29(9):1048-1054.

30. Fritscher LG, Canani S, Mottin CC, et al. Bariatric surgery in the treatment of obstructive sleep apnea in morbidly obese patients. *Respiration.* 2007;74(6):647-652.

31. Haines KL, Nelson LG, Gonzalez R, et al. Objective evidence that bariatric surgery improves obesity-related obstructive sleep apnea. *Surgery.* 2007;141(3):354-358.

32. Lankford DA, Proctor CD, Richard R. Continuous positive airway pressure (CPAP) changes in bariatric surgery patients undergoing rapid weight loss. *Obes Surg.* 2005;15(3):336-341.

33. Hallowell PT, Stellato TA, Schuster M, et al. Potentially life-threatening sleep apnea is unrecognized without aggressive evaluation. *Am J Surg.* 2007;193(3):364-367:discussion 367.

34. Sareli AE, Cantor CR, Williams NN, et al. Obstructive sleep apnea in patients undergoing bariatric surgery—A tertiary center experience. *Obes Surg.* 2009.

35. Hallowell PT, Stellato TA, Petrozzi MC, et al. Eliminating respiratory intensive care unit stay after gastric bypass surgery. *Surgery.* 2007;142(4):608-612:discussion 612 e1.

36. Fernandez Jr AZ, DeMaria EJ, Tichansky DS, et al. Experience with over 3,000 open and laparoscopic bariatric procedures: Multivariate analysis of factors related to leak and resultant mortality. *Surg Endosc.* 2004;18(2):193-197.

37. Vasquez TL, Hoddinott K. A potential complication of bi-level positive airway pressure after gastric bypass surgery. *Obes Surg.* 2004;14(2):282-284.

38. Huerta S, de Shields S, Shpiner R, et al. Safety and efficacy of postoperative continuous positive airway pressure to prevent pulmonary complications after Roux-en-Y gastric bypass. *J Gastrointest Surg.* 2002;6(3):354-358.

39. Loube DI, Loube AA, Erman MK. Continuous positive airway pressure treatment results in weight less in obese and overweight patients with obstructive sleep apnea. *J Am Diet Assoc.* 1997;97(8):896-897.

40. Redenius R, Murphy C, O'Neill E, et al. Does CPAP lead to change in BMI? *J Clin Sleep Med.* 2008;4(3):205-209.

41. Penzel T, Moller M, Becker HF, et al. Effect of sleep position and sleep stage on the collapsibility of the upper airways in patients with sleep apnea. *Sleep.* 2001;24(1):90-95.

42. Cartwright RD. Effect of sleep position on sleep apnea severity. *Sleep.* 1984;7(2):110-114.

43. Oksenberg A, Silverberg DS, Arons E, et al. Positional vs. nonpositional obstructive sleep apnea patients: Anthropomorphic, nocturnal polysomnographic, and multiple sleep latency test data. *Chest.* 1997;112(3):629-639.

44. George CF, Millar TW, Kryger MH. Sleep apnea and body position during sleep. *Sleep.* 1988;11(1):90-99.

45. Oksenberg A, Silverberg D, Offenbach D, et al. Positional therapy for obstructive sleep apnea patients: A 6-month follow-up study. *Laryngoscope.* 2006;116(11):1995-2000.

46. Jokic R, Klimaszewski A, Crossley M, et al. Positional treatment vs. continuous positive airway pressure in patients with positional obstructive sleep apnea syndrome. *Chest.* 1999;115(3):771-781.

47. Bignold JJ, Deans-Costi G, Goldsworthy MR, et al. Poor long-term patient compliance with the tennis ball technique for treating positional obstructive sleep apnea. *J Clin Sleep Med.* 2009;5(5):428-430.

48. Kushida CA, Rao S, Guilleminault C, et al. Cervical positioning for reduction of sleep-disordered breathing in mild-to-moderate OSAS. *Sleep Breath.* 2001;5(2):71-78.

49. Kushida CA, Rao S, Guilleminault C. Cervical positional effects on snoring and apneas. *Sleep Res Online.* 1999;2(1):7-10.

50. Zuberi NA, Rekab K, Nguyen HV. Sleep apnea avoidance pillow effects on obstructive sleep apnea syndrome and snoring. *Sleep Breath.* 2004;8(4):201-207.

51. Neill AM, Angus SM, Sajkov D, et al. Effects of sleep posture on upper airway stability in patients with obstructive sleep apnea. *Am J Respir Crit Care Med.* 1997;155(1):199-204.

52. McEvoy RD, Sharp DJ, Thornton AT. The effects of posture on obstructive sleep apnea. *Am Rev Respir Dis.* 1986;133(4):662-666.

53. Skinner MA, Kingshott R, Jones D, et al. Elevated posture for the management of obstructive sleep apnea. *Sleep Breath.* 2004;8(4):193-200.

54. Morgenthaler TI, Kapen S, Lee-Chiong T, et al. Practice parameters for the medical therapy of obstructive sleep apnea. *Sleep.* 2006;29(8):1031-1035.

55. Series F, Cormier Y, La Forge J, et al. Mechanisms of the effectiveness of continuous positive airway pressure in obstructive sleep apnea. *Sleep.* 1992;15(suppl 6):S47-S49.

56. Leiter JC, Knuth SL, Bartlett Jr D. The effect of sleep deprivation on activity of the genioglossus muscle. *Am Rev Respir Dis.* 1985;132(6):1242-1245.

57. White DP, Douglas NJ, Pickett CK, et al. Sleep deprivation and the control of ventilation. *Am Rev Respir Dis.* 1983;128(6):984-986.

58. Bonora M, Shields GI, Knuth SL, et al. Selective depression by ethanol of upper airway respiratory motor activity in cats. *Am Rev Respir Dis.* 1984;130(2):156-161.

59. St. John WM, Bartlett DJ, Knuth KV, et al. Differential depression of hypoglossal nerve activity by alcohol. Protection by pretreatment with medroxyprogesterone acetate. *Am Rev Respir Dis.* 1986;133(1):46-48.

60. Krol RC, Knuth SL, Bartlett Jr D. Selective reduction of genioglossal muscle activity by alcohol in normal human subjects. *Am Rev Respir Dis.* 1984;129(2):247-250.

61. Mitler MM, Dawson A, Henriksen SJ, et al. Bedtime ethanol increases resistance of upper airways and produces sleep apneas in asymptomatic snorers. *Alcohol Clin Exp Res.* 1988;12(6):801-805.

62. Dawson A, Bigby BG, Poceta JS, et al. Effect of bedtime alcohol on inspiratory resistance and respiratory drive in snoring and nonsnoring men. *Alcohol Clin Exp Res.* 1997;21(2):183-190.

63. Issa FG, Sullivan CE. Alcohol, snoring and sleep apnea. *J Neurol Neurosurg Psychiatry.* 1982;45(4):353-359.

64. Berry RB, Desa MM, Light RW. Effect of ethanol on the efficacy of nasal continuous positive airway pressure as a treatment for obstructive sleep apnea. *Chest.* 1991;99(2):339-343.

65. Scanlan MF, Roebuck T, Little PJ, et al. Effect of moderate alcohol upon obstructive sleep apnoea. *Eur Respir J.* 2000;16(5):909-913.

66. Taasan VC, Block AJ, Boysen PG, et al. Alcohol increases sleep apnea and oxygen desaturation in asymptomatic men. *Am J Med.* 1981;71(2):240-245.

67. Landolt HP, Roch C, Dijk DJ, et al. Late-afternoon ethanol intake affects nocturnal sleep and the sleep EEG in middle-aged men. *J Clin Psychopharmacol.* 1996;16(6):428-436.

68. Teschler H, Berthon-Jones M, Wessendorf T, et al. Influence of moderate alcohol consumption on obstructive sleep apnoea with and without AutoSet nasal CPAP therapy. *Eur Respir J.* 1996;9(11):2371-2377.

69. Tanigawa T, Tachibana N, Yamagishi K, et al. Usual alcohol consumption and arterial oxygen desaturation during sleep. *JAMA.* 2004;292(8):923-925.

70. Peppard PE, Austin D, Brown RL. Association of alcohol consumption and sleep disordered breathing in men and women. *J Clin Sleep Med.* 2007;3(3):265-270.

71. Kashyap R, Hock LM, Bowman TJ. Higher prevalence of smoking in patients diagnosed as having obstructive sleep apnea. *Sleep Breath.* 2001;5(4):167-172.

72. Wetter DW, Young TB, Bidwell TR, et al. Smoking as a risk factor for sleep-disordered breathing. *Arch Intern Med.* 1994;154(19):2219-2224.

73. Hedemark LL, Kronenberg RS. Flurazepam attenuates the arousal response to CO_2 during sleep in normal subjects. *Am Rev Respir Dis.* 1983;128(6):980-983.

74. Guilleminault C. Benzodiazepines, breathing, and sleep. *Am J Med.* 1990;88(3A):S25-S28.

75. Camacho ME, Morin CM. The effect of temazepam on respiration in elderly insomniacs with mild sleep apnea. *Sleep.* 1995;18(8):644-645.

76. Mendelson WB, Garnett D, Gillin JC. Flurazepam-induced sleep apnea syndrome in a patient with insomnia and mild sleep-related respiratory changes. *J Nerv Ment Dis.* 1981;169(4):261-264.

77. Cirignotta F, Mondini S, Zucconi M, et al. Zolpidem-polysomnographic study of the effect of a new hypnotic drug in sleep apnea syndrome. *Pharmacol Biochem Behav.* 1988;29(4):807-809.

78. Dolly FR, Block AJ. Effect of flurazepam on sleep-disordered breathing and nocturnal oxygen desaturation in asymptomatic subjects. *Am J Med.* 1982;73(2):239-243.

79. Lettieri CJ, Eliasson AH, Andrada T, et al. Does zolpidem enhance the yield of polysomnography? *J Clin Sleep Med.* 2005;1(2):129-131.

80. Quera-Salva MA, McCann C, Boudet J, et al. Effects of zolpidem on sleep architecture, night time ventilation, daytime vigilance and performance in heavy snorers. *Br J Clin Pharmacol.* 1994;37(6):539-543.

81. Rosenberg R, Roach JM, Scharf M, et al. A pilot study evaluating acute use of eszopiclone in patients with mild to moderate obstructive sleep apnea syndrome. *Sleep Med.* 2007;8(5):464-470.

82. Lettieri CJ, Quast TN, Eliasson AH, et al. Eszopiclone improves overnight polysomnography and continuous positive airway pressure titration: A prospective, randomized, placebo-controlled trial. *Sleep.* 2008;31(9):1310-1316.

83. Coyle MA, Mendelson WB, Derchak PA, et al. Ventilatory safety of zaleplon during sleep in patients with obstructive sleep apnea on continuous positive airway pressure. *J Clin Sleep Med.* 2005;1(1):97.

84. Walker JM, Farney RJ, Rhondeau SM, et al. Chronic opioid use is a risk factor for the development of central sleep apnea and ataxic breathing. *J Clin Sleep Med.* 2007;3(5):455-461.

85. Mogri M, Desai H, Webster L, et al. Hypoxemia in patients on chronic opiate therapy with and without sleep apnea. *Sleep Breath.* 2009;13(1):49-57.

86. Webster LR, Choi Y, Desai H, et al. Sleep-disordered breathing and chronic opioid therapy. *Pain Med.* 2008;9(4):425-432.

87. Wang D, Teichtahl H, Drummer O, et al. Central sleep apnea in stable methadone maintenance treatment patients. *Chest.* 2005;128(3):1348-1356.

88. Sharkey KM, Kurth ME, Anderson BJ, et al. Obstructive sleep apnea is more common than central sleep apnea in methadone maintenance patients with subjective sleep complaints. *Drug Alcohol Depend.* 2010;108(1-2):77-83.

89. Alattar MA, Scharf SM. Opioid-associated central sleep apnea: A case series. *Sleep Breath.* 2009;13(2):201-206.

90. Javaheri S, Malik A, Smith J, et al. Adaptive pressure support servoventilation: A novel treatment for sleep apnea associated with use of opioids. *J Clin Sleep Med.* 2008;4(4):305-310.

91. Farney RJ, Walker JM, Boyle KM, et al. Adaptive servoventilation (ASV) in patients with sleep disordered breathing associated with chronic opioid medications for non-malignant pain. *J Clin Sleep Med.* 2008;4(4):311-319.

92. Ramar K. Reversal of sleep-disordered breathing with opioid withdrawal. *Pain Pract.* 2009;9(5):394-398.

93. Veasey SC, Guilleminault C, Strohl KP, et al. Medical therapy for obstructive sleep apnea: A review by the Medical Therapy for Obstructive Sleep Apnea Task Force of the Standards of Practice Committee of the American Academy of Sleep Medicine. *Sleep.* 2006;29(8):1036-1044.

94. Andrade R, Barnes NM, Baxter G, et al. 5-Hydroxytryptamine receptors, introductory chapter. *IUPHAR database (IUPHAR-DB).* 2010-05-17 Available from http://www.iuphar-db.org/DATABASE/FamilyIntroductionForward?familyId=1:Accessed 4/5/11.

95. Veasey SC. Serotonin agonists and antagonists in obstructive sleep apnea: Therapeutic potential. *Am J Respir Med.* 2003;2(1):21-29.

96. Veasey SC, Zhan G, Fenik P, et al. Long-term intermittent hypoxia: Reduced excitatory hypoglossal nerve output. *Am J Respir Crit Care Med.* 2004;170(6):665-672.

97. Kraiczi H, Hedner J, Dahlof P, et al. Effect of serotonin uptake inhibition on breathing during sleep and daytime symptoms in obstructive sleep apnea. *Sleep.* 1999;22(1):61-67.

98. Berry RB, Yamaura EM, Gill K, et al. Acute effects of paroxetine on genioglossus activity in obstructive sleep apnea. *Sleep.* 1999;22(8):1087-1092.

99. Hanzel DA, Proia NG, Hudgel DW. Response of obstructive sleep apnea to fluoxetine and protriptyline. *Chest.* 1991;100(2):416-421.

100. Marshall NS, Yee BJ, Desai AV, et al. Two randomized placebo-controlled trials to evaluate the efficacy and tolerability of mirtazapine for the treatment of obstructive sleep apnea. *Sleep.* 2008;31(6):824-831.

101. Carley DW, Olopade C, Ruigt GS, et al. Efficacy of mirtazapine in obstructive sleep apnea syndrome. *Sleep.* 2007;30(1):35-41.

102. Brownell LG, West P, Sweatman P, et al. The role of protriptyline in obstructive sleep apnea. *Bull Eur Physiopathol Respir.* 1983;19(6):621-624.

103. Brownell LG, West P, Sweatman P, et al. Protriptyline in obstructive sleep apnea: A double-blind trial. *N Engl J Med.* 1982;307(17):1037-1042.

104. Smith PL, Haponik EF, Allen RP, et al. The effects of protriptyline in sleep-disordered breathing. *Am Rev Respir Dis.* 1983;127(1):8-13.

105. Stepanski EJ, Conway W, Young D, et al. A double-blind trial of protriptyline in the treatment of sleep apnea syndrome. *Henry Ford Hosp Med J.* 1988;36(1):5-8.

106. Whyte KF, Gould GA, Airlie MAA, et al. Role of protriptyline and acetazolamide in the sleep apnea/hypopnea syndrome. *Sleep.* 1988;11(5):463-472.

107. Espinoza H, Antic R, Thornton AT, et al. The effects of aminophylline on sleep and sleep-disordered breathing in patients with obstructive sleep apnea syndrome. *Am Rev Respir Dis.* 1987;136(1):80-84.

108. Hein H, Behnke G, Jorres RA, et al. The therapeutic effect of theophylline in mild obstructive sleep apnea/hypopnea syndrome: Results of repeated measurements with portable recording devices at home. *Eur J Med Res.* 2000;5(9):391-399.

109. Mulloy E, McNicholas WT. Theophylline in obstructive sleep apnea. A double-blind evaluation. *Chest.* 1992;101(3):753-757.

110. Saletu B, Oberndorfer S, Anderer P, et al. Efficiency of continuous positive airway pressure versus theophylline therapy in sleep apnea: Comparative sleep laboratory studies on objective and subjective sleep and awakening quality. *Neuropsychobiology.* 1999;39(3):151-159.

111. Sessler CN. Theophylline toxicity: Clinical features of 116 consecutive cases. *Am J Med.* 1990;88(6):567-576.

112. Shannon M. Predictors of major toxicity after theophylline overdose. *Ann Intern Med.* 1993;119(12):1161-1167.

113. Paloucek FP, Rodvold KA. Evaluation of theophylline overdoses and toxicities. *Ann Emerg Med.* 1988;17(2):135-144.

114. Atkinson RL, Suratt PM, Wilhoit SC. Naloxone improves sleep apnea in obese humans. *Int J Obes.* 1985;9(4):233-239.

115. Davila DG, Hurt RD, Offord KP, et al. Acute effects of transdermal nicotine on sleep architecture, snoring, and sleep-disordered breathing in nonsmokers. *Am J Respir Crit Care Med.* 1994;150(2):469-474.

116. Gothe B, Strohl K, Levin S, et al. Nicotine: A different approach to treatment of obstructive sleep apnea. *Chest.* 1985;87(1):11-17.

117. Suratt PM, Wilhoit SC, Brown ED, et al. Effect of doxapram on obstructive sleep apnea. *Bull Eur Physiopathol Respir.* 1986;22(2):127-131.

118. Chauncey JB, Aldrich MS. Preliminary findings in the treatment of obstructive sleep apnea with transtracheal oxygen. *Sleep.* 1990;13(2):167-174.

119. Farney RJ, Walker JM, Elmer JC, et al. Transtracheal oxygen, nasal CPAP and nasal oxygen in five patients with obstructive sleep apnea. *Chest.* 1992;101(5):1228-1235.

120. Landsberg R, Friedman M, Ascher-Landsberg J. Treatment of hypoxemia in obstructive sleep apnea. *Am J Rhinol.* 2001;15(5):311-313.

121. Phillips BA, Schmitt FA, Berry DT, et al. Treatment of obstructive sleep apnea. A preliminary report comparing nasal CPAP to nasal oxygen in patients with mild OSA. *Chest.* 1990;98(2):325-330.

122. Kearley R, Wynne JW, Block AJ, et al. The effect of low flow oxygen on sleep-disordered breathing and oxygen desaturation. A study of patients with chronic obstructive lung disease. *Chest.* 1980;78(5):682-685.

123. Gold AR, Schwartz AR, Bleecker ER, et al. The effect of chronic nocturnal oxygen administration upon sleep apnea. *Am Rev Respir Dis.* 1986;134(5):925-929.

124. Martin RJ, Sanders MH, Gray BA, et al. Acute and long-term ventilatory effects of hyperoxia in the adult sleep apnea syndrome. *Am Rev Respir Dis.* 1982;125(2):175-180.

125. McGinley BM, Patil SP, Kirkness JP, et al. A nasal cannula can be used to treat obstructive sleep apnea. *Am J Respir Crit Care Med.* 2007;176(2):194-200.

126. Weaver TE, Maislin G, Dinges DF, et al. Relationship between hours of CPAP use and achieving normal levels of sleepiness and daily functioning. *Sleep.* 2007;30(6):711-719.

127. Weaver TE, Chasens ER, Arora S. Modafinil improves functional outcomes in patients with residual excessive sleepiness associated with CPAP treatment. *J Clin Sleep Med.* 2009;5(6):499-505.

128. Roth T, Rippon GA, Arora S. Armodafinil improves wakefulness and long-term episodic memory in nCPAP-adherent patients with excessive sleepiness associated with obstructive sleep apnea. *Sleep Breath.* 2008;12(1):53-62.

129. Braver HM, Block AJ. Effect of nasal spray, positional therapy, and the combination thereof in the asymptomatic snorer. *Sleep*. 1994;17(6): 516-521.

130. Kiely JL, Nolan P, McNicholas WT. Intranasal corticosteroid therapy for obstructive sleep apnoea in patients with co-existing rhinitis. *Thorax*. 2004;59(1):50-55.

131. Larrain A, Kapur VK, Gooley TA, et al. Pharmacological treatment of obstructive sleep apnea with a combination of pseudoephedrine and domperidone. *J Clin Sleep Med*. 2010;6(2):117-123.

132. Strohl KP. Drug trials for obstructive sleep apnea. *J Clin Sleep Med*. 2010;6(2):124-126.

133. Larrain A, Hudson M, Dominitz JA, et al. Treatment of severe snoring with a combination of pseudoephedrine sulfate and domperidone. *J Clin Sleep Med*. 2006;2(1):21-25.

Chapter 16

Positive Airway Pressure Therapy for Obstructive Sleep Apnea

NAVEEN KANATHUR / MAX HIRSHKOWITZ / TEOFILO L. LEE-CHIONG

OVERVIEW

The human upper airway is a flexible tube; its ability to distend and collapse enables it to perform various functions in speech, deglutition, and respiration during the waking state. The generalized reduction or loss of muscle tone during sleep affects the various upper airway dilator muscles, including the genioglossus, tensor palatini, geniohyoid, and sternohyoid. This, in turn, leads to reduction in the size of the lumen of the naso-, oro-, and hypopharynx. In obstructive types of sleep-related breathing disorders, respiratory events (apneas or hypopneas) occur when forces maintaining upper airway patency (e.g., dilator muscles activation) are ineffective in counteracting factors promoting upper airway closure during sleep.[1] The critical closing pressure (P_{Crit}) is the intraluminal pressure at which collapse of the upper airway occurs. It is progressively less negative (increased collapsibility as measured by P_{Crit}) among patients along the spectrum from primary snoring to mild, moderate, or severe obstructive sleep apnea (OSA) compared to normal persons. Individuals with sleep-disordered breathing tend to have upper airways that are narrower and more vulnerable to collapse compared to those without the disorder. Repetitive upper airway compromise can manifest as snoring, respiratory effort–related arousals, hypopneas, or apneas. These respiratory events may be associated with arousals, awakenings, episodic oxyhemoglobin desaturation, and changes in heart rate and blood pressure.

Positive airway pressure (PAP) devices generally function to pneumatically splint the airway. The increased airflow helps preserve the patency of the upper airway. By increasing nasal pressure above P_{Crit}, positive airway pressure stabilizes the vulnerable portions of the naso- and oropharynx.[2] In general, PAP systems have several components: a flow generator, a patient interface, and tubing connecting the two. Most modern equipment also includes a heated humidifier that is typically integrated or articulates with the flow generator platform.

The flow generator creates airflow using a fan or turbine. The airflow is directed through a valve, and positive pressure can be controlled by altering the valve's size or altering fan speed. Over the years, advances in small motor and ball bearing technology have led to smaller, lighter, and quieter flow generators. Heated humidification was developed to reduce discomfort (chilling of nasal sinuses and nasal dryness) and thereby facilitate usage. A water reservoir (sometimes incorporating circulation baffling) mounted on a heating plate

appears to be the currently favored design. Ultimately, the generated flow is delivered using a nasal or nasal-oral interface. The interface can be a mask, nasal pillows, or a combination of the two.

A typical PAP mask is lightweight and constructed of clear plastic; however, cloth and rubberized material is sometimes used. Usually, a softer, hypoallergenic material surrounds the mask's edges to create a seal; a variety of materials and designs are used and they continue to evolve. Masks and other interfaces include a vent that allows CO_2 to escape. In the past, nonrebreathing valves and inflating bags were part of the design but their necessity has been obviated by redesign. Interfaces come in different sizes and shapes so that individual patient fitting can maximize comfort. The actual interface, be it nasal mask, nasal-oral mask, oral mask, nasal pillows, or hybrid combination, is held in place by a series of straps, clips, or Velcro tabs (headgear). Realizing that the purpose of these straps is to hold the interface in place, not to pull it forcefully up to the face, is crucial. Overtightening of the headgear is a common mistake because patients think it reduces leaks; however, more often than not, it does little more than reduce comfort. Ideally, flow should be delivered nasally; however, if a patient is an obligate mouth breather or cannot sleep with mouth closed (even with a chin strap), a full face or oral mask may be necessary. The term "full face mask" is common parlance (and will be used here); however, most of these interfaces would more accurately be described as nasal-oral interfaces. There are a couple of true full face masks but they are seldom used for nightly therapy. Nasal-oral interfaces, of course, cover the entire airway and thereby create some risk. They also are bulkier and necessitate sealing a larger surface area, making them more prone to leaks, especially if bumped at night when patients move. With the mouth open, problems with drying are more common. Using full face masks during initial titration should be discouraged unless they are really needed. Finally, full face masks should be avoided if autotitrating PAP is being used in full-range mode to explore pressure requirements. Nasal masks are smaller and lighter than full face masks and include a wide variety of designs. Nasal masks incorporating soft, form-fitting, gel materials are particularly popular at present. Since it was first introduced in the 1980s, the nasal mask has been the standard and most popular PAP interface. Nasal pillows and similar devices that are inserted directly in the nares are gaining popularity. These interfaces tend to leak less because the area requiring pneumatic sealing is small. Other advantages include being lightweight and less obtrusive than masks. However, problems can develop when therapeutic pressures are high (>12 cm H_2O) or when bilevel devices rapidly change from low to high pressures. Figure 16-1 illustrates a variety of mask and nasal pillow interfaces.

Tubing connects the flow generator to the patient interface. The most commonly used tubing is 6 ft to 8 ft long, flexible, externally ribbed, standard 22 mm in diameter, with smooth interior bore hoses with female connectors on both ends. Some devices provide optional tubing with embedded heating coils to reduce condensation inside the hose when heated humidification is used in a cool room. Smaller bore tubing with greater flexibility is available from some PAP machine manufacturers.

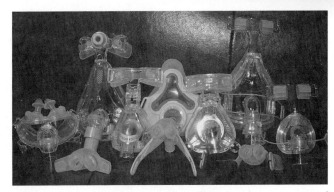

Figure 16-1 Positive airway pressure (PAP) interfaces. A variety of popular masks and nasal pillows are shown. Nasal-oral masks (so-called "full face masks") occupy the back row, nasal masks are in the middle row (with a nasal-oral hybrid shown at the far left), and nasal pillows are arrayed in front.

SLEEP-DISORDERED BREATHING EVENT DEFINITIONS

In general terms, an apnea episode is a cessation of breathing for more than two respiratory cycles, operationally defined as at least 10 seconds among adults. When the breathing cessation results from airway collapse, the event is classified as obstructive. By contrast, apnea episodes produced by lack of diaphragmatic activation or loss of respiratory drive are classified as central. Events including elements of both obstructive and central apnea are categorized as mixed. In the broadest sense, breathing events characterized by reduced airflow represent episodes of hypopnea and are not intrinsically abnormal. However, during sleep, hypopnea may produce pathophysiologic consequences, including oxyhemoglobin desaturation, central nervous system (CNS) arousal, or both. The Center for Medicare and Medicaid Services (CMS) adopted a definition for hypopnea requiring an associated 4% (or more) oxyhemoglobin desaturation even though preexisting definitions required either a 3% (or more) desaturation or a CNS arousal. The American Academy of Sleep Medicine (AASM) allows either definition; however, CMS requires testing facilities to use the identical criteria for all patients (Medicare, Medicaid, other third party carrier, or self-pay). Thus, if a laboratory evaluates even one Medicare patient, CMS criteria must, by law, be used. Consequently, hypopnea episodes associated with less than a 4% oxyhemoglobin desaturation but that are associated with a CNS arousal are typically characterized as respiratory effort–related arousals (RERA). Figure 16-2 illustrates different types of obstructive sleep-disordered breathing events and Table 16-1 for specific scoring rules.[3]

INDICATIONS FOR POSITIVE AIRWAY PRESSURE THERAPY

AASM, CMS, and various health insurance carriers established quantitative criteria for treating sleep apnea with positive airway pressure (and they do not necessarily agree). In general, criteria are based on symptoms, co-morbid illnesses, and sleep-disordered breathing severity indices. Apnea index (AI) represents the number of apnea episodes per hour of sleep (the actual time spent asleep, not the time in bed).

Apnea-hypopnea index (AHI) is the number of apnea and hypopnea episodes per hour of sleep. Respiratory disturbance index (RDI) embodies the number of apnea episodes, hypopnea episodes, and RERA per hour of sleep (note, however, recent confusion has been created by CMS redefining RDI as the number of apnea and hypopnea episodes per hour of continuous monitoring [not sleep time] when evaluation is performed using a home sleep testing device). PAP therapy is the treatment of choice for most patients with sleep-related breathing disorders, especially when the disorder is predominantly obstructive.

CMS Criteria

CMS criteria[4] approve treatment for any individual with an AHI of 15 (or more). However, treatment threshold is lower (AHI ≥5) for patients with concomitant insomnia, excessive sleepiness, or impaired cognition; or with a co-morbid condition of mood disorder, hypertension, or ischemic heart disease; or with a history of stroke. Currently, at least 2 hours of recording is required with either laboratory polysomnography or a three- (or more) channel home sleep testing device. Because Medicare criteria can change, the reader is referred to www.cms.gov for further information.

AASM Criteria

AASM criteria[5] differ mainly because of the recognition that CNS arousal (sleep disruption) signifies an important pathophysiologic event adversely affecting sleep and general health. Therefore, rather than restricting thresholds by considering only apnea and hypopnea, AASM also includes RERA. As a result, any patient with RDI of 15 or more qualifies for PAP therapy, and patients with sleepiness or relevant co-morbid conditions meet criteria with RDIs of 5 (or more) on full-night baseline polysomnographic evaluations. If diagnosis is made during the first 2 hours or more of polysomnography, and the remaining 3 hours or more of the recording procedure are used for PAP titration (a split-night protocol), an RDI of 40 (or more) is sufficient for PAP treatment. However, if the patient is sleepy, has witnessed apnea, has a body mass index (BMI) of 35 (or more), or has relevant co-morbid conditions, minimum RDI threshold for split-night polysomnography is only 20 events per hour of sleep.

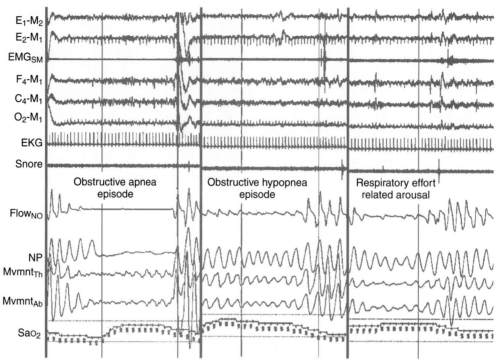

Figure 16-2 Obstructive sleep-disordered breathing events. The three panels depict 1-minute polysomnographic epochs. In the left panel, an obstructive apnea episode is characterized by airflow cessation notwithstanding continued respiratory effort. The middle panel depicts a hypopnea with reduced airflow leading to greater than 4% oxyhemoglobin desaturation. In the far right panel a respiratory effort–related arousal manifests reduced airflow and a flattening of nasal pressure, but oxyhemoglobin desaturation does not reach the 4% threshold criteria for classifying this sleep-disordered breathing event as a hypopnea. Recording notation: E_1, outer cantus of left eye; E_2, outer cantus of right eye; EMG_{SM}, submentalis electromyogram; F_4, right frontal; C_4, right central; O_2, right occipital; M_1, left mastoid; M_2, right mastoid; EKG, electrocardiogram; $Flow_{NO}$, nasal-oral airflow; NP, nasal pressure; $Mvmnt_{Th}$, thoracic movement; $Mvmnt_{Ab}$, abdominal movement; and Sao_2, oxyhemoglobin saturation.

TABLE 16-1

Definitions for Sleep-Disordered Breathing Events

Respiratory Event	Operational Definition Based on AASM Scoring Criteria
Obstructive apnea	A 10-second (or longer) 90% drop (or greater) in the nasal/oral airflow channel's peak-to-trough amplitude that persists for at least 90% of the event's duration in the presence of continued respiratory effort
Central apnea	A 10-second (or longer) 90% drop (or greater) in the nasal/oral airflow channel's peak-to-trough amplitude that persists for at least 90% of the event's duration in the absence of respiratory effort
Mixed apnea	A 10-second (or longer) 90% drop (or greater) in the nasal/oral airflow channel's peak-to-trough amplitude that persists for at least 90% of the event's duration marked by an initial lack of inspiratory effort followed by increasing respiratory effort as the individual makes an unsuccessful attempt to breath against a closed airway
Hypopnea—AASM recommended	A 10-second (or longer), 30% drop (or more) in nasal pressure signal amplitude (compared to baseline) that persists for at least 90% of the event's duration and provokes a 4% drop (or more) in oxygen saturation
Hypopnea—AASM alternate	A 10-second (or longer), 50% drop (or more) in nasal pressure signal amplitude (compared with baseline) that persists for at least 90% of the event duration and provokes either a 3% drop (or more) in O_2 saturation or a CNS arousal
Respiratory effort–related arousal	A 10-second (or longer) increased respiratory effort manifested as "flattening" in the nasal pressure channel that provokes a CNS arousal but does not meet apnea or hypopnea amplitude or oxygen saturation criteria

AASM, American Academy of Sleep Medicine; *CNS,* central nervous system.

POSITIVE AIRWAY PRESSURE MODALITIES

Treatment modalities for PAP therapy include continuous positive airway pressure (CPAP), bilevel positive airway pressure (BiPAP), autotitrating positive airway pressure (APAP), adaptive servoventilation (ASV), and noninvasive positive pressure ventilation. Figure 16-3 illustrates several different types of PAP machines. PAP therapies are principally used to treat obstructive sleep-related breathing disorders; however, they have been used, with some benefit, in patients with predominantly central and mixed (central and obstructive) episodes. For these latter patients who do not exclusively have obstructive forms of sleep-disordered breathing, adaptive servoventilation and ventilation devices are popular.

Continuous Positive Airway Pressure

CPAP devices provide a continuous and relatively constant pressure throughout the respiratory cycle. Airflow is generated by fan or turbine and then forced through a valve, which

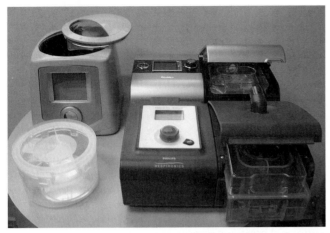

Figure 16-3 Positive airway pressure (PAP) machines. Three PAP machines are shown; all have built in heated humidification.

allows varying pressures to be selected. CPAP represents the earliest form of PAP therapy to treat sleep-disordered breathing. Initial research, development, and invention of CPAP by Colin Sullivan[6] at the Royal Prince Alfred Hospital in Sydney, Australia was followed within 5 years by commercially available devices. Pressure settings are traditionally determined during attended laboratory polysomnography. However, current technique sometimes derives a fixed therapeutic pressure from autotitrating machines (see discussion under "Determining Optimal Positive Airway Pressure"). Most modern equipment maintains flow regulation using a pressure transducer imbedded in the flow circuit. In this manner, CPAP machines can compensate for altitude changes (affecting ideal fan law properties).[7] However, rapid flow changes produced by breathing, transitioning from inhalation to exhalation, can produce pressure spikes. To better balance pressures across the respiratory cycle, some CPAP devices are equipped with an expiratory pressure relief feature that lowers the pressure at the onset of expiration. Pressure relief presumably reduces the discomfort of breathing out against high CPAP flows.

Bilevel Positive Airway Pressure

BiPAP provides two pressure levels during the respiratory cycle: a higher level during inspiration (inspiratory positive airway pressure [IPAP]) and a lower pressure during expiration (expiratory positive airway pressure [EPAP]). A transducer embedded in the airflow circuit senses the pressure change when the patient begins to exhale or inhale and automatically switches between IPAP and EPAP settings. BiPAP may increase comfort for patients who complain of significant difficulty breathing out against high CPAP flows and may reduce gastric distention secondary to aerophagia. BiPAP reportedly can help when patients have concurrent obstructive or restrictive lung disease, or hypoventilation syndrome with persistent oxygen desaturation notwithstanding CPAP therapy.[5] However, BiPAP does not significantly improve utilization in most patients, or minimize complaints regarding mask discomfort (or nasal stuffiness) compared to CPAP alone.[8] Some devices also have pressure relief systems that attempt to dampen the steep pressure rise when the machine switches from EPAP to IPAP. Some BiPAP devices are also

available with a "timed-mode" setting that alternates between EPAP and IPAP according to a set interval specified by the clinician.

Autotitrating Positive Airway Pressure

APAP devices are designed to vary pressures to meet a patient's respiratory requirements; however, the computational algorithms are device-specific and largely proprietary. In 2002, the AASM developed practice parameters for using APAP and they were updated (but were largely similar) in 2007.[9,10] APAP has several potential applications. The first possible use is for diagnosing sleep-disordered breathing (APAP Diagnosis) and is not recommended. APAP can also be used for determining a fixed pressure for subsequent treatment with CPAP (APAP Titration). The use of APAP titration is considered a guideline when the sleep evaluation is an attended polysomnographic session but is considered an option when it is unattended and necessitates close clinical follow-up to assure treatment efficacy. Furthermore, unattended APAP titration is contraindicated for patients with congestive heart failure (CHF), chronic obstructive pulmonary disease (COPD), central sleep apnea, and hypoventilation syndromes owing to potential risk and lack of safety data. Compared to conventional in-laboratory CPAP titration, APAP produces comparable reductions in AHI and arousal indices and improvements in sleep architecture, oxygenation, and nightly PAP adherence.[11] A literature meta-analysis and several randomized controlled trials report successful outcome when APAP titration was used.[12-14] Box 16-1 provides a summary of AASM guidelines for APAP.

It has long been known that pressure requirements for maintaining airway patency in some patients with sleep-disordered breathing vary from night to night as well as within a night.[15] The inter- and intranight AHI fluctuation (even when CPAP is used) can reflect changes in rapid eye movement (REM) sleep percentage, different sleep positions (supine vs. nonsupine), presence of nasal congestion, and use of alcohol, muscle relaxants, or opioids. By automatically and continually adjusting delivered pressures, APAP devices can theoretically achieve and maintain upper airway patency at lower mean airway pressures than CPAP devices.[16] AASM guidelines concerning APAP therapy for nightly use with varying pressure (APAP Treatment) require clinical follow-up, including possible standard attended CPAP titration if symptoms fail to resolve. Studies find equivalence between APAP treatment and standard CPAP therapy.[12,17,18] Although specific recommendations are not provided in the AASM practice parameters for routine management in patients for whom APAP therapy is successful, clinicians typically use the information accumulated in the machine's memory tabulating both pressure dwell times and AHI at various pressures to narrow the pressure range for subsequent nightly therapy.

Adaptive Servoventilation

With adaptive servoventilation, pressure support (difference between EPAP and IPAP) increases during hypoventilation and decreases during hyperventilation. This modality can be useful when a patient has both central and obstructive sleep-disordered breathing events. Some studies also claim efficacy for treating CPAP emergent central sleep apnea;[19] however, its application for this is controversial.

Lastly, nocturnal noninvasive positive pressure ventilation provides two pressure levels at a set rate to assist ventilation and may be used for patients with concomitant advanced respiratory disorders or hypoventilation syndromes.[20]

DETERMINING OPTIMAL POSITIVE AIRWAY PRESSURE

The Traditional Approach

Several methods are used to determine optimal CPAP or BiPAP pressure setting for subsequent nightly use at home. In patients with confirmed sleep-disordered breathing, titration during an attended full-night polysomnographic session represents the traditional technique for determining optimal pressure. Essentially, a sleep technologist gradually raises the positive airway pressure setting while monitoring changes in the respiratory pattern. The goal is to eliminate sleep-disordered breathing events (see Table 16-2 for a summary of the AASM recommended titration procedure).[21] Short of reaching this ideal, the aim is to improve breathing during sleep, as much as possible, and the overall adequacy of titration can be graded after careful inspection, review, and interpretation of the polysomnographic recording. Table 16-3 summarizes the titration adequacy grading system developed by Hirshkowitz and Sharafkhaneh[22] that was adopted by the AASM. If significant sleep-disordered breathing persists at too great a degree, the titration may not be deemed inadequate. Such cases require retitration

(possibly with higher pressures or another form of PAP) or intervention with another therapeutic approach.

Split-Night Titration

Patients with severe sleep-related breathing disorders may undergo split-night sleep study procedures that incorporate an initial diagnostic portion followed by PAP titration on the same night. Figure 16-4 shows the night summary histogram for a patient with severe sleep-related breathing disorder who was titrated using a split-night protocol. Occlusive sleep-disordered breathing events tend to be more frequent during REM sleep (that occurs in a smaller proportion in the first part of the sleep period compared to the second half); consequently, split-night studies generally underestimate sleep-disordered breathing severity.

A split-night study is generally considered appropriate if at least 2 hours of recorded sleep occur during the initial diagnostic portion of the study with an AHI during the diagnostic portion exceeding 20 events per hour in patients with significant oxygen desaturation, or 40 events per hour in patients without hypoxemia; and if at least 3 hours remain for PAP titration (with an adequate amount of REM sleep and supine-position sleep occurring to verify adequacy of titration). The goal during both full-night and split-night PAP titration studies is to identify a pressure that effectively eliminates apneas, hypopneas, snoring, and RERAs; normalizes oxygen saturation; and improves sleep architecture and quality in all body positions and during all sleep stages.

APAP Titration

In selected patients, therapeutic fixed pressure for subsequent CPAP therapy can be estimated from a trial with APAP. Individuals diagnosed with sleep apnea using traditional technique who do not have lung disease, heart disease, central sleep apnea, other forms of hypoventilation, or are status post-uvulopalatopharyngoplasty (UPPP) may qualify for APAP titration (see previous section on APAP). Although not considered an AASM "standard" according to AASM practice guidelines, unattended laboratory or home titration with APAP represents a therapeutic option.[10] The procedure involves having a patient use APAP for approximately a week or more with the pressure range set widely. The clinician then transfers and inspects the APAP machine's internally stored dwell time and AHI estimate data to determine the 90th or 95th percentile of pressure setting duration and uses this to set a fixed CPAP pressure for subsequent nightly use. By contrast, if the treatment plan is to continue using APAP in variable mode, the pressure at which sleep-related respiratory events normalize can be used as minimum pressure with the 95th percentile dwell time pressure (or slightly higher) as the maximum pressure.

BENEFICIAL EFFECTS OF POSITIVE AIRWAY PRESSURE THERAPY

Outcome studies of PAP therapy report beneficial effects on sleep quality, alertness, blood pressure control, heart function, inflammation, and mortality rate.[23,24] A meta-analysis of seven randomized controlled trials comparing CPAP to placebo or

TABLE 16-2

Steps for Successful Positive Airway Pressure Titration in Adults

Process	Step	Description
CPAP and BiPAP preparation	1	Educate the patient about CPAP before beginning titration. Allow patient to watch a video about PAP if a suitable one is available. Answer any questions the patient may have about the apparatus and equipment.
	2	Provide a "hands-on" demonstration of the PAP machine and interface.
	3	Select and fit a properly sized headgear with mask or nasal pillows. Verify proper fit with pressure applied.
	4	Have patient wear the mask or nasal pillows with positive pressure to promote acclimation to the device.
	5	Before starting titration, have the patient use a nasal decongestant if needed. If needed, use heated humidifier to prevent nasal dryness. Heated humidifiers are very strongly recommended.
CPAP and BiPAP monitoring technique	1	Use PAP device flow signal and difference between mask pressure and machine outlet to detect apnea and hypopnea episodes. Do not use a thermistor or thermocouple under the mask.
	2	Score RERAs when airflow signal flattens on inspiration and the event is terminated by a CNS arousal when detection criteria for apnea and hypopnea are not met.
CPAP titration	1	For new titrations, begin with CPAP set at 4 cm H_2O. Higher starting pressures can be used for patients with high body mass index or when performing retitration.
	2	Increase pressure 1 cm H_2O after 5 minutes if more than any of the following occur: • Two obstructive apnea episodes • Three obstructive hypopnea episodes (or 2 obstructive hypopnea episodes and one obstructive apnea episode*) • Five RERAs (or any combination of five respiratory events—apnea, hypopnea, or RERA*) • 3 minutes or longer of loud snoring
	3	Repeat CPAP titration step 2 as many times as necessary up to a pressure of 20 cm H_2O. Also, note that the goal is to reduce apnea and hypopnea to one episode or less in any given 15-minute period.*
	4	If the patient wakes up and reports the pressure is too high, lower pressure to a comfortable level, wait until the person falls back to sleep, and go back to step 2.
	5	Once the optimal pressure is reached, the patient should be allowed to go through a REM sleep episode. Ideally, there should be a 15-minute, or longer sample of breathing with CPAP while the patient sleeps in the supine position during REM sleep.
	6	A "downward" titration can be tried, at 1 cm H_2O at a time in 5-minute periods, if: • 30 minutes elapse and no events occur even in REM when the patient is sleeping supine. • Central apnea episodes begin occurring regularly and pressure is high (this is unusual at less than 10 cm H_2O, raising the question of whether the events are true central apneas).
	7	Consider switching to BiPAP if: • CPAP exceeds 12 cm H_2O and the patient begins complaining about having trouble exhaling against the pressure. In such cases, switching is discretionary and will depend on availability of BiPAP and local medical center policy. Well-tolerated CPAP should be titrated upward to 20 cm H_2O, rather than switching to BiPAP. • The patient continues having respiratory events when on CPAP at high pressures (>15 cm H_2O).
BiPAP titration	1	Begin at pressures of 8/4 (inspiratory/expiratory) cm H_2O. Higher starting pressures can be used for patients with high body mass index or when performing retitration.
	2	Increase inspiratory pressure by 1 cm H_2O after 5 minutes if more than any of the following occur: • Two obstructive apnea episodes • Three obstructive hypopnea or two obstructive hypopnea episodes and one obstructive apnea episode • Five RERAs • 3 minutes or longer of loud snoring If conducting a split-night titration, consider using inspiratory pressure increments of 2.0 to 2.5 cm H_2O.
	3	Repeat BiPAP titration step 2 as many times as necessary up to an inspiratory pressure of 30 cm H_2O. Adjust expiratory pressures as needed; however, usually it is raised as inspiratory pressure is increased. Maintain a minimum differential between inspiratory and expiratory pressures of 4 cm H_2O. Maximum differential should be 10 cm H_2O.
	4	A "downward" titration can be tried, at 1 cm H_2O at a time in 5-minute periods, if: • 30 minutes elapse and there are no events even in REM when the patient is sleeping supine • Central apnea episodes begin occurring regularly and pressure is high (this is unusual at less than 10 cm H_2O, raising the question of whether the events are true central apneas).

*Indicates additions to the AASM standard for clarification and to provide direction in situations not covered.

AASM, American Academy of Sleep Medicine; *APAP*, autotitrating positive airway pressure; *BiPAP*, bilevel positive airway pressure; *CNS*, central nervous system; *CPAP*, continuous positive airway pressure; *COPD*, chronic obstructive pulmonary disease; *OSA*, obstructive sleep apnea; *PAP*, positive airway pressure; *RERA*, respiratory effort–related arousal.

with conservative management in patients with mild to moderate OSA indicated that CPAP significantly reduced self-reported daytime sleepiness; however, the overall effect on sleepiness was interpreted as having limited clinical significance.[25] Properly titrated, PAP therapy reduces or eliminates snoring; normalizes arterial oxygen saturation and occlusive sleep-disordered breathing events; and decreases number of CNS arousals. PAP-related quality of life improvement; mood and neurocognitive function benefits, and reduced health care utilization have also been described.[23,26-28]

TABLE 16-3

PAP Titration Grading System

Grade	Label	Grading System
A	Optimal titration	In patients diagnosed with SRBD, an optimal titration reduces AHI and/or RDI to less than five events per hour of sleep. This level of reduction often is difficult to achieve. The interval during which the chosen pressure is administered must contain at least 15 minutes of sleep, contain some REM sleep, and not be continually interrupted by arousals or awakening.
B	Good titration	In patients with moderate-severe SRBD (AI, AHI, or RDI >20), a good titration must reduce AHI or RDI to 10 or less. Indices at this level are considered within the normal range. By contrast, in patients with mild SRBD with a baseline AHI <20, a good titration must reduce AHI or RDI by 50% or more. The interval during which the chosen pressure is administered must contain at least 15 minutes of sleep, contain some REM sleep, and not be continually interrupted by arousals or awakenings.
C	Adequate titration	In patients in whom normal values are not achieved (AHI or RDI ≤10) notwithstanding vastly improved sleep-related breathing, an adequate titration is one that reduces AHI or RDI by 75% or more. Such patients should be closely followed clinically, with a reevaluation as needed. Another reason for a grade C titration (adequate rather than good or optimal) is lack of occurrence of REM sleep during the best pressure. Situations in which this can arise include medication-related REM suppression, inadequate REM sleep during the sleep evaluation (so that there is not enough time for REM to recur later in the night), and satiation of REM sleep drive due to rebound earlier in the study. In such instances, the sleep specialist must rely on clinical judgment and should document the basis for deciding about titration adequacy. Such patients should be closely followed clinically, with a reevaluation as needed.
D	Unacceptable titration	An unacceptable titration is one that fails to meet even minimally adequate titration criteria. The patient should be reevaluated, or other treatment options should be applied. Sometimes an estimated positive airway pressure level can be based on a clear-cut and substantial reduction in SRBD events. If an estimate is made, close follow-up with a retitration is indicated if symptoms, including but not limited to snoring, daytime somnolence, and observed apneas during sleep, do not resolve.

AI, arousal index; *AHI,* apnea-hypopnea index; *PAP,* positive airway pressure; *RDI,* respiratory disturbance index; *REM,* rapid eye movement; *SRBD,* sleep-related breathing difficulty.

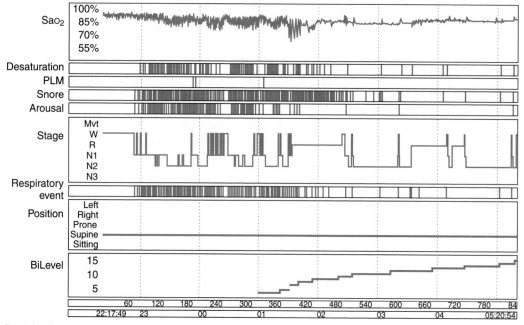

Figure 16-4 Split-night diagnostic titration sleep histogram. The figure shows the dramatic improvement in sleep-related breathing after positive airway pressure is applied and the pressures are titrated upward. Note the stabilization of oxyhemoglobin saturation (labeled SaO₂), the reduction in snoring sounds (labeled *snore*), and near elimination of respiratory events as pressure increases. A rebound in rapid eye movement (REM) sleep also occurred.

Mortality Rate

In the Sleep Heart Health Study, using a prospective cohort design, 6441 men and women were evaluated for sleep-disordered breathing (SDB) with polysomnography and followed for an average of 8.2 years. Death from any cause was recorded in this community-based cohort of individuals aged 40 years or older. Total number of deaths during the follow-up period was 1047 (female, 44%), with a crude mortality rate of 20.3 deaths per 1000 person-years. Mortality rates per 100 person-years varied with SBD severity: no SDB (AHI <5) = 16.8%; mild SDB (AHI = 5-14.9) = 21.7%; moderate SDB (AHI = 15-29.9) = 28.3%; and severe SDB (AHI ≥30) = 32.2%. All-cause death was associated with measures of sleep-related hypoxemia but not sleep fragmentation. Hazard ratios for death after adjusting for age, sex, race, smoking status, body mass index, and prevalent medical conditions were calculated. Compared to subjects without SDB, the adjusted hazard ratios (HRs) for all-cause death is progressively higher with worsening SBD (mild SDB = 0.93; moderate SDB = 1.17; and severe SDB = 1.46). Risk of death associated with severe SDB was significantly increased in subjects with mean ages 40 to 70 years (HR 2.09; 95% CI: 1.31-3.33).[29]

In an 18-year follow-up of the Wisconsin Sleep Cohort, a high mortality risk was found with untreated SDB, independent of age, sex, and body mass index. In patients who were not using CPAP, the adjusted HR (95% CI) for all-cause death with severe versus no sleep-disordered breathing was 3.8 (1.6- to 9.0) and this result was unchanged after accounting for daytime sleepiness.[30]

Blood Pressure

Lavie and colleagues noted increased blood pressure and incidence of hypertension correlated with SDB severity. They calculated that each additional apnea episode per hour of sleep, and each 10% decrease in nocturnal oxygen saturation increased the odds of hypertension by 1% and 13%, respectively.[31] SDB treatment appears to decrease blood pressure and improve hypertension control.[32-35]

Dernaika and associates conducted a retrospective chart review of 98 patients with OSA (AHI ≥5) and hypertension. Forty-two subjects had resistant hypertension, defined as daytime blood pressure of 140/90 mm Hg (or more) notwithstanding use of three or more antihypertensive medications. Hypertension was considered controlled in 56 subjects. Mean arterial pressure differed between the two groups with CPAP therapy (resistant hypertension difference = −5.6 vs. controlled hypertension difference = −0.8 mm Hg). In addition, de-escalation of required antihypertensive agents was noted after CPAP therapy in 71% of the resistant hypertension group but not in the controlled hypertension group. Interestingly, neither baseline sleep-disordered breathing severity (AHI) nor CPAP adherence (hours of CPAP use) was associated with the decrease in mean arterial pressure.[36]

PAP therapy may also alter blood pressure at night. Under normal circumstances, blood pressure decreases during sleep and is generally lower than in the morning. The term "dipping" refers to blood pressure reduction by at least 10 mm Hg systolic and 5 mm Hg diastolic blood pressure at night compared to daytime values. Absence of this blood pressure reduction is referred to as "nondipping." Patients with untreated SDB are commonly "nondippers." Akashiba and colleagues[37] reported that CPAP therapy restored the normal circadian "dipping" pattern in 68% of subjects who were "nondippers" before the start of treatment. In one placebo-controlled study, the decrease in nighttime (10 PM to 6 AM) mean arterial blood pressure was greater in patients with OSA who were given CPAP therapy; however, there was no significant difference in daytime (6 AM to 10 PM) blood pressure values between groups.[38]

A meta-analysis of randomized controlled trials evaluating CPAP-related blood pressure changes in patients with OSA searched studies from January 1980 to July 2006. Data from 16 trials representing 818 participants were examined. Mean reductions in systolic blood pressure, diastolic blood pressure, and mean arterial pressure for patients treated with CPAP were −2.46, −1.83, and −2.2 mmHg, respectively[39] when compared to control subjects.

Heart Function

CPAP-related improvements in cardiac function are reported in patients with OSA and congestive heart failure. Studies reveal CPAP therapy decreased right ventricular (RV) volumes in persons with severe obstructive sleep apnea. Magalang and associates used cardiac magnetic resonance imaging (MRI) to measure heart volumes in 15 subjects with severe untreated OSA (AHI 30-102 and mean BMI 35.3 ± 7.6) who did not have other co-morbid conditions (e.g., heart failure, coronary artery disease, unstable hypertension, or advanced lung disease). Compared to baseline values, changes in MRI at 3 months of CPAP therapy included significant decreases in RV end-systolic and end-diastolic volume indices. There were no significant differences in RV ejection fraction (EF), left ventricular (LV) volumes, LVEF, myocardial perfusion reserve index, interventricular septum thickness, and RV or LV free wall thickness.[40]

Early in-patient treatment of OSA with CPAP improved systolic heart function in hospitalized persons with acutely decompensated heart failure. In one randomized controlled trial, 46 patients hospitalized for acutely decompensated heart failure underwent polysomnography within 2 days of hospital admission.[41] Patients with AHI of 15 or more and obstructive apnea index 5 or greater were randomized to either (a) in-hospital APAP treatment of OSA and standard therapy of heart failure, or (b) standard treatment of heart failure only. Patients with central sleep apnea, hemodynamic instability, or respiratory insufficiency were excluded. Echocardiography was performed after three nights of randomization and revealed greater improvements in LVEF and LV end-systolic and end-diastolic volumes with CPAP intervention compared to control subjects.[41]

Inflammation

In a prospective case series, 52 otherwise healthy men with newly diagnosed OSA (AHI of 5 or more plus daytime symptoms) were followed for 6 months during which therapeutic adherence was monitored. Compared to less adherent subjects (mean CPAP use of 1.41 ± 1.47 hours per night), the more adherent subjects (mean CPAP use of 4.68 ± 0.56 hours nightly; $P < 0.001$) exhibited reductions in absolute count of total lymphocytes, $CD4^+$ cells, tumor necrosis factor-α (TNF-α) levels, and uric acid levels. No differences were noted in $CD8^+$, $CD19^+$ and interleukin 6 (IL-6) with CPAP therapy. No changes in these measured variables were noted in the less adherent group.[42]

Endothelial Function

Long-term CPAP therapy may improve endothelial function in persons with OSA. A prospective, controlled, observational study was completed that involved 29 men with OSA (AHI = 60.4 ± 22.1) and 17 men without OSA (AHI = 2.5 ± 0.6). After using CPAP for 6 months, subjects with OSA underwent Doppler ultrasound assessments of both endothelium-dependent flow-mediated dilation (E-DFMD) and endothelium-independent nitroglycerin-induced dilation (E-INTGD) of the brachial artery. Compared to control subjects, subjects with OSA had lower E-DFMD but similar E-INTGD. Apnea-hypopnea indices were inversely related to E-DFMD. After 6 months, E-DFMD increased in CPAP adherent subjects and a positive correlation was noted between CPAP hours of use and E-DFMD values. In contrast, no change in E-DFMD was found in CPAP nonusers.[43]

Neurocognition and Mood

Long-term CPAP therapy for OSA has been shown to produce lasting improvements in mood and to slow cognitive decline in persons with Alzheimer's disease.[44] One randomized double-blind placebo-controlled trial found CPAP-related cognitive functioning improvement in persons with concurrent Alzheimer's disease and OSA. This study involved 52 adults with OSA (AHI ≥10) and mild to moderate Alzheimer's disease but no other severe medical or psychiatric disorders. Subjects were randomized to either therapeutic CPAP for 6 weeks or placebo CPAP for 3 weeks followed by therapeutic CPAP for 3 weeks. Three weeks of therapeutic CPAP in both groups were associated with significant cognitive improvement compared to pretreatment neuropsychological test scores.[45]

ADVERSE EFFECTS OF THERAPY

Although rare, PAP-related adverse effects have been described. The most common problem is difficulty (or inability) to tolerate the mask and machine. Common complaints include nocturnal awakenings and nasal problems, including dryness, congestion, and sneezing.[46] Some patients experience gastric distention from aerophagia. The delivery interface (mask or nasal pillows) may cause skin irritation, and the pressure (or airflow leakage) can provoke sinus or ocular irritation or pain. Patients may also refuse therapy due to claustrophobia-like anxiety, chest discomfort (or tightness), or sleep disturbance from noise generated by the device.

ADHERENCE TO THERAPY

Prevalence

PAP therapy frequency and duration necessary to improve functioning and relieve SDB symptoms is not known. It is generally believed that to be optimally effective, PAP has to be used for a significant portion of sleep nightly. Unfortunately, suboptimal adherence and intermittent use of PAP therapy is common. In a large European multicenter study, therapeutic adherence was 80% (using PAP 4 or more hours per night on 70% or more nights minimum criteria).[47] In another study, CPAP was used for 94% of monitored days with a mean daily use of 7.1 ± 1.1 hours in which 60% of patients used the device nightly.[48]

Virtually all of the benefits derived from PAP therapy are rapidly lost with discontinuation of use.[49] Many factors predict the frequency and regularity of CPAP use. Usage patterns seen early frequently continued long term.[50,51] In one study, the percentage of days skipped correlated with decreased nightly usage duration.[52] Other factors correlated with long-term use include snoring history, severity of illness, self-reported sleepiness, and subjective perception of benefit.[53] Finally, adherence to CPAP therapy appears to be less among patients who underwent split-night CPAP titration compared to those who had full-night CPAP titration studies[54] and in patients with mild disease.[51]

It is essential to objectively monitor PAP adherence because self-reported usage often overestimates actual use.

In one study in which subjects were issued CPAP machines that had built-in microprocessors that can sense mask pressure and monitor usage, only 46% used CPAP for 4 or more hours on 70% of monitored days, although a majority (60%) of patients claimed to use the device regularly.[49]

Effect of Humidification

Many individuals using PAP therapy complain of nasal symptoms, including nasal dryness, rhinorrhea, nasal congestion, sneezing, and epistaxis. These problems adversely affect optimal PAP utilization.[55] Heated humidification can alleviate many of these problems and has been shown to significantly improve PAP adherence.[56] In one study, heated humidification was better than oily nose drops in patients with OSA complaining of CPAP-related upper airway dryness.[57] Heated humidification may especially benefit patients older than 60 years of age who use drying medications, who suffer from chronic mucosa disease, or who underwent uvulopalatopharyngoplasty.[58] By contrast, some investigators report conflicting results. Ryan and colleagues[59] studied 125 subjects with OSA (AHI ≥10), who were randomized to 4 weeks of dry CPAP, CPAP plus heated humidification, or CPAP plus topical nasal steroids. After 4 weeks, there were no differences between groups for CPAP adherence (dry CPAP = 5.21 ± 1.66 hours per night; CPAP plus heated humidification = 5.21 ± 1.84; and CPAP plus fluticasone = 5.66 ± 1.68). Interestingly, however, patients on CPAP plus heated humidification had fewer nasal symptoms compared to both dry CPAP and CPAP plus fluticasone.

Use of Hypnotic Agents

One-time use of a sedative-hypnotic during PAP titration reportedly improves short-term adherence to CPAP therapy. In one study, good adherence after 4 to 6 weeks of treatment (>4 hours use per night on >70% of nights) was confirmed in 56.5% of 400 subjects with newly diagnosed OSA. On average, patients used PAP therapy 78.1% of nights for 3.13 hours nightly. Improved adherence correlated with one-time use of a sedative-hypnotic during CPAP titration compared to control subjects (77% vs. 57.6%; $p < 0.0005$). The former was also associated with longer sleep times, greater sleep efficiencies during polysomnography, and lower respiratory disturbance indices on the final CPAP pressure.[60] The same research group studied the one-time use of eszopiclone, a benzodiazepine receptor agonist sedative agent during CPAP titration studies. In a randomized, double-blind, placebo-controlled trial, Lettieri and associates studied 98 patients with OSA (mean AHI of 29.2 ± 24.3) requiring PAP therapy. Subjects were randomized to either eszopiclone (3 mg) or placebo before undergoing their CPAP titration. Premedicating with eszopiclone produced greater adherence (higher percentage of nights used = $75.9 \pm 20.0\%$ vs. $60.1 \pm 24.3\%$; and more hours of use per night = 4.8 ± 1.5 vs. 3.9 ± 1.8 hours) compared with placebo. Use of eszopiclone was also associated with improved sleep efficiency and total sleep time during the CPAP titration study.[61]

Role of Education in PAP Adherence

A variety of PAP therapy education programs reportedly improve CPAP utilization. Educational approaches included outpatient group clinics designed to encourage PAP use,[62] home PAP education,[63] phone calls and providing written information about OSA and the importance of regular PAP use,[64] cognitive behavioral techniques,[65] motivational enhancement to reduce ambivalence regarding treatment,[66] and desensitization.[67]

There are several reasons individuals may poorly accept PAP therapy: (1) anxiety, (2) disbelief that PAP would help them, (3) lack of confidence that they can change their behavior and use PAP, (4) identity issues, and (5) negative feedback or miscommunication from other patients regarding its efficacy. Desensitization techniques work well in situations in which anxiety is provoked by putting a mask over the nose, over the mouth, or on the face in any way. This *phobic reaction* to the mask is often wrongly labeled claustrophobia, but this anxiety reaction is related to fear regarding breathing or smothering rather than enclosed spaces. (*Note*: claustrophobia is an anxiety disorder involving fear of enclosed or confined spaces, for example fear or panic triggered by being in an elevator.)

For individuals who do not believe PAP therapy will help them, getting them to accept this treatment can be extremely difficult. Efforts must be focused on psychoeducational issues with careful probing of why they think it will not work for them when it works for everyone else. The insistent denial of potential for benefit may be a marker for co-morbid depression. Examining disappointment with other medical treatments is also helpful. Empathy and collaboration are paramount for these patients. This is also true for individuals who lack confidence in their ability to adjust to PAP therapy. These two challenges more often adversely affect therapeutic phase adherence; however, they may also fuel lack of acceptance. The clinician must always be on guard that nonwillingness to try PAP, on the basis that it will not produce benefit or that it requires too much behavioral change, may be excuses in cases in which the real underlying issue is identity.

For some patients, the thinking may follow this kind of syllogism: If I have to use PAP nightly, then I have sleep apnea. If I have sleep apnea, then I am seriously ill. I will not consider myself a seriously ill person; therefore, I will not use a PAP device and mask. The appearance of PAP and the mistaken confusion that it is forced O_2 may magnify this thinking. Taking a medication orally can be considered acceptable or "normal" via its route, but illness requiring durable medical equipment (DME) (e.g., PAP), an injection, or an equally serious intervention are for many an acceptance of illness. A variation on this is that realizing that they are seriously ill fuels depression and then the patient may not have the will to do what is needed to improve this condition.

In cases in which a *phobic reaction* occurred that might have led to a patient refusing PAP therapy, or leaving the sleep laboratory against medical advice, PAP desensitization may be useful. This procedure, developed by Hirshkowitz and Rose,[68] involves both a session in the sleep center as well as homework. The patient comes to the sleep center and has an interview with the therapist. The purpose of the interview is to determine the nature of the problem and to some degree decide how to customize therapy, if needed. After the interview, the therapist provides some relaxation training, and has the patient practice the exercise or visualization several times. Visualization typically works best with patient-generated imagery. The mask, in many cases, is *the phobic trigger* and

should be gradually introduced. This is done while the person concentrates on remaining relaxed. The following steps proceed at the patient-desired pace:

1. An array of full face masks, nasal masks, small minimasks, nasal pillows, and nasal flow devices are presented.
2. The patient selects a mask and handles it over 5 to 10 minutes or until comfortable.
3. Eventually, the mask is brought closer and touches the face.
4. The mask is strapped into place.
5. The mask is worn around the laboratory for several hours while reading or watching television.
6. The mask is then worn in bed.
7. The mask is then worn while hooked up to an operating PAP machine.
8. Finally, the mask is worn while taking a nap.

SUMMARY

Positive airway pressure is the therapy of choice for most patients with clinically significant obstructive sleep-disordered breathing. Various treatment modalities are available and each may offer benefits for specific patient needs. PAP therapy effectively reduces or eliminates sleep-related respiratory pathophysiology in most patients. Used optimally, PAP therapy can improve sleep, enhance daytime alertness, reduce cardiovascular morbidity and mortality risks, and improve quality of life. It is important to objectively monitor adherence because efficacy depends upon regular use of the mask and machine.

REFERENCES

1. Cao MT, Guilleminault C, Kushida CA. Clinical features and evaluation of obstructive sleep apnea and upper airway resistance syndrome. In: Kryger MH, Roth T, Dement WC, eds. *Principles and Practice of Sleep Medicine*. St. Louis: Elsevier Saunders; 2011:1206-1218.
2. Smith PL, Wise RA, Gold AR, Schwartz AR, Permutt S. Upper airway pressure-flow relationships in obstructive sleep apnea. *J Appl Physiol*. 1988;64(2):789-795.
3. Iber C, Ancoli-Israel S, Chesson A, Quan SF. *for the American Academy of Sleep Medicine. The AASM Manual for the Scoring of Sleep and Associated Events: Rules, Terminology and Technical Specification*. 1st ed. Westchester, IL: American Academy of Sleep Medicine; 2007.
4. Medicare Learning Network. Continuous positive airway pressure (CPAP) Therapy for Obstructive Sleep Apnea (OSA)- JA6048. Web link available at http/www.cms.gov/ContractorLearningResources/download/JA6048.pdf; accessed on March 13, 2008.
5. Kushida CA, Littner MR, Hirshkowitz M, et al. Practice parameters for the use of continuous and bilevel positive airway pressure devices to treat adult patients with sleep-related breathing disorders. *Sleep*. 2006;29(3):375-380.
6. Sullivan CE, Issa FG, Berthon-Jones M, Eves L. Reversal of obstructive sleep apnea by continuous positive airway pressure applied through the nares. *Lancet*. 1981;1:862-865.
7. Fromm RE, Varon J, Lechin AE, Hirshkowitz M. CPAP machine performance and altitude. *Chest*. 1995;108:1577-1580.
8. Reeves-Hoche MK, Hudgel DW, Meck R, Witteman R, Ross A, Zwillich CW. Continuous versus bilevel positive airway pressure for obstructive sleep apnea. *Am J Respir Crit Care Med*. 1995;151(2 Pt 1):443-449.
9. Littner M, Hirshkowitz M, Davila D, et al. Practice parameters for the use of auto-titrating continuous positive airway pressure devices for titrating pressures and treating adult patients with obstructive sleep apnea syndrome: An American Academy of Sleep Medicine report. *Sleep*. 2002;25:143-147.
10. Morganthaler TI, Aurora RN, Brown T, et al. Practice parameters for the use of autotitrating continuous positive airway pressure devices for titrating pressures and treating adult patients with obstructive sleep apnea syndrome: An update for 2007. *Sleep*. 2008;31:141-147.

11. d'Ortho MP, Grillier-Lanoir V, Levy P, Goldenberg F, Corriger E, et al. Constant vs. automatic continuous positive airway pressure therapy: Home evaluation. *Chest*. 2000;118(4):1010-1017.

12. Ayas NT, Patel SR, Malhotra A, et al. Auto-titrating versus standard continuous positive airway pressure for the treatment of obstructive sleep apnea: Results of a meta-analysis. *Sleep*. 2004;27:249-253.

13. Senn O, Brack T, Matthews F, Russi EW, Bloch KE. Randomized short-term trial of two autoCPAP devices versus fixed continuous positive airway pressure for the treatment of sleep apnea. *Am J Respir Crit Care Med*. 2003;168:1506-1511.

14. Masa JF, Jimenez A, Duran J, et al. Alternative methods of titrating continuous positive airway pressure: A large multicenter study. *Am J Respir Crit Care Med*. 2004;170:1218-1224.

15. Meurice JC, Marc I, Series F. Efficacy of auto-CPAP in the treatment of obstructive sleep apnea/hypopnea syndrome. *Am J Respir Crit Care Med*. 1996;153(2):794-798.

16. Sharma S, Wali S, Pouliot Z, Peters M, Neufeld H, Kryger M. Treatment of obstructive sleep apnea with a self-titrating continuous positive airway pressure (CPAP) system. *Sleep*. 1996;19(6):497-501.

17. Planes C, D'Ortho MP, Foucher A, et al. Efficacy and cost of home-initiated auto-nCPAP versus conventional nCPAP. *Sleep*. 2003;26:156-160.

18. Nussbaumer Y, Bloch KE, Genser T, Thurnheer R. Equivalency in home treatment of sleep apnea. *Chest*. 2006;129:638-643.

19. Allam JS, Olson EJ, Gay PC, Morgenthaler TI. Efficacy of adaptive servoventilation in treatment of complex and central sleep apnea syndromes. *Chest*. 2007;132(6):1839-1846.

20. Piper AJ, Sullivan CE. Effects of short-term NIPPV in the treatment of patients with severe obstructive sleep apnea and hypercapnia. *Chest*. 1994;105(2):434-440.

21. Kushida CA, Chediak A, Berry RB, et al. Positive Airway Pressure Titration Task Force of the American Academy of Sleep Medicine: Clinical guidelines for the manual titration of positive airway pressure in patients with obstructive sleep apnea. *J Clin Sleep Med*. 2008;4(2):157-171.

22. Hirshkowitz M, Sharafkhaneh A. Positive airway pressure therapy of OSA. *Semin Respir Crit Care Med*. 2005;26:68-79.

23. Engleman HM, Kingshott RN, Wraith PK, Mackay TW, Deary IJ, Douglas NJ. Randomized placebo-controlled crossover trial of continuous positive airway pressure for mild sleep apnea/hypopnea syndrome. *Am J Respir Crit Care Med*. 1999;159(2):461-467.

24. Ballester E, Badia JR, Hernandez L, Carrasco E, de Pablo J, et al. Evidence of the effectiveness of continuous positive airway pressure in the treatment of sleep apnea/hypopnea syndrome. *Am J Respir Crit Care Med*. 1999;159(2):495-501.

25. Marshall NS, Barnes M, Travier N, Campbell AJ, Pierce RJ, et al. Continuous positive airway pressure reduces daytime sleepiness in mild to moderate obstructive sleep apnoea: A meta-analysis. *Thorax*. 2006;61(5):430-434:Epub 2006 Feb 7.

26. Bahammam A, Delaive K, Ronald J, Manfreda J, Roos L, Kryger MH. Health care utilization in males with obstructive sleep apnea syndrome two years after diagnosis and treatment. *Sleep*. 1999;22(6):740-747.

27. Redline S, Adams N, Strauss ME, Roebuck T, Winters M, Rosenberg C. Improvement of mild sleep-disordered breathing with CPAP compared with conservative therapy. *Am J Respir Crit Care Med*. 1998;157(3Pt1):858-865.

28. Jenkinson C, Davies RJ, Mullins R, Stradling JR. Comparison of therapeutic and subtherapeutic nasal continuous positive airway pressure for obstructive sleep apnoea: A randomised prospective parallel trial. *Lancet*. 1999;353(9170):2100-2105.

29. Punjabi NM, Caffo BS, Goodwin JL, Gottlieb DJ, Newman AB, et al. Sleep-disordered breathing and mortality: A prospective cohort study. *PLoS Med*. 2009;6(8):e1000132:Epub 2009 Aug 18.

30. Young T, Finn L, Peppard PE, Szklo-Coxe M, Austin D, et al. Sleep disordered breathing and mortality: Eighteen-year follow-up of the Wisconsin sleep cohort. *Sleep*. 2008;31(8):1071-1078.

31. Lavie P, Herer P, Hoffstein V. Obstructive sleep apnoea syndrome as a risk factor for hypertension: Population study. *BMJ*. 2000;320(7233):479-482.

32. Suzuki M, Otsuka K, Guilleminault C. Long-term nasal continuous positive airway pressure administration can normalize hypertension in obstructive sleep apnea patients. *Sleep*. 1993;16(6):545-549.

33. Faccenda JF, Mackay TW, Boon NA, Douglas NJ. Randomized placebo-controlled trial of continuous positive airway pressure on blood pressure in the sleep apnea-hypopnea syndrome. *Am J Respir Crit Care Med*. 2001;163(2):344-348.

34. Mayer J, Becker H, Brandenburg U, Penzel T, Peter JH, von Wichert P. Blood pressure and sleep apnea: Results of long-term nasal continuous positive airway pressure therapy. *Cardiology*. 1991;79(2):84-92.

35. Marin JM, Carrizo SJ, Vicente E, et al. Long-term cardiovascular outcomes in men with obstructive sleep apnoea-hypopnoea with or without treatment with continuous positive airway pressure: An observational study. *Lancet*. 2005;365:1046-1053.

36. Dernaika TA, Kinasewitz GT, Tawk MM. Effects of nocturnal continuous positive airway pressure therapy in patients with resistant hypertension and obstructive sleep apnea. *J Clin Sleep Med*. 2009;5(2):103-107.

37. Akashiba T, Minemura H, Yamamoto H, Kosaka N, Saito O, Horie T. Nasal continuous positive airway pressure changes blood pressure "non-dippers" to "dippers" in patients with obstructive sleep apnea. *Sleep*. 1999;22(7):849-853.

38. Dimsdale JE, Loredo JS, Profant J. Effect of continuous positive airway pressure on blood pressure: A placebo trial. *Hypertension*. 2000;35(1 Pt 1):144-147.

39. Bazzano LA, Khan Z, Reynolds K, He J. Effect of nocturnal nasal continuous positive airway pressure on blood pressure in obstructive sleep apnea. *Hypertension*. 2007;50(2):417-423.

40. Magalang UJ, Richards K, McCarthy B, Fathala A, Khan M, et al. Continuous positive airway pressure therapy reduces right ventricular volume in patients with obstructive sleep apnea: A cardiovascular magnetic resonance study. *J Clin Sleep Med*. 2009;5(2):110-114.

41. Khayat RN, Abraham WT, Patt B, Pu M, Jarjoura D. In-hospital treatment of obstructive sleep apnea during decompensation of heart failure. *Chest*. 2009;136(4):991-997.

42. Steiropoulos P, Kotsianidis I, Nena E, Tsara V, Gounari E, et al. Long-term effect of continuous positive airway pressure therapy on inflammation markers of patients with obstructive sleep apnea syndrome. *Sleep*. 2009;32(4):537-543.

43. Bayram NA, Ciftci B, Keles T, Durmaz T, Turhan S, et al. Endothelial function in normotensive men with obstructive sleep apnea before and 6 months after CPAP treatment. *Sleep*. 2009;32(10):1257-1263.

44. Cooke JR, Ayalon L, Palmer BW, Loredo JS, Corey-Bloom J, et al. Sustained use of CPAP slows deterioration of cognition, sleep, and mood in patients with Alzheimer's disease and obstructive sleep apnea: A preliminary study. *J Clin Sleep Med*. 2009;5(4):305-309.

45. Ancoli-Israel S, Palmer BW, Cooke JR, Corey-Bloom J, Fiorentino L, et al. Cognitive effects of treating obstructive sleep apnea in Alzheimer's disease: A randomized controlled study. *J Am Geriatr Soc*. 2008;56(11):2076-2081.

46. Hoffstein V, Viner S, Mateika S, Conway J. Treatment of obstructive sleep apnea with nasal continuous positive airway pressure: Patient compliance, perception of benefits, and side effects. *Am Rev Respir Dis*. 1992;145(4 Pt 1):841-845.

47. Pepin JL, Krieger J, Rodenstein D, Cornette A, Sforza E, et al. Effective compliance during the first 3 months of continuous positive airway pressure: A European prospective study of 121 patients. *Am J Respir Crit Care Med*. 1999;160(4):1124-1129.

48. Fleury B, Rakotonanahary D, Hausser-Hauw C, Lebeau B, Guilleminault C. Objective patient compliance in long-term use of nCPAP. *Eur Respir J*. 1996;9(11):2356-2359.

49. Kribbs NB, Pack AI, Kline LR, Getsy JE, Schuett JS, et al. Effects of one night without nasal CPAP treatment on sleep and sleepiness in patients with obstructive sleep apnea. *Am Rev Respir Dis*. 1993;147(5):1162-1168.

50. Kribbs NB, Pack AI, Kline LR, Smith PL, Schwartz AR, et al. Objective measurement of patterns of nasal CPAP use by patients with obstructive sleep apnea. *Am Rev Respir Dis*. 1993;147(4):887-895.

51. Rosenthal L, Gerhardstein R, Lumley A, Guido P, Day R, et al. CPAP therapy in patients with mild OSA: Implementation and treatment outcome. *Sleep Med*. 2000;1(3):215-220.

52. Weaver TE, Kribbs NB, Pack AI, Kline LR, Chugh DK, et al. Night-to-night variability in CPAP use over the first three months of treatment. *Sleep*. 1997;20(4):278-283.

53. McArdle N, Devereux G, Heidarnejad H, Engleman HM, Mackay TW, Douglas NJ. Long-term use of CPAP therapy for sleep apnea/hypopnea syndrome. *Am J Respir Crit Care Med*. 1999;159(4 Pt 1):1108-1114.

54. Strollo Jr PJ, Sanders MH, Costantino JP, Walsh SK, Stiller RA, Atwood Jr CW. Split-night studies for the diagnosis and treatment of sleep-disordered breathing. *Sleep*. 1996;19(Suppl 10):S255-S259.

55. Brown LK. Back to basics: If it's dry, wet it: The case for humidification of nasal continuous positive airway pressure air. *Chest*. 2000;117(3):617-619.

56. Massie CA, Hart RW, Peralez K, Richards GN. Effects of humidification on nasal symptoms and compliance in sleep apnea patients using continuous positive airway pressure. *Chest*. 1999;116(2):403-408.

57. Wiest GH, Lehnert G, Bruck WM, Meyer M, Hahn EG, Ficker JH. A heated humidifier reduces upper airway dryness during continuous positive airway pressure therapy. *Respir Med*. 1999;93(1):21-26.

58. Rakotonanahary D, Pelletier-Fleury N, Gagnadoux F, Fleury B. Predictive factors for the need for additional humidification during nasal continuous positive airway pressure therapy. *Chest.* 2001;119(2):460-465.

59. Ryan S, Doherty LS, Nolan GM, McNicholas WT. Effects of heated humidification and topical steroids on compliance, nasal symptoms, and quality of life in patients with obstructive sleep apnea syndrome using nasal continuous positive airway pressure. *J Clin Sleep Med.* 2009;5(5):422-427.

60. Collen J, Lettieri C, Kelly W, Roop S. Clinical and polysomnographic predictors of short-term continuous positive airway pressure compliance. *Chest.* 2009;135(3):704-709.

61. Lettieri CJ, Collen JF, Eliasson AH, Quast TM. Sedative use during continuous positive airway pressure titration improves subsequent compliance: A randomized, double-blind, placebo-controlled trial. *Chest.* 2009;136(5):1263-1268.

62. Likar LL, Panciera TM, Erickson AD, Rounds S. Group education sessions and compliance with nasal CPAP therapy. *Chest.* 1997;111(5):1273-1277.

63. Hoy CJ, Vennelle M, Kingshott RN, Engleman HM, Douglas NJ. Can intensive support improve continuous positive airway pressure use in patients with the sleep apnea/hypopnea syndrome? *Am J Respir Crit Care Med.* 1999;159(4 Pt 1):1096-1100.

64. Chervin RD, Theut S, Bassetti C, Aldrich MS. Compliance with nasal CPAP can be improved by simple interventions. *Sleep.* 1997;20(4):284-289.

65. Richards D, Bartlett DJ, Wong K, Malouff J, Grunstein RR. Increased adherence to CPAP with a group cognitive behavioral treatment intervention: A randomized trial. *Sleep.* 2007;30(5):635-640.

66. Aloia MS, Arnedt JT, Riggs RL, Hecht J, Borrelli B. Clinical management of poor adherence to CPAP: Motivational enhancement. *Behav Sleep Med.* 2004;2(4):205-222.

67. Rains JC. Treatment of obstructive sleep apnea in pediatric patients. Behavioral intervention for compliance with nasal continuous positive airway pressure. *Clin Pediatr (Phila).* 1995;34(10):535-541.

68. Hirshkowitz M, Rose M. PAP desensitization procedure. In: Hirshkowitz M, Kapen S, Littner M, et al. eds. *Sleep Related Breathing Disorders: Sourcebook.* Milwaukee, WI: Healthcare Analysis & Information Group; 2011.

Chapter 17

Surgical Therapy for Obstructive Sleep Apnea/Hypopnea Syndrome

MICHAEL FRIEDMAN / CHRISTOPHER W. LEESMAN / TANYA PULVER

Surgical therapy plays a vital role in the treatment of obstructive sleep apnea/hypopnea syndrome (OSAHS), despite the fact that it rarely results in complete elimination or cure of the syndrome. Surgery in general is often used to palliate symptoms, slow the progression, and reduce the severity of many diseases when complete cure is not possible. Ultimately in OSAHS, the treating physician has the responsibility to counsel patients on the risks, benefits, and limitations of surgery so that they can make an informed decision about whether or not to pursue surgical treatment.

Continuous positive airway pressure (CPAP) therapy is clearly the first-line treatment for OSAHS. However, reported rates of compliance are typically low, ranging from 35% to 95% among patients with moderate to severe sleep apnea.[1-5] The vast majority of patients with mild sleep apnea go untested and, therefore, untreated because they are reluctant to entertain the possible need for treatment with CPAP. Consequently, millions of Americans with OSAHS remain undiagnosed and untreated. The American Academy of Sleep Medicine (AASM) recommends that patients who fail CPAP and other conservative measures, such as oral appliances, can be considered candidates for surgical therapy.[6]

Surgical therapy for OSAHS fell into disfavor after early enthusiasm for uvulopalatopharyngoplasty (UPPP) was met with unexpectedly high failure rates. The high failure rates were the result of misapplication of the procedure. It is now widely recognized that obstruction in OSAHS can occur at multiple levels, namely, the nose, palate, and retrolingual area. Most patients have obstruction at more than one site. UPPP is an aggressive surgical procedure that addresses a single site of obstruction: the palate and tonsils. Thus, UPPP as an isolated procedure is likely to fail in patients whose disease is not limited to the palate and tonsils.

Fortunately, the approach to surgery for OSAHS has evolved immensely since UPPP was first introduced by Fujita and associates in 1981.[7] A number of classical surgical and minimally invasive techniques have been developed to address multilevel obstruction. These procedures can be performed simultaneously or sequentially and are often combined with nonsurgical therapy. This multilevel approach to upper airway surgery has resulted in improved outcomes for patients with OSAHS. Lin and associates[8] performed a systematic review that included 1978 patients and determined the success rate of multilevel surgery for OSAHS to be 66.4%, a noteworthy improvement from the 40% success rate found by Sher and associates for UPPP alone.[9]

This chapter will provide an overview of some of the multilevel surgical techniques available for treating OSAHS as well as the necessary preoperative considerations.

CLINICAL ASSESSMENT

Severity of disease, as evidenced by polysomnogram, symptoms, and Epworth Sleepiness Scale, does not predict surgical success.[10] Procedures must be tailored to the unique anatomic variations of individual patients. Successful treatment of OSAHS and snoring is thus predicated on a thorough history and physical examination.

A focused physical examination for surgical evaluation is paramount to determine the anatomic site or sites of upper airway obstruction unique to the surgical candidate. The sites identified, taken with relevant co-morbid conditions, will then dictate the procedures planned.

Recognizing the importance of this process has led to many attempts at formulating a way to predict the sites of obstruction likely to benefit from surgery. Examples include cephalometry, fluoroscopy, computed tomography (CT), magnetic resonance imaging (MRI), and physical examination findings. The most common method, the Mueller maneuver, utilizes flexible endoscopy to visualize any obstruction that occurs from a patient performing a negative (or reverse) Valsalva maneuver.[11] Unfortunately, there is a lack of supporting data validating any of the aforementioned methods as a tool for patient selection.

A system for the classification of difficult airways was developed in 1985 by Mallampati, an anesthesiologist. It was subsequently adapted by Friedman and associates[12] as the "modified Mallampati" system for sleep medicine. The Mallampati physical examination tool was initially introduced as a method for predicting patients in which difficult endotracheal intubation was likely.[13] The examiner, typically an anesthesiologist, would instruct the patient to protrude the tongue, and the relationship of the tongue and soft palate was thereafter noted and graded. Prior to the Friedman adaptation of a "modified Mallampati" classification in 1999, the Mallampati stages had only been studied in the context of difficult intubations. The modified Mallampati classification was thereby introduced with two major modifications for its use in sleep medicine. First, the anesthesiologist assessment in traditional Mallampati had been based on the patient sticking out the tongue; the modified Mallampati eliminated tongue protrusion. Second, the three stages of the original Mallampati classification was expanded to four in the modified Mallampati, and subsequently to five in the description of the Friedman tongue position (FTP), as highlighted later in this chapter. Thus, it is a misnomer to use the term "Mallampati classification" as it relates to sleep medicine, because the system Mallampati introduced for difficult intubations was not introduced to sleep medicine until

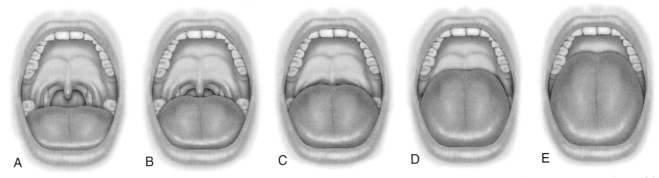

Figure 17-1 Friedman tongue position (FTP). A, FTP I permits visualization of the entire uvula and tonsils/pillars. **B,** FTP IIa permits visualization of most of the uvula, but the tonsils/pillars are obscured. **C,** FTP IIb permits visualization of the entire soft palate to the base of the uvula. **D,** FTP III permits the visualization of the proximal soft palate but not the uvula. **E,** FTP IV permits visualization of the hard palate only. (From Friedman M. *Sleep: Apnea and Snoring: Surgical and Non-Surgical Therapy.* Philadelphia, PA: WB Saunders; 2009. Reprinted with permission.)

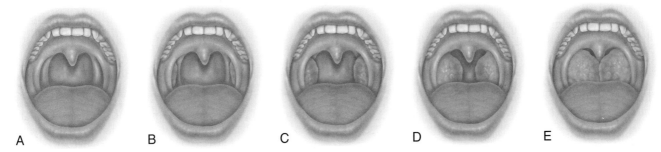

Figure 17-2 Friedman tonsil classification system. A, Tonsils, size 0, after tonsillectomy. **B,** Tonsils, size 1, within the pillars. **C,** Tonsils, size 2, extend to pillars. **D,** Tonsils, size 3, extend past pillars. **E,** Tonsils, size 4, extend to the midline. (From Friedman M. *Sleep: Apnea and Snoring: Surgical and Non-Surgical Therapy.* Philadelphia, PA: WB Saunders; 2009. Reprinted with permission.)

Friedman and associates pioneered the "modified Mallampati" classification system. There is some evidence to suggest that the Mallampati classification may be a clinical predictor of the presence of OSAHS.[14,15] However, there have been no studies to verify a role in surgical evaluation, as it is not an evaluation of obstruction, and thus is not a predictor of surgical success.

This challenge prompted Friedman and associates to devise a staging system that assists practitioners in determining the best course of therapy for individual patients.[16,17] The Friedman Anatomic Staging System acts as a way to describe the presence and relationship of palatal and hypopharyngeal obstruction. The ultimate benefit of this system is the reliable identification of procedures likely to result in success or failure in an individual patient.[16-18]

This classification system is based on three straightforward elements of the physical examination: Friedman tongue position (FTP; Fig. 17-1), the Friedman tonsil classification system (Fig. 17-2), and body mass index (BMI). The FTP is based on a modified use of the Mallampati classification and evaluates the relationship of tongue and palate in the normal resting position, as occurs during sleep. It has been shown to be an independent predictor of presence of OSAHS.[12] The addition of tonsil size helps to more accurately describe the anatomy for surgery for sleep disordered breathing.

As illustrated in Table 17-1, patients classified as stage I include those with a tongue position of I or II, large tonsils (3 or 4), and a BMI less than 40. Therapy in these patients should be directed at correcting the palate and tonsils. Patients classified as stage II or III typically require treatment of the

TABLE 17-1

Friedman Anatomic Staging System for Patients with Obstructive Sleep Apnea/Hypopnea Syndrome

Stage	Friedman Tongue Position	Tonsil Size	Body Mass Index (kg/m²)
I	I, IIa, IIb	3 or 4	<40
II	I, IIa, IIb	0, 1, or 2	<40
	III or IV	3 or 4	<40
III	III or IV	0, 1, or 2	<40
IV	Any	Any	>40

tongue base and hypopharynx in addition to or in lieu of surgery on the palate and tonsils. Treatment of these areas may be accomplished by classical or minimally invasive techniques, depending on the severity of disease.

Patients with a BMI greater than 40 or skeletal anomalies such as midface hypoplasia or retrognathia are automatically considered to be stage IV and are unlikely to benefit from multilevel upper airway surgery as the primary treatment modality. These patients should be considered for CPAP/weight reduction or orthognathic surgery, respectively.

Although the specific anatomic areas treated are determined by physical examination findings, the decision to proceed with minimally invasive procedures versus more aggressive classical techniques is dictated by the severity of disease, as measured on the polysomnogram (PSG).

PREOPERATIVE CONSIDERATIONS

Poor candidates for upper airway surgery include patients who are morbidly obese, have unstable heart or lung disease, abuse alcohol or drugs, suffer from psychiatric instability, or have unrealistic expectations. It is important for patients to understand that in order to achieve success, more than one procedure at more than one point in time may be necessary.

Patients with OSAHS have a higher risk of perioperative morbidity and death.[19-21] The major risk of surgery for individuals with OSAHS pertains to airway management. The anatomic characteristics of many sleep apnea patients, such as a short neck, long soft palate, large tongue base, and tonsillar hypertrophy, can make endotracheal intubation difficult. Thus, fiberoptic guidance is sometimes required. Postoperatively, patients with OSAHS are at higher risk for airway complications and are more susceptible to developing oversedation and respiratory depression with narcotic administration.[22,23] Thus, anesthetic technique, postoperative monitoring, and the administration of postoperative analgesia must be carefully planned. Depending on the type of surgery performed, CPAP may be indicated postoperatively. Optimization of respiratory parameters with the use of CPAP preoperatively is also recommended by some authors.[24] Steroids are often administered during and following upper airway procedures to limit the degree of edema that develops.[25-27]

SURGERY FOR CORRECTION OF PALATAL AND HYPOPHARYNGEAL OBSTRUCTION

Palatal Stiffening

Minimally invasive palatal stiffening techniques are often appropriate for patients with palatal obstruction and normal size tonsils. The pillar technique[28] is a simple procedure that can be performed in the office under local anesthesia. It consists of implanting three Dacron pillars into the soft palate, just posterior to the junction with the hard palate (Fig. 17-3).

Partial implant extrusion is a potential complication of the procedure,[28] and removal of the entire implant is required in such cases. Implant removal is a simple, office-based procedure that can be performed under local anesthesia. Although complete extrusion is theoretically possible and could potentially lead to aspiration, no such cases have been reported.

The efficacy of palatal stiffening as an isolated procedure for the treatment of OSAHS is low, as it has been shown to reduce the apnea-hypopnea index (AHI) by 26%.[29] Its main role in the treatment of sleep apnea is as an adjunctive procedure.[6] Alone, it is a valuable technique for the treatment of snoring. In one study, approximately 90% of individuals experienced a significant reduction in snoring intensity according to self-report,[28] whereas only 25% of these same subjects saw complete resolution of their OSAHS. When combined with minimally invasive treatment of nasal and retrolingual obstruction, the Pillar technique has been found to provide subjective improvement in up to 64% of patients and classical cure in 34.4%.[28]

Patients with an elongated uvula (>1.5 cm) should undergo partial uvulectomy at the same time as the Pillar technique to shorten the uvula to 1 cm. Both procedures are undertaken in the operating room under general anesthesia.

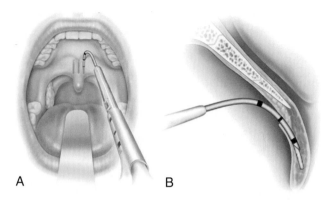

Figure 17-3 The pillar palatal stiffening technique. A, One implant is placed at the midline of the soft palate. Two additional implants are placed laterally, as close as possible to the centrally placed implant, approximately 2 mm apart. **B,** The implant is placed within the muscle layer of the soft palate. (From Friedman M. *Sleep: Apnea and Snoring: Surgical and Non-Surgical Therapy.* Philadelphia, PA: WB Saunders; 2009. Reprinted with permission.)

UVULOPALATATOPHARYNGOPLASTY AND Z-PALATOPHARYNGOPLASTY

As mentioned previously, the efficacy of UPPP as an isolated procedure has been criticized as unacceptably low following a study by Sher and associates that showed a 40% success rate in unselected patients.[9] Selective application of UPPP following appropriate staging has shown that the procedure can be highly effective. Friedman and colleagues[16] found an 80% success rate for Friedman anatomic stage I patients undergoing UPPP, including those with severe disease.

The goal of UPPP is to widen the airway in three dimensions: (1) from anterior to posterior, between the palate and the posterior pharyngeal wall; (2) vertically, between the base of the tongue and the palate; and (3) laterally, at the level of the oropharynx. The technique consists of tonsillectomy and partial resection of the soft palate (Fig. 17-4). Complications include wound dehiscence, transient velopharyngeal insufficiency (VPI), globus pharyngeus, voice and taste changes, and nasopharyngeal stenosis.[30-32]

Z-palatopharyngoplasty (ZPP) is a modification of UPPP that was developed by Friedman to treat patients with stage II and III disease according to the Friedman Anatomic Staging System.[16,17,33] Patients in this group may include those who have previously undergone tonsillectomy, have small tonsils, or have an unfavorable Friedman tongue position. This technique can also be used as salvage therapy following failed UPPP. Three studies have thus far recorded an objective cure rate around 65% for patients with stage II and III disease.[33-35]

As with UPPP, the goal of ZPP is to widen the airway in the anteroposterior, vertical, and lateral directions. ZPP differs from UPPP in that the uvula and soft palate are not resected but are instead divided along the midline and reflected laterally over the remaining intact soft palate (Fig. 17-5, *A* to *D*) such that the vectors of tension extend anterolaterally (Fig. 17-5, *E, right*) instead of anteromedially, as in UPPP (Fig. 17-5, *E, left*). As the tissue heals and begins to scar following ZPP, tension along these anterolateral vectors will increase, further widening the airway.[33]

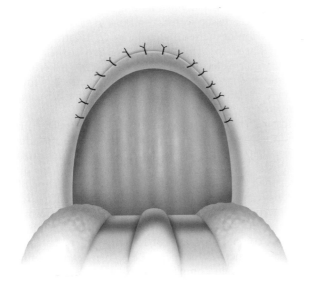

Figure 17-4 Uvulopalatopharyngoplasty (UPPP). In UPPP, the tonsils are removed, and the soft palate is partially resected. (From Friedman M. *Sleep: Apnea and Snoring: Surgical and Non-Surgical Therapy.* Philadelphia, PA: WB Saunders; 2009. Reprinted with permission.)

Similar to UPPP, significant pain and dysphagia are to be expected during the initial postoperative period following ZPP. Complications are comparable between the two procedures and include bleeding, mild dysphagia, dry throat, and globus sensation, as well as mild VPI. The rate of VPI is slightly higher for ZPP than for UPPP but rarely persists beyond 3 months.[33]

Radiofrequency tongue base reduction (RFBOT), submucosal minimally invasive lingual excision (SMILE), and other procedures that target retrolingual obstruction are often performed at the same time as UPPP or ZPP. Studies have shown higher rates of success for patients treated with ZPP and RFBOT compared to UPPP and RFBOT.[33,36-38]

TRANSPALATAL ADVANCEMENT PHARYNGOPLASTY (HARD PALATE SHORTENING)

Transpalatal advancement pharyngoplasty is indicated in cases of retropalatal obstruction but is typically reserved for cases in which UPPP has failed or is unlikely to succeed given the severity of airway narrowing. In this technique, a portion of the posterior hard palate is resected, allowing for the advancement of the intact soft palate. The upper pharyngeal airway is thus enlarged in the anteroposterior and lateral directions while maintaining the integrity of the soft palate.

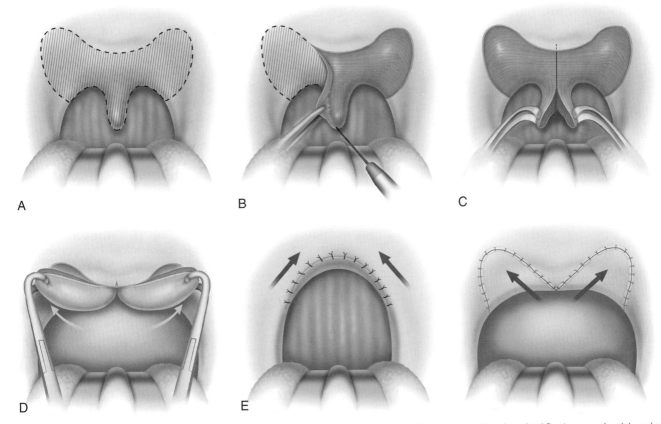

Figure 17-5 Z-palatopharyngoplasty. A, Outline of the palatal flaps, marked before incision. **B,** The mucosa overlying the palatal flap is removed and the palatal musculature is exposed. **C,** The uvula and palate are split in the midline with a cold knife. **D,** The uvular flaps, along with the soft palate, are reflected back and laterally over the soft palate. Two-layered closure is then performed. **E,** Following Z-palatopharyngoplasty (ZPP) (*right*), the vectors of tension extend anterolaterally, widening the retropharyngeal space. After uvulopalatopharyngoplasty (UPPP) (*left*), the vectors of tension are oriented anteromedially. (From Friedman M. *Sleep: Apnea and Snoring: Surgical and Non-Surgical Therapy.* Philadelphia, PA: WB Saunders; 2009. Reprinted with permission.)

Possible complications of this procedure include wound breakdown, fistula formation, nasopharyngeal reflux, VPI, and dysphagia, but they occur rarely. Most patients are able to commence a soft diet on postoperative day 1.

Woodson and associates compared this technique with UPPP and found a greater decrease in AHI among patients who had transpalatal advancement pharyngoplasty.[39] The odds ratio for success compared to UPPP in this study was 3.88. One limitation of this procedure is its minimal effect on snoring. Less scarring of the soft palate occurs following transpalatal advancement than in UPPP or ZPP. As a consequence, soft tissue flutter may persist, necessitating further treatments such as palatal implants or radiofrequency of the palate for adequate snoring reduction.

SURGERY FOR RETROLINGUAL OBSTRUCTION

Radiofrequency Reduction of the Tongue Base

Treatment of the retrolingual area could be considered in surgical candidates classified as Friedman stage II or III, regardless of OSAHS severity.[16] RFBOT is a minimally invasive technique that is generally well tolerated and can be performed in the office under local anesthesia. It is most often performed in combination with other minimally invasive or classical surgical techniques, and is currently recommended for those with mild to moderate OSAHS.[6]

In this procedure, a double-pronged probe is used to deliver radiofrequency energy to two points, 5 mm on either side of the midline at five sites between the circumvallate papillae and the vallecula (Fig. 17-6). A total of 3000 J

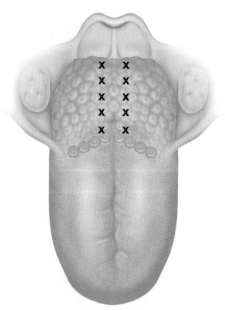

Figure 17-6 Radiofrequency tongue base reduction. Radiofrequency energy is delivered by a double probe to two points 5 mm on either side of the midline simultaneously along five sites between the circumvallate papillae and the vallecula. (From Friedman M. *Sleep: Apnea and Snoring: Surgical and Non-Surgical Therapy.* Philadelphia, PA: WB Saunders; 2009. Reprinted with permission.)

are delivered, equally divided among five sites. In the ensuing weeks, scar tissue forms, resulting in tissue contraction and expansion of the retrolingual airway. Treatment may be repeated if necessary. However, the degree of tissue reduction possible with this technique is limited. Partial glossectomy or the minimally invasive SMILE technique described in the next section is typically more appropriate for treating patients with macroglossia.

Most patients who undergo RFBOT as an isolated procedure do not require narcotics postoperatively. Return to full diet is usually within 4 days.[40] Complications are rare, but hypoglossal paralysis can occur if the electrodes are placed greater than 2 cm from the midline. Improper seating of the electrodes can also lead to mucosal burns. Although postoperative infections can occur, the incidence of abscess formation is less than 0.1%.[38] One review has estimated overall moderate/severe complication rates of 2.7%.[41]

As an adjunctive treatment, RFBOT appears to improve success rates when compared to palatal treatment alone.[38] Many authors have also found favorable outcomes for RFBOT as an isolated treatment. A 2008 meta-analysis studying the efficacy of this technique revealed a short-term respiratory disturbance index (RDI) reduction of 31% with a 45% reduction in long-term RDI.[42] More recent studies have also indicated long-term success of 33% to 56%.[43,44]

Submucosal Minimally Invasive Lingual Excision

Traditional techniques for treating macroglossia in patients with OSAHS entail removing a wedge of muscle from the tongue base along with the overlying mucosa. This can result in a protracted recovery period during which significant dysphagia and odynophagia are typical.[45] SMILE reduces tongue base mass without incurring extensive mucosal disruption. The result is less pain and impairment postoperatively.[45,46]

Multiple techniques have been described by Friedman and associates,[47] Robinson and associates,[46] Maturo and Mair,[45] Woodson and Fujita,[48] and other authors. The SMILE technique was originally developed for use in children but has been found to be appropriate for adult patients as well.[45-47] Temperature-controlled radiofrequency energy (coblation) is delivered to the submucosal tissue of tongue base via a probe inserted percutaneously through an incision in the neck or through an intraoral incision (Fig. 17-7, *A* and *B*).[45,46] Utilizing radiofrequency results in less edema and inadvertent tissue destruction than electrocautery or laser.[49] Endoscopic guidance and Doppler ultrasound may be utilized to facilitate the intraoral approach (Fig. 17-7, *C* to *E*). Possible complications include hematoma, bleeding into the airway, and hypoglossal nerve paralysis. Except during the initial postoperative period, swallowing and speech are not significantly altered.[45] There have been no reports of changes in gustation.

Limited data regarding the efficacy of this procedure are available. One small study examining the percutaneous approach reported a 40% response rate.[46] One study of 96 patients found a success rate of 65%, compared to a success rate of 41% undergoing RFBOT.[47] Additional, large-scale studies are necessary to determine the long-term efficacy of the technique.

Minimally Invasive Tongue Base Stabilization

During sleep, inadequate muscle tone within the pharynx allows the tongue base to collapse into the hypopharyngeal airway, resulting in obstruction. Tongue base suspension is a minimally invasive technique that seeks to prevent this from occurring by means of a submucosal suture looped through the base of the tongue and anchored to a screw placed along the lingual surface of the mandible (Fig. 17-8). The suture prevents passive collapse of the tongue base during sleep but does not alter the anterior movements of the tongue required for speech and swallowing. As with most therapies

for OSAHS, tongue base stabilization may be performed as an isolated treatment or as part of multilevel surgical therapy.[50]

To date, studies show success rates ranging from 20% to 57%,[50-54] though few trials have examined the long-term results of the procedure. Possible complications include transient VPI and restricted protrusive movement.[52,53] One major advantage of tongue base suspension is that it is reversible and does not preclude future surgery on the tongue base. In addition, because it is minimally invasive, morbidity associated with this procedure may be lower than for conventional glossectomy or advancement procedures. However, when compared to RFBOT as an adjunct

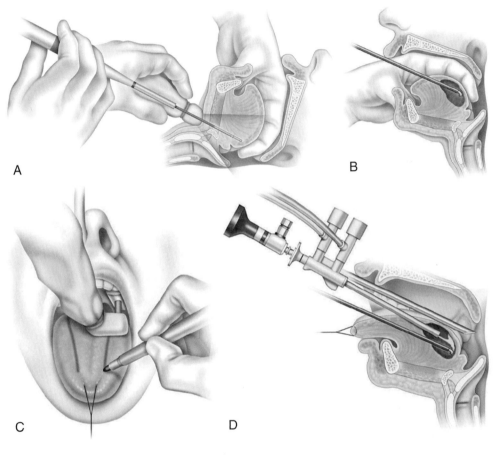

A

B

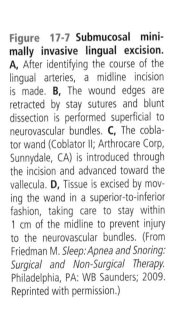

Figure 17-7 Submucosal minimally invasive lingual excision. A, After identifying the course of the lingual arteries, a midline incision is made. **B,** The wound edges are retracted by stay sutures and blunt dissection is performed superficial to neurovascular bundles. **C,** The coblator wand (Coblator II; Arthrocare Corp, Sunnydale, CA) is introduced through the incision and advanced toward the vallecula. **D,** Tissue is excised by moving the wand in a superior-to-inferior fashion, taking care to stay within 1 cm of the midline to prevent injury to the neurovascular bundles. (From Friedman M. *Sleep: Apnea and Snoring: Surgical and Non-Surgical Therapy.* Philadelphia, PA: WB Saunders; 2009. Reprinted with permission.)

C

D

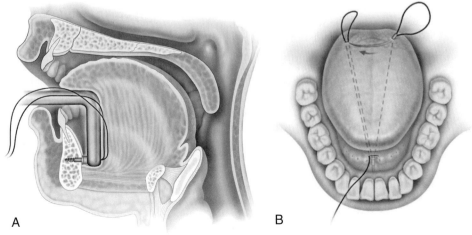

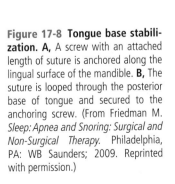

Figure 17-8 Tongue base stabilization. A, A screw with an attached length of suture is anchored along the lingual surface of the mandible. **B,** The suture is looped through the posterior base of tongue and secured to the anchoring screw. (From Friedman M. *Sleep: Apnea and Snoring: Surgical and Non-Surgical Therapy.* Philadelphia, PA: WB Saunders; 2009. Reprinted with permission.)

A

B

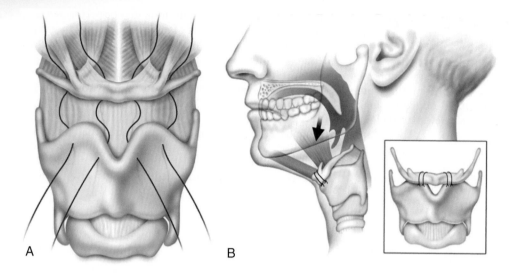

A   B

Figure 17-9 Hyoid suspension. Four nonabsorbable sutures are used to reposition the hyoid inferior and anterior to the superior border of the thyroid cartilage. (From Friedman M. *Sleep: Apnea and Snoring: Surgical and Non-Surgical Therapy.* Philadelphia, PA: WB Saunders; 2009. Reprinted with permission.)

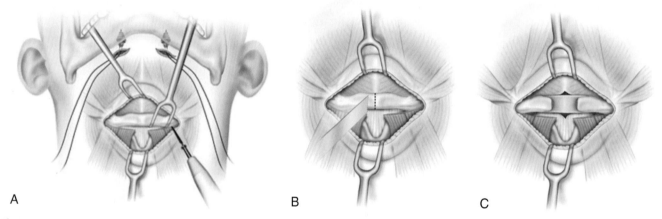

A   B   C

Figure 17-10 Hyomandibular suspension and hyoid expansion. A, After the insertion of two Repose screws into the mandible, the mandible is exposed and the infrahyoid muscles are excised via electrocautery. **B,** Hyoid distraction is accomplished with a bone cutter. **C,** The hyoid is separated and suspensed with figure of eight sutures. (From Friedman M. *Sleep: Apnea and Snoring: Surgical and Non-Surgical Therapy.* Philadelphia, PA: WB Saunders; 2009. Reprinted with permission.)

to UPPP, Fernández-Julián and associates[55] found that tongue base suspension had similar efficacy but resulted in increased morbidity, including acute submandibular sialoadenitis.

Hyoid Suspension

Anterior traction on the hyoid widens the retrolingual space. In hyoid suspension, the hyoid is repositioned anteroinferiorly and secured to the superior margin of the thyroid cartilage with permanent sutures (Fig. 17-9). The anterior repositioning prevents posterior movement of the tongue base, and the inferior displacement is an incidental effect of the procedure. In many cases, only a few millimeters of anterior movement are accomplished. Ideal candidates for this procedure have moderate to severe OSAHS and major obstruction at the tongue base without concurrent macroglossia.

Hyoid suspension is rarely effective as a single-modality treatment in patients with multilevel obstruction. Published rates of success range from 17% to 78% as a single procedure.[56-59] Most patients require additional procedures

addressing other areas of obstruction to achieve optimal results.[60-62] Postoperative pain following this procedure is lower than after UPPP. Potential complications include hematoma formation, bleeding into the airway, temporary dysphagia, and infection requiring suture removal.[56,59]

Hyomandibular Suspension and Hyoid Expansion

Hyomandibular suspension and hyoid expansion is an experimental procedure that may be performed together or alone for patients who have hypopharyngeal obstruction and suffer from severe OSAHS.[63] Hyomandibular suspension enlarges the hypopharyngeal airway by repositioning the tongue base in an anterosuperior direction, whereas hyoid expansion serves to increase the lateral dimension of the hypopharynx. In the combined procedure (Fig. 17-10), the strap muscles are dissected from the inferior border of the hyoid. The hyoid is then divided at the midline and distracted laterally. An absorbable or nonabsorbable implant may be placed between the divided edges of the hyoid to maintain separation. Anterosuperior traction is placed on the hyoid by means of a permanent suture anchored to the lingual surface of the mandible. This permits partial separation of the tongue base from the hypopharynx and can be augmented with tongue base suspension when appropriate.

Hyomandibular suspension with hyoid expansion is considered a minor procedure and is currently the only available technique for widening the hypopharyngeal airway in the lateral dimension. Complications are relatively rare but include prolonged dysphagia, odynophagia, speech alteration, infection, hematoma, and airway obstruction.

Krespi and colleagues[63] have reported a 90% subjective response as well as a mean reduction in the respiratory disturbance index from 71.2 to 28.4 after a minimum of 3 months in 52 of their patients who underwent this procedure. However, it is important to note that these results have never been replicated and, to date, no peer-reviewed reports regarding the efficacy and safety of hyoid expansion and hyomandibular suspension have been published.

SURGERY FOR NASAL AIRWAY OBSTRUCTION

Nasal surgery is an important component in a multilevel approach to OSAHS treatment. When nasal surgery is recommended for patients with OSAHS, patients should understand that it is unlikely to cure their OSAHS without correction of palatal or retrolingual obstruction. For patients willing to use CPAP, nasal surgery has been shown to improve daytime nasal function and CPAP compliance and to reduce the optimal CPAP pressure.[43]

Nasal airway obstruction is common among patients who suffer from OSAHS or snoring. Primary causes of nasal airway obstruction include septal deviation, turbinate hypertrophy, nasal polyps, and nasal valve collapse. Obstruction of the nasal airway has been identified as an independent risk factor for OSAHS,[64] but evidence of a direct causal relationship has been lacking.[65-68]

Various surgical techniques, including septoplasty and turbinate reduction via radiofrequency ablation or submucous resection, are available to help alleviate nasal airway obstruction. However, although these techniques can help to improve breathing during sleep and wakefulness and lessen or eliminate snoring, they seldom cure OSAHS. Multiple studies have examined the effects of nasal surgery on sleep apnea.[69-73] A recent review of the literature suggests that surgical correction of nasal obstruction does not have a significant impact on objective measures such as AHI, but does improve subjective measures.[74] The main benefits of nasal surgery may be a decrease in mean CPAP pressure, an increase in CPAP compliance, and improved quality of life.[69,74] Thus, while correction of nasal obstruction has limited benefit as an isolated procedure for OSAHS, it often improves patients' subjective complaints and plays a crucial role as a component of a multilevel approach to OSAHS treatment.

Nasal Valve Repair

The nasal valve, the most proximal part of the internal nasal airway, is frequently overlooked as a contributing or primary cause of nasal obstruction. Many OSAHS patients continue to experience nocturnal nasal obstruction even after undergoing nasal procedures such as turbinate reduction or correction of a deviated septum. In one series looking at 500 cases of nasal

obstruction, nasal valve incompetence was identified as the primary underlying cause in 13% of patients.[75]

Forced inspiration against an obstructed pharyngeal airway may result in collapse of the nasal valve area. Because patients with OSAHS have increased respiratory effort, it is likely that nasal valve collapse is more common in this group of patients. On the other hand, forced inspiration through an obstructed nasal airway in turn can lead to pharyngeal airway collapse. Although no study has shown a causal relationship, it is possible that OSAHS may actively contribute to valve collapse.

The nasal valve can be divided into two anatomic parts. The external nasal valve consists of the nares (nostrils) and the nasal vestibule. The internal nasal valve, typically the narrowest part of the nasal airway, consists of the area distal to the vestibule and proximal to the inferior turbinate. The anterior nostril may be narrowed by incompetence at the internal nasal valve, the external nasal valve, or both. Congenital weakness of the nasal sidewalls, aging, reduction rhinoplasty, and trauma are some of the causes of nasal valve incompetence; of these, reduction rhinoplasty is most common.[75,76]

Corrective procedures aim to increase the minimum cross-sectional area of the nasal valve through strengthening support structures. These procedures can be classified as either "opening" (increase the cross-sectional area) or "strengthening" (reinforce the lateral wall). Although most techniques have been shown to be successful, selection of the procedure will often depend on patient-specific pathology.[77] Detailed discussion of these procedures is beyond the scope of this chapter. For patients with OSAHS, the simplified approach of orbital suspension reported by Friedman has been shown to be very effective[78,79] (Fig. 17-11).

Nasal valve suspension can be performed under general or local anesthesia. The nasal valve area is examined to identify the area of collapse prior to injection of local anesthesia to avoid distortion of tissue. The Mitek Soft Tissue Anchor system (1.3-mm Micro Quick Anchor, Ethicon), which includes a drill bit, bone anchor, and attached suture, is used to anchor a suture to the orbital rim. After identifying the site of collapse and the intended site of suspension, the needle is rethreaded and passed from the caudal point toward the anchor. The suture is then secured with the amount of tension required to support the valve without distorting the external valve area. The orbital rim incisions are closed with sterile adhesive strips.

ADDITIONAL THERAPIES

Maxillomandibular Advancement

Patients with hypopharyngeal airway obstruction due to maxillomandibular deficiency may benefit from maxillomandibular advancement (MMA). MMA is an aggressive orthognathic procedure that is typically indicated for patients with severe OSAHS who have failed other medical and surgical interventions.[6] The operation is carried out under general anesthesia with nasotracheal intubation and consists of a Le Fort I osteotomy with bilateral mandibular sagittal split osteotomies followed by rigid fixation with titanium plates (Fig. 17-12). To ensure proper occlusion, intermaxillary fixation (IMF) with arch bars is required during the operation. The arch bars

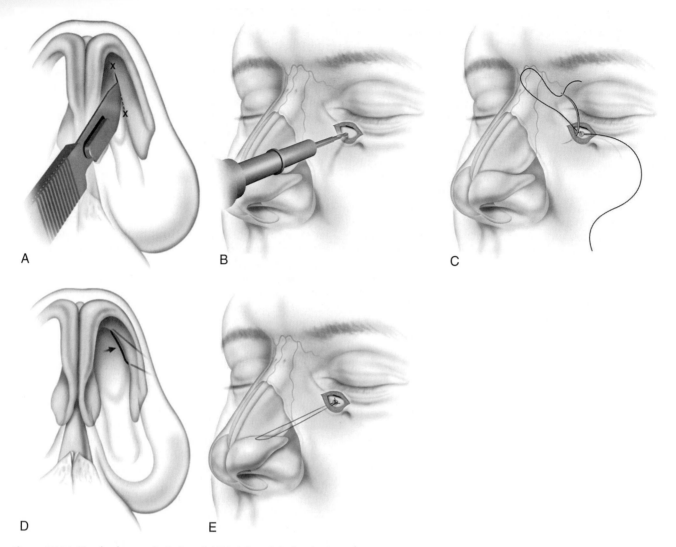

Figure 17-11 Nasal valve repair. A, A small drill hole is made in the orbital rim in preparation for insertion of the anchoring system and suture. **B,** A small infra-orbital incision is made and a hole is drilled infraorbitally into the bone to allow for the anchoring system. **C,** The suture is threaded into a curved, tapered needle and passed into the nasal valve area. **D,** The needle is then rethreaded and passed through the opening in the mucosa toward the anchor. **E,** Tension is applied, elevating and supporting the nasal valve. (From Friedman M. *Sleep: Apnea and Snoring: Surgical and Non-Surgical Therapy.* Philadelphia, PA: WB Saunders; 2009. Reprinted with permission.)

may be left in place postoperatively to maintain occlusion, though dental splints are often used instead. The degree of advancement varies among patients; however, 10 mm to 12 mm of advancement is typical. The procedure can be modified to include the resection of bone to minimize cosmetic alteration.[80] Other variations involve distraction osteogenesis[81] and autologous bone grafting.[82]

Regardless of the specific technique employed, the end result is expansion of the hypopharyngeal and pharyngeal airway. This results in a substantial improvement in objective measures as evidenced by an average AHI reduction of 87%.[29]

Intraoperative complications include bleeding and damage to the surrounding dental, neurovascular, and musculoskeletal structures. Postoperatively, this damage can manifest as malocclusion, transient dental or perioral anesthesia, hematoma formation, avascular necrosis of the palate, and mandibular weakening resulting in fracture. Airway edema is another serious complication that can occur in the immediate postoperative period. Changes in facial appearance are typical and may

be a serious drawback for some individuals. Thus, patients should be appropriately counseled prior to intervention.

Bariatric Surgery

Obesity is a co-morbid condition in 60% to 90% of patients diagnosed with OSAHS and has been identified as a significant risk factor for developing the disease.[83-86] A number of studies have shown that weight reduction can lead to improvements in AHI and subjective sleep quality.[87] For individuals unable to achieve adequate weight loss by conventional means such as diet and exercise, bariatric surgery may be indicated.

The goal of bariatric surgery is to restrict caloric intake. A variety of procedures have been developed. They can be divided into two main categories: restrictive and restrictive-malabsorptive. As the name implies, restrictive procedures reduce the amount of food the stomach can hold. A secondary result is to slow gastric emptying, which serves to prolong satiety. The most common restrictive procedure is laparoscopic

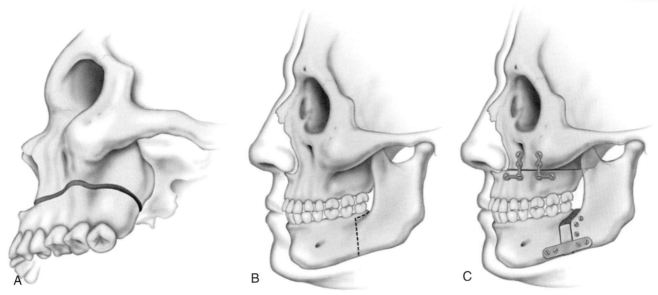

Figure 17-12 Maxillomandibular advancement. A, Le Fort I osteotomy. **B,** Bilateral sagittal split osteotomy. **C,** Maxillomandibular advancement with fixation. (From Friedman M. *Sleep: Apnea and Snoring: Surgical and Non-Surgical Therapy.* Philadelphia, PA: WB Saunders; 2009. Reprinted with permission.)

adjustable silicone gastric banding, which allows for adjustment of functional gastric capacity via a subcutaneous saline reservoir implant.

Restrictive-malabsorptive procedures, such as the Roux-en-Y gastric bypass (RYGB), divert the flow of contents through the alimentary canal from their natural course in order to reduce absorption. In RYGB, a small gastric pouch (10-30 mL) is created and anastomosed to form a gastrojejunostomy between 50 cm and 150 cm in length which is in turn anastomosed to the distal jejunum, thereby forming a conduit that bypasses the majority of the stomach, duodenum, and jejunum.

Gastric bypass may be the most effective treatment for severe obesity, leading to a 30% to 35% reduction in body weight in most individuals.[87] Long-term weight loss maintenance for 5 years has been estimated to be 60%.[88-90] Common complications include the development of deficiencies in vitamin B[12], folate, iron, calcium, and vitamin D. Lifelong supplementation with these nutrients is necessary. "Dumping syndrome" is another common side effect of this procedure. It occurs when food bypasses the stomach and rapidly enters and expands in the proximal duodenum, thereby causing nausea, vomiting, bloating, dizziness, fatigue, and diarrhea. Although usually resolving on its own over time, medication or surgery to reverse the gastric bypass may be indicated in severe cases.

Tracheostomy

Until the introduction of uvulopalatopharyngoplasty in 1981, tracheostomy was the only surgical technique available for treating obstructive sleep apnea. Given the obvious cosmetic and functional implications of the procedure, it was generally reserved for the treatment of severe and life-threatening cases of OSAHS only. Tracheostomy provides an alternate inlet for air, which bypasses the obstructed upper airway. In many cases, the stoma can be occluded or "corked" during the day and opened for nocturnal use.

With the multitude of surgical therapies available today, the number of tracheostomies performed for the treatment of

OSAHS has declined significantly. Nevertheless, tracheostomy remains a viable option for selected patients. Patients who have failed or refused nonsurgical treatment and multilevel surgical therapy may be considered for tracheostomy.[6] Often these patients are morbidly obese. The modified tracheotomy technique described by Fee and Ward[91,92] involves partial lipectomy and the creation of "defatted" skin flaps. The end result is a circumferentially skin-lined stoma that allows for better hygiene and fewer complications. The efficacy of this procedure for treatment of OSAHS is nearly 100%.[93-95] Complications, though uncommon, include granulation tissue formation, inadvertent extubation, tracheal stenosis, and chronic wound infection.

Patients must be appropriately counseled regarding the long-term postoperative care required for stomal maintenance and the potential social implications of having a tracheostomy.

POSTOPERATIVE FOLLOW-UP

Proper postoperative care is essential in the OSAHS patient. Upon adequate healing, the patient should be evaluated for objective and subjective changes. A full polysomnogram should be completed, noting primarily changes in AHI, oxygen desaturation, and secondarily arousal index and overall sleep pattern. Improvements in symptoms, including daytime and nighttime measures, should also be evaluated.

In the event of inadequate correction or relapse, options are available. Ideally, the first step includes a nonsurgical approach, either CPAP therapy or oral appliance. Owing to the changes induced by surgery, a retitration sleep study should be completed for both CPAP and any oral appliances to ensure optimization. If this step is not an option, further surgical treatment may be necessary, either through multilevel procedures or more invasive treatment.

At this time, formal recommendations on any particular strategy or timing of evaluation do not exist,[6] partly because of the difficulty of predicting the duration of improvement, as surgical gains often are not permanent.[96,97] Recurrence of OSA may be due to weight gain, other illnesses, or medication changes but may not be identifiable.[98] Thus, long-term follow-up is ideal.

SUMMARY

The modern approach to surgical therapy for OSAHS revolves around the following principles:

1. Surgery is palliative for those patients who cannot or will not use CPAP therapy.
2. The importance of identifying the site or sites of obstruction cannot be overemphasized. Typically, nasal, palatal, and retrolingual obstruction all contribute. The operative plan should include treatment of all sites, whether surgery is accomplished in one stage or multiple stages.
3. The severity of obstruction at each site must be determined by physical examination and PSG results to determine whether each site requires minimally invasive or classical surgical treatment.
4. The operative plan, nonsurgical options, and likelihood of success should be explained to the patient.

REFERENCES

1. Kim JH, Kwon MS, Song HM, et al. Compliance with positive airway pressure treatment for obstructive sleep apnea. *Clin Exp Otorhinolaryngol.* 2009;2(2):90-96.
2. Krieger J. Long-term compliance with nasal continuous positive airway pressure (CPAP) in obstructive sleep apnea patients and nonapneic snorers. *Sleep.* 1992;15(Suppl 6):S42-S46.
3. Wolkove N, Baltzan M, Kamel H, et al. Long-term compliance with continuous positive airway pressure in patients with obstructive sleep apnea. *Can Respir J.* 2008;15(7):365-369.
4. Engleman HM, Wild MR. Improving CPAP use by patients with the sleep apnoea/hypopnoea syndrome (SAHS). *Sleep Med Rev.* 2003;7(1):81-99.
5. Weaver TE, Kribbs NB, Pack AI, et al. Night-to-night variability in CPAP use over the first three months of treatment. *Sleep.* 1997;20(4):278-283.
6. Aurora RN, Casey KR, Kristo D, et al. Practice parameters for the surgical modifications of the upper airway for obstructive sleep apnea in adults. *Sleep.* 2010;33(10):1408-1413.
7. Fujita S, Conway W, Zorick F. Surgical correction of anatomic abnormalities in obstructive sleep apnea syndrome: Uvulopalatopharyngoplasty. *Otolaryngol Head Neck Surg.* 1981;89(6):923-934.
8. Lin H-C, Friedman M, Chang HW, et al. The efficacy of multilevel surgery of the upper airway in adults with obstructive sleep apnea/hypopnea syndrome. *Laryngoscope.* 2008;118(5):902-908.
9. Sher AE, Schechtman KB, Piccirillo JF. The efficacy of surgical modifications of the upper airway in adults with obstructive sleep apnea syndrome. *Sleep.* 1996;19(2):156-177.
10. Friedman M, Vidyasagar R, Bliznikas D, et al. Does severity of obstructive sleep apnea/hypopnea syndrome predict uvulopalatopharyngoplasty outcome? *Laryngoscope.* 2005;115(12):2109-2113.
11. Borowiecki BD, Sassin JF. Surgical treatment of sleep apnea. *Arch Otolaryngol.* 1983;109(8):508-512.
12. Friedman M, Tanyeri H, Rosa M, et al. Clinical predictors of obstructive sleep apnea. *Laryngoscope.* 1999;109(12):1901-1907.
13. Mallampati SR, Gatt SP, Gugino LD, et al. A clinical sign to predict difficult tracheal intubation: A prospective study. *Can Anaesth Soc J.* 1985;32(4):429-434.
14. Liistro G, Rombaux P, Belge C, et al. High Mallampati score and nasal obstruction are associated risk factors for obstructive sleep apnoea. *Eur Respir J.* 2003;21(2):248-252.
15. Nuckton TJ, Glidden DV, Browner WS, et al. Physical examination: Mallampati score as an independent predictor of obstructive sleep apnea. *Sleep.* 2006;29(7):903-908.
16. Friedman M, Ibrahim H, Joseph NJ. Staging of obstructive sleep apnea/hypopnea syndrome: A guide to appropriate treatment. *Laryngoscope.* 2004;114(3):454-459.
17. Friedman M, Ibrahim H, Bass L. Clinical staging for sleep-disordered breathing. *Otolaryngol Head Neck Surg.* 2002;127(1):13-21.
18. Li H, Chen N, Lee L, et al. Use of morphological indicators to predict outcomes of palatopharyngeal surgery in patients with obstructive sleep apnea. *ORL J Otorhinolaryngol Relat Spec.* 2004;66(3):119-123.
19. Esclamado RM, Gleen MG, McCulloch TM, et al. Perioperative complications and risk factors in the surgical treatment of obstructive sleep apnea syndrome. *Laryngoscope.* 1989;99(11):1125-1129.
20. Gentil B, de Larminat JM, Boucherez C, et al. Difficult intubation and obstructive sleep apnoea syndrome. *Br J Anaesth.* 1994;72(3):368.
21. Gupta RM, Gay PC. Postoperative complications in patients with obstructive sleep apnea syndrome undergoing hip or knee replacement: A case-control study. *Mayo Clin Proc..* 2001;76(9):897-905.
22. Riley RW, Powell NB, Guilleminault C, et al. Obstructive sleep apnea surgery: Risk management and complications. *Otolaryngol Head Neck Surg.* 1997;117(6):648-652.
23. Li KK, Powell N, Riley R. Postoperative management of the obstructive sleep apnea patient. *Oral Maxillofac Surg Clin North Am..* 2002;14(3):401-404.
24. Rennotte MT, Baele P, Aubert G, et al. Nasal continuous positive airway pressure in the perioperative management of patients with obstructive sleep apnea submitted to surgery. *Chest.* 1995;107(2):367-374.
25. Raghavendran S, Bagry H, Detheux G, et al. An anesthetic management protocol to decrease respiratory complications after adenotonsillectomy in children with severe sleep apnea. *Anesth Analg.* 2010;110(4):1093-1101.
26. Lee C-H, Peng M-J, Wu C- L. Dexamethasone to prevent postextubation airway obstruction in adults: A prospective, randomized, double-blind, placebo-controlled study. *Crit Care.* 2007;11(4):R72.
27. Meade MO, Guyatt GH, Cook DJ, et al. Trials of corticosteroids to prevent postextubation airway complications. *Chest.* 2001;120(Suppl 6):S464-S468.
28. Friedman M, Vidyasagar R, Bliznikas D, et al. Patient selection and efficacy of pillar implant technique for treatment of snoring and obstructive sleep apnea/hypopnea syndrome. *Otolaryngol Head Neck Surg.* 2006;134(2):187-196.
29. Caples SM, Rowley A, Prinsell JR, et al. Surgical modifications of the upper airway for obstructive sleep apnea in adults: A systematic review and meta-analysis. *Sleep.* 2010;33(10):1396-1407.
30. Fairbanks DN. Operative techniques of uvulopalatopharyngoplasty. *Ear Nose Throat J.* 1999;78(11):846-850.
31. Goh YH, Mark I, Fee WE. Quality of life 17 to 20 years after uvulopalatopharyngoplasty. *Laryngoscope.* 2007;117(3):503-506.
32. Riley RW, Powell NB, Guilleminault C. Obstructive sleep apnea syndrome: A review of 306 consecutively treated surgical patients. *Otolaryngol Head Neck Surg.* 1993;108(2):117-125.
33. Friedman M, Ibrahim HZ, Vidyasagar R, Pomeranz J, Joseph N. Z-palatoplasty (ZPP): A technique for patients without tonsils. *Otolaryngol Head Neck Surg: official journal of American Academy of Otolaryngology-Head and Neck Surgery.* 2004;131(1):89-100.
34. Friedman M, Duggal P, Joseph NJ. Revision uvulopalatoplasty by Z-palatoplasty. *Otolaryngol Head Neck Surg.* 2007;136(4):638-643.
35. Yi HL, Yin SK, Zhang YJ, et al. Z-palatopharyngoplasty for obstructive sleep apnea/hypopnea syndrome. *Otolaryngol Head Neck Surg.* 2009;140(5):640-645.
36. Friedman M, Ibrahim H, Lee G, Joseph N. Staging of obstructive sleep apnea/hypopnea syndrome: A guide to appropriate treatment. *Laryngoscope.* 2004;114(3):454-459.
37. Friedman M, Ibrahim H, Joseph N. Combined uvulopalatopharyngoplasty and radiofrequency tongue base reduction for treatment of obstructive sleep apnea/hypopnea syndrome. *Otolaryngol Head Neck Surg: official journal of American Academy of Otolaryngology-Head and Neck Surgery.* 2003;129(6):611-621.
38. Stuck BA, Maurer JT, Hormann K. [Tongue base reduction with radiofrequency energy in sleep apnea]. *Head Neck Otolarngol.* 2001;49(7):530-537.
39. Woodson BT, S Robinson K, Lim HJ. Transpalatal advancement pharyngoplasty outcomes compared with uvulopalatopharyngoplasty. *Otolaryngol Head Neck Surg.* 2005;133(2):211-217.
40. Friedman M, LoSavio P, Ibrahim H, et al. Radiofrequency tonsil reduction: Safety, morbidity, and efficacy. *Laryngoscope.* 2003;113(5):882-887.
41. Kezirian EJ, Goldberg AN. Hypopharyngeal surgery in obstructive sleep apnea: An evidence-based medicine review. *Arch Otolaryngol Head Neck Surg.* 2006;132(2):206-213.
42. Farrar J, Ryan J, Oliver E, et al. Radiofrequency ablation for the treatment of obstructive sleep apnea: A meta-analysis. *Laryngoscope.* 2008;118(10):1878-1883.
43. Fibbi A, Ameli F, Brocchetti F, Mignosi S, et al. Tongue base suspension and radiofrequency volume reduction: A comparison between 2 techniques for the treatment of sleep-disordered breathing. *Am J Otolaryngol.* 2009;30(6):401-406.
44. Neruntarat C, Chantapant S. Radiofrequency surgery for the treatment of obstructive sleep apnea: Short-term and long-term results. *Otolaryngol Head Neck Surg.* 2009;141(6):722-726.

45. Maturo SC, Mair EA. Submucosal minimally invasive lingual excision: An effective, novel surgery for pediatric tongue base reduction. *Ann Otol Rhinol Laryngol.* 2006;115(8):624-630.

46. Robinson S, Lewis R, Norton A, et al. Ultrasound-guided radiofrequency submucosal tongue-base excision for sleep apnoea: A preliminary report. *Clin Otolaryngol Allied Sci.* 2003;28(4):341-345.

47. Friedman M, Soans R, Gurpinar B, et al. Evaluation of submucosal minimally invasive lingual excision technique for treatment of obstructive sleep apnea/hypopnea syndrome. *Otolaryngol Head Neck Surg.* 2008;139(3):378-384:discussion 385.

48. Woodson BT, Fujita S. Clinical experience with lingualplasty as part of the treatment of severe obstructive sleep apnea. *Otolaryngol Head Neck Surg.* 1992;107(1):40-48.

49. Greene D. Radiofrequency ablation of the tongue base in obstructive sleep apnea: Rapid and effective technique using low-temperature radiofrequency molecular disassociation (coblation) for management of retroglossal obstruction. *J Otolaryngol Head Neck Surg.* 2008;37(6):777-781.

50. Miller FR, Watson D, Malis D. Role of the tongue base suspension suture with the Repose System bone screw in the multilevel surgical management of obstructive sleep apnea. *Otolaryng Head Neck Surg.* 2002;126(4):392-398.

51. Woodson BT. A tongue suspension suture for obstructive sleep apnea and snorers. *Otolaryngol Head Neck Surg.* 2001;124(3):297-303.

52. DeRowe A, Gunther E, Safaya A, et al. Tongue-base suspension with a soft tissue-to-bone anchor for obstructive sleep apnea: Preliminary clinical results of a new minimally invasive technique. *Otolaryngol Head Neck Surg.* 2000;122(1):100-103.

53. Terris DJ, Kunda LD, Gonella MC. Minimally invasive tongue base surgery for obstructive sleep apnoea. *J Laryngol Otol.* 2002;116(9):716-721.

54. Thomas AJ, Chavoya M, Terris DJ. Preliminary findings from a prospective, randomized trial of two tongue-base surgeries for sleep-disordered breathing. *Otolaryngol Head Neck Surg.* 2003;129(5):539-546.

55. Fernández-Julián E, Muñoz N, Achiques MT, et al. Randomized study comparing two tongue base surgeries for moderate to severe obstructive sleep apnea syndrome. *Otolaryngol Head Neck Surg: official journal of American Academy of Otolaryngology-Head and Neck Surgery.* 2009;140(6):917-923.

56. Bowden MT, Kezirian EJ, Utley D, et al. Outcomes of hyoid suspension for the treatment of obstructive sleep apnea. *Arch Otolaryngol Head Neck Surg.* 2005;131(5):440-445.

57. Vilaseca I, Morello A, Montserrat JM, et al. Usefulness of uvulopalatopharyngoplasty with genioglossus and hyoid advancement in the treatment of obstructive sleep apnea. *Arch Otolaryngol Head Neck Surg.* 2002;128(4):435-440.

58. Neruntarat C. Hyoid myotomy with suspension under local anesthesia for obstructive sleep apnea syndrome. *Eur Arch Otorhinolaryngol.* 2003;260(5):286-290.

59. den Herder C, van Tinteren H, de Vries N. Hyoidthyroidpexia: A surgical treatment for sleep apnea syndrome. *Laryngoscope.* 2005;115(4):740-745.

60. Jacobowitz O. Palatal and tongue base surgery for surgical treatment of obstructive sleep apnea: A prospective study. *Otolaryngol Head Neck Surg.* 2006;135(2):258-264.

61. Richard W, Kox D, den Herder C, et al. One stage multilevel surgery (uvulopalatopharyngoplasty, hyoid suspension, radiofrequent ablation of the tongue base with/without genioglossus advancement), in obstructive sleep apnea syndrome. *Eur Arch Otorhinolaryngol.* 2007;264(4):439-444.

62. Yin SK, Yi HL, Lu WY, et al. Genioglossus advancement and hyoid suspension plus uvulopalatopharyngoplasty for severe OSAHS. *Otolaryngol Head Neck Surg.* 2007;136(4):626-631.

63. Krespi Y. Hyo-mandibular suspension and hyoid expansion for obstructive sleep apnea. In: Friedman M, ed. *Sleep Apnea and Snoring: Surgical and Non-Surgical Therapy.* Philadelphia, PA: WB Saunders; 2009.

64. Lofaso F, Coste A, d'Ortho MP, et al. Nasal obstruction as a risk factor for sleep apnoea syndrome. *Eur Respir J.* 2000;16(4):639-643.

65. Kohler M, Bloch KE, Stradling JR. The role of the nose in the pathogenesis of obstructive sleep apnea. *Curr Opin Otolaryngol Head Neck Surg.* 2009;17(1):33-37.

66. Miljeteig H, Hoffstein V, Cole P. The effect of unilateral and bilateral nasal obstruction on snoring and sleep apnea. *Laryngoscope.* 1992;102(10):1150-1152.

67. Miyazaki S, Itasaka Y, Ishikawa K, et al. Influence of nasal obstruction on obstructive sleep apnea. *Acta Otolaryngol Suppl.* 1998;537:43-46.

68. Ohki M, Ushi N, Kanazawa H, et al. Relationship between oral breathing and nasal obstruction in patients with obstructive sleep apnea. *Acta Otolaryngol Suppl.* 1996;523:228-230.

69. Friedman M, Tanyeri H, Lim JW, et al. Effect of improved nasal breathing on obstructive sleep apnea. *Otolaryngol Head Neck Surg.* 2000;122(1):71-74.

70. Koutsourelakis I, Georgoulopoulos G, Perraki E, et al. Randomised trial of nasal surgery for fixed nasal obstruction in obstructive sleep apnoea. *Eur Respir J.* 2008;31(1):110-177.

71. Li H-Y, Lin Y, Chen NH, et al. Improvement in quality of life after nasal surgery alone for patients with obstructive sleep apnea and nasal obstruction. *Arch Otolaryngol Head Neck Surg.* 2008;134(4):429-433.

72. Nakata S, Noda A, Yasuma F, et al. Effects of nasal surgery on sleep quality in obstructive sleep apnea syndrome with nasal obstruction. *Am J Rhinol.* 2008;22(1):59-63.

73. Verse T, Maurer JT, Pirsig W. Effect of nasal surgery on sleep-related breathing disorders. *Laryngoscope.* 2002;112(1):64-68.

74. Rosow DE, Stewart MG. Is nasal surgery an effective treatment for obstructive sleep apnea? *Laryngoscope.* 2010;120(8):1496-1497.

75. Elwany S, Thabet H. Obstruction of the nasal valve. *J Laryngol Otol.* 1996;110(3):221-224.

76. Khosh MM, Jen A, Honrado C, Pearlman SJ. Nasal valve reconstruction: Experience in 53 consecutive patients. *Arch Facial Plast Surg.* 2004;6(3):167-171.

77. Spielmann PM, White PS, Hussain SS. Surgical techniques for the treatment of nasal valve collapse: A systematic review. *Laryngoscope.* 2009;119(7):1281-1290.

78. Friedman M, Ibrahim H, Syed Z. Nasal valve suspension: An improved, simplified technique for nasal valve collapse. *Laryngoscope.* 2003;113(2):381-385.

79. Friedman M, Ibrahim H, Lee G, Joseph NJ. A simplified technique for airway correction at the nasal valve area. *Otolaryngol Head Neck Surg.* 2004;131(4):519-524.

80. Goh YH, Lim KA. Modified maxillomandibular advancement for the treatment of obstructive sleep apnea: A preliminary report. *Laryngoscope.* 2003;113(9):1577-1582.

81. Li KK, Powell NB, Riley RW, Guilleminault C. Distraction osteogenesis in adult obstructive sleep apnea surgery: A preliminary report. *J Oral Maxillofac Surg.* 2002;60(1):6-10.

82. Powell NB, Riley RW. Facial contouring with outer-table calvarial bone. A 4-year experience. *Arch Otolaryngol Head Neck Surg.* 1989;115(12):1454-1458.

83. Rajala R, Partinen M, Sane T, et al. Obstructive sleep apnoea syndrome in morbidly obese patients. *J Intern Med.* 1991;230(2):125-129.

84. O'Keeffe T, Patterson EJ. Evidence supporting routine polysomnography before bariatric surgery. *Obes Surg.* 2004;14(1):23-26.

85. Frey WC, Pilcher J. Obstructive sleep-related breathing disorders in patients evaluated for bariatric surgery. *Obes Surg.* 2003;13(5):676-683.

86. Malhotra A, White DP. Obstructive sleep apnoea. *Lancet.* 2002;360(9328):237-245.

87. Strobel RJ, Rosen RC. Obesity and weight loss in obstructive sleep apnea: A critical review. *Sleep.* 1996;19(2):104-115.

88. MacLean LD, Rhode BM, Sampalis J, Forse RA. Results of the surgical treatment of obesity. *Am J Surg.* 1993;165(1):155-160:discussion 160–162.

89. Maggard MA, Shugarman LR, Suttorp M, et al. Meta-analysis: Surgical treatment of obesity. *Ann Intern Med.* 2005;142(7):547-559.

90. Kushner RF. Obesity management. In: Friedman M, ed. *Snoring and Sleep Apnea: Surgical and Non-Surgical Therapy.* Philadelphia, PA: WB Saunders; 2009.

91. Fee WE, Ward PH. Permanent tracheostomy: A new surgical technique. *Ann Otol Rhinol Laryngol.* 1977;86(5 Pt 1):635-638.

92. Gross ND, Cohen JI, Andersen PE, Wax MK. Defatting tracheotomy in morbidly obese patients. *Laryngoscope.* 2002;112(11):1940-1944.

93. Thatcher GW, Maisel RH. The long-term evaluation of tracheostomy in the management of severe obstructive sleep apnea. *Laryngoscope.* 2003;113(2):201-204.

94. Haapaniemi JJ, Laurikainen EA, Halme P, Antila J. Long-term results of tracheostomy for severe obstructive sleep apnea syndrome. *ORL J Otorhinolaryngol Relat Spec.* 2001;63(3):131-136.

95. Partinen M, Jamieson A, Guilleminault C. Long-term outcome for obstructive sleep apnea syndrome patients. Mortality. *Chest.* 1988;94(6):1200-1204.

96. Boot H, van Wegen R, Poublon RM, et al. Long-term results of uvulopalatopharyngoplasty for obstructive sleep apnea syndrome. *Laryngoscope.* 2000;110(3 Pt 1):469-475.

97. Walker-Engström M-L, Tegelberg A, Wilhelmsson B, Ringqvist I. 4-year follow-up of treatment with dental appliance or uvulopalatopharyngoplasty in patients with obstructive sleep apnea: A randomized study. *Chest.* 2002;121(3):739-746.

98. Levin BC, Becker GD. Uvulopalatopharyngoplasty for snoring: Long-term results. *Laryngoscope.* 1994;104(9):1150-1152.

Chapter 18

Oral Appliances in Snoring and Sleep Apnea Syndrome

ALVIN G. WEE

Although the use of continuous positive airway pressure (CPAP) devices is the recommended treatment option for patients with obstructive sleep apnea (OSA), compliance may be a concern for some patients. Patients' compliance with the CPAP device is regarded as their willingness to use the CPAP device at home for at least 1 week.[1] Compliance for patients' use of CPAP devices is defined as using it more than 4 hours per night and for more than 70% of the time assessed. This initial assessment of compliance is important, as it has been shown that patients who have been adherent during the initial 3 months are more likely to continue using the CPAP device.[2,3] Studies have shown that noncompliance of the use of the CPAP device can range initially from 5% to 50%. Approximately 12% to 25% of the remaining patients will stop using the device in 3 years.[1,4,5] Fortunately, when physicians have an appropriate follow-up visit to try to solve problems and concerns of the CPAP devices for their patients, the compliance can increase significantly to a range of 40% to 80%.[2,6-11]

For patients with enough teeth to retain an oral appliance (OA), the device is a simple, noninvasive method for the treatment of snoring and OSA.[12-15] The American Academy of Sleep Medicine recognized the use of an OA as a medical device for the management of snoring and OSA.[1,2] The OA is recognized as an option for patients with mild to moderate OSA and is also an acceptable therapy for patients with severe OSA who are unable to tolerate CPAP devices, have failed surgeries, or are snoring without apnea. The OA is also very useful for patients when they travel to remote areas where the use of a CPAP device is impractical or impossible. Unfortunately, a clinical limitation of OA therapy is the time it requires to achieve the desired therapeutic effects.

How OA therapy conceptually works is by moving the mandible forward, bringing the tongue forward so as to improve upper airway patency, especially in the oropharyngeal area. When the mandible moves forward, the palatopharyngeal and palatoglossal arches are mechanically stretched, increasing in the cross-sectional area of the velopharynx. At the same time, the oropharynx increases in the lateral dimension.[12,13] For patients who are *snoring*, the objective is to decrease the vibration of the oropharyngeal structures during mouth breathing while sleeping.

For individuals who do not have enough teeth or who are without teeth (i.e., edentulous), the use of an OA is not possible because the presence of 8 to 10 teeth in each arch is necessary for retention and stability of the OA. The use of a tongue stabilizing device (e.g., the aveoTSD) that suctions the tongue to produce more airway patency in the retroglossal region is recommended. The aveoTSD is recommended when patients do not have sufficient teeth on both arches to retain the OA.

Success with use of either CPAP or OA is defined as the individual having an apnea-hypopnea index (AHI) below a certain number of events per hour after treatment. As detailed in Table 18-1, the percentage of success with use of an OA for patients with mild to moderate OSA varies from 19% to 36% if the standard for success is an AHI below 5. The percentage of success increases to 47% to 70% if the standard of success is increased to AHI less than 10.[16-20]

Therapeutic efficacy refers to the impact of treatment on the AHI, sleep-related signs during sleep, and also related symptoms during the day. Treatment acceptability encompasses issues related to side effects, ease of use, cost impact on others (e.g., spouse), and compliance. To be a viable treatment option for sleep-related breathing disorders for the majority of patients, the treatment has to be both efficacious and acceptable (seen in the top right portion of Fig. 18-1 where the OA is positioned[20a]). Surgical therapies are positioned in the high efficacy and lower acceptability region, and the more conservative approaches (weight loss, positional therapy, and pharmacologic treatment) are positioned in the lower efficacy and high acceptability regions.

DENTAL EVALUATION AND PROGNOSIS

Because snoring and OSA are medical conditions, dentists have to collaborate with their physician colleagues in how they assess and treat their patients for these conditions. The American Academy of Sleep Medicine and the American Academy of Dental Sleep Medicine[21] have similar recommendations in terms of how the OA should assist with the management of snoring and OSA.

There are two scenarios in which dental practitioners can participate in the treatment of patients with either snoring or OSA with the use of an OA. Figure 18-2 diagrammatically illustrates the sequence and relationship of sleep-related breathing disorder screening and treatment protocol for OA therapy. First, they conduct screening as a primary care provider for their dental patients. Patients who have indicators for snoring or OSA may not realize the treatment potential of an OA to eliminate this condition. Educating these patients on the services dentists can provide to help them with their condition will be valuable. For dentists who have patients with undiagnosed sleep apnea, the dental providers can conduct valuable screening. In the United States, it is estimated that the prevalence of OSA is approximately 3.9% to 4% for males

TABLE 18-1

Clinical Outcomes with Oral Appliance (OA) Use and Continuous Positive Airway Pressure (CPAP) in Randomized Controlled Trials

N	Treatment	Mean (± SD) AHI or RDI		Percent Success		Study*
		Before	After	AHI <5	AHI <10	
20	CPAP	24 (± 17)	4 (± 2.2)	—	70%	Ferguson et al[45]
	OA	25 (± 15)	14 (± 15)	—	55%	
48	CPAP	31 (± 26)	8 (± 6)	34%	66%	Engelman et al[18]
	OA	31 (± 26)	15 (± 16)	19%	47%	
73	OA	27 (± 2)	12 (± 2)	36%		Gotsopoulos et al[17]
	Control	27 (± 2)	25 (± 2)			
80	CPAP	21 (± 1.3)	4.8 (± 0.5)	—	49%	Barnes et al[16]
	OA	21 (± 1.3)	14 (± 1.1)			
	Control	21 (± 1.3)	20 (± 1.1)			
101	CPAP	24 (± 1.9)	2.8 (± 2.5)			Lam et al[46]
	OA	21 (± 1.7)	11 (± 1.7)			
	Control	19 (± 1.9)	21 (± 2.5)			

AHI, apnea-hypopnea index; *RDI*, respiratory disturbance index.
*Studies in this table are listed in the references at the end of the chapter and are cited in the chapter text where appropriate.

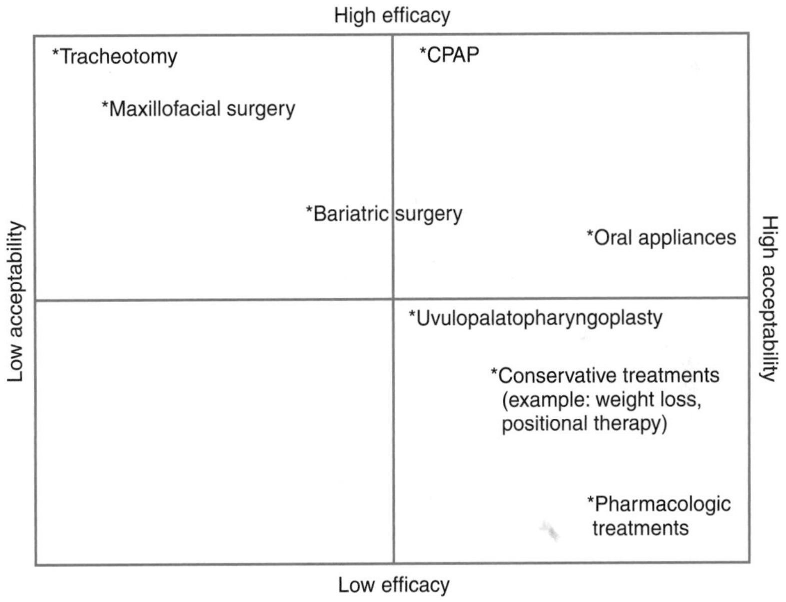

Figure 18-1 A matrix of efficacy and acceptability of various treatment options for obstructive sleep apnea. (Adapted from Cistulli PA, Grunstein RR. Medical devices for the diagnosis and treatment of obstructive sleep apnea. *Expert Rev Med Devices.* 2005;2(6):749-763.)

and 1.2% to 2% for females.[22,23] Furthermore, it is estimated that 93% of women and 82% of men with moderate to severe OSA have not been clinically diagnosed.[24]

As shown in Figure 18-2, routine screening of new patients for OSA begins by evaluating their medical risk factors, and intraoral risk factors, as detailed in Table 18-2,[24a] and by using instruments such as the Epworth Sleepiness Scale[25] and Berlin Questionnaire.[26] A discussion with the patients should follow, focusing on possible problems and how health care professionals could help alleviate the condition. If patients feel amenable to a referral to a sleep physician for a more detailed evaluation of any possible sleep-related breathing disorder, this next evaluation is then carried out. The reader can find more information in other chapters of this book about diagnosing sleep-related breathing disorders and about the Epworth Sleepiness Scale.

Berlin Questionnaire[26] has been shown to be useful as a screening tool in predicting patients that are at high risk of OSA (with a respiratory disturbance index [RDI] of higher than 5). This instrument has been shown to have sensitivity (true positive results) of 0.86, specificity (true negative results) of 0.77, and a positive predictive value (proportion of patients with positive test results who are correctly diagnosed) of 0.89.[26] The instrument has a Cronbach correlation (internal consistency) between 0.86 and 0.92.[26] The questionnaire consists of a total of 10 questions divided into three categories. These questions are related to the risk of having sleep apnea. If two of the three categories are positive, the patient is considered high risk for sleep apnea.

Bed Partner Questionnaire[27] has no psychometric properties evaluating its repeatability or reliability and only acts as a guide for the patient's bed partner to note signs during sleep

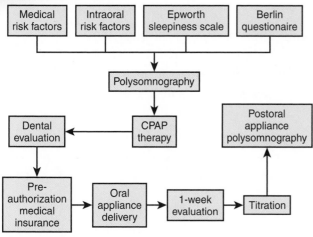

Figure 18-2 Sleep-related breathing disorder screening and treatment protocol for oral appliance therapy.

TABLE 18-2

Possible Risk Factors for Obstructive Sleep Apnea or Snoring

Extraoral/Intraoral Risk Factor

Anatomy	Sign	Possible Indication
Lips	Incompetent lip seal	Patient is possible mouth breather and likely to be a snorer
Tongue	Scalloped tongue borders	Correlation with increased risk for obstructive sleep apnea[47]
	Large tongue	Potential for occurrence of airway obstruction
	Obstructs view of airway as indicated by Mallampati score[48]	Mallampati score of II or above associated with increasing odds of having obstructive sleep apnea[28]
Uvula	Large, swollen or elongated	Potential for snorer status or occurrence of airway obstruction
Oral pharynx	Narrow airway Large tonsils as indicated by grading of tonsil size[29]	Potential for occurrence of airway obstruction

References cited in this table are listed at the end of the chapter and are cited in the chapter text where appropriate.
From Attanasio R, Bailey DR. Evaluation by the dentist. In: Attanasio R, Bailey DR, eds. *Dental Management of Sleep Disorders.* Ames, IA: Wiley-Blackwell; 2010.

of the patient. The questionnaire inquires about the relationship of the bed partner to the patient and how often have they observed the patient's sleep. Checklists of signs are included for the bed partner to mark, as detailed in Box 18-1.

Dentists can also act as a referral from physicians for patients with snoring or who have been diagnosed with OSA and need an OA for their condition. For patients with OSA, dentists should obtain a copy of the sleep study or polysomnographic evaluation from the referring physician. Information obtained from the patient's polysomnography includes the patient's sleep diagnosis, the AHI or RDI, and if the patient has positional OSA. Dentists can then examine these patients

BOX 18-1 *Bed Partner Questionnaire for Noting Signs During Patient's Sleep*

☐ Light snoring
☐ Loud snoring
☐ Occasional loud snorts
☐ Choking
☐ Pauses in breathing
☐ Limb movement every 10 to 20 seconds
☐ Awakening with pain
☐ Leg or arm twitching
☐ Leg kicking
☐ Shaking or rocking
☐ Becoming very rigid
☐ Teeth grinding
☐ Sitting up in bed
☐ Head rocking, head banging
☐ Sleepwalking
☐ Bedwetting
☐ Doing an unusual activity

to determine if an OA is an appropriate treatment option and the prognosis of the proposed OA therapy.

CLINICAL EXAMINATION

The clinical examination and information collected can be guided by using the SOAP (Subjective, Objective, Assessment, and Plan) format:

Subjective

- Chief complaint pertinent to the sleep problems
- Family and social history
  - Family situation
  - Work situation
- Medical history
  - Name of primary care physician
- Dental history
  - Name of general dentist
  - See general dentist every 6 months for checkup and cleaning
- Current medications
- History of sleep-related disorder
  - Sleep pattern
    - Hours of sleep per night
    - Sleep on the back or side
  - Signs at night by bed partner (use Bed Partner Questionnaire[27] as a guide)
    - Light or loud snoring
    - Occasional loud snorts
    - Choking
    - Pauses in breathing
    - Limb movement, twitching, kicking, or rigidity
    - Teeth grinding
    - Waking up at night, sitting in bed, walking, etc.
  - Symptoms during the day (fill out Epworth Sleepiness Scale[25])
    - Review individual situation on the scale
    - Review total score (<10 is considered normal)

- Referral sequence
  - Initial symptoms ?
  - List the health care professionals in sequence who served as referrals to the dental clinic for this condition
- Sleep study
  A copy of the sleep study
  - Date when conducted
  - Review results
  - Review the AHI of the study
- CPAP device used
  - Concern or problem with the device
  - Patient stopped using the device

Objective

- Extraoral evaluation
  - Any headaches?
  - Any jaw or head and neck muscle pain in the morning or during the day?
  - Tenderness on palpation of muscles?
  - Neck size?
  - Temporomandibular joint evaluation
    - Clicking?
    - Crepitus?
    - History of jaw locking?
- Intraoral evaluation
  - Relationship of dentition
    - Relationship of mandibular midline
    - Vertical overlap (in mm)
    - Horizontal overlap (in mm)
    - Occlusal relationship
  - Range of motion
    - Maximum opening (in mm)
    - Maximum protrusion (in mm)
    - Right excursive (in mm)
    - Left excursive (in mm)
  - Soft tissue and airway
    - Findings of oral cancer evaluation
    - Tongue size: small, moderately large, large
    - Soft palate: short, moderately long, long
    - Uvula: short, moderately long, long
    - Palatopharyngeal area: not crowded, moderately crowded, crowded
    - Mallampati score[28]
    - Grading of tonsil size[29]
  - Detailed dental evaluation
    - Any caries?
    - Occlusal contacts on the anterior or posterior teeth?
    - Wear facets on dentition: none, mild, moderate, severe?
    - Missing teeth?
    - Gingival recession: location and amount
  - Radiograph evaluation
    - Panoramic or cephalometric radiograph

Assessment

The subjective and objective information obtained from the clinical examination process will be used to formulate judgments on three parameters that will influence the prognosis

of the use of OA for the patient's sleep-related breathing disorder:

1. **Therapeutic Effect:** Will advancing the mandible forward provide successful therapeutic effect for the patient's sleep-related breathing disorder? The success of this maneuver will depend on multiple factors, including where the airway obstruction is occurring for the patient and the amount of increased airway patency that is obtained when the patient's mandible is advanced forward. Ideally, the use of imaging to predict this success would be best but is rather cost prohibitive. Use of clinical and radiographic predictors as detailed in Box 18-2 will also help in this clinical decision.
2. **Retention and pedtability:** Can the dentition provide enough retention and stability for the OA to hold the mandible in a forward position for the long term? The remaining dentition should have a good crown-to-root ratio of greater than 1:1 and well-fabricated intra- and extracoronal restorations that will not loosen when the OA adds stress to the restoration tooth junction. The patient should also have regular dental checkups and hygiene appointments that have been maintained. It is important for the dentist to confidently predict that the potential patient will continually and regularly see a dentist to maintain optimal oral health. Patients who do not follow-up with regular dental care and who have periodontal disease might experience teeth movement as a result of using OA in the long term.
3. **Tolerance:** Can the craniomandibular complex tolerate the necessary mandibular advancement so as to provide therapeutic effect for the patient's sleep-related breathing disorder? A patient with greater maximum protrusive capacity will have a lesser problem in this aspect. A minimum of 5 mm of protrusive capacity of the mandible is also required for acceptable results.[12] A patient with temporomandibular disorders may have less ability to tolerate an advanced mandibular position, reducing the prognosis of the OA's therapeutic value.

Plan

Once the clinical examination of the patient is complete, the proposed treatment plan, progress, and follow-up notes are sent to the sleep physician to ensure appropriate communication for this treatment collaboration for the patient's sleep-related breathing disorder. A preauthorization (see Fig. 18-2) is then sent to the patient's medical insurance for approval of the proposed treatment plan.

INSURANCE AND BILLING

Because OSA is a medical condition, the billing for OA therapy for this condition is billed through medical billing, rather than dental billing. The patient has to have a diagnosis of sleep apnea and the appropriate International Classification of Diseases, 9th Revision (ICD-9), codes should be used to ensure that the medical insurance provider will pay for the OA. A letter requesting pre-authorization of the patient's benefits should be sent to the patient's medical insurance provider prior to rendering treatment. In addition to the letter, the following information should also be sent: (1) polysomnogram confirming diagnosis of OSA, (2) sleep medicine physician's office notes confirming the treatment plan, (3) dentist's progress notes from the evaluation visit, and (4) if necessary, a copy of research articles to show support of the use of OA therapy for OSA or a list of them in your letter. Many medical insurance companies may require patients with moderate or severe OSA to try CPAP prior to considering the use of the OA, and an OA may be approved only if the patient cannot tolerate the use of the CPAP.

The 2010 version of the Healthcare Common Procedures Coding System (HCPCS), Medicare's level II coding system for nonphysician services and medical supplies, recommends two codes for OA as durable medical equipment, prosthetics, orthotics, and supplies (DMEPOS) codes and provided for inclusion of the appliances, as well as fitting and adjustment, as detailed in the following section. These codes were originally introduced in 2006.

Medical Codes for Oral Appliance for Sleep Apnea

E0485—Oral device/appliance used to reduce upper airway collapsibility, adjustable or nonadjustable, *prefabricated*, includes fitting and adjustment. An oral appliance is one that is first fabricated (i.e., prefabricated) in a certain size, then fitted into the patient's mouth. This prefabricated oral appliance can be purchased either off the shelf or from in a commercial laboratory. The oral appliance is then adjusted in the dental office to fit the patient's mouth, probably by relining with a particular type of dental material.

E0486—Oral device/appliance used to reduce upper airway collapsibility, adjustable or nonadjustable, *custom fabricated*, includes fitting and adjustment. A custom fabricated appliance is built to fit the patient's mouth. The dentist takes impressions of the patient's teeth and subsequently creates a bite record. The upper and lower models are mounted on an articulator and sent to the dental laboratory for the OA to be fabricated around the patient's existing oral structures (i.e., custom fabricated).

In the United States, for patients who require services related to OA for the treatment of sleep apnea to be paid by Medicare, the dentist has to enroll in the Medicare program. It is also necessary to be a participant in the Medicare Participating Physician or Supplier agreement. The dentist who applies to be in the Medicare program should submit a participation agreement to be a supplier at the same time. The procedure is detailed as follows:

1. The application enrollment form (CMS-855S) and its supporting documents are sent to the National Supplier Clearinghouse. Together with this application, submit a "Medicare Participating Physician or Supplier Agreement" (Form CMS-460).
2. National Supplier Clearinghouse reviews the application and conducts a site visit to verify compliance with all DMEPOS supplier standards.
3. After the review, National Supplier Clearinghouse notifies the applicant in writing about the enrollment decision.

Medicare claims related to fitting, initial/subsequent adjustments, and repairs of an oral device should be submitted to the appropriate Durable Medical Administrative Contractor and not as Evaluation and Management services. In addition, all services contained in the codes and payable only by the Durable Medical Administrative Contractor need to include initial patient evaluation, required imaging, all impressions, all model preparation, all fitting adjustments, and any post-fabrication adjustments.

Unfortunately, most dental insurance providers might not cover an OA for snoring. It is still encouraged to preauthorize this procedure prior to fabrication of this appliance for patients.

Dental Code for Oral Appliance for Snoring

CDT Code 5899—Unspecified, removable prosthodontic procedure by report

Preauthorization is usually obtained between 2 and 4 weeks, and then the clinical procedure to fabricate the OA should be carried out.

CLINICAL PROCEDURES FOR FABRICATION OF ORAL APPLIANCES

Before the appliance is fabricated, the patient should be informed orally and in writing of the possible health effects of sleep-related breathing disorders. The document should state whether the OA therapy is for snoring or OSA, list known side effects and possible complications of OA therapy, and note the alternative treatments for sleep-related breathing disorders. The form is signed by the patient. The patient is given a copy, and a copy is then placed in the patient's clinic record.

Once the patient is ready to proceed to fabricate an OA, good upper and lower impressions are made and poured in dental stone. A protrusive record made at approximately 60% of the maximum protrusive position is recommended, although others have recommended an estimate of 5 mm advancement.[12] Use of a George Gauge (Fig. 18-3) is recommended and convenient for this procedure. The George Gauge consists of the body and bite fork. The body has to be cold sterilized after each use, and the bite fork is disposable after

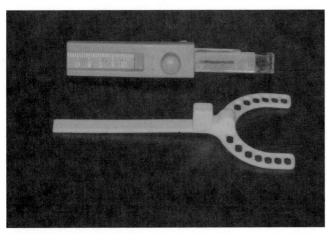

Figure 18-3 George Gauge has two components: the body with the millimeter ruler and the white 5-mm bite fork.

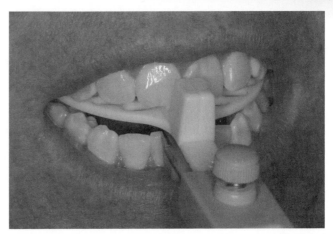

Figure 18-4 George Gauge record in the patient's mouth at established position.

each patient use. The bite fork comes in either 2- or 5-mm incisal thickness. It is recommended that the 2-mm bite fork is used when the patient has a normal occlusion. The 5-mm bite fork is used only if the patient has a deep vertical overbite or excessive anteroposterior occlusal curve. The incisal opening (either 2 or 5 mm) does not affect treatment efficacy of the OA, but an increase in vertical dimension (i.e., increasing the distance between the patient's teeth by using the 5-mm bite fork) will have an impact on patient acceptance.[30] The greater the vertical dimension, the more likely the patient will have jaw discomfort with the use of an OA.

With the George Gauge in place, the patient is asked to totally retrude the lower jaw position and a reading is made on the millimeter ruler on the body of the George Gauge. The patient is then asked to protrude the lower jaw to maximum allowable position with the George Gauge in place, and again a reading is made on the millimeter ruler on the body of the George Gauge. The distance between the most retruded position and the maximum protruded position is then calculated. The George Gauge is then set at 60% of the calculated distance.

With the George Gauge record set at the initial 60% calculated distance, it is then placed in the patient's mouth (Fig. 18-4). This final George Gauge position is then refined through clinical judgment, taking into account the following factors: (1) symptoms of discomfort; (2) ability of the patient to breathe through the nose; (3) inability to elicit snoring or "snorting" by the patient, (4) severity of patient's AHI scores, and (5) any temporomandibular joint symptoms. Once the position is finalized and the patient's skeletal midlines are aligned, the screw of the George Gauge is secured to lock the position. The protrusive jaw with the George Gauge is then formed with fast-setting vinyl polysiloxane impression material to record the position.

SELECTING AN ORAL APPLIANCE

The premise of OA therapy is based on using the upper and lower teeth to move the lower jaw forward. Thus, the most current OA is designed for individuals with teeth. There are many current OAs available today. The U.S. Food and Drug Administration (FDA) regards the OA as a class II medical device.[31] A list of current FDA-approved OAs for snoring and sleep apnea are listed in Appendix 18-1. There are basically

two types of appliance categories. Initially, in the 1980s, the OA was one piece connecting the maxillary and mandibular acrylic components. These one-piece OAs were not titratable and were fixed in position. They do not allow any mandibular movement once the OAs were delivered to the patients. These types of appliances did not allow any teeth movement (e.g., bruxism) when the OA was in place. If the position of the mandible was not in the ideal position or had to be changed, either the OA had to be remade, or the two components had to be separated and reconnected at a different position.

Most appliances developed after the 1990s have two separate maxillary and mandibular acrylic components that are connected in a unique way, according to the various manufacturers (see Appendix 18-1). These OAs allow for some lateral movements (e.g., bruxism) and incremental anteroposterior adjustments or titration for the dentist or patient to change the relationship between maxillary and mandibular arches. This balances both the therapeutic effect and the patient's comfort. An example of an OA that is titratable for sleep apnea is the Thornton Adjustable Positioners (TAP) III shown in Figures 18-5 and 18-6. Another example of a titratable OA is the Klearway (Figs. 18-7 and 18-8).

The titration appliances can be further subdivided into ones for OSA in which the titration is more refined up to 0.25 mm per titration and the ones for snoring in which the titration is grosser in 1- or 2-mm increments. Changing the length of either plastic bands or rubber bands usually provides the titration for the snoring appliances. An example for a snoring type OA is the Silent Night, as shown in Figures 18-9 and 18-10. The appliances are also generally less expensive and less robust compared to the OA for OSA.

For patients who are edentulous (without teeth), the use of an OA for mandibular advancement is not possible. The aveoTSD[28] can be used for edentulous patients. It is internationally marketed to be used for OSA and snoring, but in the United States it only has FDA approval for snoring. The aveoTSD (Fig. 18-11) has a professional fitting kit (Fig. 18-12) that includes one small, one medium, and one large aveoTSD, as well as one 4-mm and 7-mm clip-on Uni-Spacer for extra titration (i.e., increase tongue protrusion). This kit is used to determine the aveoTSD size for the patient prior to ordering the exact aveoTSD. The fitting kit can be sterilized between patients using autoclave sterilization.

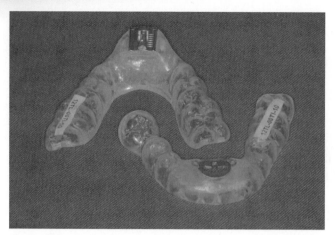

Figure 18-5 Tap III oral appliance – upper and lower appliance outside the mouth.

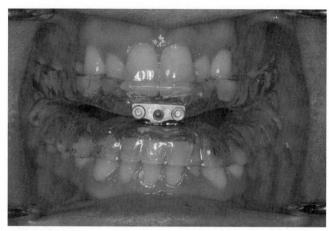

Figure 18-6 Tap III oral appliance: upper and lower appliance engaged in the mouth.

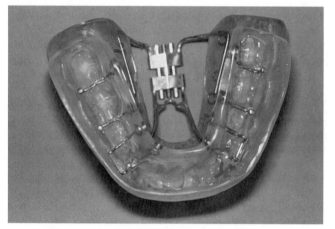

Figure 18-7 Klearway Oral Appliance outside the mouth.

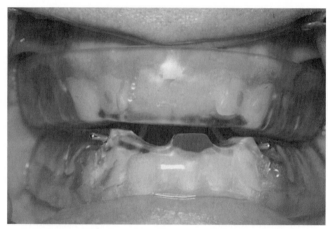

Figure 18-8 Klearway Oral Appliance engaged in the mouth.

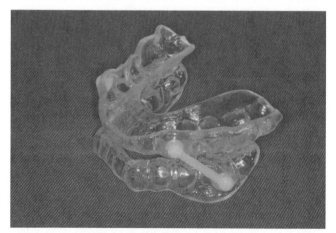

Figure 18-9 Silent Nite snoring appliance.

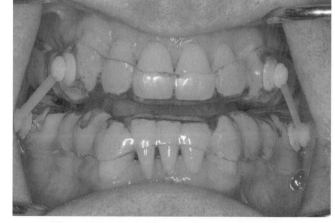

Figure 18-10 Silent Nite oral appliance used by a patient.

This was developed, recognizing the importance of keeping the tongue from blocking the airway to prevent snoring or obstructive sleep apnea. The aveoTSD is intended to stabilize and maintain the tongue in a forward position during sleep so the tongue will not collapse into the airway against the posterior pharyngeal wall. The aveoTSD has been clinically proved to treat mild and moderate OSA.[32,33] The aveoTSD can be used for edentulous patients, patients with orthodontic braces, and patients with less than 8 to 10 teeth in one arch. The aveoTSD is not related but has only historical linkages to the tongue retaining device that was developed in the 1980s.[34,35] Another possible solution for edentulous patients is to duplicate the patient's dentures and attempt to hold the lower jaw forward without causing instability of

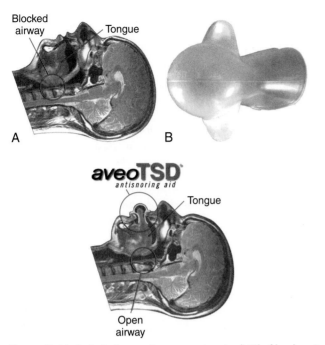

Figure 18-11 A, Sagittal magnetic resonance imaging (MRI) of head: supine position demonstrating blocked airway from the base of tongue impinging against the pharyngeal airway. **B,** Sample of an aveoTSD. **C,** Sagittal MRI of head: supine position demonstrating an upended airway from the use of the aveoTSD to maintain an advanced position of the tongue.

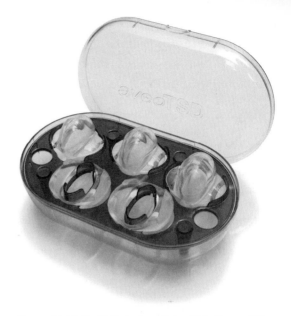

Figure 18-12 Health Professional Fitting Kit for the aveoTSD.

the duplicated denture. If the edentulous arch has a reduced alveolar ridge height, which reduces the stability of the denture, then placement of several osseointegrated dental implants (i.e., three or more) to improve retention and stability of the duplicated denture is recommended to assist in mandibular advancement.

DELIVERY AND RECALL

For the *delivery* appointment of the OA, examine the OA from the laboratory to ensure it is in good condition and without damage. With the patient in the dental chair, place the appliance in the patient's mouth and evaluate the fit and stability. Adjustments to the intaglio (teeth contacting portion of the appliance) of the OA might have to be made with an acrylic bur until the OA can be fitted comfortably in the patient's mouth. Ensure that the patient can put it in and take it out of the mouth without any difficulty.

If the OA has two components (i.e., an upper and lower component), ensure that the patient can connect the two components together either inside or outside the mouth. Adjustments might need to be done to the OA to ensure that this connection occurs. Oral and written instructions on how to take proper care of the OA are provided to the patient. The patient is also informed of possible complications that could occur with the use of the OA and to note the details of these complications. In addition to a list detailed in Table 18-3, there is a possibility of excess salivation and difficulty in swallowing with the OA. It is recommended not to wear the OA if there is any pain. The patient should note any daytime sleepiness and ask his or her bed partner to complete the Bed Partner Questionnaire[27] to evaluate signs of sleep-related breathing disorder at night.

The patient is scheduled for an initial follow-up in a week to address any concerns or symptoms following a list of categories as detailed in Table 18-3. At every dental visit after delivery of the OA, the dentist should evaluate the patient, following the list of categories. This ensures a full and comprehensive examination of the patient using the OA. Once the patient is adherent and comfortable in wearing the OA, initiation of titration can be recommended.

TITRATION

The OA should be titrated to achieve effective therapeutic results based on resolution of the patient's subjective symptoms during the day. Also considered is the patient's bed partner's report of the patient's signs of sleep-related breathing disorder at night. Using a portable monitor for objective data would be ideal.[36,37] Signs while the patient is sleeping (e.g., snoring or apnea) can be reported by the bed partner either orally or by completing the Bed Partner Questionnaire.[27] Asking the patient to utilize the Epworth Sleepiness Scale[25] at the clinical visit can also determine sleepiness during the day. There are two conceptual methods to carry out titration for OSA. The first method uses from 60% to 70% maximum protrusion position and forward titration of the OA to reach the therapeutic effective position. Second, a more recent method is to use a single night titration by polysomnography to determine the therapeutic effective position.[38,39]

The forward titration of the mandible for the patient is balanced between obtaining a therapeutic effective position (Fig. 18-13) and trying not to surpass the patient's maximum discomfort-free position. This is very dependent upon the patient's therapeutic effective position (see Fig. 18-13). Unfortunately, without an actual polysomnogram with the OA in place, it will be difficult to know where the patient's therapeutic effective position is. The clinician can only predict where the patient's therapeutic effective position is by the clinical examination and use of clinical and radiographic predictors (see Box 18-2).

TABLE 18-3

Follow-Up Evaluation after Initiation of Oral Appliance (OA) Use

Categories	Parameters	Results	Possible Actions
Nighttime signs of sleep breathing disorder*	Bed Partner Questionnaire[27]	↓ signs ↑ signs	Titration in the appropriate direction More titration needed
Daytime symptoms*	Epworth Sleepiness Scale[25]	↑ score ↓ score	More titration needed Titration in the appropriate direction
Symptoms of OA use*	Sensitivity of teeth Discomfort of craniofacial muscles Discomfort of the temporomandibular joint	↑ ↑ ↑	Titration of the OA is beyond patient's maximum discomfort-free position (see Fig. 18-13)
Weight compared with previous visit	Estimated or weight on scale	↑ weight ↓ weight	OSA might be worse OSA might improve
Adherence to OA use	How many sessions a week do you use the OA? For each session used, how long is the OA used?	<100% < All night	Counsel and adjustments as necessary
Fit of OA	Retention of OA? Too loose or too tight? Stability of OA?	Uncomfortable Not stable	Adjustments as necessary Adjustments as necessary
Intraoral examination	Any pathology due to use of OA? Occlusion different from baseline?	Pathology observed Occlusion has changed	Adjustments to OA as necessary Ensure patient is wearing the AM Aligner (see Fig. 18-16); adjustments might be necessary Orthodontic consultation
OA	Structural integrity of the OA compromised	Crack or fracture observed	Repair or adjustments if necessary

*Categories relevant to adjustment of titration for the OA.
References cited in this table are listed at the end of the chapter and are cited in the chapter text where appropriate.

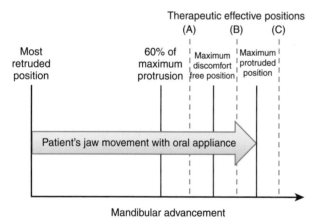

Figure 18-13 Diagram of mandibular titration.

As shown in Figure 18-13, the dentist starts the patient on the OA at approximately "60% Maximum Protrusion" position. The patient can advance the mandible forward until it reaches the "Maximum Discomfort-Free Position," which is before the "Maximum Protruded Position" is reached. If the therapeutic effective position is at A, then the use of an OA for the patient would not result in difficulty reaching this position. If the therapeutic effective position is at B, this will be beyond what the patient can tolerate, and then the patient will have symptoms of discomfort or pain from using the OA, as it has passed the "Maximum Discomfort-Free Position." The patient then must deactivate the OA to move the mandible backward to a position not causing discomfort or pain. The patient, through time, tries to regain mandibular advancement to beyond the therapeutic effective position. If the patient's therapeutic effective position is at C, the use of the OA will not be effective in helping the patient with the sleep-related breathing disorder as the

mandible cannot be advanced beyond the maximum protruded position.

Incremental advancement of the titratable OA in steps of 0.5 to 1.0 mm every week is usually recommended for patients.[40] As mentioned earlier, there are two conceptual ways to titrate the OA to the therapeutic effective position. First, self-titration by the patient to the patient's "maximum discomfort-free position." The second method is to determine that patient's therapeutic effective position by subjective data from a single night polysomnogram with the OA in place.[38,39] The use of a single night polysomnogram is attractive as it is rapid and the therapeutic effective position has been estimated with reference to the patient's maximum discomfort-free position. Unfortunately, the additional cost and the burden to the patient of the additional polysomnogram are sometimes needed. A recent study that combined both titration strategies mentioned earlier by first self-titration of the OA until symptom resolution followed by additional titration as needed during the polysomnogram.[41] The study showed that of the 49 subjects who participated in the study, 34 (69%) achieved successful treatment of the OSA with OA. Of these patients who were successful in treatment of their OSA with OA, 27 subjects (79%) were treated successfully at the self-titration stage. Seven of the 22 subjects (32%) who did not achieve successful OA self-titration were successful with a follow-up titration with a polysomnogram. Thus, a combination of the two methods might be ideal.

Once optimal therapeutic effective position is reached through titration[36,37] of the OA, the dentist then refers the patient back to his or her physician for evaluation of the use of OA for the patient's sleep-related breathing disorder, especially if the patient is diagnosed with moderate to severe OSA.[21] After OA titration polysomnography is recommended for these patients (see Fig. 18-2). For the patient being treated for snoring with OA, no follow-up physician visit is necessary. It is recommended the patient should be seen for follow-up at

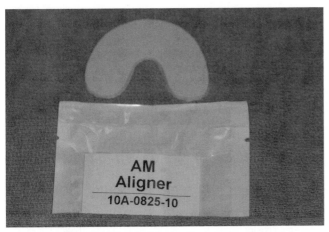

Figure 18-14 AM Aligner by Airway Management.

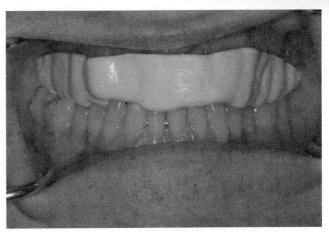

Figure 18-16 AM Aligner fitted in the patient's mouth.

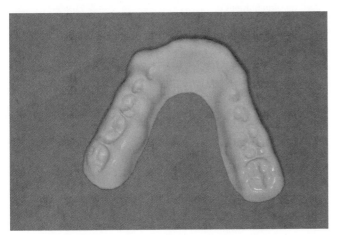

Figure 18-15 AM Aligner outside patient's mouth after fitting.

6 months after successful titration of the OA and then yearly after that appointment to assess the recommended categories again as detailed in Table 18-3.

POSSIBLE COMPLICATIONS AND SOLUTIONS

Initial transient side effects of the use of OA include excessive salivation and difficulty in swallowing with the OA in the patient's mouth. If dry mouth is a concern because the patient might be breathing through his or her mouth, the use of a humidifier is highly recommended. The dentist should also evaluate all the proposed evaluation categories as detailed in Table 18-3. In addition, regular follow-up appointments with the dentist are necessary as long-term adherence to the OA must be monitored and possible complications circumvented. The median use over the first year

of treatment is about 77% of nights.[12] Long-term adherence (76%)[42] seems to be acceptable with patients not using the OA because of side effects, wear and tear of the appliance, and reduction of the efficacy of the OA because of either snoring or daytime alertness.

Long-term complications include teeth becoming loose from the force on teeth or because the patient might have periodontal disease. The dentist has to be aware of the possibility of intra- or extracoronal restorations becoming loose from the nightly force on the teeth/restorations. There are reports of short-term and long-term bite changes from using OA. One study reported that in 70 patients who were compared visually by five orthodontists, 14.3% had no occlusal changes, 41.4% had favorable changes, and 44.3% had unfavorable changes.[43] The average time the OA in this cohort was used is 7.4 ± 2.2 years. Patients with deep bites have the smallest occlusal change for the use of OA and from devices that may reduce the force on the anterior teeth.[43, 44]

With the use of the TAP III OA device, the AM Aligner is recommended for patients using their OA. The AM Aligner from the package (Fig. 18-14) is taken out and placed in a water bath at 165° F. The plasticized AM Aligner is then placed in the patient's mouth and adapted to the upper dentition. The patient is also asked to bite down to indent into the material. Continuously adapting the material onto the upper dentition with the patient biting down until the material hardens is necessary. The hardened material is then taken out of the patient's mouth, trimmed, and made smoother (Fig. 18-15). It is then placed back in the patient's mouth (Fig. 18-16) to ensure the patient can put it in and take it out without any problems or symptoms of discomfort. Although this method has no scientific evidence in terms of stabilizing the dentition over the long term, it seems empirically promising.

APPENDIX 18-I

Current FDA-Approved Snoring and Sleep Apnea Oral Appliances*

Name of Oral Appliance	Manufacturer	Approval Date
APPROVED FOR SNORING		
Adjustable PM Positioner	Jonathan A. Parker, DDS	2/8/96
DESRA	D.S.R.A. Inc	6/15/95
Elastomeric sleep appliance	Village Park Orthodontics	6/14/95
The Equalizer airway device	Sleep Renewal Inc.	3/4/87
Full breath sleep appliance—anterior bite	Bryan Keropian, DDS	12/30/05
Full breath sleep appliance—lower	Bryan Keropian, DDS	6/24/09
Full breath sleep appliance—posterior bite and posterior bite with bumps	Bryan Keropian, DDS	1/3/06
Full breath sleep appliance with posterior tongue depressor	Bryan Keropian, DDS	5/26/06
IST snoring appliance	Dental Crafters	9/11/09
Nocturnal airway patency appliance	G-Ortho Lab	9/19/90
OSAP	Snorefree Inc.	5/9/96
PM Positioner	Jonathan A. Parker, DDS	9/15/95
Snoar open airway appliance	Kent J. Toone, DDS	5/11/88
SnoreMaster snore remedy	The SnoreMaster Co.	2/10/95
Snore-No-More	Great Lakes Orthodontics Ltd.	2/9/94
Snorenti	James P. Boyd	2/28/05
SnorEx	SnorEx (NZ) Ltd.	12/18/97
APPROVED FOR OBSTRUCTIVE SLEEP APNEA		
Acrylic Herbst splint appliance	Specialty Appliance Works Inc.	1/27/09
Adjustable soft palate lifter	Ortho Publications Inc.	2/9/90
Adjustable TheraSnore	Distar Inc.	11/12/97
AirwayEase mandibular advancement splint	Orthoplant Dental Lab	4/16/10
Anti-snoring device (ASD)	PI Medical	12/18/02
Anti-snoring/sleep apnea device	R.J. and V.K. Bird Pty Ltd.	10/27/04
Anti-snoring/sleep apnea device	Tomed Dr. Toussaint, GMBH	9/8/06
The Breathe EZ anti-snoring device	D&S Redhage	2/19/03
Dental anti-snoring device	Ortho Publications Inc.	10/18/88
Dr. B's Mouthpiece model 32129-10002	Snore-Ezzer	9/2/99
Elastic mandibular advancement appliance	Frantz Design Inc.	9/29/97
Elastic mandibular advancement-titration appliance	Frantz Design Inc.	1/9/98
EndSnor	Dockstader Orthodontic Lab Inc.	6/12/08
Hays & Meade anti-snoring device	Hays & Meade Inc.	4/14/89
Laimad	Steven Lamberg, DDS	12/14/06
Lowe Klearway	Dr. Alan A. Lowe Inc.	5/25/95
The Moses appliance	Allen J. Moses, DDS LTD	5/12/10
MPowrX snoring solution	MPowrX Health and Wellness Products Inc.	10/27/08
NorAD nocturnal oral airway dilator appliance	Dennis R. Bailey, DDS	05/28/01
Nose Breathe mouthpiece for heavy snorer	Steven K. Sue	5/28/02
Nociceptive Trigeminal Inhibition-Tension Suppression System with a Snorehook application	NTI-TSS, Inc.	5/3/05
OASYS Oral/Nasal Airway System	Mark Abramson, DDS, Inc,	8/26/03
O'Brien mandibular positioning appliance	O'Brien Dental Lab, Inc.	6/2/06
Oral sleep disorder aid	Perl-Rad Sleep Disorder Lab	9/22/99
Orthodontic bite	American Orthodontics	3/31/93
PASR/QuietNite	Exact Supplies Ltd.	6/11/10
The Quiet Sleeper	Precision Dental Laboratories Inc.	10/4/01
Removable acrylic Herbst ALLESEE Snore Appliance (ASA) and Enoch Snorinator	Sybron Dental Specialties Inc.	5/25/07
Removable Herbst appliance	University Dental AssociatesDepartment of Orthodontics	3/20/96
Repose bone screw system	Influence Inc.	8/27/99
Respironics custom I oral appliance	Respironics Inc.	2/6/04
Respironics custom II oral appliance		2/6/04
Restful Nights ISTappliance	Ottawa Dental Laboratory	3/15/04
The Silencer	Silent Knights Ventures Inc.	10/30/95
SilentNite	Glidewell Laboratories	9/18/97
Silent Partner Series OSA appliances	DreamWrx Dental Laboratory	8/9/05
Silent Sleep	Craniofacial Pain Center of Idaho	7/16/09
SleepBite	Dental Imagineers Llc.	1/30/02
Sleep Splint	Nakagawa Dental Clinic	5/19/06
Somnofit	Strategic Counsel SARL	12/18/06

APPENDIX 18-I

Current FDA-Approved Snoring and Sleep Apnea Oral Appliances*—cont'd

Name of Oral Appliance	Manufacturer	Approval Date
Somnomed Bflex	Somnomed Inc.	1/30/08
Somnomed MAS RXA	Somnomed Ltd.	7/12/05
Snore-Aid Max	Dental Imagineers LLC	12/10/02
Snore-Aid Plus		7/22/99
Snore-Cure anti-snoring appliance	Ortho-Tain Inc.	6/1/98
Snore-Ezzer	Snore-Ezzer	2/12/98
Snorefree	Scott Feldman, DDS, and Norman Shapiro, DDS	1/4/96
Snoremaster	DDS Inc.	10/2/95
The Snore Peace	The Snore Peace Group	8/24/98
Snore Tec	Marketing Technologies Inc.	4/14/97
Snoring control device	Kenneth Hilsen	1/9/98
Snor-X mouth guard	Snorex Inc.	10/17/95
The SUAD device	Strong Dental Inc.	7/8/03
Thornton adjustable positioner	Nellcor Puritan Bennett Inc.	1/24/97
Thornton adjustable positioner anti-snoring device		9/10/96
Thornton adjustable positioner II anti-snoring and obstructive sleep apnea oral appliance with attachment	Airway Management Inc.	5/17/06
Thornton adjustable positioner III anti-snoring device		12/12/06
Thornton adjustable positioner–titanium		7/12/06
TheraSnore	Dr. Thomas E. Meade	7/8/93
Thornton oral appliance	W. Keith Thornton, DDS	8/21/97
Tongue stabilizer device	University of Otago	12/21/99
Vital sleep	The Snore Reliever Company LLC	1/13/10
Zquiet mouthpiece	Sleeping Well LLC	6/22/10

FDA, U.S. Food and Drug Administration.
*As of July 2010.
U.S.A Food and Drug Administration. 510(k) premarket notification. http://www.accessdata.fda.gov/scripts/cdrh/cfdocs/cfPMN/pmn.cfm.

REFERENCES

1. Engelman HM, Wild MR. Improving CPAP use by patients with the sleep apnea/hypopnea syndrome. *Sleep Med Rev.* 2003;7:81-99.
2. Pepin JL, Krieger J, Rodenstein D, et al. Effective compliance during the first 3 months of continuous positive airway pressure. A european prospective study of 121 patients. *Am J Respir Crit Care Med.* 1999;160(4):1124-1129.
3. Kribbs NB, Pack AI, Kline LR, et al. Objective measurement of patterns of nasal CPAP use by patients with obstructive sleep apnea. *Am Rev Respir Dis.* 1993;147(4):887-895.
4. Dinges DF, Pack F, Williams K, et al. Cumulative sleepiness, mood disturbance, and psychomotor vigilance performance decrements during a week of sleep restricted to 4-5 hours per night. *Sleep.* 1997;20(4):267-277.
5. Stepnowsky Jr CJ, Moore PJ. Nasal CPAP treatment for obstructive sleep apnea: Developing a new perspective on dosing strategies and compliance. *J Psychosom Res.* 2003;54(6):599-605.
6. Massie CA, Hart RW, Peralez K, Richards GN. Effects of humidification on nasal symptoms and compliance in sleep apnea patients using continuous positive airway pressure. *Chest.* 1999;116(2):403-408.
7. Rakotonanahary D, Pelletier-Fleury N, Gagnadoux F, Fleury B. Predictive factors for the need for additional humidification during nasal continuous positive airway pressure therapy. *Chest.* 2001;119(2):460-465.
8. Sin DD, Mayers I, Man GC, Pawluk L. Long-term compliance rates to continuous positive airway pressure in obstructive sleep apnea: A population-based study. *Chest.* 2002;121(2):430-435.
9. Lewis KE, Seale L, Bartle IE, Watkins AJ, Ebden P. Early predictors of CPAP use for the treatment of obstructive sleep apnea. *Sleep.* 2004;27(1):134-138.
10. Stepnowsky Jr CJ, Bardwell WA, Moore PJ, Ancoli-Israel S, Dimsdale JE. Psychologic correlates of compliance with continuous positive airway pressure. *Sleep.* 2002;25(7):758-762.
11. Popescu G, Latham M, Allgar V, Elliott MW. Continuous positive airway pressure for sleep apnoea/hypopnoea syndrome: Usefulness of a 2 week trial to identify factors associated with long term use. *Thorax.* 2001;56(9):727-733.
12. Ferguson KA, Cartwright R, Rogers R, Schmidt-Nowara W. Oral appliances for snoring and obstructive sleep apnea: A review. *Sleep.* 2006;29(2):244-262.
13. Hoekema A, Stegenga B, De Bont LG. Efficacy and co-morbidity of oral appliances in the treatment of obstructive sleep apnea-hypopnea: A systematic review. *Crit Rev Oral Biol Med.* 2004;15(3):137-155.
14. Kushida CA, Morgenthaler TI, Littner MR, et al. Practice parameters for the treatment of snoring and obstructive sleep apnea with oral appliances: An update for 2005. *Sleep.* 2006;29(2):240-243.
15. Lim J, Lasserson TJ, Fleetham J, Wright J. Oral appliances for obstructive sleep apnoea. *Cochrane Database Syst Rev.* 2006;(1)(1):CD004435.
16. Barnes M, McEvoy RD, Banks S, et al. Efficacy of positive airway pressure and oral appliance in mild to moderate obstructive sleep apnea. *Am J Respir Crit Care Med.* 2004;170(6):656-664.
17. Gotsopoulos H, Chen C, Qian J, Cistulli PA. Oral appliance therapy improves symptoms in obstructive sleep apnea: A randomized, controlled trial. *Am J Respir Crit Care Med.* 2002;166(5):743-748.
18. Engleman HM, McDonald JP, Graham D, et al. Randomized crossover trial of two treatments for sleep apnea/hypopnea syndrome: Continuous positive airway pressure and mandibular repositioning splint. *Am J Respir Crit Care Med.* 2002;166(6):855-859.
19. Randerath WJ, Heise M, Hinz R, Ruehle KH. An individually adjustable oral appliance vs continuous positive airway pressure in mild-to-moderate obstructive sleep apnea syndrome. *Chest.* 2002;122(2):569-575.
20. Gauthier L, Laberge L, Beaudry M, Laforte M, Rompre PH, Lavigne GJ. Efficacy of two mandibular advancement appliances in the management of snoring and mild-moderate sleep apnea: A cross-over randomized study. *Sleep Med.* 2009;10(3):329-336.
20a. Cistulli PA, Grunstein RR. Medical devices for the diagnosis and treatment of obstructive sleep apnea. *Expert Rev Med Devices.* 2005;2(6):749-763.
21. American Academy of Dental Sleep Medicine. AADSM treatment protocol: Oral appliance therapy for sleep disordered breathing. www.aadsm.org. Accessed August, 2010.

22. Bixler EO, Vgontzas AN, Lin HM, et al. Prevalence of sleep-disordered breathing in women: Effects of gender. *Am J Respir Crit Care Med.* 2001;163(3 Pt 1):608-613.

23. Young T, Palta M, Dempsey J, Skatrud J, Weber S, Badr S. The occurrence of sleep-disordered breathing among middle-aged adults. *N Engl J Med.* 1993;328(17):1230-1235.

24. Young T, Evans L, Finn L, Palta M. Estimation of the clinically diagnosed proportion of sleep apnea syndrome in middle-aged men and women. *Sleep.* 1997;20(9):705-706.

24a. Attanasio R, Bailey DR. Evaluation by the dentist. In: Attanasio R, Bailey DR, eds. *Dental Management of Sleep Disorders.* Ames, IA: Wiley-Blackwell; 2010.

25. Johns MW. A new method for measuring daytime sleepiness: The epworth sleepiness scale. *Sleep.* 1991;14(6):540-545.

26. Netzer NC, Stoohs RA, Netzer CM, Clark K, Strohl KP. Using the Berlin Questionnaire to identify patients at risk for the sleep apnea syndrome. *Ann Intern Med.* 1999;131(7):485-491.

27. Talk About Sleep Inc. Bed partner questionnaire. www.talkaboutsleep.com. Accessed August, 2010.

28. Ferguson KA, Love LL, Ryan CF. Effect of mandibular and tongue protrusion on upper airway size during wakefulness. *Am J Respir Crit Care Med.* 1997;155(5):1748-1754.

29. Fairbanks DNF, Mickelson SA, Woodson BT. *Snoring and Obstructive Sleep Apnea.* 3rd ed. Philadelphia, PA: Lippincott Williams & Wilkins; 2003.

30. Pitsis AJ, Darendeliler MA, Gotsopoulos H, Petocz P, Cistulli PA. Effect of vertical dimension on efficacy of oral appliance therapy in obstructive sleep apnea. *Am J Respir Crit Care Med.* 2002;166(6):860-864.

31. Center for Device and Radiologic Health. Class II special controls guidance document: Intraoral devices or snoring and/or obstructive sleep apnea; guidance for industry and FDA. U.S. Food and Drug Administration:November 12, 2002.

31a. U.S.A Food and Drug Administration. 510(k) premarket notification. http://www.accessdata.fda.gov/scripts/cdrh/cfdocs/cfPMN/pmn.cfm. Accessed July, 2010.

32. Kingshott RN, Jones DR, Taylor DR, Robertson CJ. The efficacy of a novel tongue-stabilizing device on polysomnographic variables in sleep-disordered breathing: A pilot study. *Sleep Breath.* 2002;6(2):69-76.

33. Deane SA, Cistulli PA, Ng AT, Zeng B, Petocz P, Darendeliler MA. Comparison of mandibular advancement splint and tongue stabilizing device in obstructive sleep apnea: A randomized controlled trial. *Sleep.* 2009;32(5):648-653.

34. Cartwright R, Stefoski D, Caldarelli D, et al. Toward a treatment logic for sleep apnea: The place of the tongue retaining device. *Behav Res Ther.* 1988;26(2):121-126.

35. Cartwright RD. Predicting response to the tongue retaining device for sleep apnea syndrome. *Arch Otolaryngol.* 1985;111(6):385-388.

36. Pancer J, Al-Faifi S, Al-Faifi M, Hoffstein V. Evaluation of variable mandibular advancement appliance for treatment of snoring and sleep apnea. *Chest.* 1999;116(6):1511-1518.

37. Rogers RR. Oral appliance therapy for the management of sleep disordered breathing: An overview. *Sleep Breath.* 2000;4(2):79-84.

38. Raphaelson MA, Alpher EJ, Bakker KW, Perlstrom JR. Oral appliance therapy for obstructive sleep apnea syndrome: Progressive mandibular advancement during polysomnography. *Cranio.* 1998;16(1):44-50.

39. Petelle B, Vincent G, Gagnadoux F, Rakotonanahary D, Meyer B, Fleury B. One-night mandibular advancement titration for obstructive sleep apnea syndrome: A pilot study. *Am J Respir Crit Care Med.* 2002;165(8):1150-1153.

40. Fleury B, Rakotonanahary D, Petelle B, et al. Mandibular advancement titration for obstructive sleep apnea: Optimization of the procedure by combining clinical and oximetric parameters. *Chest.* 2004;125(5):1761-1767.

41. Krishnan V, Collop NA, Scherr SC. An evaluation of a titration strategy for prescription of oral appliances for obstructive sleep apnea. *Chest.* 2008;133(5):1135-1141.

42. Marklund M, Stenlund H, Franklin KA. Mandibular advancement devices in 630 men and women with obstructive sleep apnea and snoring: Tolerability and predictors of treatment success. *Chest.* 2004;125(4):1270-1278.

43. Almeida FR, Lowe AA, Otsuka R, Fastlicht S, Farbood M, Tsuiki S. Long-term sequellae of oral appliance therapy in obstructive sleep apnea patients: Part 2. study-model analysis. *Am J Orthod Dentofacial Orthop.* 2006;129(2):205-213.

44. Marklund M. Predictors of long-term orthodontic side effects from mandibular advancement devices in patients with snoring and obstructive sleep apnea. *Am J Orthod Dentofacial Orthop.* 2006;129(2):214-221.

45. Ferguson KA, Ono T, Lowe AA, al-Majed S, Love LL, Fleetham JA. A short-term controlled trial of an adjustable oral appliance for the treatment of mild to moderate obstructive sleep apnoea. *Thorax.* 1997;52(4):362-368.

46. Lam B, Sam K, Mok WY, et al. Randomised study of three non-surgical treatments in mild to moderate obstructive sleep apnoea. *Thorax.* 2007;62(4):354-359.

47. Weiss TM, Atanasov S, Calhoun KH. The association of tongue scalloping with obstructive sleep apnea and related sleep pathology. *Otolaryngol Head Neck Surg.* 2005;133(6):966-971.

48. Nuckton TJ, Glidden DV, Browner WS, Claman DM. Physical examination: Mallampati score as an independent predictor of obstructive sleep apnea. *Sleep.* 2006;29(7):903-908.

49. Marklund M, Cistulli PA. Oral appliance. In: Lavigne GJ, Cistulli PA, Smith MT, eds. *Sleep Medicine for Dentists.* Hanover Park, IL: Quintessence Books; 2009:77-83.

50. Marklund M, Persson M, Franklin KA. Treatment success with a mandibular advancement device is related to supine-dependent sleep apnea. *Chest.* 1998;114(6):1630-1635.

51. Eveloff SE, Rosenberg CL, Carlisle CC, Millman RP. Efficacy of a herbst mandibular advancement device in obstructive sleep apnea. *Am J Respir Crit Care Med.* 1994;149(4 Pt 1):905-909.

52. Mehta A, Qian J, Petocz P, Darendeliler MA, Cistulli PA. A randomized, controlled study of a mandibular advancement splint for obstructive sleep apnea. *Am J Respir Crit Care Med.* 2001;163(6):1457-1461.

53. Liu Y, Lowe AA, Fleetham JA, Park YC. Cephalometric and physiologic predictors of the efficacy of an adjustable oral appliance for treating obstructive sleep apnea. *Am J Orthod Dentofacial Orthop.* 2001;120(6):639-647.

Central and Mixed Sleep-Related Breathing Disorders

Chapter
19

WINFRIED J. RANDERATH

COMPLEXITY OF SLEEP-RELATED BREATHING DISORDERS

Sleep-related breathing disturbances (SRBD) present in the phenotypes of the obstructive sleep apnea syndrome (OSAS), central sleep apnea, and hypoventilation/hypoxemic syndromes[1] (Fig. 19-1). OSAS is characterized by repetitive obstruction of the upper airways leading to complete cessation or partial reduction of airflow. Predispositions include male gender, obesity, age older than 40 years, and anatomic malformations such as macroglossia, retrognathia, and large

tonsils or adenoids. Obstructive disturbances mostly occur during rapid eye movement (REM) sleep and non-REM (NREM) sleep stages 1 and 2. As a consequence, oxygen saturation decreases and sympathetic activity increases. Futile ventilatory efforts of the diaphragm and the thoracic muscles may result in a paradoxical breathing pattern of the thorax and abdomen. These events are abruptly terminated often associated with an electroencephalographic (EEG) arousal, although the causal relationship between these phenomena is ambiguous. Although most respiratory events are associated with cortical arousal and more severe events result in longer

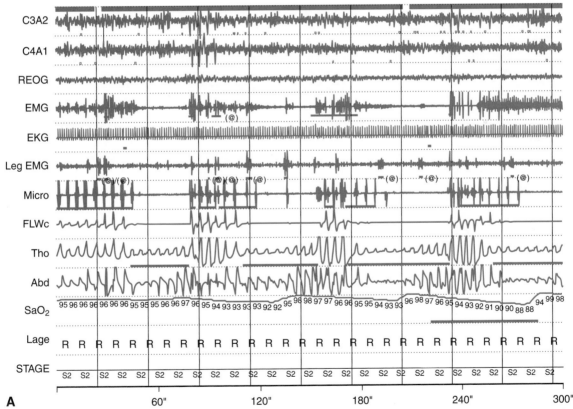

A

Figure 19-1 Polysomnographic patterns of sleep related breathing disorders. A, Obstructive sleep apnea syndrome. The microphone channel presents several events that indicate snoring. Regular inspiratory and expiratory excursions of the airflow are interrupted by cessations, which define apneas. However, thorax and abdomen show continuous ventilatory effort, which is out of phase during airflow cessation. Therefore, these events result from upper airway obstructions. The apneas are accompanied by oxygen desaturations (SpO2) and increases of the amplitude and frequency of the electroencephalogram (EEG) signals, which are called arousals from sleep. The arousals appear simultaneously with reopening of the airways (restart of airflow signals). This figure shows a 5-minute period with the following parameters from top to bottom: *C3/A2, C4A1,* electroencephalogram; *REOG,* electro-oculogram (right side); *EMG,* electromyogram; *EKG,* electrocardiogram; *FLWC,* airflow; *Tho* (thorax), *Abd* (abdomen) effort channels; *SpO2,* oxygen saturation; *Puls,* heart rate; *Micro,* snoring microphone; *Lage,* body position; *Stage,* sleep stage.

Continued

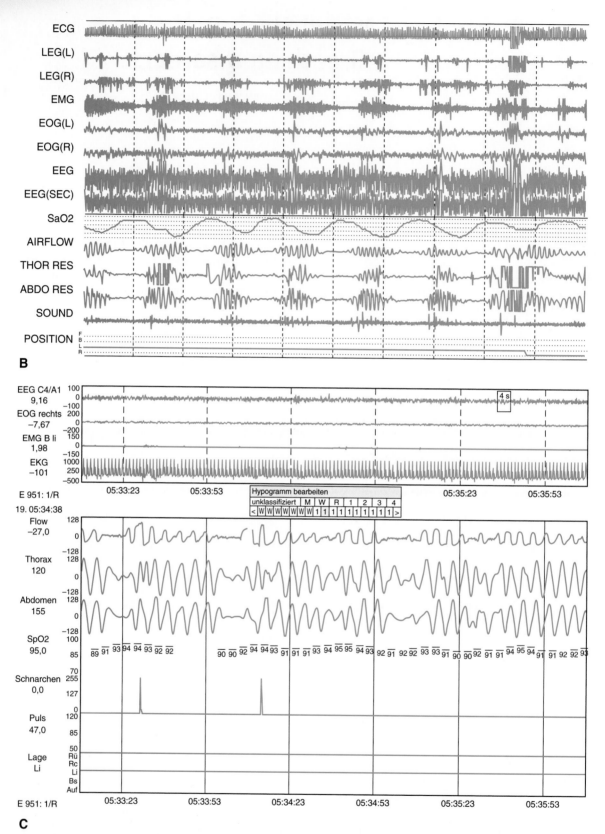

B

C

Figure 19-1, cont'd B, Central sleep apnea. Similar to the obstructive apneas (A) cessations of the airflow (apneas) are accompanied by arousals (EEG) and oxygen desaturations (SaO₂). However, in contrast to obstructive disturbances, activity in the effort channels is missing, which proves absence of ventilatory drive. This figure shows a 5-minute period of a polysomnogram with the following parameters: *ECG,* electrocardiogram; *Leg (L, R),* electromyogram left, right leg; *EMG,* electromyogram chin; *EGG (L, R),* electro-oculogram left, right eye; *EEG,* electroencephalogram; *Tho* (thorax), *Abd* (abdomen) *RES,* effort channels; *SaO₂,* oxygen saturation; sound, snoring microphone. **C,** Atactic breathing in opioid-induced sleep apnea. This figure gives a 3-minute period from a patient suffering from atactic breathing. Amplitude and frequency of inspiration send expiration differ distinctively (see text for definition of atactic breathing). *EEG C4/A1,* electroencephalogram; *EOG rechts,* electro-oculogram (right side); *EMG,* electromyogram; *EKG,* electrocardiogram; *Flow,* airflow; *Tho* (thorax), *Abd* (abdomen) effort channels; *SpO₂,* oxygen saturation; *Puls,* heart rate; *Schnarchen,* snoring; *Lage,* body position.

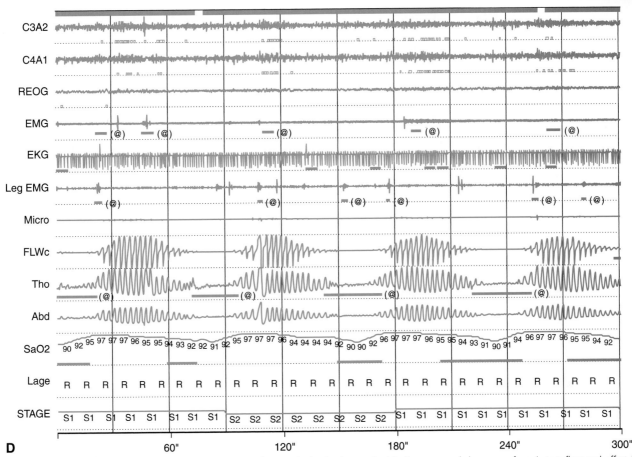

D

Figure 19-1, cont'd D, Cheyne-Stokes respiration. Cheyne-Stokes respiration is characterized by increases and decreases of respiratory flow and effort in a crescendo-decrescendo pattern. This figure shows the typical cycle length between 60 and 90 seconds. Flow, thorax, and abdomen efforts are in-phase, indicating the character of central disturbances. The arousals (EEG channel) take place at the maximum of the respiration in contrast to obstructive disturbances. *C3/A2, C4A1,* electroencephalogram; *REOG,* electro-oculogram (right side); *EMG,* electromyogram; *EKG,* electrocardiogram; *FLWC,* airflow; *Tho* (thorax), *Abd* (abdomen) effort channels; *SpO₂,* oxygen saturation; *Puls,* heart rate; *Micro,* snoring microphone; *Lage,* body position; *Stage,* sleep stage.

arousals, Younes found that inspiratory flow increased in 22% of events before arousal and was restored in 17% without an arousal.[2] In these situations combinations of stimuli, such as CO_2 and negative pressure, can activate upper airway dilator muscles during sleep and delaying of arousals may be beneficial to restore pharyngeal patency. The level of pleural pressure, generated by respiratory effort, seems to be the key trigger for inducing arousal from NREM sleep.[3] Narrowing of the airways during hypopneas and reopening after apneas cause the typical loud and irregular snoring sounds[4-7] (see Fig. 19-1, *A*).

The central sleep apnea (CSA) syndromes are defined by recurrent cessation or limitation of airflow and a simultaneous reduction of the breathing effort.[1] Ventilatory impulses generated by the brainstem are lacking. In contrast to OSAS there is no paradoxical breathing and the upper airways are not necessarily narrowed (see Fig. 19-1, *B*). However, passive or reflexive closure of the pharyngeal airways may occur.[8] The designation CSA syndromes includes primary central sleep apnea, Cheyne-Stokes breathing pattern, CSA due to high-altitude periodic breathing, and CSA due to brainstem lesions or to drugs and other substances. Opioids are the most important drugs associated with central breathing abnormalities including central apneas, periodic breathing, and Biot's breathing (atactic breathing) characterized by irregular respiratory pauses and gasping without periodicity

present during NREM sleep (see Fig. 19-1, *C*).[9-13] Similar to OSAS, the central sleep apnea syndromes can be—but do not necessarily have to be—associated with daytime sleepiness, frequent nocturnal awakenings, and insomnia. Cheyne-Stokes respiration (CSR, periodic breathing) is typically characterized by recurrent apneas and hypopneas and a crescendo-decrescendo pattern of flow and effort. The cycle length averages 60 to 90 seconds in CSR but is shorter in other forms of CSA[14] (see Fig. 19-1, *D*). Cardiovascular disorders, atrial fibrillation, heart failure, and stroke predispose to the development of CSR.[15-20]

Although these criteria may help to discriminate the sleep apnea syndromes, the complexity of sleep-related breathing disorders has come more and more to the forefront in recent years. Both from a pathophysiologic and a clinical point of view a clear separation of the entities is hardly possible:

- The majority of patients suffer from combinations of obstructive and central disturbances.
- It is often difficult to definitely allocate particular respiratory events to one of the groups based on standard polysomnography. This is especially relevant in the identification of hypopneas.
- The pathophysiologic background of obstructive and central disturbances overlaps widely. Therefore, the separation of the disturbances is more or less artificial.

PATHOPHYSIOLOGY OF CENTRAL SLEEP APNEA

Central disturbances appear predominantly during NREM sleep. Although ventilation is primarily regulated by behavioral, nonchemical factors during wakefulness, it is mainly influenced by metabolism during sleep. An increase of the $Paco_2$ stimulates ventilation, whereas ventilation is reduced during hypocapnia. Physiologically, ventilatory drive and minute ventilation are reduced during NREM sleep. The influence of the carbon dioxide 9 (CO_2) level is reduced during REM sleep owing to diminished muscle activity and arousability.[21,22]

Although the pathophysiology of sleep apnea has not as yet been completely elucidated, several crucial aspects can be described (Box 19-1):

- The loop gain of ventilatory response
- The apnea threshold
- The instability of respiratory control systems during sleep

Wellman and associates compared the ventilatory control system to the technical term *loop gain*.[23] Any disturbance of breathing (e.g., stimulation of the ventilation by acoustic arousals, pain, or cortical impulses) influences the actual $Paco_2$ via the lungs and thorax. This change may be described as the plant gain. The changes of the CO_2 level are measured at the feedback gain, which is represented by the chemoreceptors in the biologic system. The perception of these variations can be influenced by a circulatory delay. Thus, cardiovascular disorders influence the reactivity of the ventilatory system. The efferents of the chemoreceptors stimulate the respiratory control system in the brainstem, the controller gain, which urges

the plant gain to change ventilation. The term *loop gain* represents the ratio of ventilatory response to any breathing disturbances. A high loop gain results in a ventilatory overshoot with hyperventilation and hypocapnia leading to apneas and hypocapnia. Owing to the differences in muscle activity and the tendency to arousal, there is less ventilatory overshoot during REM as compared to NREM sleep. Based on these findings central sleep apnea can be characterised as a NREM disorder.[24]

The distance between the prevailing $Paco_2$ and the apnea threshold is another important aspect contributing to the instability of breathing (Fig. 19-2). The *apnea threshold* is defined by the level of the $Paco_2$ below which breathing ceases. During normal breathing the prevailing $Paco_2$ exceeds the apnea threshold. In contrast, an apnea emerges if the apnea threshold is elevated or the actual $Paco_2$ decreases below the threshold. Whenever the prevailing $Paco_2$ lies near the apnea threshold, small variations of the ventilation lead to oscillation of the $Paco_2$ above and below the apnea threshold, resulting in the pattern of periodic breathing. Xie and associates demonstrated a shift of the apnea threshold in patients suffering from central sleep apnea as compared to healthy subjects. They determined the level of the end-tidal CO_2 which was accompanied by a central apnea. Healthy subjects showed an increase of the $Paco_2$ and the apnea threshold during the wake/NREM sleep transition. In contrast, the apnea threshold increased in CSA patients while the prevailing $Paco_2$ did not relevantly change. Consequently, the distance between the $Paco_2$ and the apnea threshold narrowed, predisposing to instability of breathing.[25]

Hyperventilation can also diminish the interspace between the $Paco_2$ and the apnea threshold. Hanley and colleagues demonstrated that the CO_2 levels were chronically reduced in patients with unstable breathing both during wakefulness and during sleep.[26] This chronic hyperventilatory state is based on two important factors: (1) the stimulation of pulmonary irritant receptors and (2) a higher reactivity of the chemoreceptors.

Yu and associates injected hypertonic saline into the lungs of rabbits to stimulate pulmonary tissue receptors. This chemical irritation increased the activity of the ventilatory muscles, indicating an elevation of the central ventilatory drive. Because the reflex activation was abolished by vagotomy, the authors concluded that irritation in the periphery of the lungs was transmitted by vagal afferent nerves.[27] The irritant receptors can be stimulated in humans by inflammatory processes, for example, in pulmonary fibrosis. More commonly, pulmonary congestion in heart failure irritates intrapulmonary

---

BOX 19-1 *Factors Contributing to the Pathophysiology of Central Sleep Apnea*

- Shift of the arousal threshold
- Impairment of peripheral and central chemoreceptors
- Circulatory delay (?)
- Chronic hyperventilation
- Stimulation of pulmonary irritant receptors
- Heart failure with pulmonary congestion
- Impairment of cerebral vasoreactivity
- Arousals
- Disturbances of acid-base balance

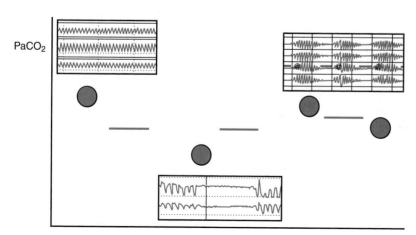

Figure 19-2 Apnea threshold. The dots represent the prevailing $Paco_2$ and the horizontal lines demonstrate the apnea threshold. If the actual $Paco_2$ exceeds the apnea threshold respiration is regular (*left part*). A central sleep apnea appears if the $Paco_2$ is below the threshold (*middle*). Periodic breathing emerges if the distance between the apnea threshold and the actual $Paco_2$ is narrow (*right part*).

receptors. Pulmonary capillary wedge (PCW) pressure serves as a measure of left ventricular failure and pulmonary congestion. Solin and co-workers showed a significant correlation between the wedge pressure and the apnea-hypopnea index (AHI). A subgroup of the study population underwent a second right-sided heart catheterization after optimizing cardiac treatment. An improvement of the PCW pressure was associated with a distinct improvement of the AHI in all patients.[17] Lorenzi-Filho and colleagues proved the correlation of the left ventricular function with the $Paco_2$—the greater the pulmonary congestion (the PCW pressure), the higher the ventilatory drive. Moreover, improvement of cardiac function reduced hyperventilation, and deterioration induced by volume application led to hyperventilation.[28]

The instability of the respiratory control system also depends on the sensitivity of the peripheral and central chemoreceptors. The sensitivity can be defined by the *hypoxic and hypercapnic ventilatory response*. Xie and associates performed hyperventilation trials to examine the apnea threshold. They calculated the response to increasing CO_2 levels after hyperventilation and found that the ventilatory response was significantly elevated in patients with central sleep apnea.[25] These findings were confirmed by Solin and associates who studied the hypercapnic ventilatory response in healthy subjects and CSA patients. Although there was no difference between healthy subjects, heart failure (HF) patients without breathing disturbances, and HF patients with obstructive sleep apnea, the response to hypercapnia was increased in HF patients with periodic breathing. Therefore, hyperreactivity of the chemoreceptors is a typical marker not of HF in general, but only if it is associated with central breathing disturbances.[29]

Based on animal trials, it has been hypothesized that a prolongation of the circulation time due to left ventricular failure might be of crucial importance in the pathophysiology of central breathing disturbances. A delayed transmission of blood gases to chemoreceptors might lead to delayed perception of changes of the CO_2 level and thus induce ventilatory overshoot and undershoot. However, the circulation time was increased to 1 minute in the animal trials, which is far from being representative for heart failure patients. Moreover, no difference between heart failure patients with or without CSR in terms of cardiac output, left ventricular ejection fraction, or lung to ear circulation time has been proved.[17,30-32]

Although apnea and hyperventilation mainly depend on the peripheral chemoreceptors, *central chemoreceptors* also seem to play a role in the pathophysiology of CSA. Interestingly, the cerebral blood flow differs between healthy subjects and CSA patients. Physiologically, increase of the $Paco_2$ augments the cerebral blood flow. However, this vasoreactivity is diminished in CSA patients as compared to control subjects.[33] The variations of the cerebral blood flow normally counterbalance changes of the H^+ concentration in the cerebral fluid. Acidosis increases cerebral blood flow and alkalosis diminishes it. If these reflexes are dampened in HF patients, cerebral alkalosis might be intensified, leading to a reduction of the ventilatory drive and central apnea. In contrast, increases of cerebral acidosis induce ventilatory overshoot and hyperventilation, both resulting in unstable breathing.

Arousals are important reactions of the brain to breathing disturbances. They restore the waking state of nonchemical control of breathing, lower the CO_2 set-point, and increase the ventilatory reactivity. As the prevailing CO_2 level during sleep is higher as compared to the new set-point in the sleep-wake transition, ventilation is rapidly elevated. In addition, arousals are associated with an increased activity of the pharyngeal muscles, which is crucial in the termination of obstructive apneas. However, patients with central sleep apnea behave differently; they are characterized by higher sensitivity of the chemoreceptors to CO_2 during sleep. Therefore, when arousals increase ventilation and reduce the CO_2 level, they induce a ventilatory overshoot, resulting in a vicious circle of hyperventilation, central apnea, and arousal. Therefore, arousals propagate periodicity and induce breathing disturbances rather than terminating instability.[22,31,34]

TREATMENT OF CENTRAL SLEEP APNEA

The therapeutic approach to patients with central breathing disturbances during sleep is based on the underlying disorder and the pathophysiologic considerations. However, the development of an evidence-based treatment algorithm is limited by the paucity of controlled clinical trials. Moreover, the most relevant clinical outcome parameters such as respiratory disturbances, quality of sleep, daytime functioning, and cardiovascular parameters are unclear. Despite this, the overwhelming majority of studies focusing on prognosis of central disturbances in patients with cardiovascular disorders show reduced survival rates in untreated CSA/CSR patients.[26,35-40] This urges the clinician to start treatment as soon as the diagnosis of central breathing disturbance has been established (Box 19-2).

Generally, treatment focuses primarily on the abolition of the underlying disorder. This includes the surgical or medical improvement of cerebral blood flow, the treatment of brain tumors, or the pharmacologic therapy of cardiac diseases. If sleep-related breathing disorders are still unresolved additional surgical or interventional approaches such as dilatation and stenting of coronary arteries, cardiac surgery, or heart transplantation can be discussed. Additional drugs that interfere with the loop gain of ventilatory response or the application of CO_2 can be considered. Finally, the application of oxygen O_2 or positive pressure treatment might be helpful (Fig. 19-3).

BOX 19-2 *Treatment Options*

- Pharmaceutical treatment of underlying cardiovascular or neurologic disorder (generally recommended despite scarce data)
- Cardiac resynchronization therapy (individual cases)
- Cardiac interventions and transplantation (individual cases)
- Application of oxygen (no general recommendation)
- Application of carbon dioxide (insufficient data for clinical use)
- Respiratory stimulants (not recommended)
- CPAP (recommended as first treatment approach; efficacy has to be proved individually)
- BPAP (insufficient data; efficacy has to be proved individually)
- Adaptive servoventilation/auto-servoventilation/anticyclic modulated ventilation (generally recommended in CPAP nonresponders)

BPAP, bilevel positive airway pressure; *CPAP,* continuous positive airway pressure.

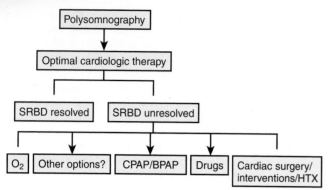

Figure 19-3 Therapeutic approach to patients with central breathing disturbances. The figure represents a recommendation for the therapeutic decisions in central sleep apnea. Treatment is based on optimization of any underlying cardiac or neurologic disorder. However, in many cases Cheyne-Stokes respiration (CSR) remains unresolved so that pharmaceutical or non-pharmaceutical options have to be considered, such as oxygen, cardiac interventions, or positive pressure therapies. *BPAP,* bilevel positive airway pressure; *CPAP,* continuous positive airway pressure; *SRBD,* sleep-related breathing disorder.

Only a few nonrandomized studies have investigated the effect of cardiac drugs in heart failure patients with breathing disturbances. Tamura and associates applied carvedilol over a period of 6 months to 16 HF patients with an ejection fraction of less than 50%.[41] They suffered from dyspnea corresponding to New York Heart Association (NYHA) class II-III and at least five central apneas/hour. Treatment with carvedilol significantly improved the left ventricular function and reduced the level of brain natriuretic peptide. Moreover, the number of central apneas was significantly reduced and there was no relevant change in obstructive apneas. Walsh and co-workers treated 12 patients with heart failure in NYHA class II-III with captopril for 1 month.[42] The authors also found a significant improvement in respiratory disturbances, sleep profile, and subjective sleep quality. Solin and co-workers studied the effect of intensive individually tailored medical therapy for 1 to 6 months in seven patients with CSR and an elevated PCW pressure. Both the PCWP and the AHI decreased under therapy with diuretics, Agiotensinconverting enzyme (ACE) inhibitors, nitrates, carvedilol, and continuous positive airway pressure.[43]

Cardiac resynchronization therapy (CRT) has proved to be an effective option to improve HF in patients with severe left ventricular systolic dysfunction. Additional indications for cardiac resynchronization therapy were electromechanical dyssynchrony and resistant heart failure symptoms despite pharmaceutical treatment. Cara and associates studied 12 patients with HF and left ventricular ejection fraction of 28 ± 2.8%. After implantation of atrial synchronized biventricular pacemakers they studied three consecutive nights, two with CRT and one without.[44] They found a significant improvement of duration and number of central disturbances in those nights with active stimulation. Moreover, the volume of mitral regurgitation significantly correlated with central sleep apnea and was improved under effective stimulation.

Oxygen Supplementation

If the treatment of the underlying cardiovascular disorders has failed to normalize respiratory disturbances, the application of oxygen may be discussed. It increases the O_2 supply of

the left ventricle and additionally may reduce the reflex activation of the peripheral chemoreceptors. Several studies have been performed to investigate the efficacy of oxygen in the treatment of CSA. Sasayama and associates compared breathing of room air and O_2 in 65 patients with moderate heart failure with a left ventricular ejection fraction (LVEF) of 45% or less and clinical NYHA class II–III. Not surprisingly, the oxygen desaturation index normalized under O_2 application but the reduction of the AHI was limited to 50%.[45] Several questions remain open in the O_2 treatment of CSA. Oxygen supplementation failed to improve sleep parameters, clinical symptoms and cognitive failure in CSA patients.[46,47] Although Sasayama showed a small but significant improvement of LVEF, the application of high inspired oxygen concentration was accompanied by an impairment of left ventricular pressure and the relaxation time.[48] There are conflicting results on the influence of O_2 on sympathetic activity. Staniforth showed a general reduction,[47] but Andreas only showed an improvement of muscular sympathetic nerve activity during voluntary apneas but not during resting ventilation in healthy subjects.[47a]

Therapeutic Application of Carbon Dioxide

The administration of CO_2 is another approach to the patient with central breathing disturbances. CO_2 not only interacts with peripheral chemoreceptors but also penetrates the blood-brain barrier and influences the regulation of breathing in the brainstem. As mentioned before, the propensity of central apneas and periodic breathing depends on the distance between the prevailing CO_2 level and the apnea threshold. The application of CO_2 enlarges this distance and therefore stabilizes breathing. Several studies have shown that the application of O_2 may avoid O_2 desaturations as compared to room air but does not sufficiently improve the total numbers of apneas and hypopneas. In contrast, the elevation of the CO_2 level by external application of CO_2 or by enlargement of the dead space normalizes ventilation in CSA patients.[49-51] Andreas and colleagues studied nine patients with heart failure and left ventricular ejection fraction of 17.8 ± 1.2%. They applied a mixture of O_2 and CO_2 in a crossover, single-blind, placebo-controlled trial for one night each. The application of CO_2 and O_2 increased the transcutaneous CO_2 level from 39 ± 2 to 43 ± 2 mm Hg and reduced the time with CSR highly significantly. However, this improvement was associated with a significant increase of sympathetic activity.[51] Because the application of CO_2 can be dangerous, safety concerns of gas application have to be solved and adverse effects have to be defined more clearly before the application of CO_2 can be recommended.

Drugs Interfering with the Ventilatory Control System

It can be hypothesized that pharmaceutical agents can influence the ventilatory loop gain by interfering with the respiratory control system in the brain. Acetazolamide is a mild diuretic and respiratory stimulant. Javaheri studied 12 patients with stable heart failure and CSR with an AHI of 15 or more episodes per hour. He applied acetazolamide in a randomized, double-blind, crossover, placebo-controlled study over six nights with a 2-week washout period between the treatment periods. The $Paco_2$ was 88 ± 11 mm Hg at baseline and increased significantly under acetazolamide to 92 ± 3 mm Hg as compared to placebo (84 ± 9 mm Hg). Although there was no change of the total and central AHI under placebo, these parameters improved significantly in subjects taking acetazolamide (total AHI at baseline 55 ± 24/hour, 57 ± 28/hour under placebo and 34 ± 20/hour under acetazolamide, $p < 0.002$, central AHI at baseline 44 ± 23/hour, 49 ± 28/hour under placebo, 23 ± 21/hour under acetazolamide, $p < 0.004$). However, a reduction of the respiratory disturbances by half is not efficacious from a clinical point of view.[52]

Andreas and associates performed a single-blind, randomized, placebo-controlled study on the efficacy of theophylline on sympathetic, hemodynamic, neurohumoral, and ventilatory parameters. The transcutaneous Pco_2 decreased in healthy subjects and HF patients under theophylline as compared to placebo. This indicates that theophylline stimulates ventilation in both groups. In contrast to healthy people, theophylline did not increase sympathetic activity in HF.[53,54]

It has been shown that arousals are not necessary for reopening of the upper airways and the maintenance of the airflow. Moreover, arousals reduce slow wave sleep and destabilize ventilation and therefore might aggravate respiratory disturbances.[2] Therefore, the question arises if the suppression of arousals may stabilize respiration. Younes and associates applied pentobarbital in a placebo-controlled animal trial. These authors demonstrated increases of genioglossus activity both at baseline and under CO_2 stimulation when the rats were sedated. The arousal threshold increased, which is a precondition to stabilize breathing. However, these authors found serious blood gas alterations with prolonged hypoxia. Data on the suppression of arousals in human beings are not yet available.[2]

Positive Airway Pressure Treatment

The application of continuous positive airway pressure (CPAP) is currently the gold standard in the treatment of central breathing disorders including CSR:

- CPAP improves ventilation-perfusion mismatches in the lungs and, therefore, increases the alveolar-arterial oxygen difference.
- It enlarges the intrapulmonary gas reservoir, which reduces the variation of the gas proportions.
- The application of positive pressure to the thorax may influence cardiac function.

There are concerns that CPAP might reduce left ventricular function. Indeed, it reduces venous return to the heart, which impairs the preload and cardiac index in healthy people. However, CPAP reduces the pleural pressure swings in HF patients and therefore improves the left ventricular transmural pressure, a marker of the left ventricular afterload. Moreover, a reduction of the pleural pressure diminishes the work of breathing and the O_2 consumption of the respiratory muscles. Both effects lead to an increase of the cardiac index. These considerations have been proved in clinical trials. Mansfield and associates and Kaneko and associates both showed significant increases of the left ventricular ejection fraction over treatment periods of 1 to 3 months of CPAP therapy as compared to placebo (Fig. 19-4).[55,56]

However, several studies from different groups consistently showed that CPAP does not allow for a complete normalization of respiratory disturbances but reduces the AHI by about 50%. Arzt and colleagues found additional improvements of

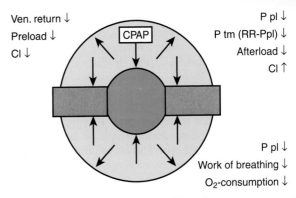

Figure 19-4 Effects of continuous positive airway pressure on the heart. The left side of the figure presents the influence of positive airway pressure on cardiac function. A significant but clinically irrelevant reduction of the cardiac index has been shown in healthy. In contrast, heart failure patients may substantially benefit from positive pressure application because it reduces oxygen demand and left ventricular transmural pressure. *CI,* cardiac index; *Ppl,* pleural pressure; *Ptm (RR-Ppl),* left ventricular transmural pressure.

respiratory disturbances after 3 months as compared to the first night of CPAP treatment.[57] This result implies that definite decisions on the efficacy should be made after a longer CPAP trial. Nevertheless, the long-term and large, controlled Canadian continuous positive airway pressure study for patients with central sleep apnoea and heart failure (CanPAP) trial confirmed the reduction of the respiratory disturbances by 50% and improvements of the minimal O_2 saturation and the left ventricular function. However, the primary outcome parameter of transplant-free survival failed.[58] Arzt and colleagues performed a post-hoc analysis of the CanPAP data. They divided the patients into those who showed a normalization of respiratory disturbances under CPAP and those with limited reduction of CSA/CSR. There was no significant difference between the CPAP nonresponders as compared to conventionally treated HF patients. In contrast, there was a clear survival benefit in those with CPAP-suppressed CSA.[59]

There are only limited data on the use of bilevel treatment (BPAP) in CSA/CSR. Dohi and colleagues applied bilevel pressure to a small group of patients who did not sufficiently respond to CPAP. The authors showed a further reduction of respiratory disturbances in nine subjects.[60] However, given the lack of controlled clinical trials on the use of bilevel pressure, this method cannot be recommended at this stage.

Adaptive Servoventilation

Most recently new devices and algorithms have been developed with the aim to more effectively improve CSA and CSR. The manufacturers have named the treatment modes "adaptive servoventilation," "autoservoventilation," or "anticyclic modulated ventilation." However, the term *adaptive servoventilation (ASV)* is frequently used to describe the principle in general.

The devices provide an expiratory positive airway pressure to eliminate obstructive apneas and hypopneas. Similarly, they modulate the inspiratory positive airway pressure to overcome central disturbances. Consequently, the devices prevent the ventilatory overshoot by avoiding both hypoxia and hypocapnia and thus stabilize respiration. The various algorithms are similar in that they analyze the patient's breathing pattern by measuring the actual patient air flow or minute ventilation.

This data is compared with the corresponding parameters in a moving average of 3 or 4 minutes throughout the night. If a predefined limit of the target parameter is not reached, additional pressure support is supplied. If it is overcome, pressure support is reduced.

The three currently available devices differ in the target parameters, backup frequency, and applicable pressure levels. One device delivers a minimum pressure support of 3 mbar (cm water [H_2O]). This device might be helpful in those patients with pure Cheyne-Stokes respiration. The other algorithms are able to apply the same pressure level during inspiration and expiration in periods of stable breathing and therefore to work as CPAP devices. This is an interesting feature in those patients with coexisting obstructive and central breathing disturbances.

Prior to the initiation of ASV the physician has to define the *minimal inspiratory pressure,* the *maximal inspiratory pressure,* and the *expiratory pressure.* The minimal inspiratory pressure describes the lower limit during inspiration which the pressure cannot fall below. The actual inspiratory pressure cannot exceed the maximum inspiratory pressure. The pressure support—the difference between the actual inspiratory pressure and the expiratory pressure—determines the tidal volume and varies within the predefined range to overcome periodic breathing.

The titration of the *expiratory pressure* differs substantially between the currently available devices. The expiratory pressure serves to sustain the upper airway patency. This level has to be defined based on a manual titration in one device. However, others combine adaptive servoventilation with automatic CPAP and pressure relief. Thus, they vary not only the pressure support but also the expiratory pressure to overcome upper airway obstruction automatically. The physician sets a maximum inspiratory pressure and a minimum end-expiratory pressure while the algorithms determine the expiratory pressure during early expiration, the inspiratory pressure, and the end-expiratory pressure.

As described before, the most important common principle of the ASV algorithms is to continuously counterbalance the ventilatory over- and undershoot. However, the devices not only increase the tidal volume during hypoventilation and reduce it during hyperventilation, but also apply mandatory breaths in a variable timed mode to cover central apneas.

The clinical pathway starts with optimizing the treatment of the underlying cardiovascular disorder. If breathing disturbances are unresolved, we recommend a CPAP trial for two reasons.

1. CPAP sufficiently suppresses respiratory disturbances in about 50% of the patients, although there are no parameters that allow the prediction of its efficacy.
2. The CPAP titration determines the expiratory pressure necessary to overcome upper airway obstruction. This pressure level is translated into the expiratory pressure of ASV.

If CPAP does not normalize central breathing disturbances the patient is switched over to ASV during the following night. The first clinical trial on the efficacy of ASV was published in 2001 by Teschler and associates.[61] They applied O_2, CPAP, BPAP, and ASV for one night each to a group of 14 patients. The study confirmed previous findings that O_2 and CPAP reduced the central apnea index (CAI) by half. BPAP showed a better improvement of the mean CAI, but the individual results varied widely. In contrast, ASV normalized the CAI in almost all patients.

Pepperell and associates performed a randomized, controlled, double-blind study comparing effective with subtherapeutic ASV for 1 month. They focused primarily on parameters regarding sleep quality and daytime performance. Subtherapeutic ASV delivered an expiratory pressure of 1.75 mbar (cm H_2O) with pressure support between 0.75 and 2.75 mbar (cm H_2O). The authors included 30 CSA patients with chronic heart failure in the NYHA class II-IV, left ventricular ejection fraction of 33% to 36%, and mainly CSR/CSA. Effective ASV improved not only respiratory disturbances but also daytime performance measured in the OSLER test and cardiovascular and sympathetic markers (brain natriuretic peptide and metadrenaline excretion).[62]

In addition, Philippe and colleagues compared the efficacy and compliance with ASV CPAP; 25 patients with CSA/CSR and stable HF in NYHA class II-IV were randomly assigned to receive one of the two treatment options for 6 months. ASV proved to be superior to CPAP in terms of AHI, left ventricular function, and compliance. Moreover, the quality of life measured by the Minnesota living with heart failure questionnaire (MLHFQ) improved significantly better with ASV as compared to CPAP. However, the study failed to show a significant improvement of daytime sleepiness (Epworth sleepiness scale). This might be due to the fact that the scores were low at baseline, giving only limited room for improvement, which is quite common in CSR patients.[63]

These studies were performed using the Adapt SV device but the efficacy of ASV has also been confirmed with the other ASV devices. Arzt and associates studied 14 patients suffering from chronic HF with an impaired left ventricular function and a portion of CSA/CSR greater than 80%. The patients were included for ASV treatment (BiPAP Auto SV) after being insufficiently treated with CPAP or BPAP for a mean period of more than 6 months. Once again, CPAP or bilevel significantly reduced the AHI by half compared to baseline. In contrast, ASV (expiratory positive airway pressure (EPAP) 8.3 ± 0.9 mbar, maximum inspiratory pressure 13.5 ± 3.0 mbar) normalized all respiratory parameters.[57]

Most of the previous studies have included patients with almost pure CSA/CSR, which is rarely found in clinical practice. Furthermore, many patients with OSAS show at least a minor proportion of central disturbances. Finally, evidence suggests CSA may emerge under positive airway pressure and persist despite continued use (CPAP persistent CSA) in a small percentage of patients.[64,65] Therefore, it is crucially important to focus on patients with coexisting OSAS and CSA/CSR and on patients with CPAP-induced CSA. For these reasons, we performed a prospective observational study on the efficacy of ASV in 10 male consecutive patients with coexisting OSAS and CSA/CSR with and without heart failure over 8 weeks. ASV (BiPAP ASV) proved to effectively suppress all types of respiratory disturbances and improve sleep quality as measured by sleep stages and arousals. The results did not differ between patients with and without cardiovascular diseases.[66] Preliminary data from a long-term CPAP controlled trial in HF patients with coexisting obstructive and central sleep apnea show a significant improvement of the total and central AHI with ASV as compared to CPAP.[67]

Most recently, the new algorithm of anticyclic modulating ventilation, which combines adaptive servoventilation and automatic CPAP, was tested in a short-term pilot study; 16 patients with greater than 20% central disturbances and less than 80% obstructive events were included. After baseline polysomnography they were adapted to the anticyclic modulating ventilation and followed for 2 weeks. The device highly significantly reduced the total AHI and both the central and obstructive AHI to normal values. Moreover, the numbers of arousals were significantly improved under treatment.

In recent years, an interesting and stimulating discussion has emerged regarding central disturbances associated with CPAP treatment. Morgenthaler and associates introduced the term *complex sleep apnea*.[65] Javaheri differentiated patients with complicated breathing patterns into three groups: CPAP-emergent CSA, CPAP-persistent CSA, and CPAP-resistant CSA. In CPAP-emergent CSA the central disturbances appear during CPAP titration but are acute and transient and disappear with continued CPAP use. The disturbances sustain in CPAP-persistent CSA. Different investigators found a portion of about 5% to 10% of CPAP-treated patients with persistent CSA. Many central disturbances exist prior to the CPAP initiation and stay unresolved under treatment. This group, CPAP-resistant CSA, includes patients with opioid use or cardiovascular diseases.[68]

Allam and associates compared the efficacy of different positive pressure modes in patients with CSA/CSR and complex sleep apnea. The diagnosis was based on a residual central AHI of 5 per hour or more after suppression of obstructive disturbances under CPAP. The total group of patients with central disturbances consisted of 100 patients and was divided into a subgroup of 63 patients with complex sleep apnea syndrome (SAS), 32 with central sleep apnea, and 90 with CSA/CSR. The authors found that ASV normalized breathing disturbances in all subgroups. It was superior to CPAP, CPAP plus O_2,

BPAP in spontaneous mode, and BPAP in continuous/timed mode.[69]

Due to a lack of controlled trials, the optimal therapeutic approach to patients with opioid-associated breathing disturbances is still under debate. Glidewell and associates presented a case study of a 41-year-old woman under long-acting opioid therapy. She presented with mild obstructive and severe CSA under CPAP and did not respond to O_2. The authors added acetazolamide at bedtime to the CPAP therapy and found a normalization of both obstructive and central disturbances.[70] Two studies focused on the use of ASV in opioid-associated sleep apnea. Farney and colleagues retrospectively analyzed the data of 22 patients treated with CPAP and ASV and failed to show sufficient efficacy with either mode.[71] In contrast, Javaheri and associates proved a good suppression of all types of respiratory disturbances with ASV as compared to CPAP in a case series of five patients.[72] The main difference between the two studies was the setting of the devices. Pressure support was much more limited in Farney and associates' study as compared to that of Javaheri and associates.

Based on these considerations a new therapeutic algorithm may be recommended at this point (Fig. 19-5). First of all, any underlying cardiovascular or neurologic disorder has to be diagnosed and optimally treated. If pharmaceutical or interventional approaches do not resolve, CPAP should be applied as the first step of positive airway pressure treatment. This decision is based on the fact that data on improvement of cardiac parameters and mortality rates have been published in general or in subgroups of CSR patients under CPAP. In contrast, there is no sufficient evidence to support bilevel pressure treatment, O_2, CO_2, or the pharmaceutical suppression of arousals. Optimal reduction of respiratory disturbances is crucial to improve mortality rate of patients with CSA and underlying cardiovascular diseases. Therefore, if CPAP

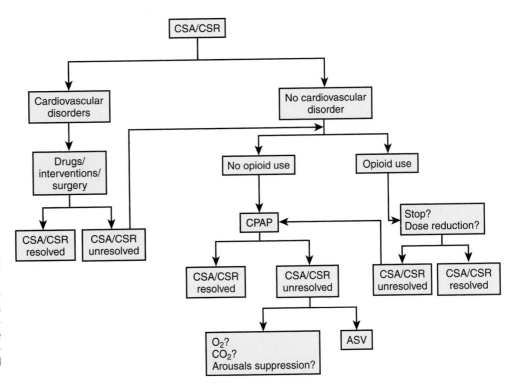

Figure 19-5 Therapeutic algorithm. The decision tree depends on the central questions of the prevalence of cardiovascular disorders, chronic use of opioids, and the efficacy CPAP. ASV seems to be the most effective treatment of different types of central breathing disturbances. However, prior to its application we recommend treating underlying cardiac disorders and reducing opioids if possible. Due to a lack of evidence, trials with oxygen are not mandatory. The application of carbon dioxide and drugs interfering with sleep cannot be recommended at the moment. *ASV,* adaptive servoventilation; *CPAP,* continuous positive airway pressure; *CSA/CSR,* central sleep apnea/Cheyne-Stokes respiration.

does not sufficiently suppress central disturbances, adaptive servoventilation should be applied.

Short-term CPAP-controlled trials and preliminary long-term data have proved that ASV is superior in the suppression of respiratory disturbances as compared to CPAP. ASV appears to be the gold standard of therapy. However, data on improvement of cardiac function and survival are still lacking.

REFERENCES

1. American Academy of Sleep Medicine. *Diagnostic and Coding Manual: International Classification of Sleep Disorders.* 2nd ed. Westchester, IL: American Academy of Sleep Medicine; 2005.
2. Younes M. Role of arousals in the pathogenesis of obstructive sleep apnea. *Am J Respir Crit Care Med.* 2004;169(5):623-633.
3. Eckert DJ, Malhotra A. Pathophysiology of adult obstructive sleep apnea. *Proc Am Thorac Soc.* 2008;5(2):144-153.
4. Schwab RJ, Pasirstein M, Pierson R, et al. Identification of upper airway anatomic risk factors for obstructive sleep apnea with volumetric magnetic resonance imaging. *Am J Respir Crit Care Med.* 2003;168(5):522-530.
5. Schwab RJ, Gefter WB, Hoffman EA, et al. Dynamic upper airway imaging during awake respiration in normal subjects and patients with sleep disordered breathing. *Am Rev Respir Dis.* 1993;148(5):1385-1400.
6. Stradling JR, Davies RJ. Sleep: 1. Obstructive sleep apnoea/hypopnoea syndrome: Definitions, epidemiology, and natural history. *Thorax.* 2004;59(1):73-78.
7. De Backer W. Obstructive sleep apnea-hypopnea syndrome. Definitions and pathophysiology. In: Randerath WJ, Sanner BM, Somers VK, eds. *Sleep Apnea.* Basel: Karger; 2006:90-96[Prog Respir Res. 2006;35:90–96].
8. Badr MS, Skatrud JB, Dempsey J. Pharyngeal narrowing/occlusion during central sleep apnea. *J Appl Physiol.* 1995;21:1839-1846.
9. Wang H, Parker JD, Newton GE, et al. Influence of obstructive sleep apnea on mortality in patients with heart failure. *J Am Coll Cardiol.* 2007;49(15):1625-1631.
10. Biot M. Contribution a l'etude de phénomène respiratoire de Cheyne Stokes. *Lyon Med.* 1876;23:517-528:561-567.
11. Webster LR, Choi Y, Desai H, et al. Sleep-disordered breathing and chronic opioid therapy. *Pain Med.* 2008;9(4):425-432.
12. Farney RJ, Walker JM, Cloward TV, et al. Sleep-disordered breathing associated with long-term opioid therapy. *Chest.* 2003;123(2):632-639.
13. Walker JM, Farney RJ, Rhondeau SM, et al. Chronic opioid use is a risk factor for the development of central sleep apnea and ataxic breathing. *J Clin Sleep Med.* 2007;3(5):455-461.
14. Hall MJ, Rutherford R, Ando S, Floras JS, Bradley TD. Cycle length of periodic breathing in patients with and without heart failure. *Am J Respir Crit Care Med.* 1996;154:376-381.
15. Bixler EO, Vgontzas AN, Ten Have T, et al. Effects of age on sleep apnea in men: I. Prevalence and severity. *Am J Respir Crit Care Med.* 1998;157(1):144-148.
16. Tkacova RHM, Liu PP, Fitzgerald FS, Bradley TD. Left ventricular volume in patients with heart failure and Cheyne-Stokes respiration during sleep. *Am J Respir Crit Care Med.* 1997;156:1549-1555.
17. Solin PBP, Richardson M, Kaye DM, Walters EH, Naughton MT. Influence of pulmonary capillary wedge pressure on central apnea in heart failure. *Circulation.* 1999;99:1574-1579.
18. Lanfranchi PA, Somers VK, Braghiroli A, et al. Central sleep apnea in left ventricular dysfunction: Prevalence and implications for arrhythmic risk. *Circulation.* 2003;107(5):727-732.
19. Nopmaneejumruslers C, Kaneko Y, Hajek V, et al. Cheyne-Stokes respiration in stroke: Relationship to hypocapnia and occult cardiac dysfunction. *Am J Respir Crit Care Med.* 2005;171(9):1048-1052.
20. Sin DD, Fitzgerald F, Parker JD, et al. Risk factors for central and obstructive sleep apnea in 450 men and women with congestive heart failure. *Am J Respir Crit Care Med.* 1999;160(4):1101-1106.
21. Phillipson EA. Control of breathing during sleep. *Am Rev Respir Dis.* 1978;118(5):909-939.
22. Bradley TD, Phillipson EA. Central sleep apnea. *Clin Chest Med.* 1992;13(3):493-505.
23. Wellman A, Malhotra A, Fogel RB, et al. Respiratory system loop gain in normal men and women measured with proportional-assist ventilation. *J Appl Physiol.* 2003;94(1):205-212.
24. Xie A, Phillipson EA, Slutsky AS, Bradley TD. Interaction of hyperventilation and arousal in the pathogenesis of idiopathic central sleep apnea. *Am J Respir Crit Care Med.* 1994;150:489-495.
25. Xie A, Skatrud JB, Puleo DS, et al. Apnea-hypopnea threshold for CO_2 in patients with congestive heart failure. *Am J Respir Crit Care Med.* 2002;165(9):1245-1250.
26. Hanly P, Zuberi N, Gray R. Pathogenesis of Cheyne-Stokes respiration in patients with congestive heart failure. Relationship to arterial Pco_2. *Chest.* 1993;104(4):1079-1084.
27. Yu J, Zhang JF, Fletcher EC. Stimulation of breathing by activation of pulmonary peripheral afferents in rabbits. *J Appl Physiol.* 1998;85(4):1485-1492.
28. Lorenzi-Filho G, Azevedo ER, Parker JD, et al. Relationship of carbon dioxide tension in arterial blood to pulmonary wedge pressure in heart failure. *Eur Respir J.* 2002;19(1):37-40.
29. Solin PRT, Johns DP, Walters EH, Naughton MT. Peripheral and central ventilatory responses in central sleep apnea with and without congestive heart failure. *Am J Respir Crit Care Med.* 2000;162:2194-2200.
30. Yumino D, Bradley TD. Central sleep apnea and Cheyne-Stokes respiration. *Proc Am Thorac Soc.* 2008;5(2):226-236.
31. Naughton M, Benard D, Tam A, et al. Role of hyperventilation in the pathogenesis of central sleep apneas in patients with congestive heart failure. *Am Rev Respir Dis.* 1993;148(2):330-338.
32. Crowell JW, Guyton AC, Moore JW. Basic oscillating mechanism of Cheyne-Stokes breathing. *Am J Physiol.* 1956;187(2):395-398.
33. Xie A, Skatrud JB, Khayat R, et al. Cerebrovascular response to carbon dioxide in patients with congestive heart failure. *Am J Respir Crit Care Med.* 2005;172(3):371-378.
34. Xie A, Wong B, Phillipson EA, et al. Interaction of hyperventilation and arousal in the pathogenesis of idiopathic central sleep apnea. *Am J Respir Crit Care Med.* 1994;150(2):489-495.
35. Lanfranchi PA, Braghiroli A, Bosimini E, et al. Prognostic value of nocturnal Cheyne-Stokes respiration in chronic heart failure. *Circulation.* 1999;99(11):1435-1440.
36. Javaheri S, Shukla R, Zeigler H, et al. Central sleep apnea, right ventricular dysfunction, and low diastolic blood pressure are predictors of mortality in systolic heart failure. *J Am Coll Cardiol.* 2007;49(20):2028-2034.
37. Andreas S, Hagenah G, Moller C, et al. Cheyne-Stokes respiration and prognosis in congestive heart failure. *Am J Cardiol.* 1996;78(11):1260-1264.
38. Roebuck T, Solin P, Kaye DM, et al. Increased long-term mortality in heart failure due to sleep apnoea is not yet proven. *Eur Respir J.* 2004;23(5):735-740.
39. Sin DD, Logan AG, Fitzgerald FS, et al. Effects of continuous positive airway pressure on cardiovascular outcomes in heart failure patients with and without Cheyne-Stokes respiration. *Circulation.* 2000;102(1):61-66.
40. Corra U, Pistono M, Mezzani A, et al. Sleep and exertional periodic breathing in chronic heart failure: Prognostic importance and interdependence. *Circulation.* 2006;113(1):44-50.
41. Tamura A, Kawano Y, Kadota J. Carvedilol reduces the severity of central sleep apnea in chronic heart failure. *Circ J.* 2009;73(2):295-298.
42. Walsh JT, Andrews R, Evans A, et al. Failure of "effective" treatment for heart failure to improve normal customary activity. *Br Heart J.* 1995;74(4):373-376.
43. Solin P, Roebuck T, Johns DP, et al. Peripheral and central ventilatory responses in central sleep apnea with and without congestive heart failure. *Am J Respir Crit Care Med.* 2000;162(6):2194-2200.
44. Kara T, Novak M, Nykodym J, et al. Short-term effects of cardiac resynchronization therapy on sleep-disordered breathing in patients with systolic heart failure. *Chest.* 2008;134(1):87-93.
45. Sasayama S, Izumi T, Seino Y, et al. Effects of nocturnal oxygen therapy on outcome measures in patients with chronic heart failure and Cheyne-Stokes respiration. *Circ J.* 2006;70(1):1-7.
46. Krachman SL, D'Alonzo GE, Berger TJ, et al. Comparison of oxygen therapy with nasal continuous positive airway pressure on Cheyne-Stokes respiration during sleep in congestive heart failure. *Chest.* 1999;116(6):1550-1557.
47. Staniforth AD, Kinnear WJ, Starling R, et al. Effect of oxygen on sleep quality, cognitive function and sympathetic activity in patients with chronic heart failure and Cheyne-Stokes respiration. *Eur Heart J.* 1998;19(6):922-928.
48. Mak S, Newton GE. The oxidative stress hypothesis of congestive heart failure: Radical thoughts. *Chest.* 2001;120(6):2035-2046.
49. Lorenzi-Filho G, Rankin F, Bies I, et al. Effects of inhaled carbon dioxide and oxygen on Cheyne-Stokes respiration in patients with heart failure. *Am J Respir Crit Care Med.* 1999;159(5 Pt 1):1490-1498.
50. Xie A, Rankin F, Rutherford R, et al. Effects of inhaled CO_2 and added dead space on idiopathic central sleep apnea. *J Appl Physiol.* 1997;82(3):918-926.

51. Andreas S, Weidel K, Hagenah G, et al. Treatment of Cheyne-Stokes respiration with nasal oxygen and carbon dioxide. *Eur Respir J*. 1998;12(2): 414-419.

52. Javaheri S. Acetazolamide improves central sleep apnea in heart failure: A double-blind, prospective study. *Am J Respir Crit Care Med*. 2006;173(2):234-237.

53. Andreas S, Reiter H, Luthje L, et al. Differential effects of theophylline on sympathetic excitation, hemodynamics, and breathing in congestive heart failure. *Circulation*. 2004;110(15):2157-2162.

54. Javaheri S, Parker TJ, Wexler L, et al. Effect of theophylline on sleep-disordered breathing in heart failure. *N Engl J Med*. 1996;335(8):562-567.

55. Mansfield DR, Gollogly NC, Kaye DM, et al. Controlled trial of continuous positive airway pressure in obstructive sleep apnea and heart failure. *Am J Respir Crit Care Med*. 2004;169(3):361-366.

56. Kaneko Y, Floras JS, Usui K, et al. Cardiovascular effects of continuous positive airway pressure in patients with heart failure and obstructive sleep apnea. *N Engl J Med*. 2003;348(13):1233-1241.

57. Arzt M, Wensel R, Montalvan S, et al. Effects of dynamic bilevel positive airway pressure support on central sleep apnea in men with heart failure. *Chest*. 2008;134(1):61-66.

58. Bradley TD, Logan AG, Kimoff RJ, et al. Continuous positive airway pressure for central sleep apnea and heart failure. *N Engl J Med*. 2005; 353(19):2025-2033.

59. Arzt M, Floras JS, Logan AG, et al. Suppression of central sleep apnea by continuous positive airway pressure and transplant-free survival in heart failure: A post hoc analysis of the Canadian Continuous Positive Airway Pressure for Patients with Central Sleep Apnea and Heart Failure Trial (CANPAP). *Circulation*. 2007;115(25):3173-3180.

60. Dohi T, Kasai T, Narui K, et al. Bi-level positive airway pressure ventilation for treating heart failure with central sleep apnea that is unresponsive to continuous positive airway pressure. *Circ J*. 2008;72(7):1100-1105.

61. Teschler H, Dohring J, Wang YM, et al. Adaptive pressure support servoventilation: A novel treatment for Cheyne-Stokes respiration in heart failure. *Am J Respir Crit Care Med*. 2001;164(4):614-619.

62. Pepperell JC, Maskell NA, Jones DR, et al. A randomized controlled trial of adaptive ventilation for Cheyne-Stokes breathing in heart failure. *Am J Respir Crit Care Med*. 2003;168(9):1109-1114.

63. Philippe C, Stoica-Herman M, Drouot X, et al. Compliance with and effectiveness of adaptive servoventilation versus continuous positive airway pressure in the treatment of Cheyne-Stokes respiration in heart failure over a six month period. *Heart*. 2006;92(3):337-342.

64. Johnson KG, Johnson DC. Bilevel positive airway pressure worsens central apneas during sleep. *Chest*. 2005;128(4):2141-2150.

65. Morgenthaler TI, Kagramanov V, Hanak V, et al. Complex sleep apnea syndrome: Is it a unique clinical syndrome? *Sleep*. 2006;29(9):1203-1209.

66. Randerath WJ, Galetke W, Stieglitz S, et al. Adaptive servo-ventilation in patients with coexisting obstructive sleep apnoea/hypopnoea and Cheyne-Stokes respiration. *Sleep Med*. 2008;9(8):823-830.

67. Randerath WNG, Anduleit N, Treml M, Schäfer T, Galetke W. Long-term efficacy of adaptive servo-ventilation (ASV) in patients with co-existing obstructive sleep apnoea (OSAS) and Cheyne-Stokes respiration (CSR). A randomised CPAP-controlled trial. *Eur Respir J*. 2009;34:S38.

68. Javaheri S, Smith J, Chung E. The prevalence and natural history of complex sleep apnea. *J Clin Sleep Med*. 2009;5(3):205-211.

69. Allam JS, Olson EJ, Gay PC, et al. Efficacy of adaptive servoventilation in treatment of complex and central sleep apnea syndromes. *Chest*. 2007;132(6):1839-1846.

70. Glidewell RN, Orr WC, Imes N. Acetazolamide as an adjunct to CPAP treatment: A case of complex sleep apnea in a patient on long-acting opioid therapy. *J Clin Sleep Med*. 2009;5(1):63-64.

71. Farney RJ, Walker JM, Boyle KM, et al. Adaptive servoventilation (ASV) in patients with sleep disordered breathing associated with chronic opioid medications for non-malignant pain. *J Clin Sleep Med*. 2008;4(4): 311-319.

72. Javaheri S, Malik A, Smith J, et al. Adaptive pressure support servoventilation: A novel treatment for sleep apnea associated with use of opioids. *J Clin Sleep Med*. 2008;4(4):305-310.

Chapter 20

Nocturnal Ventilation in Chronic Hypercapnic Respiratory Diseases

SUSHMITA PAMIDI / BABAK MOKHLESI

CHRONIC HYPOVENTILATION

Hypoventilation is either acute or chronic and can be caused by a variety of disease states. Categorically, the causes of hypoventilation syndromes can be classified into lung diseases, either due to airway obstruction or parenchymal disorders, neuromuscular diseases, conditions that cause impairment of central ventilatory control, and chest wall deformities. In Figure 20-1, the more common causes of chronic hypoventilation syndromes are listed.

Mechanisms

The respiratory system has two main functions: providing oxygen (O_2) to the pulmonary capillary bed and removing carbon dioxide (CO_2) from the blood. The partial pressure of carbon dioxide ($Paco_2$) in the blood is directly proportional to its rate of production and is inversely proportional to alveolar ventilation. This relationship is represented by the following equation: $Paco_2 = (k)(Vco_2)/V_A$, where Vco_2 is the production of CO_2, k is a constant, and V_A reflects alveolar ventilation. Alveolar ventilation is the product of minute ventilation (respiratory rate times tidal volume) and the fraction of dead space ventilation. Therefore, there are three main mechanisms by which hypercapnia can develop: (1) an increase in CO_2 production relative to elimination, (2) a decrease in minute ventilation, or (3) an increase in the fraction of dead space ventilation. The most common cause of chronic hypercapnia is ventilatory failure, which is also termed *alveolar hypoventilation*.

Sleep, although restorative and beneficial to most people, can prove to be perilous for those with underlying disease that predisposes them to hypoventilate. In normal individuals, there is decreased responsiveness of the central chemoreceptors to chemical and mechanical inputs, particularly during rapid eye movement (REM) sleep.[1-3] As a result, ventilatory responsiveness to hypoxia and hypercapnia is decreased (Fig. 20-2). Moreover, respiratory muscle function is reduced during sleep, and even more profoundly during REM sleep. The supine position also leads to lower tidal volumes due to the abdominal contents pushing the diaphragm further into the thoracic cavity. Although these ventilatory changes do not cause significant gas exchange abnormalities in normal, healthy individuals, they can cause severe oxygen desaturation in patients with preexisting ventilatory abnormalities. Hypoxemia also occurs as a result of displacement of the oxygen in the alveoli from rising CO_2 levels.

Even though the respiratory system attempts to compensate initially for the ventilatory dysfunction during sleep, muscle fatigue with and without a blunted central chemoresponsiveness leads to sustained daytime hypoventilation. Once this occurs, the end result is daytime hypercapnia, which is associated with poor outcomes.

Obesity Hypoventilation Syndrome

Patients are diagnosed with obesity hypoventilation syndrome (OHS) if they have a combination of obesity (body mass index [BMI] $\geq$ 30 kg/m^2), awake hypoventilation ($Paco_2$ > 45 mm Hg at sea level) and sleep-disordered breathing, when other causes for hypoventilation have been excluded.[4] There is a higher risk of OHS with increasing BMI and it is unlikely to occur if the BMI is below 30 kg/m^2 (Fig. 20-3). Obstructive sleep apnea (OSA) coexists with OHS in 90% of cases. In the remaining 10% of cases, the sleep-disordered breathing is manifested simply as sleep hypoventilation, with a minimum increase in $Paco_2$ of greater than 10 mm Hg.[4]

Hypercapnia in OHS is entirely due to hypoventilation because, after short-term treatment with positive airway pressure, without alterations in body weight or dead space, there is improvement in hypercapnia in the majority of patients.[5] Figure 20-4 reveals the various mechanisms that are likely involved in developing hypoventilation in obese individuals. Patients who have OHS have unique physiologic differences from those with only obesity or OSA. For example, patients with OHS tend to have increased upper airway resistance,[6] an excessive mechanical load imposed on the respiratory system by obesity, atelectasis secondary to low lung volumes that leads to ventilatory-perfusion mismatching,[7] impaired central response to hypoxemia and hypercapnia, and sleep-disordered breathing. The key features to the pathogenesis of OHS, which have the most supporting

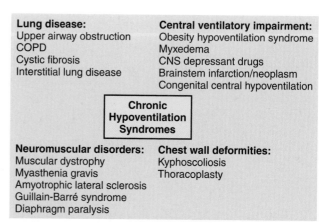

Lung disease:
Upper airway obstruction
COPD
Cystic fibrosis
Interstitial lung disease

Central ventilatory impairment:
Obesity hypoventilation syndrome
Myxedema
CNS depressant drugs
Brainstem infarction/neoplasm
Congenital central hypoventilation

Chronic Hypoventilation Syndromes

Neuromuscular disorders:
Muscular dystrophy
Myasthenia gravis
Amyotrophic lateral sclerosis
Guillain-Barré syndrome
Diaphragm paralysis

Chest wall deformities:
Kyphoscoliosis
Thoracoplasty

Figure 20-1 Common causes of chronic hypoventilation. COPD, chronic obstructive pulmonary disease; CNS, central nervous system.

evidence, are sleep-disordered breathing and a decreased central response to hypercapnia and hypoxia. In contrast to other conditions that lead to chronic hypercapnia, lung function is better preserved in patients with OHS (Fig. 20-5).[8]

Chronic Obstructive Pulmonary Disease

Respiratory diseases are a common cause of chronic hypoventilation syndromes. Most commonly, chronic obstructive pulmonary disease (COPD) can be associated with hypercapnia both in acute and chronic disease. COPD is a global problem and is one of the most common causes of death in the world.[9] COPD mortality rate is increasing and it will likely soon become the third leading cause of death worldwide.[9]

Acute exacerbations of COPD are a common scenario in which patients may become acutely hypercapnic. These patients become eucapnic once they are successfully treated and their lung function recovers. However, patients with severely reduced lung function during stable disease develop chronic ventilatory failure (defined when $Paco_2$ is persistently > 45 mm Hg at sea level) with a compensated respiratory acidosis.

In COPD, a number of mechanisms contribute to chronic hypoventilation. Owing to the mechanical disadvantage of the flattened diaphragm, the diaphragm is less effective at increasing lung volumes. During sleep, hypoxemia and hypercapnia often worsen in patients with COPD.[1] Decreased ventilatory drive, changes in ventilation-perfusion from decreased functional residual capacity, and increased airflow obstruction all

likely contribute to worsening gas exchange. REM sleep worsens hypoventilation even further because of the fall in respiratory drive and a decrease in tidal volumes. In a study of 19 patients with severe but stable COPD without significant sleep apnea, oxygen saturation (Sao_2) and transcutaneous Pco_2 ($Ptcco_2$) were monitored continuously throughout sleep. Sao_2 fell and $Ptcco_2$ increased during sleep, and these changes occurred maximally during REM sleep.[10] Loss of elastic recoil and air trapping can lead to increased intrathoracic pressure at functional residual capacity, also known as intrinsic positive end-expiratory pressure (iPEEP). This increased pressure can lead to increased inspiratory threshold load and thereby increase the work of breathing. O'Donoghue and colleagues were able to demonstrate a reduction in inspiratory muscle effort with high levels of continuous positive airway pressure (CPAP), where the extrinsic PEEP exceeded the iPEEP. CPAP or extrinsic PEEP allowed for a decrease in inspiratory threshold load and subsequent work of breathing.[11]

In contrast to patients with simple OSA, those with COPD and coexisting OSA, also known as the *overlap syndrome*, experience a more profound oxygen desaturation and a slower rate of reoxygenation during sleep. This is most likely related to the underlying lung disease leading to lower baseline oxygen saturation. Patients with overlap syndrome, therefore, are more prone to developing chronic hypoxemia, hypercapnia, and subsequent cor pulmonale compared to patients with either simple OSA or only COPD.[1] Indeed, patients with overlap syndrome develop hypercapnia at a lower BMI and apnea-hypopnea index (AHI) than OHS patients who do not have an obstructive defect on spirometry, and at a higher forced expiratory volume (FEV_1) than hypercapnic patients with pure COPD.

Chest Wall Deformities

Chest wall deformities, such as kyphoscoliosis, result in hypoventilation that is caused by a decrease in chest wall compliance from the restriction of the chest wall due to the abnormal spinal curvature. The work of breathing, therefore, tends to be higher than normal. This eventually leads to muscle fatigue and alveolar hypoventilation.[12] In addition,

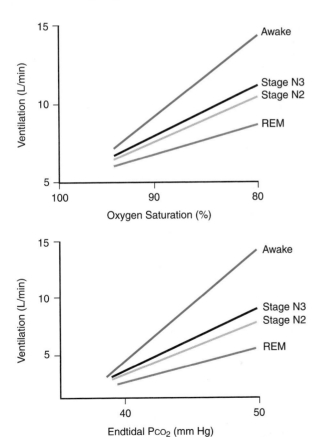

Figure 20-2 Varying responses in ventilation to hypoxia and hypercapnia depending on stage of sleep in normal subjects. Compared to wakefulness, the hypercapnic and hypoxic response is slightly blunted during non-REM sleep (stage N2 and stage N3). However, in REM sleep there is a significant reduction in the ventilatory drive. *REM,* rapid eye movement.

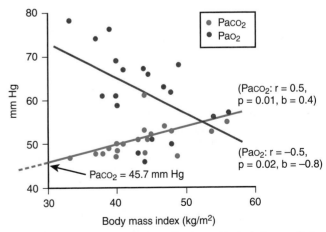

Figure 20-3 Summary of 19 case series of patients with obesity hypoventilation syndrome (OHS) in which the authors reported the mean body mass index (BMI) and arterial blood gases. The mean $Paco_2$ (*blue circles*) and Pao_2 (*gray circles*) are plotted against the BMI. Although there were no patients with BMI below 30 kg/m² in these series, if the regression line for $Paco_2$ is continued to a BMI of 30 kg/m² the $Paco_2$ would be 45.7 mm Hg. Therefore, hypercapnia is unlikely to develop if the BMI is less than 30 kg/m².

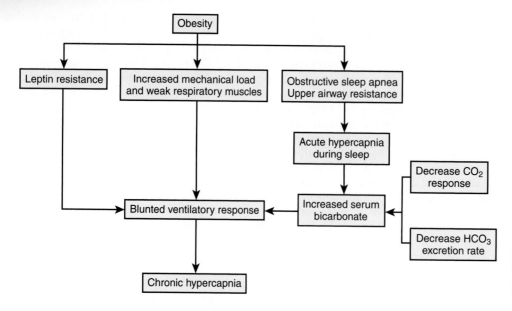

Figure 20-4 Mechanisms involved in the pathogenesis of obesity hypoventilation syndrome. CO_2: carbon dioxide, HCO_3: venous sodium bicarbonate

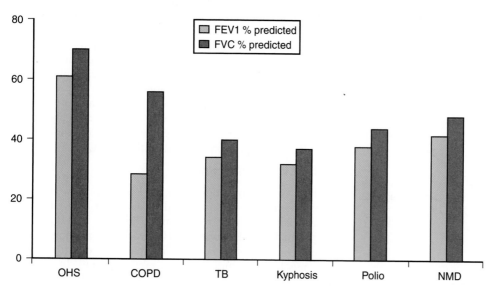

Figure 20-5 Spirometric results from patients receiving chronic noninvasive ventilation at home for hypoventilation ($n = 211$). Lung function is better preserved in OHS compared to other chronic diseases associated with hypercapnia. *KYPH*, kyphosis; *NMD*, neuromuscular disease; *OHS*, obesity hypoventilation syndrome; *TB*, post-tuberculosis. (Data from Janssens JP, Derivaz S, Breitenstein E, et al. Changing patterns in long-term noninvasive ventilation: A 7-year prospective study in the Geneva Lake area. *Chest.* 2003;123(1):67-79.)

the deformity of the chest wall also likely contributes to suboptimal function of the diaphragm owing to its mechanical disadvantage. In fact, Lisboa and colleagues measured transdiaphragmatic pressures in nine patients with kyphoscoliosis and demonstrated a positive correlation with inspiratory muscle weakness and resulting ventilatory failure.[13]

Ultimately, the end result of reduced chest wall compliance and ineffectiveness of the diaphragm is diminished tidal volume that leads to a reduction in ventilation. Although alveolar dead space is unchanged, the ratio of dead space to tidal volume (V_D/V_T) is increased as a result of the decreased tidal volumes. Most patients with kyphoscoliosis are asymptomatic, except when the curvature of the spine is most severely deformed. It remains unclear whether or not the degree of spinal curvature or muscle strength is a better determinant of disease severity.[14]

Neuromuscular Diseases

The mechanism underlying hypercapnia in patients suffering from neuromuscular disease (NMD) is not well understood, but is likely multifactorial. Some postulated mechanisms

include impairment of lung mechanics, ventilation-perfusion mismatch, a blunted central ventilatory drive, and respiratory-muscle fatigue.[15] As with many other ventilatory disorders, sleep-related hypoxemia in NMD occurs mostly in REM sleep or is more profound during REM sleep. The loss of accessory muscle contribution to breathing in the setting of diaphragmatic weakness is the main reason for worse ventilation during REM sleep.

In addition, in many NMDs, patients usually have inspiratory muscle weakness. Because the diaphragm is the most important muscle of inspiration, inspiratory muscle weakness is usually first manifested during sleep, when the patient is in the supine position. In particular, diaphragmatic weakness becomes obvious during REM sleep, when respiration is more dependent on the diaphragm. Also, with the upper airway muscles being weaker in NMD, a further decrease in neural input that occurs naturally during sleep increases the likelihood of upper airway obstruction.

Finally, NMD patients can have the added malfunction of expiratory muscle weakness, wherein the abdominal muscles

TABLE 20-1

Prevalence of Obesity Hypoventilation Syndrome in Patients with Obstructive Sleep Apnea

Study Author	N	Design	Country	Age (years)	BMI	AHI	OHS (%)
Verin[100]	218	Retrospective	France	55	34	51	10
Laaban[57]	1,141	Retrospective	France	56	34	55	11
Kessler[23]	254	Prospective	France	54	33	76	13
Resta[101]	219	Prospective	Italy	51	40	42	17
Golpe[102]	175	Retrospective	Spain	NA	32	42	14
Akashiba[103]	611	Retrospective	Japan	48	29	52	9
Mokhlesi[98]	359	Prospective	USA	48	43	62	20

Age, body mass index (BMI), and the apnea-hypopnea index (AHI) are means for all patients (OSA and OHS); values were calculated from the data provided by the study authors.
References cited in this table are listed at the end of the chapter.
Reprinted with permission from Mokhlesi B, Kryger MH, Grunstein RR. Assessment and management of patients with obesity hypoventilation syndrome. *Proc Am Thorac Soc.* 2008;5(2):218-225.

are unable to produce an effective cough. Also, swallowing function can often be compromised. Both of these consequences of NMD may not directly lead to hypoventilation, but are causes of potential respiratory failure from other mechanisms.

Prevalence

OHS is becoming more common due to the worsening epidemic in obesity. In the United States, the prevalence of obesity is approximately one third of the population, and the prevalence of extreme obesity (BMI ≥ 40 kg/m^2) has dramatically increased. In fact, there has been a fivefold increase in the prevalence of the BMI greater than or at 40 kg/m^2, resulting in 1 in 33 adults being extremely obese.[16] In various studies, the prevalence of OHS ranges between 10% and 20% in obese patients with OSA (Table 20-1), and this prevalence increases with the degree of obesity (Fig. 20-6). Although community-based studies on prevalence are lacking, the prevalence can be estimated among the general adult population in the United States. If approximately 3% of the general U.S. population has severe obesity (BMI ≥ 40 kg/m^2)[16] and half of patients with severe obesity have OSA,[17] and 10% to 20% of the severely obese patients with OSA have OHS, then a conservative estimated prevalence of OHS in the general adult population is anywhere between 0.15% to 0.3% (1.5 to 3 individuals out of 1000 adults).[18]

The prevalence of overlap syndrome (COPD and OSA) among consecutive patients with OSA has been reported to be between 10% and 15%.[19-21] The prevalence of COPD in patients with OSA, however, is similar to its prevalence in the general population.[22] There are no direct studies examining the prevalence of hypercapnic respiratory failure in patients with NMD and kyphoscoliosis.

Morbidity and Mortality Rates

If left untreated, chronic hypercapnia is associated with pulmonary hypertension and right-sided heart failure, which results in an increase in morbidity and mortality rates. In addition to these adverse cardiac consequences, chronic hypercapnia can result in daytime fatigue and hypersomnolence, as well as changes in psychological function. Prompt recognition of the disorder, in addition to urgent initiation of treatment, is pivotal for improving outcomes for hypoventilation syndromes.

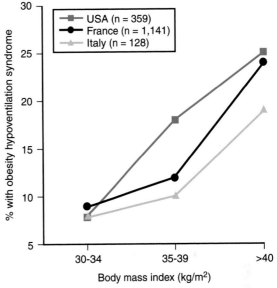

Figure 20-6 Prevalence of obesity hypoventilation syndrome (OHS) in patients with obstructive sleep apnea (OSA) by categories of body mass index (BMI) in the United States,[98] France,[57] and Italy. The data from Italy was provided by Professor Onofrio Resta from the University of Bari, Italy. In the study from the United States the mean BMI was 43 kg/m^2 and 60% of the subjects had a BMI above 40 kg/m^2. In contrast, the mean BMI in the French study was 34 kg/m^2, and 15% of the subjects had BMI above 40 kg/m^2. Consequently, OHS may be more prevalent in the United States compared to other nations because of its more exuberant obesity epidemic. (Redrawn from Mokhlesi B, Kryger MH, Grunstein RR. Assessment and management of patients with obesity hypoventilation syndrome. *Proc Am Thorac Soc.* 2008;5(2):218-225.)

A diagnosis of OHS reflects a worse prognosis than matched patients with sleep-disordered breathing who are eucapnic. OHS patients tend to be heavy users of health care resources, primarily because of the increased likelihood of suffering from severe life-threatening cardiopulmonary sequelae, such as pulmonary hypertension.[23-26] Prior to treatment, there is an increase in hospitalizations and intensive care unit (ICU) admissions among these patients when compared to obese patient control subjects.[27] In fact, Berg and colleagues demonstrated that 70% of OHS patients were admitted to the hospital at least once prior to the year of diagnosis. In contrast, after 2 years of treatment with positive airway pressure therapy,

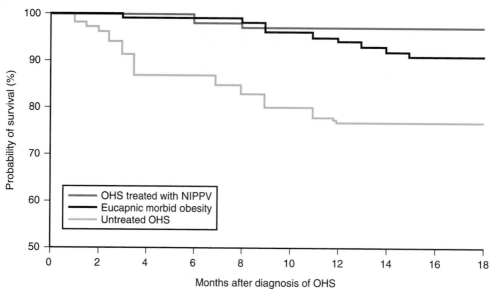

Figure 20-7 Survival curves for patients with untreated OHS ($n = 47$; mean age 55 ± 14; mean BMI 45 ± 9 kg/m²; mean $PaCO_2$ 52 ± 7 mm Hg) and eucapnic morbidly obese patients ($n = 103$; mean age 53 ± 13; mean BMI 42 ± 8 kg/m²) as reported by Nowbar and associates[28] compared to patients with OHS treated with NIPPV therapy ($n = 126$; mean age 55.6 ± 10.6; mean BMI 44.6 ± 7.8 kg/m²; mean baseline $PaCO_2$ 55.5 ± 7.7 mm Hg; mean adherence with NIPPV of 6.5 ± 2.3 h/day). Data for OHS patients treated with NIPPV was provided courtesy of Dr. Stephan Budweiser and colleagues from the University of Regensburg, Germany.[99] *BMI*, body mass index; *NIPPV*, noninvasive positive pressure ventilation; *OHS*, obesity hypoventilation syndrome. (Redrawn from Mokhlesi B, Kryger MH, Grunstein RR. Assessment and management of patients with obesity hypoventilation syndrome. *Proc Am Thorac Soc.* 2008;5(2):218-225.)

the number of hospital admissions decreased substantially to 15%. Moreover, Berg and colleagues demonstrated that patients with OHS tend to have more co-morbidities than obese control patients, including congestive heart failure, angina, and COPD.[27]

In addition to the increased morbidity rate that patients with OHS face, there is also an increased risk of death. A retrospective study reported that 46% of patients with OHS that refused long-term noninvasive positive pressure ventilation (NIPPV) therapy died during an average of a 50-month follow-up period.[21] In anther study, 47 severely obese patients were prospectively followed after hospital discharge.[28] There was an increase in the 18-month mortality rate for patients with untreated OHS when compared to the obese control group (23% vs. 9%). When adjusted for a number of factors including BMI, the hazard ratio of death in the OHS group was 4.0 in the 18-month period. Only 13% of the 47 patients were treated for OHS after hospital discharge. The difference in survival was evident as early as 3 months after hospital discharge. Figure 20-7 demonstrates these survival curves.

In COPD, chronic hypercapnia is seen when there is a severe reduction in lung function, particularly when the FEV_1 is less than 35% of predicted. The presence of chronic hypercapnia leads to a worse prognosis with approximately a 30% to 40% 2-year mortality rate.[29] In a prospective cohort study, adherence with CPAP therapy in patients with overlap syndrome was associated with higher survival rates in patients with moderate-to-severe OSA and hypoxemic COPD receiving long-term oxygen therapy.[30]

Untreated NMD associated with chronic hypoventilation also has a poor prognosis. Weakness of the respiratory muscles at diagnosis is a strong predictor of decreased quality of life in patients with amyotrophic lateral sclerosis.[31] These patients have a high propensity for respiratory failure, which often leads to death.[32]

Survival rate is decreased once patients with kyphoscoliosis develop chronic respiratory failure and hypercapnia. Those who receive long-term nocturnal ventilation have a significant improvement in survival compared to patients who simply receive nocturnal oxygen therapy. In a prospective study, Gustafson and colleagues followed 100 patients with kyphoscolisosis who received home ventilation and 144 patients who received oxygen therapy alone. Patients treated with home nocturnal ventilation experienced better survival, even when adjusting for age, gender, concomitant respiratory diseases, and blood gas levels, with a hazard ratio of 0.30 (95% confidence interval [CI], 0.18 to 0.51).[33]

VENTILATION IN SLEEP-DISORDERED BREATHING

Invasive Ventilation

Ventilation is considered invasive if it requires the presence of an endotracheal or tracheostomy tube. Noninvasive ventilation, on the other hand, occurs in the absence of either of these two interfaces.

The most common method of ventilation is positive pressure ventilation. In this technique positive airflow is forced into the patient's lungs via an endotracheal tube or mask, the latter of which is used in noninvasive ventilation. During expiration, the airflow is reduced and the lung and chest wall elastic forces allow for passive exhalation. During the poliomyelitis epidemic, negative pressure ventilation was employed in the 1940s and 1950s the "iron lung" ventilators.[34] In contrast to positive pressure ventilation, negative pressure ventilation mimics normal lung mechanics by allowing for inspiration with the creation of negative pressure around the chest wall through the use of a chamber that encloses the body but is sealed at the neck.

Expiration occurs when the negative pressure surrounding the chest is removed, thus allowing for the lung elastic recoil to allow for passive exhalation. Compared to positive pressure ventilators, negative pressure ventilators are generally less expensive and are less invasive by avoiding the need for tracheostomies.[35] However, they are generally less effective than positive pressure ventilators, and fitting of the ventilator can be challenging in patients with chest wall deformities. Additionally, they are ineffective during upper airway obstruction, or when there is aspiration risk due to poor coordination for swallowing.[36]

Invasive mechanical ventilation has been shown to be an effective therapy in NMD and chest wall deformities in which patients have daytime hypercapnia and nocturnal desaturation.[37] However, treatment of mechanical ventilation for chronic respiratory disease used to necessitate hospital admission. Gradually, home mechanical ventilation was shown to provide equal effectiveness of therapy, with the advantage of increased patient comfort, and significant psychological benefit to patients and their caregivers.[36,37] Depending on the level of nursing care, cost was also found to be decreased with home mechanical ventilation.[36] Home mechanical ventilation became more routine for patients with amyotrophic lateral sclerosis (ALS), poliomyelitis, post-tuberculosis, and severe kyphoscoliosis during the 1980s.[37,38]

Despite success in the use of invasive mechanical ventilation, the cost and invasive nature of tracheostomies, in addition to the cumbersome devices, prompted the rise in popularity of noninvasive ventilatory methods. In fact, currently, NIPPV is the predominant technique for long-term home ventilation.[39]

Noninvasive Positive Pressure Ventilation

Advantages of NIPPV over invasive ventilation include better tolerance and superior comfort, preservation of airway defenses, speech and swallowing functions, and avoidance of airway trauma. In addition, there is mounting evidence to support that NIPPV is as effective as invasive mechanical ventilation in treating patients with chronic hypoventilation syndromes.

Long-term nocturnal NIPPV should be considered the standard of care for a select group of patients with sleep-disordered breathing and chronic respiratory failure. In patients suffering from NMD and kyphoscoliosis, long-term NIPPV has demonstrated improvements in blood gases and health status and a decrease in hospitalizations for respiratory illness.[40,41] Other disease states in which sleep-disordered breathing occurs concomitantly with chronic respiratory failure, such as OHS, also demonstrate improved outcomes after treatment with nocturnal NIPPV.[21,40]

NIPPV has evolved significantly since its inception in the 1980s and has thus been gaining popularity for the treatment of both acute and chronic respiratory failure. When feasible to implement, it has assumed an important role in the management of chronic respiratory failure.

Mechanism of Action of Noninvasive Ventilation

The most common modality of NIPPV is bilevel positive airway pressure (bilevel PAP) in portable home ventilators, and it simply refers to the intermittent delivery of positive pressure during each breath cycle. The higher positive pressure that is delivered during inspiration is called inspiratory positive airway pressure (IPAP). During expiration, the positive pressure is lowered, and this is referred to as the expiratory positive airway pressure (EPAP). The difference between the IPAP and EPAP reflects the level of pressure support that the patient is receiving. Moreover, the drop in pressure during expiration enhances patient comfort because it is easier to exhale at lower pressures. In contrast, a CPAP device delivers a constant pressure throughout the respiratory cycle. CPAP is similar to EPAP that is delivered during bilevel PAP ventilation.

In the spontaneous mode without a backup rate, NIPPV devices detect inspiratory effort when a patient inhales. Once triggered, the ventilator delivers a preset IPAP during inspiration. The increase in positive airway pressure during inspiration unloads the work of the diaphragm and decreases the work of breathing. Inhalation is terminated when the flow decreases below the threshold for the machine. At that point the pressure is reduced to the preset EPAP for expiration.

NIPPV is helpful in conditions where there is progression to chronic ventilatory failure. Patients with chronic hypoventilation often present with isolated nocturnal or sleep-related hypoventilation. As a consequence of this, patients may experience symptoms such as daytime hypersomnolence, unrefreshing sleep, and morning headaches. NIPPV can offer various levels of support depending on the underlying disease. Some disease states result in complete paralysis and will require continuous support with a set backup respiratory rate (timed mode) so that the patient will not need to trigger a breath. On the other hand, in early ALS or in OHS, patients often will not require a backup respiratory rate and the patient's spontaneous breaths will be supported by positive airway pressure delivered by the NIPPV.

In various conditions, such as NMD, OHS, or COPD, there is increased work of breathing either due to respiratory muscle weakness, restrictive chest wall mechanics, or increased airway resistance. Due to the resulting ineffective ventilation from respiratory muscle fatigue and poor lung mechanics, CO_2 retention increases more than what normally occurs with sleep onset. In addition, the CO_2 retention worsens during REM sleep. Eventually, as a compensatory mechanism, CO_2 retention results in bicarbonate retention by the kidney. This increase in serum bicarbonate further decreases respiratory drive and can contribute to a vicious circle of CO_2 retention. Over time, the increase in CO_2 and concomitant hypoxemia from hypoventilation can lead to cor pulmonale and death if left untreated.

NIPPV use for as little as 4 to 5 hours per night can put a stop to and even reverse this vicious circle of CO_2 retention, hypoventilation, and decreased CO_2 responsiveness and respiratory drive. With NIPPV, gas exchange is stabilized and symptoms of hypersomnolence, daytime headaches, and poor sleep quality are relieved.[42]

The exact mechanism by which nocturnal use of NIPPV leads to resolution of daytime hypoventilation is unknown. Many have postulated that nocturnal NIPPV allows for respiratory muscle rest and recovery, which then lead to improved muscle function and ventilation during the daytime. Although the majority of studies have not been able to demonstrate improved muscle function, there have been several studies that have demonstrated an improvement or even normalization of CO_2 responsiveness and respiratory drive after several weeks of nocturnal NIPPV in patients with OHS. More than likely, there is more than just one mechanism that is responsible for the effectiveness of NIPPV.

INTRODUCTION TO EQUIPMENT

Critical Care versus Portable Ventilators

In order to ensure success with NIPPV, the settings and equipment need to be tailored to the individual patient. Unlike the ICU patient in whom sedation is used and the level of consciousness is often reduced, patients on chronic NIPPV are conscious and more sensitive to the mode of ventilation and interface used. If ineffective ventilation is provided to the patient or if the interface is uncomfortable, sleep may be disrupted even further and adherence to NIPPV will be severely compromised. Therefore, it is imperative to have an understanding of the different ventilatory modes, settings, and interfaces to choose from.

NIPPV can be given by conventional ventilators in ICUs or by portable pressure ventilators. ICU ventilators have elaborate monitoring and will allow for the detection of patient-ventilator dysynchrony based on visualization of the flow and pressure waveforms. However, these ventilators are also equipped with highly sensitive alarms that will be triggered in the presence of even minor and clinically insignificant air leaks. The bilevel PAP device is less cumbersome for long-term home ventilation because there is only a single limb circuit and single valve for inspiration and expiration, rather than separate inspiratory and expiratory limbs in the classical critical care ventilators.

Method of Ventilation

Ventilators are classified according to how they deliver gas flow, which is either pressure-cycled or volume-cycled. In the ICU, the ventilators provide both options. The portable ventilators, on the other hand, provide ventilation by either pressure-cycled mode (pressure-preset ventilation) or volume-cycled mode (volume-preset ventilation).

Pressure-preset machines deliver a preselected pressure irrespective of the lung properties of that particular patient. However, the volume delivered may be variable because it is determined by the lung mechanics, such as the compliance and resistance of the system. If there is a leak in the circuit, then there is usually a drop in the volume delivered to the patient because the preset pressure will not be achieved. However, the flow generator automatically increases flow to adjust for a certain degree of leakage in order to maintain the preset pressure. These devices cannot maintain the preset pressure with very large leaks.

Volume-preset ventilation, on the other hand, delivers a fixed tidal volume and will generate the pressure necessary to produce this volume. The pressure is variable and depends on lung mechanics, but the volume will not change despite varying patient effort. However, if there is increased impedance to inflation, then the pressures may be increased substantially in order to achieve the preset volume. The increase in pressure can be uncomfortable for patients, particularly when the impedance increases simply due to swallowing or coughing. In addition, if there is a leak during volume-preset ventilation, then there will be no increase in flow to compensate and a suboptimal volume will be delivered to the patient.

To determine if there is a significant difference between volume-preset and pressure-preset ventilation, a randomized crossover trial was conducted on 15 patients with chronic ventilatory failure who were given either a pressure-preset or volume-preset ventilator for 6 weeks and then switched to the alternate mode after this period of time.[43] The results revealed similar outcomes with respect to gas exchange. However, the variance in the peak inspiratory pressures was lower and there were fewer gastrointestinal side effects, such as gastric distention and flatulence, with pressure-preset NIPPV than volume-preset NIPPV.[43] Results from the Eurovent survey, a European prevalence study on home mechanical ventilation in 16 countries, revealed that pressure-preset ventilation was the preferred ventilator type by clinicians.[39]

Average volume-assured pressure support (AVAPS) is a newer method of ventilation, which combines the features of both pressure-preset and volume-preset ventilators. AVAPS has been shown to be effective in OHS patients.[44] Patients have the comfort of pressure-preset ventilation but the device is able to deliver a stable and consistent tidal volume. The device is able to estimate the expiratory tidal volume based on pneumotachographic inspiratory and expiratory flows. The IPAP support is variable because it is titrated in steps of 1 cm H_2O/minute in order to achieve the preset tidal volume. The EPAP on the other hand is constant and is typically set between 4 and 8 cm H_2O and occurs throughout the respiratory cycle. The respiratory backup rate can be set at 12 to 18 breaths per minute with an inspiratory/expiratory ratio (I:E) of 1:2. However, the role of a backup rate remains unclear because patients with OHS are typically tachypneic during sleep with respiratory rates ranging between 15 and 30 breaths/min. However, it is conceivable that during titration central apneas could develop with pressure support ventilation and in those instances a backup rate would be useful. Although significantly more expensive than CPAP or bilevel PAP therapy, AVAPS has been shown to be effective in a randomized controlled study of OHS patients with milder degrees of hypercapnia.[44]

Modes of Ventilation

There are three main modes of ventilation: (1) the *control* or *timed (T)* mode refers to the start and stop of the ventilator as entirely set by the clinician; (2) the *assist-control* or *spontaneous-timed (ST)* mode allows the patient to initiate a breath, but if there is absence of initiation within a preset interval of time, then the machine delivers a breath; and (3) the *assist* or *spontaneous* mode *(S)* refers to the patient controlling the initiation and cessation of all breaths. The third mode is possible only with pressure-preset ventilation.

When patients do not require a backup safety respiratory rate, then the ventilator can be set in the spontaneous mode. Patients on the spontaneous mode generally have a regular breathing pattern and do not have significant central apneas or difficulty triggering the ventilator with their spontaneous breaths. In addition, patients have control over their inspiratory and expiratory times.

If the patient needs full ventilatory support, then the control or timed mode is selected. This means that no patient effort is required to initiate breath delivery by the NIPPV machine. In acute and chronic respiratory failure, the timed modes may be used if a patient has an unreliable respiratory effort, unstable ventilatory drive or mechanics, or severe respiratory muscle weakness, or when the spontaneous mode fails to augment spontaneous breathing. The breathing frequency, however,

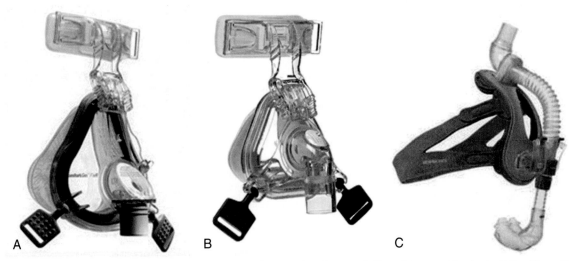

Figure 20-8 Common mask interfaces. **A,** Oronasal or full face mask. **B,** Nasal mask. **C,** Nasal pillows. (Courtesy of Respironics/Philips, Murrysville, PA.)

needs to be set slightly higher than the patient's spontaneous breathing rate in order to avoid patient-ventilatory dysynchrony. Very high respiratory rates will, on the other hand, increase patient-ventilator dysynchrony.

In the spontaneous-timed mode, the machine provides ventilatory support in response to the patient's breathing effort. However, there is a backup respiratory rate if the patient is not able to trigger the machine or if there is a central apnea. In this setting, unlike in the timed mode, the backup rate is set slightly below the spontaneous breathing rate. The percentage of breaths that will be spontaneous and the percentage that will be timed will depend on the setting of the backup rate.

Finally, if only a constant pressure is required throughout the expiratory cycle, then CPAP is used. These patients need to be able to breathe spontaneously. This setting is primarily used in cardiogenic pulmonary edema or obstructive sleep apnea. CPAP has had variable success in treating central sleep apnea or other causes of hypoxemic respiratory failure.

Triggering

To work most effectively, NIPPV ventilators should be synchronized with the patient's breathing. Ventilators can either be flow- or pressure-triggered. If the trigger is too sensitive, then there will be autotriggering. Air or mask leaks can also cause autotriggering. If the trigger is insensitive, then this can lead to an increase work of breathing for the patient since the machine is not supporting the patient's breath. A flow-triggered mechanism has been shown to decrease the work of breathing in invasive mechanical ventilation.[45]

Rise Time

The ventilator's ability to meet the flow demands of the patient is also of utmost importance in enhancing the comfort of the patient. The time to reach the preset inspiratory pressure is known as the rise time. Depending on the type of ventilator being used, the rise time may be manually adjusted. For patients with obstructive lung disease, a short rise time would be beneficial in order to maximize expiration time due to hyperinflation. On the other hand, patients with

neuromuscular disease often prefer a slightly prolonged rise time because of the decreased compliance of the chest wall.

Interfaces

A major determining factor in the success of NIPPV is the type of interface used. Not only does the interface strongly affect the patient's comfort and adherence to therapy,[46] but it also influences the effectiveness of NIPPV, depending on the amount of leak that is associated with it. If the mask fit is not optimal for a patient, problems such as pressure ulcers, rash, and eye irritation can occur.

Over the past few years, the industry has grown substantially, and now a variety of interfaces are available for patients to choose from. Full-face masks, nasal masks, and nasal pillows are the main interfaces to select from (Fig. 20-8). Advantages and disadvantages to each of these are listed in Table 20-2. Many of the newer models are less cumbersome and more comfortable for patients.

In general, the ideal interface for a particular patient depends on: (1) comfort of the fit, (2) minimization of mask leaks, and (3) ease of implementation. The ideal interface for a particular patient is dependent on the specific shape, size, and anatomy of the patient's face. Obviously, what may be right for one patient may be completely unsuitable for another patient. Moreover, if a patient is claustrophobic, a full-face mask is generally not preferable. In this situation, patients may find that the nasal pillows are a more tolerable option. Patients experiencing an acute-on-chronic exacerbation of their baseline chronic hypercapnic respiratory failure typically require a full-face mask because of significant mouth-breathing with dyspnea.

Complications

Air leaks can be a major factor in decreasing the efficacy of NIPPV. These leaks can consist of mask leaks that exist between the interface and the skin, and mouth leaks with nasal ventilation. In addition, leaks can contribute to decreased patient tolerance, increase in patient-ventilator asynchrony, and increased sleep fragmentation.[47,48] Meyer and colleagues also demonstrated that the presence of leaks diminished sleep

TABLE 20-2

Advantages and Disadvantages of Commonly Used Noninvasive Positive Pressure Ventilation Interfaces

Type of Interface	Description	Advantage(s)	Disadvantage(s)
Nasal mask	Covers the nose but not the mouth	• Easier to speak, eat, and cough • Less risk of aspiration with vomiting • Decreased claustrophobia • Decreased gastric distention	• Ineffective if patient is a mouth breather • Less effective with increased nasal resistance
Nasal pillows	Plugs inserted into the nostrils	• Good for claustrophobic patients	• Increased leak than nasal mask • Not good at higher pressures
Oronasal (full face mask)	Covers the nose and mouth	• Preferred in acute respiratory failure (patients often breathe through mouth) • If patient is a mouth breather or has increased nasal resistance	• Less patient tolerance than for nasal mask • Increased leak than nasal mask • Increased risk for aspiration if patient is vomiting
Helmet	Covers the whole head and all or part of the neck; no contact with the face or head Secured with armpit straps	• Less resistance to flow • Suitable regardless of facial shape, presence of trauma • Less need for patient cooperation	• Not good for claustrophobic patients • Poor humidification • Dry eyes

quality by increasing arousals, reducing sleep efficiency, and reducing the percentages of both REM and slow wave sleep.[49] With a pressure-preset NIPPV device, leaks can decrease the likelihood of receiving the appropriately prescribed pressure. Ensuring a tight mask-face seal is an important step in preventing leaks. However, overtightening is detrimental and can result in decreased tissue perfusion and eventual skin damage. Excessive tightening, in turn, can even further increase the degree of air leaks.

If the inspired gas in NIPPV is not humidified, the cool and dry air can lead to significant dryness of the airway epithelium because expiration is no longer able to provide moisture in the presence of unidirectional high-flow air. With time, the nasal mucosa can lose its capacity to heat and humidify the inspired air, and it progressively dries. In addition, inflammatory mediators are then released which is associated with a resultant increase in vascularity that can result in eventual problems of nasal congestion and rhinorrhea. As a result, heated humidification has become standard practice on most machines. In patients with OSA treated with CPAP, which may be extrapolated to patients on NIPPV, there was increased objective adherence with CPAP in patients who used heated humidification compared to those with cool air humidifiers or no humidification.[50] In addition, patients were more satisfied with CPAP when it was used with humidity. Side effects of dry mouth, dry nose, and dry throat were reported less frequently with the humidity.

Skin breakdown is also a major issue if the fit of the masks are too tight. It is important to get an appropriate seal on the mask without decreasing tissue perfusion. Some will advocate for rotating between different masks to decrease the risk for skin irritation.

Oxygen Supplementation

It is challenging to deliver a precise level of inspired oxygen concentration with portable ventilators. Oxygen can be added to the inspiratory circuit or the mask itself. However, the delivered oxygen concentration to the patient is often not consistent with the set oxygen flow rate or concentration. The most important reason for this is the dilution of oxygen with higher flow rates of air, but other factors such as location of leak and site of oxygen injection also affect its delivery rate.[51,52] Moreover, delivering high concentrations of oxygen is often not possible with portable ventilators. If oxygenation is severely compromised, then critical care ventilators or those with a home blender are preferred.

NONINVASIVE POSITIVE PRESSURE VENTILATION IN VARIOUS DISEASE STATES

Initiation of Noninvasive Ventilation

The criteria used for initiation of NIPPV will vary according to the underlying chronic respiratory condition. In many progressive chronic hypoventilation syndromes such as NMD, the onset of respiratory failure is typically first seen at night. *Nocturnal NIPPV* typically refers to ventilation during sleep, and does not refer to ventilation that is required for more than 12 to 24 hours per day. However, patients with progressive diseases, such as NMD, will extend the hours of use to include daytime NIPPV in addition to nocturnal therapy.

Daytime hypoventilation is defined by the following: an abnormally elevated $Paco_2$, a high serum bicarbonate level, and a relatively normal pH, which in turn is associated with a reduction in Pao_2 because of hypoventilation. When chronic daytime hypoventilation occurs, it is an indicator of worse sleep-related hypoventilation. In clinical practice, clues to hypoventilation include symptoms of orthopnea, particularly in patients with diaphragmatic weakness or dysfunction. Complaints of poor sleep quality, including insomnia and frequent arousals, can also occur. Nocturnal or early morning headaches are common complaints. Finally, patients notice daytime fatigue, drowsiness, sleepiness, loss of energy, and decrease in intellectual performance. In patients with NMD, nocturnal NIPPV is typically instituted electively as an outpatient without necessarily performing an overnight

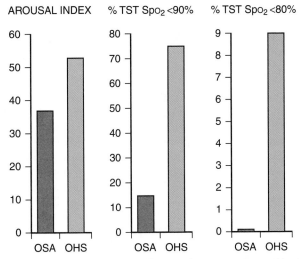

Figure 20-9 Polysomnographic differences between patients with OHS ($n = 23$) and patients with OSA ($n = 23$) matched for age, BMI, AHI, and lung function (FVC and FEV_1 % of predicted). Patients with OHS have severe nocturnal hypoxemia and spend a significant percentage of total sleep time (TST) with oxygen saturations (SpO_2) below 90% and 80%. In fact, none of the patients with eucapnic OSA had continuous oxygen saturations below 80%. Therefore, the severity of nocturnal hypoxemia is a useful tool suggesting OHS when a sleep physician is interpreting a polysomnogram of a patient not seen in clinic or when there is no additional information on blood gases. AHI, apnea-hypopnea index; BMI, body mass index; FEV, forced expiratory volume; FVC, forced vital capacity; OHS, obesity hypoventilation syndrome; OSA, obstructive sleep apnea. (Data from Banerjee D, Yee BJ, Piper AJ, et al. Obesity hypoventilation syndrome: Hypoxemia during continuous positive airway pressure. Chest. 2007;131(6):1678-184.)

polysomnogram (PSG) with positive airway pressure titration. However, if OSA or OHS is suspected, or if there is a lack of improvement in symptoms with NIPPV, an in-laboratory diagnostic PSG and positive airway titration should be strongly considered.

Overnight PSGs can help in documenting obstructive or central apneas and hypopneas in addition to nocturnal hypoventilation. With continuous recording of CO_2 (end-tidal or transcutaneous) and pulse oximetry (SpO_2), nocturnal hypoventilation can be seen throughout the study, or in the early stage, exclusively during REM sleep. A useful tool for a sleep physician interpreting a PSG of a patient they have not seen in clinic may be the percentage of total sleep time (% TST) with SpO_2 spent below 90%. In a recent meta-analysis, the mean difference of %TST with SpO_2 spent below 90% was 37.4% (56.2% for hypercapnic patients, 18.8% for eucapnic OSA patients) with very little overlap in the 95% confidence intervals.[53] In another study, Banerjee and colleagues prospectively compared sleep parameters in 23 patients with OHS (mean $PaCO_2$ 54 mm Hg) to 23 patients with eucapnic OSA by performing overnight in-laboratory polysomnography.[54] These two groups were matched for age (mean 45 vs. 43 years), BMI (58.7 vs. 59.9 kg/m²), AHI (49.6 vs. 39.4 events/hour), and forced vital capacity percentage of predicted values (69% vs. 74%). The only significant polysomnographic difference between these two well-matched groups was the severity of nocturnal hypoxemia (Fig. 20-9).

Inpatient admission may not always be necessary in order to start NIPPV for patients who develop chronic hypoventilation. A randomized controlled study demonstrated similar efficacy in either home-initiated or inpatient-initiated NIPPV in patients with NMD or chest wall deformities with chronic hypoventilation.[55]

Obesity Hypoventilation Syndrome

The main strategies for treatment of OHS include relieving upper airway obstruction and enhancing ventilation. Although no formal guidelines exist for treatment, algorithms for treatment have been proposed that suggest specific treatment approaches based on the stability of the patient, degree and acuity of respiratory acidosis, and severity of underlying obstructive sleep apnea.[4]

Positive Airway Pressure Therapy

Positive airway pressure, in the form of CPAP therapy, was first described in the treatment of OHS in 1982.[56] Although subsequent studies confirmed its efficacy, failure of CPAP in some cases has led to uncertainty whether CPAP should be attempted initially or if bilevel PAP is a better modality.[5,56-59] In a recent prospective study of outpatients with severe OHS—based on the severity of obesity, OSA, and the degree of hypercapnia—57% of patients were titrated successfully with CPAP alone, and the mean pressure required was 13.9 cm H_2O.[54] The remainder had greater than 20% of TST with an arterial O_2 saturation of less than 90%, although they also had a residual AHI of 25. The CPAP failure group was more obese, although both groups were extremely obese. Because this was a single-night titration study, the question of whether residual hypoxemia would resolve with long-term treatment was left unanswered.[60]

A recent prospective randomized study performed by Piper and associates[61] compared the long-term efficacy of bilevel PAP and CPAP. In this study, 45 consecutive patients with OHS underwent a full night of CPAP titration. Nine patients (20%) were excluded because of persistent hypoxemia—arbitrarily defined as 10 continuous minutes of SpO_2 less than 80% without frank apneas—during the CPAP titration. The remaining 36 patients who had a successful CPAP titration night were subsequently randomized to either CPAP ($n = 18$) or bilevel PAP ($n = 18$). Those randomized to bilevel PAP underwent an additional titration night to establish the effective inspiratory and expiratory pressures. Supplemental oxygen administration was necessary in three patients in the CPAP group and four in the bilevel PAP group. After 3 months, there was no significant difference between the groups in adherence with PAP therapy or in improvement in daytime sleepiness, hypoxemia, or hypercapnia. This study confirms that the majority of patients with OHS (80%) can be successfully titrated with CPAP. Their findings also suggest that as long as OSA and nocturnal hypoxemia is effectively treated with CPAP, it makes no significant difference at 3 months if patients are given bilevel PAP or CPAP therapy. Therefore, bilevel PAP is not superior to CPAP a priori; rather, treatment should be individualized to each patient. Bilevel PAP should be instituted if the patient is intolerant of higher CPAP pressures (>15 cm H_2O) that may be required to resolve apneas and hypopneas or if hypoxemia is persistent despite adequate resolution of obstructive respiratory events during the titration study.[62] During bilevel PAP titration, the IPAP should be at least 8 to 10 cm H_2O above the EPAP in order to effectively increase ventilation.[21,63-65] In the minority of patients with OHS who do not have OSA, EPAP can be set at 5 cm H_2O and IPAP can be titrated to improve ventilation.[64,65] Bilevel PAP should also be considered if the $Paco_2$ does not normalize after 3 months of therapy with CPAP.

Adherence with Positive Airway Pressure Therapy

Adherence with positive airway pressure (PAP) therapy is directly correlated with improvement in daytime arterial blood gas values. In a retrospective study of 75 outpatients with stable OHS, the $Paco_2$ decreased by 1.8 mm Hg and the Pao_2 increased by 3 mm Hg per hour of daily CPAP or bilevel PAP use during the last 30 days before a repeated measurement of arterial blood gases. Patients who used PAP therapy for more than 4.5 hours per day had a considerably greater improvement in blood gases than less adherent patients ($\Delta Paco_2$ 7.7 ± 5 vs. 2.4 ± 4 mm Hg, $p < 0.001$; ΔPao_2 9.2 ± 11 vs. 1.8 ± 9 mm Hg, $p < 0.001$). In addition, the need for daytime oxygen therapy decreased from 30% of patients to 6%.[58] There was no significant difference in improvement of hypercapnia and hypoxemia between patients on CPAP ($n = 48$) and patients on bilevel PAP therapy ($n = 27$). Improvement in blood gas values may be seen as early as 1 month after the institution of PAP therapy.[58,66,67]

The impact of long-term PAP on vital capacity and lung volumes is contradictory. Several studies have reported no change in lung volumes or forced vital capacity (FVC) after successful treatment of OHS with bilevel PAP.[21,68,69] In contrast, two studies of patients with OHS reported significant improvements in vital capacity and expiratory reserve volume after 12 months of NIPPV without any significant changes in BMI or in FEV_1/FVC ratio.[65,70]

Lack of Improvement in Hypercapnia with Positive Airway Pressure Therapy

The most common reason for persistent hypercapnia in patients with OHS is lack of adherence with PAP therapy. However, other possibilities need to be entertained if there is documented evidence of adequate adherence by objective monitoring of PAP devices such as inadequate PAP titration, CPAP failure in patients with OHS who do not have significant OSA, other causes of hypercapnia (e.g., COPD), or metabolic alkalosis due to high doses of loop diuretics.

The improvement in chronic daytime hypercapnia in patients that are adherent with PAP therapy is neither universal nor complete. In two studies,[58,61] the $Paco_2$ did not improve significantly in approximately a quarter of patients that had undergone successful PAP titration in the laboratory and were highly adherent (> 6 hours/night) with either CPAP or bilevel PAP therapy. In one study, 8 patients (23%) among the 34 patients who used PAP for at least 4.5 hours per day did not have a significant improvement in their $Paco_2$ (decrease in $Paco_2$ of less than 4 mm Hg). These nonresponders had a lower AHI compared to responders (44 ± 45 vs. 86 ± 47 per hour, $p = 0.03$). Mean adherence with PAP therapy was 7.2 ± 2.1 hours per day for nonresponders versus 6.0 ± 1.7 hours per day for responders ($p = 0.1$).[58]

In summary, there are three categories within the spectrum of OHS: (1) CPAP responders, (2) partial responders to CPAP or bilevel PAP (25% of patients), and (3) nonresponders to CPAP and bilevel PAP (pure hypoventilators without any concomitant OSA). This lack of response or partial response to PAP therapy combined with reports of persistent hypoventilation after tracheostomy[63] suggests that in a subset of patients

with OHS, factors other than sleep-disordered breathing are the driving force behind the pathogenesis of hypoventilation. These patients will most likely need more aggressive nocturnal mechanical ventilation with or without respiratory stimulants.

Positive Airway Pressure Titration Algorithms

There are two strategies for titrating NIPPV or bilevel PAP in patients with OHS. One strategy is to increase the EPAP to eliminate all obstructive events, including apneas, hypopneas, and flow limitation. At this point, IPAP can be increased with the goal of improving oxygenation or transcutaneous CO_2 (if available). With this approach, there is less room to augment ventilation by increasing the IPAP if a patient requires a high EPAP level. The second strategy consists of increasing EPAP only to eliminate obstructive apneas. Once apneas are eliminated, the IPAP is increased to eliminate hypopneas and flow limitation. A higher delta between IPAP and EPAP can be achieved with this approach leading to increased pressure support and higher tidal volumes. There are no studies that have compared these two PAP titration algorithms. However, in studies that have demonstrated return to eucapnia and normoxia after a few weeks or months of bilevel PAP treatment, the IPAP was 8 to 10 cm H_2O above the EPAP.[21,63,65] In more rare cases, in which patients do not have OSA but have only OHS, the EPAP need not be increased above 5 cm H_2O. However, the IPAP may be started at 13 cm H_2O and titrated up in order to augment tidal volume and improve ventilation and hypoxemia.

As mentioned previously in this chapter, AVAPS is an alternative hybrid mode of ventilation that provides more consistent tidal volumes. Advantages to this mode of ventilation include better patient-ventilator synchrony and a reduction in muscle workload. In a prospective study by Storre and colleagues, patients who failed CPAP therapy and then used AVAPS derived additional benefit when compared to bilevel PAP spontaneous/timed mode ventilation.[44] In particular, there was a more significant decline in transcutaneous CO_2. Among patients that failed CPAP, bilevel PAP spontaneous/time mode ventilation (with a backup rate) improved oxygenation, sleep quality, and health-related quality of life significantly more than just CPAP alone.

Intensive Care Unit Management

Given the high morbidity and mortality rates of patients with OHS, ICU admissions occur frequently when patients with OHS are admitted to the hospital. Guidelines for management of patients with OHS have not been formalized. However, in general, those with a pH below 7.30 should be monitored in an ICU setting, while those with a pH above 7.30 and without significant obtundation can be managed in a noninvasive respiratory care unit or step-down unit with close supervision.[71] Once the patient has recovered from the acute exacerbation, a full pulmonary function test (PFT) should be performed to exclude other potential causes of hypercapnia, such as severe chest wall disease, obstructive and restrictive lung disease, neuromuscular disease, CNS structural disease, and idiopathic central hypoventilation. Figure 20-10 provides a general approach to patients with OHS experiencing an acute-on-chronic exacerbation of hypercapnic respiratory failure.

The importance of careful observation of the acutely hypercapnic obese patient using NIPPV cannot be overemphasized, as potential catastrophes such as massive aspiration, unnoticed progressive respiratory failure, and even death can result

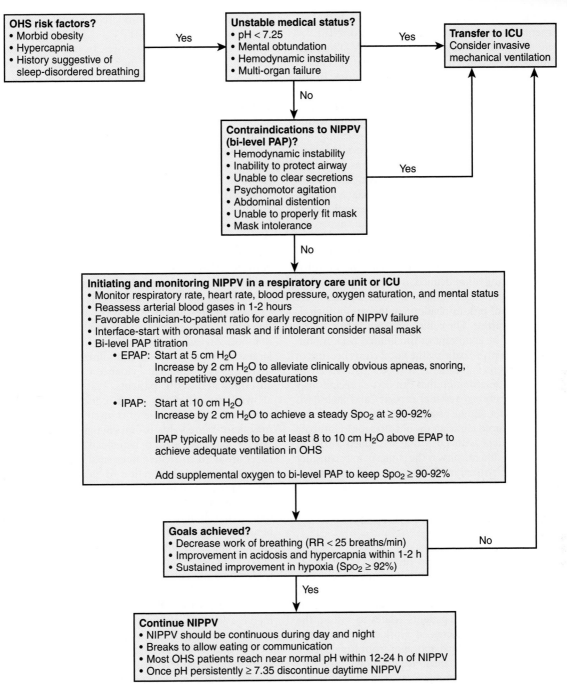

Figure 20-10 Management of patients with obesity hypoventilation syndrome (OHS) requiring hospitalization due to acute-on-chronic hypercapnic respiratory failure. *Bilevel PAP*, bilevel positive airway pressure. *EPAP*, expiratory positive airway pressure; *IPAP*, inspiratory positive airway pressure; *NIPPV*, noninvasive positive pressure ventilation; *RR*, respiratory rate; *Spo₂*, oxygen saturation by pulse oximetry. (Redrawn from Mokhlesi B, Kryger MH, Grunstein RR. Assessment and management of patients with obesity hypoventilation syndrome. *Proc Am Thorac Soc.* 2008;5(2):218-225.)

if inadequately supervised. The authors' experience is similar to prior studies in that NIPPV is as labor intensive as endotracheal intubation and invasive mechanical ventilation.[72] Therefore, a multidisciplinary approach involving skilled nurses, respiratory therapists, and intensivists are crucial to successful titration of NIPPV.[73] In addition, institutions that have successfully implemented NIPPV programs for patients with acute-on-chronic hypercapnic respiratory failure have established a centralized monitoring unit with a favorable nurse-to-patient ratio to ensure early recognition of NIPPV failure requiring invasive mechanical ventilation.

Several clinical parameters should be monitored frequently during the first hours of initiating NIPPV such as blood pressure, heart rate, mental status, evidence of respiratory distress, oxygen saturation, and arterial blood gases.[74,75] Successful alveolar ventilation will lead to tidal volumes of 8 to 10 mL/kg and will decrease the respiratory rate to less than 25 breaths per minute. Arterial blood gases should be followed closely over the first 2 hours with special attention to pH and $Paco_2$ trends. The rate of NIPPV failure in patients with COPD—not OHS—experiencing an acute hypercapnic respiratory failure has been reported between 5% and 40%.[75] The best predictor of early NIPPV failure (within the first 1-3 hours) was the lack of improvement in pH and $Paco_2$ after 1 hour of NIPPV.[76] A more recent prospective study reported a NIPPV failure rate of 36% among 33 consecutive morbidly obese patients developing acute respiratory failure due to multiple causes. In this study, a higher BMI was predictive of NIPPV failure (46.9 kg/m^2 in successful NIPPV vs. 62.5 kg/m^2 in NIPPV failure).[77] Patients with OHS should be expected to improve within 1 to 3 hours of therapy, with most OHS patients reaching near normal pH within 12 to 24 hours. Acute-on-chronic hypercapnic respiratory failure in patients with OHS resolves more rapidly compared to patients with COPD and congestive heart failure.[78] Moreover, Ortega-Gonzalez and associates did not report any cases of NIPPV failure in 17 consecutive OHS patients admitted to an ICU with acute-on-chronic hypercapnic respiratory failure.[78]

Approximately 50% of morbidly obese patients with acute respiratory failure who require emergent endotracheal intubation have a difficult intubation defined as requiring more than three attempts by experienced clinicians.[77] These patients are also at increased risk of peri-intubation complications including cardiorespiratory arrest. The clinician planning to intubate these patients should be cognizant of the limited neck mobility and the difficulty with visualizing the vocal cords because of the crowded oropharynx.[79] Furthermore, obese patients are at risk of severe oxygen desaturation that can occur precipitously owing to a lower functional residual capacity and atelectasis that is exacerbated in the supine position.[80,81] For these reasons, only the most experienced clinician should attempt to intubate a decompensated patient with OHS that has failed a trial of NIPPV. Finally, in the difficult airway the clinician may consider placing a temporary laryngeal mask device or perform intubation with the assistance of a flexible fiberoptic bronchoscope.

Chronic Obstructive Pulmonary Disease and Overlap Syndrome

The use of NIPPV is well established in acute exacerbations of COPD that lead to acute hypercapnia or acute-on-chronic hypercapnic respiratory failure. However, its use in chronic stable hypercapnic COPD is controversial. The rationale for using NIPPV in chronic stable patients relates to resting the muscles at night from the increased workload due to the mechanical disadvantage of the diaphragm from lung hyperinflation. With time, the mechanical disadvantage posed by lung hyperinflation on the diaphragm can lead to ventilatory hyporesponsiveness to increasing CO_2 levels during nocturnal hypoventilation, which is most exaggerated during REM sleep. Tidal volumes also fall during sleep, further decreasing the ventilatory capacity.

By using nocturnal NIPPV, CO_2 levels are not further increased because nocturnal hypoventilation is improved. In addition, this ideally may result in restoration of CO_2 chemoresponsiveness and prevents daytime hypoventilation. Although COPD is the most common reason for NIPPV in Europe,[39] there is controversial evidence supporting its use. An Italian multicenter study revealed that patients with chronic stable COPD with ventilatory failure ($Paco_2 > 50$ mm Hg) demonstrated benefit in those who received NIPPV (a higher average than 5 hours/night) in addition to long-term oxygen therapy (LTOT) versus LTOT alone.[82] Forty-three patients that received LTOT in addition to NIPPV had a decreased trend

in CO_2 retention when compared to patients receiving LTOT alone. In addition, the NIPPV + LTOT group had increased quality of life and dypsnea scores. In another randomized controlled trial on NIPPV in stable end-stage hypercapnic COPD with survival as the primary outcome, McEvoy and colleagues randomized 144 patients to either nocturnal NIPPV and LTOT or only nocturnal LTOT.[83] These patients had severe stable COPD (mean FEV_1 of 0.63 L or 25% predicted with awake mean $Paco_2$ of 54.8 mm Hg in the NIPPV group). The patients that received NIPPV and LTOT had improved sleep quality and sleep-related hypercapnia acutely, compared to those that received only LTOT. In addition, the patients with NIPPV and LTOT demonstrated an improvement in survival with the adjusted Cox model (adjusted hazard ratio 0.63, 95% CI 0.40 to 0.99, $p = 0.045$).[83] After 2 years, 47% of the LTOT-treated patients had died compared to 32% in the NIPPV group. By 3.5 years, however, the survival curves had come together. However, there was no change in daytime arterial blood gases or hospitalization rates after treatment in the group receiving NIPPV and LTOT. Moreover, use of NIPPV in these severely disabled COPD patients actually resulted in deterioration in general and mental health and some aspects of mood. An earlier meta-analysis that did not include the two largest above-mentioned randomized trials concluded that there was not sufficient evidence to recommend NIPPV for chronic stable COPD patients.[84] However, future clinical trials with clinical endpoints of reduced CO_2 levels overnight, perhaps through the use of transcutaneous CO_2 monitoring, may be of more value in improving quality of life.[85] Overall, NIPPV may also be more beneficial if higher inspiratory pressures are used to reduce nocturnal CO_2 levels, which would allow for increased excretion of bicarbonate and for restoration of the central respiratory drive.[85]

Patients with COPD who have both daytime and nighttime hypoxemia should receive LTOT, as there is a known survival benefit.[86,87] However, it is still unclear if oxygen therapy is beneficial in patients with COPD where there is isolated nocturnal oxygen desaturation. Chaouat and colleagues were unable to demonstrate any benefit with nocturnal oxygen therapy in these patients.[88]

In contrast to COPD, the use of PAP therapy is recommended in cases of "overlap syndrome." The "overlap syndrome" was first coined by Flenley[89] and refers to coexisting COPD and OSA. This syndrome is associated with more severe and prolonged periods of oxygen desaturation with sleep. In addition, these patients are more susceptible to pulmonary hypertension and daytime hypercapnia. The effect of CPAP on lung function in patients with the overlap syndrome remains unclear. In one study, CPAP did not improve FEV_1 and FVC.[90] In contrast, a study of 55 patients with overlap syndrome demonstrated that 6 months of treatment with CPAP led to significant reductions in $Paco_2$, with increases in Pao_2, FEV_1, and FVC.[91] Some of the mechanisms involved may relate to resting of the inspiratory muscles with CPAP therapy, and counteraction of iPEEP and subsequent relief of the inspiratory load.

Given the further predisposition to oxygen desaturation during sleep in patients with overlap syndrome, it may be beneficial to add oxygen therapy if there is sustained oxygen desaturation, particularly during REM sleep. NIPPV may also be of benefit in alleviating the sleep-disordered breathing and hypoxemia. The impact of CPAP therapy in patients with overlap syndrome was evaluated in a prospective cohort study of 95 patients with moderate to severe OSA and severe COPD receiving LTOT.[30] CPAP adherence was documented in 64% of patients. The rest of the patients were either not adherent or refused therapy. The 5-year survival rate estimate was 71% (95% CI 53-83%) in the CPAP-treated and 26% (95% CI 12-43%) in the untreated group ($p < 0.01$). After adjusting for several confounders, patients treated with CPAP showed a significantly lower risk of death with a hazard ratio of death versus untreated at 0.19 (95% CI 0.08-0.48). However, prospective randomized studies are needed to assess the effectiveness of CPAP or NIPPV with or without nocturnal oxygen supplementation in patients with the overlap syndrome.

Chest Wall Deformities

Short-term nocturnal ventilation has been shown to improve indices of respiratory failure in patients with chest wall deformities. In addition, there is a survival advantage in patients with chest wall deformities such as kyphoscoliosis who use NIPPV.[33,92] Long-term use of NIPPV has been demonstrated to improve survival, quality of life, blood gases, and sleep quality in these patients.[33,92]

Because invasive mechanical ventilation can be even more challenging in patients with chest wall deformity due to the curvature of the trachea from curving of the thoracic spine, NIPPV may be a more favorable option. In one prospective study, seven patients with daytime decompensated respiratory failure with CO_2 retention and severe kyphoscoliosis improved significantly with respect to blood gases and sleep quality after 3 months of treatment.[93] Two patients received CPAP only, while the remaining five received NIPPV. The daytime CO_2 improved from 62 ± 6 mm Hg to 49 ± 5 mm Hg in the five patients on NIPPV. In addition, it was also noted that all patients had an improvement in their respiratory muscle function, as measured by maximal inspiratory and expiratory pressures.

To determine which mode of ventilator strategy is more beneficial in this patient population, Tuggey and Elliott investigated 13 patients with chest wall deformities who underwent a 4-week single-blind randomized crossover study with either pressure-preset or volume-preset modes.[94] After 4 weeks, the minute ventilation was identical with both modes. However, there was more air leak associated with the pressure-preset than volume-preset ventilatory modes. Otherwise, there were no differences in sleep quality, daytime arterial blood gases, ventilatory drive, or daytime functioning.

Neuromuscular Disease

Respiratory failure in NMD is multifactorial in etiology, with the end result often being ventilatory failure, pneumonia, and death. Treatment with NIPPV has demonstrated that patients can be discharged from the hospital earlier, and have a lower likelihood of readmissions. There is also evidence that NIPPV improves survival.[95,96]

Respiratory muscle weakness is present in most patients with ALS at diagnosis. In fact, it is a strong predictor of quality of life.[31] Nocturnal hypoventilation can cause disruption of sleep and can result in symptoms such as morning headache, unrefreshing sleep, daytime sleepiness, lethargy, fatigue, poor concentration, and poor appetite. During sleep, patients with

NMD are also at risk for sleep-disordered breathing, including central apneas and OSA. Along with hypoventilation, sleep apnea can contribute to the development of hypercapnia and hypoxemia in the daytime.

Research by Ward and colleagues would suggest that patients with NMD and chest wall disorders such as kyphoscoliosis, with nocturnal hypercapnia but daytime eucapnia, may also benefit from nocturnal NIPPV.[97]

NIPPV should also be initiated when the presence of sleep-disordered breathing is first detected. The American Thoracic Society (ATS) published a position statement on the care of individuals with Duchenne muscular dystrophy and respiratory disease.[96] In this document, the ATS suggests investigating for subjective sleep quality and symptoms at every patient encounter, evaluating for sleep-disordered breathing when clinically indicated with an overnight polysomnogram with continuous CO_2 monitoring. Also, the American College of Chest Physicians has established that most insurers will reimburse devices for nocturnal hypoventilation if there are symptoms of sleep-disordered breathing (e.g., morning headache or daytime fatigue or dyspnea), and one of the following: (1) $Paco_2$ greater than 45 mm Hg, (2) nocturnal oximetry demonstrating oxygen saturation at 88% or less for 5 consecutive minutes, (3) a maximum inspiratory pressure of less than 60 cm H_2O, or (4) a FVC less than 50% of predicted.[95]

Nocturnal NIPPV is typically initiated either at home, in the sleep laboratory, or during a hospitalization. Although many times patients are started on NIPPV electively, some are transitioned to NIPPV after being weaned off invasive ventilation during hospitalization for severe hypercapnic respiratory failure. NIPPV is more difficult to establish in patients with significant bulbar impairment.[32]

It is not clearly defined when diurnal NIPPV should be initiated. For instance, some patients with progressive NMD, such as Duchenne muscular dystrophy, develop daytime respiratory failure despite optimal management of nocturnal hypoventilation. In this case, extending the NIPPV use to both daytime and nighttime is an option. However, given the progressive nature of the disease, some patients and families may find that it is best to allow nature to take its course and not take on any additional therapy. Finally, tracheostomy and invasive mechanical ventilation are also options. Usually, the triggers to initiate daytime support with NIPPV are diurnal hypercapnia despite maximal nocturnal ventilatory support and the development of daytime dyspnea.

In a recent Cochrane Review, it was concluded that NIPPV improves short-term hypoventilation-related clinical symptoms, nocturnal mean oxygen saturation, and daytime hypercapnia.[15] There may also be survival and quality of life benefits in the long-term, but these conclusions are less definite owing to the less rigorous nature of these studies.

REFERENCES

1. McNicholas WT. Impact of sleep in respiratory failure. *Eur Respir J.* 1997;10(4):920-933.
2. Douglas NJ, White DP, Weil JV, et al. Hypercapnic ventilatory response in sleeping adults. *Am Rev Respir Dis.* 1982;126(5):758-762.
3. Douglas NJ, White DP, Weil JV, et al. Hypoxic ventilatory response decreases during sleep in normal men. *Am Rev Respir Dis.* 1982; 125(3):286-289.
4. Mokhlesi B, Kryger MH, Grunstein RR. Assessment and management of patients with obesity hypoventilation syndrome. *Proc Am Thorac Soc.* 2008;5(2):218-225.

5. Rapoport DM, Garay SM, Epstein H, et al. Hypercapnia in the obstructive sleep apnea syndrome. A reevaluation of the "Pickwickian syndrome." *Chest.* 1986;89(5):627-635.
6. Lin CC, Wu KM, Chou CS, et al. Oral airway resistance during wakefulness in eucapnic and hypercapnic sleep apnea syndrome. *Respir Physiol Neurobiol.* 2004;139(2):215-224.
7. Piper AJ, Grunstein RR. Big breathing—The complex interaction of obesity, hypoventilation, weight loss and respiratory function. *J Appl Physiol.* 2010;108(1):199-205.
8. Janssens JP, Derivaz S, Breitenstein E, et al. Changing patterns in long-term noninvasive ventilation: A 7-year prospective study in the Geneva Lake area. *Chest.* 2003;123(1):67-79.
9. Mannino DM, Buist AS. Global burden of COPD: Risk factors, prevalence, and future trends. *Lancet.* 2007;370(9589):765-773.
10. Mulloy E, McNicholas WT. Ventilation and gas exchange during sleep and exercise in severe COPD. *Chest.* 1996;109(2):387-394.
11. O'Donoghue FJ, Catcheside PG, Jordan AS, et al. Effect of CPAP on intrinsic PEEP, inspiratory effort, and lung volume in severe stable COPD. *Thorax.* 2002;57(6):533-539.
12. Donath J, Miller A. Restrictive chest wall disorders. *Semin Respir Crit Care Med.* 2009;30(3):275-292.
13. Lisboa C, Moreno R, Fava M, et al. Inspiratory muscle function in patients with severe kyphoscoliosis. *Am Rev Respir Dis.* 1985;132(1):48-52.
14. Gonzalez C, Ferris G, Diaz J, et al. Kyphoscoliotic ventilatory insufficiency: Effects of long-term intermittent positive-pressure ventilation. *Chest.* 2003;124(3):857-862.
15. Annane D, Orlikowski D, Chevret S, et al. Nocturnal mechanical ventilation for chronic hypoventilation in patients with neuromuscular and chest wall disorders. *Cochrane Database Syst Rev.* 2007;(4):CD001941.
16. Sturm R. Increases in morbid obesity in the USA: 2000-2005. *Public Health.* 2007;121(7):492-496.
17. Lee W, Nagubadi S, Kryger MH, et al. Epidemiology of obstructive sleep apnea: A population-based perspective. *Exp Rev Respir Med.* 2008;2(3):349-364.
18. Littleton SW, Mokhlesi B. The pickwickian syndrome—Obesity hypoventilation syndrome. *Clin Chest Med.* 2009;30(3):467-478:vii-viii.
19. Resta O, Foschino Barbaro MP, Brindicci C, et al. Hypercapnia in overlap syndrome: Possible determinant factors. *Sleep Breath.* 2002;6(1):11-18.
20. Chaouat A, Weitzenblum E, Krieger J, et al. Association of chronic obstructive pulmonary disease and sleep apnea syndrome. *Am J Respir Crit Care Med.* 1995;151(1):82-86.
21. Perez de Llano LA, Golpe R, Ortiz Piquer M, et al. Short-term and long-term effects of nasal intermittent positive pressure ventilation in patients with obesity-hypoventilation syndrome. *Chest.* 2005;128(2):587-594.
22. Bednarek M, Plywaczewski R, Jonczak L, et al. There is no relationship between chronic obstructive pulmonary disease and obstructive sleep apnea syndrome: A population study. *Respiration.* 2005;72(2):142-149.
23. Kessler R, Chaouat A, Schinkewitch P, et al. The obesity-hypoventilation syndrome revisited: A prospective study of 34 consecutive cases. *Chest.* 2001;120(2):369-376.
24. Atwood Jr CW, McCrory D, Garcia JG, et al. Pulmonary artery hypertension and sleep-disordered breathing: ACCP evidence-based clinical practice guidelines. *Chest.* 2004;126(Suppl 1):S72-S77.
25. Kessler R, Chaouat A, Weitzenblum E, et al. Pulmonary hypertension in the obstructive sleep apnoea syndrome: Prevalence, causes and therapeutic consequences. *Eur Respir J.* 1996;9(4):787-794.
26. Sugerman HJ, Baron PL, Fairman RP, et al. Hemodynamic dysfunction in obesity hypoventilation syndrome and the effects of treatment with surgically induced weight loss. *Ann Surg.* 1988;207(5):604-613.
27. Berg G, Delaive K, Manfreda J, et al. The use of health-care resources in obesity-hypoventilation syndrome. *Chest.* 2001;120(2):377-383.
28. Nowbar S, Burkart KM, Gonzales R, et al. Obesity-associated hypoventilation in hospitalized patients: Prevalence, effects, and outcome. *Am J Med.* 2004;116(1):1-7.
29. Foucher P, Baudouin N, Merati M, et al. Relative survival analysis of 252 patients with COPD receiving long-term oxygen therapy. *Chest.* 1998;113(6):1580-1587.
30. Machado MC, Vollmer WM, Togeiro SM, et al. CPAP and survival in moderate-to-severe obstructive sleep apnoea syndrome and hypoxaemic COPD. *Eur Respir J.* 2010;35(1):132-137.
31. Bourke SC, Shaw PJ, Gibson GJ. Respiratory function vs. sleep-disordered breathing as predictors of QOL in ALS. *Neurology.* 2001;57(11):2040-2044.
32. Bourke SC, Bullock RE, Williams TL, et al. Noninvasive ventilation in ALS: Indications and effect on quality of life. *Neurology.* 2003;61(2):171-177.
33. Gustafson T, Franklin KA, Midgren B, et al. Survival of patients with kyphoscoliosis receiving mechanical ventilation or oxygen at home. *Chest.* 2006;130(6):1828-1833.
34. Meyer JA. A practical mechanical respirator, 1929: The "iron lung." *Ann Thorac Surg.* 1990;50(3):490-493.
35. Hill NS. Clinical applications of body ventilators. *Chest.* 1986;90(6):897-905.
36. Splaingard ML, Frates Jr RC, Harrison GM, et al. Home positive-pressure ventilation. Twenty years' experience. *Chest.* 1983;84(4):376-382.
37. Robert D, Gerard M, Leger P, et al. [Permanent mechanical ventilation at home via a tracheotomy in chronic respiratory insufficiency]. *Rev Fr Mal Respir.* 1983;11(6):923-936.
38. Sivak ED, Gipson WT, Hanson MR. Long-term management of respiratory failure in amyotrophic lateral sclerosis. *Ann Neurol.* 1982;12(1):18-23.
39. Lloyd-Owen SJ, Donaldson GC, Ambrosino N, et al. Patterns of home mechanical ventilation use in Europe: Results from the Eurovent survey. *Eur Respir J.* 2005;25(6):1025-1031.
40. Simonds AK, Elliott MW. Outcome of domiciliary nasal intermittent positive pressure ventilation in restrictive and obstructive disorders. *Thorax.* 1995;50(6):604-609.
41. Leger P, Bedicam JM, Cornette A, et al. Nasal intermittent positive pressure ventilation. Long-term follow-up in patients with severe chronic respiratory insufficiency. *Chest.* 1994;105(1):100-105.
42. Schonhofer B, Polkey MI, Suchi S, et al. Effect of home mechanical ventilation on inspiratory muscle strength in COPD. *Chest.* 2006;130(6):1834-1838.
43. Windisch W, Storre JH, Sorichter S, et al. Comparison of volume- and pressure-limited NPPV at night: A prospective randomized cross-over trial. *Respir Med.* 2005;99(1):52-59.
44. Storre JH, Seuthe B, Fiechter R, et al. Average volume-assured pressure support in obesity hypoventilation: A randomized crossover trial. *Chest.* 2006;130(3):815-821.
45. Aslanian P, El Atrous S, Isabey D, et al. Effects of flow triggering on breathing effort during partial ventilatory support. *Am J Respir Crit Care Med.* 1998;157(1):135-143.
46. Elliott MW. The interface: crucial for successful noninvasive ventilation. *Eur Respir J.* 2004;23(1):7-8.
47. Mehta S, McCool FD, Hill NS. Leak compensation in positive pressure ventilators: A lung model study. *Eur Respir J.* 2001;17(2):259-267.
48. Bach JR, Robert D, Leger P, et al. Sleep fragmentation in kyphoscoliotic individuals with alveolar hypoventilation treated by NIPPV. *Chest.* 1995;107(6):1552-1558.
49. Meyer TJ, Pressman MR, Benditt J, et al. Air leaking through the mouth during nocturnal nasal ventilation: Effect on sleep quality. *Sleep.* 1997;20(7):561-569.
50. Massie CA, Hart RW, Peralez K, et al. Effects of humidification on nasal symptoms and compliance in sleep apnea patients using continuous positive airway pressure. *Chest.* 1999;116(2):403-408.
51. Yoder EA, Klann K, Strohl KP. Inspired oxygen concentrations during positive pressure therapy. *Sleep Breath.* 2004;8(1):1-5.
52. Schwartz AR, Kacmarek RM, Hess DR. Factors affecting oxygen delivery with bi-level positive airway pressure. *Respir Care.* 2004;49(3):270-275.
53. Kaw R, Hernandez AV, Walker E, et al. Determinants of hypercapnia in obese patients with obstructive sleep apnea: A systematic review and meta-analysis of cohort studies. *Chest.* 2009;136(3):787-796.
54. Banerjee D, Yee BJ, Piper AJ, et al. Obesity hypoventilation syndrome: Hypoxemia during continuous positive airway pressure. *Chest.* 2007;131(6):1678-1684.
55. Chatwin M, Nickol AH, Morrell MJ, et al. Randomised trial of inpatient versus outpatient initiation of home mechanical ventilation in patients with nocturnal hypoventilation. *Respir Med.* 2008;102(11):1528-1535.
56. Rapoport DM, Sorkin B, Garay SM, et al. Reversal of the "Pickwickian syndrome" by long-term use of nocturnal nasal-airway pressure. *N Engl J Med.* 1982;307(15):931-933.
57. Laaban JP, Chailleux E. Daytime hypercapnia in adult patients with obstructive sleep apnea syndrome in France, before initiating nocturnal nasal continuous positive airway pressure therapy. *Chest.* 2005;127(3):710-715.
58. Mokhlesi B, Tulaimat A, Evans AT, et al. Impact of adherence with positive airway pressure therapy on hypercapnia in obstructive sleep apnea. *J Clin Sleep Med.* 2006;2(1):57-62.

59. Schafer H, Ewig S, Hasper E, et al. Failure of CPAP therapy in obstructive sleep apnoea syndrome: Predictive factors and treatment with bilevel-positive airway pressure. *Respir Med.* 1998;92(2):208-215.

60. Mokhlesi B. Positive airway pressure titration in obesity hypoventilation syndrome: Continuous positive airway pressure or bilevel positive airway pressure. *Chest.* 2007;131(6):1624-1626.

61. Piper AJ, Wang D, Yee BJ, et al. Randomised trial of CPAP vs. bilevel support in the treatment of obesity hypoventilation syndrome without severe nocturnal desaturation. *Thorax.* 2008;63(5):395-401.

62. Kushida CA, Chediak A, Berry RB, et al. Clinical guidelines for the manual titration of positive airway pressure in patients with obstructive sleep apnea. *J Clin Sleep Med.* 2008;4(2):157-171.

63. Berger KI, Ayappa I, Chatr-Amontri B, et al. Obesity hypoventilation syndrome as a spectrum of respiratory disturbances during sleep. *Chest.* 2001;120(4):1231-1238.

64. Redolfi S, Corda L, La Piana G, et al. Long-term non-invasive ventilation increases chemosensitivity and leptin in obesity-hypoventilation syndrome. *Respir Med.* 2007;101(6):1191-1195.

65. de Lucas-Ramos P, de Miguel-Diez J, Santacruz-Siminiani A, et al. Benefits at 1 year of nocturnal intermittent positive pressure ventilation in patients with obesity-hypoventilation syndrome. *Respir Med.* 2004;98(10):961-967.

66. Han F, Chen E, Wei H, et al. Treatment effects on carbon dioxide retention in patients with obstructive sleep apnea-hypopnea syndrome. *Chest.* 2001;119(6):1814-1819.

67. Piper AJ, Sullivan CE. Effects of short-term NIPPV in the treatment of patients with severe obstructive sleep apnea and hypercapnia. *Chest.* 1994;105(2):434-440.

68. Masa JF, Celli BR, Riesco JA, et al. The obesity hypoventilation syndrome can be treated with noninvasive mechanical ventilation. *Chest.* 2001;119(4):1102-1107.

69. Chouri-Pontarollo N, Borel JC, Tamisier R, et al. Impaired objective daytime vigilance in obesity-hypoventilation syndrome: Impact of non-invasive ventilation. *Chest.* 2007;131(1):148-155.

70. Heinemann F, Budweiser S, Dobroschke J, et al. Non-invasive positive pressure ventilation improves lung volumes in the obesity hypoventilation syndrome. *Respir Med.* 2007;101(6):1229-1235.

71. Lee WY, Mokhlesi B. Diagnosis and management of obesity hypoventilation syndrome in the ICU. *Crit Care Clin.* 2008;24(3):533-549;vii.

72. Nava S, Evangelisti I, Rampulla C, et al. Human and financial costs of noninvasive mechanical ventilation in patients affected by COPD and acute respiratory failure. *Chest.* 1997;111(6):1631-1638.

73. Elliott MW, Confalonieri M, Nava S. Where to perform noninvasive ventilation? *Eur Respir J.* 2002;19(6):1159-1166.

74. Plant PK, Owen JL, Elliott MW. Early use of non-invasive ventilation for acute exacerbations of chronic obstructive pulmonary disease on general respiratory wards: A multicentre randomised controlled trial. *Lancet.* 2000;355(9219):1931-1935.

75. Nava S, Ceriana P. Causes of failure of noninvasive mechanical ventilation. *Respir Care.* 2004;49(3):295-303.

76. Anton A, Guell R, Gomez J, et al. Predicting the result of noninvasive ventilation in severe acute exacerbations of patients with chronic airflow limitation. *Chest.* 2000;117(3):828-833.

77. Duarte AG, Justino E, Bigler T, et al. Outcomes of morbidly obese patients requiring mechanical ventilation for acute respiratory failure. *Crit Care Med.* 2007;35(3):732-737.

78. Ortega Gonzalez A, Peces-Barba Romero G, Fernandez Ormaechea I, et al. Evolution of patients with chronic obstructive pulmonary disease, obesity hypoventilation syndrome or congestive heart failure in a respiratory monitoring unit. *Arch Bronconeumol.* 2006;42(9):423-429.

79. Paix AD, Williamson JA, Runciman WB. Crisis management during anaesthesia: Difficult intubation. *Qual Saf Health Care.* 2005;14(3):E5.

80. Koenig SM. Pulmonary complications of obesity. *Am J Med Sci.* 2001;321(4):249-279.

81. Walz JM, Zayaruzny M, Heard SO. Airway management in critical illness. *Chest.* 2007;131(2):608-620.

82. Clini E, Sturani C, Rossi A, et al. The Italian multicentre study on non-invasive ventilation in chronic obstructive pulmonary disease patients. *Eur Respir J.* 2002;20(3):529-538.

83. McEvoy RD, Pierce RJ, Hillman D, et al. Nocturnal non-invasive nasal ventilation in stable hypercapnic COPD: A randomised controlled trial. *Thorax.* 2009;64(7):561-566.

84. Wijkstra PJ, Lacasse Y, Guyatt GH, et al. A meta-analysis of nocturnal noninvasive positive pressure ventilation in patients with stable COPD. *Chest.* 2003;124(1):337-343.

85. Elliott MW. Domiciliary non-invasive ventilation in stable COPD? *Thorax.* 2009;64(7):553-556.

86. Continuous or nocturnal oxygen therapy in hypoxemic chronic obstructive lung disease. A clinical trial. Nocturnal Oxygen Therapy Trial Group. *Ann Intern Med.* 1980;93(3):391-398.

87. Long-term domiciliary oxygen therapy in chronic hypoxic cor pulmonale complicating chronic bronchitis and emphysema. Report of the Medical Research Council Working Party. *Lancet.* 1981;1(8222):681-686.

88. Chaouat A, Weitzenblum E, Kessler R, et al. A randomized trial of nocturnal oxygen therapy in chronic obstructive pulmonary disease patients. *Eur Respir J.* 1999;14(5):1002-1008.

89. Flenley DC. Sleep in chronic obstructive lung disease. *Clin Chest Med.* 1985;6(4):651-661.

90. O'Brien A, Whitman K. Lack of benefit of continuous positive airway pressure on lung function in patients with overlap syndrome. *Lung.* 2005;183(6):389-404.

91. de Miguel J, Cabello J, Sanchez-Alarcos JM, et al. Long-term effects of treatment with nasal continuous positive airway pressure on lung function in patients with overlap syndrome. *Sleep Breath.* 2002;6(1):3-10.

92. Buyse B, Meersseman W, Demedts M. Treatment of chronic respiratory failure in kyphoscoliosis: Oxygen or ventilation? *Eur Respir J.* 2003;22(3):525-528.

93. Ellis ER, Grunstein RR, Chan S, et al. Noninvasive ventilatory support during sleep improves respiratory failure in kyphoscoliosis. *Chest.* 1988;94(4):811-815.

94. Tuggey JM, Elliott MW. Randomised crossover study of pressure and volume non-invasive ventilation in chest wall deformity. *Thorax.* 2005;60(10):859-864.

95. Clinical indications for noninvasive positive pressure ventilation in chronic respiratory failure due to restrictive lung disease, COPD, and nocturnal hypoventilation—A consensus conference report. *Chest.* 1999;116(2):521-534.

96. Finder JD, Birnkrant D, Carl J, et al. Respiratory care of the patient with Duchenne muscular dystrophy: ATS consensus statement. *Am J Respir Crit Care Med.* 2004;170(4):456-465.

97. Ward S, Chatwin M, Heather S, et al. Randomised controlled trial of non-invasive ventilation (NIV) for nocturnal hypoventilation in neuromuscular and chest wall disease patients with daytime normocapnia. *Thorax.* 2005;60(12):1019-1024.

98. Mokhlesi B, Tulaimat A, Faibussowitsch I, et al. Obesity hypoventilation syndrome: Prevalence and predictors in patients with obstructive sleep apnea. *Sleep Breath.* 2007;11(2):117-124.

99. Budweiser S, Riedl SG, Jorres RA, et al. Mortality and prognostic factors in patients with obesity-hypoventilation syndrome undergoing noninvasive ventilation. *J Intern Med.* 2007;261(4):375-383.

100. Verin E, Tardif C, Pasquis P. Prevalence of daytime hypercapnia or hypoxia in patients with OSAS and normal lung function. *Respir Med.* 2001;95(8):693-696.

101. Resta O, Foschino Barbaro MP, Bonfitto P, et al. Hypercapnia in obstructive sleep apnoea syndrome. *Neth J Med.* 2000;56(6):215-222.

102. Golpe R, Jimenez A, Carpizo R. Diurnal hypercapnia in patients with obstructive sleep apnea syndrome. *Chest.* 2002;122(3):1100-1101.

103. Akashiba T, Akahoshi T, Kawahara S, et al. Clinical characteristics of obesity-hypoventilation syndrome in Japan: A multi-center study. *Intern Med.* 2006;45(20):1121-1125.

Chapter 21

Sleep-Related Disorders in Chronic Pulmonary Disease

ALEX D. HAKIM / MICHAEL R. LITTNER

Sleep is universal and fulfills important functions in our lives. Sleep provides a respite from waking during which a number of restorative and sleep-related physiologic events occur. Although sleep of appropriate duration and quality is expected by all, the presence of pulmonary disease is often associated with disruption of sleep quantity and quality. The consequence of this disruption is varied but typically leads to complaints of insomnia, nonrestorative sleep, and a diminution of waking function such as excessive sleepiness.

Chronic pulmonary disease including chronic obstructive pulmonary disease (COPD), asthma, interstitial lung disease, and cystic fibrosis may reduce the quality of sleep as a result of diminished pulmonary function, respiratory symptoms such as shortness of breath, and nocturnal hypoxemia. Effects on sleep architecture are inconsistent and may be difficult to distinguish from typical age-related effects. There are often co-morbid conditions such as obstructive sleep apnea (OSA), which may be increased in chronic pulmonary disease and can contribute to the overall loss of sleep quality. Treatment of chronic pulmonary disease and co-morbid conditions may improve the quality of sleep and, in some cases, improve sleep architecture.

This chapter will review the interactions of sleep with COPD, asthma, interstitial lung disease (in particular, idiopathic pulmonary fibrosis), and cystic fibrosis.

NORMAL SLEEP ARCHITECTURE AND EFFECTS OF AGE

In order to better understand the effects of pulmonary disease on sleep, an appreciation of the normal sleep architecture is beneficial. Sleep architecture changes with increasing age. The trend is to less total sleep time (TST), less slow wave sleep, lower sleep efficiency, more arousals, more awakenings, more non-rapid eye movement (NREM) stage N1, and less stage N3 and stage REM (R).[1,2] The relationship of stage N2 to age is unclear. Some studies suggest an increase[1] and others a decrease.[2] The most consistent feature appears to be a reduction in total sleep time.[1-3] For example, in a study of 76 men and women, TST ranged from 446 minutes for 21- to 30-year-olds to 350 minutes for 61- to 70-year-olds.[2] In a study of 398 women, the TST ranged from 406 minutes for 20- to 40-year-olds to 364 minutes for 50- to 70-year-olds.[3] Of interest, latency to sleep onset did not appear to increase with age. Age-related changes in sleep architecture are particularly relevant for comparison in subjects with moderate to severe chronic obstructive pulmonary disease whose ages tend to average above 60 years. For example, 48 healthy elderly subjects without obstructive sleep apnea (average age 69.6 years) had arterial oxygen (O_2) saturation levels well above 90% with apparent reduced sleep efficiency, increased arousals and awakenings, increased stage N1, and reduced stage N2 and R sleep[4] (Table 21-1).

CHRONIC OBSTRUCTIVE PULMONARY DISEASE

COPD is a treatable and preventable disease that results in airflow obstruction that is not fully (i.e., is only partially) reversible.[5-7] COPD, which is primarily the result of cigarette smoking, is typically associated with either or both chronic bronchitis (chronic cough and sputum production) and emphysema. Symptoms may also include dyspnea, COPD exacerbations, and fatigue.

Spirometry documents the obstructive component of COPD. Obstruction is defined as a postbronchodilator FEV_1/FVC ratio (forced expiratory volume in 1 second divided by the forced vital capacity) of less than 0.70 (Table 21-2). Significant COPD occurs in a minority of long-time cigarette smokers. However, owing to the large number of past and current cigarette smokers, COPD is currently the fourth leading cause of death in the United States and worldwide and is projected to continue to increase for the foreseeable future.[5]

The prevalence of physician diagnosed COPD was estimated at 10 million in 2000.[8] However, based on the National Health and Nutrition Examination Survey III (NHANES III) from 1988 to 1994, which used prebronchodilator spirometry to measure pulmonary function, the estimate was 23.6 million, which would include undiagnosed as well as diagnosed patients with COPD. An estimated 2.4 million of these adults, or 1.4% of the population and 10.2% of those with COPD, had Global Initiative for Chronic Obstructive Lung Disease (GOLD)[5] stage 3 or 4, with an FEV_1 of less than 50% of the predicted value.[8] Thus, the majority of the subjects classified as having COPD by GOLD criteria have mild or moderate disease and have not been well studied with respect to sleep complaints or sleep architecture. In addition, nocturnal hypoxemia is much more likely to occur in patients with an FEV_1 below 50% predicted. For example, 49.2% of 59 COPD patients with an average FEV_1 of 37.2% predicted had an arterial O_2 desaturation below 90% by oximetry for 30% of the night.[9]

Etiology and Pathophysiology

Exposure to cigarette smoke produces neutrophil airway inflammation. Pathologically, COPD includes squamous cell metaplasia of the respiratory epithelium, respiratory ciliary loss and dysfunction, inflammation and fibrosis of airways, mucous gland hyperplasia and hypersecretion, increased airway smooth muscle, loss of alveolar attachments, and bronchoconstriction from vagally mediated release of acetylcholine.[5]

Often, there is confusion about whether a patient has asthma or COPD. The absence of reversibility to bronchodilators should *not* be the deciding factor in most cases. Asthma is often distinguished from COPD by the company it keeps, such as peripheral blood and sputum eosinophilia, early age of onset prior to substantial smoking history, elevated serum IgE levels, the presence of other allergic signs and symptoms such as hay fever and allergic rhinitis, and the absence of a significant (> 10 pack-years) smoking history. If there is strong evidence of both asthma and COPD, the diagnosis of both should be made and managed accordingly.

Apart from asthma, the differential diagnosis includes bronchiectasis, bronchiolitis, upper airway obstruction (e.g., from a tumor), postviral airway inflammation, eosinophilic bronchitis, vocal cord dysfunction, and congestive heart failure.

Laboratory studies may include, in addition to spirometry, a chest radiograph, oximetry at rest and exercise for possible hypoxemia, and a complete blood count (CBC) for polycythemia. Serum α_1-antitrypsin levels are generally recommended for COPD patients younger than 45 years with a strong family

TABLE 21-1

Studies of Typical Sleep Architecture in Healthy Adult Males and Females

Feature/Metric	Study (with Gender Distribution)				
	Sahlin[3]: All W (*N* = 152)	Sahlin[3]: All W (*N* = 120)	Sahlin[3]: All W (*N* = 126)	Phillips[4]: 27 M, 21 W (*N* = 48)	Mermigkis[110]: 11 M, 4 W (*N* = 15)
Age (years)	20-44	45-54	50-70	69.6	62.7
TIB (min)	476	473	482	401	409 (calc.)
TST (min)	409	399	364	288	320
SE %	86	85	76	71.8	78.2
N1 %	6.8	8.3	9.7	19.5*	7.4
N2 %	62	63	64	46.9	60
N3 %	11	10	9.9	21.2	16.5
R %	21	19	17	12.8	14.9
Sao$_2$ (%)	NA	NA	NA	94.5 (mean low during sleep)	95.3 (mean during sleep)
LSO (min)	22	20	25	27	NA
WASO (min)	45	54	92	86	NA
Awakenings (no./hr of sleep)	NA	NA	NA	4.9	NA
Arousals (no./hr of sleep)	NA	NA	NA	19	12.9
FEV$_1$ (L) (% pred.)	NA	NA	NA	2.5 (96.4%)	FVC (87.1)

*Data recalculated to be % of TST (awake not included).

calc., calculated from study data; *FEV$_1$*, forced expiratory volume in 1 second; *FVC*, forced vital capacity; *LSO*, latency to sleep onset from lights out; *M*, men; *N1 %*, *N2 %*, *N3 %*, stage N1, N2, and N3 non-rapid eye movement sleep as percent of TST; *NA*, not available; *% pred.*, percent of predicted value; *R %*, rapid eye movement sleep as percent of TST; *Sao$_2$*, arterial oxygen hemoglobin saturation, *SE %*, sleep efficiency as percent of TIB (TST/TIB × 100); *TIB*, time in bed from lights out to lights on; *TST*, total sleep time (which does not include wake time after sleep onset); *WASO*, wake time after sleep onset; *W*, women.
References cited in this table are listed at the end of the chapter and are cited in the chapter text where appropriate.

TABLE 21-2

Selected Measures of Pulmonary Function in Obstructive and Restrictive Lung Disease

Pulmonary Function	No Lung Disease	Obstruction	Restriction	Combined Obstruction and Restriction
FEV$_1$	80-120% predicted	Normal or reduced	Normal or reduced	Reduced
FVC	80-120% predicted	Normal or reduced	Reduced	Reduced
FEV$_1$/FVC	≤ 0.7*	Reduced	Normal or increased	Reduced
TLC	80-120% predicted	Normal or increased	Reduced	Reduced
DLcosb	80-120% predicted	Normal in chronic bronchitis, reduced in emphysema, may be increased in asthma	Normal or near normal in chest wall and neuromuscular disease, reduced in interstitial lung disease	Determined by the combination processes; may be normal or reduced

Predicted ranges are approximate and should be modified according to specific patient populations. The abnormalities of pulmonary function are generalizations; individual patients may vary.
*A rough rule of thumb that may require adjustment based on the age of the patient.
Dlcosb, single-breath diffusing capacity for carbon monoxide; *FEV1*, forced expiratory volume in 1 second; *FVC*, forced vital capacity; *TLC*, total lung capacity.
Modified from Global Initiative for Obstructive Lung Disease. Available at www.goldcopd.org; accessed Feb. 10, 2010.

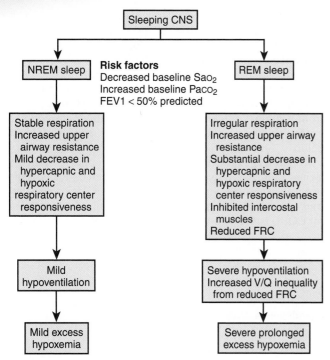

Figure 21-1 Effect of non-rapid eye movement (NREM) and rapid eye movement (REM) sleep on nocturnal arterial hemoglobin saturation in patients with severe to very severe COPD with FEV_1 generally less than 50% predicted. Boldface type indicates differences between NREM and REM sleep contributing to hypoxemia. *CNS,* central nervous system; *COPD,* chronic obstructive pulmonary disease; *FRC,* functional residual capacity (end-expiratory lung volume); $Paco_2$, partial arterial pressure of carbon dioxide; Sao_2, arterial oxygen saturation (%) of hemoglobin, usually expressed in as a percentage; $\dot{V}/\dot{Q}$, pulmonary alveolar/pulmonary capillary ventilation/perfusion inequality.

history of COPD. Arterial blood gases are generally obtained in borderline cases of hypoxemia (arterial oxygen saturation $\leq 92\%$ by pulse oximetry) and to determine the presence of hypercapnia. Patients with FEV_1 levels less than 30% predicted are most at risk of having hypercapnia.[4-6]

Co-Morbid Conditions

COPD is commonly associated with insomnia and excessive sleepiness. OSA and gastroesophageal reflux disease (GERD) may independently produce sleep complaints. Treatments for COPD such as β_2-agonists, theophylline, and inhaled and systemic corticosteroids may disrupt sleep. Treatments for smoking cessation such as varenicline, nicotine replacement therapy, and buproprion may also affect sleep.[10-12] Patients with COPD and OSA (so-called "overlap syndrome") have greater arterial oxygen desaturation, although the severity of the coexisting OSA is similar.[13] There is evidence that some OSA patients with daytime hypercapnia may have underlying COPD.[14] Apart from these co-morbid and treatment-related concerns, severe to very severe COPD itself is commonly associated with R sleep-related arterial oxygen desaturation (Fig. 21-1).

Sleep quality is markedly impaired and daytime symptoms are common in patients with COPD. For example, a prospective study of 15 women with severe COPD (FEV_1 36% predicted, average age 67.5 years) showed significant symptoms during both daytime and sleep. Such symptoms included greater

daytime fatigue, restless sleep, and rarely getting a good night's sleep, with greater nap frequency as compared to age-matched control subjects without COPD.[15] A retrospective analysis of a prospective cohort study of 734 male and female subjects (average age 73.4 years) with asthma and COPD and 1237 male and female control subjects (average age 73.9 years) was also consistent with these results.[16] Of note, arthritis and depression also independently correlated with sleep complaints in obstructive lung disease patients and it is not clear if these conditions were the main driver of the sleep complaints. In one study, patients with respiratory symptoms (cough, wheezing) had a greater prevalence of insomnia. However, diminished pulmonary function did not obviously correlate with insomnia.[17]

Sleep Architecture and Arterial Oxygen Saturation

A reduced sleep efficiency, increased time awake, increased arousals and awakenings, increased NREM stage N1 sleep, and reduced stage N3 and R sleep appear to be common in COPD patients. However, these sleep architecture results do not appear to differ markedly from individuals of similar age who do not have COPD (see Tables 21-1 and 21-3).[1-4] While there may be a general reduction in nocturnal arterial oxygen saturation, the most vulnerable period is R sleep during which prolonged arterial oxygen desaturation may occur. This desaturation is predominantly the result of a reduction in ventilation exaggerated by a reduction in resting lung volume (i.e., a reduction in functional residual capacity [FRC]). This may be the result of reduced hypercapnic and hypoxic ventilatory responsiveness combined with inhibition of contraction of the intercostal muscles[18-20] (see Figs. 21-1 and 21-2).

A randomized, placebo-controlled, crossover study of 20 patients (66 years average age) with moderate to very severe COPD ($FEV_1 < 70\%$ predicted, average of 1.18 L)[21] compared theophylline (serum levels of 6.7 to 12 mg/L serum) to albuterol 200 µg inhaled four times a day. Inhaled or oral corticosteroids were allowed if patients were already taking these medications. All patients had albuterol for rescue, as needed. No other COPD medications were allowed. Polysomnography (PSG) was performed after 12 to 16 days of therapy. There were no differences between treatments in sleep measures (see Table 21-3). There was less nocturnal wheezing with theophylline. Even though these results are consistent with a reduced sleep efficiency and fragmented sleep, there is no obvious difference between these results and those from healthy elderly subjects[1-4] (see Table 21-1). However, the patients spent a substantial amount of time with an arterial oxygen saturation level below 90% (72 minutes on albuterol, 51 minutes on theophylline, $p < 0.033$). This contrasts with the mean low arterial oxygen saturation of 94.5% in healthy elderly subjects[4] (see Tables 21-1 and 21-3).

This study is not unique.[21] Another study had similar baseline sleep architecture results (see Table 21-3) in patients with moderate to very severe COPD (average FEV_1 of 0.84 L, 32% predicted).[22] In this study, inhaled tiotropium (a long-acting inhaled anticholinergic) improved nocturnal arterial oxygen saturation compared to placebo (87.8% with placebo, 90.3% with tiotropium, $p = 0.047$). Tiotropium had no effect on sleep architecture, daytime sleepiness by the Epworth Sleepiness Scale, or subjective sleep quality recorded in diaries. A randomized crossover study also had similar baseline sleep

TABLE 21-3

Studies of Typical Sleep Architecture in Patients with Chronic Obstructive Pulmonary Disease

Feature/ Metric	Sanders[13]* (N = NA)§	Man[21]: Albuterol† (N = 20)	Man[21]: Theophylline† (N = 20)	McNicholas[22]: Baseline (N = 56)	Saaresranta[15]: Women (N = 15)	Mulloy[24]: Placebo (N = 10)	Berry[25]: Placebo (N = 12)	Ryan[23]: Placebo‡ (N = 12)
Age (years)	NA	66	66	66.4	67.5	64.2	62.8	69
TIB (min)	436 (calc)	422	424	398	401 (calc.)	394	435 (est.)	306 (calc.)
TST (min)	338	294	280	277	281	279	305 (est.)	236 (calc.)
SE %	77.5	69	66	69.6 (calc.)	70	70.8 (calc.)	70.1	77.2
N1 %	6.9	NC	NC	14.6 (calc.)	NC	29.0	19 (est.)	16.1 (calc.)
N2 %	58.9	NC	NC	57.4 (calc.)	NC	59.5	62 (est.)	52.5
N3 %	16.5	NC	NC	14.6 (calc.)	NC	0	4 (est.)	13.6
R %	17.3	NC	NC	13.6 (calc.)	NC	11.5	15 (est.)	17.8
Sao₂ (%)	NA	72 min < 90¶¶	51 min < 90¶¶	87.8 (mean during sleep for 13 placebo patients)	88.6 (mean during sleep)	88 (non-REM sleep est.) 86.2 (REM sleep est.) mean during sleep	> 90 for mean REM and non-REM activity during sleep	25.6 min < 90
LSO (min)	22	26.2	28	31ǀ	11.5	28	38.7	29ǀ
WASO (min)	76 (calc.)	102 (calc.)	116 (calc.)	90 (calc.)	122 (calc.)	59	91 (est)	41 (calc.)
Awakenings (no./hr of sleep)	NA	NA	NA	NA	NA	NA	NA	NA
Arousals (no./ hr of sleep)	18	NA	NA	NA	1	2.5	19.9	18.9
FEV₁(L) (% pred.)	NA (15.4%- 58.6%)	1.01 (NA)	1.01 (NA)	0.84 (32%)	0.73 (36%)	0.8 (31%)	1.36 (39.2%)	0.91 (39%)

*Data were obtained from unattended home polysomnogram.
†Randomized crossover study.
‡In this study, 40% of the patients were taking tiotropium and 83% were taking inhaled corticosteroid.
§Average age of patients across studies was 66.3 years, with 884 total patients with COPD.
¶¶$p < 0.033$.
ǀLSO to persistent sleep.
FEV_1, forced expiratory volume in 1 second; *LSO,* latency to sleep onset; *N1 %, N2 %, N3 %,* stage N1, N2, and N3 non-rapid eye movement sleep as percent of TST; *NC,* cannot be calculated from the study data; *REM,* rapid eye movement; *R %,* rapid eye movement sleep as percent of TST; *SE %,* sleep efficiency as percent of TIB (TST/TIB × 100); *TIB,* time in bed from lights out to lights on; *TST,* total sleep time; *WASO,* wake time after sleep onset.
References cited in this table are listed at the end of the chapter and are cited in the chapter text where appropriate.

architecture results in patients with moderate to severe COPD (FEV_1 of 0.96 L, 39% predicted).[23] In this study, inhaled salmeterol had no effect on sleep architecture, daytime sleepiness (ESS), perceived sleep quality, or quality of life by the Short Form Medical Outcomes Study Survey questionnaire (SF-36) but virtually eliminated time spent with an arterial oxygen saturation below 90% (1.8 vs. 25.6 minutes). Sleep architecture and arterial oxygen saturation in two other studies[24,25] (see Table 21-3) were also consistent with previous studies.[21-23]

Sleep architecture was studied before and after lung volume reduction surgery for pulmonary emphysema in 10 patients.[26] The baseline sleep efficiency was 45% rising to about 65% (estimated from the article's graph) and the TST increased from 184 minutes to about 250 minutes. Medical therapy had no effect on a control group of 6 emphysema patients with a similarly severely reduced FEV_1. However, the control group was not well matched for sleep efficiency or total sleep time. It can be speculated that preoperative anxiety may have influenced the markedly reduced baseline sleep efficiency (45%) in the surgical patients compared to the control group (60%).

Obstructive Sleep Apnea

OSA may occur in patients with COPD. As mentioned, this has been called the "overlap syndrome." The severity of OSA as measured by the apnea/hypopnea index (AHI) or respiratory disturbance index (RDI) is not increased, but the degree of arterial O_2 desaturation is greater. In a large study, RDI was lower and there were fewer patients with an RDI greater than 10 per hour of sleep in patients with obstructive pulmonary function.[13] However, there was a greater degree of arterial O_2 desaturation in OSA patients with obstructive pulmonary function (odds ratio of 3.36:1) compared to patients with OSA and no pulmonary obstruction.

Insomnia Treatment

As indicated by the previously reviewed studies, insomnia is a prominent symptom in patients with COPD. To date, studies have suggested that a single dose of ramelteon (a melatonin receptor 1 and 2 agonist) does not increase the AHI or arterial O_2 desaturation in patients with mild to severe COPD.[27,28] Of

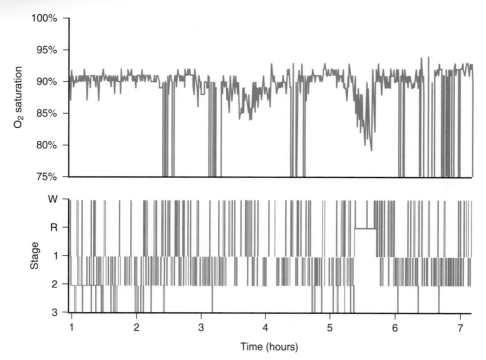

Figure 21-2 An all-night histogram of a polysomnogram from a patient with severe COPD (FEV_1 < 50% predicted) illustrating fragmented sleep with a low arterial oxygen (O_2) saturation (at or near 90% saturation with some variability to 85%) during baseline and most of the sleep period with a single prolonged episode of desaturation to a nadir below 80% during about 20 minutes of rapid eye movement (REM) sleep. Stages 1, 2, and 3 are non-rapid eye movement (NREM) sleep; *R*, REM sleep; *W*, wake.

the benzodiazepine and nonbenzodiazepine hypnotics, relatively few studies have been conducted. Zolpidem 5 and 10 mg and triazolam 0.25 mg did not reduce arterial O_2 saturation compared to placebo in a double-blind single night crossover study in 24 subjects with moderate COPD.[29] A multinight single-blind study of 8 days compared 10 mg zolpidem to baseline and post treatment placebo in 10 patients with severe to very severe COPD and did not indicate a significant deleterious effect of zolpidem on arterial O_2 saturation. However, there was a numeric increase of time spent below an arterial O_2 saturation of 90%.[30] A study comparing zolpidem to triazolam indicated that zolpidem did not reduce ventilation but triazolam did.[31]

Risk Factors

Documenting nocturnal hypoxemia in COPD patients without daytime hypoxemia requires an overnight sleep study of at least oximetry. However, less than 5% of COPD patients are estimated to be at risk for nocturnal arterial oxygen saturations below 90% for 30% of the night or more.[9] There are several predictors that increase the probability of nocturnal hypoxemia. These include daytime hypercapnia, an FEV_1 less than 50% predicted, daytime arterial oxygen saturation less than 95%, and possibly daytime sleepiness.[9,32-34] Of note, there may be no obvious impact of such nocturnal hypoxemia on outcomes such as health-related and general quality of life and, in one study, sleep-related symptoms such as daytime sleepiness.[9] The association with mortality is not well defined with at least one study suggesting an increase in mortality in patients with isolated reductions in nocturnal arterial oxygen saturation.[35]

Treatment

Treatment of COPD is primarily directed at relaxing airway smooth muscle with bronchodilators. Attempts to reduce inflammation with inhaled corticosteroids and

phosphodiesterase inhibition (e.g., theophylline) have had limited success. Nonpharmacologic therapy includes pulmonary rehabilitation, smoking cessation, and long-term oxygen therapy (LTOT). A comprehensive review of therapy and the side effects of therapy for COPD is beyond the scope of this review. (The reader is referred to the references section for more detailed information.[4-6])

Briefly, initiation of treatment is based on a combination of pulmonary function impairment (generally measured by a reduction in FEV_1), symptoms predominantly of dyspnea, and frequency of COPD exacerbations. Treatment modalities include inhaled short-acting bronchodilators, inhaled long-acting bronchodilators, and inhaled corticosteroids. Treatment generally escalates from a short-acting to a long-acting bronchodilator to a combination of more than one long-acting bronchodilator to a combination of a long-acting bronchodilator with an inhaled corticosteroid for stable COPD. Escalation is generally based on severity of symptoms, degree of reduction in FEV_1, and the potential to prevent future COPD exacerbations. Oral theophylline may be considered in patients who remain symptomatic despite inhaled therapy. Oral corticosteroids should be avoided as treatment for stable COPD.

Treatment of COPD patients with and without OSA starts with optimization of pharmacotherapy and, if necessary, simultaneous treatment of OSA, with reevaluation of the patient's daytime and nocturnal arterial O_2 saturation once treatment is optimized. Along with optimization of therapy, approaches to hypoxemia include LTOT, either continuous if daytime hypoxemia is present or nocturnal if only isolated nocturnal hypoxemia is present (Table 21-4). The effect of treatment of isolated nocturnal hypoxemia on patient outcomes is not well defined. One study of nocturnal oxygen in patients with isolated nocturnal hypoxemia had no reduction in mortality rate but the sample size was small.[36]

In some COPD patients, particularly those with hypercapnia, nocturnal noninvasive positive pressure ventilation

TABLE 21-4

Use of Positive Airway Pressure (PAP) and Oxygen for Treatment of Chronic Respiratory Failure and Hypoxemia

Modality	Clinical Target	Settings	Outcome
LTOT for all types of pulmonary disease	Arterial oxygen saturation ≥ 90% or PaO_2 ≥ 60 mm Hg	Necessary L/min flow of oxygen	Decreased mortality
Nocturnal LTOT for all types of pulmonary disease	Nocturnal arterial oxygen saturation ≥ 90%	Necessary L/min flow of oxygen monitored by oximetry during sleep	None proven; may reduce pulmonary hypertension in COPD

NIPPV ± LTOT for COPD	Pressure to relieve dyspnea, promote accessory respiratory muscle use, and reduce respiratory rate
	    Some studies titrated to tolerance only, with a fixed difference between IPAP and EPAP
	    Arterial saturation ≥ 90%
	    Most studies used only nocturnal NIPPV and used nocturnal studies to titrate
		Titrate pressure to achieve predefined endpoint
		    Pressures averaged 12-14 cm for IPAP and 3-5 cm for EPAP
			Inconsistent; may decrease mortality and reduce $PaCO_2$ on oxygen but quality of life may be reduced NIPPV when used with a timed backup rate may improve outcomes

NIPPV ± LTOT for CF	Pressure and oxygen to keep oxygen above PaO_2 of 50 mm Hg and $PaCO_2$ < 60 mm Hg or saturation ≥ 90%
	    Most studies used only nocturnal NIPPV and used nocturnal studies to titrate
		Similar to NIPPV ± LTOT	Improved arterial PaO_2 and reduced $PaCO_2$
			    Hypercapnia not improved by CPAP

COPD, chronic obstructive pulmonary disease; *CPAP*, continuous positive airway pressure; *IPAP*, inspiratory positive airway pressure; *EPAP*, expiratory inspiratory positive airway pressure; *LTOT*, long-term oxygen therapy; *NIPPV*, noninvasive positive-pressure ventilation; *PaCO₂*, partial pressure of arterial carbon dioxide; *PaO₂*, partial pressure of arterial oxygen.

(NIPPV) usually with bilevel positive airway pressure (BiPAP) and typically delivered through a nasal or full-face mask may be indicated. There have been a number of trials of the use of nocturnal NIPPV in treating stable severe hypercapnic COPD. The results of these trials are mixed with modest benefits (see Table 21-4). A recent randomized controlled trial (RCT) of NIPPV suggested an improvement in mortality rate but a reduction in quality of life.[37] A systematic review of RCTs to 2002 showed some improvements in health-related quality of life (HQOL) and dyspnea.[38] A meta-analysis of RCTs showed no obvious benefits in pulmonary function, arterial blood gases, sleep efficiency, and 6-minute walking distance.[39]

Summary

Patients with COPD have frequent complaints of insomnia which are not well correlated with sleep architecture but may be better correlated with symptoms of dyspnea and wheezing. It is unclear if COPD has a major detrimental effect on sleep architecture because many of the changes are also consistent with the age of the patients. Patients with severe to very severe COPD are at greater risk of developing R sleep-related arterial O_2 desaturation. Optimal medical treatment of the COPD may improve nocturnal O_2 saturation but does not appear to have a substantial impact on sleep architecture or daytime symptoms and quality of life. OSA may be a co-morbid condition with COPD that enhances the probability of greater nocturnal desaturation. The possibility that COPD and OSA coexist in the same patient should be considered during evaluation and management.

ASTHMA

Asthma is a chronic inflammatory disease of the airways characterized by episodic and reversible airway obstruction. The airway obstruction is the result of bronchoconstriction and airway hyperreactivity, airway edema, mucus hypersecretion,

and airway remodeling such as fibrotic changes. In 2006, asthma affected almost 23 million persons or about 7.8% of the population.[40]

In 1995 asthma accounted for more than 5000 deaths, 1.87 million emergency department visits, and more than 100 million restricted activity days. Since 1995, the number of deaths due to asthma has declined, even in the face of an increasing prevalence of the disease.[40]

A diagnosis of asthma is based on a history consistent with airway hyperreactivity (e.g., shortness of breath, cough, wheezing, or chest tightness). Objective confirmation of airway hyperreactivity is generally sought by documenting spirometrically reversible airway obstruction in response to a bronchodilator or from bronchoprovocational challenge testing such as with methacoline aerosol. Diseases such as COPD, sarcoidosis, congestive heart failure, and vocal cord dysfunction are part of the differential diagnosis. Patients may be incorrectly diagnosed and treated for asthma when they have an alternative diagnosis such as COPD.[41,42]

Inflammatory cells involved in asthma include mast cells and eosinophils. These cells release a variety of mediators such as histamine, leukotrienes, and proteins that can contribute to airway injury, smooth muscle hyperreactivity, airway edema, and airway remodeling. In addition, IgE-mediated antigen-antibody complexes often interact with the inflammatory cells to release mediators.

Transient worsening of asthma may occur as a result of internal and external stimuli such as exercise and air pollutants. More prolonged worsening is often from viral infections of the upper respiratory tract or allergen exposure.[41]

The mechanisms accounting for worsening of asthma at night may be related to circadian rhythms of epinephrine and cortisol, or an increase in airway cholinergic tone. An increase in airway inflammation at night has also been reported. In addition, GERD has been implicated in some cases of nocturnal asthma symptoms.[40-43]

Asthma Classification of Severity

Classification of asthma severity is based on *impairment*, as determined by reduction in pulmonary function and presence of symptoms such as dyspnea and nocturnal awakenings, and *risk* as reflected in number and severity of asthma exacerbations and presence of side effects from asthma treatment. Asthma is classified as intermittent or persistent. Patients with intermittent asthma have infrequent symptoms and essentially normal pulmonary function. However, such patients may have occasional exacerbations, which may be severe.[41] Persistent asthma is classified as mild, moderate, or severe. The distinction is based on the number of daytime and nocturnal symptoms, the level of reduction in pulmonary function, and the number of asthma exacerbations. *Intermittent asthma* is generally defined as normal pulmonary function, no limitation in normal activities, and symptoms and use of short-acting β_2-agonists as rescue two or fewer times a week, nighttime awakenings two or fewer times a month, and no more than one exacerbation per year. Severe persistent asthma is any one of the following: pulmonary function less than 60% of predicted, severe limitation in activities, and essentially continuous symptoms and use of rescue β_2-agonists day and night. Mild and moderate persistent asthma represent increasing reductions in pulmonary function, increasing limitation in activities, and escalating frequency of symptoms and use of β_2-agonists for rescue. A full discussion of asthma classification of severity is beyond the scope of this chapter, and the reader is referred to other sources for more detailed information.[41,42]

Management

The major objectives in management of asthma are *reduction in impairment*, such as improvement in pulmonary function and ameliorating symptoms such as nocturnal awakenings, and *reduction in risk* such as a decrease in the number of asthma exacerbations. Management of asthma also involves identification and reduction in internal and external asthma triggers, education about the cause and treatment of the disease, and an understanding of the use of pharmacotherapy to maintain asthma control and prevent exacerbations.

Pharmacotherapy is generally recommended as "step-up" and "step-down," depending on the severity of symptoms, level of pulmonary function, and response to therapy. As mentioned, short-acting β_2-agonists are used for intermittent asthma and as rescue therapy for persistent asthma. The primary target of maintenance asthma therapy for persistent asthma is to reduce airway inflammation, making anti-inflammatory agents, particularly inhaled corticosteroids, the mainstay of treatment. Long-acting β_2-agonists are added to inhaled corticosteroids in patients whose asthma is not adequately controlled, but caution must be taken because long-acting β_2-agonists have been associated with increased asthma exacerbations and increased mortality rate and should never be used as maintenance therapy without concomitant anti-inflammatory therapy. Based on a number of considerations, oral leukotriene modifiers (anti-inflammatory agents), oral theophylline, and periodic injections of anti-IgE antibody may be used to reduce or inhibit mediators that produce airway inflammation. The ultimate goal of therapy is to eliminate impairment and risk. A full discussion of treatment options is beyond the scope of this chapter, and the reader is referred to other sources for more detailed information.[41]

Sleep Disturbances and Sleep Architecture in Asthma

Asthmatic symptoms that awaken patients during the night are common and contribute to sleep disruption. A PSG study of 12 asthmatics (mean age 43 years, mean peak flow 65% predicted, suggesting at least moderate persistent asthma) with nocturnal symptoms compared to 12 subjects without asthma documented a decrease in sleep efficiency of 7%, an increase in sleep latency of 19 minutes, and an increase in time spent awake at night of 35 minutes.[44] In contrast, sleep architecture in patients with nocturnal asthma (FEV_1 67.6% predicted) did not appear to differ substantially from that shown by studies of healthy individuals of a similar age including the number of arousals per hour of sleep (see Tables 21-1 and 21-5).[1,45,46]

However, patients with asthma may have sleep complaints out of proportion to the modest disturbances in sleep architecture. For example, in a study by Janson and associates of elderly patients with asthma or COPD, sleep disturbances were greater in asthmatic patients compared to COPD patients.[16] In 267 younger (age 33 years) asthmatics with an FEV_1 of 100% predicted, sleep efficiency of 94% and sleep latency of 22 minutes (based on sleep diaries), sleep-related complaints were substantially more prevalent than in 2394 matched nonasthmatic control subjects.[47] For example, there were more complaints of difficulty falling asleep and early morning awakenings, and daytime sleepiness was increased. These problems occurred in a minority of patients (e.g., difficulty falling asleep was 12.7% vs. 6.8% of asthmatic compared to nonasthmatic patients) or were significant but modest (e.g., latency to sleep onset 22 vs. 19 minutes, sleep efficiency 94% vs. 96%). The intermittent nature and the relatively low prevalence of symptoms may make it difficult to capture disrupted sleep patterns by PSG in groups of asthmatic patients or on any given night.

Relationship of Obstructive Sleep Apnea to Asthma

A number of studies have examined coexistent OSA and asthma. One such study examined the prevalence of asthma in patients already confirmed as having OSA by PSG. The study population of 606 OSA patients had a mean age of 40 years (two thirds were male) with severe OSA on average (AHI 53.9 in asthmatics, 47.8 in nonasthmatics, $P = 0.05$) with an overall asthma prevalence of 35.1%.[48] This prevalence of asthma would appear to be higher than is typically present in the general population.[41,48]

The prevalence of OSA in asthmatic patients also appears to be increased. The study by Janson (discussed previously)[47] indicated that snoring and apneas were significantly more prevalent in asthmatic patients (snoring 14.7% vs. 9.2%, apnea 3.8% vs. 1.2%). A questionnaire study of 7469 respondents (mean age 44 years, 3920 women) indicated that 2713 had asthma-related symptoms.[49] Those with asthma-related symptoms were significantly more likely to have snoring (odds ratio [OR] 1.7) and witnessed apneas (OR 2.2). A study using the Berlin questionnaire (a questionnaire with a high positive predictive value for identifying patients with OSA) found that symptoms of OSA are significantly more prevalent in asthmatics ($n = 177$, 39.5% with symptoms of OSA) compared to patients in an internal medicine clinic without asthma ($n = 328$, 27.2%). The mean ages were 48 and 52 years

TABLE 21-5

Studies of Typical Sleep Architecture in Nocturnal Asthma

Feature/Metric	Study/Population				
	Wiegand[45]: Placebo (N = 19)[†]	Wiegand[45]: Theophylline (N = 19)[†]	Wiegand[45]: Salmeterol (N = 19)[†]	Ciftci[46]: No OSA [AHI = 4] (N = 22)	Ciftci[*46]: + OSA [AHI = 44] (N = 16)
Age	35.6	35.6	35.6	43.9	45.9
TIB (min)	402 (calc.)	412 (calc.)	399 (calc.)	NA	NA
TST (min)	356	372	344	NA	NA
SE %	88.6 (calc.)	90.4 (calc.)	86.2 (calc.)	68.9	74.1
N1 %	4.5 (calc.)	3.8 (calc.)	5 (calc.)	6.8	10.8
N2 %	53.7 (calc.)	53.7 (calc.)	52.1 (calc.)	38	45.6
N3 %	25,1 (calc.)	22.5 (calc.)	24.1 (calc.)	12.8	8
R %	16.7 (calc.)	20 (calc.)	18.7 (calc.)	14.1	15.1
SaO₂ (%)	95.7 (mean during sleep)	96.1 (mean during sleep)	95.9 (mean during sleep)	91.5 (mean during sleep)	89.1 (mean during sleep)
LSO (min)	9.8	12.8	15.9	NA	NA
WASO (min)	37 (calc.)	26 (calc.)	41 (calc.)	NA	NA
Awakenings (no./hr of sleep)	5.4	4.7	4.8	NA	NA
Arousal (no. /hr of sleep)	6.5	5.7	6.8	NA	NA
FEV₁(L) (% pred.)	3.81 (67.6%)	3.81 (67.6%)	3.81 (67.6%)	NA (65.5)	NA (70.3)

*Nocturnal asthma symptom scores were significantly improved by 2 months of CPAP.
†Randomized crossover study.
AHI, apnea-hypopnea index (events/hour of sleep); *OSA*, obstructive sleep apnea. For other abbreviations, see Tables 21-1 and 21-3.
References cited in this table are listed at the end of the chapter and are cited in the chapter text where appropriate.

(no significant difference). The asthmatic patients had more snoring and daytime sleepiness.[50] A recent PSG study of age, sex, and body mass index (BMI) matched patients with severe asthma ($n = 26$), moderate asthma ($n = 26$), and no asthma ($n = 26$) indicated that the prevalence of OSA was 88%, 58%, and 31%, respectively.[51] In contrast to these findings, one study indicated that there was no association between asthma and OSA symptoms.[52] However, OSA was not formally confirmed by sleep studies.

A review of literature exploring the relationship between asthma and OSA[53] suggested that treatment of snoring with continuous positive airway pressure (CPAP) may improve asthma control in part by eliminating nocturnal asthma symptoms. CPAP therapy also reduced bronchial hyperactivity in nonasthmatics with severe OSA and bronchial hyperreactivity. The authors[53] suggested that in asthmatics with OSA "bronchoconstriction is possibly due to the repeated stimulation of neural mechanoreceptors at the glottic inlet, laryngeal region and oropharyngeal region." A more recent study supported the concept that CPAP treatment of OSA improves nocturnal asthma symptoms.[46]

Treatment of Asthma and Sleep

Treatment of asthma can improve sleep-related daytime and nocturnal complaints. An RCT of salmeterol (long-acting β_2-agonist) ($n = 19$), theophylline ($n = 18$), and placebo ($n = 19$) in nocturnal asthma (FEV₁ 67.6% predicted)[45] was conducted. Salmeterol improved nocturnal FEV₁ and perceptions of sleep quality compared to placebo and theophylline without significant effect on sleep architecture, arousals, or awakenings.

A questionnaire study of montelukast (an oral leukotriene receptor antagonist) treatment in a prospective cohort of 9082 asthma patients was conducted for a minimum of 4 weeks. Sleep-related symptoms were common prior to montelukast therapy despite treatment with inhaled corticosteroids in 84.7% and a long-acting β_2-agonist in 60.3%. In this study 87% of the patients were 15 years of age or older, 51% were men, 45.1% had early morning awakenings, and 48.5% had difficulty sleeping because of asthma. After a mean period of 31 days of montelukast therapy, 80.2% and 87.3% of patients reported fewer early morning awakenings and less difficulty sleeping, respectively.[54]

Treatment of GERD may improve asthma symptoms but this practice is controversial. Some studies support a role for the treatment of GERD in difficult to control asthma, whereas other studies do not.[43,55,56] A proton pump inhibitor did not improve daytime or nocturnal asthma symptoms or pulmonary function but did reduce asthma exacerbations and improve some aspects of asthma-related quality of life in patients with symptomatic GERD.[55] Patients with both nocturnal asthma symptoms and symptoms of GERD had improvement in pulmonary function from a proton pump inhibitor.[43] In contrast, a study in symptomatic asthma patients with asymptomatic GERD found no benefit in treatment with a proton pump inhibitor.[56] However, a subsequent analysis[57] of that data indicated that asthmatic patients with GERD had poorer quality of life and were more likely to use oral corticosteroids, perhaps, speculatively, as a result of greater episodic worsening of asthma.

Summary

Asthmatic patients may have intermittent nocturnal symptoms of dyspnea and wheezing. These symptoms appear to produce, at most, modest changes in sleep architecture in most asthmatics and lead to significantly more complaints of difficulty falling asleep and early morning awakenings. These complaints may reduce health-related quality of life. Patients with OSA appear to have an increased prevalence of asthma, and patients with asthma appear to have an increased prevalence of OSA. CPAP treatment of OSA may improve asthma symptoms. Although GERD may be common in asthma, the impact of proton pump inhibitors on pulmonary function and daytime and nocturnal asthma symptoms is questionable. However, asthma symptoms in patients with both GERD and nocturnal asthma symptoms may be improved by treatment of GERD with acid suppressive therapy.

CYSTIC FIBROSIS

Cystic fibrosis (CF) produces obstructive pulmonary disease due to an autosomal recessive genetic disorder that is found most frequently in white people of Northern European heritage. It is the most common lethal genetic disease, affecting 1 in 2500 whites.[58] There is a genetic mutation of the CF transmembrane conductance regulator (CFTR). CFTR is found in a number of organs including the upper and lower airways, bowel, ducts of the pancreas, and reproductive tracts. The defective CFTR indirectly reduces the transport of sodium, which impairs local movement of water. This impairment leads to lower water volume and thick secretions, which impair the function of the lungs and other involved organs.[58] Average life expectancy is predicted to be greater than 50 years of age for CF patients born in 2000.[59]

Pathophysiology

Impairment of pulmonary function is the major cause of morbidity and death. The airways become chronically obstructed by abnormal secretions. This environment is ideal for bacterial growth from organisms such as *Pseudomonas aeruginosa* (including a mucoid type), *Haemophilus influenzae*, and *Staphylococcus aureus*. These organisms lead to frequent infections, the main consequence of which is bronchiectasis and remodeling of lung architecture such as an increase in mucus gland volume.[60] Even without a clinically significant infection, the lungs of a CF patient have elevated numbers of inflammatory cells that contribute to airway obstruction from increased bronchomotor tone.[61] When pulmonary function tests are followed over time, there is progressive obstructive pulmonary function with an increase in residual volume (RV) and FRC, a reduction in FEV_1, and a reduction in the FEV_1/FVC ratio.[62] Relapsing episodes of lung infections may be life threatening and can lead to bronchiectasis and scarring. The combination of bronchiectasis, progressive airway obstruction, and possibly malnutrition from pancreatic insufficiency lead to chronic hypoventilation (i.e., hypercapnia) from failure of the chest wall muscular pump, and hypoxemia from the hypoventilation combined with a ventilation-perfusion mismatch. Death often results from respiratory failure.[62]

As in the lungs, thick secretions can obstruct intrapancreatic ducts and lead to pancreatic autolysis with fatty replacement of normal pancreatic tissue. This damage can produce diabetes mellitus if enough islet cells are destroyed.[63] Both the destruction of pancreatic tissue and the obstruction of pancreatic ducts contribute to the lack of pancreatic enzyme necessary for adequate fat, protein, and fat-soluble vitamin absorption, making malnutrition and growth retardation

a significant problem.[64] In affected male patients, ductal obstruction usually occurs in the vas deferens, leading to azoospermia and infertility.[60]

Co-Morbid Sleep Conditions

CF patients commonly have reduced subjective sleep quality. Difficulty with sleep initiation is one of the most common complaints among CF patients.[65,66] There is a significant reduction in sleep quality documented by an increase in the Pittsburgh Sleep Quality Index (PSQI).[67,68] An increase in the PSQI is associated with abnormalities of sleep and pulmonary function. Actigraphy was used during sleep in 20 adult CF patients aged 26 years (Table 21-6).[67] The actigraphic sleep fragmentation index, immobile time, and mean activity score positively and significantly correlated with an increase in PSQI. However, there was no association with daytime sleepiness by the Epworth Sleepiness Scale or general quality of life by the SF-36. In another study using actigraphy, sleep diaries and questionnaires indicated a positive correlation between reduced sleep efficiency and reduced FEV_1 in a group of children with an average age of 11.9 years.[65] This study documented more awakenings for cough and bathroom usage in children with CF than for control subjects. Unlike healthy control subjects that typically micturate at night, the bathroom visits were specifically characterized as defecation, which the authors suggested was the result of the intestinal malabsorption.[65] Cough was present in CF during sleep and was an independent predictor of the degree of reduction in FEV_1.[65] In a study of 37 CF patients aged 32 years, the majority of whom had severe lung disease, a reduced FEV_1 percent predicted was associated with an increased PSQI.[68] Retrospectively, the study separated the patients into two groups: (1) "good sleepers," who had a PSQI less than or equal to 5, and (2) "bad sleepers," who had a PSQI greater than 5. The group of good sleepers had significantly better sleep efficiency and a greater percentage of R sleep during overnight PSGs. However, this study showed no statistical differences in sleep latency, duration, nocturnal arterial oxygen saturation, nocturnal transcutaneous carbon dioxide (CO_2), RDI, and the number of nocturnal arousals. Severe reductions in FEV_1 when associated with hypoxemia, including nocturnal hypoxemia, have been implicated as a major factor in the development of cor pulmonale in CF.[69,70] The unreliability for the PSQI and symptoms in general to predict the degree of nocturnal hypoxemia underscores the importance of documenting the need for nocturnal supplemental O_2.

Sleep Architecture and Gas Exchange

PSG studies are mixed (see Table 21-6), with some suggesting reduced sleep efficiency and abnormal sleep architecture, and others suggesting little reduction in sleep efficiency, little increase in arousals, or unusual percentages of NREM or R stages of sleep.[66,68,71,72] Thirty-two patients aged 32, FEV_1 36% of predicted, had essentially normal sleep architecture.[73] A study of 24 children and adolescents, average age 14.2 years, compared to 14 control subjects aged 10.7 years found that sleep was disrupted. Sleep efficiency and stage R sleep were reduced and this correlated with the severity of reduction in FEV_1.[66] A study of 44 children and adolescents, aged 11.9 years old, compared to 40 control subjects, aged 12.6 years old, had

TABLE 21-6

Studies of Sleep Architecture in Patients with Typical Cystic Fibrosis (CF) versus Control Subjects*

Feature/Metric	Study/Population					
	Jankelowitz*[67]: CF (N = 20)	Jankelowitz*[67]: Control (N = 20)	Milross[72]: CF (N = 31)	Naqvi[66]: CF (N = 24)	Naqvi[66]: Control (N = 14)	Mllross[73]: CF (N = 32)
Age	26	26	27	14.2	10.7	32
TIB (min)	457 (calc.)	432 (calc.)	427 (calc.)	NA	NA	406 (calc.)
TST (min)	389 (calc.)	369 (calc.)	354	NA	NA	353
SE %	85.2	85.4	83	75.2	86.2***	87
N1 %	NA	NA	N1 and N2 62	12.1	8.0	61, N1 and N2
N2 %	NA	NA	NA	49.7	45.8	NA
N3 %	NA	NA	19	25.1	27.8	19
R %	NA	NA	19	12.7	18.3#	21
SaO_2 (%)	NA	NA	142 min < 90	90.3 minimum during sleep	95.6# minimum during sleep	90 average during sleep
LSO (min)	13	14	15	36.9	24.5	NA
WASO (min)	NA	NA	55	NA	NA	NA
Awakenings (no./hr of sleep	NA	NA	NA	NA	NA	NA
Arousals (no./hr of sleep) or FI	FI, 31.7	FI, 18.0**	13.3	28.3	14.5	NA
FEV_1 (L) (% pred.)	NA (61)	NA	NA (37)	NA	NA	NA (36)

*Modality of study was polysomnography, except in that by Jankelowitz,[67] which used actigraphy.
** $p < 0.001$, *** $p < 0.01$, # $p < 0.05$
FI, fragmentation index (electroencephalographic events/hour of sleep). For other abbreviations, see Tables 21-1, 21-3, and 21-4.

a trend in the reduction of sleep efficiency by actigraphy that was significant only for the those with a severely reduced FEV_1 (< 40% predicted).[65] Increases in wake after sleep onset and number of awake episodes, and a reduction in sleep duration, were also significantly correlated with reductions in FEV_1. These results suggest that sleep disruption may occur and is most likely to occur in young children and adolescent CF patients, particularly those with severely reduced pulmonary function. Although CF patients have difficulty falling asleep, it does not readily correlate with latency to sleep onset by PSG.[65,66,72] However, as detailed earlier, studies of sleep architecture suggest that there is marked sleep fragmentation in many patients with CF and this finding may help explain CF patients' perception of difficulty falling asleep.

The sleep in CF patients is punctuated by respiratory events that are more frequently seen during R sleep.[68,72-74] These respiratory events are typically hypopneas with modest numbers of central, obstructive, and mixed apneic events.[73] However, R sleep appears more vulnerable with a difference in RDI between NREM and R sleep of between 11.5 and 12.6 events per hour.[72,73] A study of 32 CF patients with moderate to severe lung disease found that a decrease in expiratory muscle strength correlated with an increase in RDI during R sleep.[73] The authors suggested that, because expiratory muscle strength is a significant contributor to cough strength, a reduction in muscle strength may reduce the clearing of secretions.[73]

Nocturnal hypopneas in CF can lead to significant hypoxemia, especially during R sleep. The degree of sleep hypoxemia has been found to exceed the degree of hypoxemia from vigorous exercise in CF patients and sleep may be the most critical period for arterial O_2 desaturation.[76] In a study of 21 patients, aged 27 years,[75] 8 had significant nocturnal arterial O_2 desaturation, and these patients had greater impairment in

pulmonary function (FEV_1 31% vs. 59% predicted) and lower awake saturations (90.9% vs. 96.2%). The study concluded that the baseline arterial O_2 saturation or exercise-induced O_2 desaturation in patients who were not hypoxemic at rest were not predictive of the magnitude of sleep hypoxemia.[75] In a study of 70 CF patients aged 27 years with lung disease of a wide range of severity, 40% had arterial oxygen saturations of less than 90% for more than 5% of the night.[76] Though an FEV_1 greater than 65% demonstrated a relative resistance to nocturnal arterial oxygen desaturation (9.5% with desaturation), only about half (51%) of those patients with FEV_1 less than 65% had significant nocturnal arterial oxygen desaturation.[76] The study also concluded that nocturnal arterial O_2 desaturation is more likely if the baseline awake arterial O_2 saturation is less than 93%.[76] A study of 32 moderate to severe CF patients developed a formula for expected average nocturnal arterial O_2 saturation.[73] The authors determined that a low bedtime PaO_2 plus elevated morning $PaCO_2$ made the best combined predictor for nocturnal hypoxemia. FEV_1 and inspiratory muscle strength were also found to correlate with average overnight oxygenation.[73] No statistically significant relationship was found between FEV_1 and nocturnal oxygenation in a study of a healthier CF population with average FEV_1 of 61%, suggesting the sensitivity of this marker is reduced with less pulmonary impairment.[67] It is unclear if milder cases of CF lung disease with more normal daytime arterial O_2 saturation should be evaluated for sleep hypoxemia.

The precise cause of episodic nocturnal desaturations in CF is not fully defined, but a number of factors in combination appear to contribute. As previously mentioned, low daytime arterial O_2 saturation is a sensitive marker for further nocturnal hypoxemia, in part, because it is consistent with advanced parenchymal lung disease. In addition, because the patient is on the steep portion of the O_2 hemoglobin dissociation curve, the patient is potentially susceptible to severe hypoxemia in response to relatively brief reductions in ventilation. Because CF patients have a baseline reduction in pulmonary function with limited reserve and hyperinflated lung volumes,[77] the hypotonia of accessory ventilatory muscles during R sleep may lead to hypoventilation, a decrease in lung volume (FRC), and ventilation/perfusion mismatch similar to that of COPD. This effect is exacerbated by the greater work of breathing from requiring more respiratory effort to overcome the presence of thick secretions in the airways, which can further obstruct airflow, and the frequent malnutrition stemming from pancreatic insufficiency, which may limit respiratory muscle strength.[76]

$Paco_2$ has been found to increase during R sleep in CF patients.[66,68,71,73,74,78] Nocturnal hypercapnia was associated with significantly worse PSQI scores including global as well as sleep efficiency and sleep latency scores.[68] A study of respiratory muscle strength in adult CF patients did not find a significant correlation between respiratory muscle strength, nutritional status, and nocturnal transcutaneous Pco_2.[71] In this study, elevations in residual volume correlated significantly with an increase in nocturnal transcutaneous Pco_2. Another study found that reductions in FEV_1 and maximum respiratory expiratory pressure correlated with an increase in nocturnal transcutaneous Pco_2.[73] The significant association between these findings and nocturnal hypercapnia suggest that structural changes of the lung, specifically markers of airway obstruction, are predictors for an increase in nocturnal Pco_2. This hypoventilation appears dependent on degree of lung disease complicated by respiratory muscle weakness and is worsened during R sleep. The hypoventilation during R sleep may be explained by a study in which there was a reduced minute ventilation, an increase in $Paco_2$, and paradoxical rib cage movement during R sleep in six CF patients, who were 15 years in age.[78] The results indicate that accessory muscles of respiration, which are normally not a major contributor to resting ventilation, are actively contributing to ventilation in the face of severe obstructive lung disease but are inhibited as a natural consequence of R sleep.

Treatment

Nocturnal low-flow O_2 typically maintains arterial O_2 saturation in hypoxemic CF patients. However, O_2 does not improve[79] or may even worsen[74] nocturnal hypercapnia. R sleep was increased both in minutes and as a percentage of TST in one study of 6 patients in a randomized crossover study,[74] but there were no changes in sleep architecture in another randomized crossover study of 13 patients.[79]

Seven patients with CF and severe pulmonary impairment underwent a PSG. The group RDI was 7, and all had an R sleep RDI greater than 5 (average 25.5). Nocturnal arterial O_2 saturation and RDI frequency in NREM and R sleep was improved by CPAP in when compared to room air (four patients) or nocturnal supplemental O_2 (three patients) without CPAP.[80] Sleep architecture and hypercapnia were not improved (see Table 21-4).

A survey[81] determined that NIPPV was instituted for 7.6% of adult patients and 1.2% of pediatric patients with CF in 36 medical centers in France. NIPPV was used to treat hypercapnic exacerbations and nocturnal NIPPV was used to treat CF patients with stable daytime hypercapnia. Compliance was high (72-83%). Common complaints included difficulty sleeping with the device, feeling constrained, and a lack of perception of benefit.

There are few studies to validate the use of NIPPV in CF. Five papers analyzed nocturnal NIPPV in CF in 4 to 37 patients,[74,79,80,82,83] without long-term follow-up. BiLevel PAP, unlike low flow O_2 significantly reduced nocturnal Pco_2.[74,79] Improvement in sleep architecture was not seen with NIPPV in one study.[79] There was an improvement in R sleep minutes and percentage of total sleep time in another study.[74] Subjective assessment of sleep quality was improved in a four patient case series[82] with patients describing that the device provided rest for respiratory muscles with better cough strength and daytime function. However, the majority of patients in one study preferred low flow O_2 alone, for reasons of comfort.[74] A 6-week crossover study of 37 patients suggested that nocturnal NIPPV improves chest symptoms, exertional dyspnea, nocturnal hypoventilation, and peak exercise capacity in adult patients with stable CF.[83] A Cochrane review[84] summarized seven studies (six single session and one 6-week study) with 106 patients and concluded that NIPPV may improve sputum clearance, nocturnal saturation, and exercise performance. One prospective cohort study evaluated long-term NIPPV in CF.[85] Twelve patients with severe pulmonary disease awaiting lung transplant were followed for a mean of 5 months. NIPPV had significant progressive benefits in FEV_1, FVC, and blood gases (time of day of analysis not mentioned) with stabilization of body mass index (BMI). Subjectively, these patients described a reduction in early morning headaches and improved sleep quality and well-being.

Chest physiotherapy is routinely used in CF patients and its goal is to help clear excess mucus from the lungs using mechanical means. Such techniques include chest percussion, external vibration of the thorax, and postural drainage, which utilizes gravity to assist in clearance as well as deep breathing and controlled coughing exercises. Chest physiotherapy may be enhanced by NIPPV in acute respiratory exacerbations of CF as determined in a randomized crossover trial of 26 patients. There was improvement in inspiratory muscle function, arterial O_2 saturation, and dyspnea.[86]

Summary

Patients with severe CF often have disturbances of sleep architecture with reduced sleep efficiency and increased arousals. Patients, presumably as a result of fragmented sleep, have sleep complaints of difficulty initiating sleep, cough during sleep, and reduced sleep quality. These complaints correlate with disease severity as measured by pulmonary function. Often nocturnal hypoxemia or exaggeration of daytime hypoxemia during sleep may require nocturnal O_2 therapy. Nocturnal arterial O_2 desaturation and hypercapnia may be the result, in part, of reduced inspiratory muscle strength and is correlated with severe reductions in pulmonary function. R sleep is a vulnerable period for nocturnal desaturation and hypercapnia. Although nocturnal O_2 is recommended to correct nocturnal hypoxemia, improvements in sleep architecture are inconsistent. The use of NIPPV may improve nocturnal ventilation and daytime pulmonary function and improve quality of sleep and well-being. However, patient physical discomfort with NIPPV may limit its acceptability.

INTERSTITIAL LUNG DISEASE

Interstitial lung disease (ILD) is the result of diffuse inflammatory injury of the lung parenchyma ultimately producing fibrosis of the interstitium and alveoli. These changes lead to loss of alveoli and pulmonary capillaries. The prevalence of ILD is approximately 31.5 cases per year per 100,000 men and 26.1 cases per year per 100,000 women with the most common type being idiopathic pulmonary fibrosis (IPF), which represents about 45% of ILD cases.[87] In addition to IPF, there are over 100 disease entities caused by systemic diseases, environmental exposures, collagen vascular disorders, and drug and radiation side effects.

Pathophysiology

ILD is predominantly a restrictive pulmonary disease that ultimately results in a reduction in total lung capacity (TLC), FRC, RV, FEV_1, and FVC. Because both FEV_1 and FVC are reduced proportionally, the FEV_1/FVC ratio is preserved or slightly elevated. The combination of the preserved FEV_1/FVC ratio and a reduced TLC distinguishes restrictive from obstructive pulmonary function (see Table 21-2). Alveolar destruction, loss of alveolar surface area, and destruction of pulmonary capillaries also lead to a reduction in the single breath diffusing capacity of the lung for carbon monoxide ($DLcosb$). Arterial blood gasses may document hypoxemia. The reduction in Pao_2, particularly with exercise, results from ventilation/perfusion mismatch, diffusion impairment due to thickening of the alveolar membrane and loss of alveolar surface area, and decreased pulmonary capillary transit time.[88] The inflammatory and fibrotic processes in the lung including, when present, pulmonary hypertension and hypoxemia, stimulate a sensation of dyspnea, particularly during exercise. The dyspnea typically produces increased ventilation and a $Paco_2$ that is generally within the normal range or reduced.[89]

Clinical Presentation

The clinical presentation of ILD varies but typically includes a complaint of progressive dyspnea on exertion, which frequently is accompanied by a nonproductive cough. IPF and sarcoidosis are ILDs that can be insidious in onset and may be present for several years before diagnosis, whereas other types such as eosinophilic pneumonia, hypersensitivity pneumonitis, and cryptogenic organizing pneumonia can appear suddenly over days to weeks and thereby mimic an acute infectious process.[87] Some forms of ILD are more prevalent among younger patients and some are found more often in the elderly. Examples include Langerhans cell histiocytosis and sarcoidosis, which are classically diagnosed in patients who are 20 to 40 years old versus IPF, which presents mostly after age 50.

The treatment and prognosis of ILD are dependent, in part, on the type. Pulmonary sarcoidosis has a high rate of spontaneous remission, a generally good response to short courses of corticosteroids and a mortality rate of less than 5%.[90] This disease contrasts significantly with IPF, in which treatment results are disappointing despite use of systemic corticosteroids and cytotoxic agents such as azathioprine. For example, the long-term corticosteroid response rate ranges from 8% to 17%.[91-96] The use of N-acetylcysteine may offer some benefit when combined with a corticosteroid and azathioprine.[97]

Most IPF patients will eventually require supplemental O_2 for hypoxemia and should undergo pulmonary rehabilitation programs to maintain stamina.[98] Lung transplantation may be a therapeutic alternative in selected patients.

Apart from distinguishing IPF from other forms of ILD, the differential diagnosis includes pulmonary malignancy and congestive heart failure.

Contributing Conditions

Medical conditions potentially complicating ILD include pulmonary hypertension, emphysema, and GERD. Pulmonary hypertension occurs in 32% to 85% of IPF patients with a trend toward increasing prevalence with increased disease severity.[99-102] Patients with coexistent emphysema from cigarette smoking are more likely to have pulmonary hypertension and a severely reduced $DLcosb$.[103,104] Several limited studies have found that a majority of IPF patients have GERD and suggest that acid reflux is a potential contributing factor to IPF.[105-108]

Co-Morbid Sleep Conditions

Sleep disorders contribute to morbidity in patients with ILD. A prospective questionnaire study of subjective sleepiness in 41 IPF patients aged 68 years, including 22 men, showed more daytime sleepiness as compared to historical population control subjects. Sleep quality was measured using the PSQI and sleepiness by the Epworth Sleepiness Scale. There was a significant reduction in sleep-related quality of life and an increase in sleepiness compared to control subjects.[109] The PSQI correlated with the patients' overall quality of life, as assessed by the SF-36. However, quality of life did not correlate with disease severity based on pulmonary function testing. The use of steroids, BMI, age, smoking status, or arterial O_2 saturation during a 6-minute walk test did not correlate with degree of daytime sleepiness or sleep quality.

Daytime fatigue, quality of life, and sleepiness scores based on Fatigue Severity Scale (FSS), PSQI, Functional Outcomes in Sleep Questionnaire (FOSQ), and Epworth Sleepiness Scale were significantly impaired in IPF compared to population control subjects.[110] There were significant correlations between FOSQ and FSS and TST spent below an arterial O_2 saturation of 90%. In contrast, scores in the PSQI did not correlate with nocturnal saturations. Similar to another study,[109] there was no correlation between the various measures and daytime arterial O_2 saturation.[111] The results of these two studies suggest that nocturnal hypoxemia, rather than daytime abnormalities of pulmonary function, is a substantial contributor to a reduction in some measures of sleep-related quality of life and daytime fatigue.[109,110]

OSA is common in patients with ILD. In 18 IPF patients, OSA was present in 11 of 18 subjects, with another 3 of 18 receiving the diagnosis of upper airway resistance syndrome.[111] In 50 IPF patients (average age 64.6 years), OSA was present in 44 including 34 with an AHI greater than 15 per hour of sleep.[112] The only significant potentially contributing differences between those with and without OSA were a higher BMI and a higher Mallampati score. The Mallampati score is a measure of soft tissue crowding of the oropharynx (Fig. 21-3). Those without OSA had more severe reductions in pulmonary function.

Sleep Architecture and Arterial Oxygen Saturation

IPF is the type of ILD best studied with regard to sleep architecture. A study of 15 IPF patients aged 66.3 years[111] found that sleep architecture was substantially disturbed compared to age-matched control subjects (Table 21-7). Sleep efficiency and stage N3 sleep were reduced, and stage N1 sleep and the arousal index were increased. Arterial O_2 saturation was lower and time spent below 90% was 34.3 minutes compared to 0.9 minutes in control subjects. Sleep architecture in the control group (average age 62.7 years) was consistent with that of healthy individuals of a similar age from the literature (see Table 21-1). Eleven ILD patients demonstrated reduced R sleep percentage, increased R sleep latency, reduced arterial O_2 saturation in

R sleep, and increased arousals per hour compared to age- and sex-matched control subjects.[113] ILD patients with a daytime arterial O_2 saturation less than 90% had greater sleep fragmentation, less R sleep, and more sleep state changes.

A study of IPF in 19 patients at an altitude of 7349 ft[114] indicated that heart rate was elevated during all stages of sleep and was reduced to control levels by supplemental O_2. These patients had room air high altitude O_2 saturations of 82.3%. However, at sea level, a study of 19 patients indicated that, despite severe restrictive pulmonary function, patients with IPF with awake saturations of greater than 90% did not require supplemental O_2 during sleep to maintain an average arterial O_2 saturation greater than 90%, although there were episodes of transient hypoxemia in all the patients.[115] This finding was confirmed by another study of 48 IPF patients, but those

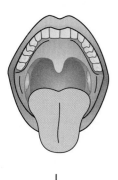 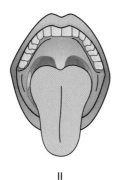 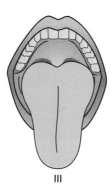 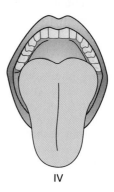

I   II   III   IV

Figure 21-3 These illustrations demonstrate the different classes of the Mallampati scoring system, which attempts to characterize the degree of oropharyngeal narrowing. Class I: Fully visible tonsils, uvula, and soft palate. Class II: Upper portion of the tonsils, most of the uvula, and hard and soft palate remain visible. Class III: Only the base of the uvula and soft and hard palates are visible. Class IV: Only the hard palate is visible.

TABLE 21-7

Studies of Typical Sleep Architecture in Patients with Interstitial Lung Disease versus Control Subjects

Feature/Metric	Study/Population					
	Mermigkis[110]: IPF (N = 15)	Mermigkis[110]: Healthy Control (N = 15)	McNicholas[115]: IPF (N = 7)	Lancaster[112]: IPF [AHI = 1.6] (N = 6)	Lancaster[112]: IPF [AHI = 39.4] (N = 34)	Mermigkis[111]: IPF + OSA/UARS [AHI = 25.2] (N = 18)
Age	66.3	62.7	59	69	64	68.1
TIB (min)	448 (calc.)	409 (calc.)	NA	NA	NA	429 (calc.)
TST (min)	291	320	284	NA	NA	270
SE %	64.9	78.2*	NA	77.2	69.8	62.9
N1 %	18.7	7.4*	27.8 (calc.)	10.4	22.3	85.2 (N1 and N2)
N2 %	59.5	60	51.1 (calc.)	70.1	63.9	NA
N3 %	10.4	16.5*	7.7 (calc.)	3.2	0.2	5.5
R %	11.3	14.9	13.4 (calc.)	16.5	12.6	8.6
Sao₂ (%)	91.6 mean during sleep, < 90 for 34.3 min	95.3 mean during sleep,* < 90 for 0.9 min†	Mean during sleep 90.4 (REM sleep) 91.0 (N3) 91.5 (N2) 92.1 (N1) 92.9 (awake)	87.3 (minimum saturation)	78.7 (minimum saturation)	17.7 min @ < 90
LSO (min)	NA	NA	NA	22.5	21.8	NA
WASO (min)	NA	NA	66	NA	NA	NA
Awakenings (no./hr of sleep)	NA	NA	NA	NA	NA	NA
Arousals (no./hr of sleep)	25.6	12.9*	NA	6.4	38.1	29.7
FVC (L) (% pred.)	NA (77.4)	NA (89.2)	NA (50)	2.2 (58)	3.0 (73)	(65.7)

*P < 0.003 compared with patients with IPF in Mermigkis study.[110]
†P < 0.05 compared with patients with IPF in Mermigkis study.[110]
IPF, idiopathic pulmonary fibrosis; *OSA*, obstructive sleep apnea; *UARS*, upper airway resistance syndrome. For other abbreviations, see Tables 21-1, 21-3, 21-4, and 21-5. Studies cited in this table are listed at the end of the chapter and are cited in the chapter text where appropriate.

authors documented a reduction in quality of life associated with the transient episodes of hypoxemia. The authors also confirmed that resting daytime arterial oxygen saturation was the best predictor of nocturnal hypoxemia,[116] whereas FVC was not. Whether treatment of the transient nocturnal hypoxemia would affect outcomes was not examined in this study. As previously indicated,[109] there was no correlation between pulmonary function testing in ILD patients and subjective measures of sleep quality. Overall, the evidence indicates that PFTs do not consistently predict the degree of sleep disruption or nocturnal arterial desaturation.

Sleep architecture in those with IPF and OSA, as expected, reflects the combination of OSA and IPF. Those with IPF and OSA have a much higher AHI, an increase in stage N1 sleep, a reduction in N3 sleep, lower nocturnal arterial O_2 saturations, and a greater number of arousals compared to IPF without OSA[111,112] (see Table 21-7). Patients with coexistent OSA should be treated as appropriate for the OSA. However, whether outcomes from ILD will be affected by treatment of OSA is unknown, because there do not appear to be studies specifically addressing the treatment of OSA in ILD patients.

The use of steroids in the treatment of ILD may contribute to the impaired sleep found in this disorder. Only one paper[111] cited in this section commented on the prevalence of use of systemic steroids in their study group for which they found no link to poorer sleep quality. However, it has been documented in other studies that corticosteroid use can decrease the amount of R sleep, increase slow wave sleep, and increase nocturnal wakefulness.[117-119] It may be an overlooked contributor to these changes. The treatment of insomnia in ILD has not been specifically addressed by any study, and the approach should take into account the potential effect of pharmacotherapy on a patient's respiratory status.

Summary

Patients with severe ILD often have disturbances of sleep architecture with reduced sleep efficiency and increased arousals. Patients, presumably as a result of fragmented sleep, have sleep complaints including daytime somnolence, reduced quality of life, and daytime fatigue. These complaints correlate with nocturnal hypoxemia but do not obviously correlate with disease severity as measured by pulmonary function or daytime arterial O_2 saturation. There is often transient hypoxemia during sleep, which is more likely the lower the daytime saturation. There appears to be an increase in prevalence of obstructive sleep apnea in patients with ILD, particularly IPF. Although nocturnal supplemental O_2 can treat hypoxemia and nocturnal hypoxemia is associated with daytime symptoms such as fatigue and sleepiness, there are no studies correlating improvement in nocturnal hypoxemia, sleep architecture, and daytime symptoms (see Table 21-4).

REFERENCES

1. Ohayon MM, Carskadon MA, Guilleminault C, Vitiello MV. Meta-analysis of quantitative sleep parameters from childhood to old age in healthy individuals: Developing normative sleep values across the human lifespan. *Sleep*. 2004;27:1255-1273.
2. Bonnet MH, Arand DL. EEG arousal norms by age. *J Clin Sleep Med*. 2007;3:271-274.
3. Sahlin C, Franklin KA, Stenlund H, Lindberg E. Sleep in women: Normal values for sleep stages and position and the effect of age, obesity, sleep apnea, smoking, alcohol and hypertension. *Sleep Med*. 2009;10:1025-1030.
4. Phillips B, Berry D, Schmitt F, et al. Sleep quality and pulmonary function in the healthy elderly. *Chest*. 1989;95:60-64.
5. Global Initiative for Obstructive Lung Disease. Available at www.goldcopd.org; Accessed Feb. 10, 2010.
6. American Thoracic Society/European Respiratory Society COPD Guidelines. Available at http://www.copd-ats-ers.org/copddoc.pdf; Accessed Feb. 10, 2010.
7. Department of Veterans Affairs/Department of Defense COPD Guidelines, Version 2.0. Available at http://www.healthquality.va.gov/Chronic_Obstructive_Pulmonary_Disease_COPD.asp; Accessed Feb. 10, 2010.
8. Mannino DM, Braman S. The epidemiology and economics of chronic obstructive pulmonary disease. *Proc Am Thorac Soc*. 2007;4:502-506.
9. Lewis CA, Fergusson W, Eaton T, et al. Isolated nocturnal desaturation in COPD: Prevalence and impact on quality of life and sleep. *Thorax*. 2009;64:133-138.
10. Williams KE, Reeves KR, Billing Jr CB, et al. A double-blind study evaluating the long-term safety of varenicline for smoking cessation. *Curr Med Res Opin*. 2007;23:793-801.
11. Garrison GD, Dugan SE. Varenicline: A first-line treatment option for smoking cessation. *Clin Ther*. 2009;31:463-491.
12. Jaehne A, Loessl B, Bárkai Z, et al. Effects of nicotine on sleep during consumption, withdrawal and replacement therapy. *Sleep Med Rev*. 2009;13:363-377.
13. Sanders MH, Newman AB, Haggerty CL, et al. Sleep Heart Health Study. Sleep and sleep-disordered breathing in adults with predominantly mild obstructive airway disease. *Am J Respir Crit Care Med*. 2003;167:7-14.
14. Bradley TD, Rutherford R, Lue F, et al. Role of diffuse airway obstruction in the hypercapnia of obstructive sleep apnea. *Am Rev Respir Dis*. 1986;134:920-924.
15. Saaresranta T, Irjala K, Aittokallio T, Polo O. Sleep quality, daytime sleepiness and fasting insulin levels in women with chronic obstructive pulmonary disease. *Respir Med*. 2005;99:856-863.
16. Bellia V, Catalano F, Scichilone N, et al. Sleep disorders in the elderly with and without chronic airflow obstruction: The SARA study. *Sleep*. 2003;26:318-323.
17. Klink ME, Dodge R, Quan SF. The relation of sleep complaints to respiratory symptoms in a general population. *Chest*. 1994;105:151-154.
18. Ballard RD, Clover CW, Suh BY. Influence of sleep on respiratory function in emphysema. *Am J Respir Crit Care Med*. 1995;151:945-951.
19. Marrone O, Salvaggio A, Insalaco G. Respiratory disorders during sleep in chronic obstructive pulmonary disease. *Int J Chron Obstruct Pulm Dis*. 2006;1:363-372.
20. Littner MR, McGinty DJ, Arand DL. Determinants of oxygen desaturation in the course of ventilation during sleep in chronic obstructive pulmonary disease. *Am Rev Respir Dis*. 1980;122:849-857.
21. Man GC, Chappman KR, Ali SH, Darke AC. Sleep quality and nocturnal respiratory function with once-daily theophylline (Uniphyl) and inhaled salbutamol in patients with COPD. *Chest*. 1996;110:648-653.
22. McNicholas WT, Calverley PM, Lee A, Edwards JC. Tiotropium Sleep Study in COPD Investigators. Long-acting inhaled anticholinergic therapy improves sleeping oxygen saturation in COPD. *Eur Respir J*. 2004;23:825-831.
23. Ryan S, Doherty LS, Rock C, et al. Effects of salmeterol on sleeping oxygen saturation in chronic obstructive pulmonary disease. *Respiration*. 2010;79:475-481.
24. Mulloy E, McNicholas. Theophylline improves gas exchange during rest, excercise, and sleep in severe chronic obstructive pulmonary disease. *Am Rev Respir Dis*. 1993;148:1030-1036.
25. Berry RB, Desa MM, Branum JP, Light RW. Effect of theophylline on sleep and sleep-disordered breathing in patients with chronic obstructive pulmonary disease. *Am Rev Respir Dis*. 1991;143:245-250.
26. Krachman SL, Chatila W, Martin UJ, et al. National Emphysema Treatment Trial Research Group. Effects of lung volume reduction surgery on sleep quality and nocturnal gas exchange in patients with severe emphysema. *Chest*. 2005;128:3221-3228.
27. Kryger M, Wang-Weigand S, Zhang J, Roth T. Effect of ramelteon, a selective MT(1)/MT (2)-receptor agonist, on respiration during sleep in mild to moderate COPD. *Sleep Breath*. 2008;12:243-250.
28. Kryger M, Roth T, Wang-Weigand S, Zhang J. The effects of ramelteon on respiration during sleep in subjects with moderate to severe chronic obstructive pulmonary disease. *Sleep Breath*. 2009;13:79-84.
29. Steens RD, Pouliot Z, Millar TW, et al. Effects of zolpidem and triazolam on sleep and respiration in mild to moderate chronic obstructive pulmonary disease. *Sleep*. 1993;16:318-326.

30. Girault C, Muir J-F, Mihaltan F, et al. Effects of repeated administration of zolpidem on sleep, diurnal and nocturnal respiratory function, vigilance, and physical performance in patients with COPD. *Chest.* 1996;110:1203-1211.

31. Murciano D, Armengaud MH, Cramer PH, et al. Acute effects of zolpidem, triazolam and flunitrazepam on arterial blood gases and control of breathing in severe COPD. *Eur Respir J.* 1993;6:625-629.

32. Vos PJ, Folgering HT, van Herwaarden CL. Predictors for nocturnal hypoxaemia (mean Sao$_2$ < 90%) in normoxic and mildly hypoxic patients with COPD. *Eur Respir J.* 1995;8:74-77.

33. Chaouat A, Weitzenblum E, Kessler R, et al. Outcome of COPD patients with mild daytime hypoxaemia with or without sleep-related oxygen desaturation. *Eur Respir J.* 2001;17:848-855.

34. Bradley TD, Mateika J, Li D, Avendano M, Goldstein RS. Daytime hypercapnia in the development of nocturnal hypoxemia in COPD. *Chest.* 1990;97:308-312.

35. Fletcher EC, Donner CF, Midgren B, et al. Survival in COPD patients with a daytime Pao$_2$ greater than 60 mm Hg with and without nocturnal oxyhemoglobin desaturation. *Chest.* 1992;101:649-655.

36. Fletcher EC, Luckett RA, Goodnight-White S, et al. A double-blind trial of nocturnal supplemental oxygen for sleep desaturation in patients with chronic obstructive pulmonary disease and a daytime Pao$_2$ above 60 mm Hg. *Am Rev Respir Dis.* 1992;145:1070-1076.

37. McEvoy RD, Pierce RJ, Hillman D, et al. Nocturnal non-invasive nasal ventilation in stable hypercapnic COPD: A randomised controlled trial. *Thorax.* 2009;64:561-566.

38. Kolodziej MA, Jensen L, Rowe B, Sin D. Systematic review of noninvasive positive pressure ventilation in severe stable COPD. *Eur Respir J.* 2007;30:293-306.

39. Wijkstra PJ, Lacasse Y, Guyatt GH, et al. A meta-analysis of nocturnal noninvasive positive pressure ventilation in patients with stable COPD. *Chest.* 2003;124:337-343.

40. http://www.cdc.gov/asthma/NHIS/05/data.htm; Accessed 2/21/10.

41. http://www.nhlbi.nih.gov/guidelines/asthma/asthgdln.htm; Accessed 2/21/10.

42. http://www.ginasthma.com; Accessed 2/21/10.

43. Kiljander TO, Harding SM, Field SK, et al. Effects of esomeprazole 40 mg twice daily on asthma: A randomized placebo-controlled trial. *Am J Respir Crit Care Med.* 2006;15:173:1091-1097.

44. Fitzpatrick MF, Engleman H, Whyte KF, et al. Morbidity in nocturnal asthma: Sleep quality and daytime cognitive performance. *Thorax.* 1991;46:569-573.

45. Wiegand L, Mende CN, Zaidel G, et al. Salmeterol vs. theophylline: Sleep and efficacy outcomes in patients with nocturnal asthma. *Chest.* 1999;115:1525-1532.

46. Ciftci TU, Ciftci B, Guven SF, et al. Effect of nasal continuous positive airway pressure in uncontrolled nocturnal asthmatic patients with obstructive sleep apnea syndrome. *Respir Med.* 2005;99:529-534.

47. Janson C, De Backer W, Gislason T, et al. Increased prevalence of sleep disturbances and daytime sleepiness in subjects with bronchial asthma: A population study of young adults in three European countries. *Eur Respir J.* 1996;9:2132-2138.

48. Alharbi M, Almutairi A, Alotaibi D, et al. The prevalence of asthma in patients with obstructive sleep apnoea. *Prim Care Respir J.* 2009;18:328-330.

49. Ekici A, Ekici M, Kurtipek E, et al. Association of asthma-related symptoms with snoring and apnea and effect on health-related quality of life. *Chest.* 2005;128:3358-3363.

50. Auckley D, Moallem M, Shaman Z, Mustafa M. Findings of a Berlin Questionnaire survey: Comparison between patients seen in an asthma clinic versus internal medicine clinic. *Sleep Med.* 2008;9:494-499.

51. Julien JY, Martin JG, Ernst P, et al. Prevalence of obstructive sleep apnea-hypopnea in severe versus moderate asthma. *J Allergy Clin Immunol.* 2009;124:371-376.

52. Karachaliou F, Kostikas K, Pastaka C, et al. Prevalence of sleep-related symptoms in a primary care population—Their relation to asthma and COPD. *Prim Care Respir J.* 2007;16:222-228.

53. Bohadana AB, Hannhart B, Teculescu DB. Nocturnal worsening of asthma and sleep-disordered breathing. *J Asthma.* 2002;39:85-100.

54. Malonne H, Lachman A, Van den Brande P. Impact of montelukast on symptoms in mild-to-moderate persistent asthma and exercise-induced asthma: Results of the ASTHMA survey: Adding Singulair Treatment to Handle symptoms in Mild to moderate Asthmatics. *Curr Med Res Opin.* 2002;18:512-519.

55. Littner MR, Leung FW, Ballard ED II, Huang B, et al. Effects of 24 weeks of lansoprazole therapy on asthma symptoms, exacerbations, quality of life, and pulmonary function in adult asthmatic patients with acid reflux symptoms. *Chest.* 2005;128:1128-1135.

56. American Lung Association Asthma Clinical Research Centers, Mastronarde JG, Anthonisen NR, et al. Efficacy of esomeprazole for treatment of poorly controlled asthma. *N Engl J Med.* 2009;360:1487-1499.

57. Dimango E, Holbrook JT, Simpson E, et al. Effects of asymptomatic proximal and distal gastroesophageal reflux on asthma severity. *Am J Respir Crit Care Med.* 2009;180(9):809-816.

58. Davies JC, Alton EW, Bush A. Cystic fibrosis. *BMJ.* 2007;335(7632):1255-1259.

59. Dodge JA, Lewis PA, Stanton M, Wilsher J. Cystic fibrosis mortality and survival in the UK: 1947-2003. *Eur Respir J.* 2007;29:522-526.

60. O'Sullivan BP, Freedman SD. Cystic fibrosis. *Lancet.* 2009;373(9678):1891-1904.

61. Hiatt P, Eigen H, Yu P, Tepper RS. Bronchodilator responsiveness in infants and young children with cystic fibrosis. *Am Rev Respir Dis.* 1988;137:119-122.

62. Davis PB. Pathophysiology of the lung disease in cystic fibrosis. In: Davis PB, ed. *Cystic Fibrosis.* New York: Marcel Dekker; 1993:193.

63. Marshall BC, Butler SM, Stoddard M, et al. Epidemiology of cystic fibrosis-related diabetes. *J Pediatr.* 2005;146:681-687.

64. Borowitz D, Baker RD, Stallings V. Consensus report on nutrition for pediatric patients with cystic fibrosis. *J Pediatr Gastroenterol Nutr.* 2002;35:246-259.

65. Amin R, Bean J, Burklow K, Jeffries J. The relationship between sleep disturbance and pulmonary function in stable pediatric cystic fibrosis patients. *Chest.* 2005;128:1357-1363.

66. Naqvi SK, Sotelo C, Murry L, Simakajornboon N. Sleep architecture in children and adolescents with cystic fibrosis and the association with severity of lung disease. *Sleep Breath.* 2008;12:77-83.

67. Jankelowitz L, Reid KJ, Wolfe L, et al. Cystic fibrosis patients have poor sleep quality despite normal sleep latency and efficiency. *Chest.* 2005;127:1593-1599.

68. Milross MA, Piper AJ, Norman M, et al. Subjective sleep quality in cystic fibrosis. *Sleep Med.* 2002;3:205-212.

69. Francis PW, Muller NL, Gurwitz D, et al. Hemoglobin desaturation: Its occurrence during sleep in patients with cystic fibrosis. *Am J Dis Child.* 1980;134:734-740.

70. Fraser KL, Tullis DE, Sasson Z, et al. Pulmonary hypertension and cardiac function in adult cystic fibrosis: Role of hypoxemia. *Chest.* 1999;115:1321-1328.

71. Bradley S, Solin P, Wilson J, et al. Hypoxemia and hypercapnia during exercise and sleep in patients with cystic fibrosis. *Chest.* 1999;116:647-654.

72. Milross MA, Piper AJ, Norman M, et al. Night-to-night variability in sleep in cystic fibrosis. *Sleep Med.* 2002;3:213-219.

73. Milross MA, Piper AJ, Norman M, et al. Predicting sleep-disordered breathing in patients with cystic fibrosis. *Chest.* 2001;120:1239-1245.

74. Gozal D. Nocturnal ventilatory support in patients with cystic fibrosis: Comparison with supplemental oxygen. *Eur Respir J.* 1997;10:1999-2003.

75. Coffey MJ, FitzGerald MX, McNicholas WT. Comparison of oxygen desaturation during sleep and exercise in patients with cystic fibrosis. *Chest.* 1991;100:659-662.

76. Frangolias DD, Wilcox PG. Predictability of oxygen desaturation during sleep in patients with cystic fibrosis: Clinical, spirometric, and exercise parameters. *Chest.* 2001;119:434-441.

77. Bell SC, Saunders MJ, Elborn JS, et al. Resting energy expenditure and oxygen cost of breathing in patients with cystic fibrosis. *Thorax.* 1996;51:126-131.

78. Tepper RS, Skatrud JB, Dempsey JA. Ventilation and oxygenation changes during sleep in cystic fibrosis. *Chest.* 1983;84:388-393.

79. Milross MA, Piper AJ, Norman M, et al. Low-flow oxygen and bilevel ventilatory support: effects on ventilation during sleep in cystic fibrosis. *Am J Respir Crit Care Med.* 2001;163:129-134.

80. Regnis JA, Piper AJ, Henke KG, et al. Benefits of nocturnal nasal CPAP in patients with cystic fibrosis. *Chest.* 1994;106:1717-1724.

81. Fauroux B, Burgel P, Boelle P, et al. Practice of noninvasive ventilation for cystic fibrosis: A nationwide survey in France. *Respir Care.* 2008;53:1482-1489.

82. Piper AJ, Parker S, Torzillo PJ, et al. Nocturnal nasal IPPV stabilizes patients with cystic fibrosis and hypercapnic respiratory failure. *Chest.* 1992;102:846-850.

83. Young AC, Wilson JW, Kotsimbos TC, Naughton MT. Randomised placebo controlled trial of non-invasive ventilation for hypercapnia in cystic fibrosis. *Thorax.* 2008;63:72-77.

84. Moran F, Bradley JM, Piper AJ. Non-invasive ventilation for cystic fibrosis. *Cochrane Database Syst Rev.* 2009(1):CD002769.

85. Hill AT, Edenborough FP, Cayton RM, Stableforth DE. Long-term nasal intermittent positive pressure ventilation in patients with cystic fibrosis and hypercapnic respiratory failure (1991-1996). *Respir Med.* 1998;92:523-526.

86. Holland AE, Denehy L, Ntoumenopoulos G, et al. Non-invasive ventilation assists chest physiotherapy in adults with acute exacerbations of cystic fibrosis. *Thorax.* 2003;58:880-884.

87. Green F. Overview of pulmonary fibrosis. *Chest.* 2002;122:S334-S339.

88. Yamaguchi K, Mori M, Kawai A, et al. Inhomogeneities of ventilation and the diffusing capacity to perfusion in various chronic lung diseases. *Am J Respir Crit Care Med.* 1997;156:86-93.

89. O'Donnell DE, Ora J, Webb KA, et al. Mechanisms of activity-related dyspnea in pulmonary diseases. *Respir Physiol Neurobiol.* 2009;167:116-132.

90. Baughman RP. Pulmonary sarcoidosis. *Clin Chest Med.* 2004;25:521-530.

91. Carrington CB, Gaensler EA, Coutu RE, et al. Natural history and treated course of usual and desquamative interstitial pneumonia. *N Engl J Med.* 1978;298:801-809.

92. Douglas WW, Ryu JH, Swensen SJ, et al. Colchicine versus prednisone in the treatment of idiopathic pulmonary fibrosis: A randomized prospective study. Members of the Lung Study Group. *Am J Respir Crit Care Med.* 1998;158:220-225.

93. Daniil ZD, Gilchrist FC, Nicholson AG, et al. A histologic pattern of nonspecific interstitial pneumonia is associated with a better prognosis than usual interstitial pneumonia in patients with cryptogenic fibrosing alveolitis. *Am J Respir Crit Care Med.* 1999;160:899-905.

94. Nicholson AG, Colby TV, Dubois RM, et al. The prognostic significance of the histologic pattern of interstitial pneumonia in patients presenting with the clinical entity of cryptogenic fibrosing alveolitis. *Am J Respir Crit Care Med.* 2000;162:2213-2217.

95. Katzenstein AL, Fiorelli RF. Nonspecific interstitial pneumonia/fibrosis: Histologic features and clinical significance. *Am J Surg Pathol.* 1994;18:136-147.

96. Yousem SA, Colby TV, Gaensler EA. Respiratory bronchiolitis-associated interstitial lung disease and its relationship to desquamative interstitial pneumonia. *Mayo Clin Proc.* 1989;64:1373-1380.

97. Demedts M, Behr J, Buhl R, et al. High-dose acetylcysteine in idiopathic pulmonary fibrosis. *N Engl J Med.* 2005;353:2229-2242.

98. Ferreira A, Garvey C, Connors GL, et al. Pulmonary rehabilitation in interstitial lung disease: Benefits and predictors of response. *Chest.* 2009;135:442-447.

99. Agarwal R, Gupta D, Verma JS, et al. Noninvasive estimation of clinically asymptomatic pulmonary hypertension in idiopathic pulmonary fibrosis. *Indian J Chest Dis Allied Sci.* 2005;47:267-271.

100. Nadrous HF, Pellikka PA, Krowka MJ, et al. Pulmonary hypertension in patients with idiopathic pulmonary fibrosis. *Chest.* 2005;128:2393-2399.

101. Lettieri CJ, Nathan SD, Barnett SD, et al. Prevalence and outcomes of pulmonary arterial hypertension in advanced idiopathic pulmonary fibrosis. *Chest.* 2006;129:746-752.

102. Hamada K, Nagai S, Tanaka S, et al. Significance of pulmonary arterial pressure and diffusion capacity of the lung as prognosticator in patients with idiopathic pulmonary fibrosis. *Chest.* 2007;131:650-656.

103. Cottin V, Nunes H, Brillet PY, et al. Combined pulmonary fibrosis and emphysema: A distinct underrecognised entity. *Eur Respir J.* 2005;26:586-593.

104. Aduen JF, Zisman DA, Mobin SI, et al. Retrospective study of pulmonary function tests in patients presenting with isolated reduction in single-breath diffusion capacity: Implications for the diagnosis of combined obstructive and restrictive lung disease. *Mayo Clin Proc.* 2007;82:48-54.

105. Raghu G. The role of gastroesophageal reflux in idiopathic pulmonary fibrosis. *Am J Med.* 2003;115(Suppl 3A):S60-S64.

106. Sweet MP, Patti MG, Leard LE, et al. Gastroesophageal reflux in patients with idiopathic pulmonary fibrosis referred for lung transplantation. *J Thorac Cardiovasc Surg.* 2007;133:1078-1084.

107. Tobin RW, Pope CE II, Pellegrini CA, et al. Increased prevalence of gastroesophageal reflux in patients with idiopathic pulmonary fibrosis. *Am J Respir Crit Care Med.* 1998;158:1804-1808.

108. Raghu G, Yang ST, Spada C, et al. Sole treatment of acid gastroesophageal reflux in idiopathic pulmonary fibrosis: A case series. *Chest.* 2006;129:794-800.

109. Krishnan V, McCormack MC, Mathai SC, et al. Sleep quality and health-related quality of life in idiopathic pulmonary fibrosis. *Chest.* 2008;134(4):693-698.

110. Mermigkis C, Stagaki E, Amfilochiou A, et al. Sleep quality and associated daytime consequences in patients with idiopathic pulmonary fibrosis. *Med Princ Pract.* 2009;18:10-15.

111. Mermigkis C, Chapman J, Golish J, et al. Sleep-related breathing disorders in patients with idiopathic pulmonary fibrosis. *Lung.* 2007;185:173-178.

112. Lancaster LH, Mason WR, Parnell JA, et al. obstructive sleep apnea is common in idiopathic pulmonary fibrosis. *Chest.* 2009;136:772-778.

113. Perez-Padilla R, West P, Lertzman M, Kryger MH. Breathing during sleep in patients with interstitial lung disease. *Am Rev Respir Dis.* 1985;132:224-229.

114. Vázquez JC, Pérez-Padilla R. Effect of oxygen on sleep and breathing in patients with interstitial lung disease at moderate altitude. *Respiration.* 2001;68:584-589.

115. McNicholas WT, Coffey M, Fitzgerald MX. Ventilation and gas exchange during sleep in patients with interstitial lung disease. *Thorax.* 1986;41:777-782.

116. Clark M, Cooper B, Singh S, et al. A survey of nocturnal hypoxaemia and health related quality of life in patients with cryptogenic fibrosing alveolitis. *Thorax.* 2001;56:482-486.

117. Fehm HL, Benkowitsch R, Kern W, et al. Influences of corticosteroids, dexamethasone and hydrocortisone on sleep in humans. *Neuropsychobiology.* 1986;16:198-204.

118. Moser NJ, Phillips BA, Guthrie G, Barnett G. Effects of dexamethasone on sleep. *Pharmacol Toxicol.* 1996;79:100-102.

119. Born J, DeKloet ER, Wenz H, et al. Gluco- and antimineralocorticoid effects on human sleep: A role of central corticosteroid receptors. *Am J Physiol.* 1991;260(2 Pt 1):E183-E188.

Central Hypersomnolence

Narcolepsy

Chapter 22

GERT JAN LAMMERS

Narcolepsy with cataplexy is usually portrayed as a syndrome characterized by excessive daytime sleepiness (EDS), cataplexy, hypnagogic hallucinations, sleep paralysis, and a disturbed nocturnal sleep.[1,2] Although this is in itself correct, simply listing these symptoms does not convey what it means to suffer from narcolepsy. The key problem of these patients, relentlessly present each and every day of their lives, is their inability to remain fully alert or even awake during longer periods of the day, paradoxically accompanied by difficulty remaining asleep during the night. In addition, the strict physiologic boundaries of specific components of wake and sleep stages are fluid. This leads to partial expressions, particularly of rapid eye movement (REM) sleep, explaining such symptoms as cataplexy, hypnagogic hallucinations, and sleep paralysis.[3,4]

Narcolepsy has an estimated prevalence of 25 to 50 per 100,000, and usually starts during adolescence, a crucial and vulnerable period in life.[5] To prevent poor performance or even dropping out of school, and to facilitate a normal emotional and social development, it is of major importance to recognize the disorder in a timely fashion and to start proper treatment as soon as possible.

SYMPTOMS

Excessive Daytime Sleepiness

Excessive daytime sleepiness is characterized both by an inability to stay awake, as well as difficulty concentrating and sustaining attention, leading to impaired performance.[6] EDS and sleep typically occur during monotonous activities such as watching television, reading, attending a meeting, or being a passenger in a car. Conversely, physical or mental activity decreases sleepiness and prevents sleep attacks. In more severe cases sleep attacks may also occur when patients are active, such as during dinner, while walking, or even when riding a bicycle. Sleep attacks tend to be short, usually less than 20 minutes, sometimes only several minutes, and refreshing for some time. The number may vary from 1 to over 10 each day, depending on the severity of the narcolepsy and the circumstances.

Narcolepsy patients generally do not spend a greater portion of their time asleep across the 24 hours of the day, when compared to people who do not have narcolepsy. This balance is mainly explained by recurring wake periods during their nocturnal sleep.[7]

Cataplexy

Cataplexy is the only specific symptom and is characterized by a sudden bilateral loss of skeletal muscle tone, with preserved consciousness, elicited by emotions.[2,8] All striated muscles can be involved, except the external sphincters and the extraocular and respiratory muscles. Cataplexy may be complete, indicating complete loss of activity of all muscle groups. But more often it is partial, only affecting control over the knees, face, and neck. Complete attacks may cause falls. Because it takes several seconds for a complete attack to build up, most patients are able to take countermeasures and prevent injury.[4,9]

Mirth is the most typical trigger, which usually involves laughing out loud. Patients may become literally "weak with laughter." Although laughter is the strongest trigger, various emotions may induce an attack including, for example, the unexpected meeting of an acquaintance and anger.[10]

The frequency of attacks varies widely from dozens a day to less than once a month. Most attacks last seconds to half a minute, sometimes up to 2 minutes, but only rarely longer. Partial attacks tend to be shorter, the majority even (much) less than 10 seconds. Patients may avoid situations in which cataplexy may occur; they may stop themselves from laughing out loud, stop visiting comedy shows, or even avoid social contacts in general.

A so-called "status catplecticus" may occur in exceptional situations, particularly after acute withdrawal of medication, such as tricyclics and mazindol, or when initiating prazosin treatment for concomitant hypertension. It is characterized by the almost continuous succession of cataplectic attacks, in part without identifiable trigger, that may last from hours to days.

Although cataplexy is the only truly specific feature of narcolepsy, it is the first symptom to appear in less than 10% of cases.[11] Usually it appears shortly after EDS has started, but it may appear months to years afterward.

Hypnagogic Hallucinations

Hypnagogic hallucinations (HHs) are very vivid, dreamlike experiences that occur during the transition between wake and sleep. The content of the hallucinations varies, but in general it is unpleasant and frightening. In 85% of the hallucinations multiple senses are simultaneously involved: visual, auditory, and tactile.[12] Sometimes the hallucinations appear so realistic that patients have difficulty telling them apart from real events after waking up. In such cases they usually can find out that it was a HH by reasoning.

Sleep Paralysis

Sleep paralysis is the inability to move any voluntary muscle at awakening or when falling asleep while being subjectively awake and conscious. The paralysis may be complete, such that patients are unable to raise as much as a little finger.

Attacks presumably last up to several minutes. Sleep paralysis may occur simultaneously with HHs.

Disturbed Nocturnal Sleep

Sleep latency in narcolepsy is typically very short. Patients usually fall asleep almost immediately. They do not stay asleep, however, which is reflected in frequent awakening. Most awakenings are brief but some may last for more than 1 hour.[4,7]

Associated Features and Co-Morbid Conditions

About 30% of patients are obese (body mass index [BMI] > 30 kg/m^2), a much higher percentage than found in the population.[13,14] Obesity in patients with narcolepsy is typically associated with hypocretin deficiency.[15] Weight gain is only partly explained by decreased activity, and probably not by increased caloric intake, suggesting a lowered basal metabolism to be the major determinant.[16]

Lack of energy or fatigue is another associated symptom in up to 60% of patients. It is important to separate this from sleepiness. Treatment with stimulants or sodium oxybate (SXB) seems to have only limited effect on this complaint.[17,18]

Sleep apnea and parasomnias are frequently present in narcolepsy, but with unclear frequency. One recent study reported the presence of obstructive sleep apnea (OSA) in 25% of the patients with narcolepsy.[19] Periodic limb movements in sleep (PLMS) have been described in up to two thirds of the subjects with narcolepsy,[20] although their contribution to the impaired quality of sleep and EDS is uncertain. REM sleep behavior disorder (RBD) has a significantly higher prevalence compared to the general population, affecting 12% to 36% of patients.[21]

Anxiety disorders, especially panic attacks and social phobias, often affect patients with narcolepsy.[22]

It can be difficult to diagnose depression as a co-morbid disorder in narcoleptics, as depression may cause complaints of EDS, disturbed nocturnal sleep, fatigue, and neurophysiologic abnormalities that resemble narcolepsy. Nevertheless, depression is considered to have a higher prevalence in narcoleptics than in the general population, but major depression is probably not more prevalent;[22] 5% to 30% of patients are reported to fulfill the criteria for depression.[23]

PATHOPHYSIOLOGY

The Hypocretin (Orexin) System

The discovery in 1999 that monogenetic forms of narcolepsy with cataplexy in dogs were caused by mutations in the hypocretin receptor-2 gene, and the report that hypocretin knockout mice have narcolepsy led to exciting new insights into the pathophysiology of human narcolepsy.[24,25] Hypocretin deficiency turned out to be the hallmark of human narcolepsy with cataplexy. The peptide is undetectable in the cerebrospinal fluid (CSF) of more than 90% of patients with cataplexy.[26] Large studies revealed that hypocretin measurement is both highly specific and sensitive for the diagnosis of narcolepsy with cataplexy.[2,26] Postmortem studies showed that the likely cause of the deficiency is a selective and almost complete loss of hypocretin-producing cells in the hypothalamus.[27,28]

Biochemical Implications of Hypocretin Deficiency

Hypocretin probably promotes wakefulness through its excitatory effects on brain regions implicated in arousal. There are particularly dense projections to histaminergic neurons of the tuberomammillary nucleus and noradrenergic neurons of the locus ceruleus, but also to dopaminergic neurons in the ventral tegmental area and serotoninergic neurons of the dorsal raphe[29,30] (Fig. 22-1). Excitation of cholinergic neurons in the basal forebrain and the laterodorsal and pedunculopontine tegmental (LDT/PPT) nuclei may also help promote wakefulness.[29]

A persistent cholinergic/aminergic imbalance may be required for the development of cataplexy.[30,31] Monoaminergic nuclei and to a lesser extent cholinergic nuclei are among the sites receiving the densest hypocretin projections. Hypocretin deficiency may thus induce an imbalance by reducing aminergic tone disproportionately.[30,31] In support of this idea, drugs that increase aminergic tone diminish the symptoms of narcolepsy; specifically, drugs that increase dopamine signaling decrease sleepiness, and drugs that increase norepinephrine or serotonin signaling reduce cataplexy.[30,31]

Genetic and Immunologic Aspects

As a rule, human narcolepsy is a sporadic disease. Only 1% to 4% of the narcolepsy cases run in families. Hypocretin deficiency is not a consequence of mutations in either hypocretin ligand or receptor genes in these sporadic cases (96-99%).[28,32] Nevertheless, a genetic susceptibility seems a prerequisite to develop narcolepsy with cataplexy.

Extensive efforts over the past 30 years to gain a better understanding of the genetic basis of the disease identified a striking association with the HLA region.[33] In nearly 100% of sporadic cases of narcolepsy with cataplexy in the white population the individual carries the *DRB1*1501-DQB1*0602* haplotype.[33] This association is thought to

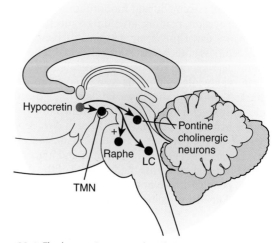

Figure 22-1 The hypocretin neurons heavily innervate neurons in the locus ceruleus (LC), raphe nuclei, tuberomammillary nucleus (TMN), and pontine cholinergic nuclei (laterodorsal and pedunculopontine tegmental nuclei). By exciting neurons in these key regions, the hypocretin system may help sustain wakefulness and regulate rapid eye movement (REM) sleep. (Courtesy of Thomas Scammell.)

represent an almost obligatory but not sufficient risk factor, because 15% to 25% of those in the healthy general population also carry the associated HLA haplotype. Together with the established selective loss of hypocretin neurons in the lateral hypothalamus in postmortem brain studies,[27,28] this information led to the hypothesis that narcolepsy is caused by an autoimmune attack targeting hypocretin-producing neurons. It is unlikely that the immune response is directed against hypocretin or preprohypocretin itself, because there is no evidence for the presence of specific autoantibodies against either neuropeptide.[34,35] However, a fascinating recent finding is the identification of tribbles homolog 2 (*Trib2*), co-localized in hypocretin-producing cells, as a possible autoantigen.[36] Antibodies against *Trib2* have been found in a higher percentage and higher concentration in patients than in control subjects. Moreover, titers were higher close to disease onset.

Very recent genome-wide association studies strengthen the autoimmune hypothesis. One study including mainly white individuals revealed an association between narcolepsy with cataplexy and the T-cell receptor alpha (*TCRA*) locus on chromosome 14, and another established a very strong protective effect of a trans-*DRB1*1301-DQB1*0603* haplotype.[37,38]

DIAGNOSIS

The International Classification of Sleep Disorders (ICSD-2)[2] distinguishes three forms of narcolepsy: (1) narcolepsy with cataplexy, (2) narcolepsy without cataplexy, and (3) narcolepsy due to medical condition.

The diagnosis of narcolepsy with cataplexy requires the presence of EDS and cataplexy, both of which must be evaluated by careful history taking, and confirmed with polysomnographic studies, including a multiple sleep latency test (MSLT) or hypocretin-1 measurement in the CSF (Box 22-1). Hypocretin measurement is particularly helpful in cases in which the presence of (typical) cataplexy is doubtful, or in patients in which the interpretation of the MSLT is hampered, as in patients using antidepressants and in children.

BOX 22-1 *Polysomnographic, Multiple Sleep Latency Test (MSLT), and Hypocretin-1 Measurement Criteria for the Diagnosis of Narcolepsy*

Polysomnography and MSLT

- The MSLT must be preceded by a nocturnal polysomnographic recoding that shows a minimum of 6 hours of sleep.
- The MSLT shows a mean sleep latency of 8 minutes or less, and two or more sleep onset REM periods.

Hypocretin-1 Measurement in CSF

- The hypocretin-1 level is 110 pg/mL or less for values that are adjusted to Stanford values.
- The concentration is one third or less of the mean normal values of the concerning laboratory.

CSF, cerebrospinal fluid; REM, rapid eye movement sleep.
From American Academy of Sleep Medicine. *International Classification of Sleep Disorders*, 2nd ed. Diagnostic and Coding Manual. Westchester, IL: American Academy of Sleep Medicine; 2005.

The clinical difference between narcolepsy with cataplexy and narcolepsy without cataplexy is, as may be expected, the absence of (typical) cataplexy in the latter form. The polysomnographic criteria for both are the same, and they have to be met to make the diagnosis of narcolepsy without cataplexy. An important difference is that hypocretin-1 levels in the CSF are normal in the majority of patients suffering from narcolepsy without cataplexy. Several explanations are possible for this difference; the most plausible is that there is less destruction of hypocretin cells in narcolepsy without cataplexy compared to narcolepsy with cataplexy. Theoretically, lesser cell loss could lead to impaired hypocretin transmission but the loss is not enough to reduce CSF hypocretin levels. Another explanation is that narcolepsy without cataplexy could be a result of various disturbances in the brain, including disturbances induced by sleep deprivation, hypocretin deficiency being just one of them.[39]

Narcolepsy due to medical condition may be accompanied by cataplexy or not. It is clinically undistinguishable from the other two subtypes but is presumed to be caused by a coexisting medical disorder. However, these medical disorders may have symptoms of their own. Examples are Parkinson's disease, head trauma, Niemann-Pick disease type C, Prader-Willi syndrome, myotonic dystrophy, and (rare) vascular, neoplastic, or inflammatory lesions confined to the lateral hypothalamic area. The same findings on ancillary investigations as described for narcolepsy with and without cataplexy are required for the diagnosis.[2]

Despite the presumed pathophysiologic differences, the management is similar for all forms, although sleep deprivation as cause should be excluded in narcolepsy without cataplexy, and in symptomatic cases treatment of the underlying disorder may be of benefit.

MANAGEMENT AND TREATMENT

For the management of narcolepsy, it is of paramount importance that patients, spouses, and family members are informed about what narcolepsy is, understand its implications, and learn to accept that it is a chronic disorder that cannot be cured. Acceptance will prevent patients from unnecessary and frustrating confrontations with their limitations, and will highly facilitate the implementation of behavioral modifications, and the adequate use of prescribed medication. A supportive social environment (e.g., patient group organizations and support groups) as well as education of relevant persons within family, school, and work environment will also add to acceptance and subsequently reduce of the burden of the disease.

Regarding treatment, there are only two treatment modalities that have proved to be effective: behavioral modification and pharmacologic therapy. As a rule, both are needed to achieve an optimal situation.

Behavioral Modification

Patients should provide themselves the opportunity to have enough nocturnal sleep, and live a regular life, that is, going to bed at the same hour each night and getting up at the same time each morning as much as possible. Scheduled daytime naps or short naps just before certain activities demanding a high degree of attention temporarily diminish sleepiness in most patients.

The optimal frequency, duration, and timing of these naps has to be established on an individual basis.[40]

Since narcoleptic patients are probably more sensitive to the sleep-inducing properties of carbohydrates, they should be advised not to eat large carbohydrate-rich meals.[41] Alcohol and sedating daytime medications should preferably be avoided for similar reasons.

Pharmacologic Treatment

General Aspects

Despite the recent advances in understanding the cause of narcolepsy, there are no treatments yet that address the underlying hypocretin deficiency. The hypocretin peptides do not easily cross the blood-brain barrier, and though alternative routes, such as nasal application, have been tried in animal studies, only one study suggests some functional benefit.[42] Therefore, it seems unlikely that this will become a clinical option in the near future. Alternatively, small molecule (i.e., nonpeptide) hypocretin agonists that cross the blood-brain barrier are worth considering, but not much progress has been made so far in the development of selective agonists.

Therefore, management focuses on improving symptoms, and no single drug or combination of drugs is effective in all. As most treatments predominantly improve either EDS or cataplexy, combinations are often needed to control both symptoms. The only available drug that may improve all major symptoms of narcolepsy is SXB. Because it is a hypnotic, it has the additional advantage that it may improve nocturnal sleep, in contrast to the other drugs.

Before initiating medications, it is important to discuss with the patient what may be expected. It must be explained that sleepiness will never be completely alleviated in any patient, whereas cataplexy may completely disappear in some. This knowledge must also guide physicians in trying new drugs or combinations of drugs and in deciding on the right balance between efficacy and side effects.

Because there are no generally accepted, objective tests to quantify the severity and the individual impact of a symptom, history taking is the main instrument to evaluate efficacy and the occurrence of side effects.

Unfortunately, there are relative large individual differences in efficacy, side effects, and tolerability of the various medications, which necessitates individually tailored treatment.

Many clinicians find the best strategy is to develop experience with a few drugs that are effective and well tolerated and only switch to others when there is an unsatisfactory response or unpleasant or hazardous side effects.

In general, it is best to start with one drug at a time, targeting the most disabling symptoms, and to explain that it may sometimes take months before an optimal situation is reached. Last, it is worth remembering that some combinations of drugs may have synergistic effects.

Treatment of Excessive Daytime Sleepiness

Stimulants are the main treatment for EDS.[43-45] These drugs include dextroamphetamine (5-60 mg/day), methamphetamine (10-50 mg/day), methylphenidate (10-60 mg/day), modafinil (100-400 mg/day), armodafinil (150-250 mg/day),

and in exceptional cases mazindol.[44,45] These drugs enhance the release and inhibit the reuptake of catecholamines and to a lesser extent of serotonin in the central nervous system and the periphery. (For more details see Chapter 6) Mazindol has been withdrawn in most countries due to severe side effects, including pulmonary hypertension and cardiac valvular regurgitation, in related drugs (fenfluramines) that suppress appetite.[46] As some patients respond better to mazindol than any other drug, it may be an option, provided that treatment is closely monitored.

Side effects and tolerance are major drawbacks in the use of stimulants. The most important side effects include irritability, agitation, headache, and peripheral sympathetic stimulation. These effects are usually dose-related. Tolerance develops in about a third of patients, leading to high dosages.[45,47] Some patients tend to increase their dosage because they prefer high alertness at the expense of an overactive mind and body. Still, addiction does not seem to be a problem in narcoleptics, though data are limited.[47] Induction or aggravation of hypertension might be expected, but seems not to be a significant problem when using normal therapeutic doses.[48] Induction of psychosis and hallucinations is rare.[47] Nocturnal sleep may be disturbed in patients who use high doses or who take stimulants in the evening.

Long-acting agents (modafinil, armodafinil, dexamphetamine, methamphetamine, and sustained release formulations of methylphenidate) seem to be tolerated better than the short-acting drugs (methylphenidate). The quick and short-acting ones can be used to good effect when "targeted" at social events or difficult periods during the day. For this reason combinations of stimulants may be tailored to the circumstances. Unfortunately, there are no studies assessing the advantages or disadvantages of combinations of stimulants.

Modafinil is usually grouped with the stimulants, but it has a different pharmacologic mode of action. Its exact mechanism has not yet been elucidated, but its therapeutic effect is probably mainly mediated by dopamine reuptake inhibition (see Chapter 6). Efficacy has been demonstrated in large randomized placebo-controlled studies and is probably comparable to that of the classical stimulants, although direct comparisons are lacking.[49,50] The advantage of modafinil over the classical stimulants probably lies in the reduction in frequency and severity of irritability and agitation[51] (also probably less sympathomimetic effects and less abuse potential). The possibility of induction of human hepatic cytochrome P-450 enzymes by modafinil should be borne in mind. Modafinil increases the metabolism of oral contraceptives and the manufacturer in the United States recommends that women of childbearing age should use an alternate or concomitant form of contraception. There are indications for an increased risk of Stevens-Johnson syndrome and other hypersensitivity syndromes, including a case of multiorgan sensitivity.[52]

Armodafinil is the dextro-enantiomer component of modafinil and has a longer elimination half-life. It seems to have a more prolonged effect during the day and may improve sleepiness in the late afternoon and early evening better than modafinil, although direct comparison is lacking.[53] The side effect profile is similar to that for modafinil. Armodafinil is currently not available in most European countries.

Recent studies with SXB have shown that it is effective in reducing EDS, particularly at dosages of 6 to 9 g per night.[54,55] Efficacy and side effects of SXB are both dose dependent. Side effects are usually mild, particularly when compared to those occurring with other drugs. Nevertheless, SXB has a black box warning because it is a potent CNS depressant with abuse potential. Although the most frequent side effect is nausea, the most disabling effects are enuresis and sleep walking. Lowering the dose may solve these problems. Weight loss can occur.[56] The effect of high dosages on EDS was similar to that of modafinil.[54] However, combination therapy with modafinil was even more effective.[54] SXB is the sodium salt of γ-hydroxybutyrate (GHB), which is a natural metabolite of γ-aminobutyrate (GABA) and acts as a hypnotic. SXB's mechanism of action has not yet been elucidated but may be mediated through the $GABA_B$ receptor.[57] It may also influence the release of dopamine and serotonin. (For a more detailed description of the role of SXB in narcolepsy see later discussion in this chapter).

Finally, selegiline, a monoamine oxidase B (MAO-B) inhibitor, and brofaromine, an MAO-A inhibitor, may alleviate EDS, but the available studies are small, and it is unclear whether the wake-promoting properties of selegiline are explained by its metabolite amphetamine.[44]

Treatment of Cataplexy, Hypnagogic Hallucination, and Sleep Paralysis

Most studies concerning the treatment of the REM sleep dissociation phenomena have focused on cataplexy, but most drugs that improve cataplexy also reduce hypnagogic hallucinations and sleep paralysis. Sodium oxybate and tricyclic antidepressants are considered the most effective treatments for cataplexy. The different tricyclic antidepressants all inhibit the reuptake of norepinephrine and serotonin and are potent REM sleep inhibitors. The most commonly used drugs are imipramine (10-100 mg/day), and clomipramine (10-150 mg/day).[43,44] Many clinicians consider low dosages of clomipramine to be the treatment of choice.[44,58] Some patients also experience some improvement of EDS when treated with clomipramine. As with stimulants, side effects and to a lesser extent tolerance are the major drawbacks. Side effects are largely due to the anticholinergic properties; the most frequently reported effects are dry mouth, increased sweating, sexual dysfunction (impotence, delayed orgasm and erection, and ejaculation dysfunction), weight gain, tachycardia, constipation, blurred vision, and urinary retention. However, in some patients very low doses may be very effective without causing significant side effects. Tricyclic antidepressants should never be stopped abruptly because of the risk of severe aggravation of cataplexy, which may even lead to status cataplecticus.

Many alternative antidepressants have been studied, especially selective serotonin reuptake inhibitors and more selective noradrenergic reuptake inhibitors such as fluoxetine, zimelidine, viloxazine, femoxitine, fluvoxamine, and paroxetine in a relative higher dosage than the tricyclic antidepressants.[31,44] All these substances appear to have anticataplectic properties and less bothersome side effects than the tricyclics. These substances seem to act mainly via less selective desmethyl metabolites, which are potent adrenergic uptake inhibitors.[59]

During recent years, venlafaxine and atomoxetine, a noradrenergic uptake inhibitor used in the treatment of attention deficit hyperactivity disorder, have become very popular in the treatment of cataplexy, although there are no randomized placebo controlled studies available.[60,61] Because venlafaxine,

particularly when used in higher dosages, may induce hypertension, blood pressure should be monitored in these patients.[62]

SXB (4.5-9 g per night) is the best studied anticataplectic drug and is a very potent inhibitor of cataplexy.[63-65] It has never been compared to any antidepressant, so it is difficult to know whether it is really more effective than these drugs in the treatment of cataplexy. However, the relatively mild side effect profile of SXB makes it a more favorable drug than antidepressants (with the exception of low-dose clomipramine) even independent of the beneficial effect of SXB on the other narcolepsy symptoms. In resistant cases, a combination of an antidepressant and SXB may be considered.

Available trials were not designed to study the effect of sodium oxybate on hypnagogic hallucinations and sleep paralysis, but these symptoms tended to improve in all studies using this drug.

Other alternatives less well studied and probably less potent are mazindol, selegiline, and brofaromine. As with SXB, these compounds may decrease sleepiness as well as the REM dissociation phenomena. Therefore, they can sometimes be used as monotherapy in patients with EDS and REM dissociation phenomena, particularly in milder forms.

Several drugs may theoretically be expected to aggravate cataplexy, but the only one for which this is reliably documented is prazosin, an α_1-antagonist used to treat hypertension.[66]

Disturbed Nocturnal Sleep

Disturbed nocturnal sleep can be a major complaint of patients. Unfortunately, treatment options are limited. SXB is the only drug with a proven long-term effect on nocturnal sleep.[67] Short-term beneficial effects of benzodiazepines have been described as well.[68] Although nocturnal sleep may sometimes be improved with benzodiazepines, improvement of EDS is uncommon.

Sodium Oxybate

The dosing and titration regimen of SXB differs from that of other drugs. Therefore, patients starting to use SXB need to be given specific instructions: two nocturnal doses are required, and eating must be avoided at least 2 hours before the first ingestion to allow optimal absorption. Patients should prepare the doses in two small containers before going to bed and take the first dose only after they have lain down in bed. The second dose must be ingested 3 to 4 hours after the first, and there must be at least 3 hours between the second dose and the scheduled wake-up time.[69] The usual starting dose is 2.25 g twice a night.[44] The dose must be gradually increased, keeping in mind that the sedating effects are immediately apparent, but it can take several weeks to see the maximal improvements in EDS and cataplexy of a given dose.[65] SXB should not be used in conjunction with other sedatives or alcohol.[70] If patients have consumed alcohol in the evening, they should omit one or both doses afterward. In patients with co-morbid obstructive sleep apnea syndrome (OSAS) or respiratory disorders, treatment should be closely monitored because SXB is a respiratory depressant. In patients with OSAS, co-treatment with continuous positive airway pressure (CPAP) is often indicated.[71,72]

In long-term follow-up studies there is no indication that tolerance develops, and abrupt cessation does not induce rebound cataplexy.[64,73] However, long-term clinical experience shows tolerance for the sleep-promoting effects in a substantial proportion of patients, but with remaining efficacy for the other symptoms.

Pharmacologic interactions are not known, and combined use with other medications involved in the treatment of EDS and cataplexy seems to be safe. The dose should be reduced in patients with hepatic failure.

Unfortunately, there is a potential for misuse. GHB is used as a party drug because it can produce a disinhibited, slightly euphoric state, and it has been used in cases of rape and theft as it can cause amnesia. Continuous use of high dosages may lead to dependence and withdrawal symptoms on cessation. Overdose can be fatal, though many deaths probably resulted from combinations of GHB with alcohol or other drugs. These risks rightly raise concerns among patients and their physicians, but it is important to realize that the drug is relatively safe with a low risk of dependence when properly used.[74]

Associated Disorders

Patients should be informed about the increased risk of obesity to prevent the occurrence as much as possible. If obesity is present, it should be managed using conventional weight loss techniques.

Lack of energy is difficult to treat. Stimulants and SXB may have some effect on this complaint.[18] There are no data on efficacy of cognitive therapy.

Treatment of associated sleep apnea usually does not improve EDS, and compliance with CPAP and other treatments can be a problem. Whether there is a medical indication for treatment is controversial.[19] Treatment with SXB may facilitate the acceptance of CPAP treatment. However, because SXB may worsen the course of sleep apnea it is important that patients are compliant with CPAP therapy.[71]

Treatment of periodic limb movements must be considered if there is coexistent restless legs syndrome (see Chapter 24).

REM sleep behavior disorder in narcolepsy can be treated, if needed, with clonazepam or melatonin (see Chapter 43).[75]

Recommendations for the Initiation of Pharmacologic Treatment

A reasonable approach is to start modafinil 200 mg as first-line therapy in patients with predominantly EDS. Depending on severity, side effects, and the experienced burden of other symptoms, adjustments can be made or other medications can be added. It is usually not helpful to increase the modafinil dose beyond 400 mg, particularly if lower doses have not been effective.

For patients with severe cataplexy, without severely disturbed nocturnal sleep, first-line treatment with a low dose of clomipramine (10-20 mg) can be very effective. Again, depending on side effects and the severity of the other symptoms, adjustments have to be made or additional medications have to be initiated. This approach and possible other initial steps, depending on the predominant complaint, are summarized in the algorithm shown in Figure 22-2. A common combination therapy that is also evidence-based is a combination of modafinil and SXB.[54]

Potential Future Treatment

Nonpharmacologic Considerations

The regulation of skin temperature is altered in narcolepsy and may worsen daytime vigilance as well as disrupt nocturnal sleep. Preliminary studies show that skin temperature manipulation

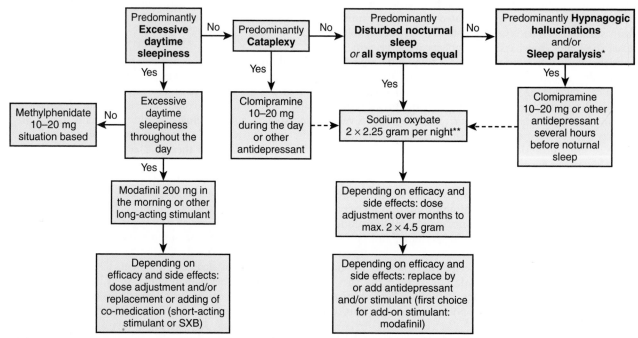

Figure 22-2 Proposed algorithm for the initiation of treatment, guided by the most symptomatic complaints. This is not an evidence-based approach, but is based on clinical experience and the European treatment guidelines. *There are no evidence-based treatment options. **Cases with concomitant obstructive sleep apnea syndrome (OSAS) should be closely monitored and co-treatment with continuous positive airway pressure may be indicated. Dashed line: if not effective or if residual complaints remain. (From Billiard M, Bassetti C, Dauvilliers Y, Dolenc-Groselj L, Lammers GJ, (EFNS Task Force). EFNS guidelines on management of narcolepsy. *Eur J Neurol.* 2006;13(10): 1035-1048.)

improves both daytime vigilance and nocturnal sleep, and further studies in nonlaboratory circumstances are needed.[76,77]

Future Pharmacologic Treatments

Emerging treatments undergoing investigation include immunotherapy, histamine (H_3) antagonists, thyrotropin (TRH) analogs, paraxanthine, hypocretin analogs, hypocretin gene therapy, and stem cell transplant.

Because autoimmune mechanisms may be responsible for the development of narcolepsy, treatments have been undertaken focusing on the immune response soon after the onset of narcolepsy. Steroids and plasmapheresis have had limited success. Intravenous immunoglobulin therapy did show improvement in several case series, particularly of cataplexy, when administrated soon after the onset of symptoms.[78] These studies were small and not blinded; possible spontaneous severity fluctuations may have influenced the outcome, and the placebo effect may be large.[79] Only randomized, double-blind, placebo-controlled studies can solve these issues.

The histaminergic system is important for promoting wakefulness. Histamine H_3 receptors are abundant in the CNS and are inhibitory autoreceptors. H_3 receptor antagonists therefore facilitate wakefulness. Several H_3 antagonists are currently being studied for the treatment of EDS with encouraging results in a first pilot study in humans.[80]

There is some evidence that thyrotropin-releasing hormone (TRH) and TRH agonists have alerting properties, thus making it a possible treatment modality for narcolepsy. TRH increases wakefulness and decreases cataplexy in dogs with narcolepsy.[81]

Paraxanthine is a metabolite of caffeine. It was recently demonstrated that paraxanthine significantly promoted wakefulness and proportionally reduced non-REM and REM sleep in both control and narcoleptic mice.[82] The wake-promoting potency of paraxanthine is greater than that of the parent compound, caffeine, and comparable to that of modafinil. It was also better tolerated than caffeine.

In view of the central role of hypocretin deficiency in narcolepsy, the best therapy might be correction of the hypocretin deficiency. Unfortunately, there still are no small molecule hypocretin agonists available that can easily cross the blood-brain barrier. An alternative could be gene therapy; although promising, it has potentially dangerous side effects.

Transplantation of hypocretin neurons might potentially provide a cure.[83] However, the current techniques need to be improved and there is the potential problem of an immune reaction to the graft in view of the autoimmune hypothesis of narcolepsy.

Ultimately, a better understanding of the pathologic process that kills the hypocretin neurons should result in effective prevention strategies.

REFERENCES

1. Dauvilliers Y, Arnulf I, Mignot E. Narcolepsy with cataplexy. *Lancet.* 2007;369:499-511.
2. American Academy of Sleep Medicine. *International Classification of Sleep Disorders: Diagnostic and Coding Manual.* 2nd ed. Westchester, IL: American Academy of Sleep Medicine; 2005.
3. Broughton R, Valley V, Aguirre M, Roberts J, Suwalski W, Dunham W. Excessive daytime sleepiness and the pathophysiology of narcolepsy-cataplexy: A laboratory perspective. *Sleep.* 1986;9:205-215.
4. Overeem S, Mignot E, van Dijk JG, Lammers GJ. Narcolepsy: Clinical features, new pathophysiologic insights, and future perspectives. *J Clin Neurophysiol.* 2001;18(2):78-105.
5. Longstreth Jr WT, Koepsell TD, Ton TG, Hendrickson AF, van Belle G. The epidemiology of narcolepsy. *Sleep.* 2007;30:13-26.
6. Fronczek R, Middelkoop HA, van Dijk JG, Lammers GJ. Focusing on vigilance instead of sleepiness in the assessment of narcolepsy: High sensitivity of the Sustained Attention to Response Task (SART). *Sleep.* 2006;29(2):187-191.
7. Broughton R, Dunham W, Newman J, Lutley K, Duschesne P, Rivers M. Ambulatory 24 hour sleep-wake monitoring in narcolepsy-cataplexy compared to matched controls. *Electroencephalogr Clin Neurophysiol.* 1988;70:473-481.
8. Anic-Labat S, Guilleminault C, Kraemer HC, Meehan J, Arrigoni J, Mignot E. Validation of a cataplexy questionnaire in 983 sleep-disorders patients. *Sleep.* 1999;22(1):77-87.
9. Vetrugno R, D'Angelo R, Moghadam KK, Vandi S, Franceschini C, et al. Behavioural and neurophysiological correlates of human cataplexy: A video-polygraphic study. *Clin Neurophysiol.* 2010;121(2):153-162.
10. Overeem S, van Nues SJ, van der Zande WL, Donjacour CE, van Mierlo P, Lammers GJ. The clinical features of cataplexy: A questionnaire study in narcolepsy patients with and without hypocretin-1 deficiency. *Sleep Med.* 2011;12(1):12-18:Epub 2010 Dec 8.
11. Cataplexy Guilleminault C. In: Guilleminault C, Dement WC, Passouant P, eds. *Narcolepsy.* New York: Spectrum; 1976:125-144.
12. Fortuyn HA, Lappenschaar GA, Nienhuis FJ, Furer JW, Hodiamont PP, et al. Psychotic symptoms in narcolepsy: Phenomenology and a comparison with schizophrenia. *Gen Hosp Psychiatry.* 2009;31(2):146-154.
13. Kok SW, Overeem S, Visscher TL, Lammers GJ, Seidell JC, et al. Hypocretin deficiency in narcoleptic humans is associated with abdominal obesity. *Obes Res.* 2003;11(9):1147-1154.
14. Poli F, Plazzi G, DiDalmazi G, Ribichini D, Vicennati V, et al. Body mass index-independent metabolic alterations in narcolepsy with cataplexy. *Sleep.* 2009;32(11):1491-1497.
15. Nishino S, Ripley B, Overeem S, Nevsimalova S, Lammers GJ, et al. Low cerebrospinal fluid hypocretin (orexin) and altered energy homeostasis in human narcolepsy. *Ann Neurol.* 2001;50(3):381-388.
16. Hara J, Beuckmann CT, Nambu T, Willie JT, Chemelli RM, et al. Genetic ablation of orexin neurons in mice results in narcolepsy, hypophagia, and obesity. *Neuron.* 2001;30(2):345-354.
17. Valko PO, Bassetti CL, Bloch KE, Held U, Baumann CR. Validation of the fatigue severity scale in a Swiss cohort. *Sleep.* 2008;31(11):1601-1607.
18. Droogleever F, Fronczek R, Smitshoek M, Overeem S, Lammers GJ, Bleijenberg G. Prevalence and correlates of severe experienced fatigue in patients with narcolepsy. (In press)
19. Sansa G, Iranzo A, Santamaria J. Obstructive sleep apnea in narcolepsy. *Sleep Med.* 2010;11(1):93-95.
20. Dauvilliers Y, Pennestri MH, Petit D, Dang-Vu T, Lavigne G, Montplaisir J. Periodic leg movements during sleep and wakefulness in narcolepsy. *J Sleep Res.* 2007;16:333-339.
21. Nightingale S, Orgill JC, Ebrahim IO, de Lacy SF, Agrawal S, Williams AJ. The association between narcolepsy and REM behavior disorder (RBD). *Sleep Med.* 2005;6:253-258.
22. Fortuyn HA, Lappenschaar MA, Furer JW, Hodiamont PP, Rijnders CA, et al. Anxiety and mood disorders in narcolepsy: A case-control study. *Gen Hosp Psychiatry.* 2010;32(1):49-56.
23. Broughton R, Ghanem Q, Hishikawa Y, Sugita Y, Nevsimalova S, Roth B. Life effects of narcolepsy in 180 patients from North America, Asia and Europe compared to matched controls. *Can J Neurol Sci.* 1981;8:299-304.
24. Lin L, Faraco J, Li R, Kadotani H, Rogers W, et al. The sleep disorder canine narcolepsy is caused by a mutation in the hypocretin (orexin) receptor 2 gene. *Cell.* 1999;98:365-376.
25. Chemelli RM, Willie JT, Sinton CM, Elmquist JK, Scammell T, et al. Narcolepsy in orexin knockout mice: Molecular genetics of sleep regulation. *Cell.* 1999;98:437-451.
26. Mignot E, Lammers GJ, Ripley B, Okun M, Nevsimalova S, et al. The role of cerebrospinal fluid hypocretin measurement in the diagnosis of narcolepsy and other hypersomnias. *Arch Neurol.* 2002;59(10):1553-1562.
27. Thannickal TC, Moore RY, Nienhuis R, Ramanathan L, Gulyani S, et al. Reduced number of hypocretin neurons in human narcolepsy. *Neuron.* 2000;27(3):469-474.
28. Peyron C, Faraco J, Rogers W, Ripley B, Overeem S, et al. A mutation in a case of early onset narcolepsy and a generalized absence of hypocretin peptides in human narcoleptic brains. *Nat Med.* 2000;6(9):991-997.
29. Peyron C, Tighe DK, Den Pol AN, de Lecea L, Heller HC, et al. l. Neurons containing hypocretin (orexin) project to multiple neuronal systems. *J Neurosci.* 1998;18:9996-10015.
30. Nishino S. Clinical and neurobiological aspects of narcolepsy. *Sleep Med.* 2007;8(4):373-399.

31. Nishino S, Mignot E. Pharmacological aspects of human and canine narcolepsy. *Prog Neurobiol*. 1997;52:27-78.

32. Mignot E. Genetic and familial aspects of narcolepsy. *Neurology*. 1998;50(2 Suppl 1):S16-22.

33. Mignot E, Lin L, Rogers W, Honda Y, Qiu X, et al. Complex HLA-DR and -DQ interactions confer risk of narcolepsy-cataplexy in three ethnic groups. *Am J Hum Genet*. 2001;68(3):686-699.

34. Tanaka S, Honda Y, Inoue Y, Honda M. Detection of autoantibodies against hypocretin, hcrtrl, and hcrtr2 in narcolepsy: Anti-Hcrt system antibody in narcolepsy. *Sleep*. 2006;29(5):633-638.

35. Overeem S, Black 3rd JL, Lammers GJ. Narcolepsy: immunological aspects. *Sleep Med Rev*. 2008 Apr;12(2):95-107.

36. Cvetkovic-Lopes V, Bayer L, Dorsaz S, Maret S, Pradervand S, et al. Elevated Tribbles homolog 2-specific antibody levels in narcolepsy patients. *J Clin Invest*. 2010;120(3):713-719.

37. Hallmayer J, Faraco J, Lin L, Hesselson S, Winkelmann J, et al. Narcolepsy is strongly associated with the T-cell receptor alpha locus. *Nat Genet*. 2009;41:708-711.

38. Hor H, Kutalik Z, Dauvilliers Y, Valsesia A, Lammers GJ, et al. Genome-wide association study identifies new HLA class II haplotypes strongly protective against narcolepsy. *Nat Genet*. 2010;42(9):786-789:Epub 2010, Aug 15.

39. Marti I, Valko PO, Khatami R, Bassetti CL, Baumann CR. Multiple sleep latency measures in narcolepsy and behaviourally induced insufficient sleep syndrome. *Sleep Med*. 2009;10:1146-1150.

40. Mullington J, Broughton R. Scheduled naps in the management of daytime sleepiness in narcolepsy-cataplexy. *Sleep*. 1993;16:444-456.

41. Bruck D, Armstrong S, Coleman G. Sleepiness after glucose in narcolepsy. *J Sleep Res*. 1994;3:171-179.

42. Deadwyler SA, Porrino L, Siegel JM, Hampson RE. Systemic and nasal delivery of orexin-A (hypocretin-1) reduces the effects of sleep deprivation on cognitive performance in nonhuman primates. *J Neurosci*. 2007;27(52):14239-14247.

43. Wise MS, Arand DL, Auger RR, Brooks SN, Watson NF. American Academy of Sleep Medicine. Treatment of narcolepsy and other hypersomnias of central origin. *Sleep*. 2007;30(12):1712-1727.

44. Billiard M, Bassetti C, Dauvilliers Y, Dolenc-Groselj L, Lammers GJ, et al. (EFNS Task Force). EFNS guidelines on management of narcolepsy. *Eur J Neurol*. 2006;13(10):1035-1048.

45. Mitler MM, Aldrich MS, Koob GF, Zarcone VP. Narcolepsy and its treatment with stimulants. ASDA standards of practice. *Sleep*. 1994;17:352-371.

46. Ryan DH, Bray GA, Helmcke F, Sander G, Volaufova J, et al. Serial echocardiographic and clinical evaluation of valvular regurgitation before, during, and after treatment with fenfluramine or dexfenfluramine and mazindol or phentermine. *Obes Res*. 1999;7:313-322.

47. Parkes JD, Dahlitz M. Amphetamine prescription. *Sleep*. 1993;16:201-203.

48. Wallin MT, Mahowald MW. Blood pressure effects of long-term stimulant use in disorders of hypersomnolence. *J Sleep Res*. 1998;7:209-215.

49. Broughton RJ, Fleming JA, George CF, Hill JD, Kryger MH, et al. Randomized, double-blind, placebo-controlled crossover trial of modafinil in the treatment of excessive daytime sleepiness in narcolepsy. *Neurology*. 1997;49:444-451.

50. U.S. Modafinil in Narcolepsy Multicenter Study Group. Randomized trial of modafinil as a treatment for the excessive daytime somnolence of narcolepsy. *Neurology*. 2000;54:1166-1175.

51. Bastuji H, Jouvet M. Successful treatment of idiopathic hypersomnia and narcolepsy with modafinil. *Prog Neuropsychopharmacol Biol Psychiatry*. 1988;12:695-700.

52. http://www.provigil.com/media/PDFs/prescribing_info.pdf; Accessed Oct.14, 2010.

53. Darwish M, Kirby M, Hellriegel ET, Robertson Jr P. Armodafinil and modafinil have substantially different pharmacokinetic profiles despite having the same terminal half-lives: Analysis of data from three randomized, single-dose, pharmacokinetic studies. *Clin Drug Investig*. 2009;29(9):613-623.

54. Black J, Houghton WC. Sodium oxybate improves excessive daytime sleepiness in narcolepsy. *Sleep*. 2006;29(7):939-946.

55. The Xyrem International Study Group. A double-blind, placebo-controlled study demonstrates that sodium oxybate is effective for the treatment of excessive daytime sleepiness in narcolepsy. *J Clin Sleep Med*. 2005;1:391-397.

56. Husain AM, Ristanovic RK, Bogan RK. Weight loss in narcolepsy patients treated with sodium oxybate. *Sleep Med*. 2009;10(6):661-663.

57. Carter LP, Koek W, France CP. Behavioral analyses of GHB: Receptor mechanisms. *Pharmacol Ther*. 2009;121(1):100-114.

58. Parkes D. Introduction to the mechanism of action of different treatments of narcolepsy. *Sleep*. 1994;17:S93-S96.

59. Nishino S, Arrigoni J, Shelton J, Dement WC, Mignot E. Desmethyl metabolites of serotonergic uptake inhibitors are more potent for suppressing canine cataplexy than their parent compounds. *Sleep*. 1993;16:706-712.

60. Mignot E, Nishino S. Emerging therapies in narcolepsy-cataplexy. *Sleep*. 2005;28(6):754-763.

61. Niederhofer H. Atomoxetine also effective in patients suffering from narcolepsy? *Sleep*. 2005;28(9):1189.

62. Mbaya P, Alam F, Ashim S, Bennett D. Cardiovascular effects of high dose venlafaxine XL in patients with major depressive disorder. *Hum Psychopharmacol*. 2007;22(3):129-133.

63. U.S. Xyrem Multicenter Study Group. A 12-month, open-label, multicenter extension trial of orally administered sodium oxybate for the treatment of narcolepsy. *Sleep*. 2003;26:31-35.

64. U.S. Xyrem Multicenter Study Group. Sodium oxybate demonstrates long-term efficacy for the treatment of cataplexy in patients with narcolepsy. *Sleep Med*. 2004;5:119-123.

65. U.S. Xyrem International Study Group. Further evidence supporting the use of sodium oxybate for the treatment of cataplexy: A double-blind, placebo-controlled study in 228 patients. *Sleep Med*. 2005;6:415-421.

66. Guilleminault C, Mignot E, Aldrich M, Quera-Salva MA, Tiberge M, Partinen M. Prazosin contraindicated in patients with narcolepsy. *Lancet*. 1988;2(8609):511.

67. Black J, Pardi D, Hornfeldt CS, Inhaber N. The nightly administration of sodium oxybate results in significant reduction in the nocturnal sleep disruption of patients with narcolepsy. *Sleep Med*. 2009;10(8):829-835.

68. Thorpy MJ, Snyder M, Aloe FS, Ledereich PS, Starz KE. Short-term triazolam use improves nocturnal sleep of narcoleptics. *Sleep*. 1992;15:212-216.

69. Lemon MD, Strain JD, Farver DK. Sodium oxybate for cataplexy. *Ann Pharmacother*. 2006;40(3):581-582:433-440; quiz.

70. Fuller DE, Hornfeldt CS, Kelloway JS, Stahl PJ, Anderson TF. The Xyrem risk management program. *Drug Saf*. 2004;27(5):293-306.

71. Feldman NT. Clinical perspective: Monitoring sodium oxybate-treated narcolepsy patients for the development of sleep-disordered breathing. *Sleep Breath*. 2010;14(1):77-79.

72. George CF, Feldman N, Inhaber N, Steininger TL, Grzeschik SM, et al. A safety trial of sodium oxybate in patients with obstructive sleep apnea: Acute effects on sleep-disordered breathing. *Sleep Med*. 2010;11(1):38-42.

73. U.S. Xyrem Multicenter Study Group. The abrupt cessation of therapeutically administered sodium oxybate (GHB) does not cause withdrawal symptoms. *J Toxicol Clin Toxicol*. 2003;41(2):131-135.

74. Lammers GJ, Bassetti C, Billiard M, Black J, Broughton R, et al. Sodium oxybate is an effective and safe treatment for narcolepsy. *Sleep Med*. 2010;11(1):105-106.

75. Billiard M. REM sleep behavior disorder and narcolepsy. *CNS Neurol Disord Drug Targets*. 2009;8(4):2642-2670.

76. Fronczek R, Raymann RJ, Overeem S, Romeijn N, van Dijk JG, et al. Manipulation of skin temperature improves nocturnal sleep in narcolepsy. *J Neurol Neurosurg Psychiatry*. 2008;79(12):1354-1357.

77. Fronczek R, Raymann RJ, Romeijn N, Overeem S, Fischer M, et al. Manipulation of core body and skin temperature improves vigilance and maintenance of wakefulness in narcolepsy. *Sleep*. 2008;31(2):233-240.

78. Dauvilliers Y. Follow-up of four narcolepsy patients treated with intravenous immunoglobulins. *Ann Neurol*. 2006;60(1):153.

79. Fronczek R, Verschuuren J, Lammers GJ. Response to intravenous immunoglobulins and placebo in a patient with narcolepsy with cataplexy. *J Neurol*. 2007;254(11):1607-1608.

80. Lin JS, Dauvilliers Y, Arnulf I, Bastuji H, Anaclet C, et al. An inverse agonist of the histamine H(3) receptor improves wakefulness in narcolepsy: Studies in orexin-/- mice and patients. *Neurobiol Dis*. 2008;30(1):74-83.

81. Riehl J, Honda K, Kwan M, Hong J, Mignot E, Nishino S. Chronic oral administration of CG-3703, a thyrotropin releasing hormone analog, increases wake and decreases cataplexy in canine narcolepsy. *Neuropsychopharmacology*. 2000;23(1):34-45.

82. Okuro M, Fujiki N, Kotorii N, Ishimaru Y, Sokoloff P, Nishino S. Effects of paraxanthine and caffeine on sleep, locomotor activity and body temperature in orexin/ataxin-3 transgenic narcoleptic mice. *Sleep*. 2010;33(7):930-942.

83. Arias-Carrión O, Murillo-Rodríguez E. Cell transplantation: A future therapy for narcolepsy? *CNS Neurol Disord Drug Targets*. 2009;8(4):309-314.

Non-Narcoleptic Hypersomnias of Central Origin

Chapter 23

MICHEL M. BILLIARD

A wide range of conditions are listed under the umbrella name of hypersomnias of central origin in the International Classification of Sleep Disorders, Second Edition (ICSD-2),[1] but only narcolepsy, idiopathic hypersomnia, and recurrent hypersomnia can be considered as genuine hypersomnias of central origin. The current therapy of narcolepsy is reported elsewhere in this volume (see Chapter 22); this chapter will focus on the treatments of idiopathic hypersomnia and recurrent hypersomnia. Although the book is intended to be a review of evidence-based management of various sleep disorders, this approach will not be the case in this chapter owing to the total lack of randomized, controlled clinical trials in the management of idiopathic hypersomnia and recurrent hypersomnia. Instead, first, evidence for the clinical definition of each type of hypersomnia will be discussed, including what is known in terms of prevalence and pathophysiology. Next will come suggestions for treatment, mainly based on retrospective evaluation of the effects of different drugs on idiopathic and recurrent hypersomnias.

IDIOPATHIC HYPERSOMNIA

Definition, Prevalence, and Pathophysiology

According to ICSD-2, there are two forms of idiopathic hypersomnia, one with and one without long sleep time. Each has six diagnostic criteria.[1]

Idiopathic hypersomnia with long sleep time is remarkable for three symptoms: a complaint of more or less constant excessive daytime sleepiness and unwanted nap(s), generally not more than one or two per day, of longer duration and less irresistible than in narcolepsy, and nonrefreshing irrespective of duration (criterion A); night sleep is abnormally prolonged and morning and nap awakenings are laborious (criterion B). In the morning, patients do not awaken to the ringing of a clock and often rely on their family members who must use vigorous and repeated procedures to wake them up. Even then, some patients are unable to begin any task, remain confused, and are unable to react adequately to external stimuli, a state referred to as "sleep drunkenness." Associated symptoms suggesting an autonomic nervous system dysfunction, such as fainting episodes, lightheadedness on standing, orthostatic hypotension, headache, and cold hands and feet, are sometimes observed. Cataplexy is never present, but hypnagogic hallucinations and sleep paralysis may occur. Nocturnal polysomnography (PSG) must exclude other causes of daytime sleepiness (criterion C). Criteria D and E provide PSG and multiple sleep latency test (MSLT) diagnostic criteria for the disorder. These criteria include nocturnal PSG demonstrating a short sleep latency and sleep duration of longer than 10 hours (criterion D); MSLT performed the next day demonstrating a mean sleep latency of less than 8 minutes with fewer than two sleep onset rapid eye movement periods (SOREMPs) (criterion E). However, a recent article comparing idiopathic hypersomnia patients with and without long sleep time provides evidence that diagnostic criteria D and E of ICSD-2 are no longer valid.[2] This study showed that the nocturnal PSG may or may not demonstrate a short sleep latency or a major sleep period that is prolonged to more than 10 hours in duration. Moreover, the MSLT performed following overnight PSG must show fewer than two SOREMPs, but not necessarily a mean sleep latency of less than 8 minutes. The hypersomnia is not better explained by another sleep disorder, medical or neurologic disorder, mental disorder, medication use, or substance use disorder (criterion F).

Idiopathic hypersomnia without long sleep time is monosymptomatic. It manifests itself as isolated excessive daytime sleepiness (criterion A). Unwanted daytime sleep episodes can be more frequent, more irresistible and more refreshing than in the form with long sleep time, similar to those of narcolepsy. Abnormally long sleep time and difficulty waking up do not belong to this form (criterion B). As in idiopathic hypersomnia with long sleep time, nocturnal PSG must exclude other causes of daytime sleepiness (criterion C). Sleep latency and total sleep time are usually normal and an MSLT following overnight PSG demonstrates a mean sleep latency of less than 8 minutes and fewer than two SOREMPs (criteria D and E). Finally, the hypersomnia is not better explained by another sleep disorder, medical or neurologic disorder, mental disorder, medication use, or substance use disorder (criterion F) (Box 23-1).

No epidemiologic study of idiopathic hypersomnias with and without long sleep time has ever been conducted, but clinical experience indicates a very low prevalence. Recent reports from large sleep disorders centers suggest a ratio of idiopathic hypersomnia to narcolepsy of 10.3 to 16.2%.[3,4] As the prevalence of narcolepsy is 20 to 50 per 100,000 in whites, the prevalence of idiopathic hypersomnia could be somewhere between 2 and 8 per 100,000. Therefore, any randomized controlled trial (RCT) should be multicentered to gather a sufficient number of patients.

Finally, predisposing factors and mechanisms of idiopathic hypersomnia with and without long sleep time are still obscure. Idiopathic hypersomnia with long sleep time is remarkable for 27% to 40% of probands reporting family members affected with the same symptoms.[4-7] An autosomal

BOX 23-1 *Idiopathic Hypersomnia*

With Long Sleep Time	Without Long Sleep Time
A. A complaint of excessive daytime sleepiness occurring almost daily for at least 3 months	A. A complaint of excessive daytime sleepiness occurring almost daily for at least 3 months
B. Prolonged nocturnal sleep time (more than 10 hours) documented by interview, actigraphy, or sleep logs Waking up in the morning or at the end of a nap is almost always laborious	B. Nocturnal sleep time of normal duration (greater than 6 hours but less than 10 hours) documented by interview, actigraphy, or sleep logs
C. PSG has excluded other causes of excessive daytime sleepiness	C. PSG has excluded other causes of excessive daytime sleepiness
D. *PSG may or may not demonstrate a short sleep latency and/or a major sleep period that is prolonged to more than 10 hours in duration*	D. PSG demonstrates a major sleep period that is normal in duration (greater than 6 hours but less than 10 hours)
E. *If an MSLT is performed after overnight PSG, mean sleep latency is variable but fewer than two SOREMPs are recorded*	E. If an MSLT is performed following overnight PSG, mean sleep latency is less than 8 minutes and fewer than two SOREMPs are recorded
F. The hypersomnia is not better explained by another sleep disorder, medical or neurologic disorder, mental disorder, medication use, or substance use disorder	F. The hypersomnia is not better explained by another sleep disorder, medical or neurologic disorder, mental disorder, medication use, or substance use disorder

MSLT, multiple sleep latency test, *PSG,* polysomnography; *SOREMPs,* sleep onset rapid eye movement sleep periods.

From the ICSD-2 (1), *italics* indicate modified ICSD-2 diagnostic criteria after the work of Vernet and Arnulf.[2]

dominant mode of inheritance has been suggested.[5] On the other hand, familial data are not available for idiopathic hypersomnia without long sleep time. Furthermore, knowledge of the mechanisms of idiopathic hypersomnia is much less advanced than it is in the case of narcolepsy. There is no natural animal model of idiopathic hypersomnia, which limits experimental approach. Almost 40 years ago, Petitjean and Jouvet reported hypersomnia with a proportional increase of non-rapid eye movement (NREM) and rapid eye movement (REM) sleep suggestive of idiopathic hypersomnia with long sleep time, after destruction of norepinephrine neurons of the rostral third of the locus ceruleus complex or of the norepinephrine bundle at the level of the isthmus in the cat.[8] Unfortunately, this experiment has not been replicated. In humans, the few neurochemical studies conducted in idiopathic hypersomnia have not distinguished patients with idiopathic hypersomnia with and without long sleep time, and none of them has been replicated.[9-11] Recently, one study has shed some light on the neurochemical basis of narcolepsy and idiopathic hypersomnia.[12] Cerebrospinal fluid (CSF) histamine levels were low in patients with narcolepsy and in patients with idiopathic hypersomnia, whereas they were relatively normal in obstructive sleep apnea-hypopnea patients, hence

the hypothesis that low histamine levels may be specific to hypersomnias of central origin. However, if histamine levels are low in both conditions, it must still be explained why narcoleptic patients have an abnormal propensity to fall asleep and idiopathic hypersomnia with long sleep time patients have an inability to wake up normally. These uncertainties of pathophysiology make it difficult to draw perspectives for new treatments.

Management of Idiopathic Hypersomnia

Although excessive daytime sleepiness is more continuous in idiopathic hypersomnia with long sleep time and more intermittent in idiopathic hypersomnia without long sleep time and in narcolepsy with or without cataplexy, the same treatments have traditionally been used for all these disorders.

No systematic study of any drug has ever been carried out in idiopathic hypersomnia patients. The only accounts we have are from a few retrospective studies, the most recent of which are those by Anderson and associates,[13] Ali and associates,[14] and Lavault and associates.[15] In the first study, 61 patients with idiopathic hypersomnia (with and without long sleep time) were treated with various drugs and followed up for a mean of 3.8 ± 2.1 years.[13] The outcome measurement was the Epworth Sleepiness Score (ESS) at every clinic visit. In the second study, 85 patients with idiopathic hypersomnia (with and without long sleep time) were also treated by various drugs and followed up for a mean of 2.4 ± 4.7 years.[14] The outcome measurement was a review of the language used by physicians or patients to report progress during the follow-up visits. Finally, in the third and last study, 104 patients with idiopathic hypersomnia, 59 with long sleep time and 45 without long sleep time, were treated by modafinil only.[15] The outcome measurements were the ESS, a visual analog scale, and patient and clinician opinions.

Pharmacologic Treatment

Amphetamines. At low doses the main effect of amphetamines is to release dopamine and to a lesser extent norepinephrine through reverse efflux, via monoaminergic transporters, the dopamine transporter (DAT) and the norepinephrine transporter (NET). At higher doses, monoaminergic depletion and inhibition of reuptake occurs.[16] The D-isomer of amphetamine is more selective for dopaminergic transmission and is a better stimulant compound. Methamphetamine is more lipophilic than D-amphetamine and therefore will have a more rapid onset of action than D-amphetamine. The elimination half-life of these drugs is between 10 and 30 hours.

In the study by Anderson and associates, of 54 patients starting modafinil, 8 switched to dexamphetamine because of adverse effects; among these 8 patients, 5 were considered as responders (drop in the ESS > 4 points).[13] In the study by Ali and associates, 7 patients received dextroamphetamine with none of them reporting a complete or partial response; whereas 5 patients received methamphetamine, and 3 of them reported a complete response.[14]

The main adverse effects of amphetamines are minor irritability, hyperactivity, mood changes, headache, palpitations, sweating, tremors, anorexia, and insomnia. However, doses greater than 120% of the maximum recommended by the American Academy of Sleep Medicine (see Chapter 6) are responsible for a significantly higher occurrence of psychosis, substance misuse, and psychiatric hospitalizations as well as tachyarrhythmias and anorexia or weight loss.[17]

Tolerance to amphetamine may develop in up to one third of narcoleptic patients.[18] There is little or no evidence of abuse and addiction in narcoleptic patients.[19] Unfortunately, there are no data in this regard for idiopathic hypersomnia patients.

The Food and Drug Administration (FDA) classifies the pregnancy risk of drugs according to their embryotoxic and teratogenic effects (see Table 58-1). Dextroamphetamine is classified as FDA Pregnancy Category D and methamphetamine as Pregnancy Category C.

Methylphenidate. Similar to the action of amphetamine, methylphenidate induces dopamine release, but in contrast, it does not have any major effect on monoamine storage. The clinical effect of methylphenidate is supposed to be similar to that of amphetamines. However, clinical experience would argue for a slight superiority of amphetamines. In comparison with amphetamine, methylphenidate has a much shorter elimination half-life (2-7 hours) and the daily dose may be divided into two or three parts. Sustained release forms are available and can be useful for some patients.

As in the case of amphetamine no systematic study of methylphenidate in idiopathic hypersomnia has been conducted. However, in the study by Ali et al. 61 patients received methyphenidate, 40 (66%) of which were still on drug at last visit.[14] Of these 40 patients, 25 (41%) reported a complete response, 13 (21%) a partial response, and 2 a poor response.

Adverse effects are the same as with amphetamines. However, methylphenidate probably has a better therapeutic index than D-amphetamine with less reduction of appetite or increase in blood pressure.[20] Moreover, in a study assessing neuronal toxicity of methamphetamine and methylphenidate, methylphenidate failed to induce sensitization to hyperlocomotion, although methamphetamine clearly induced behavioral sensitization.[21] Tolerance may develop. Abuse potential is low in narcoleptic patients. Methyphenidate is classified as FDA Pregnancy Category C.

Modafinil. Modafinil is a medication chemically unrelated to central nervous system stimulants such as amphetamine and methylphenidate. The precise mechanism through which modafinil enhances wakefulness is unclear. However, substantial evidence indicates that modafinil may exert its effects via presynaptic dopaminergic mechanisms.[22,23] In addition it has been shown that modafinil inhibits DAT.[24] Consistent with these data, modafinil administration increases the extracellular levels of DA in brain as measured by *in vivo* microdialysis[25-27] and wake-promoting actions are absent in DAT-knockout mice.[26] On the other hand, modafinil does not seem to act as an alpha agonist,[24] to have a direct effect on the reuptake of glutamate or the synthesis of γ-aminoglutamic acid (GABA) or glutamate[28] nor to require orexin/hypocretin to act on alertness.[29]

Modafinil reaches peak bioavailability within about 2 hours. The main metabolic pathway is its transformation at the hepatic level into inactive metabolites, which are eliminated at the renal level. The reported elimination half-lives range between 10 and 17 hours. The steady state is reached after 2 to 4 days.

Co-administration of modafinil with drugs such as diazepam, phenytoin, propranolol, warfarin, some tricyclic antidepressants, and selective serotonin reuptake inhibitors (SSRIs) may increase the circulatory levels of those compounds due to the inhibition of certain cytochrome P-450 (CYP) hepatic enzymes. On the other hand, modafinil may reduce plasma levels of oral contraceptives as a result of the induction of some CYP hepatic enzymes.[30] Hence, alternative nonsteroidal or concomitant methods of birth control are recommended while using modafinil.

According to the study by Anderson and associates, of 54 patients starting modafinil, 39 (72.2%) remained on this drug alone: 24 (44.4%) responded to the drug with a drop of more than 4 points on their ESS, 8 (14.8%) switched to amphetamines, and 7 reported lack of efficacy.[13] In the study by Ali and associates, 25 of the 50 patients treated with modafinil remained on the drug during the last recorded follow-up visit;[14] 18 of these individuals reported complete symptomatic relief and 4 only partial symptomatic relief. Finally, in the study by Lavault and associates, modafinil produced a similar ESS change in idiopathic hypersomnia and in narcolepsy patients (-2.6 ± 5.1) versus (-3.0 ± 5.1), with a similar benefit as estimated by the patients (6.9 ± 2.7 versus 6.5 ± 2.5) on a visual analog scale.[15] Interestingly, the ESS change was lower in the patients with long sleep time than in those without long sleep time. Sudden loss of efficacy and habituation were rare in both groups. In addition, patients with idiopathic hypersomnia reported similar but more frequent adverse effects with modafinil than narcolepsy patients: nervousness (14%), palpitations (13%), and headaches (11%). Modafinil is classified as FDA Pregnancy Category B.

Armodafinil. Armodafinil is the longer-lasting *R*-isomer of racemic modafinil. Modafinil and armodafinil have a mean single dose terminal elimination half-life of approximately 10 to 17 hours with similar mean maximum plasma drug concentration (Cmax) and median time to Cmax values. However, plasma concentrations following armodafinil administration are higher late in the day than those following modafinil administration.[31] Therefore, armodafinil might represent a valuable option for the treatment of idiopathic hypersomnia with long sleep time.

Melatonin. Anecdotally, an improvement in half of 10 idiopathic hypersomnia patients treated with melatonin (2 mg of slow release at bedtime), a medication acting on circadian rhythms, has been reported.[32]

Behavioral Treatment

Saturating the patient with sleep during weekends is generally ineffective.[33] Sleep hygiene must be recommended but may have little positive impact alone.

Future Treatment

According to the previous referred study evidencing reduced CSF histamine levels in idiopathic hypersomnia patients,[12] applying histaminomimetic compounds for the treatment of idiopathic hypersomnia can be foreseen. In a noteworthy report published in 2008, an inverse agonist of the histamine H_3 receptor has been tested in mice models of narcolepsy and in narcoleptic patients with good results.[34]

Recommendations

Given the lack of RCT and comparative studies of different drugs in patients with idiopathic hypersomnia, it is difficult to make consistent recommendations. However, because of minor adverse effects, modafinil should be recommended as the first line treatment, prescribed first at a low dose of 200 mg, and then, if well tolerated, increased up to 400 mg in two split doses. If this therapy is insufficiently effective, methylphenidate at a dose of 20 mg should be tried. In addition, taking one tablet of one of these drugs before going to bed or immediately after morning awakening may help awakening.[35]

RECURRENT HYPERSOMNIA

Definitions, Prevalence, and Pathophysiology

According to ICSD-2, recurrent hypersomnia is characterized by episodes of more or less constant sleep of 2 days' to 4 weeks' duration (criterion A), recurring at intervals of months or years (criterion B), with normal functioning between episodes (criterion C). The hypersomnia is not better explained by another sleep disorder, medical or neurologic disorder, mental disorder, medication use, or substance use disorder (criterion D).[1] The best characterized form of recurrent hypersomnia is the Kleine-Levin syndrome in which episodes of prolonged sleep are associated with behavioral abnormalities such as compulsive eating, sexual disinhibition, and odd behaviors; cognitive abnormalities such as apathy, slowness, feeling of unreality, confusion, and delusions/hallucinations; psychiatric symptoms such as depression and anxiety; dysautonomic features such as swollen or puffy face, hypotension or bradycardia, excessive perspiration, offensive body odor, or weight gain; and transient symptoms such as anorexia, elation, depression, and insomnia at the end of episodes. However, the simultaneous occurrence of all these symptoms is the exception rather than the rule. Moreover, symptoms such as compulsive eating, sexual disinhibition, and derealization, may be present only during one or two episodes and absent during other episodes. Apart from the Kleine-Levin syndrome, there is a form of recurrent hypersomnia in which the main behavioral symptom, compulsive eating, is totally absent from the first to the last episode; a form referred to as menstruation-related hypersomnia in which recurrent episodes of sleepiness and other symptoms occur in association with menarche, the menstrual cycle, or even puerperium; and a form of recurrent hypersomnia with co-morbidity, in which the co-morbidity may or may not be responsible for recurrent hypersomnia. Thus, symptoms are far from uniform and clinical variants do exist (Table 23-1).[36]

A second issue to consider in the discussion of recurrent hypersomnia is the total absence of epidemiologic study. A recent study[36] has collected 339 cases of recurrent hypersomnia in the world literature, but this study has no value for evaluating the actual prevalence of recurrent hypersomnia. In any case the prevalence is extremely low, which renders any RCT difficult to perform.

Concerning the pathophysiology, there are some emerging new data. First, there are familial cases (about 3.5%) of Kleine-Levin syndrome, as is the case with narcolepsy. Second, the hypothesis of an hypothalamic origin is now outdated.[37] Current arguments drawn from cases of recurrent hypersomnia secondary to organic insults of the central nervous system[38-42] and on single photon emission computed tomography (SPECT) studies in Kleine-Levin syndrome[43-49] speak in favor of a more complex anatomic basis with several regions such as basal ganglia; thalamus; and frontal, parietal, temporal, or occipital lobes being involved. Third, based on the generally young age of onset, the recurrence of symptoms, the frequent infectious trigger, an autoimmune cause has been suggested, although no direct evidence for this putative process has so far been documented.[50] Finally, there are hints for common mechanisms between some mood disorders, depression with atypical features, seasonal affective disorders, and recurrent hypersomnia. However, these data are much more hypothetical than evidence-based information. Therefore, in recurrent hypersomnia as well as in idiopathic hypersomnia there are obvious obstacles to systematic well-designed pharmacologic trials.

Management of Recurrent Hypersomnia

A recent Cochrane Database Systematic Review aimed at evaluating whether pharmacologic treatments for Kleine-Levin syndrome are effective and safe, and which drug or category of drugs is effective and safe, searched for RCTs and quasi-RCTs. Looking at pharmacologic interventions for Kleine-Levin

TABLE 23-1				
Recurrent Hypersomnia				
Manifestation	**K-L Syndrome**	**K-L Syndrome w/o Compulsive Eating**	**Menstruation-Related Hypersomnia**	**Recurrent Hypersomnia with Comorbidity**
Recurrent episodes of prolonged sleep (days to weeks)	+	+	+	+
Compulsive eating	+*	−	±	±
Other behaviorial abnormalities	±	±	±	±
Cognitive abnormalities	±	±	±	±
Psychiatric symptoms	±	±	±	±
Dysautonomic features	±	±	±	±
Weight gain	±	−	±	±
Transient symptoms (amnesia, elation, depression, insomnia) at the end of episodes	±	±	±	±

K-L, Kleine-Levin; w/o, without; +*, present during some episodes only.

syndrome, none was found.[51] Therefore, we are left with only individual case reports in which one or several drugs have been administered and clinically evaluated by patients' doctors.

There are two types of treatment for recurrent hypersomnia, symptomatic and prophylactic. Symptomatic treatments are mainly based on stimulants (amphetamine and methylphenidate), on the wake-promoting drug modafinil (pharmacologic characteristics discussed earlier), and due to psychotic-like symptoms, on neuroleptics and in some rare cases electroconvulsive therapy. However, proper evaluation of these drugs is rather unreliable because of the spontaneous eventual disappearance of the symptoms after a few days of evolution. Treatments aimed at preventing relapses include mood stabilizers (lithium and antiepileptic drugs including carbamazepine, sodium valproate, gabapentin, and lamotrigine). The proposed shared mechanism of these drugs is sodium channels antagonism.[52,53] Antidepressants have also been used to prevent recurrence.[54]

Carbamazepine is a tricyclic compound with a chemical structure resembling that of the tricyclic antidepressants. Plasma half-life is 25 to 65 hours, decreasing to 12 to 17 hours with repeated dosing. A major active metabolite is the 10,11-dihydroxy-10,11-epoxide with a mean half-life of approximately 7.5 hours. The most frequently reported adverse effects are rashes, vertigo, diplopia, ataxia, nystagmus, confusion, sedation, nausea, and leukopenia. The usual dosage is 400 to 800 mg per day.

Sodium valproate is another antiepileptic drug. Its elimination half-life is about 15 hours. Steady state is reached in 3 to 4 days. The main adverse effects are gastrointestinal upset, tremor, rashes, and liver toxicity. The usual dosage is 30 to 60 mg/kg/day.

Lithium, usually given as a carbonate salt, peaks in the serum in 1.5 hours; 95% is excreted in the kidney. Thus, any condition that leads to sodium loss, via disease or diuretics, poses a risk for toxicity. The elimination half-life is 24 hours, which tends to increase with age. Steady state is reached in 4 to 6 days. The most frequent adverse effects are gastrointestinal upset, tremor, polyuria, polydypsia, diabetes insipidus, and decreased thyroid function. The usual dosage range is 600 to 1400 mg per day. According to the largest study evaluating the effects of lithium therapy in five patients with Kleine-Levin syndrome, lithium carbonate at serum levels between 0.6 and 0.9 mEq/L can reduce duration and frequency of episodes.[55] In the case of menstruation-related hypersomnia, estroprogestatives are the treatment of choice.[56]

In contrast to symptomatic treatments, prophylactic treatments are easy to evaluate, based on the recurrence or not of symptomatic episodes.

Kleine-Levin Syndrome

Symptomatic Treatment. In a recent review of 186 cases in the literature, the response rate was 71% in 17 patients treated with amphetamine, 20% in 15 subjects treated with methylphenidate, and 0% in 2 subjects treated with modafinil, and neuroleptics were notably ineffective against psychotic-like symptoms.[54] In our own review of the literature[36] extending the number of cases to 239, we obtained similar results (Table 23-2).

Prophylactic Treatment. In the same review of 186 cases, the response rate was 20% in 10 patients treated with antiepileptics (mainly sodium valproate), 21% in 19 subjects treated with carbamazepine, 41% treated with lithium, and 9% in 23 subjects treated with antidepressants (tricyclics or SSRIs).[54] In our own review,[36] results were also similar except that antidepressants were mostly used as symptomatic treatments (see Table 23-2).

Kleine-Levin Syndrome without Compulsive Eating

The effects of symptomatic and prophylactic treatments were not evaluated separately from the full-blown Kleine-Levin syndrome in previous reviews. In our own review[36] the results

TABLE 23-2

Kleine-Levin Syndrome: Effect of Treatment with Various Pharmacologic Agents*

Treatment	No. of Patients	No Effect	Questionable Effect	Positive Effect	No Indication	Positive Response Rate (%)
SYMPTOMATIC						
Amphetamines	19	4	6	7	2	36
Methylphenidate	18	9	5	3	1	16
Modafinil	5	1	1	1	2	20
Antidepressants	23	11	7	2	3	11.5
Neuroleptics	14	6	5	2	1	14.2
Other treatments	7	4	2	0	1	0
No treatment	153					
PROPHYLACTIC						
Carbamazepine	27	9	7	7	4	25.9
Sodium valproate	7	2	3	2	0	28.5
Gabapentine	1	0	0	1	0	-
Lamotrigine	1	0	0	1	0	-
Lithium carbonate	41	12	12	16	0	39
Other treatments	6	4	2	0	0	0
No treatment	156					

*Unpublished data for a series of 239 patients.[36]

TABLE 23-3

Kleine-Levin Syndrome without Compulsive Eating: Effect of Treatment with Various Pharmacologic Agents*

Treatment	No. of Patients	No Effect	Questionable Effect	Positive Effect	No Indication	Positive Response Rate (%)
SYMPTOMATIC						
Amphetamines	3	3	0	0	0	0
Methylphenidate	2	1	0	0	1	0
Modafinil	2	1	1	0	0	0
Antidepressants	1	1	0	0	0	0
Neuroleptics	3	2	1	0	0	0
Other treatments	1	0	0	0	1	0
No treatment	32					
PROPHYLACTIC						
Carbamazepine	4	0	0	2	2	50
Sodium valproate	3	2	1	0	0	0
Lithium carbonate	7	1	2	4	0	57.1
Other treatments	1	0	0	0	1	0
No treatment	39					

*Unpublished data for a series of 54 patients.[36]

TABLE 23-4

Menstruation-Related Hypersomnia: Effect of Treatment with Various Pharmacologic Agents*

Treatment	No. of Patients	No Effect	Questionable Effect	Positive Effect	No Indication	Positive Response Rate (%)
SYMPTOMATIC						
Ephedrine	1	0	0	0	1	0
Methylphenidate	2	1	1	0	0	0
Pemoline	1	0	0	1	0	-
No treatment	14					
PROPHYLACTIC						
Lithium carbonate	2	0	1	1	0	50
Estroprogestative	8	1	1	6	0	75
No treatment						

*Unpublished data for a series of 18 patients.[36]

of symptomatic treatments were extremely poor, whereas those of lithium were satisfactory (Table 23-3).

Menstruation-Related Hypersomnia

Our own series[36] was limited (18 patients), but the largest ever collected from the literature. Only 4 women out of 18 were prescribed a symptomatic treatment, methylphenidate in 2, ephedrine in 1, and pemoline in 1, without any clear positive effect (Table 23-4). On the other hand, two women received lithium, with a questionable effect in one case and a positive effect in the other case. Above all, six women out of eight (75%) benefited by estroprogestatives, confirming the value of the endocrine treatment in women with menstruation-related hypersomnia.

RECOMMENDATIONS

From the results reported here, it is clear that amphetamines, methyphenidate, or modafinil have no or questionable effect on excessive daytime sleepiness and the other symptoms of

recurrent hypersomnia. Therefore, there is practically no indication for this type of treatment during symptomatic episodes, whatever the form of recurrent hypersomnia.

On the other hand, mood stabilizers, especially lithium, and to a lesser extent antiepileptic drugs, may prevent relapses in a substantial number of patients. However lithium is not free of potential adverse effects. In this context, it is advisable to prescribe lithium only in the case of a severe impact of the condition on the social life of the patient.

Finally, estroprogestatives appear as a valuable prophylactic treatment of menstruation-related hypersomnia.

SUMMARY

There is still a long way to go before one can propose satisfactory treatments, based on RCTs and a well-elucidated pathophysiology for both idiopathic and recurrent hypersomnias. The future is in well-designed RCTs in homogeneous groups of patients. Such studies must be multicentered to gather a sufficient number of patients. In addition, progress in understanding the pathophysiology of both conditions must be achieved before one can suggest etiologically oriented treatments.

REFERENCES

1. American Academy of Sleep Medicine. *International Classification of Sleep Disorders. Diagnostic and Coding Manual.* 2nd ed. Westchester, IL: American Academy of Sleep Medicine; 2005.
2. Vernet C, Arnulf I. Idiopathic hypersomnia with and without long sleep time: A controlled series of 75 patients. *Sleep.* 2009;32(6):753-759.
3. Bassetti C, Aldrich MS. Idiopathic hypersomnia. A series of 42 patients. *Brain.* 1997;120(Pt 8):1423-1435.
4. Billiard M, Dauvilliers Y. Idiopathic hypersomnia. *Sleep Med Rev.* 2001;5(5):351-360.
5. Nevsimalova-Bruhova S, Roth B. Heredofamilial aspects of narcolepsy and hypersomnia. *Schweiz Arch Neurol.* 1972;110(1):45-54.
6. Roth B. Idiopathic hypersomnia. In: Roth B, ed. *Narcolepsy and Hypersomnia.* Basel: Karger; 1980:207-227.
7. Billiard M, Merle C, Carlander B, et al. Idiopathic hypersomnia. *Psychiatr Clin Neurosci.* 1998;52(2):125-129.
8. Petitjean F, Jouvet M. Hypersomnie et augmentation de l'acide 5-hydroxy-indoleacétique cérébral par lésion isthmique chez le chat. *C R Séances Soc Biol (Paris).* 1970;164(11):2288-2293.
9. Montplaisir J, de Champlain J, Young SN, et al. Narcolepsy and idiopathic hypersomnia: Biogenic amines and related compounds in CSF. *Neurology.* 1982;32(11):1299-1302.
10. Faull KF, Guilleminault C, Berger PA, et al. Cerebrospinal fluid monoamine metabolites in narcolepsy and hypersomnia. *Ann Neurol.* 1983;13(3):258-263.
11. Faull KF, Thiemann S, King RJ, et al. Monoamine interactions in narcolepsy and hypersomnia: A preliminary report. *Sleep.* 1986;9(1 Pt 2):246-249.
12. Kanbayashi T, Kodama T, Kondo H, et al. CSF histamine contents in narcolepsy, idiopathic hypersomnia and obstructive sleep apnea syndrome. *Sleep.* 2009;32(2):175-180.
13. Anderson KN, Pilsworth S, Sharpless LD, et al. Idiopathic hypersomnia: A study of 77 cases. *Sleep.* 2007;30(10):1274-1281.
14. Ali M, Auger RR, Slocumb NL, et al. Idiopathic hypersomnia: Clinical features and response to treatment. *J Clin Sleep Med.* 2009;5(6):562-568.
15. Lavault S, Dauvilliers Y, Drouot X, et al. Benefit and risk of modafinil in idiopathic hypersomnia vs. narcolepsy with cataplexy. *Sleep Med.* 2011;12(6):550-556.
16. Seiden LS, Sabol KE, Ricaurte GA. Amphetamine: Effects on catecholamine systems and behavior. *Annu Rev Pharmacol Toxicol.* 1993;33:639-677.
17. Auger RR, Goodman SH, Silber MH, et al. Risks of high-dose stimulants in the treatment of disorders of excessive somnolence: A case-control study. *Sleep.* 2005;28(6):667-672.
18. Guilleminault C. Amphetamines and narcolepsy: Use of the Stanford data base. *Sleep.* 1993;16(3):199-201.
19. Parkes JD, Dahlitz M. Amphetamine prescription. *Sleep.* 1993;16(3):201-203.
20. Guilleminault C, Carskadon MA, Dement WC. On the treatment of rapid eye movement narcolepsy. *Arch Neurol.* 1974;30(1):90-93.
21. Narita M, Asato M, Shindo K, et al. Differences in neuronal toxicity and molecular mechanisms in methamphetamine and methylphenidate. *Seishin Yakurigaku Zasshi.* 2009;29(3):115-120.
22. Nishino S, Mao J, Sampathkumaran R, et al. Increased dopaminergic transmission mediates the wake-promoting effects of CNS stimulants. *Sleep Res Online.* 1998;1(1):49-61.
23. Minzenberg MJ, Carter CS. Modafinil: A review of neurochemical actions and effects on cognition. *Neuropsychopharmacology.* 2008;33(7):1477-1502.
24. Mignot E, Nishino S, Guilleminault C, et al. Modafinil binds to the dopamine uptake carrier site with low affinity. *Sleep.* 1994;17(5):436-437.
25. De Saint-Hilaire Z, Orosco M, Rouch C, et al. Variations in extra-cellular monoamines in the prefrontal cortex and medial hypothalamus after modafinil administration: A microdialysis study in rats. *Neuroreport.* 2001;12(16):3533-3537.
26. Wisor JP, Nishino S, Sora I, et al. Dopaminergic role in stimulant-induced wakefulness. *J Neurosci.* 2001;21(5):1787-1794.
27. Murillo-Rodriguez E, Haro R, Palomero-Rivero M, et al. Modafinil enhances extracellular levels of dopamine in the nucleus accumbens and increases wakefulness in rats. *Behav Brain Res.* 2007;176(2):353-357.
28. Ferraro I, Antonelli T, Tanganelli S, et al. The vigilance promoting drug modafinil increases extracellular glutamate levels in the medial preoptic area and the posterior hypothalamus of the conscious rat: Prevention by local GABAA receptor blockade. *Neuropsychopharmacology.* 1999;20(4):346-356.
29. Willie J, Renthal W, Chemelli RM, et al. Modafinil more effectively induces wakefulness in orexin-null mice than in wild-type littermates. *Neuroscience.* 2005;130(4):983-995.
30. Palovaara S, Kivisto KT, Tapanainen P, et al. Effect of oral contraceptive preparation containing ethinylestradiol and gestodene on CYP3A4 activity as measured by midazolam l-hydroxylation. *Br J Clin Pharmacol.* 2000;50(4):333-337.
31. Darwish M, Kirby M, Hellriegel ET, et al. Armodafinil and modafinil have substantially different pharmacokinetic profiles despite having the same terminal half-lives: Analysis of data from three randomized, single-dose, pharmacokinetic studies. *Clin Drug Investig;.* 2009;29(9):613-623.
32. Montplaisir J, Fantini L. Idiopathic hypersomnia: A diagnostic dilemna. *Sleep Med Rev.* 2001;5(5):361-362.
33. Bassetti C, Pelayo R, Guilleminault C. Idiopathic hypersomnia. In: Kryger MH, Roth T, Dement WC, eds. *Principle and Practice of Sleep Medicine.* 4th ed. 2005:791-800.
34. Lin JS, Dauvilliers Y, Arnulf I, et al. An inverse agonist of the histamine H(3) receptor improves wakefulness in narcolepsy: Studies in orexin -/- mice and patients. *Neurobiol Dis.* 2008;30(1):74-83.
35. Roth B, Nevsimalova S, Rechtschaffen A. Hypersomnia with "sleep drunkenness". *Arch Gen Psychiat.* 1972;26(5):456-462.
36. Billiard M, Jaussent I, Dauvilliers Y, et al. Recurrent hypersomnia: A review of 339 cases. *Sleep Med Rev.* 2011;15(4):247-257.
37. Mayer G, Leonhard E, Krieg J, et al. Endocrinological and polysomnographic findings in Kleine-Levin syndrome. No evidence for hypothalamic and circadian dysfunction. *Sleep.* 1998;21(3):278-284.
38. Argenta G, Bozzao L, Petruzellis MC. First CT findings in the Kleine-Levin-Critchley syndrome. *Ital J Neurol Sci.* 1981;2(1):77-79.
39. Drake Jr ME. Kleine-Levin syndrome after multiple cerebral infarctions. *Psychosomatics.* 1987;28(6):329-330.
40. Chiu HFK, Li SW, Lee S. Kleine-Levin syndrome 15 years later. *Aust N Z J Psychiatr.* 1989;23(3):425-427.
41. McGilchrist I, Goldstein LH, Jadresic D, et al. Thalamo-frontal psychosis. *Br J Psychiatry.* Jul 1993;163:113-115.
42. Kostic VS, Stefanova B, Svetel M, et al. A variant of the Kleine-Levin syndrome following head trauma. *Behav Neurol.* 1998;11(2):105-108.
43. Lu ML, Liu HC, Chen CH, et al. Kleine-Levin syndrome and psychosis: Observation from an unusual case. *Neuropsychiatr Neuropsychol Behav Neurol.* 2000;13(2):140-142.
44. Landtblom AM, Dige N, Schwerdt K, et al. A case of Kleine-Levin syndrome examined with SPECT and neuropsychological testing. *Acta Neurol Scand.* 2002;105(4):318-321.
45. Landtblom AM, Dige N, Schwerdt K, et al. Short-term memory dysfunction in Kleine-Levin syndrome. *Acta Neurol Scand.* 2003;108(5):363-367.
46. Arias M, Crespo-Iglesias IM, Perez J, et al. Syndrome de Kleine-Levin. Aportacion diagnostica de la SPECT cerebral. *Rev Neurol.* 2002;35(6):531-533.
47. Portilla P, Durand E, Chalvon A, et al. Hypoperfusion temporomésiale gauche en TEMP dans un syndrome de Kleine-Levin. *Rev Neurol (Paris).* 2002;158(5 Pt 1):593-595.
48. Huang YS, Guilleminault C, Kao PF, et al. SPECT findings in the Kleine-Levin syndrome. *Sleep.* 2005;28(8):955-960.
49. Hong SB, Joo EY, Tae WS, et al. Episodic diencephalic hypoperfusion in Kleine-Levin syndrome. *Sleep.* 2006;29(8):1091-1093.
50. Dauvilliers Y, Mayer G, Lecendreux M, et al. Kleine-Levin syndrome: An autoimmune hypothesis based on clinical and genetic analyses. *Neurology.* 2002;59(11):1739-1745.
51. Oliveira MM, Conti C, Saconato H. Pharmacological treatment for Kleine-Levin syndrome. *Cochrane Database Syst Rev.* 2009;2:1-12.
52. Bourin M, Chenu F, Hascoët M. The role of sodium channels in the mechanism of antidepressants and mood stabilizers. *Curr Drug Targets.* 2009;10(4):1052-1060.
53. Huang X, Lei Z, El-Mallakh RS. Lithium normalizes elevated cellular sodium. *Bipolar Disord.* 2007;9(3):298-300.
54. Arnulf I, Zeitzer JM, File J, et al. Kleine-Levin syndrome: A systematic review of 186 cases in the literature. *Brain.* 2005;128(Pt12):2763-2776.
55. Poppe M, Friebel D, Reuner U, et al. The Kleine-Levin syndrome-Effects of treatment with lithium. *Neuropediatrics.* 2003;34(3):113-119.
56. Billiard M, Guilleminault C, Dement WC. A menstruation linked periodic hypersomnia. Kleine-Levin syndrome or new clinical entity? *Neurology.* 1975;25(5):436-443.

Movement Disorders Affecting Sleep

Restless Legs Syndrome and Periodic Limb Movement Disorders

DAVID B. RYE / LYNN MARIE TROTTI

Restless legs syndrome (RLS) is a common sensory syndrome that is characterized by nocturnal urges to move the legs, often accompanied by unpleasant or painful calf and ankle sensations, which are triggered by rest and improved with movement. The tendency for symptoms to occur at rest results in delays in sleep onset as well as intrusion of symptoms into sedentary daily activities such as traveling in confined spaces (e.g., airplane, cars) or attending meetings. Comprehensively described in the medical literature in 1945 by Ekbom,[1] RLS was noted to have a prevalence of at least 5%, a proclivity to affect pregnant women, heritability, and favorable responses to iron supplementation and sympathectomy. We now recognize that periodic limb movements in sleep (PLMS) are present in the anterior tibialis muscles of the legs in 85% to 95% of RLS subjects, and that these movements are associated with elevations of heart rate and blood pressure that may explain the increased cardiovascular risk seen in RLS. Although the pathophysiology of RLS is not fully understood, five genetic loci in four genes have been identified that account for the majority of the population attributable risk of RLS and PLMS, and there are reductions in brain iron in a subpopulation of RLS cases. Treatments include pharmacologic agents acting at D_2 and D_3 dopamine receptors, opiates, and derivatives of gabapentin.

EPIDEMIOLOGY AND NATURAL HISTORY

RLS is defined by four cardinal features: (1) urges to move the legs that are often uncomfortable and sometimes painful; (2) worsening of symptoms at rest; (3) symptom relief, even temporary, with movement; and (4) a genuine circadian pattern with a predominance of symptoms in the evening and at night.[2-5] Variability in symptoms is common, although they tend to begin as mild and infrequent, slowly progressing to the point of diagnosis, which usually occurs in the fourth to sixth decades of life. Sensory symptoms often manifest as childhood growing pains[6,7] and are painful in 35% to 55% of adults.[8,9] Populations of European descent have RLS prevalence rates ranging from 3% to 15%,[10,11] although only 1.6% to 2.8% of these populations have RLS that is deemed to be "clinically significant," that is, frequent or severe enough to require treatment.[11] Prevalences in non-European ethnic groups are much lower: 0.1% in Singapore,[12] 0.9% in South Korea,[13] 2.0% in Ecuador,[14] 3.2% in Turkey,[15] and 3.3% in Japan.[16] A single study reported the prevalence of RLS symptoms to be similar in whites and African Americans,[17] but data are limited and have not been replicated in other studies.[18,19] The extent to which these differences reflect genetic, environmental, or sociocultural factors in expressivity or reporting is still to be

determined. However, the heritability of RLS (i.e., the proportion of phenotypic variation attributable to genes) is high at 54% to 83%,[20,21] and recently discovered genetic variants that confer risk for RLS support the idea that much of this difference in symptom burden is caused by different levels of genetic risk burden.

RLS prevalence is also influenced by age, sex, pregnancy, and common medical conditions. RLS affects 2% of school age children,[6] 3% of 30-year-olds, and 20% of those aged 80 and older.[22] Women are affected more often than men, in an approximate 2:1 ratio, and may exhibit greater night-to-night variability in PLM counts.[23] Almost one third of pregnant women develop RLS by their third trimester,[24,25] and the risk of RLS after pregnancy increases linearly with the number of live births (odds ratio [OR] = 3.57 for >3 births).[26] RLS is encountered in many common medical conditions—ostensibly "secondary" RLS—at frequencies exceeding those that would be expected by chance (see Box 24-3). In summary, the expression of RLS is strongly influenced by genetics but is further impacted by demographic, medical, environmental, and possibly additional genetic factors through mechanisms that remain poorly defined.

DIAGNOSIS

Restless Legs Syndrome

The four RLS diagnostic criteria are considered sufficient for diagnosis in adults, but several additional features may be useful in confirming the diagnosis in uncertain cases. These three features include a positive family history, a favorable response to dopaminergic therapy, and periodic limb movements of sleep (PLMS). Empiric trials of dopamine agonists or levodopa may be useful in practice and are particularly helpful in differentiating RLS from other conditions that share some common features.[27,28] Although not formally considered in the diagnostic criteria, symptom exacerbation in response to a variety of other medications, both over the counter and prescription, are also clinically useful in making the diagnosis of RLS. These drugs include antidopaminergic medications such as antipsychotics, metaclopramide, and prochlorperazine; selective serotonin and serotonin-norepinephrine reuptake inhibitors; nonspecific antihistamines (e.g., diphenhydramine); and sympathomimetics (e.g., ephedrine and pseudoephedrine).[29-32] Conflicting reports of RLS and PLMS developing after regional and spinal anesthesia may be due to the use of sympathomimetic amines to support blood pressure in these clinical scenarios.[33-37]

Self-administered questionnaires developed around the four RLS consensus criteria demonstrate sensitivities and specificities in the range of 0.75. Some of the difficulty in diagnosis arises from RLS "mimics."[38-40] These mimicking conditions include clinical entities such as radiculopathy, neuropathy, akathisia, and nocturnal leg cramps. However, careful attention to the diagnostic and supportive criteria for RLS can typically distinguish true RLS from these mimics. For example, radiculopathy may appear similar to RLS in that it is provoked by sitting or lying down, but there is no associated urge to move and no benefit from use of dopamine agonists.[41] Neuropathy can mimic RLS in having a nocturnal symptom predominance (although this is not usually as marked as that in RLS), but again, it is not associated with an urge to move and is not relieved by movement or dopaminergics.[41] Furthermore, although not part of the formal diagnostic criteria, RLS most commonly spares the feet, which are prominently involved in neuropathy. Both akathisia and RLS are associated with an urge to move, but akathisia is lacking a nocturnal predominance, a tendency to affect the legs, and leg discomfort.[42] Nocturnal leg cramps are not associated with an urge to move and do not improve with movement.[42] The syndrome of painful legs and moving toes (PLMT) is sometimes considered to be an RLS mimic, but we are of the belief, as initially proposed by Marsden and co-workers in their original descriptions of PLMT,[43,44] that PLMT is part of the phenotypic spectrum of RLS rather than a separate entity.

Periodic Leg Movements and Other Motor Stereotypies

RLS is by definition a subjective experience, and diagnostic criteria are a carefully constructed consensus tool, but do not necessarily perfectly reflect the underlying biology of the disorder. Periodic limb movements (PLMs), on the other hand, are a genetically mediated, objective, biologic phenomenon that can shed light on our understanding of RLS. PLMs are involuntary, stereotyped, repetitive movements of the legs occurring during sleep or, less commonly, wakefulness. Videographically, PLMs appear to be a Babinski or flexor-withdrawal response, implicating spinal and supraspinal circuits in their generation.[45,46] This movement manifests as extension of the big toe (i.e., extensor hallicus longus) and dorsiflexion of the ankle, although flexion of the knee or even hip may also occur. By definition, PLMs have durations of 0.5 to 10 seconds and occur between 5 and 90 seconds apart, although the typical duration between movements is most commonly around 22 seconds.[47,48] Although the exact threshold for pathology associated with PLMs has not been established, a PLMS index (PLMI; PLMs per hour of sleep) between 5 and 15 (or greater) is generally considered to be abnormal.[3,49]

Nearly all patients with RLS demonstrate PLMs, depending on how movements are measured and for how long they are sought. For instance, PLMs are seen in 80% of RLS subjects using anterior tibialis surface electrodes during routine polysomnography (PSG, using a rate of > 5/hour as positive). This increases to 88% with two consecutive nights of PSG.[50] Using ambulatory accelerometry of a single leg, 91% of RLS subjects seeking treatment demonstrate 5 or more PLMs per hour on at least one of five consecutive nights of monitoring.[23] The improvement in diagnostic sensitivity with additional nights of recording is a reflection of the nightly variability in PLMs,

which appears to be most pronounced in women, younger subjects, and those with less severe RLS symptoms. Although classically monitored at the anterior tibialis, recording over extensor hallucis longus may reveal periodic movements in an even greater proportion of RLS subjects.

Although exceedingly common in RLS subjects, PLMs are not entirely specific, occurring also in narcolepsy, in REM (rapid eye movement) sleep-behavior disorder, during antidepressant therapy, and in the otherwise asymptomatic elderly. Correlations of PLMI with the International RLS Study Group Rating Scale[51] (a measure of subjective RLS severity) are not robust (Pearson's correlations $r = 0.22\text{-}0.46$).[52-54] Despite these limitations, PLMs can improve the diagnostic accuracy of RLS, resulting in their inclusion as "supportive" criteria for RLS definition by formal consensus criteria. The addition of PLMI greater than 5 to self-reported RLS symptoms improves the positive predictive value for RLS to greater than 95%.[55] When PLMs are present at least 15 times per hour during wakefulness after sleep onset, it is a very specific sign of RLS (~90%).[56]

PLMs occurring in the absence of RLS but in association with clinical sleep disturbance or daytime fatigue are classified as periodic limb movement disorder (PLMD).[49] At present, data do not support the routine treatment of PLMD.

Prevalence estimates for PLMs range from 5% to 11% for rates at or above 5 per hour[57] to 4.3% to 9.3% for 15 per hour during a single night of PSG testing.[58] Asymptomatic PLMs have frequently been noted to predate the onset of RLS sensory symptoms,[59-62] but there are no longitudinal, population-based estimates of how many people with isolated PLMs will ultimately develop RLS. PLMs are genetically determined, occurring more commonly in relatives of RLS subjects[63] and in ethnic groups that have the highest population frequencies of RLS/PLMs risk alleles (e.g., those of European descent).[58,64] One such risk variant, in the *BTBD9* gene, is a more powerful predictor of PLMs than RLS symptoms.[38]

PLMs may be measured by routine PSG or by ambulatory actigraphy. PSG cannot capture the nightly variability of PLMs and is expensive to perform, but has the advantage of accurately distinguishing between PLMs occurring during sleep and those occurring in wake (PLMW). Actigraphic devices use miniaturized accelerometers placed on the big toe, ankle, or foot to capture limb acceleration, rather than directly measuring surface EMG activity. Actigraphy is less expensive than PSG and can be conducted in the home over multiple nights. Versions such as the PAM-RL triaxial accelerometer (Respironics; Murrysville, PA) have proved useful for diagnostic purposes and in large clinical trials, being sensitive to treatment effects.[65,66] This device provides an accurate assessment PLMI that is strongly correlated with polysomnographically measured PLMI (Pearson's correlation $r = 0.87$, $p < 0.0001$)[67] and is able to discriminate between PLMs and random nocturnal motor activity.[68] Despite these advantages, actigraphy cannot differentiate between PLMs in sleep and wake, so the use of a sleep-wake diary is helpful in distinguishing sleep and wake events.

PLMs do not occur in isolation; rather, they occur as part of a cascade of events that also includes cardiovascular and cerebrocortical arousals. In RLS subjects, they are associated with transient, repetitive elevations in heart rate[69-71] and blood pressure.[72,73] These increases are greater than those observed with either volitional leg movements (e.g., the exercise pressor reflex) or isolated, nonperiodic movements in sleep. Similar elevations in heart rate[74] and repetitive peripheral vasoconstriction occur with PLMs in subjects without RLS symptoms.[75] Such variability in sympathetic activity has been implicated in the development of cardiovascular disease[76] and stroke.[77] The increases in heart rate and blood pressure seen with PLMs are of the same magnitude as those observed with the hyperventilatory phase of sleep apnea,[78-80] and PLMs were more predictive of cardiovascular medication burden than was sleep-disordered breathing in the Bay Area Sleep Cohort.[81] Thus, PLMs with and without RLS symptoms likely share important cardiovascular consequences. It remains to be determined whether treatment of RLS or PLMs (with or without associated RLS) will decrease cardiovascular disease risk.

In addition to the spontaneous flexor-withdrawal of periodic limb movements during wake, multiple other voluntary and involuntary leg movements may be observed in RLS subjects, although a comprehensive accounting of these movements is lacking. In clinical practice, the authors frequently observe volitional foot tapping, flexion and extension of the knee, and abduction and adduction of the hip in RLS patients. In a minority of patients (~3-5% in our tertiary referral center), these movements are unequivocally nonvolitional, appearing as dyskinesia,[82] fanning or clawing of the toes, or brief myoclonic jerks in isolated muscles of the feet. We have observed such myoclonic activity in several young, unmedicated patients in whom the movements interfered with gait or coordinated activities, perhaps not dissimilar to the impairments of coordination noted by Ekbom in his original description of RLS.[1] The clinical significance of these voluntary and involuntary movements is not entirely clear, although in our experience and that of others, it appears that myoclonic, involuntary movements occur more commonly in the setting of augmentation (discussed later)[3] and may be a manifestation of opioid withdrawal in patients using opiates for treatment of RLS or pain.

HEALTH-RELATED SIGNIFICANCE OF RLS

Quality of life is poor in RLS patients, with RLS patients having lower health-related quality of life than type 2 diabetics.[83] Treatments are symptomatic, not curative, and thus the need for pharmacotherapy can be expected to be lifelong.[84] Although several effective treatments are available, 10% to 20% of subjects experience the treatment complication of augmentation, in which treatment results in more severe symptoms (discussed later).[85] Impulse control disorders potentially attributable to dopaminergic therapies have also been reported in the treatment of RLS (see later discussion). In addition to these quality of life issues, there are substantial economic costs associated with RLS, and RLS may predispose sufferers to other health problems. RLS results in sleep disruption and is associated with dramatically increased cross-sectional rates of mood, anxiety, and panic disorders.[13,86-88] An association between RLS and cardiovascular disease (CVD) has been shown by three separate, population-based studies, with odds ratios for CVD in the presence of RLS ranging from 2.07 to 2.58;[89-91] a dose effect of RLS symptom frequency was seen in two of these studies and the associations persist after controlling for other known risk factors. Among RLS subjects, those with more than 30 PLMs per hour have twice the risk of prevalent hypertension after controlling for hypertension

risk factors.[92] While the mechanisms behind these observations have yet to be determined, this growing evidence suggests that RLS confers both substantial personal and public health burden.

PATHOPHYSIOLOGY

Genetics

RLS is known to be familial and strongly heritable, and the genetic underpinnings of this disorder are beginning to emerge. Multiple linkage studies have identified regions of interest, although these studies are often limited to few families and have not always identified genes of interest.[93] Of the identified RLS linkage loci, RLS1 on chromosome 12 appears the most robust, having been implicated in families of diverse origin (e.g., French-Canadians, Icelanders, and Germans) and for which a specific gene is implicated, the neuronal nitric oxide synthase (NOS1).[94] More recently, three genome-wide association studies have revealed significant associations to five specific regions. In Icelandic and American subjects, a variant within an intron of the BTBD9 gene on chromosome 6 is associated with a 70% to 80% increased risk of RLS and PLMs.[38] This association is driven even more strongly by PLMs than by RLS sensory symptoms; the at-risk variant confers greatest risk (OR = 2.3) in RLS family members with PLMs lacking RLS or those with PLMs and atypical RLS symptoms, and somewhat less risk when considering those with classic RLS symptoms regardless of PLMI. This variant is common (present in two thirds of those of northern European descent), and so accounts for at least 50% of the population-attributable risk for RLS. The association between BTBD9 and RLS sensory symptoms was simultaneously shown in Germans and French-Canadians, in whom additional associations with the Meis1 gene on chromosome 2p14 and intergenic regions of the MAP2K5 and LBXCOR1 genes on chromosome 15q23 were also observed.[95] Unpublished data indicate that the Meis1 at-risk variant is also tightly linked with objectively measured PLMs. These three associations are robust and have been replicated in five different populations of European descent, and the effect sizes are comparable across study populations,[38,95,96] lending substantial credence to these findings. Two additional signals conferring additional risk for RLS symptoms have been identified within an intron of PTPRD (chromosome 9).[97] Together, these five genetic variants account for nearly 80% of the population attributable risk for RLS.

In addition to helping reveal the genetic underpinnings of RLS, these findings have also begun to explain some of the epidemiologic findings of RLS. For example, the common but not universal finding of iron deficiency in RLS patients has been repeatedly observed since Ekbom's original description. The BTBD9 variant demonstrates a dose-response relationship to decrements in iron stores; each copy of the BTBD9 at-risk variant predicts a 13% lower average serum ferritin.[38] Further, these at-risk variants help to explain the notable differences in worldwide RLS prevalence, as different ethnic groups have varying frequencies of the at-risk alleles that mirror each group's RLS prevalence[98] (http://www.hapmap.org).

Despite these advances, it remains unclear exactly how these at-risk variants result in RLS symptoms and PLMs, and much work remains to be done. The at-risk single nucleotide polymorphisms (SNPs) in each instance are common, being present also in people without RLS/PLMs and present within noncoding, intronic, or intergenic regions, and implicate genes that are widely expressed in the central nervous system and other organs.[98]

Functional Anatomy

Because RLS and PLMs are commonly present in the same individuals, respond to many of the same medications, share some electrophysiologic characteristics, and are mediated by some of the same risk alleles in genome-wide associations, they are assumed to share the same, or similar, pathophysiology. Multiple points along the central and peripheral nervous system may be involved in their generation, and the diversity of sites of nervous system that may be involved in RLS/PLMs highlights the need for a comprehensive neurologic examination in RLS patients. Of the portions of the nervous system involved in RLS, growing evidence suggests that the spinal cord may be the most important, largely because it is a site of convergence of both peripheral sensory afferents and central efferents for sensorimotor and autonomic function.

Spinal Cord

As discussed earlier, the movements of PLMs resemble those of the Babinski response, a primitive, pathologic spinal-level reflex designed to withdraw the limb from painful stimuli. The presence of this reflex after infancy implies heightened excitability in neural elements of the flexor-reflex arc, and in RLS patients such excitability has been demonstrated as a decreased threshold to elicit this flexor reflex during sleep and as spread of the response to muscles beyond the segmental nerve root subserving the normal reflex.[45,99] This likely reflects disruption of pre- and postsynaptic inhibitory mechanisms acting within the spinal cord, and may also be seen in PLMs occurring in the absence of sensory symptoms of RLS.[100] Later we will expand upon the multiple brain circuits that may affect disinhibition of spinal cord sensorimotor and autonomic networks. Several additional findings highlight the central role of spinal cord networks in the pathophysiology of RLS/PLMs. First, medically refractory RLS has been documented to resolve with intrathecal opiate delivery.[101-103] Second, D_3 agents are remarkably effective in treating RLS and PLMs, and the normal role of spinal D_3 dopamine receptors is to dampen the flexor reflex described previously, as well as sympathetic tone.[46,104] Third, a variety of spinal cord pathologies have been shown to elicit RLS, PLMs, or both.[105-110] The RLS and PLMs emerging in the setting of myelopathy are indistinguishable from "idiopathic" RLS and PLMs, including that they are responsive to treatment with dopamine agonists.[110] The response to treatment despite a variety of spinal lesions and spinal levels suggests that spinal networks distal to the lesion must be involved in treatment response.

Peripheral Nerves

The quality of sensory symptoms in RLS suggests that the peripheral nervous system may also be involved in pathophysiology of RLS, specifically implicating the small-caliber Aδ and C fibers that carry pain signals and mediate somatosympathetic reflexes. This concept is supported by anecdotal reports and our clinical experience that RLS can acutely worsen or lateralize to the affected side after a variety of peripheral insults, including diffuse or localized neuropathy, radiculopathy,

soft or bony tissue injury, or venous thrombosis. There is an increased risk of RLS in some hereditary neuropathies.[111,112] Yet, while associations between RLS and idiopathic, sporadic small-fiber axonopathies have been described,[113,114] including small case series of electrophysiologically or microscopically defined neuropathies,[115,116] patients with acquired neuropathies are no more likely to have RLS than are population control subjects, unless they also have a family history of RLS.[112] Thus, a patient's genetic predisposition is an important determinant of whether RLS will occur in an acquired neuropathy. Conventional electromyograms (EMGs) and nerve conduction velocities (NCVs), somatosensory evoked potentials (SEPs), and sympathetic skin responses are usually normal in idiopathic RLS,[117-121] PLMs in isolation,[122,123] and RLS with iron deficiency.[124] To the extent that a subgroup of RLS patients have symptoms triggered or worsened in association with peripheral nerve disease, the mechanisms are unknown, but can be hypothesized to involve ectopic or ephaptic excitation in damaged peripheral nerves and abnormal impulse generation in their sensory and sympathetic components.

It has also been hypothesized that the efficacy in RLS of medications classically used for neuropathic pain (e.g., gabapentin and its derivatives) might result from actions upon peripheral nerves.[125] Sympathetic mechanisms in the periphery may also turn out to be important peripheral nervous system mediators of RLS symptom control, given the complete relief from painful RLS described in three of four of Ekbom's original patients undergoing lumbar sympathetic ganglia blockade,[1] but these mechanisms need to be more formally studied.

Supraspinal Networks

In addition to spinal and peripheral nervous system influences on RLS/PLMs, additional observations support the importance of supraspinal pathways. The appearance of axial and limb movements occurring coincident with PLMs[119] necessarily implies involvement of the nervous system above the level of the spinal cord. Further, the neural hyperexcitability (indicating generalized disinhibition) that has been documented in spinal circuits in RLS/PLMs subjects[45,99,100] has also been shown to occur within the brainstem[122,126,127] and the motor cortex.[128,129] Ultimately, these supraspinal motor circuits converge upon and modulate sensorimotor function within the spinal cord. Converging lines of evidence point to a prominent role for monoaminergic pathways (i.e., noradrenergic, serotonergic, and dopaminergic) in modulating ascending sensory impulses—such as those occurring in RLS—via postsynaptic actions on dorsal horn neurons or presynaptic actions on the terminal axons of dorsal root, sensory afferents. Given the prominent clinical response to dopaminergic medications, the dopaminergic diencephalospinal pathway, which originates from the posterior hypothalamic A11 cell group, may be a particularly relevant supraspinal influence in RLS. Manipulations of this A11 cell group have been shown to reduce pain and neuropathic hypersensitivity,[130,131] and A11 lesions in animals create a phenotype reminiscent of RLS/PLMs.[132-134] These findings are entirely consistent with the finding that RLS patients exhibit static mechanical hyperalgesia (as typically seen in neuropathic pain) that derives from centrally mediated sensitization to Aδ fiber, high-threshold mechanoreceptor input.[135] Similarly, the cutaneous silent period (a spinal reflex mediated by Aδ fibers) is prolonged in RLS.[136] The interactions between reduced dopaminergic tone and pain hypersensitivity in RLS patients could alternatively involve other supraspinal circuits such as those in the basal ganglia, insular and anterior cingulate cortices, and thalamus.[137,138]

The basal ganglia and associated thalamocortical pathways have been implicated in RLS/PLMs, although there is insufficient data to establish causality. RLS and PLMs may develop following strokes or in association with multiple sclerosis, and more commonly do so when the pathologic site is subcortical (especially infratentorial).[109,139,140] Pallidotomy of the internal globus pallidus (to treat severe Parkinson's disease [PD]) has been reported to improve RLS bilaterally, although more markedly in the leg contralateral to the lesion.[141] However, bilateral subthalamic nucleus deep brain stimulation in PD patients with co-morbid RLS has been reported to produce both beneficial[142] and detrimental[143] effects on RLS symptoms. Deep brain stimulation of the thalamic ventralis intermedius nucleus for the treatment of essential tremor does not appear to improve coexisting RLS.[144]

In summary, RLS and PLMs are complex traits that are influenced by diverse nervous system networks, multiple genes, and environmental factors. A variety of peripheral and central nervous system circuits may be involved, ultimately converging on the spinal cord, and those patients with a genetic predisposition are more likely to develop symptoms. The precise interactions between the genes that confer risk and the functional anatomy of RLS/PLMs have yet to be elucidated, but will be critical in identifying novel mechanisms that can be used to develop new therapies, diagnostic tools, and preventive measures.

Iron and Dopamine Alterations

Theories about the pathophysiologic basis of RLS/PLMs focus heavily on the roles of iron and dopamine, as iron deficiency is commonly seen as a cause of "secondary" RLS and dopaminergic medications are typically effective in relieving both RLS and PLMs.[145] There exist complex interactions between iron and dopamine, as evidenced by clinical investigations, several neuroimaging modalities, analyses of autopsy tissue and cerebrospinal fluid, and experimental models of dietary iron deficiency.[145-148] However, reconsideration of these data, newer experimental findings, and evolving clinical experience challenge the monolithic construct of brain iron and dopamine deficiencies as bound to the causality of all RLS/PLMs.

Iron

Low iron stores, as measured by serum ferritin, are more frequently encountered in RLS clinical settings than they are in the general population: 25% in 113 RLS subjects in one retrospective study,[149] and 14.6% and 44.4% with values up to 15 ng/mL and up to 40 ng/mL, respectively, in our database of 437 RLS subjects. However, some of this increased frequency is likely to be a result of a selection bias for more severely affected or refractory individuals, who are more likely to present to academic centers. Although iron deficiency is clearly associated with some cases of RLS, the view that brain iron deficiency is a unifying mechanism that is causal to most or all RLS/PLMs is not upheld by clinical or epidemiologic experience. It is clear that systemic iron deficiency is neither necessary nor sufficient to produce RLS/PLMs. In one hematology clinic, for example, only 40% of those with iron deficiency

had coexisting RLS.[124] In the only large, rigorous, population-based study of RLS that probed carefully for iron deficiency using sensitive metrics (e.g., soluble transferrin receptor), no association was found with iron deficiency.[150] Although blood donors have been noted to have RLS,[151] systematic study of 2000 English blood donors (who presumably are at higher risk of iron depletion than nondonors) did not find any relationship between RLS symptoms and up to 3 units of blood donation.[152,153] The iron deficiency common in pregnancy has been implicated as a factor in the high frequency of RLS in pregnant women (occurring in nearly one third), but it is becoming clear that measured iron parameters during pregnancy do not correlate well with RLS symptoms, and pregnancy-induced RLS typically resolves shortly after delivery even though iron deficiency is more slowly corrected.[25,154-156] Results from randomized trials of iron therapy for RLS have been mixed, without consistent demonstration of benefit across studies or iron formulations;[157-161] most of these studies were not limited to subjects with documented iron deficiency, so it remains to be seen if iron therapy will be beneficial for this subgroup, but there is no evidence to suggest that iron repletion benefits all RLS subjects. Finally, although the at-risk allele in the *BTBD9* gene predicts 13% lower serum ferritin per copy, this variant accounts for only 50% of the population-attributable risk,[38] arguing that it is a potential player in at most 65% of Europeans who carry at least a single copy of this genetic variant.

In summary, systemic or brain iron deficiency is a recognizable and reversible state in a proportion, but not the entirety, of individuals with RLS. The relationship between iron and PLMs remains to be determined. In clinical practice, although screening for iron deficiency in RLS patients is a useful practice, iron parameters (or genetic at-risk variants related to iron deficiency and RLS) are not currently part of the diagnostic algorithm for RLS itself.

Dopamine

Based on the therapeutic response of both RLS and PLMs to levodopa and dopamine agonists, and the known role of the basal ganglia in the majority of both hypo- and hyperkinetic movement disorders, early hypotheses of RLS pathophysiology were focused around a hypodopaminergic state in nigrostriatal circuits. In support of this hypothesis are several findings: (1) dopamine synthesis, release, and signaling exhibit circadian rhythms with nadirs during peak times for the occurrence of RLS/PLMs symptoms;[162] (2) iron is a cofactor for tyrosine hydroxylase (TH), which is the rate-limiting enzyme in dopamine synthesis,[163,164] helping to explain the suspected associations with iron deficiency; and (3) dietary iron deficiency impairs the recycling and signaling of synaptic dopamine in the basal ganglia.[165-167] Nonetheless, concrete evidence of a hypodopaminergic state in the basal ganglia occurring independently or because of iron deficiency, and that can be generalized to the larger population of RLS patients, has not emerged despite substantial, repeated, and sustained efforts.[168] The unequivocal finding that dopaminomimetics are effective in the treatment of RLS and PLMs does not necessarily imply a hypodopaminergic state for several reasons, including the number and diversity of dopaminergic pathways that regulate sleep and wakefulness, the dose- and receptor-dependent characteristics of dopaminergic drugs, and the plasticity of the proteins involved in the synthesis, recycling, and signaling of dopamine.[162] RLS responds clinically to low doses of dopaminergic medications (in comparison to Parkinson's disease), suggesting that D_2-like (D_2, D_3, D_4) receptors may be responsible for the efficacy of these medications, as this group of receptors are autoreceptors with 10-fold higher affinities for dopamine. Newer dopamine agonist treatment of RLS (pramipexole, ropinirole, see later discussion) is based around D_3 receptor-preferring agonists. Mice lacking functional D_3 receptors exhibit behaviors and spinal electrophysiologic features[46,104,169,170] that are consistent with those observed in human RLS/PLMs. Dietary models of iron deficiency consistently demonstrate an excess in extracellular dopamine in the basal ganglia due to disordered presynaptic mechanisms governing dopamine's release (e.g., reductions in the dopamine-transporter and D_2-like receptors) as opposed to its synthesis.[165-167] Supportive of a hyper- versus hypodopaminergic state contributing to RLS are metabolic profiles of cerebrospinal fluid,[171] analyses of RLS autopsy tissue, and animals and cell lines depleted of iron,[172] and the fact that dopamine agonists efficacious in RLS reduce, rather than increase, extracellular dopamine in animals.[173,174] Thus, the mechanisms by which iron deficiency contributes to RLS and PLMs, and the extent to which this is mediated by alterations in dopamine signaling, as well as the relevant dopaminergic circuits (i.e., nigrostriatal versus diencephalospinal), have yet to be fully elucidated, and a comprehensive model accounting for iron and dopamine abnormalities in RLS is an as-yet unfulfilled goal.

ASSESSMENT AND TREATMENT

The factors that impact sensitivity and specificity of RLS diagnosis have been discussed. We now turn to practical aspects of patient assessment that impact the management and treatment of the patient (summarized in Fig. 24-1). The assessment should begin with a thorough clinical evaluation to rule out coexisting conditions that increase the likelihood of developing RLS symptoms (Box 24-1). Among these diverse medical conditions (known or unrecognized) may be the precipitating factor leading the patient to seek treatment. This is especially important to keep in mind when RLS presents acutely, or when the "ecology" of the patient is inconsistent with what is known about the clinic-epidemiologic features of the disorder (e.g., RLS appearing in a middle-aged, African-American or Asian man).

The positive or negative effects of lifestyle and diet upon RLS/PLMs have not been rigorously tested in controlled trials. That being said, insufficient sleep, tobacco, and caffeine have all been implicated in worsening of RLS[175] and should be avoided as recommended by consensus of expert opinion.[176] Although results of a national phone survey suggest that reduced alcohol consumption is associated with RLS,[177] it is our clinical experience that alcohol consumption, in particular red wine, may acutely exacerbate RLS, and alcohol consumption is associated with PLMs.[178] Those foods that are rich in vasoactive biogenic amines such as tyramine and phenylethylamines (including red wine but also aged cheeses and fermented products) are clinically noted to exacerbate RLS, and a period of abstinence from these foods should be considered. As discussed earlier, a number of medications have been implicated in worsening RLS and should be discontinued when feasible. These medications include the nonspecific antihistamines (e.g., diphenhydramine and meclizine), dopamine

antagonists (e.g., antipsychotic agents, metaclopramide, and promethazine), antidepressants, and lithium.[32,175,179,180] Of the selective serotonin (SSRI) and serotonin-norepinephrine (SNRI) reuptake inhibitors, mirtazapine appears to have the highest rate of new or worsened RLS (occurring in 28% of treated patients, versus 9% of patients treated with any SSRI or SNRI).[32] When treatment of co-morbid depression is necessary, we favor agents with the least amount of norepinephrine reuptake blockade. Bupropion, which is relatively selective for the dopamine transporter and has been anecdotally noted to improve RLS symptoms,[181,182] may be an especially good choice in this instance. Proton pump inhibitors (PPIs) also have the potential to aggravate RLS by interfering with iron absorption secondary to increased duodenal pH.[183] We have encountered such worsening of RLS symptoms within weeks of a PPI being started, suggesting that the curve describing the relationship of systemic iron availability to RLS symptom severity might be quite steep in some individuals.

Iron deficiency, while unlikely to explain all RLS, is clearly present in a substantial proportion of RLS subjects, and so should be routinely assessed at the initial evaluation and annually thereafter. Because many RLS patients who are iron deficient do not exhibit coexisting anemia (approximately two thirds of the iron-deficient patients in our RLS clinic), and ferritin is an acute-phase reactant that can be falsely elevated, a complete serum iron panel (iron, total iron binding capacity, percent transferrin saturation, and ferritin) is the screening test of choice. Although we routinely screen all RLS subjects for iron deficiency, we are particularly aware of the risk of iron deficiency in RLS patients with co-morbid gastrointestinal disorders (e.g., gastric stapling or bypass and celiac disease) in whom iron deficiency is common and may be contributory to RLS.[184-187] We also routinely assess vitamin B_{12} and folate levels in this subgroup of patients, who are prone to malabsorption , as deficiencies theoretically may interfere with dopamine synthesis through their roles in tyrosine hydroxylase functioning (both are necessary for the biosynthesis of tetrahydrobiopterin, a cofactor for tyrosine hydroxylase).[188] One small, open-label study of oral folate for RLS in subjects with folate deficiency demonstrated good results.[189] That being said, in the larger population of idiopathic RLS, folate and vitamin B_{12} deficiencies are no more common than observed in control subjects.[190,191]

Objective data supporting oral iron supplementation in RLS are mixed. A randomized trial of oral iron sulfate compared to placebo in RLS patients not stratified by iron status did not show a benefit on RLS symptoms,[160] but the subset of patients in whom RLS improved were those whose iron parameters improved substantially with treatment. A more recent randomized, controlled trial of oral iron in RLS patients with low-normal ferritin levels (15-75 ng/mL) did show a significant reduction in RLS severity.[158] Although low ferritin (≤ 50 ng/mL) does not appear to interfere with the efficacy of dopaminergic treatment,[192] very low ferritin (≤ 20 ng/mL) may increase the risk of treatment complications, specifically, augmentation.[193] In light of these findings, we concur with the RLS Foundation's consensus treatment guideline, which recommends iron repletion when ferritin is below 20 ng/mL and consideration of iron repletion on a case-by-case basis when the ferritin is between 20 and 50 ng/mL.[176]

When oral iron supplementation is implemented, patient education regarding the many factors that can interfere with

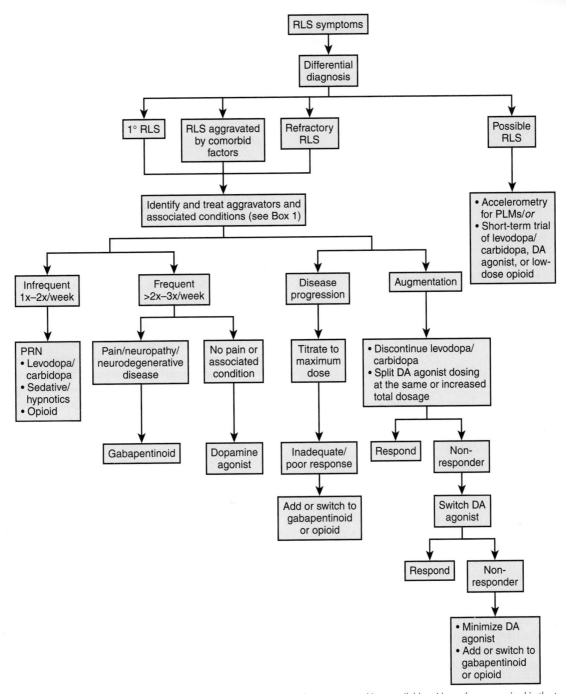

Figure 24-1 Proposed flowchart for the treatment of RLS based on clinical experience and best available evidence (as summarized in the text).

absorption of dietary or supplemental iron is critical. Dietary iron can be obtained as heme iron and nonheme iron. Heme iron is found in animal sources, especially red meat, and is efficiently absorbed because of its solubility. Nonheme iron, derived from vegetables and grains, is less efficiently absorbed. The presence of phytates, oxalates, phenols, and metallic elements (e.g., magnesium, manganese, zinc, calcium, and copper) will further impair absorption by competing with iron for absorption. Alkalinized environments limit iron absorption because they promote formation of insoluble iron complexes. For these reasons, iron supplements would ideally be ingested on an empty stomach and dosed separately from other nutritional supplements, antacids, or beverages containing tannic acid (e.g., teas, coffees, and many red wines). Vitamin C is the exception to this rule, as ascorbic acid–containing supplements, foods, and beverages significantly enhance the absorption of nonheme iron.

Both nonheme and heme iron formulations, in a variety of salts and formulations, are available for use in oral iron supplementation. Ferrous sulfate, ferrous gluconate, and ferrous fumarate preparations are all readily available, and should be dosed to provide 100 to 200 mg of elemental iron per day. (In comparison, a typical multivitamin or prenatal vitamin contains 27-65 mg of iron, and the inclusion of calcium and other elements in most multivitamins will further limit absorption.) Many iron preparations may cause gastrointestinal side effects such as constipation, diarrhea, nausea, and abdominal pain. When these side effects occur, they can be reduced by decreasing the amount of elemental iron absorbed. This can be done in several ways: taking the iron with food, lowering the total dose, or using a preparation with a relatively low amount of elemental iron such as ferrous gluconate.[194] In our clinical practice, we replete iron to a goal ferritin level of greater than 50 ng/mL and a transferrin saturation greater than 20%. The time to reach these goals is highly variable, but we typically treat for at least 6 to 8 weeks before reassessing serum iron parameters and adjusting therapy accordingly.

Clinical practice guidelines for the use of intravenous (IV) iron in RLS are not well established. In the subgroup of RLS patients with end-stage renal disease, IV iron dextran has been shown to be effective in a single randomized, controlled trial.[195] Two randomized, controlled trials of IV iron have been performed in idiopathic RLS, both using iron sucrose. In one study, subjects were not chosen based on iron status (although anemic subjects were excluded, which would tend to exclude the most severely iron-deficient subjects); this study was stopped after a prespecified interim analysis did not show superiority of the iron intervention.[157] The second study was limited to those with documented systemic iron deficiency (i.e., ferritin < 45 ng/mL), and some positive symptom benefit was demonstrable, but not at all time points.[161] In recognition that IV iron therapy outside treatment of chronic renal failure constitutes off-label use, we reserve use of IV iron for those patients with documented severe iron deficiency (e.g., ferritin < 10 ng/mL, transferrin saturations < 15%, or iron levels < 25 μg/dL [females] or 45 μg/dL [males]), *and* with refractoriness to pharmacologic interventions, *and* in whom the risks associated with RLS-related sleep deprivation to less than 3 to 4 hours of sleep per night are greater than those posed by a course of IV iron treatments. Of the available IV formulations, iron dextran has the highest rate of serious anaphylaxis (0.6-0.7%) and other adverse events, present in up to 50% of patients,[196] and we typically avoid its use. Iron sucrose and ferric gluconate have lower rates of serious anaphylaxis (0.002% and 0.04%, respectively) and adverse events (36% and 35%).[196]

When pharmacologic intervention is needed for RLS, the first-line therapy is dopaminergic agents. Several dopamine agonists have demonstrated efficacy for RLS in randomized, controlled trials (with response rates of 70-90%),[197] although many of these trials excluded subjects with iron deficiency (e.g., ferritin < 15-20 ng/mL) and were derived from clinical populations that were two thirds women, and therefore might not be generalizable to every clinician's practice. Of the dopamine agonists, the only two approved by the United States Food and Drug Administration (FDA) for treatment of RLS are pramipexole and ropinirole. No other medication, in any drug class, has an FDA approval for RLS. Pramipexole is a non-ergot-derived dopamine D_3- and D_2-receptor agonist known to be efficacious for both RLS and PLMs.[198-202] The mean effective daily dose in clinical trials ranges from 0.25 to 1 mg,[203] although in our clinical experience, particularly in older men, higher total doses (up to 1.5 mg) in divided doses may be necessary for symptom control. Pramipexole is renally excreted, so a more cautious, slower dosing titration in the setting of impaired creatinine clearances and end-stage renal disease is prudent. Ropinirole is also a non-ergot-derived dopamine agonist that preferentially acts upon D_3 and D_2 receptor subtypes and is effective for RLS and PLMs.[204-208] The mean effective daily dose of ropinirole is approximately 2 mg.[203] Ropinirole is metabolized through the CYP1A2 isoenzyme of the cytochrome P-450 (CYP) system, and therefore has important drug interactions with inhibitors and inducers (including nicotine) of this system. For example, warfarin levels can be increased by ropinirole use; thus, we prefer pramipexole as first-line therapy in those patients on warfarin. A direct comparison of these two agents has not been conducted, although one industry-sponsored meta-analysis suggests a slight superiority for pramipexole, as assessed by improvement in the International RLS Study Group's rating scale, (IRLS) and a more favorable side effect profile.[209]

Regardless of the dopamine agonist that is chosen, plasma concentrations do not peak until nearly 2 hours after ingestion, so medication should be dosed several hours prior to typical symptom onset. Treating on an as-needed basis is often less satisfactory given this 2-hour delay in symptom relief from time of medication ingestion. Divided doses (e.g., at dinner and again at bedtime) may be used to achieve sustained efficacy throughout the entire evening and sleep periods. Extended release formulations of both pramipexole and ropinirole are available (approved for use in Parkinson's disease but not RLS), but published controlled data supporting their use or superiority in RLS are not available.

Cabergoline is an ergot-derived dopamine agonist that has also been shown to be effective in RLS, and may be particularly so because of its very long elimination half-life.[210-213] However, ergot-derived dopamine agonists carry a risk for valvular heart disease and pleuropulmonary and retroperitoneal fibrosis that do not appear to be present in non-ergot-derived agents. For this reason, cabergoline is not considered a first-line therapy for RLS. Other dopamine agonists are available in transdermal formulations. The theoretical benefits of this form of medication delivery are more stable plasma levels (thereby avoiding side effects related to fluctuating levels) and better symptom coverage during daytime hours for severely affected subjects.[214,215] Randomized, controlled trial and extended open-label data support the use of rotigotine for RLS and PLMs.[215-219] However, rotigotine is currently unavailable in the United States, having been pulled from the market because of crystallization of medication within the patch substrate. Limited data also support the potential use of transdermal lisuride[214,220] for RLS and PLMs. The adverse effects associated with dopamine agonists include nausea, somnolence, headache, dizziness, rhinitis, and peripheral edema.

In addition to dopamine agonists, dopaminergic treatment of RLS can be supplied directly in the form of levodopa. However, although levodopa is effective for RLS, it appears more likely to lead to the treatment complication of augmentation (discussed later) than are the dopamine agonists, so it is not considered a first-line agent.[221] Unlike the dopamine agonists, the onset of action of levodopa is very rapid. Thus, for patients with sporadic symptoms who do not warrant daily therapy, levodopa is often a better choice for an as-needed or "rescue" medication. For this indication, doses of 100 to 200 mg are typically sufficient. Side effects of levodopa are similar to those of the dopamine agonists and include hypotension, hallucinations, sleepiness, and gastrointestinal discomfort.

Several other classes of medications are also available for the off-label treatment of RLS (Box 24-2). Based on a systematic review of available evidence, the Movement Disorders Society (MDS) task force rated gabapentin as effective for RLS,[203] and this drug is frequently used as second-line RLS therapy. The mean effective daily dose of gabapentin is approximately 1800 mg, given as two 900-mg doses after an appropriate titration period.[125] The subgroup of patients who experience their RLS symptoms as painful may be particularly responsive to gabapentin, perhaps because of its effects on neuropathic pain. Pregabalin, a related compound, also demonstrates subjective and objective (i.e., polysomnographic) benefit in RLS.[222,223] A gabapentin prodrug, gabapentin enacarbil, was recently FDA approved for treatment of moderate to severe RLS. Data from two randomized, controlled trials showed that a single daily dose can significantly improve RLS as measured by improvement in the IRLS rating scale.[224,225]

The MDS task force identified several other medications as "likely efficacious" in RLS based on the evidence supporting their use. These drugs included oxycodone, carbamazepine, valproic acid, and clonidine.[203] A detailed review of long-term use of opioid monotherapy in a single center (with 36 patients) revealed that 20 patients remained on monotherapy for an average of almost 6 years.[226] Of the 16 patients who did not remain on monotherapy, half discontinued because of side effects and seven had incomplete responses to treatment. Only one of the 36 patients developed signs of tolerance and addiction. Seven of the patients remaining on opiate monotherapy

were studied with polysomnography during therapy; of these, two developed new sleep apnea and a third showed exacerbation of previously diagnosed apnea.[226] Thus, opioids may be a useful long-term therapy for some RLS patients, with relatively low rates of tolerance and addiction, but sleep-disordered breathing may interfere with treatment. Other medications considered investigational for RLS include methadone, tramadol, clonazepam, zolpidem, and amantadine.[203]

Several nonpharmacologic or nonprescription interventions are also under investigation for use in RLS. Pneumatic sequential compression devices have been shown in a small, randomized, sham-device controlled trial to decrease RLS severity when worn for 1 hour prior to typical symptom onset.[227] In patients with both RLS and superficial venous insufficiency, endovascular laser ablation therapy significantly reduced RLS symptoms in the treatment group compared to a no-treatment control group.[228] Exercise (aerobic and lower body conditioning) has been shown to reduce RLS symptoms in a small trial,[229] but is still considered investigational.[203] Available data on acupuncture for RLS are insufficient to either support or refute its use.[230] Botulinum toxin injection initially appeared to be a promising treatment for RLS,[231] but more systematic study has not confirmed these early findings.[232] Magnesium and folate supplementation, although sometimes anecdotally effective, do not have sufficient evidence to support their use except as experimental therapy.[203] Experimental treatment of PLMs includes transcutaneous, neuromuscular stimulation of the legs for 30 minutes prior to sleep onset, which has been shown to significantly reduce PLMs and might improve in sleep continuity.[233]

BOX 24-2 *Pharmacologic Agents for Treatment of Restless Legs Syndrome (RLS)*

FIRST-LINE AGENTS

Dopamine Agonists
Pramipexole	0.25-0.75 mg
Ropinirole	0.25-4.0 mg

SECOND-LINE AGENTS
Gabapentin*	300-3000 mg
Gabapentin enacarbil	600 mg
Pregabalin*	75-450 mg
Levodopa*	100-200 mg

THIRD-LINE AGENTS*
Oxycodone	5-30 mg
Hydrocodone	5-30 mg
Carbamazepine	200-400 mg
Valproic acid	600 mg
Clonidine	0.1-0.5 mg
Transdermal rotigotine	0.5-4.0 mg
Cabergoline	0.5-2.0 mg

INVESTIGATIONAL AGENTS*
Methadone	10-40 mg
Tramadol	50-200 mg
Clonazepam	0.25-1.0 mg
Zolpidem	2.5-10.0 mg
Amantadine	100-300 mg
Transdermal lisuride	3-6 mg qod

*Use of these medications for treatment of RLS constitutes "off-label" use in the United States.

Treatment Complications: Augmentation and Impulse Control Disorders

Several complications may emerge in the course of RLS treatment. Rebound may occur late in the night or early in the morning, when symptoms recur as the drug is wearing off. Dopaminergic medications with shorter half-lives are more likely to result in symptom rebound. Such rebound can be seen in at least one fourth of RLS patients treated with levodopa,[234] although rebound does not always require modification of therapy. When rebound symptoms are severe enough to require a change in treatment, a switch to a longer-acting agent may be sufficient. Alternatively, the same agent can be used but dosing modified to include a dose immediately prior to bed (in addition to a dose taken early enough in the day to control evening symptoms).

Distinct from rebound is the phenomenon of augmentation, a problematic clinical syndrome that appears to be relatively unique to RLS. Following a period of symptom control (typically with a dopaminergic medication), patients develop tolerance (manifested as needing higher doses of medications to control symptoms) and then frank augmentation, in which RLS symptoms are more severe than in the pretreatment state. Augmentation can be identified by the occurrence of symptoms at least 4 hours earlier in the day than previously experienced, or at least two of the following: additional body parts, such as the arms, becoming affected by RLS sensations; faster symptom onset upon resting; more intense symptom character; shorter duration of response to treatment; or the appearance of PLMs while awake.[235] The appearance of RLS symptoms earlier in the day seems to be the most specific feature of augmentation, and the increase in symptom intensity the most sensitive.[221] Although not always severe, augmentation has the potential to dramatically affect patients' symptoms and quality of life, and often necessitates changes in therapy. Augmentation is primarily a problem of dopaminergic medications, although it has been reported with use of tramadol.[236] Because most clinical trials in RLS last weeks to months, yet augmentation develops over months to years, available clinical trial data may not provide accurate estimates of augmentation rates. However, data suggest high rates of augmentation for levodopa (60-73%) and relatively lower rates for pramipexole (8-56%).[85,237] Published data for augmentation rates with ropinirole are not available,[85] but in our clinical experience, augmentation appears at least as common with ropinirole as with pramipexole. In addition to medication choice, other risk factors for augmentation include a history of augmentation, a family history of RLS, and a serum ferritin level less than 20 ng/mL.[193,238]

Given the association with low iron, we routinely reevaluate serum iron stores when augmentation or tolerance develop and treat with oral iron when serum ferritin is less than 50 ng/mL. In mild cases, augmentation can be managed by moving medication dosing earlier in the day or splitting medication into divided doses, with one dose earlier in the day than previously administered.[85] If these patients are on very low doses of dopamine agonists, the total daily dose can be increased somewhat, but patients on higher doses should have the medication timing changed without increasing the total daily dose. Changing from one dopamine agonist to another in cases of augmentation is controversial but sometimes beneficial.[85,176] In more severe cases, substitution with a nondopaminergic medication is required, typically gabapentin or an opiate[85] (see Fig. 24-1). In the authors' and others'[239] experience, methadone (10-40 mg) in divided doses is an effective alternative in severe, refractory RLS, and particularly in severe cases of augmentation. To avoid the development of tolerance and augmentation, a strategy of rotation among agents from various drug classes (e.g., dopaminergics, opiates, gabapentin, and even benzodiazepines) has been advocated by some[240] but is not widespread clinical practice.

Reports of impulse control disorders (ICDs) and compulsive behaviors associated with the treatment of RLS with dopaminergic agents are limited almost solely to isolated case reports.[241-245] Cross-sectional, questionnaire based, surveys by mail[246,247] or face-to-face interview[248] of a collective of 283 RLS patients treated with a variety of dopaminergic medications suggest a rate of 8.5% of any repetitive stereotyped behavior (inclusive of impulse-control disorder/obsessions/compulsions/motor tics) and 2.8% for any increase in gambling behavior (gambling specifically noted to be "pathologic" in only a single instance). In most instances the degree of impulsivity was deemed to not be deleterious or to resolve with discontinuation or reduction in dosage.

A careful analysis of one, large controlled study comparing ICDs in sleep apnea patients and untreated RLS patients to RLS patients prescribed dopaminergic medication is particularly informative and illustrative.[249] First, while compulsive shopping and pathologic gambling were more common in RLS patients as compared to individuals with sleep apnea, only compulsive shopping appeared more common in treated versus untreated RLS patients. Second, the mean pramipexole dosage at which ICDs emerged (1.2 mg) exceeded the FDA approved dosage for RLS (0.25-0.75 mg). Third, treated RLS patients were more likely (62% vs. 37%) to have a preexisting psychiatric diagnosis. Thus, consistent with the experience that vulnerability to ICDs in Parkinson's disease is increased by high novelty-seeking personality traits, depression, male sex, substance abuse, and younger age at disease onset,[250,251] compulsive shopping in RLS may be influenced by preexistent psychiatric disease, and gambling may be reflective of an underlying diathesis to impulsivity or risk-taking that accompanies the complex RLS trait.

A recent study of 50 medication-free RLS patients and 60 age-matched control subjects confirmed higher rates of depressive symptoms in those with RLS, but not those with ICDs.[252] Patients should be alerted to this potentially serious complication, but clearly, prospective, longitudinal studies with validated measures of impulse control are needed to clarify any cause-and-effect relationship.

Treatment in Special Clinical Situations

RLS is very common in end-stage renal disease, with frequency estimates ranging from 6.6% and 62%, regardless of the method of dialysis (i.e., peritoneal versus hemodialysis).[253] RLS symptoms are typically not improved with dialysis, although they often resolve after renal transplantation.[254,255] Dopaminergic medications remain the first-line therapy in this population, with pramipexole and levodopa both having been shown to be effective.[253,256] Other medications used for idiopathic RLS that have documented efficacy in uremic patients with RLS include clonazepam, gabapentin, and clonidine.[253] As mentioned earlier, a single randomized trial

HEMATOLOGIC
Iron deficiency[124,146]
Frequent blood donation[151]

ENDOCRINE
Diabetes[260]

RHEUMATOLOGIC
Rheumatologic disorders[261]

RENAL
End-stage renal disease[253,262]

PULMONARY
Pulmonary hypertension[263]
Chronic obstructive pulmonary disease[264,265]

GASTROINTESTINAL
Hepatic disease[266]
Crohn's disease[267]
Celiac disease[186,268]
Gastric surgery[184]
Irritable bowel syndrome[185]

OBSTETRICS
Pregnancy[24,25]

NEUROLOGIC
Migraine[269,270]
Parkinson's disease[271-275]
Multiple sclerosis[276]
Myelopathy (spinal cord pathology)[110]
Charcot-Marie-Tooth disease type 2[111]
Spinocerebellar ataxias types 1, 2, and 3[276-279]
Attention deficit hyperactivity disorder[280]

supports the use of IV iron for the treatment of RLS in patients with end-stage renal disease,[159] so oral or IV iron should be considered in iron-deficient dialysis patients. Attention to renal dosing of medications is important in this population. For example, gabapentin must be dosed after dialysis rather than nightly because it is renally excreted. Pramipexole is also renally excreted.

RLS is also common during pregnancy (see Chapter 58, "Sleep in Women"), with up to one third of pregnant women experiencing RLS by their third trimester. However, safe treatment of RLS in this population is particularly difficult because of potential risks to the fetus. Medications that are commonly used for RLS in nonpregnant patients are all either FDA class C (see Chapter 58) (RLS medications in this class include ropinirole, pramipexole, levodopa, clonidine, and gabapentin) or class D or X (see Chapter 58) (these include carbamazepine and some benzodiazepines). Benzodiazepines and opiates carry the additional risk of withdrawal symptoms in newborns if these medications are taken near the end of pregnancy.[257] Thus, as with many other medical conditions during pregnancy, nonpharmacologic therapies should be used as first-line treatment. At present, these measures largely center on vitamin and mineral replacement. As with idiopathic RLS, it is recommended that iron deficiency be corrected when

present during pregnancy. Folate may play an important role in pregnancy-related RLS, as lower serum folate levels have been associated with third trimester RLS (as opposed to ferritin or vitamin B_{12})[154] and use of folate supplementation may alleviate pregnancy-related RLS.[258] Similarly, although no differences in serologic measures of ferritin, vitamin B_{12}, or folate were noted in another study of pregnant women with RLS, RLS was less frequently observed in those taking prenatal vitamins.[155] Anecdotally, magnesium may be beneficial.[259] Further safe treatment options for this common pregnancy-related condition are needed.

SUMMARY

In summary, RLS is a common sensory syndrome associated with significant personal and public health burden. As noted earlier, RLS is encountered in many common medical conditions at frequencies exceeding the expected population prevalence (Box 24-3).[260-280] The expression of RLS is strongly influenced by genetics and is further impacted by demographic, medical, environmental, and possibly additional genetic factors through mechanisms that remain poorly defined. Associated PLMs may explain some of the cardiovascular disease risk seen in RLS, although it remains to be seen whether treatment of either RLS or PLMS will decrease such risk. The pathophysiology of RLS remains incompletely understood, but recent genome-wide association studies have identified four genes that account for the majority of the population-attributable risk of RLS and PLMs, and there are reductions in brain iron in a subpopulation of RLS cases. First-line treatment is with non-ergot-derived dopamine agonists; opiates and derivatives of gabapentin are useful for second-line treatment.

REFERENCES

1. Ekbom K. Restless legs. *Acta Med Scand Suppl.* 1945;158:1-123.
2. Michaud M, Dumont M, Selmaoui B, Paquet J, Fantini M, Montplaisir J. Circadian rhythm of restless legs syndrome: Relationship with biological markers. *Ann Neurol.* 2004;55:372-380.
3. Allen R, Hening W, Montplaisir J, Picchietti D, Trenkwalder C, et al. Restless legs syndrome: Diagnostic criteria, special considerations, and epidemiology: A report from The RLS Diagnosis and Epidemiology Workshop at the National Instititutes of Health. *Sleep Med.* 2003;4:101-119.
4. Duffy J, Lowe A, Winkelman J, Czeisler C. Peak circadian occurrence of PLMs during the biological nighttime. *Sleep.* 2005;Suppl:A275 (abstract).
5. Baier P, Trenkwalder C. Circadian variation in restless legs syndrome. *Sleep Medicine.* 2007;8(6):645-650.
6. Picchietti D, Stevens H. Early manifestations of restless legs syndrome in childhood and adolescence. *Sleep Med.* 2007;22:297-300.
7. Walters AS. Is there a subpopulation of children with growing pains who really have restless legs syndrome? A review of the literature. *Sleep Med.* 2002;3(2):93-98.
8. Bassetti CL, Mauerhofer D, Gugger M, Mathis J, Hess CW. Restless legs syndrome: A clinical study of 55 patients. *Eur Neurol.* 2001;45(2):67-74.
9. Holmes R, Tluk S, Metta V, Patel P, Rao R, et al. Nature and variants of idiopathic restless legs syndrome: Observations from 152 patients referred to secondary care in the UK. *J Neural Transm.* 2007;114(7):929-934.
10. Hening W, Walters A, Allen R, Montplaisir J, Ferini-Strambi L. Impact, diagnosis and treatment of restless legs syndrome (RLS) in a primary care population: The REST (RLS epidemiology, symptoms, and treatment) primary care study. *Sleep Med.* 2004;5:237-246.
11. Allen RP, Walters AS, Montplaisir J, Hening W, Myers A, et al. Restless legs syndrome prevalence and impact: REST general population study. *Arch Intern Med.* 2005;165(11):1286-1292.

12. Tan E, Seah A, See S, Lim E, et al. Restless legs syndrome in an Asian population: A study in Singapore. *Mov Disord.* 2001;16:577-579.

13. Cho SJ, Hong JP, Hahm BJ, Jeon HJ, Chang SM, et al. Restless legs syndrome in a community sample of Korean adults: Prevalence, impact on quality of life, and association with DSM-IV psychiatric disorders. *Sleep.* 2009;32(8):1069-1076.

14. Castillo PR, Kaplan J, Lin SC, Fredrickson PA, Mahowald MW. Prevalence of restless legs syndrome among native South Americans residing in coastal and mountainous areas. *Mayo Clin Proc.* 2006;81(10):1345-1347.

15. Sevim S, Dogu O, Camdeviren H, Bugdayci R, Sasmaz T, et al. Unexpectedly low prevalence and unusual characteristics of RLS in Mersin, Turkey. *Neurology.* 2003;61(11):1562-1569.

16. Inoue Y, Ishizuka T, Arai H. Surveillance on epidemiology and treatment of restless legs syndrome in Japan. *J New Rem Clim.* 2000;49:244-254.

17. Lee HB, Hening WA, Allen RP, Earley CJ, Eaton WW, Lyketsos CG. Race and restless legs syndrome symptoms in an adult community sample in east Baltimore. *Sleep Med.* 2006;7(8):642-645.

18. Rashidzada W, Nabi SI, Romaker A, Alkhazna A, Saeed A. Racial differences in the prevalence of restless legs syndrome. *Chest.* 2009;136(4):66-67:(abstract).

19. Berger K. A message of restless legs on ethnicity. *Sleep Med.* 2006;7(8):597-598.

20. Desai A, Cherkas L, Spector T, Williams A. Genetic influences in self-reported symptoms of obstructive sleep apnoea and restless legs syndrome: A twin study. *Twin Res.* 2004;7:589-595.

21. Ondo WG, Vuong KD, Wang Q. Restless legs syndrome in monozygotic twins. *Neurology.* 2000;55(9):1404-1406.

22. Phillips B, Young T, Finn L, Asher K, Hening W, Purvis C. Epidemiology of restless legs symptoms in adults. *Arch Intern Med.* 2000;160:2137-2141.

23. Trotti LM, Bliwise D, Greer SA, Sigurdsson AP, Gudmundsdottir GB, et al. Correlates of PLMs variability over multiple nights and impact upon RLS diagnosis. *Sleep Med.* 2009;10(6):668-671.

24. Lamberg L. Sleeping poorly while pregnant may not be "normal". *JAMA.* 2006;295(12):1357-1361.

25. Manconi M, Govoni V, De Vito A, Economou N, Cesnik E, et al. Restless legs syndrome and pregnancy. *Neurology.* 2004;63:1065-1069.

26. Berger K, Luedemann J, Trenkwalder C, John U, Kessler C. Sex and the risk of restless legs syndrome in the general population. *Arch Intern Med.* 2004;164:196-202.

27. Benes H, von Eye A, Kohnen R. Empirical evaluation of the accuracy of diagnostic criteria for restless legs syndrome. *Sleep Med.* 2009;10(5):524-530.

28. Stiasny-Kolster K, Kohnen R, Moller JC, Trenkwalder C, Oertel WH. Validation of the "L-DOPA test" for diagnosis of restless legs syndrome. *Mov Disord.* 2006;21(9):1333-1339.

29. Salin-Pascual R, Galicia-Polo L, Drucker-Colin R. Sleep changes after 4 consecutive days of venlafaxine administration in normal volunteers. *J Clin Psychiatry.* 1997;58(8):348-350.

30. Yang C, White DP, Winkelman JW. Antidepressants and periodic leg movements of sleep. *Biol Psychiatry.* 2005;58(6):510-514.

31. Page II RL, Ruscin JM, Bainbridge JL, Brieke AA. Restless legs syndrome induced by escitalopram: Case report and review of the literature. *Pharmacotherapy.* 2008;28(2):271-280.

32. Rottach KG, Schaner BM, Kirch MH, Zivotofsky AZ, Teufel LM, et al. Restless legs syndrome as side effect of second generation antidepressants. *J Psychiatr Res.* 2008;43(1):70-75.

33. Fox EJ, Villanueva R, Schutta HS. Myoclonus following spinal anesthesia. *Neurology.* 1979;29(3):379-380.

34. Lee MS, Lyoo CH, Kim WC, Kang HJ. Periodic bursts of rhythmic dyskinesia associated with spinal anesthesia. *Mov Disord.* 1997;12(5):816-817.

35. Nadkarni AV, Tondare AS. Localized clonic convulsions after spinal anesthesia with lidocaine and epinephrine. *Anesth Analg.* 1982;61(11):945-947.

36. Watanabe S, Sakai K, Ono Y, Seino H, Naito H. Alternating periodic leg movement induced by spinal anesthesia in an elderly male. *Anesth Analg.* 1987;66(10):1031-1032.

37. Hogl B, Frauscher B, Seppi K, Ulmer H, Poewe W. Transient restless legs syndrome after spinal anesthesia: A prospective study. *Neurology.* 2002;59(11):1705-1707.

38. Stefansson H, Rye DB, Hicks A, Petursson H, Ingason A, et al. A genetic risk factor for periodic limb movements in sleep [see comment]. *N Engl J Med.* 2007;357(7):639-647.

39. Hening WA. Subjective and objective criteria in the diagnosis of the restless legs syndrome. *Sleep Med.* 2004;5(3):285-292.

40. Hening W, Allen R, Washburn M, Lesage S, Earley C. The four diagnostic criteria for restless legs syndrome are unable to exclude confounding conditions ("mimics"). *Sleep Med.* 2009;10(9):976-981.

41. Benes H, Walters AS, Allen RP, Hening WA, Kohnen R. Definition of restless legs syndrome, how to diagnose it, and how to differentiate it from RLS mimics. *Mov Disord.* 2007;22(suppl 18):S401-S408.

42. Chaudhuri KR, Rye DB, Muzerengi S. Differential diagnosis of RLS. In: Chaudhuri KR, Ferini-Strambi L, Rye DB, eds. *Restless Legs Syndrome.* Oxford: Oxford University Press; 2008:35-43.

43. Spillane JD, Nathan PW, Kelly RE, Marsden CD. Painful legs and moving toes. *Brain.* 1971;94(3):541-556.

44. Dressler D, Thompson PD, Gledhill RF, Marsden CD. The syndrome of painful legs and moving toes. *Mov Disord.* 1994;9(1):13-21.

45. Bara-Jimenez W, Aksu M, Graham B, Sato S, Hallett M. Periodic limb movements in sleep—State dependent excitability of the spinal flexor reflex. *Neurology.* 2000;54:1609-1615.

46. Clemens S, Rye D, Hochman S. Restless legs syndrome: Revisiting the dopamine hypothesis from the spinal cord perspective. *Neurology.* 2006;67(1):125-130.

47. Ferri R, Zucconi M, Manconi M, Plazzi G, Bruni O, Ferini-Strambi L. New approaches to the study of periodic leg movements during sleep in restless legs syndrome. *Sleep.* 2006;29(6):759-769.

48. Pennestri MH, Whittom S, Adam B, Petit D, Carrier J, Montplaisir J. PLMS and PLMW in healthy subjects as a function of age: Prevalence and interval distribution. *Sleep.* 2006;29(9):1183-1187.

49. International Classification of Sleep Disorders. *Diagnostic and Coding Manual (ICSD-2).* 2nd ed. Westchester, IL: AASM; 2005.

50. Montplaisir J, Boucher S, Poirier G, Lavigne G, Lapierre O, Lesperance P. Clinical, polysomnographic, and genetic characteristics of restless legs syndrome: A study of 133 patients diagnosed with new standard criteria. *Mov Disord.* 1997;12:61-65.

51. Walters AS, LeBrocq C, Dhar A, Hening W, Rosen R, et al. Validation of the International Restless Legs Syndrome Study Group rating scale for restless legs syndrome. *Sleep Med.* 2003;4(2):121-132.

52. Aksu M, Demirci S, Bara-Jimenez W. Correlation between putative indicators of primary restless legs syndrome severity. *Sleep Med.* 2007;8(1):84-89.

53. Garcia-Borreguero D, Larrosa O, de la Llave Y, Granizo JJ, Allen R. Correlation between rating scales and sleep laboratory measurements in restless legs syndrome. *Sleep Med.* 2004;5(6):561-565.

54. Hornyak M, Feige B, Voderholzer U, Philipsen A, Riemann D. Polysomnography findings in patients with restless legs syndrome and in healthy controls: A comparative observational study. *Sleep.* 2007;30(7):861-865.

55. Rye D, Bliwise D, Iranzo A, Thambisetty M, Freeman A, et al. A novel 2-step diagnostic approach for RLS disease classification. *Sleep.* 2004;27(suppl S):306-307.

56. Michaud M, Soucy J, Chabli A, Lavigne G, Montplaisir J. SPECT imaging of striatal pre- and postsynaptic dopaminergic status in restless legs syndrome with periodic leg movements in sleep. *J Neurol.* 2002;249:164-170.

57. Bixler E, Kales A, Vela-Bueno A, Jacoby J, Scarone S, Soldatos C. Nocturnal myoclonus and nocturnal myoclonic activity in the normal population. *Res Commun Chem Pathol Pharmacol.* 1982;36(1):129-140.

58. Scofield H, Roth T, Drake C. Periodic limb movements during sleep: Population prevalence, clinical correlates, and racial differences. *Sleep.* 2008;31(9):1221-1227.

59. Allen R, Earley C. Augmentation of the restless legs syndrome with carbidopa/levodopa. *Sleep.* 1996;19:205-213.

60. Picchietti MA, Picchietti DL. Restless legs syndrome and periodic limb movement disorder in children and adolescents. *Semin Pediatr Neurol.* 2008;15(2):91-99.

61. Santamaria J, Iranzo A, Tolosa E. Development of restless legs syndrome after dopaminergic treatment in a patient with periodic leg movements in sleep. *Sleep Med.* 2003;4:153-155.

62. Walters A, Picchietti D, Hening W, Lazzarini M. Variable expressivity in familial restless legs syndrome. *Arch Neurol.* 1990;47:1219-1220.

63. Birinyi PV, Allen RP, Hening W, Washburn T, Lesage S, Earley CJ. Undiagnosed individuals with first-degree relatives with restless legs syndrome have increased periodic limb movements. *Sleep Med.* 2006;7(6):480-485.

64. O'Brien LM, Holbrook CR, Faye Jones V, Gozal D. Ethnic difference in periodic limb movements in children [see comment]. *Sleep Med.* 2007;8(3):240-246.

65. Tuisku K, Holi M, Wahlbeck K, Ahlgren A, Lauerma H. Actometry in measuring the symptom severity of restless legs syndrome. *Eur J Neurol.* 2005;12:385-387.

66. Rye D, Allen R, Carson S, Ritchie S. Ropinirole decreases bedtime periodic leg movements in patients with RLS: Results of a 12-week US study. *Sleep.* 2005;28(suppl S):A270.

67. Sforza E, Johannes M, Claudio B. The PAM-RL ambulatory device for detection of periodic leg movements: A validation study [see comment]. *Sleep Med.* 2005;6(5):407-413.

68. Tuisku K, Holi M, Wahlbeck K, Ahlgren A, Lauerma H. Quantitative rest activity in ambulatory monitoring as a physiological marker of restless legs syndrome: A controlled study. *Mov Disord.* 2003;18:442-448.

69. Ferri R, Zucconi M, Rundo F, Spruyt K, Manconi M, Ferini-Strambi L. Heart rate and spectral EEG changes accompanying periodic and non-periodic leg movements during sleep. *Clin Neurophysiol.* 2007;118(2):438-448.

70. Sforza E, Pichot V, Cervena K, Barthelemy JC, Roche F. Cardiac variability and heart-rate increment as a marker of sleep fragmentation in patients with a sleep disorder: A preliminary study. *Sleep.* 2007;30(1):43-51.

71. Winkelman J. The evoked heart rate response to periodic leg movements of sleep. *Sleep.* 1999;22:575-580.

72. Pennestri MH, Montplaisir J, Colombo R, Lavigne G, Lanfranchi PA. Nocturnal blood pressure changes in patients with restless legs syndrome. *Neurology.* 2007;68(15):1213-1218.

73. Siddiqui F, Strus J, Ming X, Lee IA, Chokroverty S, Walters AS. Rise of blood pressure with periodic limb movements in sleep and wakefulness. *Clin Neurophysiol.* 2007;118(9):1923-1930.

74. Guggisberg AG, Hess CW, Mathis J. The significance of the sympathetic nervous system in the pathophysiology of periodic leg movements in sleep. *Sleep.* 2007;30(6):755-766.

75. Ware J, Blumoff R, Pittard J. Peripheral vasoconstriction in patients with sleep related periodic leg movements. *Sleep.* 1988;11:182-186.

76. Frattola A, Parati G, Cuspidi C, Albini F, Mancia G. Prognostic value of 24-hour blood pressure variability. *J Hypertens.* 1993;11(10):1133-1137.

77. Pringle E, Phillips C, Thijs L, Davidson C, Staessen JA, et al. Systolic blood pressure variability as a risk factor for stroke and cardiovascular mortality in the elderly hypertensive population. *J Hypertens.* 2003;21(12):2251-2257.

78. Morgan BJ, Dempsey JA, Pegelow DF, Jacques A, Finn L, et al. Blood pressure perturbations caused by subclinical sleep-disordered breathing. *Sleep.* 1998;21(7):737-746.

79. Roman MJ, Pickering TG, Schwartz JE, Pini R, Devereux RB. Relation of blood pressure variability to carotid atherosclerosis and carotid artery and left ventricular hypertrophy. *Arteriosclerosis Thrombosis Vasc Biol.* 2001;21(9):1507-1511.

80. Zakopoulos NA, Tsivgoulis G, Barlas G, Papamichael C, Spengos K, et al. Time rate of blood pressure variation is associated with increased common carotid artery intima-media thickness. *Hypertension.* 2005;45(4):505-512.

81. Bliwise D, Sleep and Aging. *Understanding Sleep: The Evaluation and Treatment of Sleep Disorders.* Washington, DC: U.S. Dept. of Health and Human Services; 1997.

82. Hening W, Walters A, Kavey N, Gidro-Frank S, Cote L, Fahn S. Dyskinesias while awake and periodic movements in sleep in restless legs syndrome: Treatment with opioids. *Neurology.* 1986;36:1363-1366.

83. Kushida C, Martin M, Nikam P, Blaisdell B, Wallenstein G, et al. Burden of restless legs syndrome on health-related quality of life. *Qual Life Res.* 2007;16(4):617-624.

84. Earley C. Restless legs syndrome. *N Engl J Med.* 2003;348:2103-2109.

85. Garcia-Borreguero D, Allen RP, Benes H, Earley C, Happe S, et al. Augmentation as a treatment complication of restless legs syndrome: Concept and management. *Mov Disord.* 2007;22(suppl 18):S476-S484.

86. Kushida CA. Clinical presentation, diagnosis, and quality of life issues in restless legs syndrome. *Am J Med.* 2007;120(suppl 1):S4-S12.

87. Lee HB, Hening WA, Allen RP, Kalaydjian AE, Earley CJ, et al. Restless legs syndrome is associated with DSM-IV major depressive disorder and panic disorder in the community. *J Neuropsychiatry Clin Neurosci.* 2008;20(1):101-105.

88. Winkelmann J, Prager M, Lieb R, Pfister H, Spiegel B, et al. "Anxietas tibiarum." Depression and anxiety disorders in patients with restless legs syndrome. *J Neurol.* 2005;252(1):67-71.

89. Winkelman JW, Finn L, Young T. Prevalence and correlates of restless legs syndrome symptoms in the Wisconsin Sleep Cohort. *Sleep Med.* 2006;7(7):545-552.

90. Winkelman JW, Shahar E, Sharief I, Gottlieb DJ. Association of restless legs syndrome and cardiovascular disease in the Sleep Heart Health Study. *Neurology.* 2008;70(1):35-42.

91. Ulfberg J, Nystrom B, Carter N, Edling C. Prevalence of restless legs syndrome among men aged 18 to 64 years: An association with somatic disease and neuropsychiatric symptoms. *Mov Disord.* 2001;16(6):1159-1163.

92. Billars L, Hicks A, Bliwise D, Sigmundsson T, Sigurdsson A, et al. Hypertension risk and PLMS in restless legs syndrome. *Sleep.* 2007;30:A297-A298.

93. Winkelmann J, Polo O, Provini F, Nevsimalova S, Kemlink D, et al. Genetics of restless legs syndrome (RLS): State-of-the-art and future directions. *Mov Disord.* 2007;22(suppl 18):S449-S458.

94. Winkelmann J, Lichtner P, Schormair B, Uhr M, Hauk S, et al. Variants in the neuronal nitric oxide synthase (nNOS, NOS1) gene are associated with restless legs syndrome. *Mov Disord.* 2008;23(3):350-358.

95. Winkelmann J, Schormair B, Lichtner P, Ripke S, Xiong L, et al. Genome-wide association study of restless legs syndrome identifies common variants in three genomic regions [see comment]. *Nat Genet.* 2007;39(8):1000-1006.

96. Vilarino-Guell C, Farrer MJ, Lin SC. A genetic risk factor for periodic limb movements in sleep. *N Engl J Med.* 2008;358(4):425-427.

97. Schormair B, Kemlink D, Roeske D, Eckstein G, Xiong L, et al. PTPRD (protein tyrosine phosphatase receptor type delta) is associated with restless legs syndrome. *Nat Genet.* 2008;40(8):946-948.

98. Mignot E. A step forward for restless legs syndrome [comment]. *Nat Genet.* 2007;39(8):938-939.

99. Aksu M, Bara-Jimenez W. State dependent excitability changes of spinal flexor reflex in patients with restless legs syndrome secondary to chronic renal failure. *Sleep Med.* 2002;3(5):427-430.

100. Rijsman R, Stam C, de Weerd A. Abnormal H-reflexes in periodic limb movement disorder: Impact on understanding the pathophysiology of the disorder. *Clin Neurophysiol.* 2005;116:204-210.

101. Jakobsson B, Ruuth K. Successful treatment of restless legs syndrome with an implanted pump for intrathecal drug delivery. *Acta Anaesthesiol Scand.* 2002;46(1):114-117.

102. Lindvall P, Ruuth K, Jakobsson B, Nilsson S. Intrathecal morphine as a treatment for refractory restless legs syndrome. *Neurosurgery.* 2008;63(6):E1209:author reply E.

103. Ross DA, Narus MS, Nutt JG. Control of medically refractory restless legs syndrome with intrathecal morphine: Case report. *Neurosurgery.* 2008;62(1):E263.

104. Clemens S, Hochman S. Conversion of the modulatory actions of dopamine on spinal reflexes from depression to facilitation in D3 receptor knock-out mice. *J Neurosci.* 2004;24:11337-11345.

105. Yokota T, Hirose K, Tanabe H, Tsukagoshi H. Sleep-related periodic leg movements (nocturnal myoclonus) due to spinal cord lesion. *J Neurol Sci.* 1991;104:13-18.

106. Dickel M, Renfrow S, Moore P, Berry R. Rapid eye movement sleep periodic leg movements in patients with spinal cord injury. *Sleep.* 1994;17(8):733-738.

107. Lee M, Choi Y, Lee S. Sleep-related periodic leg movements associated with spinal cord lesions. *Mov Disord.* 1996;11(6):719-722.

108. de Mello M, Lauro F, Silva A, Tufik S. Incidence of periodic leg movements and of the restless legs syndrome during sleep following acute physical activity in spinal cord injury subjects. *Spinal Cord.* 1996;34(5):294-296.

109. Manconi M, Rocca M, Ferini-Strambi L, Tortorella P, Agosta F, et al. Restless legs syndrome is a common finding in multiple sclerosis and correlates with cervical cord damage. *Mult Scler.* 2008;14(1):86-93.

110. Trotti LM, Rye DB. Functional anatomy and treatment of RLS/PLMS emerging after spinal cord lesions. *Sleep.* 2007;30:A306.

111. Gemignani F, Marbini A, Di Giovanni G, Salih S, Terzano MG. Charcot-Marie-Tooth disease type 2 with restless legs syndrome. *Neurology.* 1999;52(5):1064-1066.

112. Hattan E, Chalk C, Postuma R. Is there a higher risk of restless legs syndrome in peripheral neuropathy? *Neurology.* 2009;72(11):955-960.

113. Rutkove S, Matheson J, Logigian E. Restless legs syndrome in patients with polyneuropathy. *Muscle Nerve.* 1996;19(5):670-672.

114. Ondo W, Jankovic J. Restless legs syndrome: Clinicoetiologic correlates. *Neurology.* 1996;47:1435-1441.

115. Iannaccone S, Zucconi M, Marchettini P, Ferini-Strambi L, Nemni R, et al. Evidence of peripheral axonal neuropathy in primary restless legs syndrome. *Mov Disord.* 1995;10(1):2-9.

116. Polydefkis M, Allen R, Hauer P, Earley C, Griffin J, McArthur J. Subclinical sensory neuropathy in late-onset restless legs syndrome. *Neurology.* 2000;55(8):1115-1121.

117. Montplaisir J, Godbout R, Boghen D, DeChamplain J, Young S, Lapierre G. Familial restless legs with periodic movements in sleep: Electrophysiologic, biochemical, and pharmacologic study. *Neurology.* 1985;35:130-134.

118. Bliwise D, Ingham R, Date E, Dement W. Nerve conduction and creatinine clearance in aged subjects with periodic movements in sleep. *J Gerontol Med Sci.* 1989;44:M164-M167.

119. Provini F, Vetrugno R, Meletti S, Plazzi G, Solieri L, et al. Motor pattern of periodic limb movements during sleep. *Neurology.* 2001;57(2):300-304.

120. Ferreri F, Rossini P. Neurophysiological investigations in restless legs syndrome and other disorders of movement during sleep. *Sleep Med.* 2004;5:397-399.

121. Tyvaert L, Laureau E, Hurtevent J, Derambure P, Monaca C. A-delta and C-fibres function in primary restless legs syndrome. *Neurophysiol Clin.* 2009;39(6):267-274.

122. Wechsler L, Stakes J, Shahani B, Busis N. Periodic leg movements of sleep (nocturnal myoclonus): An electrophysiological study. *Ann Neurol.* 1986;19:168-173.

123. Smith R, Gouin P, Minkley P, Lyles J, Egeren LV, et al. Periodic limb movement disorder is associated with normal motor conduction latencies when studied by central magnetic stimulation—Successful use of a new technique. *Sleep.* 1992;15(4):312-318.

124. Akyol A, Kiylioglu N, Kadikoylu G, Bolaman A, Ozgel N. Iron deficiency anemia and restless legs syndrome: Is there an electrophysiological abnormality? *Clin Neurol Neurosurg.* 2003;106:23-27.

125. Garcia-Borreguero D, Larrosa O, de la Llave Y, Verger K, Masramon X, Hernandez G. Treatment of restless legs syndrome with gabapentin: A double-blind, cross-over study. *Neurology.* 2002;59:1573-1579.

126. Wechsler L, Stakes J, Shahani B, Busis N. Nocturnal myoclonus, restless legs syndrome, and abnormal electrophysiological findings. *Ann Neurol.* 1987;21:515.

127. Briellmann R, Rosler K, Hess C. Blink reflex excitability is abnormal in patients with periodic leg movements in sleep. *Mov Disord.* 1996;11(6):710-714.

128. Scalise A, Cadore IP, Gigli GL. Motor cortex excitability in restless legs syndrome. *Sleep Med.* 2004;5(4):393-396.

129. Nardone R, Ausserer H, Bratti A, Covi M, Lochner P, et al. Cabergoline reverses cortical hyperexcitability in patients with restless legs syndrome. *Acta Neurol Scand.* 2006;114(4):244-249.

130. Wei H, Viisanen H, Pertovaara A. Descending modulation of neuropathic hypersensitivity by dopamine D2 receptors in or adjacent to the hypothalamic A11 cell group. *Pharmacol Res.* 2009;59(5):355-363.

131. Fleetwood-Walker S, Hope P, Mitchell R. Antinociceptive actions of descending dopaminergic tracts on cat and rat dorsal horn somatosensory neurones. *J Physiol (Lond).* 1988;399:335-348.

132. Ondo WG, He Y, Rajasekaran S, Le WD. Clinical correlates of 6-hydroxydopamine injections into A11 dopaminergic neurons in rats: A possible model for restless legs syndrome. *Mov Disord.* 2000;15(1):154-158.

133. Qu S, Le W, Zhang X, Xie W, Zhang A, Ondo WG. Locomotion is increased in a11-lesioned mice with iron deprivation: A possible animal model for restless legs syndrome. *J Neuropathol Exp Neurol.* 2007;66(5):383-388.

134. Zhao H, Zhu W, Pan T, Xie W, Zhang A, et al. Spinal cord dopamine receptor expression and function in mice with 6-OHDA lesion of the A11 nucleus and dietary iron deprivation. *J Neurosci Res.* 2007;85(5):1065-1076.

135. Stiasny-Kolster K, Magerl W, Oertel W, Moller J, Treede R. Static mechanical hyperalgesia without dynamic tactile allodynia in patients with restless legs syndrome. *Brain.* 2004;127:773-782.

136. Han JK, Oh K, Kim BJ, Koh SB, Kim JY, et al. Cutaneous silent period in patients with restless leg syndrome. *Clin Neurophysiol.* 2007;118(8):1705-1710.

137. Rye D, Freeman A. Pain and its interaction with thalamocortical excitability states. In: Lavigne G, Choinière M, Sessle B, Soja P, eds. *Sleep and Pain.* Seattle: IASP Press; 2007:77-97.

138. Wood PB. Role of central dopamine in pain and analgesia. *Exp Rev Neurotherapeutics.* 2008;8(5):781-797.

139. Lee SJ, Kim JS, Song IU, An JY, Kim YI, Lee KS. Poststroke restless legs syndrome and lesion location: Anatomical considerations. *Mov Disord.* 2009;24:77-84.

140. Ferini-Strambi L, Filippi M, Martinelli V, Oldani A, Rovaris M, et al. Nocturnal sleep study in multiple sclerosis: Correlations with clinical and brain magnetic resonance imaging findings. *J Neurol Sci.* 1994;125:194-197.

141. Rye D, DeLong M. Amelioration of sensory limb discomfort of restless legs syndrome by pallidotomy. *Ann Neurol.* 1999;46(5):800-801.

142. Driver-Dunckley E, Evidente VG, Adler CH, Hillman R, Hernandez J, et al. Restless legs syndrome in Parkinson's disease patients may improve with subthalamic stimulation. *Mov Disord.* 2006;21(8):1287-1289.

143. Kedia S, Moro E, Tagliati M, Lang AE, Kumar R. Emergence of restless legs syndrome during subthalamic stimulation for Parkinson disease. *Neurology.* 2004;63(12):2410-2412.

144. Ondo W. VIM deep brain stimulation does not improve pre-existing restless legs syndrome in patients with essential tremor. *Parkinsonism Relat Disord.* 2006;12(2):113-114.

145. Allen R. Dopamine and iron in the pathophysiology of restless legs syndrome (RLS). *Sleep Med.* 2004;5(4):385-391.

146. Earley C, Allen R, Beard J, Connor J. Insight into the pathophysiology of restless legs syndrome. *J Neurosci Res.* 2000;62(5):623-628.

147. Allen R, Earley C. The role of iron in restless legs syndrome. *Mov Disord.* 2007;22(suppl 18):S440-S448.

148. Connor J. Pathophysiology of restless legs syndrome: Evidence for iron involvement. *Curr Neurosci Rep.* 2008;8(2):162-166.

149. Aul EA, Davis BJ, Rodnitzky RL. The importance of formal serum iron studies in the assessment of restless legs syndrome. *Neurology.* 1998;51(3):912.

150. Berger K, von Eckardstein A, Trenkwalder C, Rothdach A, Junker R, Weiland S. Iron metabolism and the risk of restless legs syndrome in an elderly general population—The MEMO study. *J Neurol.* 2002;249:1195-1199.

151. Silber M, Richardson J. Multiple blood donations associated with iron deficiency in patients with restless legs syndrome. *Mayo Clin Proc.* 2003;78:52-54.

152. Burchell BJ, Allen RP, Miller JK, Hening WA, Earley CJ. RLS and blood donation. *Sleep Med.* 2009;10(8):844-849.

153. Becker PM. Bleed less than 3: RLS and blood donation. *Sleep Med.* 2009;10(8):820-821.

154. Lee K, Zaffke M, Baratte-Beebe K. Restless legs syndrome and sleep disturbance during pregnancy: The role of folate and iron. *J Women Health Gend Based Med.* 2001;10(4):335-341.

155. Tunc T, Karadag Y, Dogulu F, Inan L. Predisposing factors of restless legs syndrome in pregnancy. *Mov Disord.* 2007;22(5):627-631.

156. Dzaja A, Wehrle R, Lancel M, Pollmacher T. Elevated estradiol plasma levels in women with restless legs during pregnancy. *Sleep.* 2009;32(2):169-174.

157. Earley CJ, Horska A, Mohamed MA, Barker PB, Beard JL, Allen RP. A randomized, double-blind, placebo-controlled trial of intravenous iron sucrose in restless legs syndrome. *Sleep Med.* 2009;10(2):206-211.

158. Wang J, O'Reilly B, Venkataraman R, Mysliwiec V, Mysliwiec A. Efficacy of oral iron in patients with restless legs syndrome and a low-normal ferritin: A randomized, double-blind, placebo-controlled study. *Sleep Med.* 2009;10(9):945-946.

159. Sloand JA, Shelly MA, Feigin A, Bernstein P, Monk RD. A double-blind, placebo-controlled trial of intravenous iron dextran therapy in patients with ESRD and restless legs syndrome. *Am J Kidney Dis.* 2004;43(4):663-670.

160. Davis BJ, Rajput A, Rajput ML, Aul EA, Eichhorn GR. A randomized, double-blind placebo-controlled trial of iron in restless legs syndrome. *Eur Neurol.* 2000;43(2):70-75.

161. Grote L, Leissner L, Hedner J, Ulfberg J. A randomized, double-blind, placebo controlled, multi-center study of intravenous iron sucrose and placebo in the treatment of restless legs syndrome. *Mov Disord.* 2009;24(10):1445-1452.

162. Freeman A, Rye D. Dopamine in behavioral state control. In: Sinton C, Perumal P, Monti J, eds. *The Neurochemistry of Sleep and Wakefulness.* Cambridge: Cambridge University Press; 2008:179-223.

163. Ramsey A, Hillas P, Fitzpatrick P. Characterization of the active site iron in tyrosine hydroxylase. Redox states of the iron. *J Biol Chem.* 1996;271:24395-24400.

164. Nagatsu I. Tyrosine hydroxylase: Human isoforms, structure and regulation in physiology and pathology. *Essays Biochem.* 1995;30:15-35.

165. Nelson C, Erikson K, Pinero D, Beard J. In vivo dopamine metabolism is altered in iron-deficient anemic rats. *J Nutr.* 1997;127:2282-2288.

166. Bianco LE, Wiesinger J, Earley CJ, Jones BC, Beard JL. Iron deficiency alters dopamine uptake and response to L-DOPA injection in Sprague-Dawley rats. *J Neurochem.* 2008;106(1):205-215.

167. Bianco L, Unger E, Earley C, Beard J. Iron deficiency alters the day-night variation in monoamine levels in mice. *Chronobiol Int.* 2009;26(3):447-463.

168. Rye DB, Trotti LM. Restless legs syndrome. In: Watts R, Obeso J, Standaert D, eds. *Movement Disorders.* 3rd ed. New York: McGraw-Hill; 2010.

169. Hue G, Decker M, Solomon I, Rye D. Increased wakefulness and hyper-responsivity to novel environments in mice lacking functional dopamine D3 receptors. *Soc Neurosci.* 2003;616:16.

170. Beckford G. The Functional Organization and Behavioral Relevance of the A11 Hypothalamospinal Dopaminergic System. Atlanta: Emory University; 2008.

171. Allen RP, Connor JR, Hyland K, Earley CJ. Abnormally increased CSF 3-ortho-methyldopa (3-OMD) in untreated restless legs syndrome (RLS) patients indicates more severe disease and possibly abnormally increased dopamine synthesis. *Sleep Med.* 2008;10(1):123.

172. Connor JR, Wang XS, Allen RP, Beard JL, Wiesinger JA, et al. Altered dopaminergic profile in the putamen and substantia nigra in restless leg syndrome. *Brain.* 2009;132(Pt 9):2403-2412.

173. Zapata A, Shippenberg TS. D(3) receptor ligands modulate extracellular dopamine clearance in the nucleus accumbens. *J Neurochem.* 2002;81(5):1035-1042.

174. Ferger B, Buck K, Shimasaki M, Koros E, Voehringer P, Buerger E. Continuous dopaminergic stimulation by pramipexole is effective to treat early morning akinesia in animal models of Parkinson's disease: A pharmacokinetic-pharmacodynamic study using in vivo microdialysis in rats. *Synapse.* 2010;64(7):533-541.

175. Hening WA. Current guidelines and standards of practice for restless legs syndrome. *Am J Med.* 2007;120(suppl 1):S22-S27.

176. Silber M, Ehrenberg B, Allen R, Buchfuhrer M, Earley C, et al. An algorithm for the management of restless legs syndrome. *Mayo Clin Proc.* 2004;79:916-922.

177. Phillips B, Young T, Finn L, Asher K, Hening WA, Purvis C. Epidemiology of restless legs symptoms in adults. *Arch Intern Med.* 2000;160(14):2137-2141:24.

178. Aldrich M, Shipley J. Alcohol use and periodic limb movements of sleep. *Alcoholism Clin Exp Res.* 1993;17(1):192-196.

179. Hornyak M, Feige B, Riemann D, Voderholzer U. Periodic leg movements in sleep and periodic limb movement disorder: Prevalence, clinical significance and treatment. *Sleep Med Rev.* 2006;10(3):169-177.

180. Urbano MR, Ware JC. Restless legs syndrome caused by quetiapine successfully treated with ropinirole in 2 patients with bipolar disorder. *J Clin Pharmacol.* 2008;28(6):704-705.

181. Kim S, Shin I, Kim J, Yang S, Shin H, Yoon J. Bupropion may improve restless legs syndrome: A report of three cases. *Clin Neuropharmacol.* 2005;28(6):298-301.

182. Lee J, Erdos J, Wilkoosz M, LaPlante R, Wagoner B. Bupropion as a possible treatment option for restless legs syndrome. *Ann Pharmacother.* 2009;43(2):370-374.

183. Smith HS, Dhingra R, Ryckewaert L, Bonner D. Proton pump inhibitors and pain. *Pain Phys.* 2009;12(6):1013-1023.

184. Banerji NK, Hurwitz LJ. Restless legs syndrome, with particular reference to its occurrence after gastric surgery. *Br Med J.* 1970;4(5738):774-775.

185. Weinstock LB, Fern SE, Duntley SP. Restless legs syndrome in patients with irritable bowel syndrome: Response to small intestinal bacterial overgrowth therapy. *Dig Dis Sci.* 2008;53(5):1252-1256.

186. Manchanda S, Davies CR, Picchietti D. Celiac disease as a possible cause for low serum ferritin in patients with restless legs syndrome. *Sleep Med.* 2009;10(7):763-765.

187. Weinstock LB, Walters AS, Mullin GE, Duntley SP. Celiac disease is associated with restless legs syndrome. *Dig Dis Sci.* 2010;55(6):1667-1673.

188. Numata Y, Kato T, Nagatsu T, Sugimoto T, Matsuura S. Effects of stereochemical structures of tetrahydrobiopterin on tyrosine hydroxylase. *Bichim Biophys Acta.* 1977;480(1):104-112.

189. Botez M, Fontaine F, Botez T, Bachevalier J. Folate-responsive neurological and mental disorders: Report of 16 cases. Neuropyschological correlates of computerized transaxial tomography and radionuclide cisternography in folic acid deficiencies. *Eur Neurol.* 1977;16(1-6):230-246.

190. O'Keeffe S, Gavin K, Lavan J. Iron status and restless legs syndrome in the elderly. *Age Ageing.* 1994;23:200-203.

191. Bachmann C, Guth N, Helmshmied K, Armstrong V, Paulus W, Happe S. Homocysteine in restless legs syndrome. *Sleep Med.* 2008;9(4):388-392.

192. Morgan JC, Ames M, Sethi KD. Response to ropinirole in restless legs syndrome is independent of baseline serum ferritin. *J Neurol Neurosurg Psychiatry.* 2008;79(8):964-965.

193. Trenkwalder C, Hogl B, Benes H, Kohnen R. Augmentation in restless legs syndrome is associated with low ferritin. *Sleep Med.* 2008;9(5):572-574.

194. Umbreit J. Iron deficiency: A concise review. *Am J Hematol.* 2005;78(3):225-231.

195. Sloand J, Shelly M, Feigin A, Bernstein P, Monk R. A double-blind, placebo-controlled trial of intravenous iron dextran therapy in patients with ESRD and restless legs syndrome. *Am J Kidney Dis.* 2004;43:663-670.

196. Silverstein SB, Rodgers GM. Parenteral iron therapy options. *Am J Hematol.* 2004;76(1):74-78.

197. Happe S, Trenkwalder C. Role of dopamine receptor agonists in the treatment of restless legs syndrome. *CNS Drugs.* 2004;18(1):27-36.

198. Montplaisir J, Nicolas A, Denesle R, Gomez-Mancilla B. Restless legs syndrome improved by pramipexole: A double-blind randomized study. *Neurology.* 1999;52:938-943.

199. Montplaisir J, Denesle R, Petit D. Pramipexole in the treatment of restless legs syndrome: A follow-up study. *Eur J Neurol.* 2000(suppl 1):27-31.

200. Winkelman JW, Sethi KD, Kushida CA, Becker PM, Koester J, et al. Efficacy and safety of pramipexole in restless legs syndrome. *Neurology.* 2006;67(6):1034-1039.

201. Ferini-Strambi L, Aarskog D, Partinen M, Chaudhuri KR, Sohr M, et al. Effect of pramipexole on RLS symptoms and sleep: A randomized, double-blind, placebo-controlled trial. *Sleep Med.* 2008;9:874-881.

202. Partinen M, Hirvonen K, Jama L, Alakuijala A, Hublin C, et al. Efficacy and safety of pramipexole in idiopathic restless legs syndrome: A polysomnographic dose-finding study—The PRELUDE study. *Sleep Med.* 2006;7(5):407-417.

203. Trenkwalder C, Hening WA, Montagna P, Oertel WH, Allen RP, et al. Treatment of restless legs syndrome: An evidence-based review and implications for clinical practice. *Mov Disord.* 2008;23(16):2267-2302.

204. Adler CH, Hauser RA, Sethi K, Caviness JN, Marlor L, et al. Ropinirole for restless legs syndrome: A placebo-controlled crossover trial. *Neurology.* 2004;62(8):1405-1407.

205. Walters AS, Ondo WG, Dreykluft T, Grunstein R, Lee D, Sethi K. Ropinirole is effective in the treatment of restless legs syndrome. TREAT RLS 2: A 12-week, double-blind, randomized, parallel-group, placebo-controlled study. *Mov Disord.* 2004;19(12):1414-1423.

206. Allen R, Becker PM, Bogan R, Schmidt M, Kushida CA, et al. Ropinirole decreases periodic leg movements and improves sleep parameters in patients with restless legs syndrome. *Sleep.* 2004;27(5):907-914.

207. Bliwise DL, Freeman A, Ingram CD, Rye DB, Chakravorty S, Watts RL. Randomized, double-blind, placebo-controlled, short-term trial of ropinirole in restless legs syndrome. *Sleep Med.* 2005;6(2):141-147.

208. Bogan RK, Fry JM, Schmidt MH, Carson SW, Ritchie SY. Ropinirole in the treatment of patients with restless legs syndrome: A US-based randomized, double-blind, placebo-controlled clinical trial. *Mayo Clin Proc.* 2006;81(1):17-27.

209. Quilici S, Abrams K, Nicolas A, Martin M, Petit C, et al. Meta-analysis of the efficacy and tolerability of pramipexole versus ropinirole in the treatment of restless legs syndrome. *Sleep Med.* 2008;9(7):715-726.

210. Stiasny-Kolster K, Benes H, Peglau I, Hornyak M, Holinka B, et al. Effective cabergoline treatment in idiopathic restless legs syndrome (RLS): A randomized, double-blind, placebo-controlled, multicenter dose-finding study followed by an open long-term extension. *Neurology.* 2004;63(12):2272-2279.

211. Benes H, Heinrich CR, Ueberall MA, Kohnen R. Long-term safety and efficacy of cabergoline for the treatment of idiopathic restless legs syndrome: Results from an open-label 6-month clinical trial. *Sleep.* 2004;27(4):674-682.

212. Oertel WH, Benes H, Bodenschatz R, Peglau I, Warmuth R, et al. Efficacy of cabergoline in restless legs syndrome: A placebo-controlled study with polysomnography (CATOR). *Neurology.* 2006;67(6):1040-1046.

213. Trenkwalder C, Benes H, Grote L, Happe S, Hogl B, et al. Cabergoline compared to levodopa in the treatment of patients with severe restless legs syndrome: Results from a multi-center, randomized, active controlled trial. *Mov Disord.* 2007;22(5):696-703.

214. Benes H. Transdermal lisuride: Short-term efficacy and tolerability study in patients with severe restless legs syndrome. *Sleep Med.* 2006;7(1):31-35.

215. Stiasny-Kolster K, Kohnen R, Schollmayer E, Moller JC, Oertel WH. Patch application of the dopamine agonist rotigotine to patients with moderate to advanced stages of restless legs syndrome: A double-blind, placebo-controlled pilot study. *Mov Disord.* 2004;19(12):1432-1438.

216. Oertel WH, Benes H, Garcia-Borreguero D, Geisler P, Hogl B, et al. One year open-label safety and efficacy trial with rotigotine transdermal patch in moderate to severe idiopathic restless legs syndrome. *Sleep Med.* 2008;9:865-873.

217. Hening WA, Allen RP, Ondo WG, Walters AS, Winkelman JW, et al. Rotigotine improves restless legs syndrome: A 6-month randomized, double-blind, placebo-controlled trial in the United States. *Mov Disord.* 2010;25(11):1675-1683.

218. Hogl B, Oertel WH, Stiasny-Kolster K, Geisler P, Benes H, et al. Treatment of moderate to severe restless legs syndrome: 2-year safety and efficacy of rotigotine transdermal patch. *BMC Neurol.* 2010;10:86.

219. Oertel WH, Benes H, Garcia-Borreguero D, Hogl B, Poewe W, et al. Rotigotine transdermal patch in moderate to severe idiopathic restless legs syndrome: A randomized, placebo-controlled polysomnographic study. *Sleep Med.* 2010;11(9):848-856.

220. Benes H, Deissler A, Rodenbeck A, Engfer A, Kohnen R. Lisuride treatment of restless legs syndrome: First studies with monotherapy in de novo patients and in combination with levodopa in advanced disease. *J Neural Transm.* 2006;113(1):87-92.

221. Paulus W, Trenkwalder C. Less is more: Pathophysiology of dopaminergic-therapy-related augmentation in restless legs syndrome. *Lancet Neurol.* 2006;5(10):878-886.

222. Allen R, Chen C, Soaita A, Wohlberg C, Knapp L, et al. A randomized, double-blind, 6-week, dose-ranging study of pregabalin in patients with restless legs syndrome. *Sleep Med.* 2010;11(6):512-519.

223. Garcia-Borreguero D, Larrosa O, Williams AM, Albares J, Pascual M, et al. Treatment of restless legs syndrome with pregabalin: A double-blind, placebo-controlled study. *Neurology.* 2010;74(23):1897-1904.

224. Kushida C, Walters A, Thein S, Perkins A, Roth T, et al. A randomized, double-blind, placebo-controlled, crossover study of XP1351/GSK183262 in the treatment of patients with primary restless legs syndrome. *Sleep.* 2009;32(2):159-168.

225. Kushida CA, Becker PM, Ellenbogen AL, Canafax DM, Barrett RW. Randomized, double-blind, placebo-controlled study of XP13512/GSK1838262 in patients with RLS. *Neurology.* 2009;72(5):439-446.

226. Walters AS, Winkelmann J, Trenkwalder C, Fry JM, Kataria V, et al. Long-term follow-up on restless legs syndrome patients treated with opioids. *Mov Disord.* 2001;16(6):1105-1109.

227. Lettieri CJ, Eliasson AH. Pneumatic compression devices are an effective therapy for restless legs syndrome: A prospective, randomized, double-blinded, sham-controlled trial. *Chest.* 2009;135(1):74-80.

228. Hayes CA, Kingsley JR, Hamby KR, Carlow J. The effect of endovenous laser ablation on restless legs syndrome. *Phlebology.* 2008;23(3):112-117.

229. Aukerman MM, Aukerman D, Bayard M, Tudiver F, Thorp L, Bailey B. Exercise and restless legs syndrome: A randomized controlled trial. *J Am Board Fam Med.* 2006;19(5):487-493.

230. Cui Y, Wang Y, Liu Z. Acupuncture for restless legs syndrome. *Cochrane Database Syst Rev.* 2008(4):CD006457.

231. Rotenberg JS, Canard K, Difazio M. Successful treatment of recalcitrant restless legs syndrome with botulinum toxin type A. *J Clin Sleep Med.* 2006;2(3):275-278.

232. Nahab FB, Peckham EL, Hallett M. Double-blind, placebo-controlled, pilot trial of botulinum toxin A in restless legs syndrome. *Neurology.* 2008;71(12):950-951.

233. Kovacevic-Ristanovic R, Cartwright RD, Lloyd S. Nonpharmacologic treatment of periodic leg movements in sleep. *Arch Phys Med Rehabil.* 1991;72(6):385-389.

234. Guilleminault C, Cetel M, Philip P. Dopaminergic treatment of restless legs and rebound phenomenon. *Neurology.* 1993;43(2):445.

235. Garcia-Borreguero D, Allen RP, Kohnen R, Hogl B, Trenkwalder C, et al. Diagnostic standards for dopaminergic augmentation of restless legs syndrome: Report from a World Association of Sleep Medicine—International Restless Legs Syndrome Study Group consensus conference at the Max Planck Institute. *Sleep Med.* 2007;8(5):520-530.

236. Earley CJ, Allen RP. Restless legs syndrome augmentation associated with tramadol. *Sleep Med.* 2006;7(7):592-593.

237. Garcia-Borreguero D, Kohnen R, Hogl B, Ferini-Strambi L, Hadjigeorgiou GM, et al. Validation of the augmentation severity rating scale (ASRS). *Sleep Med.* 2007;8:455-463.

238. Ondo W, Romanyshyn J, Vuong K, Lai D. Long-term treatment of restless legs syndrome with dopamine agonists. *Arch Neurol.* 2004;61:1393-1397.

239. Ondo WG. Methadone for refractory restless legs syndrome. *Mov Disord.* 2005;20(3):345-348.

240. Kurlan R, Richard I, Deeley C. Medication tolerance and augmentation in restless legs syndrome: The need for drug class rotation. *J Gen Intern Med.* 2006;21(12):C1-C4.

241. Tippmann-Peikert M, Park JG, Boeve BF, Shepard JW, Silber MH. Pathologic gambling in patients with restless legs syndrome treated with dopaminergic agonists. *Neurology.* 2007;68(4):301-303.

242. Quickfall J, Suchowersky O. Pathological gambling associated with dopamine agonist use in restless legs syndrome. *Parkinsonism Relat Disord.* 2007;13(8):535-536.

243. Evans AH, Stegeman JR. Punding in patients on dopamine agonists for restless legs syndrome. *Mov Disord.* 2009;24(1):140-141.

244. Salas RE, Allen RP, Earley CJ, Gamaldo CE. A case of compulsive behaviors observed in a restless legs syndrome patient treated with a dopamine agonist. *Sleep.* 2009;32(5):587-588.

245. Kolla BP, Mansukhani MP, Barraza R, Bostwick JM. Impact of dopamine agonists on compulsive behaviors: A case series of pramipexole-induced pathological gambling. *Psychosomatics.* 2010;51(3):271-273.

246. Driver-Dunckley ED, Noble BN, Hentz JG, Evidente VG, Caviness JN, et al. Gambling and increased sexual desire with dopaminergic medications in restless legs syndrome. *Clin Neuropharmacol.* 2007;30(5):249-255.

247. Pourcher E, Remillard S, Cohen H. Compulsive habits in restless legs syndrome patients under dopaminergic treatment. *J Neurol Sci.* 2010;290(1-2):52-56.

248. Ondo WG, Lai D. Predictors of impulsivity and reward seeking behavior with dopamine agonists. *Parkinsonism Relat Disord.* 2008;14(1):28-32.

249. Cornelius JR, Tippmann-Peikert M, Slocumb NL, Frerichs CF, Silber MH. Impulse control disorders with the use of dopaminergic agents in restless legs syndrome: A case-control study. *Sleep.* 2010;33(1):81-87.

250. Voon V, Thomsen T, Miyasaki JM, de Souza M, Shafro A, et al. Factors associated with dopaminergic drug-related pathological gambling in Parkinson disease. *Arch Neurol.* 2007;64(2):212-216.

251. Potenza MN, Voon V, Weintraub D. Drug insight: Impulse control disorders and dopamine therapies in Parkinson's disease. *Nat Clin Pract Neurol.* 2007;3(12):664-672.

252. Bayard S, Yu H, Langenier MC, Carlander B, Dauvilliers Y. Decision making in restless legs syndrome. *Mov Disord.* 2010;25(15):2634-2640.

253. Kavanagh D, Siddiqui S, Geddes CC. Restless legs syndrome in patients on dialysis. *Am J Kidney Dis.* 2004;43(5):763-771.

254. Winkelmann J, Stautner A, Samtleben W, Trenkwalder C. Long-term course of restless legs syndrome in dialysis patients after kidney transplantation. *Mov Disord.* 2002;17(5):1072-1076.

255. Molnar MZ, Novak M, Ambrus C, Szeifert L, Kovacs A, et al. Restless legs syndrome in patients after renal transplantation. *Am J Kidney Dis.* 2005;45(2):388-396.

256. Miranda M, Kagi M, Fabres L, Aguilera L, Alvo M, et al. Pramipexole for the treatment of uremic restless legs in patients undergoing hemodialysis. *Neurology.* 2004;62(5):831-832.

257. Chesson Jr AL, Wise M, Davila D, Johnson S, Littner M, et al. Practice parameters for the treatment of restless legs syndrome and periodic limb movement disorder. An American Academy of Sleep Medicine Report. Standards of Practice Committee of the American Academy of Sleep Medicine. *Sleep.* 1999;22(7):961-968.

258. Botez M, Lambert B. Folate deficiency and restless legs syndrome in pregnancy. *N Engl J Med.* 1977;297(12):670.

259. Bartell S, Zallek S. Intravenous magnesium sulfate may relieve restless legs syndrome in pregnancy. *J Clin Sleep Med.* 2006;2(2):187-188.

260. Merlino G, Fratticci L, Valente M, Del Giudice A, Noacco C, et al. Association of restless legs syndrome in type 2 diabetes: A case-control study. *Sleep.* 2007;30(7):866-871.

261. Hening WA, Caivano CK. Restless legs syndrome: A common disorder in patients with rheumatologic conditions. *Semin Arth Rheum.* 2008;38(1):55-62.

262. Winkelman JW, Chertow GM, Lazarus JM. Restless legs syndrome in end-stage renal disease. *Am J Kidney Dis.* 1996;28(3):372-378.

263. Minai OA, Malik N, Foldvary N, Bair N, Golish JA. Prevalence and characteristics of restless legs syndrome in patients with pulmonary hypertension. *J Heart Lung Transplant.* 2008;27(3):335-340.

264. Kaplan Y, Inonu H, Yilmaz A, Ocal S. Restless legs syndrome in patients with chronic obstructive pulmonary disease. *Can J Neurol Sci.* 2008;35(3):352-357.
265. Lo Coco D, Mattaliano A, Lo Coco A, Randisi B. Increased frequency of restless legs syndrome in chronic obstructive pulmonary disease patients. *Sleep Med.* 2009;10(5):572-576.
266. Franco RA, Ashwathnarayan R, Deshpandee A, Knox J, Daniel J, et al. The high prevalence of restless legs syndrome symptoms in liver disease in an academic-based hepatology practice. *J Clin Sleep Med.* 2008;4(1):45-49.
267. Weinstock LB, Bosworth BP, Scherl EJ, Li E, Iroku U, et al. Crohn's disease is associated with restless legs syndrome. *Inflamm Bowel Dis.* 2010;16(2):275-279.
268. Weinstock LB, Walters AS, Mullin GE, Duntley SP. Celiac disease is associated with restless legs syndrome. *Dig Dis Sci.* 2010;55(6):1667-1673.
269. Cologno D, Cicarelli G, Petretta V. d'Onofrio F, Bussone G. High prevalence of dopaminergic premonitory symptoms in migraine patients with restless legs syndrome: A pathogenetic link? *Neurol Sci.* 2008;29(suppl 1):S166-S168.
270. Rhode AM, Hosing VG, Happe S, Biehl K, Young P, Evers S. Comorbidity of migraine and restless legs syndrome—A case-control study. *Cephalalgia.* 2007;27(11):1255-1260.
271. Poewe W, Hogl B. Akathisia, restless legs, and periodic limb movements in sleep in Parkinson's disease. *Neurology.* 2004;63(suppl 3):S12-S16.
272. Nomura T, Inoue Y, Miyake M, Yasui Y, Nakashima K. Prevalence and clinical characteristics of restless legs syndrome in Japanese patients with Parkinson's disease. *Mov Disord.* 2006;21(3):380-384.
273. Gomez-Esteban JC, Zarranz JJ, Tijero B, Velasco F, Barcena J, et al. Restless legs syndrome in Parkinson's disease. *Mov Disord.* 2007;22(13):1912-1916.
274. Calzetti S, Negrotti A, Bonavina G, Angelini M, Marchesi E. Absence of comorbidity of Parkinson disease and restless legs syndrome: A case-control study in patients attending a movement disorders clinic. *Neurol Sci.* 2009;30:119-122.
275. Lee J, Shin H, Kim K, Sohn Y. Factors contributing to the development of restless legs syndrome in patients with Parkinson disease. *Mov Disord.* 2009;24(4):579-582.
276. Manconi M, Fabbrini M, Bonanni E, Filippi M, Rocca M, et al. High prevalence of restless legs syndrome in multiple sclerosis. *Eur J Neurol.* 2007;14(5):534-539.
277. Abele M, Burk K, Laccone F, Dichgans J, Klockgether T. Restless legs syndrome in spinocerebellar ataxia types 1, 2, and *3. J Neurol.* 2001;248(4):311-314.
278. Schöls L, Haan J, Riess O, Amoiridis G, Przuntek H. Sleep disturbance in spinocerebellar ataxias. Is the SCA3 mutation a cause of restless leg syndrome? *Neurology.* 1998;51:1603-1607.
279. Tuin I, Voss U, Kang JS, Kessler K, Rub U, et al. Stages of sleep pathology in spinocerebellar ataxia type 2 (SCA2). *Neurology.* 2006;67(11):1966-1972.
280. Oner P, Dirik EB, Taner Y, Caykoylu A, Anlar O. Association between low serum ferritin and restless legs syndrome in patients with attention deficit hyperactivity disorder. *Tohoku J Exp Med.* 2007;213(3):269-276.

Chapter 25

Sleep-Related Bruxism

NOSHIR R. MEHTA / STEVEN J. SCRIVANI / LEOPOLDO P. CORREA / JEAN K. MATHESON

Sleep-related bruxism is a nonfunctional oral activity characterized by clenching and grinding of the teeth during sleep often associated with arousal. Formerly considered a parasomnia, the International Classification of Sleep Disorders, Second Edition (ICSD-2) now classifies nocturnal bruxism as a sleep-related movement disorder.[1]

Bruxism itself is divided into two main types: sleep-related bruxism and awake bruxism. Sleep-related bruxism (SB) involves both grinding, which is a back-and-forth, side-to-side motion of the lower teeth rubbing against the upper teeth, creating a characteristic grinding sound, and clenching, which is a rocking motion of the lower teeth against the upper teeth without the teeth actually making the side-to-side motion. Although grinding typically occurs only during sleep, clenching frequently occurs during both wake and sleep.[2] Both grinding and clenching are "parafunctional activities," as they are not part of a normal chewing and swallowing function. Parafunctional behaviors can begin in early childhood and persist throughout adulthood.[2]

SB can be either a primary or secondary disorder. Primary SB has no identifiable cause, whereas secondary SB is associated with medical problems including other sleep disorders, drug abuse, and a wide range of neurologic disease. Bruxism may also be iatrogenically induced by medications, especially those with a serotoninergic mechanism, stimulants, and neuroleptics.[3,4]

DEMOGRAPHICS

SB is common in the general population. Using a clinical questionnaire based on the minimal set of criteria from the ICSD, Ohayon and associates[5] interviewed more than 13,000 subjects in Europe. These authors report that 8.2% of respondents reported grinding of teeth at night at least once a week and that 4.4% met ICSD criteria for SB (see later discussion of diagnostic criteria). There was a slightly higher rate of SB in women (4.9%) compared to men (4.1%). SB is more common in children, with estimates as high as 10% to 20%, and decreases with age. In the Ohayon study only 1.1% of subjects over the age of 65 met criteria for SB.

DENTAL PATHOPHYSIOLOGY

Normal chewing has been shown to apply forces of around 25 lb to 50 lb on the molar teeth. Parafunctional clenching or grinding, on the other hand, has been shown to create forces as high as 250 lb during sleep.[6,7] During normal chewing, teeth come into contact only approximately 25 to 30 minutes in a 12-hour day. During SB, however, teeth may be in contact as much as 40 minutes per hour of sleep. The increase in both force and contact between teeth is impressive and can lead to a variety of dental conditions.[8]

During the day, the individual has some ability to control such parafunctional activities. During sleep, however, this ability is lost. As such, the majority of diagnoses and treatments are aimed at reducing sleep-related bruxism. Because most adults will grind teeth in their sleep at some time in their life, SB has been considered by some to be a physiologic release mechanism for stress. This view leads these authors to view SB as a positive symptom and to discourage treatment.[9] Although this may be true of bruxism in the milder form, as the duration and severity of grinding increases, there is more concern about such forces causing damage to the masticatory system of teeth, bones, muscles, and nerves.

The damage from daytime clenching and nighttime bruxism primarily affects the dental structures. Here a concept of the "weak link theory" comes into effect. The weak link theory[7] relies on the principle that bruxism causes damage to the (1) teeth, (2) the gums and supporting bones, or (3) the temporomandibular jaw joints and supporting muscles, but very rarely all three. Whichever area is the weakest will be the first to be affected by bruxism, and what is affected can vary from patient to patient. This situation often leads to misdiagnoses, as some dentists have been trained to look for only one manifestation of bruxism (Box 25-1).[7,10,11]

Dental Damage

Dental damage is usually noticed by the dentist as wear of the tooth structures (enamel and dentin) between regularly scheduled dental visits. This is evidenced by wear on the lower anterior teeth that matches the edges of the upper anterior teeth in anterior and lateral excursive movements.[11]

Dentists look at worn or flattened teeth as a sign of active bruxism (Fig. 25-1). However, the wear could have been created at an earlier age. Teeth once worn will always show the wear unless new fillings or crowns cover the worn surfaces. The only reliable clinical method to determine whether active grinding is ongoing is by eliciting a report of sounds consistent with bruxism from the patient or an observer.[12]

Depending on the severity of the bruxing, fracture lines or tiny chips breaking from the grinding surfaces can be seen on dental examination. Excessive forces can sometimes lead to the need for a root canal if the wear reaches the inner surfaces of the teeth, causing an inflammation of the pulp of the tooth. Forces on the teeth can sometimes cause a torque of the tooth

BOX 25-1 *Important Signs and Symptoms of Sleep-Related Bruxism*

- Rhythmic crunching or grating noises resembling that associated with chewing on crackers or ice
- Headaches and stiffness of the neck on awakening in the morning
- Muscle pain in the jaw muscles or a feeling of tightness in the jaws
- Masseter hypertrophy
- Awakening with the teeth clenched together
- Temporomandibular joint pain and clicking sounds
- Chronic facial pain
- Ear pain, stuffiness or even ringing of the ears
- Increased tooth sensitivity, especially in the morning, that slowly abates as the day progresses
- Wearing of the teeth, chipping or fractures to the teeth in the absence of trauma
- Chewing of the inner aspects of the cheeks or biting of the tongue
- Teeth that are loose or moveable
- Inability to chew without tightening and fatigue of jaw muscles
- Tiredness and sleepiness in the daytime

Data from Mehta NR, Forgione AG, Maloney G, Greene R. Different effects of nocturnal parafunction on the masticatory system: The Weak Link Theory. *Cranio.* 2000;18(4):280-286; Arnold M. Bruxism and the occlusion. *Dent Clin North Am.* 1981;25(3):395-407.

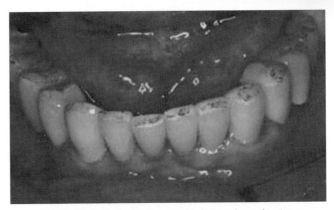

Figure 25-1 Image showing worn teeth secondary to bruxism.

BOX 25-2 *SRB Criteria from ICSD-2*[1]

A. The patient reports or is aware of tooth-grinding sounds or tooth clenching during sleep.

B. One or more of the following is present:
  a. Abnormal wear of teeth
  b. Jaw muscle discomfort, fatigue, or pain and jaw lock upon awakening.
  c. Masseter muscle hypertrophy upon voluntary forceful clenching.

C. The jaw muscle activity is not better explained by another current sleep disorder, medical or neurological disorder, medication use, or substance use disorder.

at the gingival margin. If the torque is buccal, there is a shearing of the enamel tooth structure called an *abfraction.*[13] An abfraction is a shiny, smooth, scooped out gouge on the outer surface of a tooth, usually in the premolar and molar teeth, caused by rocking forces.

Periodontal and Bone Damage

In the presence of existing gum inflammation (gingivitis) or infection (periodontal disease) bony changes can occur when there are excessive forces on teeth over an extended period of time. This has been termed *trauma from occlusion,* and is a potential consequence of bruxism. This can lead further to bone loss, loosening of the teeth, mobility of the teeth or even tooth movement related to the reduction of the bone support for the tooth.[14,15]

Temporomandibular Joint and Muscle Damage

If the teeth do not wear and the surrounding bone is strong, then the forces of bruxism can cause damage to the muscles and the joints of the jaw. Clicking, popping, and grating sounds are indicators of internal damage to the temporomandibular joints and can possibly lead to dental instability and difficulty chewing. Pain in the muscles of jaw and tension of the neck muscles leading to headaches and neck pain are also common consequences of nighttime bruxism. Chronic clenching and grinding have also been known to trigger nerve-related pain and sometimes appear as sharp shooting pains mimicking trigeminal neuralgia, or tooth pain such as atypical odontalgia.[2,16]

DIAGNOSIS

SB is a clinical diagnosis. The current criteria listed in ICSD-2[1] are listed in Box 25-2.

Polysomnographic (PSG) criteria have been suggested as well.[17,18] Jaw muscle contractions, referred to as *rhythmic masticatory muscle activity (RMMA),* are normal during sleep. In SB these contractions are excessive (higher amplitude and frequency) and are, at times, associated with teeth grinding. Bruxism episodes may take the form of rhythmic repetitive contractions, isolated tonic contractions, or a combination of both, with or without teeth grinding.[19] Electromyogram (EMG) of the masseter muscles plus audiovisual recordings can be used to monitor bruxism episodes. Classification of severity is based on a scoring system that, among other metrics, quantifies episodes of SB per hour as the SB index. Patients with SB typically demonstrate an SB index of 4 to 8, up to three times the index of normal control subjects.[1,3,19] Studies such as these are primarily obtained at specialty centers and for research, but can be obtained during standard polysomnography with the addition of masseter electrodes and audio recording.[3] A sleep study is not required for the diagnosis of SB.[1] However, bruxism is frequently identified incidentally in routine polysomnographic study as evidenced by rhythmic or tonic EMG activity in chin leads and contaminating the electroencephalograph (EEG) recording with muscle artifact (Fig. 25-2). *The AASM Manual for the Scoring of Sleep and Associated Events* provides rules for scoring bruxism during polysomnography[18] (Box 25-3). Portable systems are available for study in the patient's home but are less sensitive than in-laboratory studies. Most often, SB occurs in sleep stages Stage N1 and

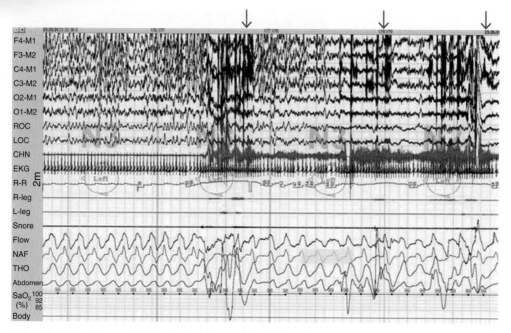

Figure 25-2 Bruxism as identified on routine polysomnography with both rhythmic and tonic features. Rhythmic electromyographic (EMG) activity is identified in the chin leads and contaminating the electroencephalographic (EEG) leads with muscle artifact. Tonic elevation of chin EMG is noted between runs of rhythmic bursts *(arrows)*. Subtle flow limitation *(bar)* may contribute to the bruxism (2-minute window).

BOX 25-3 *AASM Manual for the Scoring of Sleep and Associated Events: Scoring Bruxism*

- Bruxism may consist of brief (phasic) or sustained (tonic) elevations of chin EMG activity of amplitude at least twice that of background EMG.
- Brief elevations of chin EMG activity are scored as bruxism if they are 0.25 to 2.0 seconds in duration and if at least three such elevations occur in a regular sequence.
- Sustained elevations of chin EMG activity are scored as bruxism if the duration is more than 2 seconds.
- A period of at least 3 seconds of stable background chin EMG must occur before a new episode of bruxism can be scored.
- Bruxism can be scored reliably by audio in combination with polysomnography by a minimum of two audible tooth-grinding episodes or two nights of polysomnography in the absence of epilepsy.

AASM, American Academy of Sleep Medicine; *EMG*, electromyography.
From Iber C, American Academy of Sleep Medicine. *The AASM Manual for the Scoring of Sleep and Associated Events: Rules, Terminology and Technical Specifications.* Westchester, IL: American Academy of Sleep Medicine; 2007.

Stage N2[20] and can occur in the rapid eye movement (REM) stage.[17] Sleep architecture is surprisingly normal.[17]

ETIOLOGY AND RISK FACTORS

The underlying mechanisms that promote SB are unknown. The commonly held belief that SB is a manifestation of anxiety, stress, or a task-oriented personality type is not consistently upheld in the literature.[21] Similarly, theories that occlusal abnormalities are responsible for inducing SB are controversial.[21,22]

The relationship of SB to arousals during sleep is an active subject of study.[23] RMMAs have been noted to occur following evidence of apparently spontaneous physiologic arousal with signs of increased sympathetic tone (heart rate) and cortical activation (EEG) preceding the SB, but are also induced by exogenous arousal stimuli such as sound or light.[19] These findings suggest that SB could represent an excessive response to arousal during sleep. It follows that endogenous or exogenous causes of arousal during sleep could precipitate events in predisposed patients.

OSA is a common cause of nocturnal arousal and a risk factor for SB.[24] Ohayon and associates[5] reported that patients with symptoms of OSA by questionnaire had an odds ratio of 1.8 of reporting symptoms of SB. The occurrence of episodes of SB following the termination of an apnea is a common clinical observation.[25] Bruxism is more common in the supine position,[26,27] a posture that is more likely to compromise the airway during sleep. Lavigne and associates[19] notes that RMMA may function to increase airway patency. Recent studies demonstrating improvement in bruxism (see later discussion) with the use of mandibular advancement appliances (MAA) (devices designed for the treatment of sleep apnea), even in patients without demonstrated underlying sleep apnea, suggest that compromised airway patency could be an important predisposing factor.[25]

A number of medications and recreational drugs are reported to increase bruxism, but most reports are anecdotal or include only a small number of patients. Selective serotonin reuptake inhibitors (SSRIs), selective serotonin and norepinephrine uptake inhibitors (SNRIs), stimulants, and antidopaminergic drugs (neuroleptics) are the most consistently implicated.[4] Ohayon and associates[5] questionnaire study of 13,057 subjects in Europe reported an increased odds ratio for bruxism of 1.8 for heavy drinkers, 1.4 for smokers, and 1.3 for caffeine uses.

Bruxism has been reported in a wide variety of neurologic diseases including seizures,[28] coma, and movement disorders such as parkinsonism, Huntington's disease, and Tourette's syndrome.[3] An interview study showed a higher prevalence of bruxism in restless legs syndrome patients.[29] Bruxism has been reported as an associated feature of a variety of parasomnias.[3]

TREATMENT

The literature on the management of bruxism is hampered by variable definitions of the outcomes measured; there are few well-done randomized controlled trials (RCTs) and multiple types of therapies. No known curative treatment exists and clinicians approaching the care of patients need to be clear as to goals of therapy. Sleep disruption is uncommon[17] with bruxism and is not generally considered a primary target of therapy. On the other hand, consequences of bruxism such as tooth grinding noise (often a problem for the sleep partner), tooth wear, and jaw muscle and joint symptoms (e.g., temporomandibular pain, masseter pain and hypertrophy, early morning temporal headaches, and stiffness) prompt patients to seek therapy.[30]

Treatment modalities are divided into three main categories: (1) dental occlusive therapies that encompass both use of a wide variety of appliances and permanent procedural interventions, (2) pharmacologic interventions, and (3) behavioral treatments such as biofeedback using aversive methods. Lobbezoo and colleagues[31] point out that the trends in therapy have evolved from the 1960s, with early studies focusing on behavioral therapies and later ones on occlusal and pharmacologic modalities.

Mild bruxism is widespread in the normal population and does not generally need treatment unless the dentist sees the beginnings of damage to the masticatory system. For those patients with more moderate or severe bruxism, the three principle approaches just mentioned have been tried and are discussed next.

Occlusal Interventions

These interventions can be divided into permanent or true occlusal interventions and the use of occlusal appliances.

Permanent Interventions

A wide variety of procedures have been described but none has demonstrated efficacy in well-done studies. So-called *occlusal equilibrium, rehabilitation,* and *orthodontic therapies* have been touted since 1970[32] but have been questioned as to their efficacy.[33] Lobbezoo and associates[31] could find only one RCT on buccal separator therapy (an orthodontic technique).[34] That study evaluated 21 patients with bruxism treated with either a separator, placebo (separator initially placed but immediately removed), or nothing. All three groups were monitored with a 12-item questionnaire, physical examination, and EMG. No significant differences were found in any of the modalities measured in any group.

These therapies are irreversible and are not recommended by experts.[35,36] Based on the scant literature and lack of evidence suggesting efficacy, permanent occlusal intervention is not recommended.

Oral Appliances

Oral appliances typically include soft mouth guards and a variety of hard occlusal splints[31] (Fig. 25-3). More recently, MAAs designed to treat snoring and sleep apnea have also been tried in patients with SB.[25,37] Soft mouth guards are generally only used for a short time because they degrade. Most studies focus on hard occlusal splints (see Fig. 25-3). These devices can prevent or limit dental damage in patients with bruxism and are widely used for that purpose. However, whether they are

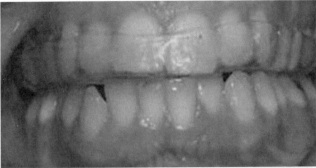
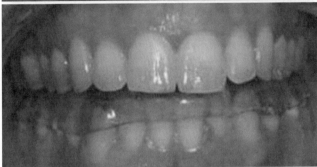

Figure 25-3 Image showing hard acrylic occlusal splints on the upper and lower teeth.

useful to treat bruxism itself is not clear. Here the literature is particularly difficult to analyze because of the wide variety of devices available to dentists.

The Cochrane Collaboration published a comprehensive review of the utility of occlusal splints for the treatment of bruxism.[38] They found 32 potentially relevant RCTs but only five that could be used in meta-analysis. This study analyzed the efficacy of occlusal splints as compared to no treatment, pharmacologic therapies, behavioral therapy, and other types of appliances such as a palatal splint. The primary endpoint analyzed was arousal index. They concluded that "the evidence is insufficient for affirming that the occlusal splint is effective for treating sleep bruxism." Huynh and associates[39] used another method of assessing efficacy and analyzed studies comparing the number needed to treat (NNT). They conclude that occlusal splints, MAAs, and clonidine (see later discussion) are effective therapies. This paper uses a bruxism index to evaluate efficacy, as opposed to the arousal index used by Cochrane, and thus these are not comparable analyses.

Klasser and Greene[40] reviewed this subject recently as well. They point out that observational studies suggest that occlusal splints are effective in reducing sleep muscle activity as measured by EMG, but that this activity returns to baseline once the devices are not used, indicating that they have no lasting impact on SB itself. Moreover, there may be individual variation and in some patients increased EMG activity is noted with occlusal splints in place.[37,41] Klasser makes the point that occlusal splints are analogous to crutches in orthopedic injuries in preventing dental damage and pain, but that their utility in treating bruxism must be reconsidered.

MAAs have been studied in SB patients with and without sleep apnea.[25,37] In a short-term crossover randomized controlled study of 12 patients comparing custom-made MAA with an occlusal splint as the active control arm, the MAA significantly decreased the number of SB episodes per hour but this improvement was not significantly different than the occlusal splint, and the MAA was less well tolerated.[37] A similar study in patients without sleep apnea using a "boil and bite" MAA showed comparable improvement in SB episodes. Therefore, MAA devices appear to be effective in reducing bruxism but have not been tried in long-term studies and may not be well tolerated.[25] These devices may be particularly appropriate in patients who require treatment for both sleep apnea and bruxism, but further studies are necessary. On the other hand, one study showed worsening of respiratory measures in sleep apnea patients using a standard occlusal splint for bruxism.[42] Of note, positive airway pressure has been reported to improve bruxism in a patient with sleep apnea in a single case report.[43]

In summary, there is consensus opinion that oral devices limit and prevent teeth damage.[31] However, there is no conclusive evidence that oral devices are effective in treating the spectrum of clinical symptoms and signs associated with SB.

Pharmacologic Interventions

With the understanding that central mechanisms may be involved in the pathogenesis of bruxism,[31,19] the use of pharmacologic treatments to treat the underlying cause of bruxism has emerged in the past decade. Again, as with occlusal therapies, most studies are case reports, with only a few well conducted RCTs. Winocur and associates[4] wrote a critical review of drug therapy in 2003 and concluded that there were insufficient evidence- based studies on which to base a firm conclusion as to efficacy of any specific treatment.

Huynh and associates[39] reviewed data from trials with bromocriptine, propranolol, clonidine, L-dopa, amitriptyline, clonazepam, and tryptophan for bruxism. All were RCTs except for the study of clonazepam, which was a single blinded study. A variety of outcomes were measured, treatment duration was short, and all studies had few subjects. Among these agents only clonidine appeared to be effective based on a calculation of NNT to benefit. Clonidine resulted in a reduction in the sleep bruxism index by 61% in one study. However, this was a short-term study and resulted in significant morning hypotension.[44] Another small study demonstrated that clonidine reduced RMMA.[45]

Muscle relaxants such as methocarbamal have been tried but have not been adequately studied using modern study designs.[31] Botulinum toxin has been reported in case reports of severe cases (such as patients with autism and Huntington's disease).[31] Tan and Jankovic[46] tried botulinum toxin injections (botulinum toxin type A [BTX-A], mean dose 61.7 ± 11.1 mouse units [MU] [range 25-100 MU] per side for the masseter muscles) in 18 patients with bruxism and, although it was effective, concluded it should be reserved for the most severe cases.

Saletu and colleagues[47] studied the effect of clonazepam in 21 patients with bruxism using a single blinded method. They demonstrated a reduction in the SB index as well as a reduction in the arousal index. Because this was a short study and was not randomized, further studies are needed to corroborate these results.

Further research into the mechanisms of SB is required before better pharmacologic therapies can be evaluated. Larger RCTs for longer periods of time are also required before any specific recommendations on pharmacologic therapy can be offered.

Behavioral Therapies

Multiple behavioral therapies have been tried in bruxism.[31] These treatments range from hypnosis to biofeedback. Relaxation techniques, meditation, and improvement in sleep hygiene have all been tried but no well-done trials exist supporting any specific intervention. Biofeedback has been most widely studied. The techniques described use mostly aversive therapies such as a sound blast or a capsule filled with an aversive substance that is released when patients clench their jaws. Vibration has also been tried. These techniques suffer from the fact that they also cause arousal from sleep, although a recent study using electric pulses to inhibit jaw muscles did not cause sleep disruption.[48]

SUMMARY

Mild bruxism does not require treatment. Moderate and severe bruxism may be treated with an occlusal splint to protect the teeth and potentially to improve orofacial pain and headache. Medications reported to exacerbate bruxism (e.g., SSRIs, SNRIs) should be reviewed for clinical necessity. Underlying sleep disorders should be considered and treated. MAA may be appropriate for patients with co-morbid sleep apnea, especially if first-line treatment with positive airway pressure has failed. At the present time there is no proven benefit to any specific pharmacologic or behavioral therapy. There is no role for permanent occlusal therapies. Further research is needed to advance the field.

REFERENCES

1. American Academy of Sleep Medicine. *The International Classification of Sleep Disorders: Diagnostic and Coding Manual.* 2nd ed. Westchester, IL: American Academy of Sleep Medicine; 2005.
2. Glaros AG. Bruxism. In: Mostofsky DI, Forgione AG, Giddon DB, eds. *Behavioral Dentistry.* Ames, IA: Blackwell; 2006:127-137.
3. Kryger MH, Roth T, Dement WC, eds. *Principles and Practice of Sleep Medicine.* 5th ed. Philadelphia: Saunders/Elsevier; 2011:1128–1139.
4. Winocur E, Gavish A, Voikovitch M, Emodi-Perlman A, Eli I. Drugs and bruxism: A critical review. *J Orofac Pain.* 2003;17(2):99-111.
5. Ohayon MM, Li KK, Guilleminault C. Risk factors for sleep bruxism in the general population. *Chest.* 2001;119(1):53-61.
6. Bruxism Graf H. *Dent Clin North Am.* 1969;13(3):659-665.
7. Mehta NR, Forgione AG, Maloney G, Greene R. Different effects of nocturnal parafunction on the masticatory system: The weak link theory. *Cranio.* 2000;18(4):280-286.
8. Park BK, Tokiwa O, Takezawa Y, Takahashi Y, Sasaguri K, Sato S. Relationship of tooth grinding pattern during sleep bruxism and temporomandibular joint status. *Cranio.* 2008;26(1):8-15.
9. Magnusson T, Egermarki I, Carlsson GE. A prospective investigation over two decades on signs and symptoms of temporomandibular disorders and associated variables. A final summary. *Acta Odontol Scand.* 2005;63(2):99-109.
10. Arnold M. Bruxism and the occlusion. *Dent Clin North Am.* 1981; 25(3):395-407.
11. Forgione AG. A simple but effective method for quantifying bruxing behavior. *J Dental Res.* 1974;53:127.
12. Pau AK, Croucher R, Marcenes W. Prevalence estimates and associated factors for dental pain: A review. *Oral Health Prev Dent.* 2003;1(3):209-220.
13. Mehta NR, Forgione AG, Rosenbaum RS, Holmberg R. "TMJ" triad of dysfunctions: A biologic basis of diagnosis and treatment. *J Mass Dent Soc.* 1984;33(4):173-176:212-213.
14. Rossetti LM, Rossetti PH, Conti PC, de Araujo Cdos R. Association between sleep bruxism and temporomandibular disorders: A polysomnographic pilot study. *Cranio.* 2008;26(1):16-24.
15. Carlsson GE, Egermark I, Magnusson T. Predictors of bruxism, other oral parafunctions, and tooth wear over a 20-year follow-up period. *J Orofac Pain.* 2003;17(1):50-57.

16. Matsumoto MA, Matsumoto W, Bolognese AM. Study of the signs and symptoms of temporomandibular dysfunction in individuals with normal occlusion and malocclusion. *Cranio.* 2002;20(4):274-281.

17. Lavigne GJ, Rompre PH, Montplaisir JY. Sleep bruxism: Validity of clinical research diagnostic criteria in a controlled polysomnographic study. *J Dent Res.* 1996;75(1):546-552.

18. Iber C, American Academy of Sleep Medicine. *The AASM Manual for the Scoring of Sleep and Associated Events: Rules, Terminology and Technical Specifications.* Westchester, IL, American Academy of Sleep Medicine. 2007.

19. Lavigne GJ, Kato T, Kolta A, Sessle BJ. Neurobiological mechanisms involved in sleep bruxism. *Crit Rev Oral Biol Med.* 2003;14(1):30-46.

20. Macaluso GM, Guerra P, Di Giovanni G, Boselli M, Parrino L, Terzano MG. Sleep bruxism is a disorder related to periodic arousals during sleep. *J Dent Res.* 1998;77(4):565-573.

21. Huynh N, Lavigne GJ, Okura K, Yao D, Adachi K. Sleep bruxism. *Handbook Clin Neurol.* 2011;99:901-911.

22. Lavigne GJ, Khoury S, Abe S, Yamaguchi T, Raphael K. Bruxism physiology and pathology: An overview for clinicians. *J Oral Rehabil.* 2008;35(7):476-494.

23. Huynh N, Kato T, Rompre PH, Okura K, Saber M, et al. Sleep bruxism is associated to micro-arousals and an increase in cardiac sympathetic activity. *J Sleep Res.* 2006;15(3):339-346.

24. Okeson JP, Phillips BA, Berry DT, Cook YR, Cabelka JF. Nocturnal bruxing events in subjects with sleep-disordered breathing and control subjects. *J Craniomandib Disord.* 1991;5(4):258-264.

25. Landry ML, Rompre PH, Manzini C, Guitard F, de Grandmont P, Lavigne GJ. Reduction of sleep bruxism using a mandibular advancement device: An experimental controlled study. *Int J Prosthodont.* 2006;19(6):549-556.

26. Miyawaki S, Lavigne GJ, Pierre M, Guitard F, Montplaisir JY, Kato T. Association between sleep bruxism, swallowing-related laryngeal movement, and sleep positions. *Sleep.* 2003;26(4):461-465:15.

27. Okeson JP, Phillips BA, Berry DT, Cook Y, Paesani D, Galante J. Nocturnal bruxing events in healthy geriatric subjects. *J Oral Rehabil.* 1990;17(5):411-418.

28. Meletti S, Cantalupo G, Volpi L, Rubboli G, Magaudda A, Tassinari CA. Rhythmic teeth grinding induced by temporal lobe seizures. *Neurology.* 2004;62(12):2306-2309.

29. Lavigne GJ, Montplaisir JY. Restless legs syndrome and sleep bruxism: Prevalence and association among Canadians. *Sleep.* 1994;17(8):739-743.

30. Kato T, Lavigne GJ. *Sleep Bruxism: A Sleep-Related Movement Disorder Sleep Medicine Clinics.* New York: Elsevier; 20109–35.

31. Lobbezoo F, van der Zaag J, van Selms MK, Hamburger HL, Naeije M. Principles for the management of bruxism. *J Oral Rehabil.* 2008;35(7):509-523.

32. Butler JH. Occlusal adjustment. *Dent Dig.* 1970;76(10):422-426.

33. Greene CS, Klasser GD, Epstein JB. "Observations" questioned. *J Am Dent Assoc.* 2005;136(7):856:858.

34. Abraham J, Pierce C, Rinchuse D, Zullo T. Assessment of buccal separators in the relief of bruxist activity associated with myofascial pain-dysfunction. *Angle Orthodont.* 1992;62(3):177-184.

35. Clark GT, Adler RC. A critical evaluation of occlusal therapy: Occlusal adjustment procedures. *J Am Dent Assoc.* 1985;110(5):743-750.

36. Okeson JP, de Kanter RJ. Temporomandibular disorders in the medical practice. *J Fam Pract.* 1996;43(4):347-356.

37. Landry-Schonbeck A, de Grandmont P, Rompre PH, Lavigne GJ. Effect of an adjustable mandibular advancement appliance on sleep bruxism: A crossover sleep laboratory study. *Int J Prosthodont.* 2009;22(3):251-259.

38. Macedo CR, Silva AB, Machado MA, Saconato H, Prado GF. Occlusal splints for treating sleep bruxism (tooth grinding). *Cochrane Database Syst Rev.* 2007:(4):CD005514.

39. Huynh N, Manzini C, Rompre PH, Lavigne GJ. Weighing the potential effectiveness of various treatments for sleep bruxism. *J Can Dent Assoc.* 2007;73(8):727-730.

40. Klasser GD, Greene CS. Role of oral appliances in the management of sleep bruxism and temporomandibular disorders. *Alpha Omegan.* 2007;100(3):111-119.

41. Clark GT, Beemsterboer PL, Solberg WK, Rugh JD. Nocturnal electromyographic evaluation of myofascial pain dysfunction in patients undergoing occlusal splint therapy. *J Am Dent Assoc.* 1979;99(4):607-611.

42. Gagnon Y, Mayer P, Morisson F, Rompre PH, Lavigne GJ. Aggravation of respiratory disturbances by the use of an occlusal splint in apneic patients: A pilot study. *Int J Prosthodont.* 2004;17(4):447-453.

43. Oksenberg A, Arons E. Sleep bruxism related to obstructive sleep apnea: The effect of continuous positive airway pressure. *Sleep Med.* 2002;3(6):513-515.

44. Huynh N, Lavigne GJ, Lanfranchi PA, Montplaisir JY, de Champlain J. The effect of 2 sympatholytic medications—propranolol and clonidine—on sleep bruxism: Experimental randomized controlled studies. *Sleep.* 2006;29(3):307-316.

45. Carra MC, Macaluso GM, Rompre PH, Huynh N, Parrino L, et al. Clonidine has a paradoxical effect on cyclic arousal and sleep bruxism during NREM sleep. *Sleep.* 2010;33(12):1711-1716.

46. Tan EK, Jankovic J. Treating severe bruxism with botulinum toxin. *J Am Dent Assoc.* 2000;131(2):211-216.

47. Saletu A, Parapatics S, Anderer P, Matejka M, Saletu B. Controlled clinical, polysomnographic and psychometric studies on differences between sleep bruxers and controls and acute effects of clonazepam as compared with placebo. *Eur Arch Psychiatry Clin Neurosci.* 2010;260(2):163-174.

48. Jadidi F, Castrillon E, Svensson P. Effect of conditioning electrical stimuli on temporalis electromyographic activity during sleep. *J Oral Rehabil.* 2008;35(3):171-183.

Chapter 26

Sleep Disorders in Parkinson's Disease and Parkinsonian Syndromes

HLYNUR GEORGSSON / BRIAN J. MURRAY

Parkinson's disease (PD) and the parkinsonian syndromes are a group of chronic, progressive neurodegenerative diseases affecting approximately 1% of those older than 60 years.[1] In PD degeneration of dopamine neurons, most prominently in the substantia nigra (SN) of the brainstem, is recognized as a characteristic pathologic finding; dopamine replacement has been the standard therapy. Deterioration of nondopaminergic pathways is now recognized as contributing greatly to these disorders, especially the nonmotor symptoms such as neuropsychiatric problems, dysautonomia, fatigue, and sleep disorders.[2]

In *An Essay on the Shaking Palsy*, written in 1817, James Parkinson described most of the features of the disease we still recognize today. These features include resting tremor, rigidity, bradykinesia, and gait disturbance. In addition to the motor symptoms, he also described cases of sleep disturbance: "…the sleep becomes much disturbed. The tremulous motion of the limbs occur during sleep, and augment until they awaken the patient, and frequently with much agitation and alarm."[3] Parkinson also noted the consequences of this sleep disruption, "…constant sleepiness, with slight delirium, and other marks of extreme exhaustion."[3]

PD patients are indeed susceptible to a variety of sleep problems, whether related to disease-specific symptoms and co-morbidities, sleep disorders related to neurodegeneration of pathways involved in sleep regulation, or treatment side effects. These associations are being increasingly appreciated as major targets for improving quality of life. Understanding sleep changes in PD is also helping us better understand the neurobiology of the condition.

Recent evidence suggests that deterioration of nondopaminergic pathways may in fact occur earlier in the course of PD than deterioration of dopaminergic systems, and that associated sleep disorders may predate the appearance of classic PD motor symptoms.[4,5] This realization is especially important in relation to the ongoing search for neuroprotective therapies that could hypothetically be instituted many years prior to the onset of overt motor symptoms and thus delay clinical PD.[6]

DEFINITIONS

Parkinson's Disease

PD is a chronic, progressive neurodegenerative disease of unknown etiology most commonly diagnosed in the elderly. The cardinal symptoms of PD (resting tremor, rigidity, bradykinesia, and gait disturbance) can be traced to dopamine depletion in the SN and the resulting dysfunction of striatonigral pathways of the basal ganglia.[7,8] This group of symptoms is referred to as *parkinsonism*, but also occurs in disorders other than PD. A majority of PD patients also develop a variety of characteristic symptoms (Box 26-1) such as dysautonomia, dementia, and sleep disorders, which, in advanced disease, often cause much greater disability than the classical motor symptoms.[9]

Motor symptoms of PD are treated with oral dopaminergic drugs. As the disease progresses it becomes increasingly difficult to maintain appropriate drug effect throughout the day. This leads to two types of motor complications referred to as *on-off phenomenon* and *dyskinesias*. "On-off" refers to the unpredictable and dramatic motor responses that rise and fall with each dose. Dyskinesias describe involuntary movements aside from tremor that advanced PD patients may experience with relatively higher levodopa concentrations. These motor complications affect up to 90% of PD patients after 5 to 10 years of levodopa (L-dopa) therapy and cause considerable disability.[4]

Parkinson Plus Syndromes

In addition to PD, there are a number of less common but clinically related disorders referred to as the *parkinson plus* or *parkinsonian plus syndromes (P+)*, which possess elements of parkinsonism but have other characteristic features (Table 26-1). These features include dementia with Lewy bodies (DLB), corticobasal degeneration (CBD), multiple system atrophy (MSA), progressive supranuclear palsy (PSP), and other disorders. The similarities of these syndromes to PD, especially in early stages of disease, can make accurate diagnosis difficult.

In general, the most helpful signs for distinguishing between PD and P+, and which should lead one to consider a diagnosis other than PD, are: (1) symmetry of signs at onset, (2) absence of resting tremor, and (3) absence of response to levodopa (L-dopa), The presence of dysautonomia and prominent falls early in the disease, as well as rapid progression of symptoms, are atypical for PD and should raise concern for a P+ disease.[10,11] A period of clinical observation and follow-up is usually required before making a diagnosis, and even so, autopsy studies have shown that PD diagnoses are incorrect in about a quarter of cases.[12] Patients who demonstrate rapid eye movement (REM) sleep behavior disorder (RBD) (see Chapter 43) tend to have synuclein-based pathology,[13] such as PD and MSA, in contrast to other degenerative conditions associated with prominent tau pathology such as progressive supranuclear palsy or CBD.

Dementia with Lewy Bodies

DLB is the second most common cause of neurodegenerative dementia after Alzheimer's disease. DLB is characterized by dementia with fluctuating cognition, prominent visual hallucinations, parkinsonism, RBD, falls, and autonomic dysfunction. Importantly, DLB patients are exquisitely sensitive to neuroleptic medications; these drugs can significantly worsen symptoms and should be avoided. Despite the fact that approximately 40% of PD patients also eventually develop dementia, clinical differentiation between PD and DLB is often possible by considering the timing of dementia onset, with DLB motor symptoms usually occurring after cognitive impairment becomes obvious.[11,14]

Multiple System Atrophy

MSA is the term for a set of syndromes previously known separately as *olivopontocerebellar atrophy, striatonigral degeneration,* and *Shy-Drager syndrome.* In addition to asymmetrical parkinsonism, MSA commonly presents with varying degrees of dysautonomia, cerebellar involvement, and pyramidal signs, although these can be subtle in early disease. A relative lack of cognitive decline and a poorly sustained response to levodopa are also associated features.[15] MSA shares with PD an association with RBD and sleep-disordered breathing. Uniquely, some MSA patients may demonstrate life-threatening diurnal and nocturnal stridor secondary to degeneration of brainstem nuclei controlling laryngeal function.[16]

Corticobasal Degeneration

CBD is a rare, sporadic parkinsonian disorder that resembles PD clinically in that it can present with asymmetrical parkinsonism including bradykinesia, postural instability, and prominent limb rigidity.[17] Characteristic cortical features such as alien limb phenomenon (involuntary movements of an arm typically of which the patient is unaware), aphasia, and apraxia should raise suspicion of this disorder. A distinct rhythmic type of myoclonus (a sudden, brief, jerk-like, involuntary movement) is present in about half of CBD patients, occurring unilaterally in an affected arm more commonly than in a leg. This myoclonus is activated by movement or in reaction to somatosensory stimulation, suggesting a cortical origin.[18]

Progressive Supranuclear Palsy

Also known as *Steele-Richardson-Olszewski syndrome,* this disorder is typically a more rapidly progressive parkinsonian syndrome that presents with symmetrical bradykinesia and rigidity, but rarely with tremor.[19] Distinctive, but not invariant, features are a supranuclear vertical gaze palsy and prominent postural instability with unexplained backward falls early in the disease course. A characteristic wide-eyed appearance accompanies the gaze palsy. Pseudobulbar palsy develops in a majority of patients, with dysphagia and a spastic dysarthria.

BOX 26-1 *Manifestations of Parkinson's Disease Aside from Traditional Motor Dysfunction*

Sleep Complaints and Disorders
Excessive daytime sleepiness
Insomnia
Restless legs syndrome and periodic limb movements
Sleep-disordered breathing
Parasomnias: nightmares, vivid dreams
Rapid eye movement (REM) sleep behavior disorder (RBD)

Sensory Symptoms
Pain
Olfactory disturbance
Visual changes—blurring, contrast, color vision
Ageusia—loss of taste

Autonomic Symptoms
Orthostatic hypotension
Hyperhydrosis, hypersalivation
Seborrhea
Dry eyes
Nausea, reflux, vomiting
Dysphagia, choking
Constipation, fecal incontinence
Urinary disturbances: urgency, frequency, nocturia
Sexual dysfunction
Hypersexuality (dopaminergic drug effect)

Neuropsychiatric Symptoms
Cognitive impairment and dementia
Anhedonia, depression, apathy, anxiety
Hallucinations, illusions, delusions
Impulse control disorders (dopaminergic drug effect)

Modified from Chaudhuri KR, Schapira AH. Non-motor symptoms of Parkinson's disease: dopaminergic pathophysiology and treatment. *Lancet Neurol.* 2009;8:464-474.

TABLE 26-1

Major Parkinsonian Syndromes

Syndrome	Classic Features	Synucleinopathy?
Dementia with Lewy bodies	Dementia, hallucinations, fluctuations, RBD	Yes
Corticobasal degeneration	Alien limb phenomenon, cortical features such as aphasia and apraxia, myoclonus	No
Multiple system atrophy	Autonomic dysfunction, cerebellar involvement, pyramidal weakness, nocturnal and/or diurnal stridor, RBD	Yes
Progressive supranuclear palsy	Restricted vertical gaze, dysarthria, dysphagia, dementia, falls	No
Parkinsonism associated with other neurodegenerative disorders	Late-stage Alzheimer's and Huntington's disease presentations, frontotemporal dementia with parkinsonism linked to chromosome 17, spinocerebellar ataxia with prominent ataxia symptoms	No
Vascular parkinsonism	"Lower-half" parkinsonism with prominent gait difficulties, sudden onset	No

RBD, rapid eye movement sleep behavior disorder.
Modified from Lang AE, Lozano AM. Parkinson's disease. First of two parts. *N Engl J Med.* 1998;339:1044-1053.

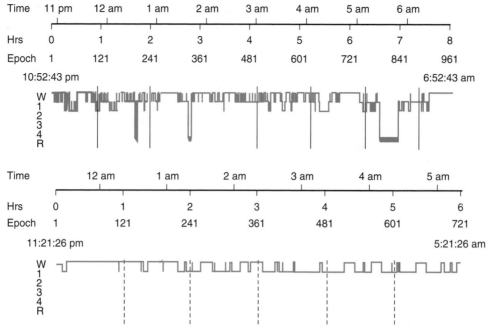

Figure 26-1 Hypnograms of patients with advanced parkinsonism showing marked sleep fragmentation with frequent awakenings.

RBD is rarely seen in these patients. Neuropsychiatric problems are common and many suffer from a frontal dementia before succumbing to the disease, usually within 10 years of identifiable disease onset. Response to levodopa is poor.[20,21]

Other Neurodegenerative Disorders

Parkinsonism can be a feature of various other neurodegenerative diseases including late-stage Alzheimer's and Huntington's disease. Other rare conditions include frontotemporal dementia with parkinsonism linked to chromosome 17 (FTDP-17) and the spinocerebellar ataxias.[14] Parkinsonism may also be seen with vascular disease of the brain. This "lower-half" parkinsonism is characterized by prominent gait disturbance, sometimes of sudden onset, and is poorly responsive to levodopa. Neuroimaging in this case will reveal evidence of cerebral ischemia.[22]

EPIDEMIOLOGY OF PARKINSON'S DISEASE

PD is the second most common neurodegenerative disease after Alzheimer's disease, with an estimated prevalence in industrialized countries of 0.3%. PD is rare before age 50 years, but its prevalence increases with age, reaching 1% and higher in people over 60 years of age. Several causative monogenetic mutations have been described, but known familial cases account for only a minority of cases. The remaining 90% of cases are sporadic and most likely result from the interplay of as-yet undiscovered genetic susceptibility loci and unknown environmental factors.[1]

SLEEP COMPLAINTS IN PARKINSON'S DISEASE AND RELATED SYNDROMES

Sleep disturbances and excessive daytime sleepiness (EDS) are very common in PD and their prevalence correlates with disease severity, use of PD medications, and depression.[23]

Nearly all PD patients (98%) have nocturnal symptoms that can disrupt sleep and lead to fatigue and sleepiness during the day.[24] In one community-based prevalence study, 44% of PD patients reported feeling excessive daytime fatigue compared to 18% of healthy elderly control subjects.[25]

Sleep disturbances in PD can arise from a variety of causes including the disease itself and treatment-related factors, physiologic alterations in circadian rhythms, changes in sleep architecture associated with advancing age, dementia or depression, and increased prevalence of primary sleep disorders such as restless legs syndrome (RLS) (see Chapter 24) and RBD (see Chapter 43).[26]

Approximately two thirds of PD patients report some form of sleep fragmentation while at least a quarter have clinically overt sleep disorders.[27] In one community-based survey the reported prevalence of sleep symptoms among PD patients (60%) was significantly higher than in control groups of diabetic patients (46%) and healthy elderly control subjects (33%). Also, frequent (38.9%) or early (23.4%) awakenings were twice as common in PD patients as in other groups.[28] Affected PD patients typically report two to five nighttime awakenings (twice the rate in control subjects), which keep them awake for an average of 30% to 40% of the night (Fig. 26-1). Altered dreams were prevalent in one study of PD (48%) and were associated with sleep fragmentation and hallucinations.[29] RBD, a disorder in which the normal atonia of REM sleep is lost and patients subsequently enact dreams, is common in PD and may antedate motor symptoms by many years.[30] This condition is present in 15% to 60% of patients with PD and is seen in even greater prevalence in other neurodegenerative synucleinopathies such as DLB (86%) and MSA (90%).[31]

Sleep difficulties contribute to the increased use of hypnotics, which PD patients use substantially more than the general elderly population.[23] Hypnotic use is of particular concern in this population because these medications are associated with an increased risk of falls and cognitive impairment in the elderly.[32]

PATHOPHYSIOLOGY

Classical Pathophysiology of Parkinson's Disease

PD is characterized by the progressive loss of numerous neuronal populations along with the accumulation of intracellular inclusions known as *Lewy bodies*. These inclusions contain α-synuclein, a presumed toxic protein. Dopaminergic neurons of the SN are prominently involved and their degeneration is a neuropathologic hallmark of the disorder. This loss of neurons contributes to the overt motor symptoms of PD. Neurodegenerative changes occur in other regions of the brain even earlier and proceed in a stereotyped fashion ascending from brainstem nuclei to temporal cortex and progressing to further cortical regions.[33]

Pathophysiology of Sleep Disorders in Parkinson's Disease

Dopamine is known to have a complex role in sleep and arousal. Dopaminergic neurons in the ventral tegmental area are part of the basal ganglia-thalamocortical limbic circuitry, and project to the prefrontal cortex and striatum, thus possibly regulating arousal.[34] More recent evidence points to dopaminergic cells in the ventral periaqueductal gray matter of rats as having extensive connections with the sleep-wake regulatory systems.[35]

Degeneration of nondopaminergic pathways in various areas of the brainstem and basal ganglia have been recognized as integral to PD. These areas include the cholinergic nucleus basalis of Meynert and pedunculopontine nucleus (PPN), noradrenergic neurons in the locus ceruleus, serotoninergic neurons in the raphe, and orexinergic neurons in the hypothalamus.[31] Many of these pathways have been closely linked to arousal and sleep functions.

Significant overlap and interaction exist between the neuroanatomic substrates of motor and nonmotor symptoms. Pathways from key dopaminergic areas of the brain (substantia nigra pars compacta, ventral tegmental area) project extensively and thus contribute to a variety of nonmotor functions such as cognition, arousal, and pain.[35,36] In addition, positron emission tomography (PET) scan evidence in PD demonstrates dopaminergic dysfunction in the hypothalamus, an area that contains key regulatory centers for many nonmotor modalities such as sleep, endocrine, and autonomic function.[37]

RBD is closely linked to PD and other synucleinopathic neurodegenerative diseases. Using animal model studies in rats[38] and cats[39] as well as neuroimaging data from the few published human cases of RBD associated with structural lesions in the brainstem, Boeve and associates[13] have recently summarized anatomic considerations in RBD.

The orexin/hypocretin system, which is known to be abnormal in narcolepsy (see Chapter 22), has been implicated as a possible cause of daytime sleepiness in PD. A recent study by Siegel and colleagues[40] demonstrates reduced hypocretin neurons in the hypothalamus of PD brains. This finding correlated with disease severity and

may account for some of the profound sleepiness seen in advanced PD.[40]

The brainstem PPN, a region that promotes REM sleep, is relevant in linking PD to sleep/arousal mechanisms. This nucleus receives widespread inputs from the subthalamic nucleus (STN) and globus pallidus interna (GPi), which are heavily affected by PD, and projects to the SN and thalamus via cholinergic pathways, which are themselves affected early in the neuropathologic course of PD.[23]

TREATMENT OF PARKINSON'S DISEASE

Levodopa/Carbidopa

L-dopa, a precursor of dopamine, was introduced for the treatment of PD more than 40 years ago and is still the mainstay of treatment. It acts by replacing deficient dopamine in the striatum. Because L-dopa can cross the blood-brain barrier and dopamine cannot, L-dopa is coadministered with a peripheral decarboxylase inhibitor (either carbidopa or benserazide) to prevent peripheral conversion of L-dopa to dopamine. This combination reduces peripheral dopamine side effects and maximizes central nervous system (CNS) L-dopa availability. Catechol-*O*-methyltransferase (COMT) or monoamine oxidase B (MAO-B) inhibitors (see later discussion) can be administered separately and act by further impeding L-dopa or dopamine catabolism, thus prolonging the therapeutic effect.

In addition to the common side effects of nausea and postural hypotension, long-term L-dopa therapy is often associated with the development of motor fluctuations and dyskinesias. These complications affect up to half of all patients within 5 years of treatment. Younger PD patients are especially prone to develop dyskinesias and thus treatment is often delayed or a dopamine agonist in used in this population.[41,42] Controversy persists regarding whether L-dopa is actually toxic, and some have wondered whether dopaminergic agonists may have a similar problem at comparable clinically effective doses.

It is important to match the level of therapy to the patient's need. A careful log of patient complaints relative to dosing timing is helpful for titrating the optimal dopaminergic load and schedule for each patient. This scheduling is especially crucial for patients experiencing disruptive nighttime symptoms. For best absorption, L-dopa should not be taken with high-protein foods, which limits timing options.[43]

Dopamine Agonists

Nonergot dopaminergic agonists (DAs), such as ropinirole, and pramipexole, are commonly used as L-dopa–sparing strategies. Although dopamine agonists may have less potency than L-dopa, DAs can be used in early PD to effectively delay the clinical need for levodopa therapy given the possibility of L-dopa toxicity in chronic use. Therefore, the direct dopamine agonists may play a role in delaying some of the inevitable motor complications that develop with chronic L-dopa use. This strategy is appropriate in younger cognitively intact PD patients who are less prone to the neuropsychiatric side effects of DAs such as hallucinations and vivid dreams. In older patients, DAs may be slowly titrated as tolerated as an adjunct to L-dopa to provide more consistent dopaminergic stimulation.[4]

These drugs will be familiar to the sleep clinician because they are also used for the treatment of RLS, though the dosage in PD is typically much higher than that typically used in the management of RLS—up to an order of magnitude greater.[44] The ergot-derived dopamine agonists bromocriptine and pergolide are no longer used because of serious side effects, including pleuropulmonary and cardiac valvular fibrosis.[45] DA therapy, particularly at higher doses, is occasionally associated with an increased risk of impulse control disorders such as pathologic gambling and compulsive sexual behavior. DAs have also been linked to unintended sleep episodes in PD patients, though many of these patients were sleepy to begin with and become sleepier still with a variety of medications used to treat PD.[46-48]

Catechol-*O*-methyltransferase Inhibitors

Despite peripheral blockade by coadministration of carbidopa, only about 5% to 10% of oral L-dopa reaches the brain. COMT inhibitors further prolong the plasma half-life of L-dopa by blocking another important catabolic pathway of L-dopa, mainly peripherally. These agents become especially helpful in more advanced disease when prominent motor fluctuations call for more consistent drug levels in the CNS.[49] Entacapone is the first-line agent for this purpose and is administered orally with each L-dopa dose. Tolcapone, while considerably more potent, now requires strict laboratory monitoring and is reserved only for exceptional situations given its association with severe hepatic toxicity.[50]

Monoamine Oxidase B Inhibitors

MAO-B inhibitors act centrally, by blocking the oxidation of dopamine in the synapse. In addition to mild symptomatic benefit, these agents (especially rasagiline) are thought to possess neuroprotective effects unrelated to their primary mechanism of action. Although this effect is controversial, these agents are often started early in the course of PD. Selegiline is given once or twice daily, avoiding doses later than noon due to the possible sleep-disrupting effects of its amphetamine metabolites. The more potent and MAO-B–specific rasagiline does not produce amphetamine metabolites and is undergoing trials designed specifically to ascertain its neuroprotective profile.[4,51]

Anticholinergics

Cholinergic drugs exacerbate and anticholinergic drugs improve parkinsonian symptoms. Although anticholinergics are helpful for tremor-predominant parkinsonism in younger patients, side effects (memory impairment, confusion, and hallucinations) limit anticholinergic use in elderly or cognitively impaired persons.[52]

Amantadine

Amantadine is an antiviral agent with mild antiparkinsonian activity. It increases dopamine release, inhibits dopamine reuptake, and stimulates dopamine receptors by an unknown mechanism. It antagonizes *N*-methyl-D-aspartic acid (NMDA) receptors and may also exert central anticholinergic effects. Amantadine is more effective than anticholinergic drugs for kinesis and rigidity and is generally better tolerated. Its effects, however, are transient in some patients. It is best used as short-term monotherapy in mild disease but may also temporarily reduce motor complications when added to L-dopa in advanced disease.[52] The medication can be associated with significant neuropsychiatric disturbances, particularly in the context of drug interactions.

Deep Brain Stimulation

There has been a recent revitalized interest in surgical treatments for advanced PD. Building on neurosurgical advances (stereotactic procedures, microelectrode recording techniques) and an improved understanding of the basal ganglia, deep brain stimulation (DBS) through surgical implantation of electrodes has emerged as a potent and relatively safe treatment for advanced PD.

Current common sites of stimulation, ventral intermediate (VIM) thalamic nucleus, GPi, and STN, mirror the sites of the early ablative surgeries for PD. DBS has demonstrated equal potency without the irreversible collateral damage common with surgical ablation. The STN is currently the most widely targeted site of stimulation. STN stimulation has been demonstrated to improve most features of PD. Numerous studies have noted consistent and sustained motor improvements with STN DBS, including a reduction in dyskinesia, daily off-periods, and L-dopa requirements, all in the range of 56% to 70%.[53]

DBS of the STN has also been shown to substantially decrease nocturnal motor symptoms and sleep fragmentation, improving total sleep time and sleep architecture.[54] One study (10 patients) showed that nighttime akinesia was reduced by 60% and early morning dystonia was completely suppressed during DBS. Total sleep time increased by 47% when stimulation was "on" compared to "off." However, periodic limb movements and RBD are not improved.[55] Daytime sleepiness remains problematic despite a significant reduction in dopaminergic medications.[56]

Other promising novel stimulation sites, including the PPN, are being evaluated.[4] A study of patients undergoing unilateral PPN stimulation showed a near doubling of nocturnal REM sleep between the DBS "off" and DBS "on" states, suggesting that DBS of specific regions can selectively modulate human sleep.[57] Fortunately, cataplexy has not been noted with this treatment, which was a concern given the possibility of inducing REM-like atonia during waking hours.

CLASSIFICATION OF SLEEP DISORDERS IN PARKINSON'S DISEASE

Motor Symptoms

The phenomenon of nocturnal akathisia, which often accompanies bradykinesia and stiffness in PD, is often due to underdosage or wearing-off of dopaminergic therapy. It is characterized by a subjective sensation of restlessness causing an urge for repetitive movement. However, this disorder differs from RLS in that it can occur at any time of day and is often not relieved by movement. Similar symptoms may occur as a side effect of neuroleptic medications.[4,58]

PD patients may experience marked fluctuations in their motor symptoms over the course of the day, especially as their disease becomes more advanced. These fluctuations can be especially pronounced and troublesome during the night, as the effects of medications wear off. Motor symptoms during the night can be manifest as slowed movements, difficulties turning in bed, nocturnal and early morning dystonia, and pain, as well as tremor and cramps, and result in frequent awakenings, most commonly in the lighter stages of sleep. The number of awakenings and sleep latency increase proportionally with the severity of daytime parkinsonian symptoms.[58,59]

The tremor of PD typically disappears with progression of sleep but may reappear with arousals, movements, and sleep stage changes including the onset/offset of REM and during phasic bursts of REM. When tremor is present, the amplitude is reduced. Tremor is typically absent during delta and tonic REM sleep, but can nonetheless cause considerable sleep disruption.[58]

Sleep benefit (SB), coined by Marsden and colleagues[60] in 1981, refers to the phenomenon in PD of transiently lessened disability upon waking from sleep in the morning. Between 33% and 55% of PD patients experience this sleep-related improvement in symptoms, typically lasting from 0.5 to 3 hours, often allowing patients to skip or delay their first morning medication dose.[61-63] Studies have shown inconsistent results as to what subset of patients is likely to experience sleep benefit. The SB phenomenon does not seem to relate to any evident sleep, disease, or treatment variable.[64]

Co-Morbid Nonmotor Symptoms

PD patients experience a wide array of nonmotor symptoms (NMS) (see Box 26-1). These nonmotor symptoms become increasingly debilitating as the disease progresses, typically more so than even the motor complications. For example, neuropsychiatric complications of PD such as delirium/dementia and hallucinations are the leading cause of institutionalization among PD patients.[65]

Depression is very common in PD, even more so than in other chronic disabling diseases.[66] Approximately 40% of PD patients experience depression over the course of their disease, with both exogenous as well as endogenous disease-related factors involved.[4] Depression has a well-known association with insomnia in otherwise healthy adults and has also been shown to correlate significantly with sleep disorders in PD patients.[67] Depression is likely a further contributing factor to excessive daytime sleepiness and fatigue.[68]

Early morning awakening is typically considered a marker of depression and is often prominent in elderly patients with depression, as aging is associated with an advanced sleep phase. However, sleep-disordered breathing may also manifest with early morning awakening due to the worsening of sleep apnea in REM sleep, which is more common in the early morning. Depression is sometimes suspected on polysomnography when a reduced REM latency is observed.[69]

Conservative estimates put the frequency of *dementia* in PD at 30% to 60%, and the presence of dementia predicts the presence of other neuropsychiatric problems such as depression (58%), apathy (54%), anxiety (49%), and hallucinations (44%).[70,71] These features all correlate with sleep disruption in PD. Indeed, one study found that 82% of PD patients with hallucinations also experienced sleep disturbances.[4,29] Polysomnography can help distinguish between depression and dementia in older adults, as the latter show reductions in REM sleep proportional to the degree of cognitive impairment, and the former shows increased REM sleep.[69]

Hallucinations in PD are typically visual, nonthreatening images of a familiar person or animal. Patients are usually aware that what they are witnessing is a hallucination, although this insight is often lost with progressing disease, at which point more frank psychosis may also become evident.[4] The onset of hallucinations early in the course of PD, or a sensitivity to this complication of levodopa treatment, is predictive for the subsequent development of dementia.[72] Dopaminergic drugs may improve RBD symptoms, though they frequently exacerbate vivid dreams and hallucinations in PD patients.[4] In fact, dopaminergic therapy is likely the major modifiable cause of altered dreams and hallucinations in PD. This effect was demonstrated by Sharf and associates,[73] who found that the new onset of vivid dreams (23%) and nightmares (6%) in a group of 88 PD patients correlated with the duration of chronic L-dopa therapy but not to age or severity of disease. Hallucinations and dream phenomena have been clearly associated with sleep fragmentation[29] and may herald the future development of RBD.[58,74] Indeed, PD patients with RBD have a threefold higher frequency of hallucinations than do PD patients without RBD.[31,75] Furthermore, some have considered whether the hallucinations in PD represent intrusions of REM sleep into wakefulness, similar to the hypnagogic hallucinations of narcolepsy.[76]

EDS is common in PD. One study showed EDS in 76% of PD patients assessed using the Epworth Sleepiness Scale (ESS) versus 47% of age-matched control subjects. A quarter of these PD patients had serious EDS, with ESS scores judged to be in the range of those seen in narcolepsy.[77] This degree of sleepiness could be related to the loss of orexin neurons in PD, similar to that seen in narcolepsy.[40]

The multiple sleep latency test (MSLT) is used to objectively measure sleepiness. Patients who are truly sleepy will show reduced sleep latency (< 10 minutes), and may demonstrate sleep-onset REM periods (SOREMPS), or the onset of REM sleep within 15 minutes of falling asleep.[78] Although sleep studies have indicated that PD patients sleep just over half the number of hours that are typically required, evaluations of daytime sleepiness using MSLT in 27 PD patients did not correlate with the quantity or quality of the previous night's sleep. This finding suggests that daytime sleepiness may in part be a specific feature of PD itself rather than simply a function of impaired nocturnal sleep.[79] Arnulf and associates[106] has shown that routine polysomnography and MSLT of PD patients reveals significant sleep pathology that may account for daytime sleepiness: a 15% prevalence of periodic limb movements, 20% prevalence of obstructive sleep apnea (OSA), and 40% prevalence of "secondary narcolepsy."[80] The mean sleep latency was less than 5 minutes in 37% of a separate study of 30 patients with PD, though sleep onset REM periods were not seen.[81]

Nocturia is often cited as the most common nonmotor cause of sleep disturbance in PD reported by up to 80% of patients.[24] Although PD-related dysautonomia is likely a factor, the contribution of the diuretic and arousing effects of sleep-disordered breathing must also be recognized and dealt with accordingly.[82]

Treatment-Related Side Effects

Dopamine has a complex role in sleep and arousal, and dopaminergic therapies for PD have dose-dependent side effects. Dopamine agonists can have biphasic effects on arousal, with sleep-disrupting effects during the night and sedative properties during the day. Indeed, attention has recently focused on the possible role of dopamine agonists in the exacerbation of EDS. A paper from 1999 of eight PD patients reported that extreme EDS in patients taking certain dopamine agonists was associated with "sleep attacks" or unintended sleep episodes while driving.[46] A subsequent controlled study of 100 consecutive PD patients found that 21% had experienced unintended sleep episodes while driving, compared to 6% of age-matched control subjects.[77] However, those who had experienced sleep episodes had a daily dopaminergic load almost twice that of patients who had not, with all dopaminergics including L-dopa being implicated.

To what degree dopaminergic drugs contribute to the phenomenon of general EDS is still debated. An 8-year longitudinal study showed a steady increase in the rate of EDS in PD patients (from 5.6% at baseline to 22.5% at 4 years and 44.9% at 8 years) irrespective of whether they were on DA therapy or not.[83] Another study showed that the combination of L-dopa and dopamine agonist had little effect on MSLT scores compared to those on L-dopa alone.[84] These results indicate that factors other than dopaminergic treatment are involved in the mechanism of EDS in PD patients.

Many patients with PD and depression are treated with antidepressant medication. Selective serotonin reuptake inhibitors (SSRIs) are effective antidepressants but are also alerting agents that may cause arousal. Antidepressants, especially SSRIs and serotonin-norepinephrine reuptake inhibitors (SNRIs), can also induce or worsen RBD and RLS.[85]

Nocturia is sometimes treated with anticholinergic agents that can cause or aggravate hallucinations and nightmares in PD patients.

Selegiline, an MAO-B inhibitor with amphetamine metabolites, and amantadine have stimulatory effects and may contribute to insomnia. They should be avoided after noon, particularly in patients with prominent sleep initiation or maintenance insomnia.[4]

Common Primary Sleep Disorders

Patients with PD may have coincidental common sleep disorders that require treatment just as they would without the diagnosis of PD. Full details of diagnosis and management can be found in their respective chapters in this textbook. A few common and important conditions with specific relevance to PD and parkinsonian disorders are outlined here.

Parasomnias are undesirable behaviors occurring during sleep, such as vivid dreams, nightmares, hallucinations, and RBD. They are frequently seen in PD patients and may be idiopathic or occur secondary to the disease process itself or its treatment. Most prominent among these in our discussion is RBD.

RBD (see Chapter 43) was first described by Schenck and associates[86] in 1986. It is characterized by a loss of normal skeletal muscle atonia during REM sleep (Fig. 26-2), allowing patients to act out dreams through vocalizations and vigorous movements, sometimes with violently injurious consequences. A third of unselected PD patients were found to

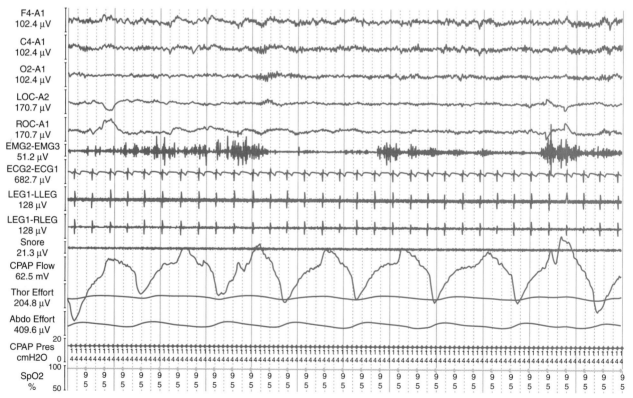

Figure 26-2 Thirty seconds of a polysomnogram (PSG) demonstrating elevated axial phasic motor tone in rapid eye movement (REM) sleep, consistent with REM sleep behavior disorder (RBD).

have RBD on polysomnography in one study.[87] RBD is closely associated with PD and other synucleinopathies (MSA, DLB), but also often predates onset of clinical symptoms.[31] One study found that close to 40% of men with idiopathic RBD were later diagnosed with a parkinsonian disorder with a mean interval of 3.7 ± 1.4 (standard deviation [SD]) years from the time of diagnosis of RBD and 12.7 ± 7.3 years from the time of onset of RBD symptoms. Follow-up suggests that the percentage of patients who go on to develop a parkinsonian disorder is even higher over time.[30,88]

The prospect of early recognition of patients likely to develop neurodegenerative disease has sparked interest among researchers looking for neuroprotective agents. If such agents were discovered, their use could be instituted hypothetically earlier in the disease process, delaying the development of overt neurodegenerative disease.

Interestingly, motor and vocal performance in PD patients is observed to improve dramatically during RBD activity. The mechanism for this improvement is unknown but seems to represent a temporary reinstitution of the basal ganglia loop or a REM sleep-related uncoupling of the pyramidal and extrapyramidal systems.[89]

RLS (see Chapter 24) is a common disorder characterized by uncomfortable sensations in the legs (and sometimes other body parts), accompanied by an urge to move, which occurs while sedentary, worsens at night, and is improved by movement.[90] The elderly are especially prone to this disorder (at least 5-15% prevalence), with most studies showing a slightly increased prevalence among PD patients (12-20.8%), although symptoms may be masked by concurrent treatment with dopaminergic agents. Antidepressant medications and antihistamines may worsen RLS. RLS is generally of mild severity in PD patients, but can contribute especially to sleep initiation difficulties.[91-93]

Approximately 90% of patients with RLS have associated periodic leg movements of sleep (PLMS), but PLMS can also occur in isolation. The prevalence of PLMS is correlated with age but is also more common in PD. A polysomnographic study involving mildly affected PD patients with no medications showed a markedly increased PLMS arousal index (45/hour) compared to age-matched healthy control subjects (3/hour).[94]

Dysfunction of dopaminergic systems is postulated as a cause of RLS, supported by the clinical effectiveness of dopaminergic therapies. There is some debate, however, as to whether RLS in PD represents a relative deficit of dopamine stimulation during the evening and night, which would be amenable to replacement therapy, or whether excess dopamine stimulation during the day leads to a rebound phenomenon during the night, which might benefit from a more paced dopaminergic strategy during the day.[31]

Other evidence has supported the idea that brain iron deficiency (more specifically deficient iron in the SN) is a contributor to dopamine dysfunction in RLS,[95-98] given that iron is a rate-limiting step in the synthesis of dopamine and is necessary for proper dopamine transporter function. Curiously, this is in contrast to the hypothesis that primary elevation of neuronal iron could lead to neurodegeneration in PD.[99]

PD patients have a higher prevalence of *sleep-disordered breathing* than age-matched control subjects.[100] Several studies have documented respiratory problems in wakefulness in PD[58] including respiratory incoordination and abnormal tone in upper airways,[101] abnormal movements of glottic and supraglottic structures,[102] and abnormal respiratory drive.[103]

Studies of sleeping PD patients demonstrated central and obstructive apneas and episodes of hypoventilation, the severity of which was greater in patients with autonomic disturbance or more advanced disease.[104,105] A more recent study showed that 20% of unselected PD patients had moderate to severe predominantly obstructive sleep apnea on polysomnography despite a normal body mass index.[106] Another group studied 15 patients and confirmed that obstructive sleep-related breathing disorders were common in PD, though generally mild with respect to hypoxia, and that respiratory events appeared to correlate with the severity of disease.[100] It is important to identify sleep-disordered breathing, given the potential contribution to PLMS, nocturia, and daytime sleepiness,[82] and the ability to treat the problem with interventions such as continuous positive airway pressure or simple positional therapy.

DIAGNOSIS OF SLEEP PROBLEMS IN PARKINSON'S DISEASE

History

Nonmotor symptoms of PD, including sleep disorders, are often overlooked during routine neurology consultations. A report by Shulman and associates[107] demonstrated that nonmotor symptoms are not identified by neurologists in over half of consultations, and sleep disruption goes unrecognized in more than 40% of PD patients.[108]

As always, a detailed history is crucial. Information regarding the patient's general motor function, ability to turn over in bed, the presence of nocturia, the occurrence of nightmares or other parasomnias, and excessive daytime sleepiness should be assessed. The contribution of a patient's bed partner or caregiver is necessary when taking a history as the patient may be unaware, forgetful, or accustomed to his/her nighttime symptoms or arousals. Snoring and symptoms of restless legs are particularly relevant, and further clarification may be gained by the use of a sleep log, home diary, or actigraphy,[4] though this technique can be problematic in patients with movement disorders.

Circadian fluctuations are significant in this condition and a few carefully documented 24-hour logs can be extremely helpful in sorting out the effects of medication administration and napping on motor function, sleep quality, and sleepiness.

Subjective Measures

The Unified Parkinson's Disease Rating Scale[109] is a rating tool used to follow the longitudinal course of PD. It is conducted by an interviewer and evaluates three domains: (1) mentation, behavior, and mood, (2) activities of daily living, and (3) motor performance, but of 31 items only one is related to sleep. A revision has recently been proposed.[110]

Although self-reporting of sleep issues is often inherently unreliable, several questionnaires have been designed to assess for the presence of sleep disorders. The Pittsburgh Sleep Quality Index (PSQ) is a commonly used scale to detect sleep disorders, but it does not specifically address the sleep disturbances of PD such as restless legs or motor disturbances specific to PD.[111] The ESS is a self-administered questionnaire designed for the evaluation of daytime sleepiness based on the patient's estimation of the likelihood that he/she would fall asleep in eight different sedentary situations. The ESS is the most commonly used scale for subjective sleepiness, and it has been shown to correlate to some degree with the gold standard MSLT.[112] Unfortunately, sleep state misperception and sleepiness state misperception interfere with its use, and subjects may provide biased responses in various clinical scenarios, such as for the purpose of retaining driving privileges. A version modified for PD has been developed.[48]

Objective Measures

The objective tools used in sleep clinics for diagnosing sleep disorders are described elsewhere in this volume. Those most relevant to PD patients are mentioned here along with their common findings.

Polysomnography (PSG) is the gold standard for diagnosing sleep disorders and is ideal for demonstrating many of the nighttime disruptions PD patients experience but may not report. Patients often tolerate these recordings better than expected, and even severely disabled patients and patients with dementia are often able to complete overnight studies with a family member present.

As one might expect, frequent awakenings and a decreased total sleep time are the most common findings on polysomnography in PD patients. Sleep architecture is altered, showing diminished slow wave sleep (common in the elderly) and a loss of the normal REM/NREM cycling.[63,94,113] Observers have noted a reduction in the amplitude and frequency of sleep spindles and K complexes in stage N2 sleep. Tremor may be obvious on video/electromyographic recording, particularly in light sleep. Repeated blinking or blepharospasm may occur at the onset of sleep and before individual REM episodes. REMs may rarely appear during slow wave sleep,[114] consistent with state dissociation as seen in conditions such as narcolepsy. PLMS are often markedly increased. RBD may be obvious. REM sleep without atonia without behavioral correlate may also be seen and has been shown to correlate with disease severity.[115] This finding might also be helpful in confirming a suspected diagnosis of parkinsonism where clinical features are not otherwise definitive.

Interpreting a recording with an active deep brain stimulator is particularly challenging. Altered filter settings may be required when there is significant artifact. A view of the electroencephalogram (EEG) may be difficult over the stimulator leads but re-referencing to assess EEG leads not directly over the stimulator may be helpful. Review of the video and other polysomnographic variables will help clarify events and behavioral state.

OSA has polysomnographic characteristics not mentioned further here, but it is important to note the presence of inspiratory stridor, a high-pitched sound due to upper airway obstruction in the larynx, which is common in MSA.[16] This life-threatening airway obstruction was observed in 42% of unselected MSA patients in a recent polysomnographic series.[116] One polysomnographic study of 19 consecutive MSA patients demonstrated that all MSA patients tested snored and displayed RBD features and 37% had sleep apnea. Interestingly, episodes of stridor were not associated with marked hypoxia. Also, in a reversal to the norm, the mean respiratory disturbance index (RDI) was observed to be higher during NREM sleep than during REM sleep, and oxygenation was not worse during REM sleep.[116]

The MSLT is an objective measure of a patient's tendency to fall asleep when given the opportunity. It is performed during the day in a sleep laboratory and the patient is encouraged to sleep in four or five, 20-minute nap periods at 2-hour intervals. The latency to sleep and presence of REM sleep in each nap is recorded. A normal result is a sleep latency greater than10 minutes with no more than one sleep onset REM period.[78] Patients with PD have a higher daytime sleep propensity and have a higher number of sleep onset REM periods, similar to narcolepsy. This finding is particularly interesting given the presence of hallucinations in these patients.[76]

The maintenance of wakefulness test (MWT) is perhaps a better test of alertness from a face validity perspective. The patient is instructed to remain awake while sitting in a comfortable chair in a quiet, dimly lit room. Sleep stage is monitored four to five times in 20- or preferably 40-minute sessions separated by 2 hours during the day to detect whether the patient falls asleep. Improved alertness is positively correlated with sleep latency on this test.

TREATMENT OF SLEEP PROBLEMS IN PARKINSON'S DISEASE

The management of coincidental sleep disorders and RBD is reviewed elsewhere in this book (see Chapter 43). The following is a discussion of PD-specific treatment strategies for relevant sleep disorders. Commonly used medications are summarized in Table 26-2. It should be noted that the literature regarding treatment of sleep disorders in PD patients is sparse, and does not allow for a strictly evidence-based approach in most cases, though a recent review outlined existing evidence and emphasized the need for further objective studies.[117]

Motor Symptoms

A variety of PD motor symptoms may re-emerge during the night or early morning as dopaminergic drug effects wear off, causing discomfort and sleep fragmentation. Nocturnal tremor, painful rigidity, and bradykinesia or akinesia can make it difficult to get comfortable, and can hamper bed movements such as turning over. Some patients may experience nighttime dyskinesias or dystonias related to their medications.

An optimal dosing strategy will aim to maintain dopaminergic effect during the night, while avoiding the dose-dependent sleep-disrupting side effects of excessive dopaminergic stimulation. This balancing task becomes more difficult with advanced disease that requires more intensive therapy to maintain constant dopaminergic levels.

To extend nighttime antiparkinsonian efficacy, patients may benefit from bedtime dosing of a sustained-release levodopa formulation or addition of a COMT inhibitor. Patients with advanced PD may require even more sustained dopaminergic stimulation to avoid wearing-off phenomena, and subcutaneous infusion of apomorphine has been used successfully in some countries.[118] Newer developments include extended release once-daily oral formulations of ropinirole and pramipexole, and a transdermal patch of the dopamine agonist rotigotine designed to provide continuous 24-hour delivery,[4] However, rotigotine has recently been unavailable due to inconsistencies in the patch's drug delivery system.

TABLE 26-2

Commonly Used Medications in the Treatment of Parkinson's Disease

Symptoms and Signs	Category	Drug	Typical Doses
MOTOR SYMPTOMS			
	Peripheral decarboxylase inhibitor with dopamine precursor	Carbidopa-levodopa	25/100 mg, 1 or 2 tablets up to four times a day; controlled-release preparation occasionally used at bedtime: 50/200 mg
	Dopamine agonist	Pramipexole	Maximum of 1.5 mg three times a day to facilitate titration or extended-release preparations to a maximum of 4.5 mg/day
	Dopamine agonist	Ropinirole	Maximum of 8 mg three times a day to facilitate titration or extended-release preparations to a maximum of 24 mg/day
	Monoamine oxidase inhibitor	Selegiline	Usually 5 mg in AM, up to 5 mg twice a day
	Monoamine oxidase inhibitor	Rasagiline	0.5-1 mg/day
	COMT inhibitor	Entacapone	200 mg/dose; taken with each dose of levodopa to a maximum of 1600 mg/day
	NMDA antagonist; dopamine releaser	Amantadine	100-400 mg/day; in divided doses, preferably avoiding late day dosing
CO-MORBID NONMOTOR SYMPTOMS			
Depression	SSRI	Sertraline	50 mg/day
Depression	Other antidepressant	Trazodone	25-50 mg at bedtime
Depression	Other antidepressant	Bupropion	Up to 100 mg, three times a day maximum to facilitate titration, or longer-acting preparations
Hallucinations	Neuroleptic	Clozapine	6.25-50 mg at bedtime
Hallucinations	Neuroleptic	Quetiapine	12.5-50 mg at bedtime
EDS and fatigue	Wake-promoting agents	Modafinil	200 mg in AM, occasionally with an additional noon dose of 100-200 mg
EDS and fatigue	Stimulants	Methylphenidate	20 mg long-acting in AM or 5 mg immediate-release as needed through the day, every 3-5 hours, with maximum daily total dose of 60 mg
COMMON PRIMARY SLEEP DISORDERS			
RBD	Benzodiazepine	Clonazepam	Usually 0.25-2 mg, occasionally up to 4 mg, at bedtime
RBD	Dopamine agonist	Pramipexole	Typically 0.75 mg at night
RBD	Hormone for REM sleep behavior	Melatonin	3-12 mg at night
RLS	Dopamine agonist	Pramipexole	0.125-0.375 mg taken 2 hours before bedtime, avoiding higher doses if possible to prevent augmentation
RLS	Dopamine agonist	Ropinirole	0.25-0.5 mg at night, avoiding higher doses if possible to prevent augmentation
RLS	Anticonvulsant	Gabapentin	300-1200 mg taken at night, with additional doses earlier in the day as needed

COMT, catechol-*O*-methyltransferase; *EDS*, excessive daytime sleepiness; *NMDA*, N-methyl-D-aspartate; *RBD*, rapid eye movement sleep behavior disorder; *REM*, rapid eye movement sleep; *RLS*, restless legs syndrome; SSRI, selective serotonin reuptake inhibitor.

Co-Morbid Nonmotor Symptoms

Symptoms of depression and anxiety may coexist or overlap. Both may fluctuate with motor symptoms, being more prominent during "off" periods. Successful treatment of PD motor symptoms is thus the first consideration in treating these patients. Interestingly, the dopamine agonists pramipexole and ropinirole and the MAO-B inhibitor selegiline have demonstrated antidepressant properties, although only a few studies have examined this effect specifically in PD.[119,120] Although benzodiazepines should generally be avoided, clonazepam (with effective doses often of 0.5 mg) can be considered in the context of anxiety, particularly if there is also evidence of RBD. Sleep-disordered breathing should be addressed prior to adding benzodiazepines and other sedating medications that may specifically relax upper airway muscles.

SSRIs are the mainstay of antidepressant therapy in PD and are used in the same doses as for other causes of depression, though a low dose and slow increase is generally advised in elderly patients. These agents are effective and generally better tolerated than tricyclic antidepressants (TCAs) due a relative lack of anticholinergic side effects. However, SSRIs, SNRIs, and TCAs are associated with exacerbation of PLMS and RBD.[121,122] Trazodone is sometimes used as a sleep aid in depressed patients. Bupropion is relatively alerting, and could thus be considered in situations in which depression is accompanied by daytime somnolence. This drug may be potentially helpful in PD due to its inhibition of dopamine reuptake.

Neuroleptics are avoided where possible to avert motor complications from dopamine blockade. However, hallucinations sometimes necessitate that these drugs be used. Low-dose atypical neuroleptics are sometimes effective against hallucinations and often permit the use of higher levodopa dosing without complication. Clozapine, quetiapine, olanzapine, or risperdone given at bedtime are generally well tolerated, although some demented patients may demonstrate a paradoxical worsening of psychosis. The dose is generally much lower than that used in patients with schizophrenia.[123] Ondansetron, a 5-HT$_3$ receptor antagonist seems to also provide a benefit to hallucinating PD patients and can be given parenterally.[124] Clozapine is the most effective agent in the setting of hallucinations, though the presence of blood dyscrasias and need for frequent blood monitoring severely compromise routine use.[4] Unfortunately, the atypical neuroleptics have recently been noted to be associated with an increased risk of metabolic syndromes (likely with an increase in sleep-disordered breathing)[125] and death.

EDS cannot be explained by sleep disruption alone[79] and is likely, in part, an independent feature of the PD phenotype related to disruption of arousal pathways in the brain.[40] Management should include counseling on the associated risks of EDS and unintended sleep episodes, especially in relation to driving. The quality of sleep should be maximized by addressing sleep hygiene, as well as optimizing treatment of nighttime PD symptoms, and addressing concurrent sleep disorders. It is also important to rule out possible medical or neuropsychiatric contributors to sleepiness (e.g., hypothyroidism or depression). All medications should be reviewed, and the lowest effective dose used to avoid soporific side effects as seen with commonly used dopaminergic, benzodiazepine, and antidepressant medications. Drugs with an activating profile (selegiline or amantadine) should be given earlier in the day.[23]

Symptomatic treatment of daytime sleepiness includes wake-promoting agents such as modafinil which has been studied in PD[126] and is well tolerated though not associated with dramatic objective response on multiple sleep latency testing.[127] Traditional stimulants such as methylphenidate[80] could be considered, though insomnia may be a problem if they are taken too close to bedtime. Long-acting preparations given in the morning and at noon are a common approach. Tonic dopamine stimulation is probably easier to manage in these situations, though short-acting agents can be used intermittently at times in the day where patients are particularly sleepy.

In the context of nocturia, condom catheters, urinals, or bedside commodes can be used to minimize the need for nighttime toilet trips. Peripheral acting anticholinergics such as tolterodine or oxybutynin, which also has prominent antispasmodic effects, reduce bladder hyperreflexia, but can cause vivid nightmares and awakenings. Lastly, desmopressin nasal spray may reduce urine production during the night.[4]

Treatment-Related Side Effects

Levodopa

Dopaminergic agents can cause a host of sleep-related side effects, as discussed in previous sections (sedation, and hallucinations suggestive of REM sleep). Decreased sleep fragmentation has been reported with increasing doses of levodopa within the range of 50 to 1625 mg per day, likely due to better control of PD symptoms.[58,128] Higher L-dopa doses with advancing disease may still benefit sleep overall if their beneficial effects on motor symptoms outweigh their arousing side effects.[63] The rule of thumb is to always use the lowest effective dose.

Dopaminergic Agonists

In PD patients with daytime fatigue or sleepiness, dopaminergic drugs should be minimized to the degree that motor function permits. A decision to start therapy with a DA should always be discussed thoroughly with the patient and weighed against the possible adverse effects. Patients with EDS should be made fully aware of the possible dangers of unintended sleep episodes, especially while driving, though this is really applicable to all PD medications. DAs are also more prone than L-dopa to cause neuropsychiatric problems, such as hallucinations and nightmares, especially in the elderly or those with cognitive impairment, and should be avoided where possible in these subgroups.[4]

Antidepressants

As outlined previously, antidepressant medications are frequently associated with PLMS and RBD. Further investigation of bupropion would be warranted given the fact that one of its effects is dopamine reuptake inhibition. Particular consideration should be given to timing of the medication and selection of an agent that is alerting or sedating, depending on the clinical context.

Anticholinergics

Because anticholinergics often induce confusion and hallucinations, these drugs should be used with caution and discontinued if those symptoms become problematic.

Selegiline

This medication should be avoided beyond late afternoon to minimize insomnia from the amphetamine metabolites.

Deep Brain Stimulation

DBS is relatively uncommon but increasingly useful. Although the parameters of effective stimulation continue to be mapped out, consideration will also eventually be directed to whether different stimulation settings during the night may be helpful for restoration of normal sleep. Different target sites may also benefit sleep disorders.

Common Primary Sleep Disorders

The treatment of primary sleep disorders including insomnia, sleep apnea, and circadian rhythm abnormalities in the elderly are covered elsewhere in this volume. Given the sleep benefit phenomenon, restoration of good sleep quality from underlying common sleep disorders, such as apnea, is important. The following is a discussion of specific treatment considerations in the PD population.

Although there are no randomized controlled trials of any drug treatment for RBD (see Chapter 43), the benzodiazepine clonazepam (usually 0.25-2 mg, up to 4 mg nightly) has long been the treatment of choice, although its mechanism of action is not known. It is well tolerated and effective in close to 90% of patients.[129,130] For patients resistant or intolerant of clonazepam, for example, due to aggravation of sleep apnea, melatonin is an alternate therapy, having shown some effectiveness in several limited uncontrolled trials with doses from 3 to 12 mg per day.[131-133] Dopaminergic medications such as levodopa and pramipexole may have some effect against RBD symptoms as well.[31,134,135] However, one recent study of PD patients with RBD showed no improvement in RBD when pramipexole was added to a stable L-dopa regimen.[136] Several small studies of the acetylcholinesterase inhibitors donepezil and rivastigmine have indicated possible reduction of

RBD symptoms, but polysomnographic confirmation was not obtained and the results have not been supported by larger studies of patients with RBD in the context of DLB.[130,137]

In addition to pharmacologic treatment, preventive measures to avoid patients injuring themselves or their partners should be implemented, such as sleeping in separate beds and putting loose or dangerous objects out of reach. Medications known to aggravate RBD (MAO inhibitors, selegiline, and antidepressants, especially TCAs, SSRIs, and SNRIs) should be reduced or discontinued if necessary.[130,138]

RLS (see Chapter 24) can be secondary to various medical conditions such as iron deficiency, end-stage renal failure, and polyneuropathy, which may be common in the PD age group and amenable to specific therapies. Indeed, PD patients with RLS were found to have lower ferritin levels than those without RLS.[31,92] Iron supplementation may be helpful in the appropriate clinical context.[139]

The dopamine agonists pramipexole and ropinirole are the first-line therapies for both RLS and PLMS in PD patients, and response is often dramatic. Increasing the evening or bedtime L-dopa dose or using a sustained-release preparation is another option.[4] The phenomenon of augmentation, in which RLS symptoms begin earlier with greater severity and more widespread anatomic distribution, has been strongly associated with L-dopa use, but also with higher doses of dopaminergic agonists.[140,141] In these cases, other nondopaminergic agents like low-dose gabapentin, clonazepam, or opiates could be tried (see Chapter 24). Removing aggravating agents such as SSRIs SNRIs, or TCAs where possible is an important consideration.

Therapy, typically positive airway pressures devices, should be offered to patients with PD and OSA (see Chapter 16) or central and mixed sleep breathing disorders (see Chapter 19). Restricted motor function may limit the ability to adjust the positive pressure mask in the night, so as simple an apparatus as possible should be used. Special attention to mask seal must be considered if there is orofacial weakness. Patients with multiple system atrophy and stridor may be managed long term with continuous positive airway pressure,[142] but if this is not successful, tracheostomy should be considered. Tracheostomy may not prevent sudden death in patients with stridor.[143] Central hypoventilation is sometimes observed and could be managed with mechanical ventilation.

SUMMARY

PD and parkinsonian syndromes are uniquely associated with an array of sleep disorders and complaints, most notably REM sleep behavior disorder and excessive daytime sleepiness. In the evaluation of sleep disorders in PD patients, a careful history of both patient and bed partner, combined with a detailed assessment using questionnaires and objective polysomnography and alertness testing, is crucial to establishing a correct diagnosis. The various ways in which PD symptoms and sleep/arousal physiology interact can make treatment of these sleep disorders complicated. In general, the following form the foundations for effectively treating PD patients with sleep disorders: (1) optimizing the dopaminergic therapy of motor symptoms using the lowest and most strategically timed dosing, (2) recognizing and addressing common yet frequently overlooked nonmotor symptoms, and

(3) diagnosing and treating common sleep disorders. Special consideration must be given to timing of medications and patient needs at various times of the day. Fortunately, there are a wide variety of treatment options and many patients can benefit significantly from a thoughtful sleep assessment.

REFERENCES

1. de Lau LM, Breteler MM. Epidemiology of Parkinson's disease. *Lancet Neurol.* 2006;5:525-535.
2. Forno LS. Neuropathology of Parkinson's disease. *J Neuropathol Exp Neurol.* 1996;55:259-272.
3. Parkinson J. An essay on the shaking palsy. *J Neuropsychiatry Clin Neurosci.* 1817;2002(14):223-236:discussion 222.
4. Olanow CW, Stern MB, Sethi K. The scientific and clinical basis for the treatment of Parkinson disease. *Neurology.* 2009;72:S1-S136.
5. Boeve BF. REM sleep behavior disorder: Updated review of the core features, the REM sleep behavior disorder-neurodegenerative disease association, evolving concepts, controversies, and future directions. *Ann N Y Acad Sci.* 2010;1184:15-54.
6. Iranzo A, Santamaria J, Tolosa E. The clinical and pathophysiological relevance of REM sleep behavior disorder in neurodegenerative diseases. *Sleep Med Rev.* 2009;13(6):385-401.
7. Lang AE, Lozano AM. Parkinson's disease. First of two parts. *N Engl J Med.* 1998;339:1044-1053.
8. Lang AE, Lozano AM. Parkinson's disease. Second of two parts. *N Engl J Med.* 1998;339:1130-1143.
9. Hely MA, Morris JG, Reid WG, Trafficante R. Sydney Multicenter Study of Parkinson's disease: Non-l-dopa-responsive problems dominate at 15 years. *Mov Disord.* 2005;20:190-199.
10. Wenning GK, Ben-Shlomo Y, Hughes A, Daniel SE, Lees A, Quinn NP. What clinical features are most useful to distinguish definite multiple system atrophy from Parkinson's disease?. *J Neurol Neurosurg Psychiatry.* 2000;68:434-440.
11. Christine CW, Aminoff MJ. Clinical differentiation of parkinsonian syndromes: Prognostic and therapeutic relevance. *Am J Med.* 2004;117:412-419.
12. Gelb DJ, Oliver E, Gilman S. Diagnostic criteria for Parkinson disease. *Arch Neurol.* 1999;56:33-39.
13. Boeve BF, Silber MH, Saper CB, et al. Pathophysiology of REM sleep behaviour disorder and relevance to neurodegenerative disease. *Brain.* 2007;130:2770-2788.
14. Chou K. Diagnosis of Parkinson disease. In: Basow D, ed. *UpToDate.* Waltham, MA: UpToDate; 2009.
15. Gilman S, Low PA, Quinn N, et al. Consensus statement on the diagnosis of multiple system atrophy. *J Neurol Sci.* 1999;163:94-98.
16. Ghorayeb I, Yekhlef F, Chrysostome V, Balestre E, Bioulac B, Tison F. Sleep disorders and their determinants in multiple system atrophy. *J Neurol Neurosurg Psychiatry.* 2002;72:798-800.
17. Rebeiz JJ, Kolodny EH, Richardson Jr EP. Corticodentatonigral degeneration with neuronal achromasia. *Arch Neurol.* 1968;18:20-33.
18. Thompson PD, Day BL, Rothwell JC, Brown P, Britton TC, Marsden CD. The myoclonus in corticobasal degeneration. Evidence for two forms of cortical reflex myoclonus. *Brain.* 1994;117(Pt 5):1197-1207.
19. Williams DR, Lees AJ, Wherrett JR, Steele JC. J. Clifford Richardson and 50 years of progressive supranuclear palsy. *Neurology.* 2008;70:566-573.
20. Verny M, Jellinger KA, Hauw JJ, Bancher C, Litvan I, Agid Y. Progressive supranuclear palsy: A clinicopathological study of 21 cases. *Acta Neuropathol.* 1996;91:427-431.
21. Litvan I, Campbell G, Mangone CA, et al. Which clinical features differentiate progressive supranuclear palsy (Steele-Richardson-Olszewski syndrome) from related disorders? A clinicopathological study. *Brain.* 1997;120(Pt 1):65-74.
22. Winikates J, Jankovic J. Clinical correlates of vascular parkinsonism. *Arch Neurol.* 1999;56:98-102.
23. Simuni T, Sethi K. Nonmotor manifestations of Parkinson's disease. *Ann Neurol.* 2008;64(Suppl 2):S65-S80.
24. Lees AJ, Blackburn NA, Campbell VL. The nighttime problems of Parkinson's disease. *Clin Neuropharmacol.* 1988;11:512-519.
25. Tandberg E, Larsen JP, Karlsen K. Excessive daytime sleepiness and sleep benefit in Parkinson's disease: A community-based study. *Mov Disord.* 1999;14:922-927.
26. Barone P, Amboni M, Vitale C, Bonavita V. Treatment of nocturnal disturbances and excessive daytime sleepiness in Parkinson's disease. *Neurology.* 2004;63:S35-S38.

27. Porter B, Macfarlane R, Walker R. The frequency and nature of sleep disorders in a community-based population of patients with Parkinson's disease. *Eur J Neurol.* 2008;15:50-54.
28. Tandberg E, Larsen JP, Karlsen K. A community-based study of sleep disorders in patients with Parkinson's disease. *Mov Disord.* 1998;13:895-899.
29. Pappert EJ, Goetz CG, Niederman FG, Raman R, Leurgans S. Hallucinations, sleep fragmentation, and altered dream phenomena in Parkinson's disease. *Mov Disord.* 1999;14:117-121.
30. Schenck CH, Bundlie SR, Mahowald MW. Delayed emergence of a parkinsonian disorder in 38% of 29 older men initially diagnosed with idiopathic rapid eye movement sleep behaviour disorder. *Neurology.* 1996;46:388-393.
31. De Cock VC, Vidailhet M, Arnulf I. Sleep disturbances in patients with parkinsonism. *Nat Clin Pract Neurol.* 2008;4:254-266.
32. Bloem BR, Grimbergen YA, Cramer M, Willemsen M, Zwinderman AH. Prospective assessment of falls in Parkinson's disease. *J Neurol.* 2001;248:950-958.
33. Braak H, Del Tredici K, Rub U, de Vos RA, Jansen Steur EN, Braak E. Staging of brain pathology related to sporadic Parkinson's disease. *Neurobiol Aging.* 2003;24:197-211.
34. De Keyser J, Ebinger G, Vauquelin G. Evidence for a widespread dopaminergic innervation of the human cerebral neocortex. *Neurosci Lett.* 1989;104:281-285.
35. Lu J, Jhou TC, Saper CB. Identification of wake-active dopaminergic neurons in the ventral periaqueductal gray matter. *J Neurosci.* 2006;26:193-202.
36. Chaudhuri KR, Schapira AH. Non-motor symptoms of Parkinson's disease: Dopaminergic pathophysiology and treatment. *Lancet Neurol.* 2009;8:464-474.
37. Politis M, Piccini P, Pavese N, Koh SB, Brooks DJ. Evidence of dopamine dysfunction in the hypothalamus of patients with Parkinson's disease: An in vivo 11C-raclopride PET study. *Exp Neurol.* 2008;214:112-116.
38. Boissard R, Fort P, Gervasoni D, Barbagli B, Luppi PH. Localization of the GABAergic and non-GABAergic neurons projecting to the sublaterodorsal nucleus and potentially gating paradoxical sleep onset. *Eur J Neurosci.* 2003;18:1627-1639.
39. Sastre JP, Jouvet M. [Oneiric behavior in cats.] *Physiol Behav.* 1979;22:979-989.
40. Thannickal TC, Lai YY, Siegel JM. Hypocretin (orexin) cell loss in Parkinson's disease. *Brain.* 2007;130:1586-1595.
41. Lewitt PA. Levodopa for the treatment of Parkinson's disease. *N Engl J Med.* 2008;359:2468-2476.
42. Oertel WH, Wolters E, Sampaio C, et al. Pergolide versus levodopa monotherapy in early Parkinson's disease patients: The PELMOPET study. *Mov Disord.* 2006;21:343-353.
43. Tarsy D. Motor fluctuations and dyskinesia in Parkinson disease. In: Basow D, ed. *UpToDate.* Waltham, MA: UpToDate; 2009.
44. Garcia-Borreguero D, Odin P, Serrano C. Restless legs syndrome and PD: A review of the evidence for a possible association. *Neurology.* 2003;61:S49-S55.
45. Schade R, Andersohn F, Suissa S, Haverkamp W, Garbe E. Dopamine agonists and the risk of cardiac-valve regurgitation. *N Engl J Med.* 2007;356:29-38.
46. Frucht S, Rogers JD, Greene PE, Gordon MF, Fahn S. Falling asleep at the wheel: Motor vehicle mishaps in persons taking pramipexole and ropinirole. *Neurology.* 1999;52:1908-1910.
47. Razmy A, Lang AE, Shapiro CM. Predictors of impaired daytime sleep and wakefulness in patients with Parkinson disease treated with older (ergot) vs newer (nonergot) dopamine agonists. *Arch Neurol.* 2004;61:97-102.
48. Hobson DE, Lang AE, Martin WR, Razmy A, Rivest J, Fleming J. Excessive daytime sleepiness and sudden-onset sleep in Parkinson disease: A survey by the Canadian Movement Disorders Group. *JAMA.* 2002;287:455-463.
49. Kurth MC, Adler CH. COMT inhibition: A new treatment strategy for Parkinson's disease. *Neurology.* 1998;50:S3-S14.
50. Olanow CW, Watkins PB. Tolcapone: An efficacy and safety review. *Clin Neuropharmacol.* 2007;(30):287-294.
51. Hauser RA, Lew MF, Hurtig HI, Ondo WG, Wojcieszek J, Fitzer-Attas CJ. Long-term outcome of early versus delayed rasagiline treatment in early Parkinson's disease. *Mov Disord.* 2009;24:564-573.
52. Tarsy D. Pharmacologic treatment of Parkinson disease. In: Basow D, ed. *UpToDate.* Waltham, MA: UpToDate; 2009.
53. Kleiner-Fisman G, Herzog J, Fisman DN, et al. Subthalamic nucleus deep brain stimulation: Summary and meta-analysis of outcomes. *Mov Disord.* 2006;21(Suppl 14):S290-S304.
54. Iranzo A, Valldeoriola F, Santamaria J, Tolosa E, Rumia J. Sleep symptoms and polysomnographic architecture in advanced Parkinson's disease after chronic bilateral subthalamic stimulation. *J Neurol Neurosurg Psychiatry.* 2002;72:661-664.
55. Arnulf I, Bejjani BP, Garma L, et al. Improvement of sleep architecture in PD with subthalamic nucleus stimulation. *Neurology.* 2000;55:1732-1734.
56. Hjort N, Ostergaard K, Dupont E. Improvement of sleep quality in patients with advanced Parkinson's disease treated with deep brain stimulation of the subthalamic nucleus. *Mov Disord.* 2004;19:196-199.
57. Lim AS, Moro E, Lozano AM, et al. Selective enhancement of rapid eye movement sleep by deep brain stimulation of the human pons. *Ann Neurol.* 2009;66:110-114.
58. Pal PK, Calne S, Samii A, Fleming JA. A review of normal sleep and its disturbances in Parkinson's disease. *Parkinsonism Relat Disord.* 1999;5:1-17.
59. Friedman A. Sleep pattern in Parkinson's disease. *Acta Med Pol.* 1980;21:193-199.
60. Marsden CD, Parkes J, Quinn N. Fluctuations of disability in Parkinson's disease: Clinical aspects. In: Marsden CD, ed. *Movement Disorders.* London: Butterworth Scientific; 1981:96.
61. Currie LJ, Bennett Jr JP, Harrison MB, Trugman JM, Wooten GF. Clinical correlates of sleep benefit in Parkinson's disease. *Neurology.* 1997;48:1115-1117.
62. Merello M, Hughes A, Colosimo C, Hoffman M, Starkstein S, Leiguarda R. Sleep benefit in Parkinson's disease. *Mov Disord.* 1997;12:506-508.
63. Diederich NJ. Sleep disturbances in Parkinson's disease. In: Chokroverty SHW, Walters AS, eds. *Sleep and Movement Disorders.* Boston: Butterworth-Heinemann; 2002:478-488.
64. Hogl BE, Gomez-Arevalo G, Garcia S, et al. A clinical, pharmacologic, and polysomnographic study of sleep benefit in Parkinson's disease. *Neurology.* 1998;50:1332-1339.
65. Goetz CG, Stebbins GT. Risk factors for nursing home placement in advanced Parkinson's disease. *Neurology.* 1993;43:2227-2229.
66. Ehmann TS, Beninger RJ, Gawel MJ, Riopelle RJ. Depressive symptoms in Parkinson's disease: A comparison with disabled control subjects. *J Geriatr Psychiatry Neurol.* 1990;3:3-9.
67. Borek LL, Kohn R, Friedman JH. Mood and sleep in Parkinson's disease. *J Clin Psychiatry.* 2006;67:958-963.
68. Whitney CW, Enright PL, Newman AB, Bonekat W, Foley D, Quan SF. Correlates of daytime sleepiness in 4578 elderly persons: The Cardiovascular Health Study. *Sleep.* 1998;21:27-36.
69. Buysse DJ. Insomnia, depression and aging. Assessing sleep and mood interactions in older adults. *Geriatrics.* 2004;59:47-51;quiz 52.
70. Aarsland D, Zaccai J, Brayne C. A systematic review of prevalence studies of dementia in Parkinson's disease. *Mov Disord.* 2005;20:1255-1263.
71. Aarsland D, Bronnick K, Ehrt U, et al. Neuropsychiatric symptoms in patients with Parkinson's disease and dementia: Frequency, profile and associated caregiver stress. *J Neurol Neurosurg Psychiatry.* 2007;78:36-42.
72. Stern Y, Marder K, Tang MX, Mayeux R. Antecedent clinical features associated with dementia in Parkinson's disease. *Neurology.* 1993;43:1690-1692.
73. Sharf B, Moskovitz C, Lupton MD, Klawans HL. Dream phenomena induced by chronic levodopa therapy. *J Neural Transm.* 1978;43:143-151.
74. Mahowald MW, Schenck CH. NREM sleep parasomnias. *Neurol Clin.* 1996;14:675-696.
75. Pacchetti C, Manni R, Zangaglia R, et al. Relationship between hallucinations, delusions, and rapid eye movement sleep behavior disorder in Parkinson's disease. *Mov Disord.* 2005;20:1439-1448.
76. Arnulf I, Bonnet AM, Damier P, et al. Hallucinations, REM sleep, and Parkinson's disease: A medical hypothesis. *Neurology.* 2000;55:281-288.
77. Brodsky MA, Godbold J, Roth T, Olanow CW. Sleepiness in Parkinson's disease: A controlled study. *Mov Disord.* 2003;18:668-672.
78. Carskadon MA, Dement WC, Mitler MM, Roth T, Westbrook PR, Keenan S. Guidelines for the multiple sleep latency test (MSLT): A standard measure of sleepiness. *Sleep.* 1986;9:519-524.
79. Rye DB, Bliwise DL, Dihenia B, Gurecki P. Fast Track: Daytime sleepiness in Parkinson's disease. *J Sleep Res.* 2000;9:63-69.
80. Rye DB, Jankovic J. Emerging views of dopamine in modulating sleep/wake state from an unlikely source: PD. *Neurology.* 2002;58:341-346.
81. Poryazova R, Benninger D, Waldvogel D, Bassetti CL. Excessive daytime sleepiness in Parkinson's disease: Characteristics and determinants. *Eur Neurol.* 2010;63:129-135.
82. Pressman MR, Figueroa WG, Kendrick-Mohamed J, Greenspon LW, Peterson Nocturia DD. A rarely recognized symptom of sleep apnea and other occult sleep disorders. *Arch Intern Med.* 1996;156:545-550.

83. Gjerstad MD, Alves G, Wentzel-Larsen T, Aarsland D, Larsen JP. Excessive daytime sleepiness in Parkinson disease: Is it the drugs or the disease? *Neurology.* 2006;67:853-858.

84. Arnulf I. Excessive daytime sleepiness in parkinsonism. *Sleep Med Rev.* 2005;9:185-200.

85. Wilson S, Argyropoulos S. Antidepressants and sleep: A qualitative review of the literature. *Drugs.* 2005;65:927-947.

86. Schenck CH, Mahowald MW. REM sleep behavior disorder: Clinical, developmental, and neuroscience perspectives 16 years after its formal identification in SLEEP. *Sleep.* 2002;25:120-138.

87. Gagnon JF, Bedard MA, Fantini ML, et al. REM sleep behavior disorder and REM sleep without atonia in Parkinson's disease. *Neurology.* 2002;59:585-589.

88. Schenck C, Bundlie S, Mahowald MW. REM behavior disorder (RBD): Delayed emergence of parkinsonism and/or dementia in 65% of older men initially diagnosed with idiopathic RBD, and an analysis of the minimum and maximum tonic and/or phasic electromyographic abnormalities found during REM sleep. *Sleep.* 2003;26:A316.

89. De Cock VC, Vidailhet M, Leu S, et al. Restoration of normal motor control in Parkinson's disease during REM sleep. *Brain.* 2007;130:450-456.

90. Allen RP, Picchietti D, Hening WA, Trenkwalder C, Walters AS, Montplaisi J. Restless legs syndrome: Diagnostic criteria, special considerations, and epidemiology. A report from the restless legs syndrome diagnosis and epidemiology workshop at the National Institutes of Health. *Sleep Med.* 2003;4:101-119.

91. Hening W, Allen RP, Tenzer P, Winkelman JW. Restless legs syndrome: Demographics, presentation, and differential diagnosis. *Geriatrics.* 2007;62:26-29.

92. Ondo WG, Vuong KD, Jankovic J. Exploring the relationship between Parkinson disease and restless legs syndrome. *Arch Neurol.* 2002;59:421-424.

93. Loo HV, Tan EK. Case-control study of restless legs syndrome and quality of sleep in Parkinson's disease. *J Neurol Sci.* 2008;266:145-149.

94. Wetter TC, Collado-Seidel V, Pollmacher T, Yassouridis A, Trenkwalder C. Sleep and periodic leg movement patterns in drug-free patients with Parkinson's disease and multiple system atrophy. *Sleep.* 2000;23:361-367.

95. Turjanski N, Lees AJ, Brooks DJ. Striatal dopaminergic function in restless legs syndrome: 18F-dopa and 11C-raclopride PET studies. *Neurology.* 1999;52:932-937.

96. Allen RP, Barker PB, Wehrl F, Song HK, Earley CJ. MRI measurement of brain iron in patients with restless legs syndrome. *Neurology.* 2001;56:263-265.

97. Connor JR, Boyer PJ, Menzies SL, et al. Neuropathological examination suggests impaired brain iron acquisition in restless legs syndrome. *Neurology.* 2003;61:304-309.

98. Matheson JK, Saper CB. REM sleep behavior disorder: A dopaminergic deficiency disorder? *Neurology.* 2003;61:1328-1329.

99. Oakley AE, Collingwood JF, Dobson J, et al. Individual dopaminergic neurons show raised iron levels in Parkinson disease. *Neurology.* 2007;68:1820-1825.

100. Maria B, Sophia S, Michalis M, et al. Sleep breathing disorders in patients with idiopathic Parkinson's disease. *Respir Med.* 2003;97:1151-1157.

101. Hovestadt A, Bogaard JM, Meerwaldt JD, van der Meche FG, Stigt J. Pulmonary function in Parkinson's disease. *J Neurol Neurosurg Psychiatry.* 1989;52:329-333.

102. Vincken WG, Gauthier SG, Dollfuss RE, Hanson RE, Darauay CM, Cosio MG. Involvement of upper-airway muscles in extrapyramidal disorders. A cause of airflow limitation. *N Engl J Med.* 1984;311:438-442.

103. Feinsilver SH, Friedman JH, Rosen JM. Respiration and sleep in Parkinson's disease. *J Neurol Neurosurg Psychiatry.* 1986;49:964.

104. Apps MC, Sheaff PC, Ingram DA, Kennard C, Empey DW. Respiration and sleep in Parkinson's disease. *J Neurol Neurosurg Psychiatry.* 1985;48:1240-1245.

105. Hardie RJ, Efthimiou J, Stern GM. Respiration and sleep in Parkinson's disease. *J Neurol Neurosurg Psychiatry.* 1986;49:1326.

106. Arnulf I, Konofal E, Merino-Andreu M, et al. Parkinson's disease and sleepiness: An integral part of PD. *Neurology.* 2002;58:1019-1024.

107. Shulman LM, Taback RL, Rabinstein AA, Weiner WJ. Non-recognition of depression and other non-motor symptoms in Parkinson's disease. *Parkinsonism Relat Disord.* 2002;8:193-197.

108. Chaudhuri KR, Martinez-Martin P, Schapira AH, et al. International multicenter pilot study of the first comprehensive self-completed non-motor symptoms questionnaire for Parkinson's disease: The NMSQuest study. *Mov Disord.* 2006;21:916-923.

109. Fahn S, Elton RL, UPDRS program members. Unified Parkinson's Disease Rating Scale. In: Fahn S, Marsden CD, Goldstein M, Calne DB, eds. *Recent Developments in Parkinson's Disease.* vol. 2. Florham Park, NJ: Macmillan Healthcare Information; 1987:153-163, 293-304.

110. Goetz CG, Tilley BC, Shaftman SR, et al. Movement Disorder Society-sponsored revision of the Unified Parkinson's Disease Rating Scale (MDS-UPDRS): Scale presentation and clinimetric testing results. *Mov Disord.* 2008;23:2129-2170.

111. Buysse DJ, Reynolds 3rd CF, Monk TH, Berman SR, Kupfer DJ. The Pittsburgh Sleep Quality Index: A new instrument for psychiatric practice and research. *Psychiatry Res.* 1989;28:193-213.

112. Johns MW. A new method for measuring daytime sleepiness: The Epworth sleepiness scale. *Sleep.* 1991;14:540-545.

113. Askenasy JJ, Yahr MD. Parkinsonian tremor loses its alternating aspect during non-REM sleep and is inhibited by REM sleep. *J Neurol Neurosurg Psychiatry.* 1990;53:749-753.

114. Mouret J. Differences in sleep in patients with Parkinson's disease. *Electroencephalogr Clin Neurophysiol.* 1975;38:653-657.

115. Postuma RB, Gagnon JF, Rompre S, Montplaisir JY. Severity of REM atonia loss in idiopathic REM sleep behavior disorder predicts Parkinson disease. *Neurology.* 2010;74:239-244.

116. Vetrugno R, Provini F, Cortelli P, et al. Sleep disorders in multiple system atrophy: A correlative video-polysomnographic study. *Sleep Med.* 2004;5:21-30.

117. Zesiewicz TA, Sullivan KL, Arnulf I, et al. Practice Parameter: Treatment of nonmotor symptoms of Parkinson disease: Report of the Quality Standards Subcommittee of the American Academy of Neurology. *Neurology.* 2010;74:924-931.

118. Reuter I, Ellis CM, Ray Chaudhuri K. Nocturnal subcutaneous apomorphine infusion in Parkinson's disease and restless legs syndrome. *Acta Neurol Scand.* 1999;100:163-167.

119. Lemke MR, Brecht HM, Koester J, Kraus PH, Reichmann H. Anhedonia, depression, and motor functioning in Parkinson's disease during treatment with pramipexole. *J Neuropsychiatry Clin Neurosci.* 2005;17:214-220.

120. Barone P, Scarzella L, Marconi R, et al. Pramipexole versus sertraline in the treatment of depression in Parkinson's disease: A national multicenter parallel-group randomized study. *J Neurol.* 2006;253:601-607.

121. Teman PT, Tippmann-Peikert M, Silber MH, Slocumb NL, Auger RR. Idiopathic rapid-eye-movement sleep disorder: Associations with antidepressants, psychiatric diagnoses, and other factors, in relation to age of onset. *Sleep Med.* 2009;10:60-65.

122. Yang C, White DP, Winkelman JW. Antidepressants and periodic leg movements of sleep. *Biol Psychiatry.* 2005;58:510-514.

123. Ruggieri S, De Pandis MF, Bonamartini A, Vacca L, Stocchi F. Low dose of clozapine in the treatment of dopaminergic psychosis in Parkinson's disease. *Clin Neuropharmacol.* 1997;20:204-209.

124. Zoldan J, Friedberg G, Livneh M, Melamed E. Psychosis in advanced Parkinson's disease: treatment with ondansetron, a 5-HT3 receptor antagonist. *Neurology.* 1995;45:1305-1308.

125. Newcomer JW. Second-generation (atypical) antipsychotics and metabolic effects: A comprehensive literature review. *CNS Drugs.* 2005;(19 Suppl 1):1-93.

126. Nieves AV, Lang AE. Treatment of excessive daytime sleepiness in patients with Parkinson's disease with modafinil. *Clin Neuropharmacol.* 2002;25:111-114.

127. Ondo WG, Fayle R, Atassi F, Jankovic J. Modafinil for daytime somnolence in Parkinson's disease: Double blind, placebo controlled parallel trial. *J Neurol Neurosurg Psychiatry.* 2005;76:1636-1639.

128. van Hilten JJ, Weggeman M, van der Velde EA, Kerkhof GA, van Dijk JG, Roos RA. Sleep, excessive daytime sleepiness and fatigue in Parkinson's disease. *J Neural Transm Park Dis Dement Sect.* 1993;5:235-244.

129. Schenck CH, Mahowald MW. Long-term, nightly benzodiazepine treatment of injurious parasomnias and other disorders of disrupted nocturnal sleep in 170 adults. *Am J Med.* 1996;100:333-337.

130. Gagnon JF, Postuma RB, Montplaisir J. Update on the pharmacology of REM sleep behavior disorder. *Neurology.* 2006;67:742-747.

131. Kunz D, Bes F. Melatonin as a therapy in REM sleep behavior disorder patients: An open-labeled pilot study on the possible influence of melatonin on REM-sleep regulation. *Mov Disord.* 1999;14:507-511.

132. Boeve BF, Silber MH, Ferman TJ. Melatonin for treatment of REM sleep behavior disorder in neurologic disorders: Results in 14 patients. *Sleep Med.* 2003;4:281-284.

133. Takeuchi N, Uchimura N, Hashizume Y, et al. Melatonin therapy for REM sleep behavior disorder. *Psychiatry Clin Neurosci.* 2001;55:267-269.

134. Fantini ML, Gagnon JF, Filipini D, Montplaisir J. The effects of prami-pexole in REM sleep behavior disorder. *Neurology*. 2003;61:1418-1420.

135. Tan A, Salgado M, Fahn S. Rapid eye movement sleep behavior disorder preceding Parkinson's disease with therapeutic response to levodopa. *Mov Disord*. 1996;11:214-216.

136. Kumru H, Iranzo A, Carrasco E, et al. Lack of effects of pramipexole on REM sleep behavior disorder in Parkinson disease. *Sleep*. 2008;31:1418-1421.

137. Ringman JM, Simmons JH. Treatment of REM sleep behavior disorder with donepezil: A report of three cases. *Neurology*. 2000;55:870-871.

138. Dhawan V, Healy DG, Pal S, Chaudhuri KR. Sleep-related problems of Parkinson's disease. *Age Ageing*. 2006;35:220-228.

139. Earley CJ. The importance of oral iron therapy in restless legs syndrome. *Sleep Med*. 2009;10(9):945-946.

140. Earley CJ, Allen RP. Pergolide and carbidopa/levodopa treatment of the restless legs syndrome and periodic leg movements in sleep in a con-secutive series of patients. *Sleep*. 1996;19:801-810.

141. Winkelman JW, Johnston L. Augmentation and tolerance with long-term pramipexole treatment of restless legs syndrome (RLS). *Sleep Med*. 2004;5:9-14.

142. Iranzo A, Santamaria J, Tolosa E, et al. Long-term effect of CPAP in the treatment of nocturnal stridor in multiple system atrophy. *Neurology*. 2004;63:930-932.

143. Silber MH, Levine S. Stridor and death in multiple system atrophy. *Mov Disord*. 2000;15:699-704.

Sleep Disruption from Movement Disorders

LIUDMILA LYSENKO / PHILIP A. HANNA / SUDHANSU CHOKROVERTY

The purpose of this chapter is to present information on movement disorders during sleep in a way that would facilitate diagnosis and treatment strategies. Because few of these disorders have been subjected to randomized controlled trials (RCTs), treatment recommendations are largely based on expert consensus.

Movement disorders during sleep include daytime movement disorders that persist in sleep (such patients are mostly seen by movement disorder specialists) as well as the sleep disorders associated with abnormal movements (such patients are traditionally seen by sleep specialists). Movement disorders of sleep are diverse in their etiology and clinical presentation. They can occur predominantly in specific sleep stages, for example, rapid eye movement behavior disorder (RBD) in rapid eye movement (REM) sleep (see Chapter 43), somnambulism in non–rapid eye movement (NREM) sleep (see Chapter 44), or movements persisting through multiple stages of sleep and daytime abnormal movements persisting in sleep (e.g., palatal myoclonus/tremor). Age is also a very important factor in the epidemiology of movement disorders during sleep. There appears to be a bimodal distribution of sleep-associated movement disorders. Arousal disorders such as sleep walking, sleep terrors, and confusional arousals as well as sleep talking and rhythmic movement disorders tend to prevail during childhood and disappear by adulthood or adolescence, perhaps due to the immaturity of regulatory system.[1] The second peak occurs later in life when sleep-related movement disorders such as RBD, restless legs syndrome (RLS), periodic limb movements in sleep (PLMS) (see Chapter 24), nocturnal leg cramps, and neurodegenerative disorders become manifest. The authors have not used strictly the International Classification of Sleep Disorders[2] here, as different motor disturbances are found in its various sections. Instead we propose a classification taking into consideration behavioral aspects manifested by a variety of motor activities during sleep to facilitate an approach to categorical analysis of the motor disturbances in sleep (Box 27-1). Movement disorders during sleep can be classified into physiologic and pathologic types. Physiologic motor activity during sleep includes postural shifts, body and limb movements, and physiologic fragmentary myoclonus. Pathologic movements that occur during sleep include motor parasomnias, sleep-related movement disorders, isolated sleep-related motor symptoms (apparently normal variants), nocturnal seizures (see Chapter 50) (traditionally not classified with movement disorders), miscellaneous nocturnal motor activities, and

diurnal involuntary movements that persist into sleep. Nocturnal seizures (see Chapter 50), Parkinson's disease (see Chapter 26), RLS-PLMS (see Chapter 24), NREM parasomnias (see Chapter 44), REM parasomnias (see Chapter 43), sleep talking (see Chapter 45), and bruxism (see Chapter 25) are discussed in other chapters.

MOTOR PARASOMNIAS

Motor parasomnias are abnormal movements intruding into sleep without generally disturbing sleep architecture. Motor parasomnias include NREM parasomnias, REM parasomnias, and other parasomnias not related to any specific sleep stage. Most of these parasomnias have been described in other chapters (see, among others, Chapters 43 to 45).

SLEEP-RELATED MOVEMENT DISORDERS

These disorders include rhythmic movement disorders, nocturnal leg cramps, RLS-PLMS, and sleep-related bruxism (see Chapter 24).

Rhythmic Movement Disorders

Rhythmic movement disorders mostly become manifest before 18 months of age (see Chapter 25). The movements include head banging, head rolling, body rolling, and body rocking occurring immediately before sleep during relaxed wakefulness and they continue into light sleep.[2,3] These are stereotyped repetitive movements of large muscles (usually of head and neck, but leg rolling and leg banging have also been described). The rhythmic movements usually occur at a rate between 0.5 and 2 oscillations per second. A cluster of movements can last a few minutes, but sometimes last up to 30 minutes or longer.[2,4] The patients are usually unresponsive during the episodes and have no memory of the episodes on awakening. The cause of rhythmic movements is usually unknown, although an abnormality of basal ganglia has been suggested.[5] Sometimes rhythmic disorders are associated with mental retardation, especially when these persist into older age.

Differential diagnosis of rhythmic movement disorders includes bruxism, thumb sucking, and rhythmic sucking of a pacifier. Rhythmic movement disorders can be diagnosed clinically; polysomnography (PSG) can be used to differentiate a rhythmic movement disorder from an epileptic disorder.

BOX 27-1 *Classification of Motor Activities During Sleep*

PHYSIOLOGIC (NORMAL) MOTOR ACTIVITY DURING SLEEP
Postural shifts, body and limb movements during sleep
Physiologic fragmentary myoclonus

PATHOLOGIC (ABNORMAL) MOTOR ACTIVITY DURING SLEEP
Motor Parasomnias
Non–rapid eye movement (NREM) sleep parasomnias
Confusional arousals
Sleep walking
Sleep terror
Rapid eye movement (REM) sleep parasomnias
REM sleep behavior disorder
Nightmare disorder
Recurrent isolated sleep paralysis
Other motor parasomnias
Sleep-related eating disorder
Sleep-related groaning (catathrenia)
Sleep-related dissociative disorders

Sleep-Related Movement Disorders
Restless legs syndrome (RLS)
Periodic limb movements in sleep (PLMS)
Sleep-related leg cramps
Sleep-related bruxism
Sleep-related rhythmic movement disorder

Isolated Sleep-Related Motor Symptoms (apparently normal variants)
Sleep talking
Hypnic jerks (sleep starts)
Benign sleep myoclonus of infancy
Hypnagogic foot tremor
Alternating-leg muscle activation
Propriospinal myoclonus at sleep onset
Excessive fragmentary myoclonus

Nocturnal Seizures
True nocturnal seizures
Tonic seizure
Benign rolandic seizure

Nocturnal frontal lobe epilepsy (NFLE)
　Nocturnal paroxysmal dystonia
　Paroxysmal arousals and awakenings
　Episodic nocturnal wanderings
Autosomal dominant nocturnal frontal lobe epilepsy (ADNFLE)
Nocturnal temporal lobe epilepsy
Continuous spike waves during slow wave sleep (CSWS) or electrical status epilepticus in sleep (ESRS)
Nocturnal and diurnal seizures
Juvenile myoclonic epilepsy
Generalized tonic-clonic seizures on awakening
Infantile spasms (West's syndrome)
Generalized tonic-clonic seizures
Partial complex seizures
Frontal lobe seizures
Epilepsia partialis continua

Miscellaneous Nocturnal Motor Hyperactivity
Drug-induced nocturnal dyskinesias
Nocturnal jerks and shakes in obstructive sleep apnea syndrome
Nocturnal panic attacks
Post-traumatic stress disorder
Fatal familial insomnia

Involuntary Diurnal Movement Disorders
Usually persisting during sleep
Palatal myoclonus/palatal tremor
Frequently persisting during sleep
Spinal myoclonus
Tics in Tourette's syndrome
Hemifacial spasms
Hyperekplexia
Sometimes persisting during sleep
Tremor
Chorea
Dystonia
Hemiballismus

Treatment

Rhythmic movement disorders are benign and the patient usually outgrows the movements by the second or third year of life. Although persistence of the symptoms beyond 4 years of age is unusual, movements can sometimes be seen in adolescence and adulthood. Young infants and children do not require treatment. Treatment is indicated when the condition persists into adolescence or adulthood. Behavior therapy should be the first line of treatment and includes overpracticing the activity during wakefulness, hypnosis, avoidance of emotional stress, and lack of environmental stimuli. In severe cases short-acting benzodiazepines can be helpful.[6] Clonazepam (at a dose of 0.5-1.0 mg nightly) was shown to be effective.[6] Imipramine at a dose of 10 mg per day has been reported to be effective in a case that had not responded to clonazepam;[7] L-dopa was also tried and found to be effective in one adult case.[8] For children who suffer from particularly violent movements the use of protective padding around the bed as well as use of a protective helmet can be of benefit. Improvement of symptoms was reported after use of waterbeds in two cases[9] and controlled sleep restriction.[10]

Nocturnal Leg Cramps

Nocturnal leg cramps are painful muscle contractions associated with the sensation of muscle tightness occurring during sleep. They mostly occur unilaterally in calf muscles, but they can also involve the foot and the thigh.[11,12] Cramps usually last for a few seconds, but sometimes persist for several minutes and remit spontaneously. During the cramp the muscle feels firm on palpation; this remits after the cramp but muscle tenderness remains for at least half an hour. Typically episodes occur one or two times per night. Nocturnal cramps usually cause awakening from sleep, leading to sleep fragmentation. Leg cramps can also sometimes occur during the daytime.

This disorder occurs in about 16% of healthy individuals; the male-female ratio is 1:1. They occur more often with advanced age. Sedentary activity can predispose to leg cramps, but in some patients they occur during or immediately after exercising.[13] Familial forms of nocturnal leg cramps have been described with an autosomal dominant pattern of inheritance.[12]

The etiology of nocturnal leg cramps is unknown, although abnormal calcium metabolism and electrolyte abnormalities have been postulated as a possible cause.[14] Muscle membrane overexcitability has been suggested as a mechanism for nocturnal cramps. Extracellular volume depletion and dialysis may predispose to leg cramps. Pregnancy-related cramps may be associated with low serum magnesium and were shown to respond to magnesium supplementation.[15] Other disorders of metabolism may predispose to leg cramps: hyperglycemia and hypoglycemia, alcoholism, nonalcoholic cirrhosis, bariatric surgery, lead poisoning, hypothyroidism, and renal failure requiring hemodialysis.[16] Medications such as lipid-lowering drugs, antihypertensives, diuretics, beta agonists, insulin, oral contraceptives, raloxifene, cisplatin, and vincristine chemotherapy have been associated with muscle cramps.[16] Structural disorders such as hypermobility syndrome, flat feet, and genu recurvatum can predispose to nocturnal leg cramps. Nocturnal leg cramps often accompany myopathies, myotonias, myokymia, neuropathies, radiculopathies, motor neuron disorders, and disorders with reduced mobility such as Parkinson's disease and arthritis. Peripheral vascular disease and various neuropathies are the most frequent co-morbidities associated with muscle cramps. Most commonly nocturnal leg cramps are idiopathic.

Differential diagnosis of nocturnal leg cramps includes tetany (due to low calcium or magnesium), compartment syndrome, muscle contractures related to chronic myopathies and peripheral neuropathies, akathisia, RLS, and muscular pain fasciculation syndrome.

Diagnosis is usually clinical. Metabolic disorders can be ruled out by obtaining complete metabolic profile, calcium level, magnesium level, thyroid-stimulating hormone (TSH), and other biochemical tests depending on suspected cause. Usually the disorder has a benign course as the episodes remit spontaneously.

Treatment

Nonpharmacologic measures should be tried as the first line of treatment. Local massage or movement of the limbs (for instance, foot dorsiflexion in calf cramps) usually relieves the cramps. Avoidance of foot plantar flexion in bed may help as a prophylactic measure as well as frequent passive stretching of affected muscles.[17,14] Sedentary patients may benefit from using a stationary bicycle before bedtime. Quinine sulfate had been used effectively in many patients in the past, but because of conflicting results from several drug trials[18,19] and an adverse side effect profile, the Food and Drug Administration (FDA) ordered a stop to marketing of quinine in the United States for nocturnal leg cramps treatment. Vitamin E has been tried for nocturnal leg cramps, but the data on its efficacy are equivocal.[20-22] Verapamil 120 mg at bedtime was shown to be beneficial in older patients who did not respond to quinine.[23] Diphenhydramine 25 to 50 mg at bedtime and procainamide 250 mg three times a day may also be beneficial.[24]

Gabapentin 600 mg daily and higher doses were tried in an open label trial with benefit.[25] Herbal medication derived from white peony and licorice root (shakuyaku-kanzo-to) taken during hemodialysis sessions was shown to be helpful in relieving muscle cramps.[26]

ISOLATED SLEEP-RELATED MOTOR SYMPTOMS

Hypnagogic Foot Tremor

Hypnagogic foot tremor is classified as an isolated sleep-related motor symptom associated with involuntary rhythmic contractions of the foot and leg described by Broughton in 1988 as an incidental PSG finding.[27,28] These movements represent coarse tremor of one or both feet observed mostly in the predormitum (a period of relaxed wakefulness before sleep); they persist in stages N1 and N2 and during the transition from sleep to wakefulness. The origin of this activity is unknown.

PSG shows 0.3 to 4 Hz rhythmic contractures of the leg in series lasting for a few seconds. The duration of individual movement varies between 100 and 1000 ms.[29] At least four movements in a row must be present to make a diagnosis.[4]

Differential diagnosis includes RLS and PLMS. However, the time between the onsets of consecutive bursts on the electromyogram (EMG) in PLMS is 5 to 90 seconds, and in hypnagogic foot tremor it ranges between 0.25 and 3.33 seconds.

This condition is considered benign, and no treatment is usually required.[29,30]

Alternating Leg Muscle Activation

First described by Chervin and associates,[31] alternating leg muscle activation (ALMA) represents a quickly alternating pattern of anterior tibialis activations. This phenomenon occurs in all stages of sleep, but particularly during arousals. It is sometimes considered to be a variant of hypnagogic foot tremor. Chervin and associates[31] speculated that ALMA represents a transient facilitation of a spinal central pattern generator for locomotion, perhaps due to serotoninergic effects of antidepressant medications, which many of their patients were taking.

The pattern of ALMA in PSG recording is somewhat similar to hypnagogic foot tremor: diagnostic criteria include a minimum of four alternating bursts of leg muscle activity in a row, with a frequency range of 0.5 to 3 Hz. The usual duration of bursts is 100 to 500 ms and each series of activations typically lasts several (up to 20) seconds. The range of time between the onsets of consecutive EMG bursts was reported in the above mentioned series to be 0.33 to 2 seconds.

Differential diagnosis includes PLMS, which can also occur in alternating legs, but the time between the onset of consecutive bursts in the EMG in PLMS is 5 to 90 seconds.

This condition is usually benign and there is no convincing evidence of definite clinical consequences of these movements. Pramipexole in one patient reduced ALMA and improved sleep.[32]

Propriospinal Myoclonus

Propriospinal myoclonus (PSM) is a type of spinal myoclonus originating from a myoclonic generator (hyperexcitable myelomere) usually located in the midthoracic region with propagation up and down the spinal cord via the slowly conducting propriospinal pathways (2-16 m/second).[33-35] PSM can be idiopathic or can occur after cervical and thoracic spinal cord lesions due to trauma, ischemic myelopathy, surgery, degenerative joint disease with cord compression and cord section, demyelinating disease, thoracic herpes zoster, hemangioblastoma, arachnoid cysts, and syringomyelia. It has also been described in drug use, malignancy, and infection.[33] The myoclonic jerks involve predominantly the axial muscles with possible extension into the limbs and exclude the cranial muscles.

Although classic PSM occurs in wakefulness and may persist in sleep, in a special type of isolated propriospinal myoclonus jerks occur exclusively in the predormitum.[36] This subtype is usually termed "propriospinal myoclonus at sleep onset." Characteristic of this form of the disorder, myoclonus can be abolished either by shifting to sleep or wakefulness. In this condition[37,38] myoclonic jerks occur every 10 to 20 seconds, preventing the patient from falling asleep, causing significant sleep-onset insomnia. Propriospinal myoclonus at sleep onset also interferes with sleep maintenance as it reappears during intrasleep wakefulness. As opposed to some cases of classic PSM, this type of myoclonus is not precipitated by sensory and auditory stimuli, and is inhibited by mental activity and sensory stimulation in relaxed wakefulness. Recumbence during sleep is not associated with jerking.

Moreover, EEG/EMG correlation study has shown that myoclonic jerks are present only in association with the alpha rhythm on electroencephalogram (EEG) and disappear with EEG desynchronization or with the appearance of sleep spindles.[37] It has been suggested that changes in supraspinal control specific to the predormitum stage set the spinal generator responsible for PSM into motion.[38]

The diagnosis of PSM during relaxed wakefulness preceding sleep onset is based on polymyography during PSG recording (see following discussion). Jerk-locked back-averaging (EEG/EMG correlation) shows no time-locked cortical potentials preceding the spontaneous jerks.

Differential diagnosis includes the following:
- Intensified hypnic jerks or physiologic hypnic jerks (see later discussion): Hypnic jerks occur as soon as the patient falls asleep (and are often associated with the appearance of vertex waves in the EEG) in contrast to propriospinal myoclonus at sleep onset, which disappears as the patient goes into sleep or reverses into alert wakefulness by mental or physical activity. Hypnic jerks usually involve the whole body and not just axial muscles.
- Hyperekplexia (see later discussion): myoclonic jerks occur not only in sleep/wake transition, but also persist into sleep, and can be brought on by external stimuli.
- PLMS (see Chapter 24): These movements occur mostly during NREM sleep but may appear in the predormitum.
- Spinal segmental myoclonus (see later): These contractions are restricted to a few spinal segments only.
- Propriospinal psychogenic myoclonus: These contractions are voluntary; readiness potential (Bereitschaftspotential) seen on the EEG preceding the myoclonic jerks is pathognomonic, but requires back-averaging (i.e., EMG/EEG correlation) techniques.
- Cortical myoclonus: This type of myoclonus involves mainly distal limb and facial muscles. EEG/EMG correlation (back-averaging technique) shows that cortical

discharges precede the jerk by about 20 ms in the distal upper extremities and by about 35 to 40 ms in the distal lower extremities.
- Magnetic resonance imaging (MRI) of the spinal cord: Usually propriospinal myoclonus is idiopathic and patients have no structural lesions on spinal cord imaging (70-80%), but it can also be secondary to a structural lesion.[33]
- PSG: The sleep architecture in all patients in one small series of propriospinal myoclonus at sleep onset revealed an increased proportion of light stages of sleep and sleep fragmentation resulting in decreased sleep efficiency. Sleep latency was increased.[38]

Treatment

The treatment of PSM can be challenging, and symptomatic drug therapy is often disappointing. Clonazepam 1 to 2 mg at bedtime and other benzodiazepines showed mild to moderate improvement in a number of cases, so they could be suggested as a first line of therapy, though there are no clear guidelines.[34,37,40] Zonisamide is an alternative add-on therapy for patients with PSM. It was shown to have significant benefit at a dose of 100 to 200 mg daily in some cases refractory to treatment with other medications.[33] Other antiepileptic drugs (valproic acid, primidone, levetiracetam, carbamazepine, oxcarbazepine, topiramate, and pregabalin) as well as some non-antiepileptic drugs (amitriptyline, ropinirole, morphine, baclofen, piracetam) have been tried.[33] Of these other drugs, valproic acid has been tried most frequently with some improvement in isolated patients.[40] Etiologic treatment of the lesion was helpful in one case.[41] Treatment with ciprofloxacin and transcutaneous electrical nerve stimulation (TENS) has been described in the literature[42,43] with some improvement.

Benign Sleep Myoclonus of Infancy

Benign sleep myoclonus of infancy (previously known as *benign neonatal sleep myoclonus*) manifests during the first few weeks of life (usually within the first 15 days) and resolves within months (hence the change in terminology). Myoclonic jerky flexion, extension, abduction, and adduction movements are observed in the extremities and sometimes in the trunk and face, and they often occur in clusters.[44] The movements are brief, asynchronous, and repetitive; they can be focal, multifocal, or generalized. The typical frequency is 1 Hz lasting 40 to 300 ms in clusters of four to five.[45]

The myoclonic jerks occur only during sleep; they are mostly seen in NREM sleep, but can also occur in REM sleep and they usually do not cause arousals. The movements are not continuous, and when not present, they can be brought on by rocking the infant or by gentle restraint during sleep. They cease abruptly on awakening. No movements are observed during wakefulness and no EEG abnormalities are associated with these movements.

The pathogenesis of benign sleep myoclonus of infancy is not well understood. It has been suggested that a disturbance of the reticular activating system could play a role.[46] Genetic factors may also contribute. The condition is benign and usually subsides before 6 to 7 months of age; no associated developmental abnormalities have been reported. Sometimes this condition runs in families. However, there is a broad differential diagnosis for myoclonus in this age group, including convulsive and nonconvulsive conditions. Epileptic conditions include neonatal seizures secondary to asphyxia, metabolic disturbances, infection, benign neonatal seizures, pyridoxine-dependent seizures, and infantile spasms. EEG is helpful to rule out an epileptic origin of myoclonus. Nonepileptic conditions include hyperekplexia, phasic REM twitches, excessive fragmentary myoclonus, and hypnic jerks.

Benign infantile myoclonus does not require treatment. In fact, it was reported that myoclonus can be exacerbated by treatment with anticonvulsants and benzodiazepines.[45,47]

Hypnic Jerks

Hypnic jerks are sudden nonstereotyped myoclonic contractions of all or most body muscles (especially the axial and most proximal muscles) occurring during quiet wakefulness in individuals trying to fall asleep and during light sleep.[48] They are often associated with sensations of tripping, falling through space, or electric shock. Vocalizations can be associated with hypnic jerks.

On the PSG hypnic jerks are recorded during quiet wakefulness and stage N1, and they disappear during N3 and REM sleep. Hypnic jerks are frequently associated with the appearance of vertex sharp waves on EEG. PSG also registers the signs of sympathetic activation associated with hypnic jerks (tachypnea, tachycardia) and they cause transient lightening of sleep. Hypnic jerks tend to be intensified by caffeine and other stimulants and by anxiety.

Intensified hypnic jerks represent an unusual variant, when hypnic jerks become excessive in amplitude, frequency, or both, interfering with sleep onset and causing insomnia.

Differential diagnosis includes propriospinal myoclonus (which only occurs in the predormitum and does not persist into sleep), PLMS, epileptic myoclonus, and hyperekplexia in children.

There is no clear indication for treatment of hypnic jerks or intensified hypnic jerks. Avoidance of caffeine and other stimulants and avoidance of physical and mental stress as well as relaxation techniques at bedtime should be tried first. Clonazepam can be tried in severe cases but no adequately studied data are available.

Physiologic Hypnic Fragmentary Myoclonus

Physiologic hypnic fragmentary myoclonus (PHM) describes asynchronous, asymmetrical, and aperiodic muscle twitches resembling fasciculations observed in muscles of distal body parts (face, lips, fingers, and toes) with occasional movement in the involved segment (lips or fingers).[2,49] PHM is more prominent in babies and infants.

EMG shows random phasic bursts of one or several motor units discharging asynchronously or in small clusters, usually lasting less than a second and often resembling fasciculations. The twitches occur in stage N1 and REM sleep, decreasing progressively in sleep stages N2 and N3. These movements are physiologic and do not disrupt sleep patterns.

There are several theories on where PHM originates. Animal models have suggested reticulospinal tract,[50] or pontine tegmentum;[51] alternatively, the confinement of myoclonic jerks to distal muscles has been taken to suggest a cortical/subcortical origin.[49]

Excessive Fragmentary Myoclonus

This entity is believed to represent pathologic intensification of physiologic hypnic (fragmentary) myoclonus. The term *excessive fragmentary myoclonus (EFM)* describes intense partial myoclonus sustained through all sleep stages with short contractions (less then 150 ms) of the limbs (predominantly distally, but movements can involve larger joints such as knees or hips) and face in an asynchronous and aperiodic pattern. The twitches are absent in wakefulness preceding sleep, appear abruptly at sleep onset, and persist unchanged through NREM and REM sleep.[52]

The EMG pattern consists of brief, sharp, asynchronous potentials occurring randomly on both sides of the body, accompanied by brief prominent local twitches. They are not associated with any specific EEG changes, so it is unlikely that they originate from the cortex. This condition theoretically may arise due to inadequate inhibitory drive from higher centers or due to excessive activation of higher centers during sleep. It has been observed predominantly in men and often coexists with a variety of primary sleep disorders, such as obstructive sleep apnea (OSA), narcolepsy, and PLMS, and is possibly facilitated by nocturnal hypoxemia. Excessive fragmentary myoclonus can cause sleep fragmentation. It has been associated with daytime sleepiness and insomnia even in patients without any other associated sleep disorders.[53] More evidence, however, is needed to prove that excessive fragmentary myoclonus has any biologic consequence.

Differential diagnosis includes physiologic hypnic myoclonus, hypnic jerks, propriospinal myoclonus at sleep onset, epileptic myoclonus, and minipolymyoclonus; the latter is characterized by multiple, small, jerky, involuntary movements of the fingers and was originally described in spinal muscular atrophy but was later also described in Alzheimer's disease patients.

For the diagnosis at least 20 minutes of NREM sleep with the characteristic EMG pattern should be recorded and at least 5 EMG potentials per minute should be registered in the PSG.[4]

The need for treatment of EFM is unclear. Clonazepam and carbamazepine have been found to be useful in reducing EFM.[54]

DIURNAL INVOLUNTARY MOVEMENT DISORDERS

Many of the abnormal movements seen in traditional daytime movement disorder patients may persist into sleep.[55] This discussion includes the disorders that *usually* persist in sleep (palatal myoclonus/palatal tremor), those that *frequently* persist in sleep (spinal and propriospinal myoclonus, tics in Tourette's syndrome, hemifacial spasms, and hyperekplexia), and those that *infrequently* persist during sleep (tremor, chorea, dystonia, and hemiballismus).

Involuntary Movement Disorders Usually Persisting During Sleep

Palatal Tremor (Palatal Myoclonus)

Palatal tremor (palatal myoclonus) is a term that describes involuntary rhythmic movements of the soft palate and pharynx at a typical rate of 100 to 150 per minute, with rates ranging from 20 to 600 per minute.[56] These movements are sometimes associated with rhythmic ocular, buccal, lingual, laryngeal, and diaphragmatic movements and sometimes also with the movements of the limbs. Patients with palatal tremor usually complain of a clicking noise in the ears due to rhythmic movement of the eustachian tube during the contraction of pharyngeal muscles, which can be heard by the examiner by placing minimicrophones in the external auditory canals. Palatal tremor usually persists throughout the day and night for the remaining lifespan of the patient. Palatal tremor was found to persist in sleep and during anesthesia in most of the cases, albeit with shifts in amplitude and frequency.[57] Two types have been described: a primary (essential) type and a secondary (symptomatic) type resulting from brainstem lesions of different etiologies.[56] Patients with essential palatal tremor mostly complain of clicking noise in the ear (unilateral or bilateral), which can be quite disabling. Their MRI is usually unremarkable. Patients with symptomatic palatal tremor usually develop symptoms beginning from 1 day to 30 months after the occurrence of anatomic lesions in Guillain-Mollaret triangle (see next paragraph), which can be seen on the MRI. These patients usually have multiple associated complaints resulting from the lesions (ataxia of the trunk or limbs, oscillopsia, oculomotor impairment, dysarthria).

Palatal tremor results from an involvement of the Guillain-Mollaret triangle, which is formed by the cerebellar dentate nucleus and its outflow tract in the superior cerebellar peduncle crossing over to the contralateral side in the vicinity of the red nucleus and descending ipsilaterally along the central tegmental tract to the inferior olivary nucleus with a final connection from the inferior olivary nucleus back to the contralateral dentate nucleus. The lesions are usually found in the dentate nucleus or in the central tegmental tract. In the rare case of unilateral palatal tremor, the lesions are noted in the contralateral central tegmental tract or inferior olivary nucleus or in the ipsilateral dentate nucleus and its outflow tract. A characteristic pathologic finding is olivary hypertrophy, a pathologic response of the cells of the inferior olive, which can be identified on MRI.

Treatment. Palatal tremor (especially symptomatic type) is generally refractory to medical treatment. Botulinum toxin injections of the levator veli palatini or tensor veli palatini were suggested as the initial treatment because they were shown to be effective with low side effect profile and less invasive than surgical treatment.[58]

There is some evidence of palatal tremor responding to treatment with clonazepam 1 mg daily (complete recovery of essential palatal myoclonus was described) and sumatriptan 6 mg subcutaneously (partial response in a case of palatal myoclonus secondary to infarct was shown).[59]

Baclofen, valproic acid, piracetam (2.4 mg daily), carbamazepine (400 mg daily), L-dopa, lamotrigine (125 mg twice daily),[60] 5-hydroxytryptophan (5-HTP), ceruletide (a potent analog of cholecystokinin octapeptide), phenytoin, tetrabenazine, and trihexyphenidyl were also reported to be effective in some cases.[61,62]

Surgical treatment includes veli palatini tenotomy and occlusion of eustachian tube for patients with disabling ear clicking refractory to medical management.[63] Radiofrequency ablation of palate (another destructive treatment) has also been successful in some cases.[64]

Involuntary Movement Disorders Frequently Persisting During Sleep

Spinal Myoclonus (Segmental Spinal Myoclonus)

Similar to palatal myoclonus, spinal myoclonus is a type of segmental myoclonus. It results from discharges from a myoclonic generator located in one or more contiguous segments of the spinal cord affecting the muscles supplied by the corresponding segments. Spinal myoclonus clinically presents with rhythmic myoclonic movements of one or both limbs and trunk. The movements can sometimes be asynchronous, and stimulus sensitive; they frequently persist during sleep.

In most cases of segmental spinal myoclonus an underlying structural lesion is found on neuroimaging. The etiology is diverse including degenerative joint disease, herpes zoster myelitis, demyelinating myelopathy, arteriovenous malformation, intrathecal medications, and spinal anesthesia.

Spinal myoclonus shows a good response to clonazepam (up to 6 mg daily). Alternative choices include levetiracetam, botulinum toxin injections, carbamazepine, diazepam, and tetrabenazine.[61,62]

Tics in Tourette's Syndrome

Gilles de la Tourette's syndrome involves multiple motor tics with vocalizations. Tourette's syndrome patients frequently suffer from associated behavior disorders, including attention deficit hyperactivity disorder (ADHD) and obsessive-compulsive disorder (OCD). This disorder usually begins in childhood and adolescence and it may subside with age. Motor tics and sometimes vocalizations tend to occur in all sleep stages as was documented in 11 of 12 Tourette's patients.[65] Tourette's patients were also noticed to have increased frequency of associated insomnia, enuresis, somnambulism, night terrors, and bruxism.[66] They tend to have difficulty falling asleep, increased number of awakenings, and early morning awakenings, especially if the patients have associated ADHD.[67] Bodily movements are generally increased in Tourette's patients. There were conflicting PSG data, which was probably due to methodologic difference in the sleep laboratory evaluation. Severity of the syndrome during the day is an important predictor of sleep alteration in these patients.[68]

Treatment. The pharmacologic treatment of Tourette's syndrome and associated disorders (ADHD and OCD) has diverse effects on sleep. In general, treatment with neuroleptics reduced overall nocturnal movements, normalized stage N3 sleep and increased REM sleep latency and sleep efficiency.[69] Haloperidol and pimozide, however, tended to increase evening fatigue.[70] Risperidone tended to improve sleep quality and quantity.[71] Of all neuroleptics fluphenazine appears to have the lowest incidence of sedation compared to other neuroleptics, but this has not been specifically studied. As was reported by Jankovic and colleagues, treatment with tetrabenazine (a monoamine depleting and dopamine receptor blocking agent) showed significant decrease in the percentage of total sleep, number of awakenings, and number of tics during sleep and in the daytime.[72] Clonidine was also helpful in improving sleep as well as tics in some patients, reducing the REM sleep and sleep latency.[73,74] Selective serotonin reuptake inhibitors (SSRIs) used in the treatment of OCD increased REM latency and nocturnal awakenings while reducing REM sleep and overall sleep time and sleep efficiency.[75] SSRI use was also associated with nocturnal bruxism.[76]

Hemifacial Spasm

Hemifacial spasm is an intermittent contraction of one side of the face that can be repetitive and jerklike or sustained. It is believed to arise from irritation to the facial nerve or nucleus. Hemifacial spasm persists during the lighter stages of sleep, decreasing significantly in N3 and REM sleep. PSG shows prolonged sleep latencies and frequent awakenings. EMG shows highly synchronous discharges in upper and lower facial muscles.

Treatment. The treatment options include botulinum toxin injections into affected muscles[77] (injections should be repeated approximately every 3 months); antiepileptic drugs such as carbamazepine, gabapentin, and pregabalin; as well as benzodiazepines (clonazepam) and muscle relaxants. Surgical treatment such as vascular decompression of facial nerve is also used in refractory cases.[78]

Hyperekplexia

Hyperekplexia denotes a group of movements associated with increased startle response consisting of rapid stereotyped motor response and a variety of motor behaviors and vocalizations, autonomic changes, and emotions. Hyperekplexia can be classified as primary (without other neurologic abnormalities) and secondary or symptomatic (occurs in the setting of other neurologic disorders). Primary hyperekplexia can be familial or idiopathic (Box 27-2). Hereditary hyperekplexia is inherited as an autosomal dominant pattern in most of the cases and rarely sporadic cases result from recessive mutations in the gene encoding for the α_1 subunit of the receptor for the inhibitory neurotransmitter glycine (*GLYRA1*). In addition to exaggerated startle response the patients with hereditary hyperekplexia exhibit marked muscle stiffness during infancy. During sleep the infants with hereditary hyperekplexia often experience apneas, which can lead to sudden infant death in the neonatal period (especially in the first 24 hours). The leading hypothesis[79] of the cause of apneas in this disorder proposes that infants have episodic spasm of the trunk and respiratory tract muscles either spontaneously or induced by external stimuli (e.g., repetitive nose tapping). The other theory postulates a deficiency of central regulation of respiration (possibly glycinergic), leading to dyscoordination of oropharyngeal and respiratory musculature.[80] The EEG does not show any abnormalities. Adults with hereditary hyperekplexia often exhibit nocturnal jerks on falling asleep and during sleep that may cause arousals. Those jerks as described in early reports could be triggered by external stimuli (noise, turning the light on) as well as by events in dreams.[81] The pathogenesis of sleep jerks in patients with hyperekplexia is not very clear. Secondary (symptomatic) hyperekplexia (occurs with other neurologic abnormalities, including brainstem and thalamic lesions, drugs, hypoxic ischemic encephalopathy, Tourette's syndrome, and post-traumatic stress disorder [PTSD]). Those patients also exhibit nocturnal jerks and infantile apneas. Differential diagnosis includes a group of disorders associated with exaggerated startle response, for example, jumping Frenchmen of Maine syndrome, myriachit (observed in Siberia), latah (observed in Malaysia). Those disorders are often associated with echolalia and echopraxia, which are not observed in hyperekplexia. Startle epilepsy occurs in the setting of perinatal anoxic encephalopathy, characterized by focal and generalized seizures occurring as a startle response.

Treatment. In infants it has been shown that treatment with clonazepam (0.1 to 0.2 mg/kg/day) reduces the incidence of apneas as well as muscle stiffness and exaggerated startle response. The need for immediate monitoring of at-risk infants, observation for signs of hyperekplexia, and initiation of clonazepam in these patients has been emphasized.[79,82] Clonazepam has also been useful in adult hyperekplexia.[61,83]

Involuntary Movements Sometimes Persisting During Sleep

Many involuntary movement disorders (parkinsonian tremor, tics, dystonia, chorea, hemiballism) are shown to persist into sleep stage N1 and rarely into stage N2; they usually disappear during stage N3 and can occasionally reappear in REM sleep.[84] They tend to reappear on transition from sleep to awakening. Those movements that occur during sleep without awakenings are usually preceded by arousal phenomena and, rarely, by sleep spindles or slow waves. Physiologic motor activity during sleep shows a similar pattern, suggesting that both normal and abnormal movements in sleep are modulated similarly either due to the general suppression of both centers for physiologic and pathologic movements, or by suppression of descending pathways,[85] although most abnormal motor activity is believed to be generated in higher motor centers above the brainstem.

Tremor

Tremor is defined as a rhythmic, involuntary oscillatory movement of a body part that involves alternating or synchronous contractions of reciprocally innervated agonist and antagonist muscles. Tremor can be divided into physiologic and pathologic types. Tremor can be further classified into those occurring at rest and those occurring with action. Action tremor can be divided into postural (occurring while maintaining a certain posture) and intentional or kinetic (with goal-directed movements). Tremors can be central or peripheral in origin. All primary tremors tend to diminish or disappear in sleep.

Rest Tremor (Parkinsonian Tremor). Rest tremor is seen most frequently in Parkinson's disease and secondary parkinsonism in addition to other basal ganglia symptoms. The frequency of the tremor is 3 to 5 Hz. It usually starts in the limb on one side, and later it can manifest in the other limbs.

BOX 27-2 *Hyperekplexia: Classification*

PRIMARY
Hereditary
Idiopathic

SECONDARY (SYMPTOMATIC)
Structural lesions (brainstem, thalamus)
Drugs (amphetamine, cocaine)
Hypoxic-ischemic encephalopathy
Post-traumatic stress disorder (PTSD)
Tourette's syndrome

The tremor is present at rest and it disappears with movement, but can reappear with a static posture (re-emergent tremor). Rest tremor tends to persist in drowsiness, and occasionally occurs in stage N1 sleep; it is rarely seen in stage N3 and is usually not observed in REM sleep. However, it can reappear on arousals, awakenings, and during sleep transitions to stage N1 and stage N2. The exact location of the oscillator is unknown.

Management of rest tremor is similar to management of Parkinson's disease and consists of anticholinergic drugs (trihexyphenidyl, benztropine) or other antiparkinsonian agents such as amantadine, dopamine agonists, and L-dopa (see Chapter 26).

Exaggerated Physiologic Tremor. Physiologic tremor is a fine, 8- to 13-Hz tremor that is best seen in the fingers when the arms are outstretched. It tends to be bilaterally symmetrical. Physiologic tremor becomes exaggerated with anxiety, fatigue, exercise, thyrotoxicosis, hypoglycemia, excessive use of caffeine or other stimulant drugs, and withdrawal from alcohol or sedative agents. The origin of the tremor is unknown, but there may be a component from an 8- to 13-Hz central oscillator in this condition.[86]

Eliminating tremor "triggers" such as caffeine and other stimulants from the diet is often recommended in treating exaggerated physiologic tremor.

Essential Tremor. Essential tremor (ET) is a common disorder affecting about 4% of the population. It is frequently familial with autosomal-dominant inheritance. It can manifest in childhood or later in life (third to fourth decades). ET is an action tremor (with both postural and intention components) with the frequency of 5 to 8 Hz and is usually bilaterally symmetrical. There is often an associated component of physiologic tremor (8-13 Hz). It gets exaggerated by the same conditions as physiologic tremor. ET is typically alleviated by alcohol. ET disappears in sleep, but reappears with rebound on awakening. The origin of ET is believed to be central. The cerebellum and cerebellar circuits seem to be involved, the inferior olivary nucleus being the potential candidate.[87]

Propranolol is first line of treatment for ET.[61] There is less evidence for the efficacy of other beta blockers in the treatment of ET. Primidone is effective for the treatment of ET, and other anticonvulsants (e.g., gabapentin and topiramate) are also used. Benzodiazepines are sometimes used in the treatment of ET with caution due to addictive potential. Botulinum toxin injections have modest benefit in the treatment of ET. Both deep brain stimulation and unilateral thalamotomy are effective for the treatment of medically refractory ET.[61]

Cerebellar Tremor. Cerebellar tremor can be postural and kinetic. The lesions can be in the cerebellum or cerebellar pathways. The frequency of cerebellar tremor is usually 2.5 to 4 Hz. Cerebellar tremor decreases and disappears in sleep. Cerebellar tremor typically does not respond to medical treatment.

Patients with rubral tremor showing a characteristic wing-beating component may receive some relief using L-dopa, anticholinergic drugs, or a high dose of isoniazid.[88] Patients with severe tremor and little or no ataxia can be helped by deep brain stimulation of the ventral intermediate nucleus of the thalamus.

Chorea and Ballismus

Chorea represents nonstereotypical, nonsustained involuntary movements with variable speed and direction. Random muscles throughout the body are affected at random times. The movements can be brief or prolonged. Ballismus represents large amplitude violent choreic movements (called *hemiballismus* if present on one side of the body, which is usually associated with the damage to the contralateral subthalamic nucleus). During sleep chorea generally persists to some extent (especially in light sleep), but with decreased severity. Ballistic movements progressively diminish in intensity and frequency from stage NI to N3 and REM sleep. These findings are documented in patients with ballismus secondary to basal ganglia stroke.[89,90] Disrupted sleep and prolonged sleep latency are also reported.[91]

Successful treatment with haloperidol improved sleep. Tetrabenazine, neuroleptics, and amantadine are used in the treatment of chorea.[61] Anticonvulsants (e.g., levetiracetam and topiramate) have been reported to improve chorea in some cases.[61] Benzodiazepine can be used intermittently when there has been temporary worsening of chorea in stressful situations.

Dystonia

Dystonia is characterized by sustained muscle contractions causing twisting and repetitive movements or abnormal postures. The types of dystonia include generalized dystonia, writer's cramp, spasmodic torticollis, and blepharospasm. In sleep, dystonic movements decrease markedly from stage N1 to stage N2 and are absent in N3 and REM sleep. Some studies in patients with severe torsion dystonia (a generalized dystonia) showed increased sleep latency, frequent awakenings, decreased REM sleep, and reduced total sleep time and sleep efficiency indicating severe sleep disturbance at night.[92] Other studies suggested that the cause of sleep disruption by dystonia is persistent muscular activity, as shown by electromyographic findings in stage N1 in patients with cervical dystonia. Pain also contributes to increased sleep latency.[93,94]

Medications used for the treatment of dystonia include levodopa (for dopa-responsive dystonia), and anticholinergic medications (trihexyphenidyl).[61] Other medications used in the treatment of dystonia without sufficient evidence of benefit include tetrabenazine, clonazepam, and baclofen.[61]

SLEEP DYSFUNCTION IN PARKINSON'S PLUS SYNDROME

Parkinson's disease is discussed in a separate chapter (see Chapter 26). Parkinson's plus syndrome includes multiple system atrophy (MSA), progressive supranuclear palsy (PSP), corticobasal ganglionic degeneration (CBGD), and diffuse Lewy body disease with dementia (DLBD).[84,95]

Multiple System Atrophy

MSA is a neurodegenerative disease with multiple overlapping clinical features.[96] In addition to parkinsonism it is characterized by autonomic disturbances and cerebellar and pyramidal features. When autonomic features predominate, the condition is typically referred to as

Shy-Drager syndrome. When the extrapyramidal features are mainly prominent, the condition is called *striatonigral degeneration* or *MSA-P* and when cerebellar dysfunction predominates, the term *olivopontocerebellar atrophy (OPCA)* or *MSA-C* is used.

Median age of onset of MSA is about 55 years (range of 33 to 76). It affects men slightly more than women. The pathologic features of MSA include degenerative cell loss and gliosis in the basal ganglia, brainstem, cerebellum, and spinal cord with characteristic glial cytoplasmic inclusions due to the accumulation of the protein α-synuclein.

MSA is associated with multiple respiratory abnormalities as well as REM sleep behavior disorder. The most characteristic sleep-related breathing problem is nocturnal laryngeal stridor, which represents a coarse, high-pitched snore sound. Laryngeal stridor can also occur during the day. The possible pathogenesis of this phenomenon includes atrophic paralysis of laryngeal abductor muscles or sleep-related hyperactivity of adductors. This condition can potentially cause sudden respiratory death.

MSA is frequently associated with RBD, which often occurs early in the course of MSA and precedes other symptoms. The pathogenesis of RBD in MSA is believed to be due to degeneration of pontine tegmentum. The clinical features of RBD are described in Chapter 43.

Patients with MSA were also reported to have an increased incidence of PLMS.[95,96] In addition, MSA patients have sleep disturbance secondary to stiffness and pain, causing reduced sleep efficiency and total sleep time.[95,96]

Treatment

Continuous positive airway pressure (CPAP) can help in many mild to moderate cases of laryngeal dysfunction,[95,96] but more severe cases (especially when daytime stridor is present) may require tracheostomy.[97] Those measures, however, do not completely eliminate the possibility of sudden respiratory death. Another possible surgical approach includes vocal cord lateralization reported in one patient.[98] A limited study of unilateral injection of botulinum toxin to thyroarytenoid muscle showed improvement of stridor confirmed by the EMG in three out of four patients.[99] Respiratory failure can also occur in MSA patients from central alveolar hypoventilation. In that case nocturnal ventilation through nasal mask with oxygen supplementation should be considered. Other respiratory sleep problems in MSA patients include OSA, central apneas, and sometimes periodic breathing. All MSA patients and their bed partners should be asked about stridor, snoring and witnessed apnea events during the interview.

The gold standard treatment for RBD is clonazepam (see Chapter 43), but benzodiazepines should be used with caution in patients with MSA because they can precipitate obstructive and central respiratory events.

Progressive Supranuclear Palsy

PSP is a neurodegenerative disease that is characterized by parkinsonism, supranuclear vertical gaze palsy, pseudobulbar palsy, and frontal lobe dementia.[95,84] Parkinsonian syndrome in PSP is characterized by prominent axial rigidity and a poor response to levodopa. The mean age of onset of PSP is 60 years. The median survival time from onset is 5.3 to 5.6 years. This disorder belongs to the group of tauopathies and its pathologic features include neurofibrillary tangles, neuropil threads, neuronal loss, and gliosis in the basal ganglia and brainstem with relative sparing of cortex and hippocampus. The most common sleep-related complaints in patients with PSP are frequent nocturnal awakenings and sleep maintenance insomnia, which correlate with the severity of motor involvement. Sleep dysfunction tends to be more pronounced in PSP compared to Parkinson's disease. RBD and PLMS are described in PSP, but RBD is less prevalent in PSP compared with synucleinopathies. PSG shows decreased sleep time, decreased sleep efficiency (about 50-58%), increased stages N1 and N2 sleep, and decreased REM sleep.[100,101] Reduction in spindle density and amplitude was also noted.

The pathophysiologic basis of sleep disturbance in this disorder is believed to be due to involvement of locus ceruleus or other pontomesencephalic nuclei. The reduction in spindles could be explained by disruption of tegmental pathways connecting thalamic nucleus reticularis and pontine nuclei. Little is known about treatment of sleep dysfunction in this condition.

Treatment

Dopa and dopamine agonists (with poor response) and antidepressants are used for the treatment of PSP. Sleep maintenance insomnia is treated symptomatically by hypnotics (eszopiclone zolpidem). Tricyclic antidepressants with sedative potential (e.g., amitriptyline) could potentially help with insomnia and motor symptoms.[102]

Corticobasal Ganglionic Degeneration

CBGD is a neurodegenerative disease characterized by parkinsonism and cortical signs including apraxia, cortical sensory disturbances, alien limb phenomenon, and dementia.[84] Pathologically it belongs to the group of tauopathies. Intracytoplasmic inclusion bodies, neuronal loss, and gliosis are found in the cortex and substantia nigra. RBD was described in a single case of CBGD.[103] Other sleep disturbances have not been specifically reported.

Diffuse Lewy Body Disease with Dementia

DLBD is a neurodegenerative disease characterized by dementia with pronounced visual-spatial abnormalities closely followed by parkinsonism without the characteristic rest tremor.[84,95] These symptoms are associated with visual hallucinations, delusions, and autonomic instability. There is a significant fluctuation in cognitive symptoms in DLBD. RBD is very common in DLBD and it can appear years before other symptoms manifest. Disturbance of circadian rhythm is also common, causing sleep fragmentation and daytime sleepiness in DLBD patients.[95]

The etiology of DLBD is not known. Rare cases of familial DLB have been reported.

Pathologic findings include Lewy bodies (clumps of α-synuclein and ubiquitin protein) in the neurons of substantia nigra, other brainstem structures (locus ceruleus, nucleus raphe), limbic regions, and cerebral cortex; senile plaques and neurofibrillary tangles are also present. DLBD belongs to the group of synucleinopathies.

Treatment

Patients with DLBD do not respond very well to dopaminergic medications. The treatment is symptomatic. For RBD in DLBD low doses of clonazepam can be effective. Melatonin is also effective and can also be prescribed as a more natural alternative. Dopaminergic drugs (L-dopa, pramipexole) are occasionally useful (see Chapter 43).

MISCELLANEOUS NOCTURNAL MOTOR HYPERACTIVITY

Drug-Induced Movement Disorders During Sleep

Drug-induced abnormal movements are predominantly seen in daytime. They can persist into sleep with decreased severity and they are mostly prominent on sleep transition and in light stages of sleep.[104]

Abnormal Movements Associated with Levodopa in Parkinson's Disease Patients

Dopa-related dyskinesias are characterized by choreiform and dystonic movements.

All dopaminergic drugs used in the treatment of Parkinson's disease can produce these effects, which are more pronounced for catechol-O-methyl transferase (COMT) inhibitors, than for direct dopamine agonists.[104]

- High dopa dyskinesias (HDD) occur above a specific plasma L-dopa threshold, continue to worsen as plasma concentration increases, and disappear when plasma L-dopa concentration declines below a certain (usually lower) threshold. HDD is the most common type of dyskinesia that occurs during the day, but dyskinesias can also be present in some patients in sleep, especially with high and frequent L-dopa doses and when L-dopa is taken in the evening or during the night (some patients with severe bradykinesia take controlled release L-dopa at that time to help them sleep). The choreic movements were reported in the lighter stages of sleep. These movements in some cases caused awakenings and sleep maintenance insomnia, but in the other cases they did not disrupt sleep architecture.[104]
- Low dopa dyskinesias (LDD) begin at a certain L-dopa threshold and then disappear above another higher threshold L-dopa concentration, when the "on" effect of a particular dose sets in. LDD also represent choreiform and dystonic movements that occur as the "end dose" effect after the last dose of L-dopa taken during the day when the plasma concentration of L-dopa has dropped, but not yet approached zero. LDD can occur at sleep onset if the last dose of L-dopa is taken several hours before bedtime, or they can occur later in the night if the doses were taken before bedtime or during the night. LDDs are the most severe and longest lasting of all L-dopa-associated abnormal movements: they can last 4 to 5 hours continuously. Sometimes it is helpful to add a dopamine agonist to the last evening L-dopa dose to minimize the duration and severity of those movements.
- L-dopa in Parkinson's disease patients can also cause kicking and flailing of the arms during sleep, which can get rather hazardous to a sleep partner. These movements are commonly associated with nightmares and sleeptalking. There is no recollection of the event the next morning.[104] These patients can also exhibit hallucination and psychosis. Night time L-dopa doses should be reduced in some patients.
- L-dopa-induced nighttime myoclonus has been described with chronic L-dopa use. Methysergide was reported to decrease L-dopa-induced myoclonus.[104]
- Other L-dopa-related abnormal movements that can occur during sleep include dyskinetic breathing patterns with gasping for air, painful dystonia with the cramping of legs and feet, and akathisia, when the patient feels the need to get out of bed and walk during the night.[104] Laryngeal stridor associated with cranial and cervical dystonia has been reported as the late effect of the last L-dopa dose.[105]

Abnormal Movements Associated with Other Medications

The frequency of abnormal movements associated with medications other than L-dopa is not high. The information is based on anecdotal reports frequently written by physicians not trained in movement disorders. The information on abnormal movements associated with other medications is presented in Boxes 27-3 to 27-12.

Nocturnal Jerks and Body Movements in Obstructive Sleep Apnea Syndrome

Apneas and hypopneas of OSA syndrome can be associated with flailing and jerking movements of body and limbs. These movements occur at the termination of apneas/hypopneas and on restoration of normal breathing. Overnight PSG helps to correlate the movements to respiratory events to differentiate

---

BOX 27-3 *Medications Noted to Cause/Exacerbate Myoclonus*

Opiates (myoclonus is most commonly caused by opioids)
  Meperidine
  Morphine
  Methadone
  Oxycodone
Lithium
Trazodone
Buspirone
Verapamil
Nifedipine
Cocaine
Lithium
Monoamine oxidase inhibitors
L-Tryptophan
Tricyclic antidepressants
Monoamine reuptake inhibitors
Neuroleptics
Penicillin
Cephalosporins

Adapted from Sage JI. Drug-related movement disorders during sleep. In: Chokroverty S, Hening WA, Walters AS, eds. *Sleep and Movement Disorders.* Philadelphia: Elsevier Science; 2003:430-435.

BOX 27-4 *Medications Noted to Cause Chorea*

Methsuximide
Phenobarbital
Primidone
Ethosuximide
Phenytoin
Carbamazepine
Cocaine
Methylphenidate
Amphetamine
Lithium
Imipramine
Neuroleptics
Pemoline
Digoxin
Oxymetholone
Flecainide
Disulfiram
Trazodone
Anticholinergics
Cimetidine
Oral contraceptives

Adapted from Sage JI. Drug-related movement disorders during sleep. In: Chokroverty S, Hening WA, Walters AS, eds. *Sleep and Movement Disorders.* Philadelphia: Elsevier Science; 2003:430-435.

BOX 27-6 *Medications Noted to Cause Dystonia*

Doxepin
Amitriptyline
Neuroleptics
Prochlorperazine
Promethazine
Metoclopramide
Molindone
Phenytoin
Chloroquine
Amodiaquine
Disulfiram
Diazepam
Cimetidine
Histamine H$_2$ receptor blockers
Verapamil
Cinnarizine
Flunarizine
Cocaine
Amphetamine
Tranylcypromine
Amoxapine

Adapted from Sage JI. Drug-related movement disorders during sleep. In: Chokroverty S, Hening WA, Walters AS, eds. *Sleep and Movement Disorders.* Philadelphia: Elsevier Science; 2003:430-435.

BOX 27-5 *Medications Noted to Cause Tremor*

Lithium
Monoamine reuptake inhibitors
Monoamine oxidase inhibitors
Dopamine receptor–blocking drugs
Dopamine-depleting drugs
Stimulants (e.g., amphetamines)
Beta agonists (e.g, terbutaline, epinephrine)
Valproic acid

Adapted from Sage JI. Drug-related movement disorders during sleep. In: Chokroverty S, Hening WA, Walters AS, eds. *Sleep and Movement Disorders.* Philadelphia: Elsevier Science; 2003:430-435.

BOX 27-7 *Medications Noted to Cause Akathisia*

Neuroleptics (most likely agents to cause akathisia)
Midazolam
Cyproheptadine
Methysergide
Buspirone
Diltiazem
Cinnarizine
Flunarizine
Alcohol
Amoxapine
Promethazine
Droperidol
Metoclopramide
Prochlorperazine

Adapted from Sage JI. Drug-related movement disorders during sleep. In: Chokroverty S, Hening WA, Walters AS, eds. *Sleep and Movement Disorders.* Philadelphia: Elsevier Science; 2003:430-435.

BOX 27-8 *Medications Noted to Cause Tics*

Carbamazepine
Cocaine
Pemoline
Levodopa
Methylphenidate
Amphetamine
Tricyclic antidepressants
Neuroleptics

Adapted from Sage JI. Drug-related movement disorders during sleep. In: Chokroverty S, Hening WA, Walters AS, eds. *Sleep and Movement Disorders.* Philadelphia: Elsevier Science; 2003:430-435.

BOX 27-9 *Medications Noted to Cause Oral/Facial Dyskinesias*

Neuroleptics
Metoclopramide
Prochlorperazine
Antihistamines
Chlorpheniramine
Brompheniramine
Phenindamine
Verapamil
Ethanol withdrawal
Anticholinergics

Adapted from Sage JI. Drug-related movement disorders during sleep. In: Chokroverty S, Hening WA, Walters AS, eds. *Sleep and Movement Disorders.* Philadelphia: Elsevier Science; 2003:430-435.

BOX 27-11 *Medications Noted to Worsen Periodic Leg Movements in Sleep (PLMS) and Restless Legs Syndrome (RLS)*

Tricyclic antidepressants
Selective serotonin and serotonin-norepinephrine reuptake inhibitors (SSRIs, SNRIs)
Levodopa
Lithium
Caffeine
Terbutaline
Nifedipine
Antihistamines

Adapted from Sage JI. Drug-related movement disorders during sleep. In: Chokroverty S, Hening WA, Walters AS, eds. *Sleep and Movement Disorders.* Philadelphia: Elsevier Science; 2003:430-435.

BOX 27-10 *Medications Noted to Cause Somnambulism*

Thioridazine
Lithium
Diphenhydramine
Chlorpromazine
Thioxanthene
Methylphenidate
Chlorprothixene
Methaqualone
Propranolol
Triazolam
Zolpidem

Adapted from Sage JI. Drug-related movement disorders during sleep. In: Chokroverty S, Hening WA, Walters AS, eds. *Sleep and Movement Disorders.* Philadelphia: Elsevier Science; 2003:430-435.

BOX 27-12 *Medications Noted to Cause or Worsen Bruxism*

Dopaminergic agonists (especially in patients with Parkinson's disease)
Tricyclic antidepressants
Alcohol
Cocaine
Amphetamines

Adapted from Sage JI. Drug-related movement disorders during sleep. In: Chokroverty S, Hening WA, Walters AS, eds. *Sleep and Movement Disorders.* Philadelphia: Elsevier Science; 2003:430-435.

these movements from other motor abnormalities during sleep, such as PLMS. Respiratory-related PLMS are noted frequently in OSA syndrome at the end of apneas with associated arousal responses and true PLMS are also noted independently of apnea episodes.[106] Sleep walking is more common in individuals suffering from OSA syndrome.[107]

Sleep-Related Panic Attacks

About 30% of patients who have panic attacks during the daytime can also have panic attacks during sleep.[108] Pure sleep-associated panic attacks have also been described.[109] Panic attacks usually are manifest in adolescence (15-19 years) or middle age.[110] Panic attacks usually wake the patients up during transition from stage N2 to N3 sleep. Similar to daytime panic attacks, the patients experience intense anxiety, shortness of breath, choking, palpitations, dizziness, trembling, and the fear of imminent death. The mean duration of panic attacks is about 24 minutes,[110] but they can be shorter. The patients with panic attacks often have coexistent insomnia and fear of going to bed or falling asleep. Most patients with nocturnal panic attacks also tend to experience panic attacks

during the daytime. PSG of patients with panic attacks showed short duration body movements (2.5-15 seconds) during NREM sleep. Unlike PTSD and major depression, REM sleep density was not increased in patients with panic attacks.[111]

The differential diagnosis of nocturnal panic attacks includes sleep terrors, nocturnal seizures, and nightmares. Unlike those who experience sleep terrors, patients with panic attacks tend to recall the episodes of panic attacks very well, and they tend to last longer than nocturnal seizures. Overnight PSG with seizure montage can help in differential diagnosis in complicated cases (see Chapter 50).

The treatment of panic disorder includes psychotherapy and pharmacologic treatment. Four classes of medications are useful and significantly more effective than placebo: SSRIs, serotonin-norepinephrine reuptake inhibitors (SNRIs) (venlafaxine), tricyclic antidepressants (TCAs), and benzodiazepines[108,112]

Fatal Familial Insomnia

Fatal familial insomnia (FFI) is an autosomal dominant prion disease, although sporadic cases have also been reported.[96] Clinical features of this disorder include loss of circadian rhythm (circadian dysrhythmia), autonomic dysfunction, and neuroendocrine dysfunction in addition to cognitive, behavioral manifestations and focal neurologic deficits (ataxia, myoclonus, upper motoneuron dysfunction and tremor). Severe progressive insomnia is frequently the predominant complaint. PSG shows severe disorganization of sleep pattern with short periods of REM sleep lasting seconds to minutes without the normal muscle atonia. Those short REM periods were associated with complex movements and gestures (similar to enacting the dreams in RBD). During those episodes the patients are completely unresponsive to the environment.

The disease usually becomes manifest in middle age, but a younger age of onset has also been described.[113] Men and women are equally affected. The primary pathologic change is degeneration of dorsomedial and anteroventral thalamic nuclei. This disorder is relentlessly progressive and fatal (mean duration is 18.4 ± 17.3 months).[96,114]

FFI remains an untreatable disease at present. Gamma-hydroxybutyrate provided some symptomatic relief of insomnia in one case.[115]

Post-Traumatic Stress Disorder

PTSD is characterized by re-enactment of severely traumatic or life-threatening past experiences. Patients experience flashbacks and nightmares. PTSD patients suffer from chronic insomnia and hyperarousal. Physiologic movements and PLMS tend to be increased in these patients.[116] PSG findings include decreased total sleep time, reduced slow wave sleep, increased REM density,[117] increased number of awakenings, and decreased sleep efficiency.

Treatment

The treatment of PTSD encompasses multiple psychotherapeutic modalities.[108] Pharmacotherapy is primarily aimed at flashbacks and nightmares. SSRIs are currently the first line therapy as per American Psychiatric Association[118] and have been most studied, generally with positive results in RCTs and open label studies, but with poorer response in returning combat veterans. The American Academy of Sleep Medicine Standards of Practice Committee recommended prazosin for PTSD-associated nightmares on the basis of three RCTs and other less rigorous trials demonstrating moderate to strong efficacy of prazosin in combination with other psychotropic medications.[119] Tricyclic antidepressants, venlafaxine, mirtazapine, and nefazodone have also been shown in some trials to be better than placebo.[118] In one RCT alprazolam (a benzodiazepine anxiolytic) was helpful in decreasing anxiety and improving insomnia in these patients, but was ineffective in targeting specific PTSD symptoms.[120] Moreover, because patients with PTSD frequently suffer from co-morbid substance abuse, benzodiazepines should generally be avoided. Anticonvulsant drugs (tiagabine and valproic acid) have been studied in a limited number of RCTs and open-label studies with mixed results.[118] Novel antipsychotics risperidone and olanzapine have been studied in RCTs as adjunctive therapy in patients refractory to other therapies with suggestive positive results for risperidone.[121,122]

CLINICAL APPROACH TO PATIENTS WITH MOVEMENT DISORDERS DURING SLEEP

The approach to a patient complaining of abnormal movements and behaviors during sleep should start with a detailed sleep history.[55] It is important to get the detailed description of the movements and behaviors, frequency and pattern, and the time of onset during the night or at the transition between wakefulness and sleep. A complete history of current or previous medical, neurologic, and psychiatric illnesses and history of drug and alcohol consumption as well as family history are important. Video recording of the events by family members is very helpful (e.g., in diagnosing PLMS, arousal disorders, and nocturnal seizures during sleep). Excessive daytime sleepiness should be addressed because it can be suggestive of sleep fragmentation. Several scales have been developed for objective measuring of daytime sleepiness. Sleep log and sleep diary are helpful to get an accurate history and keep the interview more efficient. Psychiatric history and psychological factors such as stress at work, home, or school should also be addressed.

The possibility of daytime involuntary movements persisting in sleep should be kept in mind. The clues to nocturnal seizures (e.g., tongue biting, nocturnal enuresis, vocalization, and risk factors for seizures) should be considered. It is important to obtain a detailed physical examination with specific attention to the nervous system.

Laboratory Assessment

Laboratory assessment is performed if indicated after detailed history and physical examination. The diagnosis of typical parasomnias is clinical and does not require PSG. Video PSG is helpful to correlate abnormal movements and behaviors with the stage of sleep, and to rule out OSA and nocturnal seizures. When nocturnal seizures are suspected, overnight PSG with seizure montage with more EEG leads is required. Daytime routine EEG, 24-hour ambulatory or video EEG, should be considered for those patients about whom there is a strong clinical suspicion. For patients with suspected RBD, EMG recordings from four limbs are required as there is often dissociation in the activities among cranial, upper limb, and lower limb muscles in these patients. PSGs with polymyographic montages are important in the differential diagnosis of different types of myoclonus.

For evaluation of myoclonic movements a daytime polymyographic recording is used to characterize the movement and locate the site of the generator based on the pattern of progression; the addition of EEG/EMG back-averaging may help to differentiate between cortical, psychogenic, and subcortical myoclonus.

Actigraphy is a technique of motion detection. The actigraphic instrument is a small device worn on a wrist for 1 to 2 weeks. In combination with the sleep log, actigraphic recordings help to objectively assess the time the patients spend in sleep and wakefulness and the specific sleep-wake patterns. Actigraphy is especially helpful in diagnosing circadian rhythm disorders, paradoxical insomnia, and PLMS and for assessing patients with abnormal movement disorders during sleep at night.

Neuroimaging studies (preferably MRI) should be considered to rule out structural brain lesions as a possible cause for the abnormal movements.

GENERAL APPROACH TO THERAPY OF MOVEMENT DISORDERS DURING SLEEP

Depending on the diagnosis therapy should be aimed at the primary movement disorder or primary sleep disorder associated with abnormal movements. If the sleep disorder is caused by some medical or psychiatric problem, the problem should also be addressed. For example, treating OSA will improve jerky movements, which are sometimes associated with it. Treating depression is required in insomnia secondary to depression. Sleep hygiene is important in the treatment of primary sleep disorders.

Pharmacologic therapy should be aimed at specific movement and sleep disorders. Doses should be titrated prudently in elderly patients. It is important to avoid continuous use of sedative-hypnotics and polypharmacy. Benzodiazepines could be substituted for antihistamines such as diphenhydramine or anticholinergic antidepressants such as amitriptyline which may induce more prominent anticholinergic side effects in this age group. However, benzodiazepines are indicated as a chronic treatment for some movement disorders during sleep such as RBD, jerks related to hyperekplexia, and myoclonus in order to prevent injuries to self or others.[61,83]

REFERENCES

1. Frank MG, Heller HC. The ontogeny of mammalian sleep: A reappraisal of alternative hypotheses. *J Sleep Res.* 2003;12:25-34.
2. American Academy of Sleep Medicine. *The International Classification of Sleep Disorders: Diagnostic and Coding Manual.* 2nd ed. Westchester, IL: American Academy of Sleep Medicine; 2005.
3. Sallustro F, Atwell CW. Body rocking, head banging, and head rolling in normal children. *J Pediatr.* 1978;93:704-708.
4. Iber C, Ancoli-Israel S, Chesson A, Quan SF. *The AASM Manual for the Scoring of Sleep and Associated Events: Rules, Terminology and Technical Specifications.* Westchester, IL: American Academy of Sleep Medicine; 2007.
5. Freund HJ, Hefter H. The role of basal ganglia in rhythmic movement. *Adv Neurol.* 1993;60:88-92.
6. Thorpy MJ, ed. *Handbook of Sleep Disorders.* New York: Marcel Dekker; 1990.
7. Alves RS, Aloe F, Silva AB, Tavares SM. Jactatio capitis nocturna with persistence in adulthood. Case report. *Arq Neuropsiquiatr.* 1998;56:655-657.
8. Rosenfeld DS, Nazir N. Rhythmic movement disorder: Treatment with L-dopa. *Sleep Res.* 1997;26:485.
9. Garcia J, Rosen G, Mahowald MW. Waterbeds in treatment of rhythmic movement disorders: Experience with 2 cases. *Sleep Res.* 1996;25:243.
10. Etzioni T, Katz N, Hering E, et al. Controlled sleep restriction for rhythmic movement disorder. *J Pediatr.* 2005;147:393-395.
11. Layzer RB, Rowland LP. Cramps. *N Engl J Med.* 1971;285:31-40.
12. Jacobsen JH, Rosenberg RS, Huttenlocher PR, Spire JP. Familial nocturnal cramping. *Sleep.* 1986;9:54-60.
13. Schwellnus MP. Muscle cramping in the marathon: Etiology and risk factors. *Sports Med.* 2007;37:364-367.
14. Weiner IH, Weiner HL. Nocturnal leg muscle cramps. *JAMA.* 1980;244:2332-2333.
15. Dahle LO, Berg G, Hammar M, et al. The effect of oral magnesium substitution on pregnancy-induced leg cramps. *Am J Obstet Gynecol.* 1995;173:175-180.
16. Maquirriain J, Merello M. The athlete with muscular cramps: Clinical approach. *J Am Acad Orthop Surg.* 2007;15:425-431.
17. Daniell HW. Simple cure for nocturnal leg cramps. *N Engl J Med.* 1979;301:216.
18. Man-Son-Hing M, Wells G. Meta-analysis of efficacy of quinine for treatment of nocturnal leg cramps in elderly people. *BMJ.* 1995;310:13-17.
19. Man-Son-Hing M, Wells G, Lau A. Quinine for nocturnal leg cramps: A meta-analysis including unpublished data. *J Gen Intern Med.* 1998;13:600-606.
20. Roca AO, Jarjoura D, Blend D, et al. Dialysis leg cramps. Efficacy of quinine versus vitamin E. *ASAIO J.* 1992;38:M481-M485.
21. Connolly PS, Shirley EA, Wasson JH, Nierenberg DW. Treatment of nocturnal leg cramps. A crossover trial of quinine vs. vitamin E. *Arch Intern Med.* 1992;152:1877-1880.
22. Walton T, Kolb KW. Treatment of nocturnal leg cramps and restless leg syndrome. *Clin Pharm.* 1991;10:427-428.
23. Baltodano N, Gallo BV, Weidler DJ. Verapamil vs. quinine in recumbent nocturnal leg cramps in the elderly. *Arch Intern Med.* 1988;148:1969-1970.
24. Cutler P. Cramps in the legs and feet. *JAMA.* 1984;252:98.
25. Serrao M, Rossi P, Cardinali P, et al. Gabapentin treatment for muscle cramps: An open-label trial. *Clin Neuropharmacol.* 2000;23:45-49.
26. Hyodo T, Taira T, Takemura T, et al. Immediate effect of Shakuyaku-kanzo-to on muscle cramp in hemodialysis patients. *Nephron Clin Pract.* 2006;104:C28-C32.
27. Broughton R. Pathological fragmentary myoclonus, intensified hypnic jerks and hypnagogic foot tremor: Three unusual sleep-related movement disorders. In: Koella WP, Obal F, Schultz H, Visser P, eds. *Sleep' 86.* Stuttgart: Gustav Fischer Verlag; 1988:240-242.
28. Broughton RJ. Field studies of sleep/wake patterns and performance: A laboratory experience. *Can J Psychol.* 1991;45:240-253.
29. Wichniak A, Tracik F, Geisler P, et al. Rhythmic feet movements while falling asleep. *Mov Disord.* 2001;16:1164-1170.
30. Walters AS. Clinical identification of the simple sleep-related movement disorders. *Chest.* 2007;131:1260-1266.
31. Chervin RD, Consens FB, Kutluay E. Alternating leg muscle activation during sleep and arousals: A new sleep-related motor phenomenon? *Mov Disord.* 2003;18:551-559.
32. Cosentino FI, Iero I, Lanuzza B, et al. The neurophysiology of the alternating leg muscle activation (ALMA) during sleep: Study of one patient before and after treatment with pramipexole. *Sleep Med.* 2006;7:63-71.
33. Roze E, Bounolleau P, Ducreux D, et al. Propriospinal myoclonus revisited: Clinical, neurophysiologic, and neuroradiologic findings. *Neurology.* 2009;72:1301-1309.
34. Brown P, Thompson PD, Rothwell JC, et al. Axial myoclonus of propriospinal origin. *Brain.* 1991;114(Pt 1A):197-214.
35. Chokroverty S, Walters A, Zimmerman T, Picone M. Propriospinal myoclonus: A neurophysiologic analysis. *Neurology.* 1992;42:1591-1595.
36. Critchley M. *[The pre-dormitum.] Rev Neurol (Paris).* 1955;93:101-106.
37. Vetrugno R, Provini F, Meletti S, et al. Propriospinal myoclonus at the sleep-wake transition: A new type of parasomnia. *Sleep.* 2001;24:835-843.
38. Montagna P, Provini F, Plazzi G, et al. Propriospinal myoclonus upon relaxation and drowsiness: A cause of severe insomnia. *Mov Disord.* 1997;12:66-72.
39. Okuma Y, Fujishima K, Machida Y, et al. Propriospinal negative myoclonus. *Eur Neurol.* 2001;46:99-101.
40. Chokroverty, S. Propriospinal myoclonus Clinical Neuroscience 1995;3:219-222.
41. Capelle HH, Wohrle JC, Weigel R, et al. Propriospinal myoclonus due to cervical disc herniation. Case report. *J Neurosurg Spine.* 2005;2:608-611.
42. Maltete D, Verdure P, Roze E, et al. TENS for the treatment of propriospinal myoclonus. *Mov Disord.* 2008;23:2256-2257.
43. Post B, Koelman JH, Tijssen MA. Propriospinal myoclonus after treatment with ciprofloxacin. *Mov Disord.* 2004;19:595-597.
44. Hanna P, Walters A, eds. *Benign neonatal sleep myoclonus.* Philadelphia: Butterworth Heinemann; 2003.
45. Daoust-Roy J, Seshia SS. Benign neonatal sleep myoclonus. A differential diagnosis of neonatal seizures. *Am J Dis Child.* 1992;146:1236-1241.
46. Coulter DL, Allen RJ. Benign neonatal sleep myoclonus. *Arch Neurol.* 1982;39:191.
47. Reggin JD, Johnson MI. Exacerbation of benign neonatal sleep myoclonus by benzodiazepines. *Ann Neurol.* 1989;26:455.
48. Chokroverty S, Gupta D. Hypnic jerks. In: Thorpy M, Plazzi G, eds. *The Parasomnia and Other Sleep-Related Movement Disorders.* Cambridge: Cambridge University Press; 2010:229-236.
49. Dagnino N, Loeb C, Massazza G, Sacco G. Hypnic physiological myoclonias in man: An EEG-EMG study in normal and neurological patients. *Eur Neurol.* 1969;2:47-58.
50. Gassel MM, Marchiafava PL, Pompeiano O. Phasic changes in muscular activity during desynchronized sleep in unrestrained cats. An analysis of the pattern and organization of myoclonic twitches. *Arch Ital Biol.* 1964;102:449-470.
51. Gastaut H. [Semeiology of myoclonus and analytic nosology of myoclonic syndromes]. *Rev Neurol (Paris).* 1968;119:1-30.
52. Lins O, Castonguay M, Dunham W, et al. R. Excessive fragmentary myoclonus: Time of night and sleep stage distributions. *Can J Neurol Sci.* 1993;20:142-146.

53. Broughton R, Tolentino MA, Krelina M. Excessive fragmentary myoclonus in NREM sleep: A report of 38 cases. *Electroencephalogr Clin Neurophysiol.* 1985;61:123-133.

54. Vetrugno R, Plazzi G, Provini F. Excessive fragmentary hypnic myoclonus: Clinical and neurophysiological findings. *Sleep Med.* 2002;3:73-76.

55. Chokroverty S, Hening W, Walters A, eds. *An Approach to a Patient with Movement Disorders During Sleep and Classification.* Philadelphia: Butterworth/Heinemann; 2003.

56. Deuschl G, Toro C, Valls-Sole J, et al. Symptomatic and essential palatal tremor. 1. Clinical, physiological and MRI analysis. *Brain.* 1994;117 (Pt 4):775-788.

57. Chokroverty S, Barron KD. Palatal myoclonus and rhythmic ocular movements: A polygraphic study. *Neurology.* 1969;19:975-982.

58. Cho JW, Chu K, Jeon BS. Case of essential palatal tremor: Atypical features and remarkable benefit from botulinum toxin injection. *Mov Disord.* 2001;16:779-782.

59. Fabiani G, Teive HA, Sa D, et al. Palatal myoclonus: Report of two cases. *Arq Neuropsiquiatr.* 2000;58:901-904.

60. Nasr A, Brown N. Palatal myoclonus responding to lamotrigine. *Seizure.* 2002;11:136-137.

61. Fahn S, Jankovic J. *Principles and Practice of Movement Disorders.* Philadelphia: Churchill-Livingstone/Elsevier; 2007.

62. Pappert EJ, Goetz CG. Treatment of myoclonus. In: Kurlan, ed. *Treatment of Movement Disorders.* Philadelphia: Lippincott; 1995:247-336.

63. Ensink RJ, Vingerhoets HM, Schmidt CW, Cremers CW. Treatment for severe palatoclonus by occlusion of the eustachian tube. *Otol Neurotol.* 2003;24:714-716.

64. Aydin O, Iseri M, Ozturk M. Radiofrequency ablation in the treatment of idiopathic bilateral palatal myoclonus: A new indication. *Ann Otol Rhinol Laryngol.* 2006;115:824-826.

65. Glaze DG, Frost Jr JD, Jankovic J. Sleep in Gilles de la Tourette's syndrome: Disorder of arousal. *Neurology.* 1983;33:586-592.

66. Hanna P, Jankovic J. Sleep and tic disorders. In: Chokroverty S, Hening WA, Walters AS, eds. *Sleep and Movement Disorders.* Philadelphia: Butterworth Heinemann; 2003:464-471.

67. Comings DE, Comings BG. A controlled study of Tourette syndrome. VI. Early development, sleep problems, allergies, and handedness. *Am J Hum Genet.* 1987;41:822-838.

68. Cohrs S, Rasch T, Altmeyer S, et al. Decreased sleep quality and increased sleep related movements in patients with Tourette's syndrome. *J Neurol Neurosurg Psychiatry.* 2001;70:192-197.

69. Maixner S, Tandon R, Eiser A, et al. Effects of antipsychotic treatment on polysomnographic measures in schizophrenia: A replication and extension. *Am J Psychiatry.* 1998;155:1600-1602.

70. Nicholson AN, Pascoe PA. Dopaminergic transmission and the sleep-wakefulness continuum in man. *Neuropharmacology.* 1990;29:411-417.

71. Dursun SM, Patel JK, Burke JG, Reveley MA. Effects of typical antipsychotic drugs and risperidone on the quality of sleep in patients with schizophrenia: A pilot study. *J Psychiatry Neurosci.* 1999;24:333-337.

72. Jankovic J, Glaze DG, Frost Jr JD. Effect of tetrabenazine on tics and sleep of Gilles de la Tourette's syndrome. *Neurology.* 1984;34:688-692.

73. Kenney C, Kuo SH, Jimenez-Shahed J. Tourette's syndrome. *Am Fam Physician.* 2008;77:651-658.

74. Gentili A, Godschalk MF, Gheorghiu D, et al. Effect of clonidine and yohimbine on sleep in healthy men: A double-blind, randomized, controlled trial. *Eur J Clin Pharmacol.* 1996;50:463-465.

75. Vasar V, Appelberg B, Rimon R, Selvaratnam J. The effect of fluoxetine on sleep: A longitudinal, double-blind polysomnographic study of healthy volunteers. *Int Clin Psychopharmacol.* 1994;9:203-206.

76. Ellison JM, Stanziani P. SSRI-associated nocturnal bruxism in four patients. *J Clin Psychiatry.* 1993;54:432-434.

77. Kenney C, Jankovic J. Botulinum toxin in the treatment of blepharospasm and hemifacial spasm. *J Neural Transm.* 2008;115:585-591.

78. Sindou MP. Microvascular decompression for primary hemifacial spasm. Importance of intraoperative neurophysiological monitoring. *Acta Neurochir (Wien).* 2005;147:1019-1026.

79. Nigro MA, Lim HC. Hyperekplexia and sudden neonatal death. *Pediatr Neurol.* 1992;8:221-225.

80. Floeter MK, Hallett M. Hyperekplexia and sleep disorders. In: Chokroverty S, Hening WA, Walters AS, eds. *Sleep and Movement Disorders.* Philadelphia: Butterworth-Heinemann; 2003:472-477.

81. Gastaut H, Villeneuve A. The startle disease or hyperekplexia. Pathological surprise reaction. *J Neurol Sci.* 1967;5:523-542.

82. Giacoia GP, Ryan SG. Hyperekplexia associated with apnea and sudden infant death syndrome. *Arch Pediatr Adolesc Med.* 1994;148:540-543.

83. Andermann F, Keene DL, Andermann E, et al. Startle disease or hyperekplexia: Further delineation of the syndrome. *Brain.* 1980;103:985-997.

84. Hening WA, Allen RP, Walters AS, Chokroverty S. Motor functions and dysfunctions of sleep. In: Chokroverty S, ed. *Sleep Disorders Medicine: Basic Science, Technical Considerations and Clinical Aspects.* Philadelphia: Saunders/Elsevier; 2009:397-435.

85. Fish DR, Sawyers D, Allen PJ, et al. The effect of sleep on the dyskinetic movements of Parkinson's disease, Gilles de la Tourette syndrome, Huntington's disease, and torsion dystonia. *Arch Neurol.* 1991;48:210-214.

86. Hallett M. Classification and treatment of tremor. *JAMA.* 1991;266:1115-1117.

87. Hallett M, Dubinsky RM. Glucose metabolism in the brain of patients with essential tremor. *J Neurol Sci.* 1993;114:45-48.

88. Koch M, Mostert J, Heersema D, De Keyser J. Tremor in multiple sclerosis. *J Neurol.* 2007;254:133-145.

89. Mano T, Shiozawa Z, Sobue I. Extrapyramidal involuntary movements during sleep. *Electroencephalogr Clin Neurophysiol Suppl.* 1982;35:431-442.

90. Dyken ME, Rodnitzky RL. Periodic, aperiodic, and rhythmic motor disorders of sleep. *Neurology.* 1992;42:68-74.

91. Silvestri R, De Domenico P, Di Rosa AE, et al. The effect of nocturnal physiological sleep on various movement disorders. *Mov Disord.* 1990;5:8-14.

92. Jankel WR, Niedermeyer E, Graf M, Kalsher M. Polysomnography of torsion dystonia. *Arch Neurol.* 1984;41:1081-1083.

93. Chan J, Brin MF, Fahn S. Idiopathic cervical dystonia: Clinical characteristics. *Mov Disord.* 1991;6:119-126.

94. Claypool DW, Duane DD, Ilstrup DM, Melton III LJ. Epidemiology and outcome of cervical dystonia (spasmodic torticollis) in Rochester, Minnesota. *Mov Disord.* 1995;10:608-614.

95. Chokroverty S. Sleep and neurodegenerative diseases. *Semin Neurol.* 2009;29:445-466.

96. Chokroverty S, Montagna P. Sleep and breathing in neurological disorders. In: Chokroverty S, ed. *Sleep Disorders Medicine.* Philadelphia: Saunders/Elsevier; 2009:436-498.

97. Miyamoto M, Miyamoto T, Katayama S, Hirata K. [Effective nasal CPAP therapy for heavy snoring and paradoxical respiration during sleep in a case of multiple system atrophy.]. *Rinsho Shinkeigaku.* 1998;38:1059-1063.

98. Kenyon GS, Apps MC, Traub M. Stridor and obstructive sleep apnea in Shy-Drager syndrome treated by laryngofissure and cord lateralization. *Laryngoscope.* 1984;94:1106-1108.

99. Merlo IM, Occhini A, Pacchetti C, Alfonsi E. Not paralysis, but dystonia causes stridor in multiple system atrophy. *Neurology.* 2002;58:649-652.

100. Montplaisir J, Petit D, Decary A, et al. Sleep and quantitative EEG in patients with progressive supranuclear palsy. *Neurology.* 1997;49:999-1003.

101. Aldrich MS, Foster NL, White RF, et al. Sleep abnormalities in progressive supranuclear palsy. *Ann Neurol.* 1989;25:577-581.

102. Nieforth KA, Golbe LI. Retrospective study of drug response in 87 patients with progressive supranuclear palsy. *Clin Neuropharmacol.* 1993;16:338.

103. Kimura K, Tachibana N, Aso T, et al. Subclinical REM sleep behavior disorder in a patient with corticobasal degeneration. *Sleep.* 1997;20:891-894.

104. Sage JI. Drug-related movement disorders during sleep. In: Chokroverty S, Hening WA, Walters AS, eds. *Sleep and Movement Disorders.* Philadelphia: Elsevier; 2003:430-435.

105. Corbin DO, Williams AC. Stridor during dystonic phases of Parkinson's disease. *J Neurol Neurosurg Psychiatry.* 1987;50:821-822.

106. Fry JM, DiPhillipo MA, Pressman MR. Periodic leg movements in sleep following treatment of obstructive sleep apnea with nasal continuous positive airway pressure. *Chest.* 1989;96:89-91.

107. Guilleminault C, Kirisoglu C, Bao G, Arias V, Chan A, Li KK. Adult chronic sleepwalking and its treatment based on polysomnography. *Brain.* 2005;128(Pt 5):1062-1069.

108. Ramsawh H, Stein MB, Mellman TA. Anxiety disorders. In: Kryger MH, Roth T, Dement WC, eds. *Principles and Practice of Sleep Medicine.* Philadelphia: Elsevier/Saunders; 2011:1473.

109. Rosenfeld DS, Furman Y. Pure sleep panic: Two case reports and a review of the literature. *Sleep.* 1994;17:462-465.

110. Von Korff MR, Eaton WW, Keyl PM. The epidemiology of panic attacks and panic disorder. Results of three community surveys. *Am J Epidemiol.* 1985;122:970-981.

111. Insel TR, Gillin JC, Moore A, et al. The sleep of patients with obsessive-compulsive disorder. *Arch Gen Psychiatry*. 1982;39:1372-1377.

112. http://www.psychiatryonline.com/pracGuide/PracticePDFs/PanicDisorder_2e_Practice Guideline.pdf. pp 54–61. Accessed 1-1-11.

113. Harder A, Gregor A, Wirth T, et al. Early age of onset in fatal familial insomnia. Two novel cases and review of the literature. *J Neurol*. 2004;251:715-724.

114. Montagna P, Cortelli P, Avoni P, et al. Clinical features of fatal familial insomnia: Phenotypic variability in relation to a polymorphism at codon 129 of the prion protein gene. *Brain Pathol*. 1998;8:515-520.

115. Reder AT, Mednick AS, Brown P, et al. Clinical and genetic studies of fatal familial insomnia. *Neurology*. 1995;45:1068-1075.

116. Mellman TA, Kulick-Bell R, Ashlock LE, Nolan B. Sleep events among veterans with combat-related posttraumatic stress disorder. *Am J Psychiatry*. 1995;152(1):110-115.

117. Ross RJ, Ball WA, Dinges DF, et al. Rapid eye movement sleep disturbance in posttraumatic stress disorder. *Biol Psychiatry*. 1994;35:195-202.

118. http://www.psychiatryonline.com/content.aspx?aID=156498&;searchStr=post-traumatic+stress+disorder. Accessed 1-1-11.

119. Aurora RN, Zak RS, Auerbach SH, Casey KR, Chowdhuri S, et al. Best practice guide for the treatment of nightmare disorder in adults. *J Clin Sleep Med*. 2010;6(4):389-401.

120. Braun P, Greenberg D, Dasberg H, Lerer B. Core symptoms of posttraumatic stress disorder unimproved by alprazolam treatment. *J Clin Psychiatry*. 1990;51(6):236-238.

121. Institute of Medicine (U.S.). *Committee on Treatment of Posttraumatic Stress Disorder. Treatment of Posttraumatic Stress Disorder: An Assessment of the Evidence*. Washington, DC: National Academies Press; 2008.

122. Pae CU, Lim HK, Peindl K, Ajwani N, Serretti A, et al. The atypical antipsychotics olanzapine and risperidone in the treatment of posttraumatic stress disorder: A meta-analysis of randomized, double-blind, placebo-controlled clinical trials. *Int Clin Psychopharmacol*. 2008;23(1):1-8.

Circadian Rhythm Disorders

Overview of the Circadian Timekeeping System and Diagnostic Tools for Circadian Rhythm Sleep Disorders

Chapter 28

STEVEN W. LOCKLEY

Circadian rhythm sleep disorders (CRSDs) represent about 10% of the approximately 75 clinical sleep disorders that are formally recognized,[1-3] although nearly everyone will experience a circadian sleep disorder at some time in life. CRSDs are characterized by sleep being attempted or occurring at an abnormal time relative to the internal circadian rhythm for sleep propensity (Box 28-1). There is only a narrow window within the daily circadian cycle when sleep can easily be initiated and maintained, and attempting to sleep outside this window of time will result in difficulty with falling asleep or staying asleep. Some of these disorders are largely self-induced, for example, shift work disorder and jet lag disorder, such as when individuals voluntarily choose to sleep and wake at an adverse circadian phase, whereas others are caused by misalignment between the biologic drive for sleep and the 24-hour solar or social day (delayed sleep phase disorder [DSPD], advanced sleep phase disorder [ASPD], non-24-hour sleep-wake disorder [N24HSWS]). Sleep patterns which do not show a regular 24-hour cycle are also classified as CRSDs (irregular sleep-wake rhythm [ISWR]) and include those associated with a medical or neurologic condition such as dementia, for example.

Although the current clinical criteria rely largely on subjective reports of sleep timing or complaints of insomnia or sleepiness, a more thorough examination of how sleep timing relates to internal circadian phase is warranted if we are to understand the fundamental cause of circadian rhythm sleep disorders and develop appropriate treatments. There likely exist subtypes of disorders within the current categories that have different genetic and physiologic bases but are currently grouped under a limited sleep phenotype that cannot distinguish between them. More sophisticated diagnostic criteria and methodologies are required in order to ensure correct diagnoses and to develop optimal individualized therapies. Before discussing these issues, a brief review of human circadian organization is required.

THE CIRCADIAN SYSTEM

Many aspects of human physiology, metabolism, and behavior are dominated by 24-hour cycles including the sleep-wake cycle, alertness and performance patterns, core body temperature rhythms, and the production of hormones such as melatonin and cortisol. In mammals, including humans, endogenous near-24-hour rhythms are generated spontaneously by the suprachiasmatic nuclei (SCN) of the anterior hypothalamus. The cells in these nuclei generate rhythms with a period close to, but not exactly, 24 hours and in order for

the circadian pacemaker to ensure that physiology and behavior are appropriately timed to anticipate events in the outside world, environmental time cues must be able to reset this internal clock. The major environmental time cue that resets the internal clock in mammals is the 24-hour light-dark cycle, which in turn synchronizes the physiology, metabolism, and behavior controlled by the clock. The circadian system has traditionally been described by three components: an intrinsic circadian pacemaker, input pathways providing information about environmental time to the clock, and output pathways sending circadian signals to other brain areas. Although there is emerging evidence for additional brain and organ-specific circadian pacemakers, this simple model remains useful in conceptualizing the basis of CRSDs.

Defining Circadian Rhythms

The time taken to complete one cycle of a circadian ("about a day") rhythm is defined as the period (τ). A fixed point within a single cycle is termed the phase (φ) and is usually measured from the peak (maximum) or trough (minimum) of the rhythm, but any phase marker can be used if defined. The peak of a rhythm fitted using a sine function is termed the acrophase. The *circadian period* is therefore defined as the duration of time between one phase and the next. The *amplitude of a rhythm* is defined as half of the maximum to minimum oscillation of the rhythm.

By definition, a circadian rhythm is one that persists in the absence of external time cues, that is, it occurs in constant conditions. Strictly speaking, therefore, any 24-hour rhythm that is measured in the presence of time cues (e.g., the light-dark cycle, sleep-wake cycle, standard meal times, social interactions) is not circadian but usually either diurnal (peaking in the day) or nocturnal (peaking at night). This definition has important consequences, as some outcomes appear rhythmic under ambulatory conditions but do not persist when the external cues are removed (e.g., growth hormone), or only reveal their rhythmicity under controlled conditions but not when measured in normal conditions (e.g., thyroid-stimulating hormone)[4-6] (Fig. 28-1). Most rhythmic markers are altered or "masked" to some extent by environmental time cues, and therefore, understanding the basis of apparent rhythms and the effect of experimental conditions on rhythmic variables is vital when trying to measure circadian rhythms clinically (see discussion under "Measurement of Circadian Rhythms in the Diagnosis of CRSD").

The gold standard to measure circadian phase and amplitude is the constant routine (CR) procedure, which removes or minimizes external influences that might affect expression of the endogenous circadian rhythm or, if this is not possible, distributes them evenly across all circadian phases so that any effect of the masking stimulus is effectively averaged out. This method requires subjects to be assessed for at least 24 hours (usually 30 hours or more) in constant conditions; subjects remain awake during continuous semirecumbent bed rest in constant dim light (< 15 lux or lower) with no activity and regular (e.g., hourly) identical meals and fluids. Using these techniques, it has been possible to make a systematic review of endogenous circadian rhythms and the phase resetting effects of potential time cues, for example, in response to light, as outlined in the next section.[7]

Measurement of circadian period requires a longer assessment than can be achieved during a CR procedure. Even though a CR can sometimes last two and rarely three circadian cycles (48-72 hours), the small number of cycles is insufficient to assess circadian period accurately. Although numerous techniques have been used to measure period in the laboratory, the forced desynchrony protocol, pioneered by Nathanial Kleitman in the 1930s, represents the best developed method for the accurate and reliable measurement of circadian period. The technique requires that subjects live on a scheduled day-length (called a *T-cycle*) that is outside the range of entrainment of the circadian pacemaker (i.e., a T-cycle so different from 24 hours that the circadian pacemaker cannot entrain to it and consequently reverts to its intrinsic period).[8] Examples of forced desynchrony T-cycles include 20-, 28-, 30-, and 42.85-hour "days" and a 2:1 wake:sleep ratio.[9-12] Under these conditions, the circadian pacemaker of healthy adults exhibits an average period of approximately 24.2 hours with a range from 23.5 to 24.7 hours.[8] Similar non-24-hour periods have been observed in subjects living in darkness or under dim light in the laboratory.[13] Ultrashort sleep-wake cycles, for example, 20-minute or 90-minute "days," are also a type of forced desynchrony, but these very short T-cycles cannot be sustained for more than a few days.[14-16]

A canonical property of circadian rhythms is their ability to be reset by external time cues. In order for the circadian pacemaker to remain entrained to environmental time, a daily phase shift is required that opposes the daily "drift" in phase as determined by the intrinsic period of the pacemaker. For example, if the endogenous period of an individual is 24.5 hours, then a phase shift of 0.5 hour per day is required

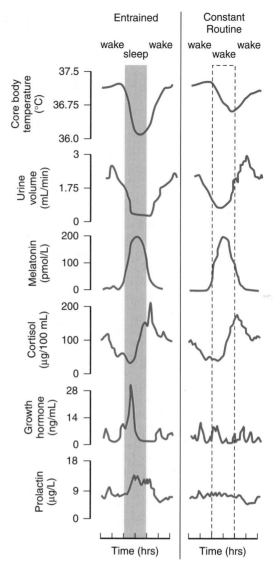

Figure 28-1 Measuring circadian rhythms. This figure shows the relative profiles of temperature, urine volume, and a number of common endocrine markers under normal baseline 16-hour wake/8-hour sleep/16-hour wake (W-S-W) conditions (*left panels*, sleep shown by dark shaded area) and under constant routine (CR) conditions in which subjects remain awake in a time-free environment, under dim light, and in a semirecumbent posture with hourly snacks for 30 hours or longer. Melatonin (*third panel*) and cortisol (*fourth panel*) profiles are relatively unchanged by sleep, except that there is a small wake-dependent rise in cortisol in the morning not seen during CR conditions. Controlled dim light exposure is necessary to maintain melatonin levels under CR conditions, however, because light directly suppresses melatonin. There is a large sleep-dependent increase in the amplitude of core body temperature (*top panel*) and a lowering of the temperature minimum reached due to the direct hypothermic effect of sleep in addition to the circadian decline in temperature at night. Growth hormone (*fifth panel*) and, to a lesser extent, prolactin (*bottom panel*) have a sleep-dependent increase in levels such that production of these hormones is greatly reduced if sleep is absent (*right panels*). These examples serve to underscore the importance of potential masking effects when assessing circadian phase (see text). (Adapted with permission from Figure 1 in Maywood ES, O'Neill JS, Chesham JE, Hastings MH. Minireview: The circadian clockwork of the suprachiasmatic nuclei—Analysis of a cellular oscillator that drives endocrine rhythms. *Endocrinology*. 2007;148:5624-5634.)

to maintain entrainment. As this shift requires a shortening of the period, causing the circadian cycle to be completed in a shorter time, the direction of shift is termed an advance shift. If the period (τ) = 23.8 hours, then a phase delay shift of 0.2 hour per day is required, lengthening the period and delaying the time taken to complete one circadian cycle. Light is the most powerful and well-studied resetting stimulus and, as outlined in the following section, can either phase advance or phase delay the clock, depending on the time of exposure.[17]

LIGHT AND CIRCADIAN RHYTHMS

Light, and specifically the light-dark cycle, plays a major role in the etiology of CRSDs. Light is also a potential therapy for CRSDs, so it is therefore useful to understand some of the properties of light that affect photic circadian resetting.

Light information is captured exclusively by the eyes using specialized retinal photoreceptors and transduced directly to the SCN via a dedicated neural pathway, the retinohypothalamic tract (RHT). Bilateral enucleation or transection of the RHT (but not other tracts of the optic nerve) abolish all circadian responses to light. The specialized "circadian" photoreceptors are not located in the outer retinal layer where traditional rod and cone photoreceptors that are used for vision are located, but are found in the ganglion cell layer of the eye. A small fraction of retinal ganglion cells (< 0.3%) are intrinsically photosensitive and respond directly to light *in vivo* and *in vitro*.[18-20] They contain a novel opsin photopigment, melanopsin, which is most sensitive to short-wavelength blue visible light ($\lambda_{max} \sim 480$ nm) and they project directly to brain areas involved in "nonvisual" responses to light, with the majority projecting to the SCN via the RHT.[21,22] All circadian effects of light are mediated by these photosensitive ganglion cells, but not necessarily by melanopsin. Rod- and cone-based photoreception can stimulate circadian responses under certain circumstances, and circadian responses to light are still obtained in melanopsin-knockout animals, albeit with a reduced efficacy.[23] These rod and cone signals are mediated solely through the specialized ganglion cells independently of melanopsin; however, if this subset of ganglion cells are killed, all circadian responses to light are abolished, even in an otherwise intact eye.[24]

As might be expected, circadian resetting and other "nonvisual" responses to light such as melatonin suppression, acute alerting responses, and the pupillary reflex, are most sensitive to blue light in humans, primates, and other mammals.[25] Using classical photobiology techniques, action spectra have been generated for a number of responses and species, including melatonin suppression in humans, and exhibit a peak sensitivity in the short-wavelength (blue) range (446-477 nm) that does not match the action spectra for human scotopic (rod) or photopic color (cone) vision, and is close to that of melanopsin (Fig. 28-2, *A*).[26,27] Although full action spectra are not yet available for circadian phase-shifting in humans, comparisons of equal photon density exposures of monochromatic 460-nm and 555-nm light have shown that the circadian system is also more sensitive to short-wavelength 460 nm light, confirming that the three-cone photopic photoreceptor system (which has a peak sensitivity at 555 nm) is not the primary photoreceptor system mediating the resetting effects of light, at least at night, and is consistent with the concept of a nonrod, noncone photoreceptor system in the human eye.[28,29]

The circadian photoreception system is not optimized to detect light with the same sensitivity as the visual system but rather represents a relatively insensitive irradiance detector. This irradiance detection system predates vision in evolutionary terms[30] and both the anatomic location of the photoreceptors, distributed sparsely in a network across the eye, and the properties of the system, particularly the ability to integrate light information over a long duration of time, reflect this specific role.

Role of Blindness

Given that circadian responses to light are mediated exclusively via the eyes, an obvious question is what happens to circadian organization in visually impaired or blind people? First, individuals without eyes, either through bilateral enucleation or as a result of developmental disorders, are unable to entrain their circadian pacemaker to the 24-hour light-dark cycle. Similarly, the majority of totally blind individuals who retain their eyes but cannot consciously perceive light also exhibit circadian rhythms that are not entrained to the 24-hour light-dark cycle.[31] As a result of light information failing to reach the SCN to synchronize the clock and its outputs, the pacemaker reverts to its endogenous non-24-hour period and non-24-hour sleep-wake syndrome develops. Disorders of the visual system do not always attenuate the circadian effects of light, however, demonstrating a functional separation of the visual and circadian photoreception systems. The majority of legally blind individuals who retain some degree of light perception, even with very little usable vision in some cases, have normally entrained circadian rhythms.[32] Color blindness, a more specific lesion of the three-cone photopic visual system, also does not attenuate circadian responses to bright light, as measured by acute suppression of pineal melatonin.[33] Finally, and most definitively, it has been demonstrated that some totally visually blind people retain normal circadian phase-shifting and melatonin suppression responses to white light even in the absence of any normal visual response, as assessed by conscious ability to detect light, visually evoked potentials, or electroretinogram, and exhibit normally entrained 24-hour rhythms and do not report sleep disorders.[34,35] Exposure to bright blue, but not green, light also stimulates these responses, suggesting that the melanopsin system is intact and functional in the absence of visual photoreception.[36]

Properties of Light for Circadian Phase Resetting

Light wavelength is not the only factor of significance; light timing, intensity, duration, pattern, and history of exposure affect the stimulus strength for photic phase resetting (see Fig. 28-2).[17] These factors have been largely studied separately in order to confirm their individual contribution to the resetting effects of light, although their interactions are beginning to be examined. Under real-world conditions, of course, many of these factors will apply simultaneously to the net phase resetting effects of light.

Timing

A primary factor determining the phase resetting effects of light, which is particularly important when considering light therapy for CRSD, is the timing of the light exposure.

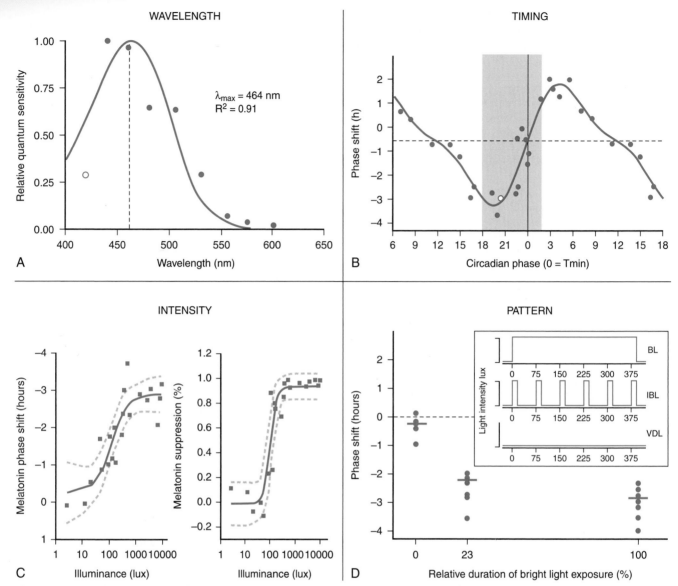

Figure 28-2 Four major properties of light affecting circadian photic resetting. A, The wavelength (color) sensitivity of light-induced melatonin suppression during a 90-minute night-time exposure. Each point in the action spectrum (*blue and white dots*) represents the half-saturation constant of the dose-response function for one wavelength, normalized to the maximum response. The solid curve shows the best-fit template for a vitamin A1 retinaldehyde photopigment and predicts a maximal response to visible blue light (λ_{max} 464 nm, range 446-477 nm).

B, Type 1 phase response curve (PRC) following exposure to a single 6.7-hour bright light (10,000 lux) stimulus at night. The magnitude and direction of the phase shifts are plotted against the initial phase of the stimulus (0 = Tmin, equivalent to ~6 A.M. under normal conditions). The gray bar represents a typical 8-hour sleep episode. Light exposure before Tmin causes a delay shift of the circadian pacemaker to a later phase (negative value on ordinate) whereas light after Tmin causes a phase advance (positive value). The circadian timing of light is an important consideration when using light to correct circadian misalignment; inappropriately timed light can shift the clock in the wrong direction and make the disorder worse.

C, Intensity-response curve for the phase delaying and melatonin suppression effects of a 6.5- hour nighttime bright light exposure (10,000 lux). Each subject was exposed to a different intensity of light. The four-parameter logistic model used to fit the data predicts an inflection point of the phase resetting curve (i.e., the half-saturation constant) at 119 lux and saturation of the response at ~550 lux (*left panel*). Similar results were obtained for melatonin suppression (*right panel*). These data show that relatively dim light exposure, equivalent to that experienced indoors, is capable of shifting the circadian pacemaker and inducing neuroendocrine responses.

D, Effects of exposure to bright light (10,000 lux) given intermittently (6 × 15 minutes, each separated by an hour; IBL) as compared to continuous bright light (BL, 10,000 lux) or continuous very dim light (VDL, <1 lux) (*insert*). Despite representing only 23% of the total light exposure duration, intermittent bright light caused approximately 75% of the phase shift as compared to continuous bright light exposure.

(*A,* Adapted with permission from Figure 5 in Brainard GC, Hanifin JP, Greeson JM, et al. Action spectrum for melatonin regulation in humans: evidence for a novel circadian photoreceptor. *J Neurosci.* 2001;21(16):6405-6412; *B,* Adapted with permission from Figure 3 in Khalsa SB, Jewett ME, Cajochen C, Czeisler CA. A phase response curve to single bright light pulses in human subjects. *J Physiol.* 2003;549[Pt 3]:945-952; *C,* Redrawn with permission from Figure 2 in Zeitzer JM, Dijk DJ, Kronauer R, Brown E, Czeisler C. Sensitivity of the human circadian pacemaker to nocturnal light: Melatonin phase resetting and suppression. *J Physiol.* 2000;526[Pt 3]:695-702; *D,* Adapted with permission from Figures 2 *(insert)* and 4 in Gronfier C, Wright KP Jr, Kronauer RE, Jewett ME, Czeisler CA. Efficacy of a single sequence of intermittent bright light pulses for delaying circadian phase in humans. *Am J Physiol Endocrinol Metab.* 2004;287[1]:E174-181.)

Light can either phase advance or phase delay the circadian system, depending on the timing of exposure.[37-39] Under normal conditions, light exposure in the later day/early night (~ 6 PM to 6 AM), before the core body temperature minimum (Tmin; Fig. 28-2B) causes a phase delay of the pacemaker to a later time, whereas light exposure in the late night/early day (~ 6 AM to 6 PM), after Tmin, will phase advance the clock to an earlier time. The relationship between the timing of a stimulus and the direction and magnitude of the resultant, shift is described in a phase response curve (PRC) (see Fig. 28-2B). Two types of light PRCs have been described across many organisms, including humans; a low amplitude PRC with maximum shifts of several hours (type 1 or weak resetting; see Fig. 28-2, B) and a high amplitude PRC with maximal shifts of 12 hours (type 0 or strong resetting).[40] In practice, most phase shifts experienced by humans are type 1 shifts as very particular timing of the light is required to achieve type 0 resetting. The type 1 PRC provides an essential tool in calculating when to time light therapy for treatment of CRSD with mistiming of light shifting the clock in the opposite direction to that required, making the sleep disorder worse (see Fig. 28-2, B). For example, in treating DSPD, "morning" light therapy designed to phase advance the circadian pacemaker needs to be timed to the individual's circadian phase (i.e., given after the individual's Tmin), which may vary considerably between patients. Light therapy starting at 8 AM would be appropriate for someone with a Tmin of 8 AM or earlier but would be mistimed for someone with a Tmin later than 8 AM and would cause a delay shift, exacerbating the DSPD.

Intensity

The intensity of light is a vital property when considering the resetting strength of the light exposure. There is a nonlinear relationship between the intensity of light and its circadian phase resetting effects such that exposure to relatively dim indoor room light (~ 100 lux) for 6.5 hours at night can stimulate 50% of the maximum effect of an equal-duration exposure with 10- to 100-fold greater illuminance (see Fig. 28-2, C).[41] Light levels commonly experienced from artificial indoor illumination are able to induce considerable resetting effects on the clock and may potentially undo the beneficial effect of light therapy at other times if not controlled.

Duration and Pattern

The duration of light exposure interacts nonlinearly with the magnitude of phase resetting such that shorter exposures induce greater effects than would be predicted by a simple linear relationship. When continuous exposures are compared to intermittent patterns, a nonlinear interaction is also observed. As compared to a single continuous 6.5-hour bright light exposure (~ 10,000 lux) at night, an intermittent exposure pattern consisting of six 15-minute bright light pulses separated by 60 minutes of very dim light (< 1 lux) caused approximately 75% of the phase shifting response (3.0-hour vs. 2.3-hour delay, respectively) despite representing only 23% of the total duration (see Fig. 28-2, D).[42,43] The ability of the circadian system to integrate light information over time presents potential advantages when developing light therapy programs, as most of the potential benefit can be realized without requiring prolonged continuous exposure.

Photic History

The effect of a light stimulus on circadian resetting depends not just on the current light intensity but also on the contrast with prior light history. The circadian photoreception system exhibits adaptation such that the current stimulus will have a greater effect if preceded by dimmer light rather than equivalent or higher light levels.[45] Again, this factor might be important to consider when developing light therapy regimens.

Melatonin

The major biochemical correlate of the light-dark cycle is provided by the pineal melatonin rhythm.[47] Under normal light-dark conditions, melatonin is produced only during the night and provides an internal representation of the environmental photoperiod, specifically night-length (scotoperiod). The synthesis and timing of melatonin production requires an afferent signal from the SCN, which projects to the pineal gland via the paraventricular nucleus and the superior cervical ganglion. Ablation of this pathway, as occurs in some people due to spinal damage at the upper cervical level, completely abolishes melatonin production, although other circadian rhythms not requiring this projection, for example, the cortisol, temperature, and sleep-wake rhythms, persist.[48,49] Light exposure during the night also inhibits melatonin production acutely and provides an indirect assessment of light input to the SCN via the RHT. Given the close temporal relationship between the SCN and melatonin production, the melatonin rhythm is often used as a marker of circadian phase and the melatonin suppression response as a proxy for RHT-SCN integrity and sensitivity.

REGULATION OF SLEEP-WAKE CYCLES

The two-process model of sleep regulation, first formally proposed by Alexander Borbély in 1982, remains the cornerstone on which our understanding of sleep-wake timing and structure is built.[50,51] The model proposes that two oscillatory processes, an hourglass-like homeostat and the endogenous 24-hour circadian pacemaker, interact to determine the timing, duration, and structure of sleep and the time course of daytime sleepiness and cognitive functioning.

It is well understood that it is easier to fall asleep at 1 AM in the morning compared to 1 PM in the afternoon. This 24-hour rhythm in sleep propensity is determined by the endogenous near-24-hour pacemaker, defined as *Process C*, which predicts maximum sleep propensity at approximately 6 AM, close to habitual wake time (assumed to be ~ 8 AM in this example) and minimum sleep propensity at approximately 9 PM, prior to habitual bedtime (~ midnight) and just before the onset of melatonin production (the wake maintenance zone; see later discussion) (Fig. 28-3). It is also intuitively understood that it is easier to fall asleep the longer one has been awake, and easier to wake up the longer one has been asleep. This homeostatic determinant of sleep propensity is defined as *Process S* and is best represented physiologically by the amount of slow wave activity during sleep (SWS or stage N3) or measured in the electroencephalograph (EEG) during wake (delta activity, 0.5-5.0 Hz).[52] Process S predicts maximum sleep propensity at the end of the waking day just before habitual bedtime, and minimal propensity for sleep just before wake time. Under normal circumstances, these two processes oscillate in opposition in order to maintain a long bout of consolidated wakefulness during the day and a long bout of consolidated sleep at night.[53] The progressive increase in the circadian alerting signal through the day is counteracted by the increasing homeostatic pressure for sleep with longer time awake, permitting a prolonged consolidated wake episode. Conversely, the increasing circadian drive for sleep through the night is opposed by the reduction in homeostatic drive for sleep that decreases during the sleep episode, the sleep effectively "releasing" the sleep pressure built up during the day.

Distinguishing the relative contribution of these processes on sleep is not usually possible, as sleep always occurs at a particular part of the circadian cycle and generally after the same

number of hours awake.[54] The forced desynchrony protocol, however, forcibly desynchronizes sleep from its endogenous circadian rhythm, allowing an examination of the effect of circadian phase on sleep structure. Under these circumstances, the role of the circadian clock on sleep is revealed. Importantly, it is clear that sleep duration depends on the circadian timing of sleep;[55] there is only a narrow window of time where sleep can continue for a long duration and remain uninterrupted (see Fig. 28-3). Sleeping outside this circadian "window" causes difficulties with falling asleep if sleep occurs too early, or difficulties staying asleep if the sleep opportunity is too late; this is the underlying cause of CRSDs. Regarding sleep structure, Rapid Eye Movement (REM) sleep is highly controlled by the circadian system with a distinct rhythm peaking in the early morning. Non-REM sleep particularly SWS, is much less under the control of the circadian system but is more influenced by the homeostatic Process S, and exhibits a strong sleep-dependent decline with increasing time asleep.[52] These processes also interact such that the circadian influence on sleep structure increases with increasing time asleep; as the homeostatic sleep pressure is reduced, the relative influence of the circadian system increases.[56]

The forced desynchrony protocol also reveals the "wake maintenance zone" (WMZ), or the forbidden zone for sleep, which is a 2- to 3-hour window of reduced sleep propensity that occurs immediately prior to the evening onset of melatonin secretion and, under normal conditions, occurs several hours prior to bedtime. The WMZ results from the interaction of circadian and homeostatic processes such that the increased circadian drive for alertness in the early evening is not yet fully countered by the increase in homeostatic sleep pressure, resulting in higher levels of alertness. The onset of melatonin secretion marks the start of the biologic night and is closely associated with a decreasing circadian wake-promoting

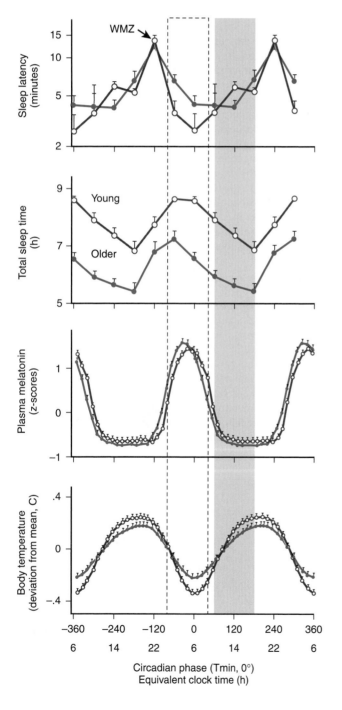

Figure 28-3 Circadian rhythm in sleep propensity and sleep duration. This figure shows the variation in sleep latency and total sleep time (*top panels*) as a function of circadian phase in young (21-30 years, *white dots*) and older men (64-74 years, *blue dots*). Subjects in these studies lived on a scheduled 28-hour "day" (18:40 hours wake: 9:20 hours sleep) for several weeks in order to schedule sleep and wake uniformly across all circadian phases. Circadian phase is expressed in degrees (one circadian cycle = 360°) and was measured under controlled laboratory conditions using core body temperature minimum (Tmin = 0°) and plasma melatonin. Data are double-plotted to aid visualization of the rhythms. The open bar represents the timing of a normal 8-hour sleep period (~ 0:00-8:00 hours) if Tmin occurs at approximately 6:00 A.M. Sleep latency is the duration of time taken to fall asleep at the start of each sleep opportunity and total sleep time is the duration spent asleep in each 9:20-hour scheduled sleep opportunity.

There is a distinct circadian rhythm in the propensity to fall asleep (sleep latency) with shortest sleep latencies (*top panel*) during the biologic night when melatonin is produced. The longest sleep latencies are observed several hours before habitual sleep time, and illustrate the "wake maintenance zone" (WMZ). Total sleep time also shows a distinct circadian rhythm with the highest sleep duration obtained during the biologic night in both young and older subjects, although overall sleep duration is lower in the older adults (*second panel*). The "window" of time when sleep duration is maximal is also narrower for the older subjects. Sleeping completely outside this circadian "window," for example, as experienced by shift workers and during jet lag, makes it very difficult to fall asleep and decreases total sleep time (*shaded bar*). (Adapted with permission from Figure 7 in Dijk DJ, Duffy JF, Czeisler CA. Contribution of circadian physiology and sleep homeostasis to age-related changes in human sleep. *Chronobiol Int.* 2000;17[3]:285-311.)

signal, ending the WMZ and opening the "sleep gate"[13,14,57] (see Fig. 28-3).

The relationship between the timing of sleep and the circadian system is an important factor in determining sleep quality and the risk of CRSDs. First, the period of the circadian clock varies among individuals, causing their sleep phase to be set relatively early or relatively late. Those with a clock that cycles relatively quickly tend to be more "morning-type" and prefer to go to sleep earlier, and those with a longer period clock tend to be more "evening type" and prefer to sleep and wake later[58] (Fig. 28-4). Furthermore, not everyone sleeps at the same circadian phase—the relative timing, or phase angle, between sleep and circadian phase also varies widely between individuals. For example, there might be as much as 5 to 6 hours difference in the circadian phase of sleep among a

group of young healthy subjects, and the gap is likely wider in less healthy groups.[59,60] Older people tend to go to sleep earlier than younger people, and they sleep and wake at a relatively earlier circadian phase (see Fig. 28-4); young morning types also go to sleep earlier than young evening types, but their sleep occurs at a relatively later circadian phase (see Fig. 28-4). This difference in the circadian timing of sleep due to circadian period, age, or other factors is a key factor in determining the duration and quality of sleep; trying to go to sleep too early in the circadian cycle will coincide with the WMZ and make it very difficult to fall asleep. Sleeping at too late a circadian phase will make it easy to fall asleep but difficult to stay asleep for a long time, however, as the end of the sleep episode will coincide with the increased circadian drive for alertness in the morning (see Fig. 28-3). Only by sleeping at the correct circadian phase can long, consolidated sleep be achieved routinely.

CIRCADIAN RHYTHM SLEEP DISORDERS

CRSDs are caused by people sleeping at the wrong circadian phase and can be self-induced, environmentally induced, or due to an intrinsic disorder in the circadian organization of sleep. Current clinical criteria do not differentiate between these underlying causes in determining either the diagnosis or most appropriate treatment for CRSD, but there are enormous potential benefits in beginning to do so. The current criteria rely largely on subjective reports of sleep timing or complaints of insomnia or sleepiness which, while defining the patient complaint, do not adequately describe the cause of the sleep disorder. Most other sleep disorders require a more detailed examination of the physiology or psychology underlying the complaint and CRSD should not be different in this regard. Moreover, many people may suffer from a CRSD but not report subjective symptoms and would therefore not currently qualify for a diagnosis. Although sleepiness and insomnia are the primary symptoms of these disorders, there may be long-term health risks of untreated CRSD not related to the sleep symptoms which should also be addressed (see "Other consequences of Circadian Rhythm Sleep Disorders"). Detailed discussions of these criteria are presented in the individual chapters for each CRSD (see Chapters 29 to 32) but are reviewed briefly here.

Shift Work Disorder and Jet Lag Disorder

Shift work disorder and jet lag disorder are self-induced disorders, at least in clinical terms, and are similar in their underlying cause (see Chapters 29 and 30). In both conditions, individuals choose to sleep and wake at an adverse circadian phase: In shift work disorder, patients work during the night and then try to sleep during the day, and in jet lag disorder, patients attempt to sleep at night in the new time zone before they have adapted to it, which often coincides with daytime in their home time zone. As shown in Figure 28-3, attempting to sleep during the biologic day is likely to result in insomnia due to difficulty falling asleep, difficulty maintaining sleep, and reduced sleep duration—the circadian drive for alertness wakes them up. Sleepiness symptoms arise from both inadequate sleep duration and trying to stay awake during the biologic night, when the circadian drive for sleepiness is high.

In both shift work disorder and jet lag disorder, the underlying source of the symptoms is the failure of the internal

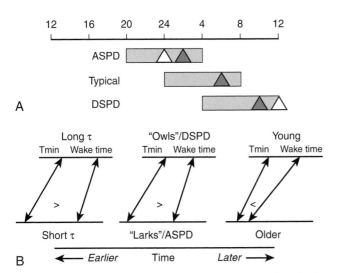

Figure 28-4 **Timing of sleep and circadian phase in circadian rhythm sleep disorders (CRSD). A,** Relative timing of sleep (*blue bars*) in advanced (ASPD) and delayed sleep phase disorder (DSPD) with patients reporting falling asleep earlier or later than typically desired, respectively. Although not routinely measured for making an outpatient diagnosis, core body temperature minimum (Tmin, *gray triangle*) is shown as a circadian marker to illustrate the normal temporal relationship between sleep and circadian phase and usually occurs approximately 2.3 hours before wake time. This normal phase relationship is maintained in some patients with ASPD and DSPD (*gray triangle*). Some patients, have an abnormal phase angle of entrainment such that their Tmin occurs at an abnormal time relative to sleep (*white triangle*), either relatively early in the sleep episode (ASPD) or relatively late (DSPD).
B, Relative differences in the timing of circadian phase (as indicated by Tmin) and wake time in three different comparative groups. As might be predicted, young morning types (Larks) have an earlier circadian phase and earlier wake time than young evening types (Owls) (*middle panel*). The phase relationship between sleep timing and circadian phase is not the same, however, i.e., the lines are not parallel. The time between Tmin and wake time is longer (>) in morning, as compared to evening types, indicating that morning types wake at a relatively later phase of their circadian cycle. Similar phase angle disorders are observed in some ASPD and DSPD patients, waking at a relatively later or earlier circadian phase, respectively. These differences could theoretically be driven by differences in endogenous circadian period between these groups (*left panel*).
This internal phase relationship changes with aging, however (*right panel*). Older adults, who usually tend to be more morning type, do indeed have an earlier circadian phase and earlier wake time than young subjects. Unlike young morning types, however, older subjects wake at a relatively earlier circadian phase (<), closer to their Tmin than young subjects.
(Adapted with permission from Figure 4 in Dijk DJ, Lockley SW. Integration of human sleep-wake regulation and circadian rhythmicity. *J Appl Physiol.* 2002;92:852-862.)

circadian pacemaker to remain synchronized with the rapid change in the environmental light-dark cycle. Shift-workers' and travelers' schedules (and therefore the light-dark cycle) change more rapidly than the circadian system can adapt to, resulting in wake (work) and sleep occurring at an inappropriate circadian phase. A general "rule of thumb" is that the circadian system takes a day to shift by approximately an hour; thus, a 12-hour shift from day shift to night shift, or a 12-hour time zone change, will take approximately 12 days to adapt to. Under most shift work schedules, however, the shifts are often changed again before full adaptation has been achieved, making it virtually impossible for the circadian system to adapt. A different approach is to have a rotating shift system that is so rapid (e.g., only 1 day on each shift) that it does not induce major shifts in circadian phase. This system, however, requires workers to be on shift at night in a fully unadapted state when the risk of accidents is highest. Jet lag is slightly different in this regard as most episodes are isolated and the magnitude and direction of the phase shift required to adapt is generally predictable. It is possible, therefore, to design light-dark exposure schedules to facilitate circadian adaptation and reduce the number of days taken to re-entrain to the new time zone. Such schedules require consideration of the PRC for light in order to time light and dark exposure appropriately (see Chapter 30).

These two disorders bring up the question of whether expression of normal physiology should be designated a disorder. It is perfectly normal, and expected, that a shift worker trying to sleep in the day and stay awake at night would suffer from insomnia and sleepiness. There is not an intrinsic disorder, *per se*, but simply expression of a natural physiologic response. The sleepiness symptoms, however, could be considered a disorder in that the safety and health consequences arising from the symptoms are very real;[61] just because the sleepiness is expected does not make the drowsy shift worker driving home any less of a hazard to himself or the public.

Delayed Sleep Phase Disorder and Advanced Sleep Phase Disorder

DSPD and ASPD are disorders in which sleep is misaligned with the social day or the desired sleep time (see Chapter 31). In DSPD sleep occurs later than desired, and in ASPD sleep occurs earlier than desired (see Fig. 28-4, *A*). According to the current clinical criteria, any misalignment between a patient's sleep pattern and one's desired time for sleep may qualify for a diagnosis; *in extremis*, this could mean that someone who wanted to go to sleep at 7 PM but could not fall asleep until 11 PM would qualify for DSPD, even though the sleep pattern might be considered "normal." Similarly, someone who wanted to go to sleep at 5 AM but fell asleep naturally at midnight could be diagnosed with ASPS, despite perfectly normal physiology. Of course, the clinical criteria were not developed to identify such cases and are meant to target those patients who want to go to sleep at a normal social time but find that they fall asleep very early (ASPD) or cannot go to sleep until very late (DSPD). Clarification of what is considered clinically "abnormal" would be helpful, however, in order to differentiate disorders resulting from a natural physiologic response or intrinsic disorders of sleep timing.

DSPD and ASPD can be can be self-induced, environmentally induced, or due to an intrinsic disorder in the circadian organization of sleep. For example, repeated late-night light exposure will cause a phase delay shift and make it difficult to sleep at a normal time, whereas repeated early morning light exposure will cause a phase advance and make it difficult to stay awake in the evening. There are also age-related changes in the timing of sleep relative to circadian phase. Young adults tend to have a higher incidence of DSPD, which reflects a tendency for a phase delay shift in the circadian clock during adolescents. Conversely, older adults tend to phase advance with increasing age and have a higher incidence of ASPD. Finally, polymorphisms in a number of circadian clock genes have been associated with either ASPD or DSPD, suggesting an intrinsic basis to abnormal sleep timing in some individuals.[62,63]

Although patients with ASPD or DSPD are identified by their sleep timing phenotype, there are differences between sleep timing and circadian phase (phase angle) within each disorder, suggesting that subtypes of these disorders may exist. In DSPD, for example, many patients have a normal phase angle, with both sleep and circadian phase becoming delayed in parallel.[64] Some patients, however, while having a delayed sleep pattern, have an even greater phase delay shift in their circadian clock, resulting in a disordered phase angle of entrainment[54,65,66] (see Fig. 28-4, *B*). This phase angle difference may be caused by social constraints (i.e., despite a delayed circadian clock, sleep is curtailed relatively early by school or college requirements) or an intrinsic difference in the homeostatic and circadian control of sleep between individuals. As a result, DSPD patients tend to sleep and wake at a relatively earlier circadian phase than normal subjects, resulting in prolonged sleep latency (due to attempting to go to sleep during the WMZ) and poor alertness and performance early in the wake episode (see Fig. 28-4, *B*). ASPD patients can have the opposite problem, with a greater advance in circadian phase, causing sleep to occur at a relatively later circadian phase, resulting in short sleep latencies and a higher than normal level of alertness upon waking.[54] Defining these subtypes may be important when trying to associate these disorders with underlying genotypes or when developing specific therapies.

Non-24-Hour Sleep-Wake Syndrome and Irregular Sleep-Wake Rhythm

N24HSWS and ISWR have a reduced prevalence compared to the other CRSD categories but impose a high patient burden for those suffering from these disorders. Detailed descriptions of these conditions are provided in Chapter 32, but are reviewed briefly herein.

N24HSWS is also known as "circadian rhythm disorder, nonentrained type" or sometimes "free-running type." It is characterized by symptoms of insomnia or excessive sleepiness caused by the sleep-wake cycle running on a non-24-hour pattern in the presence of a 24-hour day.[67] This mismatch occurs because the endogenous circadian pacemaker, which controls the timing of sleep, becomes desynchronized from the 24-hour light-dark cycle or social day.[31] In many cases, a cyclic sleep-wake disorder is apparent, characterized by periods of good sleep followed by periods of poor sleep and excessive daytime sleepiness, followed by good sleep, as the internal non-24-hour circadian period cycles in and out of phase with the 24-hour social day.[67]

Two groups emerge with a particular risk of N24HSWS. In sighted patients, N24HSWS tends to be associated with psychiatric disorders and is likely caused by inappropriate behavioral exposure to light which repeatedly and progressively delays the circadian pacemaker.[68] It usually begins during adolescence and is often preceded by DSPD, supporting the idea that alteration of light exposure may play a role. It is also highly prevalent (> 50%) in *totally* blind individuals—those who have neither visual nor melanopsin-based photoreception—due to a physical inability to detect light at the eye, causing the circadian pacemaker to revert to its intrinsic non-24-hour period.[32,67] Not all totally blind patients get the disorder, however; about 20% develop ASPD or DSPD and the remainder are normally phased, most of whom are synchronized by nonphotic time cues. Only a small fraction of totally visually blind subjects retain melanopsin-based circadian photoreception. When N24HSWS is present in the blind, however, one may consider the disorder an intrinsic, physical, irreversible (but treatable) disorder, whereas in the sighted, it is behaviorally induced, may be associated with a psychiatric disorder, and is transient and reversible. Even though the current clinical definitions for N24HSWS are the same for both groups, the disorders have different sleep pattern phenotypes and require different treatment approaches. For example, resynchronizing the sleep-wake cycle using timed light therapy may be possible for sighted patients, whereas blind patients must be treated with a nonphotic therapy, for example, appropriately timed melatonin treatment (see Chapter 32).

ISWR is a CRSD during which sleep becomes multiphasic, characterized by multiple (at least three), irregular, shorter (1-4 hours) bouts across the day. Unlike other CRSDs that are primarily disorders of circadian phase, ISWR is postulated to be a disorder of reduced circadian amplitude, although the current clinical criteria are not specific in this regard. Most cases of ISWR occur in association with neurodegenerative or developmental disorders and may be categorized as "CRSD due to medical condition." ISWR associated with dementia is the most studied example and is thought to be caused, in part, by cell loss in the SCN (see Chapter 32). Enhancement of sleep-wake consolidation using increased daytime light exposure holds promise for treating both the sleep-wake disorder and cognitive deficits associated with dementia.[69]

Other Consequences of Circadian Rhythm Sleep Disorders

In addition to the primary complaints about insomnia and sleepiness caused by CRSD, other longer-term health risks that require greater attention are emerging. Given that the circadian system mediates many aspects of human physiology, metabolism, and behavior, disorders of circadian rhythms are likely to have widespread consequences on physical and mental health and well-being. At this time the sleep medicine field is primarily concerned with the classification of sleep sequelae, but the role of sleep and circadian rhythms on cardiovascular and metabolic function is gaining interest and is extremely relevant to CRSD.[70]

Over the past decade, circadian rhythms have been identified in peripheral tissues in addition to the SCN, and most tissues studied have the molecular machinery required to generate endogenous circadian rhythms. In nonhuman mammals, circadian rhythms have been identified *in vitro* and often *in vivo* in liver, lung, kidney, heart, stomach, ovary, and multiple other tissues,[71] and in humans, circadian rhythms have been identified *in vivo* in the heart, lung, kidney, pancreas, adipose tissue, and a range of metabolic responses.[72-75] The disruption to normal circadian organization that induces sleep disorders will also cause disorders in these other systems, leading to suboptimal function and potentially long-term health problems. Understanding the role of medication timing, for example, to address the nighttime increase in asthma attacks, or the morning increase in heart attacks, or to improve the side effects, tolerability, and efficacy of chemotherapy, is of increasing interest and requires an understanding of the role of circadian rhythms and how to measure them. There are two examples outlined below that illustrate how understanding the widespread impact of circadian rhythm disorders (distinct from the sleep symptoms) may be important in assessing and improving health.

Shift Work and Cardiometabolic Disease

When sleep-wake behavior becomes misaligned from circadian timing in shift work disorder and jet lag disorder, meal timing also becomes misaligned from its normal circadian timing, as meal schedules tend to follow sleep-wake schedules. It is well established that the circadian timing of meals greatly affects our ability to digest and metabolize nutrients; meals taken during the biologic night, at an inappropriate circadian phase (e.g., 1:30 AM), result in increased postprandial circulating levels of insulin, glucose, and fats as compared to when the same meal is taken during the day (e.g., 1:30 PM)[75-79] (Fig. 28-5). Shift workers' and transmeridian travelers' circadian systems are rarely fully adapted to their sleep-wake and meal schedule, causing repeated misalignment of meal timing and potentially chronically elevated insulin, glucose, and fats. Furthermore, shift workers also suffer from chronic sleep deficiency, which has also been shown to affect metabolic function.[80-82] The resultant chronic elevation of insulin, glucose, and fats are well-established risk factors for type 2 diabetes and cardiovascular disease,[82,83] both of which have a high prevalence in shift workers.

Shift Work and Cancer

In 2007, the World Health Organization International Agency for Research on Cancer formally ruled that "shift work that involves circadian disruption is probably carcinogenic to humans," placing shift work alongside ultraviolet light, diesel fumes, and 55 other agents considered type 2A probable carcinogens.[84] While the exact mechanisms increasing the risk of cancer in shift workers are unknown, shift workers' sleep-wake cycles and light exposure patterns are thought to play a major role.[85] First, the repeated disruption of sleep and circadian cycles inherent in shift work has been shown to promote tumor growth in animal models,[86] possibly through disruption of cell cycles, which are under circadian control. Second, working at night requires exposure to light at night, which suppresses production of the pineal hormone melatonin. In animal models, suppression of melatonin by exposure to constant light, or removal of the pineal gland, will increase mammary tumorigenesis in rodents.[87] Melatonin administration will inhibit proliferation of human breast cancer cells in culture and also inhibit rat hepatoma and human breast

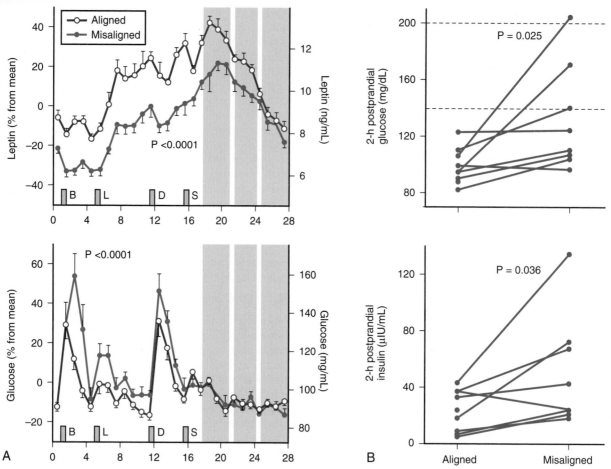

Figure 28-5 **Effects of circadian misalignment on metabolism. A,** Data from subjects who lived on a 28-hour day for a week whose sleep and meal times were shifted by 4 hours later each day. After 3 days, subjects were eating their meals approximately 12 hours later than normal. When compared to eating at normal circadian phase (aligned), eating during the biologic night (misaligned) increased glucose by 6% (*bottom panel*), increased insulin by 22% (not shown), and reduced leptin by 17% (*top panel*). Leptin helps suppress appetite, and therefore, lower leptin stimulates appetite and decreases energy expenditure, and may contribute to the risk of obesity. High glucose levels in the presence of high insulin indicated decreased insulin sensitivity, which is a risk factor for diabetes.
B, The extent to which circadian misalignment reduced glucose tolerance and insulin sensitivity. For 2 hours after eating breakfast at approximately 9 AM, glucose (*top panel*) and insulin (*bottom panel*) levels are significantly increased when compared to eating at a normal circadian phase. The dotted lines represent when glucose levels would be considered prediabetic (140 mg/dL) or diabetic (200 mg/dL).
(Redrawn with permission from Figures 4 and 5 in Scheer FA, Hilton MF, Mantzoros CS, Shea SA. Adverse metabolic and cardiovascular consequences of circadian misalignment. *Proc Natl Acad Sci U S A.* 2009;106[11]:4453-4458.)

tumor xenograph growth.[88] Melatonin is also a potent free radical scavenger and therefore may also play a role in preventing cancerous cell damage and proliferation.[89] Although the epidemiological and animal data suggest a strong association between light exposure, melatonin, and cancer, there is as yet no direct evidence in humans proving that alteration of melatonin levels alters cancer risk, or that taking synthetic melatonin has any effect on cancer risk or proliferation.

The current clinical criteria for diagnosis and treatment of CRSD do not address the potentially serious health consequences associated with the disorders and tend to try and alleviate sleepiness or insomnia without necessarily attempting to correcting the underlying circadian misalignment causing the disorder in the first place. Notwithstanding the fact that sleepy individuals often underestimate their own sleepiness or level of performance impairment,[90] treating circadian rhythm disorders even in the absence of sleep-related symptoms would be beneficial. For example, while treatment for obstructive sleep apnea (OSA) primarily addresses the sleepiness symptoms, there is increasing recognition of the need to treat OSA

to address the longer-term cardiovascular and metabolic consequences of untreated OSA in their own right; a similar approach is required for CRSD. One could make an argument that every night-shift worker suffers from shift work disorder based on the metabolic desynchrony alone, and the circadian misalignment should be addressed, even if the patient does not report insomnia or sleepiness. A re-evaluation of the strategies to diagnose and treat the widespread consequences of CRSD is therefore required.

MEASUREMENT OF CIRCADIAN RHYTHMS IN THE DIAGNOSIS OF CRSD

If symptom assessment for CRSD needs to go beyond subjective sleep-related complaints, a method of assessing circadian rhythms, and therefore circadian desynchrony, is required. As yet, there are no clinical standards for measuring circadian phase. The "gold standard" for assessing circadian phase and amplitude is the constant routine protocol (see "Defining Circadian

Rhythms") but this approach is too cumbersome for clinical use. There are two less onerous approaches, however, that have been used in research studies that have potential clinical utility in an outpatient setting, and these are described here.

The decision about which outcome to use to measure circadian phase is important, as each marker is affected differently or "masked" by environmental factors, which can confound the integrity of the assessment. Traditionally, candidate circadian phase markers in laboratory experiments have included rectal, oral, and tympanic temperature and plasma, salivary, or urinary measures of cortisol and melatonin and their metabolites. Under controlled laboratory conditions, most circadian markers are highly correlated, as they are all considered "hands of the clock," reflecting a common central circadian control but having different relative phases and variability.[91] For example, the timing of core body temperature minimum is highly correlated with melatonin peak but occurs approximately 3 hours later (see Fig. 28-1). The sleep-wake or rest-activity cycle has also been used as a proxy marker of circadian phase. Each of these has advantages and disadvantages when considered for use in an outpatient setting. First, temperature is unsuitable for outpatient use because it is easily affected by external factors such as activity and meal times, which acutely elevate temperature, or sleep which suppresses temperature (see Fig. 28-1, *top row*). Phase estimates using temperature in an ambulatory setting can be extremely inaccurate, and may be off by as much as 12 hours.[92] The sleep-wake cycle has similar problems as a marker of internal circadian phase in that there are many external factors that affect sleep timing in addition to the intrinsic circadian rhythm; even in very healthy young subjects who are asked to maintain a strict sleep-wake schedule, there is a 5-hour range in circadian phase[59] which is too large an error for clinical circadian phase assessment.

Salivary Melatonin and Cortisol Rhythms

Hormonal measures such as cortisol and melatonin are more robust markers of circadian phase, although the choice of body fluid becomes important. Although plasma may provide the most sensitive measure of melatonin or cortisol, repeated blood draws are impractical in an outpatient setting. Melatonin and cortisol can both be measured in saliva, however, which provides an attractive noninvasive alternative to blood, although there are some additional considerations when measuring salivary hormones. First, hormone levels are relatively low in saliva (about 30% of that in plasma) and therefore sensitive assays are required for accurate measurement. Second, saliva can only be collected when the patient is awake which may raise issues of sleep deprivation or practicality. Third, when assessing circadian phase, a reasonable time series and sample frequency are required to ensure that the data can be interpreted accurately. While sampling over 24 hours would be ideal, this would again be impractical for an outpatient setting. For the melatonin rhythm, a reliable phase marker is the onset of melatonin production as levels change very rapidly from near-undetectable levels during the biologic day to peaks up to 20 to 30 pg/mL in saliva. Given that melatonin is suppressed acutely by light, however, accurate assessment of the onset requires that patients are studied in dim room light, ideally less than 15 lux, and the dim light melatonin onset (DLMO) has become a standard measure of circadian phase.[93] Salivary DLMO is most commonly defined as the point at which melatonin levels reach a threshold,

using at 3 or 5 pg/mL, which requires a high sensitivity assay. Under normal circumstances, DLMO occurs approximately 2 to 3 hours before sleep in the late evening.[59,60] In order to quantify DLMO reliably, the time course of melatonin production has to be observed for several hours before and several hours after DLMO occurs. A typical outpatient study may therefore ask subjects to begin collecting saliva every hour from early evening (e.g., 5 PM) until 2 hours after their habitual bedtime (e.g., 2 AM) to ensure an adequate duration. Subjects would remain in dim light and would also be asked to refrain from eating or drinking for at least 30 minutes before each sample to avoid contamination, wash their mouths with water at that time, and avoid using substances that may affect the assay such as caffeine, lipstick, and Chapstick. Maintaining a seated posture for 15 minutes before each sample would also be desirable, as posture can affect circulating melatonin levels. Saliva can be collected by simply spitting into a plastic tube, or commercial kits are available that include a swab that is placed in the mouth for a set time to soak up sufficient saliva for assay. Several milliliters are needed for each sample for assay purposes, and the sample should be frozen at −20° C as soon as possible after sampling. These measures can easily be performed in the sleep laboratory and have also been used in the patients' homes. The risks with this method are that salivary levels may be too low to measure and that the DLMO may be "missed" in a significant proportion of the population if the assessment window does not coincide with the DLMO time. The risk of missing the DLMO will depend on the CRSD being studied; ASPD patients may need to start sampling earlier in the day (e.g., 3 PM) and DSPD may need to continue until later than normal (e.g., 5 AM) to ensure that the DLMO is detected. Circadian phase assessments using salivary melatonin in shift work disorder, jet lag disorder, and N24HSWS are very challenging, however, unless a full 24-hour assessment is completed, given the difficulty in predicting where the DLMO might occur in these disorders.

Salivary cortisol has been used less extensively as a phase marker. As with plasma cortisol, the pulsatile nature of cortisol production may make discrete samples difficult to interpret. Potential stressors are also of concern because they would raise cortisol levels acutely and not reflect the endogenous circadian rhythm.[4,94] The acute effect of light is less of a concern than with salivary melatonin, although light may have small acute effects on cortisol production. The main issue with salivary cortisol is choosing which part of the profile to measure and which phase marker to take. Some researchers have used the postsleep decline in cortisol as a potential marker, but the onset and offset of cortisol production are not as easy to determine as compared to melatonin (a DLCO has not been defined) and therefore there are no commonly accepted procedures for assessing cortisol phase in saliva.

Note that with both melatonin and cortisol, care should be taken to ensure that patients are not taking medications that would affect their levels, for example, synthetic melatonin, beta blockers, SSRIs, and monoamine oxidase inhibitors for melatonin, and steroids for cortisol.

Urinary Melatonin and Cortisol Rhythms

Another noninvasive method for assessing circadian phase under outpatient conditions is to use urinary hormones; both cortisol and 6-sulfatoxymelatonin (aMT6S), the major metabolite of melatonin, exhibit robust circadian rhythms.[47,95-97]

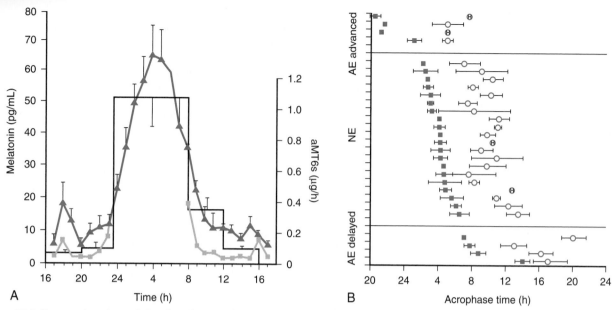

Figure 28-6 Hormonal markers of circadian phase. A, The relationship between plasma melatonin *(blue triangles)*, salivary melatonin *(light blue squares)*, and urinary 6-sulfatoxymelatonin (aMT6S; —) illustrates the strong correlations between the measures. Saliva data are only shown during wake times (assuming sleep from 11:30 PM to 8 AM) and illustrate the shortcoming of having to wake individuals to collect saliva during the sleep episode. An indwelling cannula can permit plasma sampling without waking the subject. Pooled urine sampling (every ~ 4 hours while awake and ~8 hours overnight/during sleep) does not have this limitation and permits coverage of the entire 24-hour rhythm. Cosinor analysis of the urinary data (ng/hour versus midpoint of collection episode) provides a peak (acrophase) phase that is highly correlated with plasma.

B, The relationship between the peak timing of urinary aMT6S *(blue squares)* and urinary cortisol *(white circles)* across a range of circadian phases in 28 visually impaired subjects (normally entrained (NE), *n* = 20; abnormally entrained (AE) advanced, *n* = 4; AE delayed, *n* = 4). Urine was collected approximately every 4 to 8 hours for 48 hours per week for 4 weeks. aMT6S and cortisol were measured in the same samples and data from each week were fitted with a cosine function to estimate the peak time and averaged over 4 weeks (mean ± SD shown). Cortisol and aMT6S rhythms were highly correlated ($r = 0.81$), although the cortisol rhythm was more variable. The cortisol peak occurred an average of 5.7 hours later than aMT6S (9.9 hours versus 4.2 hours, respectively) in normally entrained subjects.

(A, Redrawn with permission from Figure 7.4b in Arendt J. *Melatonin and the Mammalian Pineal Gland.* London: Chapman & Hall; 1995; *B,* Redrawn with permission from Figure 1 in Skene DJ, Lockley SW, James K, Arendt J. Correlation between urinary cortisol and 6-sulphatoxymelatonin rhythms in field studies of blind subjects. *Clin Endocrinol (Oxford).* 1999;50[6]:715-719.)

Urinary aMT6S levels correlate highly with circulating plasma levels, although the fitted peak occurs approximately 1 to 2 hours later on average[96] (Fig. 28-6, *A*). Urinary cortisol can also be used if the patient is taking drugs that affect melatonin,[97,98] and although the pulsatile nature of cortisol production is less apparent in urine sampling, phase estimates are more variable than aMT6S[97] (Fig. 28-6, *B*).

Urine is usually collected for 48 hours and at least 36 hours and, depending on the suspected CRSD, on multiple occasions. All urine produced over this time is collected in approximately 4-hour episodes while awake plus an 8-hour overnight collection, although more frequent collection times are acceptable if increased assay costs are not limiting. The sample times and total urine volumes are also recorded in order to calculate hourly rates for each collection episode: (ng/mL × total sample volume)/total sample hours. This rate should be plotted versus the midpoint of the time over which the sample was collected. Normality of phase can be assessed either from the observed peak time of the plotted data or after being fit to a simple cosine function to calculate the acrophase, or peak time, of aMT6S production. This method has been used successfully in prior studies of shift workers on North Sea oil rigs,[99-101] in shift working nurses,[102] in shift workers living in Antarctica,[103,104] to confirm ASPD, DSPD and N24HSWS in blind patients[32,67] and N24HSWS in schizophrenic patients,[105] during jet lag simulation in the laboratory,[106] and in many other clinical populations and experimental protocols.[107-110]

The choice of method for outpatient circadian phase assessment depends on a number of factors. Although saliva provides a reasonable proxy of plasma patterns, it is a difficult fluid to work with, requiring several milliliters each time, often requiring centrifugation prior to aliquoting to remove contaminants, and needs to be frozen shortly after collection. It is sensitive to the pulsatile release of cortisol and a dim light environment is mandatory for assessment of melatonin. Saliva is therefore most appropriate in a more controlled laboratory setting, rather than a home-based setting. This assessment need not be overnight, but should at least run from late afternoon (5 PM) to the early hours of the morning (2 AM), depending on the disorder, in order to detect DLMO (see "Salivary Melatonin and Cortisol Rhythms," earlier).

Under nonlaboratory conditions, urinary measures are generally preferable. Urine is easier to collect and work with and it is stable at room temperature for at least 5 days[95] and therefore does not need to be frozen immediately, and assay volumes are generally small. Assays also need to be less sensitive as aMT6S is measured in nanograms rather than picograms and has a very large day-night difference that is simple to detect. A particular advantage of collecting urine over 24 or more hours is that the entire circadian rhythm is assessed, minimizing the risk of "missing" the circadian phase, which can occur if saliva or plasma samples are mistimed. Moreover, this technique, compared to saliva or plasma measures, is least affected by environmental light (melatonin) or pulsatile secretion (cortisol), as collecting integrated urine samples reduces the impact of these masking effects on the overall rhythm, although this remains to be tested systematically.

Also note that, when core body temperature minimum has been used as a phase marker under controlled laboratory conditions to establish the fundamental properties of the circadian system (e.g., for example in defining the PRC for light [see Fig. 28-2, *B*] or phase angle of entrainment [see Fig. 28-4, *B*]), an appropriate conversion is required to relate these data to a different phase marker if one is used in the field. For example, the PRC to light (see Fig. 28-2, *B*) is plotted using temperature minimum (Tmin) as the phase marker and predicts that light given in the 12 hours before Tmin will cause a delay and light given in the 12 hours after Tmin will cause an advance. If melatonin DLMO were used as the phase marker instead of Tmin, the definition of how to time the light exposure would also change: DLMO occurs approximately 7 hours before Tmin,[39] and therefore light given from 5 hours before to 7 hours after DLMO would cause a phase delay, whereas light given 7 to 19 hours after DLMO would cause an advance.

FUTURE CONSIDERATIONS

Although the methods available to assess circadian phase are relatively simple, clinicians often express concern about the burden of collecting serial urine or saliva samples on both the clinic and the patients. They also question the value of these measures in view of the lack of clinical guidelines on how to interpret the data for diagnostic and treatment purposes. The lack of reimbursement for these procedures also hinders their use in clinical settings and most data to date have been collected in research studies that some argue do not reflect a typical outpatient environment. Although these are valid concerns, they can be addressed. First, the research community needs to conduct high-quality randomized clinical trials of patients with CRSD using outpatient circadian phase markers to help diagnose the disorders and to time light or melatonin therapy appropriately. These data will also begin to permit better differentiation of potential subtypes of disorders by classifying both circadian phase and the relative phase angle between sleep and circadian phase, and will provide better phenotypes in understanding the potential genetic bases of these disorders. This approach will also help to reduce false positive diagnoses.[111] Such information can then be included in clinical criteria, along with detailed guidelines of how to measure and interpret circadian rhythm data which, along with high-quality demonstrations of the clinical utility of circadian rhythm information, will help to build the case for reimbursement. Finally, clinics should develop circadian assessment programs for CRSD (and eventually for other nonsleep conditions; see "Other Consequences of Circadian Rhythm Sleep Disorders") and will discover that it is not difficult or prohibitively costly and will bring a better understanding of the disorders. For example, when compared to the time, training, manpower, cost, and subject burden required for the overnight polysomnography assessment required for many sleep disorders, a 9-hour saliva test program in the laboratory, or collection of 10 urine samples over 2 days at home, require fewer resources. Moving beyond subjective complaints and simple assessments of sleep timing will bring new depth to our understanding of the causes, consequences, and management of the circadian rhythm sleep disorders that affect many millions of people.

REFERENCES

1. American Academy of Sleep Medicine. *The International Classification of Sleep Disorders, Diagnostic and Coding Manual*. 2nd ed. Westchester, IL: American Academy of Sleep Medicine; 2005.
2. Sack RL, Auckley D, Auger RR, Carskadon MA, Wright Jr KP, et al. Circadian rhythm sleep disorders: Part I, basic principles, shift work and jet lag disorders. An American Academy of Sleep Medicine review. *Sleep*. 2007;30(11):1460-1483.
3. Sack RL, Auckley D, Auger RR, Carskadon MA, Wright Jr KP, et al. Circadian rhythm sleep disorders: Part II, advanced sleep phase disorder, delayed sleep phase disorder, free-running disorder, and irregular sleep-wake rhythm. An American Academy of Sleep Medicine review. *Sleep*. 2007;30(11):1484-1501.
4. Czeisler CA. Circadian rhythmicity and its disorders. In: Nicholson AN, Welbers IB, eds. *Sleep and Wakefulness: Pharmacology and Pathology*. Ingelheim-am-Rhein: Boehringer Ingelheim; 1986:1-49.
5. Czeisler CA, Klerman EB. Circadian and sleep-dependent regulation of hormone release in humans. *Rec Prog Horm Res*. 1999;54:97-132.
6. Hastings M, O'Neill JS, Maywood ES. Circadian clocks: Regulators of endocrine and metabolic rhythms. *J Endocrinol*. 2007;195(2):187-198.
7. Duffy JF, Dijk DJ. Getting through to circadian oscillators: Why use constant routines? *J Biol Rhythms*. 2002;17(1):4-13.
8. Czeisler CA, Duffy JF, Shanahan TL, Brown EN, Mitchell JF, et al. Stability, precision, and near-24-hour period of the human circadian pacemaker. *Science*. 1999;284:2177-2181.
9. Boivin DB, Czeisler CA, Dijk DJ, Duffy JF, Folkard S, et al. Complex interaction of the sleep-wake cycle and circadian phase modulates mood in healthy subjects. *Arch Gen Psychiatry*. 1997;54:145-152.
10. Wyatt JK, Ritz-De Cecco A, Czeisler CA, Dijk DJ. Circadian temperature and melatonin rhythms, sleep, and neurobehavioral function in humans living on a 20-h day. *Am J Physiol Regul Integr Comp Physiol*. 1999;277:R1152-R1163.
11. Wyatt JK, Cajochen C, Ritz-De Cecco A, Czeisler CA, Dijk DJ. Low-dose repeated caffeine administration for circadian-phase-dependent performance degradation during extended wakefulness. *Sleep*. 2004;27(3):374-381.
12. Grady S, Aeschbach D, Wright Jr KP, Czeisler CA. Effect of modafinil on impairments in neurobehavioral performance and learning associated with extended wakefulness and circadian misalignment. *Neuropsychopharmacology*. 2010;35(9):1910-1920.
13. Dijk DJ, Duffy JF, Czeisler CA. Contribution of circadian physiology and sleep homeostasis to age-related changes in human sleep. *Chronobiol Int*. 2000;17(3):285-311.
14. Lavie P. Ultrashort sleep-waking schedule III. "Gates" and "forbidden zones" for sleep. *Electroenceph Clin Neurophysiol*. 1986;63:414-425.
15. Nakagawa H, Isaki K, Sack RL, Lewy AJ. Free-running melatonin, sleep propensity, cortisol and temperature rhythms in a totally blind person. *Jpn J Psychiatry Neurol*. 1992;46(1):210-212.
16. Burgess HJ, Revell VL, Eastman CI. A three pulse phase response curve to three milligrams of melatonin in humans. *J Physiol*. 2008;586(2):639-647.
17. Czeisler CA, Gooley JJ. Sleep and circadian rhythms in humans. *Cold Spring Harbor Symp Quant Biol*. 2007;72:579-597.
18. Berson DM, Dunn FA, Takao M. Phototransduction by retinal ganglion cells that set the circadian clock. *Science*. 2002;295:1070-1073.
19. Dacey DM, Liao HW, Peterson BB, Robinson FR, Smith VC, et al. Melanopsin-expressing ganglion cells in primate retina signal colour and irradiance and project to the LGN. *Nature*. 2005;433(7027):749-754.
20. Peirson S, Foster RG. Melanopsin: Another way of signaling light. *Neuron*. 2006;49(3):331-339.
21. Gooley JJ, Lu J, Chou TC, Scammell TE, Saper CB. Melanopsin in cells of origin of the retinohypothalamic tract. *Nat Neurosci*. 2001;4(12):1165.
22. Provencio I, Rollag MD, Castrucci AM. Photoreceptive net in the mammalian retina. *Nature*. 2002;415:493.
23. Hattar S, Lucas RJ, Mrosovsky N, Thompson S, Douglas RH, et al. Melanopsin and rod-cone photoreceptive systems account for all major accessory visual functions in mice. *Nature*. 2003;424(6944):76-81.
24. Güler AD, Ecker JL, Lall GS, Haq S, Altimus CM, et al. Melanopsin cells are the principal conduits for rod-cone input to non-image-forming vision. *Nature*. 2008;453(7191):102-105.
25. Brainard GC, Hanifin JP. Photons, clocks, and consciousness. *J Biol Rhythms*. 2005;20(4):314-325.
26. Brainard GC, Hanifin JP, Greeson JM, Byrne B, Glickman G, et al. Action spectrum for melatonin regulation in humans: Evidence for a novel circadian photoreceptor. *J Neurosci*. 2001;21(16):6405-6412.

27. Thapan K, Arendt J, Skene DJ. An action spectrum for melatonin suppression: Evidence for a novel non-rod, non-cone photoreceptor system in humans. *J Physiol*. 2001;535(1):261-267.

28. Lockley SW, Brainard GC, Czeisler CA. High sensitivity of the human circadian melatonin rhythm to resetting by short wavelength light. *J Clin Endocrinol Metab*. 2003;88(9):4502-4505.

29. Gooley JJ, Rajaratnam SMW, Brainard GC, Kronauer RE, Czeisler CA, Lockley SW. Spectral responses of the human circadian system depend on the irradiance and duration of exposure to light. *Sci Transl Med*. 2010;2(31):31ra33.

30. Peirson SN, Halford S, Foster RG. The evolution of irradiance detection: Melanopsin and the non-visual opsins. *Philos Trans R Soc Lond B Biol Sci*. 2009;364(1531):2849-2865.

31. Lockley SW, Arendt J, Skene DJ. Visual impairment and circadian rhythm disorders. *Dialog Clin Neurosci*. 2007;9(3):301-314.

32. Lockley SW, Skene DJ, Arendt J, Tabandeh H, Bird AC, Defrance R. Relationship between melatonin rhythms and visual loss in the blind. *J Clin Endocrinol Metab*. 1997;82(11):3763-3770.

33. Ruberg FL, Skene DJ, Hanifin JP, Rollag MD, English J, et al. Melatonin regulation in humans with color vision deficiencies. *J Clin Endocrinol Metab*. 1996;81(8):2980-2985.

34. Czeisler CA, Shanahan TL, Klerman EB, Martens H, Brotman DJ, et al. Suppression of melatonin secretion in some blind patients by exposure to bright light. *N Engl J Med*. 1995;332(1):6-11.

35. Klerman EB, Shanahan TL, Brotman DJ, Rimmer DW, Emens JS, et al. Photic resetting of the human circadian pacemaker in the absence of conscious vision. *J Biol Rhythms*. 2002;17:548-555.

36. Zaidi FH, Hull JT, Peirson SN, Wulff K, Aeschbach D, et al. Short-wavelength light sensitivity of circadian, pupillary, and visual awareness in humans lacking an outer retina. *Curr Biol*. 2007;17(24):2122-2128.

37. Honma K, Honma S. A human phase response curve for bright light pulses. *Jpn J Psychiatry Neurol*. 1988;42(1):167-168.

38. Minors DS, Waterhouse JM, Wirz-Justice A. A human phase-response curve to light. *Neurosci Lett*. 1991;133:36-40.

39. Khalsa SBS, Jewett ME, Cajochen C, Czeisler CA. A phase response curve to single bright light pulses in human subjects. *J Physiol (Lond)*. 2003;549(Pt 3):945-952.

40. Jewett ME, Kronauer RE, Czeisler CA. Phase-amplitude resetting of the human circadian pacemaker via bright light: A further analysis. *J Biol Rhythms*. 1994;9(3-4):295-314.

41. Zeitzer JM, Dijk DJ, Kronauer RE, Brown EN, Czeisler CA. Sensitivity of the human circadian pacemaker to nocturnal light: Melatonin phase resetting and suppression. *J Physiol (Lond)*. 2000;526.3:695-702.

42. Rimmer DW, Boivin DB, Shanahan TL, Kronauer RE, Duffy JF, Czeisler CA. Dynamic resetting of the human circadian pacemaker by intermittent bright light. *Am J Physiol Regul Integr Comp Physiol*. 2000;279(5):R1574-R1579.

43. Gronfier C, Wright Jr KP, Kronauer RE, Jewett ME, Czeisler CA. Efficacy of a single sequence of intermittent bright light pulses for delaying circadian phase in humans. *Am J Physiol Endocrinol Metab*. 2004;287: E174-E181.

44. Hébert M, Martin SK, Lee C, Eastman CI. The effects of prior light history on the suppression of melatonin by light in humans. *J Pineal Res*. 2002;33:198-203.

45. Smith KA, Schoen MW, Czeisler C. Adaptation of human pineal melatonin suppression by recent photic history. *J Clin Endocrinol Metab*. 2004;89(7):3610-3614.

46. Chang AM, Scheer FA, Czeisler CA. The human circadian system adapts to prior photic history. *J Physiol*. 2011;589(Pt 5):1095-1102.

47. Arendt J. *Melatonin and the Mammalian Pineal Gland*. 1st ed. London: Chapman and Hall; 1995.

48. Kneisley LW, Moskowitz MA, Lynch HJ. Cervical spinal cord lesions disrupt the rhythm in human melatonin excretion. *J Neural Transm*. 1978;13(suppl):311-323.

49. Zeitzer JM, Ayas NT, Shea SA, Brown R, Czeisler CA. Absence of detectable melatonin and preservation of cortisol and thyrotropin rhythms in tetraplegia. *J Clin Endocrinol Metab*. 2000;85:2189-2196.

50. Borbély AA. A two process model of sleep regulation. *Hum Neurobiol*. 1982;1:195-204.

51. Daan S, Beersma DGM, Borbély AA. Timing of human sleep: Recovery process gated by a circadian pacemaker. *Am J Physiol*. 1984;246: R161-R183.

52. Dijk DJ. Regulation and functional correlates of slow wave sleep. *J Clin Sleep Med*. 2009;5(2):S6-S15.

53. Dijk DJ, Czeisler CA. Paradoxical timing of the circadian rhythm of sleep propensity serves to consolidate sleep and wakefulness in humans. *Neurosci Lett*. 1994;166(1):63-68.

54. Lockley SW, Dijk DJ, Kosti O, Skene DJ, Arendt J. Alertness, mood and performance rhythm disturbances associated with circadian sleep disorders in the blind. *J Sleep Res*. 2008;17(2):207-216.

55. Czeisler CA, Weitzman ED, Moore-Ede MC, Zimmerman JC, Knauer RS. Human sleep: Its duration and organization depend on its circadian phase. *Science*. 1980;210:1264-1267.

56. Dijk DJ, Czeisler CA. Contribution of the circadian pacemaker and the sleep homeostat to sleep propensity, sleep structure, electroencephalographic slow waves, and sleep spindle activity in humans. *J Neurosci*. 1995;15(5):3526-3538.

57. Aeschbach D, Matthews JR, Postolache TT, Jackson MA, Giesen HA, Wehr TA. Dynamics of the human EEG during prolonged wakefulness: Evidence for frequency-specific circadian and homeostatic influences. *Neurosci Lett*. 1997;239(2-3):121-124.

58. Dijk DJ, Lockley SW. Integration of human sleep-wake regulation and circadian rhythmicity. *J Appl Physiol*. 2002;92:852-862.

59. Wright Jr KP, Gronfier C, Duffy JF, Czeisler CA. Intrinsic period and light intensity determine the phase relationship between melatonin and sleep in humans. *J Biol Rhythms*. 2005;20(2):168-177.

60. Sletten TL, Vincenzi S, Redman JR, Lockley SW, Rajaratnam SMW. Timing in sleep and its relationship with the endogenous melatonin rhythm. *Front Neurol*. 2010;1:137.

61. Folkard S, Lombardi DA, Tucker PT. Shiftwork: Safety, sleepiness and sleep. *Ind Health*. 2005;43(1):20-23.

62. von Schantz M, Archer SN. Clocks, genes and sleep. *J R Soc Med*. 2003;96(10):486-489.

63. Dijk DJ, Archer SN. PERIOD3, circadian phenotypes, and sleep homeostasis. *Sleep Med Rev*. 2010;14(3):151-160.

64. Chang AM, Reid KJ, Gourineni R, Zee PC. Sleep timing and circadian phase in delayed sleep phase syndrome. *J Biol Rhythms*. 2009;24(4): 313-321.

65. Shibui K, Uchiyama M, Okawa M. Melatonin rhythms in delayed sleep phase syndrome. *J Biol Rhythms*. 1999;14(1):72-76.

66. Wyatt JK. Delayed sleep phase syndrome: Pathophysiology and treatment options. *Sleep*. 2004;27(6):1195-1203.

67. Uchiyama M, Lockley SW. Non-24-hour sleep–wake syndrome in sighted and blind patients. *Sleep Med Clin*. 2009;4(2):195-211.

68. Hayakawa T, Uchiyama M, Kamei Y, Shibui K, Tagaya H, et al. Clinical analyses of sighted patients with non-24-hour sleep-wake syndrome: A study of 57 consecutively diagnosed cases. *Sleep*. 2005;28(8):945-952.

69. Riemersma-van der Lek RF, Swaab DF, Twisk J, et al. Effect of bright light and melatonin on cognitive and noncognitive function in elderly residents of group care facilities: A randomized controlled trial. *JAMA*. 2008;299(22):2642-2655.

70. Cappuccio FP, Miller MA, Lockley SW, eds. *Sleep, health and society: From Aetiology to Public Health*. Oxford: Oxford University Press; 2010.

71. Hastings MH, Reddy AB, Maywood ES. A clockwork web: Circadian timing in brain and periphery, in health and disease. *Nat Rev Neurosci*. 2003;4(8):649-661.

72. Spengler CM, Czeisler CA, Shea SA. An endogenous circadian rhythm of respiratory control in humans. *J Physiol (Lond)*. 2000;526(3):683-694.

73. Hilton MF, Umali MU, Czeisler CA, Wyatt JK, Shea SA. Endogenous circadian control of the human autonomic nervous system. *Comput Cardiol*. 2000;27:197-200.

74. Shea SA, Hilton MF, Orlova C, Ayers RT, Mantzoros CS. Independent circadian and sleep/wake regulation of adipokines and glucose in humans. *J Clin Endocrinol Metab*. 2005;90:2537-2544.

75. Scheer FA, Hilton MF, Mantzoros CS, Shea SA. Adverse metabolic and cardiovascular consequences of circadian misalignment. *Proc Natl Acad Sci U S A*. 2009;106(11):4453-4458.

76. Ribeiro D, Hampton SM, Morgan L, Deacon S, Arendt J. Altered postprandial hormone and metabolic responses in a simulated shift work environment. *J Endocrinol*. 1998;158:305-310.

77. Hampton SM, Morgan LM, Lawrence N, Anastasiadou T, Norris F, et al. Postprandial hormone and metabolic responses in simulated shift work. *J Endocrinol*. 1996;151:259-267.

78. Lund J, Arendt J, Hampton SM, English J, Morgan LM. Postprandial hormone and metabolic responses amongst shift workers in Antarctica. *J Endocrinol*. 2001;171:557-564.

79. Morgan L, Arendt J, Owens D, Folkard S, Hampton S, et al. Effects of the endogenous clock and sleep time on melatonin, insulin, glucose and lipid metabolism. *J Endocrinol*. 1998;157:443-451.

80. Spiegel K, Leproult R, Van Cauter E. Impact of sleep debt on metabolic and endocrine function. *Lancet.* 1999;354:1435-1439.
81. Spiegel K, Tasali E, Penev P, Van Cauter E. Brief communication: Sleep curtailment in healthy young men is associated with decreased leptin levels, elevated ghrelin levels, and increased hunger and appetite. *Ann Intern Med.* 2004;141(11):846-850.
82. Broussard J, Knutson KL. Sleep and metabolic disease. In: Cappuccio FP, Miller MA, Lockley SW, eds. *Sleep, Health and Society: From Aetiology to Public Health.* Oxford: Oxford University Press; 2010: 111-140.
83. Spiegel K, Knutson K, Leproult R, Tasali E, Van Cauter E. Sleep loss: A novel risk factor for insulin resistance and type 2 diabetes. *J Appl Physiol.* 2005;99(5):2008-2019.
84. Straif K, Baan R, Grosse Y, Secretan B, El Ghissassi F, et al. Carcinogenicity of shift-work, painting, and fire-fighting. *Lancet Oncol.* 2007;8(12):1065-1066.
85. Stevens RG, Blask DE, Brainard GC, Hansen J, Lockley SW, et al. Meeting report: The role of environmental lighting and circadian disruption in cancer and other diseases. *Environ Health Perspect.* 2007;115(9):1357-1362.
86. Filipski E, Delaunay F, King VM, Wu MW, Claustrat B, et al. Effects of chronic jet lag on tumor progression in mice. *Cancer Res.* 2004;64(21): 7879-7885.
87. Blask DE, Dauchy RT, Sauer LA, Krause JA, Brainard GC. Light during darkness, melatonin suppression and cancer progression. *Neuroendocrinol Lett.* 2002;23(suppl 2):52-56.
88. Blask DE, Brainard GC, Dauchy RT, Hanifin JP, Davidson LK, et al. Melatonin-depleted blood from premenopausal women exposed to light at night stimulates growth of human breast cancer xenografts in nude rats. *Cancer Res.* 2005;65(23):11174-11184.
89. Reiter RJ. Oxidative damage in the central nervous system: Protection by melatonin. *Prog Neurobiol.* 1998;56:359-384.
90. Van Dongen HPA, Maislin G, Mullington JM, Dinges DF. The cumulative cost of additional wakefulness: Dose-response effects on neurobehavioral functions and sleep physiology from chronic sleep restriction and total sleep deprivation. *Sleep.* 2003;26(2):117-126.
91. Klerman EB, Gershengorn HB, Duffy JF, Kronauer RE. Comparisons of the variability of three markers of the human circadian pacemaker. *J Biol Rhythms.* 2002;17:181-193.
92. Klerman EB, Lee Y, Czeisler CA, Kronauer RE. Linear demasking techniques are unreliable for estimating the circadian phase of ambulatory temperature data. *J Biol Rhythms.* 1999;14(4):260-274.
93. Wright KP, Drake CL, Lockley SW. Diagnostic tools for circadian rhythm sleep disorders. In: Kushida CA, ed. *Handbook of Sleep Disorders.* 2nd ed. New York: Informa Healthcare; 2009:147-173.
94. Czeisler CA, Moore-Ede MC, Regestein QR, et al. Episodic 24-hour cortisol secretory patterns in patients awaiting elective cardiac surgery. *J Clin Endocrinol Metab.* 1976;42(2):273-283
95. Bojkowski CJ, Arendt J, Shih MC, Markey SP. Melatonin secretion in humans assessed by measuring its metabolite, 6-sulfatoxymelatonin. *Clin Chem.* 1987;33:1343-1348.
96. Bojkowski CJ, Arendt J. Factors influencing urinary 6-sulphatoxymelatonin, a major melatonin metabolite, in normal human subjects. *Clin Endocrinol.* 1990;33:435-444.
97. Skene DJ, Lockley SW, James K, Arendt J. Correlation between urinary cortisol and 6-sulphatoxymelatonin rhythms in field studies of blind subjects. *Clin Endocrinol.* 1999;50:715-719.
98. Lockley SW, Skene DJ, James K, Thapan K, Wright J, Arendt J. Melatonin administration can entrain the free-running circadian system of blind subjects. *J Endocrinol.* 2000;164:R1-R6.
99. Barnes RG, Deacon SJ, Forbes MJ, Arendt J. Adaptation of the 6-sulphatoxymelatonin rhythm in shiftworkers on offshore oil installations during a 2-week 12-h night shift. *Neurosci Lett.* 1998;241:9-12.
100. Barnes RG, Forbes MJ, Arendt J. Shift type and season affect adaptation of the 6-sulphatoxymelatonin rhythm in offshore oil rig workers. *Neurosci Lett.* 1998;252:179-182.
101. Gibbs M, Hampton S, Morgan L, Arendt J. Adaptation of the circadian rhythm of 6-sulphatoxymelatonin to a shift schedule of seven nights followed by seven days in offshore oil installation workers. *Neurosci Lett.* 2002;325:91-94.
102. Dumont M, Benhaberou-Brun D, Paquet J. Profile of 24-h light exposure and circadian phase of melatonin secretion in night workers. *J Biol Rhythms.* 2001;16(5):502-511.
103. Midwinter MJ, Arendt J. Adaptation of the melatonin rhythm in human subjects following night-shift work in Antarctica. *Neurosci Lett.* 1991;122(2):195-198.
104. Ross JK, Arendt J, Horne J, Haston W. Night-shift work in Antarctica: Sleep characteristics and bright light treatment. *Physiol Behav.* 1995; 57(6):1169-1174.
105. Wulff K, Joyce E, Middleton B, Dijk DJ, Foster RG. The suitability of actigraphy, diary data, and urinary melatonin profiles for quantitative assessment of sleep disturbances in schizophrenia: A case report. *Chronobiol Int.* 2006;23(1-2):485-495.
106. Deacon SJ, Arendt J. Phase-shifts in melatonin, 6-sulphatoxymelatonin and alertness rhythms after treatment with moderately bright light at night. *Clin Endocrinol.* 1994;40:413-420.
107. Skene DJ, Bojkowski CJ, Currie JE, Wright J, Boulter PS, Arendt J. 6-Sulphatoxymelatonin production in breast cancer patients. *J Pineal Res.* 1990;8:269-276.
108. Tzischinsky O, Shlitner A, Lavie P. The association between the nocturnal sleep gate and nocturnal onset of urinary 6-sulfatoxymelatonin. *J Biol Rhythms.* 1993;8(3):199-209.
109. Girotti L, Lago M, Ianovsky O, Elizari MV, Dini A, et al. Low urinary 6-sulfatoxymelatonin levels in patients with severe congestive heart failure. *Endocrine.* 2003;22(3):245-248.
110. Montagnese S, Middleton B, Mani AR, Skene DJ, Morgan MY. Sleep and circadian abnormalities in patients with cirrhosis: Features of delayed sleep phase syndrome? *Metab Brain Dis.* 2009;24(3):427-439.
111. Lockley SW. Timed melatonin treatment for delayed sleep phase syndrome: The importance of knowing circadian phase. *Sleep.* 2005;28(10): 1214-1216.

Chapter 29

Shift Work Disorder

SUZANNE FTOUNI / TRACEY L. SLETTEN / LAURA K. BARGER / STEVEN W. LOCKLEY / SHANTHA M.W. RAJARATNAM

Shift work disorder is a circadian rhythm sleep disorder caused by an intentional misalignment of the sleep-wake cycle from the circadian rhythm of sleep propensity. The International Classification of Sleep Disorders has described shift work disorder based on four main criteria (Box 29-1)[1] and the adverse consequences of shift work have also been recognized in the Diagnostic and Statistical Manual of Mental Disorders (DSM-IV), which classifies shift work disorder as a dyssomnia of the primary circadian rhythm sleep disorders.[2]

Shift work disorder is described as a disruption of the endogenous circadian sleep/wake cycle due to the conflict between the natural pattern of sleep and wakefulness, and the desired pattern of sleep and wakefulness required by shift work schedules.[3] It is characterized by complaints of insomnia or excessive sleepiness associated with recurring shift work schedules that take place during usual sleep times.[1,2] Symptoms experienced typically involve shorter sleep durations and frequent disturbances in sleep continuity.[3-6] Symptoms are most typically present in workers on night shift schedules and early morning schedules.[7] The DSM-IV also highlights the higher degree of sleep disturbance associated with slow and counterclockwise rotating shift schedules.[2,7] There are few reports with empirical data assessing the prevalence of shift work disorder. Some have reported a 5% to 10% prevalence in shift workers,[1,8] and others have reported up to 60% prevalence in night shift workers, with the disorder typically persisting for as long as the individual works the shift schedule.[2]

BOX 29-1 *Diagnostic Criteria for Circadian Rhythm Sleep Disorder, Shift Work Type*

Shift Work Disorder

A. There is a complaint of insomnia or excessive sleepiness that is temporally associated with a recurring work schedule that overlaps the usual time for sleep.

B. The symptoms are associated with the shift work schedule over the course of at least 1 month.

C. Sleep log or actigraphy monitoring (with sleep diaries) for at least 7 days demonstrates disturbed circadian and sleep time misalignment.

D. The sleep disturbance is not better explained by another current sleep disorder, medical or neurologic disorder, mental disorder, medication use, or substance use disorder.

From American Academy of Sleep Medicine. *The International Classification of Sleep Disorders; Diagnostic and Coding Manual, (ICSD-2),* 2nd ed. Westchester, IL: American Academy of Sleep Medicine; 2005.

SHIFT WORK

The prevalence of shift work varies among industries and occupations. In 2004, 17.7% of the workforce in the United States was undertaking shift work.[9] Similar proportions are reported in Japan (22.7%),[10] Australia (16%),[11] the United Kingdom (18.1%), and France (13%).[12] The demand for growth in productivity and round-the-clock availability of services is likely to stimulate an increase in the need for shift work in our increasingly 24-hour society. The proportion of individuals employed in shift work varies between industries and occupational groups. For example, in Australia, the mining industry has the highest prevalence of shift work, followed by health care and hospitality.[11]

Shift work refers to a system of nonstandard working hours whereby the daily hours of operation are split into at least two sets of work periods, or shifts, over the 24-hour day.[13,14] There is great variability in the hours of shift work among individuals, occupations, and industries. Generally, there are three broad shift types: the standard, conventional day shift; afternoon or evening shift; and the night shift.[3,13] Day shift hours extend from the early morning into the late afternoon/early evening, typically occurring between 7 AM and 6 PM.[13,15] Early morning shifts are also common, often occurring between 6 AM and 2 PM.[7,16,17] Evening shifts generally begin in the mid to late afternoon and end late in the evening (e.g., 3 PM to 11 PM) or early morning,[15,18] and night shifts generally cover the remaining hours from the end of the evening shift until the beginning of the day shift (e.g., 10 PM to 7 AM).[7,19,20]

Shift systems can differ based on a number of characteristics including the type and duration of shifts worked; and the length, speed, and direction of a shift cycle.[13,15,21] Workers on a shift system can be employed on permanent or rotating shift cycles.[7,13,15,21] Permanent shift systems involve working one primary shift type, commonly an evening or night shift, with scheduled days off.[18] Day shifts can be worked permanently, yet are generally not considered as shift work unless they are worked as part of a rotating shift schedule,[18] or unless they involve particularly early start times. Rotating shift systems involve cycling through various shift types periodically in either a clockwise or counterclockwise direction. *Clockwise rotations,* also known as *phase delay rotations,* involve working through shifts from day, to evening, to night shifts. Alternatively, *counterclockwise rotations,* or *phase advance rotations,* work on backward rotations in which shift cycles progress from night shifts through to day shifts (Fig. 29-1).[13,22,23] The rate of a shift cycle rotation can be described as either rapid or slow. Rapid rotations typically involve 2 to 3 days worked

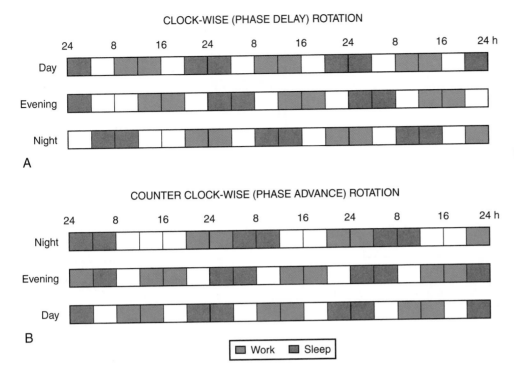

Figure 29-1 Diagrammatic representation of phase delay and phase advance shift rotations. A, Example of a clockwise (or phase delay) shift rotation in which shifts are worked from day, to evening, to night shifts with progressively later start times. This pattern allows for greater time between shifts to allow for sufficient sleep opportunity. **B,** Example of a counterclockwise (or phase advance) shift rotation in which shifts are worked from nights to evenings to day shifts with shift start times beginning progressively earlier. This arrangement provides less sleep opportunity when switching to the next shift type.

consecutively on one particular type of shift before moving on to another shift type or scheduled days off.[18,24,25] Slow rotations usually incorporate 5 to 7 days consecutively on one type of shift before rotating to another shift or days off. The length of these cycles may depend on the duration of the shifts involved, commonly between 8 and 12 hours.[11] Longer shifts of 12 hours or more usually allow for a compressed work week with fewer shifts worked and more days off following a series of shifts.

SLEEP AND CIRCADIAN DISRUPTION

The sleepiness experienced by shift workers can be explained by four physiologic determinants: circadian phase (time of day), duration of continuous wakefulness (acute sleep deprivation), habitual sleep duration (sleep deficiency), and sleep inertia (Fig. 29-2).[19] Shift workers commonly suffer from impaired alertness and neurobehavioral performance during wake time due to a combination of these factors.

Circadian Phase

The endogenous circadian pacemaker, located in the suprachiasmatic nuclei (SCN) of the hypothalamus, generates oscillations of alertness and performance which cycle approximately every 24 hours.[20,26-28] Light is the major environmental time cue that synchronizes the circadian pacemaker to the solar day-night cycle.[20,28-30] Alertness and performance are at their highest as the pacemaker promotes wakefulness during the biologic day and are worst during the biologic night, in particular between 3 AM and 6 AM.[31] This circadian alertness rhythm results in impaired performance (and therefore impaired safety and productivity) when work is scheduled during the biologic night. The circadian pacemaker also functions to facilitate consolidated sleep during the night and to promote and maintain wakefulness during the day.[32] When

a person is required to work at night, sleep during the daytime hours is strongly negatively affected as the circadian drive for wakefulness during the biologic day results in shorter and more disturbed sleep.[32,33] Circadian misalignment is therefore experienced by night and early morning shift workers because they are required to sleep and wake at times of day that oppose the endogenous circadian cycle.

The type of shift rotation worked can influence an individual's ability to adapt to shift work according to fundamental characteristics of endogenous circadian rhythms.[34] Although circadian rhythms are disrupted by both clockwise and counterclockwise rotations, it is argued that clockwise (delaying) rotations are associated with more rapid adjustment and reduced adverse consequences. This effect is due to the natural tendency for the circadian pacemaker to delay in most individuals because the average circadian period has a cycle length that is slightly longer than 24 hours.[14,17,23,35] Despite greater disruption to the circadian cycle, however, counterclockwise shift systems are popular among shift workers as they result in less time between shifts and therefore may compress the working week, allowing more time off.[24,36]

Intuitively one would expect slow rotating shift systems to be biologically preferable because they allow time for circadian adaptation. With a higher number of consecutive shifts worked, an individual can begin to adjust his or her endogenous circadian rhythms.[18] Slow rotating schedules, however, can cause great disruption because just as the circadian system adapts to a shift type, the next shift type is to begin[17,24] or a day off is scheduled. Full adaptation to the change in sleep and wake time may not occur under these circumstances, however, as even a small amount of sun exposure at an inappropriate time (for instance when attempting sleep during the day following a night shift) is enough to prevent the circadian pacemaker from readily changing to the different time schedule.[18,37] Additionally, shift workers often revert to "day shift" schedules on days off from night shift rotations (e.g., to

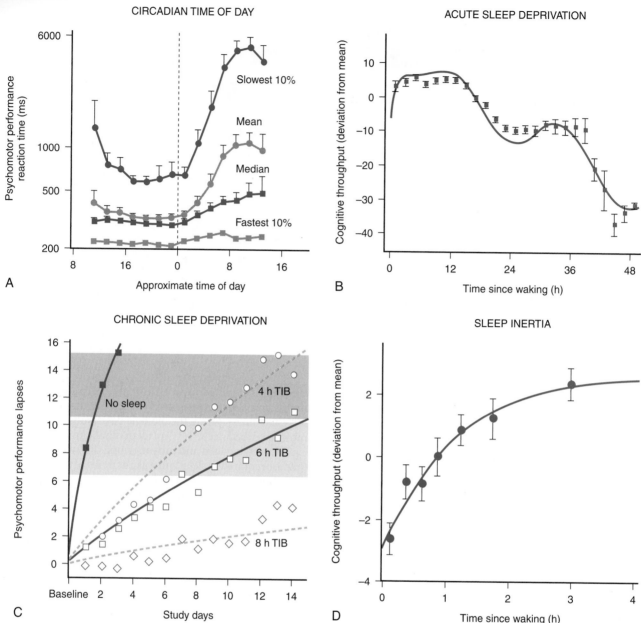

Figure 29-2 Data from laboratory-based investigations illustrating the four physiologic determinants of sleepiness. A, The endogenous circadian rhythm in visual psychomotor performance over a 32-hour constant routine ($n = 10$). Performance is poorest toward the end of the biologic night but then improves slightly owing to the drive for alertness emanating from the endogenous circadian pacemaker. **B,** The effects of 48 hours of continuous wakefulness on mean ($\pm$ SEM) cognitive throughput, as measured by a simple addition test ($n = 94$). Cognition declines across all circadian phases with increasing time awake. The line represents a model prediction of cognition under these conditions. **C,** A representation of how different amounts of chronic partial sleep deprivation affect psychomotor performance. The figure compares the time course of average daily lapses in attention over 2 weeks in subjects with an 8-hour (open diamond, $n = 9$), 6-hour (open square, $n = 13$), and 4-hour (open circle, $n = 13$) time-in-bed (TIB) sleep opportunity each day and 88 hours of continuous sleep deprivation (closed square, $n = 13$). Performance deteriorated in the 6- and 4-hour sleep groups such that after 14 days the participants in the 6-hour sleep group performed at an equivalent level to those kept awake for 24 hours continuously and members of the 4-hour group were performing at the same level as someone kept awake for 3 entire days. **D,** The time course of sleep inertia in cognitive throughput over the first 4 hours of wakefulness after a normal 8-hour sleep for 3 days. Although there is an exponential improvement in performance over time, it takes at least 2 hours to reach maximal performance and there is a high risk of a fatigue-related error in the first 30 minutes after waking. (**A,** Data from Cajochen C, Khalsa SB, Wyatt JK, et al. EEG and ocular correlates of circadian melatonin phase and human performance decrements during sleep loss. *Am J Physiol.* 1999;277(3 Pt 2):R640-649. **B,** Data from Jewett ME, Dijk DJ, Kronauer RE, et al. Sigmoidal decline of homeostatic component in subjective alertness and cognitive throughput. *Sleep.* 1999;22(Suppl):S94-S95. **C,** Data from Van Dongen HP, Maislin G, Mullington JM, et al. The cumulative cost of additional wakefulness: Dose-response effects on neurobehavioral functions and sleep physiology from chronic sleep restriction and total sleep deprivation. *Sleep.* 2003;26(2):117-126. **D,** Data from Jewett ME, Wyatt JK, Ritz-De Cecco A, et al. Time course of sleep inertia dissipation in human performance and alertness. *J Sleep Res.* 1999;8(1):1-8.)

accommodate family commitments) making complete adaptation to night work more difficult. These considerations mean that, in practice, shift workers on rapidly rotating shift schedules rarely adapt[24] and experience acute sleep and alertness problems when working at night, as described previously.

Duration of Wakefulness: Acute Sleep Deprivation

Shift workers often experience prolonged periods of wakefulness or acute sleep deprivation, in particular prior to the first of a sequence of night shifts. Homeostatic pressure for sleep builds with sustained wakefulness and consequently has a negative impact on neurocognitive performance.[38-42] The effects of acute sleep deprivation become apparent during work periods as alertness and performance gradually diminish with the increase in the duration of wakefulness.[19,39,40,43] This can have significant effects on an individual's speed and accuracy, working memory, short-term memory, and in particular, sustained attention or vigilance.[39-41] Lapses in performance during sleep deprivation have been associated with attenuated brain activation in frontoparietal regions, extrastriate visual cortex, and the thalamus.[44] Sleep-deprived individuals show decreased task-related brain activation compared to well-rested individuals, resulting in slower, less accurate, and more variable performance on tasks.[44] The effects of sleep deprivation on neurobehavioral performance are comparable to the effects of alcohol intoxication.[45-48] After 17 to 19 hours of wakefulness, performance on tests of vigilance and perceptual coding decrease to levels equivalent to, or worse than, that seen in individuals with a blood alcohol concentration (BAC) of 0.05%.[46,47,49] After 24 hours or more of extended wakefulness, cognitive motor performance can decrease to levels similar to that of BAC levels of 0.1%.[46] Shift workers often report remaining awake for at least 24 hours by the end of the first scheduled night shift,[50] and report being awake for at least 8 hours before commencing the next night shift.[18] Commuting times also have to be taken into consideration when determining work-related continuous wake hours, particularly for individuals with long-distance commutes or slow travel times.

Sleep Duration: Chronic Sleep Deficiency

Shift workers can accumulate a chronic sleep debt over time when an inadequate amount of sleep is obtained over consecutive days as a result of shortened sleep duration between successive shifts.[51,52] A survey by the American National Sleep Foundation reported that 58% of shift workers spend less than 6 hours in bed or sleeping between successive shifts, and 63% believed that this was due to their work hours not allowing them to achieve adequate sleep.[53] The duration of sleep obtained by a shift worker varies with the type of shift. A meta-analysis of the effects of permanent and rotating shift work schedules on sleep length based on 36 primary shift work studies demonstrated that permanent night shift workers reported an average sleep duration of 6.6 hours of per night.[17] This decreased to an average of 5.9 hours per day between successive night shifts. Slow rotating schedules allowed greater sleep opportunity with an average of 6.4 hours of sleep between night shifts, while those on rapidly rotating shift cycles obtained on average 5.7 hours of sleep between

night shifts.[17] Among the analyzed studies was an investigation of paper mill shift workers by Torsvall and colleagues,[6] who reported that total sleep time decreased by 2 hours in those working night shifts compared to those working day shifts. Particularly during periods when work load was low and while sitting, electroencephalogram (EEG) recordings revealed that 20% of workers had sleep episodes during night shift work periods.[6] Laboratory studies have demonstrated dose-dependent cumulative effects of sleep restriction on neurobehavioral performance. Restricting sleep to 3 to 7 hours per night for seven consecutive nights affects alertness and sleepiness, frequency and duration of lapses, and feelings of fatigue and stress, equivalent to levels observed after two nights of total sleep deprivation.[40,52,54]

Sleep Inertia

Another physiologic determinant of sleepiness is sleep inertia, defined as the grogginess and substantial impairment in performance experienced immediately upon waking.[55] The effects of sleep inertia dissipate exponentially with time, yet are detectable for up to 2 to 4 hours following waking.[56,57] This impairment is exacerbated following sleep deprivation[55,58] and when the individual is awakened during the biologic night during the circadian nadir.[59] Wertz and colleagues[58] found that cognitive performance immediately on awakening was significantly worse than performance following 26 hours of sleep deprivation. Sleep inertia may also be experienced following short sleep episodes, or naps.[60] Hofer-Tinguely and colleagues[60] observed greater levels of impairment in performance following afternoon naps, as compared to performance following periods of awake-rest or activity. This is particularly important in night shift workers who often nap prior to or during a shift, or in occupations that include on-call duty, such as physicians and firefighters who often make critical decisions within minutes of waking. Sleep inertia following a nap taken in the work place setting may result in impaired performance for several hours, exposing the worker (and potentially the public) to increased risks of accidents, injuries, and errors.

OCCUPATIONAL SAFETY AND HEALTH RISKS

Of the individuals who experienced a work-related injury or illness in Australia during 2006, 27% were working under shift arrangements.[61] The Sleep in America Poll reported that among workers who reported at least one accident in the past year, 23% were achieving less than 6 hours of sleep during work days.[53] As described in the previous section, disruption to sleep and circadian rhythmicity is a consequence of shift work. This mismatch between the endogenous circadian system and environmental cues, and the resultant sleep disruption, can have a severe impact on many aspects of health and well-being, as well as performance and safety during working hours, including the ability to drive to and from work safely.[19,30,40,43,51,62,63] Shift work therefore impacts both long-term health in affecting the risk of developing certain chronic diseases (cardiovascular disease, diabetes, cancer) and short-term health in increasing the risk of a sleepiness-related accident and injury. It should also be recognized that the short-term health and safety consequences of shift work are not limited to the shift workers themselves; workplace accidents may put fellow workers at risk in addition to members of the public (for example, by crashing into them or harming them with a medical error) or society at large (e.g., large-scale industrial accidents such as those at Chernobyl, Three-Mile Island, and Bhopal).

Occupational Performance and Safety

Circadian disruption and sleep deficiency associated with shift work can negatively impact occupational safety and performance.[64] As discussed earlier, alertness and neurobehavioral performance are impaired during the biologic night as the endogenous circadian pacemaker is promoting sleep at this time. This is particularly important in night shift workers because they are required to work at this time, when the risks of workplace errors and accidents and motor vehicle crashes are known to increase.[19,65]

Sleep disruption and fatigue associated with shift work have been observed in a number of occupational settings, including train and railway traffic controllers,[66] oil rig workers,[4] fire fighters,[67] and pilots.[65] For example, police officers engaged in shift work report worse sleep quality and reduced sleep duration,[68-70] which are associated with impaired vigilance and attention on the job[68] and increased occurrence of critical incidents, compared to non-shift working police officers.[71-73]

A number of studies have assessed the risks associated with different work schedules in health care settings, with greater error rates and risks of self-harm and patient harm evident in shift working nurses, resident anesthetists, interns, and physicians.[74-78] A meta-analysis of the effects of sleep loss on performance in physicians and nonphysicians revealed that sleep loss impaired cognitive performance by nearly one standard deviation.[79] The rate of percutaneous injuries was twice as high during night shift periods compared to day periods and were significantly increased during extended hours following on call night shifts.[80] Lapses in concentration and fatigue were the two most commonly reported contributing factors.[80] Nurses working extended night shift hours often experience fatigue and sleepiness and thus may also make errors in clinical judgment or medication administration and fail to intercept errors made by others.[74,81] Extended duration shifts have been associated with an increased risk of medical errors,[82] adverse events[76] and attentional failures in medical interns,[77] and increased rates of accidental blood or fluid exposure in residents.[83] In nurses, the likelihood of making an error also increased with longer working hours.[75]

Driving Risks

Drowsy Driving

While shift work and safety concerns tend to focus on workplace accidents and injuries, driving to and from work also contributes to occupational risk. In 2002, an estimated 1715 people died in fatal motor vehicle crashes (MVCs) on Australian roads.[84] During 2002 in the United States, over 42,000 fatalities were due to MVCs, and there were 2778 in Canada and 3423 in the United Kingdom.[84] Sleepiness and fatigue are among the most common causes of preventable MVCs.[85] In Australia, approximately 20% of fatal MVCs are reportedly a result of sleepiness- or fatigue-related driving.[84] In the United States, 16.5% of fatal highway crashes are attributed to driver

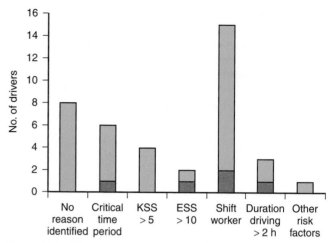

Figure 29-3 **Comparison of risk factors contributing to sleepiness in sleep related and not sleep related collisions.** Risk factors contributing to sleepiness between collisions defined as sleep related by Australian Transport and Safety Bureau (ATSB) criteria *(blue)* and not sleep related *(gray)*. *ESS,* Epworth sleepiness score; *KSS,* Karolinska sleepiness score. (Redrawn from Crummy F, Cameron PA, Swann P, et al. Prevalence of sleepiness in surviving drivers of motor vehicle collisions. *Intern Med J.* 2008;38[10]:769-775.)

sleepiness.[86] MVCs associated with sleepiness and fatigue are often underestimated, however. Because of the multifactorial nature of many crashes, it can be difficult to identify sleep or fatigue as the cause. There is often an association with drug and alcohol consumption, and thus many are not regarded as a sleepiness- or fatigue-related accident (despite sleepiness being a major component of drug- and alcohol-related accidents). Determining that the cause of an accident is due to driver sleepiness is difficult because there is no widely used objective and reliable test or "breathalyzer" for sleepiness.[85,87,88] Furthermore, variations in the estimates are also attributable to the lack of a universal definition of sleepiness- or fatigue-related collisions.[85] The Australian Transport Safety Bureau (ATSB) has developed an operational definition of fatigue- (or sleepiness-) related crashes based on police and coroner reports on fatal road crashes.[85] Sleepiness-related crashes are identified as single vehicle collisions that occur between the critical periods for sleepiness-related crashes (midnight to 6 AM and 2 PM to 4 PM), or head-on collisions that occur at any time where neither vehicle was overtaking. This definition excludes all crashes involving unlicensed drivers, pedestrians, speed limits less than 50 mph, and a driver with a BAC above the legal limit (0.05 g/100 mL). Despite this effort to establish a system to identify sleepiness-related crashes, however, the definition is unable to entirely encompass all such cases.[89] A crash investigation study by Crummy and colleagues[89] used the preceding definition to identify collisions that could be attributed to sleepiness but of the crashes deemed as sleepiness-related by the study's questionnaire, only 25% were identified as such by the ATSB definitions (Fig. 29-3). This study demonstrates that the proportion of MVCs attributed to driver sleepiness may be grossly underestimated in the population.

Factors Influencing Motor Vehicle Collision Risk

Feelings of drowsiness and fatigue while driving can affect a driver's ability to safely maintain control of a vehicle as the driver's vigilance deteriorates and performance is impaired.[46,47,49,87] With increased sleepiness, drivers show

Comparison of Shift Workers and Non-Shift Workers*

Sleep-Related Activity/Condition[†]	Self-Reported Frequency	
	Shift Workers	Non-Shift Workers
Spending less than 6 hours in bed on work days	58%	13%
Sleeping less than 6 hours on work days	33%	15%
Being diagnosed with sleep apnea	18%	8%
Driving drowsy at least once a month in the past year	48%	30%

*For this survey, a shift worker was classified as someone who began shifts after 6 PM but before 6 AM. Of a total of 1000 respondents, 7% were classified as shift workers.

[†]More common in shift workers than in non-shift workers.

Data from National Sleep Foundation, *Sleep in America Poll.* Washington, DC: National Sleep Foundation; 2008.

an increased likelihood of experiencing "micro-sleeps", periods of inattention, longer and more frequent eye closures, and falling asleep at the wheel.[87,90] Night shift workers are at an increased risk of involvement in sleepiness-related MVCs due to the combination of circadian drive for sleep, decreased sleep duration, and extended time awake.[89-92] A recent poll by the National Sleep Foundation found that in a sample of 1000 U.S. drivers, 32% reported experiencing at least one instance of drowsy driving per month in the past year.[53] Of these drivers, 48% were shift workers (Table 29-1). Crash investigation studies have found that in a sample of 31 drivers involved in MVCs, 48% were night shift workers, and of these crashes, 33% had worked a night shift immediately prior to the incident.[89] A nationwide survey by Barger and colleagues[92] investigated the risk of MVCs on the drive home following extended work shifts (≥ 24 hours) in first-year postgraduate medical interns: 40% of all reported MVCs occurred on the commute following work. The odds ratio of reporting an MVC or near-miss while driving after an extended work shift was 2.3 and 5.9, respectively, compared to that following non-extended shifts.[92]

The higher incidence of sleepiness-related collisions that occur between the critical period of midnight and 6 AM, and more modestly between 2 PM and 4 PM,[5,48,89,91,93-98] are explained by the circadian drive for sleep during the night and a secondary increase in sleepiness in the afternoon.[32,62,95] Investigation of crash data in England during 1987 to 1992 found three clear peak periods of sleepiness-related MVCs at 6 AM, 4 PM, and the major peak at 2 AM.[94] Owing to the nature of night shift start and end times, peak commute times for shift workers are often during the peak in the circadian rhythm of sleepiness. Investigation into shift working drivers found that 54% of shift workers reported driving home between the hours of 2 PM to 4 PM, and 14% reported driving home between 2 AM and 5 AM, whereas non-shift workers reported an average time for their commute following work of 2 PM.[99]

Sleep deficiency is a major contributor to the risk of experiencing a sleepiness-related MVC.[48,91,100] Drivers with 5 hours sleep or less in the preceding 24 hours are at a significantly higher risk of being involved in a sleep-related MVC.[48,91,98] Simulator studies have demonstrated the effects of sleep

deprivation on driving performance, with drivers deprived of sleep for 20 hours having more instances of lane drifting, slower reaction time to on-road events, unintentional changes in speed, and jerking motions of the wheel.[87,98,101] A study by Philip and colleagues[102] assessed the effects of sleep restriction on on-road driving performance. Findings indicated that drivers restricted to 2 hours of sleep had 8.1 times more inappropriate line crossings while driving compared to the well-rested drivers.[102] When a sleep-restricted individual was driving, the co-pilot in the front passenger seat was required to intervene 61 times in order to maintain safety of the drive.[102]

Time on task and sleep deprivation (acute and chronic) substantially impact the ability to maintain safe driving. Long distance driving increases the risk of MVCs due to increasing levels of drowsiness and the subsequent effects on driver performance.[5,91,100,102] Simulator studies demonstrate that subjective feelings of sleepiness and fatigue progressively increase on a linear scale over the first 80 minutes of driving.[103,104] In an on-road drowsy driver study, well-rested drivers were able to drive for over 1000 km (621 miles), from 9 AM to 7 PM with rest stops without experiencing significant performance decrements.[102] After sleep restriction, however, drivers showed clear deficits in driving performance after a relatively short duration of driving (1-2 hours).[102] Shift workers often report feelings of increased sleepiness during driving, which is also observed through physiologic indicators, such as blink rate, which demonstrate increased sleepiness levels at the beginning and a progressive increase throughout the drive.[90,104] Driving performance declines throughout the drive with greater lateral lane deviation with increased time driving,[90,104] and these performance impairments are associated with increasing sleepiness levels.[105]

Long-Term Health Risks

Disturbances to the circadian system, chronic sleep deficiency, and exposure to light in the evening can increase a shift worker's risk of experiencing a range of health problems[106,107] (Fig. 29-4). Disturbances in psychological well-being and mental health have also been documented in shift workers, with night shift nurses reporting greater feelings of depression and poorer global sleep than permanent day shift nurses.[106,108-110] Associations have been made between shift work and higher incidences of adverse endocrine and immune system responses,[43] gastrointestinal complaints and diseases such as peptic ulcers,[111,112] diabetes,[113-116] and higher body mass index.[117]

Cardiovascular disease is overrepresented in shift worker populations.[43,106,118] Working at night is associated with increases in heart rate and blood pressure, and the normal circadian rhythm of heart rate variability is strongly modified by physical activity during the night shift.[62,119] Knutsson and colleagues[118] showed that shift work was associated with increased risk of myocardial infarctions in both men and women. A previous study by this group demonstrated that the relative risk of ischemic heart disease increased with increasing exposure to shift work over time.[114,120] Although occupational stress associated with shift work has been linked with the increased risk of cardiovascular disease,[106] other studies suggest that job strain may not be the major cause.[118] Although the mechanisms underlying the association between shift work and cardiovascular disease are presently unclear, a

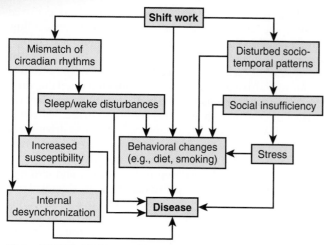

Figure 29-4 Model of the possible mechanisms contributing to disease in shift workers. (Redrawn from Knutsson A. Health disorders of shift workers. *Occup Med (Lond)*. 2003;53[2]:103-108.)

number of possibilities exist including the direct effect of sleep deficiency on metabolic function and inflammation,[121-123] disrupted circadian rhythms in cardiac function,[124] elevation of circulating lipids and impairment of glucose metabolism due to eating during the biologic night,[59,125,126] and cardiovascular disease associated with undiagnosed sleep apnea.[127]

Relatively recent reports have linked shift work to cancer, in particular breast cancer in female shift workers.[128-130] Shift work that involves circadian desynchrony has been categorized as a probable carcinogen by the World Health Organization (WHO).[128] A number of factors associated with shift work may contribute to this increased risk,[131] including circadian disruption,[132] disrupted sleep,[7] and suppression of melatonin by light.[131,133]

TREATMENTS AND COUNTERMEASURES FOR MANAGING SHIFT WORK DISORDER AND SHIFT WORK

The American Academy of Sleep Medicine[134] has put forward guidelines for the treatment of shift work disorder (SWD), including timed light exposure, melatonin administration, management of sleep/wake scheduling, and use of wake-promoting medication.

Modafinil (Provigil) is a wake-promoting agent approved by the U.S. Food and Drug Administration (FDA) to treat excessive sleepiness associated with narcolepsy, obstructive sleep apnea, and SWD.[134-136] The precise mechanisms of action of modafinil are currently unclear,[137-139] although they are believed to differ substantially from those of conventional stimulants, such as amphetamine, by localizing brain activation to wakefulness-promoting regions[139-141] (see Chapter 6). The use of modafinil to treat excessive sleepiness in SWD has been validated in a double-blind, placebo-controlled field study by Czeisler and associates.[135] Patients with SWD were administered modafinil (200 mg, $N = 96$) or placebo ($N = 108$) 30 to 60 minutes before each scheduled shift over 3 months. Patients were evaluated at baseline and at three time points, 1 month apart, during an overnight, laboratory-simulated shift following

three consecutive night shifts. At the final visit, patients who received modafinil had significant reductions in the frequency and duration of lapses of attention during a nighttime psychomotor vigilance task, as compared to baseline levels and the placebo group. Sleepiness levels and sleep latency also improved significantly at the final visit compared to baseline levels and the placebo group (Fig. 29-5). During worked shifts and the commute home, the treatment group also reported lower maximum levels of sleepiness, and 25% fewer patients reported accidents or near accidents. Overall, of those receiving treatment, 74% of the patients had improvement in their clinical symptoms compared to 36% on placebo. The use of modafinil has also been found to improve overall well-being, including functional status and quality of life.[136] Although the use of modafinil has been successful in improving alertness levels during night work, it has not been found to restore alertness to regular daytime levels.[135]

As described earlier, night shift work causes daytime sleep disruption by a failure of the circadian clock to synchronize with the inverted light-dark cycle. Appropriately timed exposure to bright light and melatonin administration are circadian phase-dependent countermeasures that can accelerate adaptation to shifted sleep-wake and light-dark schedules and thus improve sleep duration and quality during the daytime hours. Timed exposure to bright light during night work can reset the timing of the circadian pacemaker by shifting circadian phase.[142,143] The human circadian system responds to light in a nonlinear dose-response relationship: 100 lux exposure achieves about half the phase-shifting response induced by about 10,000 lux despite representing only 1% of the intensity.[144] Appropriate timing of the light exposure is a crucial consideration in treatment protocols, as light and the relative timing of light and dark have the ability to advance or delay the circadian system depending on the time of exposure.[62] For example, Santhi and colleagues[145] found that sleep/dark scheduled from 2 PM to 10 PM prior to a night shift phase advanced the system, while sleep/dark exposure following a night shift (8 AM to 2 PM) caused phase delay shifts.

Melatonin is secreted by the pineal gland at night and is thought to play a role in the regulation of sleep timing.[146] Administration of melatonin promotes sleep particularly during the biologic day when endogenous levels of the hormone are typically low.[146,147] Melatonin is, therefore, a potential treatment for SWD to improve sleep quality and duration when sleep occurs at an adverse circadian phase.[148-151] Melatonin administration can also shift circadian phase, with the magnitude and direction of shifts depending on the circadian time of administration,[152,153] although the magnitude of effect of melatonin is generally less than that of exposure to bright light.[154] In order to phase-advance the system, melatonin should be administered prior to the onset of the endogenous melatonin rise (late afternoon/evening hours in an individual with a normal sleep-wake cycle). Phase-delays in response to melatonin treatment are reported to occur in the morning hours in normally synchronized subjects, coinciding broadly with cessation of endogenous melatonin production.[152,153]

Management strategies such as changes to shift schedules and napping can help minimize sleepiness due to circadian rhythm disturbance and sleep loss. Workers often desire rapidly rotating, counterclockwise shift systems as it compresses the work week by minimizing time between shifts,

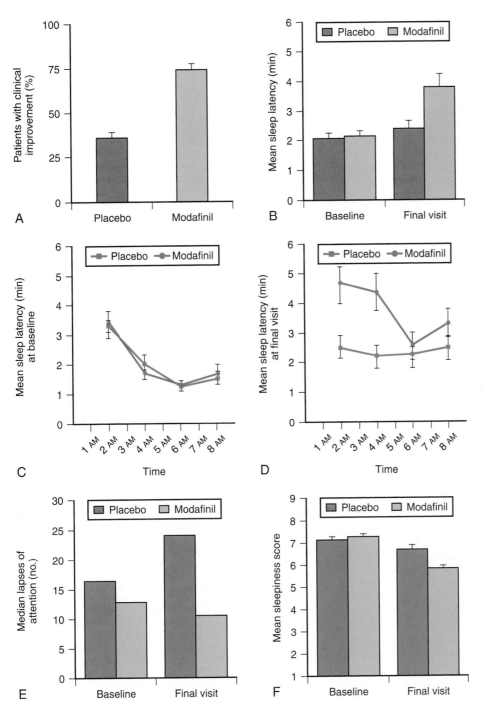

Figure 29-5 Improvement in efficacy measures used to assess the effects of modafinil versus placebo in patients with shift work disorder. A, A greater percentage of patients on the treatment showed improvement on self-rated symptoms. B, Mean sleep latency, as measured by the multiple sleep latency test (MSLT), was significantly higher at the final visit, compared to baseline and placebo. C and D, The difference in change in mean MSLT from baseline to the final visit for modafinil compared to placebo was statistically significant at 2 AM and 4 AM. E, Median lapses of attention in the Psychomotor Vigilance Task was significantly lower at the final visit in the treatment group when compared to baseline and placebo. F, Significantly lower levels of self-reported sleepiness, as measured on the Karolinska sleepiness scale (KSS), in the modafinil group at the final visit compared to levels at baseline and in the placebo group. (Redrawn from Czeisler CA, Walsh JK, Roth T, et al. Modafinil for excessive sleepiness associated with shift-work sleep disorder. *N Engl J Med.* 2005;353[5]:476-486.)

thus allowing shifts to be worked through more rapidly.[36] Although often desirable to workers, this type of shift system has a negative impact on sleep, particularly its timing, duration, and quality, and in turn can increase neurobehavioral performance impairment during the waking hours. Furthermore, circadian adaptation to counterclockwise shift rotations can take longer than for clockwise rotations.[23] Scheduling shifts in a clockwise rotation is believed to assist in faster adaptation by delaying circadian phase.[23] Scheduled napping during night shifts has been suggested as a countermeasure for sleepiness experienced on the job.[134] Naps of less than 1 hour were found to improve alertness and sleepiness levels when taken during a night shift.[155,156] Naps of less than

20 minutes were found to improve reaction time and increase alertness.[157] Despite the positive effects of napping during night shifts, caution must be taken to avoid the effects of sleep inertia.[158,159] Limiting the duration of the naps to between 10 and 20 minutes may help prevent impairments associated with sleep inertia.[160] The stimulant effects of caffeine may also be used to improve alertness levels and decrease the physiologic sleep tendency during night shift.[161-163] A number of studies have combined scheduled naps and caffeine to counteract the sleepiness experienced. A study by Schweitzer and colleagues[161] found that the combination of napping and caffeine during simulated and field night shifts improved alertness and psychomotor performance.

SUMMARY

Shift work is increasingly prevalent in society as the result of the demand of 24-hour productivity and services. Although the type of shift work systems can vary between industries and companies, the negative consequences are largely similar because of the underlying factors of circadian misalignment and sleep deficiency inherent in all shift work patterns. These factors impair a shift worker's ability to perform and remain alert during the biologic night and cause difficulty initiating and maintaining sleep during the biologic day. Furthermore, circadian disruption and sleep deficiency also adversely affect the medical and mental health of shift workers, increasing the risk of cardiovascular disease, cancer, and psychological disturbance. Safety of both shift workers and the public at large are also substantially affected by shift work, with the risk of accidents and MVCs while commuting to and from shifts increased considerably. Procedures to reduce the incidence of these preventable sleepiness-related accidents are required, along with a fuller appreciation of the legal responsibilities and consequences that shift workers accept when working overnight. A focused reexamination of whether all shift work is necessary is required, especially in the context of public safety, so that society can review the tradeoff between the demand for 24-hour services with the increased safety risk and health burden that shift work brings.

REFERENCES

1. American Academy of Sleep Medicine. *The International Classification of Sleep Disorders (ICSD-2)*. 2nd ed. Westchester, IL: American Academy of Sleep Medicine; 2005.
2. American Psychiatric Association. *Diagnostic and Statistical Manual of Mental Disorders (IV-TR)*. 4th ed. Washington, DC: American Psychiatric Association; 2000.
3. Akerstedt T. Shift work and disturbed sleep/wakefulness. *Occup Med (Lond)*. 2003;53:89-94.
4. Waage S, Moen BE, Pallesen S, et al. Shift work disorder among oil rig workers in the North Sea. *Sleep*. 2009;32(4):558-565.
5. Mitler MM, Miller JC, Lipsitz JJ, et al. The sleep of long-haul truck drivers. *N Engl J Med*. 1997;337(11):755-761.
6. Torsvall L, Akerstedt T, Gillander K, et al. Sleep on the night shift: 24-hour EEG monitoring of spontaneous sleep/wake behavior. *Psychophysiology*. 1989;26(3):352-358.
7. Akerstedt T. Shift work and disturbed sleep/wakefulness. *Sleep Med Rev*. 1998;2(2):117-128.
8. Drake CL, Roehrs T, Richardson G, et al. Shift work sleep disorder: Prevalence and consequences beyond that of symptomatic day workers. *Sleep*. 2004;27(8):1453-1462.
9. McMenamin TM. A time to work: Recent trends in shift work and flexible schedules. *Mon Labor Rev*. 2007;130(12):3-15.
10. Dochi M, Suwazono Y, Sakata K, et al. Shift work is a risk factor for increased total cholesterol level: A 14-year prospective cohort study in 6886 male workers. *Occup Environ Med*. 2009;66(9):592-597.
11. Australian Bureau of Statistics. *Working time arrangements*. Sydney, Australia: Australian Bureau of Statistics; 2009.
12. Wedderburn A. Statistics and news. In: *Bulletin of European Studies on Time*. Dublin: European Foundation for the Improvement of Living and Working Conditions; 1996.
13. Driscoll TR, Grunstein RR, Rogers NL. A systematic review of the neurobehavioural and physiological effects of shiftwork systems. *Sleep Med Rev*. 2007;11(3):179-194.
14. Akerstedt T, Wright Jr KP. Sleep loss and fatigue in shift work and shift work disorder. *Sleep Med Clin*. 2009;4(2):257-271.
15. Costa G. The problem: Shiftwork. *Chronobiol Int*. 1997;14(2):89-98.
16. Australian Bureau of Statistics. *Australian labour market statistics*. Sydney, Australia: Australian Bureau of Statistics; 2010.
17. Pilcher JJ, Lambert BJ, Huffcutt AI. Differential effects of permanent and rotating shifts on self-report sleep length: A meta-analytic review. *Sleep*. 2000;23(2):155-163.
18. Pilcher JJ. Shift work. In: Kushida CA, ed. *Sleep deprivation: Basic Science, Physiology and Behavior*. New York: Marcel Dekker; 2005:157-166.
19. Barger LK, Lockley SW, Rajaratnam SMW, et al. Neurobehavioral, health, and safety consequences associated with shift work in safety-sensitive professions. *Curr Neurol Neurosci Rep*. 2009;9(2):155-164.
20. Refinetti R. *Circadian Physiology*. Boca Raton, FL: CRC Press; 2000.
21. Knauth P. Changing schedules: Shiftwork. *Chronobiol Int*. 1997;14(2):159-171.
22. Turek FW. Circadian principles and design of rotating shift work schedules. *Am J Physiol*. 1986;251(3 Pt 2):R636-R638.
23. Czeisler CA, Moore-Ede MC, Coleman RM. Rotating shift work schedules that disrupt sleep are improved by applying circadian principles. *Science*. 1982;217(4558):460-463.
24. Signal TL, Gander PH. Rapid counterclockwise shift rotation in air traffic control: Effects on sleep and night work. *Aviat Space Environ Med*. 2007;78(9):878-885.
25. Fischer FM, Bruni ADC, Berwerth A, et al. Do weekly and fast rotating shiftwork schedules differentially affect duration and quality of sleep? *Int Arch Occup Environ Health*. 1997;69(5):354-360.
26. Borbely AA. A two process model of sleep regulation. *Hum Neurobiol*. 1982;1(3):195-204.
27. Daan S, Beersma DGM, Borbely AA. Timing of human sleep: Recovery process gated by a circadian pacemaker. *Am J Physiol*. 1984;246:R161-R178.
28. Moore RY. Circadian rhythms: Basic neurobiology and clinical applications. *Annu Rev Med*. 1997;48:253-266.
29. Panda S, Hogenesch JB, Kay SA. Circadian rhythms from flies to human. *Nature*. 2002;417(6886):329-335.
30. Klerman EB. Clinical aspects of human circadian rhythms. *J Biol Rhythms*. 2005;20(4):375-386.
31. Dijk DJ, Duffy JF, Czeisler CA. Circadian and sleep/wake dependent aspects of subjective alertness and cognitive performance. *J Sleep Res*. 1992;1(2):112-117.
32. Dijk DJ, Czeisler CA. Paradoxical timing of the circadian rhythm of sleep propensity serves to consolidate sleep and wakefulness in humans. *Neurosci Lett*. 1994;166(1):63-68.
33. Knauth P, Rutenfranz J. Duration of sleep related to the type of shift work. In: *Fifth International Symposium on Night and Shift Work*. Rouen, France: Scientific Committee on Shift Work of the Permanent Commission and International Association on Occupational Health (PCIAOH); 1980.
34. Sallinen M, Kecklund G. Shift work, sleep, and sleepiness—Differences between shift schedules and systems. *Scand J Work Environ Health*. 2010;36(2):121-133.
35. Czeisler CA, Duffy JF, Shanahan TL, et al. Stability, precision, and near-24-hour period of the human circadian pacemaker. *Science*. 1999;284(5423):2177-2181.
36. Cruz C, Detwiler C, Nesthus T, et al. Clockwise and counterclockwise rotating shifts: Effects on sleep duration, timing, and quality. *Aviat Space Environ Med*. 2003;74(6):597-605.
37. Folkard S. Do permanent night workers show circadian adjustment? A review based on the endogenous melatonin rhythm. *Chronobiol Int*. 2008;25(2-3):215-224.
38. Borbely AA, Achermann P. Sleep homeostasis and models of sleep regulation. *J Biol Rhythms*. 1999;14(6):559-568.
39. Alhola P, Polo-Kantola P. Sleep deprivation: Impact on cognitive performance. *Neuropsychiatr Dis Treat*. 2007;3(5):553-567.
40. Van Dongen HP, Maislin G, Mullington JM, et al. The cumulative cost of additional wakefulness: Dose-response effects on neurobehavioral functions and sleep physiology from chronic sleep restriction and total sleep deprivation. *Sleep*. 2003;26(2):117-126.
41. Frey DJ, Badia P, Wright Jr KP. Inter- and intra-individual variability in performance near the circadian nadir during sleep deprivation. *J Sleep Res*. 2004;13(4):305-315.
42. Cohen DA, Wang W, Wyatt JK, et al. Uncovering residual effects of chronic sleep loss on human performance. *Sci Transl Med*. 2010;2(14):14ra3.
43. Banks S, Dinges DF. Behavioral and physiological consequences of sleep restriction. *J Clin Sleep Med*. 2007;3(5):519-528.
44. Chee MW, Tan JC, Zheng H, et al. Lapsing during sleep deprivation is associated with distributed changes in brain activation. *J Neurosci*. 2008;28(21):5519-5528.
45. Czeisler CA. The Gordon Wilson Lecture: Work hours, sleep and patient safety in residency training. *Trans Am Clin Climatol Assoc*. 2006;117:159-188.

46. Dawson D, Reid K. Fatigue, alcohol and performance impairment. *Nature*. 1997;388(6639):235.

47. Arnedt JT, Owens J, Crouch M, et al. Neurobehavioral performance of residents after heavy night call vs. after alcohol ingestion. *JAMA*. 2005;294(9):1025-1033.

48. Connor J, Norton R, Ameratunga S, et al. Driver sleepiness and risk of serious injury to car occupants: Population based case control study. *BMJ*. 2002;324(7346):1125.

49. Williamson AM, Feyer AM. Moderate sleep deprivation produces impairments in cognitive and motor performance equivalent to legally prescribed levels of alcohol intoxication. *Occup Environ Med*. 2000;57(10):649-655.

50. Akerstedt T, Landstrom U. Work place countermeasures of night shift fatigue. *Int J Ind Ergon*. 1998;21(3-4):167-178.

51. Van Dongen HP, Rogers NL, Dinges DF. Sleep debt: Theoretical and empirical issues. *Sleep Biol Rhythms*. 2003;1(1):5-13.

52. Belenky G, Wesensten NJ, Thorne DR, et al. Patterns of performance degradation and restoration during sleep restriction and subsequent recovery: A sleep dose-response study. *J Sleep Res*. 2003;12(1):1-12.

53. National Sleep Foundation. *Sleep in America poll*. Washington, DC: National Sleep Foundation; 2008.

54. Dinges DF, Pack F, Williams K, et al. Cumulative sleepiness, mood disturbance, and psychomotor vigilance performance decrements during a week of sleep restricted to 4-5 hours per night. *Sleep*. 1997;20(4):267-277.

55. Balkin TJ, Badia P. Relationship between sleep inertia and sleepiness: Cumulative effects of our nights of sleep disruption/restriction on performance following abrupt nocturnal awakenings. *Biol Psychol*. 1988;27(3):245-258.

56. Jewett ME, Wyatt JK, Ritz-De Cecco A, et al. Time course of sleep inertia dissipation in human performance and alertness. *J Sleep Res*. 1999;8(1):1-8.

57. Achermann P, Werth E, Dijk DJ, et al. Time course of sleep inertia after nighttime and daytime sleep episodes. *Arch Ital Biol*. 1995;134(1):109-119.

58. Wertz AT, Ronda JM, Czeisler CA, et al. Effects of sleep inertia on cognition. *JAMA*. 2006;295(2):163-164.

59. Scheer FAJL, Shea TJ, Hilton MF, et al. An endogenous circadian rhythm in sleep inertia results in greatest cognitive impairment upon awakening during the biological night. *J Biol Rhythms*. 2008;23(4):353-361.

60. Hofer-Tinguely G, Achermann P, Landolt HP, et al. Sleep inertia: Performance changes after sleep, rest and active waking. *Brain Res Cogn Brain Res*. 2005;22(3):323-331.

61. Australian Bureau of Statistics. *Work-related injuries*. Sydney: Australian Bureau of Statistics; 2006.

62. Rajaratnam SMW, Arendt J. Health in a 24-h society. *Lancet*. 2001;358(9286):999-1005.

63. Åkerstedt T. Sleepiness and circadian rhythm sleep disorders. *Sleep Med Clin*. 2006;1(1):17-30.

64. Folkard S, Lombardi DA. Modeling the impact of the components of long work hours on injuries and "accidents." *Am J Ind Med*. 2006;49(11):953-963.

65. Morris TL, Miller JC. Electrooculographic and performance indices of fatigue during simulated flight. *Biol Psychol*. 1996;42(3):343-360.

66. Härmä M, Sallinen M, Ranta R, et al. The effect of an irregular shift system on sleepiness at work in train drivers and railway traffic controllers. *J Sleep Res*. 2002;11:141-151.

67. Elliott DL, Kuehl KS. *Effects of sleep deprivation on fire fighters and EMS responders*. Fairfax, VA: International Association of Fire Chiefs (IAFC) and the United States Fire Administration (USFA); 2007.

68. Neylan TC, Metzler TJ, Henn-Haase C, et al. Prior night sleep duration is associated with psychomotor vigilance in a healthy sample of police academy recruits. *Chronobiol Int*. 2010;27(7):1493-1508.

69. Charles LE, Burchfiel CM, Fekedulegn D, et al. Shift work and sleep: The Buffalo police health study. *Policing: Int J Police Strategies Management*. 2007;30(2):215-227.

70. Garbarino S, Nobili L, Beelke M, et al. Sleep disorders and daytime sleepiness in state police shiftworkers. *Arch Environ Health*. 2002;57(2):167-173.

71. Neylan TC, Metzler TJ, Best SR, et al. Critical incident exposure and sleep quality in police officers. *Psychosom Med*. 2002;64:345-352.

72. Garbarino S, De Carli F, Nobili L, et al. Sleepiness and sleep disorders in shift workers: A study on a group of Italian police officers. *Sleep*. 2002;25(6):642-647.

73. Vila B, Kennedy DJ. Tired cops: The prevalence and potential consequences of police fatigue. *Natl Inst Justice J*. 2002;248:16-21.

74. Rothschild JM, Landrigan CP, Cronin JW, et al. The Critical Care Safety Study: The incidence and nature of adverse events and serious medical errors in intensive care. *Crit Care Med*. 2005;33(8):1694-1700.

75. Rogers AE, Hwang WT, Scott LD, et al. The working hours of hospital staff nurses and patient safety. *Health Aff (Millwood)*. 2004;23(4):202-212.

76. Barger LK, Ayas NT, Cade BE, et al. Impact of extended-duration shifts on medical errors, adverse events, and attentional failures. *PLoS Med*. 2006;3(12):2440-2448.

77. Lockley SW, Cronin JW, Evans EE, et al. Effect of reducing interns' weekly work hours on sleep and attentional failures. *N Engl J Med*. 2004;351(18):1829-1837.

78. Bartel P, Offermeier W, Smith F, et al. Attention and working memory in resident anaesthetists after night duty: Group and individual effects. *Occup Environ Med*. 2004;61(2):167-170.

79. Philibert I. Sleep loss and performance in residents and nonphysicians: A meta-analytic examination. *Sleep*. 2005;28(11):1392-1402.

80. Ayas NT, Barger LK, Cade BE, et al. Extended work duration and the risk of self-reported percutaneous injuries in interns. *JAMA*. 2006;296(9):1055-1062.

81. Rothschild JM, Hurley AC, Landrigan CP, et al. Recovery from medical errors: The critical care nursing safety net. *Jt Comm J Qual Patient Saf*. 2006;32(2):63-72.

82. Landrigan CP, Rothschild JM, Cronin JW, et al. Effect of reducing interns' work hours on serious medical errors in intensive care units. *N Engl J Med*. 2004;351(18):1838-1848.

83. Green-McKenzie J, Shofer FS. Duration of time on shift before accidental blood or body fluid exposure for housestaff, nurses, and technicians. *Infect Control Hosp Epidemiol*. 2007;28(1):5-9.

84. RoadFacts Austroads. *2005: An overview of the Australian and New Zealand road systems*. Sydney: Austroads Inc; 2005.

85. Australian Transport Safety Bureau. Fatigue-related crashes: An analysis of fatigue-related crashes on Australian roads using an operational definition of fatigue. In *Road Safety Research Report*. Canberra, Australia: Commonwealth Department of Transport and Regional Services; 2002:1-30.

86. Teff BC. *Asleep at the wheel: The prevalence and impact of drowsy driving*. Washington, DC: AAA Foundation for Traffic Safety; 2010.

87. Lyznicki JM, Doege TC, Davis RM, et al. Sleepiness, driving, and motor vehicle crashes. *JAMA*. 1998;279(23):1908-1913.

88. Akerstedt T, Czeisler CA, Dinges DF, et al. Accidents and sleepiness: A consensus statement from the International Conference on Work Hours, Sleepiness and Accidents, Stockholm, 8-10 Sept 1994. *J Sleep Res*. 1994;3(4):195.

89. Crummy F, Cameron PA, Swann P, et al. Prevalence of sleepiness in surviving drivers of motor vehicle collisions. *Intern Med J*. 2008;38(10):769-775.

90. Akerstedt T, Peters B, Anund A, et al. Impaired alertness and performance driving home from the night shift: A driving simulator study. *J Sleep Res*. 2005;14(1):17-20.

91. Stutts JC, Wilkins JW, Osberg SJ, et al. Driver risk factors for sleep-related crashes. *Accid Anal Prev*. 2003;35(3):321-331.

92. Barger LK, Cade BE, Ayas NT, et al. Extended work shifts and the risk of motor vehicle crashes among interns. *N Engl J Med*. 2005;352(2):125-134.

93. Lenne MG, Triggs TJ, Redman JR. Time of day variations in driving performance. *Accid Anal Prev*. 1997;29(4):431-437.

94. Horne JA, Reyner LA. Sleep related vehicle accidents. *BMJ*. 1995;310(6979):565-567.

95. Horne JA, Reyner LA. Vehicle accidents related to sleep: A review. *Occup Environ Med*. 1999;56(5):289-294.

96. Leger D. The cost of sleep-related accidents: A report for the National Commission on Sleep Disorders Research. *Sleep*. 1994;17(1):84-93.

97. Maycock G. Sleepiness and driving: The experience of U.K. car drivers. *Accid Anal Prev*. 1997;29(4):453-462.

98. Reyner LA, Horne JA. Falling asleep whilst driving: Are drivers aware of prior sleepiness? *Int J Legal Med*. 1998;111(3):120-123.

99. Di Milia L. Shift work, sleepiness and long distance driving. Part F: Traffic Psychology and Behaviour. *Transportation Res.*. 2006;9(4):278-285.

100. Cummings P, Koepsell TD, Moffat JM, et al. Drowsiness, countermeasures to drowsiness, and the risk of a motor vehicle crash. *Inj Prev*. 2001;7(3):194-199.

101. Arnedt JT, Wilde GJ, Munt PW, et al. Simulated driving performance following prolonged wakefulness and alcohol consumption: Separate and combined contributions to impairment. *J Sleep Res.*. 2000;9(3):233-241.

102. Philip P, Sagaspe P, Moore N, et al. Fatigue, sleep restriction and driving performance. *Accid Anal Prev*. 2005;37(3):473-478.

103. Nilsson T, Nelson TM, Carlson D. Development of fatigue symptoms during simulated driving. *Accid Anal Prev.* 1997;29(4):479-488.

104. Anund A, Kecklund G, Kircher A, et al. The effects of driving situation on sleepiness indicators after sleep loss: A driving simulator study. *Ind Health.* 2009;47(4):393-401.

105. Phipps-Nelson J, Redman JR, Schlangen LJM, et al. Blue light exposure reduces objective measures of sleepiness during prolonged nighttime performance testing. *Chronobiol Int.* 2009;26(5):891-912.

106. Spurgeon A, Harrington JM, Cooper CL. Health and safety problems associated with long working hours: A review of the current position. *Occup Environ Med.* 1997;54(6):367-375.

107. Puttonen S, Kivimäki M, Elovainio M, et al. Shift work in young adults and carotid artery intima-media thickness: The Cardiovascular Risk in Young Finns study. *Atherosclerosis.* 2009;205(2):608-613.

108. Ruggiero JS. Correlates of fatigue in critical care nurses. *Res Nurs Health.* 2003;26(6):434-444.

109. Suzuki K, Ohida T, Kaneita Y, et al. Mental health status, shift work, and occupational accidents among hospital nurses in Japan. *J Occup Health.* 2004;46(6):448-454.

110. Bara AC, Arber S. Working shifts and mental health-Findings from the British Household Panel Survey (1995-2005). *Scand J Work Environ Health.* 2009;35(5):361-367.

111. Angersbach D, Knauth P, Loskant H, et al. A retrospective cohort study comparing complaints and diseases in day and shift workers. *Int Arch Occup Environ Health.* 1980;45(2):127-140.

112. Knutsson A, Bøggild H. Gastrointestinal disorders among shift workers. *Scand J Work Environ Health.* 2010;36(2):85-95.

113. Kawachi I, Colditz GA, Stampfer MJ, et al. Prospective study of shift work and risk of coronary heart disease in women. *Circulation.* 1995;92(11):3178-3182.

114. Scheer FAJL, Hilton MF, Mantzoros CS, et al. Adverse metabolic and cardiovascular consequences of circadian misalignment. *Proc Natl Acad Sci U S A.* 2009;106(11):4453-4458.

115. Kroenke CH, Spiegelman D, Manson J, et al. Work characteristics and incidence of type 2 diabetes in women. *Am J Epidemiol.* 2007;165(2):175-183.

116. Morikawa Y, Nakagawa H, Miura K, et al. Effect of shift work on body mass index and metabolic parameters. *Scand J Work Environ Health.* 2007;33(1):45-50.

117. Suwazono Y, Dochi M, Sakata K, et al. A longitudinal study on the effect of shift work on weight gain in male Japanese workers. *Obesity.* 2008;16(8):1887-1893.

118. Knutsson A, Hallquist J, Reuterwall C, et al. Shiftwork and myocardial infarction: A case-control study. *Occup Environ Med.* 1999;56(1):46-50.

119. Ito H, Nozaki M, Maruyama T, et al. Shift work modifies the circadian patterns of heart rate variability in nurses. *Int J Cardiol.* 2001;79(2-3):231-236.

120. Knutsson A, Akerstedt T, Jonsson BG, et al. Increased risk of ischemic-heart-disease in shift workers. *Lancet.* 1986;2(8498):89-91.

121. Miller MA, Cappuccio FP. Sleep, inflammation, and disease. In: Cappuccio FP, Miller MA, Lockley SW, eds. *Sleep, Health and Society.* Oxford, England: Oxford University Press; 2010.

122. Spiegel K, Leproult R, Van Cauter E. Impact of sleep debt on metabolic and endocrine function. *Lancet.* 1999;354(9188):1435-1439.

123. Knutson KL, Spiegel K, Penev P, et al. The metabolic consequences of sleep deprivation. *Sleep Med Rev.* 2007;11(3):163-178.

124. Muller JE, Stone PH, Turi ZG, et al. Circadian variation in the frequency of onset of acute myocardial infarction. *N Engl J Med.* 1985;313(21):1315-1322.

125. Ribeiro DCO, Hampton SM, Morgan L, et al. Altered postprandial hormone and metabolic responses in a simulated shift work environment. *J Endocrinol.* 1998;158(3):305-310.

126. Hampton SM, Morgan LM, Lawrence N, et al. Postprandial hormone and metabolic responses in simulated shift work. *J Endocrinol.* 1996;151(2):259-267.

127. Kales A, Bixler EO, Cadieux RJ. Sleep apnoea in a hypertensive population. *Lancet.* 1984;2(8410):1005-1008.

128. Straif K, Baan R, Grosse Y, et al. Carcinogenicity of shift-work, painting, and fire-fighting. *Lancet Oncol.* 2007;8(12):1065-1066.

129. Davis S, Mirick DK. Circadian disruption, shift work and the risk of cancer: A summary of the evidence and studies in Seattle. *Cancer Causes Control.* 2006;17(4):539-545.

130. Pesch B, Harth V, Rabstein S, et al. Night work and breast cancer—Results from the German GENICA study. *Scand J Work Environ Health.* 2010;36(2):134-141.

131. Stevens RG, Blask DE, Brainard GC, et al. Meeting report: The role of environmental lighting and circadian disruption in cancer and other diseases. *Environ Health Perspect.* 2007;115(9):1357-1362.

132. Filipski E, Subramanian P, Carrière J, et al. Circadian disruption accelerates liver carcinogenesis in mice. *Mutation Res Genetic Toxicol Environmental Mutagenesis.* 2009;680(1-2):95-105.

133. Davis S, Mirick DK, Stevens RG. Night shift work, light at night, and risk of breast cancer. *J Natl Cancer Inst.* 2001;93(20):1557-1562.

134. Sack RL, Auckley D, Auger RR, et al. Circadian rhythm sleep disorders: Part I, basic principles, shift work and jet lag disorders: An American Academy of Sleep Medicine review. *Sleep.* 2007;30(11):1460-1483.

135. Czeisler CA, Walsh JK, Roth T, et al. Modafinil for excessive sleepiness associated with shift-work sleep disorder. *N Engl J Med.* 2005;353(5):476-486.

136. Erman MK, Rosenberg R. Modafinil for excessive sleepiness associated with chronic shift work sleep disorder: Effects on patient functioning and health-related quality of life. *Primary Care Companion J Clin Psychiatry.* 2007;9(3):188-194.

137. Kumar R. Approved and investigational uses of modafinil: An evidence-based review. *Drugs.* 2008;68(13):1803-1839.

138. Ballon JS, Feifel D. A systematic review of modafinil: Potential clinical uses and mechanisms of action. *J Clin Psychiatry.* 2006;67(4):554-566.

139. Scammell TE, Estabrooke IV, McCarthy MT, et al. Hypothalamic arousal regions are activated during modafinil-induced wakefulness. *J Neurosci.* 2000;20(22):8620-8628.

140. Lin JS, Hou Y, Jouvet M. Potential brain neuronal targets for amphetamine-, methylphenidate-, and modafinil-induced wakefulness, evidenced by c-fos immunocytochemistry in the cat. *Proc Natl Acad Sci U S A.* 1996;93(24):14128-14133.

141. Lin JS, Roussel B, Akaoka H, et al. Role of catecholamines in the modafinil and amphetamine induced wakefulness, a comparative pharmacological study in the cat. *Brain Res.* 1992;591(2):319-326.

142. Czeisler CA, Allan JS, Strogatz SH. Bright light resets the human circadian pacemaker independent of the timing of the sleep-wake cycle. *Science.* 1986;233(4764):667-671.

143. Dawson D, Campbell SS. Timed exposure to bright light improves sleep and alertness during simulated night shifts. *Sleep.* 1991;14(6):511-516.

144. Zeitzer JM, Dijk DJ, Kronauer R, et al. Sensitivity of the human circadian pacemaker to nocturnal light: Melatonin phase resetting and suppression. *J Physiol.* 2000;526(Pt 3):695-702.

145. Santhi N, Duffy JF, Horowitz TS, et al. Scheduling of sleep/darkness affects the circadian phase of night shift workers. *Neurosci Lett.* 2005;384(3):316-320.

146. Arendt J, Rajaratnam SMW. Melatonin and its agonists: An update. *Br J Psychiatry.* 2008;193(4):267-269.

147. Wyatt JK, Dijk DJ, Ritz-de Cecco A, et al. Sleep-facilitating effect of exogenous melatonin in healthy young men and women is circadian-phase dependent. *Sleep.* 2006;29(5):609-618.

148. Sack RL, Hughes RJ, Edgar DM, et al. Sleep-promoting effects of melatonin: At what dose, in whom, under what conditions, and by what mechanisms? *Sleep.* 1997;20(10):908-915.

149. Sharkey KM, Fogg LF, Eastman CI. Effects of melatonin administration on daytime sleep after simulated night shift work. *J Sleep Res.* 2001;10(3):181-192.

150. Sharkey KM, Eastman CI. Melatonin phase shifts human circadian rhythms in a placebo-controlled simulated night-work study. *Am J Physiol Regul Integr Comp Physiol.* 2002;282:R454-R463.

151. Folkard S, Arendt J, Clark M. Can melatonin improve shift workers' tolerance of the night shift? Some preliminary findings. *Chronobiol Int.* 1993;10(5):315-320.

152. Burgess HJ, Revell VL, Molina TA, et al. Human phase response curves to three days of daily melatonin: 0.5 mg versus 3.0 mg. *J Clin Endocrinol Metab.* 2010;95(7):3325-3331.

153. Lewy AJ, Ahmed S, Jackson JM, et al. Melatonin shifts human circadian rhythms according to a phase-response curve. *Chronobiol Int.* 1992;9(5):380-392.

154. Dawson D, Encel N, Lushington K. Improving adaptation to simulated night shift: Timed exposure to bright light versus daytime melatonin administration. *Sleep.* 1995;18(1):11-21.

155. Sallinen M, Härmä M, Åkerstedt T, et al. Promoting alertness with a short nap during a night shift. *J Sleep Res.* 1998;7(4):240-247.

156. Bonnefond A, Muzet A, Winter-Dill AS, et al. Innovative working schedule: Introducing one short nap during the night shift. *Ergonomics.* 2001;44(10):937-945.

157. Purnell MT, Feyer AM, Herbison GP. The impact of a nap opportunity during the night shift on the performance and alertness of 12-h shift workers. *J Sleep Res*. 2002;11(3):219-227.

158. Muzet A, Nicolas A, Tassi P, et al. Implementation of napping in industry and the problem of sleep inertia. *J Sleep Res*. 1995;4(S2):67-69.

159. Kubo T, Takahashi M, Takeyama H, et al. How do the timing and length of a night-shift nap affect sleep inertia? *Chronobiol Int*. 2010;27(5): 1031-1044.

160. Brooks A, Lack L. A brief afternoon nap following nocturnal sleep restriction: Which nap duration is most recuperative? *Sleep*. 2006;29(6): 831-840.

161. Schweitzer PK, Randazzo AC, Stone K, et al. Laboratory and field studies of naps and caffeine as practical countermeasures for sleep-wake problems associated with night work. *Sleep*. 2006;29(1):39-50.

162. Muehlbach MJ, Walsh JK. The effects of caffeine on simulated night-shift work and subsequent daytime sleep. *Sleep*. 1995;18(1):22-29.

163. Walsh JK, Muehlbach MJ, Humm TM, et al. Effect of caffeine on physiological sleep tendency and ability to sustain wakefulness at night. *Psychopharmacology (Berl)*. 1990;101(2):271-273.

Chapter 30

Jet Lag and Its Prevention

VICTORIA L. REVELL / CHARMANE I. EASTMAN

DEFINING JET LAG AND ITS RISKS

In the days following a flight across several time zones our sleep patterns, level of alertness, and general state of well-being are frequently in disarray. The assortment of symptoms that we experience is known collectively as *jet lag* and this syndrome occurs because the circadian clock, which drives daily rhythms in virtually all aspects of physiology and behavior, cannot be instantaneously set to the new time zone. The rate at which the clock resets to local time, and accordingly our sleep and functioning normalize, is dependent upon a number of parameters including the direction of the flight, the number of time zones crossed, and the light exposure experienced before and upon arrival. When flying long distances north and south there may be travel fatigue from long flights and sleep deprivation, but individuals usually recover from this within a day or two. Jet lag occurs only when crossing time zones (eastward and westward travel) (Box 30-1) and lasts much longer, although travel fatigue may also accompany flights east and west. This chapter will review the causes of jet lag, situations that can prolong its occurrence, and methods to minimize or even avoid it entirely. Diagnostic criteria according to the American Academy of Sleep Medicine[1] are listed in Box 30-1.

Jet lag is caused by a self-imposed misalignment between the circadian clock and desired sleep/wake schedule. The resulting constellation of symptoms experienced will gradually dissipate as the clock becomes aligned with the local sleep/wake (dark/light) cycle. Perhaps the most prevalent and debilitating symptom of jet lag is the disruption to sleep, including sleep onset insomnia (inability to fall asleep when required) and sleep maintenance insomnia (waking earlier than desired) along with the problem that the sleep that is obtained is often of poor quality and short duration. In addition, during waking hours the traveler will often feel sleepy, not alert, and unable to perform cognitive or manual tasks; these decrements result from accumulated fatigue, due to the lack of sufficient nocturnal sleep, and frequently because the misaligned circadian clock may be at its lowest point for driving alertness during the daytime. The quality, timing, and duration of our sleep is determined by an interaction between the circadian clock and the sleep homeostat, which builds up with time awake and dissipates with sleep.[2] Thus, if the clock is not correctly aligned with local time, it will promote wake and sleep at inappropriate social times. An estimate of when jet lag will be entirely dissipated is when the minimum of the core body temperature rhythm (Tmin), the sleepiest time of day and a marker of the circadian clock, once again coincides with the major sleep episode, as this will usually ensure that sleep is of sufficient duration and quality, and that alertness will be maximal during the local daytime.

In addition to disruptions to sleep and daytime functioning, many travelers will also suffer gastrointestinal distress in the days following a flight, which some call "gut lag." It is now well established that a master circadian clock is situated in the brain, in the suprachiasmatic nuclei (SCN) of the hypothalamus, and drives rhythmic events in the body.[3] However, it appears that there are in fact clocks in every cell in the body, with peripheral clocks in all organs and tissues.[4,5] The SCN are necessary for the appropriate synchronization of all these local clocks to the external day as well as to each other.[6] Thus, upon arrival in a new time zone many of the physiologic disruptions observed will be attributable to disorganization between clocks in different organs and tissues as they resynchronize at different rates. In mice, following a 6-hour phase advance, even though the SCN appeared to be resynchronized by day 3, the peripheral tissues (thymus, lung, spleen, esophagus) adjusted at very different rates and were not all correctly synchronized until day 8.[7] This internal dissociation was first observed many years ago, and Aschoff and associates[8] reviewed the many examples of different rhythmic variables re-entraining at different rates in animals and in humans in laboratory experiments and after jet flights.

The occurrence and duration of jet lag has a number of implications for health. Repeated circadian misalignment, as would be experienced by pilots and cabin crew on long haul flights, has been associated with menstrual disturbance, temporal lobe atrophy, cognitive defects, and increased risk of cancer, cardiovascular disease, and diabetes.[9-12] Indeed, in mice, chronic jet lag (10 days of shifting 8 hours earlier every 2 days) accelerated the growth and progression of tumors.[13] The serious repercussions of jet lag were highlighted in another study in mice which either experienced no change in schedule or were shifted 6 hours earlier or 6 hours later, simulating crossing six time zones east or west, respectively, once a week for 8 weeks.[14] The survival of aged mice was significantly affected by these schedules; after 8 weeks only 47% of animals shifted eastward had survived compared to 68% shifted westward and 83% in the unchanged group. The rate of death was increased when the schedule was shifted every 4 days instead of every 7 days.

In addition to disruptions of circadian rhythms being detrimental to health, the short sleep episodes associated with jet lag could also have health implications. Chronic sleep restriction (4 hours per night for 6 nights) has been shown to impair glucose tolerance, with a reduced glucose clearance rate, lowered acute insulin response, and diminished thyrotropin levels.[15] Moreover, after only 2 days of sleeping 4 hours per night there is an elevation of ghrelin (appetite stimulating hormone) and reduction of leptin (satiety hormone).[16] These altered metabolic responses and the potential increased food intake are all risk factors for the development of obesity, diabetes, and the metabolic syndrome.

LIGHT AND MELATONIN PHASE RESPONSE CURVES

To understand how and why the circadian clock adapts, or does not, to a new time zone it is essential to appreciate the influence of exogenous stimuli. The circadian clock does not run at exactly 24 hours, but either slightly more or slightly less, and therefore to remain appropriately synchronized or entrained to the 24-hour day, the clock requires a daily adjustment. This adjustment is achieved by exposure to daily environmental stimuli that prevent the clock from drifting along at its own internal circadian period (or tau) and maintain it on a 24-hour rhythm. Depending on the individual circadian period or the direction of shift required, external environmental signals must be able to both advance and delay the clock, depending on the time of day of the exposure. The relationship between the timing of a stimulus and the magnitude and direction (earlier or later) of the phase shift (change in timing) can be illustrated with a phase response curve (PRC). A shift to an earlier time is termed a phase advance, whereas a shift to a later time is a phase delay. On average, the endogenous human clock runs at slightly longer than 24 hours[17-19] and therefore requires a daily phase advance to remain synchronized to the 24-hour solar day.

The most potent environmental stimulus for synchronizing the clock to the 24-hour day is the light/dark cycle. Nonphotic stimuli, such as exercise and mealtimes, are also able to shift human circadian timing but to a lesser extent,[20] and the most studied nonphotic stimulus is treatment with exogenous melatonin. The hormone melatonin is produced in a circadian fashion by the pineal gland in the brain with low levels during the daytime hours and high levels during the nighttime.[21] The duration of the nocturnal secretion mirrors the duration of the dark phase of the 24-hour day (scotoperiod), which has given melatonin the name "darkness hormone." The robust and reproducible circadian rhythm of melatonin production has led to its widespread use as a marker of the circadian clock both in laboratory and in field-based studies as well as in the clinic. In addition, the ability of light to suppress nocturnal levels of melatonin acutely has been used as a tool to identify the integrity and properties of human nonvisual photoreception.[22-24] Treatment with synthetic melatonin has been demonstrated to have the capacity to phase shift the circadian clock[25-27] and has been successfully used to entrain the clock of nonentrained, totally blind individuals[28,29] (see Chapter 32).

Figure 30-1 represents how light and melatonin can shift the timing of the clock relative to an individual's typical sleep schedule and internal circadian phase. When light is presented before the Tmin, in the late evening and the beginning of sleep under normal conditions, the clock is phase delayed. When light is administered after the Tmin, at the end of sleep or early morning, the clock is phase advanced. Light does not have an equal effect across the phase delay or phase advance region; the optimal time of exposure (maximum phase shift achieved) will depend upon the parameters of the light stimulus such as wavelength, duration, and intensity as well as the protocol used to generate the data. For example, in mice both the amplitude and width of the phase advance and delay regions are influenced by the duration of the light stimulus. As the duration of the light pulse increases from 1 to 9 hours, the width of the "dead zone" (the time in the middle of the day when light has no phase-shifting effect) decreases and the amplitude of the PRC increases.[30]

The timing of the phase advance and delay regions for light shown in Figure 30-1 is based on a preliminary light PRC generated with 2-hour light pulses delivered from small commercially available light boxes.[31] Other light PRCs have also been generated, but these used much longer light pulses (e.g., 6.7 hours) and large lighting fixtures (e.g., ceiling or wall banks).[32,33] Such lighting regimens and equipment would not be feasible in practical schedules designed to reduce or eliminate jet lag. Further, research is needed to generate PRCs to single light boxes using intermittent bright light mimicking the way it is usually received at home.

Figure 30-1 shows that, under conditions of normal entrainment, melatonin treatment in the afternoon/early evening is capable of phase advancing the circadian clock, whereas melatonin at the end of sleep and in the morning induces phase delays. Similar to light, melatonin is not uniformly effective across the advance and delay regions with the optimal administration time being highly dependent on dose. Current estimates for the optimal times for advances are 5 to 9 hours before sleep onset for 3 mg and 5 to 7 hours before sleep onset for 0.5 mg.[27]

FACTORS THAT DETERMINE THE DURATION OF JET LAG

Directional Asymmetry

The number of days that a traveler will experience jet lag is dependent upon a number of factors, including the direction of travel, the number of time zones crossed, and behavior before the flight and upon arrival. The greater the number of time zones crossed, the greater the phase shift that will be required to adapt to local time, and hence, there will be an increased number of days when the clock is misaligned. Human circadian period is on average longer than 24 hours and when left to its own devices in constant conditions, the clock will delay each day. This natural delay is at least one reason why most people generally find it easier to adjust to flying westward, which requires a phase delay for adaptation to the new time zone, and this observation has been called the "asymmetry effect."[8] In a survey of 507 business travelers, 49%

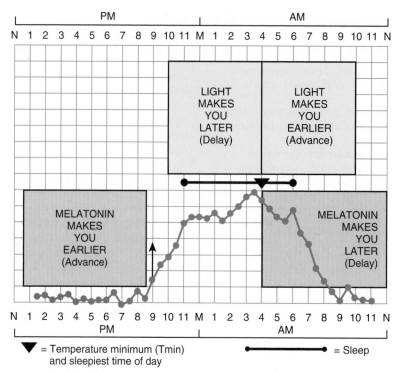

▼ = Temperature minimum (Tmin)
and sleepiest time of day

●———● = Sleep

Figure 30-1 The phase-shifting effect of light and melatonin on the human circadian clock. These diagrams represent simplified versions of phase response curves (PRCs). The horizontal line with circles on each end indicates a typical sleep schedule for an individual (11 PM to 6 AM). The triangle represents the temperature minimum (Tmin), which is the sleepiest time of day, a marker of the timing of the circadian clock, and an approximate indicator of the transition from when light causes phase delays to advances. A typical endogenous melatonin profile is superimposed (blue line with points every half hour). The onset of nocturnal melatonin production (as indicated by the upward arrow) occurs approximately 2 to 3 hours before the start of sleep time.
The blue boxes indicate time periods when light has the largest phase shifting effects. Light at other times has much less of an effect. There is no dramatic change at the borders of the boxes, but rather a gradual change. The width of the boxes will depend on the intensity and duration of light exposure and on other details of the procedure such as whether the sleep/dark period is shifted, which contributes to the phase shift of the clock. These boxes were drawn based on estimates of phase shifts that can be expected from relatively short durations of exposure using a single light box at home.[31] The gray boxes indicate the time periods when exogenous melatonin has the largest phase-shifting effects. Again, the boxes show when melatonin is most likely to produce a phase shift, but there is no dramatic drop-off at the borders. The width and placement of the boxes depends on the dose. These boxes encompass the times that phase shifts are most likely for two popular doses of melatonin, 0.5 or 3.0 mg.[26,27]

reported fatigue during their trips, and of these, fatigue was an important factor for 25% on westward flights and for 59% for eastward flights,[34] re-enforcing the asymmetry associated with the direction of shift. The time of arrival of the flight will also be key in determining the duration of jet lag as it will strongly influence the timing and type of light exposure received upon arrival as well as the timing and type of behavior (e.g., sleep or stay awake), which will further influence light/dark exposure patterns and affect the direction and rate of adaptation.

Effects of Age

It should be noted that the age of the traveler may also have an impact on the severity of jet lag. It has been demonstrated that older people are less phase tolerant and find it more difficult to sleep at the "wrong" circadian phase,[35] meaning that during the days following a flight an older individual could obtain less sleep than a younger traveler. In contrast, however, it has been shown that older individuals exhibit less sleepiness, performance decrements, and unintentional sleep episodes than younger individuals when staying awake all night.[36] Thus, older people may be less tolerant at sleeping at the wrong circadian phase but more tolerant for being awake at the wrong circadian phase. So far, laboratory studies on the rate the circadian clock phase-shifts with or without artificial bright

light have found only minor differences between young, middle–aged, and older people.[37-39] More research is therefore needed to study jet lag and aging.

FLYING EAST ACROSS SEVERAL TIME ZONES:

We will now consider six individuals who fly from Los Angeles (LA) to London (eight time zones east). Their home sleep schedule, their preflight and postflight behavior, and the timing of the flight will all contribute to the severity and duration of their jet lag symptoms. Although flights from LA to London are used as examples, the general principles will apply to any flight east across several time zones, and the last example (see Fig. 30-8 later in chapter) will also apply to flying west.

THREE EXAMPLES OF JET LAG

The Circadian Clock Advances After Landing

Nicole's flight is shown in Figure 30-2. While in London, she wants to maintain the same sleep schedule that she has at home (11 PM to 6 AM). To phase advance her clock upon arrival, she exposes herself to outdoor light in the estimated phase advance region of her PRC (after estimated Tmin) while remaining indoors in dim light during her phase delay region

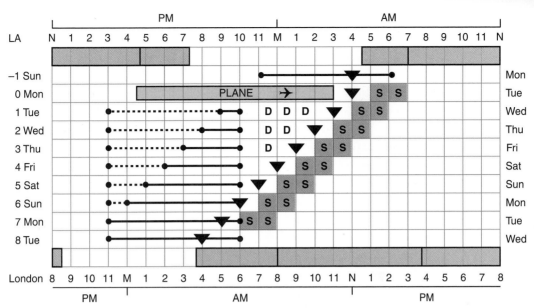

Figure 30-2 Nicole takes a flight from Los Angeles to London, eight time zones east. The line at the top shows the time in Los Angeles (from noon [N] to noon with midnight [M] in the middle), and the time line on the bottom shows the equivalent time in London (8 hours ahead). The rectangle on day 0 shows the time of the flight, which leaves on Monday afternoon LA time and lands on Tuesday morning London time. Note that the day of the week listed on the right side of each row is 1 day later than on the left because the day changes at midnight. The blue horizontal bars show the maximum duration of the photoperiod (light portion of the day) at the summer solstice, and the vertical lines within the bars show the minimum duration of the photoperiod at the winter solstice. This schedule shows what might happen to Nicole, who usually sleeps from 11 PM to 6 AM and maintains the same schedule while in London. Times in bed are represented by the horizontal lines and dots. The triangles represent the temperature minima (Tmin). The goal is for the Tmin to occur within the sleep period, as this will permit a consolidated bout of good quality sleep of sufficient duration, and move the sleepiest time of day out of the waking portion of the day. Nicole does not do any preparation to avoid jet lag until after landing in London. On arrival, however, she is careful to get the ideal light exposure pattern to help phase advance her circadian clock to London time according to the light phase response curve (PRC), as described in Figure 30-1. She gets bright light after her Tmin by going outside, and avoids bright light before her Tmin by staying indoors. S indicates outdoor sunlight exposure and Ds indicate times to stay indoors and avoid bright light or, if it is necessary to go out, to wear very dark sunglasses. Nicole's circadian clock phase advances by 1 hour per day (orthodromic re-entrainment shown by the triangles). This is the classic average for phase shifts after eastward flights calculated by Aschoff and associates.[8] The dotted lines show when poor sleep is expected because the time in bed is so far from the Tmin. Nicole has sleep onset insomnia, which gradually improves as her Tmin gets closer to her time in bed. Regardless of how much sleep she obtains at night, however, she will be sleepy during the day, especially in the hours around her Tmin, the sleepiest time of day. Her Tmin falls within the sleep episode by day 7, and by then she should be over her jet lag. Despite her best efforts, jet lag due to circadian misalignment is pronounced during the first few days after landing, and she will experience sleepiness, especially in the mornings, and insomnia at night.

(before estimated Tmin). For the first 5 days in London, she will struggle to fall asleep at 11 PM, as this time is too far away from her Tmin, and on days 4 to 6 she will struggle to wake up in the mornings as her wakeup time is too close to the Tmin. By day 7 her Tmin is occurring in her desired sleep period and she should have a good, consolidated night of sleep. If she does not sleep on the plane, she may be able to sleep on the first night in London because of increased sleep pressure due to sleep deprivation but would experience difficulty sleeping the next night. While Nicole's clock is adapting, her daytime functioning and alertness will be significantly impaired because of the accumulated fatigue from sleeping so little at night plus having the circadian peak for sleepiness (equivalent to Tmin) occurring during the day. Although her clock is shifting in the correct phase advance direction to adapt to an eastward flight (orthodromic re-entrainment), previous studies indicate that only an average phase advance of approximately 1 hour per day would be achieved.[8] If factors such as inclement weather or scheduled indoor events interfere with the planned light/dark schedule, then the phase advances might average less than 1 hour per day, making adaptation even slower.

More research is needed to assess both circadian phase and light exposure before and after real flights. There are several computer programs and commercial devices that attempt

to tell the traveler when to seek and when to avoid outdoor light to help reduce jet lag. Most of them assume phase shifts greater than 1 hour per day, however,[40] and overestimation of the shift achieved may lead to light being timed inadvertently during the phase delay part of the PRC, reversing the therapeutic effect.

The Circadian Clock Delays After Landing

Clyde's flight is scheduled for earlier in the day such that he arrives in London very early in the morning (Fig. 30-3). This means that when he lands, he will be exposed to light before his Tmin, causing a phase delay, the opposite of that required, rather than a phase advance; such adaptation in the wrong direction is known as antidromic re-entrainment. Phase shifting in the "wrong" direction can prolong the duration and severity of jet lag, as it did for Clyde (see Fig. 30-3) compared to Nicole (see Fig. 30-2). Because transcontinental flights often arrive early in the morning, bright light may be experienced for several hours before the Tmin and promote delays. Unfortunately, many review papers and websites advise travelers to seek outdoor light in the morning in the new time zone after flying east, which can be the wrong advice, depending on the time of arrival, as illustrated in Figure 30-3. In a study of

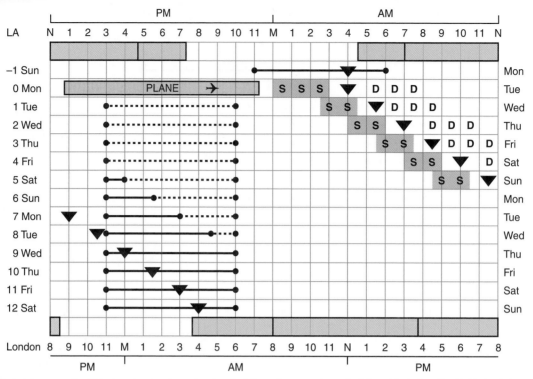

Figure 30-3 Clyde takes an earlier flight from Los Angeles to London. He follows the same sleep schedule as Nicole (see Fig. 30-2). Symbols are the same as in Figure 30-2. Upon landing he is exposed to bright outdoor light before his Tmin (▼) and is not exposed to bright light after his Tmin. This pattern continues for several days and makes his circadian clock phase shift in the wrong direction; it delays instead of advancing (antidromic reentrainment shown by the triangles). It delays by 1.5 hours per day, which is the classic average for phase delay shifts after flights calculated by Aschoff and associates.[8] He has severe insomnia for the first few days, which changes into sleep maintenance insomnia (waking early and being unable to fall back asleep) and finally better sleep as his Tmin gets closer to his time in bed. He will be completely adapted by about day 9.

people flying from Tokyo, one out of six individuals arriving in LA (eight time zones east) and seven out of eight individuals arriving in New York (11 time zones east) demonstrated antidromic re-entrainment as assessed by their plasma melatonin rhythm.[41,42] This illustrates the principle that the more time zones crossed when flying east, the more likely that antidromic re-entrainment will occur. In fact, if many time zones are being crossed, then it may be quicker to adapt via antidromic re-entrainment as, following a flight, a daily phase advance of 1 hour per day is expected compared to a delay of 1.5 hours per day[8] if no additional intervention is performed. Theoretically, an eastward flight of 11 time zones is equivalent to a westward flight across 13 time zones, and therefore, orthodromic re-entrainment would be completed in 11 days (1 hour advance per day) compared to antidromic re-entrainment, which would be completed after 8.7 days (1.5 hours delay per day). The study from Tokyo to NY found an average phase delay of 65 minutes per day when endogenous melatonin was sampled at baseline and on the fifth day in NY,[42] which is less than the classic 1.5 hours per day estimate given by Aschoff and associates.[8]

The Circadian Clock Gets Stuck After Landing

Rodney takes the same flight as Clyde but his erratic light exposure, sometimes before and sometimes after Tmin, means that his clock cannot adapt to the new time zone (Fig. 30-4). The clock is advanced on some days and delayed on others so that overall he remains adapted to home time. Although this "zigzag" pattern is theoretical and has not been documented, lack of adaptation has been observed; the melatonin rhythm

of an individual traveling from Tokyo to LA (eight time zones east) remained entrained to Tokyo time 5 days after arriving in LA.[41] In addition, a laboratory study demonstrated that bright light at inappropriate times can prevent the clock from shifting even after the sleep/dark period was shifted 9 hours for several days.[43] Figure 30-4 is included to reinforce the idea that the rates of phase advances and phase delays predicted in Figures 30-2 and 30-3 could easily be attenuated by outdoor light exposure.

Rodney (see Fig. 30-4) will suffer from nighttime insomnia, as his sleep occurs too far from Tmin, and daytime sleepiness throughout his trip. He will get some sleep at night due to a buildup of homeostatic pressure through the day, but this sleep will not be of good quality or sufficient duration. Upon return home he should not suffer greatly from jet lag because his circadian system has remained on home time, although he will probably be exhausted from days of chronic sleep deprivation.

THREE APPROACHES TO ELIMINATE OR REDUCE JET LAG

Advancing the Circadian Clock Before the Flight

Cynthia decides to set her circadian clock to her destination time zone before she flies to minimize the duration and severity of jet lag (Fig. 30-5). When bright light exposure is indicated, intermittent exposure is recommended for convenience (the light pulses can be interspersed with taking showers,

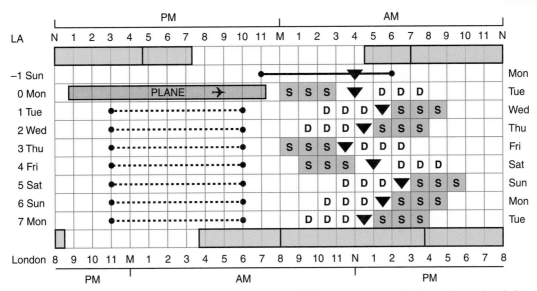

Figure 30-4 Rodney takes the same flight from LA to London as Clyde (see Fig. 30-3) and follows the same sleep schedule, but his circadian clock gets stuck and does not adjust to the new time zone because of his variable light/dark exposure. Bright light first pushes his circadian clock in one direction and then the other. Symbols are the same as in Figure 30-2.

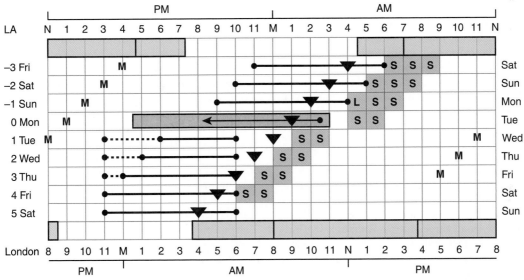

Figure 30-5 Cynthia takes the same flight from LA to London as Nicole in Figure 30-2, but she uses bright light and melatonin at home to help phase advance her circadian clock before the flight. She has the same sleep schedule as Nicole, from 11 PM to 6 AM, but she goes to bed and wakes up 1 hour earlier each day for 2 days before the flight. She takes 3 mg melatonin (M) 7 hours before her usual bedtime on day −3, and then 1 hour earlier each day. She exposes herself to bright light in the morning as soon as she can after she wakes up. She goes outside when she can to get sunlight (S) but uses a light box (L) when her wake time is before sunrise or it is inconvenient to go outside. Sunlight is always preferable to a light box because it is brighter and will be more powerful for shifting the circadian clock. She gets intermittent bright light exposure during the times indicated. By following this regimen her circadian clock advances by about 1 hour per day. On the first day after landing, her Tmin (▼) is much closer to the time for sleep than it was for Nicole (see Fig. 30-2), so she has less circadian misalignment, better sleep, and much lower risk of phase delaying (antidromic re-entrainment). Furthermore, her jet lag is completely eliminated 3 days sooner than Nicole's. If she wanted to completely eliminate jet lag, she could advance her sleep with melatonin and bright light for more than 3 days before the flight. The more days of preparation before the flight, the less jet lag will be experienced after the flight. The left pointing arrow in the flight rectangle means she can go to sleep as early as she wants, which is true for all sleep episodes while on an advancing schedule. In the first few hours after taking melatonin, caution should be observed and driving should be avoided because melatonin induces sleepiness.

getting dressed, making breakfast, etc.). Laboratory studies have show that light duration has a nonlinear relationship with phase resetting capacity such that intermittent light pulses are almost as powerful for producing phase shifts as continuous exposure.[30,44-46] The amount of intermittent bright light that is needed before flight in a schedule such as in Figure 30-5 can be adjusted as needed as the days progress. If Cynthia finds

it difficult to fall asleep or wake up as early as planned, then she should get more morning light the next day. The exact duration and intensity of light that an individual needs to help produce the maximum phase shift cannot be specified because it will depend on the individual's light exposure history, which affects his or her light sensitivity,[47] internal period, shape of the PRC, and perhaps sensitivity to social cues. Anecdotal reports suggest that it is not difficult to fall asleep and wake up earlier when following a pre-flight schedule such as in Fig. 30-5, but that the change in schedule limits social and family activities. This temporary inconvenience needs to be balanced against the importance of reducing jet lag.

For Cynthia, upon landing in London the outdoor light exposure she receives will fall upon the phase advance region of her PRC and continue to advance her clock as desired. On day 1 in London, Cynthia's Tmin is closer to the desired sleep period than it was for Nicole (see Fig. 30-2) and will reduce sleep disruption, and when she wakes, she will continues to be exposed to outdoor light at a time that promotes phase advances. In addition, she can continue to take melatonin in the first few evenings following her arrival (until her sleep normalizes) to advance the clock more rapidly. Her Tmin will fall within sleep by day 3 of her trip and she will experience less jet lag than if she had not started to adapt before the flight. In addition, by preparing herself before she flies, Cynthia is much less likely to receive phase delaying light upon arrival, and therefore, she minimizes her risk of antidromic re-entrainment and prolonged jet lag.

Laboratory Studies of Bright Light and Melatonin for Phase Advancing

A side effect of taking exogenous melatonin, which must be considered in preflight schedules, is induction of sleepiness. There is evidence both for and against exogenous melatonin inducing sleepiness and its soporific influence is likely to depend upon an individual's sensitivity, based on factors such as metabolism and pharmacokinetics, as well as the time of day that it is consumed and the dose. In a protocol similar to that shown in Figure 30-5 (days −3 to −1) sleepiness was assessed (Stanford Sleepiness Scale [SSS]) in the early evening hours approaching bedtime. Individuals either ingested 3.0 mg melatonin (7 hours before bedtime on night 1) or 0.5 mg (5 hours before bedtime on night 1) or placebo; the timing of the pills was advanced 1 hour earlier each day. Sleepiness gradually increased in the hours after pill ingestion (in the 7 hours before bed) in all three groups. Although the individuals were a little sleepier with the 3.0-mg dose compared to the 0.5-mg dose, there were no statistically significant differences among the three groups.[48] A further study assessed the impact of 5.0 mg melatonin taken at 4:30 PM on driving performance and sleepiness ($n = 20$)[49] and demonstrated an enhancement of subjective sleepiness but no significant impact on body sway or 15 of 16 variables on a driving performance test battery. Morning (9:45 AM) melatonin (6.0 mg, sustained release) increased subjective sleepiness but did not adversely impact performance in the subsequent 7 hours[50] unlike shorter lasting (zaleplon) and longer lasting (zopiclone, temazepam) hypnotics.

By contrast, administration of higher doses of melatonin (10-80 mg) at 11:45 AM revealed a dose-dependent impairment of neurobehavioral performance.[51] A 5-mg dose of melatonin administered at 12:30 PM induced decrements in neurobehavioral performance that paralleled the salivary melatonin profile[52] and when administered at 7 AM resulted in an impairment of cognitive function for the subsequent 6 hours.[53] Subjective assessment of sleepiness may not accurately reflect underlying changes in cognitive function; after administration of 5 mg melatonin, measurable electroencephalographic

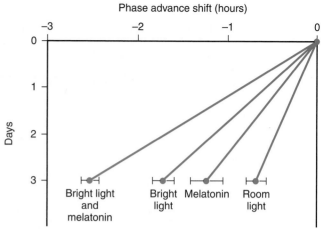

Figure 30-6 Phase advance shifts in the timing of the circadian clock measured by the dim light melatonin onset (DLMO) when using a preflight adjustment protocol for an eastward flight. The sleep schedule was advanced by 1 hour per day for 3 days. This advancing sleep schedule was combined with intermittent morning bright light and afternoon melatonin, administered for 3 days. The magnitude of the cumulative phase advance attained over 3 days with an advancing sleep schedule alone (room light) is increased progressively by utilizing afternoon melatonin only, morning intermittent bright light only, and morning intermittent bright light and afternoon melatonin together. The phase-shifting effects of afternoon melatonin and morning bright light appear to be additive.

(EEG) changes were observed almost immediately before any subjective soporific effects were identified.[54] Interestingly, these changes in the theta/alpha power were more visible when melatonin was administered during the day (1 PM or 6 PM) compared to the evening (8:40 PM). Posture is also a contributing factor to feelings of alertness with both subjective and objective measures of sleepiness being suppressed when posture changed from supine to standing.[54] The observed variation in the soporific effect of exogenous melatonin highlights that a degree of caution should be exercised when scheduling melatonin consumption into a phase shifting program.

In the past, we have recommended 0.5 mg melatonin in our preflight schedules to minimize the possibility of unwanted sleepiness.[55] However, since then our melatonin PRC studies have shown that the 3.0-mg dose is likely to produce more reliable phase shifts than the 0.5-mg dose, even though the average size of the phase shifts is similar.[27] Thus, if possible, we would recommend the 3.0-mg dose or, if this is not appropriate, then a lower dose could be used with increased morning bright light exposure.

We have tested preflight interventions for eastward travel in the laboratory using bright light and melatonin administered at the optimal times to promote phase shifts (see Fig. 30-6). When only the sleep schedule was advanced, with only ordinary dim room light upon awakening and no melatonin administered, circadian phase shifted very little (0.7 ± 0.1 hour; mean ± SEM, $n = 20$).[46,56] The addition of an afternoon melatonin 3.0-mg dose, 7 hours before baseline bedtime on the first day and advanced in conjunction with the sleep schedule, increased the phase advance to 1.2 ± 0.2 hours ($n = 11$) (updated from Crowley and associates[56]). When the advancing sleep schedule was combined with morning intermittent bright light (30 minutes bright light ~ 5000 lux alternating with 30 minutes room lighting < 60 lux for 3.5 hours) (no melatonin) a phase advance of 1.6 ± 0.7 hours ($n = 26$) was achieved.[46,48] The greatest phase advance (2.5 ± 0.1 hours,

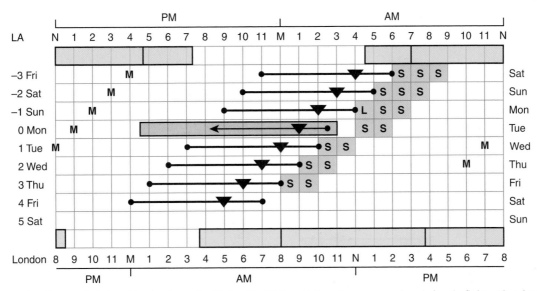

Figure 30-7 Kim takes the same flight from LA to London as Cynthia (see Fig. 30-5) and follows the same procedures before the flight, with melatonin in the afternoon and intermittent bright light in the morning. After landing she does not try to sleep at her usual time in London (11 PM to 6 AM). Instead, she gradually advances her sleep times by 1 hour per day. The first night (day 1) she sleeps from 3 AM to 10 AM, then 2 AM to 9 AM (day 2), etc. In this way her Tmin (▼) stays within sleep and she does not experience any jet lag. If she wanted to be on her usual sleep schedule of 11 PM to 6 AM sooner, she could do more than 2 days of advancing her sleep before the flight. Alternatively, she could keep a later sleep schedule (e.g., 1 AM to 8 PM) while in London to be completely adjusted sooner.

$n = 29$) was attained when morning intermittent bright light and afternoon melatonin were combined. The 3.0-mg and 0.5-mg doses were given at their optimal times (3.0 mg 7 hours before and 0.5 mg 5 hours before baseline bedtime) and advanced 1 hour per day along with the sleep schedule. There was no difference in phase shift between the two doses of melatonin.[48] It should be noted that the combination of advancing sleep, bright light, and melatonin achieves just under 1 hour advance per day such that the clock remains suitably aligned with the sleep schedule. We recommend using the combination of morning bright light, afternoon melatonin, and an advancing sleep schedule to attain the maximal phase advance and minimize the probability of suffering from jet lag.

It is probably not advisable to advance the sleep schedule much more than 1 hour per day; a previous laboratory study comparing advances of sleep of 1 hour per day and 2 hours per day combined with intermittent morning bright light demonstrated that the 2 hours per day advance did not significantly increase the phase advance compared to 1 hour per day. Thus, the 2 hours per day advance of sleep was too rapid for the clock to adapt to resulting in the melatonin onset occurring after sleep and the Tmin occurring after wake time, which is problematic for both falling asleep and waking up.[57] Further research is needed to test other combinations designed to phase advance the circadian clock, such as advancing the sleep schedule 1.5 hours per day and adding afternoon melatonin in addition to morning bright light.

Advancing the Circadian Clock Before and After the Flight

Kim (Fig. 30-7) takes the same flight and conducts the same preflight preparation as Cynthia (see Fig. 30-5), but she manages to eliminate jet lag completely by maintaining alignment between her circadian clock and her sleep/wake schedule after arrival. To do this she gradually advances her sleep schedule by 1 hour per day, such that her Tmin remains in sleep, until

she is sleeping 11 PM to 6 AM in London. Often, travelers are advised to sleep at the destination time as soon as possible in order to reduce jet lag, but as Figure 30-7 shows, this is not always the best strategy.

In this example, Kim completes 3 days of preflight phase advance, but she could do more days of shifting before the flight and then less after if desired. If she is crossing a large number of time zones, then it may be more beneficial to complete more days before the flight to minimize the number of days of adaptation upon arrival. Those flying to important events, such as athletes, business people, diplomats, and musicians, may be more motivated to complete greater preflight adaptation. For example, astronauts use bright light to shift their circadian rhythms before launch to prepare for shifted sleep schedules on space shuttle missions.[58]

Delaying the Circadian Clock Before Eastward or Westward Flights

For very late chronotypes it may be easier and quicker to phase delay rather than advance to adapt to an eastward flight (antidromic re-entrainment). Therefore, in the week leading up to the flight, Larry gradually delays himself by using bright light before bedtime and shifting his sleep times 1.5 hours later each day (Fig. 30-8). He plans to sleep for most of the flight and upon arrival he will be adapted to an 11 PM to 6 AM sleep schedule in the new time zone and will therefore not experience any jet lag.

This type of schedule can also be used to phase delay the circadian clock before flying west. The number of days of phase delay before the flight can be adjusted, taking into account the number of time zones to be crossed and how much the individual wants to be adjusted before flying west. When a delaying schedule is used before flying east or west, it can interfere with morning activities, however, making it difficult for those with set working hours. This type of schedule can also be used as chronotherapy[59,60] for night owls and delayed sleep

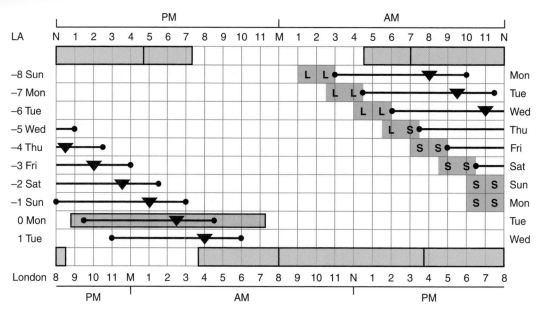

Figure 30-8 Larry is a night owl, not going to bed until 2 AM or 3 AM and he wants to be on an earlier sleep schedule in London, so he decides to delay his circadian clock instead of advancing it before the flight to London. He delays his sleep schedule by 1.5 hours per day and uses intermittent bright light in the 2 hours before bed. His Tmin (▼) always stays within sleep and he does not have any jet lag. On the first day in London, he is sleeping much earlier than at home, and he plans to stay on that schedule (11 PM to 6 AM) while in London. He has completely eliminated jet lag and is on a more desirable sleep schedule in London. Meals should also be delayed along with the sleep schedule and a nap is desirable in the middle of each waking period, if possible. Scheduling meals to shift along with the sleep schedule is also a good idea for advancing schedules (see Figs. 30-5 and 30-7), but naps are not recommended when advancing because building homeostatic sleep pressure can help when going to bed earlier.

phase disorder patients to get on an earlier sleep schedule (see Chapter 31), although we do not recommend delaying the sleep schedule more than 2 hours per day or attempting this procedure without having a light box or outdoor light available.

There are limited data on the rate of adaptation with gradually delaying sleep schedules and light boxes designed for home use. We have showed that when the sleep schedule was delayed 2 hours per day for 13 days and light boxes (~ 2000-4000 lux) were used during the 2 hours before bed, the temperature rhythm of 14 of 19 subjects was entrained to the 26-hour schedule, and thus, delays of about 2 hours per day were produced.[61] In a more recent study with 2-hour delays of sleep and bright light (4000-5000 lux) in the 2 hours before bed for 4 days, the melatonin rhythm delayed an average of about 1 hour per day.[62] Another study with a single 2-hour bright light exposure (~ 4000 lux) and a 4-hour delay of sleep produced a delay of about 1.5 hours in 1 day.[63] In Figure 30-8, we chose a 1.5 hours per day delay of the sleep schedule, assuming the circadian clock will be shifted about 1.5 hours per day, but a 1-hour or 2-hour delay could also be used in some cases, depending on the individual and the circumstances. In our current example, if Larry's circadian clock does not delay as fast as the sleep schedule delay of 1.5 hours per day, then his Tmin will gradually move earlier within the sleep period (see the triangles in Fig. 30-8). This will turn night owl Larry into an early bird, feeling very sleepy at bedtime and waking up alert, bright, and cheerful. The worst outcome, which would only appear after several days, is that he would have trouble staying awake until bedtime and would wake up earlier than planned. In contrast, the consequences of advancing a sleep schedule faster than the clock advances are more serious, because bright light intended to help advance can more easily occur before the Tmin and promote delays.

OTHER METHODS OF REDUCING JET LAG

Using Melatonin Only

If it is not possible to utilize morning bright light exposure before a flight then melatonin can be used alone in a preflight program. The sleep schedule and the time for taking melatonin should be advanced by only 30 minutes per day to retain alignment with the circadian clock as the combination of melatonin and an advancing sleep schedule produces an average phase shift of only 1.2 ± 0.2 hours over 3 days, or about 24 minutes per day (modified from Crowley and associates[56]). Upon arrival, the regimen can be continued and augmented with properly timed outdoor light if possible until the desired sleep/wake schedule is attained.

A number of field studies have assessed the efficacy of melatonin, taken at local bedtime for a few days after the flight, to hasten adaptation to a new time zone. This strategy takes advantage of both the sleep-promoting and phase-shifting effects of melatonin. As can be seen in Figure 30-1, advancing the sleep schedule by several hours, which happens after flying east, places the bedtime into the phase advance portion of the melatonin PRC, and delaying it by several hours, which happens after flying west, places bedtime in the delay portion of the PRC. Indeed, there was a 50% reduction in subjective assessment of jet lag following use of melatonin ($n = 474$) compared to placebo ($n = 126$).[64] A set of studies using the internal melatonin rhythm as a marker of circadian phase showed that taking a 3.0 mg melatonin dose at bedtime (11 PM) for 3 days following an eastward flight across eight time zones promoted orthodromic re-entrainment in all six travelers, whereas two of them had showed antidromic re-entrainment on a previous trip between the same destinations but without melatonin.

Furthermore, melatonin enhanced the rate of re-entrainment in the four subjects who advanced during both trips from 67 minutes per day to 82 minutes per day.[65] For six individuals whose rhythms delayed after a flight east across 11 time zones evening melatonin (3.0 mg) increased the degree of phase delay.[66]

The effectiveness of using melatonin at local bedtime, however, will be dependent upon whether the administration time coincides with optimal times in the phase advance or delay regions on the PRC. The number of time zones crossed as well as the bedtime at home and at the destination will determine the usefulness of melatonin in promoting appropriate adaptation, and thus, the use of melatonin should be carefully considered. The soporific effect alone of melatonin treatment may still be beneficial at bedtime to reduce sleep onset insomnia, even in the absence of a phase resetting effect.

Availability of Light Boxes and Melatonin

Exogenous melatonin and bright light boxes are the most effective mechanism of adapting to the local light/dark cycle. In the United States melatonin is sold over the counter as a food supplement in a variety of different doses. As with any supplement, it is essential that the purity and dose are reliable and only a trusted source should be used. In most other countries, melatonin is a prescription-only drug. Prior to using melatonin on a flight, it would be advisable to assess safety by taking a "test dose" prior to travel when there are no requirements to be alert after taking it or restrictions on sleep.

A wide range of bright light boxes are commercially available with a variety of designs tailored to suit different situations, such as small, portable devices for travelers and narrow boxes to use next to computers. However, if the weather, time of day, and season permit, going outside in bright sunlight at the appropriate time of day will be the most effective mechanism of shifting the clock.

Coping with Short Trips

In certain situations, such as business trips, individuals may travel several time zones for a very short time, only 2 or 3 days. To maximize performance on short trips, when preadaptation is not possible, scheduling important meetings at times when sleep occurs at the home time zone should be avoided. For example, in Nicole's example (see Fig. 30-2), it would be best to avoid scheduling important events until at least 3 PM at her destination (1 hour after usual home wake time of 6 AM). If it is necessary to schedule meetings earlier, then a partial advance by 1 or 2 hours before the trip should allow better alertness. Alternatively, if scheduling permits, the sleep time at the new destination could remain on the home time zone, with no adaptation attempted (e.g., from 7 AM to 2 PM; see Fig. 30-2). Deciding whether to reset the circadian clock to the destination time zone partially or fully before the flight will depend on schedule commitments before and after the flight, and on how important it is to be fully functional at the destination or on the return home.

Sleeping Pills and Stimulants

Some individuals may choose to take sleeping medication at night and stimulants during the day to overcome the insomnia and sleepiness, respectively. These drugs will only attempt to treat the symptoms of jet lag, however, not the underlying cause of the problem, which is circadian misalignment. The degree of improvement obtained using these "masking" approaches cannot match that which is obtained by maintaining the proper alignment between sleep and circadian rhythms. Furthermore, sleeping pills and stimulants have side effects and "hangover" effects that can interfere with performance or sleep.[67,68] For example, following eastward flight over seven time zones, travelers were administered 300 mg slow-release caffeine at 8 AM for 5 days.[69] Although daytime sleepiness was alleviated under the caffeine treatment, compared to a group receiving placebo, the subjects were still sleepier than before the flight. The newer stimulants (modafinil and armodafinil) are increasingly being prescribed (off-label) for jet lag.[70] One study found that 600 mg caffeine (similar to a Starbucks grande) was as effective as 400 mg modafinil for improving performance on the psychomotor vigilance task (PVT). The pills were given in the middle of the second night without sleep. In the example in Figure 30-2, this treatment would be equivalent to taking the drugs in London at 10 AM on day +1 after not sleeping at all since day -1. Caffeine produced more side effects, such as jitteriness and nausea, than modafinil, but modafinil caused more headaches.[71] Although hypnotics can improve sleep in the new time zone, they do not shift the circadian dip in alertness and performance around the Tmin, which may still coincide with wake times. A large study of frequent flyers showed that zolpidem 10 mg taken for 3 to 4 days after eastward travel across five to nine time zones improved sleep compared to placebo, but there was no improvement in daytime alertness and functioning.[72]

Light also has acute alerting effects in addition to its phase resetting effects and therefore can also be used to boost alertness, mood, and performance,[73] for example, by using a light box at one's desk, by sitting next to a window, or taking walks outside.

SUMMARY

In conclusion, the examples discussed here have utilized the model of an eastward flight across eight time zones to explain the circadian principles of jet lag and the mechanisms by which light and melatonin can phase shift the clock to minimize the occurrence and severity of jet lag. It is recommended that travelers preadapt before they fly to minimize or eliminate jet lag. For eastward flights, a phase shift earlier (advance) is required and can be achieved by advancing sleep 1 hour per day using intermittent bright light for 2 to 3 hours after waking and taking 3 mg melatonin 7 hours before home sleep onset and 1 hour earlier each day. For westward flights, a phase delay shift later is required and can be achieved by delaying sleep 1.5 hours per day and using intermittent bright light for 2 hours before bed. Using such schedules can reduce the debilitating effects of jet lag.

Acknowledgments
This work is supported in part by NIH grants R01 NR07677 and R01 HL086934 to CIE. The content is solely the responsibility of the authors and does not necessarily represent the official views of the National Institutes of Health, the National Institute of Nursing Research, or the National Heart, Lung and Blood Institute. VLR is currently supported by the 6th Framework project EUCLOCK (018741).

REFERENCES

1. American Academy of Sleep Medicine. *International Classification of Sleep Disorders: Diagnostic and Coding Manual.* 2nd ed. Westchester, IL: American Academy of Sleep Medicine; 2005.
2. Borbely AA. A two process model of sleep regulation. *Hum Neurobiol.* 1982;1(3):195-204.
3. Ralph MR, Foster RG, Davis FC, Menaker M. Transplanted suprachiasmatic nucleus determines circadian period. *Science.* 1990;247(4945):975-978.
4. Balsalobre A, Brown SA, Marcacci L, et al. Resetting of circadian time in peripheral tissues by glucocorticoid signaling. *Science.* 2000;289(5488):2344-2347.
5. Yamazaki S, Numano R, Abe M, et al. Resetting central and peripheral circadian oscillators in transgenic rats. *Science.* 2000;288(5466):682-685.
6. Yoo SH, Yamazaki S, Lowrey PL, et al. PERIOD2:LUCIFERASE real-time reporting of circadian dynamics reveals persistent circadian oscillations in mouse peripheral tissues. *Proc Natl Acad Sci U S A.* 2004;101(15):5339-5346.
7. Davidson AJ, Castanon-Cervantes O, Leise TL, Molyneux PC, Harrington ME. Visualizing jet lag in the mouse suprachiasmatic nucleus and peripheral circadian timing system. *Eur J Neurosci.* 2009;29(1):171-180.
8. Aschoff J, Hoffmann K, Pohl H, Wever R. Re-entrainment of circadian rhythms after phase-shifts of the Zeitgeber. *Chronobiologia.* 1975;2(1):23-78.
9. Cho K. Chronic "jet lag" produces temporal lobe atrophy and spatial cognitive deficits. *Nat Neurosci.* 2001;4(6):567-568.
10. Pukkala E, Aspholm R, Auvinen A, et al. Incidence of cancer among Nordic airline pilots over five decades: Occupational cohort study. *BMJ.* 2002;325(7364):567.
11. Rafnsson V, Tulinius H, Jonasson JG, Hrafnkelsson J. Risk of breast cancer in female flight attendants: A population-based study (Iceland). *Cancer Causes Control.* 2001;12(2):95-101.
12. Reynolds P, Cone J, Layefsky M, Goldberg DE, Hurley S. Cancer incidence in California flight attendants (United States). *Cancer Causes Control.* 2002;13(4):317-324.
13. Filipski E, Delaunay F, King VM, et al. Effects of chronic jet lag on tumor progression in mice. *Cancer Res.* 2004;64(21):7879-7885.
14. Davidson AJ, Sellix MT, Daniel J, Yamazaki S, Menaker M, Block GD. Chronic jet-lag increases mortality in aged mice. *Curr Biol.* 2006;16(21):R914-R916.
15. Spiegel K, Leproult R, Van Cauter E. Impact of sleep debt on metabolic and endocrine function. *Lancet.* 1999;354(9188):1435-1439.
16. Spiegel K, Tasali E, Penev P, Van Cauter E. Brief communication: Sleep curtailment in healthy young men is associated with decreased leptin levels, elevated ghrelin levels, and increased hunger and appetite. *Ann Intern Med.* 2004;141(11):846-850.
17. Burgess HJ, Eastman CI. Human tau in an ultradian light-dark cycle. *J Biol Rhythms.* 2008;23(4):374-376.
18. Czeisler CA, Duffy JF, Shanahan TL, et al. Stability, precision, and near-24-hour period of the human circadian pacemaker. *Science.* 1999;284(5423):2177-2181.
19. Middleton B, Arendt J, Stone BM. Human circadian rhythms in constant dim light (8 lux) with knowledge of clock time. *J Sleep Res.* 1996;5(2):69-76.
20. Mistlberger RE, Skene DJ. Nonphotic entrainment in humans? *J Biol Rhythms.* 2005;20(4):339-352.
21. Arendt J. The pineal gland: Basic physiology and clinical implications. In: Groot D, ed. *Endocrinology.* 3rd ed. Philadelphia: WB Saunders; 1993:432-443.
22. Brainard GC, Hanifin JP, Greeson JM, et al. Action spectrum for melatonin regulation in humans: Evidence for a novel circadian photoreceptor. *J Neurosci.* 2001;21(16):6405-6412.
23. Thapan K, Arendt J, Skene DJ. An action spectrum for melatonin suppression: Evidence for a novel non-rod, non-cone photoreceptor system in humans. *J Physiol.* 2001;535(Pt 1):261-267.
24. Revell VL, Skene DJ. Light-induced melatonin suppression in humans with polychromatic and monochromatic light. *Chronobiol Int.* 2007;24(6):1125-1137.
25. Lewy AJ, Bauer VK, Ahmed S, et al. The human phase response curve (PRC) to melatonin is about 12 hours out of phase with the PRC to light. *Chronobiol Int.* 1998;15(1):71-83.
26. Burgess HJ, Revell VL, Eastman CI. A three pulse phase response curve to three milligrams of melatonin in humans. *J Physiol.* 2008;586(2):639-647.
27. Burgess HJ, Revell VL, Molina TA, Eastman CI. Human phase response curves to three days of daily melatonin: 0.5 mg versus 3.0 mg. *J Clin Endocrinol Metab.* 2010;95(7):3325-3331.
28. Lockley SW, Skene DJ, James K, Thapan K, Wright J, Arendt J. Melatonin administration can entrain the free-running circadian system of blind subjects. *J Endocrinol.* 2000;164(1):R1-R6.
29. Sack RL, Brandes RW, Kendall AR, Lewy AJ. Entrainment of free-running circadian rhythms by melatonin in blind people. *N Engl J Med.* 2000;343(15):1070-1077.
30. Comas M, Beersma DG, Spoelstra K, Daan S. Phase and period responses of the circadian system of mice (*Mus musculus*) to light stimuli of different duration. *J Biol Rhythms.* 2006;21(5):362-372.
31. Revell VL, Eastman CI. How to trick mother nature into letting you fly around or stay up all night. *J Biol Rhythms.* 2005;20(4):353-365.
32. Khalsa SB, Jewett ME, Cajochen C, Czeisler CA. A phase response curve to single bright light pulses in human subjects. *J Physiol.* 2003;549(Pt 3):945-952.
33. Kripke DF, Elliott JA, Youngstedt SD, Rex KM. Circadian phase response curves to light in older and young women and men. *J Circadian Rhythms.* 2007;5:4.
34. Leger D, Badet D, de La Giclais B. The prevalence of jet lag among 507 travelling businessmen. *Sleep Res.* 1993;22:409.
35. Dijk DJ, Duffy JF, Riel E, Shanahan TL, Czeisler CA. Aging and the circadian and homeostatic regulation of human sleep during forced desynchrony of rest, melatonin and temperature rhythms. *J Physiol.* 1999;516(Pt 2):611-627.
36. Duffy JF, Willson HJ, Wang W, Czeisler CA. Healthy older adults better tolerate sleep deprivation than young adults. *J Am Geriatr Soc.* 2009;57(7):1245-1251.
37. Campbell SS. Effects of timed bright-light exposure on shift-work adaptation in middle-aged subjects. *Sleep.* 1995;18(6):408-416.
38. Klerman EB, Duffy JF, Dijk DJ, Czeisler CA. Circadian phase resetting in older people by ocular bright light exposure. *J Investig Med.* 2001;49(1):30-40.
39. Monk TH. Aging human circadian rhythms: Conventional wisdom may not always be right. *J Biol Rhythms.* 2005;20(4):366-374.
40. Houpt TA, Boulos Z, Moore-Ede MC. MidnightSun: Software for determining light exposure and phase-shifting schedules during global travel. *Physiol Behav.* 1996;59(3):561-568.
41. Takahashi T, Sasaki M, Itoh H, et al. Re-entrainment of circadian rhythm of plasma melatonin on an 8-h eastward flight. *Psychiatry Clin Neurosci.* 1999;53(2):257-260.
42. Takahashi T, Sasaki M, Itoh H, et al. Re-entrainment of the circadian rhythms of plasma melatonin in an 11-h eastward bound flight. *Psychiatry Clin Neurosci.* 2001;55(3):275-276.
43. Mitchell PJ, Hoese EK, Liu L, Fogg LF, Eastman CI. Conflicting bright light exposure during night shifts impedes circadian adaptation. *J Biol Rhythms.* 1997;12(1):5-15.
44. Gronfier C, Wright Jr KP, Kronauer RE, Jewett ME, Czeisler CA. Efficacy of a single sequence of intermittent bright light pulses for delaying circadian phase in humans. *Am J Physiol Endocrinol Metab.* 2004;287(1):E174-E181.
45. Rimmer DW, Boivin DB, Shanahan TL, Kronauer RE, Duffy JF, Czeisler CA. Dynamic resetting of the human circadian pacemaker by intermittent bright light. *Am J Physiol Regul Integr Comp Physiol.* 2000;279(5):R1574-R1579.
46. Burgess HJ, Crowley SJ, Gazda CJ, Fogg LF, Eastman CI. Preflight adjustment to eastward travel: 3 days of advancing sleep with and without morning bright light. *J Biol Rhythms.* 2003;18(4):318-328.
47. Hebert M, Martin SK, Lee C, Eastman CI. The effects of prior light history on the suppression of melatonin by light in humans. *J Pineal Res.* 2002;33(4):198-203.
48. Revell VL, Burgess HJ, Gazda CJ, Smith MR, Fogg LF, Eastman CI. Advancing human circadian rhythms with afternoon melatonin and morning intermittent bright light. *J Clin Endocrinol Metab.* 2006;91(1):54-59.
49. Suhner A, Schlagenhauf P, Tschopp A, Hauri-Bionda R, Friedrich-Koch A, Steffen R. Impact of melatonin on driving performance. *J Travel Med.* 1998;5(1):7-13.
50. Paul MA, Gray G, Kenny G, Pigeau RA. Impact of melatonin, zaleplon, zopiclone, and temazepam on psychomotor performance. *Aviat Space Environ Med.* 2003;74(12):1263-1270.
51. Dollins AB, Lynch HJ, Wurtman RJ, et al. Effect of pharmacological daytime doses of melatonin on human mood and performance. *Psychopharmacology (Berl).* 1993;112(4):490-496.
52. Rogers NL, Phan O, Kennaway DJ, Dawson D. Effect of daytime oral melatonin administration on neurobehavioral performance in humans. *J Pineal Res.* 1998;25(1):47-53.

53. Graw P, Werth E, Kräuchi K, Gutzwiller F, Cajochen C, Wirz-Justice A. Early morning melatonin administration impairs psychomotor vigilance. *Behav Brain Res.* 2001;121(1-2):167-172.

54. Cajochen C, Krauchi K, Wirz-Justice A. The acute soporific action of day-time melatonin administration: Effects on the EEG during wakefulness and subjective alertness. *J Biol Rhythms.* 1997;12(6):636-643.

55. Eastman CI, Burgess HJ. How to travel the world without jet lag. *Sleep Med Clin.* 2009;4(2):241-255.

56. Crowley SJ, Smith MR, Munoz J, Eastman CI. Advancing circadian rhythms with afternoon melatonin and a gradually advancing sleep/dark schedule. *Sleep.* 2010;33:A64.

57. Eastman CI, Gazda CJ, Burgess HJ, Crowley SJ, Fogg LF. Advancing circadian rhythms before eastward flight: A strategy to prevent or reduce jet lag. *Sleep.* 2005;28(1):33-44.

58. Stewart KT, Eastman CI. The light stuff: Shiftwork, circadian rhythms, and manned spaceflight. In: Holick MF, Jung EG, eds. *Biologic Effects of Light 1995.* Berlin: Walter de Gruyter & Co.; 1996:340-347.

59. Czeisler CA, Richardson GS, Coleman RM, et al. Chronotherapy: Resetting the circadian clocks of patients with delayed sleep phase insomnia. *Sleep.* 1981;4(1):1-21.

60. Weitzman ED, Czeisler CA, Coleman RM, et al. Delayed sleep phase syndrome: A chronobiological disorder with sleep-onset insomnia. *Arch Gen Psychiatry.* 1981;38(7):737-746.

61. Eastman CI, Miescke KJ. Entrainment of circadian rhythms with 26-h bright light and sleep-wake schedules. *Am J Physiol.* 1990;259(6 Pt 2): R1189-R1197.

62. Smith MR, Eastman CI. Phase delaying the human circadian clock with blue-enriched polychromatic light. *Chronobiol Int.* 2009;26(4):709-725.

63. Canton JL, Smith MR, Choi HS, Eastman CI. Phase delaying the human circadian clock with a single light pulse and moderate delay of the sleep/dark episode: No influence of iris color. *J Circadian Rhythms.* 2009;7:8.

64. Arendt J, Skene DJ, Middleton B, Lockley SW, Deacon S. Efficacy of melatonin treatment in jet lag, shift work, and blindness. *J Biol Rhythms.* 1997;12(6):604-617.

65. Takahashi T, Sasaki M, Itoh H, et al. Effect of 3 mg melatonin on jet lag syndrome in an 8-h eastward flight. *Psychiatry Clin Neurosci.* 2000; 54(3):377-378.

66. Takahashi T, Sasaki M, Itoh H, et al. Melatonin alleviates jet lag symptoms caused by an 11-hour eastward flight. *Psychiatry Clin Neurosci.* 2002; 56(3):301-302.

67. Morris 3rd HH, Estes ML. Traveler's amnesia. Transient global amnesia secondary to triazolam. *JAMA.* 1987;258(7):945-946.

68. Mitler MM, O'Malley MB. Wake-promoting medications: Efficacy and adverse effects. In: Kryger MH, Roth T, Dement WC, eds. *Principles and Practices of Sleep Medicine.* 4th ed. St Louis: Elsevier; 2005:484-498.

69. Beaumont M, Batejat D, Pierard C, et al. Caffeine or melatonin effects on sleep and sleepiness after rapid eastward transmeridian travel. *J Appl Physiol.* 2004;96(1):50-58.

70. McCarty DE. Ready for takeoff? A critical review of armodafinil and modafinil for the treatment of sleepiness associated with jet lag. *Nature and Science of Sleep.* 2010;2010(2):85-94.

71. Killgore WD, Rupp TL, Grugle NL, Reichardt RM, Lipizzi EL, Balkin TJ. Effects of dextroamphetamine, caffeine and modafinil on psychomotor vigilance test performance after 44 h of continuous wakefulness. *J Sleep Res.* 2008;17(3):309-321.

72. Jamieson AO, Zammit GK, Rosenberg RS, Davis JR, Walsh JK. Zolpidem reduces the sleep disturbance of jet lag. *Sleep Med.* 2001;2(5):423-430.

73. Cajochen C, Zeitzer JM, Czeisler CA, Dijk DJ. Dose-response relationship for light intensity and ocular and electroencephalographic correlates of human alertness. *Behav Brain Res.* 2000;115(1):75-83.

Chapter 31

Delayed and Advanced Sleep Phase Disorders

JAMES K. WYATT / JAMIE A. CVENGROS

Delayed sleep phase disorder (DSPD) and advanced sleep phase disorder (ASPD) may be conceptualized as two of the intrinsic circadian rhythm sleep disorders. In contrast to the extrinsic circadian rhythm sleep disorders, which are due to intentional misalignment of one's sleep-wake schedule and circadian phase (jet lag and shift work disorder), the intrinsic disorders are presumably due to a malfunction of the circadian system itself or its interaction with sleep-generating systems. In DSPD and ASPD, the circadian system maintains a near 24-hour oscillation, but its phase is misaligned with the desired sleep-wake schedule. In DSPD, a patient's internal circadian clock is significantly delayed, or "set later" than the desired sleep schedule. In ASPD, the internal clock is significantly advanced, or "set earlier" than the desired sleep schedule. This chapter will review clinical diagnosis, diagnostic tools, and treatment options for DSPD and ASPD. In addition, this chapter will also review nondiagnosis associated features (e.g., genetics) and issues in differential diagnosis (e.g., co-morbid/secondary conditions) of DSPD and ASPD.

CLINICAL DIAGNOSIS

Delayed Sleep Phase Disorder

Common presenting complaints among patients with DSPD are difficulty falling asleep at night, difficulty waking in the morning, and excessive daytime sleepiness.[1] Specifically, patients often complain of prolonged sleep onset latencies, often as long as 2 or more hours past desired bedtime. Patients will also commonly report significant difficulty waking in the morning at their desired wake time. Often the desired bedtime and wake time are dictated by daytime commitments such as work or school. The combination of prolonged sleep onset and early wake time leads to decreased total sleep time and contributes to subsequent excessive daytime sleepiness. When their sleep-wake schedule is not dictated by daytime commitments, such as during weekends or vacations, patients report little difficulty falling asleep at later bedtimes and arising at later wake times. Thus, on these ad lib schedules, they have adequate total sleep times and minimal daytime sleepiness. Research has suggested that normal-sleeping adolescents and young adults experience a delay in circadian rhythm relative to young children.[2] This may explain why DSPD, perhaps itself an extreme of this normal phase delay, is more common among this younger population. A summary of key diagnostic features in DSPD is presented in Box 31-1 and the precise diagnostic criteria are listed in Box 31-2.

Advanced Sleep Phase Disorder

In contrast to DSPD, common presenting complaints in ASPD are difficulty staying awake in the evening and waking too early in the morning.[1] Specifically, patients endorse significant sleepiness in the evening and an inability to stay awake until the desired bedtime. In addition, patients report early morning awakenings, often 2 to 3 hours before desired wake time. This excessive evening sleepiness can significantly impact social functioning, as patients are unable to participate in desired evening social activities. Unlike with DSPD, the advanced sleep-wake patterns in ASPD do not usually vary with patient's daytime commitments. Although prevalence data are limited, ASPD appears to be more common among older adults and may represent an extreme of normal advancement of circadian rhythm that occurs with aging.[3] A summary of key diagnostic features in ASPD is presented in Box 31-1, and the precise diagnostic criteria are listed in Box 31-2.

Diagnostic Tools

The practice parameters for the diagnosis and treatment of circadian rhythm disorders published in 2007[4] and the two accompanying review papers[5,6] provided recommendations for the use of diagnostic tools and treatment protocols for management of the circadian rhythm sleep disorders. Recommendations at the level of standard are "generally accepted patient-care strategies with a high degree of clinical certainty." Recommendations at the level of guideline are patient-care strategies with a "moderate degree of clinical certainty." Recommendations at the level of option are strategies with "uncertain clinical use."[4] Several diagnostic tools and treatment protocols (critically evaluated in this chapter) were reviewed for use in patients with DSPD and ASPD.

Sleep Diaries

Daily sleep diaries or sleep logs are recommended at the level of guideline in the diagnosis of DSPD and ASPD.[4] Patients use sleep diaries prospectively to record several sleep and wake variables including bedtime, sleep onset latency, time and duration of nocturnal awakenings, final wake time, and time out of bed. From these variables, total sleep time and sleep efficiency (i.e., percentage of time in bed spent sleeping) can be computed, typically by the patient. Sleep diaries can take a variety of formats including a tabular format, in which patients write in sleep variables, or a graphic format, in which patients "X-out" blocks of sleep time. Sleep diaries can also

> **BOX 31-1** *Key Diagnostic Features in Delayed Sleep Phase Disorder (DSPD) and Advanced Sleep Phase Disorder (ASPD)*
>
> | DSPD | ASPD |
> | --- | --- |
> | Difficulty falling asleep at desired time | Difficulty staying awake until desired time |
> | Difficulty waking at desired time | Excessive evening sleepiness |
> | Excessive daytime sleepiness | |
> | No difficulty sleeping if allowed to sleep on free schedule | |

> **BOX 31-2** *Diagnostic Criteria for Circadian Rhythm Sleep Disorder, Delayed and Advanced Sleep Phase Types*
>
> Circadian Rhythm Sleep Disorder, Delayed Sleep Phase Type
>
> A. There is a delay in the phase of the major sleep period in relation to the desired sleep time and wake-up time, as evidenced by a chronic or recurrent complaint of inability to fall asleep at a desired conventional clock time together with the inability to awaken at a desired and socially acceptable time.
> B. When allowed to choose their preferred schedule, patients will exhibit normal sleep quality and duration for age and maintain a delayed, but stable, phase of entrainment to the 24-hour sleep-wake pattern.
> C. Sleep log or actigraphy monitoring (including sleep diary) for at least 7 days demonstrates a stable delay in the timing of the habitual sleep period. (NOTE: In addition, a delay in the timing of other circadian rhythms, such as the nadir of the core body temperature rhythm or DLMO, is useful for confirmation of the delayed phase.)
> D. The sleep disturbance is not better explained by another current sleep disorder, medical or neurologic disorder, mental disorder, medication use, or substance use disorder.
>
> Circadian Rhythm Sleep Disorder, Advanced Sleep Phase Type
>
> A. There is an advance in the phase of the major sleep period in relation to the desired sleep time and wake-up time, as evidenced by a chronic or recurrent complaint of inability to stay awake until the desired conventional clock time, together with an inability to remain asleep until the desired and socially acceptable time for awakening.
> B. When patients are allowed to choose their preferred schedule, sleep quality and duration are normal for age with an advanced, but stable, phase of entrainment to the 24-hour sleep-wake pattern.
> C. Sleep log or actigraphy monitoring (including sleep diary) for at least 7 days demonstrates a stable advance in the timing of the habitual sleep period. (NOTE: In addition, an advance in the timing of other circadian rhythms, such as the nadir of the core body temperature rhythm or DLMO, is useful for confirmation of the advanced circadian phase.)
> D. The sleep disturbance is not better explained by another current sleep disorder, medical or neurologic disorder, mental disorder, medication use, or substance use disorder.
>
> *DLMO,* dim light melatonin onset.
> From American Academy of Sleep Medicine. *The International Classification of Sleep Disorders; Diagnostic and Coding Manual,* 2nd ed. Westchester, IL: American Academy of Sleep Medicine; 2005.

include space for patients to provide a daily rating of daytime sleepiness (e.g., propensity to fall asleep) and daytime fatigue (e.g., somatic or cognitive fatigue). Diaries may also include space for patients to record daytime naps and any factors that may impact sleep onset latency, such as alcohol or nicotine use before bedtime.

For the diagnosis of DSPD, at least 1 week of sleep diary use is recommended. This time allows for recording on days when patients have mandated early bedtimes and wake times, usually during the week, and on days when patients have unrestricted bedtimes and wake times, usually on the weekend. A sample sleep diary for a patient with DSPD is shown in Figure 31-1. In this diary, the patient has a desired bedtime of 11:30 PM on Tuesday through Thursday nights with sleep onset latencies that range from 90 minutes to 3 hours. On Wednesday through Friday, the patient has a mandated wake time of 7:30 AM, which yields total sleep times that range from 4 to 6 hours. On these days, the patient endorses significant sleepiness and fatigue. On Friday and Saturday nights, the patient has a much delayed bedtime of 3 AM or later with sleep onset latencies of less than 30 minutes. Wake times on Saturday and Sunday morning are also delayed and allow for total sleep times of 8 and 9 hours. Ratings of sleepiness and fatigue are much improved on these days. Note as well that the patient's calculation of total sleep time is not always correct.

In the diagnosis of ASPD, sleep diaries will likely reflect patients' presenting complaint of difficulty staying awake with sleep times much earlier than desired. Bedtimes may be as early as 6 PM or 7 PM Wake times will also be much earlier than desired and may be as early as 3 AM or 4 AM. Patients with ASPD may remain in bed in the morning after waking, which may contribute the development of other sleep disorders (see discussion of "insomnias" in Section 4).

Actigraphy

Actigraphy is also recommended at the level of a guideline in the diagnosis of DSPD and ASPD.[4] An actigraph is a small accelerometer worn like a wrist watch. The actigraph records movement throughout the day and night and provides a record of rest and activity periods throughout the day. Often, actigraphs have an event marker that patients can use to indicate specific events, such as time getting into bed and time getting out of bed. Using various algorithms, rest and activity periods are interpreted as sleep and wake periods, respectively. A variety of parameters similar to those in a sleep diary

(e.g., bedtime, sleep onset latency, nocturnal awakenings, wake time, total sleep time, and sleep efficiency) can be calculated from actigraphy data.

In the diagnosis of DSPD, actigraphy should be recorded for at least 1 week, to span a period of schedule-restricted bedtimes and wake times as well as period of unrestricted bedtimes and wake times. An example of actigraphy data from a patient with DSPD is shown in Figure 31-2. These actigraphy data demonstrate late sleep onset times, along with fixed early wake times and decreased total sleep time on weekdays, except for one morning of sleeping in past the alarm. On the weekend, bedtime and wake time are shifted later with normal

⦿RUSH

SLEEP DIARY

Sleep Disorders Service and Research Center
Rush University Medical Center

Patient: _____   Week Ending: _____/_____/_____   Next Appointment: _____/_____/_____   at ___ AM/PM with Dr. _____

SLEEPINESS AND FATIGUE RATING SCALE: (AVERAGE RATING FOR <u>THE WHOLE DAY</u> FOLLOWING A GIVEN SLEEP EPISODE)					
	0	25	50	75	...100
SLEEPINESS:	Extremely sleepy	Somewhat sleepy	Neither	Somewhat alert	Very alert
FATIGUE:	Extremely fatigued	Somewhat fatigued	Neither	Somewhat energetic	Very energetic

←		COMPLETE AFTER GETTING OUT OF BED							→	← NEXT DAY →	
Day and Date	Naps: time and sleep time	Unusual stressors, alcohol, and medications for sleep	Time you went to bed	Time it took you to fall asleep	No. of awakenings	Amount of time* awake	Time you got up for the day	Total sleep time	Sleepiness Rating	Fatigue Rating
Mon 2/7/11	None	Studying for math test	11:30p	3 hrs	0	0	7:45a	5 hrs	20	25
Tues 2/8/11	None		11:45p	2.5 hrs	1	5 min	7:30a	4 hrs	10	10
Wed 2/9/11	None		11:30p	3 hrs	0	0	8:00a	5.5 hrs	15	30
Thurs 2/10/11	5 pm 1 hr		12:00a	1.5 hrs	0	0	7:30a	6 hrs	30	25
Fri 2/11/11	None	Out with friends	3:00a	15 min	1	15 min	11:30a	8 hrs	50	50
Sat 2/12/11	None	Out late at party	3:15a	15 min	0	0	12:00p	9 hrs	60	75
Sun 2/13/11	None		11:30p	3 hrs	0	0	7:30a	5 hrs	10	15

*This is all the time you spent awake during the night, from the first time you awakened to the time you got out of bed.
It does not include the time it took you to fall asleep initially.

Figure 31-1 A sample sleep diary for a patient with delayed sleep phase disorder (DSPD).

sleep onset latencies and adequate total sleep times. In the diagnosis of ASPD, actigraphy data can provide corroboration of patient's complaint of falling asleep earlier than desired in the evening and waking too early in the morning.

Dim Light Melatonin Onset

Using the timing of the dim light melatonin onset (DLMO)[7] as an objective marker of circadian phase is recommended at the level of an option in the diagnosis of DSPD and ASPD.[4] Endogenous melatonin, a circadian phase–dependent sleep-promoting hormone, is secreted by the pineal gland approximately 2 hours before habitual bedtime. In DLMO assessment, patients are kept in dimly lit room, and blood or saliva samples are collected every 30 to 60 minutes from late afternoon to the time of habitual bedtime or slightly beyond. The time when melatonin begins to rise beyond a predetermined threshold is considered dim light melatonin onset. DLMO can be estimated from sleep diary data,[8,9] although with variable confidence.[10] Given the expense of the testing procedure and lack of reimbursement, DLMO is not routinely measured in making

the diagnosis of DSPD and ASPD. However, measurement of DLMO or other reliable circadian phase markers is important for optimal treatment response to melatonin or phototherapy treatment, as will be discussed later.

In patients with DSPD, DLMO is significantly delayed as compared to healthy sleepers.[9] For example, DLMO in a healthy sleeper with a habitual bedtime of 10:30 PM may be 8:30 PM, whereas DLMO in a patient with DSPD may be 1 AM, suggesting a habitual bedtime of 3 AM. In patients with ASPD, DLMO is significantly advanced as compared to healthy sleepers.[11,12] For example, a patient with ASPD may have a DLMO of 5 PM, suggesting a habitual bedtime of 7 PM. Given that melatonin secretion is suppressed by exposure to bright light, behavioral factors must be considered in the diagnosis of DSPD and ASPD. Late night activities among younger adults that include exposure to light, such as working on a computer or watching television in a brightly lit room, may contribute to the delayed circadian rhythm in patients with DSPD. Conversely, limited exposure to light in the evening due to decreased social activity among older adults and increased

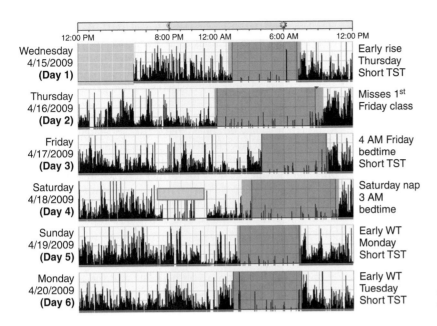

12:00 PM	8:00 PM	12:00 AM	6:00 AM	12:00 PM

Wednesday 4/15/2009 **(Day 1)** — Early rise Thursday Short TST

Thursday 4/16/2009 **(Day 2)** — Misses 1st Friday class

Friday 4/17/2009 **(Day 3)** — 4 AM Friday bedtime Short TST

Saturday 4/18/2009 **(Day 4)** — Saturday nap 3 AM bedtime

Sunday 4/19/2009 **(Day 5)** — Early WT Monday Short TST

Monday 4/20/2009 **(Day 6)** — Early WT Tuesday Short TST

Figure 31-2 An example of actigraphy data from a patient with delayed sleep phase disorder (DSPD). TST, total sleep time; WT, wake time.

early morning light exposure because of difficulty maintaining sleep may contribute to the advanced circadian rhythm in patients with ASPD.

Polysomnography

Polysomnography is not indicated in the diagnosis of DSPD or ASPD.[4] However, polysomnography can be useful in the differential diagnosis to rule out other sleep disorders that may present with similar symptoms. For example, excessive daytime sleepiness suggestive of DSPD or difficulty remaining awake in the evening suggestive of ASPD may be in part due to obstructive sleep apnea (OSA) or periodic limb movement disorder.

NONDIAGNOSTIC ASSOCIATED CLINICAL FEATURES

Although not utilized in diagnosis, certain associated clinical features have been examined with respect to DSPD and ASPD. For example, research has examined chronotype or "morningness/eveningness" in the development of DSPD and ASPD. Recent research has also focused on genetic factors that may contribute to the development of DSPD and ASPD. Finally, differences in phase angle have been implicated in relation to DSPD, ASPD, and psychological disorders.

Chronotype

Initially described by Horne and Östberg,[13] chronotype refers to individual differences in timing of peak physical activity, alertness, and other physiologic functions throughout the day. Individuals who show a preference for earlier bedtimes and wake times and demonstrate highest levels of activity and alertness earlier in the day are referred to as morning-types, or "larks." Individuals who show a preference for later bedtimes and wake times and show greatest activity and alertness later in the day are referred to as evening-types, or "owls." Indicated as an option in the diagnosis of DSPD and ASPD, the Morningness-Eveningness Questionnaire (MEQ)[13] is a subjective assessment of chronotype. The MEQ includes self-report

questions that ask respondents about their desired sleep-wake habits and preferred or most productive time for completing activities (e.g., exercise, cognitive challenges). Higher scores are indicative of a morning type, and lower scores are indicative of an evening type. MEQ scores have been shown to correlate with objective markers of circadian phase.[13,14]

Genetic Factors

Recent research has identified several genes implicated in the circadian timekeeping system and the development of circadian rhythm sleep disorders. Of particular relevance to the development of DSPD and ASPD are the *Per3* and *Per2* genes, respectively. *Per3* gene length has been found to correlate with morningness and eveningness as assessed with the MEQ.[15] Specifically, the longer allele of *Per3* is significantly associated with morningness while the shorter allele is significantly associated with eveningness. Furthermore, a diagnosis of DSPD is highly correlated with being homozygous with the shorter allele.[15] In contrast, in a prospective study of participants selected by *Per3* polymorphism, markers of circadian phase were not statistically different between those with 4/4 versus 5/5 polymorphism of *Per3*. However, participants with the 5/5 *Per3* polymorphism did demonstrate shorter sleep onset latency and greater percentage of slow wave sleep, as compared to those with the 4/4 *Per3* polymorphism,[16] suggestive of a role of *Per3* in regulation of sleep homeostasis and not merely the circadian system.[17] *Per2* has been implicated in ASPD. In a study of three families with ASPD, Jones and associates found that a mutation in *Per2* was found in those family members affected with ASPD and absent in those unaffected.[11]

Phase Angle Disorders

Circadian phase angle is defined as the relationship between two or more circadian markers, such as DLMO, cortisol secretion, and midpoint of the sleep period. A larger phase angle indicates that the two markers are more "out of phase" with each other; that is, at a particular point in time, one marker may be closer to its peak level while the other marker maybe closer to its nadir level. A smaller phase angle indicates that the two markers are more "in phase" with each other. Phase angle has been found to be associated with a variety of outcomes. For example, a larger phase angle between DLMO and cortisol secretion has been found among patients with major depressive disorder as compared to nondepressed control subjects.[18] In addition, recent studies suggest that a smaller phase angle between DLMO and the midpoint of the sleep period is associated with mood disorders.[19] An abnormality of phase angle between ambulatory (and hence, masked) core body temperature and the habitual sleep schedule has been reported,[20] but a more recent publication failed to find any difference in phase angle between laboratory assessment of DLMO on three separate assessments and sleep timing in DSPD patients relative to normal-sleeping control subjects.[9]

TREATMENT OF DELAYED SLEEP PHASE DISORDER

Chronotherapy

In 1981, Czeisler and colleagues[21] proposed chronotherapy, the first treatment for DSPD. They reported on a series of five patients who had a history of symptoms for longer than 4 years. The authors hypothesized that because the patients had a delayed-but-stable timing of their sleep episode, they must have had a circadian system capable of entraining to the 24-hour light-dark cycle; patients with DSPD were thought to be capable of the small phase advance required each day to adapt to a 24-hour light-dark cycle despite having an intrinsic period ("tau") slightly longer than 24 hours. However, it was hypothesized that the patients could not accomplish the extra phase advancing required to move their delayed sleep episode to an earlier hour. Note that this observation was made prior to the demonstration of the phase shifting effect of artificial bright light in humans. In normal sleepers the "range of entrainment," or the ability of the circadian system to adjust the sleep-wake schedule to non-24-hour sleep-wake cycles, was suggested to range from 23 to 27 hours[22]. Hence, the rationale for chronotherapy was that patients with DSPD could take advantage of tau being longer than 24 hours, and the range of entrainment in normal sleepers allowing adaptation for up to 27 hours. Thus "chronotherapy" involved scheduling the patients with DSPD to a 3-hour progressive delay in the sleep-wake schedule each sleep-wake cycle until they had rotated their schedule to the desired timing. Four patients were treated in the laboratory and one was treated in his home. Following treatment, patients kept sleep diaries and were educated about the need to adhere strictly to the new sleep schedule and to avoid napping. Follow-up data showed very good maintenance of treatment gain.

Intermittent case reports have been published in the intervening years, though typically as part of multicomponent treatments. Ito and colleagues[23] reported successful treatment in three patients with DSPD with chronotherapy alone and in three patients with chronotherapy followed by triazolam. In 1-year follow-up, all six patients showed some degree of return of symptoms.

Czeisler and colleagues[21] also suggested that phase advance chronotherapy might also be an effective treatment for DSPD, by shifting the sleep-wake schedule 15 minutes earlier per day.

However, this treatment approach was not utilized in their early report. Two decades later Yanagida and colleagues[24] reported on a 19-year-old female with DSPD, who had previously failed phototherapy, being treated with chronotherapy with a 1-hour advance of her sleep schedule per week.

There has been a report of free-running disorder developing after chronotherapy for DSPD in three patients.[25] Although this may be considered a risk associated with chronotherapy, there have been other case reports of patients who may alternate between DSPD and free-running symptoms,[26,27] thus highlighting the need for further research into the potential overlap between these two circadian rhythm sleep disorders. There is also a case report of failure of multiple attempts at chronotherapy in a case of DSPD following a closed head injury,[28] further supporting the need for more research into the pathophysiology of this disorder and the possibility of multiple causal factors.

Given the paucity of published data and the low levels of evidence, the American Academy of Sleep Medicine (AASM) has ranked chronotherapy, as a form of sleep scheduling, an "option" in the recent standard of practice paper.[5,29] We have also speculated that the mechanism of action for chronotherapy is unknown, and that it is unlikely that the circadian system successfully phase delays 3 hours each day with only manipulation of the sleep-wake schedule without precise application of phototherapy.[30]

Phototherapy

Although it had been shown in a mammal in 1960 that exposure to artificial bright light could shift the circadian system earlier or later depending on time of exposure relative to the rest-activity cycle,[31] it took until the 1980s to demonstrate this same phase shifting effect of light in the human, and that this phase shifting effect was independent of the timing of the sleep-wake cycle.[32,33] Subsequently there have been multiple publications showing the shift in circadian phase to bright light exposure (phototherapy) and the dependence on the timing of light exposure relative to circadian phase.[34-36] A consistent finding is that light exposure following the trough of core body temperature (approximately 1.5-3 hours prior to routine wake time) results in a circadian phase advance. This is important for understanding the optimal timing of phototherapy to phase advance the circadian system in DPSD patients. However, it is also important to appreciate that light exposure in the late evening and early nighttime hours will phase delay the circadian system. Thus, regardless of treatment option used in DSPD, it is important for the patient to avoid significant light exposure several hours prior to bedtime, lest an inadvertent phase delay be promoted.

The classic report of phototherapy treatment for DSPD was published by Rosenthal and colleagues[37] in 1990. Twenty patients with DSPD were studied in a crossover design. The active treatment consisted of exposure to 2500 lux of light for a 2-hour interval between 6 AM and 9 AM and light-attenuating goggles worn from 4 PM until after sundown. The control condition consisted of exposure to 300 lux of light for the same 2-hour interval between 6 AM and 9 AM, and goggles that did not attenuate light were worn, also from 4 PM until after sundown. Each treatment lasted 2 weeks and was separated by a washout delay until relapse. The active condition produced a 1 hour 25 minute advance of the core body temperature rhythm, as opposed to a 10-minute advance in the control condition. Though statistically significant for the active condition, this degree of phase advance is unlikely to be clinically significant for a patient whose circadian system and sleep schedule may be delayed by many hours. Further, the core body temperature assessments were conducted in the presence of sleep episodes and multiple sleep latency testing, thus introducing significant confounding influences to the circadian phase assessment from core body temperature. Finally, it is possible that the timing of light exposure may have been prior to the trough of core body temperature for many of the patients; thus some may have phase advanced and lowered the overall group mean effect.

Watanabe and colleagues[38] reported on phototherapy treatment for six patients with DSPD. Though light intensity was not stated, the report does document that a 3-hour pulse of light was delivered starting 1.5 hours after the minimum of core body temperature (collected under ambulatory and hence masked conditions). Treatment lasted for 5 days. Sleep onset was advanced by 1 hour 25 minutes and morning awakening was advanced by 3 hours 17 minutes. Core temperature was also said to have advanced, but the data are not reported in this paper.

Phototherapy treatment for DSPD has also been tested in delivery via a bright light mask[39] producing 2700 lux of white light in the active condition, and only 0.1 lux in the control condition. Over a 26-day treatment phase, participants wore the mask during sleep episodes. The mask was programmed to increase illumination progressively starting 4 hours prior to scheduled wake-up time, increased to full intensity over the first hour, and remained at full intensity for the next 3 hours until scheduled wake-up time. As part of both treatment arms, the sleep-wake schedule was advanced by approximately 1 hour or more per week. The authors reported that they estimated that only 57 lux of light reached the surface of the eye after attenuation by the eyelid, and hence, per the dose response curve for light[40,41] one would not expect significant phase shifting relative to the more typically light levels (thousands of lux) typically used in these experiments. Consistent with this limitation, the results failed to show a treatment effect of the active treatment relative to the control condition. A subset of patients in each treatment condition even phase delayed during the home treatment. However, a subset in the active condition who had a more pronounced phase delay at baseline (as measured by urinary 6-sulfatoxymelatonin collected in 2-hour intervals only during wakefulness) advanced by 1 hour 38 minutes in the active condition versus only 29 minutes in the control condition.

Though publications of phototherapy treatment for DSPD are limited in number, given the higher evidence levels based on the sophistication of the methodology the AASM has recommended that phototherapy is indicated as treatment at the "guideline" level.[5,29]

Melatonin

Many treatment studies in DSPD address the efficacy of exogenous melatonin. Like light, exogenous melatonin can phase shift the circadian system according to a phase response curve (PRC).[42-45] However, the effect is nearly opposite that found with light: maximal phase advancing from melatonin administration comes from afternoon dosing (approximately 5 hours prior to the DLMO) and maximal phase delay

region coincides with morning awakening or just after (approximately 11 hours after DLMO).[42] Thus, for DSPD, optimal administration would occur 5 hours prior to DLMO. DLMO has been reported to occur, on average, 11 hours prior to habitual wake time in DSPD patients.[9] Though DLMO does not correlate as well with bedtime as it does with wake time, DLMO typically occurs approximately 2.5 hours prior to bedtime.[46] Thus, for maximal phase advancing in DSPD, melatonin would be administered approximately 7.5 hours prior to habitual bedtime. This risks sleepiness during the wake episode, however, as melatonin will suppress the wake-promoting drive from the circadian system (as reviewed by Wyatt and associates[47]) in addition to its phase shifting effect. Patients should also be advised to avoid sleepiness-sensitive activities (e.g., driving or operating machinery) in the interval between dosing and bedtime. Further, the optimal protocol would be to measure DLMO to have an objective circadian phase marker, in order to map the timing of exogenous melatonin to the phase response curve for melatonin.

A 1991 publication by Dahlitz and colleagues[48] reports the effects of 4 weeks' treatment with 5 mg melatonin or placebo given 5 hours prior to habitual sleep onset time in eight patients with DSPD in a double-blind, randomized, crossover design. The melatonin condition showed an 82-minute advance of sleep onset and a 117-minute advance of wake time relative to the placebo condition. It was noted that a return of the phase delay typically began within 2 days of stopping the melatonin, suggesting a lack of durability of the treatment effect or that melatonin administration would have to be a long-term treatment. Also relative to the information on the melatonin PRC given previously, the timing of melatonin administration was suboptimal in this report.

Administration of 5 mg melatonin has also been reported to advance sleep onset by nearly 2 hours after 1 month of treatment.[49] However, in this case series, there was no placebo control, no blinding, and the time of melatonin administration was fixed in the 5 PM to 7 PM window based on estimation of when DLMO would have occurred, itself based on the self-reported sleep onset times of the six patients. As with the previous study, this 1994 publication did not optimize the timing of melatonin administration for the maximal phase advance.

Nagtegaal and colleagues[50] administered 5 mg melatonin or placebo 5 hours prior to measured DLMO in a group of 25 patients with DSPD in a double-blind, crossover study. Though treatment lasted only 2 weeks per condition, there was a significant advance of sleep onset assessed via actigraphy, and DLMO was advanced 1 hour 38 minutes. However, core body temperature was not advanced and the offset of nocturnal melatonin was not advanced, leading the authors to posit that circadian advance may not have occurred, and that the efficacy of melatonin may have been due to a sleep-promoting effect of melatonin. This group subsequently reported significant improvement on most scales of a standard questionnaire assessing quality of life in patients with DSPD treated with melatonin administration.[51]

A relatively large group of 61 patients with DSPD were treated with 5 mg melatonin taken at a fixed time, 10 PM, for 6 weeks.[52] Objective measures of treatment response were not presented, nor was there a control condition. However, 97% of the patients reported positive effect of melatonin treatment in a questionnaire sent to them 12 to 18 months after treatment. Interestingly, as with the Dahlitz and associates paper,[48] relapse was high after melatonin discontinuation, with 29% having relapse within 1 week and 92% having relapse within 1 year. In a group of 20 patients given 5 mg of melatonin or placebo in the 7 PM to 9 PM window for 4 weeks in a double-blind crossover design, melatonin was associated with a significant decrease in sleep latency in sleep episodes restricted to the midnight to 8 AM window.[53]

Mundey and colleagues,[54] in one of the most recent clinical trials of melatonin administration, examined two doses of melatonin, 0.3 mg and 3.0 mg, relative to placebo for treatment of DSPD. They also varied the timing of melatonin administration, ranging from 6.5 hours to 1.5 hours prior to measured DLMO. The study does not appear to be powered to detect a difference between the two doses of melatonin, and the authors collapsed the data across the melatonin conditions. Sleep onset time did not advance significantly, but DLMO advanced by 1.75 hours and core body temperature by 1.63 hours after 4 weeks of treatment. The results suggested that earlier administration of melatonin was associated with larger phase advances of DLMO, consistent with the predictions of the PRC for melatonin.

In contrast to the treatment failure of chronotherapy in post-traumatic DSPD noted earlier, there is a report of successful treatment with 5 mg of melatonin prior to measured nocturnal onset in a teenage girl with DSPD following a closed head injury.[55]

To summarize this section, there are a number of publications on melatonin administration for DSPD. Many have shown improvements in sleep latency or advancement of sleep onset time or DLMO. However, when measured, relapse tends to occur very soon after treatment is discontinued, and several authors have questioned whether the phase advance observed, if any, was in fact responsible for earlier sleep onset times. This raises the possibility that some degree of treatment efficacy comes from the demonstrated circadian phase–dependent hypnotic property of melatonin.[47,56-59] Based on the strength of the publications reviewed by the expert panel, the AASM recommended that melatonin is indicated for treatment of DSPD at the "guideline" level.

Vitamin B$_{12}$

In 1983, there was a published case report from the National Institutes of Health of a patient with a DSPD history but who later developed symptoms of free-running disorder.[60] This patient failed multiple treatments including thyroxin administration for suspected "partially compensated hypothyroidism." According to the publication, the patient later self-medicated with vitamin B$_{12}$, based on reports of deficiency of vitamin B$_{12}$ in hypothyroidism. Per his self-report, he was able to phase advance his sleep-wake schedule and even develop a consistent sleep schedule. Subsequently, there was a case report of vitamin B$_{12}$ supplementation improving symptoms in a 55-year-old patient who had DSPD symptoms since age 18[61] and in a 15-year-old girl with DSPD.[62] In a multisite, placebo-controlled, double-blind study, 27 patients with DSPD received vitamin B$_{12}$ and 23 ingested placebo for 4 weeks, three times a day after meals.[63] In contrast to a previous open-label trial,[64] this study failed to document improvement in clinical symptoms or sleep diary variables. Given these findings, the AASM did not recommend vitamin B$_{12}$ as a treatment for DSPD.[29]

Combination Treatments

There have been a variety of cases reports and case series publications reporting on multicomponent treatments for DSPD.[65,66] Given the inability to attribute treatment efficacy to individual treatment components and the relatively small samples, combination treatment studies will not be discussed in this chapter. However, it may be noted that combination treatments have shown robust effects in other areas of sleep medicine, such as multicomponent cognitive-behavioral treatment for insomnia, or stimulant medication and scheduled napping in narcolepsy.

TREATMENT OF ADVANCED SLEEP PHASE DISORDER

Chronotherapy

Moldofsky and colleagues[67] reported the case of a 62-year-old man with ASPD, who had a habitual bedtime of 6:30 PM and a wake time of 3 AM. Every 2 days, his sleep schedule was advanced by 3 hours, allowing him to maintain an 11 PM to 6 AM sleep schedule, as verified at follow-up 5 months later. Complicating the case was a significant history of depression, a significantly reduced latency to rapid eye movement (REM) sleep, and untreated OSA. Given the paucity of published data and the lack of sophisticated clinical trials, the AASM has given chronotherapy as a form of sleep scheduling an indication as a treatment for ASPD, but only at the option level.[29]

Phototherapy

Given the circadian phase advance thought to underlie ASPD, phototherapy given in the early evening hours, prior to the trough of core body temperature, would presumably phase delay the circadian system. Unfortunately, most of the phototherapy publications in this area have focused on older adults with a complaint of insomnia, many of whom have been diagnosed with primary insomnia instead of ASPD. Thus, the AASM has recommended that phototherapy is indicated for the treatment of ASPD, but only at the option level.[29] Results have also been conflicting. Campbell and colleagues[68] reported improvement in wake after sleep onset and increased stage 2, slow wave sleep, and REM sleep in a group of 16 older adults with sleep maintenance insomnia treated with evening phototherapy for 12 days. In 2002, however, the same investigator failed to replicate the result in a similar experiment, noting that the smaller circadian phase delay and lack of improvement in sleep may have been related to less extensive adherence monitoring.[69] Exposure to increased light levels for 2 to 3 hours in the evening for nearly a month failed to show a delay in circadian phase but did mildly improve subjective symptoms in a group of ASPD patients,[70] though the intensity of evening light exposure was relatively low (approximately 265 lux) and may have been insufficient to produce a robust phase delay.

Consideration must also be given to prevention of bright light exposure during the phase advance region of the PRC to light. It has been reported that compared to younger adults, older adults are exposed to brighter light during the daytime hours, including in the first 8 hours after awakening.[71] Older adults also have more difficulty sleeping past the circadian phase position of the trough of core body temperature, and hence awaken at an earlier circadian phase corresponding to the maximal phase advance region of the PRC to light.[72] Thus, it is possible that this exposure to brighter light levels may maintain a phase advance in older adults in general, not merely in patients with ASPD. Prevention of exposure to light in the phase advance region of the PRC may eventually be found to be a key component in any treatment of ASPD.

Melatonin

Though the AASM has recommended melatonin administration as an indicated treatment for ASPD at the option level,[29] it has been pointed out that this is recommended despite a lack of an evidence base.[73] A follow-up letter clarified that perhaps the practice parameter should have refrained from recommending melatonin for ASPD, even though there was consensus of opinion from the expert panel that the melatonin PRC provided guidance on the timing of melatonin administration to achieve a phase delay in this clinical population.[74]

Summary

Much has been learned over the past three decades about the human circadian system and its influence on the timing of sleep and wakefulness. However, the mechanisms of pathophysiology for DSPD and ASPD remain elusive. Genetic studies have started to be applied to these circadian disorders, but findings are preliminary and clearly genetic variation alone is unlikely to explain the full pathophysiology of either disorder. Phase angle between sleep and the circadian system might be abnormal in DSPD, for example, thus lowering confidence in being able to trust proxy measures of DLMO, such as habitual wake time. However, much of the data suggesting a phase relationship abnormality in DSPD has come from flawed designs, such as ambulatory collection of core body temperature with sleep episodes allowed, as opposed to more precise measurement under constant routine conditions.[75] There are relatively simple methods for measuring circadian phase, such as the DLMO, yet phase is not routinely measured in either disorder due to the lack of reimbursement and the fact that most sleep clinicians lack expertise in collecting or analyzing these data. Insurance companies are unlikely to endorse reimbursement for measuring DLMO as a diagnosis tool or to time administration of melatonin or phototherapy until there is an increase in the level of evidence demonstrating that measuring DLMO affects diagnostic precision, treatment planning, or response to treatment.

Much has been learned about the impact of sleep scheduling, phototherapy, and melatonin administration on sleep and circadian phase in normal sleepers. Much less is known about the strengths and weaknesses of these interventions as treatment options for DSPD and ASPD. The result has been lukewarm indications for these treatments, based on comprehensive review of the literature. In short, significant basic and clinical research is required in these disorders, at levels from genetics, through pharmacology and systems neurobiology, up to the psychological and social factors that may play important roles in the development, maintenance, and treatment of these two circadian rhythm sleep disorders.

REFERENCES

1. American Academy of Sleep Medicine. *International Classification of Sleep Disorders. Diagnostic and Coding Manual.* 2nd ed. Westchester, IL: American Academy of Sleep Medicine; 2005.
2. Carskadon MA, Wolfson AR, Acebo C, Tzischinsky O, Seifer R. Adolescent sleep patterns, circadian timing, and sleepiness at a transition to early school days. *Sleep.* 1998;21:871-881.
3. Duffy JF, Zeitzer JM, Rimmer DW, Klerman EB, Dijk DJ, Czeisler CA. Peak of circadian melatonin rhythm occurs later within the sleep of older subjects. *Am J Physiol Endocrinol Metab.* 2002;282:E297-E303.
4. Morgenthaler TI, Lee-Chiong T, Alessi C, et al. Practice parameters for the clinical evaluation and treatment of circadian rhythm sleep disorders. An American Academy of Sleep Medicine report. *Sleep.* 2007;30:1445-1459.
5. Sack RL, Auckley D, Auger RR, et al. Circadian rhythm sleep disorders: Part II. Advanced sleep phase disorder, delayed sleep phase disorder, free-running disorder, and irregular sleep-wake rhythm. An American Academy of Sleep Medicine review. *Sleep.* 2007;30:1484-1501.
6. Sack RL, Auckley D, Auger RR, et al. Circadian rhythm sleep disorders: Part I. Basic principles, shift work and jet lag disorders. An American Academy of Sleep Medicine review. *Sleep.* 2007;30:1460-1483.
7. Lewy AJ, Sack RL. The dim light melatonin onset as a marker for circadian phase position. *Chronobiol Int.* 1989;6:93-102.
8. Burgess HJ, Savic N, Sletten T, Roach G, Gilbert SS, Dawson D. The relationship between the dim light melatonin onset and sleep on a regular schedule in young healthy adults. *Behav Sleep Med.* 2003;1:102-114.
9. Wyatt JK, Stepanski EJ, Kirkby J. Circadian phase in delayed sleep phase syndrome: Predictors and temporal stability across multiple assessments. *Sleep.* 2006;29:1075-1080.
10. Wright Jr KP, Gronfier C, Duffy JF, Czeisler CA. Intrinsic period and light intensity determine the phase relationship between melatonin and sleep in humans. *J Biol Rhythms.* 2005;20:168-177.
11. Jones CR, Campbell SS, Zone SE, et al. Familial advanced sleep-phase syndrome: A short-period circadian rhythm variant in humans. *Nat Med.* 1999;5:1062-1065.
12. Satoh K, Mishima K, Inoue Y, Ebisawa T, Shimizu T. Two pedigrees of familial advanced sleep phase syndrome in Japan. *Sleep.* 2003;26:416-417.
13. Horne JA, Östberg O. A self-assessment questionnaire to determine morningness-eveningness in human circadian rhythms. *Int J Chronobiol.* 1976;4:97-110.
14. Taillard J, Philip P, Chastang JF, Bioulac B. Validation of Horne and Ostberg morningness-eveningness questionnaire in a middle-aged population of French workers. *J Biol Rhythms.* 2004;19:76-86.
15. Archer SN, Robilliard DL, Skene DJ, et al. A length polymorphism in the circadian clock gene Per3 is linked to delayed sleep phase syndrome and extreme diurnal preference. *Sleep.* 2003;26:413-415.
16. Viola AU, Archer SN, James LM, et al. PER3 polymorphism predicts sleep structure and waking performance. *Curr Biol.* 2007;17:613-618.
17. Dijk DJ, Archer SN. PERIOD3, circadian phenotypes, and sleep homeostasis. *Sleep Med Rev.* 2010;14:151-160.
18. Buckley TM, Schatzberg AF. A pilot study of the phase angle between cortisol and melatonin in major depression—A potential biomarker? *J Psychiatr Res.* 2010;44:69-74.
19. Lewy AJ. Circadian misalignment in mood disturbances. *Curr Psychiatry Rep.* 2009;11:459-465.
20. Ozaki S, Uchiyama M, Shirakawa S, Okawa M. Prolonged interval from body temperature nadir to sleep offset in patients with delayed sleep phase syndrome. *Sleep.* 1996;19:36-40.
21. Czeisler CA, Richardson GS, Coleman RM, et al. Chronotherapy: Resetting the circadian clocks of patients with delayed sleep phase insomnia. *Sleep.* 1981;4:1-21.
22. Wever R. *The Circadian System of Man.* New York: Springer-Verlag; 1979.
23. Ito A, Ando K, Hayakawa T, et al. Long-term course of adult patients with delayed sleep phase syndrome. *Jpn J Psychiatry Neurol.* 1993;47:563-567.
24. Yanagida H, Nakajima T, Kajimura N, et al. Physical symptoms under forced-phase advance treatment in a patient with delayed sleep phase syndrome: A case report. *Psychiatry Clin Neurosci.* 2002;56:219-220.
25. Oren DA, Wehr TA. Hypernyctohemeral syndrome after chronotherapy for delayed sleep phase syndrome. *N Engl J Med.* 1992;327:1762.
26. Boivin DB, Caliyurt O, James FO, Chalk C. Association between delayed sleep phase and hypernyctohemeral syndromes: A case study. *Sleep.* 2004;27:417-421.
27. Mukai M, Uchimura N, Takeuchi N, et al. Therapeutic progress of two sibling cases exhibiting sleep-wake rhythm disorder. *Psychiatry Clin Neurosci.* 2000;54:354-355.

28. Patten SB, Lauderdale WM. Delayed sleep phase disorder after traumatic brain injury. *J Am Acad Child Adolesc Psychiatry*. 1992;31:100-102.

29. Morgenthaler TI, Lee-Chiong T, Alessi C, et al. Practice parameters for the clinical evaluation and treatment of circadian rhythm sleep disorders. An American Academy of Sleep Medicine report. *Sleep*. 2007;30(11): 1445-1459.

30. Wyatt JK. Delayed sleep phase syndrome: Pathophysiology and treatment options. *Sleep*. 2004;27:1195-1203.

31. De Coursey PJ. Daily light sensitivity rhythm in a rodent. *Science*. 1960;131:33-35.

32. Czeisler CA, Richardson GS, Zimmerman JC, Moore-Ede MC, Weitzman ED. Entrainment of human circadian rhythms by light-dark cycles: A reassessment. *Photochem Photobiol*. 1981;34:239-247.

33. Czeisler CA, Allan JS, Strogatz SH, et al. Bright light resets the human circadian pacemaker independent of the timing of the sleep-wake cycle. *Science*. 1986;233:667-671.

34. Honma K, Honma S. A human phase response curve for bright light pulses. *Jpn J Psychiatry Neurol*. 1988;42:167-168.

35. Minors DS, Waterhouse JM, Wirz-Justice A. A human phase-response curve to light. *Neurosci Lett*. 1991;133:36-40.

36. Khalsa SB, Jewett ME, Cajochen C, Czeisler CA. A phase response curve to single bright light pulses in human subjects. *J Physiol*. 2003;549: 945-952.

37. Rosenthal NE, Joseph-Vanderpool JR, Levendosky AA, et al. Phase-shifting effects of bright morning light as treatment for delayed sleep phase syndrome. *Sleep*. 1990;13:354-361.

38. Watanabe T, Kajimura N, Kato M, Sekimoto M, Takahashi K. Effects of phototherapy in patients with delayed sleep phase syndrome. *Psychiatry Clin Neurosci*. 1999;53:231-233.

39. Cole RJ, Smith JS, Alcala YC, Elliott JA, Kripke DF. Bright-light mask treatment of delayed sleep phase syndrome. *J Biol Rhythms*. 2002;17: 89-101.

40. Boivin DB, Duffy JF, Kronauer RE, Czeisler CA. Sensitivity of the human circadian pacemaker to moderately bright light. *J Biol Rhythms*. 1994;9:315-331.

41. Boivin DB, Duffy JF, Kronauer RE, Czeisler CA. Dose-response relationships for resetting of human circadian clock by light. *Nature*. 1996;379:540-542.

42. Burgess HJ, Revell VL, Eastman CI. A three pulse phase response curve to three milligrams of melatonin in humans. *J Physiol*. 2008;586:639-647.

43. Burgess HJ, Revell VL, Molina TA, Eastman CI. Human phase response curves to three days of daily melatonin: 0.5 mg versus 3.0 mg. *J Clin Endocrinol Metab*. 2010;95:3325-3331.

44. Lewy AJ, Ahmed S, Jackson JML, Sack RL. Melatonin shifts human circadian rhythms according to a phase-response curve. *Chronobiol Int*. 1992;9:380-392.

45. Lewy AJ, Bauer VK, Ahmed S, et al. The human phase response curve (PRC) to melatonin is about 12 hours out of phase with the PRC to light. *Chronobiol Int*. 1998;15:71-83.

46. Burgess HJ, Eastman CI. The dim light melatonin onset following fixed and free sleep schedules. *J Sleep Res*. 2005;14:229-237.

47. Wyatt JK, Dijk DJ, Ritz-De Cecco A, Ronda JM, Czeisler CA. Sleep facilitating effect of exogenous melatonin in healthy young men and women is circadian-phase dependent. *Sleep*. 2006;29:609-618.

48. Dahlitz M, Alvarez B, Vignau J, English J, Arendt J, Parkes JD. Delayed sleep phase syndrome response to melatonin. *Lancet*. 1991;337: 1121-1124.

49. Oldani A, Ferini-Strambi L, Zucconi M, Stankov B, Fraschini F, Smirne S. Melatonin and delayed sleep phase syndrome: Ambulatory polygraphic evaluation. *Neuroreport*. 1994;6:132-134.

50. Nagtegaal JE, Kerkhof GA, Smits MG, Swart AC, van der Meer YG. Delayed sleep phase syndrome: A placebo-controlled cross-over study on the effects of melatonin administered five hours before the individual dim light melatonin onset. *J Sleep Res*. 1998;7:135-143.

51. Nagtegaal JE, Laurant MW, Kerkhof GA, Smits MG, van der Meer YG, Coenen AM. Effects of melatonin on the quality of life in patients with delayed sleep phase syndrome. *J Psychosom Res*. 2000;48:45-50.

52. Dagan Y, Yovel I, Hallis D, Eisenstein M, Raichik I. Evaluating the role of melatonin in the long-term treatment of delayed sleep phase syndrome (DSPS). *Chronobiol Int*. 1998;15:181-190.

53. Kayumov L, Brown G, Jindal R, Buttoo K, Shapiro CM. A randomized, double-blind, placebo-controlled crossover study of the effect of exogenous melatonin on delayed sleep phase syndrome. *Psychosom Med*. 2001;63:40-48.

54. Mundey K, Benloucif S, Harsanyi K, Dubocovich ML, Zee PC. Phase-dependent treatment of delayed sleep phase syndrome with melatonin. *Sleep*. 2005;28:1271-1278.

55. Nagtegaal JE, Kerkhof GA, Smits MG, Swart AC, van der Meer YG. Traumatic brain injury-associated delayed sleep phase syndrome. *Funct Neurol*. 1997;12:345-348.

56. Tzischinsky O, Lavie P. Melatonin possesses time-dependent hypnotic effects. *Sleep*. 1994;17:638-645.

57. Shochat T, Luboshitzky R, Lavie P. Nocturnal melatonin onset is phase locked to the primary sleep gate. *Am J Physiol*. 1997;273:R364-R370.

58. Cajochen C, Krauchi K, Wirz-Justice A. Role of melatonin in the regulation of human circadian rhythms and sleep. *J Neuroendocrinol*. 2003;15:432-437.

59. Sack RL, Hughes RJ, Edgar DM, Lewy AJ. Sleep-promoting effects of melatonin: At what dose, in whom, under what conditions, and by what mechanisms? *Sleep*. 1997;20:908-915.

60. Kamgar-Parsi B, Wehr TA, Gillin JC. Successful treatment of human non-24-hour sleep-wake syndrome. *Sleep*. 1983;6:257-264.

61. Okawa M, Mishima K, Nanami T, et al. Vitamin B_{12} treatment for sleep-wake rhythm disorders. *Sleep*. 1990;13:15-23.

62. Ohta T, Ando K, Iwata T, et al. Treatment of persistent sleep-wake schedule disorders in adolescents with methylcobalamin (vitamin B_{12}). *Sleep*. 1991;14:414-418.

63. Okawa M, Takahashi K, Egashira K, et al. Vitamin B_{12} treatment for delayed sleep phase syndrome: A multi-center double-blind study. *Psychiatry Clin Neurosci*. 1997;51:275-279.

64. Yamadera H, Takahashi K, Okawa M. A multicenter study of sleep-wake rhythm disorders: Therapeutic effects of vitamin B_{12}, bright light therapy, chronotherapy and hypnotics. *Psychiatry Clin Neurosci*. 1996;50: 203-209.

65. Weyerbrock A, Timmer J, Hohagen F, Berger M, Bauer J. Effects of light and chronotherapy on human circadian rhythms in delayed sleep phase syndrome: Cytokines, cortisol, growth hormone, and the sleep-wake cycle. *Biol Psychiatry*. 1996;40:794-797.

66. Okawa M, Uchiyama M, Ozaki S, Shibui K, Ichikawa H. Circadian rhythm sleep disorders in adolescents: Clinical trials of combined treatments based on chronobiology. *Psychiatry Clin Neurosci*. 1998;52: 483-490.

67. Moldofsky H, Musisi S, Phillipson EA. Treatment of a case of advanced sleep phase syndrome by phase advance chronotherapy. *Sleep*. 1986;9: 61-65.

68. Campbell SS, Dawson D, Anderson MW. Alleviation of sleep maintenance insomnia with timed exposure to bright light. *J Am Geriatr Soc*. 1993;41:829-836.

69. Suhner AG, Murphy PJ, Campbell SS. Failure of timed bright light exposure to alleviate age-related sleep maintenance insomnia. *J Am Geriatr Soc*. 2002;50:617-623.

70. Palmer CR, Kripke DF, Savage Jr HC, Cindrich LA, Loving RT, Elliott JA. Efficacy of enhanced evening light for advanced sleep phase syndrome. *Behav Sleep Med*. 2003;1:213-226.

71. Scheuermaier K, Laffan AM, Duffy JF. Light exposure patterns in healthy older and young adults. *J Biol Rhythms*. 2010;25:113-122.

72. Duffy JF, Dijk DJ, Klerman EB, Czeisler CA. Later endogenous circadian temperature nadir relative to an earlier wake time in older people. *Am J Physiol*. 1998;275:R1478-R1487.

73. Zee PC. Melatonin for the treatment of advanced sleep phase disorder. *Sleep*. 2008;31:923.

74. Morgenthaler TI, Lee-Chiong T, Alessi C, et al. Response to Zee PC. Melatonin for the treatment of advanced sleep phase disorder. *Sleep*. 2008;31:925:[Sleep. 2008;31:923.].

75. Duffy JF, Dijk DJ. Getting through to circadian oscillators: Why use constant routines? *J Biol Rhythms*. 2002;17:4-13.

Other Circadian Rhythm Disorders:
Non-24-Hour Sleep-Wake Disorder and Irregular Sleep-Wake Disorder

STEVEN W. LOCKLEY / DANIEL COHEN / DAVID G. HARPER /
MAKOTO UCHIYAMA

In addition to advanced and delayed sleep phase disorders (see Chapter 31), shift work disorder (see Chapter 29), and jet lag disorder (see Chapter 30) the International Classification of Sleep Disorders (ICSD)[1] describes five other circadian rhythm sleep disorders (CRSDs): (1) nonentrained type; (2) irregular sleep-wake type; (3) CRSD due to a medical condition; (4) CRSD due to drug or substance use; and (5) CRSD due to reasons "not otherwise specified" (NOS). In this chapter, we will review what is understood about the etiology of these other CRSDs and review treatment possibilities where known. Readers are referred to Chapter 28 for a general overview of circadian organization in humans.

Non-24-Hour Sleep-Wake Syndrome in Sighted Patients

Definitions and Basic Description

"Circadian rhythm disorder, nonentrained type" is otherwise known as non-24-hour sleep-wake syndrome (N24HSWS), or sometimes "free-running type." The disorder is characterized by symptoms of insomnia or excessive sleepiness that occur because the endogenous circadian pacemaker is not synchronized to the 24-hour light-dark cycle and exhibits a non-24-hour period.[1] The sleep pattern of classical N24HSWS features a chronic steady pattern of approximately 1-hour delays in spontaneous sleep onset and wake times in individuals living under normal environmental conditions (Fig. 32-1). Other reports, however, have suggested that the nonentrained sleep may also exhibit other more variable patterns including a delayed and irregular sleep phase mingled with a nonentrained pattern lasting for several days,[2] a "scalloping" pattern consisting of predictable transitions between episodes of relatively advanced and delayed sleep sometimes with a series of larger "phase jumps,"[3,4] or sometimes an absence of a distinct nonentrained sleep pattern but with a clear non-24-hour pattern in strong markers of circadian phase such as melatonin or cortisol[2] (see later discussion of N24HSWS in totally blind patients).

Clinical Diagnostic Criteria

The formal diagnostic criteria are shown in Box 32-1. In practice, patients often exhibit cyclic episodes lasting several weeks or months in which they experience nocturnal insomnia and daytime sleepiness, followed by relatively good sleep, followed by bad sleep and so on due to the mismatch between their attempt to live on a 24-hour day and the internal non-24-hour circadian clock period. The cyclic nature of these symptoms is sometimes not recognized, leading to a delay in diagnosis or a misdiagnosis and inappropriate treatment. For example, if the period of the circadian pacemaker is close to 24 hours, the episodes of good and bad sleep will be long and will not appear cyclic (see later discussion), sometimes resulting in a misdiagnosis of insomnia and inappropriate treatment with stimulants and hypnotics. As noted, some patients do not always exhibit cyclic sleep disorders despite an underlying nonentrained circadian pacemaker. Nocturnal activities related to lifestyle preference can contribute to a nonentrained rhythm as well as to misdiagnosis. For example, indiscriminate light exposure at night from computer and video game use by adolescents, the most at-risk group for this disorder, can lead to an incorrect diagnosis of insomnia related to Inadequate Sleep Hygiene (see Chapters 10 and 11).

Demographics

N24HSWS is a rare condition in sighted individuals, although there have been a considerable number of reports,[4-6] with a recent review indicating that the disorder may be more common than previously thought in individuals in their teens and twenties.[6] The basic clinical characteristics of this disorder in sighted patients remain to be elucidated. It appears to be more prevalent in males (4:1 ratio) and the onset of the nonentrained sleep pattern tends to occur when patients are in their teens or twenties. Virtually all patients have a history of disturbed social functioning due to inability to attend school or work regularly. A quarter of patients also have a psychiatric disorder, with reports of N24HSWS preceded by schizophrenia, bipolar disorder, depression, obsessive-compulsive disorder, or schizoid personality. Although it is possible that a common neural deficit causes psychiatric symptoms and an inability to be entrained by light, it is more likely that social isolation and the nonuniform or erratic day-night behavior associated with some of these disorders could induce N24HSWS as a result of repeated exposure to inappropriately timed light-dark patterns. A minority of N24HSWS patients may exhibit delayed sleep phase disorder (DSPD) prior to developing a nonentrained sleep pattern, suggesting these two disorders may share a common pathology, or that the abnormal timing of light exposure in *response* to a delayed sleep-wake rhythm systematically promotes repetitive phase delays. The adolescent onset of N24HSWS, an age at which the circadian pacemaker naturally delays (see Chapter 31), also supports this idea.

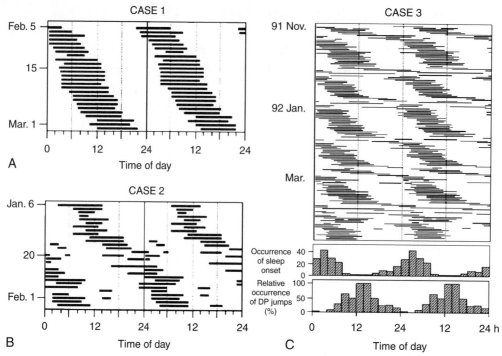

Figure 32-1 Non-24-hour sleep-wake syndrome in three sighted patients. This figure shows the sleep-wake patterns in three sighted patients with non-24-hour sleep-wake syndrome: a 26-year-old female (Case 1), a 22-year-old male (Case 2), and a 30-year-old male (Case 3). Sleep times (■) are double-plotted for clarity according to time of day (abscissa) and study day (ordinate). All three cases exhibit non-24-hour sleep-wake rhythms, although sleep tends to occur most during the night (e.g., Case 3, middle panel), reflecting the fact that most patients generally attempt to live on a 24-hour social day. Case 1 clearly exhibits a non-24-hour sleep rhythm (24.8 hours), which remains relatively consistent. Case 2 exhibits a 24.7 sleep rhythm on average, although the rhythm becomes more disrupted for about a week around January 20. This change in rhythmicity is more clearly illustrated in Case 3, who has episodes of regularly free-running sleep (24.6 hours) interspersed regularly (about every 4 weeks) with episodes in which the sleep pattern delays more quickly and becomes more disrupted. These "delay phase jumps" occur at a particular circadian phase (Case 3, lower panel) and are similar to those seen in studies of subjects living in temporal isolation who have access to artificial light, and are most likely caused when light exposure occurs at a particular phase of the circadian cycle (Redrawn from Uchiyama M, Lockley SW. Non-24-hour sleep-wake syndrome in sighted and blind patients. *Sleep Med Clin.* 2009;4:195-211.)

BOX 32-1 *Diagnostic Criteria for Circadian Rhythm Sleep Disorder, Nonentrained Type*

A. There is a complaint of insomnia or excessive sleepiness related to abnormal synchronization between the 24-hour light-dark cycle and the endogenous circadian rhythm of sleep and wake propensity.
B. Sleep log or actigraphy monitoring (with sleep diaries) for at least 7 days demonstrates a pattern of sleep and wake times that typically delays each day with a period longer than 24 hours.
C. The sleep disturbance is not better explained by another current sleep disorder, medical or neurologic disorder, mental disorder, medication use, or substance use disorder.

From American Academy of Sleep Medicine. *The International Classification of Sleep Disorders: Diagnostic and Coding Manual,* 2nd ed. Westchester, IL: American Academy of Sleep Medicine; 2005.

Conversely, N24HSWS may predispose patients to develop psychiatric disorders; approximately a third of patients without psychiatric problems before the onset of N24HSWS develop major depression thereafter, with depression symptoms sometimes worsening when their sleep is out of phase with the 24-hour day and maximally disrupted.

Clinical Treatments

Therapeutic interventions for N24HSWS should be aimed at resynchronizing the patient's circadian pacemaker, and therefore sleep-wake cycle, to the 24-hour day.[7] Case studies in sighted N24HSWS patients using bright light exposure or melatonin administration have been reported but there have been no large-scale randomized clinical trials to date.[4,7]

Light Therapy

In humans and other mammals, appropriately timed exposure to light can reset the phase, or relative timing, of human circadian rhythms and is the major environment time cue that entrains the internal near-24-hour circadian pacemaker to the solar day. The magnitude and direction of phase shifts are described by a phase response curve (PRC),[8,9] with phase delays (shifting circadian phase to a later time) generally occurring when light exposure is timed before core body temperature minimum, and phase advances (shifting circadian phase earlier) occurring after temperature minimum. Since in healthy subjects the minimum core body temperature occurs approximately 2 to 3 hours before the habitual wake time (usually about 5-6 AM), the most sensitive portion of PRC to light coincides with the last hours of sleep, and therefore the timing of sleep itself is a major gateway in determining light input to the pacemaker,[5,10] which is mediated exclusively by the eyes (see later discussion).

Most patients with N24HSWD have a circadian period longer than 24 hours (i.e., a daily delay) and therefore need a daily phase advance to correct their disorder. As outlined previously, light therapy after core body temperature minimum is required and, under normally entrained circumstances, this would coincide with the early morning (after 6 AM). These patients, however, have a nonentrained circadian pacemaker, so determining the correct treatment time based on knowledge of the PRC is not straightforward. Ideally, clinicians would evaluate circadian phase to determine treatment time and begin morning light therapy when the sleep is at a normal part of the cycle and occurs at night, and the circadian pacemaker is normally phased with respect to the solar day (see Chapter 28). If circadian phase information is not available, then starting treatment just as the patient is "slipping out" of a normal sleep phase would be a practical, although not optimal, approach. In both cases, patients should keep to a fixed sleep-wake schedule, and use light therapy at the same time each day for at least a week. Failure to time the light appropriately, however, may lead to the disorder becoming worse, at least initially, if morning light exposure happens to fall prior to the core body temperature minimum. Such timing would lead to phase delays rather than advances, potentially delaying entrainment by several weeks. Further investigations are warranted, both on the methodology to assess circadian phase in outpatients (see Chapter 28) and for optimizing light duration, timing, intensity, wavelength, and pattern.[11]

As noted previously, it has been suggested that N24HSWS in sighted subjects may be in part due to inappropriate exposure to light in the phase delay portion of the PRC, systematically delaying the clock each day.[4] Avoidance of evening light, and particularly short-wavelength blue light (see Chapter 28), for example, by using specific filters, may therefore be an effective adjunct to timed light therapy.

Pharmacologic Treatment

Melatonin is emerging as the treatment of choice in blind and sighted individuals with N24HSWS.[7] Melatonin also has a PRC that is generally opposite that for light;[12] under normal phase conditions, melatonin administered in the evening, prior to the natural melatonin onset, induces a phase advance, and when administered near or after the melatonin maximum it causes a phase delay. In individuals entrained to a normal sleep-wake schedule, maximum advances and delays occur at approximately 7 PM and 7 AM, respectively. Sighted patients with DSPD or N24HSWS have been treated successfully with melatonin administration, although without placebo control in the N24HSWS patients.[5,13-18] Again, assessing circadian phase prior to treatment is important to ensure appropriate timing and a successful clinical outcome,[14-16] but if circadian phase information is not available, as for light therapy, melatonin treatment should be started when the sleep episode occurs at the normal local time. Perhaps the most important aspect of treatment is that it should occur on a strict 24-hour cycle (i.e., at a fixed clock time each night) so that even if it is started at a suboptimal phase, entrainment should eventually occur. The clock time should also take advantage of the sleepiness-inducing properties of melatonin and occur in the mid to late evening (e.g., 9 PM), after which the patient does not expect to do anything requiring alertness, such as driving. Studies in the blind (see the next section) suggest that 0.5 mg is the most appropriate dose. Long-term safety data are not available for melatonin, although research studies suggest that it is a relatively safe drug in most patient groups.[19,20]

A number of melatonin agonists are approved or in development for other sleep disorders and have been shown to cause a phase advance of the circadian pacemaker.[21,22] These drugs therefore have high potential to treat N24HSWS but have yet to be tested. Vitamin B_{12} has been reported to be effective in treating nonentrained type,[23,24] although the efficacy and mechanism are unknown.

Benzodiazepines or other hypnotic medications have not been studied systematically for N24HSWS, although there are several anecdotal reports.[7,25] Generally, conventional hypnotics seem to have limited property to synchronize or phase-shift the circadian pacemaker and simply "mask" the underlying circadian sleep-wake disorder (as do stimulants), although the sleep-wake state, or the light-dark changes associated with the sleep-wake cycle, may serve as circadian time cues. Echizenya and associates[26] reported two sighted adolescents suffering from N24HSWS in whom paradoxical arousal occurred after taking conventional benzodiazepine-related hypnotic agents (case 1, triazolam and brotizolam, and case 2, zolpidem) and suggested that the use of hypnotic agents in adolescent patients with N24HSWS required consideration of the possible occurrence of paradoxical reactions.

NON-24-HOUR SLEEP-WAKE SYNDROME IN TOTALLY BLIND PATIENTS

Definitions and Basic Description

The clinical definition for N24HSWS in blind patients is the same as that for sighted patients (see Box 32-1), but the disorder is much more common in totally blind patients. Given the central role of light in entraining the circadian pacemaker to the 24-hour day, it is not surprising that those lacking light detection for the circadian system experience problems with maintaining entrainment, and sleep and other rhythm disorders have been recognized in the blind for more than 60 years.[27] Although the clinical definitions for N24HSWS are currently the same for blind and sighted patients, the disorders often present differently and have different underlying causes. In totally blind people, the disorder is caused by an inability of the circadian pacemaker to be entrained by light because of the lack of a functional retina–retinohypothalamic tract (RHT)–suprachiasmatic nuclei (SCN) pathway (see Chapter 28). In sighted subjects, this pathway is likely functional but the patient is generally not exposed to an appropriate 24-hour light-dark cycle and becomes nonentrained. One may consider the disorder in the blind an intrinsic, physical, irreversible (but treatable) disorder that is not associated with any psychiatric condition, whereas in the sighted, it is behaviorally induced, may be associated with a psychiatric disorder, and is transient and reversible (see Fig. 32-4). As outlined in this section, the differences in the etiology between these patient groups result in a different expression of the sleep problem and affect possible treatments.

Clinical Diagnostic Criteria

N24HSWS is very common in totally blind patients with as many as half having a nonentrained circadian pacemaker.[27] The physical inability of the circadian pacemaker to be entrained by ocular light information causes it to revert to its endogenous non-24-hour period, in many cases causing a chronic, cyclic sleep-wake disorder characterized by periods of good sleep followed by periods of poor sleep and excessive daytime sleepiness, followed by good sleep *ad infinitum*, as the internal non-24-hour circadian period cycles in and out of phase with the 24-hour social day.

The research on this disorder has tended to use measurements of a non-24-hour period in strongly circadian physiologic markers such as melatonin or its metabolites, cortisol, or body temperature, either in the laboratory or at home,[27-30] rather than the clinical complaint of insomnia or sleepiness.[1] The average circadian period of these markers is approximately 24.5 hours (range 23.8-25.1 hours), but such a distinct period is generally not observed in the sleep pattern.[31] The sleep tends to show "relative coordination" rather than

a clear nonentrained rhythm, a competition of sorts set up between the underlying non-24-hour circadian clock and nonphotic time cue exposure from the patient's desire keep a 24-hour social sleep pattern (Fig. 32-2). Consequently, many (but not all) of those with non-24-hour rhythms have sleep complaints[32] and many, but not all, also exhibit non-24-hour sleep-wake rhythms[31] (see Fig. 32-2). This is in contrast to sighted subjects with N24HSWS who tend to have a clearly "free-running" sleep-wake cycle with a longer circadian period of about 25 hours. Laboratory studies have shown that such long periods are observed when sighted individuals have free access to light and unrestricted sleep opportunity, as individuals tend to go to sleep and expose themselves to light until later than usual, during the phase delay portion of the PRC, causing a daily systematic delay of their circadian pacemaker and an apparent 25 hour sleep-wake period[4,33] (see Fig. 32-1).

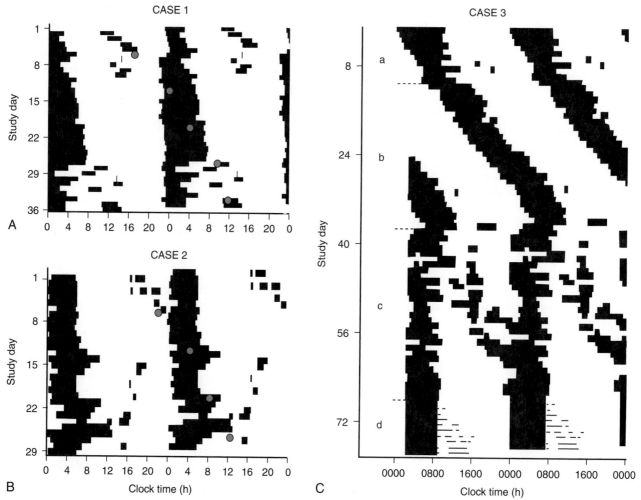

Figure 32-2 Non-24-hour sleep-wake syndrome in three totally blind patients. These sleep-wake patterns in three totally blind men with non-24-hour sleep-wake syndrome are plotted as shown in Figure 32-1. The peak time of the urinary 6-sulfatoxymelatonin (aMT6s) rhythm, collected each week, is also plotted where available (●). Case 1 is a 66-year-old totally blind man with one eye and no light perception due to ocular trauma. Case 2 is a 35-year-old bilaterally enucleated (retinoblastoma) male. Both exhibited a 24.7-hour melatonin rhythm and a non-24-hour sleep-wake pattern when measured for a month while living freely at home, with characteristic recurrent episodes of disturbed nighttime sleep and many daytime naps when nighttime sleep was attempted at an adverse circadian phase. Most sleep still occurred during the social night, however, and the extent of disruption varied between patients. Case 3 shows the sleep-wake pattern of a 28-year-old male who lost his light perception at birth due to retinopathy of prematurity. Sections a and c represent his sleep while living freely at home and Section B shows sleep during an "ad-lib" inpatient study when the subject was free to sleep as he pleased. During Section d, an unsuccessful attempt was made to entrain his cycle via strict 24-hour scheduling of sleep, meals, and activity. While living freely in the laboratory (b), his sleep-wake, plasma cortisol, alertness, performance, and urinary electrolyte rhythms all exhibited a circadian period of 24.9 hours. This rhythm persisted when living at home (c) but was modulated by attempting to live on a social 24-hour day, as in Cases 1 and 2. (Redrawn from Uchiyama M, Lockley SW. Non-24-hour sleep-wake syndrome in sighted and blind patients. *Sleep Med Clin.* 2009;4:195-211.)

Given that complaints of insomnia or excessive daytime sleepiness are required for a diagnosis of N24HSWS, it could be argued that a totally blind individual with a non-24-hour circadian pacemaker but who did not have any sleep complaints or who had a 24-hour sleep pattern, could not be formally diagnosed with N24HSWS. This would be a mistake, however, owing to potential disorders of other systems governed by the circadian system (e.g., cognitive function, mood, metabolism), which would still be affected by the non-24-hour circadian period even in the apparent absence of sleep complaints. For example, it is well established that the time course of alertness, mood, and a range of different cognitive functions are determined by the phase relationship between the sleep-wake cycle and circadian phase,[34-36] including in the blind.[37,38] Waking at an inappropriate circadian phase, even if the sleep had been relatively good, may still result in daytime dysfunction.[38] It is also becoming clear that a number of peripheral organs have the ability to generate local circadian rhythms (e.g., the liver, lungs, heart, kidneys, ovaries), affecting the temporal relationship of local functions.[39] This has important implications for metabolism, as it is known that eating at an inappropriate circadian phase (i.e., during the biologic night) impairs postprandial metabolism such that glucose, insulin, and lipids stay higher for longer as compared to when the same meal is eaten in the daytime,[40] and likely underlies some of the increased risk of heart disease and diabetes seen in shift workers (see Chapter 29). Again, even in the absence of a sleep complaint, desynchrony between the SCN, peripheral clocks, and the 24-hour meal schedule is likely to increase the risk of underlying health problems. Linking the diagnosis of the entire disorder to just sleep and sleepiness may miss other important sequelae and hopefully these nuances will be addressed in the next revision of the ICSD.[1]

Demographics

Although representative studies have not been performed, based on measurements of endogenous circadian markers, N24HSWS is likely to afflict between one third and two thirds of the totally blind population (which represents about 1% of the visually impaired population). Of the remaining totally blind patients who do not exhibit sleep-wake or other circadian rhythm disorders, most are entrained to the 24-hour social day (not the 24-hour light-dark cycle) via nonphotic time cues including strict scheduling of activities, exercise, mealtimes and social interaction.[29,41,42] In a small proportion of cases (about 5%), patients may retain circadian photoreception in the absence of visual function.[43-45] Non-24-hour sleep-wake disorder is rare in visually impaired patients who retain at least minimal light perception, with only a handful of such cases in the literature.[27]

Onset can occur at any age, from birth onward, and usually coincides with or follows shortly after loss of light perception or loss or surgical removal of the eyes.[27] There may be age-related differences in recognizing a cyclic sleep-wake complaint and reporting N24HSWS, however, such that middle-aged adults may tend to recognize the sleep complaint more readily than younger adults. The type of blindness does not ultimately affect risk of N24HSWS; complete loss of visual and circadian photoreceptive function due to any ocular disorder will abolish light-dark input to the circadian pacemaker and prevent entrainment to the light-dark cycle. Eye disorders that damage the ganglion cell layer (e.g., glaucoma), affect the optic nerve (e.g., retinopathy of prematurity), or require removal of the eye entirely (e.g., retinoblastoma, trauma) are more likely to result in total blindness, prevent circadian entrainment, and increase the likelihood of N24HSWS.

Clinical Treatments

Pharmacologic Treatment

Given the inability of light to treat this disorder in the blind, use of melatonin for N24HSWS remains the most promising therapeutic strategy in this population.[27] Although the soporific properties of melatonin have been shown to "stabilize" the sleep-wake cycle in blind patients even without entrainment of the circadian pacemaker,[46] entrainment of the circadian pacemaker, and therefore the sleep rhythm, is necessary to treat N24HSWS appropriately. After the initial demonstrations that a 5-mg[47] or 10-mg[48] dose could entrain circadian rhythms in the blind, several studies have shown that lower doses (≤ 0.5 mg) appear to be equally effective, if not more so,[49,50] at entraining the clock, maybe through providing a more discreet temporal signal than higher doses. Given melatonin's soporific properties, treatment should be administered at the same time each day close to the desired bedtime to ensure the alignment of the circadian and social day. Regarding the circadian time of administration, while low doses (≤ 0.5 mg-) initiated at any circadian phase will eventually cause entrainment of the circadian pacemaker,[49-52] there may be a lag in experiencing beneficial effects until the time of administration coincides with the phase advance part of the PRC. If treatment can be timed initially to induce a phase advance, entrainment should occur within a few days and the patient will perceive immediate benefit (Fig. 32-3). If timed inappropriately, entrainment can take longer, on the order of weeks, or may not occur at all.[47,49] The individual's circadian period may also affect the likelihood of entrainment with melatonin,[53] as those subjects with periods furthest from 24 hours may be outside the range of entrainment for this relatively weak synchronizing time cue.

Other pharmacologic treatments to reset the pacemaker have been tried (e.g., triazolam) but without success. Nonpharmacologic treatments, such as scheduling, regular mealtimes, and exercise, have also been tried but they tend to be complicated and onerous and appear to have minimal effect.

IRREGULAR SLEEP-WAKE RHYTHM

Definitions and Basic Description

Irregular sleep-wake rhythm (ISWR) is characterized by multiple (at least three), irregular bouts of sleep distributed across a 24-hour cycle[1] (Box 32-2). Sleep bouts are usually 1 to 4 hours in duration.[54] In contrast to most circadian disorders in which there is misalignment between the phase of the endogenous circadian sleep-wake rhythm and the desired sleep-wake schedule, ISWR is postulated to be a condition in which there is greatly reduced amplitude of circadian rhythms.[55] Normally, sleep-wake timing is regulated by sleep homeostatic and circadian processes.[10] Sleep homeostatic mechanisms reflect an increasing drive to sleep with increasing time awake, with rapid dissipation of homeostatic sleep pressure during sleep.[56] In order to maintain long consolidated bouts of wakefulness and sleep, however, the endogenous circadian sleep propensity

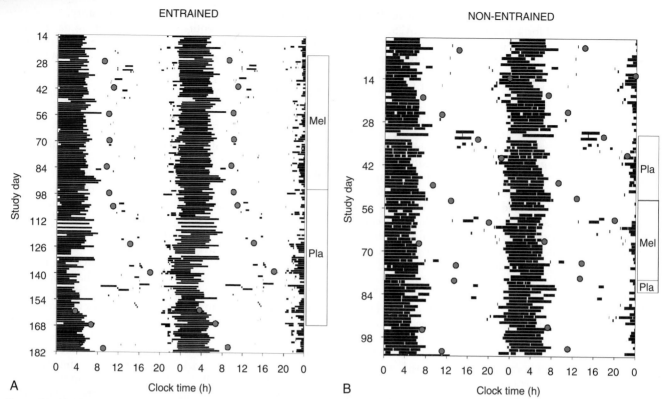

Figure 32-3 Melatonin treatment of non-24-hour sleep-wake syndrome in the blind. This figure shows the double-plotted sleep timing (■) and urinary cortisol peak times (●) for two totally blind men treated with 5 mg fast-release melatonin (Mel) or placebo (Pla) given orally at 9 PM over at least one circadian cycle in a single-blind design.[47] Sequential study days are plotted on the ordinate and clock time is double-plotted on the abscissa. Panel A shows a subject who was entrained by melatonin treatment (S17). He exhibited a nonentrained cortisol rhythm (24.3 hours) during placebo treatment but was entrained at a normal circadian phase by the melatonin treatment (mean ± SD urinary cortisol peak time = 9.9 ± 0.7 hour). The entrained sleep-wake cycle observed during melatonin treatment becomes immediately disrupted upon cessation of treatment and reverts to the characteristic non-24-hour cyclic pattern. Panel B shows a subject who failed to entrain to 5 mg melatonin treatment (S45), and a persistent cyclic non-24-hour sleep-wake disorder is clearly apparent throughout both the placebo and melatonin treatment. (Reproduced in part from Lockley SW, Skene DJ, James K, et al. Melatonin administration can entrain the free-running circadian system of blind subjects. *J Endocrinol.* 2000;164:R1-R6.)

BOX 32-2 *Diagnostic Criteria for Circadian Rhythm Sleep Disorder, Irregular Sleep-Wake Type*

A. There is a chronic complaint of insomnia, excessive sleepiness, or both.
B. Sleep log or actigraphy monitoring (including sleep diaries) for at least 7 days demonstrates multiple irregular sleep bouts (at least three) during a 24-hour period.
C. Total sleep time per 24-hour period is essentially normal for age.
D. The sleep disturbance is not better explained by another current sleep disorder, medical or neurologic disorder, mental disorder, medication use, or substance use disorder.

From American Academy of Sleep Medicine. *The International Classification of Sleep Disorders: Diagnostic and Coding Manual,* 2nd ed. Westchester, IL: American Academy of Sleep Medicine; 2005.

---

rhythm counters the effects of homeostatic sleep pressure, with an increasing drive for alertness throughout the day, peaking several hours prior to habitual bedtime, and a decrease in alertness during the night, reaching minimal alertness around 3 AM to 6 AM.[10] If this circadian influence is removed in animals, for example by lesioning the SCN or using specialized light exposures, sleep becomes arrhythmic but has the same total sleep duration per 24 hours as in intact individuals, illustrating continued homeostatic regulation of sleep.[57,58] An analogous situation is assumed in individuals with ISWR—an absent or greatly reduced circadian amplitude in sleep propensity does little to counteract the homeostatic regulation of sleep, resulting in multiple sleep and wake bouts but normal sleep duration for age per 24 hours.[54] In practice, although individual sleep bouts tend to be less than 4 hours in duration and are scattered across the day and night, the longest sleep period still tends to occur overnight in most individuals,[55] which may reflect some residual, albeit weak, circadian rhythm expression or the result of socially enforced wakefulness during the day, which increases homeostatic sleep pressure at night.

A variety of mechanisms can cause a reduction in the amplitude of circadian rhythms, including the loss of a critical population of SCN neurons,[59] disruption of circadian output pathways affecting the behavioral expression of some biologic rhythms despite intact pacemaker activity,[60] or a functional disruption within the SCN that reduces the coherence of individual cellular oscillators,[61,62] leading to phase cancellation effects. It has also been demonstrated that precisely timed light exposure in healthy humans can suppress the circadian amplitude of body temperature or cortisol rhythms, at least for brief periods.[63] This finding suggests that, at least for some individuals with ISWR, the functional activity of the endogenous circadian pacemaker and the amplitude of the sleep-wake rhythm can be modulated and perhaps restored by traditional circadian treatments.

Clinical Diagnostic Criteria

The disorder is characterized by lack of a clear 24-hour rhythm in sleep and wake cycles, with symptoms of insomnia or excessive daytime sleepiness depending on the time of day. As for the other CRSD, there are no specific criteria for abnormalities in timing or amplitude of other circadian rhythms, such as body temperature, cortisol, or melatonin, although ICSD-II states that "other circadian rhythms…may also show a loss of clear circadian rhythmicity."[1] Theoretically, therefore, an individual with an intact and normally functioning circadian system but with a post-SCN interruption of SCN efferents to the sleep centers, blocking the 24-hour control of sleep and wake, could also be diagnosed with ISWR (Fig. 32-4).

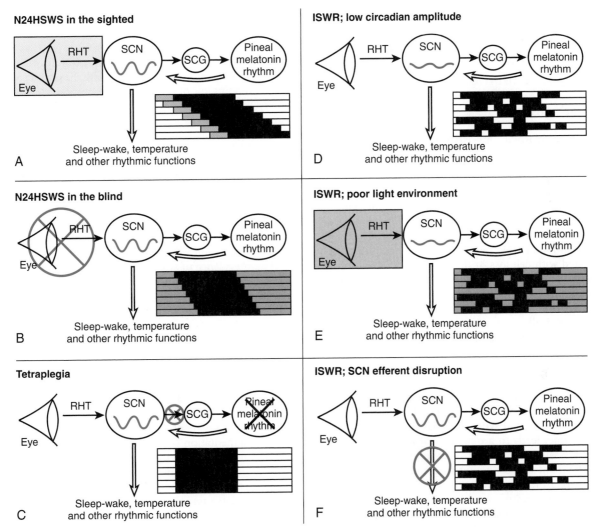

Figure 32-4 Anatomic basis of sleep and circadian rhythm disruption. Shown here are the mechanisms by which compromises in circadian organization may underlie non-24-hour sleep-wake syndrome (N24HSWS) and irregular sleep-wake rhythm (ISWR). The basic organization of the circadian system comprises three parts; an endogenous near-24-hour oscillator located in the suprachiasmatic nuclei (SCN) which is synchronized via light-dark input from the retina-retinohypothalamic tract (RHT)-SCN pathway, which then sends efferent signals to the pineal gland and other brain areas to control the timing of melatonin and sleep-wake rhythms, respectively, among others. **A,** In sighted patients with N24HSWS, the endogenous circadian pacemaker is intact and functional but is likely systematically phase delayed by inappropriate exposure to light *(blue bars)*, resulting in an approximately 25-hour sleep-wake cycle. **B,** In blind patients, the pacemaker is also functionally intact but reverts to its near 24-hour endogenous periodicity (about 24.5 hours) due to a nonfunctional RHT. **C,** By comparison, tetraplegic patients have no melatonin production due to a post-SCN cervical lesion that blocks the signal from the SCN to the pineal gland required for melatonin secretion but have otherwise normal circadian cortisol and temperature rhythms, and relatively normal sleep, as direct SCN efferents to other brain areas are not affected by the cervical lesion.[122,123] The anatomic etiology of ISWR is not known but several possibilities exist. **D,** The amplitude of the endogenous circadian pacemaker may be reduced, for example, by loss of SCN neurons in dementia, leading to a weakened circadian signal to all SCN efferent targets, including sleep-wake control. **E,** Reduced SCN amplitude may be further exacerbated if the SCN receives weak light-dark cycle information *(gray bars)* caused by living in a poorly lit care home or eye disorders such as cataract, and the reduced light may lead to inappropriate entrainment, for example, the phase delay described in some Alzheimer's disease patients. **F,** "Circadian" sleep-wake rhythm disturbance could arise when the endogenous circadian clock is functional but if the sleep centers are unable to receive the circadian signal, for example, due to disrupted SCN efferents. Analogous to the tetraplegia patients' lack of melatonin production, a disrupted circadian output marker does not necessarily indicate a circadian clock disorder. (Adapted with permission from Arendt J. *Melatonin and the Mammalian Pineal Gland.* London: Chapman and Hall; 1995.)

Demographics

Most reported cases of presumed or explicitly defined ISWR occur in the setting of neurologic disease such as neurodegenerative diseases or developmental disorders in children and are therefore more appropriately categorized as "CRSD due to a medical condition" (see next section).

Clinical Treatments

There are no clinical treatments specific to ISWR that are not described for CRSD due to a medical condition (see next section).

CIRCADIAN RHYTHM SLEEP DISORDER DUE TO A MEDICAL CONDITION

Alzheimer's Disease

Definitions and Basic Description

The most studied CRSD due to a medical condition is the irregular sleep wake rhythm seen in dementia patients (see Chapter 52). The prevalence of dementia increases with age, with up to 50% of those aged 85 years or older affected. Approximately two thirds of cases are due to Azheimer's disease (AD), the leading cause of dementia, followed by vascular dementia. Although other neurodegenerative conditions may be associated with cell loss in the SCN and a low-amplitude circadian rhythm, circadian abnormalities have been studied most often in AD and will be the focus of this section.

AD is a debilitating, progressive neurodegenerative disorder. It is clinically characterized by a steady and progressive loss of neurocognitive and functional abilities. Patients diagnosed with AD frequently also have profound behavioral changes including increases in agitation, depression, apathy, anxiety, and many other troubling symptoms. Initially, complaints can be mild and involve difficulty encoding new declarative (fact-based) memories. These early deficits, composing a prodromal syndrome that frequently, with the passage of time, leads to a diagnosis of AD, do not generally interfere with activities of daily living but can lead to some curtailment of tasks requiring intense cognitive activity. Declarative memory gradually becomes more impaired as the neurodegenerative syndrome progresses. This initial impairment can be accompanied by deficits in frontal executive functioning and visuoconstructional impairments that are characterized by an inability to plan and organize. When these deficits begin to interfere with the patient's functional abilities, the diagnosis of AD can be made. As the disease progresses from the mild to the moderate stage, cognitive domains become affected, and semantic and phonemic fluencies degrade, spatial disorientation increases, and previously learned skilled movements (e.g., tool use) become impaired, leading to a much greater loss of functional abilities. Recognition of familiar people and places also becomes difficult and occasional false recognition leads to increasing confusion and loss of orientation. Behavioral symptoms increase as brain areas affecting mood, behavioral inhibition, sleep, and many others are affected by the progressive degeneration. These symptoms then become more and more disruptive and dangerous to patients and those helping care for them.

Of these impaired behaviors, it is the sleep-wake disturbance that is most disruptive to caregivers,[64] especially since it is frequently accompanied by agitated pacing, confusion, wandering, and other disruptive behavior. This disruption is one of the major reasons for institutionalization of a patient[65] and therefore treating the sleep disturbance that accompanies mid- to late-stage AD could yield significant benefits in decreasing the stress on caregivers and ultimately delaying institutionalization.

Clinical Diagnostic Criteria

There are no specific criteria for CRSD due to a medical condition beyond the general description (Box 32-3) as the sleep disturbances can be specific for that medical disorder.

Sleep disturbances in AD increase with the severity of dementia[66-68] and this loss of sleep likely impacts both global cognitive ability[69] and memory consolidation,[70] a process that is particularly vulnerable in patients with AD. AD patients have a greater reduction of non–rapid eye movement (NREM) slow wave sleep (SWS) than healthy older people[71-74] and a reduction in sleep spindles.[73,74] Latency to rapid eye movement (REM) sleep is longer in AD than in aged control subjects[75] and AD patients have shorter mean duration of REM episodes, likely due to the degeneration seen in cholinergic neurons in early AD. The changes in REM sleep are severity-specific[76] with patients with mild AD showing few changes but those with moderate to severe AD becoming quite different from normal control subjects.

The prevalence of sleep-disordered breathing (SDB) is up to three times higher in advanced dementia than in the normal geriatric population,[77] estimated between 35% and 63%,[78-80] which further limits SWS beyond that observed in dementia patients who do not have SDB.[81]

Sleep-wake (or more properly rest-activity) disturbances based on wrist actigraphy[82] show that interdaily stability (IS), a measurement of rhythm stability from day to day,[83] is significantly lowered in patients with moderate to severe AD but not in patients with mild AD[67,84-86] (Fig. 32-5). IS changes are also closely correlated with cognitive decline.[87] Intradaily variability (IV), an assessment of hour-to-hour variability of activity or the fragmentation of rest-activity patterns, is not as clearly affected across the severity spectrum of AD, although it trends toward greater disturbance in patients[85,88] (although this may be due to the presence of other dementia diagnoses in the sample of AD patients).[68,88] The rest-activity cycle also appears to be more phase delayed in AD,[68,84,88-90] although the extent to which this timing reflects internal circadian phase is arguable.

Measurements of strongly endogenous circadian markers such as core body temperature also show a significant phase delay in the temperature rhythm under ambulatory conditions[84] that is highly specific to AD[88] and more profound with increasing severity of illness.[67,68] When measured under more controlled conditions, when the effects of environmental factors on temperature have been removed, AD patients exhibit a weakened endogenous amplitude circadian rhythm and a profound phase delay compared to both normal elderly subjects and young control subjects to an even greater degree than that observed under real-world conditions.[91] Consistent with a phase delay, multiple sleep latency test (MSLT) shows an AD severity-specific shortening of sleep latency, especially in the morning hours.[92]

Clinical Treatments

Therapeutic interventions for CRSD in AD are aimed at consolidating the stability and amplitude of the rest-activity and sleep-wake cycle, and correcting any phase delay. In addition

---

> **BOX 32-3** *Diagnostic Criteria for Circadian Rhythm Sleep Disorder Due to a Medical Condition*
>
> A. There is a complaint of insomnia or excessive sleepiness related to alterations of the circadian time-keeping system or a misalignment between the endogenous circadian rhythm and exogenous factors that affect the timing or duration of sleep.
> B. An underlying medical or neurologic disorder predominantly accounts for the circadian rhythm sleep disorder.
> C. Sleep log or actigraphy monitoring (with sleep diaries) for at least 7 days demonstrates disturbed or low amplitude circadian rhythmicity.
> D. The sleep disturbance is not better explained by another current sleep disorder, mental disorder, medication use, or substance use disorder.
>
> From American Academy of Sleep Medicine. *The International Classification of Sleep Disorders: Diagnostic and Coding Manual,* 2nd ed. Westchester, IL: American Academy of Sleep Medicine; 2005.

---

to improving sleep and daytime alertness, improvements in mood and cognition may also be possible. If treated during the early stages of AD when the patient still lives at home, these treatments may also reduce caregiver disruption and delay admission into institutional care. Given these aims, options include bright light therapy and melatonin treatment in an attempt to treat the underlying chronobiologic disturbance. There are some barriers to the effective delivery of treatment in these patients, however, and potential to exacerbate a circadian phase delay if the treatments are timed inappropriately[91] (see earlier discussion).

Light Therapy. Two naturalistic studies first demonstrated that patients with mild and moderate-severe dementia received less light than cognitively intact individuals living under similar conditions.[89,93] Light box therapy either in the evening (1500-2000 lux) or morning (3000-3500 lux for 2 hours) was shown to improve nurse-rated sleep and disruptive behavior (sundowning) or sleep measures,[94] although a later randomized, placebo-controlled crossover study found the effect to be restricted to those patients with a non-AD dementia.[95]

Compliance with light therapy delivered via a light box is potentially difficult in AD patients, however, particularly in those with advanced dementia or significant agitation. Providing light therapy by improving ambient exposure is a more promising approach. Increasing the intensity of ambient

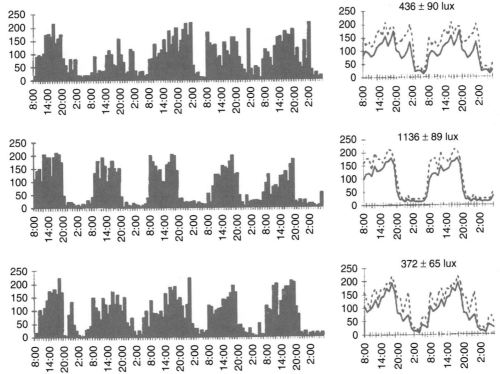

Figure 32-5 Light treatment for irregular sleep-wake rhythm (ISWR) in dementia patients. Patients with Alzheimer's disease (*n* = 16), multi-infarct dementia (*n* = 3), dementia associated with alcoholism (*n* = 2), and normal pressure hydrocephalus (*n* = 1) were studied in a nursing home environment for about 10 weeks each. After a 2-week baseline (average light levels ± SEM, 436 ± 90 lux), bright lights were installed in the ceiling and remained for 4 weeks (1136 ± 89 lux), when they were removed again for 4 weeks (baseline 2; 372 ± 65 lux). Patients rest-activity and light-dark exposure was assessed using wrist actigraphy during the baseline, during the last 2 weeks of light therapy, and during the last 2 weeks of normal light (baseline 2). Raw activity data of a patient with Alzheimer's disease are shown in the left panel for 5 days before (*top*), during (*middle*), and after (*bottom*) light treatment. The right panels show double plots of the average 24-hour activity level (*solid line*) + 1 SD (*dashed line*). On average, the variability of the rest-activity rhythm was reduced and its stability improved during the light exposure as compared to the pooled pre- and postbaseline levels. These effects were not observed in patients with severe visual impairment. (Redrawn from Van Someren EJ, Kessler A, Mirmiran M, Swaab DF. Indirect bright light improves circadian rest-activity rhythm disturbances in demented patients. *Biol Psychiatry.* 1997;41[9]:955-963.)

illumination in common areas of a care home to approximately 1100 lux (790-2100 lux) at eye level is effective at improving the stability and consolidation of the rest-activity pattern[96] (see Fig. 32-5). Increasing environmental light has also showed efficacy in promoting stability of circadian phase,[97] consolidating sleep and wakefulness,[98] increasing nighttime sleep,[99] and reducing agitation[100] (although not in all cases).[101] Morning bright light has also been found to improve depressive symptoms in institutionalized patients with dementia.[102]

The inconsistent but generally positive results from these trials offer encouraging evidence for using light therapy in patients with moderate-severe dementia. Several caveats remain, however, for example, the lack of blinding affecting the subjective ratings. A more significant issue is the use of clock time, rather than circadian time, to time light therapy, which could result in mistimed treatment[91] as for other CRSD (see previous discussion).

Pharmacologic Treatment. Evening melatonin had been shown to be efficacious in a small, placebo-controlled, double-blind study for improving nighttime sleep and cognitive and noncognitive symptoms of AD.[103] In a large, multicenter, double-blind, placebo-controlled trial of melatonin at 2.5 and 10 mg 1 hour before sleep for the treatment of insomnia in patients with AD, no significant effects were seen on the objective measures of sleep, although positive trends were apparent, including in caregiver ratings.[104] There were no differences in adverse events between active and placebo conditions. Open-label studies of melatonin have also showed promising responses in treating both behavioral and sleep disturbances in AD.[105,106]

Combination Therapy. More recently, two promising clinical trials have moved to a combination therapy employing both melatonin and light. The first, employing morning light and evening melatonin, while not showing any significant differences in nighttime sleep, showed significant reductions in daytime sleep, improved diurnal activity, and more consolidated circadian activity.[107] A second study treated care-home patients with 2.5 mg evening melatonin or placebo while increasing indoor lighting availability from around 300 lux to 1000 lux from 10 AM. The combination therapy showed significant improvements in a large number of domains including a significant slowing in the decline of cognitive and day-to-day functioning; improved clinical ratings of depression; improved sleep; and lowered complaints of aggressive behavior, irritability, dizziness, headache, constipation, and inability to sleep;[108] and was clearly superior to either treatment given alone. (Melatonin alone had an adverse effect on caregiver ratings of positive and negative affect and increased withdrawn behavior.) Importantly, the benefits obtained in cognitive symptoms from the combined therapy were equivalent to those observed with clinically-approved cholinesterase inhibitors.

While the exact mechanism of action of the combined therapy is unknown, light has acute alerting properties in addition to its circadian phase resetting effects and therefore better daytime lighting may directly improve arousal and cognitive function. A more robust light-dark cycle will also stabilize sleep-wake patterns, which in itself may help slow the decline in cognitive function, and may help to stabilize other behaviors such

as social interaction and medication compliance. Light also has mood elevating and even clinical antidepressant effects in some conditions (e.g., seasonal affective disorder), which may account for the reduction in depression ratings. This promising therapeutic effect needs to be replicated, and cognitive endpoints should be added to chronotherapeutic trials in patients with dementia. Although not a panacea for all symptoms of dementia, the approach is relatively simple, inexpensive, and noninvasive (if light therapy alone is used), and will help patients to get better sleep, which has myriad health benefits. This approach is not only limited to those with dementia; reinforcing robust daily light-dark exposure in all elderly people, especially those who may not be mobile and are unable get outside daily, is likely to be of benefit, as is reinforcing good light-dark exposure for hospitals and other care facilities, schools and colleges, and other environments, including our own homes.

Other Neurologic Disorders

Clinical Diagnostic Criteria

In addition to neurodegenerative illnesses (see Chapters 26 and 52), other neurologic populations have been described to have irregular or erratic sleep-wake behavior. These reports predominantly included individuals with neurodevelopmental disorders (NDD) arising in infancy or early childhood from a variety of insults, including suspected asphyxia, birth injury, central nervous system infections, genetic abnormalities, and syndromes of unknown etiology. Although formal diagnostic criteria have rarely been used, however, ISWR has been inferred in many of these cases, often based on sleep log information filled out by parents or actigraphy.

While these methods are practical in clinical populations and are recommended by a recent position paper from the American Academy of Sleep Medicine,[109] the lack of reliably measured circadian phase and amplitude information may lead to incorrect assumptions about the underlying circadian disorder. For example, in a pediatric sample of 14 individuals with a variety of neurologic insults, 3 were described as having sleep that was "dispersed" within small bouts over a 24-hour period, suggestive of ISWR. When hourly rectal temperature was recorded, however, only one of these individuals with dispersed sleep had a low amplitude rhythm.[110] Similarly, in a population of 12 children with chronic fatigue, 5 were described as having an irregular sleep-wake rhythm on the basis of actigraphy measures of daytime compared to nighttime activity.[111] However, these individuals were also more likely to have extremely long sleep bouts (defined as a sleep interval longer than 10 hours) and may have had a nonentrained rather than a low-amplitude rhythm (see discussion earlier of N24HSWS). In a population of children with Smith-Magenis syndrome, in which a chromosomal deletion is associated with severe cognitive impairment and sleep disruption, the circadian peak in a urinary melatonin metabolite occurs at an abnormal time but has normal amplitude,[112] demonstrating a disorder of circadian phase but not amplitude. Finally, in a group of 6 children with septo-optic dysplasia but with normal light perception, one patient had an actigraphy pattern compatible with ISWR but with normal serum melatonin. In contrast, two other patients with prolonged nocturnal awakenings but without an ISWR pattern did not have detectable 24-hour melatonin rhythms.[113]

Similar difficulties occur in assessment of adult populations. Of 42 patients with mild traumatic brain injury (TBI) and complaints of insomnia, 15 were suspected of having a circadian disorder and were studied in more detail.[114] Salivary melatonin and oral temperature were measured every 2 hours for 24 hours in the sleep laboratory. Seven individuals had a sleep-wake pattern consistent with formal criteria of ISWR.[1] Three of these individuals did not show a 24-hour periodicity for oral temperature but did show a rhythmic pattern of expression for melatonin. Furthermore, there were no melatonin amplitude differences between the ISWR group and the eight additional patients who were diagnosed with delayed sleep phase syndrome.

These studies illustrate the difficulty in measuring and interpreting circadian rhythms in the diagnosis of circadian disorders (see Chapter 28). There are several potential problems with these measures. For example, oral temperature is a weak measure of endogenous circadian phase and amplitude because it is so easily masked by environmental factors such as air temperature, eating and drinking, activity, sleep-wake state, and others. It is no surprise, therefore, that there can be inconsistencies between oral temperature and melatonin measurements, which, when assessed under dim light, is a much more reliable marker of circadian phase. Moreover, the clinical criteria for diagnosing CRSD are based primarily on sleep complaints and tend to be upheld even in the face of evidence from circadian markers that the diagnosis is unsound.[115] For example, the lack of melatonin amplitude difference between the TBI ISWR and DPSD patients may simply be due to interindividual variation, or could reflect the lack of an intrinsic circadian disorder in the ISWR patients (see Fig. 32-4). The lack of consistency between the interpretation of sleep and melatonin measures in diagnosing ISWR in the children with septo-optic dysplasia is also problematic.

Clinical Treatments

Light Therapy. Light therapy (≥ 4000 lux from 7-7:45 AM) has been studied in an uncontrolled trial in 14 children (ages 9 months to 4 years) with moderate to severe developmental cognitive impairment and severe sleep disturbances.[116] Sleep logs of a 3-year-old girl demonstrated no consistent 24-hour pattern to the longest sleep period, while the remaining individuals generally had a longest sleep period between 8 PM and midnight, with sleep otherwise scattered across the 24-hour cycle in bouts of 15 to 80 minutes. Five children were considered light-responders, including the child without a discernible 24-hour sleep-wake rhythm, with a group average increase in nocturnal sleep time from 3.4 to 7.1 hours.

Pharmacologic Treatment. Melatonin has been used to improve the sleep of children with NDD, with a recent systematic review concluding that melatonin 0.5 to 7.5 mg can improve sleep latency by 30 minutes but without a significant increase in total nocturnal sleep time.[117] Only three studies were considered suitable for inclusion, however, and these studies did not specifically include individuals with ISWR. For example, one of these studies using 1 week of actigraphy to characterize baseline sleep specifically stated that "none of the patients demonstrated obvious circadian-based sleep disturbances such as free running."[118] In contrast to the conclusions from the systematic review, a randomized, placebo-controlled crossover trial including 51 patients with NDD demonstrated

that melatonin 5 mg (1 mg instant release, 4 mg sustained release) improved nocturnal total sleep time by 31 minutes,[119] although it is not clear whether any of these individuals would satisfy criteria for ISWR.

In an uncontrolled study with two children with Rett syndrome, one child had a very low amplitude melatonin rhythm and scattered bouts of sleep during the daytime though retained a dominant sleep period overnight.[120] A 3-mg dose of melatonin appeared more effective than a 5-mg dose, suggesting that the optimal dose may vary across individuals. Finally, in five children with severe neurodevelopmental cognitive impairment and short, interrupted sleep bouts across the day and night, three of the individuals had urinary melatonin metabolite measurements and all of them showed a markedly reduced melatonin amplitude as well as an abnormally timed peak.[121] Melatonin 3 mg at 6:30 PM increased nocturnal total sleep time from 5.9 to 7.3 hours, with an increase in sleep efficiency from 69.3% to 88.3%; daytime sleep decreased from 3.2 hours to 1.7 hours, and total 24-hour sleep time remained the same at 9 hours. Two of these individuals were able to discontinue treatment with sustained benefits, although the mechanisms of sustained action are unknown.

SUMMARY

This review highlights that the mechanisms underlying nonentrained, unusual or fragmented sleep-wake rhythms may vary considerably. Although sleep logs and actigraphy remain clinically practical, rigorous research criteria assessing multiple phase markers in conditions of dim light (for melatonin assessments) and controlled activity (for temperature recordings) can improve our understanding of the pathophysiology of these disorders, lead to refined clinical diagnostic criteria, and improve the ability to individualize therapy or predict treatment responses.

REFERENCES

1. American Academy of Sleep Medicine. *International Classification of Sleep Disorders: Diagnostic and Coding Manual.* 2nd ed. Westchester, IL: American Academy of Sleep Medicine; 2005.
2. Hashimoto S, Nakamura K, Honma S, Honma K. Free-running circadian rhythm of melatonin in a sighted man despite a 24-hour sleep pattern: A non-24-hour circadian syndrome. *Psychiatry Clin Neurosci.* 1997;51(3):109-114.
3. Uchiyama M, Okawa M, Ozaki S, et al. Delayed phase jumps of sleep onset in a patient with non-24-hour sleep-wake syndrome. *Sleep.* 1996;19:637-640.
4. Uchiyama M, Lockley SW. Non-24-hour sleep-wake syndrome in sighted and blind patients. *Sleep Med Clin.* 2009;4:195-211.
5. Okawa M, Uchiyama M. Circadian rhythm sleep disorders: Characteristics and entrainment pathology in delayed sleep phase and non-24-h sleep-wake syndrome. *Sleep Med Rev.* 2007;11(6):485-496.
6. Hayakawa T, Uchiyama M, Kamei Y, et al. Clinical analyses of sighted patients with non-24-hour sleep-wake syndrome: A study of 57 consecutively diagnosed cases. *Sleep.* 2005;28:945-952.
7. Reid KJ, Zee PC. Circadian disorders of the sleep-wake cycle. In: Kryger MH, Roth T, Dement WC, eds. *Principles and Practice of Sleep Medicine.* 5th ed. Philadelphia: Elsevier Saunders; 2011:470-482.
8. Khalsa SB, Jewett ME, Cajochen C, Czeisler CA. A phase response curve to single bright light pulses in human subjects. *J Physiol.* 2003;549 (Pt 3):945-952.
9. Honma KI, Honma S. A human phase response curve for bright light pulses. *Jap J Psych Neurol.* 1988;42(1):167-168.
10. Dijk DJ, Lockley SW. Integration of human sleep-wake regulation and circadian rhythmicity. *J Appl Physiol.* 2002;92(2):852-862.
11. Lockley SW. Circadian rhythms: Influence of light in humans. In: Squire LR, ed. *Encyclopaedia of Neuroscience.* Oxford: Academic Press; 2009:971-986.

12. Lewy AJ, Ahmed S, Jackson JM, et al. Melatonin shifts human circadian rhythms according to a phase-response curve. *Chronobiol Int.* 1992;9:380-392.

13. Kamei Y, Hayakawa T, Urata J, et al. Melatonin treatment for circadian rhythm sleep disorders. *Psychiatry Clin Neurosci.* 2000;54:381-382.

14. Pandi-Perumal SR, Smits M, Spence W, et al. Dim light melatonin onset (DLMO): A tool for the analysis of circadian phase in human sleep and chronobiological disorders. *Prog Neuropsychopharmacol Biol Psychiatry.* 2007;31:1-11.

15. Arendt J. Does melatonin improve sleep? Efficacy of melatonin. *Br Med J.* 2006;332:550.

16. Mundey K, Benloucif S, Harsanyi K, et al. Phase-dependent treatment of delayed sleep phase syndrome with melatonin. *Sleep.* 2005;28:1271-1278.

17. Van der Heijden KB, Smits MG, van Someren EJ, et al. Prediction of melatonin efficacy by pretreatment dim light melatonin onset in children with idiopathic chronic sleep onset insomnia. *J Sleep Res.* 2005;14:187-194.

18. Carter KA, Lettieri CJ, Peña JM. An unusual cause of insomnia following IED-induced traumatic brain injury. *J Clin Sleep Med.* 2010;6(2):205-206.

19. Arendt J. Safety of melatonin in long-term use(?). *J Biol Rhythms.* 1997;12(6):673-681.

20. Buscemi N, Vandermeer B, Hooton N, et al. Efficacy and safety of exogenous melatonin for secondary sleep disorders and sleep disorders accompanying sleep restriction: Meta-analysis. *BMJ.* 2006;332(7538):385-393.

21. Richardson GS, Zee PC, Wang-Weigand S, Rodriguez L, Peng X. Circadian phase-shifting effects of repeated ramelteon administration in healthy adults. *J Clin Sleep Med.* 2008;4(5):456-461.

22. Rajaratnam SM, Polymeropoulos MH, Fisher DM, Roth T, Scott C, et al. Melatonin agonist tasimelteon (VEC-162) for transient insomnia after sleep-time shift: Two randomised controlled multicentre trials. *Lancet.* 2009;373(9662):482-491.

23. Kamgar-Parsi B, Wehr TA, Gillin JC. Successful treatment of human non-24-hour sleep-wake syndrome. *Sleep.* 1983;6:257-264.

24. Okawa M, Mishima K, Nanami T, Shimizu T, et al. Vitamin B12 treatment for sleep-wake rhythm disorders. *Sleep.* 1990;13:15-23.

25. Yamadera H, Takahashi K, Okawa M. A multicenter study of sleep-wake rhythm disorders: Clinical features of sleep-wake rhythm disorders. *Psychiatry Clin Neurosci.* 1996;50:195-201.

26. Echizenya M, Iwaki S, Suda H, Shimizu T. Paradoxical reactions to hypnotic agents in adolescents with free-running disorder. *Psychiatry Clin Neurosci.* 2009;63(3):428.

27. Lockley SW, Arendt J, Skene DJ. Visual impairment and circadian rhythm disorders. *Dialogues Clin Neurosci.* 2007;9(3):301-314.

28. Sack RL, Lewy AJ, Blood ML, et al. Circadian rhythm abnormalities in totally blind people: Incidence and clinical significance. *J Clin Endocrinol Metab.* 1992;75:127-134.

29. Lockley SW, Skene DJ, Arendt J, et al. Relationship between melatonin rhythms and visual loss in the blind. *J Clin Endocrinol Metab.* 1997;82:3763-3770.

30. Skene DJ, Lockley SW, Thapan K, et al. Effects of light on human circadian rhythms. *Reprod Nutr Dev.* 1999;39:295-304.

31. Lockley SW, Skene DJ, Butler LJ, et al. Sleep and activity rhythms are related to circadian phase in the blind. *Sleep.* 1999;22(5):616-623.

32. Tabandeh H, Lockley SW, Buttery R, et al. Disturbance of sleep in blindness. *Am J Ophthalmol.* 1998;126(5):707-712.

33. Czeisler CA, Duffy JF, Shanahan TL, et al. Stability, precision, and near-24-hour period of the human circadian pacemaker. *Science.* 1999;284(5423):2177-2181.

34. Boivin DB, Czeisler CA, Dijk DJ, et al. Complex interaction of the sleep-wake cycle and circadian phase modulates mood in healthy subjects. *Arch Gen Psychiat.* 1997;54(2):145-152.

35. Wyatt JK, Ritz-De Cecco A, Czeisler CA, Dijk DJ. Circadian temperature and melatonin rhythms, sleep, and neurobehavioral function in humans living on a 20-h day. *Am J Physiol.* 1999;277(4 Pt 2):R1152-R1163.

36. Kerkhof GA. The 24-hour variation of mood differs between morning- and evening-type individuals. *Percept Mot Skills.* 1998;86:264-266.

37. Miles LE, Raynal DM, Wilson MA. Blind man living in normal society has circadian rhythms of 24.9 hours. *Science.* 1977;198(4315):421-423.

38. Lockley SW, Dijk DJ, Kosti O, Skene DJ, Arendt J. Alertness, mood and performance rhythm disturbances associated with circadian sleep disorders in the blind. *J Sleep Res.* 2008;17(2):207-216.

39. Hastings MH, Reddy AB, Maywood ES. A clockwork web: Circadian timing in brain and periphery, in health and disease. *Nat Rev Neurosci.* 2003;4(9):649-661.

40. Morgan L, Hampton S, Gibbs M, Arendt J. Circadian aspects of postprandial metabolism. *Chronobiol Int.* 2003;20(5):795-808.

41. Klerman EB, Rimmer DW, Dijk DJ, et al. Nonphotic entrainment of the human circadian pacemaker. *Am J Physiol.* 1998;274(4 Pt 2):R991-R996.

42. Mistlberger RE, Skene DJ. Nonphotic entrainment in humans? *J Biol Rhythms.* 2005;20(4):339-352.

43. Czeisler CA, Shanahan TL, Klerman EB, et al. Suppression of melatonin secretion in some blind patients by exposure to bright light. *N Engl J Med.* 1995;332(1):6-11.

44. Klerman EB, Shanahan TL, Brotman DJ, et al. Photic resetting of the human circadian pacemaker in the absence of conscious vision. *J Biol Rhythms.* 2002;17(6):548-555.

45. Zaidi FH, Hull JT, Peirson SN, et al. Short-wavelength light sensitivity of circadian, pupillary, and visual awareness in humans lacking an outer retina. *Curr Biol.* 2007;17(24):2122-2128.

46. Arendt J, Skene DJ, Middleton B, et al. Efficacy of melatonin treatment in jet lag, shift work, and blindness. *J Biol Rhythms.* 1997;12(6):604-617.

47. Lockley SW, Skene DJ, James K, et al. Melatonin administration can entrain the free-running circadian system of blind subjects. *J Endocrinol.* 2000;164:R1-R6.

48. Sack RL, Brandes RW, Kendall AR, et al. Entrainment of free-running circadian rhythms by melatonin in blind people. *N Engl J Med.* 2000;343:1070-1077.

49. Hack LM, Lockley SW, Arendt J, et al. The effects of low-dose 0.5 mg melatonin on the free-running circadian rhythms of blind subjects. *J Biol Rhythms.* 2003;18(5):420-429.

50. Lewy AJ, Bauer VK, Hasler BP, et al. Capturing the circadian rhythms of free-running blind people with 0.5 mg melatonin. *Brain Res.* 2001;918:96-100.

51. Lewy AJ, Emens JS, Lefler BJ, et al. Melatonin entrains free-running blind people according to a physiological dose-response curve. *Chronobiol Int.* 2005;22(6):1093-1106.

52. Lewy AJ, Emens JS, Bernert RA, et al. Eventual entrainment of the human circadian pacemaker by melatonin is independent of the circadian phase of treatment initiation: Clinical implications. *J Biol Rhythms.* 2004;19(1):68-75.

53. Lewy AJ, Hasler BP, Emens JS, et al. Pretreatment circadian period in free-running blind people may predict the phase angle of entrainment to melatonin. *Neurosci Lett.* 2001;313:158-160.

54. Sack RL, Auckley D, Auger RR, et al. Circadian rhythm sleep disorders: Part II, advanced sleep phase disorder, delayed sleep phase disorder, free-running disorder, and irregular sleep-wake rhythm. An American Academy of Sleep Medicine review. *Sleep.* 2007;30:1484-1501.

55. Zee PC, Vitiello MV. Circadian rhythm sleep disorder: Irregular sleep wake rhythm type. *Sleep Med Clin.* 2009;4:213-218.

56. Borbély AA, Baumann F, Brandeis D, Strauch I, Lehmann D. Sleep deprivation: Effect on sleep stages and EEG power density in man. *Electroencephalogr Clin Neurophysiol.* 1981;51:483-495.

57. Larkin JE, Yokogawa T, Heller HC, Franken P, Ruby NF. Homeostatic regulation of sleep in arrhythmic Siberian hamsters. *Am J Physiol.* 2004;287:R104-R111.

58. Edgar DM, Dement WC, Fuller CA. Effect of SCN lesions on sleep in squirrel monkeys: Evidence for opponent processes in sleep-wake regulation. *J Neurosci.* 1993;13:1065-1079.

59. Harper DG, Stopa EG, Kuo-Leblanc V, et al. Dorsomedial SCN neuronal subpopulations subserve different functions in human dementia. *Brain.* 2008;131:1609-1617.

60. Cheng MY, Bullock CM, Li C, et al. Prokineticin 2 transmits the behavioural circadian rhythm of the suprachiasmatic nucleus. *Nature.* 2002;417:405-410.

61. Schwartz MD, Congdon S, de la Iglesia HO. Phase misalignment between suprachiasmatic neuronal oscillators impairs photic behavioral phase shifts but not photic induction of gene expression. *J Neurosci.* 2010;30:13150-13156.

62. Meng QJ, Maywood ES, Bechtold DA, et al. Entrainment of disrupted circadian behavior through inhibition of casein kinase 1 (CK1) enzymes. *Proc Natl Acad Sci USA.* 2010;107:15240-15245.

63. Jewett ME, Kronauer RE, Czeisler CA. Light-induced suppression of endogenous circadian amplitude in humans. *Nature.* 1991;350:59-62.

64. Pollak CP, Perlick D. Sleep problems and institutionalization of the elderly. *J Geriatr Psychiatry Neurol.* 1991;4(4):204-210.

65. Banerjee S, Murray J, Foley B, et al. Predictors of institutionalisation in people with dementia. *J Neurol Neurosurg Psychiatry*. 2003;74(9): 1315-1316.

66. Bliwise DL, Hughes M, McMahon PM, Kutner N. Observed sleep/wakefulness and severity of dementia in an Alzheimer's disease special care unit. *J Gerontol A Biol Sci Med Sci*. 1995;50(6):M303-M306.

67. Volicer L, Harper DG, Manning BC, Goldstein R, Satlin A. Sundowning and circadian rhythms in Alzheimer's disease. *Am J Psychiatry*. 2001;158(5):704-711.

68. Harper DG, Stopa EG, McKee AC, et al. Dementia severity and Lewy bodies affect circadian rhythms in Alzheimer's disease. *Neurobiol Aging*. 2004;25(6):771-781.

69. Durmer JS, Dinges DF. Neurocognitive consequences of sleep deprivation. *Semin Neurol*. 2005;25(1):117-129.

70. Walker MP, Stickgold R. Sleep, memory, and plasticity. *Annu Rev Psychol*. 2006;57:139-166.

71. Feinberg I, Koresko RL, Heller N. EEG sleep patterns as a function of normal and pathological aging in man. *J Psychiatr Res*. 1967;5(2): 107-144.

72. Loewenstein RJ, Weingartner H, Gillin JC, et al. Disturbances of sleep and cognitive functioning in patients with dementia. *Neurobiol Aging*. 1982;3(4):371-377.

73. Prinz PN, Vitaliano PP, Vitiello MV, et al. Sleep, EEG and mental function changes in senile dementia of the Alzheimer's type. *Neurobiol Aging*. 1982;3(4):361-370.

74. Reynolds III CF, Kupfer DJ, Taska LS, et al. EEG sleep in elderly depressed, demented, and healthy subjects. *Biol Psychiatry*. 1985;20(4):431-442.

75. Bliwise DL, Tinklenberg J, Yesavage JA, et al. REM latency in Alzheimer's disease. *Biol Psychiatry*. 1989;25(3):320-328.

76. Vitiello MV, Bokan JA, Kukull WA, et al. Rapid eye movement sleep measures of Alzheimer's-type dementia patients and optimally healthy aged individuals. *Biol Psychiatry*. 1984;19(5):721-734.

77. Reynolds III CF, Kupfer DJ, Taska LS, et al. Sleep apnea in Alzheimer's dementia: Correlation with mental deterioration. *J Clin Psychiatry*. 1985;46(7):257-261.

78. Hoch CC, Reynolds III CF, Kupfer DJ, et al. Sleep-disordered breathing in normal and pathologic aging. *J Clin Psychiatry*. 1986;47(10):499-503.

79. Ancoli-Israel S, Klauber MR, Butters N, Parker L, Kripke DF. Dementia in institutionalized elderly: Relation to sleep apnea. *J Am Geriatr Soc*. 1991;39(3):258-263.

80. Gehrman PR, Martin JL, Shochat T, et al. Sleep-disordered breathing and agitation in institutionalized adults with Alzheimer's disease. *Am J Geriatr Psychiatry*. 2003;11(4):426-433.

81. Cooke JR, Liu L, Natarajan L, et al. The effect of sleep-disordered breathing on stages of sleep in patients with Alzheimer's disease. *Behav Sleep Med*. 2006;4(4):219-227.

82. Ancoli-Israel S, Clopton P, Klauber MR, Fell R, Mason W. Use of wrist activity for monitoring sleep/wake in demented nursing-home patients. *Sleep*. 1997;20(1):24-27.

83. Witting W, Kwa IH, Eikelenboom P, Mirmiran M, Swaab DF. Alterations in the circadian rest-activity rhythm in aging and Alzheimer's disease. *Biol Psychiatry*. 1990;27(6):563-572.

84. Satlin A, Volicer L, Stopa EG, Harper D. Circadian locomotor activity and core-body temperature rhythms in Alzheimer's disease. *Neurobiol Aging*. 1995;16(5):765-771.

85. Van Someren EJ, Hagebeuk EE, Lijzenga C, et al. Circadian rest-activity rhythm disturbances in Alzheimer's disease. *Biol Psychiatry*. 1996;40(4):259-270.

86. Hatfield CF, Herbert J, van Someren EJ, Hodges JR, Hastings MH. Disrupted daily activity/rest cycles in relation to daily cortisol rhythms of home-dwelling patients with early Alzheimer's dementia. *Brain*. 2004;127(Pt 5):1061-1074.

87. Carvalho-Bos SS, Riemersma-van der Lek RF, Waterhouse J, Reilly T, Van Someren EJ. Strong association of the rest-activity rhythm with well-being in demented elderly women. *Am J Geriatr Psychiatry*. 2007;15(2):92-100.

88. Harper DG, Stopa EG, McKee A, et al. Differential circadian rhythm disturbances in men with Alzheimer's disease and frontotemporal degeneration. *Arch Gen Psychiatry*. 2001;58(4):353-360.

89. Ancoli-Israel S, Klauber MR, Jones DW, et al. Variations in circadian rhythms of activity, sleep, and light exposure related to dementia in nursing-home patients. *Sleep*. 1997;20(1):18-23.

90. Gehrman P, Marler M, Martin JL, et al. The timing of activity rhythms in patients with dementia is related to survival. *J Gerontol A Biol Sci Med Sci*. 2004;59(10):1050-1055.

91. Harper DG, Volicer L, Stopa EG, et al. Disturbance of endogenous circadian rhythm in aging and Alzheimer's disease. *Am J Geriatr Psychiatry*. 2005;13(5):359-368.

92. Bonanni E, Maestri M, Tognoni G, et al. Daytime sleepiness in mild and moderate Alzheimer's disease and its relationship with cognitive impairment. *J Sleep Res*. 2005;14(3):311-317.

93. Campbell SS, Kripke DF, Gillin JC, Hrubovcak JC. Exposure to light in healthy elderly subjects and Alzheimer's patients. *Physiol Behav*. 1988;42(2):141-144.

94. Mishima K, Okawa M, Hishikawa Y, et al. Morning bright light therapy for sleep and behavior disorders in elderly patients with dementia. *Acta Psychiatr Scand*. 1994;89(1):1-7.

95. Mishima K, Hishikawa Y, Okawa M. Randomized, dim light controlled, crossover test of morning bright light therapy for rest-activity rhythm disorders in patients with vascular dementia and dementia of Alzheimer's type. *Chronobiol Int*. 1998;15(6):647-654.

96. Van Someren EJ, Kessler A, Mirmiran M, Swaab DF. Indirect bright light improves circadian rest-activity rhythm disturbances in demented patients. *Biol Psychiatry*. 1997;41(9):955-963.

97. Dowling GA, Hubbard EM, Mastick J, et al. Effect of morning bright light treatment for rest-activity disruption in institutionalized patients with severe Alzheimer's disease. *Int Psychogeriatr*. 2005;17(2):221-236.

98. Ancoli-Israel S, Gehrman P, Martin JL, et al. Increased light exposure consolidates sleep and strengthens circadian rhythms in severe Alzheimer's disease patients. *Behav Sleep Med*. 2003;1(1):22-36.

99. Sloane PD, Williams CS, Mitchell CM, et al. High-intensity environmental light in dementia: Effect on sleep and activity. *J Am Geriatr Soc*. 2007;55(10):1524-1533.

100. Skjerve A, Holsten F, Aarsland D, et al. Improvement in behavioral symptoms and advance of activity acrophase after short-term bright light treatment in severe dementia. *Psychiatry Clin Neurosci*. 2004;58(4): 343-347.

101. Ancoli-Israel S, Martin JL, Gehrman P, et al. Effect of light on agitation in institutionalized patients with severe Alzheimer's disease. *Am J Geriatr Psychiatry*. 2003;11(2):194-203.

102. Hickman SE, Barrick AL, Williams CS, et al. The effect of ambient bright light therapy on depressive symptoms in persons with dementia. *J Am Geriatr Soc*. 2007;55(11):1817-1824.

103. Asayama K, Yamadera H, Ito T, et al. Double blind study of melatonin effects on the sleep-wake rhythm, cognitive and non-cognitive functions in Alzheimer's-type dementia. *J Nippon Med Sch*. 2003;70(4):334-341.

104. Singer C, Tractenberg RE, Kaye J, et al. A multicenter, placebo-controlled trial of melatonin for sleep disturbance in Alzheimer's disease. *Sleep*. 2003;26(7):893-901.

105. Jean-Louis G, von Gizycki H, Zizi F. Melatonin effects on sleep, mood, and cognition in elderly with mild cognitive impairment. *J Pineal Res*. 1998;25(3):177-183.

106. Cardinali DP, Brusco LI, Liberczuk C, Furio AM. The use of melatonin in Alzheimer's disease. *Neuro Endocrinol Lett*. 2002;23(Suppl 1):20-23.

107. Dowling GA, Burr RL, Van Someren EJ, et al. Melatonin and bright-light treatment for rest-activity disruption in institutionalized patients with Alzheimer's disease. *J Am Geriatr Soc*. 2008;56(2):239-246.

108. Riemersma-van der Lek RF, Swaab DF, Twisk J, et al. Effect of bright light and melatonin on cognitive and noncognitive function in elderly residents of group care facilities: A randomized controlled trial. *JAMA*. 2008;299(22):2642-2655.

109. Morgenthaler TI, Lee-Chiong T, Alessi C, et al. Practice parameters for the clinical evaluation and treatment of circadian rhythm sleep disorders. An American Academy of Sleep Medicine report. *Sleep*. 2007;30:1445-1459.

110. Okawa M, Sasaki H, Takahashi K. Disorders of circadian body temperature rhythm in severely brain-damaged patients. *Chronobiol Int*. 1984;1:67-71.

111. Ohinata J, Suzuki N, Araki A, et al. Actigraphic assessment of sleep disorders in children with chronic fatigue syndrome. *Brain Dev*. 2008;30: 329-333.

112. Potocki L, Glaze D, Tan DX, et al. Circadian rhythm abnormalities of melatonin in Smith-Magenis syndrome. *J Med Genet*. 2000;37:428-433.

113. Webb EA, O'Reilly MA, Orgill J, et al. Rest-activity disturbances in children with septo-optic dysplasia characterized by actigraphy and 24-hour plasma melatonin profiles. *J Clin Endocrinol Metab*. 2010;95: E198-E203.

114. Ayalon L, Borodkin K, Dishon L, Kanety H, Dagan Y. Circadian rhythm sleep disorders following mild traumatic brain injury. *Neurology*. 2007;68:1136-1140.

115. Lockley SW. Timed melatonin treatment for delayed sleep phase syndrome: The importance of knowing circadian phase. *Sleep*. 2005;28(10):1214-1216.

116. Guilleminault C, McCann CC, Quera-Salva M, Cetel M. Light therapy as treatment of dyschronosis in brain impaired children. *Eur J Pediatr*. 1993;152:754-759.

117. Phillips L, Appleton RE. Systematic review of melatonin treatment in children with neurodevelopmental disabilities and sleep impairment. *Dev Med Child Neurol*. 2004;46:771-775.

118. McArthur AJ, Budden SS. Sleep dysfunction in Rett syndrome: A trial of exogenous melatonin treatment. *Dev Med Child Neurol*. 1998;40:186-192.

119. Wasdell MB, Jan JE, Bomben MM, et al. A randomized, placebo-controlled trial of controlled release melatonin treatment of delayed sleep phase syndrome and impaired sleep maintenance in children with neurodevelopmental disabilities. *J Pineal Res*. 2008;44:57-64.

120. Miyamoto A, Oki J, Takahashi S, Okuno A. Serum melatonin kinetics and long-term melatonin treatment for sleep disorders in Rett syndrome. *Brain Dev*. 1999;21:59-62.

121. Pillar G, Shahar E, Peled N, et al. Melatonin improves sleep-wake patterns in psychomotor retarded children. *Pediatr Neurol*. 2000;23:225-228.

122. Zeitzer JM, Ayas NT, Shea SA, Brown R, Czeisler CA. Absence of detectable melatonin and preservation of cortisol and thyrotropin rhythms in tetraplegia. *J Clin Endocrinol Metab*. 2000;85(6):2189-2196.

123. Scheer FA, Zeitzer JM, Ayas NT, et al. Reduced sleep efficiency in cervical spinal cord injury; Association with abolished nighttime melatonin secretion. *Spinal Cord*. 2006;44(2):78-81.

Therapy in Pediatric Sleep-Related Disorders

Sleep Apnea in Children

CAROL L. ROSEN

The basic treatment recommendations have changed little since the American Academy of Pediatrics (AAP) published their classic evidence and expert consensus based Clinical Practice Guideline in 2002 for diagnosis and management of childhood obstructive sleep apnea (OSA) syndrome in otherwise healthy children (Box 33-1).[1,2]

This chapter provides updated evidence for those original expert recommendations, provides more information about treatment options in medically complex children, and describes some newer adjunctive measures with limited prospective data. The reader is directed to several comprehensive reviews that discuss treatment options in more detail.[3-9] Treatment options can be categorized into four groups, as per Box 33-2 and as discussed here.

LEVELS OF EVIDENCE TO SUPPORT TREATMENT OPTIONS

Conventional therapies (adenotonsillectomy, continuous positive airway pressure [CPAP]) have sufficient evidence to support their general use in children with OSA. The alternative respiratory support therapies (nasal insufflation, supplemental oxygen) minimize OSA severity and may be appropriate in some patients, but only limited data are available. Specialty surgeries may be appropriate for complex patients: they bypass the upper airway obstruction (tracheostomy), target specific craniofacial or anatomic abnormalities, or eliminate co-morbid conditions (bariatric surgery). A number of adjunctive treatments address modifiable risk factors for OSA: optimal management of nasal allergies; avoidance of the supine sleep position; avoidance of environmental tobacco smoke, allergens, and other irritants; dental therapies; and weight loss. These adjunctive therapies have limited or no prospective data to support their use in children, but some may be appropriate for individual patients.

BOX 33-1 *AAP Guidelines for Management of Childhood Obstructive Sleep Apnea[1,2]*

1. **Adenotonsillectomy**
   First-line treatment for an otherwise healthy child with OSA symptoms and adenotonsillar hypertrophy
2. **Continuous positive airway pressure (CPAP)**
   Option for children who are not candidates for adenotonsillectomy or who do not respond the surgery
3. **Referral to specialists for evaluation and management of OSA**
   For high-risk, medically complex children

AAP, American Academy of Pediatrics.
1. Clinical practice guideline. Diagnosis and management of childhood obstructive sleep apnea syndrome. *Pediatrics.* 2002;109(4):704-712.
2. Schechter MS. Technical report: Diagnosis and management of childhood obstructive sleep apnea syndrome. *Pediatrics.* 2002;109(4):e69.

BOX 33-2 *Treatment Options for Pediatric Obstructive Sleep Apnea*

CONVENTIONAL THERAPIES FOR OTHERWISE HEALTHY CHILDREN
- Adenotonsillectomy
- Positive airway pressure (PAP) therapy

ALTERNATIVE SUPPORTIVE RESPIRATORY THERAPIES
- High-flow nasal cannula
- Supplemental oxygen

ALTERNATIVE SURGICAL THERAPIES FOR MEDICALLY COMPLEX PATIENTS
- Targeted surgical treatments
  - Septoplasty and turbinectomy with nonadenoidal nasal obstruction
  - Uvulopalatopharyngoplasty for redundant lateral pharyngeal tissue
  - Tongue reduction for macroglossia
  - Maxillary advancement for midface hypoplasia
  - Genioglossal advancement
  - Mandibular distraction for retro- or micrognathia
- Tracheostomy for severe OSA refractory to conventional therapies
- Bariatric surgery

ADJUNCTIVE THERAPIES
- Dental and orthodontic therapies
  - Rapid maxillary expansion for narrow upper jaw
  - Oral appliances that advance the mandible
- Pharmacotherapy to reduce nasal obstruction or lymphoid hyperplasia
  - Nasal steroids
  - Leukotriene antagonists
  - Antibiotics
  - Systemic corticosteroids
- Weight loss
- Positional therapy to prevent supine sleep
- Avoidance of environmental tobacco smoke and other irritants or allergens

CONVENTIONAL TREATMENTS

Adenotonsillectomy

The surgical treatment of OSA focuses on relieving airway obstruction in the retroglossal region, the nose, and the retropalatal region. Adenotonsillectomy potentially addresses all three areas of obstruction. Despite the lack of randomized controlled data, several evidence-based reviews have concluded that adenotonsillectomy is effective, safe, and the first-line treatment for most uncomplicated cases of childhood OSA associated with adenotonsillar hypertrophy.[1,2,10,11]

The 2002 AAP clinical practice guideline estimated that adenotonsillectomy was associated with resolution of OSA based on reduction of the apnea-hypopnea index (AHI) seen in overnight polysomnography (PSG) in 75% to 100% of otherwise healthy children undergoing the procedure (where AHI is the total number of complete cessations [apneas] and partial obstructions [hypopneas] of breathing occurring per hour of sleep).[1] A 2006 meta-analysis of pooled data on 355 otherwise healthy children from 14 uncontrolled cases series reported that using a variable of "success" threshold (AHI from < 1 to < 5), PSG results improved in 83% and the summary AHI was reduced by almost 14.[10] However, using an AHI less than 1 to defined "success," several more recent large case series have reported lower success rates for adenotonsillectomy.[12,13]

In otherwise healthy children, obesity, family history, genetic background, anatomic variations, chronic asthma, and higher baseline AHI values all contribute to higher risk of residual OSA after surgery. Tauman and associates[12] assessed 110 children with OSA (age 6 ± 4 years, obstructive AHI 22 ± 29; 52% obese) before and after adenotonsillectomy. Mean AHI declined to 5.6, but complete "normalization" of the AHI was observed in only 25% of subjects, 46% had a residual AHI between 1 and 5, and 29% still had a postadenotonsillectomy AHI over 5. Obese participants were more likely to have residual OSA. Guilleminault and associates[13] also reported relatively high rates of persistent PSG abnormalities with 92 (46%) of 199 subjects demonstrating an AHI of 1 or more. Multivariate analyses indicated that a "crowded" airway on visual inspection, retroposition of mandible, enlargement of nasal inferior turbinates, and deviated septum were all associated with residual abnormal polysomnographic (PSG) findings. A 2009 meta-analysis of four studies pooled data from 110 obese children with OSA (mean body mass index Z score, 2.8) (studied before and after adenotonsillectomy) and found, in these very obese children, the mean pre- and postoperative AHI was 29 and 10, respectively.[14] Almost one half of the children had a postoperative AHI less than 5, one quarter had a postoperative AHI less than 2, and 12% had a postoperative AHI less than 1.[14] A recent multicenter collaborative retrospective study that reviewed all nocturnal PSGs performed both pre- and postoperatively on 578 otherwise healthy children (mean age 7 ± 4 years, 50% obese) found that, of the 578 children, only 157 (27.2%) had complete resolution of OSA with postsurgical AHI less than 1. Older age and higher body mass index Z-score were the strongest predictors of higher postsurgery AHI values with modest contribution from asthma and presurgical AHI values in nonobese children. These authors suggested that in a nonobese child with presurgical findings of OSA, the presence of asthma or presurgical findings of severe OSA are indications for obtaining a postsurgical PSG to confirm resolution

of OSA.[15] Other studies suggest that adenotonsillectomy may be less effective in obese children or in those who gain weight after surgery.[16-18] Finally, in a prospective observational family cohort study of 577 children, predictors of residual OSA (AHI ≥ 5) included African-American heritage, obesity, and family history of OSA.[19] These same investigators found that African-American children were less likely to have undergone adenotonsillectomy, but more likely to have residual OSA, after surgery.

Given the increasing rates of childhood obesity, clinicians will need to be increasingly vigilant in monitoring for residual OSA in this high-risk group.[18,20] Although children with co-morbid or complex medical conditions may also benefit from adenotonsillectomy when adenotonsillar hypertrophy is present, these children are at even greater risk for residual OSA related to their underlying conditions. In this high-risk group, objective documentation of OSA presence and severity at baseline and after intervention becomes even more important in determining optimal management.[4]

Decisions for adenotonsillectomy must balance the potential risks, side effects, and benefits of surgery. The main risk of adenotonsillectomy is postoperative hemorrhage, which has a rate of 3.5%.[21] The mortality rate is 1 in 25,000, due to bleeding, airway obstruction, or anesthesia.[22] Careful preoperative evaluation is essential, especially in medically complex patients. Numerous authors have demonstrated that pediatric patients with OSA are at increased risk for peri- and postoperative respiratory complications.[23] These patients can be more sensitive to opiates and inhalational anesthetic agents and are more likely to experience postoperative hypoxemia. Rarely, children can develop pulmonary edema that results from the sudden loss of the positive end-expiratory pressure they experienced secondary to the airway obstruction. With relief of the obstruction, a transudate and pulmonary edema can develop.[24] The rates for postoperative complications vary widely, depending on the proportions of co-morbid conditions present in the patient populations.

The major risk factors for postoperative respiratory complications in children with OSA (Box 33-3) include young age (younger than 3 years),[25] high preoperative AHI, low nadir oxygen saturation (< 70-80%), obesity, and presence of concurrent medical problems or craniofacial disorders.[2,23,26] Rare but late complications of adenotonsillectomy include nasopharyngeal stenosis and velopharyngeal incompetence.[27]

Benefit data for nonrespiratory outcomes after adenotonsillectomy are limited, and randomized controlled studies are not available. Case series have reported postoperative improvements in measures of attention, behavior, sleepiness, and quality of life, and nocturnal enuresis.[4,9] A recent meta-analysis of the literature on growth or growth biomarker changes after adenotonsillectomy found significant increases in weight and height Z scores and in serum levels of insulin-like growth factor 1 (IGF-1) and insulin-like growth factor-binding protein 3 (IGFBP-3).[28]

Children scheduled for adenotonsillectomy often have mild-to-moderate OSA and significant neurobehavioral morbidity, including hyperactivity, inattention, attention deficit hyperactivity disorder, and excessive daytime sleepiness, all of which tend to improve by 1 year after surgery. In terms of neurocognitive dysfunction that has been attributed to OSA, polysomnographic parameters do not predict which children will have neuropsychologic problems or which children will improve after surgery.[29] The lack of better correspondence between OSA measures and neurobehavioral outcomes suggests the need for better measures or improved understanding of underlying causal mechanisms. An important caveat for the clinician to consider is that there is still a lack of consensus on the level of severity of OSA that justifies treatment in children.

Continuous Positive Airway Pressure

Indications for use of CPAP in children for treatment of OSA are listed in Box 33-4 and described here. Children of any age who fail to improve following adenotonsillectomy or are poor surgical candidates for other surgeries or treatments should be considered for CPAP therapy. CPAP therapy is indicated when a child is confirmed to have moderate to severe OSA that persists despite prior adenotonsillectomy and is not a candidate for other surgeries. It may also be indicated when a child needs stabilization of severe OSA until surgery can be scheduled. A "diagnostic" trial of positive airway pressure (PAP) therapy can be considered in a child with milder OSA to see if nocturnal treatment reduces daytime dysfunction thought to be attributable to the OSA. In general, children requiring CPAP treatment are medically complex and have not had an optimal response to adenotonsillectomy because of additional underlying structural, neurologic, neuromuscular, or respiratory disorders. With the obesity epidemic, morbidly obese children are becoming the fastest growing group of pediatric patients who can benefit from this therapy.

Effective and safe use of CPAP for the treatment of childhood OSA has been demonstrated in several large case series with success rates ranging from 74% to 97%.[30-35] Side effects, such as mask leak, skin irritation, and pressure sores, are generally mild, self-limited, and easily addressed by adjusting or refitting the interface. Nasal dryness or congestion can be addressed with use of a heated humidifier. Serious short-term side effects are uncommon apart from rare reports of pneumothorax in children with underlying neuromuscular disorders.[36] The development of midface hypoplasia following prolonged use of nasal CPAP has been reported as a rare long-term complication.[37] Maxillomandibular growth should be monitored carefully and regularly in children on long-term PAP therapy.

CPAP therapy should be titrated during PSG to determine effective pressures, and children on CPAP therapy should be followed regularly to ensure compliance and proper fit of the mask interface. Specific guidelines for conduct of PAP titrations in children have been developed.[38] CPAP in children may be customized in several ways based on the clinical circumstances of individual patients. A variety of interface options are available, including nasal masks, full face masks, and nasal pillows.

The successful initiation and continued effective treatment with CPAP requires a unique and specialized approach to the pediatric patient and their family.[39] Nearly, half of children needing CPAP will be uncooperative upon initial exposure to this unusual treatment. Best practices for PAP therapy in children require a child- and family-focused, chronic disease/health management team approach with coordinated services from clinicians, nurses, respiratory therapist, sleep laboratory personnel, the durable medical equipment provider, and office staff. Successful CPAP therapy also requires a team with expert trouble-shooting strategies to maximize initial and ongoing compliance with prescribed therapy. Clinicians desiring more detailed information about operating a comprehensive and successful pediatric CPAP program for their pediatric patients who will benefit from CPAP therapy are referred to Kirk and O'Donnell's review[39] on ways to maximize compliance.

A child's adherence with long-term CPAP therapy may be influenced by multiple factors. Children who are old enough to perceive improvement of symptoms on treatment or who otherwise recognize and accept the importance of therapy often achieve consistent long-term use, particularly when appropriate parental support is present. Even infants and developmentally disabled older children with limited ability to cooperate may also successfully entrain to long-term use once acclimated. Sustained parental effort and implementation of behaviorally based desensitization programs are sometimes helpful in improving compliance for children whose tolerance of CPAP is initially poor. Availability of behavioral therapy support services may facilitate adherence.[40]

CPAP adherence data in children are scant. Published reports indicate that treatment is associated with a high dropout rate. Even in the adherent children, nightly use is suboptimal considering the long sleep hours in children.[41-43] A randomized control trial comparing continuous and bilevel positive airway pressure in 29 children found that both PAP treatments were highly efficacious in pediatric OSA.[43] New technologic innovations (downloadable and wireless monitoring) that document adherence and provide troubleshooting information are now readily available from durable medical equipment providers and should be used in all pediatric patients. Together with regular face-to-face clinical follow-up, these can be used to monitor therapy and assure that treatment goals are met. Adherence data are now required to determine reimbursement for equipment and services. Clinicians and practice managers need to be knowledgeable about third-party payor requirements for documentation in order to ensure continued access to therapy for their patients.

The PAP interface can also be a conduit for noninvasive nocturnal respiratory support in children with nonobstructive sleep-disordered breathing with hypoventilation, or OSA with sleep-related respiratory insufficiency, associated with other co-morbid conditions including obesity hypoventilation syndrome, neuromuscular weakness, or thoracic cage deformity. Equipment that provides bilevel PAP therapy also allows setting of a backup rate and provides an option to add ventilatory assistance to the respiratory muscle pump in the form of inspiratory pressure support above the expiratory pressure needed to relieve upper airway obstruction. These features are especially important for patients with sleep-related hypoventilation caused by muscle weakness, neurologic disease, or obesity. Data regarding use of CPAP and bilevel PAP in the treatment of nonobstructive sleep-disordered breathing are extremely limited, but successful use of bilevel PAP has been reported in small case series of children with sleep-related hypoventilation caused by congenital central alveolar hypoventilation syndrome or Duchenne's muscular dystrophy.[44-46]

ALTERNATIVE RESPIRATORY SUPPORT THERAPIES

Nasal Insufflation

Although CPAP is a very effective treatment for OSA, some children, especially those with limited ability to cooperate, are unable to tolerate this therapy. A single case series of the effect of using high flow, warm humidified air delivered through an open nasal cannula, so-called "nasal insufflation," was evaluated in children with OSA with and without adenotonsillectomy.[47] Twelve participants (age 10 ± 1 years; BMI 35 ± 14 kg/m^2) with obstructive apnea-hypopnea syndrome ranging from mild to severe (AHI range 2-36 events per hour) were administered 20 L/minute of air through a nasal cannula in a hospital setting. PSG measures were assessed at baseline, on nasal insufflation, and on CPAP. On nasal insufflation therapy, inspiratory flow limitation and respiratory rate were reduced, oxygen stores improved, arousals decreased, and obstructive apnea decreased from 11 ± 3 to 5 ± 2 events per hour ($P < 0.01$). Nasal insufflation may be an alternative to therapy to CPAP in children with mild-to-severe sleep apnea. Additional studies are needed to determine the treatment efficacy.

Oxygen

In patients with limited ability to tolerate PAP therapy or who are not candidates for more aggressive surgical therapies, supplemental oxygen therapy can reduce or abolish the desaturation episodes associated with OSA. However, it does not treat the underlying obstruction and may worsen hypoventilation.[48]

ALTERNATIVE SURGICAL THERAPIES FOR COMPLEX PATIENTS

Procedures that remove or reduce nonlymphoid tissue of the upper airway are sometimes effective in alleviating obstruction, but have received limited study in the pediatric age group. Septoplasty and turbinectomy may improve nasal airflow in older children with significant nonadenoidal obstruction.[3,13] Concerns about facial growth tend to limit extensive nasal surgery in young children, although turbinate reduction appears to be less problematic.

Children with abnormal craniofacial anatomy or abnormalities of neuromotor tone may require additional (beyond the standard therapies) or alternate treatments for persistent or residual OSA; these may include pharyngeal surgery, craniofacial surgery, and even tracheostomy.[23,49] Uvulopharyngopalatoplasty (UPPP) is sometimes performed in children with high Mallampati scores (a scale that rates the degree of pharyngeal crowding based on the appearance of soft palate, uvula, tonsils, and tonsillar pillars) or redundant lateral pharyngeal tissue. UPPP includes resection of the uvula and part of the soft palate and tonsillar pillars. The addition of UPPP to adenotonsillectomy, with the goal of addressing retropalatal obstruction, has been advocated in neurologically impaired children such as those with cerebral palsy and trisomy 21. Several small case series have reported clinical improvement in children with trisomy 21 and other developmental disabilities treated with UPPP, but surgical outcomes in otherwise healthy children have not been assessed.[50-53]

Soft tissue reduction surgery to address retroglossal obstruction, including radiofrequency reduction of the tongue base or soft palate and lingual tonsillectomy, are rarely performed in children. One study using magnetic resonance imaging (MRI) compared the presence or absence of lingual tonsils in children. They found that they were absent in 100% of control subjects but present in 33% of children with residual OSA after adenotonsillectomy and in 50% of children with OSA and Down syndrome, suggesting that tongue base procedures may be underutilized in this population.[54] Tongue reduction surgery may be considered for patients with obstructive macroglossia. Flap takedown can be performed for children with sleep-related airway obstruction after pharyngeal flap surgery for velopharyngeal insufficiency.[55]

Craniofacial procedures, such as mandibular distraction/advancement, genioglossus advancement, and midfacial advancement, have been used to treat OSA resulting from craniofacial structural abnormalities,[56] but are rarely performed in children outside specialty craniofacial centers. In a group of five children whose severe micrognathia had been previously treated with mandibular distraction surgery, significant residual OSA was identified in only one case.[57] Additional case reports have documented OSA improvements for children following treatment with mandibular distraction and with mandibular midline osteotomy.[58,59] Maxillary advancement procedures are sometimes performed in children with significant maxillary hypoplasia, but impact of the procedure on associated OSA has not been systematically assessed. If these medically complex patients have life-threatening OSA, then a temporizing tracheotomy may be necessary even if these aggressive surgeries are considered in the future.

Tracheostomy is only undertaken when a child's OSA is severe and refractory to less drastic forms of therapy (Box 33-5). The procedure is highly effective for alleviation of upper airway obstruction, but adverse impact on quality of life is well documented.[60-62] The procedure also necessitates ongoing stoma care and risk for bacterial colonization and infection. Because of these significant tradeoffs, aggressive use of CPAP or alternative surgical techniques has been advocated.[61]

Bariatric surgery (such as gastric banding or bypass to aid weight reduction) may be a supportive surgical treatment option in morbidly obese children, but data are limited. In the Cincinnati bariatric cohort,[63] 17 adolescents with OSA have been followed and a resolution of OSA was seen in 13 (77%) of these patients after bariatric surgery. Among the three adolescents with persistent OSA, the severity of OSA was reduced substantially, to AHI values less than 10, but not to values less than 5.

ADJUNCTIVE SUPPORTIVE CARE

Dental and Orthodontic Therapies for Childhood Sleep-Related Breathing Disorders

Children who suffer with chronic snoring, mouth breathing, or OSA commonly exhibit disturbances of craniofacial morphology. A significant number have nasal obstruction associated with a narrow maxilla, and maxillary constriction may increase nasal resistance and alter the tongue posture, leading to narrowing of the retroglossal airway and OSA. Dental and orthodontic procedures may play a complementary or even primary role in the evaluation and management of these patients, but scant pediatric outcome data are available.

Rapid maxillary expansion is being investigated as a possible treatment for OSA in children with narrow upper jaws. The procedure involves a fixed oral appliance that is gradually expanded to open the midpalatal suture with the goal of widening the maxilla and maintaining it in this position until the suture reossifies. In a group of 31 children with OSA and narrow maxillas but no adenoidal hypertrophy, rapid maxillary expansion (RME) resulted in a reduction of the mean AHI from 12.2 to 0.4, with all treated subjects having a post-treatment AHI of less than 1.[64] In a recent review article, these same investigators describe their experience in 60 children, mean age 7 years (range 6 to 13 years), with a case histories of oral breathing, snoring, and nighttime apneas (AHI 6 to 22). The authors report that, following comprehensive dental and radiographic evaluations and then treatment by RME, improvements in various outcome measures were found.[8] In addition to restoration of nasal airflow in most children, PSG findings also improved (SpO_2 nadir, AHI level, duration of obstructive events) with greatest improvement in the milder patients. More studies are needed to determine the role of this treatment in the management of children with obstructive signs and symptoms.

Oral appliances, such as mandibular advancing devices and tongue retainers, are rarely used in children with OSA because of concern that this treatment might have the potential to cause orthodontic problems. This concern notwithstanding, two small case series have reported improvements in AHI for children with OSA following 6 months of treatment with an oral appliance.[65,66]

Pharmacologic Treatments

Nasal steroids can be used to treat rhinitis if nasal obstruction is thought to be making a substantial contribution to OSA. Six weeks of nasal steroid resulted in improvement of mean AHI from 8.4 to 1.2 in 14 preadolescent children with allergic rhinitis and OSA.[67] In a prospective, randomized, double-blind study, 13 children with mild to moderate OSA were treated with a 6-week course of nasal corticosteroids. The treatment group showed moderate improvement characterized by concomitant decreases of approximately 50% in the desaturation index and the movement arousal index (the number of desaturations of 4% or greater, or the number of movements associated with EEG arousal, per hour of sleep). In contrast, the placebo group did not show any improvement.[68] A 6-week treatment with nasal steroids effectively reduced both the severity of very mild OSA syndrome (mean AHI < 4) and the magnitude of the underlying adenoidal hypertrophy, and these effects persisted for at least 8 weeks after cessation of therapy. These findings justify the use of topical steroids as the initial therapeutic option in otherwise healthy children with mild OSA.[69] The only long-term nasal steroid data relate to a nonrandomized longitudinal study in 27 children that found modest improvements in AHI (reduction in AHI from 5.2 to 3.2) after 4 weeks of nasal steroids. The clinical effect was maintained as evidenced by a further reduction in symptom scores 9 months after treatment.[70] Because post-treatment AHI values remained abnormal for many of the children in these studies, and because long-term trials assessing safety and effectiveness have not been performed, nasal steroids cannot yet be recommended as *sole* treatment for most childhood OSA.

In an open-labeled study, the leukotriene receptor antagonist montelukast was found to be clinically effective in reducing disease severity in children with mild OSA.[71] In a subsequent study, a combination of intranasal steroids and leukotriene modifier was found to be useful in children with residual OSA after adenotonsillectomy.[72]

Other pharmacotherapies for childhood OSA have received only limited study. Five days of oral corticosteroid therapy was found to be ineffective in treating OSA in seven children with adenotonsillar hypertrophy.[73] Broad-spectrum antibiotics may offer temporary improvement, particularly if snoring and obstruction occur intermittently and are associated with recurrent tonsillitis or adenoiditis,[74] but antibiotics do not obviate the need for surgery in most cases with adenotonsillar hypertrophy.[75]

Weight Loss

Although the American Academy of Pediatrics clinical practice guideline included weight loss as a treatment modality for obese children with OSA,[1] systematic studies on the effect of weight loss on the severity of OSA are scant. Weight loss was reported to be effective in improving nocturnal oxygen saturation in a morbidly obese 8-year-old placed on a calorie-restricted diet.[76] One study examined the effect of regular aerobic exercise in 111 overweight children aged 7 to 11 years, and found that regular exercise improved snoring and reduced

---

BOX 33-6 *Research Areas in Obstructive Sleep Apnea Requiring Further Investigation*

- Assess the extent to which PSG measures, neurobehavioral outcomes, and other indicators of OSA-related morbidity improve after various treatments.
- Determine thresholds for treatment associated with improved health outcomes.
- Identify risk groups for incomplete resolution of OSA after adenotonsillectomy.
- Test strategies to improve PAP adherence in children.
- Determine the role of nasal insufflation in pediatric OSA management.
- Determine the role of dental therapies in pediatric OSA management.
- Determine safety and efficacy of nasal steroids and leukotriene receptor antagonists for adjunctive OSA management.

PAP, positive airway pressure; *PSG*, polysomnography.

---

the risk of OSA, as assessed by a questionnaire.[77] In obese children, weight management strategies should be long-term goals, but should not delay implementation of known effective therapies (adenotonsillectomy, CPAP), as appropriate for the patient.

Other Adjunctive Therapies

Most other adjunctive measures in the treatment of childhood OSA have not been prospectively evaluated. Avoidance of environmental tobacco smoke and other indoor pollutants, avoidance of indoor allergens, and positional therapy may be helpful. Positional therapy, in which a patient is prevented from comfortably assuming a supine position during sleep, has been reported to be helpful in adults with position-dependent OSA[78] but has not been studied in children.

SUMMARY

Adenotonsillectomy is an effective treatment in most uncomplicated cases of obstructive sleep apnea in childhood. Results from the on-going NIH sponsored Childhood Adenotonsillectomy Study (CHAT) should help to inform best practices for using adenotonsillectomy for OSA in children.[79] Given the obesity epidemic, clinicians need to be increasingly familiar with implementation of CPAP therapy in youth. More complex cases of OSA will require involvement of specialty service with pediatric expertise in the evaluation and management at health centers with appropriate support facilities. More randomized clinical trials or comparative effectiveness research is needed to guide present-day management and determine future directions (Box 33-6).

REFERENCES

1. Clinical practice guideline. Diagnosis and management of childhood obstructive sleep apnea syndrome. *Pediatrics*. 2002;109(4):704-712.
2. Schechter MS. Technical report: Diagnosis and management of childhood obstructive sleep apnea syndrome. *Pediatrics*. 2002;109(4):e69.
3. Guilleminault C, Lee JH, Chan A. Pediatric obstructive sleep apnea syndrome. *Arch Pediatr Adolesc Med*. 2005;159(8):775-785.
4. Hoban TF, Chervin RD. Sleep-related breathing disorders of childhood: Description and clinical pictures, diagnosis, and treatment approaches. *Sleep Med Clin*. 2007;2:445-462.
5. Halbower AC, McGinley BM, Smith PL. Treatment alternatives for sleep-disordered breathing in the pediatric population. *Curr Opin Pulm Med*. 2008;14(6):551-558.
6. Capdevila OS, Kheirandish-Gozal L, Dayyat E, Gozal D. Pediatric obstructive sleep apnea: Complications, management, and long-term outcomes. *Proc Am Thorac Soc*. 2008;5(2):274-282.
7. Au CT, Li AM. Obstructive sleep breathing disorders. *Pediatr Clin North Am*. 2009;56(1):243-259:xii.
8. Pirelli P, Saponara M, De Rosa C, Fanucci E. Orthodontics and obstructive sleep apnea in children. *Med Clin North Am*. 2010;94(3):517-529.
9. Powell S, Kubba H, O'Brien C, Tremlett M. Paediatric obstructive sleep apnoea. *BMJ*. 2010;340:c1918.
10. Brietzke SE, Gallagher D. The effectiveness of tonsillectomy and adenoidectomy in the treatment of pediatric obstructive sleep apnea/hypopnea syndrome: A meta-analysis. *Otolaryngol Head Neck Surg*. 2006;134(6):979-984.
11. Robb PJ, Bew S, Kubba H, Murphy N, Primhak R, et al. Tonsillectomy and adenoidectomy in children with sleep related breathing disorders: Consensus statement of a UK multidisciplinary working party. *Clin Otolaryngol*. 2009;34(1):61-63.
12. Tauman R, Gulliver TE, Krishna J, Montgomery-Downs HE, O'Brien LM, et al. Persistence of obstructive sleep apnea syndrome in children after adenotonsillectomy. *J Pediatr*. 2006;149(6):803-808.
13. Guilleminault C, Huang YS, Glamann C, Li K, Chan A. Adenotonsillectomy and obstructive sleep apnea in children: A prospective survey. *Otolaryngol Head Neck Surg*. 2007;136(2):169-175.
14. Costa DJ, Mitchell R. Adenotonsillectomy for obstructive sleep apnea in obese children: A meta-analysis. *Otolaryngol Head Neck Surg*. 2009;140(4):455-460.
15. Bhattacharjee R, Kheirandish-Gozal L, Spruyt K, et al. Adenotonsillectomy outcomes in treatment of obstructive sleep apnea in children: A multicenter retrospective study. *Am J Respir Crit Care Med*. 2010;182(5):676-683.
16. Shine NP, Coates HL, Lannigan FJ. Obstructive sleep apnea, morbid obesity, and adenotonsillar surgery: A review of the literature. *Int J Pediatr Otorhinolaryngol*. 2005;69(11):1475-1482.
17. Apostolidou MT, Alexopoulos EI, Chaidas K, Ntamagka G, Karathanasi A, et al. Obesity and persisting sleep apnea after adenotonsillectomy in Greek children. *Chest*. 2008;134(6):1149-1155.
18. Amin R, Anthony L, Somers V, Fenchel M, McConnell K, et al. Growth velocity predicts recurrence of sleep-disordered breathing 1 year after adenotonsillectomy. *Am J Respir Crit Care Med*. 2008;177(6):654-659.
19. Morton S, Rosen C, Larkin E, Tishler P, Aylor J, Redline S. Predictors of sleep-disordered breathing in children with a history of tonsillectomy and/or adenoidectomy. *Sleep*. 2001;24(7):823-829.
20. Ievers-Landis CE, Redline S. Pediatric sleep apnea: Implications of the epidemic of childhood overweight. *Am J Respir Crit Care Med*. 2007;175(5):436-441.
21. Lowe D, van der Meulen J, Cromwell D, Lewsey J, Copley L, et al. Key messages from the National Prospective Tonsillectomy Audit. *Laryngoscope*. 2007;117(4):717-724.
22. Lee KL. *Essential Otolaryngology: Head and Neck Surgery*. 9th ed. New York: McGraw-Hill; 2008.
23. Schwengel DA, Sterni LM, Tunkel DE, Heitmiller ES. Perioperative management of children with obstructive sleep apnea. *Anesth Analg*. 2009;109(1):60-75.
24. Blum RH, McGowan Jr FX. Chronic upper airway obstruction and cardiac dysfunction: Anatomy, pathophysiology and anesthetic implications. *Paediatr Anaesth*. 2004;14(1):75-83.
25. Statham MM, Elluru RG, Buncher R, Kalra M. Adenotonsillectomy for obstructive sleep apnea syndrome in young children: Prevalence of pulmonary complications. *Arch Otolaryngol Head Neck Surg*. 2006;132(5):476-480.
26. Ye J, Liu H, Zhang G, Huang Z, Huang P, Li Y. Postoperative respiratory complications of adenotonsillectomy for obstructive sleep apnea syndrome in older children: Prevalence, risk factors, and impact on clinical outcome. *J Otolaryngol Head Neck Surg*. 2009;38(1):49-58.
27. Marcus CL. Sleep-disordered breathing in children. *Am J Respir Crit Care Med*. 2001;164(1):16-30.
28. Bonuck KA, Freeman K, Henderson J. Growth and growth biomarker changes after adenotonsillectomy: Systematic review and meta-analysis. *Arch Dis Child*. 2009;94(2):83-91.
29. Chervin RD, Ruzicka DL, Giordani BJ, Weatherly RA, Dillon JE, et al. Sleep-disordered breathing, behavior, and cognition in children before and after adenotonsillectomy. *Pediatrics*. 2006;117(4):e769-e778.

30. Massa F, Gonsalez S, Laverty A, Wallis C, Lane R. The use of nasal continuous positive airway pressure to treat obstructive sleep apnoea. *Arch Dis Child*. 2002;87(5):438-443.

31. Downey 3rd R, Perkin RM, MacQuarrie J. Nasal continuous positive airway pressure use in children with obstructive sleep apnea younger than 2 years of age. *Chest*. 2000;117(6):1608-1612.

32. Waters KA, Everett FM, Bruderer JW, Sullivan CE. Obstructive sleep apnea: The use of nasal CPAP in 80 children. *Am J Respir Crit Care Med*. 1995;152(2):780-785.

33. McNamara F, Sullivan CE. Obstructive sleep apnea in infants and its management with nasal continuous positive airway pressure. *Chest*. 1999;116(1):10-16.

34. Guilleminault C, Pelayo R, Clerk A, Leger D, Bocian RC. Home nasal continuous positive airway pressure in infants with sleep-disordered breathing. *J Pediatr*. 1995;127(6):905-912.

35. Marcus CL, Ward SL, Mallory GB, Rosen CL, Beckerman RC, et al. Use of nasal continuous positive airway pressure as treatment of childhood obstructive sleep apnea. *J Pediatr*. 1995;127(1):88-94.

36. Simonds AK. Pneumothorax: An important complication of non-invasive ventilation in neuromuscular disease. *Neuromuscul Disord*. 2004;14(6):351-352.

37. Li KK, Riley RW, Guilleminault C. An unreported risk in the use of home nasal continuous positive airway pressure and home nasal ventilation in children: Mid-face hypoplasia. *Chest*. 2000;117(3):916-918.

38. Kushida CA, Chediak A, Berry RB, Brown LK, Gozal D, et al. Clinical guidelines for the manual titration of positive airway pressure in patients with obstructive sleep apnea. *J Clin Sleep Med*. 2008;4(2):157-171.

39. Kirk VG, O'Donnell AR. Continuous positive airway pressure for children: A discussion on how to maximize compliance. *Sleep Med Rev*. 2006;10(2):119-127.

40. Koontz KL, Slifer KJ, Cataldo MD, Marcus CL. Improving pediatric compliance with positive airway pressure therapy: The impact of behavioral intervention. *Sleep*. 2003;26(8):1010-1015.

41. O'Donnell AR, Bjornson CL, Bohn SG, Kirk VG. Compliance rates in children using noninvasive continuous positive airway pressure. *Sleep*. 2006;29(5):651-658.

42. Uong EC, Epperson M, Bathon SA, Jeffe DB. Adherence to nasal positive airway pressure therapy among school-aged children and adolescents with obstructive sleep apnea syndrome. *Pediatrics*. 2007;120(5):e1203-e1211.

43. Marcus CL, Rosen G, Ward SL, Halbower AC, Sterni L, et al. Adherence to and effectiveness of positive airway pressure therapy in children with obstructive sleep apnea. *Pediatrics*. 2006;117(3):e442-e451.

44. Tibballs J, Henning RD. Noninvasive ventilatory strategies in the management of a newborn infant and three children with congenital central hypoventilation syndrome. *Pediatr Pulmonol*. 2003;36(6):544-548.

45. Migliori C, Cavazza A, Motta M, Bottino R, Chirico G. Early use of Nasal-BiPAP in two infants with congenital central hypoventilation syndrome. *Acta Paediatr*. 2003;92(7):823-826.

46. Fanfulla F, Berardinelli A, Gualtieri G, Zoia MC, Ottolini A, et al. The efficacy of noninvasive mechanical ventilation on nocturnal hypoxaemia in Duchenne's muscular dystrophy. *Monaldi Arch Chest Dis*. 1998;53(1):9-13.

47. McGinley B, Halbower A, Schwartz AR, Smith PL, Patil SP, Schneider H. Effect of a high-flow open nasal cannula system on obstructive sleep apnea in children. *Pediatrics*. 2009;124(1):179-188.

48. Marcus CL, Carroll JL, Bamford O, Pyzik P, Loughlin GM. Supplemental oxygen during sleep in children with sleep-disordered breathing. *Am J Respir Crit Care Med*. 1995;152(4 Pt 1):1297-1301.

49. Sterni LM, Tunkel DE. Obstructive sleep apnea in children: An update. *Pediatr Clin North Am*. 2003;50(2):427-443.

50. Kerschner JE, Lynch JB, Kleiner H, Flanary VA, Rice TB. Uvulopalatopharyngoplasty with tonsillectomy and adenoidectomy as a treatment for obstructive sleep apnea in neurologically impaired children. *Int J Pediatr Otorhinolaryngol*. 2002;62(3):229-235.

51. Kosko JR, Derkay CS. Uvulopalatopharyngoplasty: Treatment of obstructive sleep apnea in neurologically impaired pediatric patients. *Int J Pediatr Otorhinolaryngol*. 1995;32(3):241-246.

52. Seid AB, Martin PJ, Pransky SM, Kearns DB. Surgical therapy of obstructive sleep apnea in children with severe mental insufficiency. *Laryngoscope*. 1990;100(5):507-510.

53. Strome M. Obstructive sleep apnea in Down syndrome children: A surgical approach. *Laryngoscope*. 1986;96(12):1340-1342.

54. Fricke BL, Donnelly LF, Shott SR, Kalra M, Poe SA, et al. Comparison of lingual tonsil size as depicted on MR imaging between children with obstructive sleep apnea despite previous tonsillectomy and adenoidectomy and normal controls. *Pediatr Radiol*. 2006;36(6):518-523.

55. Maturo SC, Mair EA. Submucosal minimally invasive lingual excision: An effective, novel surgery for pediatric tongue base reduction. *Ann Otol Rhinol Laryngol*. 2006;115(8):624-630.

56. Sundaram S, Bridgman SA, Lim J, Lasserson TJ. Surgery for obstructive sleep apnoea. *Cochrane Database Syst Rev*. 2005(4):CD001004.

57. Lin SY, Halbower AC, Tunkel DE, Vanderkolk C. Relief of upper airway obstruction with mandibular distraction surgery: Long-term quantitative results in young children. *Arch Otolaryngol Head Neck Surg*. 2006;132(4):437-441.

58. Cohen SR, Holmes RE, Machado L, Magit A. Surgical strategies in the treatment of complex obstructive sleep apnoea in children. *Paediatr Respir Rev*. 2002;3(1):25-35.

59. Guilleminault C, Li KK. Maxillomandibular expansion for the treatment of sleep-disordered breathing: Preliminary result. *Laryngoscope*. 2004;114(5):893-896.

60. Guilleminault C, Korobkin R, Winkle R. A review of 50 children with obstructive sleep apnea syndrome. *Lung*. 1981;159(5):275-287.

61. Cohen SR, Simms C, Burstein FD, Thomsen J. Alternatives to tracheostomy in infants and children with obstructive sleep apnea. *J Pediatr Surg*. 1999;34(1):182-186;discussion 187.

62. McNamara F, Sullivan CE. Treatment of obstructive sleep apnea syndrome in children. *Sleep*. 2000;23(Suppl 4):S142-S146.

63. Kalra M, Inge T. Effect of bariatric surgery on obstructive sleep apnoea in adolescents. *Paediatr Respir Rev*. 2006;7(4):260-267.

64. Pirelli P, Saponara M, Guilleminault C. Rapid maxillary expansion in children with obstructive sleep apnea syndrome. *Sleep*. 2004;27(4):761-766.

65. Cozza P, Gatto R, Ballanti F, Prete L. Management of obstructive sleep apnoea in children with modified monobloc appliances. *Eur J Paediatr Dent*. 2004;5(1):24-29.

66. Villa MP, Bernkopf E, Pagani J, Broia V, Montesano M, Ronchetti R. Randomized controlled study of an oral jaw-positioning appliance for the treatment of obstructive sleep apnea in children with malocclusion. *Am J Respir Crit Care Med*. 2002;165(1):123-127.

67. Mansfield LE, Diaz G, Posey CR, Flores-Neder J. Sleep disordered breathing and daytime quality of life in children with allergic rhinitis during treatment with intranasal budesonide. *Ann Allergy Asthma Immunol*. 2004;92(2):240-244.

68. Brouillette RT, Manoukian JJ, Ducharme FM, Oudjhane K, Earle LG, et al. Efficacy of fluticasone nasal spray for pediatric obstructive sleep apnea. *J Pediatr*. 2001;138(6):838-844.

69. Kheirandish-Gozal L, Gozal D. Intranasal budesonide treatment for children with mild obstructive sleep apnea syndrome. *Pediatrics*. 2008;122(1):e149-e155.

70. Alexopoulos EI, Kaditis AG, Kalampouka E, Kostadima E, Angelopoulos NV, et al. Nasal corticosteroids for children with snoring. *Pediatr Pulmonol*. 2004;38(2):161-167.

71. Goldbart AD, Goldman JL, Veling MC, Gozal D. Leukotriene modifier therapy for mild sleep-disordered breathing in children. *Am J Respir Crit Care Med*. 2005;172(3):364-370.

72. Kheirandish L, Goldbart AD, Gozal D. Intranasal steroids and oral leukotriene modifier therapy in residual sleep-disordered breathing after tonsillectomy and adenoidectomy in children. *Pediatrics*. 2006;117(1):e61-e66.

73. Al-Ghamdi SA, Manoukian JJ, Morielli A, Oudjhane K, Ducharme FM, Brouillette RT. Do systemic corticosteroids effectively treat obstructive sleep apnea secondary to adenotonsillar hypertrophy? *Laryngoscope*. 1997;107(10):1382-1387.

74. Sclafani AP, Ginsburg J, Shah MK, Dolitsky JN. Treatment of symptomatic chronic adenotonsillar hypertrophy with amoxicillin/clavulanate potassium: Short- and long-term results. *Pediatrics*. 1998;101(4 Pt 1):675-681.

75. Don DM, Goldstein NA, Crockett DM, Ward SD. Antimicrobial therapy for children with adenotonsillar hypertrophy and obstructive sleep apnea: A prospective randomized trial comparing azithromycin vs placebo. *Otolaryngol Head Neck Surg*. 2005;133(4):562-568.

76. Kudoh F, Sanai A. Effect of tonsillectomy and adenoidectomy on obese children with sleep-associated breathing disorders. *Acta Otolaryngol Suppl*. 1996;523:216-218.

77. Davis CL, Tkacz J, Gregoski M, Boyle CA, Lovrekovic G. Aerobic exercise and snoring in overweight children: A randomized controlled trial. *Obesity (Silver Spring)*. 2006;14(11):1985-1991.

78. Permut I, Diaz-Abad M, Chatila W, Crocetti J, Gaughan JP, et al. Comparison of positional therapy to CPAP in patients with positional obstructive sleep apnea. *J Clin Sleep Med*. 2010;6(3):238-243.

79. Redline S, Amin R, Beebe DW, et al. The childhood adenotonsillectomy trial (CHAT): Rationale, design and challenges of a randomized controlled trial evaluating a standard surgical procedure in a pediatric population. *Sleep*. Accepted for publication.

Chapter 34

Disorders of Central Respiratory Control During Sleep in Children

ELIOT S. KATZ

OVERVIEW OF RESPIRATORY CONTROL

Breathing is regulated to maintain oxygen (O_2), carbon dioxide (CO_2), and acid-base balance within a narrow range, under conditions of changing state, airway resistance, and energy expenditure. The central respiratory pattern generator network is located in the brainstem and receives input from the lung, chemoreceptors (central/peripheral), and upper airway. This chapter will focus on disorders of central respiratory control in children resulting in decreased respiratory drive.

Anatomy and Physiology

The respiratory pattern generator consists of a small group of neurons in the ventrolateral medulla termed the pre-Botzinger complex. Signals generated in the pre-Botzinger complex project both to the dorsal respiratory group in the nucleus tractus solitarius (NTS) and the ventral respiratory group in the medulla. The NTS also receives afferent inputs that modulate respiration from peripheral arterial chemoreceptors, the upper airway, and lungs. The various respiratory rhythm inputs are integrated in the NTS and project to respiratory motor neurons including the hypoglossal (upper airway) and the phrenic (diaphragm) nerves. Wakefulness also imparts an excitatory influence on ventilation, which is lost at sleep onset.

Central chemoreceptors are located on the ventral surface of the medulla and respond primarily to the acidity of the cerebrospinal fluid. CO_2 rapidly equilibrates into the cerebrospinal fluid and alters the pH accordingly. Ventilation is inversely related to pH. The central chemoreceptors are believed to contribute to ventilatory homeostasis with a time constant of a few minutes. The peripheral chemoreceptors are located at the bifurcation of the common carotid artery and on the aortic arch. The peripheral chemoreceptors are sensitive to both O_2 and CO_2 tensions in the arterial blood, and they provide afferent information to the NTS with a short time constant, allowing breath-by-breath modulation of breathing. The primary determinant of steady state ventilation is central chemoreceptor activity, whereas the peripheral chemoreceptors are believed to be more important in the response to acute changes in arterial gas tensions.

Influence of Sleep on Ventilation

During wakefulness, breathing is controlled by a combination of behavioral inputs (feeding, speech, exercise) in addition to chemical inputs (principally CO_2, and to a lesser extent O_2, tension). The carotid chemoreceptors also respond to alterations in CO_2 and pH, and are thought to play a role in respiratory control stability and arousal from sleep in response to hypoxemia and hypercapnia. The contribution of peripheral O_2 chemoreceptor to eupneic ventilation can be quantified by measuring the ventilatory reduction in response to a single breath of 100% oxygen (Dejour test). The Dejour test response of preterm infants, term infants, and adults are 45%, 30%, and 6%, respectively.[1] Thus, O_2 tension has an important contribution to respiratory drive, especially in premature infants.

During sleep, there is a reduction in the metabolic rate, ventilatory responsiveness to CO_2 and O_2, and minute ventilation. On balance, the CO_2 level increases 3 to 7 torr during sleep. In non–rapid eye movement sleep (NREM) breathing is typically regular and principally regulated by chemical regulation. By contrast, in rapid eye movement (REM) sleep breathing is highly irregular and influenced by central REM processes, rather than primarily chemical drive. Respiratory pauses of 8 to 10 seconds are common during sleep in children, particularly during REM sleep, and frequently follow sighs or body movements. Respiratory pauses are more frequent during sleep (versus wakefulness), during REM sleep (versus NREM sleep), and at younger ages.

CENTRAL APNEA

Definition

The proper classification of centrally mediated apnea requires an understanding of the various patterns of decreased respiratory drive and the context of age-specific normative data. The term *respiratory pause* is defined exclusively by an arbitrary threshold duration. Brief respiratory pauses in the 3- to 20-second range are normal occurrences in all age groups, and commonly occur following sighs, body movements, and during REM sleep.[2] These brief events are generally not associated with sleep disruption or gas exchange abnormalities and are not considered pathologic. Longer pauses, in the 20- to 30-second range, are also occasionally observed in otherwise normal infants.[3] The term *central apnea* in infants and children is defined as a respiratory pause lasting 20 seconds or greater, or a respiratory pause lasting at least two missed breaths that is associated with an electrocortical arousal or oxygen desaturation of at least 3%.[4] Central apnea is deemed clinically important when it results in chronic intermittent hypoxemia or bradycardia, which may adversely affect neurocognitive development or cardiovascular function. In preterm infants, the definition of a "pathologic" central apnea is often tied to a clinically significant outcome, such as an O_2 desaturation below 85% or to bradycardia less than 80 beats per minute (see discussion under "Apnea of Prematurity"). This nomenclature may lead to confusion in the setting of parenchymal lung disease or low lung volumes (such as obesity) in which rapid O_2 desaturation may occur with brief respiratory pauses. In this context, respiratory pauses of normal duration would be scored as central apneas due to decreased O_2 reserve.

In the typical form of respiratory pauses and central apneas described earlier, expiration is a passive process resulting in a gradual return toward the passive end-expiratory volume. However, additional patterns of central apnea have been described. In *mixed apnea*, airway closure occurs toward the end of the central apneic events, resulting in respiratory efforts against a closed airway.[5,6] Mixed apneas are generally longer than central apneas and are associated with more profound O_2 desaturation.[7] *Apneustic breathing* is a different pattern, characterized by a prolonged end-inspiratory pause in breathing. *Biot's breathing* is a dysrhythmic breathing pattern first described in patients with tuberculous meningitis. It is characterized by an irregular pattern of variable respiratory pauses separated by periods of tachypnea. It has been reported in children with hypoxic-ischemic encephalopathy or central nervous system tumor.[8] *Periodic breathing* has a regular crescendo-decrescendo pattern and is normally observed in preterm and term infants (Fig. 34-1). *Prolonged expiratory apnea with cyanosis* usually occurs during wakefulness, typically after a startle or crying. In this condition, active expiration lowers lung volumes below functional residual capacity (FRC) and may induce intrapulmonary shunting, resulting in profound hypoxemia that is poorly responsive to positive pressure ventilation. Conditions associated with central apnea in children are listed in Box 34-1.

In interpreting a polysomnogram, it is important to distinguish between central apneas that are scored due to a prolonged respiratory pause (> 20 seconds) versus those consisting of a normal respiratory pause (8-12 seconds) that are associated with O_2 desaturation. The former may suggest a brainstem abnormality such as a Chiari malformation

or brain tumor. By contrast, rapid O_2 desaturation associated with normal, brief respiratory pauses would be consistent with decreased oxygen reserve, including parenchymal lung disease or obesity.

Normative Data for Central Apneas in Infants

Fetal breathing is highly irregular with bursts of respiratory efforts separated by long central pauses. After birth, infants continue to have extremely irregular breathing patterns, especially during the first few months of life. The coefficient of variation of minute ventilation is highest in preterm infants (39%) compared to term infants (25%) and adults (14%).[9] Some of the variability in infant breathing patterns relates to the proportion of time spent in REM sleep, which is 60% at term, and 30% by 1 year of age. Normative data for respiratory pauses and central apnea in infants is predicated on the event definition, gestational age, postconceptional age, and duration of monitoring:

1. Ramanathan and associates[3] prospectively studied 306 healthy term infants continuously during sleep in

---

BOX 34-1 *Conditions Associated with Central Sleep Apnea in Children*

- Congenital central hypoventilation syndrome
- Chiari malformation
- Leigh syndrome
- Joubert syndrome
- Brain/brainstem tumor
- Rett syndrome
- Medications (narcotics, anesthetics)
- Achondroplasia
- Post-CNS infection
- Respiratory syncytial virus infection
- Hypoxic-ischemic encephalopathy

CNS, central nervous system.

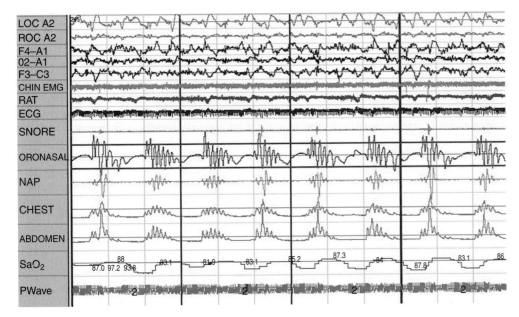

Figure 34-1 Periodic breathing in a 1-month-old infant, associated with intermittent oxygen desaturation. Dark vertical bars mark 30-second intervals. *EMG,* electromyogram; *LOC,* left outer canthus; *NAP,* nasal air pressure; *PWAVE,* oximeter pulse wave; *RAT,* right anterior tibial EMG; *ROC,* right outer canthus.

the first 6 months of life; 43% were observed to have *conventional events* (apnea 20 seconds and mild brady-cardia), and 2% had *extreme events* (apnea 30 seconds and marked bradycardia).[10] Importantly, these events are not associated with an apparent acute morbidity, though there is greater heart rate and respiratory variability preceding the apnea events. Conventional events are accompanied by a median O_2 desaturation of 20% to 30%. The apneas had a partially obstructive component (mixed apnea) in 50% of conventional events and 70% of extreme events.[3] By contrast, of 367 asymptomatic preterm infants in the same study, 64% had one or more conventional event, and 20% had one or more extreme events during the first 6 months of life.[3] The preterm infant's risk of extreme events was evident only until 43 weeks' postconceptional age.[3] There was an association between five or more conventional events with lower Bayley Scales of Infant Development at 1 year of age, though causality has not been established.

2. Hoppenbrouwers and colleagues[11] studied term infants at 0.25, 1, 2, 3, 4, and 6 months of age, and tabulated respiratory pauses of 6 seconds or longer. In active sleep, they observed an average of 12 such pauses per hour at 1 week, 7 per hour at 1 month, and 5 per hour at 2 to 6 months. In NREM sleep, pauses occurred at a rate of approximately 1.5 per hour between 0.25 and 6 months of age.

3. Kahn and associates[12] studied healthy infants over the gestational age range of 25 to 43 weeks (average 38.5 weeks) at an average of 55.6 weeks' postconceptional age (range 34-91 weeks), and tabulated respiratory pauses of 4 seconds or longer. Before 45 weeks' postconceptional age respiratory pauses occurred at a rate of approximately 9 per hour in active sleep (90th percentile, 26/hour) and 2.6 per hour in NREM sleep (90th percentile, 8.5/hour). Beyond 60 weeks' postconceptional age the rate of respiratory pauses was approximately 5.4 per hour in active sleep (90th percentile, 11/hour) and 1.7 per hour in NREM sleep (90th percentile, 3.9/hour).

4. Stein and associates[13] studied 250 healthy term infants during the first 3 days of life and observed a respiratory pause of 15 seconds or longer in 27% of infants, and 20 seconds or longer in 5% of infants.

Acute decreases in O_2 saturation (> 10%) during sleep are observed in most otherwise normal infants.[14] These events are most common in the first 2 months of life, and are usually associated with periodic breathing (79%) or isolated respiratory pauses (16%).[14] The end-expiratory volume is the principal determinant of the rate at which O_2 desaturation occurs during an apnea.[15,16] At birth, the high compliance of the chest wall results in very low end-expiratory volume and therefore low O_2 reserve. The lung volumes in infants decrease approximately 30% during REM sleep (active sleep), rendering them particularly vulnerable to O_2 desaturation.[17] Consequently, O_2 desaturations are commonly observed even with brief respiratory pauses during REM sleep. By contrast, older infants (beyond 0.5-1 year) have lower chest wall compliance, a higher end-expiratory volume, and therefore sufficient O_2 reserve to sustain O_2 saturations during most normal respiratory pauses.[18-21] There is a further reduction in the end-expiratory volume during respiratory pauses in infants,

thereby increasing the likelihood of O_2 desaturation.[15] When respiratory pauses are grouped, such as in periodic breathing, the O_2 desaturation rate is greater during the later apneas. In addition to lung volume, the determinants of O_2 desaturation rate include baseline arterial O_2 tension, metabolic rate, and mixed venous O_2 content (influenced by cardiac output and hemoglobin concentration). The baseline O_2 saturation during sleep in a healthy term infant has a median of 97.9% and a lower 10th percentile of 95.2%.[14] However, 59% of infants had at least one 3-minute epoch with a baseline O_2 saturation less than 90%.[14] The median O_2 saturation nadir in a healthy term infant is 83% with the 10th percentile 78%.[14]

Normative Data for Central Apneas in Children

Normative data for respiratory pauses has also been well established after infancy. Older children rarely have scorable central apneas, though respiratory pauses of 8 to 10 seconds are commonly observed, and isolated central apneas lasting up to 25 seconds may be seen.[21,22] Breathing, both in terms of respiratory frequency and tidal volume, is generally less variable in older children. Carskadon and associates[23] reported that healthy 12-year-old children have approximately 17.2 ± 11.4 respiratory pauses of 5 seconds or more per night of sleep.[23] Forty-two percent of these pauses lasted longer than 10 seconds (maximum 25 seconds).[23] The incidence of respiratory pauses was highest in stage N1 sleep, intermediate in REM sleep, and lowest in stages N2 and N3/N4 sleep. Poets and associates[21] reported respiratory pauses of 15 to 19.9 seconds in 43 of 70 children, and over 20 seconds in 12 of 70 children between 2 and 16 years of age. O_2 desaturation was rarely observed during these respiratory pauses, especially in older children.[21] Similarly, Moss and associates[22] reported that 26% of children (age 10.1 ± 0.7) had a central apnea lasting 20 seconds or longer, though only 18% experienced an O_2 desaturation below 90%. Overall, central apneas defined as 20 seconds or longer or associated with a 4% O_2 desaturation are generally recorded less than once per hour in normal children.[24,25] Scorable central apneas are more common during REM sleep,[24] in keeping with the greater likelihood of oxygen desaturation. Thus, occasional brief O_2 desaturations associated with respiratory pauses are commonly observed in older children.

Apnea of Prematurity

There is no clear consensus on the definition of *apnea of prematurity (AOP)* or the severity level that requires treatment. The general approach is to consider neonatal central apneas as pathologic if they last 20 seconds or more, or if they are associated with bradycardia or hypoxemia. Clinically, infants appear limp, cyanotic, and unresponsive. In most cases, AOP is diagnosed and treated by neonatologists without involving the sleep laboratory or sleep medicine physicians. Nevertheless, there are instances in which the AOP is resistant to therapy or prolonged beyond the point of discharge from the nursery and a polysomnogram is requested to clarify the breathing pattern.

The frequency of AOP is inversely related to gestational age, affecting nearly 100% of infants weighing less than 1000 g.[26,27] In infants born between 28 and 35 weeks of gestation, central apnea usually resolves by 38 to 40 weeks' postconceptual age.[28] However, infants born before 28 weeks of gestation often have clinical apnea that persists until 40 to 44 weeks' postconceptual age.[29] AOP is rarely observed in infants born after 36 weeks of gestation. The term "apnea of infancy" is often used to describe episodes of central apnea that begin to occur after 37 weeks' postconceptional age. Prolonged episodes of pathologic central apnea in infants have been associated with adverse neurodevelopmental outcomes.[30]

AOP is observed during a 3- to 4-month developmental window and resolves spontaneously between 36 and 44 weeks' postconceptional age. Nevertheless, the marked bradycardia and hypoxemia that characterize AOP warrant treatment. The prone position has been shown to reduce, but not eliminate, the frequency of central apnea in premature infants.[31] In addition, the prone position is associated with increases in lung volume and higher oxygenation in preterm infants between 26 and 32 weeks' postconceptional age, and in older preterm infants with respiratory distress.[32] As the infants approach discharge, the increased risk of sudden infant death syndrome (SIDS) mandates that infants be placed supine during sleep.[33] Continuous positive airway pressure (CPAP) delivered via nasal prongs is highly effective in reducing AOP and improves oxygenation in preterm infants, likely by increasing the functional residual capacity.[34] The mainstay of treatment for AOP is oral caffeine, which improves diaphragmatic function and increases respiratory drive.[35] In addition to reducing AOP, caffeine therapy in doses of 5 to 10 mg/kg per day after a 20 mg/kg loading dose has been associated with a reduction in the duration of positive pressure therapy/O_2, a decrease in the rate of bronchopulmonary dysplasia, and a lower incidence of cerebral palsy/cognitive deficits.[36,37] In most infants, the caffeine is discontinued by 36 weeks' postconceptual age, but may be needed longer in infants born before 28 weeks of gestation.[38] Importantly, other than a few case reports, there is insufficient data to support the use of caffeine as a respiratory stimulant for central apnea in older children.

Apparent Life-Threatening Events (ALTEs)

Suspected apnea in a newborn is a frequent cause for referral to the pediatric sleep laboratory. The term *apparent life-threatening event (ALTE)* refers to an episode that is "frightening to the observer and that is characterized by some combination of apnea (central or occasionally obstructive), color change (usually cyanotic or pallid but occasionally erythematous or plethoric), marked change in muscle tone (usually marked limpness), choking, or gagging."[39] ALTEs are reported in 0.2 to 0.9% of infants,[40,41] though recognized long-term sequelae are rare. Though the pathophysiology of ALTEs is variable, central apnea is a prominent feature in most cases. The physical examination is typically normal. The differential diagnosis of an ALTE in infants is listed in Box 34-2. There are no polysomnographic differences in the incidence of central apnea in infants with an ALTE compared to those without.[3]

The management and workup of an ALTE is predicated on the perceived severity based on the clinical history. In most cases, a period of cardiorespiratory monitoring is indicated, including oximetry, heart rate, and respiratory rate. More concerning ALTEs warrant a complete blood count, serum glucose and electrolytes, and a venous blood gas. Additional testing may be indicated if there is a strong suspicion of trauma (head imaging), gastroesophageal reflux (impedance/pH

monitoring), seizures (electroencephalogram [EEG]), hypoxemia or respiratory distress (chest radiograph), or stridor (direct laryngoscopy). A polysomnogram might be indicated if there are repeated ALTEs of unknown etiology, documented hypoxemia, a clear suspicion of central apnea, excessive periodic breathing, or concerns for airway obstruction. An extended EEG montage may be added to the polysomnogram to help identify epileptiform activity.

Home cardiorespiratory monitors have limited utility because they do not detect obstructive sleep apnea (OSA) or hypoxemia and are prone to false alarms. Though most bradycardia events are associated with O_2 desaturation,[42] significant hypoxemia can occur without bradycardia.[43] These monitors may be helpful to document the frequency and duration of respiratory pauses in certain patients including children with known central apnea, infants being weaned off of caffeine, or infants and older children with known brainstem dysfunction. In rare circumstances a documenting oximeter may be indicated if there are concerns for abnormal ventilatory control, impaired respiratory mechanics, or parenchymal lung disease. Home monitoring has not been demonstrated to prevent SIDS.

BOX 34-2 *Differential Diagnosis for Apparent Life-Threatening Event (ALTE) in Infants*

Neurologic
- Seizures
- Infection
- Intracranial hemorrhage/hydrocephalus
- Congenital central hypoventilation syndrome
- Chiari malformation
- Asphyxia
- Brain tumor

Infectious
- Respiratory syncytial virus infection
- Sepsis

Gastrointestinal
- Gastroesophageal reflux
- Direct aspiration

Cardiac
- Arrhythmias
- Right-to-left shunting

Pulmonary
- Craniofacial abnormalities
- Laryngomalacia
- Tracheomalacia

Metabolic
- Inborn errors of metabolism
- Hypoglycemia
- Electrolyte disturbancess

Other
- Ingestion
- Medication effect
- Trauma
- Laryngomalcia
- Subglottic stenosis
- Obstructive sleep apnea
- Breath-holding spell

Some practitioners prescribe a home monitor to allay parental fears, though the frequent false alarms may actually provoke anxiety in caregivers.[44]

Periodic Breathing

Periodic breathing (PB) is defined as a series of three or more respiratory pauses lasting 3 seconds or longer separated by 20 seconds or more of normal breathing[4] (see Fig. 34-1). The apneic interval is typically 5 to 8 seconds, and the ventilatory phase is 7 to 10 seconds. PB is minimal in the first week of life, peaks at 2 to 4 weeks of age, is markedly reduced by 4 months of age, and rarely occurs after 6 months of age in normal infants.[18,45] PB is observed in nearly 100% of preterm infants weighing less than 1000 g at birth, and in 30% to 80% of term infants during sleep.[26,27] PB as a percentage of total sleep time ranges from 8% to 15% in preterm, and 0% to 5% in term infants. PB that is markedly elevated during infancy, or present in older children, may require further investigation, such as central nervous system imaging.

PB occurs during both REM and NREM sleep. In NREM sleep periodic breathing is characterized a regular pattern of pauses separated by consistent intervals of respiratory efforts, whereas in REM sleep PB has an irregular configuration of both. During the ventilatory phase of the cycle there is a reduction in CO_2. If the CO_2 tension decreases below the apneic threshold (1.5 torr below the baseline level in infants, 5 torr below in adults), a respiratory pause ensues. During the apneic phase of the cycle the CO_2 increases and the O_2 tension decreases, thus driving subsequent hyperventilation. Because of the close proximity of the apneic threshold to baseline breathing in infants, brief perturbations can induce PB, including sighs or body movements. PB is also associated with low lung volumes, which predispose toward decreased O_2 reserve and increased intrapulmonary shunting. O_2 desaturations frequently occur during sleep in infants, and 80% of these desaturations are associated with PB.[14]

PB is often presents with documented hypoxemia in the newborn nursery, during assessment for an apparent life-threatening event, or as a parental observation. The majority of documented cases of PB are benign and do not require treatment. However, therapy is indicated in the presence of significant sleep disruption, bradycardia, or hypoxemia. There is no consensus on the threshold level of hypoxemia that requires treatment. Therapy with O_2 via nasal cannula is highly effective in both eliminating the hypoxemia and reducing the frequency of PB.[46,47] Increasing lung volumes with prone positioning, CPAP therapy, or externally applied negative pressure improves oxygenation, thereby reducing the frequency of PB.[48,49] However, CPAP is often poorly tolerated in infants and prone positioning is discouraged in infants. Methylxanthines, such as caffeine or theophylline, are also effective in reducing PB,[50] but their side effects make them a less desirable form of therapy.

CONGENITAL CENTRAL HYPOVENTILATION SYNDROME

Congenital central hypoventilation syndrome (CCHS) is a rare disorder characterized by alveolar hypoventilation that is particularly pronounced during sleep. CCHS patients have a diminished responsiveness to changes in CO_2 tension by the medullary chemoreceptors in the absence of any structural brainstem lesion, parenchymal lung disease, cardiac disease, or neuromuscular weakness. Patients with CCHS present with life-threatening hypercapnia and hypoxemia. The clinical features of CCHS are summarized in Box 34-3. Life-long ventilatory support is necessary and the sleep laboratory is an important resource for ensuring optimal ventilator settings. A comprehensive Consensus Statement on the diagnosis and health care needs of CCHS patients was published in 2010.[51]

Genetics

The disease-defining gene for CCHS is the paired-like homeobox 2B (*PHOX2B*) gene located on chromosome 4.[52,53] *PHOX2B* encodes for a transcription factor that effects neural crest development, including the autonomic nervous system. Transmission is autosomal dominant, with 85% to 90% of identified cases de novo mutations. Asymptomatic mosaicism is found in 5% to 10% of parents of infants with CCHS. About 90% of CCHS patients are heterozygous for a polyalanine expansion mutation in exon 3 of the *PHOX2B* gene. The remaining 10% of CCHS patients are heterozygotes for various insertion or deletion mutations.

The normal polyalanine repeat sequence in exon 3 of the *PHOX2B* gene is 20 alanines on both chromosomes (20/20). Heterozygous polyalanine repeat expansion mutations ranging between 20/24 to 20/33 are typically observed in CCHS, with 20/25, 20/26, and 20/27 being by far the most common.[54] Germline polyalanine mutations larger than 20/25 are fully penetrant, whereas some 20/24 and 20/25 mutations have been reported with decreased penetrance.

BOX 34-3   *Clinical Features of Congenital Central Hypoventilation Syndrome (CCHS)*

Ophthalmologic
- Strabismus
- Decreased pupillary reflex

Respiratory
- Elevated P_{CO_2}*
- Breath-holding spells

Cardiac
- Asystole
- Syncope/staring spells

Gastrointestinal
- Esophageal dysmotility
- Hirschsprung's disease

Neurocognitive
- Intellectual impairment
- Mood disorders

Autonomic
- Temperature instability
- Pain insensitivity
- Diaphoresis

Miscellaneous
- Neural crest tumors

*P_{CO_2}, carbon dioxide partial pressure

The spectrum of severity of CO_2 responsiveness and some ancillary features of CCHS are related to the underlying genotype. Generally, longer polyalanine repetitions are associated with more severe disease. Late-onset CCHS in childhood[55] and adults is most often reported with the 20/24[55] and 20/25[56-58] genotype. Approximately 10% of CCHS cases have a 20/20 genotype, with a missense, nonsense, or frameshift mutation in the *PHOX2B* gene (*nonpolyalanine repeat expansion mutations*). Most of these are de novo mutations and tend to have a very severe phenotype with neural crest tumors and Hirschsprung's disease as well as a round-the-clock 24-hour ventilator requirement.

Presentation

The majority of recognized cases of CCHS are diagnosed in the newborn period. Presentations in older infants, toddlers,[55] adolescents,[56] and adults[57,58] are termed *late-onset* CCHS. Typically these late-onset cases will present during anesthesia, after intake of central nervous system depressants, or during the course of a lower respiratory tract infection. A special subset of late-onset central hypoventilation features a form of hypothalamic dysfunction, termed *rapid-onset obesity with hypothalamic dysfunction, hypoventilation, and autonomic dysregulation* (see section on *ROHHAD;* discussed later), and is not caused by a recognized mutation in *PHOX2B*.

The diagnosis of CCHS requires testing of the *PHOX2B* gene for mutations. An initial screen by gel electrophoresis is recommended to identify polyalanine repeat expansion mutations (*PHOX2B* Screening Test, see www.genetests.org). If negative, the *PHOX2B* gene may be sequenced to identify the nonpolyalanine expansion mutations. A referral to a tertiary care center with experience in managing CCHS patients is recommended. Parents of CCHS patients should be screened for *PHOX2B* mutations or mosaicism.

Respiratory Abnormalities

Children with CCHS who can maintain a CO_2 below 45 torr during wakefulness generally do not need daytime (i.e., awake time) ventilatory support. CCHS genotypes are highly predictive of the requirement for ventilatory support only during sleep versus continuous mechanical ventilation. Individuals with the 20/24 genotype often present as late-onset cases, and typically need nocturnal ventilation alone. The 20/25 genotype usually presents at birth, but also generally requires only nocturnal ventilation. The 20/26 genotype frequently requires additional daytime ventilatory assistance in the setting of exercise or illness. Finally, the 20/27 to 20/33 genotypes mostly require 24-hour per day mechanical ventilation. Most CCHS patients with the nonpolyalanine repeat expansion mutations also need uninterrupted 24-hour ventilatory assistance. Overall, approximately one third of children with CCHS need 24-hour a day ventilatory support. Though exercise does stimulate breathing to some extent in CCHS patients, hypoventilation may become apparent during moderate exercise.[59]

To ensure optimal neurocognitive development, it is essential to maintain proper oxygenation and ventilation. The ventilatory needs of a patient with CCHS should be established during resting wakefulness, exercise, and sleep. Comprehensive monitoring is indicated in each of these states using respiratory inductance plethysmography, oximetry, end-tidal CO_2,

and electrocardiogram. Serum chemistries may reveal an elevation of the hematocrit due to chronic hypoxemia or elevation of serum bicarbonate, related to hypercapnia. Overnight polysomnography with continuous end-tidal CO_2 monitoring is recommended twice per year. It is important to note that although supplemental O_2 alone will correct the oxygenation deficit, it does not reverse the underlying hypoventilation, which will eventually result in pulmonary hypertension. The target end-tidal CO_2 during sleep ranges between 35 and 40 torr, with normal oxygenation. Some authors recommend maintaining the sleeping CO_2 at or below 35 torr, in order to facilitate daytime ventilation.[60] Careful attention to monitoring alarms during sleep, as well as having emergency plans including availability of an electrical backup source for the ventilator, is essential. The recent clinical policy statement of the American Thoracic Society on care for CCHS patients recommends continuous monitoring by a trained nurse with knowledge of ventilator management.[51] It is important that a monitor be placed *before* sleep onset, as hypoventilation can occur fulminantly immediately after sleep onset. A standard impedance-type cardioapnea monitor should not be used in CCHS, because it will not detect hypoventilation or sinus arrests. Rather, patients with CCHS should sleep with a documenting oximeter (alarm set at 85%) and end-tidal CO_2 monitor (alarm set at 55 torr) at all times.

The mainstay of therapy for young children with CCHS is positive pressure ventilation through a tracheostomy. Pressure-cycled ventilation using a portable, battery-powered, continuous flow ventilator using a small tracheostomy tube is typically sufficient during the first 6 years of life. Patients with CCHS should have an extra tracheostomy tube and ventilation bag with them at all times, including visits to the sleep laboratory. Noninvasive ventilation is an option in older children with CCHS (after 6-8 years of age) who require ventilatory support only during sleep. Typically, a nasal mask with a fixed leak is utilized in combination with a bilevel ventilator in the *timed* or *spontaneously timed* mode. Strict adherence to the aforementioned monitoring regimen is also essential with noninvasive ventilation.

Some children requiring daytime ventilation may consider diaphragmatic pacing to free themselves from a more cumbersome ventilator.[60] Diaphragmatic pacing involves bilateral thoracoscopic placement of phrenic nerve electrodes that activate the diaphragm and thus provide ventilatory support. The external device is small and easily portable. Diaphragmatic pacing should be limited to 12 to 15 hours per day due to concerns regarding diaphragmatic fatigue. Thus, an alternative form of respiratory support will be necessary for those patients requiring continuous ventilation. Diaphragmatic pacer settings are determined during continuous monitoring and should be tested one or two times per year.[60] Both the respiratory rate and tidal volume (electrode voltage) can be set. The same monitoring and nursing requirements apply to patients with CCHS who have diaphragmatic pacers implanted. In addition, a backup transmitter is desirable. Though large datasets are not available, it is believed that at least 50% of children utilizing diaphragmatic pacers exclusively at night will tolerate decannulation.[60] Some children with diaphragmatic pacers develop obstructive apnea during sleep. Insertion and care of diaphragmatic pacers should be limited to institutions with particular experience in the technique. In the event of a pacing malfunction, noninvasive or tracheostomy ventilation will be necessary emergently. Patients with a diaphragmatic pacer cannot obtain an magnetic resonance imaging (MRI) scan.

Children with CCHS are vulnerable to acute respiratory failure during anesthesia, intercurrent viral illnesses, and the use of respiratory depressants. Viral upper respiratory illnesses pose a considerable risk to CCHS patients because they are unable to perceive elevations of CO_2 that may accompany parenchymal lung disease or soft tissue swelling of the upper airway. Similarly, great caution should be taken during swimming because patients with CCHS lack the perception of asphyxia and are at risk of drowning. Alcohol and illicit drugs are known to be respiratory depressants, and death or coma has been reported in adolescents with CCHS after ingesting alcohol.[61] Patients with CCHS should be counseled regarding the risks of substance abuse. A recent report on two female CCHS patients documented a restoration of CO_2 chemosensitivity in response to the progestin contraceptive desogestrel.[62] Progestins are known to augment ventilatory drive and chemosensitivity. This concept requires further evaluation.

Cardiac Abnormalities

CCHS is associated with abnormal cardiac autonomic regulation, including decreased baroreflex activity,[63] decreased heart rate variability,[64] sinus bradycardia, and asystole.[65] Holter monitoring often reveals isolated prolonged R-R intervals (> 3 seconds) in CCHS patients, particularly with the genotype 20/26 (19% affected) and 20/27 (87% affected).[66] The CCHS 20/25 genotype tends to have a normal R-R interval during childhood, but adults with the 20/25 genotype may also develop asystoles.[58] In one important report of three children with both CCHS and at least one R-R interval greater than 3 seconds, and who did not receive a pacemaker, two died suddenly and unexpectedly.[66] All children with CCHS have a prolonged corrected QT interval, though this does not seem to vary with genotype. A 72-hour Holter monitor is recommended annually to screen for life-threatening arrhythmias, particularly with genotypes 20/26 and 20/27. Because of the risk of sudden death, it is recommended that a pacemaker be implanted in children with CCHS if they are having R-R intervals greater than 3 seconds, even if they are asymptomatic.[66] Right ventricular hypertrophy and pulmonary hypertension may also be present. Screening for unrecognized hypoxemia and pulmonary hypertension should include a yearly hematocrit and echocardiogram. Children with CCHS may develop complete heart block when exposed to anesthetic agents.[67]

Neural Crest Abnormalities

CCHS patients have a diverse constellation of abnormalities related to aberrant neural crest development that warrant enhanced clinical suspicion. Neural crest tumors, such as ganglioneuroma, neuroblastoma, and ganglioneuroblastoma, are commonly observed in nonpolyalanine repeat expansion mutations, and rarely with the 20/29 to 20/33 genotypes. Because these genotypes are generally not seen in cases of late-onset CCHS, tumors are rare in this population. MRI scans of the chest and abdomen are recommended approximately every 2 years for CCHS patients with 20/29 to 20/33 genotypes, as well as with nonpolyalanine expansion mutations.

Hirschsprung's disease is characterized by an aganglionic section of the distal bowel and usually presents with constipation. A barium enema demonstrates the luminal narrowing; a rectal biopsy revealing a lack of ganglion cells is diagnostic. The standard therapy is resection of the affected colon and a "pull-through" procedure using proximal bowel. Hirschsprung's disease is usually present in nonpolyalanine repeat expansion mutations (> 87% of cases), and occasionally with 20/27 and longer genotypes (15% of cases). Severe constipation may be present in CCHS even without Hirschsprung's disease.

CCHS is associated with additional symptoms of autonomic nervous system dysfunction including breath-holding spells, temperature instability, and sporadic profuse diaphoresis. Individuals with CCHS frequently have a characteristic facial phenotype including a short, flat face, increased nasal tip protrusion, decreased nasolabial angle, decreased upper lip height, and inferior inflection of the vermilion border of the upper lip.[68] Many children with CCHS have developmental delay and learning disabilities. Whether the neurocognitive impairment is an integral part of CCHS or secondary to hypoxemia has not been established. Subtle abnormalities of neurocognitive function should be proactively identified with an individual education program (IEP). A careful ophthalmologic examination should be performed regularly to screen for strabismus and pupillary abnormalities.

RAPID-ONSET OBESITY WITH HYPOTHALAMIC DYSFUNCTION, HYPOVENTILATION, AND AUTONOMIC DYSREGULATION

Rapid-onset obesity with hypothalamic dysfunction, hypoventilation, and autonomic dysregulation (ROHHAD) is a distinct syndrome of late-onset central hypoventilation that generally becomes clinically apparent between 1.5 and 7 years of age.[69,70] The essential characteristics of ROHHAD are an apparently normal growth and development in the first 1 to 2 years of life followed by a marked, rapid weight gain over a 4- to 6-month interval. The rapid onset of obesity is the first recognized symptom in 80% of cases. There is considerable variability in the occurrence of the other manifestations including hypothalamic dysfunction (average 3 years), autonomic dysfunction (3.6 years), and hypoventilation (6.2 years).[70] Similarly, another large study confirmed that rapid-onset obesity was the initial symptom, and hypoventilation was apparent a median of 1.5 years later.[71]

Tumors of neural crest origin are observed at some time in their lives in 30% to 40% of patients and include ganglioneuroblastoma and ganglioneuroma.[70,71] Hypothalamic dysfunction includes water balance abnormalities, hyperprolactinemia, hypothyroidism, growth hormone deficiency, adrenal insufficiency, and puberty timing abnormalities. Disordered thirst (increased or decreased) has been frequently reported.[71] Autonomic irregularities include strabismus, pupillary sensitivity, gastrointestinal dysmotility, temperature instability, decreased pain sensation, and an irregular heart rate. Neurocognitive deficits are common, including 30% to 40% with some developmental delay, and 50% to 60% with behavioral disorders.[70,71]

Many children with ROHHAD present after undergoing anesthesia or during an upper respiratory infection. Cardiorespiratory arrest is commonly reported in these children before their hypoventilation is recognized and properly treated. Strabismus and scoliosis are also frequently observed.

Approximately 50% to 60% of ROHHAD patients will require mechanical ventilation only during sleep and are typically managed with a nasal interface. The remainder of children will require 24 hours per day respiratory support. The profound hypoventilation has been reported to precipitate seizures, respiratory arrest, and even death in many cases. Despite the clinical similarity of ROHHAD with late-onset CCHS, testing for *PHOX2B* mutations have been consistently negative in ROHHAD. One report (still unpublished at the time of this writing) of identical twins discordant for ROHHAD has led to speculation that epigenetic factors may be important.

Treatment considerations for ROHHAD are similar to those for CCHS as discussed in CCHS section earlier in chapter. A thorough assessment of ventilation during wakefulness, sleep, and exercise is critically important to determine the necessary respiratory support. Patients must take special care in the setting of anesthesia, intercurrent viral illnesses, and ingesting medications and other substances known to depress ventilation. Routine MRI surveillance of the chest and abdomen (every 1-1.5 years for the first decade of life, then every 2 years thereafter) for evidence of neural crest tumors is recommended. A high index of suspicion for the development of endocrinopathies should be maintained. Weight loss is an important objective to improve pulmonary mechanics and facilitate ventilator support.

RETT SYNDROME

Rett syndrome (RS) is a heterogeneous disorder affecting females and is caused by a mutation of the *MECP2* gene on the X chromosome. Clinical onset is typically between 6 and 18 months of age. The respiratory characteristics of RS are summarized in Box 34-4. Breathing abnormalities usually begin after 2 years of age and are often confined to wakefulness[72] but may also occur during sleep[73] (Fig. 34-2). The apneustic breathing pattern predominates in the first 10 years of life. Older individuals also frequently demonstrate Valsalva breathing, central apnea, and shallow breathing.[72] The sleep abnormalities are frequently observed at sleep onset transitions, but prolonged central apneas have been reported in all stages of sleep. Typically, RS patients have normal sleep architecture and NREM breathing, with an occasional prolonged central apnea during REM sleep.[74] Parenchymal lung disease on the basis of gastroesophageal reflux and oropharyngeal dysfunction may contribute to the hypoxemia observed during respiratory pauses.

Hyperventilation is associated with hypocarbia, and apnea produces hypercarbia and hypoxemia. Hypocapnic alkalosis may result in vasoconstriction, reducing cerebral and coronary artery perfusion. Sudden death has been reported.[72] During hyperventilation episodes there is widespread activation of the ventrolateral medulla, including autonomic excitation. Autonomic symptoms often include flushing, pupillary dilatation, and cold extremities. Breath-holding spells are often interspersed with hyperventilation. Brief, nonepileptic staring episodes, termed "vacant spells," may be associated with respiratory dysrhythmias. During Valsalva maneuvers, forced expiration against a closed glottis increases intrapleural pressure, which impairs systemic venous return, and leads to arterial hypotension. Dystonic posturing or repetitive movements are frequently seen during breathing dysrhythmias, although epileptiform discharges are rare. Impairment in parasympathetic circuitry gives rise to exaggerated sympathetic responses and an increased

> **BOX 34-4** *Dysrhythmic Breathing Patterns in Rett Syndrome*
>
> - Hyperventilation
> - Irregular respiratory rate
> - Central apnea
> - Valsalva breathing: expiration against a closed glottis
> - Apneustic breathing
>   - Fast full inspiration followed by breath hold until fast expiration
>   - End-inspiratory breath hold after normal tidal breath
>   - Prolonged inspiration
> - Exaggerated deep breathing
> - Shallow breathing (slow or rapid)
> - Biot's breathing: abrupt apnea followed by abrupt regular breathing
> - Periodic breathing

risk of cardiac arrhythmias. Aerophagia has been reported to occur during hyperventilation and breath-holding episodes resulting in gastric distention that may interfere with respiratory gas exchange. Successful treatment of the gastric distention may require gastrostomy tube placement.[75] The termination of inspiration is serotonin-dependent and agonists to serotonin 1A receptors have been used to treat apneustic breathing in RS.[76]

PRADER-WILLI SYNDROME

Prader-Willi syndrome (PWS) is characterized by dysfunction of the hypothalamus, peripheral chemoreceptors, and autonomic nervous system. The gene defect is found on paternal chromosome 15 and, less commonly, through maternal uniparental disomy or imprinting errors. Symptoms of hypothalamic and autonomic dysfunction include pain insensitivity, temperature instability, diminished salivation, poor satiety, excessive daytime sleepiness, and an altered sleep-wake cycle.

Excessive Daytime Sleepiness

Children with PWS have a central abnormality of sleep-state cycling including REM sleep fragmentation, sleep-onset REM cycles, and increased cyclic alternating pattern.[77] Over half of children with PWS report excessive daytime sleepiness (EDS) that is more severe than in other developmental disabilities.[78] Children with PWS are both objectively[79] and subjectively[78] sleepy. EDS in PWS may arise from OSA, from obesity, or as a primary feature of PWS. Some PWS patients have objective EDS based on multiple sleep latency testing (MSLT), even in the absence of obesity or OSA.[77,80,81] Thus, sleepiness in PWS is indicative of a primary hypothalamic dysfunction. Low cerebrospinal fluid hypocretin levels were reported in two PWS patients with objective sleepiness but minimal OSA.[82] A wakefulness-promoting agent, such as modafinil, may perhaps prove helpful in reducing the level of sleepiness in PWS.

Sleep-Disordered Breathing

Children with PWS have multiple risk factors for sleep-related breathing disturbances including respiratory muscle weakness, obesity, midfacial hypoplasia, micrognathia, pharyngeal

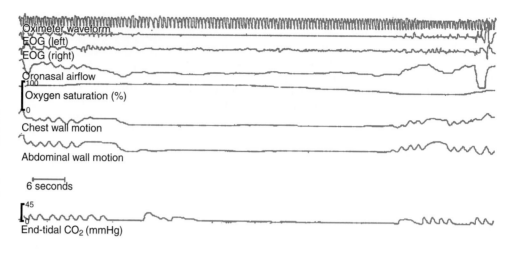

Figure 34-2 Patient with Rett syndrome during wakefulness. After a period of hyperventilation, a 41-second central apnea is observed associated with marked oxygen desaturation. (Redrawn from Marcus CL, Carroll JL, McColley SA, et al. *EOG,* electrooculogram. Polysomnographic characteristics of patients with Rett syndrome. *J Pediatr.* 1994;125:218-224, used with permission.)

muscle weakness, impaired peripheral chemoreceptors, and scoliosis. Hyperphagia ensues after approximately 1 year of age, resulting in marked weight gain and often obesity. Peripheral chemoreceptor function is impaired in all individuals, but the central hypercapnic ventilatory response is impaired only in obese PWS patients. Thus, the obesity per se is responsible for considerable cardiopulmonary morbidity and death.[80] Longstanding OSA in PWS may lead to pulmonary hypertension, behavioral disturbances,[83] and cognitive impairment.[84] Pulmonary hypertension is a major contributor to death in PWS patients.

Lean patients with PWS (matched for gender, age, birth weight, and gestational age) frequently demonstrate O_2 desaturation associated with normal, brief respiratory pauses and also during REM sleep.[85] PWS patients have more respiratory pauses longer than 2 seconds, but not more obstructive apnea than control subjects.[85] Most studies in PWS children have demonstrated little or no OSA in the absence of obesity.[80] However, O_2 desaturations are commonly related to respiratory muscle weakness. OSA in PWS tends to be mild and occurs equally in male and female patients.[80] It is hypothesized that the fat distribution in PWS is more central (female pattern) rather than visceral (male pattern), accounting for the small effect that body mass index (BMI) has on OSA severity. Children with PWS may be particularly vulnerable to OSA during intercurrent viral respiratory infections in which airway resistance increases due to peripherally chemoreceptor dysfunction.[86-88]

PWS patients with severe sleep-disordered breathing and daytime respiratory failure have been successfully treated with nocturnal bilevel ventilation, resulting in normalization of daytime gas exchange.[89] The hypercapnic ventilatory drive has been documented to increase after tracheostomy in an obese PWS patient. Weight reduction has also been documented to improve both alveolar ventilation and OSA in PWS, but not EDS.[81,90] Treating the OSA in PWS patients with adenotonsillectomy or CPAP reduces the EDS in some patients.[91]

Influence of Growth Hormone on Sleep Apnea

Growth hormone (GH) therapy in PWS may improve behavior, physical activity, hypersomnolence, respiratory muscle strength, hypercapnic ventilatory responsiveness, and basal ventilation.[92,93] The long-term outcome after treatment with GH remains to be established. Safety concerns were raised by a series of case reports of sudden death after starting GH in PWS.[94] These deaths occurred mostly during sleep within 4 months of starting therapy, and OSA was suspected as a contributor. GH replacement only rarely produces OSA in GH-deficient patients. However, GH may contribute to worsening OSA by inducing adenotonsillar hypertrophy, increasing the basal metabolic rate, or altering the body fluid balance. The adverse effects of GH might be mediated by insulin growth factor-1 (IGF-1) that may result in adenotonsillar hypertrophy. IGF-1 levels have been previously correlated with the AHI in PWS patients.[88] Also, there are several reports of OSA worsening in PWS patients during an intercurrent viral illness.[86,88] Children with PWS may be particularly vulnerable to the effects of increased upper airway resistance, given their peripheral chemoreceptor dysfunction.

Three prospective trials of GH in children with PWS have not demonstrated a consistent worsening of OSA on therapy.[86,88,95] Miller and associates[88] studied 25 PWS patients (average age 13 years) before and 6 weeks after initiation of GH therapy. The AHI decreased in 19 patients and increased in 6 patients but, overall, the AHI was not significantly different after GH. Of the patients whose OSA worsened after starting GH, 4 had an intercurrent viral illness at the time of the follow-up polysomnogram.[88] Festen and associates[86] studied 53 prepubertal PWS patients (median age 5.4 years) before and after 6 months of GH therapy. There was no change in the AHI following GH therapy. However, one child died unexpectedly during a mild upper respiratory infection despite having a normal polysomnogram before and after GH treatment. Haqq and colleagues[95] studied 12 PWS patients (age 9.7 ± 3.3 years) before and after 6 months of GH and observed, at baseline, a slightly higher incidence of apnea/hypopnea in PWS children with and without obesity; they found no significant increase in the apnea/hypopnea following 6 months of GH treatment.

There are numerous cases of documented sudden death in PWS patients who were *not* on GH.[96,97] The authors of a study of a large cohort of PWS deaths in patients with and without GH therapy concluded that sudden death is twice as common in males with or without GH; that deaths were most often associated with intercurrent viral infections in both groups; and that 75% of the deaths in the GH group were in the first 9 months (median 3 months) of GH therapy (and therefore the possibility that GH may predispose toward sudden death could not be fully eliminated).[97] In summary, there is little data implicating GH in exacerbating OSA in children with OSA. Intercurrent viral respiratory illnesses seem to be an important trigger to OSA worsening and, perhaps through this mechanism, may be a precipitant of sudden death.

There is no clear consensus on the optimal serial screening protocol for OSA in PWS children treated with GH, but practice guidelines from an expert panel are available.[98] Before starting GH therapy, a detailed clinical sleep history, physical examination, and overnight polysomnography is recommended. If OSA is present, treatment is initiated before beginning GH. PWS children treated with GH should have repeat polysomnography after 2 months initially, and every 6 months thereafter. A routine clinical history and airway examination should be performed every 3 months. GH therapy is started in low doses and gradually increased over several months. Symptoms of OSA should prompt an immediate reevaluation, including polysomnography, airway physical examination, and measurement of weight and serum IGF-1 levels. GH therapy should be discontinued in the setting of worsening OSA. Given the beneficial effects of GH in PWS, treatment in PWS children with OSA that is adequately treated with positive pressure is generally recommended. PWS patients started on GH should be placed on a strict dietary regimen to ensure that weight gain does not accompany GH usage. Following the OSA screening, there should be a low threshold for adenotonsillectomy in suitable patients. The first 3 to 4 months of GH therapy appear to at greatest risk for sudden death and heightened vigilance during this time is recommended.

CHIARI MALFORMATIONS

Chiari malformations (CMs) are characterized by congenital or acquired herniations of the cerebellum or brainstem through the foramen magnum, potentially causing symptoms of brainstem compression. CMs are common (1:1000) and may present as an isolated finding or be associated with hydrocephalus and myelomeningocele.[99] The sleep-disordered breathing observed in CM associated with myelomeningocele may be complicated by vocal cord paralysis, dysphagia, aspiration, scoliosis, and respiratory muscle weakness. Symptomatic CMs are usually accompanied by headache, neck pain, ataxia, or oculomotor disturbances. Occasionally, asymptomatic children may present with sudden death due to an unrecognized CM.[100] Because the brainstem regulates central respiratory drive, upper airway motor control, and arousal from sleep, a combination of central apnea, obstructive apnea, and hypoventilation may be observed (Fig. 34-3). In one series 25% of the children with CM had central apnea and 35% had obstructive apnea.[101] The incidence of central apnea increases to 57% if the CM is associated with myelomeningocele.[99] The central apnea seen with CM may occur in infancy and is usually associated with myelomeningocele and hydrocephalus, but occasionally occurs as an isolated finding.[102] Most cases of isolated CM present in later childhood or in the adult. Children with CM with myelomeningocele may also demonstrate prolonged expiratory apnea with cyanosis (PEAC)[99,103,104] and have parenchymal lung disease (Box 34-5). Individual events may resolve spontaneously or patients may require resuscitation; occasionally deaths occur.[104] PEAC events do not resolve with surgical decompression and may be fatal, even after tracheotomy and mechanical ventilation.

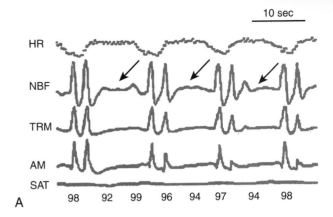

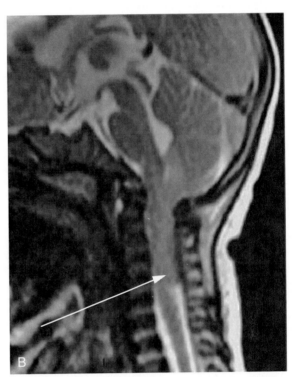

Figure 34-3 A 4-month-old infant with a Chiari type I malformation presenting with inspiratory stridor and respiratory pauses. **A,** A 60-second epoch demonstrating a series of central apneas (central apnea index 228/hour). Arrows indicate a sequence of central apneas. **B,** Brain MRI demonstrating a displacement of the cerebellar tonsils through the foramen magnum to the level of C5 *(arrow). AM,* abdominal movement; *HR,* heart rate; *MRI,* magnetic resonance imaging; *NBF,* nasobuccal flow; *SAT,* oxygen saturation; *TRM,* thoracic respiratory movement. (Modified from Van den Broek MJA, Arbues AS, Chalard F, et al. Chiari type I malformation causing central apnoeas in a 4-month-old boy. *Eur J Pediatr Neurol.* 2009;13:463-465, used with permission.)

From a surgical perspective, older children with a new onset of brainstem dysfunction often respond to craniocervical decompression, whereas the response of infants is more variable. Some case series of early decompression surgery reported improvement in brainstem dysfunction, while others have not.[105-109] In our experience, infants are most often asymptomatic at birth; instead, they develop symptoms of brainstem dysfunction over time and then do respond to decompression, although some residual central apnea remains.

The early recognition and treatment of symptoms of brainstem compression is critical in preserving function. Patients with CMs undergoing repair are at high-risk of worsening respiratory failure in the postoperative period, likely related to swelling of the brainstem.[101] Even following successful decompression surgery, a relapse of brainstem compression symptoms are common, often in the first 2 to 3 years, and central apnea may be an early sign.[110] Thus, close follow-up is essential. Shunt malfunction in myelomeningocele may lead to sudden brainstem compression and respiratory arrest.[111] Infants who are symptomatic at birth and those with bilateral vocal cord paralysis have a poor prognosis with irreversible damage to the brainstem and often require tracheostomy.

The choice of medical therapies depends in part on the consequences of the central apnea observed, including hypoxemia, hypercapnia, and EEG arousal. Patients with hypercapnia will likely need positive pressure ventilation in the spontaneous/timed or timed mode. Patients with isolated episodes of hypoxemia may benefit from supplemental oxygen alone. Oxygen may also regularize cyclic breathing patterns in some cases. Patients who are unresponsive to supplemental oxygen, or who are experiencing frequent sleep fragmentation, will also need positive pressure ventilation. The optimal settings should be established by performing a titration

study during overnight polysomnography. In the majority of cases there will be coexisting obstructive sleep apnea that may respond to continuous positive airway pressure. An adenotonsillectomy is frequently unsuccessful in resolving OSA, suggesting impairment in pharyngeal motor control. By eliminating the opening and closing of the airway, CPAP contributes to ventilatory stability.

MISCELLANEOUS CONDITIONS ASSOCIATED WITH CENTRAL APNEA

In addition to CM, there are many other causes of brainstem injury or compression that have been associated with prolonged central apneas, including tumors, infections, and metabolic disorders. Brainstem tumors may be associated with pathologic apnea,[112,113] and death has been reported (Fig. 34-4). Some improvement in the severity of central apnea has been reported following surgical resection, but considerable residual respiratory dysrhythmia is expected.[112] Children with pathologic central apnea associated with a brain tumor frequently require long-term ventilation during sleep. Apneustic breathing may respond to a serotonin 1A receptor agonist.[114,115]

Leigh syndrome is a mitochondrial disorder with brainstem involvement that results in prolonged central apneas and apneusis.[116,117] Treatment with the opioid antagonist naltrexone was reported to decrease central apnea in three children with Leigh syndrome.[118] Children with achondroplasia have foramen magnum stenosis and occasionally experience symptoms of brainstem compression, including central or obstructive sleep apnea.[119] Joubert syndrome is characterized by structural abnormalities of the hindbrain commonly associated with central apnea during sleep. Narcotic agents may produce central apnea in otherwise normal children, or exacerbate apnea in children with underlying conditions such as OSA, CCHS, CM, or brain tumors.[120] Propofol has been associated with temporary central apnea at a rate of 31 per 10,000 administrations.[121]

> **BOX 34-5** *Respiratory Complications of Chiari Malformation and Myelomeningocele*
>
> - Vocal cord paralysis
> - Obstructive sleep apnea
> - Central respiratory control dysfunction
>   - Central apnea
>   - Obstructive apnea
>   - Prolonged expiratory apnea with cyanosis
> - Dysphagia
> - Scoliosis
> - Respiratory muscle weakness
> - Ineffective cough

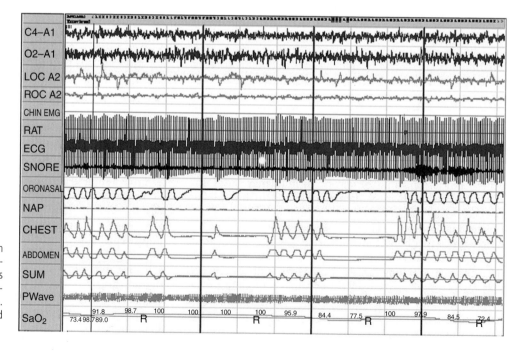

Figure 34-4 A 2-year-old child with a brainstem tumor demonstrating frequent grouped respiratory pauses between 12 and 22 seconds associated with marked oxygen desaturation. Dark vertical bars mark 30-second intervals.

SUMMARY

Disorders of central respiratory control may arise from congenital or acquired abnormalities of the brainstem or peripheral chemoreceptors. A thorough understanding of age-specific normative data, specifically respiratory pauses, periodic breathing, and oxygenation, is essential for properly interpreting polysomnograms. Several respiratory control disorders resolve with maturity including apnea of prematurity and periodic breathing. Others, such as congenital central hypoventilation syndrome, remain stable throughout life. A multitude of disorders that result in brainstem compression can give rise to central apnea including tumors, Chiari malformations, infectious processes, and mitochondrial disorders. Prader-Willi syndrome is unique in that it is characterized by peripheral chemoreceptor dysfunction that renders an individual vulnerable to acute changes in gas exchange parameters. Establishing a clear diagnosis and respiratory pattern in these various disorders allows physicians to select the appropriate ventilatory support during sleep and to follow established guidelines regarding co-morbid conditions.

REFERENCES

1. Al-Matary A, Kutbi I, Qurashi M, et al. Increased peripheral chemoreceptor activity may be critical in destabilizing breathing in neonates. *Semin Perinatol.* 2004;28:264-272.
2. Fukumizu M, Kohyama J. Central respiratory pauses, sighs, and gross body movements during sleep in children. *Physiol Behav.* 2004;82:721-726.
3. Ramanathan R, Corwin MJ, Hunt CE, et al. Cardiorespiratory events recorded on home monitors: Comparison of healthy infants with those at increased risk for SIDS. *JAMA.* 2001;285:2199-2207.
4. Iber C, Ancoli-Israel S, Chesson AL, Quan SFfor the American Academy of Sleep Medicine. *The AASM Manual for the Scoring of Sleep and Associated Events: Rules, Terminology, and Technical Specifications.* Westchester, IL: American Academy of Sleep Medicine; 2007.
5. Dransfeld DA, Spitzer AR, Fox WM. Episodic airway obstruction in premature infants. *Am J Dis Child.* 1983;137:441-443.
6. Milner AD, Boon AW, Saunders RA, Hopkin IE. Upper airways obstruction and apnoea in preterm babies. *Arch Dis Child.* 1980;55:22-25.
7. Al-Sufayan F, Bamehrez M, Kwiatkowski K, Alvaro RE. The effects of airway closure in central apneas and obstructed respiratory efforts in mixed apneas in preterm infants. *Pediatr Pulmonol.* 2009;44:253-259.
8. Kuna ST, Smickley JS, Murchison LC. Hypercarbic breathing during sleep in a child with a central nervous system tumor. *Am Rev Resp Dis.* 1990;142:880-883.
9. Al-Hathlol K, Idiong N, Hussain A, et al. A study of breathing pattern and ventilation in newborn infants and adult subjects. *Acta Paediatr.* 2000;89:1420-1425.
10. Hunt CE, Corwin MJ, Baird T, et al. Cardiorespiratory events detected by home memory monitoring and one-year neurodevelopmental outcome. *J Pediatr.* 2004;145:465-471.
11. Hoppenbrouwers T, Hodgman JE, Harper RM, Hofmann E, Sterman MB, McGinty DJ. Polygraphic studies of normal infants during the first six months of life: III. Incidence of apnea and periodic breathing. *Pediatrics.* 1977;60:418-425.
12. Kahn A, Franco P, Kato I, et al. Breathing during sleep in infancy. In: Loughlin GM, Marcus CL, Carroll JL, eds. *Sleep and Breathing in Children—A Developmental Approach.* New York: Marcel Dekker; 2000:405-422.
13. Stein IM, Fallon M, Merisalo RL, Kennedy JL. The frequency of apnea and bradycardia in a population of healthy, normal infants. *Neuropediatrics.* 1983;14:73-75.
14. Hunt CE, Corwin MJ, Lister G, et al. Longitudinal assessment of hemoglobin oxygen saturation in healthy infants during the first 6 months of age. *J Pediatr.* 1999;134:580-586.
15. Poets CF, Rau GA, Neuber K, Gappa M, Seidenberg J. Determinants of lung volume in spontaneously breathing preterm infants. *Am J Respir Crit Care Med.* 1997;155:649-653.
16. Henderson-Smart DJ. Vulnerability to hypoxaemia in the newborn. *Sleep.* 1980;3:331-342.
17. Henderson-Smart DJ, Read DJC. Reduced lung volume during behavioral active sleep in the newborn. *J Appl Phys.* 1979;46:1081-1085.
18. Stebbens VA, Poets CF, Alexander JR, Arrowsmith WA, Southall DP. Oxygen saturation and breathing patterns in infancy. 1: Full term infants in the second month of life. *Arch Dis Child.* 1991;66:569-573.
19. Poets CF, Stebbens VA, Alexander JR, Arrowsmith WA, Salfield SA, Southall DP. Oxygen saturation and breathing patterns in infancy. 2: Preterm infants at discharge from special care. *Arch Dis Child.* 1991;66:574-578.
20. Poets CF, Stebbens VA, Southall DP. Arterial oxygen saturation and breathing movements during the first year of life. *J Dev Physiol.* 1991;15:341-345.
21. Poets CF, Stebbens VA, Samuels MP, Southall DP. Oxygen saturation and breathing patterns in children. *Pediatrics.* 1993;92:686-690.
22. Moss D, Urschitz MS, Bodman AV, et al. Reference values for nocturnal home polysomnography in primary school children. *Pediatr Res.* 2005;58:958-965.
23. Carskadon MA, Harvey K, Dement WC, Guilleminault C, Simmons FB, Anders TF. Respiration during sleep in children. *West J Med.* 1978;128:477-481.
24. Uliel S, Tauman R, Greenfeld M, Sivan Y. Normal polysomnographic respiratory values in children and adolescents. *Chest.* 2004;125:872-878.
25. Verhulst SL, Schrauwen N, Haentjens D, Van Gaal L, De Backer WA, Desager KN. Reference values for sleep-related respiratory variables in asymptomatic European children and adolescents. *Pediatr Pulmonol.* 2007;42:159-167.
26. Fenner A, Schalk U, Hoenicke H, Wendenburg A, Roehling T. Periodic breathing in premature and neonatal babies: Incidence, breathing pattern, respiratory gas tensions, response to changes in the composition of ambient air. *Pediatr Res.* 1973;7:174-183.
27. Glotzbach SF, Baldwin MA, Lederer NE, Tansey PA, Ariagno RL. Periodic breathing in preterm infants: Incidence and characteristics. *Pediatrics.* 1989;84:785-792.
28. Henderson-Smart DJ. The effect of gestational age on the incidence and duration of recurrent apnoea in newborn babies. *Aust Pediatr J.* 1981;17:273-276.
29. Eichenwald EC, Aina A, Stark AR. Apnea frequently persists beyond term gestation in infants delivered at 24 to 28 weeks. *Pediatrics.* 1997;100:354-359.
30. Cheung PY, Barrington KJ, Finer NN, Robertson CMT. Early childhood neurodevelopment in very low birth weight infants with predischarge apnea. *Pediatr Pulmonol.* 1999;27:14-20.
31. Heimler R, Langlois J, Hodel DJ, Nelin LD, Sasidharan P. Effect of positioning on the breathing pattern of preterm infants. *Arch Dis Child.* 1992;67:312-314.
32. Kassim Z, Donaldson N, Khetriwal B, et al. Sleeping position, oxygen saturation, and lung volume in convalescent, prematurely born infants. *Arch Dis Child Fetal Neonatal Ed.* 2007;92:347-350.
33. Poets CF, von Bodman A. Placing pretern infants for sleep. First prone, then supine. *Arch Dis Child Fetal Neonatal Ed.* 2007;92:F331-F332.
34. Speidel BD, Dunn PM. Use of nasal continuous positive airway pressure to treat severe recurrent apnoea in very preterm infants. *Lancet.* 1976;2:658-660.
35. Aranda JV, Gorman W, Bergsteinsson H, Gunn T. Efficacy of caffeine in treatment of apnea in the low-birth-weight infant. *J Pediatr.* 1977;90:467-472.
36. Schmidt B, Roberts RS, Davis P, et al. Caffeine therapy for apnea of prematurity. *N Engl J Med.* 2006;354:2112-2121.
37. Schmidt B, Roberts RS, Davis P, et al. Long-term effects of caffeine therapy for apnea of prematurity. *N Engl J Med.* 2007;357:1893-1902.
38. Eichenwald EC, Aina A, Stark AR. Apnea frequently persists beyond term gestation in infants delivered at 24 to 28 weeks. *Pediatrics.* 1997;100:354-359.
39. National Institutes of Health Consensus Development Conference on Infantile Apnea and Home Monitoring, Sept. 29 to Oct. 1, 1986. *Pediatrics.* 1987;79:292-299.
40. Mitchell EA, Thompson JM. Parental reported apnea, admissions to hospital and sudden infant death syndrome. *Acta Paediatr.* 2001;90:417-422.
41. Kiechl-Kohlendorfer U, Hof D, Peglow UP, Traweger-Ravanelli B, Kiechl S. Epidemiology of apparent life threatening events. *Arch Dis Child.* 2005;90:297-300.

42. Hunt CE, Corwin MJ, Lister G, et al. Precursors of cardiorespiratory events in infants detected by home memory monitor. *Pediatr Pulmonol.* 2008;43:87-98.

43. Poets CF, Stebbens VA, Richard D, Southall DP. Prolonged episodes of hypoxemia in preterm infants undetectable by cardiorespiratory monitors. *Pediatrics.* 1995;95:860-863.

44. Abendroth D, Moser DK, Dracup K, Doering LV. Do apnea monitors decrease emotional distress in parents of infants at high risk for cardiopulmonary arrest?. *J Pediatr Health Care.* 1999;13:50-57.

45. Poets CF, Stebbens VA, Lang JA, O'Brien LM, Boon AW, Southall DP. Arterial oxygen saturation in healthy term neonates. *Eur J Pediatr.* 1996;155:219-223.

46. Simakajornboon N, Beckerman RC, Mack C, Sharon D, Gozal D. Effect of supplemental oxygen on sleep architecture and cardiorespiratory events in preterm infants. *Pediatrics.* 2002;110:884-888.

47. Weintraub Z, Alvaro R, Kwiatkowski K, Cates D, Rigatto H. Effects of inhaled oxygen (up to 40%) on periodic breathing and apnea in preterm infants. *J Appl Phys.* 1992;72:116-120.

48. Thibeault DW, Wong MM, Auld PAM. Thoracic gas volume changes in premature infants. *Pediatrics.* 1967;40:403-411.

49. Heimler R, Langlois J, Hodel DJ, Nelin LD, Sasidharan P. Effect of positioning on the breathing pattern of preterm infants. *Arch Dis Child.* 1992;67:312-314.

50. Kelly DH, Shannon DC. Treatment of apnea and excessive periodic breathing in the full-term infant. *Pediatrics.* 1981;68:183-186.

51. Weese-Mayer DE, Berry-Kravis EM, Ceccherini I, et al. An official ATS clinical policy statement: Congenital central hypoventilation syndrome: Genetic basis, diagnosis, and management. *Am J Resp Crit Care Med.* 2010;181:626-644.

52. Amiel J, Laudier B, Attie-Bitach T, et al. Polyalanine expansion and frameshift mutations of the paired-like homeobox gene PHOX2B in congenital central hypoventilation syndrome. *Nat Genet.* 2003;33: 459-461.

53. Weese-Mayer DE, Berry-Kravis EM, Zhou L, et al. Idiopathic congenital central hypoventilation syndrome: Analysis of genes pertinent to early autonomic nervous system embryologic development and identification of mutations in PHOX2b. *Am J Med Genet.* 2003;123A:267-278.

54. Weese-Mayer DE, Rand CM, Berry-Kravis EM, et al. Congenital central hypoventilation syndrome from past to future: Model for translational and transitional autonomic medicine. *Pediatr Pulmonol.* 2009;44: 521-535.

55. Repetto GM, Corrales RJ, Abara SG, et al. Later-onset congenital central hypoventilation syndrome due to a heterozygous 24-polyalanine repeat expansion mutation in the PHOX2B gene. *Acta Paediatr.* 2009;98: 190-198.

56. Fine-Goulden MR, Manna S, Durward A. Cor pulmonale due to congenital central hypoventilation syndrome presenting in adolescence. *Pediatr Crit Care Med.* 2009;10:E41-E42.

57. Weese-Mayer DE, Berry-Kravis EM, Zhou L. Adult identified with congenital central hypoventilation syndrome-mutation in PHOX2B gene and late-onset CHS. *Am J Resp Crit Care Med.* 2005;171:88.

58. Antic NA, Malow BA, Lange N, et al. PHOX2B mutation-confirmed congenital central hypoventilation syndrome: Presentation in adulthood. *Am J Resp Crit Care Med.* 2006;174:923-927.

59. Silvestri JM, Weese-Mayer DE, Flanagan EA. Congenital central hypoventilation syndrome: Cardiorespiratory responses to moderate exercise, simulating daily activity. *Pediatr Pulmonol.* 1995;20:89-93.

60. Chen ML, Tablizo MA, Kun S, Keens TG. Diaphram pacers as a treatment for congenital central hypoventilation syndrome. *Expert Rev Med Devices.* 2005;2:577-585.

61. Chen ML, Turkel SB, Jacobson JR, Keens TG. Alcohol use in congenital central hypoventilation syndrome. *Pediatr Pulmonol.* 2006;41: 283-285.

62. Straus C, Trang H, Becquemin MH, Touraine P, Similowski T. Chemosensitivity recovery in Ondine's curse syndrome under treatment with desogestrel. *Respir Physiol Neurobiol.* 2010;171(2):171-174.

63. Trang H, Girard A, Laude D, Elghozi JL. Short-term blood pressure and heart rate variability in congenital central hypoventilation syndrome (Ondine's curse). *Clin Sci.* 2005;108:225-230.

64. Woo MS, Woo MA, Gozal D, Jansen MT, Keens TG, Harper RM. Heart rate variability in congenital central hypoventilation syndrome. *Pediatr Res.* 1992;31:291-296.

65. Silvestri JM, Hanna BD, Volgman AS, Jones PJ, Barnes SD, Weese-Mayer DE. Cardiac rhythm disturbances among children with idiopathic congenital central hypoventilation syndrome. *Pediatr Pulmonol.* 2000;29:358.

66. Gronli JO, Santucci BA, Leurgans SE, Berry-Kravis EM, Weese-Mayer DE. Congenital central hypoventilation syndrome: PHOX2B genotype determines risk for sudden death. *Pediatr Pulmonol.* 2008;43:77-86.

67. Sochala C, van Deenen D, de Ville A, Govaerts MJM. Heart block following propofol in a child. *Paediatr Anaesth.* 1999;9:349-351.

68. Todd ES, Weinberg SM, Berry-Kravis EM, et al. Facial phenotype in children and young adults with PHOX2B-determined congenital central hypoventilation syndrome: Quantitative pattern of dysmorpholohy. *Pediatr Res.* 2006;59:39-45.

69. Katz ES, McGrath S, Marcus CL. Late-onset central hypoventilation with hypothalamic dysfunction: A distinct clinical syndrome. *Pediatr Pulmonol.* 2000;29:62-68.

70. Ize-Ludlow D, Gray JA, Sperling MA, et al. Rapid-onset obesity with hypothalamic dysfunction, hypoventilation, and autonomic dysregulation presenting in childhood. *Pediatrics.* 2007;120:E179-E188.

71. De Pontual L, Trochet D, Caillat-Zucman S, et al. Delineation of late onset hypoventilation associated with hypothalamic dysfunction syndrome. *Pediatr Res.* 2008;64:689-694.

72. Julu POO, Kerr AM, Apartopoulos F, et al. Characterization of breathing and associated central autonomic dysfunction in the RETT disorder. *Arch Dis Child.* 2001;85:29-37.

73. d'Orsi G, Demaio V, Scarpelli F, Calvario T, Minervini MG. Central sleep apnoea in Rett syndrome. *Neurol Sci.* 2009;30:389-391.

74. Marcus CL, Carroll JL, McColley SA, et al. Polysomnographic characteristics of patients with Rett syndrome. *J Pediatr.* 1994;125:218-224.

75. Anzai Y, Ohya T. A case of effective gastrostomy for severe abdominal distention due to breathing dysfunction of Rett's syndrome: A treatment of autonomic disorder. *Brain Dev.* 2001;23:S240-S241.

76. Kerr AM, Julu POO, Hansen S, Apartopoulos F. Serotonin and breathing dysrhythmia in Rett syndrome. In: Perat MV, ed. *New Developments in Child Neurology.* Bologna: Monduzzi Editore; 1998:191-195.

77. Priano L, Grugni G, Miscio G, et al. Sleep cycling alternating pattern (CAP) expression is associated with hypersomnia and GH secretory pattern in Prader-Willi syndrome. *Sleep Med.* 2006;7:627-633.

78. Cotton S, Richdale A. Brief report: Parental descriptions of sleep problems in children with autism, Down syndrome, and Prader-Willi syndrome. *Res Dev Disabilities.* 2003;27:151-161.

79. Hertz G, Cataletto M, Feinsliver SH, Angulo M. Sleep and breathing patterns in patients with Prader-Willi syndrome (PWS): Effects of age and gender. *Sleep.* 1993;16:366-371.

80. Hertz G, Cataletto M, Feinsilver SH, Angulo M. Developmental trends of sleep-disordered breathing in Prader-Willi syndrome. *Am J Med Gen.* 1995;56:188-190.

81. Harris JC, Allen RP. Is excessive daytime sleepiness characteristic of Prader-Willi syndrome? The effects of weight change. *Arch Pediatr Adolesc Med.* 1996;150:1288-1293.

82. Nevsimalova S, Vankova J, Stepanova I, Seemanova E, Mignot E, Nishino S. Hypocretin deficiency in Prader-Willi syndrome. *Eur J Neurol.* 2005;12:70-72.

83. O'Donoghue F, Camfferman D, Kennedy J, et al. Sleep-disordered breathing in Prader-Willi syndrome and its associations with neurobehavioral abnormalities. *J Pediatr.* 2005;147:823-829.

84. Festen DAM, Wevers M, De Weerd AW, et al. Psychomotor development in infants with Prader-Willi syndrome and associations with sleep-related breathing disorders. *Pediatr Res.* 2007;62:221-224.

85. Schluter B, Buschatz D, Trowitzsch E, Aksu F, Andler W. Respiratory control in children with Prader-Willi syndrome. *Eur J Pediatr.* 1997;156:65-68.

86. Festen DAM, de Weerd AW, van den Bossche RAS, Joosten K, Hoeve H, Hokken-Koelega ACS. Sleep-related breathing disorders in prepubertal children with Prader-Willi syndrome and effects of growth hormone treatment. *J Clin Endocrinol Metab.* 2006;91:4911-4915.

87. Arens R, Gozal D, Burrell BC, et al. Arousal and cardiorespiratory responses to hypoxia in Prader-Willi syndrome. *Am J Respir Crit Care Med.* 1996;153:283-287.

88. Miller J, Silverstein J, Shuster J, Driscoll DJ, Wagner M. Short-term effects of growth hormone on sleep abnormalities in Prader-Willi syndrome. *J Clin Endocrinol Metab.* 2006;91:413-417.

89. Smith IE, King MA, Siklos PWL, Shneerson JM. Treatment of ventilatory failure in the Prader-Willi syndrome. *Eur Respir J.* 1998;11: 1150-1152.

90. Vgontzas AN, Bixler EO, Kales A, Vela-Bueno A. Prader-Willi syndrome: Effects of weight loss on sleep-disordered breathing, daytime sleepiness and REM sleep disturbance. *Acta Pediatr.* 1995;84:813-814.

91. Clift S, Dahlitz M, Parkes JD. Sleep apnoea in the Prader-Willi syndrome. *J Sleep Res.* 1994;3:121-126.

92. Carrel AL, Myers SE, Whitman BY, Allen DB. Growth hormone improves body composition, fat utilization, physical strength and agility, and growth in Prader-Willi syndrome: A controlled study. *J Pediatr.* 1999;134:215-221.

93. Lindgren AC, Hellstrom LG, Ritzen EM, Milerad J. Growth hormone treatment increases CO_2 response, ventilation and central inspiratory drive in children with Prader-Willi syndrome. *Eur J Pediatr.* 1999;158:936-940.

94. Eiholzer U, Nordmann Y. L'Allemand. Fatal outcome of sleep apnoea in PWS during the intial phase of growth hormone treatment. A case report. *Horm Res.* 2002;58:24-26.

95. Haqq AM, Stadler DD, Jackson RH, Rosenfeld RG, Purnell JQ, LaFranchi SH. Effects of growth hormone on pulmonary function, sleep quality, behavior, cognition, growth velocity, body composition, and resting energy expenditure in Prader-Willi syndrome. *J Clin Endocrinol Metab.* 2003;88:2206-2212.

96. Nagai T, Obata K, Tonoki H, et al. Cause of sudden, unexpected death of Prader-Willi syndrome patients with or without growth hormone treatment. *Am J Med Gene.* 2005;136A:45-48.

97. Tauber M, Diene G, Molinas C, Hebert M. Review of 64 cases of death in children with Prader-Willi syndrome (PWS). *Am J Med Genet.* 2008;146A:887.

98. Goldstone AP, Holland AJ, Hauffa BP, Hokken-Koelega AC, Tauber M. on behalf of speakers and contributors at the Second Expert Meeting of the Comprehensive Care of Patients with PWS. Recommendations for the diagnosis and management of Prader-Willi syndrome. *J Clin Endocrinol Metab.* 2008;93:4183-4197.

99. Waters KA, Forbes P, Morielli A, et al. Sleep-disordered breathing in children with myelomeningocele. *J Pediatr.* 1998;132:672-681.

100. Martinot A, Hue V, Leclerc F, Vallee L, Closset M, Pruvo JP. Sudden death revealing chiari type 1 malformation in two children. *Intensive Care Med.* 1993;19:73-74.

101. Dauilliers Y, Stal V, Abril B, et al. Chiari malformation and sleep related breathing disorders. *J Neurol Neurosurg Psychiatry.* 2007;78:1344-1348.

102. Van den Broek MJA, Arbues AS, Chalard F, et al. Chiari type I malformation causing central apnoeas in a 4-month-old boy. *Eur J Paediatr Neurol.* 2009;13:463-465.

103. Ward SLD, Jacobs RA, Gates EP, Hart LD, Keens TG. Abnormal ventilatory patterns during sleep in infants with myelomeningocele. *J Pediatr.* 1986;109:631-634.

104. Cochrane DD, Adderley R, White CP, Norman M, Steinbok P. Apnea in patients with myelomeningocele. *Pediatr Neurosurg.* 1990;16:232-239.

105. Murray C, Seton C, Prelog K, Fitzgerald DA. Arnold-Chiari type 1 malformation presenting with sleep disordered breathing in well children. *Arch Dis Child.* 2006;91:342-343.

106. Park TS, Hoffman HJ, Hendrick EB, Humpheys RP. Experience with surgical decompression of the Arnold-Chiari malformation in young infants with myelomeningocele. *Neurosurgery.* 1983;13:147-152.

107. Pollack IF, Kinnunen D, Albright AL. The effect of early craniocervical decompression on functional outcome in neonates and young infants with myelodysplasia and symptomatic Chiari II malformations: Results from a prospective series. *Neurosurgery.* 1996;38:703-710.

108. Bell WO, Charney EB, Bruce DA, Sutton LN, Schut L. Symptomatic Arnold-Chiari malformation: Review of experience with 22 cases. *J Neurosurg.* 1987;66:812-816.

109. Gagnadoux F, Meslier N, Svab I, Menei P, Racineux JL. Sleep-disordered breathing in patients with Chiari malformation: Improvement after surgery. *Neurology.* 2006;66:136-138.

110. Zolty P, Sanders MH, Pollack IF. Chiari malformation and sleep-disordered breathing: A review of diagnostic and management issues. *Sleep.* 2000;23:1-7.

111. Tomita T, McClone DG. Acute respiratory arrest: A complication of malformation of the shunt in children with myelomeningocele and Arnold-Chiari malformation. *Am J Dis Child.* 1983;137:142-144.

112. Hui SHL, Wing YK, Poon W, Chan YL, Buckley TA. Alveolar hypoventilation syndrome in brainstem glioma with improvement after surgical resection. *Chest.* 2000;118:266-268.

113. Rosen GM, Bendel AE, Neglia JP, Moertel CL, Mahowald M. Sleep in children with neoplasms of the central nervous system: Case review of 14 children. *Pediatrics.* 2003;112:E46-E54.

114. Wilken B, Lalley P, Bischoff AM, et al. Treatment of apneustic respiratory disturbance with a serotonin-receptor agonist. *J Pediatr.* 1997;130:89-94.

115. Saito Y, Hashimoto T, Iwata H, et al. Apneustic breathing in children with brainstem damage due to hypoxic-ischemic encephalopathy. *Dev Med Child Neurol.* 1999;41:560-567.

116. Yasaki E, Saito Y, Nakano K, et al. Characteristics of breathing abnormality in Leigh and its overlap syndromes. *Neuropediatrics.* 2001;32:299-306.

117. Huntsman RJ, Sinclair DB, Bhargava R, Chan A. Atypical presentations of Leigh syndrome: A case series and review. *Pediatr Neurol.* 2005;32:334-340.

118. Myer EC, Morris DL, Brase DA, Dewey WL, Zimmerman AW. Naltrexone therapy of apnea in children with elevated cerebrospinal fluid B-endorphin. *Ann Neurol.* 1990;27:75-80.

119. Mogayzel PJ, Carroll JL, Loughlin GM, Hurko O, Francomano CA, Marcus CL. Sleep-disordered breathing in children with achondroplasia. *J Pediatr.* 1998;132:667-671.

120. Waters KA, McBrien F, Stewart P, Hinder M, Wharton S. Effects of OSA, inhalational anesthesia, and fentanyl on the airway and ventilation of children. *J Appl Phys.* 2002;92:1987-1994.

121. Cravero JP, Beach ML, Blike GT, Gallagher SM, Hertzog JH. The incidence and nature of adverse events during pediatric sedation/anesthesia with propofol for procedures outside the operating room: A report from the pediatric sedation research consortium. *Anesth Analg.* 2009;108:795-804.

Chapter 35

Pediatric Insomnia and Behavioral Interventions

BRETT R. KUHN / BRANDY M. ROANE

Basic sleep physiology differs little across the human lifespan. The clinical presentation and manifestation of *disordered* sleep may vary greatly, however, depending on one's age or developmental status. Adults with sleep-related breathing disorders (SRBDs), for example, typically experience excessive daytime sleepiness (EDS), whereas children may present with restless sleep, mouth breathing, and inattention. The etiology of SRBD in children is more often associated with craniofacial abnormalities, neuromuscular disorders, and adenotonsillar hypertrophy than with obesity.[1] As opposed to the sleepiness and lethargy experienced by adults, sleep deprivation in children may produce "paradoxical" manifestations such as hyperactivity, aggression, or risk-taking behavior. Narcolepsy in children can be a diagnostic challenge, particularly in young children who still nap or who have not yet developed cataplexy, sleep paralysis, or hypnagogic hallucinations.[2,3]

Although the term "insomnia" has been used indiscriminately across the entire lifespan, the clinical manifestations, evaluation methods, and treatment options for infants and children are clearly distinct from adults.[4-10] These differences are widely recognized by pediatric sleep specialists who have recently proposed developmentally modified definitions and diagnostic criteria for children.[11-13]

Why is the presentation of insomnia in children, and in young children in particular, so different? First of all, parents or caregivers are usually the ones who define whether or not the child's sleep is a "problem." This determination can vary greatly depending on cultural practices, parental expectations, and the child's developmental status.[7,14,15] Frequently the primary caregivers suffer the most from a sleepless child and therefore they often initiate the clinic referral in hopes of reducing their own level of frustration, sleepiness, or even marital conflict. Second, adults with insomnia frequently go to bed earlier in hopes of capturing additional sleep, while young children often resist going to bed and may purposefully resist sleep. In other words, adults with insomnia complain of difficulty falling asleep despite their best efforts, but young children may actively resist falling to sleep despite their parents' best efforts. Third, a number of intrinsic factors have been linked to the development and course of adult insomnia, but children tend to be more susceptible to extrinsic factors that disrupt sleep.[16-19] Finally, adults are usually in a position to dictate their own sleep schedule, whereas it is the parents who usually determine the child's bedtime, wake time, and nap time. This obvious but important fact increases the likelihood that some children will be placed into bed when they are not physiologically prepared to fall asleep.

INFANTS, TODDLERS, AND PRESCHOOLERS

Sleep problems are a common occurrence in early childhood,[20] and their presence can affect virtually every realm of child and family functioning.[21-25] At infant, toddler, and preschool stages of development, the predominant clinical presentation consists of an extrinsic dyssomnia involving difficulty settling to sleep at bedtime and nap times and frequent awakenings during the night. These two symptoms often coexist, and treatments targeting one symptom will often generalize to the other. This can be explained by the fact that the process of initiating sleep takes place not just at bedtime, but also following brief nighttime awakenings that are a normal part of a child's sleep cycle. Children who initiate sleep in the presence of nonadaptive sleep associations (e.g., feeding, rocking, parental presence) cannot recreate these familiar associations themselves upon awakening, and therefore signal parents to gain assistance several times each night. There are a host of biologic and psychosocial factors that can adversely impact children's sleep, yet the strongest predictors of pediatric insomnia in the early years are parent management practices during sleep initiation and in response to nighttime waking.[26-28] These predictive practices are listed in Box 35-1.[29-34]

Even after children develop the habit of falling asleep independently, the transition from the crib to a toddler bed may present a considerable challenge. Disassembling the infant crib leaves parents without their "toddler containment device," which immediately tests their ability to establish and enforce effective behavioral limits during sleep times. Bedtime problems at this age often include frequent requests, crying, tantrums, and leaving the bedroom. Most of these behaviors function to gain parental presence and attention, to delay going to bed, or to avoid separation from the parent. Disruptive bedtime behavior then results in delayed sleep onset, reduced sleep time, and possibly negative parent-child interactions during the day and night.

A wide range of treatment modalities have been proposed to address pediatric sleep disturbances, including pharmacologic agents,[35] nutritional adjustments,[36] chiropractic manipulation,[37] massage therapy,[38] and aromatherapy.[39] However, the combined evidence supporting the effectiveness of these therapies does not approach that of short-term behavioral therapy. Behaviorally based interventions rely on the clinical application of fundamental principles of learning to bring about changes in a child's sleep-related skills, habits, and behaviors. Parents typically serve as the active agents of change in their children.[40,41] For example, parents may be taught (or actively coached) to alter previously established connections between specific cues (such as parental presence, physical contact, or other actions) and the desired outcome (sleep), or to modify the relationship (contingency) between specific behaviors and their reinforcing consequences.

The intervention outcome research on pediatric insomnia is heavily weighted toward the younger end of the age spectrum. In fact, the large majority of studies have focused on infants and children 5 years old and younger. Specific behavioral interventions targeting this age group are described first and are listed in Box 35-2.

Parent Education and Problem Prevention

Providing early intervention to prevent sleep disturbances from occurring in the first place presents an enticing alternative to treating sleep problems after they are firmly established. Teaching parents to instill healthy sleep habits appears to be the most effective, economical, and time-efficient approach to behaviorally based pediatric sleep problems. Most parent education programs target soon-to-be-parents or parents of newborns during the prenatal through 6-month postnatal period. The primary aim of these programs is the promotion of positive sleep habits by educating parents on how to develop bedtime routines, sleep schedules, and appropriate sleep associations. The universal message to parents derives from the research on parental handling; place the infant in bed "drowsy, but awake." The overarching goal is to teach children to initiate sleep independently at bedtime, which affords them the ability to reinitiate sleep following naturally occurring nighttime awakenings.

Possibly the most impressive outcomes using this approach were reported by Symon and colleagues,[42] who randomly assigned 268 infants to early intervention or control at 2 to 3 weeks of age. The intervention involved nothing more than a single, 45-minute consultation to teach parental handling skills and promote independent sleep initiation skills. By 6 weeks of age, infants in the treatment group averaged 1.3 hours more sleep each day than control infants, resulting in 9 more hours of sleep per week!

Extinction

Using behavioral extinction to address pediatric sleep disturbance has been referred to as "sleep training," "systematic ignoring," or the "cry-it-out approach." However, using extinction does not necessitate any of these things. Extinction, rather, involves terminating the reinforcing consequence that maintains a behavior, which reduces the frequency of that behavior over time.[43] Learning theory posits that inappropriate behaviors are acquired through classical or operant conditioning and are maintained by their reinforcing consequences. Sleep-related problem behaviors (e.g., bedtime tantrums, dawdling) may be negatively reinforced if they result in the removal (escape, avoidance) of an unpleasant event (e.g., bedtime, separation from parents). Alternatively, behaviors may be positively reinforced if they produce a preferred event. With very few attempts many children learn to misbehave (e.g., crying, screaming, demanding) or come up with "creative" requests to gain a desired response at bedtime. Although some children may indeed desire to have three or four glasses of water not only delivered to their bedroom but specially prepared—"cold water, with ice, crushed not cubed, shaken not stirred"—these requests usually function to secure parents' attention or physical presence in the bedroom. The behavior is then maintained over time as long as the behaviors are reinforced at least some of the time. Extinction reduces the inappropriate behavior by simply removing the reinforcing consequence. In using extinction for bedtime problems, parents are typically asked to establish a regular prebedtime routine, place the child into bed, then leave the bedroom and ignore inappropriate child behavior until the morning. Possible exceptions to ignoring would include illness, danger of harming oneself, and property destruction.

In the treatment of pediatric insomnia, unmodified extinction is second only to parent education and prevention when it comes to research support,[7] and boasts an impressive treatment effect size.[44] There are, however, several inherent problems with the use of extinction-based interventions that must be considered:

- *Extinction can be difficult to execute.* Success relies on parents' ability to consistently ignore a child's disruptive bedtime behavior, sometimes for long periods of time. Parents can easily fall into the trap of selectively reinforcing more unique or severe occurrences of behavior, including a child's behavioral persistence, which only strengthens the child's behavior and makes it more resistant to future intervention. Clinicians are strongly advised to identify a family's previous treatment attempts[45] because a child's learning history will play a big role in their response to the introduction or reintroduction of extinction-based interventions.
- *Initial increase or later return of symptom; undesirable responses.* Although extinction is usually nonproblematic,

on occasion one may see an extinction burst (a temporary increase in frequency, duration, or magnitude of the behavior) or extinction-induced emotional outbursts or aggression.[46] Parents should be informed about these potential reactions, including the possibility that sleep-related behavior problems may reappear "spontaneously," even after treatment success, with any changes in the environment (bed, bedroom, routine, or caregivers).[47]

- *Extinction may be viewed poorly by some parents.* The treatment acceptability literature indicates that parents tend to prefer positive interventions such as praise and reinforcement, which are designed to increase adaptive child behaviors, as opposed to punishment procedures, which are intended to decrease problem behaviors.[48]

Critics have argued that prolonged crying in response to extinction-based sleep treatments may produce deleterious effects on children's health, attachment, or emotional security. Although this is an empirical question, one could contend that over the long run the frequency and duration of a child's crying would actually decrease following the introduction of effective treatment. For instance, an irritable, sleep-disturbed toddler who cries for 30 minutes per night (perhaps 15 minutes at bedtime and 5 minutes at each of three awakenings) may spend 210 minutes crying per week (not counting any crying during the day). If the child's crying is placed on extinction, parents would likely note a temporary burst in crying (let's say 90 minutes or three times the pretreatment level) the first night. Crying would likely reduce by half across each successive intervention night (not an unreasonable expectation), reaching near zero by the seventh night or sooner. The treatment protocol then is associated with approximately 25 minutes of crying per night over the first week, less than the untreated child's weekly average of 30 minutes. After 1 week, the untreated child continues to cry an average of 210 minutes per week, while the treated child is now going to bed cooperatively without crying, resulting in an overall "savings" of 840 minutes (14 hours) of crying each month of the year. Thus, the crying in response to effective treatments (like extinction) may represent a very small amount compared to long-term duration of crying in children who remain untreated. Granted, hypothetical numbers were chosen for this example, but this question begs to be answered by a long-term clinical outcome study.

Graduated Extinction

Because of some of the problems associated with extinction, sleep experts have gone to great lengths to develop modifications. Graduated extinction (GE), or graduated systematic ignoring, has the strongest evidence base of these modified versions. The protocol has experienced widespread popularity since the publication of the first edition of Ferber's (1985) self-help book, *Solve Your Child's Sleep Problems.*[49] A number of variations in technique have been developed that still fall under the realm of GE.[50] The goal of GE is to gradually reduce parental presence or parental attention to inappropriate bedtime behaviors interfering with sleep initiation. Most often this is accomplished by combining extinction with scheduled parent "check-ins" that are faded over time. These check-ins involve parents making planned but brief (e.g., 15- to 60-secomd) visits into the child's bedroom to ensure that the child is physically okay and to reassure the child that the parents are

still close by), while minimizing social interactions and attention. The duration of time between check-ins often needs to be fine-tuned during treatment. The intervals may be individualized depending on the child's age, temperament, past learning history, or parents' estimate of how long they can tolerate the child crying. Two common variations of GE involve the use of fixed and graduated time schedules.

A fixed time schedule establishes a specific duration of time (e.g., 5 minutes) that remains constant across parent checks. For instance, if parents indicated that they could tolerate listening to their child cry for no more than 5 minutes, they would implement extinction while interspersing check-ins after each 5-minute period has elapsed. A graduated schedule progressively increases the duration between parent checks. For instance, parents might implement extinction for 5 minutes before the first check, but lengthen the intervals across successive checks by 5 minutes (to 10 minutes, 15 minutes, and so on). This version is sometimes referred to as "incremental" graduated extinction. Advantages of GE over other treatments include the convenience of maintaining the child's regular bedtime and the reassurance that some parents find with the integrated check-ins. One potential disadvantage stems from this very advantage, as parents may inadvertently shape longer bouts of crying (behavioral persistence) if the duration and intensity of parent-child interactions increase across successive check-ins.

Extinction with Parental Presence

This variation of extinction calls for the parent to implement extinction (planned ignoring) from within the child's bedroom. As with unmodified extinction, extinction with parental presence (E/PP) requires parents to ignore inappropriate behavior unless the child is feeling ill or is in danger. The main modification with this procedure is that the parent remains in the child's bedroom, feigning sleep in a separate cot or bed. The parent may leave the room each night after the child falls asleep. The procedure is carried out for up to 1 week, or until the child learns to fall asleep independently and sleep through the night. The parent then moves back to sleep in his or her own bedroom and uses unmodified extinction from that point on.

By using E/PP, consistent (noncontingent) parental presence in the child's bedroom lessens the concern that poorly timed parental check-ins may inadvertently reinforce peak levels or more persistent child behavior. France[51] contends that children's awareness of parent presence reduces separation anxiety, making E/PP a more gentle approach for young children. Indeed, there is evidence that E/PP resolves sleep problems more effectively and with less crying than both unmodified and graduated extinction.[52] Another possibility is that E/PP reduces the parent's level of anxiety due to the continued presence in the child's bedroom. On the other hand, some parents may find it more difficult to effectively ignore a screaming child while in close proximity. Parents implementing E/PP must also be willing to temporarily alter their own sleeping arrangements.

The Bedtime Pass

A more recent modification to extinction is the bedtime pass (BP). The BP specifically targets children at least 3 years old who have mastered the skill of independent sleep initiation, but nonetheless exhibit bedtime struggles such as calling out or coming out of the bedroom.[53] First, parents assist the child in choosing or creating an object (decorated index card, small toy) to serve as the bedtime pass. The child is informed that the BP may be "traded" for one trip out of the bedroom or one small request that takes less than 3 minutes to complete. Parents immediately respond favorably to the child's request (e.g., hug, drink of water, question) and collect the pass from the child. The BP is an extinction-based procedure, as once the pass is surrendered parents are to ignore subsequent problematic bedtime behaviors. Research suggests that the BP is effective in reducing bedtime resistance for typically developing toddlers and school age children.[54-56] The protocol appears to minimize postextinction response bursts and tends to be perceived highly by consumers.

Scheduled Awakenings

Unlike extinction-based protocols, the scheduled awakening (SA) allows parents to provide their usual caregiving behaviors, but in a manner that disconnects them from the child's signaling during nighttime awakenings. The procedure first requires close monitoring to establish a baseline pattern of the timing of all nocturnal awakenings (e.g., 12:30 AM, 2:30 AM, and 4:30 AM). Once this pattern is determined, parents begin waking the child 15 to 30 minutes prior to each anticipated awakening (e.g., 12:15 AM, 2:15 AM, and 4:15 AM). The infant or child can be provided immediate access to all the usual, preferred caregiving activities (e.g., rocking, patting, feeding) until sleep is reinstated. The time of each awakening is gradually delayed (later) as the child sleeps uninterrupted for longer stretches and eventually sleeps through the night. SA represents an effective treatment option for children who, for various reasons, may be resistant to extinction-based procedures or who engage in self-harming behaviors upon awakening. As with any intervention, there are potential drawbacks to SA. Compared to extinction-based treatments, SA is a more complicated protocol that requires long-term adherence to achieve success. In addition, the self-imposed disruptions to parents' own sleep schedule may make SA more difficult for parents to maintain treatment adherence. Finally, the intervention does not address independent sleep initiation skills, potentially limiting its usefulness with children who present with both nighttime awakenings and bedtime resistance. Although some have questioned the mechanism of effect, SA appears to represent a form of noncontingent reinforcement (NCR) with schedule thinning, which behavioral analysts have successfully used to treat a variety of problem behaviors in individuals with developmental disabilities.[57]

Positive Routines

The positive routines (PR) procedure shifts the focus of treatment from reducing problem behaviors to reinforcing, and therefore increasing appropriate presleep behaviors. The method begins with parents temporarily delaying the child's bedtime to more closely match the time the child falls asleep naturally. Parents initiate a sequential "chain" of four to seven activities, lasting no longer than 20 minutes, leading up to the child's bedtime. These activities serve as presleep cues (positive sleep associations) for sleep onset, and may include going to the bathroom, putting on pajamas, brushing teeth,

and reading a story. Successful completion of each activity is met with positive reinforcement, usually in the form of verbal praise. If the child begins to tantrum or resist during the routine, parents are instructed to leave the child alone for 15 minutes before returning to pick up the chain where it had been broken. Once the behavioral chain is well established and the child is falling asleep quickly without resistance, the entire routine gradually is moved earlier in the evening until reaching a pre-established bedtime goal.[58,59] Compared to graduated extinction, PR appear to produce more noticeable reductions in the frequency and duration of bedtime tantrums, and parents report that the protocol is easier to understand.[59]

Faded Bedtime with (or without) Response Cost

Like PR, the faded bedtime with response cost (FB/RC) protocol requires parents to temporarily delay their child's bedtime to facilitate rapid sleep onset. While PR matches the new bedtime to the child's usual sleep onset time, the FB procedure delays the bedtime 30 minutes after the average pretreatment sleep onset time. FB/RC requires no alterations in the nature or frequency of parent-child interactions during bedtime, as parents may interact with or respond to their child in the same manner as they did prior to treatment. The addition of the response cost procedure involves removing children from bed and keeping them awake for 1 hour if they do not fall to sleep within 15 minutes of the prescribed bedtime.[60,61] The sleep schedule is managed tightly and children are not allowed to sleep outside the prescribed sleep times in order to prevent them from making up for poor night sleep by sleeping late in the morning or napping during the day. An exception can be made for young children of napping age (e.g., 4 years and under) for whom disallowing a normal amount of daytime sleep may be developmentally inappropriate.[62] Fading the bedtime involves adjusting the child's nightly bedtime based on the sleep onset time from the previous evening. If the child falls to sleep within 15 minutes of being placed in bed, then bedtime is moved 30 minutes earlier the following night. If the child does not fall asleep within 15 minutes, bedtime is moved 30 minutes later the next night. When FB is combined with response cost, the protocol closely reflects the combination of sleep restriction therapy and stimulus control therapy, both highly effective treatments for primary and co-morbid insomnia in adults.

The FB/RC and PR protocols are similar in many ways. Both procedures circumvent many of the problems associated with extinction by combining sleep scheduling and stimulus control. Both procedures help parents shift their focus from removing unwanted behaviors to establishing positive sleep associations. FB/RC and PR place the child in bed at a time when sleep onset is highly probable. Circadian process and homeostatic sleep pressure increase to the point that a child's desire to sleep overcomes the desire for parental attention or engaging in other activities. Both protocols gradually fade the bedtime earlier once the child learns to fall asleep cooperatively and quickly.

The FB/RC and PR protocols differ, however, in how much emphasis is placed on altering parent-child interactions. Other than removing a sleepless child from bed, FB/RC does not require parents to alter their normal bedtime interactions with the child. The focus instead is placed on increasing the reinforcement value of sleep itself through strict management of the child's sleep schedule. In addition to the bedtime routine, PR incorporates contingency management procedures (e.g., differential reinforcement) to target the child's bedtime behavior. Parents using PR begin ignoring ("cease social interaction") once the child is placed in bed, and repeatedly return the child to the bed if he or she comes out. At face value, FB/RC appears to present a less complicated procedure to implement, yet it has proved effective in reducing a range of sleep-related problems (e.g., undesirable co-sleeping, difficulty falling asleep, frequent nighttime awakenings, early morning awakening). The primary drawback is that parents must be willing to monitor and accept night-to-night fluctuations in their child's bedtime. Further studies of FB/RC are needed to identify the active ingredients and determine if the addition of the response-cost procedure improves outcomes. To date, the majority of studies have targeted children with special needs residing in institutionalized settings, utilizing trained professionals to implement the FB/RC procedure. Further research is needed to demonstrate the usefulness of FB with typically developing children in their own homes.

Obviously clinicians who evaluate and treat young children with insomnia have a number of behavioral treatment options at their disposal. Although choosing among these options may be confusing, there is some guidance for clinicians practicing evidence-based medicine. A task force appointed by the American Academy of Sleep Medicine reviewed the literature on the clinical management of bedtime struggles and night awakenings in children under 5 years of age, establishing the first pediatric practice parameters.[7,63] The task force reviewed 52 treatment studies using Sackett criteria for evidenced-based support. The review concluded that behavioral interventions produce reliable and durable change, with 94% of the published studies reporting that intervention was efficacious. Specific interventions tagged as *Standard Treatments*, supported by well-designed randomized trials and overwhelming support from randomized trials, include *unmodified extinction* and *preventive parent education about sleep*. Interventions considered *Guideline Treatments*, or interventions with support from randomized trials or nonrandomized concurrently controlled studies, include GE, PR/FB, and SA. There was insufficient evidence to recommend standardized bedtime routines or positive reinforcement as stand-alone therapies. The findings of this task force were generally consistent with two previous reviews utilizing criteria[64] adopted by the field of clinical psychology to identify efficacious treatments.[44,65]

Notably, the task force found no evidence of adverse outcomes associated with behavioral treatments. In fact, no fewer than 15 studies concluded that behavioral treatment of pediatric sleep disturbance reduces child irritability, crying, and detachment and enhances their overall well-being.[7,66,67] Neutral to positive outcomes have been reported on infant security, predictability, feeding and daily fluid intake, and daytime behavior. Parents themselves report improved mood, enhanced marital satisfaction, and reduced stress.[68] Even if side effects are associated with certain behavioral interventions, clinicians must consider the magnitude of these side effects against those of alternative treatments (e.g., pharmacologic) as well as the potential long-term impact of failing to treat.

MIDDLE CHILDHOOD

Parents continue to report bedtime problems in 15% to 30% of school-age children.[69,70] The prevalence of pediatric insomnia in school children that goes beyond bedtime refusal, however, is relatively low (1-6%) in the general population.[12] Thanks to the strong opposing forces of clock-dependent alertness and homeostatic sleep drive, middle childhood is typically a developmental period accompanied by good sleep.[71,72] School-aged children have usually developed increased confidence initiating and reinitiating sleep, and most have successfully mastered separation from their primary caregiver. They can turn off their own lights, read a book, or simply remain quietly in bed until they drift off to sleep. Some children may have developed the ability to recognize their internal signs of sleepiness and begin to initiate their own bedtimes and wake times. A child's interests at this stage tend to center around academics, extracurricular activities, and peer relationships; therefore, parental attention becomes less central in motivating their (mis-) behavior.

When children do present with insomnia at this age, the evaluation process becomes more challenging because the list of possible causes expands well beyond parental limit setting to include a host of environmental, psychiatric, medical, and psychosocial factors[73] (see Chapters 41 to 43). In our experience, insomnia during middle childhood is most often found in association with other medical, neurodevelopmental, and psychiatric co-morbidities. (Circadian considerations, such as delayed sleep phase syndrome (DSPS), are important as well, though usually not as problematic here as in adolescence; see Chapter 37.) Conditions in which insomnia frequently co-occurs include, but are not limited to, attention deficit hyperactivity disorder (ADHD), oppositional defiant disorder, autism/pervasive developmental disorders, anxiety, and depression. Secondary insomnia becomes a consideration at this age, especially when it comes to psychosocial stressors and the use of certain medications such as the psychostimulants and the selective serotonin reuptake inhibitors (SSRIs).

Unlike the mature treatment outcome literature for infants and preschool children, there is little research on the treatment of insomnia in school-aged children.[70,74] The few studies evaluating behavioral insomnia treatments for school-age children have relied on contingency management techniques, differential reinforcement, and other fundamental principles of behavior change. Three interventions described above, PR, FB/RC, and the BP, are intended to be used with school-age children. Of course, healthy sleep practices should always be promoted and include limiting caffeinated beverages, maintaining appropriate sleep schedules, and monitoring late night use of electronics. Finally, clinicians working with preadolescent populations can begin to borrow interventions from the adult insomnia literature (e.g., sleep restriction therapy or stimulus control therapy as discussed in the next section for adolescents and in Chapters 10 to 14), but with school-age children the focus must remain on the family unit as the mechanism of treatment delivery and for monitoring adherence.

ADOLESCENCE

Insomnia in older children and adolescents may present much like it does in adults. The key features of primary and co-morbid insomnia still include difficulties falling or staying asleep and daytime impairment; but unlike the behavioral insomnias of younger children, the older child or adolescent may report these concerns directly rather than through the parent. Adolescents largely complain of sleep onset and/or sleep maintenance insomnia; however, some will report early-morning awakening insomnia. Daytime impairment depends on the individual and ranges from feeling fatigued during the day to mood instability. Frequency, duration, and precipitating factors help to determine the specific type of insomnia. For instance, insomnia associated with a chronic pain disorder is considered co-morbid insomnia, whereas a complaint of insomnia independent of medical or psychological illness and not linked to an immediate stressor would be considered a primary insomnia. Similarly, insomnia can be of an acute nature and time-limited, or it may persist as a more chronic and enduring illness.

Connections have been made between insomnia and circadian rhythm disorders. For instance, research evaluating body temperature, one of the circadian rhythm markers, found adults with sleep onset insomnia experience a 2.5-hour delay in their body temperature drop.[8] In addition, one criterion for diagnosing DSPS is the presence of sleep onset insomnia. Adolescents represent a unique population in that they are also experiencing biologic changes that are associated with changes in their circadian rhythm. Specifically, previous research has shown a connection between puberty and biologic delays in the circadian rhythm.[75] Circadian rhythm disorders very commonly cause, or at least complicate, many of the insomnia presentations seen in adolescents; full explorations of the connections between insomnia and circadian rhythm disorders are discussed elsewhere in this book (see Chapters 28, 31, 32, and 37).

However, it is also important to point out the potential misdiagnoses that may be made between DSPS and insomnia. Johnson and associates[76] explored the overlap between insomnia and DSPS and found roughly 2% of the adolescents in the sample met criteria for DSPS within the previous 2 weeks. When DSPS was evaluated by insomnia status, findings showed 1.6% of the adolescents without insomnia and 4.2% of the adolescents with insomnia met criteria for DSPS. Comparisons between groups reflected no significant relationship between insomnia and DSPS status.

Point-prevalence rates of adolescent insomnia range from 4% to 39%, new onset rates range from 5% to 23%, rates of chronic insomnia range from 2% to 20%, and remission rates range from 5.9% to 6.2%.[76-81] Despite these numbers, only one treatment outcome study for insomnia in adolescents has been published to date. Bootzin and Stevens[82] utilized *stimulus control therapy (SCT), bright light therapy, cognitive therapy, mindfulness-based stress reduction (MBSR) therapy,* and *sleep hygiene (SH)* to treat adolescents with co-morbid insomnia and substance abuse. Significant improvements were noted in the sleep-related variables with actigraphy data supporting subjective reports of improvements in total sleep time and sleep onset latency. All participants reported a reduction in sleepiness, worry, and mental health distress. In addition, adolescents who completed the treatment reported a decrease in long-term drug use compared to adolescents who did not complete the treatment program.

Clinicians working with older children and adolescents have little guidance from the literature on specific interventions for insomnia in these populations; therefore, they have

---

BOX 35-3 *Cognitive-Behavioral Therapies for Insomnia in the Adolescent*

- **Stimulus control therapy (SCT)**[83]
- **Sleep restriction therapy (SRT)**[84-86]
- **Progressive muscle relaxation (PMR)**[85,86]
- **Cognitive therapy**
- **Sleep hygiene (SH)**

SCT, SRT, and PMR are the primary behavioral mono-therapeutic approaches. All five items together make up the standard polytherapeutic intervention—namely, cognitive-behavioral therapy for insomnia (CBTi).

---

generally relied upon empirical support for treatments in adults with insomnia. As such, the behavioral treatments outlined in this section will reflect this trend. Primary monotherapeutic behavioral interventions include *SCT,*[83] *SRT,*[84-86] and *progressive muscle relaxation (PMR).*[85,86] Standard polytherapeutic intervention—namely *cognitive-behavioral therapy for insomnia (CBTi)*—combines *SCT, SRT,* and *PMR* with *cognitive therapy* and *SH.*[87] These therapeutic approaches are listed in Box 35-3 and described in the following paragraphs.

Cognitive-behavioral therapy for insomnia. CBTi combines both behavioral and cognitive therapies in order to effectively address the multifactorial nature of insomnia. Behavioral interventions apply the theories of classical and operant conditioning to increase or decrease the occurrence of a behavior, and cognitive therapies operate under the assumption that altering thoughts and beliefs will produce a positive impact on emotions and behaviors. Theoretically, pairing mono- and polytherapeutic treatments helps to impact multiple aspects of a disorder that cannot always be addressed using only one approach.

CBTi utilizes approaches rooted in either behavioral or cognitive perspectives in order to more comprehensively treat insomnia. The goal of CBTi is to decrease the discrepancy between time in bed and total sleep time, increase the association between bed and sleep, provide education on sleep and its impact on daytime functioning, and decrease dysfunctional beliefs about sleep.[87] Initial treatment sessions typically focus on SCT and SRT with the introduction of cognitive therapy, relaxation techniques, and SH in subsequent sessions.

Numerous studies have found CBTi to be effective at improving insomnia,[85] and recent research indicates CBTi is cost effective, has enduring effects, and is nonaddictive in comparison to pharmaceutical therapy in adults.[88,89] CBTi has been found to be as effective as pharmacologic treatments in the short term, and has been more effective in the long term.[86,89-91]

Stimulus control therapy. SCT strengthens the association between sleep and the bedroom by removing incompatible associations and thereby increasing the likelihood of the individual falling asleep in bed.[83] Often, in individuals with insomnia, the bed or bedroom no longer serve as cues for sleepiness, but become generalized to numerous activities. In order to remove these competing cues, access to the bed is made contingent on being sleepy. If the individual is not sleepy, he or she is not to enter the bed. Through the repeated

---

BOX 35-4 *Stimulus Control Therapy: Five Key Instructions*

- Go to bed only when sleepy
- Get out of bed when unable to sleep
- Use the bed for sleep only
- Awaken at the same time each morning
- No daily naps

BOX 35-5 *Goals of Cognitive Therapy for Treatment of Insomnia*

- Alter unidimensional explanations of insomnia
- Alter misattributions to or amplifications of the consequences of insomnia
- Change unrealistic explanations regarding sleep
- Decrease performance anxiety

---

experience of falling asleep quickly in bed, the bed and bedroom are reestablished as cues for sleep.

SCT consists of five key instructions as listed in Box 35-4 and described here: The first three instructions focus on strengthening the association between sleep and the bedroom and the last two reestablish a consistent sleep/wake schedule. When providing these instructions, the clinician should problem-solve with the individual to find reasonable ways to carry out these instructions.

Ideally, the only activity occurring in the bedroom would be sleep; however, for adolescents, leaving the room may not always be feasible. Thus, alternative ways to remove non-sleep-compatible cues from the bed and bedroom should be explored. For instance, establish a set place within the bedroom that is the "go-to" spot for the adolescent if unable to fall asleep. This arrangement reduces the associated cues with the bed itself, but works within the reality that the teen may not have another location to go to. Another alteration may include establishing an *electronics-off* time in which the adolescent agrees to turn off all electronics for the evening. In some instances, this may require the adolescent to relinquish the electronics to parents in order to reduce temptation to continue use (texting, etc.). This practice provides a time buffer between engaging in stimulating activities and the bedroom.

Sleep restriction therapy. SRT increases the likelihood of falling asleep quickly by reducing a person's allowable time in bed.[84] Individuals with insomnia frequently report poor sleep efficiency (their actual sleep time as a percent of their total time in bed trying to sleep) because they are spending more time in bed than required to meet their individual sleep need. By restricting the total time in bed, homeostatic sleep pressure continues to build throughout the day because the individual is required to maintain wakefulness for a longer period of time prior to going to bed. The increased sleep pressure, paired with a reduced allowable time in bed, results in quicker sleep onset and reduced sleep fragmentation. Thus, SRT facilitates a quicker sleep onset and fewer night awakenings.

A prescribed total sleep time and wake-up time is established based on pretreatment sleep diary data and required wake-up time to accomplish the day's events. The average total sleep time is determined from the sleep diary data and guides the recommendations for the allowable time in bed, which should not be less than 5 to 5.5 hours for adults.[84] Knowledge of the required wake-up time allows a better determination of the window when time in bed should occur. Individuals are encouraged to spend no more than the prescribed total time in bed and not sleep any later than the prescribed wake-up time on both weekdays and weekends. Each week an average sleep efficiency (100 times the total sleep time divided by total time in bed) of 85% or greater is achieved, the total time in bed is increased by 15 minutes until the optimal total time in bed is achieved. Any week the sleep efficiency is less than 85%, the total time in bed is decreased by 15 to 30 minutes. Optimal time in bed is achieved once the total time in bed cannot be extended without the sleep efficiency dipping and remaining below 85%.

Progressive muscle relaxation therapy. PMR is the most common relaxation technique used; others include diaphragmatic breathing (or deep breathing), visual imagery, meditation, and biofeedback. Of the various treatment modalities available, PMR has the most evidence to support its effectiveness in the treatment of insomnia compared to placebo, wait-list, and no-treatment control subjects.[85,86] PMR involves first tensing and then relaxing different muscle groups including the forehead, face, jaw, neck, shoulders, chest, arms, hands, abdomen, buttocks, thighs, calves, feet, and toes. Patients are taught to discriminate between muscle tension and muscle relaxation. Being able to differentiate between these feelings allows patients to recognize when they are feeling tension and to consciously relax. This skill requires practice to master and is best practiced when the person is not feeling particularly tense (e.g., during a middle of the night awakening). Initially, patients are encouraged to practice this skill at bedtime and during the day. Once they learn to differentiate, they can progress to using the skill when they are feeling tense.

Sleep hygiene. SH focuses on reducing or eliminating behaviors that may interfere with sleep (e.g., nicotine, alcohol, and caffeine use, exercise timing). These guidelines reflect practices that are usually present in "good" sleepers. Unfortunately, sleep hygiene has been shown to be ineffective as a stand-alone treatment.[92,93] In addition, studies manipulating the elements of sleep hygiene have been inconclusive as to whether these practices really influence sleep, at least in baseline good sleepers.[92] Nevertheless, improving sleep hygiene is frequently part of a therapeutic program, and such recommendations are almost always included in multicomponent treatment protocols.

Cognitive therapy. CT focuses on identifying dysfunctional beliefs and replacing these dysfunctional beliefs with more adaptive substitutes.[87] Interventions with a CT component require a certain level of cognitive development and maturation to be effective. Most older children and adolescents have acquired the necessary cognitive maturation required for the cognitive therapy component of CBTi. The four goals of cognitive therapy are listed in Box 35-5.

The first step of cognitive therapy is to identify any dysfunctional beliefs about sleep an individual may possess by interview and standardized assessment tools such as the *Dysfunctional Belief and Attitudes About Sleep Scale (DBAS)*.[94] The next step is to replace them with more adaptive alternatives by providing education about sleep and the true impact of sleepiness.

SUMMARY

The clinical manifestations, evaluation methods, and interventions for children presenting with insomnia are clearly distinct from those used with adults. There is extensive research supporting the effectiveness of behavioral interventions for insomnia in infants, toddlers, and preschool children. Little attention has been paid, however, to the evaluation and treatment of insomnia in school age children; this area is in need of further research and development. In recent years, the field of sleep medicine has turned some of its attention to helping adolescents with insomnia. Clinical outcome studies are now being conducted and promising interventions are on the horizon. In the meantime, clinicians treating adolescents may rely on components of CBTi that have proven successful with adults including CT, SH (including sleep schedule normalization), SCT, SRT, and PMR.

REFERENCES

1. Hoban TF, Chervin RD. Pediatric sleep-related breathing disorders and restless legs syndrome: How children are different. *Neurologist.* 2005;11:325-337.
2. Kotagal S. Narcolepsy in childhood. In: Sheldon SH, Ferber R, Kryger M, eds. *Principles and Practice of Pediatric Sleep Medicine.* Philadelphia: Elsevier Saunders; 2005:171-182.
3. Stores G. The protean manifestations of childhood narcolepsy and their misinterpretation. *Dev Med Child Neurol.* 2006;48:307-310.
4. Robinson PD, Waters K. Are children just small adults? The differences between paediatric and adult sleep medicine. *Intern Med J.* 2008;38:719-731.
5. Sheldon SH. Diagnostic methods in pediatric sleep medicine. *Sleep Med Clin.* 2007;2:343-351.
6. Kuhn BR, Weidinger D. Interventions for infant and toddler sleep disturbance: A review. *Child Fam Behav Ther.* 2000;22:33-50.
7. Mindell JA, Kuhn B, Lewin DS, Meltzer LJ, Sadeh A. Behavioral treatment of bedtime problems and night wakings in infants and young children. *Sleep.* 2006;29:1263-1276.
8. Owens JA, Rosen CL, Mindell JA. Medication use in the treatment of pediatric insomnia: Results of a survey of community-based pediatricians. *Pediatrics.* 2003;111:E628-E635.
9. Schnoes CJ, Kuhn BR, Workman E, Ellis C. Pediatric prescribing practices of clonidine and other psychopharmacological agents for pediatric sleep disturbances. *Clin Pediatr (Phila).* 2006;45:229-238.
10. Owens JA, Rosen CL, Mindell JA, Kirchner HL. Use of pharmacotherapy for insomnia in child psychiatry practice: A national survey. *Sleep Med.* 2010;11:692-700.
11. Glaze DG, Rosen CL, Owens JA. Toward a practical definition of pediatric insomnia. *Curr Ther Res.* 2002;63:B4-B17.
12. Mindell JA, Emslie G, Blumer J, et al. Pharmacologic management of insomnia in children and adolescents: Consensus statement. *Pediatrics.* 2006;117:E1223-E1232.
13. Anders TF, Dahl RE. Classifying sleep disorders in infants and toddlers. In: Narrow WN, First MB, Sivoratka P, Regier DA, eds. *Age and Gender Considerations in Psychiatric Diagnosis: A Research Agenda for DSM-V.* Arlington: American Psychiatric Association; 2007:215-226.
14. Goodlin-Jones B, Tang K, Liu J, Anders TF. Sleep problems, sleepiness and daytime behavior in preschool-age children. *J Child Psychol Psychiatry.* 2009;50:1532-1540.
15. Jenni OG, O'Connor BB. Children's sleep: An interplay between culture and biology. *Pediatrics.* 2005;115:204-216.
16. Adair R, Bauchner H, Philipp B, Levenson S, Zuckerman B. Night waking during infancy: Role of parental presence at bedtime. *Pediatrics.* 1991;87:500-504.
17. Anders TF, Halpern LF, Hua J. Sleeping through the night: A developmental perspective. *Pediatrics.* 1992;90:554-560.
18. Anuntaseree W, Mo-Suwan L, Vasiknanonte P, Kuasirikul S, Ma-A-Lee A, Choprapawan C. Night waking in Thai infants at 3 months of age: Association between parental practices and infant sleep. *Sleep Med.* 2008;9:564-571.

19. Fehlings D. Frequent night awakenings in infants and preschool children referred to a sleep disorders clinic: The role of non-adaptive sleep associations. *Child Health Care.* 2001;30:43-55.
20. Owens J. Epidemiology of sleep disorders during childhood. In: Sheldon SH, Ferber R, Kryger MH, eds. *Principles and Practice of Pediatric Sleep Medicine.* New York: Elsevier Saunders; 2005:27-33.
21. Quach J, Hiscock H, Canterford L, Wake M. Outcomes of child sleep problems over the school-transition period: Australian population longitudinal study. *Pediatrics.* 2009;123:1287-1292.
22. Gregory AM, Caspi A, Moffitt TE, Poulton R. Sleep problems in childhood predict neuropsychological functioning in adolescence. *Pediatrics.* 2009;123:1171-1176.
23. Martin J, Hiscock H, Hardy P, Davey B, Wake M. Adverse associations of infant and child sleep problems and parent health: An Australian population study. *Pediatrics.* 2007;119:947-955.
24. Fallone G, Owens JA, Deane J. Sleepiness in children and adolescents: Clinical implications. *Sleep Med Rev.* 2002;6:287-306.
25. Smedje H, Broman JE, Hetta J. Associations between disturbed sleep and behavioural difficulties in 635 children aged six to eight years: A study based on parents' perceptions. *Eur Child Adolesc Psychiatry.* 2001;10:1-9.
26. Sadeh A, Tikotzky L, Scher A. Parenting and infant sleep. *Sleep Med Rev.* 2010;14:89-96.
27. Mindell JA, Sadeh A, Kohyama J, How TH. Parental behaviors and sleep outcomes in infants and toddlers: A cross-cultural comparison. *Sleep Med.* 2010;11:393-399.
28. Hiscock H. Rock-a-bye baby? Parenting and infant sleep. *Sleep Med Rev.* 2010;14:85-87.
29. Hale L, Berger LM, LeBourgeois MK, Brooks-Gunn J. Social and demographic predictors of preschoolers' bedtime routines. *J Dev Behav Pediatr.* 2009;30:394-402.
30. Mindell JA, Telofski LS, Wiegand B, Kurtz ES. A nightly bedtime routine: Impact on sleep in young children and maternal mood. *Sleep.* 2009;32:599-606.
31. Adair R, Zuckerman B, Bauchner H, Philipp B, Levenson S. Reducing night waking in infancy: A primary care intervention. *Pediatrics.* 1992;89:585-588.
32. Pinilla T, Birch LL. Help me make it through the night: Behavioral entrainment of breast-fed infants' sleep patterns [see comments]. *Pediatrics.* 1993;91:436-444.
33. Mindell JM, Babu M, Sekartini R, Sadeh A. *How to Breastfeed and Sleep: It May Not Be Whether You Nurse, But Whether You Nurse to Sleep.* Denver, CO: 5th Annual Conference on Pediatric Sleep Medicine; Oct. 2010.
34. Ramos KD. Intentional versus reactive cosleeping. *Sleep Res Online.* 2003;5:141-147.
35. Owens JA, Moturi S. Pharmacologic treatment of pediatric insomnia. *Child Adolesc Psychiatr Clin North Am.* 2009;18:1001-1016.
36. Cubero J, Narciso D, Terron P, et al. Chrononutrition applied to formula milks to consolidate infants' sleep/wake cycle. *Neuroendocrinol Lett.* 2007;28:360-366.
37. Jamison JR, Davies NJ. Chiropractic management of cows milk protein intolerance in infants with sleep dysfunction syndrome: A therapeutic trial. *J Manipulative Physiol Ther.* 2006;29:469-474.
38. Forbes EA. Behavioral and massage treatments for infant sleep problems. *Med Health R I.* 2006;89:97-99.
39. Williams TI. Evaluating effects of aromatherapy massage on sleep in children with autism: A pilot study. *Evidence-Based Compl Alt.* 2006;3:373-377.
40. Owens JA. When child can't sleep, start by treating the parents. *Curr Psychiatr.* 2006;5:21-22:27-30.
41. Sadeh A. Cognitive-behavioral treatment for childhood sleep disorders. *Clin Psychol Rev.* 2005;25:612-628.
42. Symon BG, Marley JE, Martin AJ, Norman ER. Effect of a consultation teaching behaviour modification on sleep performance in infants: A randomised controlled trial. *Med J Aust.* 2005;182:215-218.
43. Lerman DC, Iwata BA. Developing a technology for the use of operant extinction in clinical settings: An examination of basic and applied research. *J Appl Behav Anal.* 1996;29:345-382:discussion 83-85.
44. Kuhn BR, Elliott AJ. Treatment efficacy in behavioral pediatric sleep medicine. *J Psychosom Res.* 2003;54:587-597.
45. Kuhn BR. Sleep disorders. In: Hersen M, Thomas JC, eds. *Handbook of Clinical Interviewing with Children.* New York: Sage Publications; 2007:420-447.

46. Iwata BA, Pace GM, Cowdery GE, Miltenberger RG. What makes extinction work: An analysis of procedural form and function. *J Appl Behav Anal*. 1994;27:131-144.

47. Didden R, Sigafoos J, Lancioni GE. Unmodified extinction for childhood sleep disturbance. In: Perlis M, Aloia M, Kuhn BR, eds. *Behavioral Treatments for Sleep Disorders: A Comprehensive Primer of Behavioral Sleep Medicine Interventions*. Boston: Elsevier/Academic Press; 2010:257-264.

48. Reimers TM, Wacker D, Cooper LJ. Evaluation of the acceptability of treatments for children's behavioral difficulties: Ratings by parents receiving services in an outpatient clinic. *Child Fam Behav Ther*. 1991;13:53-71.

49. Ferber R. *Solve your child's sleep problems*. New York: Simon & Schuster; 1985.

50. Meltzer LJ, Mindell JA. Graduated extinction: Behavioral treatment for bedtime problems and night wakings in young children. In: Perlis M, Aloia M, Kuhn BR, eds. *Behavioral Treatments for Sleep Disorders: A Comprehensive Primer of Behavioral Sleep Medicine Interventions*. Boston: Elsevier/Academic Press; 2010:265-274.

51. France KG. Extinction with parental presence. In: Perlis M, Aloia M, Kuhn BR, eds. *Behavioral Treatments for Sleep Disorders: A Comprehensive Primer of Behavioral Sleep Medicine Interventions*. Boston: Elsevier/Academic Press; 2010:275-284.

52. France KG, Blampied NM. Modifications of systematic ignoring in the management of infant sleep disturbance: Efficacy and infant distress. *Child Fam Behav Ther*. 2005;27:1-16.

53. Kuhn BR. The excuse-me drill for bedtime problems. In: Perlis M, Aloia M, Kuhn BR, eds. *Behavioral Treatments for Sleep Disorders: A Comprehensive Primer of Behavioral Sleep Medicine Interventions*. Boston: Elsevier/Academic Press; 2010:299-310.

54. Freeman K. Treating bedtime resistance with the bedtime pass: A systematic replication and component analysis with 3-year-olds. *J Appl Behav Analysis*. 2006;39:423-428.

55. Friman PC, Hoff KE, Schnoes C, Freeman KA, Woods DW, Blum N. The bedtime pass: An approach to bedtime crying and leaving the room. *Arch Pediatr Adolesc Med*. 1999;153:1027-1029.

56. Moore BA, Friman PC, Fruzzetti AE, MacAleese K. Brief report: Evaluating the bedtime pass program for child resistance to bedtime: A randomized, controlled trial. *J Pediatr Psychol*. 2007;32:283-287.

57. Carr JE, Severtson JM, Lepper TL. Noncontingent reinforcement is an empirically supported treatment for problem behavior exhibited by individuals with developmental disabilities. *Res Dev Disabil*. 2009;30:44-57.

58. Milan MA, Mitchell ZP, Berger MI, Pierson DF. Positive routines: A rapid alternative to extinction for elimination of bedtime tantrum behavior. *Child Behav Ther*. 1981;3:13-25.

59. Adams LA, Rickert VI. Reducing bedtime tantrums: Comparison between positive routines and graduated extinction. *Pediatrics*. 1989;84:756-761.

60. Piazza CC, Fisher WW. A faded bedtime with response cost protocol for treatment of multiple sleep problems in children. *J Appl Behav Anal*. 1991;24:129-140.

61. Piazza CC, Fisher WW. Bedtime fading in the treatment of pediatric insomnia. *J Behav Ther Exp Psychiatry*. 1991;22:53-56.

62. Kodak T, Piazza CC. Bedtime fading with response cost for children with multiple sleep problems. In: Perlis M, Aloia M, Kuhn BR, eds. *Behavioral Treatments for Sleep Disorders: A Comprehensive Primer of Behavioral Sleep Medicine Interventions*. Boston: Elsevier/Academic Press; 2010:285-292.

63. Morgenthaler TI, Owens J, Alessi C, et al. Practice parameters for behavioral treatment of bedtime problems and night wakings in infants and young children. *Sleep*. 2006;29:1277-1281.

64. Chambless DL, Sanderson WC, Shoham V, et al. An update on empirically validated therapies. *Clin Psychol*. 1996;49:5-18.

65. Mindell JA. Empirically supported treatments in pediatric psychology: Bedtime refusal and night wakings in young children. *J Pediatr Psychol*. 1999;24:465-481.

66. Hall WA, Clauson M, Carty EM, Janssen PA, Saunders RA. Effects on parents of an intervention to resolve infant behavioral sleep problems. *Pediatr Nurs*. 2006;32:243-250.

67. Hiscock H, Bayer JK, Hampton A, Ukoumunne OC, Wake M. Long-term mother and child mental health effects of a population-based infant sleep intervention: Cluster-randomized, controlled trial. *Pediatrics*. 2008;122: E621-E627.

68. Crncec R, Cooper E, Matthey S. Treating infant sleep disturbance: Does maternal mood impact upon effectiveness? *J Paediatr Child Health*. 2010;46:29-34.

69. Blader JC, Koplewicz HS, Abikoff H, Foley C. Sleep problems of elementary school children. A community survey. *Arch Pediatr Adolesc Med*. 1997;151:473-480.

70. Owens JA, Spirito A, McGuinn M, Nobile C. Sleep habits and sleep disturbance in elementary school-aged children. *J Dev Behav Pediatr*. 2000;21:27-36.

71. Dement WC. *The Promise of Sleep*. New York: Dell; 1999.

72. Ferber R. Introduction. *Pediatrician*. 1990;17:2-4.

73. Sadeh A, Raviv A, Gruber R. Sleep patterns and sleep disruptions in school-age children. *Dev Psychol*. 2000;36:291-301.

74. Tikotzky L, Sadeh A. The role of cognitive-behavioral therapy in behavioral childhood insomnia. *Sleep Med*. 2010;11:686-691.

75. Carskadon MA, Vieira C, Acebo C. Association between puberty and delayed phase preference. *Sleep*. 1993;16:258-262.

76. Johnson EO, Roth T, Schultz L, Breslau N. Epidemiology of DSM-IV insomnia in adolescence: Lifetime prevalence, chronicity, and an emergent gender difference. *Pediatrics*. 2006;117:E247-E256.

77. Roberts RE, Roberts CR, Duong HT. Chronic insomnia and its negative consequences for health and functioning of adolescents: A 12-month prospective study. *J Adolesc Health*. 2008;42:294-302.

78. Ohayon MM, Roberts RE, Zulley J, Smirne S, Priest RG. Prevalence and patterns of problematic sleep among older adolescents. *J Am Acad Child Adolesc Psychiatry*. 2000;39:1549-1556.

79. Patten CA, Choi WS, Gillin JC, Pierce JP. Depressive symptoms and cigarette smoking predict development and persistence of sleep problems in US adolescents. *Pediatrics*. 2000;106:E23.

80. Roberts RE, Lewinsohn PM, Seeley JR. Symptoms of DSM-III-R major depression in adolescence: Evidence from an epidemiological survey. *J Am Acad Child Adolesc Psychiatry*. 1995;34:1608-1617.

81. Roane BM, Taylor DJ. Natural course of adolescent insomnia: Patterns and consequences. In preparation.

82. Bootzin RR, Stevens SJ. Adolescents, substance abuse, and the treatment of insomnia and daytime sleepiness. *Clin Psychol Rev*. 2005;25:629-644.

83. Bootzin RR. Stimulus Control Treatment for Insomnia. *Proceedings of the 80th Annual Convention of the American Psychological Association*. 1972:395-396.

84. Spielman AJ, Saskin P, Thorpy MJ. Treatment of chronic insomnia by restriction of time in bed. *Sleep*. 1987;10:45-56.

85. Morgenthaler T, Kramer M, Alessi C, et al. Practice parameters for the psychological and behavioral treatment of insomnia: An update. An American Academy of Sleep Medicine report. *Sleep*. 2006;29:1415-1419.

86. Morin CM, Bootzin RR, Buysse DJ, Edinger JD, Espie CA, Lichstein KL. Psychological and behavioral treatment of insomnia: Update of the recent evidence (1998-2004). *Sleep*. 2006;29:1398-1414.

87. Sloan EP, Hauri P, Bootzin R, Morin C, et al. The nuts and bolts of behavioral therapy for insomnia. *J Psychosom Res*. 1993;37:19-37.

88. Espie CA. Cognitive behaviour therapy as the treatment of choice for primary insomnia. *Sleep Med Rev*. 1999;3:97-99.

89. Smith MT, Perlis ML, Park A, et al. Comparative meta-analysis of pharmacotherapy and behavior therapy for persistent insomnia. *Am J Psychiatry*. 2002;159:5-11.

90. Morin CM, Hauri PJ, Espie CA, Spielman AJ, Buysse DJ, Bootzin RR. Nonpharmacologic treatment of chronic insomnia. An American Academy of Sleep Medicine review. *Sleep*. 1999;22:1134-1156.

91. Sivertsen B, Omvik S, Pallesen S, et al. Cognitive behavioral therapy vs. zopiclone for treatment of chronic primary insomnia in older adults: A randomized controlled trial. *JAMA*. 2006;295:2851-2858.

92. Stepanski EJ, Wyatt JK. Use of sleep hygiene in the treatment of insomnia. *Sleep Med Rev*. 2003;7:215-225.

93. Taylor DJ, Bramoweth AD. Patterns and consequences of inadequate sleep in college students: Substance use and motor vehicle accidents. *J Adolesc Health*. 2010;46:610-612.

94. Morin CM, Vallières A, Ivers H. Dysfunctional beliefs and attitudes about sleep (DBAS): Validation of a brief version (DBAS-16). *Sleep*. 2007;30:1547-1554.

Sleep Pharmacotherapeutics for Pediatric Insomnia:

FDA-Approved and Off-Label Evidence

Chapter 36

ELIZABETH R. SUPER / KYLE P. JOHNSON

Although the Food and Drug Administration (FDA) has not approved any medications for the treatment of pediatric insomnia, physicians are ordering prescription medications and recommending nonprescription medications at increasing rates. More than 75% of primary care pediatricians surveyed recommended nonprescription medications for pediatric insomnia and greater than 50% had prescribed a medication specifically for sleep. The clinical situations in which these medications were most commonly used were acute pain and travel, closely followed by children with special needs such as mental retardation, autism, and attention deficit hyperactivity disorder (ADHD).[1] A more recently published survey of child and adolescent psychiatrists reveals that prescription or nonprescription medications are frequently used to manage insomnia in the following disorders: primary insomnia, depression, bipolar affective disorder, anxiety, post-traumatic stress disorder, delayed sleep phase syndrome, ADHD, autism spectrum disorder, chronic pain, oppositional disorder, and mental retardation/developmental delay.[2]

Antihistamines were the *nonprescription* medications most commonly recommended for treatment of insomnia in children, and alpha agonists (such as clonidine) were the medications most frequently *prescribed*. Choice of medications was somewhat dependent on clinical presentation: thus, whereas alpha agonists were the most commonly prescribed insomnia medications for children with ADHD, trazodone was the medication most widely prescribed to treat insomnia in children suffering with mood or anxiety disorders.

Only quite recently has there been published research on pharmacotherapy for pediatric sleep disorders. This chapter will summarize the use of medications for sleep disorders in children and adolescents.

OFF-LABEL USE OF MEDICATIONS IN PEDIATRICS IN GENERAL

In the 1990s, special legal regulations were put in place to encourage development of pediatric medications.[3] These regulations allowed evidence of drug efficacy in children to be derived from data about drug efficacy in adults if convincing proof of similarity in psychopathologic features and pharmacologic response existed across the age groups.[4] Even with new regulations, only approximately 11% of all medications with patent protection by the FDA granted for pediatric studies are neuropharmacologic medications.[5]

Thus, unfortunately, there is still a lack of progress in development and testing of hypnotic medications for pediatric populations. Nevertheless, off-label pharmaceutical use is widespread among pediatric providers, despite the absence of much data regarding long-term effects, even in the adult studies. There is no substitute for clinical research in children. Yet, in order to aid primary care providers, a task force was formed through the American Academy of Sleep Medicine to formulate a rational approach to the pharmacologic treatment of pediatric insomnia. Clinical guidelines for implications, target populations, and parameters for use of hypnotics in children were published in 2005.[6]

Although children's responses to drugs have much in common with the responses in adults, there may be important differences. Children are not small adults. There may be age-dependent differences in pharmacodynamics (the effects of drugs and their mechanisms of action), drug metabolism, and drug receptor sensitivity, which may affect both desired actions and adverse events. Programming by drugs (i.e., permanent effects resulting from a drug administered during a *critical window* in development) is a phenomenon almost exclusive to early life (especially fetal and neonatal periods). Different pathophysiologies, different disease variants, different pharmacodynamics, different "host" responses, and different adverse drug reactions can all explain why some drugs behave differently in children.[7]

All these considerations add considerable complexity to decision making regarding prescribing to the pediatric population. The clinician is left to decide several important issues: what are the clinical indications for drug treatment, and what are the drugs of choice, the doses, the dosing schedules, the contraindications, and the potential (short- and long-term) side effects? Pharmacology references, such as *Micromedex*, contain citations that may simply report that "safety and effectiveness in pediatric patients have not been established." Unfortunately, guidance for pediatric clinicians is often largely anecdotal. Clinical teaching suggests caution: "start low and go slow."

MEDICATIONS FOR INSOMNIA

The regulation of sleep involves multiple redundant neuropathways that involve many neurotransmitters, including γ-aminobutyric acid (GABA), histamine, melatonin, and norepinephrine, and the medications used to treat insomnia act at the receptors of these neurotransmitters. Benzodiazepines and other benzodiazepine receptor agonists bind to the benzodiazepine receptor site, leading to modulation of the GABA receptor and its chloride ion channels. Antidepressants (e.g., amitriptyline, trazodone, and mirtazapine) exert sedative effects through anticholinergic and antihistaminergic mechanisms. Antihistamines, available in a wide variety of compounds, are sedating and often used to treat pediatric insomnia. α-Adrenergic agonists such as clonidine and guanfacine, impact noradrenergic tone and are often prescribed for their sedative qualities.

Insomnia can be primary or a symptom of a number of medical and psychiatric conditions as well as other sleep disorders. When treating children with insomnia, it is paramount to use sedating pharmacologic agents only when behavioral interventions have been thoroughly tried and found to be noneffective (see Chapter 35). The underlying diagnosis contributing to insomnia should influence the choice of medication. In many cases, treating the underlying condition will lead to improvement and resolution of insomnia. For example, use of a selective serotonin reuptake inhibitor (SSRI) in a child with major depressive disorder may be all that is necessary to treat the child's insomnia. However, the insomnia associated with a medical or psychiatric condition may be severe enough to warrant its own pharmacologic treatment, at least in the short term (see Chapter 42). Patients and their parents need to understand that there are no FDA-approved drugs for pediatric insomnia, and therefore, medicines prescribed for this purpose are being used *off-label*. A careful discussion of the risks, benefits, and alternatives is imperative.

The next section will discuss specific pharmacologic agents that are often used to treat pediatric insomnia, whether or not the insomnia is associated with a medical or psychiatric condition or a sleep disorder (Tables 36-1 and 36-2).

Melatonin Receptor Agonists

Melatonin

In the United States, melatonin is a widely sold nutritional supplement, not a licensed drug. To date, there have been more placebo-controlled trials for melatonin in the treatment of pediatric insomnia than there have been for drugs licensed by the FDA.[8-10] Melatonin is widely prescribed by pediatricians and child psychiatrists, particularly for children with ADHD and autism spectrum disorders.[1,2,11]

Melatonin is an indolamine with chronobiotic and sleep-promoting properties. Chronobiotic properties are those that influence the timing of sleep. In the United States, synthetic melatonin has been available as an over-the-counter medication since 1993. Melatonin has been used to treat insomnia in a number of pediatric populations including typically developing children with initial insomnia, children with ADHD and co-morbid insomnia, children with neurodevelopmental disabilities, children with autism spectrum disorder, and adolescents with delayed sleep phase syndrome.[9,10,12-16]

Melatonin is relatively short acting, with a half-life of approximately 1 hour. For this reason, it is much more effective in treating initial insomnia rather than sleep maintenance insomnia or terminal insomnia. For the treatment of initial insomnia, melatonin should be administered approximately 30 minutes before desired time of sleep onset. Melatonin

is thought to be sedating in dosages of 1 mg and greater. Research studies typically give doses of 2.5 mg to 10 mg when treating initial insomnia. One potential strategy in treating initial insomnia with melatonin is to start with a dose of 1.5 mg and to increase in 1.5-mg increments every 4 to 5 days as indicated.[17] Researchers have used doses as high as 10 to 15 mg in children with severe neurodevelopmental disabilities without evidence of significant adverse events.[12]

If melatonin is to be used to alter the circadian sleep-wake cycle, it can be given in smaller doses. In these cases, the timing of the administration is even more important. For example, in the treatment of delayed sleep phase syndrome, there is evidence that low-dose melatonin (e.g., 0.3 mg) is effective if given approximately 4 to 5 hours before the current usual time of falling asleep, which may differ considerably from the desired bedtime. This low dose of melatonin then can be given progressively earlier as the sleep phase is moved earlier (advanced).

One particular use of low-dose melatonin is in children with total blindness. These children do not have access to the light/dark cycle; therefore, they tend to *free run*, with their sleep-wake schedule progressively delaying over time. This delay leads to periods of mismatch between the body and the external clocks: the children are left extremely sleepy during the day, more awake and alert at night, and significantly impaired. Low-dose melatonin can be used to help entrain their circadian rhythms as demonstrated in adults.[18]

Overall, adverse effects from melatonin have been minimal. There are reports of enuresis, depression, and excessive daytime somnolence, with one report noting increased seizures in children with profound mental retardation, epilepsy, and sleep-wake cycle disorders.[19]

Ramelteon

Ramelteon is the first in a new class of hypnotic medication FDA approved for the treatment of initial insomnia in adults. The labeling of ramelteon lists no limitation for duration of use. Ramelteon is a potent melatonin receptor agonist with higher affinity for melatonin MT_1 and MT_2 receptors than the MT_3 receptor. The selective binding to these receptors induces sleep and maintains the circadian rhythm underlying the normal sleep-wake cycle. Time to peak concentration is 0.75 hour. Ramelteon has an active metabolite, M-II. The half-life is approximately 1 to 2.6 hours for the parent compound and 2 to 5 hours for the active metabolite. It comes only in 8 mg tablet strength.

Common side effects of ramelteon include dizziness, nausea, somnolence, fatigue, and depression. In addition, a precaution listed in the labeling states that, given the possible effect of this medicine on the endocrine system, reproductive development in children or adolescents may be affected. The SSRI fluvoxamine is a major inhibitor of the cytochrome P-450 system enzyme CYP1A2; therefore, co-administration of ramelteon should not be prescribed because concurrent use of these two medicines can lead to significant increases in ramelteon plasma concentrations.

Sedative-Hypnotics

Benzodiazepines

Benzodiazepines act on the specific sites of GABA type A receptors ($GABA_A$) and produce anxiolytic, anticonvulsant, myorelaxant, and hypnotic effects. Benzodiazepines approved

TABLE 36-1

Pharmacology of Selected Medications Used for Pediatric Insomnia

Class	Drug	Half-Life ($t_{1/2}$)	Onset of Action/Peak Level (min)	Mechanism of Action	Metabolism	Drug-Drug Interaction(s)	Effect(s) on Sleep Architecture
BZD	Clonazepam (Klonopin)	19-60 hr	Rapid absorption slowed by food	Bind to central GABA receptors	Hepatic	ETOH/barbiturates increase CNS depression	Suppresses SWS; reduces frequency of nocturnal arousals
	Flurazepam (Dalmane)	48-120 hr	20-60				
	Quazepam (Doral)	48-120 hr	20-45				
	Temazepam (Restoril)	3-25 hr	20-45				
	Estazolam (Prosom)	8-24 hr	45-60				
	Triazolam (Halcion)	8-24 hr	15-30				
			15-30				
Alpha-receptor agonist	Clonidine (Catapres) Guanfacine (Tenex)	6-24 hr	Rapid absorption; bioavailability 100%; onset action within 1 hr; peak effects 2-4 hr	Alpha-adrenergic receptor agonists (guanfacine more selective); decrease NE release	50%-80% of dose excreted unchanged in urine	Reports of serious CNS effects with coadministration with psychostimulants	Decreases SOL
Pyrimidine derivatives	Zolpidem (Ambien)	2.5 hr	90	BZD-like	Hepatic, no active metabolites	ETOH, CNS depressants may potentiate effects	Decreases SOL, little effect on sleep architecture
	Zolpidem CR	2.8 hr	90				
	Zaleplon (Sonata)	1 hr	30-60				
	Eszopiclone (Lunesta)	6 hr	60				
Atypical antidepressant	Trazodone (Desyrel)	7 hr	30-120	5-HT, serotonin agonist	Hepatic	Potentiates effects of ETOH, CNS depressants, digoxin, phenytoin, and antihypertensives	Decreases SOL; improves sleep continuity, decreases REM sleep, increases SWS
Hormone analog	Melatonin	30-50 min	30-60 (sustained-release peak level: 4 hr)	Main effect circadian; weak hypnotic	Hepatic	Largely unknown; NSAID, ETOH, caffeine, BZD may interfere with normal melatonin production	Decreases SOL; main effect on circadian rhythm
Tetracyclic antidepressant	Mirtazapine (Remeron)	Females: 37 hr; males: 26 hr	Rapid and complete	Largely unknown 5-HT$_2$, 5-HT$_3$ antagonist, moderate muscarinic antagonist, potent H$_1$ antagonist	Hepatic	Probable with: Clonidine Fluoxetine Fluvoxamine Olanzapine Procarbazine Tramadol Venlafaxine	Decreases SOL
Antihistamines	Diphenhydramine (Benadryl)	4-6 hr	Rapid absorption and onset of action; peak levels at 2-4 hr	H$_1$ agonists; first-generation drugs cross blood-brain barrier	Hepatic	ETOH/CNS depressants (barbiturates, opiates)	Decreases SOL, may impair sleep quality
	Brompheniraine	4-6 hr					
	Chlorpheniramine	4-6 hr					
	Hydroxyzine (Atarax)	6-24 hr					

BZD, benzodiazepine; *CNS*, central nervous system; *CR*, controlled release; *ETOH*, ethyl alcohol; *GABA*, γ-aminobutyric acid; *H$_1$*, histamine H$_1$ receptor subtype; *5-HT$_2$, 5-HT$_3$*, 5-hydroxytryptamine (serotonin) receptor subtypes 2, 3; *NE*, norepinephrine; *NSAID*, nonsteroidal anti-inflammatory drug; *REM*, rapid eye movement; *SOL*, sleep onset latency; *SWS*, slow wave sleep (stage N3).
Adapted with permission from Owens JA, Babcock, D, Blumer J, et al. The use of pharmacotherapy in the treatment of pediatric insomnia in primary care: Rational approaches. A Consensus Meeting Summary. *J Clin Sleep Med.* 2005;1:49-59.

by the FDA for the treatment of insomnia in adults include temazepam, estazolam, quazepam, flurazepam, and triazolam. These medications vary mainly in their elimination half-life, presence of active metabolites, and affinity for the benzodiazepine receptor subtype.

Benzodiazepines are lipophilic, highly bound to plasma membranes, and eliminated by hepatic enzymes. Their effects on sleep architecture include increase of sleep spindles and stage N2 sleep, suppression of slow wave sleep (stage N3), mild suppression of rapid eye movement (REM) sleep, and reduction in frequency of nocturnal arousals.

Tolerance, rebound insomnia, next-day sedation, anterograde amnesia, cognitive and psychomotor impairments, and tolerance are known side effects of benzodiazepines. There are no pediatric clinical trials of benzodiazepines for insomnia and therefore no established data on their safety and effectiveness for this clinical indication. All benzodiazepines have abuse potential, and should be used only with great caution, especially in the pediatric population (Table 36-2).

Nonbenzodiazepine Benzodiazepine Receptor Agonists

The nonbenzodiazepine benzodiazepine receptor agonists include zolpidem, zaleplon, and eszopiclone. These medications bind preferentially to the ω1-benzodiazepine receptor of the GABA$_A$ receptor complex. This preferential binding may explain the relative absence of anticonvulsant and myorelaxant effects as well as the preservation of stage N3 sleep (slow wave sleep). These medications are FDA approved for the treatment of insomnia in adults only. Although the FDA approved indication is for short-term insomnia, these medicines are often used long term in adults with chronic, severe insomnia. These three medications differ primarily in their half-lives.

Although there is little published research on the use of these medications in the treatment of insomnia in children or adolescents, there may be a role for their use *off-label* in certain cases of severe incapacitating insomnia.

New warnings have been issued regarding the sedative-hypnotic medications. In March 2007, the FDA requested that all manufacturers of sedative-hypnotic medications change their product labeling to include the risks of severe allergic reactions and complex sleep-related behaviors including sleep-driving and sleep-eating.

Zolpidem. Zolpidem (Ambien) was the first benzodiazepine receptor agonist released in the United States. A non-controlled-release formulation (referred to from here forward as *zolpidem*) was first released. The non-controlled-release formulation is now available as a generic drug. Zolpidem has an onset of action of less than 30 minutes and a half-life of approximately 2.5 hours. The most common side effects experienced by adults in clinical trials included nausea, myalgia, dizziness headache, and somnolence. There have been reports of parasomnias in adults taking zolpidem including sleepwalking and sleep-eating. It is very important that patients are instructed to take this medicine just as they are getting in bed with the intention to fall asleep. In 2009, the first study was published evaluating the effectiveness and safety of zolpidem in children and adolescents (ages 6-17) with insomnia associated with ADHD.[20] At a dose of 0.25 mg/kg (maximum 10 mg), zolpidem failed to reduce

latency to persistent sleep on polysomnography after 4 weeks of treatment.

More recently, a controlled-release formulation of zolpidem has been released (referred to from here forward as *zolpidem CR*). This controlled release formulation was designed as a two-layer tablet, allowing biphasic absorption and a prolonged duration of effect. This design makes zolpidem CR effective for both initial and maintenance (middle-of-the-night) insomnia. It comes in 6.25 mg and 12.5 mg tablet strengths. The most common side effects in adults taking zolpidem CR are headaches, somnolence, and dizziness.

Zaleplon. Zaleplon (Sonata) is FDA approved for the short-term treatment of insomnia in adults. It has a very short half-life of 1 hour, making it particularly effective for initial insomnia. It also has a unique role as an *as-needed* medicine for middle-of-the-night insomnia. Adult data suggest that it can be taken if the patient can stay in bed for at least 4 hours. Typical doses are 5 mg and 10 mg, but adults can take a dose up to 20 mg. It comes in capsule strengths of 5 mg and 10 mg. Common side effects include headache, dizziness, and somnolence.

Eszopiclone. Eszopiclone (Lunesta) is a racemic isomer of zopiclone, a sedative-hypnotic used in Europe for many years. The precise mechanism of action is not known, but it is suspected to work at the benzodiazepine receptor of the GABA$_A$ receptor complex, much like zolpidem and zaleplon. Eszopiclone is FDA approved for the treatment of insomnia in adults, without the disclaimer that it should be used only short term. It comes in 1 mg, 2 mg, and 3 mg tablet strengths. The half-life is 6 hours, which is significantly longer than zolpidem or zaleplon, potentially making eszopiclone an attractive medicine to treat insomnia in children. However, as with zolpidem and zaleplon, there are no significant pediatric studies.

While more data on the use of the nonbenzodiazepine benzodiazepine receptor agonists in children are gathered, a conservative approach is warranted. One should consider referring children who may be candidates for treatment with these medications to a sleep specialist.

Antihistamines

Antihistamines are often recommended or prescribed to treat pediatric insomnia. Of the antihistamines, diphenhydramine hydrochloride, available over the counter, is the most commonly recommended to induce sleep in children. Hydroxyzine hydrochloride is another antihistamine that has often been prescribed for insomnia. Despite clinical trials demonstrating some efficacy with the use of these medicines, they are not ideal. Next-day sedation is often experienced owing to their relatively long half-lives and negative impact on sleep quality. Side effects include constipation, nausea, loss of appetite, and even vomiting or diarrhea. Other anticholinergic side effects such as dry mouth are common and there is a risk of confusion and paradoxical agitation, especially in vulnerable children. It is our recommendation that these medications not be used to treat significant insomnia in children. The only potential role that we see for them in children is as one- or two-night therapy in cases of transient insomnia.

TABLE 36-2

Clinical Properties of Selected Medications Used for Pediatric Insomnia

Drug	Adult Dose Range (mg)	Formulation	Side Effects	Tolerance/ Withdrawal Effects	Safety Profile/ Overdose	Comment(s)
Clonazepam Flurazepam Quazepam Temazepam Estazolam Triazolam	0.5-2 15-30 7.5-30 15-30 1-2 0.125-0.25	Tablets	Residual daytime sedation, rebound insomnia on discontinuation, psychomotor/ cognitive impairment, anterograde amnesia (dose-dependent); impaired respiratory function	Yes, especially with shorter acting BZD; withdrawal effects include seizures	Marked abuse potential	Also used to control partial arousal parasomnias (night terrors, sleep walking), use short half-life BZD for sleep onset; longer-half-life agent for sleep maintenance
Clonidine Guanfacine	0.025-0.3 (maximum daily dose of 0.8 mg); increase by 0.05-mg increments 0.5-2	Tablet, transdermal patch	Dry mouth, bradycardia, hypotension, rebound hypertension on discontinuation		Narrow therapeutic index *Overdose*: bradycardia, decreased consciousness, hypotension	Also used in daytime treatment of ADHD
Zolpidem Zolpidem CR Zaleplon Eszopiclone	5-10 6.25-12.5 5-10 1-3	Pill, sublingual tab, oral spray	Headache, retrograde amnesia, few residual next-day effects, insomnia on discontinuation	May develop tolerance/ adaptations with extended use; may develop rebound	Well tolerated in adults *Overdose*: CNS depression, hypotension	Little clinical experience in children, not found to be effective in children with ADHD
Trazodone	25-50	Tablet	Dizziness, CNS overstimulation, cardiac arrhythmias, hypotension, priapism		*Overdose*: hypotension, cardiac effects	May be used with co-morbid depression
Melatonin	0.3-6	Tablet—various strengths	Largely unknown		Unknown	Used in children with developmental disabilities, mental retardation, autism, pervasive development disorders, neurologic impairment, blindness, jet lag
Mirtazapine	7.5-15	Oral tablet and disintegrating	Increased appetite, weight gain, constipation, dry mouth		Mild clinical symptoms with tachycardia, disorientation, drowsiness	FDA indication for major depressive disorder only, used at low doses for somnolence effect
Diphenhydramine Brompheniramine Chlorpheniramine Hydroxyzine	25-50 (should not exceed total daily dose of 300 mg) 4 4 25-100 (*children*: 0.6 mg/kg)	Tablet, capsule, syrup, injectable	Daytime drowsiness, gastrointestinal (appetite loss, nausea/vomiting, constipation, dry mouth), paradoxical excitation		*Overdose*: hallucination, seizures, excessive stimulation	Weak soporifics; high level of parental/ practitioner acceptance

ADHD, attention deficit hyperactivity disorder; *BZD*, benzodiazepine; *CNS*, central nervous system; *FDA*, U.S. Food and Drug Administration.
Adapted with permission from Owens JA, Babcock, D, Blumer J, et al. The use of pharmacotherapy in the treatment of pediatric insomnia in primary care: Rational approaches. A Consensus Meeting Summary. *J Clin Sleep Med.* 2005;1:49-59.

Other Medications with Sedative-Hypnotic Properties

Chloral Hydrate

Chloral hydrate was one of the first synthetic agents used as a hypnotic. Although it is more commonly used as a preoperative anxiolytic/sedative, it has been prescribed to children with severe, persistent insomnia. Chloral hydrate has a poor safety profile and should not be used to treat insomnia in children. It has a long half-life, is habit-forming, and is associated with tolerance.

Antidepressants

Research evidence supporting the use of sedating antidepressants in the treatment of pediatric insomnia is lacking. Although an argument can be made for treating insomnia associated with clinical depression with a sedating antidepressant, it may not be the best choice (see Chapter 42). It may be more safe and efficacious to treat the depression with a SSRI and adding a sedating medication such as melatonin, a benzodiazepine, or a nonbenzodiazepine benzodiazepine receptor agonist in the short term as the depression resolves. (see Chapter 42).

Trazodone. According to data in 2002, trazodone, a triazolopyridine antidepressant, is the second most commonly prescribed agent for the treatment of insomnia in adults.[21] Trazodone is FDA approved only for the treatment of depression. Its popularity for managing insomnia may be related to its perceived lack of risk and its availability as an unscheduled generic agent with lack of restriction on prescription duration. Of community-based pediatricians who had prescribed at least one medication for sleep in the previous 6 months, 16% prescribed an antidepressant (SSRI, tricyclic antidepressant, or trazodone).[1]

In 2005 a review of the literature[22] assessed the efficacy and side effects of trazodone when prescribed for insomnia. Of the 18 studies reviewed from 1980 to 2003, most studies were small, conducted in populations of depressed patients, with design issues lack of objective efficacy measures. Evidence for the efficacy of trazodone in treating insomnia was found to be limited.

Side effects associated with trazodone are not insignificant. The most common adverse events ($\geq 10\%$) seen at doses of 75 to 500 mg per day include drowsiness, dizziness, dry mouth, nausea/vomiting, constipation, headache, hypotension, and blurred vision.[23] However, it is unclear what trazodone's adverse effect profile is at the lower doses typically used to treat insomnia, since so few studies have been conducted on the use of trazodone in nondepressed insomnia populations. There is also some evidence of tolerance related to use of trazodone, although this has not been systematically evaluated.

Of note, for use in the adolescent male population, priapism is a potential side effect of trazodone, with the incidence reported to be between 1 in 1000 and 1 in 10,000.[24] The mechanism is theorized to be due to α-adrenergic blocking properties of the drug. The majority of the cases have occurred at doses of 50 to 150 mg per day, with onset usually within the first 28 days of treatment.[25] Because of the difficulties treating medication-associated priapism, and the need for possible surgical intervention, it has been our practice to avoid prescribing trazodone to male adolescents, and to encourage discontinuation if a patient, seen in consultation, already has been prescribed trazodone.

Mirtazapine. Mirtazapine is a tetracyclic piperazino-azepine antidepressant medication sometimes used in adults to treat co-morbid symptoms of insomnia. It, like other antidepressants, carries the warning of increased risk of suicidal thinking and behavior (suicidality) in children and adolescents, and there is even less experience using this medication in children than there is with many of the other antidepressants; thus, there is little reason to consider its use in pediatric insomnia.

Antipsychotic Medications

There is no evidence supporting the use of antipsychotics in the treatment of pediatric insomnia, unless the insomnia is associated with a psychotic disorder. The potential risks far outweigh the benefits when considering use of an antipsychotic to treat primary insomnia or insomnia not associated with psychosis. This class of agents will not be discussed further here.

Alpha Agonists

According to recent surveys of pediatricians and child psychiatrists,[1,2] α_2-adrenergic agonists are the class of drugs most *prescribed* for pediatric insomnia despite limited research data supporting their use and problematic safety profiles. Two case series suggest the efficacy of clonidine in treating insomnia associated with neurodevelopmental disorders such as ADHD.[26,27] The mean dosage at bedtime in the case series of children with ADHD was approximately 0.15 mg.[26] An open-label, retrospective study of clonidine in the treatment of insomnia in 19 children with autism spectrum disorder demonstrated efficacy in reducing sleep initiation latency and night awakenings.[28] There are no placebo-controlled studies using α_2-adrenergic agonists to treat pediatric insomnia.

Sodium Oxybate

Sodium oxybate (Xyrem), also known as gamma-hydroxybutyrate (GHB), is an FDA-approved drug for the treatment of narcolepsy in adults. It is available only through a centralized pharmacy as a schedule III controlled substance. The drug is tightly controlled owing to a history of diversion and abuse. Sodium oxybate activates the $GABA_B$ receptors and suppresses dopaminergic neuronal activity, leading to an increase in slow wave sleep and a decrease in awakenings at night. Improved sleep efficiency is the end result. Although not FDA approved for children, it has been reported to be effective in treating severe childhood narcolepsy-cataplexy.[29] Sodium oxybate should be used only in children and adolescents with documented narcolepsy with cataplexy, or narcolepsy with significant excessive daytime sleepiness, and should probably be prescribed to children only by sleep specialists experienced in treating narcolepsy. There is no indication for its use in otherwise treating childhood insomnia.

RESEARCH DIRECTIONS

As is clear from this review, there is a need for research in the area of pharmacologic management of pediatric sleep disorders. In particular, clinical trials of hypnotics in children and adolescents are needed. A recent conference consensus statement called for initial concentration to be on neuropsychiatric

TABLE 36-3

Pharmacology and Clinical Properties of Selected Herbal Preparations Used for Pediatric Insomnia

Common Name	Scientific Name	Mechanism of Action	Sleep Architecture Effect(s)	Usual Dose	Comment(s)
Valerian	*Valeriana officinalis*	Binds BZD receptors	Decreases SOL, improves sleep continuity; ?increases SWS	2-3 g in tea every day to tid; extract equivalent to 2-3 g	Reported toxicity rare; effects may take several weeks
German chamomile	*Matricaria recutita*	Binds BZD receptors	?Decreases SOL	1-3 g in tea tid	Weak hypertensive effect; may cause contact allergies
Kava	*Piper methysticum*	CNS depressant	Improves sleep quality	60-120 mg every day	May have anxiolytic effects; does not appear to potentiate alcohol, BZD effects
Lavender	*Lavandula angustifolia*	CNS depressant	Improves sleep quality, decreases restless sleep	Essential oil, inhalation	May potentiate effects of alcohol

BZD, benzodiazepine; *CNS*, central nervous system; *SOL*, sleep onset latency; *SWS*, slow wave sleep.
Adapted with permission from Owens JA, Babcock, D, Blumer J, et al. The use of pharmacotherapy in the treatment of pediatric insomnia in primary care: Rational approaches. A Consensus Meeting Summary. *J Clin Sleep Med.* 2005;1:49-59.

disorders with the highest priority set on autism spectrum disorders followed by attention deficit hyperactivity disorder, mood disorders, and anxiety disorders.[30] There also was a call to study medical disorders with co-morbid insomnia as well as primary sleep disorders.

Combined behavioral and pharmacologic treatments should be studied against behavioral treatment alone and pharmacologic treatment alone. Combined treatment may be the most efficacious. Appropriate doses of medications need to be determined for children and adolescents, potentially based on weight for the younger children. Different formulations such as liquid suspensions and chewable tablets need to be developed, making medications easier to use, especially in children with special needs. Appropriate use (if any) of herbal preparations should be determined as well, and Table 36-3 lists properties of four of them that have been used in the treatment of insomnia.

Future research should use objective measures of sleep including polysomnography (PSG) and actigraphy. PSG is an important tool that allows accurate measurement of sleep architecture at baseline and clinical endpoints. Actigraphy is less expensive and less invasive than PSG and can be used to determine sleep patterns that may change with treatment.

REFERENCES

1. Owens J, Rosen CL, Mindell JA. Medication use in the treatment of pediatric insomnia: Results of a survey of community-based pediatricians. *Pediatrics.* 2003;111(5):E628-E635.
2. Owens JA, Rosen CL, Mindell JA, Kirchner HL. Use of pharmacotherapy for insomnia in child psychiatry practice: A national survey. *Sleep Med.* 2010;11:692-700.
3. Vitiello B, Heiligenstein JH, Riddle MA, et al. The interface between publicly funded and industry funded research in pediatric psychopharmacology: Opportunities for integration and collaboration. *Biol Psychiatry.* 2004;56:3-9.
4. Food and Drug Administration. Specific requirements on content and format of labeling for human prescription drugs: Revision of pediatric use subsection in the labeling. *Fed Reg.* 1994;59:64240-64250.
5. Food and Drug Administration. Approved moieties to which FDA has granted pediatric exclusivity for pediatric studies under section 505A of the Federal Food. *Drug and Cosmetic Act.* 2003. Available at http://www.fda.gov/cder/pediatric/exgrant.htm.

6. Owens JA, Babcock D, Blumer J, Chervin R, Ferber R, et al. The use of pharmacotherapy in the treatment of pediatric insomnia in primary care: Rational approaches. A consensus meeting summary. *J Clin Sleep Med.* 2005;1(1):49-59.
7. Stephenson T. How children's responses to drugs differ from adults. *Br J Clin Pharmacol.* 2005;59(6):670-673.
8. Smits MG, Nagtegaal EE, van der Heijden J, Coenen AML, Kerkhof GA. Melatonin for chronic sleep onset insomnia in children: A randomized placebo-controlled trial. *J Child Neurol.* 2001;16:86-92.
9. Smits MG, van Stel HF, van der Heijden K, Meijer AM, Coenen AM, Kerkhof GA. Melatonin improves health status and sleep in children with idiopathic chronic sleep-onset insomnia: A randomized placebo-controlled trial. *J Am Acad Child Adolesc Psychiatry.* 2003;42:1286-1293.
10. Weiss MD, Wasdell MB, Bomben MM, Rea KJ, Freeman RD. Sleep hygiene and melatonin treatment for children and adolescents with ADHD and initial insomnia. *J Am Acad Child Adolesc Psychiatry.* 2006;45:512-519.
11. Clark A. Incidences of new prescribing by British child and adolescent psychiatrists: A prospective study over 12 months. *J Psychopharmacol.* 2004;18(1):115-120.
12. Jan JE, Freeman RD. Melatonin therapy for circadian rhythm sleep disorders in children with multiple disabilities: What have we learned in the last decade? *Dev Med Child Neurol.* 2004;46:776-782.
13. Garstang J, Wallis M. Randomized controlled trial of melatonin for children with autistic spectrum disorders and sleep problems. *Child Care Health Dev.* 2006;32(5):585-589.
14. Andersen IM, Kaczmarska J, McGrew SG, Malow BA. Melatonin for insomnia in children with autism spectrum disorders. *J Child Neurol.* 2008;23(5):482-485.
15. Braam W, Didden R, Maas AP, Korzilius H, Smits MG, Curfs LM. Melatonin decreases daytime challenging behaviour in persons with intellectual disability and chronic insomnia. *J Intellect Disabil Res.* 2010;54(1):52-59.
16. Szeinberg A, Borodkin K, Dagan Y. Melatonin treatment in adolescents with delayed sleep phase syndrome. *Clin Pediatr.* 2006;45:809-818.
17. Jan JE, Wasdell MB, Reiter RJ, Weiss MD, Johnson KP, et al. Melatonin therapy of pediatric sleep disorders: Recent advances, why it works, who are the candidates and how to treat. *Curr Pediatr Rev.* 2007;3:214-224.
18. Lewy AJ, Emens JS, Lefler BJ, Yuhas K, Jackman AR. Melatonin entrains free-running blind people according to a physiological dose-response curve. *Chronobiol Int.* 2005;22(6):1093-1106.
19. Sheldon SH. Proconvulsant effects of oral melatonin in neurologically disabled children. *Lancet.* 1998;351:1254.
20. Blumer JL, Findling RL, Shih WF, Soubrane C, Reed MD. Controlled clinical trial of zolpidem for the treatment of insomnia associated with attention-deficit/hyperactivity disorder in children 6 to 17 years of age. *Pediatrics.* 2009;123(5):E770-E776.
21. IMS Health National Prescription Audit Plus, 2002.
22. Mendelson W. A review of the evidence for the efficacy and safety of trazodone in insomnia. *J Clin Psychiatry.* 2005;66(4):469-476.

23. Maxmen JS. Antidepressants. In: Maxmen JS, Ward NC, eds. *Psychotropic Drugs: Fast Facts.* New York: WW Norton; 1991:57-97.

24. Haria M, Fitton A, McTavish D. Trazodone: A review of its pharmacology, therapeutic use in depression and therapeutic potential in other disorders. *Drugs Aging.* 1994;4:331-335.

25. Warner MD, Peabody CA, Whiteford HA, et al. Trazodone and priapism. *J Clin Psychiatry.* 1987;48:244-245.

26. Prince JB, Wilens TE, Biederman J, Spencer TJ, Wozniak JR. Clonidine for sleep disturbances associated with attention-deficit hyperactivity disorder: A systematic chart review of 62 cases. *J Am Acad Child Adolesc Psychiatry.* 1996;35:599-605.

27. Ingrassia A, Turk J. The use of clonidine for severe and intractable sleep problems in children with neurodevelopmental disorders: A case series. *Eur Child Adolesc Psychiatry.* 2005;14(1):34-40.

28. Ming X, Gordon E, Kang N, Wagner GC. Use of clonidine in children with autism spectrum disorders. *Brain Dev.* 2008;30(7):454-460.

29. Murali H, Kotagal S. Off-label treatment of severe childhood narcolepsy-cataplexy with sodium oxybate. *Sleep.* 2006;29:1025-1029.

30. Mindell JA, Emslie G, Blumer J, Genel M, Glaze D, et al. Pharmacologic management of insomnia in children and adolescents: Consensus statement. *Pediatrics.* 2006;117(6):E1223-E1232.

ADDITIONAL READING

Kuhn BR, Elliott AJ. Treatment efficacy in behavioral pediatric sleep medicine. *J Psychosom Res.* 2003;54(6):587-597.

Mindell JA. Empirically supported treatments in pediatric psychology: Bedtime refusal and night wakings in young children. *J Pediatr Psychol.* 1999;24:465-481.

Mindell JA, Kuhn B, Lewin DS, Meltzer LJ, Sadeh A. Behavioral treatment of bedtime problems and night wakings in infants and young children. *Sleep.* 2006;29:1263-1276.

Miyazaki S, Uchida S, Mukai J, Nishihara K. Clonidine effects on all-night human sleep: Opposite action of low- and medium-dose clonidine on human NREM-REM sleep proportion. *Psychiatry Clin Neurosci.* 2004;58:138-144.

Wilens TE, Biederman J, Spencer T. Clonidine for sleep disturbances associated with attention-deficit hyperactivity disorder. *J Am Acad Child Adolesc Psychiatry.* 1994;33:424-426.

Circadian Rhythm Disorders in Children

Chapter 37

GERALD ROSEN

BACKGROUND

Circadian rhythms are woven into the fabric of our lives and together with the homeostatic drive determine how quickly we fall asleep at night, the quality and duration of our sleep, the ease with which we awaken in the morning, and our degree of daytime alertness. The circadian rhythm is a clock-like, endogenously generated signal that is almost entirely independent of sleep. Effectively all physiologic systems show circadian effects. For alertness and sleepiness the effects are (1) an increasing degree of alertness across the day from the time of spontaneous awakening until reaching a maximum during the "wake maintenance zone" about 1 hour before the habitual time of sleep onset; and (2) an increasing propensity to sleep over the course of the night until reaching a maximum during the hour or two before the time of spontaneous waking.[1-3]

The circadian rhythm provides an alerting counterweight to the homeostatic drive, which—under usual circumstances—is entirely sleep/wake dependent, building during wakefulness and dissipated only by sleep.[4] (This drive can be modified by illness or medication.) When the homeostatic and circadian processes are properly aligned and synchronized in a child, these two opposing forces create a delicate balance that results in a stable 24-hour sleep/wake rhythm leading to a rapid transition to sleep at bedtime, high sleep efficiency, an adequate sleep duration, spontaneous awakening in the morning, a high level of daytime alertness, and age-appropriate nap times. The opponent process model of sleep regulation,[5] shown in Figure 37-1, describes the relationship between the homeostatic and circadian processes. When the circadian and homeostatic systems are misaligned or desynchronized, the result is a circadian rhythm disorder: a delayed or advanced sleep phase as illustrated in Figure 37-2, a nonentrained rhythm, or an irregular sleep/wake rhythm. Circadian rhythm disorders[6] typically result in some degree of sleep insufficiency; they may also lead to irritability, sleep onset insomnia, nighttime awakenings, difficulty waking in the morning at the desired time, and excessive daytime sleepiness (EDS).

Circadian rhythms are well established by 6 months of age.[7] Clear sleep phase preferences of morningness (larks) or eveningness (owls) are often apparent even in toddlers and appear to have a genetic basis. In most children, however, these preferences are not striking. These are stable behavioral traits that persist throughout childhood and into adolescence. During adolescence, regardless of what the preadolescent circadian phase preference was, the intrinsic free-running circadian period (almost always longer than 24 hours) lengthens further, and the sleep phase will become delayed, resulting in a later preferred sleep onset time and later wake time.[8] Children who were larks as toddlers are likely to remain larks as they age. As adolescents, they will likely shift to a later preferred sleep onset time, but will remain larks relative to their peers. Similarly, children who were owls as toddlers are likely to remain owls as they grow. As adolescents, these children often develop a delayed sleep phase because their tendency toward a late circadian sleep phase becomes more pronounced not only because of the biologic changes that take place in adolescence but also because of behavioral and social realities that occur: increased opportunities for adolescents to engage in late night activities, decreased parental controls over adolescents' bedtime and waking schedules, and adolescents' increasing ability and choice to sleep in on the weekends if given the opportunity, all of which tends to phase shift their sleep time to a later clock time.

The homeostatic drive to sleep is a powerful force in children, especially in young children. However, the rate of rise of the homeostatic pressure during daytime wakefulness slows during adolescence.[9] This results in teens being less sleepy at the end of their day, contributing to increased difficulty at sleep onset and making a delayed sleep phase syndrome (DSPS) a very common problem in adolescents.

Understanding how much sleep a child needs to be well rested is an important topic in pediatric sleep medicine, separate, though related to, the circadian and homeostatic factors. The circadian and homeostatic processes follow a predictable developmental trajectory, which determines the timing and duration of nighttime sleep and daytime naps. As children age, their total sleep requirement decreases. By age 5 most children are no longer taking regular naps. The trend of total sleep duration described in a population-based epidemiologic study of normal Swiss children ages 1 to 16 in the Zurich Longitudinal Study is summarized in Figure 37-3.[10] This study describes a wide range in total sleep times in normal children at each age. For example, as illustrated in Figure 37-3, for a 5-year-old child at the 50th percentile for sleep requirement, the mean total sleep time is about 11¼ hours, but at the 2nd percentile it is only 9½ hours, and at the 98th percentile it is 13 hours. So, when the parent of a 5-year-old child asks, "How much sleep does my 5-year-old need?" the answer should be: "It depends, probably between 9½ and 11¼ hours." To get a better estimate of how much sleep this particular child needs to be well rested it is necessary to gather more information. The best estimate of a child's sleep need is based on the child's historical sleep duration when given the opportunity to sleep *ad lib*, in an environment that was conducive to sleep and free from scheduling constraints. In most children, scheduling constraints are more common as the children get older and are involved in more activities, so their sleep duration at a younger age is often a better indication of their true sleep need than their current sleep duration. However, many American children have never been allowed to sleep *ad lib*, so it may be difficult to deduce their sleep need. Sleep insufficiency, it should be remembered, is defined by comparing the amount of sleep a child gets relative to their sleep need, not how much sleep they get relative to an age-based norm. As children mature, their sleep duration decreases but does tend to remain on the same percentile relative to their age-matched peers over time. This means that children who were long (or short) sleepers as infants tend to remain long (or short) sleepers as preschoolers and adolescents. So, one way to estimate a child's current sleep need is to determine the sleep duration at a younger age based on the parents' history, identify what percentile that corresponds to from Figure 37-3, and check the value at the child's current age on that same percentile.

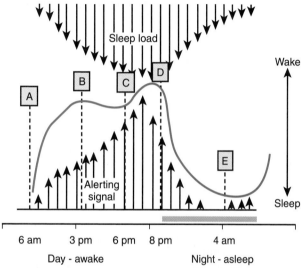

Figure 37-1 Opponent-process model of sleep regulation. The curve follows the relationship between the homeostatic and circadian processes. Point A is spontaneous wake time at 6 AM, and from this point rising circadian alertness (*alerting signal*) is unopposed by homeostatic load (*sleep load*). Point B is afternoon siesta time (*sleep load* has grown and *alerting signal* is still not very strong); point C is the beginning of the wake maintenance zone (*alerting signal* is now very strong); and point D is the habitual sleep onset time when the circadian *alerting signal* dramatically decreases. Point E is at 4 AM, the time of body temperature minimum, about 2 hours before spontaneous wake time at 6 AM (when *sleep load* has been fully dissipated). The dark underscore bar represents sleep time. (Modified from Beersma DGM, Gordijn MCM. Circadian control of the sleep-wake cycle. *Physiol Behav.* 2007;90(2-3):190-195.)

PHASE DELAY/PHASE ADVANCE

Figure 37-2 is a schematic representation of circadian misalignments leading to a delayed sleep phase and an advanced sleep phase. If a child has a 10-hour sleep need, and the child's parents would like him to sleep from 8 PM to 6 AM, and the child falls asleep easily in bed at 8 PM in a quiet, dark, comfortable, safe environment and spontaneously awakens at 6 AM, the sleep is considered to be at a *normal* sleep phase. The sleep phase would be considered *delayed* if the child were put to bed at 8 PM, but was unable to fall asleep until 11 PM even if the environment was conducive for sleep, and would spontaneously awaken at 9 AM if given the opportunity to sleep in. The sleep phase would be considered *advanced* if the child would prefer to fall asleep at 5 PM if given the opportunity and would spontaneously awaken at 3 AM. In all three scenarios, the child would sleep for 10 hours if allowed to sleep on his preferred sleep schedule. Circadian rhythm disorders are always defined as a misalignment between the desired sleep time and the circadian determined time of greatest sleep propensity. It is only if the schedule of one's sleep conflicts with the schedule of one's life that a circadian sleep disorder exists. So, for example, an adolescent with a 9-hour sleep need, whose preferred bedtime is 2 AM and preferred wake time is 11 AM, does not have a circadian rhythm disorder if it is summer and he does not need to awaken for any scheduled activities. This sleep schedule would be typical of a delayed sleep phase if he is expected to fall asleep at 9 PM and to awaken at 6 AM to catch the school bus.

As a consequence of the circadian misalignment in children with delayed sleep phase, the following occurs:
1. Bedtime is scheduled during the child's "wake maintenance zone," making sleep onset very difficult unless there is a very large homeostatic sleep drive.
2. Arousal in the morning is attempted while the child is in the midst of his normal nighttime sleep interval, making awakening very difficult and, if successful, occurs before the homeostatic sleep debt has been fully dissipated.

As a consequence of the circadian misalignment in children with advanced sleep phase the following occurs:
1. In the evening, prior to the planned bedtime, the child is sleep deprived, often irritable, and may fall asleep if placed in a low stimulation setting.
2. Spontaneous awakening occurs in the early morning, hours before the parents want the child to awaken and usually before the entire homeostatic sleep need has been dissipated.

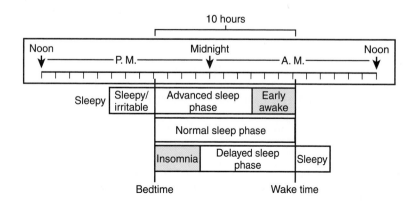

Figure 37-2 Advanced sleep phase and delayed sleep phase are defined as circadian misalignment. The "normal" desired sleep phase is between 8 PM and 6 AM, providing 10 hours available for sleep; the sleep phase is *advanced* if the child wishes to go to bed at 5 PM and is spontaneously awakening at 3 AM; the sleep phase is *delayed* if the child is unable to fall asleep until 11 PM and would spontaneously awaken at 9 AM, if allowed.

Both of these scenarios lead to sleep insufficiency and as a result are often associated with daytime sleepiness, irritability, mood lability, and inattentiveness. Because parents are usually the ones to schedule their (nonadolescent) children's bedtimes and waking, if the schedule chosen is inappropriate and inconsistent, a circadian rhythm disorder may result.

ISSUES IMPORTANT IN THE EVALUATION AND TREATMENT OF CIRCADIAN RHYTHM DISORDERS

Circadian rhythm disorders in children all are easy to recognize and can be successfully treated if one is attentive to the following issues:

1. There are developmental changes that occur normally in sleep physiology, autonomy, and anxiety from infancy through adolescence.
2. Stimulation and light from electronics such as television, computers, video games, and cell phones may have important effects on the ability to fall asleep and the timing of sleep.
3. Anxiety, depression, and a heightened level of arousal may have important effects on sleep.
4. Parents and children need good information to avoid and to treat circadian rhythm disorders.
5. Bedtime is commonly where behavioral problems present during the day are played out, with problem sleep the result. Parents without effective behavior management strategies for dealing with daytime misbehavior are rarely able to develop an effective behavior management strategies on their own to deal with related problem sleep behaviors.
6. A delayed sleep phase (although physiologic in nature) may be behaviorally induced and behaviorally corrected.
7. Motivation of all affected parties is necessary for change to occur.

Evaluation of Sleep Problems in Children

Fundamental to any treatment strategy for sleep disorders is a full understanding of all of the factors that may be contributing to and sustaining the sleep problem in the first place.

There are four main presentations of problems with sleep and alertness (relevant to this discussion) that children can experience:[11]

1. Inability to fall asleep at the desired bedtime
2. Nighttime awakening
3. Inability to awaken in the morning at the desired wake time
4. Excessive daytime sleepiness

Though any of these sleep problems may be attributable to a circadian rhythm disorder, there are also other sleep disorders that will lead to the same complaints. Often the presenting sleep problem is the result of the confluence of several very different causes that are all aligned in such a way as to both cause and sustain the sleep complaint. Failure to recognize and treat the other contributing factors, or co-morbidities, in addition to the circadian rhythm disorder, will affect the success of treatment.

Psychosocial and Developmental Issues Affecting Children's Sleep

Though sleep is a physiologic process, it occurs in a behavioral/psychological context. Consequently psychosocial issues, particularly those affecting arousal, attachment, and anxiety, are important. In typically developing children, attachment to primary caregivers occurs in the first year of life and is the core task of children and parents.[12] However, in special settings such as adoption, attachment may continue to be an important issue until much later. Separation anxiety is a very functional emotional response that children appropriately experience when separated from a caregiver. It typically becomes apparent around 9 months of age, though it may begin as early as 5 months; it peaks between 18 months and 2 years of age and lessens thereafter. Children with heightened separation anxiety or sensory integration disorder often experience difficulties at bedtime, at the transition between wake and sleep, and this can lead to consistent delays in sleep onset, which, in children predisposed to a later rise time, can lead to a shift in their entire sleep schedule to a later clock time and the development of a delayed sleep phase. Autonomy and limit setting are important issues for toddlers and adolescents, and problems in these areas are frequently manifested at bedtime.

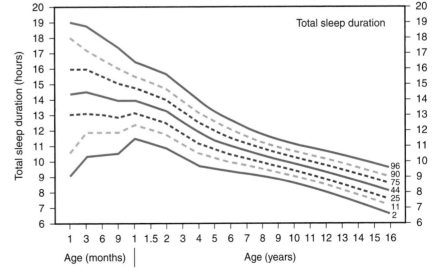

Figure 37-3 The trend of total sleep duration described in a population-based epidemiologic study of normal Swiss children ages 1 to 16 in the Zurich Longitudinal Study. Percentiles of total and nighttime sleep duration (time in bed) per 24 hours in 493 healthy children studied longitudinally from age 1 month to 16 years. (Redrawn from Iglowstein I, Jenni O, Molinari L, et al. Sleep duration from infancy to adolescence: Reference values and generational trends. *Pediatrics.* 2003;111:302-307.)

Understanding these issues and addressing them within the context of whatever intervention is recommended is important if the intervention is to be successful.

Clinical Evaluation of Sleep Problems in Children

The goals of the initial clinical visit, when evaluating a child for a sleep problem, are to establish the correct diagnosis and identify all of the contributing factors, develop a therapeutic relationship with the child and family, educate the child and family regarding the problem, and to begin a plan. All of these elements are woven together into the clinical interview.

Clinical evaluation of children for a suspected circadian disorder requires several kinds of information:

1. Complete medical, neurologic, and sleep history (Box 37-1)
2. Current sleep log (Fig. 37-4) prospectively filled out

For older children, a detailed history of sleep duration at a younger age, when the parents likely had more control over the child's sleep schedule and there were likely fewer scheduling constraints placed on the child, will help identify children who are either long or short sleepers. This is important because long sleepers and short sleepers may have sleep patterns that mimic some elements of a circadian rhythm disorders.

The best way to collect the current sleep history is by having the child describe in detail the sequence of a typical school day

---

BOX 37-1 *Essential Elements of Sleep History in Evaluating Suspected Circadian Rhythm Disorders in Children*

- Current sleep schedule for weekend/weekday/recent vacation (when the child was allowed to sleep *ad libitum*)
- Past sleep schedule (sleep onset times and spontaneous wake times) as a toddler, preschooler, and school-aged child, especially at times when no scheduling constraints were placed on the child
- Caffeine/energy drink consumption: time of day, quantity
- Drug use, past and present: prescription (stimulants), over-the-counter, recreational drugs, alcohol, marijuana, nicotine
- Previous use of melatonin or sedative-hypnotics and their effectiveness. For melatonin: dose and timing; strictness of control of light exposure and sleep schedule
- School information
  - Academic demands and performance
  - Scheduled start time
  - Peer and teacher relations
  - Number of days late (tardy) per week, present and past; typical number of minutes late
  - Number of days absent per week, present and past; time of awakening on days of school absence; consequences (if any) of missing school for child
  - History of truancy proceedings at school
  - Possibility that the inability to awaken in the morning is a symptom of school avoidance behavior, to be addressed before initiation of treatment for the delayed sleep phase syndrome
- Daytime sleepiness assessment
  - Questionnaires: Pediatric Epworth Sleepiness Scale,[23] Pediatric Daytime Sleepiness Scale (PDSS),[24] Cleveland Adolescent Sleepiness Questionnaire (CASQ),[25] Pediatric Sleep Questionnaire (PSQ)[26]
  - Occurrences of daytime sleep:
    On the way to and from school?
    During quiet activities?
    While watching television or videos?
    During social activities?
    While traveling in a vehicle?
  - Scheduled naps:
    Frequency, timing, and duration
    Age at which regular naps were discontinued
    Age at which naps were restarted (if applicable)
- Electronics use: television, computer, video games, cell phones; time and duration of use, especially in the evening
- Bedroom environment
  - Amount of light in the bedroom (natural, artificial); use of shades
  - Location of bedroom in the home

- At sleep onset
  - Presence of restless legs, sleep paralysis, hypnagogic hallucinations, fears
  - Customary or required presence of another family member at bedtime and selection of that person by parent or by child
  - Sleep onset latency: average length; number of days per week with latencies of:
    < 30 minutes
    > 30 minutes
    30-60minutes
    > 60 minutes
    > 90 minutes
- Arousals during sleep: description, causes, frequency, duration
- Other sleep problems: snoring, sleep apnea, frequent leg movements, enuresis, parasomnias (night terrors, sleepwalking)
- At morning waking
  - Difficulty awakening, morning headaches
  - Manner of awakening: spontaneous, alarm, parents
  - Consequences to the child (if any) if he or she cannot be awakened or refuses to respond to arousal efforts
- Underlying neuropsychiatric conditions: autism, attention deficit disorder, school refusal, depression, anxiety, bipolar disorder
- Medical review of systems
  - Hospitalizations
  - Allergies
  - Eyes: visual impairment
  - Ears, nose, throat: ear infections, enlarged tonsils and adenoids, streptococcal infections, sinusitis, chronic mouth breathing, difficulty swallowing, aspiration/choking on food
  - Cardiopulmonary: asthma, pneumonia, heart disease, heart disease
  - Gastroenterologic: reflux, vomiting, abdominal pain, constipation, diarrhea
  - Neurologic: headaches, seizures, hypotonia, hypertonia, cataplexy, developmental/cognitive/behavioral problems, pain; school-related: grade, academic performance, behavior
  - Endocrine: hormone deficiencies, replacement therapy
- Level of motivation of parents and child to change the sleep-wake schedule
- Previous treatments attempted and results
- Significant family stressors (which may interfere with adherence to recommendations)
- Number of hours per week child works at a paid job
- Family history of circadian rhythm or other sleep disorder symptoms in parent, grandparent, or another relative

and a typical weekend day, with particular attention to timing. After the child has been given the opportunity to describe the sleep schedule, ask the parent for their perspective. Giving the child (if old enough) the first opportunity to provide the sleep history is important because it sends the message to parent and child that the child's opinion is important. Often one has to gently prevent the parent from interrupting the child. Children as young as 5 years can give a very accurate sleep history and generally do not edit the history as thoroughly as their parents might.

The clinical history and sleep log together generally provide the information necessary to establish the diagnosis and to identify those factors that might have contributed to and sustain the circadian rhythm disorder. It should also identify co-morbidities and other factors that may prevent the parents and child from following through on the recommendations. Actigraphy can provide an objective measure of sleep/wake schedule if the sleep log is not considered to be reliable. Actigraphy (where information from a digital motion sensor that a child wears for several weeks can be downloaded to give a good estimate of actual sleep times) is particularly helpful in the evaluation of adolescents with sleep state misperception who may not be able to provide accurate sleep logs.

Establishing the diagnosis of a circadian rhythm disorder is generally straightforward; designing a successful treatment intervention strategy is the step that takes the time and clinical skills.

TREATMENT FOR CIRCADIAN RHYTHM DISORDERS

Several tools are available and effective for treatment of circadian rhythm disorders in children:
1. Education
2. Light exposure and restriction
3. Sleep/wake scheduling
4. Sleep deprivation leading to an increased homeostatic drive
5. Behavioral management techniques
6. Melatonin

The key to successful treatment of circadian rhythm disorders involves using these tools correctly. Treatment of circadian rhythm disorders always begins by educating a child (adolescent) and parent regarding the physiology of the circadian timing system. Because the predisposition toward morningness or eveningness is often a familial trait, it is common that one or both parents experienced similar problems as a child or adolescent. The core elements of the education regarding circadian rhythm disorders includes the following:
1. The difficulties with sleep arise because of the misalignment of the schedule imposed on an individual, such as school start times, with the child's natural sleep/wake rhythm. There is no good or bad sleep/wake schedule if the sleep schedule fits and supports the demands of one's life, is appropriately regular, and provides for an adequate duration of sleep.

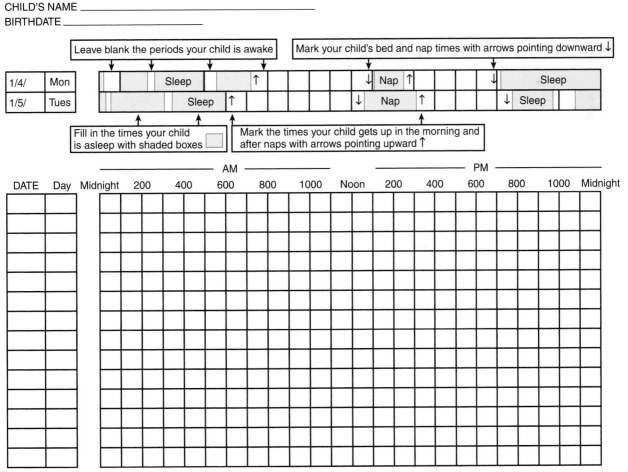

Figure 37-4 **Sleep log.** Parents can use this chart to track all sleeping and waking periods of the child.

2. These rhythms are movable but they have a preferred setting and, if left alone, will usually settle into their preferred setting.

3. Light exposure through open eyes at the beginning and end of the sleep period is the most powerful influence on the establishment of sleep/wake rhythms and can help to normalize the circadian rhythms (if the light exposure is correctly timed) or to undermine treatment (when the light is incorrectly timed).

4. Melatonin can be helpful, and may be useful in resetting these rhythms, but melatonin will be ineffective unless there is adequate control of light exposure.

5. The homeostatic drive is a powerful tool for adjusting the timing of sleep onset but can only be harnessed by sleep scheduling and sleep restriction.

There are no pharmacologic agents that have been approved for the treatment of insomnia in children. In the author's experience, sedative hypnotic agents are rarely effective for the treatment of insomnia that is associated with a delayed sleep phase. Light is the most potent force for the realignment of the circadian sleep/wake rhythm. However light can phase advance, phase delay, or have no effect on the circadian sleep/wake rhythm depending on when it occurs during the circadian sleep cycle.[13] The relationship between the light and the effect on the circadian sleep/wake rhythm is described by the phase response curve for light (see Chapter 28). Light will phase delay the circadian sleep onset time if the exposure occurs near but prior to the core body temperature minimum; it will phase advance the circadian sleep onset time if the exposure is near but after the core body temperature minimum; and it will have very little effect on the circadian rhythm if the exposure is far from the core body temperature minimum, such as during the middle of the physiologic day.[14,15] In a research setting, circadian rhythms, core body temperature, and other circadian phase markers can be precisely measured. However, in a clinical setting one usually must estimate when the tipping point is likely to be between phase advance and phase delay portions of the phase response curve. If the sleep/wake schedule is regular, the core body temperature minimum usually occurs about 2 hours before the circadian wake-up time. When using this value, it is important to use the circadian (which is probably close to the spontaneous) wake time, not the scheduled wake time.

The phase response curve for exogenously administered melatonin is similar to but opposite in direction to the phase response curve of light. So, light in the morning has the same effect as melatonin in the evening, and light in the evening has the same effect as melatonin in the morning.[14,15]

Delayed Sleep Phase Syndrome

Treatment of a delayed sleep phase syndrome is described in the following lists. Studies in children are few. Where evidence is available to support these recommendations it is referenced, but otherwise the recommendations are based on the author's clinical experience:

1. Establish the correct diagnosis.
2. Assess the child's family's motivation for change.
3. Recognize co-morbidities and those factors that have led to, and are likely to sustain, the problem sleep behavior and address them.
4. Based on sleep logs or actigraphy, make the best estimate of the child's circadian sleep/wake schedule: the time of preferred sleep onset (earliest time of consistent ability to fall asleep), the time of spontaneous awakening, and the sleep need.
   a. Then, beginning at the current spontaneous wake time, advance the wake-up time 30 minutes a day until the desired wake time is achieved (Fig. 37-5).[16]
   b. Expose the child, on being wakened, to bright natural sunlight (or artificial light if natural light in not available) for least 20 minutes.
      i. In preadolescent children, in whom the needed shift is usually just 1 to 3 hours, one can often simply

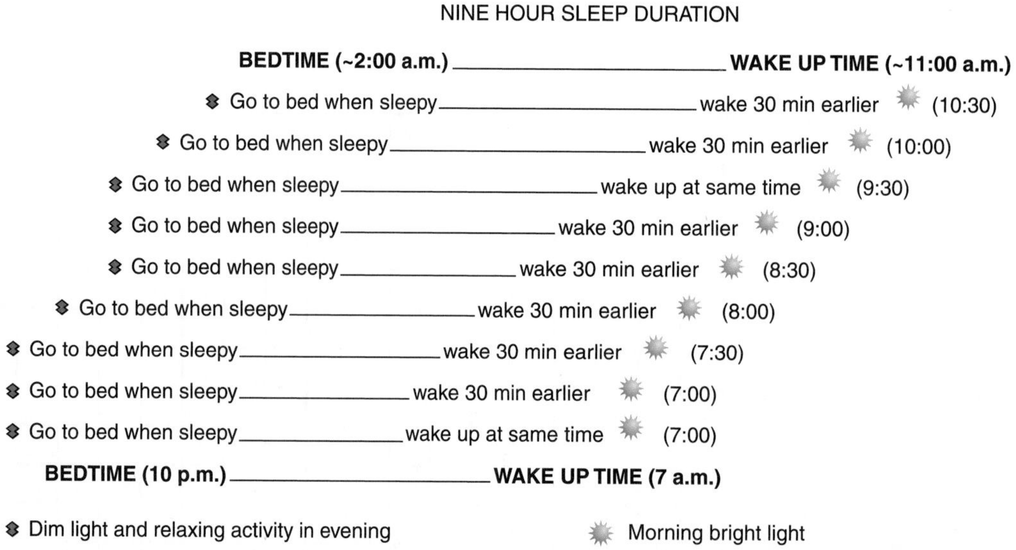

NINE HOUR SLEEP DURATION

BEDTIME (~2:00 a.m.) _____ **WAKE UP TIME (~11:00 a.m.)**

♠ Go to bed when sleepy_____wake 30 min earlier ※ (10:30)

♠ Go to bed when sleepy_____wake 30 min earlier ※ (10:00)

♠ Go to bed when sleepy_____wake up at same time ※ (9:30)

♠ Go to bed when sleepy_____wake 30 min earlier ※ (9:00)

♠ Go to bed when sleepy_____wake 30 min earlier ※ (8:30)

♠ Go to bed when sleepy_____wake 30 min earlier ※ (8:00)

♠ Go to bed when sleepy_____wake 30 min earlier ※ (7:30)

♠ Go to bed when sleepy_____wake 30 min earlier ※ (7:00)

♠ Go to bed when sleepy_____wake up at same time ※ (7:00)

BEDTIME (10 p.m.) _____ **WAKE UP TIME (7 a.m.)**

♠ Dim light and relaxing activity in evening   ※ Morning bright light

Figure 37-5 Sleep scheduling for treatment of delayed sleep phase. The progressive phase advance in the time of arousal is necessary to minimize the chance that the morning wakeup and light exposure will occur before the body temperature minimum. This is important because morning light will lead to a phase delay if it occurs before the body temperature minimum and a phase advance, which is desired, if it occurs after the body temperature minimum. (Redrawn from Lack LL, Wright HR, Bootzen RR. Delayed sleep phase disorder. *Sleep Med Clin.* 2009;4(2):229-240.

establish the preferred wake-up time without this gradual phase advance.

  ii. The advantage of progressively phase advancing the wake-up time when a large shift is needed is to ensure that the morning wake-up time and light exposure occur during the phase advance portion of the child's phase response curve. (For example, if a child's spontaneous wake time is 12 noon, and he is awakened at 6 AM, light exposure at that hour would likely be before the temperature minimum and the effect of the light on the circadian sleep system would be a further phase delay instead of a phase advance. Scheduling the wake-up time and light exposure 30 minutes before the spontaneous wake time and then advancing the wake time by 30 minutes each day minimizes the likelihood that this will occur.)

5. If the child is school age or older, discontinue naps.

6. There should be avoidance of alcohol, recreational drugs, and nicotine.

7. Do not allow caffeine after 3 PM.

8. If the child is taking long-acting stimulant medication, only administer in the morning and have the parent awaken the child before 8 AM or 30 minutes before he needs to be awakened for school to give him the medication. Then allow the child to return to sleep until the desired wake time. This strategy is intuitive, and has proved useful for the author, though it has never been formally evaluated. Awakening the child with a DSPS in the morning is often the most difficult part of the treatment plan for the parents. This approach, in conjunction with the gradual phase advance of the sleep schedule, is usually successful in helping the child start the day.

9. If the child is taking short-acting stimulants in the morning, awaken him 30 minutes before the desired wake time to administer the medication, and then allow the child to return to sleep until the desired awakening time. The last dose of short-acting stimulants should be before 3 PM.

10. Encourage physical activity, especially in the midafternoon during the child's afternoon "siesta" time (and avoid quiet activities, such as TV, at this time), so inappropriate naps do not occur.

11. Plan a pleasant evening routine.

12. All electronics should be discontinued by 8 to 9 PM including television, video games, computers, and cell phones.

13. Evening light should be as low as possible. Use low-intensity clip-on LED lights for reading.

14. If anxiety is an issue or if the child engages in rumination at bedtime, these issues need to be identified and addressed. In mild cases, simply instructing parents and children to set aside a specific worry time in the early afternoon, possibly with journaling, may be an effective strategy for displacing the anxious time away from sleep time. If anxiety is more severe, or is thought to be associated with school avoidance, then referral for psychological treatment may be necessary before fully addressing the DSPS (which, at least for the older child, requires his or her motivation and cooperation).

15. At bedtime, advise the child not to get in bed until sleepy. Bedtime initially should not be based on the clock time one wants to reach after correction. Once in bed, if not asleep within 15 minutes, the child should be instructed to get out of bed and do some quiet, nonstimulating activity until sleepy. The next night start with bedtime later (it is important to find a late enough bedtime so sleep onset can occur quickly, before one considers advancing it).

16. If the child is in school and sleep is substantially delayed with spontaneous wake time well into the school day, then working with the school to provide for accommodation during the initial treatment is necessary. Schools are generally required to provide accommodation for medical conditions. One needs to make it clear to the child and parent that you are not providing an open-ended excuse for missing school. The accommodation is for a limited period (typically 1 to 2 weeks), excused lateness will be allowed until the sleep phase is advanced, and all the missed schoolwork needs to be made up.

17. Once the desired wake time is established, the schedule needs to be maintained. If the child is allowed to sleep in more than 1 ½ to 2 hours past the school week wake times on both days of the weekend, the sleep phase delay will likely recur.

18. After the DSPS has been corrected one can negotiate with the child and parent about allowing 1 day per week for the child to sleep in up to 1 ½ hours past the school week wake-up time. How much sleeping in on the weekends can be done without triggering a recurrence of the delayed sleep phase is variable in different children so the schedule requires monitoring and adjustment.

19. Discuss with the adolescent that treatment may only be necessary during the school year when the child must adhere to a fixed schedule. During the summer, the family may choose to allow the child to phase shift back to the preferred sleep schedule. This is not necessarily a problem, except the schedule will need to be reset prior to the next school year and, until that happens, the child and parent may not have much awake time that overlaps.

20. Discuss the risks of excessive daytime sleepiness, especially the risk of drowsy driving, with the adolescent and the parents. Adolescents may need to have driving privileges restricted for safety reasons.

If the child and parents are willing to do strict sleep scheduling, then melatonin can be offered as an adjunct. It is important that melatonin not be thought of as a quick fix because melatonin treatment alone, without the sleep hygiene measures described here, is unlikely to be effective. If the parent and adolescent are not inclined to use melatonin, that decision should be supported.

Numerous protocols for melatonin administration have been shown to be helpful in the treatment of delayed sleep phase syndrome:

1. Low-dose (0.5 mg) melatonin given 5 hours before the desired sleep onset time[14-17] has been shown to be the most effective strategy to induce a phase advance of sleep onset.

2. Split-dose (0.5 mg given 5 hours before the desired sleep time and 3 mg given at bedtime) melatomin.

3. Bedtime dose of 3 mg[15,17] takes advantage of both the phase advancement and the sedating effects of melatonin.

There have been numerous different protocols put forward for the use of melatonin in the treatment of insomnia.[14-22] The success of melatonin for the treatment of insomnia depends on both a phase-shifting effect as well as a direct soporific effect. Consequently, the response to melatonin can be quite variable in children, depending on what the cause of their insomnia is; as a result different children respond better to different protocols. When melatonin is used to phase shift the circadian sleep schedule in a child with a DSPS, it is best given 4 to 5 hours before the desired sleep onset time.[14-17] In children with neurodevelopmental delays, melatonin is generally given at bedtime.[18] The decision about which protocol to use depends on the child and family schedule and the child's response to medication. Adolescents often are not home 4 to 5 hours before bedtime and may not be able to consistently take medication without some parental supervision. If the child is at home in the evening, beginning with the trial of low-dose melatonin 4 to 5 hours before bedtime is often the best first step. If, after 1 week, there is no significant improvement, and the child is adhering to all of the sleep hygiene guidelines, then adding 3 mg at bedtime is the next step. As noted previously, without strict sleep scheduling and control of light exposure, melatonin alone is unlikely to be effective. Some children are very sensitive to low doses of melatonin, and only a bedtime dose is necessary.

Chronotherapy, or progressive phase advance of the sleep schedule (i.e., going to bed and waking 3 hours later each day until the sleep schedule is moved, around-the-clock, to the desired time), is an intervention for delayed sleep phase that has been shown to be effective in a well-controlled laboratory research setting where light can be controlled. Unfortunately, it does not apply well to a home setting, because of the difficulty, especially in adolescents, in preventing light exposure in the evening during the phase delay portion of the phase response curve.

Successful treatment of children, especially adolescents with delayed sleep phase, requires their active involvement. They need to believe there is a problem, understand what the problem is, and be willing to participate in the solution. This is why education and motivation are so important for a successful treatment outcome. Many adolescents with a delayed sleep phase do not feel there is a problem and are not interested in solving what, for them, is someone else's problem. The approach to this situation should be straightforward. Providing the child and parent with correct information regarding delayed sleep phase is useful, even if they are not interested in addressing it at that time. Explore if there are any consequences of the DSPS that the adolescent is unhappy about. Is truancy an issue? How severe is the associated EDS, and if severe does it pose a risk to safe driving? Should driving privileges be made contingent on successful treatment of the DSPS because of the risks of EDS? If the parents/adolescent chooses not to follow the recommendations to correct the delayed sleep phase, they should always be offered the opportunity to return at some time in the future when they are willing to work on it.

Occasionally, even when the interventions described here are followed, the delayed sleep phase cannot be adequately corrected. If this is the case, then alternative school placements should be considered. In many school districts, on-line high schools are available. This is an option that is attractive to some adolescents; however, exploring with the family the nonacademic elements of school is important before they make this choice. The importance of the teen establishing a regular sleep schedule and receiving an adequate amount of sleep continues to be important regardless of what sleep schedule the youngster ultimately adopts. This may need to be emphasized to the family. A simple instruction sheet (Fig. 37-6) should be given to the family after the first clinic visit, describing the agreed-upon treatment strategy. This information can be framed as a contract with the adolescent.

Advanced Sleep Phase Disorder

Advanced sleep phase is most often seen in younger children. The symptom that parents will generally complain about is the early morning awakening when the child is unable to return to sleep, even if the child is allowed to co-sleep with the parents. Because of the sleep insufficiency that invariably accompanies circadian rhythm disorders, parents will often complain of their child's daytime irritability, especially in the late afternoon. An advanced sleep phase is a mismatch between a physiologic and a desired schedule.[19] Although it reflects a biologic tendency, it is usually easy to correct. It is not a symptom of an underlying behavioral problem. However, in older children, especially in those without a prior history of an advanced sleep schedule when the child was young, be suspicious regarding possible depression as a cause of the early morning awakening and daytime irritability.

Treatment for advanced sleep phase is as follows:
1. Evening light, natural if it is available, or artificial light if not, until 30 minutes before the desired bedtime. In young children this can most easily be accomplished during the summer by simply having the family go outdoors after dinner to the park or for a walk until 30 minutes before bedtime. In many cases this is the only intervention that is necessary.
2. Consider low-dose melatonin 0.5 mg given to the child upon spontaneous wake time in the morning, especially if schedule change alone does not appear to be working (monitor for daytime sedation). There have been no well-controlled trials on the use of melatonin for the treatment of advanced sleep phase. However, melatonin has been used successfully in this manner by the author and this approach is also described in review articles.[19]
3. Shield the child from bright morning light.
4. If the child is still at an age for napping, daytime naps may be necessary to enable the child to get to a later bedtime. For the same reason, lengthening afternoon naps can be encouraged.

Nonentrained Sleep/Wake Rhythm

Light is the primary factor that anchors the timing of the circadian sleep/wake schedule. Consequently, the majority of individuals who are blind experience a non-24-hour sleep/wake syndrome.[20] The symptoms they experience may include both insomnia and hypersomnia. The problem arises because, in the absence of light perception, the circadian propensity to sleep is free running and is entirely desynchronized from the sleep/wake schedule the individual is trying to adhere to. In this setting, melatonin is the only treatment that is able to phase shift the circadian pacemaker. The timing of melatonin needs to be adjusted based on its effect but generally a single dose 1 to 5 hours before bedtime is effective. A trial of melatonin administration at different times will identify the optimal time of administration for an individual child. Long-term use is usually necessary to maintain a consistent sleep schedule.[20]

Irregular Sleep/Wake Rhythm

This is a common problem, especially in young children who are short sleepers and in families who have difficulties setting limits and enforcing rules on their children. Four weeks of

Evening Routine:

- Decrease evening light; eliminate exposure to brightly lit areas.
- TV, video, computer, cell phone should be removed from bedroom and OFF_____ pm.
- No use of caffeine (soda, energy drinks, coffee, chocolate) after 3 PM.
- A low intensity light may be used such as a clip-on book reading light.
- Get in bed when tired, if not asleep in 20 minutes get out of bed until tired.
- Other: _____

Melatonin: _____ mg at ___PM

  _____ mg at ___PM

  _____ none

Morning Routine:

- Early morning bright light exposure helps to reset the biologic clock. Open curtains and shades to allow the daylight to help awaken you.
- Advance your wake-up time by 30 minutes a day from your spontaneous wake time, until you reach your desired wake time.

  Current wake time_____,
  Wake time day 1_____
  Wake time day 2_____
  Wake time day 3_____
  Wake time day 4_____
  Wake time day 5_____
  Wake time day 6_____
  Wake time day 7_____

- After reaching desired wake time regular wake up time 7 days a week at _____.
- Other: _____

School:

You may need an excused lateness for school when beginning this protocol.

General Guidelines:

- Do not take naps.
- Do not drink caffeine before noon or after 3 PM.
- If using stimulant prescription medications (e.g., methylphenidate or amphetamine), have parent administer medication before 8 AM, if this is before scheduled wake time go back to sleep after the medication is given.

Safety:

Driving requires a high level of alertness. Limitations of this privilege may be necessary. Do not drive drowsy.

Figure 37-6 Guidelines for treatment of delayed sleep phase in children: A sample patient handout. This instruction sheet can be modified as needed and provided for the patient and family. (Based on the author's clinical experience and reports of clinical experience at adult sleep centers.)

sleep logs are important to gather as a baseline for establishing the diagnosis and beginning treatment. It is common that this sleep problem occurs in conjunction with behavioral insomnia (sleep onset association disorder). If this is the case, the solution of the behavioral problem often will need to precede treatment of the circadian rhythm disorder. For both problems, the use of strict sleep scheduling and sleep restriction is a very powerful and effective tool that needs to be used consistently. Co-morbidities, such as autism and sensory integration disorder, need to be addressed before or during the treatment for the circadian sleep disorder.

Treatment for an irregular sleep/wake rhythm involves the following steps:

1. Based on the 4-week sleep log, average the number of hours of sleep per night the child has been getting.
2. Ask the parents when they wish the child to awaken. The wake time is then fixed and provides the anchor for the remainder of the sleep/wake schedule. The importance of a consistent wake time with bright natural light exposure needs to be emphasized.
3. Bedtime is scheduled by counting back, from the desired wake time, the average number of hours the child sleeps per night. This is the earliest time that the child should be put to bed. However, instruct the parents that if the child does not appear ready to go to bed at this time, the child should (initially) be allowed to stay up later.
4. The evening routine should be quiet and pleasant in low light conditions. Conflicts need to be avoided around bedtime.
5. All electronics—TV, video games, cell phones—should be discontinued by 8 to 9 PM depending on the age of the child.
6. The child should not allowed to go to bed before the scheduled bedtime regardless of how tired the child may appear.
7. Upon awakening in the morning the child should be exposed to bright, natural sunlight if available; artificial light may be necessary if it is dark outside at the desired wake time.

8. Depending on the child's age daytime naps may need to be eliminated or restricted to a specific nap window. The child is allowed to nap during any part of the nap window, but is not allowed to nap outside this window.

9. In children with neurodevelopmental disorders such as autism, the use of a bedtime dose of melatonin, in addition to the sleep hygiene measures discussed here, may be necessary.

This schedule invariably leads to significant initial sleep restriction with sleep insufficiency. This lack in turn will lead to an increase is the homeostatic sleep drive, which is a force that will ultimately help the child to fall asleep easily and remain asleep during the child's nighttime sleep period. This process needs to be explicitly discussed with the parents. Parents need to understand that the sleep restriction is temporary but necessary in order to achieve the desired goal of a rapid and easy transition to sleep at bedtime. Once sleep is consolidated during the night, bedtime and wake times are gradually adjusted to allow the child to receive an adequate amount of sleep. Once the child is both falling asleep quickly and sleeping through the night without much wakefulness, the parents can begin easing the sleep restriction at whichever end of the sleep period they choose (with an earlier bedtime or a later waking). The opening of the sleep window should be gradual, 15 minutes at a time, and should only be done as long as the nighttime sleep consolidation remains good. Parents require a great deal of encouragement to use sleep restriction. They need to understand that sleep restriction is a short-term tool, and they may need reminding that even if the child is being put to bed later, the actual number of hours of sleep the child is getting, based on the sleep log of how much sleep he had before treatment, is not less than before, and that the sleep is better consolidated. If parents are unable to enforce these bedtime rules, they may need some explicit coaching by a behavioral psychologist. Parents who are unable to establish limits and rules regarding daytime behaviors are rarely able to set them around bedtime. Parents' ability to set and enforce limits in the examination room during the office visit is often an indicator of their ability to set and enforce limits at home.

Many of the problems described in this chapter are chronic and may require long-term treatment with melatonin. It is important to have a frank discussion with parents and adolescents regarding this issue. If the parents use the Internet to gather information, they will likely come across information advising against long-term use of melatonin, and warnings of its risks. There have been studies of short-term use, of up to 3 months,[21,22] but there have not been reports of long-term use in the literature.

SUMMARY

Circadian rhythm disorders are common in children and adversely impact the quality of lives of parents and their children. They are easy to recognize, and they are easy to treat if the provider is able to create a therapeutic alliance with the parents and child. A systematic approach to evaluation, along with flexibility, good humor, and creativity in the treatment is the key. These disorders are generally very obvious to recognize if one asks the right questions, and they are easy to treat if one understands the problem and the family context in which they occur.

REFERENCES

1. Gilette MU, Abbott SM. Biologic timekeeping. *Sleep Med Clin.* 2009;4(2):99-100.
2. Jenni O, Carskadon M. Sleep behavior and sleep regulation from infancy through adolescence: Normative aspects. *Sleep Med Clin.* 2007;2(3):3231-3331.
3. Borbely AA, Baumann F, Brandeis D, et al. Sleep deprivation: Effect on sleep stages and EEG power density in man. *EEG Clin Neurophysiol.* 1981;51:483-493.
4. Strogatz SH, Kronauer RE, Czeisler CA. Circadian pacemaker interferes with sleep onset at specific times each day: Role in insomnia. *Am J Physiol.* 1987;253:172-178.
5. Edgar DM, Dement WC, Fuller CA. Effect of SCN lesions on sleep in squirrel monkeys: Evidence of opponent process in sleep regulation. *J Neurosci.* 1993;13:1065-1079.
6. Hauri P, Sateia M. *The International Classification of Sleep Disorders: Diagnostic and Coding Manual.* 2nd ed. Westchester, IL: AASM; 2005.
7. Rivkees S. The development of circadian rhythms: From animals to humans. *Sleep Med Clin.* 2007;2(3):331-341.
8. Carskadon M, Viera C, Acebo C. Association between puberty and delayed sleep phase preference. *Sleep.* 1993;16(3):258-262.
9. Jenni OJ, Achermann P, Carskadon MA. Homeostatic sleep regulation in to adolescents. *Sleep.* 2005;28(11):1446-1454.
10. Iglowstein I, Jenni O, Molinari L, et al. Sleep duration from infancy to adolescence: Reference values and generational trends. *Pediatrics.* 2003;111:302-307.
11. Rosen G. Evaluation of the patient who has sleep complaints: A case based method using the sleep process matrix. *Prim Care Clin Office Pract.* 2005;32:319-328.
12. Hagan JF, Shaw JS, Duncan PM, eds. *Bright Futures: Guidelines for Health Supervision of Infants, Children, and Adolescents.* 3rd ed. Elk Grove Village, IL: American Academy of Pediatrics; 2008:45.
13. Duffy JF, Czeisler CA. Effect of light on human circadian physiology. *Sleep Med Clin.* 2009;4(2):165-177.
14. Bjorvatn B, Pallesen S. A practical approach to circadian rhythm sleep disorders. *Sleep Med Rev.* 2009;13:47-60.
15. Rajaratnam S, Cohen D, Rogers N. Melatonin and melatonin analogues. *Sleep Med Clin.* 2009;4(2):179-193.
16. Lack LL, Wright HR, Bootzen RR. Delayed sleep phase disorder. *Sleep Med Clin.* 2009;4(2):229-240.
17. Mundey K, Benloucif K, Dubocovich ML, et al. Phase dependent treatment of delayed sleep phase syndrome with melatonin. *Sleep.* 2005;28(10):1271-1276.
18. Johnson KP, Malow BA. Assessment and pharmacologic treatment of sleep disturbance in autism. *Child Adol Psych Clin North Am.* 2008;17:773-785.
19. Auger RR. Advanced-related sleep complaints and advanced sleep phase disorder. *Sleep Med Clin.* 2009;4(2):219-227.
20. Uchiyama M, Lockley SW. Non-24-hour sleep wake syndrome in sighted and blind patients. *Sleep Med Clin.* 2009;4(2):195-211.
21. Buscemi N, Vandermeer B, Pandya R, et al. Efficacy and safety of exogenous melatonin for secondary sleep disorders and sleep disorders accompanying sleep restriction: Meta-analysis. *Br Med J.* 2006;332:385-393.
22. Buscemi N, Vandermeer B, Hooton N, et al. The efficacy and safety of exogenous melatonin for primary sleep disorders a meta-analysis. *J Gen Intern Med.* 2005;20:1151-1158.
23. Melendres CS, Lutz JM, Rubin ED, Marcus CL. Daytime sleepiness and hyperactivity in children with suspected sleep-disordered breathing. *Pediatrics.* 2004;114:768-775.
24. Drake C, Nickel C, Burduvali E, Roth T, Jefferson C, Pietro B. The Pediatric Daytime Sleepiness Scale (PDSS): Sleep habits and school outcomes in middle-school children. *Sleep.* 2003;26(4):455-458.
25. Spilsbury JC, Drotar D, Rosen CL, Redline S. The Cleveland Adolescent Sleepiness Questionnaire: A new measure to assess excessive daytime sleepiness in adolescents. *J Clin Sleep Med.* 2007;3(6):603-612.
26. Chervin RD, Hedger K, Dillon JE, Pituch KJ. Pediatric Sleep Questionnaire (PSQ): Validity and reliability of scales for sleep-disordered breathing, snoring, sleepiness, and behavioral problems. *Sleep Med.* 2000;1(1):21-32.

Parasomnias, Periodic Limb Movements, and Restless Legs in Children

SURESH KOTAGAL

PARASOMNIAS

Definition

Parasomnias are episodic phenomena that intrude onto sleep. Sleep quality in general remains unaffected but the events can lead to significant worry for the parents (as in confusional arousals and sleep terrors). They show a familial predisposition. The events are most common in preschool age-children, with gradual resolution over time.[1] An overview of common childhood parasomnias will be presented here.

Prevalence

Petit and associates,[2] in a prospective study of parasomnias in childhood, followed approximately 1000 Quebec children between the ages of 2.5 years and 6 years. They found an overall prevalence rate for sleepwalking of 14.5%, for sleep terrors 39.8%, and for sleep enuresis 25%. The prevalence rates for bruxism (teeth grinding) and rhythmic movements such as head banging were 45.6% and 9.2%, respectively. The occurrence of parasomnias in preschool age-children was found to be quite ubiquitous—88% of the cohort manifested at least one parasomnia during the study period.

Pathophysiology

Parasomnias are the consequence of the incomplete dissociations of the states of wakefulness, non–rapid eye movement (NREM) sleep, and rapid eye movement (REM) sleep from each other, often at least partially because of a genetic predisposition, with behaviors characteristic of one state becoming superimposed on another.[3] During the transitions between waking and sleep, these patterns appear as hypnic starts or rhythmic movements (waking and NREM sleep) or as sleep paralysis (waking and REM sleep); during the transitions from NREM sleep to waking (or perhaps to REM sleep), they become manifest as confusional arousals, sleep terrors, sleepwalking, or bruxism.

Parasomnias such as bruxism and some forms of sleepwalking are composed of stereotyped patterns of motor behavior most likely associated with activation of central pattern generators (CPGs). These generators are groups of interneurons in the brainstem or spinal cord that have connections with ventral motor neurons.[4,5] Activation of these CPGs is known to trigger stereotypical behavior patterns consistent with their neuroanatomic location (Fig. 38-1). Glutamate and serotonin are key neurotransmitters within CPGs.[6,7] The favorable response of most parasomnias to treatment with benzodiazepines *suggests* an alteration of the inhibitory neurotransmitters such as γ-hydroxybutyric acid (although other mechanisms are possible). Most typical childhood parasomnias subside by the second decade, presumably owing to progressive maturation of descending cortical inhibitory projections on the brainstem and spinal cord.

Parasomnias Occurring at the Transition from Wakefulness to Sleep

Hypnic Starts

Hypnic starts are the most common sleep-onset parasomnia observed during childhood. Also termed *sleep starts*, these are isolated, quick jerks of the extremities that occur at the time of sleep onset and may be accompanied by a sensation of falling, a dream-like feeling, or a flashing sensation.[8] Hypnic starts are only infrequently bothersome to the child, but may be mistaken as seizures by the parents. They are benign, occur at all ages, and most likely represent a release phenomenon that is mediated at the level of the brainstem or spinal cord due to a transient loss of cortical inhibition. They can even occur in a brief cluster in normal children. In neurologically impaired children, however, they may occur in more prominent and repetitive clusters, with the time between jerks ranging from a few seconds to a minute or so. Even though there may be a history of epilepsy, these events do not show epileptiform electroencephalographic (EEG) correlates.[9]

Isolated Sleep Paralysis

The term *isolated sleep paralysis (ISP)* refers to isolated or recurrent episodes of transient inability to move the body as one is drifting off to sleep or (more commonly, in normal, non-narcoleptic subjects) immediately upon awakening from REM sleep. (The paralysis is real and is only what normally occurs within REM sleep during normal periods of dreaming, albeit without conscious awareness.) The individual remains conscious during episodes of sleep paralysis and fully aware of the surroundings. There is a (sometimes terrifying) feeling of inability to move, typically lasting seconds but occasionally up to several minutes. Hallucinatory experience, such as sensing the presence of others nearby, feeling pressure on one's chest, or hearing footsteps, may coexist.[10] Approximately 20% of young adults with anxiety disorder may manifest ISP on occasion.[11] Sleep deprivation in otherwise healthy teenagers is also a common trigger. The differential diagnosis includes partial seizures and periodic paralysis. Isolated events are generally due to sleep deprivation and do not require treatment. Recurrent episodes may be very bothersome to the patient. Studies of treatments of ISP in the child have not been done. It is the experience of the author, however, that ISP can be treated with REM-suppressing agents, such as low doses of tricyclic agents, or by medications such as clonidine 0.1 to 0.2 per day in two divided doses, or clonazepam 0.125 to 0.5 mg at bedtime.

Rhythmic Movement Disorder

Rhythmic movements in infants and toddlers at or near the time of sleep onset are physiologic, and generally resolve spontaneously by the age of 3 to 4 years. Rhythmic movements may occur in drowsy wakefulness and during the transition from wakefulness to light NREM sleep; they sometimes also occur during deeper stages of NREM sleep (although this is fairly uncommon).[12] The movements may recur, or only appear, in the middle of the night after the child has awakened and is attempting to fall back to sleep. The three common types of rhythmic movements are side-to-side head rolling, head banging (into pillow or headboard), and body rocking. Rhythmic movement *disorder* is identified when the movements lead to significant consequences such as self-injury. There is a 4:1 male predominance.[12] The child generally has little or no recollection of the event upon awakening the next morning (depending upon how much takes place in wakefulness). The rhythmic

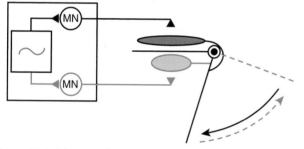

Central Pattern Generator (CPG)

Figure 38-1 Schematic of a CPG in the spinal cord. A central circuit of interneurons generates rhythmic output to pools of motor neurons (MN) that innervate antagonist groups of muscle, leading to rhythmic patterns such as stereotyped walking movements. (Adapted with permission from Marder E, Bucher D. Central pattern generators and the control of rhythmic movements. *Curr Biol.* 2001;11:R986-R996).

movements around the time of sleep onset should be distinguished from those seen in autism and pervasive developmental disorders, which tend to appear during full wakefulness as well.

There is no one satisfactory treatment. Anecdotal therapies include reducing time in bed by the amount of time spent in these behaviors (especially if time in bed is clearly excessive), creating intentional and extraneous rhythmic movements before bedtime, adding rhythmic sounds to the sleeping environment, and the use of antihistamines. On occasion, short-term benzodiazepine therapy may be justified,[13] and padding the sides of the crib may help prevent injury.

Parasomnias of Non–Rapid Eye Movement Sleep

The following are by far the most problematic parasomnias for which families generally seek medical attention.

Arousal Parasomnias: Confusional Arousals, Sleep Terrors, and Sleepwalking

These three related occurrences are the key NREM parasomnias.[12-14] They are termed *arousal parasomnias* as they appear during partial arousals from NREM sleep. Typically, they occur at the time of transition from deep NREM sleep (stage N3) to the lighter stages of NREM sleep or to waking, and are most common in the first third of night sleep when N3 sleep is most abundant and deep. Table 38-1 summarizes the characteristics of these three arousal parasomnias.

Pathophysiology. A genetic predisposition may lead to arousal parasomnias as may acquired disturbances that trigger shifts from slow wave sleep toward the lighter stages of sleep or waking. The latter may occur both with physiologic events, such as sleep-disordered breathing, periodic limb movements (PLMs), or gastroesophageal reflux (GER), and with behaviorally mediated events, such as getting up nightly to be rocked or to change beds (particularly when combined with an age vulnerability, generally 2-12 years). Separation anxiety may be a predisposing factor for both sleep terrors and sleepwalking.[2] Sleep deprivation and fever can trigger all three forms of arousal parasomnia. Often, however, no trigger or predisposition can be identified.

Cyclic alternating patterns (CAPs) are periodic EEG events of NREM sleep characterized by spontaneous high-voltage bursts that recur at regular intervals of up to 2 minutes.[15]

TABLE 38-1

Comparison of Arousal Parasomnias

Clinical Feature	Confusional Arousals	Sleep Terrors	Sleepwalking
Typical age at onset	2-10 years	2-10 years	4-10 years
Usual frequency	3-4/week to 1-2/month	3-4/week to 1-2/month	3-4/week to 1-2/month
Peak time of occurrence	First third of night's sleep	First third of night's sleep	First third of night's sleep
Behaviors during event	Whimpering, some articulation, sitting up in bed, inconsolable	Screaming, agitation, flushed face, sweating, inconsolable	Walking about the room or house May be quiet or agitated, unresponsive to verbal commands
Concurrent polysomnographic findings	Deep NREM (N3) sleep with rhythmic theta or delta activity	N3 sleep with rhythmic theta or delta activity	N3 sleep with rhythmic theta or delta activity
Typical duration	2-30 minutes	5-30 minutes	5-30 minutes

NREM, non–rapid eye movement.

CAPs are one marker of unstable sleep and may be increased during the slow wave sleep of children with sleep terrors.[15]

Confusional Arousals. This NREM parasomnia is most common in 2- to 10-year–olds,[12,16] although it may be seen in infants (certainly those as young as 6 months) and may persist or recur through adolescence. The onset of symptoms is typically within 2 to 3 hours of sleep onset. The child generally will sit up in bed, whimper, cry, or moan, and may utter words or phrases like "No," "Stop it!" or "Go away." He or she may appear distressed and remain inconsolable regardless of efforts at soothing. There is generally no truly stereotypic motor behavior. The child usually remains in the bed. The duration of the event is usually 2 to 30 minutes, though it may last up to 45 minutes. A simultaneously recorded EEG may show generalized, high-amplitude rhythmic delta or theta activity, at least at the start, with progressive mixing of delta EEG patterns typical of deep sleep, theta activity of light sleep, and alpha or theta activity of waking. The following morning, the patient awakens feeling normally alert and refreshed, and has no recollection of the event whatsoever. Paradoxically, it is the sleep of parents and other family members that may be disrupted—from worry about the child. In those children with sleep-disordered breathing or periodic limb movements as a trigger, there may be preexisting sleep disruption and hence possibly associated daytime behavioral manifestations such as hyperactivity and mood swings.

Sleep Terrors. The typical age of occurrence is between 2 and 10 years, although sleep terrors may certainly be seen in adolescents. The events usually occur during the first third of night sleep. The child awakens abruptly from sleep with a blood-curdling scream, agitation, tachycardia, and facial flushing and sweating. The child may jump out of bed as if running away from an unseen threat[16] and remain unresponsive to parental efforts at calming down. A simultaneously obtained EEG may show patterns as described for confusional arousals (discussed previously). There is a strong genetic predisposition. Most patients show gradual, spontaneous resolution over months to years.

Sleepwalking. The age of onset, time of occurrence, and the frequency of spells are similar to those for confusional arousals and sleep terrors. During mild episodes, a toddler may sit up and crawl around the bed, or a child may walk quietly in sleep to the bedside of the parents. If the child remains in his room, episodes may go unnoticed by others.[13,16] During more intense episodes, children may become agitated and run around the house. Patients have injured themselves, for example, by bumping into furniture; truly dangerous behaviors—like jumping out of a second story window—may occur but are fortunately uncommon, especially before adolescence. Children may unknowingly risk injury, for example, by walking out of the house on a cold winter night with consequent exposure to accidental hypothermia. Autonomic dysfunction may occur in the form of sweating and flushing of the face. Some patients exhibit a combination of sleep terrors and sleepwalking (as perhaps is the case with the most dangerous behaviors), though one manifestation or another usually predominates.

Differential Diagnosis of Arousal Parasomnias. Nocturnal seizures can mimic the arousal parasomnias because disorganized bodily movements, staring, unresponsiveness, vocalizations, and confused behavior are common to both groups of disorders. Table 38-2 summarizes features that help distinguish seizures from arousal parasomnias. Nocturnal frontal lobe epilepsy (NFLE) is due to mutations in the genes *CHRNA2*, *CHRNA4*, or *CHRNB2*, which regulate the expression of nicotinic acetylcholine receptors.[17-19] The seizures in NFLE show abrupt onset, last only a few seconds, may be accompanied by hypermotor thrashing or dystonic posturing of the limbs, and have a clear point of termination. A full EEG montage should be incorporated into the polysomnogram (PSG) for the investigation of any nocturnal events suspected to be seizures.[20,21] Home video recordings of the spells by the parents may be an invaluable aid in diagnosis, as may in-hospital long-term EEG/video monitoring (because a 1- or 2-night stay in the artificial environment of the sleep laboratory will not consistently capture the nocturnal events).

Management. The management of parasomnias in children is summarized in Table 38-3. Infrequently occurring (one or two times per month) confusional arousals, sleep terrors, and sleepwalking (without dangerous behaviors) most often do not need to be treated, especially in young children. Parents should be informed about the benign and self-limiting nature of the disturbance, with likely spontaneous resolution over 1 to 2 years. Toddlers should receive adequate napping time during the day, as sleep deprivation may be a trigger, and be on a regular and appropriate schedule. Unnecessary nighttime behaviors, such as bed switching or frequent calling for

TABLE 38-2

Distinction Between Arousal Parasomnias and Nocturnal Seizures

Feature	Arousal Parasomnias	Nocturnal Seizures
Age at onset	Preschool age and childhood	Infancy, preschool age, childhood, and adolescence
Family history of similar events	Generally positive	May or may not be positive
Usual time of occurrence	First third of night sleep	Randomly through the night
Most common sleep stage at occurrence	Stage N3	Stage N1, N2
Duration of event	5-30 minutes	0.5-5 minutes
Concurrent electroencephalographic features	Rhythmic theta or delta activity	Normal/spikes or sharp waves over a focal or generalized distribution
Usual daytime behavior	Normal (unless complicated by sleep related breathing disturbance or restless legs/periodic limb movement disorder)	May be irritable and sleepy; seizures may also occur during the day

TABLE 38-3

Management of Parasomnias

Concept	Specific Measures
Ensuring patient safety	Installing dead bolts and motion sensors in the house for sleep walkers, padded bed rails for head banging
Decreasing activation of central pattern generators	Adenotonsillectomy/nasal corticosteroids for obstructive sleep apnea; iron replacement if indicated for restless legs syndrome/periodic limb movement disorder; histamine (H_2) receptor antagonist such as ranitidine for gastroesophageal reflux
Anticipatory awakening (scheduled awakening)	Deliberate interruption of sleep of the patient by the parent, usually 15-20 minutes before the usual time of occurrence of the parasomnia
Pharmacotherapy	Clonazepam, 0.125 to 0.5 mg at bedtime (for most NREM and REM sleep parasomnias); melatonin 1-3 mg at bedtime for REM sleep behavior disorder

NREM, non–rapid eye movement; *REM*, rapid eye movement

interventions, should be eliminated, if possible, because they can become almost automatic at times of nighttime wakings with inappropriate behavior occurring when the waking is incomplete (as may happen when the child's waking is from deep sleep). In the case of sleepwalking, environmental safety issues should be discussed with the parents. Unless the child is at risk of injury, parents should be advised not to restrain or try to awaken the child, as this may exacerbate the disturbance. Nocturnal polysomnography and specific pharmacologic measures should be considered when arousal parasomnias become associated with daytime mood or behavioral disturbance (suggesting an underlying trigger such as obstructive sleep apnea [OSA] or restless legs syndrome [RLS]/periodic limb movement disorder [PLMD]), when the safety of the child becomes a concern, when medicolegal issues are present (as when events start after an injury), when events are atypical in timing, frequency, or appearance, or when the sleep of other family members becomes regularly disrupted. If OSA, PLMD, or GER are identified as triggers, treatment efforts should be directed at these underlying issues. If no specific underlying triggers are found and the parasomnias remain problematic, treatment with a low dose of a benzodiazepine usually works well, such as clonazepam in a dose of 0.125 to 0.5 mg at bedtime (at least in children of school age).[22] Typically treatment is necessary for 6 to12 months, occasionally longer, with attempts at tapering to be considered after any 3-month period with few or no events.

Anticipatory awakening (scheduled awakening) is a behavioral technique that can be utilized to prevent arousal parasomnias.[23,24] As the occurrence of these events is generally time-locked to the first third of the night, momentary awakening of the child by the parent, 15 to 20 minutes prior to the usual time of occurrence may alter the sleep state and thereby abort the event. During the scheduled awakening attempt, the parent comforts the child and generally behaves as he/she would when awakened by the child. The technique may be

worth trying, particularly if the family is inclined toward non-pharmacologic management. However, attempts to waken the child may only trigger a parasomnia event or postpone the spontaneous event to later in the night.

Benign Neonatal Sleep Myoclonus

This condition is characterized by symmetrical or asymmetrical jerks of extremities during NREM sleep that are first observed in the newborn period. The movements cease upon awakening. They can be mistaken for seizures, but the movements have no epileptiform correlates on a simultaneously obtained video-EEG. The entity is benign and resolves spontaneously over weeks to months.[25,26]

Parasomnias of Rapid Eye Movement Sleep

Because patient reporting of dream content is key to establishing a diagnosis of disorders in this group, these parasomnias are most often recognized in school age-children.

Nightmares

Nightmares are bad dreams that awaken the dreamer. The International Classification of Sleep Disorders defines nightmares as "recurrent episodes of awakening from sleep with recall of intensely disturbing dream mentation, usually involving fear or anxiety, but also anger, sadness, disgust, and other dysphoric emotions." There is generally full alertness and dream recall immediately upon awakening after a nightmare. Additionally, there may be delayed return to sleep after the episode.[27] Because REM sleep is preponderant during the second half of the night, and increasingly intense as the night goes on, nightmares generally occur during the early hours of the morning.

The historical origin of the suffix *mare*, from the proto-Germanic *maron*, refers to demons, more specifically incubi, who were believed to sit on the chest of sleepers and cause a feeling of pressure or weight[28] as portrayed in a 1781 painting by Henry Fuseli.[29]

There is adequate recall of dream content in children who are sufficiently verbal. The description of dreams in preschool age-children is usually short and simple, but older children may embellish the dream content with fantasy. In children with post-traumatic stress disorder (PTSD), the dream content may be distressing, with themes of inflicted violence, death, or separation involving close family members. As muscle tone and mobility are actively inhibited during REM sleep, body movements are rare during a nightmare. Autonomic manifestations like sweating and flushing of the face are minimal. There may be mild tachycardia. The duration of the event (at least the scary part of the dream) is generally a few minutes, though the wakening that follows, with persisting memory of the upsetting dream, may be prolonged. Polysomnography is not routinely indicated for the investigation of nightmares.

Management

The recommendations for the management of recurrent nightmares in children are based on observations from small, nonrandomized case series.[30] Some nightmares may subside simply with reassurance. Rescripting techniques in which children are taught to create a new, more pleasant ending to a recurring nightmare may minimize their distress. Desensitization techniques may also help alleviate the fear of nightmares.[31] Some therapists have found it useful to encourage

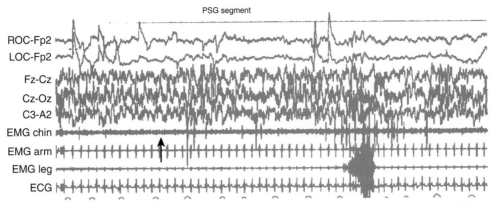

Figure 38-2 Nocturnal polysomnogram (one minute segment) during rapid eye movement (REM) sleep on a patient with REM sleep behavior disorder. The patient (a 14-year-old girl) had manifested repetitive yelling and thrashing behavior during sleep at night. The chin electromyogram (EMG) channel shows persistence of tonic electromyographic activity, characteristic of REM sleep without atonia. Channels 1-2, electro-oculogram; 3-5, electroencephalogram; 6-8, chin and limb electromyogram; 9, electrocardiogram.

the child to write down the content of the nightmare, or draw pictures of the object(s) they encounter during the nightmare, as this may help make the experience less scary. Hauri and associates[32] have reported that one or two sessions of hypnotherapy will help adults and children with nightmares, with 5 of 7 (71%) remaining spell-free or much improved at 18 months and 4 of 6 (67%) remaining spell-free after 5 years. Pharmacologic therapy is rarely indicated.

REM Sleep Behavior Disorder

Physically aggressive motor behavior during a dream (apparent dream enactment), such as kicking, punching, banging on the bedroom wall, and attacking the bed partner, is generally seen in adults with degenerative neurologic disorders, such as Parkinson's disease and idiopathic Lewy body disease, and as a side effect of certain medications.[33] It apparently occurs because of lack of normal REM-associated motor suppression or exaggerated tonic and phasic motor activity. REM sleep behavior disorder is possibly under-recognized in childhood, though certainly it is uncommon in the otherwise normal individual. Nevsimalova and colleagues have reported two girls aged 7 and 9 years with combined REM sleep behavior disorder and narcolepsy-cataplexy.[34] The nocturnal PSG shows EMG evidence of loss of the normal physiologic REM atonia in submental leads and excessive phasic twitching in REM sleep in limb leads[35] (Fig. 38-2). Events captured on videotape may show yelling, agitation, or flailing of the limbs. The significance and long-term outcome of childhood REM sleep behavior disorder is unknown.

Management

As in adults, the disorder may respond to treatment with benzodiazepines such as clonazepam, 0.125 to 0.5 mg at bedtime or to melatonin, 1 to 3 mg at bedtime.[36]

PERIODIC LIMB MOVEMENTS IN SLEEP AND PERIODIC LIMB MOVEMENT DISORDER

Definition

PLMs are electromyographically recorded jerks of the muscles of the extremities, generally four or more, that last 0.5 to 10 seconds and occur at intervals of 5 to 90 seconds.[37] They are observed most commonly during NREM sleep and are linked to sleep fragmentation. Periodic limb movements in sleep (PLMS) refer to a disturbance that is observed only on the PSG unaccompanied by clinical manifestations, and thus is likely an epiphenomenon. On the other hand, PLMD is a condition that is associated with clinical symptoms of sleep-wake disruption.

Prevalence

A PLM index (PLMI, the number of leg movements per hour of sleep) of 5 or more has been conventionally extrapolated from adult literature to define significant PLMS in childhood.[38] In a retrospective study of 591 children of median age 7.9 years, Kirk and Bohn[39] found a PLM prevalence rate of 5.6%. Another survey reported a prevalence of 11.9% in a community sample of children and in 8.4% of a sleep center population.[40] Certain special populations of children may exhibit a higher prevalence. Thus, in a study of 118 children aged 2 to 18 years old with sleep-disordered breathing, Chervin and Archbold[41] found a prevalence rate of 26%; and in a different study, Scofield and associates[42] found PLMS occurring with a frequency greater than 15 per hour of sleep seemed to be more common in white children than in African-American children.

About 80% of adult patients with RLS have coexisting PLMs, thus suggesting the latter constitutes an important clinical feature of RLS. Not all subjects with RLS manifest PLMs on PSG however, possibly due to night-to-night variability in the occurrence of PLMs,[43] or perhaps suggesting that PLMs are not truly an essential component of RLS. In preschool and elementary school children, the diagnosis of RLS may often be missed because of these children's inability to clearly express symptoms of RLS, even if present. If this were true, the number of children diagnosed with PLMS/PLMD *without* RLS would be artefactually large. This possibility remains to be explored.

Pathophysiology

The origin of PLMS is likely at the level of the spinal cord, due to activation of CPGs[4] (as was described previously and in Fig. 38-1 for rhythmic movement disorder and other parasomnas), those circuits of interneurons that generate a rhythmic drive to motor neurons in the ventral spinal cord that trigger coordinated, rhythmic output.[4,5] Generators of stereotyped bodily movements are located at various levels of the neuraxis, including the brainstem and spinal cord. In mammals, the end result of activation of CPGs depends upon the locus of activation and may be manifested as coordinated swimming, walking, and running behaviors.[44,45] The stereotyped movements of flexion at the ankle, knee, and hip that characterize PLMs are likely indicative of activation of a set of spinal CPGs.[4] The spinal cord origin of CPGs for PLMs can also be assumed from the fact that these movements persist after lesions that have severed connections between the brain and spinal cord.

There is a strong genetic predisposition to PLMs, which is likely transmitted in an autosomal dominant manner.[46] Using whole genome analysis, Stefansson and associates[47] studied a group of patients and first-degree relatives with PLMs from Iceland and the United States. PLMs were ascertained using a wristwatch accelerometer that was attached to the ankle. A total of 306 subjects and 15,664 control subjects were tested for 306,937 single nucleotide polymorphism (SNP) markers. There was a strong association between PLMs and an intronic variant on allele A of SNP rs3923809. The odds ratio for having allele A of marker rs3923809 increased with the number of periodic limb movements and ranged from 1.0 in the group with 5 or fewer movements to 2.0 in the group with 21 or more movements. Also, patients without allele A exhibited 13% higher levels of serum ferritin than heterozygotes for the allele, and they, in turn, had higher ferritin levels than those who were homozygous for the allele. The association of the *BTBD9* (*broad complex, tram trac, and bric-a-brac*) genes with PLMs was also established independently at about the same time as the Stefansson study by Winkelmann and associates.[48] The *BTBD9* genes are localized to chromosome 6p. They are widely expressed in the amygdala, cerebellum, caudate nuclei, and the subthalamic nuclei. In *Drosophila melanogaster*, they are required for embryonic development, cell fate determination, metamorphosis, and pattern formation in the limbs.[48,49] Their role in humans is at this point unclear.

The association of iron deficiency with PLMs has also been well studied. Simakajornboon and colleagues[50] prospectively evaluated complete blood count, serum iron, and ferritin levels in a group of 39 children with a mean age of 7.5 years. Twenty-eight of 39 (71.8%) of the subjects had serum ferritin levels below 50 µg/L. The PLMI in subjects with serum ferritin levels below 50 µg/L was higher than in those with ferritin levels above 50 µg/L, though the trend did not reach statistical significance ($p = 0.09$). On the other hand, serum iron levels correlated significantly and inversely with PLMI those with serum iron levels less than 50 µg/L had higher PLMI (mean PLMI 42.8, ± 18.3) than did those with higher iron levels (mean PLMI 23.1, ± 10.1) ($p = 0.02$). Further, supplementation with iron increased the serum ferritin level and reduced the PLMI (Fig. 38-3). Iron is a co-factor for tyrosine hydroxylase, which serves as the rate-limiting step in the synthesis of dopamine. A deficiency of dopamine might underlie PLMD, just as it does in RLS. The favorable response of PLMs to treatment with dopamine receptor agonists further supports the assumption of an underlying dopamine deficiency state.[51]

Are there subtypes of PLMs? Clearly, there are subjects with increased PLMs who exhibit a concurrent sleep-related

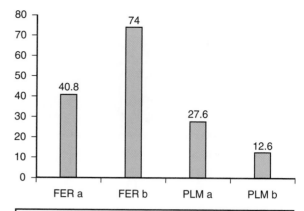

Fer a = serum ferritin (µg/mL) before iron therapy
Fer b = serum ferritin (µg/mL) after iron therapy
PLM a = periodic limb movement index before iron therapy
PLM b = periodic limb movement index after iron therapy

Figure 38-3 A comparison of serum ferritin levels and the periodic limb movement index in children before and after treatment with iron. There is an increase in values of the mean serum ferritin after treatment with iron and a corresponding decrease in the periodic limb movement index ($n = 25$). (Redrawn from Simakajornboon N, Gozal D, Vlasic V, et al. Periodic limb movements in sleep and iron status in children. *Sleep.* 2003;26(6):735-738.)

breathing disturbance. In mild OSA, coinciding with resolution of the respiratory disturbance, the periodic movements also seem to resolve.[52] In these patients, there is likely nonspecific activation by apnea or oxygen desaturation of the spinal CPGs that mediate stereotyped leg movements, with amelioration of the respiratory disturbance also lessening activation of CPG generators. On the other hand, when PLMs occur in the absence of somatic triggers, they are likely primary, linked to genetic factors or systemic iron deficiency.[46]

Another approach to classification based upon polysomnography has been to segregate PLMs into those with cortical arousals (PLMA) and without (PLMS). Although this method is often utilized in clinical practice, the significance is not clear. For instance, increases in heart rate and systolic and diastolic blood pressure that reflect activation of subcortical autonomic regions are observed in both PLMS and PLMA.[53,54] Larger, population-based studies are needed to determine whether PLMS/PLMA predispose to essential hypertension.

Diagnosis

PLMs can be readily recognized on nocturnal PSG. One needs to be aware of the night-to-night variability that might exist in the PLMI, especially in mild cases in which the index may fluctuate just below or above the cutoff of 5 movements per hour of sleep.[55] Sforza and associates[56] have developed an automated analysis using an ambulatory monitor. Using PSG as the standard, the sensitivity and specificity of this ambulatory device for PLMI greater than 10 was 0.88 and 0.76, respectively, with the receiver operator curve having an area under the curve of 0.86. With the ambulatory device, it is difficult to distinguish secondary PLMs, for example, those triggered by respiratory events, from those that are primary. Checking for reduced levels of serum ferritin—below 50 µg/L—should always be considered.

Treatment

Isolated PLMs are not associated with clinical symptoms, and thus do not need treatment. PLMD associated with systemic iron deficiency should be treated with iron supplementation. In older patients with refractory sleep-wake disturbance, dopamine receptor agonists can be used as in adults with PLMD, but with appropriate dosage adjustment and on an off-label basis (see Chapter 25). Because the treatment aspects are similar to those of RLS, they are dealt with in the next section of this chapter.

RESTLESS LEGS SYNDROME

RLS is a common presenting complaint among children who experience difficulty initiating or maintaining sleep. As previously stated, the condition is likely under-recognized in preschool and elementary school age-children because they are unable to clearly articulate the nature of their symptoms.

History

In 1832, Duchamp[57] observed that children may suffer aches and pains around puberty and labeled them as "growing pains." In 1994, Walters and associates[46] first described RLS in a mother and her three children aged 6, 4, and 1 years as well as a 16-year-old from an unrelated family. The disorder exhibited autosomal transmission. The patients experienced leg discomfort and nocturnal motor restlessness, with temporary relief by voluntary movement. Walters and associates[46] had also observed that children with RLS showed PLMS on nocturnal PSG.

Definition

The 2003 National Institutes of Health Consensus Conference recognized definite and probable forms of RLS.[58] The *definite* form consists of an urge to move the limbs that appears in the evening, worsening of the sensation with immobility, relief with movement, and presence of a sleep disturbance. The child must express the discomfort in his or her own words—often that means descriptive terms such as *owwies, ouchies,* or *tickles.* Owing to the subjective nature of the sleep complaints, a higher level of evidence needs to be established before making a definitive diagnosis. Unlike in adults, therefore, PSG documentation of more than five PLMs per hour of sleep is used as a diagnostic criterion. Owing to the autosomal dominant nature of the condition, a positive family history of RLS is also helpful in diagnosis.

The term *probable RLS* is applied when the patient meets some, but not all, of the diagnostic criteria. It is likely that *probable* and *definite* RLS define the same entity.

Prevalence

In a tertiary care sleep center, RLS constituted about 5% of the children seen.[59] In a large population-based survey of over 10,000 families from the United States and the United Kingdom, Picchietti and associates[60] observed an approximately 2% incidence. There may be higher prevalence in special populations; Chervin and associates[61] found that approximately 17% of hyperactive children had symptoms of coexisting RLS. The disorder seems equally common in boys and girls.

Pathophysiology

In adults, primary and secondary forms of RLS have been identified. In the primary form there is a strong genetic predisposition, onset is generally before age 45, and there are one or more close relatives also manifesting symptoms of RLS.[62] Cerebrospinal fluid levels of ferritin are also lower in adults with age of onset younger than 45 years.[63] In children with RLS, for reasons that are unclear, mothers have been found to be the affected parent more often than fathers.[59] Whether this represents a sampling artifact or indeed reflects an inherent predisposition is yet to be determined. Winkelmann and associates[64] carried out complex segregation analysis on 238 predominantly adult patients with RLS and 537 relatives. The lower end of the age range in their study was 12 years. They found that those with age of onset of symptoms below age 30 years most likely had autosomal dominant transmission with a multifactorial component. In those with onset after age 30 years, no genetic predisposition could be established. The role of environmental factors in influencing the development of RLS can also be gleaned from RLS studies on twins.[65] Ondo and associates[66] described the demographic, phenotypic, and serologic findings in 12 pairs of identical twins with RLS. A high concordance rate of 83% was seen, but the age of onset of symptoms varied markedly, which points to significant phenotypic variability. The genetics of RLS is closely linked with that of PLMs, which are found in about 80% of RLS subjects.

As in PLMD, the role of iron and dopamine deficiency is central in both primary and secondary forms of RLS.[67] Secondary RLS is diagnosed less often in childhood than in adults but may be associated with antipsychotic agents, antidepressant medications, pregnancy, lithium, peripheral neuropathy, uremia, and spinal cord lesions.[68-73] Systemic iron deficiency, manifested as a serum ferritin level below 50 µg/L, is observed in both primary and secondary forms of RLS. In a series of 32 children, Kotagal and Silber[59] found that 75% of subjects had low levels of serum ferritin. Chronic gastrointestinal disorders such as celiac disease, malabsorption syndromes, and (possibly) longstanding treatment of GER with proton pump inhibitors may also impair iron absorption.[74]

Gender and age are important determinants of the serum ferritin levels in adolescents, with reference values in females lower than those of age-matched males. In a longitudinal survey of dietary habits, physical activity, energy metabolism, iron status, and body composition, in Sweden, Samuelson and associates[75] reported that the mean serum ferritin level was lower in both boys and girls at age 15 than at age 17 years. For boys, the means serum ferritin level at age 15 was 36.3 µg/L (SD = 17.8; $n = 103$) while at age 17 the mean serum ferritin level was 53.6 µg/L (SD = 32.8, $n = 103$). For girls, the mean serum ferritin level at age 15 was 30 µg/L (SD = 19, $n = 124$) while at 17 years it had risen to 33 µg/L (SD = 30.6, $n = 124$). Unfortunately age and gender differences in serum ferritin have not been adequately considered in the study of childhood RLS and PLMD.

There is close correspondence between the serum and intracellular levels of ferritin level and total body iron stores. There is however no correlation between serum ferritin and hematologic indices of iron deficiency (low hemoglobin, hematocrit, and red blood cell mean corpuscular volume) as ferritin levels have to generally drop below 10 µg/L before bone marrow stores of iron are affected.[75,76]

The sensory discomfort in RLS appears to be mediated at the level of the central nervous system (brain or spinal cord) and less likely in the peripheral nerves. In a study of 10 adults with idiopathic RLS (mean time since disease onset 11.4 years), Tyvaert and associates[77] did not find evidence of disturbance of A delta or C small fibers or the spinothalamic tracts. Increased central sensitization to pain is likely with iron deficiency. Compared to mice fed on a normal diet, iron-deficient mice seem to show increased responses when exposed to a hot plate or to formalin. The increased responses were of expression of c-Fos immunoreactivity at the level of the dorsal horns of the spinal cord, suggesting increased activity of this pain-mediating region.[78] Activation of the spinal cord may activate the central pattern generators as well, which manifests clinically in the form of periodic limb movements.[79]

Clinical Features

Sleep Initiation and Maintenance Difficulty

Onset of the symptoms may be during infancy or early childhood[59] (Box 38-1). Parents may find that only rocking or patting the infant provides relief, thus sometimes giving a misleading impression of a behavioral insomnia of childhood, sleep onset association type.

Sensation of Discomfort

The school age child may complain of a creeping or crawling feeling or similar uncomfortable sensations in either the upper or lower extremities that is worse while resting and relieved partially by movement. Leading questions may need to be asked in order to extract this history. Some younger children may be able to provide graphic depictions of the sensory disturbance through drawing (as mentioned previously in the section on nightmares).[80]

NREM Sleep Parasomnias

The sensory discomfort of periodic limb movements accompanying RLS may trigger partial arousals that can be manifested clinically as sleepwalking or confusional arousals.

Nonrestorative Sleep

The child may awaken in the morning feeling tired and unrefreshed, probably on account of increased fragmentation of night sleep from RLS

Neurobehavioral Disturbance

Attention deficit hyperactivity disorder (ADHD) may coexist with RLS,[59] and the child with RLS may also experience difficulty sitting still in the afternoon in the classroom owing to an overwhelming urge to move the limbs. In such cases, treatment of ADHD with psychostimulants may only lead to a partial improvement in symptoms such as inattention and hyperactivity; however, after successful treatment of RLS symptoms, there may be additional improvement.

Periodic Limb Movements

A PSG will demonstrate PLMs in a majority of children with RLS. As described earlier, PLMS should be distinguished from PLMD. PLMS are an epiphenomenon, not accompanied a feeling of nonrestorative sleep, whereas PLMD is indeed associated with a sleep disturbance, especially feeling tired upon awakening in the morning.

BOX 38-1 *Diagnostic Criteria for Adult and Childhood Restless Legs Syndrome (RLS)*

Essential Diagnostic Criteria for Adult RLS
1. An urge to move the legs, usually accompanied or caused by uncomfortable and unpleasant sensations in the legs
2. The urge to move or unpleasant sensations begin or worsen during periods of rest or inactivity such as lying down or sitting
3. The urge to move or unpleasant sensations are partially or totally relieved by movement, such as walking or stretching, at least as long as the activity continues
4. The urge to move or unpleasant sensations are worse in the evening or night than during the day, or only occur during the evening or night

Definite Childhood RLS
1. The child meets all four essential adult criteria, *and*
2. The child relates a description in his or her own words that is consistent with leg discomfort

OR

The child meets all four essential adult criteria *and* has two or three of the following:
1. Sleep disturbance for age
2. Biologic parent or sibling with definite RLS
3. Polysomnographically documented periodic limb movement index of 5 or more per hour of sleep

Probable Childhood RLS
1. The child meets all four essential adult criteria for RLS except criterion 4 (the urge to move or sensations are worse in the evening or at night than during the day), *and*
2. The child has a biologic parent or sibling with definite RLS

OR

1. The child is observed to have behavioral manifestations of lower extremity discomfort when sitting or lying, accompanied by motor movement of the affected limbs; the discomfort has characteristics of adult criteria 2,3, and 4, *and*
2. The child has a biologic parent or sibling with definite RLS

Adapted from Allen RP, Picchietti D, Hening WA, et al. Restless legs syndrome: Diagnostic criteria, special considerations, and epidemiology. A report from the restless legs syndrome diagnosis and epidemiology workshop at the National Institutes of Health. *Sleep Med.* 2003;4(2): 101-119.

RLS Severity Scale Value

Although the subjective nature of the symptoms and the variable expressive ability of children have posed difficulty in the development of a validated severity scale for children, such a scale has recently been developed through a multicenter study conducted by pediatric RLS experts with publication in late 2010.[80]

Diagnosis

In older children, the diagnosis can be established on clinical grounds alone, but nocturnal polysomnography might be needed for documentation of periodic limb movements in children below the age of 8 to 10 years who are not good historians. Some PLMs are associated with cortical arousals, whereas others are not. There is no data in children to support the likelihood that PLMs associated with arousal manifest greater morbidity than PLMs without arousal. When scoring PLMs, it is important to exclude leg movements that may due to a sleep-related breathing disturbance.

The serum ferritin level should be checked in all patients with suspected RLS, with levels below 50 μg/L having an association with RLS/PLMD.[43,59] A caveat about ferritin testing is the fact that this acute phase reactant may be spuriously elevated when there is coexisting systemic inflammation or fever. In such instances, one can resort to checking the serum-soluble transferrin, which is not impacted by acute illness, and shows elevation with iron deficiency.

Management

All treatment measures for childhood onset RLS are based upon empiric observations. The lack of a validated scale for assessing RLS severity has hindered conducting rigorous clinical trials. Iron supplementation is a key empiric treatment measure, however. In infants and young children who are unable to swallow tablets, liquid oral iron preparations such as ferrous sulfate drops, 15 mg/mL can be provided in a dose of 1 mL once or twice a day. The treatment needs to be continued for a few months till the serum ferritin level has risen above 50 μg/L.[43,50] It is important to indicate to the parent or guardian that improvement in sleep-wake function will be slow, and might take many weeks. Side effects of oral iron therapy include constipation and abdominal discomfort. The discomfort can be minimized by providing the medication with food. A bulk laxative may be needed for constipation. For iron supplementation in older children, tablet formulations can be used, such as ferrous sulfate or ferrous gluconate, 200 mg, once or twice a day with food. Monitoring of serum ferritin levels every 2 to 3 months is recommended during the period of iron therapy until the serum ferritin level has risen above 50 μg/L. Contraindications to systemic iron therapy have not been definitively established, but might include a family history of hemachromatosis or mitochondrial disorders.

Gabapentin, 50 to 100 mg at bedtime, has been helpful in alleviating the uncomfortable sensory disturbance. This finding has been confirmed in a randomized controlled trial in adults.[81] The response is likely related to the antineuropathic pain effects of the medication.

Dopamine receptor agonists such as pramipexole or ropinirole can be prescribed in refractory cases, especially if the patient is a young adult or teenager.[43,59] The usual dose is 0.125 to 0.5 mg of pramipexole or 0.25 to 0.75 mg of ropinirole. Potential side effects include nausea, sudden onset of sleep, hallucinations, and the development of compulsive behaviors such as tics. A positive family history of melanoma may be a relative contraindication to using these agents.

Nonpharmacologic measures such as exercise in the evening should also be stressed because anecdotal reports suggest they may have a salutary effect upon RLS symptoms.

Conclusion

The discovery of a link between the *BTBD9* homeobox gene complex and periodic limb movements was a significant milestone in sleep medicine.[47,48] It will likely spur large population-based, whole-genome analysis-based searches for genetic markers of other rhythmic or automatic nocturnal phenomena such as bruxism and sleepwalking.[4] As we move from phenomenology to physiology, the central role played by central pattern generators in pathogenesis of many parasomnias may receive more attention. Study of biophysiologic markers of unstable sleep such as cyclic alternating patterns seen on polysomnography may gain more acceptance among sleep clinicians.[79] The publication of a validated scale for assessing the severity of restless legs syndrome in children will facilitate clinical trials in children with this disorder.[80] Do children outgrow RLS? This question remains unanswered.

REFERENCES

1. Klackenberg G. Incidence of parasomnias in children in a general population. In: Guilleminault C, ed. *Sleep and Its Disorders in Children*. New York: Raven Press; 1987:99-113.
2. Petit D, Touchette E, Tremblay RE, et al. Dyssomnias and parasomnias in early childhood. *Pediatrics*. 2007;119:e1016-e1025.
3. Mahowald MW, Schenck CH. Dissociated states of wakefulness and sleep. *Neurology*. 1992;42(suppl 6):44-51.
4. Kotagal S. Parasomnias in childhood. *Sleep Med Rev*. 2009;13(2):157-168.
5. Grillner S, Wallen P, Saitoh K, et al. Neural bases of goal directed locomotion in vertebrates—An overview. *Brain Res Rev*. 2008;57(1):2-12.
6. Cazalets JR, Sqalli-Houssaini Y, Clarac F. Activation of the central pattern generators for locomotion by serotonin and excitatory amino acids in neonatal rats. *J Physiol*. 1992;455(9):187-204.
7. Gezelius H, Wallen-Mackenzie A, Enjin A, et al. Role of glutamate in locomotor rhythm generating neural circuitry. *J Physiol (Paris)*. 2006;100 (5-6):297-303.
8. American Academy of Sleep Medicine. Sleep starts. In: *The International Classification of Sleep Disorders: Diagnostic and Coding Manual*, 2nd ed. Westchester, IL: American Academy of Sleep Medicine; 2005:208-210.
9. Fusco L, Pachatz C, Cusmai R, et al. Repetitive sleep starts in neurologically impaired children. An unusual non-epileptic manifestation in otherwise epileptic subjects. *Epileptic Disord*. 1999;1:63-67.
10. Mason TBA, Pack AJ. Pediatric parasomnias. In: Marcus CL, Carroll JL, Donnely DF, Loughlin GM, eds. *Sleep in Children*. New York: Informa Healthcare; 2008:223-241.
11. Otto M, Simon NM, Powers M, et al. Rates of isolated sleep paralysis in outpatients with anxiety disorders. *J Anxiety Disord*. 2006;20(5):687-693.
12. Sheldon SH. Parasomnias in childhood. *Pediatr Clin North Am*. 2004;51(1):69-88.
13. Stores G. Parasomnias of childhood and adolescence. *Sleep Med Clin*. 2007;2:405-417.
14. Kotagal S. Parasomnias of childhood. *Curr Opin Pediatr*. 2008;20(6): 659-665.
15. Bruni O, Ferri R, Novelli L, et al. NREM sleep instability in children with sleep terrors: The role of slow-wave interruptions. *Clin Neurophysiol*. 2008;119(9):985-992.
16. Rosen GM, Mahowald MW. Disorders of arousal in children. In: Sheldon SH, Ferber R, Kryger MH, eds. *Principles and Practice of Pediatric Sleep Medicine*. Philadelphia: Elsevier Saunders; 2005:293-304.
17. Aridon P, Marini C, Di Resta C, et al. Increased sensitivity of the neuronal nicotinic receptor alpha 2 subunits causes familial epilepsy with nocturnal wandering and ictal fear. *Am J Hum Genet*. 2006;79(2):342-359.
18. Steinlein OK, Mulley JC, Propping P, et al. A missense mutation in the neuronal nicotinic acetylcholine receptor alpha 4 subunit is associated with autosomal dominant nocturnal frontal lobe epilepsy. *Nat Genet*. 1995;11(2):201-203.
19. Diaz-Otero F, Quesada M, Morales-Cirraliza J, et al. Autosomal dominant nocturnal frontal lobe epilepsy with a mutation in the CHRNB2 gene. *Epilepsia*. 2008;49(3):516-520.
20. Tinuper P, Provini F, Bisulli F, et al. Movements in sleep guidelines for differentiating sleep from nonepileptic motor phenomena arising from sleep. *Sleep Med Rev*. 2007;11(4):255-267.
21. Nobili L. Nocturnal frontal lobe epilepsy and non rapid eye movement sleep parasomnias: Differences and similarities. Guest editorial. *Sleep Med Rev*. 2007;11(4):251-254.
22. Pelayo R, Dubik M. Pediatric sleep pharmacology. *Semin Pediatr Neurol*. 2008;15(2):79-90.
23. Johnson MC, Lerner M. Amelioration of infant sleep disturbances: Effects of scheduled awakenings by compliant parents. *Infant Ment Health J*. 1985;6:21-30.
24. Tobin JD. Treatment of somnambulism with anticipatory awakening. *J Pediatr*. 1991;122:426-427.

25. Walters AS. Clinical identification of simple sleep-related movement disorders. *Chest*. 2007;131(4):1260-1266.

26. Ramelli GP, Sozzo AB, Vella S, et al. Benign neonatal sleep myoclonus: An under-recognized, non-epileptic condition. *Acta Pediatr*. 2005;94(7): 962-963.

27. The International Classification of Sleep Disorders. *Diagnostic and Coding Manual*. 2nd ed. Westchester, IL: American Academy of Sleep Medicine; 2005.

28. Bjordvand H, Lindeman FO. Våre Arveord. Oslo: Novus; 2007.

29. Powell N. *Fuseli: The Nightmare*. London: Allen Lane; 1973.

30. Sadeh A. Cognitive behavioral treatment for childhood sleep disorders. *Clin Psychol Rev*. 2005;25(5):612-628.

31. Halliday G. Treating nightmares in children. In: Schafer CE, ed. *Clinical Handbook of Sleep Disorders in Children*. Northvale, NJ: Aronson; 1995:149-175.

32. Hauri PJ, Silber MH, Boeve BF. The treatment of parasomnias with hypnosis: A 5-year follow-up study. *J Clin Sleep Med*. 2007;3(4):369-373.

33. Mahowald MW, Schenck CH. Insights from studying human sleep disorders. *Nature*. 2005;437(7063):1279-1285.

34. Nevsimalova S, Prihodiva I, Kemlink D, et al. REM behavior disorder (RBD) can be one of the first symptoms of childhood narcolepsy. *Sleep Med*. 2007;8(7-8):784-786.

35. Schenck CH, Mahowald MW. Motor dyscontrol in narcolepsy: Rapid-eye-movement (REM) sleep without atonia and REM sleep behavior disorder. *Ann Neurol*. 1992;32(1):3-10.

36. Stores G. Rapid eye movement sleep behaviour disorder in children and adolescents. *Dev Med Child Neurol*. 2008;50(10):728-732.

37. Iber C, Ancoli-Israel S, Chesson A, Quan SFfor the American Academy of Sleep Medicine. *The AASM Manual for the Scoring of Sleep and Associated Events: Rules, Terminology, and Technical Specifications*. 1st ed. Westchester, IL: American Academy of Sleep Medicine; 2007.

38 Coleman RM, Pollack C, Weitzman ED. Periodic movements in sleep (nocturnal myoclonus): Relation to sleep-wake disorders. *Ann Neurol*. 1980;8(4):416-421.

39. Kirk VG, Bohn S. Periodic limb movements in children: Prevalence in a referred population. *Sleep*. 2004;27(2):313-315.

40. Crabtree VM, Ivanenko A, O'Brien LM, et al. Periodic limb movement disorder of sleep in children. *J Sleep Res*. 2003;12(1):73-81.

41. Chervin RD, Archbold KH. Hyperactivity and polysomnographic findings in children evaluated for sleep disordered breathing. *Sleep*. 2001;24(3):313-320.

42. Scofield H, Roth T, Drake C. Periodic limb movements during sleep: Population prevalence, clinical correlates and racial differences. *Sleep*. 2008;31(9):1221-1227.

43. Picchietti MA, Picchietti DL. Restless legs syndrome and periodic limb movement disorder in children and adolescents. *Semin Pediatr Neurol*. 2008;15(2):91-99.

44. Cramer NP, Keller A. The whisking rhythm generator: A novel mammalian network for the generation of movement. *J Neurophysiol*. 2007;97(3):2148-2158.

45. Mor Y. Analysis of rhythmic patterns produced by spinal neural networks. *J Neurophysiol*. 2007;98(5):2807-2817.

46. Walters AS, Picchietti DL, Ehrenberg BL, Wagner ML. Restless legs syndrome in childhood and adolescence. *Pediatr Neurol*. 1994;11(3): 241-245.

47. Stefansson H, Rye DB, Hicks A, Petursson H, et al. A genetic risk factor for periodic limb movements in sleep. *N Engl J Med*. 2007;357(7): 639-647.

48. Winkelmann J, Schormair B, Lichtner P, Ripke S, et al. Genome-wide association study of restless legs syndrome identifies common variants in three genomic regions. *Nat Genet*. 2007;39(8):1000-1006.

49. Chu J, Dong PD, Panganiban G. Limb type-specification of bric a brac contributes to morphologic diversity. *Development*. 2002;129(3):695-704.

50. Simakajornboon N, Gozal D, Vlasic V, et al. Periodic limb movements in sleep and iron status in children. *Sleep*. 2003;26(6):735-738.

51. Manconi M, Ferri R, Feroah TR, et al. Defining the boundaries of the response of sleep leg movements to a single dose of dopamine agonist. *Sleep*. 2008;31(9):1229-1237.

52. Baran AS, Richert AC, Douglas AB, et al. Change in periodic limb movement index during treatment of obstructive sleep apnea with continuous positive airway pressure. *Sleep*. 2003;26(6):717-720.

53. Siddiqui F, Strus JM, Lee IA, et al. Rise of blood pressure with periodic limb movements in sleep and wakefulness. *Clin Neurophysiol*. 2007;118(9):1923-1930.

54. Walters AS, Rye DB. Review of the relationship of restless legs syndrome and periodic limb movements in sleep to hypertension, heart disease and stroke. *Sleep*. 2009;32(5):589-597.

55. Picchietti MA, Picchietti DL, England SJ, et al. Children show individual night to night variability of periodic limb movements in sleep. *Sleep*. 2009;32(4):530-535.

56. Sforza E, Johannes M, Claudio B. The PAM-RL ambulatory device for detection of periodic leg movements: A validation study. *Sleep Med*. 2005;6(5):407-413.

57. Duchamp M. Maladies de la croissance. In: Levrault FG, ed. *Memories de Medicine Practique*. Paris: Jean-Frederic Lobstein; 1832.

58. Allen RP, Picchietti D, Hening WA, et al. Restless legs syndrome: Diagnostic criteria, special considerations, and epidemiology. A report from the restless legs syndrome diagnosis and epidemiology workshop at the National Institutes of Health. *Sleep Med*. 2003;4(2):101-119.

59. Kotagal S, Silber MH. Childhood-onset restless legs syndrome. *Ann Neurol*. 2004;56(6):803-807.

60. Picchietti D, Allen RP, Walters AS, et al. Restless legs syndrome: Prevalence and impact in children and adolescents. The Peds REST study. *Pediatrics*. 2007;120(2):253-266.

61. Chervin RD, Hedger-Archbold K, Dillon JE, et al. Associations between symptoms of inattention, hyperactivity, restless legs, and periodic limb movements. *Sleep*. 2002;25(2):213-218.

62. Allen RP, Buda MC, Becker P, et al. Family history study of the restless legs syndrome. *Sleep Med*. 2002(Suppl 3):S3-S7.

63. Early CJ, Connor JR, Beard JL, et al. Ferritin levels in the cerebrospinal fluid and restless legs syndrome: Effects of different clinical phenotypes. *Sleep*. 2005;28(9):1069-1075.

64. Winkelmann J, Muller-Myhsok B, Wittchen HU, et al. Complex segregation analysis of restless legs syndrome provides evidence for an autosomal dominant mode of inheritance in early at onset families. *Ann Neurol*. 2002;52(3):297-302.

65. Rao S, Winkelmann J, Wang QK. Genetics of restless legs syndrome. In: Ondo WG, ed. *Restless Legs Syndrome: Diagnosis and Treatment*. New York: Informa Healthcare; 2007:111-123.

66. Ondo WG, Vuong KD, Wang Q. Restless legs syndrome in monozygotic twins: Clinical correlates. *Neurology*. 2000;55(9):1404-1406.

67. Ondo WG. Iron deficiency associated restless legs syndrome. In: Ondo WG, ed. *Restless Legs Syndrome: Diagnosis and Treatment*. New York: Informa Healthcare; 2007:211-218.

68. Kavanaugh D, Siddiqui S, Gedds CC. Restless legs syndrome in patients on dialysis. *Am J Kidney Dis*. 2004;43(5):763-771.

69. Gemignani F, Marbini A. Restless legs syndrome and peripheral neuropathy. *J Neurol Neurosurg Psychiatry*. 2002;72(4):555.

70. Mindell JA, Jacobson BJ. Sleep disturbances during pregnancy. *J Obstet Gynecol Neonat Nurs*. 2000;29(6):590-597.

71. Wetter TC, Brunner J, Bronisch T. Restless legs syndrome probably induced by risperidone treatment. *Pharmacopsychiatry*. 2002;35(3): 109-111.

72. Hargrave R, Beckley DJ. Restless legs syndrome exacerbated by sertraline. *Psychosomatics*. 1998;39(2):177-178.

73. Brown LK, Heffner JE, Obbens EA. Transverse myelitis associated with restless legs syndrome and periodic movements of sleep responsive to an oral dopaminergic agent but not to intrathecal baclofen. *Sleep*. 2000;23(5):591-594.

74. Paul SP, Taylor TM, Barnard P. Severe iron deficiency as a manifestation of celiac disease: A case report and literature review. *J Family Health Care*. 2010;20(2):56-59.

75. Samuelson G, Lonnerdal B, Kempe B, et al. A follow-up study of serum ferritin and transferrin receptor concentrations in Swedish adolescents at age 17 years compared to age 15. *Acta Pediatr*. 2000;89(10):1162-1168.

76. Harrison PM, Arosio P. The ferritins: Molecular properties, iron storage function and cellular regulation. *Biochem Biophys Acta*. 1996;1275(3): 161-203.

77. Tyvaert L, Lareau E, Hurtevent JP, et al. A-delta and C-fibers function in primary restless legs syndrome. *Neurophysiol Clin*. 2009;39(6):267-274.

78. Dowling P, Klinker F, Amaya F, et al. Iron deficiency sensitizes mice to acute pain stimuli and formalin induced nociception. *J Nutr*. 2009;139(11):2087-2092.

79. Tassinari CA, Cantalupo G, Hogl B, et al. Neuroethological approach to frontolimbic epileptic seizures and parasomnias: The same central pattern generators for the same behaviors. *Rev Neurol*. 2009;165(10): 762-768.

80. Arbuckle R, Abetz L, Durmer JS, et al. The development of the Pediatric Restless Legs Syndrome Severity Scale (P-RLS-SS): A patient reported outcome measure of pediatric RLS symptoms and impact for sleep medicine. *Sleep Med*. 2010;11(9):897-906.

81. Garcia-Borreguero D, Larossa O, de la Llave O, et al. Treatment of restless legs syndrome with gabapentin: A double blind cross-over study. *Neurology*. 2002;59(10):1573-1579.

Narcolepsy in Children

SHANNON S. SULLIVAN / RAFAEL PELAYO

Chapter 39

THERAPY IN SLEEP MEDICINE

The evaluation and treatment of a sleepy child can be very challenging. Sleepiness may be due simply to sleep deprivation from poor habits or it can be caused by a life-threatening brain tumor; thus, there is a wide range of diagnostic possibilities with little room for diagnostic error. Thankfully, a thorough history, careful physical examination, and appropriate laboratory studies should narrow this range and allow for accurate diagnosis and prompt initiation of proper treatment. Circadian, behavioral, respiratory, and sleep hygiene issues are discussed in other chapters. This chapter will review the pediatric presentation and management of narcolepsy.

NARCOLEPSY

Narcolepsy is a chronic neurologic disorder in which the boundaries between the awake, sleeping, and dreaming brain are blurred. It is characterized by excessive daytime sleepiness, disturbed nocturnal sleep, and cataplexy, as well as by other pathologic manifestations related to rapid eye movement (REM) sleep such as hypnagogic/hypnopompic hallucinations and sleep paralysis. The human form of this disease is caused by the loss of 70,000 or so hypothalamic neurons that produce the neuropeptide variously named hypocretin or orexin.[1-3] Both sporadic and familial forms exist in humans, with the sporadic form much more common (95%).[4]

The disease is associated with human leukocyte antigen (HLA) allele DQB1*0602.[5-7] Like other HLA-associated diseases, the cause of narcolepsy is likely autoimmune, which is supported by recent work showing that hypocretin deficiency is highly associated with certain T-cell receptor alpha polymorphisms and that *Streptococcus* infections are possible triggers for narcolepsy.[8,9] Immunizations against H1N1 flu have been associated with narcolepsy predominately in Europe.[10] Narcolepsy patients have been found to have higher serum levels of immune complexes of autoantibodies directed against hypocretin.[11] Specific autoantibodies have also been found to appear close in time to the onset of cataplexy.[12-14] Further discussion can be found in Chapter 22.

Clinical Characteristics

The cardinal features of narcolepsy-cataplexy are daytime somnolence, cataplexy, sleep paralysis, and hypnagogic hallucinations.[15] Not all four of these symptoms are necessarily present in all patients. In addition, all of these symptoms—with the exception of cataplexy—can be seen in association with other sleep disorders or sleep deprivation. The latter is a particular clinical concern among adolescents. The primary features of narcolepsy-cataplexy syndrome are listed in Box 39-1.

Daytime sleepiness in narcolepsy may be described as a feeling of being sleep deprived, excessively fatigued, or "run down," or it may present as unwanted episodes of sleep (*sleep attacks*) during the day. Narcoleptic patients typically wake up in the morning or after naps feeling more refreshed, and there is a refractory period until sleepiness again mounts.

Cataplexy is an abrupt and reversible decrease or loss of muscle tone, most frequently provoked by strong emotion, such as laughter.[16] Consciousness remains intact during the episodes, which typically last 30 seconds to 2 minutes. Cataplexy may involve certain or most voluntary muscles (although the diaphragm and muscles of eye movements are spared). Most commonly the jaw sags, the head falls forward, the arms drop to the side, and the knees buckle. The severity and extent of cataplectic attacks can range from a state of absolute powerlessness, which seems to involve the entire body, to little more than a fleeting sensation of weakness. Uncommonly, cataplectic attacks involve complete loss of muscle tone, which may result in falls and possible injuries. The attacks may also be too subtle to be noticed by an observer. *Status cataplecticus* is a rare presentation in which an episode of cataplexy lasts hours.

Sleepiness is typically the first symptom to develop in the child, with the onset of cataplexy following within the next 5 years in two thirds of cases. However, in one report by Aran and associates[17] of an analysis of 51 cases of pediatric narcolepsy-cataplexy, cataplexy reportedly occurred within 2 months of onset of sleepiness 82% of the time, with similar data for pre-, peri-, and postpubertal subgroups. In this particular series the onset of cataplexy was quite rapid; longer intervals are usually seen clinically. Although sleepiness typically appears first, in up to 15% of children cataplexy, sleep paralysis, or hypnagogic hallucinations is the presenting symptom.

Certain features of narcolepsy may be classified as REM sleep phenomena that occur at the transitions to and from sleep. *Hypnagogic hallucinations* reflect dreaming that occurs just prior to sleep onset while the person still feels awake; *hypnopompic hallucinations* are similar but occur during awakening. The hallucinations may be visual or auditory. *Sleep paralysis* is a true inability to move, speak, or exert voluntary control over certain muscles (as normally occurs in REM sleep). It too occurs at the transition to and from sleep, possibly (but not necessarily) in association with hallucinations. Individuals typically describe this feeling of paralysis at

> **BOX 39-1** *CHESS: A Mnemonic for the Cardinal Symptoms of Narcolepsy-Cataplexy Syndrome*
>
> **C**ataplexy
> **H**ypnagogic hallucinations
> **E**xcessive daytime sleepiness
> **S**leep attacks
> **S**leep paralysis

least as disconcerting if not actually terrifying. During these events, individuals are fully aware of what is happening, and events typically last up to a few minutes. In pediatric narcolepsy-cataplexy patients, 66% report hypnagogic hallucinations and 55% report sleep paralysis (however, for children with postpubertal onset, these numbers are 89% and 78%).[17] The symptoms of hypnagogic hallucinations, hypnopompic hallucinations, and sleep paralysis may, on occasion, be experienced in non-narcolepsy conditions, even in otherwise completely normal individuals. Up to 5% of the general population may have had episodes of sleep paralysis.

Excessive weight gain may be a symptom present at onset of narcolepsy-cataplexy; in the series of 51 pediatric cases at Stanford University, 86% gained at least 4 kg within 6 months of the appearance of symptoms.[17] Other clinical features that have been reported with narcolepsy-cataplexy include gestural, ambulatory, or speech automatisms, disturbed nighttime sleep—possibly punctuated by periodic limb movements or motor activity suggestive of a REM sleep behavior disorder (see Chapter 43) — and secondary impairments in school, work, or social function. If patients are seen soon after symptom onset, it may be possible to obtain a history of a preceding streptococcal throat infection (as reported recently by Longstreth and associates).[18]

Because symptoms may begin gradually in younger populations, even with increased attention it may be several years before the diagnosis is made. Along the way, young individuals in particular may be misdiagnosed with seizures, attention deficit problems, or behavior problems.[19-21] However, not all sleepiness is narcolepsy-cataplexy. In a series of 125 children with a complaint of hypersomnolence reported by Vendrame and colleagues,[22] 72% had sleep disordered breathing and 17% had delayed sleep phase syndrome; only 16% had narcolepsy (defined by the mean sleep latency test, as discussed later in the Diagnosis section), and only three individuals had narcolepsy-cataplexy.

Epidemiology

The prevalence of narcolepsy is about 1 per 2000 of the general population.[23] Age at onset varies from early childhood to the fifth decade, but there is a peak in the second decade; thus, symptoms most commonly begin in childhood or early adolescence.[24] An early report observed that about half of patients had onset prior to age 15, with less than 10% prior to age 5.[25] More recently, researchers at the *Stanford Center for Narcolepsy* found, after reviewing of 1219 cases of narcolepsy, that although only 10% of these patients were younger than 18 years of age at the time of evaluation, 40% reported symptom onset before the age of 15 years, and 2.1% had onset before the age of 5. Only 1.1% had cataplexy before age 5.[17]

Thus, the time from symptom onset to diagnosis can be quite long. Early reports described a median delay between onset and diagnosis of greater than 10 years.[26] However, with increased awareness of, and more focused attention to, this disorder, cases are being diagnosed with less delay: in a recent series of children with narcolepsy-cataplexy, diagnosis was commonly made less than 2 years from symptom onset.[17]

Diagnosis

To diagnose narcolepsy-cataplexy in a child clinically (i.e., without supportive laboratory study), there must be three elements: sleepiness (by patient or family report), absence of other disorders (medical or sleep) that could cause sleepiness, and presence of clear-cut cataplexy. Cataplexy, considered the *sine qua non* for a clinical diagnosis of narcolepsy-cataplexy, may be hard to recognize in children in general and in young subjects in particular. A recent report by Serra and associates[27] emphasized that cataplexy can be polymorphic and difficult to diagnose close to sleep onset. Unless cataplexy is unequivocally present, an overnight polysomnogram followed by daytime multiple sleep latency test (MSLT) is necessary to establish the diagnosis. In practice, these studies are probably indicated even if cataplexy is present because narcolepsy is a life-long condition. Cataplexy is usually diagnosed only by report, and all uncertainty in diagnosis should be eliminated as much as possible.

The overnight polysomnogram should last at least 6 hours and confirm that no other sleep disorders are present or untreated. The MSLT is a daytime study, usually done following the polysomnogram, whereby the patient is recorded polygraphically during four or five nap opportunities at 2-hour intervals; the number of sleep periods, the mean latency to sleep, and the number of REM periods that occur are documented. An MSLT with a mean sleep latency (MSL) of up to 8 minutes plus two or more sleep onset REM periods (or SOREMPs, defined as periods of REM sleep within 20 minutes of sleep onset) is considered to be consistent with the diagnosis of narcolepsy;[28] however, there is ongoing debate about the diagnostic certainty of MSLT results. Some patients with sleep-disordered breathing have been shown to have MSLT results similar to those of narcoleptics,[29] and occasionally even normal subjects can have two or more SOREMPs, even without clinical symptoms of sleepiness.[30,31] Additionally, not all patients with clinically certain narcolepsy meet MSLT criteria for that diagnosis.[32,33] Finally, despite the routine use of the MSLT in the workup of pediatric patients with suspected narcolepsy, the test has not been validated for those younger than 8 years of age.[28] Recent pediatric data show that in prepubertal children with undetectable cerebrospinal fluid (CSF) hypocretin and *bona fide* cataplexy (i.e., certain narcolepsy), MSLT is less likely to be positive than in older children, and may even be in the normal range (MSLT > 8 minutes, no SOREMPs) when studied within a year after onset of symptoms.[17] Although every effort should be made to discontinue all medications that may affect MSLT results, starting at least 2 weeks or 4 half-lives prior to the study, as a practical matter this is not always possible (e.g., in youngsters being treated for seizures or depression). For all of these reasons, caution must be used in MSLT interpretation, and a diagnosis of narcolepsy must not be made based on MSLT results alone. One must carefully consider presenting clinical features, sleep and nonsleep co-morbidities, medications, and (when needed) adjunctive testing as described below.

Other electrophysiologic and imaging studies, such as electroencephalogram (EEG) and magnetic resonance imaging (MRI), are not typically abnormal in primary narcolepsy (but may have been performed as part of prior workup to rule out other disorders). However, certain additional nonelectrophysiologic testing has become available in recent years that may be useful in the workup of sleepy patients in whom the diagnosis of narcolepsy is suspected but still uncertain.

Genetic testing can aid in the process of establishing (or helping to rule out) the diagnosis of narcolepsy-cataplexy. HLA DQB1*0602 is the most specific genetic marker for narcolepsy across all ethnic groups. Almost all patients with narcolepsy-cataplexy are positive for HLA subtype DQB1*0602, compared to 40% of those with narcolepsy without cataplexy and 12% to 25% in most control populations.[28] An HLA-negative result, therefore, can help rule out the possibility of narcolepsy-cataplexy, although not narcolepsy without cataplexy (see later discussion).

The discovery of hypocretin/orexin, a neuropeptide important for stabilizing sleep-wake states, in CSF has led to further characterization of narcolepsy in the last decade. Although two subtypes of the hypocretin neuropeptide are known, hypocretin-1 has been shown to be deficient in the human form of narcolepsy-cataplexy. Lumbar puncture to obtain CSF for hypocretin-1 measurement may be used in certain cases to confirm the diagnosis of narcolepsy-cataplexy.[34,35] CSF hypocretin-1 levels below 110 ng/L have a high positive predictive value (94%) for narcolepsy with cataplexy.[35,36] The major limitations of this test are that it involves an invasive procedure (lumbar puncture) and testing is not yet widely available (currently it is generally available only in certain research settings). To date, no serologic or salivary testing is available for hypocretin-1.

The International Classification of Sleep Disorders-2 (ICSD-2) includes diagnostic categories for both narcolepsy with cataplexy (the classic form of the disorder) and narcolepsy without cataplexy (with sleepiness and short MSLT sleep latencies but without [yet] the existence of the cardinal symptom of cataplexy).[28] It is not fully clear to what extent these two diagnostic categories have similar, overlapping, or differing pathophysiologic underpinnings of disease. Around 10% of cases of narcolepsy without (yet demonstrating) cataplexy have low hypocretin levels in the CSF (< 110 pg/mL); almost all of these individuals are HLA DQB1*0602 positive. On the other hand, HLA DQB1*0602 negative cases of narcolepsy without cataplexy almost always have normal hypocretin levels.[28]

Secondary Narcolepsy

In addition to the classic form of narcolepsy-cataplexy, for which evidence continues to grow suggesting etiologic autoimmune destruction of specialized hypocretin-producing neurons in the hypothalamus, secondary forms of the disorder have also been reported; and the ICSD-2 includes the diagnostic category of narcolepsy (with or without cataplexy) secondary to a medical condition.[28] Medical disorders that have been shown to be associated with *bona fide* cataplexy include lesions of the hypothalamus (tumors, multiple sclerosis plaques, sarcoidosis), paraneoplastic syndrome with anti-Ma2 antibodies, Neimann-Pick type C disease, and possibly Coffin-Lowry syndrome. Challamel and associates reported a high frequency of secondary cases in their series of

97 cases of pediatric narcolepsy: 12 had Niemann-Pick type C, a disorder associated with cataplexy; 2 had diencephalic tumors; and 2 had unspecified neurologic abnormalities.[37] In a meta-analysis of 116 symptomatic cases of secondary narcolepsy with excessive daytime sleepiness (EDS), reduced CSF hypocretin-1 was found in most; however, there was reversal in the symptom of EDS, and CSF hypocretin-1 levels increased, when there was a corresponding improvement in the primary neurologic disorder.[38,39] Low CSF hypocretin levels have also been reported in multiple sclerosis patients with hypothalamic lesions and sleepiness; here, too, when the disease improved, CSF hypocretin levels were found to return to normal and daytime sleepiness disappeared.[39] In primary (presumably autoimmune) narcolepsy with low CSF hypocretin, there are no documented cases of CSF hypocretin levels returning to normal after the disease is established.

Secondary narcolepsy *without* cataplexy has been reported with head trauma, alpha-synucleinopathies, and myotonic dystrophy; some of these disorders have been associated with obstructive sleep apnea as well and must first be ruled out before a diagnosis of narcolepsy can be made.[28]

Treatment Strategies

Given emerging evidence of its autoimmune underpinnings, there has been increased interest in early diagnosis of narcolepsy-cataplexy, which would allow for the possibility of immunomodulators that may reduce the destruction of hypocretin-producing hypothalamic neurons and reduce or eliminate the burden of this disease. However, most trials of steroid administration, plasmapheresis, or intravenous immunoglobulin therapy (IVIG) have so far been shown to be of little or no value, although a few reports described decreased cataplexy or sleepiness with the IVIG treatment.[40-45]

At present, there is no cure for narcolepsy-cataplexy, only control of symptoms and optimization of lifestyle and psychosocial function. Therefore, it is important to assess and address any treatable causes of sleepiness such as circadian rhythm disorders, sleep apnea, poor sleep hygiene, sleep deprivation, and other conditions that may coexist with narcolepsy (Box 39-2). Patient education about lifestyle and behavioral adaptation to narcolepsy-cataplexy is crucial. In our experience, short 15- to 30-minute naps at scheduled times two to three times during the day are helpful, especially in older children (short naps in older children and adults with narcolepsy are typically refreshing and alerting); at times longer naps may be needed, especially in younger individuals. At all ages, it is also important to maintain a regular sleep-wake schedule and good sleep hygiene. There are few limitations on career plans, but counseling should suggest avoidance of shift work, transportation-related occupations (trucker, pilot), and occupations requiring frequent time zone shifts. A child with narcolepsy may have difficulty maintaining attention in quiet situations without breaks, and schools should be contacted to help ensure reasonable accommodations are available for scheduled naps (perhaps during lunch or in lieu of study period) and arrangements made for breaks during test-taking (which may occasionally be necessary). Finally, given the frequently long duration from symptom onset to diagnosis (sometimes over a decade), the changes in alertness and energy levels that will be present, and the occurrence of cataplexy, the child's quality of life, social relationships, and function at school or work may suffer. Development of reactive depression or maladaptive behaviors that develop in response to symptoms should be discussed with patients with suspected narcolepsy and their families. Information about patient-oriented support groups such as the Narcolepsy Network may be provided.

Pharmacotherapy targeted to treating daytime sleepiness and cataplexy is the mainstay of narcolepsy treatment. While many studies have been performed in adults, no double-blind placebo-controlled trials of medication have been specifically conducted on children with narcolepsy. Nonetheless, treatment of children is necessary because the disease commonly presents in childhood; thus, one is forced to generalize from the adult narcolepsy data and from pediatric data for drug usage in other disorders. The evidence as it stands will be presented. Table 39-1 lists medications commonly used in the treatment of daytime sleepiness; Table 39-2 lists those commonly used for cataplexy. A brief description of the most frequently used agents follows.

Treatment of Daytime Sleepiness

Central nervous system (CNS) stimulants have been the drugs most widely used in the treatment of narcolepsy, and amphetamines were first proposed in 1935.[46] A number of side effects, including irritability, anxiety, nervousness, headache, psychosis, tachycardia, hypertension, nocturnal sleep disturbances, tolerance, and drug dependence, may arise. The use of methylphenidate was later encouraged because of a shorter half-life and lower incidence of similar side effects.

Methylphenidate. Methylphenidate is a stimulant that was first patented in the United States in 1954. It is a dopamine and catecholamine reuptake inhibitor, thereby increasing the amount of time these neurotransmitters are in the synaptic cleft. Methylphenidate may also enhance serotonin transmission.[47] In adults methylphenidate doses between 10 and 100 mg are used. Randomized trials of methylphenidate in children with narcolepsy are not available. However, the widespread use of this medication for children with attention deficit hyperactivity disorder (ADHD) provides dosing guidelines. The American Academy of Child and Adolescent Psychiatry (AACAP) recommends that treatment for ADHD with immediate-release methylphenidate be initiated with 5 mg dosed twice daily, in the morning and around noon, owing to its short half-life.[48] The same general dosing guidelines are used in pediatric narcolepsy (however, in some narcoleptic

children an additional dose may need to be added after school if scheduled naps have not provided an adequate response). Therapy should be optimized with upward titration by 5 to 10 mg/day at weekly intervals up to a maximum total dose of 60 mg/day. However, no single dose should exceed 25 mg. In children weighing less than 25 kg, the methylphenidate dose should not exceed 45 mg/day. Several formulations of methylphenidate are available, including immediate release and extended release options that can allow for individual adjustments to be made based on the clinical situation. Extended release preparations do not have specific dosing guidelines for narcolepsy, but generally pediatric ADHD guidelines may be helpful in guiding initiation and titration. Extended release preparations of methylphenidate should also not exceed 60 mg/day, and quite often lower doses are adequate. Skin patch preparations as well as enantiomers of methylphenidate are also available.[47]

Side effects with methylphenidate include insomnia, weight loss, decreased appetite, stomach ache, and dry mouth. Though less common, palpitations, elevation of blood pressure, and pulse changes can occur. Cardiovascular risk is greater in children with known cardiac disease. Motor tics can emerge. Tolerance can occur, requiring dose adjustments.[47] In the authors' experience, these side effects have made methylphenidate a less attractive treatment option in children with narcolepsy as newer therapeutic agents have become available.

Modafinil. Today, modafinil is considered a first-line therapy for EDS associated with narcolepsy in adults.[46,49] In children, more caution is necessary, especially at younger ages, owing to reports of serious adverse events at elevated modafinil doses.[50,51] The mechanism of this wake-promoting drug is unknown, but it seems different from that of amphetamines and is hypothesized to work on hypothalamic wake-promoting circuits. The results of several multicenter trials have demonstrated improvements in objective measures of sleepiness and improved wakefulness in narcoleptic adult patients, and additive effects have been demonstrated when used with gamma-hydroxybutyrate (GHB).[52-54] Total daily doses of 200 to 400 mg are typically used, usually once a day, but sometimes split between morning and noon administration. Elimination half-life is 10 to 12 hours. It is important to know that modafinil can reduce the effectiveness of oral contraceptives, and therefore, patients should be advised to use additional forms of contraception. Abuse potential for this medication is low and discontinuation of modafinil is not associated with rebound hypersomnolence; nor is there evidence of tolerance. As with methylphenidate, there is support in the literature for modafinil in the treatment of ADHD in children. In general it is reported to be effective and well tolerated in these studies, although it remains an off-label indication.[51,55-58]

Armodafinil is the *R*-enantiomer of modafinil with a longer duration of action, approved in 2007 for the treatment of EDS in narcolepsy. At daily doses of 150 to 250 mg, armodafinil has been shown to improve EDS throughout the day with improved scores on MSLT in randomized double-blind, placebo-controlled trials in adults.[59]

Although neither modafinil nor armodafinil is approved for use in children, modafinil has been reported to be useful in the treatment of EDS in narcoleptic children.[60] The possibility of significant drug reactions at high doses is a concern

Pharmacologic Treatment of Excessive Daytime Sleepiness in Pediatric Narcolepsy

Drug	Dose	Timing	Comments
Modafinil	50-400 mg per day *For children*: 50-200 mg; *For adolescents*: 200-400 mg	qAM or in divided doses given in morning and at noon	100-, 200-mg tablets *For children*: Start with 50 mg qAM; then add 50 mg increments to the morning dose or at noon as needed *For adolescents*: same, but use 100 mg as starting dose and increment Manufacturer recommends against use in younger children (see text)
Sodium oxybate	4.5-9 g per night (2.25-4.5 g/dose) *For children*: 6 g/night is typical, with lower dose in younger children; *For adolescents*: may need up to 9 g (full adult dose)	*Twice a night*: At bedtime and typically after 2-4 hours of sleep; timing of second dose is individualized	0.5 g/mL *For younger children*: start at 1.5-2 g twice nightly; titrate up by 0.25 g per dose *For older children and adolescents*: start at 2.25 g twice nightly; titrate up slowly by 0.75 g/dose as needed Initial increases at 5-7 days up to 3 g/dose; then further increases at 7- to 14-day intervals Even though medication may help with sleepiness, titration is usually based on control of cataplexy May worsen sleep-disordered breathing
Methylphenidate, immediate-release	*For children*: < 25 kg: 10-45 mg/day; ≥ 25 kg: 20-60 mg/day	*2-3 times daily*: In morning and at noon, before meals, plus after school if needed (see text)	2.5-, 5-, 10-, 20-mg tablets or capsules; 5-10 mg/tsp of liquid *For children*: start with 5 mg in morning and at noon; titrate up in 5-mg increments weekly as needed; an after-school dose may be necessary (e.g., to complete school work) *For adolescents*: start at 10 mg/dose and increase by 10 mg/dose as needed Medication should be adjusted after other measures to improve sleepiness (e.g., adequate nocturnal sleep, scheduled naps, and treatment of coexisting OSA) are in place See text regarding potential side effects
Methylphenidate, extended-release: Ritalin LA, Ritalin SR, Metadate ER, Metadate CD, Methylin ER	20-60 mg/day (drug availability depends on specific trade preparation) *For patients ≥ 6 years old*: guidelines similar to those for ADHD;	In the morning on an empty stomach	10-, 20-, 30-, 40-mg tablets and capsules *For older children*: may be used in lieu of shorter-acting formulations May replace immediate-release formulations at (approximately) the same total dose, once the total daily dose is titrated (e.g., on titration to 10 mg of immediate-release formulation bid/tid, patient may be switched to 20 mg extended-release qAM); *or* start with 20 mg qAM extended-release and increase at weekly intervals by 10 to 20 mg
Methylphenidate, extended-release: Concerta	*For patients 6-12 years old*: 18-54 mg/day; *For patients 13-17 years old*: 36-72 mg/day (Adapted from pediatric ADHD dosing)	In the morning on an empty stomach	18-, 27-, 36-, 54-mg tablets Start at 18 mg qAM; may be adjusted weekly in 18-mg increments
Atomoxetine	20-100 mg/day (Adapted from pediatric ADHD dosing)	In the morning with or without food	10-, 18-, 25-, 40-, 60-, 80-, 100-mg capsules *For children > 6 years and < 70 kg*: starting dose is 0.5 mg/kg/day; increase every 3-7 days as needed; typical final dose 1.2 mg/kg/day (*maximum*: 1.4 mg/kg/day) *For children > 70 kg*, start at 40 mg; typical final dose 80 mg (*maximum*: 100 mg) Drug is a norepinephrine reuptake inhibitor May reduce cataplexy as well as sleepiness (anticataplexy effect usually seen by 40-60 mg in adults) Often used as adjunctive agent with other drugs when additional alerting or anticataplectic activity needed.

ADHD, attention deficit hyperactivity disorder; *OSA*, obstructive sleep apnea.

in children, and the clinician must be aware that the manufacturer recommends against use of, these agents in younger children. During the pivotal trials skin reactions, including one case of possible erythema multiforme/Stevens-Johnson syndrome, were reported.[51]

Gamma-Hydroxybutyrate/Sodium Oxybate. Sodium oxybate (γ-hydroxybutyrate, GHB) is FDA-approved for both the treatment of cataplexy and EDS of narcolepsy in adults. GHB is an endogenous central nervous system metabolite with highest concentrations in the hypothalamus and basal

TABLE 39-2

Pharmacologic Treatment of Cataplexy in Pediatric Narcolepsy*

Drug	Dose	Timing	Comments
Sodium oxybate	See Table 39-1	See Table 39-1	Not associated with rebound cataplexy at discontinuation Titrated for effect on cataplexy, which may take weeks or months to fully manifest, so slow titration upward is recommended May require additional anticataplexy medication during initiation phase
Venlafaxine, extended-release formulation only	37.5-150 mg XR (no established dosing for treating cataplexy in pediatrics)	qAM with food	37.5-, 75-, 150-mg capsules *For children*: start at 37.5 mg; titrate up in 37.5-mg increments *For adolescents*: start at 75 mg; titrate up in 37.5- to 75-mg increments Potent inhibitor of neuronal serotonin and norepinephrine reuptake and weak inhibitors of dopamine reuptake May have some positive impact on alertness in addition to anticataplexy activity, but anticataplexy effects seem to occur at lower doses Antidepressants work more quickly than sodium oxybate for cataplexy but, unlike sodium oxybate, may produce rebound cataplexy if discontinued too abruptly
Selective serotonin reuptake inhibitors (SSRIs) (e.g., fluoxetine)	Fluoxetine: 10-60 mg; 20 mg typical to control cataplexy *Maximum dose*: 30 mg in preadolescents, 60 mg in adolescents (based on pediatric psychiatry dosing for children age 7 and older)	Once daily	10, 20 mg—fluoxetine Start at 10 mg; increase in 10-mg increments SSRIs work more quickly on cataplexy than does sodium oxybate Anticataplexy dose typically is lower than antidepressant dose; hence, maximal dose not often needed May produce rebound cataplexy when discontinued
Atomoxetine	See Table 39-1	See Table 39-1	See Table 39-1
Tricyclic antidepressants (TCAs) (e.g., clomipramine)	Clomipramine: 10-100 mg *Maximum dose*: 100 mg or 3 mg/kg (information on dosing in children younger than 10 years not available for this agent)	Once daily; may be given at night to reduce daytime sedation	10, 25, 50, 75 mg—clomipramine Start at 10-25 mg; titrate up to 25 mg; then increase in 25-mg increments TCAs work more quickly on cataplexy than does sodium oxybate Anticataplexy dose typically is lower than antidepressant dose; hence, maximal dose not often needed May cause sedation; may produce rebound cataplexy when discontinued Although TCAs are highly effective for cataplexy, side effects may limit long-term use (see text)

*No medications have been FDA approved to treat cataplexy in patients younger than 16 years.

ganglia. It is considered a neuromodulator/neurotransmitter affecting dopamine, serotonin, γ-aminobutyric acid (GABA), and endogenous opioids; it is also considered to be a GABA$_B$ receptor agonist.[61,62] As a therapeutic agent in narcolepsy-cataplexy, its mechanisms of action are incompletely understood, but clinically it has been shown to dramatically reduce cataplexy as well as treat daytime sleepiness and improve the sleep fragmentation and disturbed sleep typical of narcolepsy-cataplexy (at least in the adult).[52,63-65] The improvement in cataplexy is much more rapid than is the effect on daytime sleepiness, which may take up to 6 to 8 weeks, an important fact since titrating up too quickly in an attempt to control daytime sleepiness is a common mistake. Some have suggested that the time course for improvements in cataplexy and daytime sleepiness indicates differing mechanisms of action of GHB on these two dimensions; additionally, another GABA$_B$ agonist, baclofen, has been shown to lead to similar polysomnographic improvement as GHB but, unfortunately, not to impact cataplexy or daytime sleepiness, suggesting that non-GABAB mechanisms are involved.[66]

GHB has powerful central nervous system depressant effects and has been shown to increase slow wave (stage N3) sleep. It has a short half-life (90-120 minutes), so the first dose is taken at bedtime and a second dose is most commonly taken 2.5 to 4 hours later, though timing may vary between patients. The recommended starting dose in adults is 4.5 g/day divided into two equal doses of 2.25 g. Dosing may be gradually increased over 8 weeks or longer, with a typical adult dose goal of 6 to 9 g, which has been shown to be effective for improvements in EDS and nocturnal sleep.[67] Until the full alerting effects of GHB are fully manifest, other alerting agents may be used. Side effects include disorientation in the middle of the night, grogginess upon awakening, enuresis, and nausea (especially at initiation and at higher doses). Use of this medication also confers a significant sodium load, which may be limiting for those with fluid retention, congestive heart failure, or hypertension.

Although this novel agent is considered by some to be the treatment of choice in narcolepsy-cataplexy, targeting multiple dimensions of the disorder, it is expensive and access is only through a centralized mail-order pharmacy. In 2007, 80% of private insurance plans covered GHB. In addition, the product's package insert does not recommend using this medication in patients younger than age 16 years, and little is published about use of sodium oxybate in pediatric narcolepsy. Nonetheless, it is used in treatment of pediatric narcolepsy at some centers. In the pediatric narcolepsy series reported from Stanford, 85% of children (with similar rates for pre-, peri-, and postpubertal children) were treated with sodium oxybate with a high retention rate (79%) and a reportedly high positive effect on daytime sleepiness, disturbed nighttime sleep, and cataplexy. Irritability and nausea were commonly reported side effects, and the report found no impact of the use of sodium oxybate on the occurrence of subsequent puberty. The authors also reported that sodium oxybate alone, or in association with one other drug, modafinil, was sufficient treatment in half of prepubertal cases of narcolepsy-cataplexy.[17]

Treatment of Cataplexy

Although recently published data from Stanford describes the use of GHB as a useful medication for treatment of pediatric cataplexy, a body of clinical experience supports treatment with a host of other medications that are used off-label with significant impact on cataplexy.[17] Older tricyclic antidepressants such as imipramine, which block presynaptic reuptake of catecholamines, were at one time commonly used, but they are now considered something of a last resort, owing to their considerable side effect profile. They are also associated with robust rebound cataplexy at discontinuation.

Selective serotonin reuptake inhibitors such as fluoxetine have also been used. Newer antidepressants with selective noradrenergic/serotoninergic uptake inhibition are considered better choices, with respect to both side effect profile and efficacy for cataplexy, sleep paralysis, and hypnagogic/hynopompic hallucinations. The most commonly used drug in this class in venlafaxine at typical doses of 75 to 150 mg daily (as low as 37.5 mg in younger pediatric patients). Newly reported data in children with narcolepsy-cataplexy demonstrate reasonable retention rate (68%) and good efficacy for cataplexy, with frequent side effects of irritability and weight gain reported both in prepubertal (18%) and peri-/postpubertal (29%) groups.

Atomoxetine, a highly specific noradrenergic reuptake blocker, has also been effective for treatment of cataplexy as well as EDS in adults and children, and may be useful in treating resistant cataplexy at 18 to 100 mg given as a single dose, or divided into two doses, daily.[68]

Investigational Agents

There is interest in a variety of novel approaches to treating narcolepsy, including hypocretin replacement, hypocretin gene therapy, stem cell transplant, and new pharmaceutical agents active on thryotropin (TRH) and histamine (H_3) systems to promote alertness. Much additional work is still needed to allow these ideas to achieve fruition as clinical therapies. Because the vast majority of narcolepsy-cataplexy patients are deficient in CNS hypocretin ("ligand deficient"), hypocretin replacement therapy is theoretically an especially attractive way to treat both sleep problems and cataplexy. However logical this approach may be, hypocretin-1 does not readily cross the blood-brain barrier and had little therapeutic effect when given intravenously or, in fact, intrathecally, in ligand-deficient canines; however, improvements in daytime sleepiness were reported in a murine model when the peptide was delivered via the intracerebroventricular route.[69-71] Early reports of gene therapy in murine models also demonstrate some promise.[71-73] Intranasal administration of hypocretin-1 may prove useful, as this would potentially deliver the drug directly without requiring passage via the blood-brain barrier.[74,75]

CONCLUSION

Narcolepsy is a challenging clinical problem in children. Although narcolepsy is less common than other sleep disorders in children, such as insomnia and sleep apnea, it does allow for a greater understanding of overall sleep physiology and CNS pathophysiology. Narcolepsy is predominately a disorder that begins in childhood or adolescence. Clinicians need to be aware of this condition because misdiagnosis of the initial symptoms can occur. Randomized clinical trials are necessary to further advance our ability to care for these children. With the increased awareness of narcolepsy, one should be optimistic that some day, instead of ameliorating treatments, therapeutic approaches will be available for prevention and cure.

REFERENCES

1. Peyron C, Faraco J, Rogers W, et al. A mutation in a case of early onset narcolepsy and a generalized absence of hypocretin peptides in human narcoleptic brains. *Nat Med.* 2000;6:991-997.
2. Thannickal TC, Moore RY, Nienhuis R, et al. Reduced number of hypocretin neurons in human narcolepsy. *Neuron.* 2000;27:469-474.
3. Cao M. Advances in narcolepsy. *Med Clin North Am.* 2010;94:541-555.
4. Mignot E, Wang C, Rattazzi C, et al. Genetic linkage of autosomal recessive canine narcolepsy with a mu immunoglobulin heavy-chain switch-like segment. *Proc Natl Acad Sci U S A.* 1991;88:3475-3478.
5. Mignot E, Kimura A, Lattermann A, et al. Extensive HLA class II studies in 58 non-DRB1*15 (DR2) narcoleptic patients with cataplexy. *Tissue Antigens.* 1997;49:329-341.
6. Matsuki K, Grumet FC, Lin X, et al. DQ (rather than DR) gene marks susceptibility to narcolepsy. *Lancet.* 1992;339:1052.
7. Mignot E, Lin L, Rogers W, et al. Complex HLA-DR and -DQ interactions confer risk of narcolepsy-cataplexy in three ethnic groups. *Am J Hum Genet.* 2001;68:686-699.
8. Hallmayer J, Faraco J, Lin L, et al. Narcolepsy is strongly associated with the T-cell receptor alpha locus. *Nat Genet.* 2009;41:708-711.
9. Aran A, Lin L, Nevsimalova S, et al. Elevated anti-streptococcal antibodies in patients with recent narcolepsy onset. *Sleep.* 2009;32:979-983.
10. Dauvilliers Y, Montplaisir J, Cochen V, et al. Post-H1N1 narcolepsy-cataplexy. *Sleep.* 2010;33:1428-1430.
11. Deloumeau A, Bayard S, Coquerel Q, et al. Increased immune complexes of hypocretin autoantibodies in narcolepsy. *PLoS One.* 2010;5:e13320.
12. Kawashima M, Lin L, Tanaka S, et al. Anti-Tribbles homolog 2 (TRIB2) autoantibodies in narcolepsy are associated with recent onset of cataplexy. *Sleep.* 2010;33:869-874.
13. Lim AS, Scammell TE. The trouble with Tribbles: Do antibodies against TRIB2 cause narcolepsy? *Sleep.* 2010;33:857-858.
14. Toyoda H, Tanaka S, Miyagawa T, Honda Y, Tokunaga K, Honda M. Anti-Tribbles homolog 2 autoantibodies in Japanese patients with narcolepsy. *Sleep.* 2010;33:875-878.
15. Guilleminault C, Pelayo R. Narcolepsy in children: A practical guide to its diagnosis, treatment and follow-up. *Paediatr Drugs.* 2000;2:1-9.
16. Vetrugno R, D'Angelo R, Moghadam KK, et al. Behavioural and neurophysiological correlates of human cataplexy: A video-polygraphic study. *Clin Neurophysiol.* 2010;121:153-162.
17. Aran A, Einen M, Lin L, Plazzi G, Nishino S, Mignot E. Clinical and therapeutic aspects of childhood narcolepsy-cataplexy: A retrospective study of 51 children. *Sleep.* 2010;33:1457-1464.
18. Longstreth Jr WT, Ton TG, Koepsell TD. Narcolepsy and streptococcal infections. *Sleep.* 2009;32:1548.
19. Guilleminault C, Pelayo R. Narcolepsy in prepubertal children. *Ann Neurol.* 1998;43:135-142.
20. Plazzi G, Tonon C, Rubboli G, et al. Narcolepsy with cataplexy associated with holoprosencephaly misdiagnosed as epileptic drop attacks. *Mov Disord.* 2010;25:780-782.
21. Hirst J, Mignot E, Stein MT. Episodic hypersomnia and unusual behaviors in a 14-year-old adolescent. *J Dev Behav Pediatr.* 2010;31:S18-S20.
22. Vendrame M, Havaligi N, Matadeen-Ali C, Adams R, Kothare SV. Narcolepsy in children: A single-center clinical experience. *Pediatr Neurol.* 2008;38:314-320.

23. Silber MH, Krahn LE, Olson EJ, Pankratz VS. The epidemiology of narcolepsy in Olmsted County, Minnesota: A population-based study. *Sleep.* 2002;25:197-202.

24. Okun ML, Lin L, Pelin Z, Hong S, Mignot E. Clinical aspects of narcolepsy-cataplexy across ethnic groups. *Sleep.* 2002;25:27-35.

25. Yoss RE, Daly DD. Narcolepsy in children. *Pediatrics.* 1960;25:1025-1033.

26. Morrish E, King MA, Smith IE, Shneerson JM. Factors associated with a delay in the diagnosis of narcolepsy. *Sleep Med.* 2004;5:37-41.

27. Serra L, Montagna P, Mignot E, Lugaresi E, Plazzi G. Cataplexy features in childhood narcolepsy. *Mov Disord.* 2008;23:858-865.

28. *International Classification of Sleep Disorders.* 2nd ed. Westchester, IL: American Academy of Sleep Medicine; 2005.

29. Aldrich MS. The neurobiology of narcolepsy-cataplexy. *Prog Neurobiol.* 1993;41:533-541.

30. Singh M, Drake CL, Roth T. The prevalence of multiple sleep-onset REM periods in a population-based sample. *Sleep.* 2006;29:890-895.

31. Bishop C, Rosenthal L, Helmus T, Roehrs T, Roth T. The frequency of multiple sleep onset REM periods among subjects with no excessive daytime sleepiness. *Sleep.* 1996;19:727-730.

32. Moscovitch A, Partinen M, Guilleminault C. The positive diagnosis of narcolepsy and narcolepsy's borderland. *Neurology.* 1993;43:55-60.

33. Dauvilliers Y, Gosselin A, Paquet J, Touchon J, Billiard M, Montplaisir J. Effect of age on MSLT results in patients with narcolepsy-cataplexy. *Neurology.* 2004;62:46-50.

34. Nishino S, Ripley B, Overeem S, Lammers GJ, Mignot E. Hypocretin (orexin) deficiency in human narcolepsy. *Lancet.* 2000;355:39-40.

35. Mignot E, Lammers GJ, Ripley B, et al. The role of cerebrospinal fluid hypocretin measurement in the diagnosis of narcolepsy and other hypersomnias. *Arch Neurol.* 2002;59:1553-1562.

36. Dauvilliers Y, Arnulf I, Mignot E. Narcolepsy with cataplexy. *Lancet.* 2007;369:499-511.

37. Challamel MJ, Mazzola ME, Nevsimalova S, Cannard C, Louis J, Revol M. Narcolepsy in children. *Sleep.* 1994;17:S17-S20.

38. Nishino S, Kanbayashi T. Symptomatic narcolepsy, cataplexy and hypersomnia, and their implications in the hypothalamic hypocretin/orexin system. *Sleep Med Rev.* 2005;9:269-310.

39. Kanbayashi T, Shimohata T, Nakashima I, et al. Symptomatic narcolepsy in patients with neuromyelitis optica and multiple sclerosis: New neurochemical and immunological implications. *Arch Neurol.* 2009;66:1563-1566.

40. Lecendreux M, Maret S, Bassetti C, Mouren MC, Tafti M. Clinical efficacy of high-dose intravenous immunoglobulins near the onset of narcolepsy in a 10-year-old boy. *J Sleep Res.* 2003;12:347-348.

41. Dauvilliers Y, Carlander B, Rivier F, Touchon J, Tafti M. Successful management of cataplexy with intravenous immunoglobulins at narcolepsy onset. *Ann Neurol.* 2004;56:905-908.

42. Dauvilliers Y. Follow-up of four narcolepsy patients treated with intravenous immunoglobulins. *Ann Neurol.* 2006;60:153.

43. Fronczek R, Verschuuren J, Lammers GJ. Response to intravenous immunoglobulins and placebo in a patient with narcolepsy with cataplexy. *J Neurol.* 2007;254:1607-1608.

44. Plazzi G, Poli F, Franceschini C, et al. Intravenous high-dose immunoglobulin treatment in recent onset childhood narcolepsy with cataplexy. *J Neurol.* 2008;255:1549-1554.

45. Dauvilliers Y, Abril B, Mas E, Michel F, Tafti M. Normalization of hypocretin-1 in narcolepsy after intravenous immunoglobulin treatment. *Neurology.* 2009;73:1333-1334.

46. Littner M, Johnson SF, McCall WV, et al. Practice parameters for the treatment of narcolepsy: An update for 2000. *Sleep.* 2001;24:451-466.

47. Peterson PC, Husain AM. Pediatric narcolepsy. *Brain Dev.* 2008;30:609-623.

48. Greenhill LL, Pliszka S, Dulcan MK, et al. Practice parameter for the use of stimulant medications in the treatment of children, adolescents, and adults. *J Am Acad Child Adolesc Psychiatry.* 2002;41:26S-49S.

49. Wise MS, Arand DL, Auger RR, Brooks SN, Watson NF. Treatment of narcolepsy and other hypersomnias of central origin. *Sleep.* 2007;30:1712-1727.

50. Spiller HA, Borys D, Griffith JR, et al. Toxicity from modafinil ingestion. *Clin Toxicol (Phila).* 2009;47:153-156.

51. Rugino T. A review of modafinil film-coated tablets for attention-deficit/hyperactivity disorder in children and adolescents. *Neuropsychiatr Dis Treat.* 2007;3:293-301.

52. Black J, Houghton WC. Sodium oxybate improves excessive daytime sleepiness in narcolepsy. *Sleep.* 2006;29:939-946.

53. Randomized trial of modafinil as a treatment for the excessive daytime somnolence of narcolepsy. U.S. Modafinil in Narcolepsy Multicenter Study Group. *Neurology.* 2000;54:1166-1175.

54. Broughton RJ, Fleming JA, George CF, et al. Randomized, double-blind, placebo-controlled crossover trial of modafinil in the treatment of excessive daytime sleepiness in narcolepsy. *Neurology.* 1997;49:444-451.

55. Kahbazi M, Ghoreishi A, Rahiminejad F, Mohammadi MR, Kamalipour A, Akhondzadeh S. A randomized, double-blind and placebo-controlled trial of modafinil in children and adolescents with attention deficit and hyperactivity disorder. *Psychiatry Res.* 2009;168:234-237.

56. Biederman J, Pliszka SR. Modafinil improves symptoms of attention-deficit/hyperactivity disorder across subtypes in children and adolescents. *J Pediatr.* 2008;152:394-399.

57. Amiri S, Mohammadi MR, Mohammadi M, Nouroozinejad GH, Kahbazi M, Akhondzadeh S. Modafinil as a treatment for attention-deficit/hyperactivity disorder in children and adolescents: A double blind, randomized clinical trial. *Prog Neuropsychopharmacol Biol Psychiatry.* 2008;32:145-149.

58. Wigal SB, Biederman J, Swanson JM, Yang R, Greenhill LL. Efficacy and safety of modafinil film-coated tablets in children and adolescents with or without prior stimulant treatment for attention-deficit/hyperactivity disorder: Pooled analysis of 3 randomized, double-blind, placebo-controlled studies. *Prim Care Companion J Clin Psychiatry.* 2006;8:352-360.

59. Lankford DA. Armodafinil: A new treatment for excessive sleepiness. *Expert Opin Investig Drugs.* 2008;17:565-573.

60. Ivanenko A, Tauman R, Gozal D. Modafinil in the treatment of excessive daytime sleepiness in children. *Sleep Med.* 2003;4:579-582.

61. Pelayo R, Dubik M. Pediatric sleep pharmacology. *Semin Pediatr Neurol.* 2008;15:79-90.

62. Lammers GJ, Bassetti C, Billiard M, et al. Sodium oxybate is an effective and safe treatment for narcolepsy. *Sleep Med.* 2010;11:105-106:author reply 6–8.

63. Lammers GJ, Arends J, Declerck AC, Ferrari MD, Schouwink G, Troost J. Gamma-hydroxybutyrate and narcolepsy: A double-blind placebo-controlled study. *Sleep.* 1993;16:216-220.

64. The U.S. Xyrem Multicenter Study Group. Sodium oxybate demonstrates long-term efficacy for the treatment of cataplexy in patients with narcolepsy. *Sleep Med.* 2004;5:119-123.

65. The U.S. Xyrem Multicenter Study Group. A randomized, double blind, placebo-controlled multicenter trial comparing the effects of three doses of orally administered sodium oxybate with placebo for the treatment of narcolepsy. *Sleep.* 2002;25:42-49.

66. Huang YS, Guilleminault C. Narcolepsy: Action of two gamma-aminobutyric acid type B agonists, baclofen and sodium oxybate. *Pediatr Neurol.* 2009;41:9-16.

67. Scharf MB, Lai AA, Branigan B, Stover R, Berkowitz DB. Pharmacokinetics of gamma-hydroxybutyrate (GHB) in narcoleptic patients. *Sleep.* 1998;21:507-514.

68. Billiard M. Narcolepsy: Current treatment options and future approaches. *Neuropsychiatr Dis Treat.* 2008;4:557-566.

69. Fujiki N, Yoshida Y, Ripley B, Mignot E, Nishino S. Effects of IV and ICV hypocretin-1 (orexin A) in hypocretin receptor-2 gene mutated narcoleptic dogs and IV hypocretin-1 replacement therapy in a hypocretin-ligand-deficient narcoleptic dog. *Sleep.* 2003;26:953-959.

70. Schatzberg SJ, Cutter-Schatzberg K, Nydam D, et al. The effect of hypocretin replacement therapy in a 3-year-old Weimaraner with narcolepsy. *J Vet Intern Med.* 2004;18:586-588.

71. Mieda M, Willie JT, Hara J, Sinton CM, Sakurai T, Yanagisawa M. Orexin peptides prevent cataplexy and improve wakefulness in an orexin neuron-ablated model of narcolepsy in mice. *Proc Natl Acad Sci U S A.* 2004;101:4649-4654.

72. Liu M, Thankachan S, Kaur S, et al. Orexin (hypocretin) gene transfer diminishes narcoleptic sleep behavior in mice. *Eur J Neurosci.* 2008;28:1382-1393.

73. Nishino S. Clinical and neurobiological aspects of narcolepsy. *Sleep Med.* 2007;8:373-399.

74. Dhuria SV, Hanson LR, Frey 2nd WH. Intranasal drug targeting of hypocretin-1 (orexin-A) to the central nervous system. *J Pharm Sci.* 2009;98:2501-2515.

75. Deadwyler SA, Porrino L, Siegel JM, Hampson RE. Systemic and nasal delivery of orexin-A (hypocretin-1) reduces the effects of sleep deprivation on cognitive performance in nonhuman primates. *J Neurosci.* 2007;27:14239-14247.

Sleep and Sleep Problems in Children with Neurologic Disorders

MADELEINE M. GRIGG-DAMBERGER

Chapter
40

NEURODEVELOPMENTAL DISORDERS

Sleep problems in children with neurodevelopmental disorders are often much more common, frequent, severe, and persistent compared to the general population. In many children with particular neurodevelopmental disorders, sleep problems are so highly prevalent as to be considered a behavioral phenotype. Complex and often reciprocal relationships among cognitive function, learning, problematic behaviors, and sleep problems are common in children with neurologic disorders.[1,2]

Down Syndrome

Down syndrome (DS) is the most common genetic cause of mental retardation. The incidence ranges from 1 per 1000 births in mothers younger than 40 years to 1 in 50 births for mothers 40 years or older,[3,4] and DS accounts for approximately 30% of all cases of moderate to severe intellectual disability (ID).[5] DS is usually caused by the presence of an extra copy of chromosome 21 (trisomy 21); less often it is due to a translocation of the proximal q22 segment of chromosome 21 to another chromosome (4% of cases). The region of chromosome 21 that contains the main genes responsible for the clinical expression and pathogenesis of DS are located proximal to 21q22.3. The phenotypic expression of the trisomy 21 genotype shows great interindividual variability, seemingly modified by allelic variation, genomic imbalances, and epigenetic and environmental factors.[6] Genetic factors alone no longer determine the best cognitive outcome a child with DS can achieve; early intervention programs and parental nurturing may significantly contribute to better cognitive outcomes for children with DS.[6]

Delayed maturation of non–rapid eye movement (NREM) sleep architecture and abnormalities in rapid eye movement (REM) sleep have been reported in DS. Thus, the *trace alternant* pattern of quiet sleep (that is normal in full-term newborns) disappears at an average of 55 days of life in DS infants compared to 33 days in control subjects;[7] sleep spindles first appear later and are less abundant in the first year of life than normal;[8] and in older DS children, there may be prolongation of REM latency, reduction in mean numbers of rapid eye movements during REM sleep (REM density), and a decrease in the percentage of sleep time spent in REM sleep, with the more severe abnormalities correlating with lower intelligence quotients (IQs).[8-11]

Children with DS have significantly more sleep problems compared to the general pediatric population.[12] For example,

a community prevalence study of 100,000 U.K. children by Carter and associates[12] found that the 58 children with DS (mean age 8.6 years, range 0.7 to 17.9 years) had significantly greater bedtime resistance and sleep anxiety and more frequent night wakings, parasomnias, sleep-disordered breathing (SDB), and excessive daytime sleepiness. They further found that of the DS children 4 years or older, 66% rarely fell asleep in their own beds, 55% were always restless during sleep, 40% usually woke at least once during the night, and 78% seemed tired during the day at least 2 days per week.

The prevalence of *obstructive sleep apnea(OSA)* in individuals with DS ranges from 30% to 60% compared with 2% to 3% of the general pediatric population.[13] The risk factors for SDB in children with DS are summarized in Box 40-1. Uong and colleagues[14] found that children with DS (mean age 3.2 ± 1.4 years) have smaller airway volumes, smaller midface and lower face skeletons, shorter hard palates, and smaller mandible volumes compared with age-matched control subjects. However, the volume of their adenoids and tonsils, and even the size of their tongues, was *not* larger than that of control subjects, but these soft tissues caused crowding of their upper airways because of small midface and lower face dimensions. A retrospective review of 23 children with DS (mean age 1.8 years) referred to a pediatric otolaryngology service found upper airway obstruction in infants with DS younger than 1 month was most often related to laryngomalacia,[15] whereas adenotonsillar hypertrophy (complicated by gastroesophageal reflux disease in nearly two thirds) was more likely the cause of upper airway obstruction in the DS children older than 2 years.[15]

Some researchers argue that OSA is so common in young children with DS that polysomnography (PSG) should be done on all of them between ages 3 and 4 years.[16] A prospective cohort overnight PSG study of 65 DS children found OSA in 57% (mean age 42 months), increasing to 80% if cases of upper airway resistance (snoring, increased work of breathing, triggering frequent arousals) were included.[16] OSA (defined as an *apnea-hypopnea index [AHI]* > 1.5) was found in 59% of 22 DS children compared with 32% of children with snoring but without DS.[17] Another prospective study found OSA in 79% of 19 unselected children with DS (mean AHI 6.0).[18]

OSA in children with DS tends to be more severe (with significantly higher AHI) than OSA present in otherwise normal children.[13] Also, parents of DS children both under- and overestimated the likelihood their child would have OSA on a PSG.[16] This apparent inability to recognize OSA in their DS children may explain the reason 62% of DS children with PSG-confirmed OSA were not reported to habitually snore.[19]

> **BOX 40-1** *Risk Factors for Sleep-Disordered Breathing in Children with Down Syndrome*
>
> - Midface and mandibular hypoplasia
> - Narrow palate
> - Glossoptosis
> - Relatively large and/or posteriorly placed tongue in relatively small oral cavity
> - Reduced pharyngeal tone
> - Laryngomalacia and/or tracheomalacia
> - Tracheal abnormalities
> - Adenotonsillar hypertrophy
> - Increased secretions
> - Axial hypotonia
> - Obesity
> - Pulmonary arterial hypertension
> - Hypothyroidism
> - Atlantoaxial subluxation and/or cervical ligament laxity
> - Reduced hypoxic drive

As in normal children, adenotonsillectomy (AT) is the initial treatment of choice for DS children with OSA and relatively enlarged tonsils and adenoids. Before surgery, however, cervical radiographs in extension and lateral flexion are recommended to screen for atlantoaxial subluxation or cervical ligament instability (present in 10-20% of infants and children with DS).[20] AT under endoscopic guidance may be useful to ensure maximal removal of their adenoidal tissue.[21] Because of the small airways in children with DS, when intubating a child with DS one should consider selecting an endotracheal tube that is at least two sizes smaller than would be used in a child of the same age without DS.[22]

Children with DS in general, and particularly those with SDB, are at increased risk for postoperative respiratory complications. A retrospective survey by Goldstein and colleagues[23] found respiratory complications occurred in 25% of 87 children with DS following AT compared to 5% in age-matched "uncomplicated" control subjects. They found the children with DS had longer lengths of stay following AT than did control subjects (mean 1.6 days vs. 0.8 days). Moreover, 25% of the DS children required airway management or observation in the pediatric intensive care unit (compared to none of the control subjects). Because of this increased incidence of postoperative complications, at least overnight hospitalization for DS children undergoing upper airway surgery should be considered.

A repeat PSG should be considered 2 to 3 months after AT in children with DS because significant residual OSA may be found on postoperative study despite parental reports of subjective "cure."[16] AT usually lessens OSA severity in children with DS, but often it does not normalize their SDB, and the improvement is less than seen after AT in children without DS.[24,25] A small case-control study by Shete and associates,[25] comparing PSG findings in children with and without DS, found that although the AHI improved both in children with and without DS, it improved less in the children with DS. Furthermore, the oxygen saturation nadir and AHI during REM sleep did not significantly change following AT in the children with DS, but all respiratory parameters improved following surgery in the children without DS. OSA resolved sufficiently so that no further treatment was required in only 27% of the

children with DS, but 73% required further treatment (continuous or bilevel positive airway pressure or oxygen) for significant residual obstruction.

Residual (or recurrent) OSA following AT in a child with DS warrants evaluation for the presence of lingual tonsils or regrowth of adenoidal tissue.[26-29] Donnelly and associates,[26] using cine magnetic resonance imaging (MRI) under sedation in 27 children with DS who had persistence or recurrence of OSA following AT (mean age 9.9 years),[26] found multiple causes for their OSA: macroglossia (74%), glossoptosis (63%), adenoidal regrowth (63%), and enlarged lingual tonsils (30%). Other studies have found lingual tonsils in 35% to 50% of DS children who had persistent or recurrent OSA following palatine tonsillectomy.[28,29] Enlarged lingual tonsils can be visualized on flexible nasopharyngoscopy or identified using cine MRI.[27]

Persistent OSA in a child with DS following removal of all adenoidal and tonsillar tissues warrants consideration of continuous positive airway pressure (CPAP) (or bilevel positive airway pressure [BiPAP], if needed to improve tolerance or treat hypoventilation). Nasal or oronasal CPAP is an effective treatment for OSA in those who can tolerate it.[30] Extensive mask desensitization using play therapy is often required in this group to achieve satisfactory PAP compliance.[31,32] Oral aversion, common in children with DS, often contributes to their difficulty tolerating PAP.[33] Oral appliances should be considered for older children with DS who will not tolerate or use PAP,[32] but there are similar issues of compliance.[34] Weight management, good dental care, and medical treatment of rhinitis and allergies may also help when indicated clinically.[34-37] For infants and young children with DS who have severe persistent OSA and severe retrognathia, midface hypoplasia, or macroglossia, but do not tolerate PAP, upper airway surgeries such as mandibular distraction osteogenesis, tongue base reduction, maxillary/midface advancement, or tracheostomy may be considered.[38-41]

Prader-Willi Syndrome

Prader-Willi syndrome (PWS) is the most frequent cause of *secondary* obesity in children, occurring in about 1 in 15,000 births.[42] During infancy, PWS is characterized by severe central hypotonia with poor suck, weak cry, decreased movement, and lethargy. Between ages 1 and 6 years, symptoms of hyperphagia and insatiable appetite develop and lead to morbid central obesity. Short stature is usually present as well (50% are at or below the third percentile for age). The main clinical features of PWS are summarized in Box 40-2.[42,43]

PWS has a genetic basis: in 70% there is a sporadic microdeletion on the long arm of the paternal chromosome 15 at q11q13, and in 20% both copies of chromosome 15 are inherited from the mother (maternal uniparental disomy).[42] The origin of this particular region of chromosome 15 is important because it is subject to parent-of-origin imprinting (i.e., only one copy of the gene is expressed while the other is silenced). For the genes affected in PWS it is the paternal copy that is usually expressed, while the maternal copy is silenced. Molecular genetic testing confirms the particular parent-specific methylation abnormality in more than 99% of individuals with PWS. Genetic testing is particularly helpful in diagnosing those with atypical features or too young to make the diagnosis on clinical grounds.

- Severe central hypotonia at birth with a poor suck, weak cry, lethargy, and decreased movement during infancy
- Delayed language development
- Delayed motor milestones
- Characteristic facies (almond-shaped eyes, strabismus, narrow bifrontal diameter, thin upper lip, down-turned mouth)
- Small hands and feet
- Short stature
- Hyperphagia and insatiable appetite by age of 1 to 6 years, morbid obesity by age of 4 years
- Fat storage in the abdomen, buttocks, and thighs even in nonobese patient
- Hypothalamic hypogonadism (genital hypoplasia, incomplete pubertal development, and, in most cases, infertility)
- Stubbornness, temper tantrums, self-injury, skin-picking, food foraging, impulsivity, mood lability, repetitive speech
- Learning difficulties, poor academic performance, mean IQ 60s to 70s
- Impaired social cognition, literal-mindedness, cognitive inflexibility
- Sleep-disordered breathing (especially sleep-related hypoventilation, often mild obstructive sleep apnea)
- Hypothalamic dysfunction with central hypersomnia
- Impaired growth hormone secretion and low serum insulin-like growth factor-I levels

SDB is common in PWS, even in those without sleep/wake complaints. Sleep-related hypoventilation is the most common pattern of SDB in PWS, with the risk for it increased by hypotonia and obesity.[44-51] Nevertheless, 10% to 50% of PWS patients will have OSA on overnight PSG,[52-54] but most often findings are mild with obstructive AHI of less than 10.[53-55] In one study of 30 PWS patients (mean age 7 ± 4 years) the AHI averaged only 6 ± 4 events per hour of sleep and desaturation events occurred at a rate of only 8 ± 7 per hour, but the lowest oxygen saturation value seen during PSG was more striking, namely 77 ± 10%.[54] Another study found that neither the severity nor type(s) of SDB could be predicted by the body mass index (BMI) Z score, Epworth sleepiness scale score, or the particular genetic mutation in patients with PWS;[50] for these reasons, the investigators argued there should be a low threshold for obtaining PSG to evaluate SDB in PWS.

Compared with healthy control subjects, children with PWS have PSG findings of a shorter REM latency, decreased duration of NREM stage N3 sleep, and increased NREM instability.[44,56,57] Most respiratory events in children with PWS are central apneas (although, as mentioned previously, obstructive hypopneas are seen with considerable frequency).[58] The sleep-related hypercapnia often present in patients with PWS will go undetected unless there is reliable CO_2 monitoring.

Sleep hypoventilation in PWS is usually treated by BiPAP, sometimes requiring a timed or backup rate. Treating SDB in children with PWS reportedly improves their cognitive function, daytime performance, and sleep quality.[46] If significant OSA is found on the PSG, AT can be considered if there are findings of adenotonsillar hypertrophy (ATH); the clinician should be aware, however, that there is increased risk for postoperative complications, and residual SDB may remain and require CPAP treatment.[49,59]

Central Hypersomnia in Prader-Willi Syndrome

Hypersomnia often remains in patients with PWS after successful treatment of both SDB and obesity, and this symptom is thought to be central in origin related to hypothalamic dysfunction.[60,61] Multiple sleep latency test (MSLT) studies done in PWS patients with hypersomnia are often abnormal (with mean sleep latencies of < 5 minutes in 50% of patients, and sleep onset REM periods in some).[61] Other factors that may contribute to hypersomnia in PWS are obesity-hypoventilation, impaired respiratory drive, and to a lesser extent, OSA. Skeletal axial hypotonia improves over time, but PWS adults remain mildly hypotonic and are often prone to scoliosis (which may add a pulmonary restrictive component to their SDB).

The most common sleep/wake complaint in adults with PWS is excessive daytime sleepiness.[62] Higher levels of fasting plasma adiponectin (an adipose tissue–derived hormone) in children with PWS was recently found to correlate with excessive daytime sleepiness and AHI values.[63] A recent review by Bruni and associates[64] found that central hypothalamic dysfunction may contribute to obesity and hypersomnia in PWS, findings that are made worse by the presence of OSA and obesity-hypoventilation. Hypersomnia that occurs without concomitant SDB or that persists after successful treatment of SDB warrants consideration of trials of modafinil (or armodafinil) and other central nervous system (CNS) stimulants.

Risks and Benefits of Exogenous Growth Hormone in Children with Prader-Willi Syndrome

Exogenous growth hormone (GH) treatment is increasingly recommended to increase height and the ratio of lean muscle to body fat composition in PWS. A randomized placebo-controlled trial found that PWS children aged 4 to 16 treated with GH showed significantly increased height velocity, decreased mean body fat, increased mean lean body mass, improved physical strength, and increased respiratory muscle function,[65,66] prompting a recommendation for its use in PWS,[67] preferably started before age 3 years.[68]

A randomized controlled trial of GH (1 mg/m^2/day) in 91 prepubertal children (infancy to 14 years) found that GH administration significantly improved height and BMI, normalized head circumference, and improved body proportions and body fat percentage.[69] Another recently published study found 21 PWS children treated with GH for 6 years (beginning at age 13 ± 6 months) had lower body fat (mean 36% vs. 45%), greater height (131 vs. 114 cm), greater motor strength, and better lipid profiles compared to 27 children of a similar age (ages 5-9 years) prior to GH treatment.[70]

A recent prospective study evaluated the effects of 3 years of GH treatment on 36 children (ages 1-15 years) with PWS. Over the 3-year treatment period, children treated with GH gained 1.2 standard deviations in height, and lean body mass increased significantly each treatment year, total body fat decreased (by 5.4% in the first year, 1.2% the second), and lipid profiles improved. Before treatment 23% had glucose intolerance, but none did after the 3-year treatment. Other studies also support the efficacy of GH use in children with PWS,[69,71-73,74,75] especially when started before age 3 years.[68]

It is crucial to identify and treat other endocrine deficiencies common in children with PWS, many of which may contribute to their predisposition for obesity, hypersomnia, and SDB. Diene and associates[76] recently reported that 80% of 142 PWS children (median age 7.1 years) in the French National PWS pediatric database had GH deficiency (87% of them were being treated with GH), but 49% also had hypogonadism, 24% hypothyroidism, and 4% glucose intolerance (although none had diabetes mellitus). Because of their obesity, PWS children are predisposed to develop metabolic syndrome, and identifying and treating this disorder are also important.[77]

Increased Risk for Sudden or Premature Death in Prader-Willi Syndrome

Individuals with PWS have an annual death rate of 3% and are at increased risk for sudden or premature death.[44] A large case series found respiratory failure and infections, the most common cause of death in PWS patients, present in 61% of 64 PWS children.[58] Childhood sudden death in PWS is often associated with respiratory infection and high temperature.[44,58] Impaired central (hypothalamic) body temperature regulation may contribute to sudden death in PWS infants and children when they are sick. Sudden death in infants with PWS is more often secondary to milk aspiration; viral infections seem to be the most common association in older children and adolescents; respiratory failure, pulmonary embolism, and cellulitis or other complications of morbid obesity are the most common causes of death in adults with PWS.[58]

Initial reports raised great concern that exogenous GH therapy contributed to or caused sudden death in PWS. More recent studies refute this. Exogenous GH treatment does not worsen SDB in PWS.[44] Festen and colleagues[44] found a mean AHI of 5.4 in 53 prepubertal PWS children (mean age 5.4 years) before receiving GH (1 mg/m^2) and a mean AHI of 4.8 after 6 months of treatment. More than half of the respiratory events (2.8/hour) in the pretreatment PSG were central apneas (mean duration 15 seconds); the rest were hypopneas. Central apneas did not correlate with BMI, but did decrease with age. One child died unexpectedly during a mild upper respiratory tract infection (although he had a nearly normal PSG). Miller and associates[78] found no significant effect on SDB in 20 infants with PWS (aged 2 to 21 months) 6 weeks after starting GH therapy. However, 12 had an increase in the frequency of obstructive events associated with either gastroesophageal reflux or an upper respiratory infection at the time of the second sleep study, which normalized on repeat PSG studies.

Central adrenal insufficiency during stress may be the crucial factor predisposing people with PWS to unexpected death.[79-81] Researchers from the Netherlands hypothesized that PWS patients might suffer from central adrenal insufficiency during stressful conditions.[81] They showed that 60% of 25 randomly selected patients with PWS (mean age 9.7 years) had central adrenal insufficiency with adrenocorticotropic hormone (ACTH) levels remaining below 33 pmol/L at 7:30 AM after receiving metyrapone (a pharmacologic stressor) at a dose of 30 mg/kg at 11:30 PM the night before.[80] The authors suggested that the high percentage of central adrenal insufficiency in PWS might explain the high rate of sudden death in these patients, particularly during infection-related stress. Based on their data, they recommended treating PWS patients during acute illnesses with stress doses of hydrocortisone (unless central adrenal insufficiency has recently been ruled out with a metyrapone test).[80]

The same investigators found SDB was worse in 10 healthy PWS children (median age 8.4 years) who also had findings consistent with central adrenal insufficiency (with ACTH levels during the metyrapone test < 33 pmol/L at 7:30 AM).[79] They also found the median central apnea index (number of central apneas per hour of sleep) increased from 2.2 to 5.2 after metyrapone administration, and the increase was significantly higher among the children with central adrenal insufficiency (2.8 vs. 1.0). PSG performed before the metyrapone stress test showed that PWS children with central adrenal insufficiency had significantly higher central apnea indices and lower nadir Spo$_2$ values than did those without it. Identifying central adrenal insufficiency under stress in children with PWS may identify those at increased risk for sudden unexpected death (however, a recent case series found central adrenal insufficiency in only a fraction of PWS patients).[82]

Rett Syndrome

Rett syndrome (RS) is a progressive neurodevelopmental disorder that almost exclusively affects females because it is transmitted as an X-linked dominant trait; the homozygous mutation is lethal, with most males carrying the mutation dying shortly after birth.[83] More than 95% of cases of typical RS are due to sporadic (de novo) mutations in the methyl-CpG-binding protein 2 (*MECP2*) gene located on the X chromosome (Xq28). The *MECP2* gene codes for the MECP2 protein that turns off transcription of certain other genes, including brain-derived neurotrophic factor, which is important for neural plasticity, learning, and memory.[83] Familial cases of RS have been reported in which the mutation was inherited from a normal or mildly affected mother with either a gonadal mosaicism or favorable inactivation of the X chromosome.[84-87]

RS develops in 1 of every 10,000 to 20,000 female births and is the second most common cause of genetic mental retardation in females (after DS). After normal or near normal development for the first 6 to 18 months of life, slowing or stagnation of skill acquisition occurs, and then autistic features and truncal hypotonia appear,[88] followed by regression with loss of communication skills, eye contact, and purposeful hand use. Head growth slows and repetitive stereotyped hand movements (e.g., hand washing) and jerky truncal ataxia or gait ataxia appear.[89] Social withdrawal, early epileptic seizures, bruxism, panic-like attacks, progressive kyphosis or scoliosis, decreased somatic growth, small and cold hands and feet, and impaired cardiac, respiratory and gastrointestinal autonomic regulation are all common symptoms or findings.[90,91]

Episodic hyperventilation interspersed with breath holding is common in individuals with RS when *awake*; these problems begin spontaneously (not preceded by hypoxemia) and are interspersed with periods of prolonged breath holding (with apneas often lasting >19 seconds) accompanied by Valsalva maneuvers, severe hypocapnia, and sometimes arterial oxygen desaturations to values below 50%.[92]

More than 80% of patients with RS have sleep problems; often they are severe and persistent.[89] The most common sleep problems reported in 202 subjects with RS were nocturnal laughter (59%), bruxism (55%), long spells of screaming (36%), nocturnal seizures (26%), sleep terrors (18%), and sleep talking (18%). Up to age 7, 54% had frequent nocturnal awakenings; this number decreased to 40% at age 18. Daytime napping was common; 75% of those 8 years and older took daytime naps (70% of 8- to 12-year-olds, 73% of 13- to 17-year-olds, and 85% of the those older than 18 years old).[89] Nocturnal seizures peaked between ages 13 and 17, and nocturnal screaming decreased to 30% in those older than 18 years.[89]

Another study of 83 RS subjects found a nocturnal sleep latency of 31 minutes, a sleep efficiency of 90%, and total 24-hour sleep time of 10.75 hours (including 0.8 hour of daytime sleep) across 7 days of actigraphy monitoring.[93]

Compared with age-matched control subjects, girls with RS did not exhibit the age-related decrease in total sleep time and daytime sleep time seen in normal children. However, a case-controlled study found sleep architecture, sleep efficiency, and breathing were normal in 30 RS patients (median age 7 years) compared to age-matched control subjects.[94] Thus, unless there are clinical symptoms suggestive of SDB (e.g., scoliosis, which is present in 65% of patients), the diagnostic yield of PSG is low in patients with RS.[94]

The majority of RS patients (81-94%) suffer from epilepsy, particularly when young.[95,96] The median age of onset of seizures is 4 years (18% start before 1 year of age, 4% after age 12).[95] The seizures are often nocturnal. An electroencephalogram (EEG) pattern of rhythmical theta (4-5 or 5-6 Hz) activity over the central regions is characteristic, particularly during NREM sleep, and is often accompanied by central spikes.[97] Patients with RS have a higher incidence of sudden unexplained death compared with age-matched control subjects, which may reflect their loss of heart rate variability and impaired cardiac autonomic regulation.[98]

Treating Insomnia in Children with Rett Syndrome

Oral melatonin is often effective in treating sleep problems in girls with RS.[87,99] A double-blind, placebo-controlled, crossover trial of oral melatonin (2.5-7.5 mg based upon body weight) prescribed nightly in 9 girls with RS (mean age 10.1 years) reduced their mean sleep latency from 42 ± 12 minutes to 19 ± 5 minutes without adverse effects or loss of efficacy over 10 weeks.[75] Abnormalities in melatonin secretion were observed in two girls with RS, the effectiveness of oral melatonin (3 mg nightly) was maintained over 2 years of nightly treatment, and sleep disorders recurred when melatonin was withheld.[99] Problematic nighttime behaviors in RS may also respond to graduated extinction and other behavioral treatments.[100] Other symptomatic and supportive treatments for RS, summarized in Box 40-3, can greatly improve the quality of life, health, and well-being for these children.[91,101-104]

Angelman Syndrome

Angelman syndrome (AS) is characterized by frequent laughter, jerky movements, a peculiar gait (so-called *happy puppet*), developmental delay, lack of speech, severe intellectual disability, brachy-microcephaly, and often medically refractory epilepsy with multiple seizure types and a characteristic EEG.[105,106] AS is a genetic disorder, occurs in 1 in 20,000 people, and is caused by a deletion of the maternal allele at chromosome 15q11-13 domain (70%) or, less often, by a *UBE3A* gene mutation (10-15%), a methylation imprinting mutation (3-5%), or inheritance of both alleles of the gene from the father (unilateral paternal disomy, 2-3%).

BOX 40-3 *Symptomatic and Supportive Treatments (Other than Melatonin) for Girls with Rett Syndrome*

- L-Carnitine (improves patient sense of well-being and quality of life; it also increases heart rate variability, thereby possibly reducing risk for sudden death)
- Magnesium (reduces episodes of hyperventilation in awake state)
- Soft elbow splints (may reduce repetitive hand washing movements)
- Gastrostomy tube (often useful to supplement inadequate caloric intake secondary to persistence of immature chewing and swallowing patterns)
- Encouragement of communication (through eye movements, finger pointing, gesture, body language, or communication devices)
- Bracing and, if needed, surgery for scoliosis
- Avoidance of drugs that may prolong QT intervals
- Prolonged video-EEG monitoring (to distinguish epileptic from nonepileptic behaviors)
- Bilateral ankle orthoses (for tight Achilles tendons and toe-walking)
- Parent support group and psychosocial support for caregivers

EEG, electroencephalography.

Children and adults with AS often have significant and persistent problems falling asleep and staying asleep; there are also complaints of reduced sleep duration, frequent nocturnal awakenings, and increased wake time after sleep onset.[107-111] Patients are easily awakened by loud noises, disoriented when aroused, rely heavily upon sleep facilitators, and are beset by parasomnias (sleepwalking, sleep terrors, bruxism, periodic limb movements, and sleep-related epilepsy).[107-111] Their sleep problems tend to persist past midpuberty and adversely affect caregivers' coping strategies.[109] Low-dose oral melatonin (0.3 mg 30-60 minutes before the patient's habitual bedtime) promoted and reduced motor activity during sleep in 13 AS children (aged 2-10 years).[112]

Smith-Magenis Syndrome

Smith-Magenis syndrome (SMS) occurs in 1 of 25,000 births and is characterized by the presence of short stature, scoliosis, a distinctive face (bradycephaly, midfacial hypoplasia, and prognathia with a cupid bow-shaped mouth), a hoarse deep voice, peripheral neuropathy, and developmental delay with later IQs in 40 to 60 range.[113-115] SMS is most often caused by a small 3.5 Mb interstitial deletion of chromosome 17p11.2 in the retinoic acid induced (*RAI1*) gene. This tiny deletion is easily overlooked when suspicion of SMS is not listed on the requisition.

SMS children and adults often have a behavioral phenotype characterized by self-injury (hitting, biting, skin picking, inserting foreign objects into body orifices, yanking nails) and a low sensitivity to pain, motor stereotypies (spasmodic upper body self-hugging, and lick and flip behavior—compulsive finger licking and book or magazine page flipping), temper tantrums, other emotional outbursts, attention-seeking or repetitive behaviors, disobedience, aggression, attention deficit hyperactivity disorder (ADHD), and sleep problems.[116] SMS infants have hypotonia and hyporeflexia and are often described as lethargic, constantly sleeping, and needing to be awakened to feed. One case series of 39 SMS subjects (mean age 10.5 years) found varying sleep problems in 65% to 100%, including difficulty falling asleep, shortened sleep cycles, frequent and prolonged nocturnal awakenings, excessive daytime sleepiness, daytime napping, snoring, and nocturnal enuresis.[117]

An extraordinary inversion of melatonin secretion with peaking in the day (instead of normally at night) was first reported by De Leersnyder and associates[118] in nine children with SMS (aged 4-17 years) and subsequently confirmed in two large cohorts, with 96% having inverted endogenous melatonin secretion.[119,120] However, multiple daytime samplings of salivary melatonin are needed to confirm the daytime elevation (lessening the clinical utility of such measurements as a diagnostic test).[121] The inverted melatonin secretion and maladaptive sleep behaviors of SMS have been treated by giving both a selective β_1-adrenergic antagonist (10 mg of acebutolol in the early morning to suppress the daytime melatonin secretion) and an evening dose of melatonin (to replace the normal nighttime peak).[118,120,122] This treatment regimen improved daytime behavior and concentration, delayed sleep onset, increased hours of sleep at night, and delayed waking.[118] Melatonin alone may not sufficiently improve the insomnia, and cognitive behavioral insomnia therapy may also be needed.[123] A recently published retrospective review queried parents and caregivers of 62 individuals with SMS regarding which medications best helped the disruptive behaviors and difficulty sleeping.[124]

Williams Syndrome

Williams syndrome (WS) is another genetic disorder that is characterized by a distinctive facies (full cheeks and lips, broad nasal tip, widely spaced teeth), a particular cognitive profile (visual spatial deficits, relatively preserved expressive language, and IQs in the 60s and 70s), a distinctive personality (social, friendly, gregarious, empathetic, loquacious, difficulty interpreting social cues, and prone to worries and fears), and various cardiovascular, skeletal, connective tissue, growth, and endocrine abnormalities.[125,126] Feeding difficulties often lead to failure to thrive as infants. Hypotonia and hyperextensible joints can result in delayed motor milestones. WS is caused by a hemizygous deletion of between 1.55-1.8 Mb of chromosome 7q11.23.[127] It occurs in 1 in 7500 births and is caused by a contiguous gene microdeletion in the region of the elastin (ELN) gene. The diagnosis is confirmed by finding the gene mutation (present in > 90% of individuals with the clinical phenotype).

A recently published study compared sleep difficulties in 64 children with WS (aged 6-12 years) and 92 age-matched healthy control subjects.[128] The study found 97% of parents of children with WS reported that their children had sleep problems: greater bedtime resistance, sleep anxiety, night waking, and daytime sleepiness. Other sleep disorders that have been reported in patients with WS include sleep onset and sleep maintenance insomnia, restless legs, periodic limb movements during sleep, SDB, daytime sleepiness, and nocturnal anxieties, phobias, and fears.[126] A study using actigraphy, sleep questionnaires, and diaries confirmed that 23 adolescents

and adults with WS (mean age 25 ± 8 years) who were often described as excessively sleepy slept a mean of 9 hours nightly but had reduced mean sleep efficiencies (74%), prolonged sleep latencies (38 minutes), increased wake time after sleep onset (WASO) (56 min), and an elevated movement index (14 movements per hour).[126] A case-control study recorded overnight PSG in 9 adolescents and young adults with WS and 9 healthy control subjects[129] and found the WS subjects had decreased sleep time, decreased sleep efficiency, increased WASO, decreased percentage of REM sleep, increased numbers of leg movements, and irregular sleep cycles. A study by Arens and colleagues[130] recorded in-laboratory PSG in 16 WS children (mean age 4 ± 2 years) who were reported to have excessive movements when sleeping. They found that the children with WS had significantly more periodic limb movements per hour of sleep compared with age-matched control subjects (15/hour vs. 3/hour), and periodic limb movements in the WS children often caused arousals or awakenings. Clonazepam was prescribed for five of these children and parents reported improved sleep quality in four.

Fragile X Syndrome

Fragile X syndrome (FXS) is the most common cause of genetically acquired intellectual disability and is due to a mutation in the fragile X mental retardation 1 gene (FMR1) on the X chromosome at Xq23.7. FXS occurs in 1 per 250 to 810 males and 1 per 130 to 250 females in the general population.[131] The severity of the phenotype is significantly influenced by the length of the CGG triplet repeats in the gene (a normal repeat number is 5 to 44, carriers of the mutation have 55 to 200 repeats, and the full FXS mutation typically have more than 200 CGG repeats). The FMR1 gene codes for the FMR1 protein (FMRP), and absence of this protein leads to failed inhibition and subsequent up-regulation of proteins involved in synaptic maturation and plasticity, especially in the metabotropic glutamate receptor 5 system (mGluR5).

Individuals with FXS often have excessive arousal responses to sensory stimuli (and enhanced sympathetic nerve activity) that may manifest as social anxiety, agitation, and outbursts of physical or verbal aggression.[132] They may also have inattention and mood swings, and 30% have symptoms consistent with autism spectrum disorder.[133] Characteristic clinical features of FXS are summarized in Box 40-4. Males with fragile X syndrome have mild to severe intellectual disability: IQs

---

BOX 40-4 *Clinical Features in Children with Fragile X Syndrome*

- Long face, large ears, prominent jaw
- High-arched palate
- Poor eye contact, autistic behaviors
- Unusual motor behaviors (biting, hand flapping)
- Excessive arousal responses to sensory stimuli (social anxiety, agitation, aggressive physical or verbal outbursts)
- Attention deficit, hyperactivity, mood swings.
- Large testicles (two to three times normal adult size)
- Flat feet
- Double-jointed or hyperextensible finger joints
- Variable cognitive impairment

greater than 70 present in only 15%, and higher IQs have been found to correlate with higher levels of FMRP.[134] By contrast, 40% of women with the full fragile X mutation are cognitively normal, 35% have borderline intelligence, and only 25% have an IQ below 70.

Sleep problems are common in children with FXS. A recently published study surveyed the parents of 1295 children and adolescents with FXS regarding sleep problems: 32% were experiencing sleep problems at the time of the survey, most often difficulty falling asleep or frequent nocturnal awakenings.[135] An earlier study by the same investigators found 47% of 90 FXS children had sleep problems and that 19% had been treated with medications to improve sleep.[136] One case-control study of adolescents with FXS (mean age 13.1 years) found those with FXS had reduced time in bed, a higher percentage of NREM stage N1 sleep, a lower percentage of REM sleep, and more disrupted sleep compared to age-matched control subjects and children with DS.[137] Experimental studies in *Drosophila* have shown the fragile X gene appears to regulate sleep need.[138]

One study found boys with FXS had higher peak melatonin levels and greater concentration-time curves between 10:00 PM and 8 AM compared to control subjects, findings that were attributed to overactivity of the sympathetic nervous system in FXS.[139] A 4-week, randomized, double-blind controlled trial of 18 subjects (mean age 5.5 ± 3.6 years) with FXS by Wirojanan and associates[140] found that 3 mg of melatonin given for 2 weeks resulted in a significantly longer mean sleep duration and reductions of the mean sleep latency (to 28 minutes) and in-bed time (by 42 minutes).

Behavioral insomnias in FRX children who also have autism spectrum disorder can improve by educating their parents on how to develop more effective bedtime rituals, providing clear (verbal or, when needed, nonverbal) bedtime instructions, and applying behavioral therapies such as graduated extinction and reinforcement techniques[141] (see the following section and Chapter 35).

Autism Spectrum Disorders

The 4th edition of the Diagnostic and Statistical Manual of Mental Disorders (DSM-IV) defines autism as a spectrum disorder that include autistic disorder, pervasive developmental disorder not otherwise specified, Asperger syndrome, childhood disintegrative disorder, and RS.[142,143] The core features of autism spectrum disorder (ASD) are impaired social interaction, limited communication, and a restricted repertoire of motor behaviors, interests, and activities.[142,143] The 2007 National Survey of Children's Health estimated the prevalence of parent-reported ASD among U.S. children aged 3 to 17 years as 110 per 10,000 children (673,000 children overall), with ASD being four times more common in boys than girls.[144]

The neuropathologic basis of autism continues to unfold. A recently published longitudinal case-control study found early brain overgrowth during infancy and the toddler years, in autistic boys and girls, followed by an accelerated rate of decline in size or perhaps degeneration, from adolescence to late middle age.[145] Neuropathologic studies in autism have found cortical dysgenesis, misorientation of pyramidal neurons, and increased cell packing density.[146] ASD probably has a genetic basis (based on findings of a higher risk for the disorder in monozygotic and dizygotic twins and siblings), but inheritance is most likely polygenetic.[147-151] Brain autoantibodies, proinflammatory cytokine abnormalities, and altered T-cell function in some individuals with ASD suggest that complex gene-environmental interactions may also contribute.[152-158] Additional research is needed to understand how glutamate neurotoxicity, low melatonin production, and proinflammatory cytokines contribute to the symptoms and development of ASD.

Sleep problems are very common in children with ASD, reportedly occurring in 44% to 83% of children with ASD (according to one study)[159] compared to 11% to 37% of normally developing children.[160,161] Insomnia is the most commonly reported sleep problem in children with ASD, and may present as problems with sleep onset or sleep maintenance.[162,163] Thus, ASD children often take more than an hour to fall asleep, and many have nocturnal awakenings that may last as long as 2 to 3 hours.[163] These problems are often associated with poor sleep hygiene and maladaptive sleep associations.[164]

Another study of 167 ASD children found 86% had at least one sleep/wake problem including parasomnias (53%), suspected SDB (25%), difficulty awakening in morning (45%), and excessive daytime sleepiness (31%).[165] A cross-sectional study, using standardized sleep questionnaires and sleep diaries coupled with 10 days of actigraphy, found 66% of 59 children (aged 4-10 years) with ASD had sleep problems compared to 45% of 40 normally developing control subjects.[162] A population-based study found parents reported at least one sleep problem in 53% of 529 ASD children (aged 2-5 years) compared with 46% of 63 children with non-ASD developmental delays and 32% of 163 normally developing children.[166] Actigraphy and PSG confirmed that those children with ASD who were rated by their parents as being poor sleepers had longer sleep latencies, reduced sleep efficiency, and increased sleep fragmentation than did ASD children described by their parents as good sleepers.[167]

There has been the suggestion that the higher prevalence of sleep problems in children with ASD is primarily related to the level of intellectual disability; thus, one study found more frequent and severe sleep problems in ASD children with moderate to severe intellectual disability compared to those with only mild intellectual dysfunction.[159] However, sleep problems (particularly decreased sleep durations and increased sleep latencies, sleep anxieties, and parasomnias) were reported in 78% of 37 high-functioning ASD children without intellectual disabilities compared to 26% of 44 normally developing children.[168] Risk factors for sleep problems in children with ASD are summarized in Box 40-5.[165]

BOX 40-5 *Risk Factors for Sleep Problems in Children with Autism Spectrum Disorders*

- Hypersensitivity to environmental stimuli
- Family history of sleep problems
- Young age
- Co-sleeping
- Epilepsy
- Developmental regression (typically at age 2 to 3 years)
- Interictal epileptiform activity during sleep

Disturbed circadian rhythms (irregular sleep/wake schedules, free-running rhythms, delayed sleep phase) have been observed in some children with ASD.[164,169-172] One study found that sleep problems varied with the season in more than 10% of children with ASD, rapidly increasing in severity in the fall and spring (especially in those with a history of developmental regression).[173]

Anomalies in clock genes (that control the function of the circadian timing system) may explain circadian rhythm disorders common in children with ASD.[174,175] Low nocturnal melatonin levels, for example, may reflect certain of these anomalies and contribute the abnormal circadian timing observed in some children with ASD.[176] Thus, 24-hour monitoring of serum melatonin levels have shown that individuals with ASD often have lower nocturnal melatonin levels than control subjects,[177-179] a finding attributed to low activity of acetyl-serotonin O-methyltransferase (ASMT).[178,179] ASMT is the last enzyme in the melatonin synthesis pathway, and the gene that codes for ASMT may be involved in the development of ASD. As a result, nocturnal urinary excretion of 6-sulfatoxymelatonin (6-SM), the major urinary metabolite of melatonin, is also often low in individuals with ASD compared with age-matched healthy control subjects. A recently published case series of 23 children (mean age 5.7 years) with ASD, with two nights of in-laboratory PSG and one night of overnight 6-SM collection,[180] found the children with ASD as a group had low urinary 6-SM excretion rates but the levels varied widely among individuals. They found a greater percent of time spent in stage N3 sleep, less time in stage N2 sleep, and decreased parent-reported daytime sleepiness in the subset of ASD with relatively higher (i.e., more normal) 6-SM levels.

Diagnostic Sleep Studies in Children with Autism Spectrum Disorder

Diagnostic studies confirming altered sleep architecture and sleep/wake cycles in children in ASD are sparse (in part because of the recording challenges many of these children present). Buckley and associates[181] compared overnight PSG in three cohorts: children with ASD, those with non-ASD developmental delay, and normally developing age- and gender-matched control subjects. They found that children with ASD had shorter total sleep time, greater percentage of stage N3 sleep, and much less time spent in REM sleep than did children with non-ASD developmental delay or normally developing children. There were no significant differences in sleep architecture between the children with non-ASD developmental delay and the control group.

A small case-control PSG study by Elia and colleagues[182] found that 17 children with ASD (including 7 with mental retardation and fragile X syndrome) had less total sleep time, less time in bed, less sleep period time, a lower percentage of N1 sleep, less time in bed, and shorter REM latency than 5 age-matched control subjects. Another PSG study in 31 children with ASD found significantly reduced time in bed, total sleep time, sleep period time, and REM latency, and increased NREM instability compared with control subjects.[183] Diomedi and colleagues[184] found reduced REM density, inappropriate markers of REM sleep in NREM sleep, and excessive phasic activity during REM sleep in children with ASD and marked intellectual disability. A cross-sectional study by Bruni and associates,[185] comparing PSG findings in

8 children with Asperger's syndrome, 10 with autism, and 12 healthy age-matched control subjects, found only minor sleep architecture differences among the three groups, but cyclic alternating pattern analysis showed abnormalities consistent with NREM instability in the affected children.

Malow and colleagues[186] recorded two nights of PSG in 21 children with ASD (10 identified by their caregivers as good sleepers, 11 as poor sleepers) and 10 children with normal development. The ASD poor sleepers had longer sleep latencies, reduced sleep efficiency, and more sleep fragmentation on their first night PSG compared with the ASD good sleepers and control group. No differences in sleep architecture were found between the ASD good sleepers and the control subjects.

Approximately a third of children with ASD have regression of language and social behavior (most often occurring between ages 2 and 3 years).[187-189] These children are much more likely to have interictal epileptiform discharge (IED) activity in their NREM sleeping EEGs (present in 20-50% of patients).[190,191] Approximately 10% to 15% of children with ASD have epilepsy and another 8% to 10% will have asymptomatic IEDs (i.e., without associated seizures).[190,191] However, the likelihood of finding IEDs during sleep in a child with ASD without history of regression is low. Given all this, an EEG with sleep is warranted if a child with ASD also has a history of autistic regression, especially after age 2.[192]

Sleep disturbances affect daytime functioning in ASD. The amount of daytime inattention, hyperactivity, and repetitive or restricted behaviors correlates with the amount of sleep fragmentation found at night.[167] Similarly, stereotypic behaviors, social skill deficits, overall autism scores, and nocturnal screaming were all increased in ASD children sleeping too little at night.[193] Sleep problems in children with ASD were also associated with more self-injurious compulsive ritualistic behaviors during the day, especially in those with more significant cognitive impairments.[194] Also, treating these sleep disorders in children (or adults) with ASD can help their daytime behavior and cognitive functioning.[163,186,195-197]

Diagnosing and Treating Behavioral Insomnia in Children with Autism Spectrum Disorder

Sleep disorders in children with ASD can be divided into two principal groups: insomnias and paroxysmal nocturnal behaviors.[167] Treatment of insomnia in individuals with ASD begins with a comprehensive history and physical examination, sleep diaries, and sleep questionnaires (specifically validated for ASD).[186,196,198,199]

Actigraphy, when available, may help clarify when and how much the youngster is actually sleeping. It is crucial to identify and treat concomitant epilepsy, gastroesophageal reflux, iron deficiency, or other primary sleep disorders (e.g., OSA, periodic limb movements, circadian rhythm disorder).[200] Children with ASD are occasionally referred to sleep specialists to determine whether their paroxysmal nocturnal behaviors are epileptic seizures, NREM arousal disorders, rhythmic movement disorder, or REM sleep behavior disorder. Video-PSG with expanded EEG montages and extra electromyogram (EMG) electrodes to the wrist extensor muscles should be used when evaluating parasomnias in children with ASD.[192] REM sleep without atonia and REM sleep behavior disorder was observed in the PSG of 5 of 11 children with ASD, many of whom also had OSA.[201] Complaints of excessive motor restlessness, frequent limb jerks, or restless legs, or the PSG finding of periodic limb movements of sleep (PLMS), should prompt an evaluation of serum ferritin levels. Decreased iron and ferritin levels have been observed in children with ASD and should be treated with supplemental iron (taken with orange juice with vitamin C to improve absorption).[202,203]

Behavioral treatments for insomnia (usually coupled with parent or caregiver education) are the next step.[141,204-206] Teaching parents of children with ASD how to establish good sleep hygiene and positive bedtime rituals is crucial.[207,208] Use of storybooks is to be encouraged[209] and excessive computer game or television exposure before bedtime discouraged.[210] Treatment strategies for behavioral therapy in children with ASD are discussed in greater detail in Chapter 35 and are listed in Box 40-6.

If the insomnia in children with ASD remains problematic after trying behavioral strategies, consider initiating sleep-promoting agents while continuing behavioral treatments. Several studies have recently reported the efficacy of oral melatonin before bed to treat insomnia in children with ASD who have not responded to behavioral treatments. Andersen and associates[211] found that sleep problems resolved completely in 25% and improved in 60% of 107 children with ASD (ages 2-18 years) treated with oral doses of melatonin ranging from 0.75 to 6 mg (coupled with sleep hygiene education for the caregivers). Sleep worsened in only one child treated with melatonin. Adverse effects in 3 children included morning sleepiness and nocturnal enuresis. A recently published double-blind randomized controlled crossover trial of oral melatonin (up to 10 mg) of 22 children with ASD found melatonin significantly improved sleep latency (by an average of 47 minutes) and total sleep time (by 52 minutes) but did not lessen nocturnal awakenings.[212] The side effect profile was low and not significantly different between melatonin and the placebo. A small randomized double-blind, placebo-controlled crossover design study by Wirojanan and associates[140] found that mean sleep duration increased 21 minutes and sleep-onset time moved 42 minutes earlier in 12 children with ASD (mean age 5.5 years) taking 3 mg of melatonin before desired bedtime. A retrospective study by Galli-Carminati and colleagues[213] found that melatonin in doses of 3 to 9 mg before nocturnal bedtime improved sleep in six adults with ASD and severe circadian rhythm disorders.

Melatonin is an important synchronizer of many physiologic processes in the brain and body. Dysfunction in melatonin receptors, mutant melatonin genes, and abnormal melatonin synthesis may be primary contributor to the pathogenesis of ASD.[177,179,212,214,215] Shah and associates[216] found that melatonin harvested from pills or capsules can be mixed in a variety of liquids and foods (water, orange juice, semi-skimmed milk, strawberry yogurt, and strawberry jam) and remains stable for up to 6 hours at room temperature, useful in children who have difficulty swallowing pills. Box 40-7 provides a summary of current considerations when prescribing melatonin in children with ASD.

Other Medications Used to Treat Autism Spectrum Disorder

Medications used to treat other symptoms of ASD can help, or worsen, the symptoms of insomnia or daytime sleepiness. Hyperarousal behaviors (hyperactivity, stereotyped body movements, self-stimulation, hypervigilance, and impulsivity) in ASD may respond to treatment with α_2-adrenergic receptor agonists (clonidine or guanfacine) or selective norepinephrine reuptake inhibitors (atomoxetine).[217-221] A weekly transdermal patch of clonidine reportedly helped daytime behaviors, but sleepiness and fatigue were particularly common during the first 2 weeks of treatment.[220] A open-label retrospective review of 19 children with ASD found that oral clonidine (0.1-0.2 mg) given 30 minutes before bed promoted sleep, especially in ASD children who were overly aroused or mildly anxious at bedtime.[218] The authors reported clonidine reduced sleep latency, lessened nocturnal awakenings, and (to a lesser extent) may have improved daytime symptoms of ADHD, mood instability, and aggressiveness. Guanfacine (3 mg by mouth) significantly improved aberrant behaviors and lessened hyperactivity in 5 of 11 children with ASD but caused some drowsiness and irritability.[221]

Anxiety, obsessive-compulsive repetitive behaviors, irritability, and behavioral rigidity may respond to treatment with selective serotonin reuptake inhibitors (SSRIs) such as fluoxetine or fluvoxamine.[222-225] Repetitive behaviors in ASD may

---

BOX 40-6 *Treatment Strategies for Behavioral Insomnia in Children with Autism Spectrum Disorders*

- Develop consistent bedtime ritual.
- Adhere to consistent and appropriate bedtimes and wake times.
- Provide quiet, comfortable, safe place to sleep, darkened (or dim nightlight).
- Reinforce sleep time by turning the lights out just before "time to go to sleep" and turning them on again as soon as the child awakens in the morning.
- Remove television and other electronic distractions from bedroom.
- Avoid stimulating activities during the hour before bed.
- Ensure adequate daily exercise.
- Introduce graduated extinction techniques as appropriate (see Chapter 35).
- If behavioral strategies alone are unsuccessful, consider adding sleep-promoting agents (see Chapter 36).

BOX 40-7 *Current Considerations in Prescribing Oral Melatonin in Children with Autism Spectrum Disorders*

- Dose at 1 mg one-half hour before bedtime; increase by 3 mg every 1-2 weeks as needed (usual dose, 3 to 6 mg; maximum, 6 to 9 mg).
- Avoid over-the-counter formulations of melatonin, which may contain other active ingredients.
- Extended-release melatonin may be useful for children with sleep maintenance difficulties.
- Wean slowly 6 weeks after a sleep cycle is established.
- Capsules may be dissolved or mixed into water, orange juice, part-skim milk, or strawberry jam or yogurt (melatonin will remain stable in solution for 6 hours at room temperature).

respond to divalproex sodium[226] or low-dose liquid fluoxetine (mean final dose 10 ± 4 mg/day).[224] A recently published 12-week randomized double-blind placebo-controlled trial demonstrated the efficacy of oral divalproex sodium in treating irritability in 55 children (mean age 9.5 ± 2.5 years). Overall, 63% of divalproex subjects were responders, compared to only 9% of placebo subjects. There was a trend for responders to have higher valproate blood levels compared with nonresponders. An earlier 8-week double-blind placebo-controlled trial showed oral divalproex was effective in treating repetitive behaviors in 13 children with ASD.[226]

Because SSRIs may cause insomnia or sleepiness, timing of dosing may need adjustment, for example, depending on whether the insomnia is in the morning or evening. SSRIs may also trigger sleepwalking, and can worsen periodic limb movements or symptoms of restless legs. Insomnia caused by SSRIs may respond to clonazepam (0.25-1 mg 30 minutes before bed) but can cause disinhibition in some children. Antidepressants are sometimes used to treat insomnia, particularly the tetracyclic agent trazodone.[227,228] Trazodone can be associated with priapism thought to result from unopposed α-adrenergic blockade;[229,230] therefore, its use should be avoided in pubertal males who cannot communicate the occurrence of such symptoms.

Symptoms of aggression, irritability, self-injury, and explosive outbursts in children with ASD often respond to aripiprazole[231-235] or risperidone, but weight gain remains a major adverse effect (as it does, to varying degrees, for all atypical neuroleptics)[184-188] and can lead to the subsequent development of childhood obesity and OSA. A recently published double-blind placebo-controlled parallel-group trial by Marcus and colleagues confirmed the short-term efficacy and safety of aripiprazole to treat tantrums, aggression, and self-injurious behaviors in 218 children and adolescents with ASD (ages 6-17 years).[234] Aripiprazole was dosed at 5, 10, or 15 mg per day and was well tolerated (sedation was the most common adverse event leading to discontinuation). Another randomized double-blind placebo-controlled trial of aripiprazole found extrapyramidal symptom-related adverse event rates were 15% for aripiprazole and 8% for placebo; mean weight gain was 2.0 kg on aripiprazole and 0.8 kg on placebo at week 8.[233]

Physicians and families should be encouraged to take advantage of online resources for ASD.[236] Different behavioral therapies are primary for deficient and excessive behaviors in ASD and should be started when the condition is first recognized to improve outcomes.[237,238] Families and patients should be encouraged to find a medical source that provides them accessible, continuous, comprehensive, compassionate, culturally sensitive family-centered care. Delivery of family-centered services improves both patient and family outcomes.[236,239,240] The Centers for Disease Control and Prevention website provides useful information, autism-specific diagnostic tools, and autism awareness materials for families and physicians.[241] The American Academy of Pediatrics also has a website providing guidelines and a tool kit to help physicians and families identify ASD.[242] There are powerful ASD support groups, such as Autism Speaks[243] and the Autism Network that provide help, and parent-based sleep education programs have had some success as well by providing suggestions to help reduce symptoms of insomnia in children with ASD.[205]

OTHER PEDIATRIC NEUROLOGIC DISORDERS

Intellectual Disability

In a study by Didden and associates[244] 16% of children with mild to profound intellectual disability (ID) had at least one type of sleep problem, namely severe settling problems (4%), night wakings (11%), or early morning awakening in (4%). Severe sleep problems were seen more often in children who were younger, needed medication more often, or had cerebral palsy, epilepsy, more severe ID, daytime sleepiness with napping, and daytime problem behaviors (aggression, hyperactivity, and opposition).[244] Sleep problems in children with severe ID tend to be persistent; thus, sleep problems present in 44% of 209 ID children had existed for 7 ± 4 years.[245] Robinson and Richdale[246] summarized data from two studies of children (aged 3-18 years) with ID (n = 149 and n = 243, respectively). The prevalence rates of sleep problems in the two studies were 26% and 36%. Sleep problems tended to be persistent (the reported average durations were 6 and 9 years).

A case-control study found successful application of cognitive behavioral insomnia therapy and education for caregivers improved sleep of ID children and increased sense of control and reduced stress among caregivers.[247] Oral melatonin may be effective in treating insomnia in children with intellectual disability.[248,249] Oral melatonin at a dose of 5 mg (or 2.5 in subjects younger than 6 years) significantly reduced challenging daytime behaviors, sleep latency, number and duration of nighttime awakenings, and advanced the timing of their nocturnal rise in melatonin measured by salivary dim light melatonin onset (DLMO) in 49 ID patients (mean age 18.2 ± 17.1 years) with chronic insomnia and challenging daytime behaviors.[248] The same investigators reported in an earlier study that oral melatonin compared with placebo significantly advanced mean sleep onset time by 34 minutes, decreased mean sleep latency by 29 minutes, increased mean total sleep time by 48 minutes, decreased the mean duration of nighttime awakenings by 17 minutes, and advanced the endogenous melatonin onset at night by an average of 2 hours in 51 adolescent and adult ASD subjects.[249]

Cerebral Palsy

Sleep disorders are common in children with cerebral palsy (CP). Forty-four percent of 173 children with CP (mean age 8.8 years) had at least one sleep problem compared to 5% of the general pediatric population.[198] Nineteen percent of the CP children had excessive daytime sleepiness, 15% had SDB, and 8% had NREM arousal disorders.[250] The risk for a sleep disorder was 21 times higher if the child had dyskinetic CP, 17 times greater with active epilepsy, and 13 times greater with either spastic quadriplegia or visual impairment.[250] Other studies have found that children with CP are more likely to have poor quality sleep, altered sleep architecture, increased arousals, delayed REM sleep latency, decreased numbers of gross body movements, fewer body position shifts, and decreased duration of REM sleep compared to age-matched healthy control subjects.[251,252]

Repeated pulmonary aspiration, airway colonization with pathogenic bacteria, bronchiectasis, and SDB are major contributors to death and morbidity in individuals with CP.[253] SDB in children with severe CP is often more severe compared to children with suspected sleep apnea without chronic medical conditions.[252] SDB in children with CP often consists of varying combinations of obstructive and central apneic events, and central or obstructive hypoventilation with hypoxemia during REM sleep. Children with severe CP and spastic quadriparesis had far fewer body position changes (0.3/hour) than did control subjects (6.6/hour) even when their oxygen saturation values fell as low as 70%.[252]

Treating Sleep-Disordered Breathing in Children with Cerebral Palsy

OSA in children with CP is often treated by initial tonsillectomy and adenoidectomy. Children with moderate to severe CP (especially those with spastic quadriparesis or epilepsy) are more likely to suffer postoperative respiratory complications, be left with residual OSA, and have lower "cure rates" following AT.[254-256] In 27 children with CP, 25 had tonsillar or adenoidal hyperplasia documented on physical examination or lateral neck radiographs.[257] Nineteen were treated for their OSA by tonsillectomy and adenoidectomy, 3 additionally had uvulectomy. Symptoms of OSA remitted in 19 of 25 when seen in follow-up of 34 months, while 6 patients required further surgeries, but 4 children still later required tracheotomy to control their OSA.[257] Another study compared the likelihood of residual OSA following upper airway surgeries in children with "uncomplicated" OSA and those with complex co-morbidities.[255] The authors' findings were similar and led to the suggestion that a postoperative PSG should be considered 2 to 3 months following surgery because residual OSA is likely to remain.

For clinically significant SDB not (successfully) treatable by AT, CPAP titration (or BiPAP if better tolerated) can be undertaken but often would need to be preceded by a PAP desensitization trial.[31,258] Other choices are possible and include otolaryngologic/oral-surgical reevaluation for other airway surgeries (including mandibular distraction and skeletal expansion);[257,259-261] aggressive treatment of co-morbidities such as excessive oral secretions, swallowing problems, epilepsy, and reflux;[262] use of nocturnal postural devices[263] or oral appliances;[264] and botulinum toxin injections of submandibular salivary glands to reduce hypersalivation.[265] Fitzgerald and colleagues[253] summarized treatment strategies for managing OSA and respiratory complications in CP. Treating OSA in 51 children with CP (by AT or PAP) significantly improved their quality of life (especially sleep disturbances, caregiver concerns, and daytime functioning) compared to children for whom treatment was refused.[266]

Epilepsy

Seizures are a common neurologic problem in childhood, affecting 4% to 10% of children before age of 16 years. From 5% to 10% of children have seizures exclusively or primarily during sleep. NREM sleep is an activator of seizures and IEDs, especially those with frontal lobe foci,[267,268] but both seizures and IEDs are usually suppressed during REM (presumably reflecting the synchronizing functions of thalamo-cortical oscillations). In fact, most unsuspected or previously undiagnosed epileptic seizures in sleeping children represent nocturnal frontal lobe epilepsy (NFLE).[269-271]

Incidental (often asymptomatic) spike-wave discharges emanating from the central or occipital regions are found in 1.45% of pediatric PSGs.[272] Most often these are central-midtemporal *benign rolandic* spike-wave discharges. Miano and co-workers found unexpected IEDs in 18 (14.2%) of 127 children with OSA: 9 were centrotemporal, 5 were temporo-occipital, and 4 were frontocentral;[273] however, no IEDs were found in 40 children studied who only had primary snoring. The investigators also found lower REM sleep time and less cyclic alternating patterns in the children with IEDs. The finding of unanticipated IEDs in a child's PSG warrants concern of current or eventual seizures or epilepsy. Some of the children who have central rolandic spikes will have auditory language-processing difficulties that warrant clinical correlation. When IEDs are observed in a PSG, confirmation of their presence and character by standard EEG with sleep should follow, along with a formal neurologic evaluation. Figure 40-1 shows runs of focal

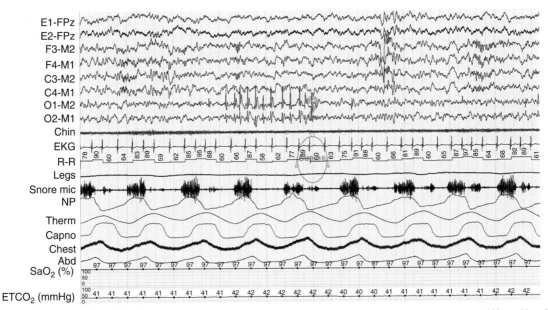

Figure 40-1 30-second PSG epoch showing runs of bi-occipital spike-wave discharges during stage N2 (light NREM) sleep in a 4-year-old boy with asthma and loud snoring. Channels 1-2, electro-oculogram; 3-8, EEG; 9, Chin EMG; 10-11, EKG, R-R interval, and heart rate; 12, leg EMG; 13, snore; 14, nasal pressure; 15, oronasal thermistor; 16, capnogram; 17-18, chest and abdominal excursion; 19-20, oxygen saturation and end-tidal carbon dioxide.

spike-wave discharges emanating from the occipital regions in a 4-year-old boy without any cognitive dysfunction or epilepsy.

Children with epilepsy have significantly more sleep problems than their siblings or healthy control subjects.[274] More bedtime difficulties, sleep fragmentation, daytime drowsiness, and parasomnias were reported in children with idiopathic epilepsy, especially those whose seizures were poorly controlled.[274] Poor sleep quality correlated with daytime inattention in children with epilepsy.[275] Children with epilepsy compared with control subjects had more daytime sleepiness and less on-task behavior and attentional abilities.[276] Another case-control parental-report study of 43 children with rolandic epilepsy (ages 6-16 years) found the children with epilepsy had significantly shorter sleep duration and more frequent parasomnias and daytime sleepiness than the control subjects.[277] Unfortunately, sleep complaints in children with epilepsy are rarely discussed at pediatric visits and thus the problems are often undiagnosed or misdiagnosed.[278]

Children with epilepsy who have "sleep problems" often have OSA.[274,275,279,280] One case-control study found 43% of 40 children with epilepsy referred for various sleep complaints had OSA on overnight PSG.[280] OSA on overnight PSG was more severe in the children with epilepsy and OSA compared to 11 children with "uncomplicated" moderate OSA: the children with epilepsy and OSA had significantly higher BMI (29 vs. 21.5), were more often obese (BMI > 95th percentile 62% vs. 18%), and had longer sleep latencies (51 vs. 16 minutes), higher arousal indices (49/hour vs. 21/hour of sleep), and lower nadirs of oxygen saturation (86% vs. 90%), despite having a lower mean AHI (3.4)

Vagal nerve stimulation (a treatment for medically refractory epilepsy) can worsen or unmask OSA in children with epilepsy. Decreases in airflow and respiratory effort, or frank obstructive events, during the period of vagal nerve activation (typically 30 seconds every 5 minutes) have been observed in children and adults,[281-284] but reducing the pulse width of the vagal nerve stimulation can sometimes lessen the effect upon breathing during sleep. In 26 children using vagal nerve stimulation, OSA was found in 15% and subsequently developed in another 15%, but such children responded successfully to AT or CPAP.[281]

Diagnostic Issue: Epileptic and Nonepileptic Parasomnias

Most children with epilepsy referred to sleep specialists arrive with the diagnosis of epilepsy already made. The referral may be to determine whether certain nocturnal behaviors represent a different type of epileptic seizure or a (nonepileptic) parasomnia. Parasomnias are unusual or undesirable behavioral events that occur predominantly during, or while emerging from, sleep; they are potentially injurious to the child or to those who attempt to intervene, and if sufficiently frequent they may disrupt sleep/wake schedules and family functioning[285] (see Chapters 38 and 43 to 45). The most common of these parasomnias (sleepwalking, sleep terrors, confusional arousals) are NREM sleep disorders of arousal and typically occur 90 to 180 minutes after sleep onset (when the first cycle in deep NREM is ending).

During a disorder of arousal, the child shows certain features also seen in seizures, namely confusion, disorientation, automatic behaviors, and sympathetic activation with little or no responsiveness to the external environment. Events last minutes and are followed by a return to sleep with little or no subsequent recall. There is commonly a familial or genetic predisposition: 60% have a first-degree relative with parasomnias versus 30% of the general population.[286] The incidence of NREM arousal parasomnias is higher in individuals and families with nocturnal frontal lobe epilepsy.[287] Many different medications can trigger or increase these events, including antipsychotics, antidepressants, antihistamines, sedative-hypnotics, and antiseizure drugs.[288-290]

Clinical features that should raise suspicion of a possible ictal origin include the following: events are very stereotyped; multiple episodes occur each night; events happen more than 2 or 3 nights per week; events may occur any time of the night, including the second half of the night or shortly before morning waking; there are occasional occurrences during wakefulness or a brief nap; there is associated impairment of daytime functioning or the presence of excessive daytime sleepiness; and there is a poor response to conventional (parasomnia) therapy.[192]

A PSG is *not* needed if the nocturnal behavior events are typical, noninjurious, infrequent, and not disruptive to the child or family.[285] However, if any of the atypical features listed here are present, of if the history suggests OSA, a sleep study should be done. OSA was found in 58% of 84 children with frequent arousal parasomnias, and tonsillectomy eliminated OSA and arousals in those who had tonsillectomy.[291] Insufficient sleep is another important trigger. For a fuller description of parasomnias in children (see Chapter 38).

If undiagnosed epileptic seizures are suspected, a routine video-EEG with partial sleep deprivation should be obtained. A prospective study of routine EEG done on 534 children referred for possible epilepsy reported epileptiform activity was found in 37% of the children with definite epilepsy, and 13% of clinically suspected cases.[292] Adding video when recording routine EEGs an average duration of only 26 minutes helped confirmed the diagnosis in 45% of children referred for frequent paroxysmal events and in 55% of the children with cognitive impairment.[293] Using video helped to confirm the nature of many nonepileptic events including staring spells, tics, motor stereotypies, tremor, paroxysmal eye movements, and breath-holding or cyanotic spells.

To evaluate nocturnal events that are unusual or atypical (of the sort described above), then, if the initial clinical evaluation and the results of a standard EEG are inconclusive, an in-laboratory video-PSG (V-PSG) is recommended.[285] If the goal is to differentiate epileptic seizures from nonepileptic events, especially frontal lobe seizures, 18 channels of EEG are recommended.[294] Home video recording of events in question may be possible and helpful, if they are frequent and long enough,[295,296] although, unfortunately, the beginning of the events likely will be missed.

Treating Sleep Disorders in Children with Epilepsy

Studies suggest that nocturnal melatonin levels may be lower in children with epilepsy, especially those with medically intractable epilepsy.[297,298] A recently published study evaluated melatonin every 3 hours using a radioactive immune assay on 74 children with various types of medically refractory epilepsy and 37 children without epilepsy.[297] Melatonin levels were lower in the children with medically refractory epilepsy. The daily rhythm of melatonin secretion in the study group was maintained, with a peak shift of melatonin secretion especially visible in the subgroup with generalized symptomatic refractory epilepsy in the age group between 6 months and 3 years of age. Another recent study of 40 children found significantly lower salivary peak melatonin levels (at 4 AM) in children with febrile seizures compared to control subjects.[298]

Of note, oral melatonin used to treat insomnia in children with epilepsy may also have anticonvulsant effects.[299-302] Anticonvulsive effects of melatonin have been demonstrated in several different animal models of epilepsy.[303-310]

Three randomized double-blind placebo control studies of bedtime oral melatonin in children with epilepsy have shown positive effects on sleep.[299,311,312] One study of 31 (3-12 years old) children with epilepsy found that oral melatonin improved sleep latency and sleep quality and reduced the percentage of parasomnias by a mean of 60%.[311] Another report of 23 children with medically refractory epilepsy treated nightly with melatonin described significant improvements in bedtime resistance, sleep duration, sleep latency, nocturnal arousals, sleepwalking, nocturnal enuresis, daytime sleepiness, and even seizure frequency.[299] A third study of 25 children with epilepsy, mental retardation, and sleep/wake disorders (mean age 10.5 years) reported significantly improved sleep latency with treatment with fast-release synthetic oral melatonin (3 mg increased weekly to 9 mg as needed).[312] Another recently published study gave 10 children with severe medically intractable epilepsy 3 mg of oral melatonin before bed nightly for 3 months, then placebo for 3 months.[302] Sleep efficiency among patients who received melatonin was significantly higher than among those given the placebo, with fewer nighttime awakenings. Better control of convulsions was also observed.

Certain antiepileptic medications are sedating for some children with epilepsy (e.g., topiramate, carbamazepine, gabapentin, pregabalin), and therefore, if a child is overly sleepy in the daytime, adjusting the dosing regimen (largest or only dose at night) is reasonable. On the other hand, if an antiepileptic agent (e.g., lamotrigine) seems to contribute to the child's insomnia, switching to an extended release formula in the morning, or selection of another medication, may be helpful.

Sleep disorders and seizures may be interrelated. Thus, treating sleep disorders (including OSA) in patients with epilepsy leads to modest improvements in seizure control for some patients; and, improved seizure control can lead to improvements in sleep quality and daytime functioning.[313-316]

If a child with epilepsy has excessive daytime sleepiness, or impaired daytime functioning is present, general recommendations for assessment and treatment include use of a sleep diary (and possibly actigraphy), improved sleep hygiene, and consideration (and treatment) of the effects of the child's antiepileptic medications, sleep habits, nocturnal seizures, and possible coexisting sleep disorders (snoring and OSA, periodic limb movement disorder, parasomnias).[313-316]

Chiari Malformation, Spina Bifida, and Meningomyelocele

The craniocervical junction (CCJ) is an intricate pathway of interlocking muscles, ligaments, and skeletal components that act in concert to preserve neurologic function. Infants and children with CCJ disorders are at increased risk for sleep apnea, prolonged breath holding, and sudden death. Early diagnosis and prevention of neurologic compromise is crucial. Combinations of inspiratory stridor and central sleep apnea (with or without coexisting OSA) are often present in patients with CCJ disorders and may be the sole manifestation of potentially life-threatening cervical medullary junction compression.[317-326]

Youngsters with Chiari malformations (CMs) are particularly likely to develop CCJ disorders. CM is often associated with varying combinations of spina bifida (SB), meningomyelocele (MM), bilateral abductor landmark vocal cord paralysis, SDB, and sudden unexplained death.[319,327-333] A study in 1974 found that 26 infants with SB had life-threatening apnea or stridor accompanied by profound bradycardia, particularly during phasic periods of REM sleep.[333] When these events occurred in an infant, the child would sometimes be slow (or fail) to self-resuscitate.

SDB occurs much more often in children with MM than in the general pediatric population: 62% of 83 children attending a MM clinic had SDB (moderate to severe in 20%, mild in 42%, and normal in 37%).[329] Among the 17 patients with moderately/severely abnormal SDB, 12 patients had predominantly central apneas and 5 had predominantly obstructive apnea. The risk for finding SDB on a PSG in a child or adolescent with MM was increased 11.6 times if the child also had abnormal pulmonary function tests, 9.2 times if there were thoracic spinal cord lesions, 3.5 times with a history of a previous posterior fossa decompression, and 3.0 times in those with Chiari 2 (as opposed to milder Chiari 1) malformations.[329] Another study found 41% of 73 children with MM had moderate to severe OSA (mean obstructive AHI of 17), 34% had central sleep apnea (16.6 events per hour), 16% had central sleep-related hypoventilation (peak endotracheal tube P_{CO_2} 67 ± 11 mm Hg), and 8% had sleep-exacerbated restrictive lung disease that caused nocturnal hypoxemia with apnea or hypercapnea (nadir oxygen saturation $67 \pm 14\%$).[331] Another study of 20 children with CM found sleep apnea in 60% (35% obstructive, 25% central).[328] The investigators found the central apnea index was best predicted by age, CM severity, and the finding of vocal cord paralysis. Clinical symptoms of CCJ compression are summarized in Box 40-8.

BOX 40-8 *Clinical Symptoms of Cervical-Medullary Compression*

- Neck or occipital pain (in 85%)
- Myelopathy (either mono-, hemi-, para-, or quadriparesis), which may develop acutely after a seemingly mild head or neck injury
- Abnormal sensation in hands or feet (manifested in an infant or young child by constant rubbing of affected limbs)
- Basilar migraine (in 25%)
- Transient visual field deficits, vertigo, altered consciousness, or confusional states (sometimes provoked or reproduced by neck extension or rotation of the head or neck)
- Unilateral or bilateral paralysis or dysfunction of soft palate or pharynx
- Downbeat nystagmus
- Hearing loss
- Various combinations of inspiratory stridor and obstructive or central sleep apnea
- Severe breath-holding or apneic episodes during awake periods
- Sudden death in sleep

The most common clinical symptom of CCJ compression is neck or occipital pain, present in 85%. Basilar migraine is present in 25% of children with CCJ with medullary compression.[334,335] Other clinical signs of CCJ compression include myelopathy (mono-, hemi-, para-, or quadriparesis), which may develop acutely following a seemingly mild head or neck injury; abnormal sensation in hands or feet (possibly presenting in an infant or young child as constant rubbing of the affected limbs); transient visual field deficits, vertigo, altered consciousness, or confusional states (sometimes provoked by neck extension or rotation); uni- or bilateral paralysis or dysfunction of soft palate or pharynx; and downbeat nystagmus, hearing loss, and SDB with apneic episodes, breath holding, or sudden death in sleep.

Heightened awareness of the need to screen children at risk for CCJ compression disorders is needed. Kirk and associates[330] sent questionnaires to 212 SB clinics in the United States and Canada: 41% responded.[330] Although 67% of these clinics had the ability to monitor children with SB for SDB, only 8% of the patients with SB/MM had received cardiorespiratory studies, and 3.1% were diagnosed with SDB. Death during sleep had been reported in 13% and sudden unexplained death in 9%. The investigators raised the possibility of SDB being the missed diagnosis contributing to sudden expected death when sleeping.

Chiari 1 Malformations

Chiari 1 malformation (CM1) is defined as a caudal herniation of the cerebellar tonsils 5 mm below the foramen magnum.[334,335] Symptoms usually present in the second or third decade of life (younger in those with syringomyelia). Typical symptoms of cervicomedullary compression in CM1 include suboccipital headache (which may increase with coughing, sneezing, or bowel movement), neck pain (continuous burning, deep-seated discomfort in the shoulders, nape, chest, or arms that often worsens with Valsalva maneuvers), vertigo (especially positional or triggered by head movements, often with tinnitus, aural fullness, and sometimes mild sensorineural hearing loss), and symptoms of medullary or cervical spinal compression. Syringomyelia (a central cavitation or tubular fluid-filled cavity in several spinal cord segments) is present in 40% to 75% of cases of CM1 (occurring as early as 12 months); and 90% of patients with syringomyelia have CMs. CM1 is thought to arise from abnormal cerebrospinal fluid (CSF) flow dynamics through the central spinal canal.

Presenting symptoms of 130 symptomatic CM1 patients (mean age 11 years, 58% with syringomyelia) were head or neck pain (38%), migraine-like headaches (22%), progressive scoliosis (18%), dysphagia (15%), ataxia (9%), apnea or bradypnea (8%), hoarseness (5%), and drop attacks (2%).[335] Physical signs of CM1 include a short neck, levoscoliosis (in those with syringomyelia), motor neuron signs (initially generalized hyperreflexia, spasticity, plantar extensor responses; later atrophy, weakness, fasciculations, areflexia), lower cranial nerve dysfunction (abductor vocal cord paralysis, soft palate weakness, lingual atrophy, cricopharyngeal achalasia, facial hypoesthesia, absent gag reflexes), central spinal cord syndrome (in those with syringomyelia), and cerebellar symptoms (ataxia, nystagmus, dysmetria). CM1 children with symptomatic cervicomedullary compression may present with only SDB,[319] rarely with persistent nocturnal enuresis.[317]

Chiari 2 Malformations

Chiari 2 malformation (CM2) is a caudal herniation of the brainstem, caudal cerebellar vermis, and fourth ventricle through the foramen magnum into the cervical spinal canal.[336] Compression of the cervicomedullary junction in CM2 is often complicated by problems including mechanical compression of the medulla by a vermian peg (most often at the level of the atlas), caudal displacement of the brainstem into the spinal canal (by a small posterior fossa and obstructive hydrocephalus), and bilateral adductor vocal cord paralysis (with inspiratory stridor and progressive airway obstruction but near-normal phonation).[337] There may also be central or obstructive apneic episodes when asleep, severe breath-holding spells when awake, and sudden death.

Diagnostic Approach to Evaluating Sleep-Related Breathing Disorders in Chiari Malformations

A diagnostic approach to evaluating sleep-associated breathing disorders in CM begins with a thorough medical and sleep history and neurologic examination followed by neuroimaging, beginning with cervical radiographs in flexion and extension.[334,338] Computed tomography (CT) scan of the CCJ is useful for evaluating bony structures. Static or dynamic MRI of CCJ evaluates soft tissue structures, ligaments, and brain. Comprehensive overnight PSG with CO_2 monitoring evaluates for OSA, central sleep apnea, stridor, central or obstructive sleep-related hypoventilation, and pulmonary restrictive disease. Somatosensory evoked potentials assesses for impaired conduction through the CCJ.

Treating Sleep-Disordered Breathing in Chiari Malformations and Meningomyelocele

Posterior fossa decompression in 130 patients with symptomatic CM1 resulted in improvement or stabilization of symptoms: sleep apnea resolved in 100%, headache in 90%, and scoliosis improved in 43% (but motor or sensory deficits present before surgery were likely to persist).[335] Syrinxes would usually stabilize (and sometimes decrease) in size. Acute hydrocephalus sometimes develops in the immediate postoperative period, heralded by worsening of the SDB, and better outcomes are found if decompression is performed when symptoms have been present less than 2 years.

Posterior fossa decompression in symptomatic CM2 may reverse obstructive hydrocephalus, vocal cord paralysis, and central sleep apnea.[328] Potentially irreversible causes of SDB in infants or children with CM2 include developmentally immature brainstem networks and respiratory centers, lower brainstem cranial nerve nuclei aplasia or hypoplasia, ischemic or hemorrhagic changes in the brainstem, and chronic chemical meningitis and arachnoiditis.

OSA may be present in a child with both adenotonsillar hypertrophy and CM (with/without MM). Excluding symptomatic posterior fossa compression is crucial before proceeding with pharyngeal surgery. In these youngsters, OSA often persists following AT but can be satisfactorily treated with CPAP. Central sleep apnea or central sleep hypoventilation may be effectively treated using a stepwise approach of supplemental oxygen (with or without oral methylxanthines), adding nasal positive pressure ventilation when needed.

Achondroplasia

Achondroplasia (AC) is the most common cause of short-limbed dwarfism, affects more than 250,000 individuals worldwide, and occurs in 1 of 10,000 to 40,000 live births. AC is due to a heterozygous mutation in the *FGFR3* gene on chromosome 4p16.3 that codes for production of the FGFR3 (fibroblast growth receptor-3) protein.[339] FGFR3 protein is a negative regulator of linear bone growth inhibiting chondrocyte proliferation. The *FGFR3* mutant gene causes a gain of function by increasing FGFR3 protein activity that severely inhibits bone and cartilage growth. Phenotypic expression of the mutant gene in AC is 100%.

Patients with AC have short stature (average adult height 4 feet), large heads with frontal bossing set on a short cranial base, short squat long bones, and short proximal limbs.[340] Intelligence is usually normal. AC infants usually have some degree of thoracolumbar kyphosis (gibbus) attributed to a combination of a large head, cervical ligamentous laxity, and delayed motor milestones. AC infants exhibit poor head control, which improves by 3 to 4 months of age. Lumbar kyphosis is usually replaced by an exaggerated lumbar lordosis once the children begin to walk (typically by 24-36 months).

Infants, children, and young adults with AC have higher mortality rates compared with the age-matched general population. Most deaths in AC children younger than 4 years of age are sudden and unexpected, and half of these are due to brain stem compression.[341] Foramen magnum stenosis in AC infants can cause brainstem compression with apnea and sudden death.[341-344] Other possible causes of sudden death include compression of the pontomedullary junction, obstruction of the sylvian aqueduct, ischemic injury to vital brainstem nuclei, and craniocervical dislocations from minor trauma with poor neck support. A 42-year follow-up study of mortality rate in 793 subjects with AC found that young adults continued to have a higher incidence of accidental, neurologic, and cardiac-related deaths, and a life expectancy 10 years less than the general population, despite advances in their medical care.[345]

Various factors predispose children with AC to SDB (these factors are summarized in Box 40-9). SDB is present in 38% to 42% of children or adults with AC and is characterized by varying combinations of pulmonary restrictive disease, OSA, central sleep apnea, and abnormal activity of accessory muscles.[346-351] Early studies found 48% of 88 children with AC (1 month to

12.6 years) seen in a skeletal dysplasia clinic had abnormal PSGs, most commonly due to nocturnal hypoxemia (44% were related to pulmonary restrictive disease; a minority also had severe central or obstructive sleep apnea).[349] Another study found OSA in 38% of 95 AC children (mean age 3.7 years).[352] Symptoms most predictive of OSA were snoring, observed apnea, glottal stops, and apneic episodes awake. Physical findings, including severe tonsillar hypertrophy, were of little predictive value. A recent study of young infants with AC (mean age 1.5 ± 0.5 months) found that 67% had a respiratory disturbance index (RDI) above 5 (mean 14 ± 11) versus 2 ± 1 in control subjects.[353] AC infants also had fewer spontaneous or respiratory-related arousals (12/hour) compared to control subjects (19/hour). Sleep architecture did not differ between AC infants and control subjects, and the investigators found no correlation between foramen magnum size and either SDB or arousal frequency.

Treatment Strategies for Achondroplasia

Assessment and management of infants or children with AC include growth measurements using AC-specific weight, height, head circumference, and upper-to-lower limb segment ratio growth charts; screening for symptoms and signs of SDB or CCJ dysfunction; possible orthodontic evaluation for dental malocclusion or crowding; weight control; and treatment of the commonly frequent middle ear infections to avoid conductive hearing loss.[354-357] Proper neck support in hypotonic AC infants can prevent cervicomedullary compression that otherwise may follow minor head or cervical injuries. Thoracolumbar kyphosis in AC resolves in 90% of AC children once they start walking, but the remaining 10% need braces until the curvature is 10 degrees or less; only 4% will need spinal surgery or fusion by age 15.

Infants and children with AC are at risk for cervicomedullary compression and need for decompression should be assessed in children with cervical or occipital pain, cranial nerve dysfunction, paresis, ankle clonus, hyperreflexia, hypotonia, or abnormal central sleep apneas.[358] Poor feeding, transient visual deficits, syncope, and basilar migraine are other possible indications. Evaluation for foramen magnum stenosis is recommended before AT in AC children with OSA, even those without central sleep apnea on PSG. A retrospective review of cervicomedullary MRI conducted on 22 AC children referred to a tertiary pediatric otolaryngology clinic found 50% had sufficient foramen magnum stenosis to warrant decompressive surgery before undergoing AT.[355]

The current surgery of choice for symptomatic cervicomedullary decompression in AC is a suboccipital craniectomy with C1 laminectomy and division of fibrous extradural bands.[354] Central sleep apnea present in 12 AC patients who underwent decompressive surgeries improved in all but one (whose sleep apnea improved after repeat decompressive surgery).[354] Patients with AC often need repeat decompression (11% had repeat surgery, done at a mean age of 5.5 years), and the need is often heralded by return of their central sleep apnea.[354]

Patients with AC may also have OSA, often requiring CPAP therapy (or BiPAP therapy if concomitant pulmonary restrictive disease is present). Successful treatment strategies for OSA in one study of 17 AC patients (median age 6.6 years) with OSA were CPAP (13 patients), AT (3 patients), and weight loss (1 patient).[359] Individuals with AC undergoing surgeries for OSA are at increased risk for perioperative

---

BOX 40-9 *Factors That Predispose Children with Achondroplasia to Sleep-Disordered Breathing*

- Recurrent infections (especially in the first 5 to 6 years of life, probably secondary to eustachian tube dysfunction and faulty bone development)
- Small upper airway, relative adenotonsillar hypertrophy
- Hypotonia of airway muscles
- Narrow trunk with small thoracic cage
- Obesity (present in 13% to 42%)
- Brainstem compression and cervical spinal canal stenosis (due to small foramen magnum)

complications.[352] Affected children and infants typically have small-caliber airways, which may be difficult to visualize, and may have concomitant pulmonary restrictive disease. Another study found 61% of 98 AC adolescents or young adults who underwent lumbar decompressive surgery had at least one perioperative complication (with neurologic complications in 23%).[360] One study recommended PSG recording before and following surgery in AC children and reported successfully treating a variety of SDB disorders found in these patients with BiPAP, assisted ventilation, or supplemental oxygen after hospital discharge.[361] Two patient and family support groups helpful to families with AC children are *Little People of America* (www.lpaonline.org) and the *Magic Foundation for Children's Growth* (www.magicfoundation.org).

Neuromuscular Disorders

Sleep-related breathing disorders are common in children with neuromuscular disease (NMD). Respiratory muscle weakness predisposes to hypoventilation. NMD patients with diaphragmatic weakness depend upon their intercostal and accessory respiratory muscles to breathe adequately, and because these muscles are inhibited in REM sleep, hypoventilation is first seen in the REM sleep stage. Weak cough reflexes, kyphoscoliosis, obesity, impaired central respiratory control, restrictive pulmonary disease, medication effects, malnutrition, and obesity will, when present, further predispose to SDB.

Nocturnal or *sleep-related hypoventilation* is defined in the second edition of the International Classification of Sleep Disorders (ICSD-2) as a rise in arterial carbon dioxide partial pressure ($Paco_2$) to values greater than 45 mm Hg (torr) or to disproportionately increased levels relative to those present during wakefulness.[362] *Sleep-induced hypoxemia* is defined as an oxygen saturation less than 90% for 5 minutes or longer with a nadir below 85%, or greater than 30% of the total sleep time with oxygen saturation below 90%. In 2007, the American Academy of Sleep Medicine published sleep scoring guidelines that defined *sleep-related hypoventilation* in children as greater than 25% of the total sleep time with a $Paco_2$ more than 50 mm Hg, and a 10 mm Hg or greater rise in $Paco_2$ in sleep compared to wakefulness in adults.[363]

Symptoms that suggest sleep-related hypoventilation in slowly progressive NMD are summarized in Box 40-10.[364-366] However, symptoms are poorly predictive of which children with NMD will have SDB, even when using a structured sleep questionnaire.[364-366] Many NMD patients with moderate to severe sleep-related hypoventilation seem to breathe normally when awake because they have little to tax their respiratory systems once they are wheelchair-bound. Assessing patients for paradoxical breathing should be routine. In children, paradoxical breathing in a child with NMD, as a sign of diaphragmatic weakness, is not obvious until diaphragmatic strength is less than 25% of normal.

The prevalence of SDB in children with NMD is greater than 40%, 10 times higher than in the general pediatric population.[367] Duchenne muscular dystrophy (DMD) is one of the most common muscular dystrophies presenting in childhood and is due to mutation in the short arm of the X chromosome (Xp21) leading to absence of dystrophin (a muscle protein). DMD occurs almost exclusively in males with an incidence of 1 in 3500.[368] A study of 32 DMD patients referred for suspected SDB found OSA in 31% (median age 8 years) and sleep-related hypoventilation in 32% (median age 13 years).[369] Based on these findings, the authors suggested that SDB in patients with DMD often has a bimodal presentation with OSA in the first decade of life, sleep-related hypoventilation later on. Boys with DMD usually become wheelchair-bound around 12 years of age.[369-374] Once ambulation is lost, kyphoscoliosis accelerates. Forced vital capacity (FVC) falls approximately 4% for each 10 degrees of increase in the thoracic spine curvature. Sleep-related central hypoventilation is also the pattern of SDB in children with spinal muscular atrophies,[375] myotonic dystrophy,[376] limb girdle muscular dystrophies,[377] or childhood-onset acid maltase deficiency.[378]

Predicting Sleep-Disordered Breathing in Children with Neuromuscular Disease

Serial monitoring of lung function is mandated for all children with NMD once they are able to perform them (usually age 5 years).[379,380] Pulmonary function test abnormalities help predict (more reliably than do symptoms) which NMD patients are most likely to have sleep-related hypoventilation.[381] Sleep hypoventilation is likely once FVC falls below 40% of predicted.[382] Daytime $Paco_2$ greater than 40 mm Hg and inspiratory vital capacity (IVC) less than 40% were two other measures with over a 90% predictive sensitivity (with specificities of 72% and 88%) in 49 children and adolescents with NMD (mean age 11.3 ± 4.4 years).[383] Another study of 42 patients with primary myopathies found hypopneas during REM sleep when IVC was less than 60% predicted, REM sleep hypoventilation when IVC was less than 40%, hypoventilation during both NREM and REM sleep when IVC was less than 30%, and respiratory failure when IVC was below 25%.[384] Sleep-related hypoventilation was similarly predicted with high sensitivity and specificity in 27 children with congenital and limb girdle muscular dystrophies by a vital capacity below 40%;[377] however, hypoventilation during REM sleep may develop at an IVC less than 60% in children with NMD who are obese, have concomitant lung disease, or are suffering an acute respiratory infection.

Not unsurprisingly, respiratory failure or pneumonia is often the cause of death in NMD. The American College of Physicians recommends treating sleep-related hypoventilation in patients with NMD when they have symptoms (morning headache, fatigue, or dyspnea) and $Paco_2$ greater than 45 mm Hg, nocturnal oxygen saturation less than 88% for longer than 5 minutes, maximal inspiratory pressure (MIP)

BOX 40-10 *Most Common Symptoms of Sleep-Related Hypoventilation in Slowly Progressive Neuromuscular Disorders*

- Morning headache
- Nocturnal arousals
- Need for frequent repositioning
- Restless sleep
- Daytime fatigue
- Difficulty awakening from sleep
- Impaired concentration
- Orthopnea
- A decline in academic performance

below 60 cm H_2O, or forced vital capacity less than 50% predicted.[385] PSG should be considered in children with NMD when wheelchair use becomes necessary, the FVC drops to less than 40% (< 60% if the children are obese or have concomitant pulmonary disease or respiratory symptoms), the maximal inspiratory pressure is less than 60%, or the daytime $Paco_2$ is greater than 40 mm Hg.[385]

Common Polysomnographic Findings in Children with Neuromuscular Diseases

Common PSG findings in NMD are summarized in Box 40-11. Some NMD patients have no apneas or hypopneas, only nocturnal hypercapnia with or without hypoxemia. Others have apneas or short hypopneas that may occur only during REM sleep; usually most are central, or combinations of central, mixed, and obstructive hypopneas. However, patients with severe REM sleep-related hypoventilation can have ominous prolonged hypopneas which last longer than 30 to 70 seconds, causing arterial oxygen desaturations to values below 70%.

Managing Sleep-Related Hypoventilation in Neuromuscular Disorders

As reviewed earlier, sleep-related hypoventilation in NMD is most often central in type, and best treated by either BiPAP therapy or nocturnal intermittent positive pressure ventilation (NIPPV).[369,375,378,386-391] Assessment of effectiveness during PSG requires continuous monitoring of end-tidal or transcutaneous CO_2. If capnography is unavailable (or malfunctions) during the PSG, an arterial blood gas can be drawn upon awakening.

The American Thoracic Society published a consensus statement in 2004 regarding respiratory care of patients with DMD.[379] They recommended that patients with DMD should visit a physician specializing in pediatric sleep every 6 months once wheelchair-bound, if there is a fall in vital capacity to less than 80% predicted, or when the child has reached age 12 years. Quality of sleep and symptoms of SDB should be discussed at every patient encounter, and overnight PSG with CO_2 monitoring should be done at least annually once DMD patients are wheelchair-bound.

BOX 40-11 *Common Polysomnographic Findings in Patients with Neuromuscular Disorders*

- Sleep-related drop in baseline SpO_2 and rise in ET Pco_2, transcutaneous Pco_2, or arterial Pco_2, especially during REM sleep
- Periods of nonapneic oxygen desaturation, intermittent periodic or shallow breathing
- Tachycardia and tachypnea
- Reduced, absent, or fragmented REM sleep; arousals from REM sleep after SpO_2 drops and/or ET Pco_2 rises in transition to REM sleep
- Elevated mean ET Pco_2 and low mean SpO_2, both initially present only during REM sleep
- Progressive fall in the baseline SaO_2 and rise in ET Pco_2 as REM sleep proceeds
- Apneas and hypopneas not necessarily present

ET, endotracheal tube; *REM*, rapid eye movement; *Sao$_2$*, arterial oxygen saturation; *Spo$_2$*, oxygen saturation as measured by pulse oximetry.

Home pulse oximetry can help monitor effectiveness of airway clearance during respiratory illnesses and identify DMD patients needing hospitalization. Repetitive clusters of "sawtooth" desaturations suggest OSA, whereas prolonged periods of desaturation suggest hypoventilation. Home capnography would be useful (as CO_2 monitoring is necessary to assess for hypoventilation, and, in some children, even to recognize OSA) but is not yet routinely available.[392]

Expiratory muscles in patients with DMD are first to become weak, and associated weak coughing abilities may lead to atelectasis and infection. Mechanical insufflator-exsufflators to simulate a cough are particularly useful in preventing hospitalization or tracheostomy in patients with peak cough expiratory flows around 160 L/minute, especially when scoliosis prevents optimal use of manual assisted cough. Treatment of nocturnal hypoventilation with noninvasive ventilator support can improve quality of life and reduce morbidity and mortality risks. Supplemental oxygen alone (without ventilatory assistance) should not be used to treat sleep-related hypoventilation unless it can be shown that it is not associated with unacceptable further increases in CO_2. Daytime ventilation should be considered when waking Pco_2 exceeds 50 mm Hg or when waking oxygen saturation is below 92%. Tracheostomy should be considered when contraindications, or patient aversion, to noninvasive ventilation are present, or when noninvasive ventilation is not feasible owing to bulbar weakness or dysfunction.

Home noninvasive nocturnal ventilation has contributed to longer survival in NMD patients with hypercapnic hypoventilation with the mean age of survival in DMD increasing from 19 to 25 years[393] and in spinal muscular atrophy type 1 (SMA-1, Werdnig-Hoffman disease) from 10 ± 4 months to 65 ± 46 months.[394] The benefits of nasal NIPPV in patients with severe kyphoscoliosis and chronic alveolar hypoventilation due to neuromuscular disease, spinal cord injury, or skeletal deformity include improved daytime and nighttime arterial blood gases,[395] fewer hospitalizations,[395] fewer nocturnal desaturations,[395] and improved exercise capacity.[396] A longitudinal study of 14 children with NMD treated with BiPAP ($n = 13$) or CPAP ($n = 1$) followed an average of 30 months (range 6-84) found symptoms of daytime sleepiness and morning headache lessened, hospitalization rates and health care costs decreased, and quality of life remained stable despite disease progression.[386]

Another longitudinal prospective study of treating SDB in 30 young patients (12 ± 4 years) with various inherited NMD found NIPPV reduced their nocturnal transcutaneous Pco_2 from 54 to 42 mm Hg and diurnal arterial Pco_2 from 48 to 41 mm Hg, decreased arousals from sleep, reduced nocturnal heart rates, and improved respiratory disturbance index and sleep architecture. Effects persisted over 25 ± 13 months.[389]

A case-control study found NIPPV improved quality of life and longevity, and avoided or delayed the need for tracheostomy among 48 patients with DMD.[387] Treating SDB in 10 of 15 patients with different types of spinal muscular atrophy with NIPPV increased stage N3 sleep, reduced mean nocturnal heart rate by 12 beats per minute, normalized sleep architecture, and was associated with improved concentration and appetite and fewer morning headaches.[375] Ninety percent of the DMD patients in the untreated control group developed diurnal hypercapnia or respiratory complications.

Serial Adjustments of Nocturnal Ventilation in Treatment of Sleep-Related Hypoventilation

Patients with progressive NMD need close follow-up, reassessment, and repeat titration of their nocturnal ventilation treatments. A retrospective review of 61 sleep studies recorded over a 12-month period in 45 children with NMD (median age 8.3 years, 27 boys) found changes in sleep-related respiratory support were needed in 66% of the studies,[391] but none of the clinical parameters monitored predicted which of the children these would be.

Another longitudinal study of 20 patients with NMD initially treated their sleep-related hypoventilation with BiPAP using a spontaneous mode in 18.[390] One patient required his BiPAP set to a timed rate 1 year later. The mean inspiratory positive airway pressure (IPAP) in these adolescents and young adults was 11.5 (range 9 to 14) cm H_2O, and expiratory positive airway pressure (EPAP) was 4.5 (range 4 to 5) cm H_2O. Over the 3.5-year follow-up period, supplemental oxygen (0.5-1.0 L/minute) was added to positive pressure ventilation in three patients, and three others switched to nasal volume controlled NIPPV. However, if hypersomnia persists in individuals with myotonic dystrophy after controlling their SDB, a trial of wakefulness-promoting agents (e.g., modafinil) may be considered. Modafinil has been reported to reduce subjective hypersomnia in adults with myotonic dystrophy type 1.[397-400] However, a recently published multicenter randomized double-blind controlled study of 28 adults with myotonic dystrophy type 1 found modafinil did not improve objective measures of hypersomnia on maintenance of wakefulness tests.[401]

CONCLUSION

Children and adolescents with neurologic disorders frequently have complex sleep disorders that need to be treated. A night of restful sleep is a wanted and elusive desire of their caregivers, but only half seek treatment for the child's sleep problems.[204,245] Treatment strategies are available and are often effective for most of these problems. Awareness of them is crucial toward improving health-related quality of life, longevity, and well-being for the patients and their caregivers.

REFERENCES

1. Dorris L, Scott N, Zuberi S, Gibson N, Espie C. Sleep problems in children with neurological disorders. *Dev Neurorehabil.* 2008;11(2):95-114.
2. Didden R, Curfs LM, van Driel S, de Moor JM. Sleep problems in children and young adults with developmental disabilities: Home-based functional assessment and treatment. *J Behav Ther Exp Psychiatry.* 2002;33(1):49-58.
3. Habayeb O, Goodburn S, Chudleigh T, et al. The NTplus method of screening for Down syndrome: Achieving the 2010 targets? *Prenat Diagn.* 2010;30(5):434-437.
4. Allen EG, Freeman SB, Druschel C, et al. Maternal age and risk for trisomy 21 assessed by the origin of chromosome nondisjunction: A report from the Atlanta and national Down syndrome projects. *Hum Genet.* 2009;125(1):41-52.
5. Rachidi M, Lopes C. Molecular and cellular mechanisms elucidating neurocognitive basis of functional impairments associated with intellectual disability in Down syndrome. *Am J Intellect Dev Disabil.* 2010;115(2):83-112.
6. Lott IT, Dierssen M. Cognitive deficits and associated neurological complications in individuals with Down's syndrome. *Lancet Neurol.* 2010;9(6):623-633.
7. Ellingson RJ, Peters JF. Development of EEG and daytime sleep patterns in trisomy-21 infants during the first year of life: Longitudinal observations. *Electroencephalogr Clin Neurophysiol.* 1980;50(5-6):457-466.
8. Fukuma E, Umezawa Y, Kobayashi K, Motoike M. Polygraphic study on the nocturnal sleep of children with Down's syndrome and endogenous mental retardation. *Folia Psychiatr Neurol Jpn.* 1974;28(4):333-345.
9. Castaldo V. Down's syndrome: A study of sleep patterns related to level of mental deficiency. *Am J Ment Defic.* 1969;74(2):187-190.
10. Castaldo V, Krynicki V. Sleep pattern and intelligence in functional mental retardation. *J Ment Defic Res.* 1973;17(3):231-235.
11. Castaldo V, Krynicki V. Sleep and eye movement patterns in two groups of retardates. *Biol Psychiatry.* 1974;9(3):231-244.
12. Carter M, McCaughey E, Annaz D, Hill CM. Sleep problems in a Down syndrome population. *Arch Dis Child.* 2009;94(4):308-310.
13. Fitzgerald DA, Paul A, Richmond C. Severity of obstructive apnoea in children with Down syndrome who snore. *Arch Dis Child.* 2007;92(5):423-425.
14. Uong EC, McDonough JM, Tayag-Kier CE, et al. Magnetic resonance imaging of the upper airway in children with Down syndrome. *Am J Respir Crit Care Med.* 2001;163(3 Pt 1):731-736.
15. Mitchell RB, Call E, Kelly J. Diagnosis and therapy for airway obstruction in children with Down syndrome. *Arch Otolaryngol Head Neck Surg.* 2003;129(6):642-645.
16. Shott SR, Amin R, Chini B, et al. Obstructive sleep apnea: Should all children with Down syndrome be tested? *Arch Otolaryngol Head Neck Surg.* 2006;132(4):432-436.
17. Ng DK, Hui HN, Chan CH, et al. Obstructive sleep apnoea in children with Down syndrome. *Singapore Med J.* 2006;47(9):774-779.
18. Dyken ME, Lin-Dyken DC, Poulton S, Zimmerman MB, Sedars E. Prospective polysomnographic analysis of obstructive sleep apnea in Down syndrome. *Arch Pediatr Adolesc Med.* 2003;157(7):655-660.
19. Ng DK, Chan CH, Cheung JM. Children with Down syndrome and OSA do not necessarily snore. *Arch Dis Child.* 2007;92(11):1047-1048.
20. Harley EH, Collins MD. Neurologic sequelae secondary to atlantoaxial instability in Down syndrome. Implications in otolaryngologic surgery. *Arch Otolaryngol Head Neck Surg.* 1994;120(2):159-165.
21. Schaffer SR, Wong GH. Endoscopic visualization facilitates adenoidectomy. *Otolaryngol Head Neck Surg.* 2007;136(3):510.
22. Shott SR. Down syndrome: Analysis of airway size and a guide for appropriate intubation. *Laryngoscope.* 2000;110(4):585-592.
23. Goldstein NA, Armfield DR, Kingsley LA, et al. Postoperative complications after tonsillectomy and adenoidectomy in children with Down syndrome. *Arch Otolaryngol Head Neck Surg.* 1998;124(2):171-176.
24. Tauman R, Gulliver TE, Krishna J, et al. Persistence of obstructive sleep apnea syndrome in children after adenotonsillectomy. *J Pediatr.* 2006;149(6):803-808.
25. Shete MM, Stocks RM, Sebelik ME, Schoumacher RA. Effects of adeno-tonsillectomy on polysomnography patterns in Down syndrome children with obstructive sleep apnea: A comparative study with children without Down syndrome. *Int J Pediatr Otorhinolaryngol.* 2010;74(3):241-244.
26. Donnelly LF, Shott SR, LaRose CR, Chini BA, Amin RS. Causes of persistent obstructive sleep apnea despite previous tonsillectomy and adenoidectomy in children with Down syndrome as depicted on static and dynamic cine MRI. *AJR Am J Roentgenol.* 2004;183(1):175-181.
27. Shott SR, Donnelly LF. Cine magnetic resonance imaging: Evaluation of persistent airway obstruction after tonsil and adenoidectomy in children with Down syndrome. *Laryngoscope.* 2004;114(10):1724-1729.
28. Fricke BL, Donnelly LF, Shott SR, et al. Comparison of lingual tonsil size as depicted on MR imaging between children with obstructive sleep apnea despite previous tonsillectomy and adenoidectomy and normal controls. *Pediatr Radiol.* 2006;36(6):518-523.
29. Guimaraes CV, Kalra M, Donnelly LF, et al. The frequency of lingual tonsil enlargement in obese children. *AJR Am J Roentgenol.* 2008;190(4):973-975.
30. Marcus CL, Rosen G, Ward SL, et al. Adherence to and effectiveness of positive airway pressure therapy in children with obstructive sleep apnea. *Pediatrics.* 2006;117(3):E442-E451.
31. Kirk VG, O'Donnell AR. Continuous positive airway pressure for children: A discussion on how to maximize compliance. *Sleep Med Rev.* 2006;10(2):119-127.
32. Rains JC. Treatment of obstructive sleep apnea in pediatric patients. Behavioral intervention for compliance with nasal continuous positive airway pressure. *Clin Pediatr (Phila).* 1995;34(10):535-541.

33. Shore S, Lightfoot T, Ansell P. Oral disease in children with Down syndrome: Causes and prevention. *Community Pract.* 2010;83(2):18-21.

34. Waldman HB, Hasan FM, Perlman S. Down syndrome and sleep-disordered breathing: The dentist's role. *J Am Dent Assoc.* 2009;140(3):307-312.

35. Ng DK, Chan CH. Obesity is an important risk factor for sleep disordered breathing in children with Down syndrome. *Sleep.* 2004;27(5):1023-1024:author reply 1025.

36. Sato K, Shirakawa T, Niikuni N, Sakata H, Asanuma S. Effects of oral care in Down syndrome children with obstructive sleep apnea. *J Oral Sci.* 2010;52(1):145-147.

37. Trois MS, Capone GT, Lutz JA, et al. Obstructive sleep apnea in adults with Down syndrome. *J Clin Sleep Med.* 2009;5(4):317-323.

38. Bell RB, Turvey TA. Skeletal advancement for the treatment of obstructive sleep apnea in children. *Cleft Palate Craniofac J.* 2001;38(2):147-154.

39. Miloro M. Mandibular distraction osteogenesis for pediatric airway management. *J Oral Maxillofac Surg.* 2010;68(7):1512-1523.

40. Brooker GE, Cooper MG. Airway management for infants with severe micrognathia having mandibular distraction osteogenesis. *Anaesth Intensive Care.* 2010;38(1):43-49.

41. Guimaraes CV, Donnelly LF, Shott SR, Amin RS, Kalra M. Relative rather than absolute macroglossia in patients with Down syndrome: Implications for treatment of obstructive sleep apnea. *Pediatr Radiol.* 2008;38(10):1062-1067.

42. Cassidy SB. Prader-Willi syndrome. In: Pagon RA, Dolan CR, Stephens K, eds. *Gene Reviews.* Seattle: University of Washington; 2009.

43. Holm VA, Cassidy SB, Butler MG, et al. Prader-Willi syndrome: Consensus diagnostic criteria. *Pediatrics.* 1993;91(2):398-402.

44. Festen DA, de Weerd AW, van den Bossche RA, et al. Sleep-related breathing disorders in prepubertal children with Prader-Willi syndrome and effects of growth hormone treatment. *J Clin Endocrinol Metab.* 2006;91(12):4911-4915.

45. Festen DA, Wevers M, de Weerd AW, et al. Cognition and behavior in pre-pubertal children with Prader-Willi syndrome and associations with sleep-related breathing disorders. *Am J Med Genet A.* 2008;146A(23):3018-3025.

46. Festen DA, Wevers M, de Weerd AW, et al. Psychomotor development in infants with Prader-Willi syndrome and associations with sleep-related breathing disorders. *Pediatr Res.* 2007;62(2):221-224.

47. Lin HY, Lin SP, Lin CC, et al. Polysomnographic characteristics in patients with Prader-Willi syndrome. *Pediatr Pulmonol.* 2007;42(10):881-887.

48. Miller J, Silverstein J, Shuster J, Driscoll DJ, Wagner M. Short-term effects of growth hormone on sleep abnormalities in Prader-Willi syndrome. *J Clin Endocrinol Metab.* 2006;91(2):413-417.

49. Pavone M, Paglietti MG, Petrone A, et al. Adenotonsillectomy for obstructive sleep apnea in children with Prader-Willi syndrome. *Pediatr Pulmonol.* 2006;41(1):74-79.

50. Williams K, Scheimann A, Sutton V, Hayslett E, Glaze DG. Sleepiness and sleep disordered breathing in Prader-Willi syndrome: Relationship to genotype, growth hormone therapy, and body composition. *J Clin Sleep Med.* 2008;4(2):111-118.

51. O'Donoghue FJ, Camfferman D, Kennedy JD, et al. Sleep-disordered breathing in Prader-Willi syndrome and its association with neurobehavioral abnormalities. *J Pediatr.* 2005;147(6):823-829.

52. Clift S, Dahlitz M, Parkes JD. Sleep apnoea in the Prader-Willi syndrome. *J Sleep Res.* 1994;3(2):121-126.

53. Hertz G, Cataletto M, Feinsilver SH, Angulo M. Sleep and breathing patterns in patients with Prader-Willi syndrome (PWS): Effects of age and gender. *Sleep.* 1993;16(4):366-371.

54. Lin HY, Lin SP, Lin CC, et al. Polysomnographic characteristics in patients with Prader-Willi syndrome. *Pediatr Pulmonol.* 2007;42(10):881-887.

55. Kaplan J, Fredrickson PA, Richardson JW. Sleep and breathing in patients with the Prader-Willi syndrome. *Mayo Clin Proc.* 1991;66(11):1124-1126.

56. Priano L, Grugni G, Miscio G, et al. Sleep cycling alternating pattern (CAP) expression is associated with hypersomnia and GH secretory pattern in Prader-Willi syndrome. *Sleep Med.* 2006;7(8):627-633.

57. Joo EY, Hong SB, Sohn YB, et al. Plasma adiponectin level and sleep structures in children with Prader-Willi syndrome. *J Sleep Res.* 2009;19:248-254.

58. Tauber M, Diene G, Molinas C, Hebert M. Review of 64 cases of death in children with Prader-Willi syndrome (PWS). *Am J Med Genet A.* 2008;146(7):881-887.

59. Tanna N, Choi SS. Efficacy and safety of adenotonsillectomy for pediatric obstructive sleep apnea in Prader-Willi syndrome. *Ann Otol Rhinol Laryngol.* 2009;118(4):267-269.

60. Harris JC, Allen RP. Is excessive daytime sleepiness characteristic of Prader-Willi syndrome? The effects of weight change. *Arch Pediatr Adolesc Med.* 1996;150(12):1288-1293.

61. Manni R, Politini L, Nobili L, et al. Hypersomnia in the Prader-Willi syndrome: Clinical-electrophysiological features and underlying factors. *Clin Neurophysiol.* 2001;112(5):800-805.

62. Maas AP, Sinnema M, Didden R, et al. Sleep disturbances and behavioural problems in adults with Prader-Willi syndrome. *J Intellect Disabil Res.* 2010;54(10):906.

63. Joo EY, Hong SB, Sohn YB, et al. Plasma adiponectin level and sleep structures in children with Prader-Willi syndrome. *J Sleep Res.* 2010;19 (1 Pt 2):248-254.

64. Bruni O, Verrillo E, Novelli L, Ferri R. Prader-Willi syndrome: Sorting out the relationships between obesity, hypersomnia, and sleep apnea. *Curr Opin Pulm Med.* 2010;16(6):568-573.

65. Carrel AL, Myers SE, Whitman BY, Allen DB. Growth hormone improves body composition, fat utilization, physical strength and agility, and growth in Prader-Willi syndrome: A controlled study. *J Pediatr.* 1999;134(2):215-221.

66. Myers SE, Carrel AL, Whitman BY, Allen DB. Physical effects of growth hormone treatment in children with Prader-Willi syndrome. *Acta Paediatr Suppl.* 1999;88(433):112-114.

67. Davies PS. Body composition in Prader-Willi syndrome: Assessment and effects of growth hormone administration. *Acta Paediatr Suppl.* 1999;88(433):105-108.

68. Nyunt O, Harris M, Hughes I, et al. Benefit of early commencement of growth hormone therapy in children with Prader-Willi syndrome. *J Pediatr Endocrinol Metab.* 2009;22(12):1151-1158.

69. Festen DA, de Lind van Wijngaarden R, van Eekelen M, et al. Randomized controlled GH trial: Effects on anthropometry, body composition and body proportions in a large group of children with Prader-Willi syndrome. *Clin Endocrinol (Oxford).* 2008;69(3):443-451.

70. Carrel AL, Myers SE, Whitman BY, Eickhoff J, Allen DB. Long-term growth hormone therapy changes the natural history of body composition and motor function in children with Prader-Willi syndrome. *J Clin Endocrinol Metab.* 2010;95(3):1131-1136.

71. de Lind van Wijngaarden RF, Siemensma EP, Festen DA, et al. Efficacy and safety of long-term continuous growth hormone treatment in children with Prader-Willi syndrome. *J Clin Endocrinol Metab.* 2009;94(11):4205-4215.

72. de Lind van Wijngaarden RF, Festen DA, Otten BJ, et al. Bone mineral density and effects of growth hormone treatment in prepubertal children with Prader-Willi syndrome: A randomized controlled trial. *J Clin Endocrinol Metab.* 2009;94(10):3763-3771.

73. de Lind van Wijngaarden RF, de Klerk LW, Festen DA, et al. Randomized controlled trial to investigate the effects of growth hormone treatment on scoliosis in children with Prader-Willi syndrome. *J Clin Endocrinol Metab.* 2009;94(4):1274-1280.

74. Colmenares A, Pinto G, et al. "Effects on growth and metabolism of growth hormone treatment for 3 years in 36 children with Prader-Willi syndrome." *Hormone research in paediatrics.* 2011;75(2):123-130.

75. Sode-Carlsen R, Farholt S. "Growth hormone treatment for two years is safe and effective in adults with Prader-Willi syndrome." *Growth hormone & IGF research : official journal of the Growth Hormone Research Society and the International IGF Research Society.* 2011.

76. Diene G, Mimoun E, Feigerlova E, et al. Endocrine disorders in children with Prader-Willi syndrome—Data from 142 children of the French database. *Horm Res Paediatr.* 2010;74(2):121-128.

77. Brambilla P, Crinò A, Bedogni G, et al. Metabolic syndrome in children with Prader-Willi syndrome: The effect of obesity. *Nutrition, metabolism, and cardiovascular diseases NMCD.* 2011;21(4):269-276.

78. Miller JL, Shuster J, Theriaque D, Driscoll DJ, Wagner M. Sleep disordered breathing in infants with Prader-Willi syndrome during the first 6 weeks of growth hormone therapy: A pilot study. *J Clin Sleep Med.* 2009;5(5):448-453.

79. de Lind van Wijngaarden RF, Joosten KF, van den Berg S, et al. The relationship between central adrenal insufficiency and sleep-related breathing disorders in children with Prader-Willi syndrome. *J Clin Endocrinol Metab.* 2009;94(7):2387-2393.

80. de Lind van Wijngaarden RF, Otten BJ, Festen DA, et al. High prevalence of central adrenal insufficiency in patients with Prader-Willi syndrome. *J Clin Endocrinol Metab.* 2008;93(5):1649-1654.

81. Connell NA, Paterson WF, Wallace AM, Donaldson MD. Adrenal function and mortality in children and adolescents with Prader-Willi syndrome attending a single centre from 1991-2009. *Clin Endocrinol (Oxford)*. 2010;73(5):686-688.
82. Farholt S, Sode-Carlsen R, Christiansen JS, Ostergaard JR, Hoybye C. Normal cortisol response to high-dose synacthen and insulin tolerance test in children and adults with Prader-Willi syndrome. *J Clin Endocrinol Metab*. 2011;96(1):E173-E180.
83. Matijevic T, Knezevic J, Slavica M, Pavelic J. Rett syndrome: From the gene to the disease. *Eur Neurol*. 2009;61(1):3-10.
84. Tsai SJ. Zinc sulfate could be potential agent for the treatment of Rett syndrome through increasing central BDNF levels. *Med Hypotheses*. 2007;68(1):230-231.
85. Wilfong AA, Schultz RJ. Vagus nerve stimulation for treatment of epilepsy in Rett syndrome. *Dev Med Child Neurol*. 2006;48(8):683-686.
86. Tsai SJ. Lithium and antidepressants: Potential agents for the treatment of Rett syndrome. *Med Hypotheses*. 2006;67(3):626-629.
87. Yamashita Y, Matsuishi T, Murakami Y, Kato H. Sleep disorder in Rett syndrome and melatonin treatment. *Brain Dev*. 1999;21(8):570.
88. Nomura Y. Early behavior characteristics and sleep disturbance in Rett syndrome. *Brain Dev*. 2005;27(Suppl 1):S35-S42.
89. Young D, Nagarajan L, de Klerk N, et al. Sleep problems in Rett syndrome. *Brain Dev*. 2007;29(10):609-616.
90. Williamson SL, Christodoulou J. Rett syndrome: New clinical and molecular insights. *Eur J Hum Genet*. 2006;14(8):896-903.
91. Weaving LS, Ellaway CJ, Gecz J, Christodoulou J. Rett syndrome: Clinical review and genetic update. *J Med Genet*. 2005;42(1):1-7.
92. Southall DP, Kerr AM, Tirosh E, et al. Hyperventilation in the awake state: Potentially treatable component of Rett syndrome. *Arch Dis Child*. 1988;63(9):1039-1048.
93. Ellaway C, Peat J, Leonard H, Christodoulou J. Sleep dysfunction in Rett syndrome: Lack of age related decrease in sleep duration. *Brain Dev*. 2001;23(Suppl 1):S101-S103.
94. Marcus CL, Carroll JL, McColley SA, et al. Polysomnographic characteristics of patients with Rett syndrome. *J Pediatr*. 1994;125(2):218-224.
95. Steffenburg U, Hagberg G, Hagberg B. Epilepsy in a representative series of Rett syndrome. *Acta Paediatr*. 2001;90(1):34-39.
96. Jian L, Nagarajan L, de Klerk N, et al. Predictors of seizure onset in Rett syndrome. *J Pediatr*. 2006;149(4):542-547.
97. Niedermeyer E, Naidu SB, Plate C. Unusual EEG theta rhythms over central region in Rett syndrome: Considerations of the underlying dysfunction. *Clin Electroencephalogr*. 1997;28(1):36-43.
98. Sekul EA, Moak JP, Schultz RJ, et al. Electrocardiographic findings in Rett syndrome: An explanation for sudden death? *J Pediatr*. 1994;125(1):80-82.
99. Miyamoto A, Oki J, Takahashi S, Okuno A. Serum melatonin kinetics and long-term melatonin treatment for sleep disorders in Rett syndrome. *Brain Dev*. 1999;21(1):59-62.
100. Piazza CC, Fisher W, Moser H. Behavioral treatment of sleep dysfunction in patients with the Rett syndrome. *Brain Dev*. 1991;13(4):232-237.
101. Ellaway C, Williams K, Leonard H, et al. Rett syndrome: Randomized controlled trial of L-carnitine. *J Child Neurol*. 1999;14(3):162-167.
102. Egger J, Hofacker N, Schiel W, Holthausen H. Magnesium for hyperventilation in Rett's syndrome. *Lancet*. 1992;340(8819):621-622.
103. Motil KJ, Schultz RJ, Abrams S, Ellis KJ, Glaze DG. Fractional calcium absorption is increased in girls with Rett syndrome. *J Pediatr Gastroenterol Nutr*. 2006;42(4):419-426.
104. Didden R, Korzilius H, Smeets E, et al. Communication in individuals with Rett syndrome: An assessment of forms and functions. *J Dev Phys Disabil*. 2010;22(2):105-118.
105. Laan LA, Vein AA. Angelman syndrome: Is there a characteristic EEG? *Brain Dev*. 2005;27(2):80-87.
106. Boyd SG, Harden A, Patton MA. The EEG in early diagnosis of the Angelman (happy puppet) syndrome. *Eur J Pediatr*. 1988;147(5):508-513.
107. Bruni O, Ferri R, D'Agostino G, et al. Sleep disturbances in Angelman syndrome: A questionnaire study. *Brain Dev*. 2004;26(4):233-240.
108. Conant KD, Thibert RL, Thiele EA. Epilepsy and the sleep-wake patterns found in Angelman syndrome. *Epilepsia*. 2009;50(11):2497-2500.
109. Didden R, Korzilius H, Smits MG, Curfs LM. Sleep problems in individuals with Angelman syndrome. *Am J Ment Retard*. 2004;109(4):275-284.
110. Pelc K, Cheron G, Boyd SG, Dan B. Are there distinctive sleep problems in Angelman syndrome? *Sleep Med*. 2008;9(4):434-441.
111. Walz NC, Beebe D, Byars K. Sleep in individuals with Angelman syndrome: Parent perceptions of patterns and problems. *Am J Ment Retard*. 2005;110(4):243-252.
112. Zhdanova IV, Wurtman RJ, Wagstaff J. Effects of a low dose of melatonin on sleep in children with Angelman syndrome. *J Pediatr Endocrinol Metab*. 1999;12(1):57-67.
113. Elsea SH, Girirajan S. Smith-Magenis syndrome. *Eur J Hum Genet*. 2008;16(4):412-421.
114. Smith AC, Magenis RE, Elsea SH. Overview of Smith-Magenis syndrome. *J Assoc Genet Technol*. 2005;31(4):163-167.
115. Shelley BP, Robertson MM. The neuropsychiatry and multisystem features of the Smith-Magenis syndrome: A review. *J Neuropsychiatry Clin Neurosci*. 2005;17(1):91-97.
116. Smith AC, Dykens E, Greenberg F. Behavioral phenotype of Smith-Magenis syndrome (del 17p11.2). *Am J Med Genet*. 1998;81(2):179-185.
117. Smith AC, Dykens E, Greenberg F. Sleep disturbance in Smith-Magenis syndrome (del 17 p11.2). *Am J Med Genet*. 1998;81(2):186-191.
118. De Leersnyder H, de Blois MC, Vekemans M, et al. Beta(1)-adrenergic antagonists improve sleep and behavioural disturbances in a circadian disorder, Smith-Magenis syndrome. *J Med Genet*. 2001;38(9):586-590.
119. Boudreau EA, Johnson KP, Jackman AR, et al. Review of disrupted sleep patterns in Smith-Magenis syndrome and normal melatonin secretion in a patient with an atypical interstitial 17p11.2 deletion. *Am J Med Genet A*. 2009;149A(7):1382-1391.
120. De Leersnyder H, de Blois MC, Bresson JL, et al. [Inversion of the circadian melatonin rhythm in Smith-Magenis syndrome]. *Rev Neurol (Paris)*. 2003;159(Suppl 11):S21-S26.
121. Chik CL, Rollag MD, Duncan WC, Smith AC. Diagnostic utility of daytime salivary melatonin levels in Smith-Magenis syndrome. *Am J Med Genet A*. 2010;152A(1):96-101.
122. Carpizo R, Martinez A, Mediavilla D, et al. Smith-Magenis syndrome: A case report of improved sleep after treatment with beta1-adrenergic antagonists and melatonin. *J Pediatr*. 2006;149(3):409-411.
123. De Leersnyder H. Inverted rhythm of melatonin secretion in Smith-Magenis syndrome: From symptoms to treatment. *Trends Endocrinol Metab*. 2006;17(7):291-298.
124. Laje G, Bernert R, Morse R, Pao M, Smith AC. Pharmacological treatment of disruptive behavior in Smith-Magenis syndrome. *Am J Med Genet C Semin Med Genet*. 2010;154C(4):463-468.
125. Morris CA. Introduction: Williams syndrome. *Am J Med Genet C Semin Med Genet*. 2010;154C(2):203-208.
126. Goldman SE, Malow BA, Newman KD, Roof E, Dykens EM. Sleep patterns and daytime sleepiness in adolescents and young adults with Williams syndrome. *J Intellect Disabil Res*. 2009;53(2):182-188.
127. Morris CA. The behavioral phenotype of Williams syndrome: A recognizable pattern of neurodevelopment. *Am J Med Genet C Semin Med Genet*. 2010;154C(4):427-431.
128. Annaz D, Hill CM, Ashworth A, Holley S, Karmiloff-Smith A. Characterisation of sleep problems in children with Williams syndrome. *Res Dev Disabil*. 2011;32(1):164-169.
129. Gombos F, Bodizs R, Kovacs I. Atypical sleep architecture and altered EEG spectra in Williams syndrome. *J Intellect Disabil Res*. 2011;55(3):255-262.
130. Arens R, Wright B, Elliott J, et al. Periodic limb movement in sleep in children with Williams syndrome. *J Pediatr*. 1998;133(5):670-674.
131. Hagerman RJ, Hall DA, Coffey S, et al. Treatment of fragile X-associated tremor ataxia syndrome (FXTAS) and related neurological problems. *Clin Interv Aging*. 2008;3(2):251-262.
132. Miller LJ, McIntosh DN, McGrath J, et al. Electrodermal responses to sensory stimuli in individuals with fragile X syndrome: A preliminary report. *Am J Med Genet*. 1999;83(4):268-279.
133. Farzin F, Perry H, Hessl D, et al. Autism spectrum disorders and attention-deficit/hyperactivity disorder in boys with the fragile X premutation. *J Dev Behav Pediatr*. 2006;27(Suppl 2):S137-S144.
134. Loesch DZ, Huggins RM, Hagerman RJ. Phenotypic variation and FMRP levels in fragile X. *Ment Retard Dev Disabil Res Rev*. 2004;10(1):31-41.
135. Kronk R, Bishop EE, Raspa M, et al. Prevalence, nature, and correlates of sleep problems among children with fragile X syndrome based on a large scale parent survey. *Sleep*. 2010;33(5):679-687.
136. Kronk R, Dahl R, Noll R. Caregiver reports of sleep problems on a convenience sample of children with fragile X syndrome. *Am J Intellect Dev Disabil*. 2009;114(6):383-392.
137. Miano S, Bruni O, Elia M, et al. Sleep phenotypes of intellectual disability: A polysomnographic evaluation in subjects with Down syndrome and fragile-X syndrome. *Clin Neurophysiol*. 2008;119(6):1242-1247.

138. Bushey D, Tononi G, Cirelli C. The Drosophila fragile X mental retardation gene regulates sleep need. *J Neurosci.* 2009;29(7):1948-1961.

139. Gould EL, Loesch DZ, Martin MJ, et al. Melatonin profiles and sleep characteristics in boys with fragile X syndrome: A preliminary study. *Am J Med Genet.* 2000;95(4):307-315.

140. Wirojanan J, Jacquemont S, Diaz R, et al. The efficacy of melatonin for sleep problems in children with autism, fragile X syndrome, or autism and fragile X syndrome. *J Clin Sleep Med.* 2009;5(2):145-150.

141. Weiskop S, Richdale A, Matthews J. Behavioural treatment to reduce sleep problems in children with autism or fragile X syndrome. *Dev Med Child Neurol.* 2005;47(2):94-104.

142. American Psychiatric Association. *Electronic DSM-IV-TR plus.* Washington, DC: American Psychiatric Association; 2000.

143. Rapin I, Tuchman RF. Autism: Definition, neurobiology, screening, diagnosis. *Pediatr Clin North Am.* 2008;55(5):1129-1146:viii.

144. Kogan MD, Blumberg SJ, Schieve LA, et al. Prevalence of parent-reported diagnosis of autism spectrum disorder among children in the US. *Pediatrics.* 2007;124(5):1395-1403:2009.

145. Courchesne E, Campbell K, Solso S. Brain growth across the life span in autism: Age-specific changes in anatomical pathology. *Brain Res.* 2011;1380:138-145.

146. DiCicco-Bloom E, Lord C, Zwaigenbaum L, et al. The developmental neurobiology of autism spectrum disorder. *J Neurosci.* 2006;26(26):6897-6906.

147. Stilp RL, Gernsbacher MA, Schweigert EK, Arneson CL, Goldsmith HH. Genetic variance for autism screening items in an unselected sample of toddler-age twins. *J Am Acad Child Adolesc Psychiatry.* 2010;49(3):267-276.

148. Nishiyama T, Taniai H, Miyachi T, Ozaki K, Tomita M, Sumi S. Genetic correlation between autistic traits and IQ in a population-based sample of twins with autism spectrum disorders (ASDs). *J Hum Genet.* 2009;54(1):56-61.

149. Mazefsky CA, Goin-Kochel RP, Riley BP, Maes HH. Genetic and environmental influences on symptom domains in twins and siblings with autism. *Res Autism Spectr Disord.* 2008;2(2):320-331.

150. Betancur C, Leboyer M, Gillberg C. Increased rate of twins among affected sibling pairs with autism. *Am J Hum Genet.* 2002;70(5):1381-1383.

151. Greenberg DA, Hodge SE, Sowinski J, Nicoll D. Excess of twins among affected sibling pairs with autism: Implications for the etiology of autism. *Am J Hum Genet.* 2001;69(5):1062-1067.

152. Zimmerman AW, Connors SL, Matteson KJ, et al. Maternal antibrain antibodies in autism. *Brain Behav Immun.* 2007;21(3):351-357.

153. Singer HS, Morris CM, Williams PN, Yoon DY, Hong JJ, Zimmerman AW. Antibrain antibodies in children with autism and their unaffected siblings. *J Neuroimmunol.* 2006;178(1-2):149-155.

154. Ashwood P, Krakowiak P, Hertz-Picciotto I, Hansen R, Pessah I, Van de Water J. Elevated plasma cytokines in autism spectrum disorders provide evidence of immune dysfunction and are associated with impaired behavioral outcome. *Brain Behav Immun.* 2011;25(1):40-45.

155. Parker-Athill EC, Tan J. Maternal immune activation and autism spectrum disorder: Interleukin-6 signaling as a key mechanistic pathway. *Neurosignals.* 2010;18(2):113-128.

156. Goines P, Van de Water J. The immune system's role in the biology of autism. *Curr Opin Neurol.* 2010;23(2):111-117.

157. Careaga M, Van de Water J, Ashwood P. Immune dysfunction in autism: A pathway to treatment. *Neurotherapeutics.* 2010;7(3):283-292.

158. Blaylock RL, Strunecka A. Immune-glutamatergic dysfunction as a central mechanism of the autism spectrum disorders. *Curr Med Chem.* 2009;16(2):157-170.

159. Richdale AL, Schreck KA. Sleep problems in autism spectrum disorders: Prevalence, nature, and possible biopsychosocial aetiologies. *Sleep Med Rev.* 2009;13(6):403-411.

160. Fricke-Oerkermann L, Pluck J, Schredl M, et al. Prevalence and course of sleep problems in childhood. *Sleep.* 2007;30(10):1371-1377.

161. Sadeh A, Gruber R, Raviv A. Sleep, neurobehavioral functioning, and behavior problems in school-age children. *Child Dev.* 2002;73(2):405-417.

162. Souders MC, Mason TB, Valladares O, et al. Sleep behaviors and sleep quality in children with autism spectrum disorders. *Sleep.* 2009;32(12):1566-1578.

163. Cortesi F, Giannotti F, Ivanenko A, Johnson K. Sleep in children with autistic spectrum disorder. *Sleep Med.* 2010;11(7):659-664.

164. Wiggs L, Stores G. Sleep patterns and sleep disorders in children with autistic spectrum disorders: Insights using parent report and actigraphy. *Dev Med Child Neurol.* 2004;46(6):372-380.

165. Liu X, Hubbard JA, Fabes RA, Adam JB. Sleep disturbances and correlates of children with autism spectrum disorders. *Child Psychiatry Hum Dev.* 2006;37(2):179-191.

166. Krakowiak P, Goodlin-Jones B, Hertz-Picciotto I, Croen LA, Hansen RL. Sleep problems in children with autism spectrum disorders, developmental delays, and typical development: A population-based study. *J Sleep Res.* 2008;17(2):197-206.

167. Goldman SE, Surdyka K, Cuevas R, Adkins K, Wang L, Malow BA. Defining the sleep phenotype in children with autism. *Dev Neuropsychol.* 2009;34(5):560-573.

168. Couturier JL, Speechley KN, Steele M, Norman R, Stringer B, Nicolson R. Parental perception of sleep problems in children of normal intelligence with pervasive developmental disorders: Prevalence, severity, and pattern. *J Am Acad Child Adolesc Psychiatry.* 2005;44(8):815-822.

169. Hayashi E. Seasonal changes in sleep and behavioral problems in a pubescent case with autism. *Psychiatry Clin Neurosci.* 2001;55(3):223-224.

170. Takase M, Taira M, Sasaki H. Sleep-wake rhythm of autistic children. *Psychiatry Clin Neurosci.* 1998;52(2):181-182.

171. Oyane NM, Bjorvatn B. Sleep disturbances in adolescents and young adults with autism and Asperger syndrome. *Autism.* 2005;9(1):83-94.

172. Glickman G. Circadian rhythms and sleep in children with autism. *Neurosci Biobehav Rev.* 2010;34(5):755-768.

173. Giannotti F, Cortesi F, Cerquiglini A, et al. An investigation of sleep characteristics, EEG abnormalities and epilepsy in developmentally regressed and non-regressed children with autism. *J Autism Dev Disord.* 2008;38(10):1888-1897.

174. Nicholas B, Rudrasingham V, Nash S, Kirov G, Owen MJ, Wimpory DC. Association of Per1 and Npas2 with autistic disorder: Support for the clock genes/social timing hypothesis. *Mol Psychiatry.* 2007;12(6):581-592.

175. Szarfarc SC, de Souza SB. Prevalence and risk factors in iron deficiency and anemia. *Arch Latinoam Nutr.* 1997;47(2)(Suppl 1):35-38.

176. Bourgeron T. The possible interplay of synaptic and clock genes in autism spectrum disorders. *Cold Spring Harb Symp Quant Biol.* 2007;72:645-654.

177. Chaste P, Clement N, Mercati O, et al. Identification of pathway-biased and deleterious melatonin receptor mutants in autism spectrum disorders and in the general population. *PLoS One.* 2010;5(7):E11495.

178. Jonsson L, Ljunggren E, Bremer A, et al. Mutation screening of melatonin-related genes in patients with autism spectrum disorders. *BMC Med Genomics.* 2010;3:10.

179. Melke J, Goubran Botros H, Chaste P, et al. Abnormal melatonin synthesis in autism spectrum disorders. *Mol Psychiatry.* 2008;13(1):90-98.

180. Leu RM, Beyderman L, Botzolakis EJ, Surdyka K, Wang L, Malow BA. Relation of melatonin to sleep architecture in children with autism. *J Autism Dev Disord.* 2011;41(4):427-433.

181. Buckley AW, Rodriguez AJ, Jennison K, et al. Rapid eye movement sleep percentage in children with autism compared with children with developmental delay and typical development. *Arch Pediatr Adolesc Med.* 2010;164(11):1032-1037.

182. Elia M, Ferri R, Musumeci SA, et al. Sleep in subjects with autistic disorder: A neurophysiological and psychological study. *Brain Dev.* 2000;22(2):88-92.

183. Miano S, Bruni O, Elia M, et al. Sleep in children with autistic spectrum disorder: A questionnaire and polysomnographic study. *Sleep Med.* 2007;9(1):64-70.

184. Diomedi M, Curatolo P, Scalise A, Placidi F, Caretto F, Gigli GL. Sleep abnormalities in mentally retarded autistic subjects: Down's syndrome with mental retardation and normal subjects. *Brain Dev.* 1999;21(8):548-553.

185. Bruni O, Ferri R, Vittori E, et al. Sleep architecture and NREM alterations in children and adolescents with Asperger syndrome. *Sleep.* 2007;30(11):1577-1585.

186. Malow BA, Marzec ML, McGrew SG, Wang L, Henderson LM, Stone WL. Characterizing sleep in children with autism spectrum disorders: A multidimensional approach. *Sleep.* 2006;29(12):1563-1571.

187. Davidovitch M, Glick L, Holtzman G, Tirosh E, Safir MP. Developmental regression in autism: Maternal perception. *J Autism Dev Disord.* 2000;30(2):113-119.

188. Goldberg WA, Osann K, Filipek PA, et al. Language and other regression: Assessment and timing. *J Autism Dev Disord.* 2003;33(6):607-616.

189. Baird G, Charman T, Pickles A, et al. Regression, developmental trajectory and associated problems in disorders in the autism spectrum: The SNAP study. *J Autism Dev Disord.* 2008;38(10):1827-1836.

190. Tharp BR. Epileptic encephalopathies and their relationship to developmental disorders: Do spikes cause autism?. *Ment Retard Dev Disabil Res Rev.* 2004;10(2):132-134.

191. Canitano R. Epilepsy in autism spectrum disorders. *Eur Child Adolesc Psychiatry.* 2007;16(1):61-66.

192. Grigg-Damberger M. Evaluating children who seize during sleep. *Pediatr Ann.* 2008;37(7):472-480.

193. Schreck KA, Mulick JA, Smith AF. Sleep problems as possible predictors of intensified symptoms of autism. *Res Dev Disabil.* 2004;25(1):57-66.

194. Yaouyanc G, Jonville AP, Yaouyanc-Lapalle H, Barbier P, Dutertre JP, Autret E. Seizure with hyponatremia in a child prescribed desmopressin for nocturnal enuresis. *J Toxicol Clin Toxicol.* 1992;30(4):637-641.

195. Malow BA. Sleep disorders, epilepsy, and autism. *Ment Retard Dev Disabil Res Rev.* 2004;10(2):122-125.

196. Malow BA, Crowe C, Henderson L, et al. A sleep habits questionnaire for children with autism spectrum disorders. *J Child Neurol.* 2009;24(1):19-24.

197. Eldevik S, Jahr E, Eikeseth S, Hastings RP, Hughes CJ. Cognitive and adaptive behavior outcomes of behavioral intervention for young children with intellectual disability. *Behav Modif.* 2010;34(1):16-34.

198. Malow BA. Searching for autism symptomatology in children with epilepsy—A new approach to an established comorbidity. *Epilepsy Curr.* 2006;6(5):150-152.

199. McGrew S, Malow BA, Henderson L, Wang L, Song Y, Stone WL. Developmental and behavioral questionnaire for autism spectrum disorders. *Pediatr Neurol.* 2007;37(2):108-116.

200. Malow BA, McGrew SG, Harvey M, Henderson LM, Stone WL. Impact of treating sleep apnea in a child with autism spectrum disorder. *Pediatr Neurol.* 2006;34(4):325-328.

201. Thirumalai SS, Shubin RA, Robinson R. Rapid eye movement sleep behavior disorder in children with autism. *J Child Neurol.* 2002;17(3):173-178.

202. Dosman CF, Brian JA, Drmic IE, et al. Children with autism: Effect of iron supplementation on sleep and ferritin. *Pediatr Neurol.* 2007;36(3):152-158.

203. Dosman CF, Drmic IE, Brian JA, et al. Ferritin as an indicator of suspected iron deficiency in children with autism spectrum disorder: Prevalence of low serum ferritin concentration. *Dev Med Child Neurol.* 2006;48(12):1008-1009.

204. Wiggs L, France K. Behavioural treatments for sleep problems in children and adolescents with physical illness, psychological problems or intellectual disabilities. *Sleep Med Rev.* 2000;4(3):299-314.

205. Reed HE, McGrew SG, Artibee K, et al. Parent-based sleep education workshops in autism. *J Child Neurol.* 2009;24(8):936-945.

206. Moon EC, Corkum P, Smith IM. Case Study: A case-series evaluation of a behavioral sleep intervention for three children with autism and primary insomnia. *J Pediatr Psychol.* 2011;36(1):47-54.

207. Mindell JA, Telofski LS, Wiegand B, Kurtz ES. A nightly bedtime routine: Impact on sleep in young children and maternal mood. *Sleep.* 2009;32(5):599-606.

208. Mindell JA, Meltzer LJ, Carskadon MA, Chervin RD. Developmental aspects of sleep hygiene: Findings from the 2004 National Sleep Foundation Sleep in America poll. *Sleep Med.* 2009;10(7):771-779.

209. Burke RV, Kuhn BR, Peterson JL. Brief report: a "storybook" ending to children's bedtime problems—The use of a rewarding social story to reduce bedtime resistance and frequent night waking. *J Pediatr Psychol.* 2004;29(5):389-396.

210. Dworak M, Schierl T, Bruns T, Struder HK. Impact of singular excessive computer game and television exposure on sleep patterns and memory performance of school-aged children. *Pediatrics.* 2007;120(5):978-985.

211. Andersen IM, Kaczmarska J, McGrew SG, Malow BA. Melatonin for insomnia in children with autism spectrum disorders. *J Child Neurol.* 2008;23(5):482-485.

212. Wright B, Sims D, Smart S, et al. Melatonin versus placebo in children with autism spectrum conditions and severe sleep problems not amenable to behaviour management strategies: A randomised controlled crossover trial. *J Autism Dev Disord.* 2011;41(2):175-184.

213. Galli-Carminati G, Deriaz N, Bertschy G. Melatonin in treatment of chronic sleep disorders in adults with autism: A retrospective study. *Swiss Med Wkly.* 2009;139(19-20):293-296.

214. Nir I, Meir D, Zilber N, Knobler H, Hadjez J, Lerner Y. Brief report: Circadian melatonin, thyroid-stimulating hormone, prolactin, and cortisol levels in serum of young adults with autism. *J Autism Dev Disord.* 1995;25(6):641-654.

215. Chamberlain RS, Herman BH. A novel biochemical model linking dysfunctions in brain melatonin, proopiomelanocortin peptides, and serotonin in autism. *Biol Psychiatry.* 1990;28(9):773-793.

216. Shah T, Tse A, Gill H, et al. Administration of melatonin mixed with soft food and liquids for children with neurodevelopmental difficulties. *Dev Med Child Neurol.* 2008;50(11):845-849.

217. Arnold LE, Aman MG, Cook AM, et al. Atomoxetine for hyperactivity in autism spectrum disorders: Placebo-controlled crossover pilot trial. *J Am Acad Child Adolesc Psychiatry.* 2006;45(10):1196-1205.

218. Ming X, Gordon E, Kang N, Wagner GC. Use of clonidine in children with autism spectrum disorders. *Brain Dev.* 2008;30(7):454-460.

219. Koshes RJ, Rock NL. Use of clonidine for behavioral control in an adult patient with autism. *Am J Psychiatry.* 1994;151(11):1714.

220. Fankhauser MP, Karumanchi VC, German ML, Yates A, Karumanchi SD. A double-blind, placebo-controlled study of the efficacy of transdermal clonidine in autism. *J Clin Psychiatry.* 1992;53(3):77-82.

221. Handen BL, Sahl R, Hardan AY. Guanfacine in children with autism and/or intellectual disabilities. *J Dev Behav Pediatr.* 2008;29(4):303-308.

222. Posey DI, Litwiller M, Koburn A, McDougle CJ. Paroxetine in autism. *J Am Acad Child Adolesc Psychiatry.* 1999;38(2):111-112.

223. Anagnostou E, Esposito K, Soorya L, et al. Divalproex versus placebo for the prevention of irritability associated with fluoxetine treatment in autism spectrum disorder. *J Clin Psychopharmacol.* 2006;26(4):444-446.

224. Hollander E, Phillips A, Chaplin W, et al. A placebo controlled crossover trial of liquid fluoxetine on repetitive behaviors in childhood and adolescent autism. *Neuropsychopharmacology.* 2005;30(3):582-589.

225. DeLong GR, Teague LA, McSwain Kamran M. Effects of fluoxetine treatment in young children with idiopathic autism. *Dev Med Child Neurol.* 1998;40(8):551-562.

226. Hollander E, Soorya L, Wasserman S, et al. Divalproex sodium vs. placebo in the treatment of repetitive behaviours in autism spectrum disorder. *Int J Neuropsychopharmacol.* 2006;9(2):209-213.

227. Zavesicka L, Brunovsky M, Horacek J, et al. Trazodone improves the results of cognitive behaviour therapy of primary insomnia in non-depressed patients. *Neuro Endocrinol Lett.* 2008;29(6):895-901.

228. Bon OL. Low-dose trazodone effective in insomnia. *Pharmacopsychiatry.* 2005;38(5):226.

229. Kem DL, Posey DJ, McDougle CJ. Priapism associated with trazodone in an adolescent with autism. *J Am Acad Child Adolesc Psychiatry.* 2002;41(7):758.

230. Carson III CC, Mino RD. Priapism associated with trazodone therapy. *J Urol.* 1988;139(2):369-370.

231. Pardini M, Guida S, Gialloreti LE. Aripiprazole treatment for coprophagia in autistic disorder. *J Neuropsychiatry Clin Neurosci.* 2010;22(4):451.

232. Aman MG, Kasper W, Manos G, et al. Line-item analysis of the aberrant behavior checklist: Results from two studies of aripiprazole in the treatment of irritability associated with autistic disorder. *J Child Adolesc Psychopharmacol.* 2010;20(5):415-422.

233. Owen R, Sikich L, Marcus RN, et al. Aripiprazole in the treatment of irritability in children and adolescents with autistic disorder. *Pediatrics.* 2009;124(6):1533-1540.

234. Marcus RN, Owen R, Kamen L, Manos G, McQuade RD, Carson WH, et al. A placebo-controlled, fixed-dose study of aripiprazole in children and adolescents with irritability associated with autistic disorder. *J Am Acad Child Adolesc Psychiatry.* 2009;48(11):1110-1119.

235. Erickson CA, Stigler KA, Posey DJ, McDougle CJ. Aripiprazole in autism spectrum disorders and fragile X syndrome. *Neurotherapeutics.* 2010;7(3):258-263.

236. Carbone PS, Farley M, Davis T. Primary care for children with autism. *Am Fam Physician.* 2010;81(4):453-460.

237. Rogers SJ, Vismara LA. Evidence-based comprehensive treatments for early autism. *J Clin Child Adolesc Psychol.* 2008;37(1):8-38.

238. Eldevik S, Hastings RP, Hughes JC, Jahr E, Eikeseth S, Cross S. Meta-analysis of early intensive behavioral intervention for children with autism. *J Clin Child Adolesc Psychol.* 2009;38(3):439-450.

239. Brachlow AE, Ness KK, McPheeters ML, Gurney JG. Comparison of indicators for a primary care medical home between children with autism or asthma and other special health care needs: National survey of children's health. *Arch Pediatr Adolesc Med.* 2007;161(4):399-405.

240. Bitterman A, Daley TC, Misra S, Carlson E, Markowitz J. A national sample of preschoolers with autism spectrum disorders: Special education services and parent satisfaction. *J Autism Dev Disord.* 2008;38(8):1509-1517.

241. Centers for Disease Control and Prevention, http://www.cdc.gov/ncbdd/autism.

242. American Academy of Pediatrics, http://www.medicalhomeinfo.org/health.autism.htm.

243. Autism Speaks, http://autismspeaks.org.

244. Didden R, Korzilius H, van Aperlo B, van Overloop C, de Vries M. Sleep problems and daytime problem behaviours in children with intellectual disability. *J Intellect Disabil Res.* 2002;46(Pt 7):537-547.

245. Wiggs L, Stores G. Severe sleep disturbance and daytime challenging behaviour in children with severe learning disabilities. *J Intellect Disabil Res.* 1996;40(Pt 6):518-528.

246. Robinson AM, Richdale AL. Sleep problems in children with an intellectual disability: Parental perceptions of sleep problems, and views of treatment effectiveness. *Child Care Health Dev.* 2004;30(2):139-150.

247. Wiggs L, Stores G. Behavioural treatment for sleep problems in children with severe intellectual disabilities and daytime challenging behaviour: Effect on mothers and fathers. *Br J Health Psychol.* 2001;6(Pt 3):257-269.

248. Braam W, Didden R, Maas AP, Korzilius H, Smits MG, Curfs LM. Melatonin decreases daytime challenging behaviour in persons with intellectual disability and chronic insomnia. *J Intellect Disabil Res.* 2010;54(1):52-59.

249. Braam W, Didden R, Smits M, Curfs L. Melatonin treatment in individuals with intellectual disability and chronic insomnia: A randomized placebo-controlled study. *J Intellect Disabil Res.* 2008;52(Pt 3):256-264.

250. Newman CJ, O'Regan M, Hensey O. Sleep disorders in children with cerebral palsy. *Dev Med Child Neurol.* 2006;48(7):564-568.

251. Hayashi M, Inoue Y, Iwakawa Y, Sasaki H. REM sleep abnormalities in severe athetoid cerebral palsy. *Brain Dev.* 1990;12(5):494-497.

252. Kotagal S, Gibbons VP, Stith JA. Sleep abnormalities in patients with severe cerebral palsy. *Dev Med Child Neurol.* 1994;36(4):304-311.

253. Fitzgerald DA, Follett J, Van Asperen PP. Assessing and managing lung disease and sleep disordered breathing in children with cerebral palsy. *Paediatr Respir Rev.* 2009;10(1):18-24.

254. Biavati MJ, Manning SC, Phillips DL. Predictive factors for respiratory complications after tonsillectomy and adenoidectomy in children. *Arch Otolaryngol Head Neck Surg.* 1997;123(5):517-521.

255. Wiet GJ, Bower C, Seibert R, Griebel M. Surgical correction of obstructive sleep apnea in the complicated pediatric patient documented by polysomnography. *Int J Pediatr Otorhinolaryngol.* 1997;41(2):133-143.

256. Kerschner JE, Lynch JB, Kleiner H, Flanary VA, Rice TB. Uvulopalatopharyngoplasty with tonsillectomy and adenoidectomy as a treatment for obstructive sleep apnea in neurologically impaired children. *Int J Pediatr Otorhinolaryngol.* 2002;62(3):229-235.

257. Magardino TM, Tom LW. Surgical management of obstructive sleep apnea in children with cerebral palsy. *Laryngoscope.* 1999;109(10):1611-1615.

258. O'Donnell AR, Bjornson CL, Bohn SG, Kirk VG. Compliance rates in children using noninvasive continuous positive airway pressure. *Sleep.* 2006;29(5):651-658.

259. Preciado DA, Sidman JD, Sampson DE, Rimell FL. Mandibular distraction to relieve airway obstruction in children with cerebral palsy. *Arch Otolaryngol Head Neck Surg.* 2004;130(6):741-745.

260. Cohen SR, Holmes RE, Machado L, Magit A. Surgical strategies in the treatment of complex obstructive sleep apnoea in children. *Paediatr Respir Rev.* 2002;3(1):25-35.

261. Cohen SR, Simms C, Burstein FD, Thomsen J. Alternatives to tracheostomy in infants and children with obstructive sleep apnea. *J Pediatr Surg.* 1999;34(1):182-186:discussion 187.

262. Cohen SR, Lefaivre JF, Burstein FD, et al. Surgical treatment of obstructive sleep apnea in neurologically compromised patients. *Plast Reconstr Surg.* 1997;99(3):638-646.

263. Hill CM, Parker RC, Allen P, Paul A, Padoa KA. Sleep quality and respiratory function in children with severe cerebral palsy using nighttime postural equipment: A pilot study. *Acta Paediatr.* 2009;98(11):1809-1814.

264. Yoshida K. Elastic retracted oral appliance to treat sleep apnea in mentally impaired patients and patients with neuromuscular disabilities. *J Prosthet Dent.* 1999;81(2):196-201.

265. Sriskandan N, Moody A, Howlett DC. Ultrasound-guided submandibular gland injection of botulinum toxin for hypersalivation in cerebral palsy. *Br J Oral Maxillofac Surg.* 2010;48(1):58-60.

266. Hsiao KH, Nixon GM. The effect of treatment of obstructive sleep apnea on quality of life in children with cerebral palsy. *Res Dev Disabil.* 2008;29(2):133-140.

267. Crespel A, Coubes P, Baldy-Moulinier M. Sleep influence on seizures and epilepsy effects on sleep in partial frontal and temporal lobe epilepsies. *Clin Neurophysiol.* 2000;111(Suppl 2):S54-S59.

268. Herman ST, Walczak TS, Bazil CW. Distribution of partial seizures during the sleep-wake cycle: Differences by seizure onset site. *Neurology.* 2001;56(11):1453-1459.

269. Zucconi M, Oldani A, Ferini-Strambi L, Bizzozero D, Smirne S. Nocturnal paroxysmal arousals with motor behaviors during sleep: Frontal lobe epilepsy or parasomnia? *J Clin Neurophysiol.* 1997;14(6):513-522.

270. Provini F, Plazzi G, Tinuper P, et al. Nocturnal frontal lobe epilepsy. A clinical and polygraphic overview of 100 consecutive cases. *Brain.* 1999;122(Pt 6):1017-1031.

271. Lugaresi E, Cirignotta F, Montagna P. Nocturnal paroxysmal dystonia. *J Neurol Neurosurg Psychiatry.* 1986;49(4):375-380.

272. Capdevila OS, Dayyat E, Kheirandish-Gozal L, Gozal D. Prevalence of epileptiform activity in healthy children during sleep. *Sleep Med.* 2008;9(3):303-309.

273. Miano S, Paolino MC, Peraita-Adrados R, et al. Prevalence of EEG paroxysmal activity in a population of children with obstructive sleep apnea syndrome. *Sleep.* 2009;32(4):522-529.

274. Cortesi F, Giannotti F, Ottaviano S. Sleep problems and daytime behavior in childhood idiopathic epilepsy. *Epilepsia.* 1999;40(11):1557-1565.

275. Stores G, Wiggs L, Campling G. Sleep disorders and their relationship to psychological disturbance in children with epilepsy. *Child Care Health Dev.* 1998;24(1):5-19.

276. Didden R, de Moor JM, Korzilius H. Sleepiness, on-task behavior and attention in children with epilepsy who visited a school for special education: A comparative study. *Res Dev Disabil.* 2009;30(6):1428-1434.

277. Tang SS, Clarke T, Owens J, Pal DK. Sleep behaviour disturbances in rolandic epilepsy. *J Child Neurol.* 2011;26(2):239-243.

278. Nunes ML. Sleep disorders. *J Pediatr (Rio J).* 2002;78(Suppl 1):S63-S72.

279. Maganti R, Hausman N, Koehn M, et al. Excessive daytime sleepiness and sleep complaints among children with epilepsy. *Epilepsy Behav.* 2006;8(1):272-277.

280. Kaleyias J, Cruz M, Goraya JS, et al. Spectrum of polysomnographic abnormalities in children with epilepsy. *Pediatr Neurol.* 2008;39(3):170-176.

281. Khurana DS, Reumann M, Hobdell EF, et al. Vagus nerve stimulation in children with refractory epilepsy: Unusual complications and relationship to sleep-disordered breathing. *Childs Nerv Syst.* 2007;23(11):1309-1312.

282. Malow BA, Edwards J, Marzec M, Sagher O, Fromes G. Effects of vagus nerve stimulation on respiration during sleep: A pilot study. *Neurology.* 2000;55(10):1450-1454.

283. Marzec M, Edwards J, Sagher O, Fromes G, Malow BA. Effects of vagus nerve stimulation on sleep-related breathing in epilepsy patients. *Epilepsia.* 2003;44(7):930-935.

284. Nagarajan L, Walsh P, Gregory P, Stick S, Maul J, Ghosh S. Respiratory pattern changes in sleep in children on vagal nerve stimulation for refractory epilepsy. *Can J Neurol Sci.* 2003;30(3):224-227.

285. Kushida CA, Littner MR, Morgenthaler T, et al. Practice parameters for the indications for polysomnography and related procedures: An update for 2005. *Sleep.* 2005;28(4):499-521.

286. Hublin C, Kaprio J, Partinen M, Koskenvu M. Parasomnias: Co-occurrence and genetics. *Psychiatr Genet.* 2001;11(2):65-70.

287. Bisulli F, Vignatelli L, Naldi I, et al. Increased frequency of arousal parasomnias in families with nocturnal frontal lobe epilepsy: A common mechanism? *Epilepsia.* 2010;51(9):1852-1860.

288. Zolpidem. sleepwalking and automatic behaviours. *Prescrire Int.* 2007;16(91):200.

289. Lange CL. Medication-associated somnambulism. *J Am Acad Child Adolesc Psychiatry.* 2005;44(3):211-212.

290. Yang W, Dollear M, Muthukrishnan SR. One rare side effect of zolpidem—sleepwalking: A case report. *Arch Phys Med Rehabil.* 2005;86(6):1265-1266.

291. Guilleminault C, Palombini L, Pelayo R, Chervin RD. Sleepwalking and sleep terrors in prepubertal children: What triggers them? *Pediatrics.* 2003;111(1):E17-E25.

292. Aydin K, Okuyaz C, Serdaroglu A, Gucuyener K. Utility of electroencephalography in the evaluation of common neurologic conditions in children. *J Child Neurol.* 2003;18(6):394-396.

293. Watemberg N, Tziperman B, Dabby R, et al. Adding video recording increases the diagnostic yield of routine electroencephalograms in children with frequent paroxysmal events. *Epilepsia.* 2005;46(5):716-719.

294. Foldvary-Schaefer N, De Ocampo J, Mascha E, et al. Accuracy of seizure detection using abbreviated EEG during polysomnography. *J Clin Neurophysiol.* 2006;23(1):68-71.

295. Woody RC. Home videorecording of "spells" in children. *Pediatrics.* 1985;76(4):612-613.

296. Sheth RD, Bodensteiner JB. Effective utilization of home-video recordings for the evaluation of paroxysmal events in pediatrics. *Clin Pediatr (Phila).* 1994;33(10):578-582.

297. Paprocka J, Dec R, Jamroz E, Marszal E. Melatonin and childhood refractory epilepsy—A pilot study. *Med Sci Monit.* 2010;16(9):CR389-CR396.

298. Ardura J, Andres J, Garmendia JR, Ardura F. Melatonin in epilepsy and febrile seizures. *J Child Neurol.* 2010;25(7):888-891.

299. Elkhayat HA, Hassanein SM, Tomoum HY, et al. Melatonin and sleep-related problems in children with intractable epilepsy. *Pediatr Neurol.* 2010;42(4):249-254.

300. Scorza FA, Colugnati DB, Arida RM, et al. Cardiovascular protective effect of melatonin in sudden unexpected death in epilepsy: A hypothesis. *Med Hypotheses.* 2008;70(3):605-609.

301. Sanchez-Forte M, Moreno-Madrid F, Munoz-Hoyos A, et al. The effect of melatonin as anti-convulsant and neuron protector. *Rev Neurol.* 1997;25(144):1229-1234.

302. Uberos J, Augustin-Morales MC, Molina Carballo A, et al. Normalization of the sleep-wake pattern and melatonin and 6-sulphatoxy-melatonin levels after a therapeutic trial with melatonin in children with severe epilepsy. *J Pineal Res.* 2011;50(2):192-196.

303. Fenoglio-Simeone K, Mazarati A, Sefidvash-Hockley S, et al. Anticonvulsant effects of the selective melatonin receptor agonist ramelteon. *Epilepsy Behav.* 2009;16(1):52-57.

304. Molina-Carballo A, Munoz-Hoyos A, Sanchez-Forte M, et al. Melatonin increases following convulsive seizures may be related to its anticonvulsant properties at physiological concentrations. *Neuropediatrics.* 2007;38(3):122-125.

305. Yahyavi-Firouz-Abadi N, Tahsili-Fahadan P, Riazi K, et al. Melatonin enhances the anticonvulsant and proconvulsant effects of morphine in mice: Role for nitric oxide signaling pathway. *Epilepsy Res.* 2007;75(2-3):138-144.

306. Yildirim M, Marangoz C. Anticonvulsant effects of melatonin on penicillin-induced epileptiform activity in rats. *Brain Res.* 2006;1099(1):183-188.

307. Yahyavi-Firouz-Abadi N, Tahsili-Fahadan P, Riazi K, et al. Involvement of nitric oxide pathway in the acute anticonvulsant effect of melatonin in mice. *Epilepsy Res.* 2006;68(2):103-113.

308. Ray M, Mediratta PK, Reeta K, Mahajan P, Sharma KK. Receptor mechanisms involved in the anticonvulsant effect of melatonin in maximal electroshock seizures. *Methods Find Exp Clin Pharmacol.* 2004;26(3):177-181.

309. Mevissen M, Ebert U. Anticonvulsant effects of melatonin in amygdala-kindled rats. *Neurosci Lett.* 1998;257(1):13-16.

310. Lapin IP, Mirzaev SM, Ryzov IV, Oxenkrug GF. Anticonvulsant activity of melatonin against seizures induced by quinolinate, kainate, glutamate, NMDA, and pentylenetetrazole in mice. *J Pineal Res.* 1998;24(4):215-218.

311. Gupta M, Aneja S, Kohli K. Add-on melatonin improves sleep behavior in children with epilepsy: Randomized, double-blind, placebo-controlled trial. *J Child Neurol.* 2005;20(2):112-115.

312. Coppola G, Iervolino G, Mastrosimone M, et al. Melatonin in wake-sleep disorders in children, adolescents and young adults with mental retardation with or without epilepsy: A double-blind, cross-over, placebo-controlled trial. *Brain Dev.* 2004;26(6):373-376.

313. Parisi P, Bruni O, Pia Villa M, et al. The relationship between sleep and epilepsy: The effect on cognitive functioning in children. *Dev Med Child Neurol.* 2010;52(9):805-810.

314. Matos G, Andersen ML, do Valle AC, Tufik S. The relationship between sleep and epilepsy: Evidence from clinical trials and animal models. *J Neurol Sci.* 2010;295(1-2):1-7.

315. Manni R, Terzaghi M. Comorbidity between epilepsy and sleep disorders. *Epilepsy Res.* 2010;90(3):171-177.

316. Kothare SV, Kaleyias J. Sleep and epilepsy in children and adolescents. *Sleep Med.* 2010;11(7):674-685.

317. Brown BJ, Habelt S, Koral K, et al. Secondary nocturnal enuresis caused by central sleep apnea from Chiari malformation type 1. *J Pediatr Urol.* 2010;6(3):265-269.

318. Gosalakkal JA. Sleep-disordered breathing in Chiari malformation type 1. *Pediatr Neurol.* 2008;39(3):207-208.

319. Murray C, Seton C, Prelog K, Fitzgerald DA. Arnold-Chiari type 1 malformation presenting with sleep disordered breathing in well children. *Arch Dis Child.* 2006;91(4):342-343.

320. Hershberger ML, Chidekel A. Arnold-Chiari malformation type I and sleep-disordered breathing: An uncommon manifestation of an important pediatric problem. *J Pediatr Health Care.* 2003;17(4):190-197.

321. Yoshimi A, Nomura K, Furune S. Sleep apnea syndrome associated with a type I Chiari malformation. *Brain Dev.* 2002;24(1):49-51.

322. Miyamoto M, Miyamoto T, Hirata K, Katayama S. A case of Arnold-Chiari type I malformation presenting with dysrhythmic breathing during sleep. *Psychiatry Clin Neurosci.* 1998;52(2):212-216.

323. Shiihara T, Shimizu Y, Mitsui T, Saitoh E, Sato S. Isolated sleep apnea due to Chiari type I malformation and syringomyelia. *Pediatr Neurol.* 1995;13(3):266-267.

324. Najjar JA, Peitersen SE, Carter LP. Craniocervical stenosis and apnea spells in a 2-month-old baby with achondroplasia. *J Child Neurol.* 1995;10(6):484-486.

325. Keefover R, Sam M, Bodensteiner J, Nicholson A. Hypersomnolence and pure central sleep apnea associated with the Chiari I malformation. *J Child Neurol.* 1995;10(1):65-67.

326. Levitt P, Cohn MA. Sleep apnea and the Chiari I malformation: Case report. *Neurosurgery.* 1988;23(4):508-510.

327. Cochrane DD, Adderley R, White CP, Norman M, Steinbok P. Apnea in patients with myelomeningocele. *Pediatr Neurosurg.* 1990;16(4-5):232-239.

328. Dauvilliers Y, Stal V, Abril B, et al. Chiari malformation and sleep related breathing disorders. *J Neurol Neurosurg Psychiatry.* 2007;78(12):1344-1348.

329. Waters KA, Forbes P, Morielli A, et al. Sleep-disordered breathing in children with myelomeningocele. *J Pediatr.* 1998;132(4):672-681.

330. Kirk VG, Morielli A, Brouillette RT. Sleep-disordered breathing in patients with myelomeningocele: The missed diagnosis. *Dev Med Child Neurol.* 1999;41(1):40-43.

331. Kirk VG, Morielli A, Gozal D, et al. Treatment of sleep-disordered breathing in children with myelomeningocele. *Pediatr Pulmonol.* 2000;30(6):445-452.

332. Holinger PC, Holinger LD, Reichert TJ, Holinger PH. Respiratory obstruction and apnea in infants with bilateral abductor vocal cord paralysis, meningomyelocele, hydrocephalus, and Arnold-Chiari malformation. *J Pediatr.* 1978;92(3):368-373.

333. Wealthall SR, Whittaker GE, Greenwood N. The relationship of apnoea and stridor in spina bifida to other unexplained infant deaths. *Dev Med Child Neurol.* 1974;16(6)(Suppl 32):107-116.

334. Fernandez AA, Guerrero AI, Martinez MI, et al. Malformations of the craniocervical junction (Chiari type I and syringomyelia: Classification, diagnosis and treatment). *BMC Musculoskelet Disord.* 2009;10(Suppl 1):S1.

335. Tubbs RS, McGirt MJ, Oakes WJ. Surgical experience in 130 pediatric patients with Chiari I malformations. *J Neurosurg.* 2003;99(2):291-296.

336. Teo C, Parker EC, Aureli S, Boop FA. The Chiari II malformation: A surgical series. *Pediatr Neurosurg.* 1997;27(5):223-229.

337. Choi SS, Tran LP, Zalzal GH. Airway abnormalities in patients with Arnold-Chiari malformation. *Otolaryngol Head Neck Surg.* 1999;121(6):720-724.

338. Menezes AH, Vogel TW. Specific entities affecting the craniocervical region: Syndromes affecting the craniocervical junction. *Childs Nerv Syst.* 2008;24(10):1155-1163.

339. Nahar R, Saxena R, Kohli S, Puri R, Verma IC. Molecular studies of achondroplasia. *Indian J Orthop.* 2009;43(2):194-196.

340. Shirley ED, Ain MC. Achondroplasia: Manifestations and treatment. *J Am Acad Orthop Surg.* 2009;17(4):231-241.

341. Hecht JT, Francomano CA, Horton WA, Annegers JF. Mortality in achondroplasia. *Am J Hum Genet.* 1987;41(3):454-464.

342. Pauli RM, Horton VK, Glinski LP, Reiser CA. Prospective assessment of risks for cervicomedullary-junction compression in infants with achondroplasia. *Am J Hum Genet.* 1995;56(3):732-744.

343. Bland JD, Emery JL. Unexpected death of children with achondroplasia after the perinatal period. *Dev Med Child Neurol.* 1982;24(4):489-492.

344. Kato I, Franco P, Groswasser J, et al. Incomplete arousal processes in infants who were victims of sudden death. *Am J Respir Crit Care Med.* 2003;168(11):1298-1303.

345. Wynn J, King TM, Gambello MJ, Waller DK, Hecht JT. Mortality in achondroplasia study: A 42-year follow-up. *Am J Med Genet A.* 2007;143A(21):2502-2511.

346. Nelson FW, Hecht JT, Horton WA, Butler IJ, Goldie WD, Miner M. Neurological basis of respiratory complications in achondroplasia. *Ann Neurol.* 1988;24(1):89-93.

347. Onodera K, Niikuni N, Chigono T, et al. Sleep disordered breathing in children with achondroplasia. Part 2. Relationship with craniofacial and airway morphology. *Int J Pediatr Otorhinolaryngol.* 2006;70(3):453-461.

348. Onodera K, Sakata H, Niikuni N, et al. Survey of the present status of sleep-disordered breathing in children with achondroplasia. Part I. A questionnaire survey. *Int J Pediatr Otorhinolaryngol.* 2005;69(4):457-461.

349. Mogayzel Jr PJ, Carroll JL, Loughlin GM, et al. Sleep-disordered breathing in children with achondroplasia. *J Pediatr.* 1998;132(4):667-671.

350. Zucconi M, Weber G, Castronovo V, et al. Sleep and upper airway obstruction in children with achondroplasia. *J Pediatr.* 1996;129(5):743-749.

351. Waters KA, Everett F, Sillence D, Fagan E, Sullivan CE. Breathing abnormalities in sleep in achondroplasia. *Arch Dis Child.* 1993;69(2):191-196.

352. Sisk EA, Heatley DG, Borowski BJ, Leverson GE, Pauli RM. Obstructive sleep apnea in children with achondroplasia: Surgical and anesthetic considerations. *Otolaryngol Head Neck Surg.* 1999;120(2):248-254.

353. Ednick M, Tinkle BT, Phromchairak J, et al. Sleep-related respiratory abnormalities and arousal pattern in achondroplasia during early infancy. *J Pediatr.* 2009;155(4):510-515.

354. King JA, Vachhrajani S, Drake JM, Rutka JT. Neurosurgical implications of achondroplasia. *J Neurosurg Pediatr.* 2009;4(4):297-306.

355. Collins WO, Choi SS. Otolaryngologic manifestations of achondroplasia. *Arch Otolaryngol Head Neck Surg.* 2007;133(3):237-244.

356. Baujat G, Legeai-Mallet L, Finidori G, et al. Achondroplasia. *Best Pract Res Clin Rheumatol.* 2008;22(1):3-18.

357. Hoover-Fong JE, Schulze KJ, McGready J, Barnes H, Scott CI. Age-appropriate body mass index in children with achondroplasia: Interpretation in relation to indexes of height. *Am J Clin Nutr.* 2008;88(2):364-371.

358. Danielpour M, Wilcox WR, Alanay Y, Pressman BD, Rimoin DL. Dynamic cervicomedullary cord compression and alterations in cerebrospinal fluid dynamics in children with achondroplasia. Report of four cases. *J Neurosurg.* 2007;107(Suppl 6):504-507.

359. Waters KA, Everett F, Sillence DO, Fagan ER, Sullivan CE. Treatment of obstructive sleep apnea in achondroplasia: Evaluation of sleep, breathing, and somatosensory-evoked potentials. *Am J Med Genet.* 1995;59(4):460-466.

360. Ain MC, Chang TL, Schkrohowsky JG, et al. Rates of perioperative complications associated with laminectomies in patients with achondroplasia. *J Bone Joint Surg Am.* 2008;90(2):295-298.

361. Ottonello G, Villa G, Moscatelli A, Diana MC, Pavanello M. Noninvasive ventilation in a child affected by achondroplasia respiratory difficulty syndrome. *Paediatr Anaesth.* 2007;17(1):75-79.

362. The International Classification of Sleep Disorders. *Diagnostic and Coding Manual.* 2nd ed. Westchester, IL: American Academy of Sleep Medicine; 2005.

363. Iber C, Ancoli-Israel S, Chesson A, Quan SF. For the American Academy of Sleep Medicine. *The AASM Manual for the Scoring of Sleep and Associated Events: Rules, Terminology and Technical Specifications.* 1st ed. Westchester, IL: American Academy of Sleep Medicine; 2007.

364. Birnkrant DJ, Bushby KM, Amin RS, et al. The respiratory management of patients with duchenne muscular dystrophy: A DMD care considerations working group specialty article. *Pediatr Pulmonol.* 2010;45(8):739-748.

365. Cheng G, Bach JR. Noninvasive ventilation for continuous critical care and long-term ventilatory support. *Pediatr Emerg Care.* 2009;25(1):59-60.

366. Bach JR, Alba AS. Management of chronic alveolar hypoventilation by nasal ventilation. *Chest.* 1990;97(1):52-57.

367. Katz SL. Assessment of sleep-disordered breathing in pediatric neuromuscular diseases. *Pediatrics.* 2009;123(Suppl 4):S222-S225.

368. Velazquez-Wong AC, Hernandez-Huerta C, Marquez-Calixto A, et al. Identification of duchenne muscular dystrophy female carriers by fluorescence in situ hybridization and RT-PCR. *Genet Test.* 2008;12(2):221-223.

369. Suresh S, Wales P, Dakin C, Harris MA, Cooper DG. Sleep-related breathing disorder in Duchenne muscular dystrophy: Disease spectrum in the paediatric population. *J Paediatr Child Health.* 2005;41(9-10):500-503.

370. Brooke MH, Fenichel GM, Griggs RC, et al. Duchenne muscular dystrophy: Patterns of clinical progression and effects of supportive therapy. *Neurology.* 1989;39(4):475-481.

371. Manni R, Ottolini A, Cerveri I, et al. Breathing patterns and HbSaO$_2$ changes during nocturnal sleep in patients with Duchenne muscular dystrophy. *J Neurol.* 1989;236(7):391-394.

372. Khan Y, Heckmatt JZ. Obstructive apnoeas in Duchenne muscular dystrophy. *Thorax.* 1994;49(2):157-161.

373. Smith PE, Calverley PM, Edwards RH. Hypoxemia during sleep in Duchenne muscular dystrophy. *Am Rev Respir Dis.* 1988;137(4):884-888.

374. Barbe F, Quera-Salva MA, McCann C, et al. Sleep-related respiratory disturbances in patients with Duchenne muscular dystrophy. *Eur Respir J.* 1994;7(8):1403-1408.

375. Mellies U, Dohna-Schwake C, Stehling F, Voit T. Sleep disordered breathing in spinal muscular atrophy. *Neuromuscul Disord.* 2004;14(12):797-803.

376. Quera Salva MA, Blumen M, Jacquette A, et al. Sleep disorders in childhood-onset myotonic dystrophy type 1. *Neuromuscul Disord.* 2006;16(9-10):564-570.

377. Dohna-Schwake C, Ragette R, Mellies U, Straub V, Teschler H, Voit T. Respiratory function in congenital muscular dystrophy and limb girdle muscular dystrophy 2I. *Neurology.* 2004;62(3):513-514.

378. Nabatame S, Taniike M, Sakai N, et al. Sleep disordered breathing in childhood-onset acid maltase deficiency. *Brain Dev.* 2009;31(3):234-239.

379. Finder JD, Birnkrant D, Carl J, et al. Respiratory care of the patient with Duchenne muscular dystrophy: ATS consensus statement. *Am J Respir Crit Care Med.* 2004;170(4):456-465.

380. Myers SM, Challman TD, Bock GH. End-stage renal failure in Smith-Magenis syndrome. *Am J Med Genet A.* 2007;143A(16):1922-1924.

381. Kennedy JD, Martin AJ. Chronic respiratory failure and neuromuscular disease. *Pediatr Clin North Am.* 2009;56(1):261-273:xii.

382. Wallgren-Pettersson C, Bushby K, Mellies U, Simonds A. Ventilatory support in congenital neuromuscular disorders—Congenital myopathies, congenital muscular dystrophies, congenital myotonic dystrophy and SMA (II). 117th ENMC Workshop, 4-6 April 2003, Naarden, The Netherlands. *Neuromuscul Disord.* 2004;14(1):56-69.

383. Mellies U, Ragette R, Schwake C, et al. Daytime predictors of sleep disordered breathing in children and adolescents with neuromuscular disorders. *Neuromuscul Disord.* 2003;13(2):123-128.

384. Ragette R, Mellies U, Schwake C, Voit T, Teschler H. Patterns and predictors of sleep disordered breathing in primary myopathies. *Thorax.* 2002;57(8):724-728.

385. Benditt JO. Initiating noninvasive management of respiratory insufficiency in neuromuscular disease. *Pediatrics.* 2009;123(Suppl 4):S236-S238.

386. Young HK, Lowe A, Fitzgerald DA, et al. Outcome of noninvasive ventilation in children with neuromuscular disease. *Neurology.* 2007;68(3):198-201.

387. Ward S, Chatwin M, Heather S, Simonds AK. Randomised controlled trial of non-invasive ventilation (NIV) for nocturnal hypoventilation in neuromuscular and chest wall disease patients with daytime normocapnia. *Thorax.* 2005;60(12):1019-1024.

388. Edwards EA, Hsiao K, Nixon GM. Paediatric home ventilatory support: The Auckland experience. *J Paediatr Child Health.* 2005;41(12):652-658.

389. Mellies U, Ragette R, Dohna Schwake C, et al. Long-term noninvasive ventilation in children and adolescents with neuromuscular disorders. *Eur Respir J.* 2003;22(4):631-636.

390. Guilleminault C, Philip P, Robinson A. Sleep and neuromuscular disease: Bilevel positive airway pressure by nasal mask as a treatment for sleep disordered breathing in patients with neuromuscular disease. *J Neurol Neurosurg Psychiatry.* 1998;65(2):225-232.

391. Tan E, Nixon GM, Edwards EA. Sleep studies frequently lead to changes in respiratory support in children. *J Paediatr Child Health.* 2007;43(7-8):560-563.

392. Kirk VG, Batuyong ED, Bohn SG. Transcutaneous carbon dioxide monitoring and capnography during pediatric polysomnography. *Sleep.* 2006;29(12):1601-1608.

393. Eagle M, Baudouin SV, Chandler C, et al. Survival in Duchenne muscular dystrophy: Improvements in life expectancy since 1967 and the impact of home nocturnal ventilation. *Neuromuscul Disord.* 2002;12(10):926-929.

394. Bach JR. Medical considerations of long-term survival of Werdnig-Hoffmann disease. *Am J Phys Med Rehabil.* 2007;86(5):349-355.

395. Bach JR, Robert D, Leger P, Langevin B. Sleep fragmentation in kyphoscoliotic individuals with alveolar hypoventilation treated by NIPPV. *Chest.* 1995;107(6):1552-1558.

396. Fuschillo S, De Felice A, Gaudiosi C, Balzano G. Nocturnal mechanical ventilation improves exercise capacity in kyphoscoliotic patients with respiratory impairment. *Monaldi Arch Chest Dis.* 2003;59(4):281-286.

397. Wintzen AR, Lammers GJ, van Dijk JG. Does modafinil enhance activity of patients with myotonic dystrophy? A double-blind placebo-controlled crossover study. *J Neurol.* 2007;254(1):26-28.

398. Talbot K, Stradling J, Crosby J, Hilton-Jones D. Reduction in excess daytime sleepiness by modafinil in patients with myotonic dystrophy. *Neuromuscul Disord*. 2003;13(5):357-364.

399. MacDonald JR, Hill JD, Tarnopolsky MA. Modafinil reduces excessive somnolence and enhances mood in patients with myotonic dystrophy. *Neurology*. 2002;59(12):1876-1880.

400. Damian MS, Gerlach A, Schmidt F, Lehmann E, Reichmann H. Modafinil for excessive daytime sleepiness in myotonic dystrophy. *Neurology*. 2001;56(6):794-796.

401. Orlikowski D, Chevret S, Quera-Salva MA, et al. Modafinil for the treatment of hypersomnia associated with myotonic muscular dystrophy in adults: A multicenter, prospective, randomized, double-blind, placebo-controlled, 4-week trial. *Clin Ther*. 2009;31(8):1765-1773.

Sleep and Sleep Problems in Children with Medical Disorders

Chapter 41

MADELEINE M. GRIGG-DAMBERGER

Sleep disorders occur frequently in children, but in children with certain medical disorders, they occur more frequently and are often more persistent and severe.[1] The coexistence of sleep and medical problems further impairs quality of life (QoL) for both the child and caregivers. Not only may medical disorders lead to poorer quality sleep, but primary sleep disorders may worsen many medical disorders. Recent research even shows that chronically insufficient or fragmented sleep may increase the likelihood of developing certain medical conditions.

THE IMPACT OF INSUFFICIENT SLEEP OR SHORT SLEEP DURATION ON MEDICAL DISORDERS IN CHILDREN

Prepubertal children should sleep at least 9 to 10 hours per night and adolescents should have 8.5 to 9.25 hours. Cross-sectional population surveys have shown a significant association between reported short sleep and increased body mass index (BMI) and obesity in children, adolescents, and even infants.[2-7] Using actigraphy, Nixon and associates[2] found that sleeping less than 9 hours a night in 591 Australian 7-year-olds was associated with a 3.3 odds ratio (OR) for being overweight or obese and a 3.3% increase in body fat, effects not explained by increased television watching or decreased physical activity. They also found that short sleep duration was associated with a lower intelligence quotient (IQ) and higher emotional lability and attention deficit hyperactivity disorder (ADHD) scores.

Another study, by Shi and colleagues,[3] found the OR for obesity for children sleeping less than 9 hours a night was 2.23 for boys and 1.70 for girls, compared to those sleeping 10 or more hours, in a representative random sample of 3495 Australian children (aged 5-15 years, mean age 10.7 years). A cross-sectional study of 529 U.S. adolescents found that 90% of those with a BMI Z score above the 85th percentile averaged less than 8 hours of sleep on school nights and 19% averaged less than 6 hours.[8] Compared with students sleeping more than 8 hours, the age- and gender-adjusted OR of being overweight was 8.5 for those sleeping less than 5 hours, 2.8 for those sleeping 5 to 7 hours, and 1.3 for those getting 7 to 8 hours.

Insulin resistance and systemic arterial hypertension are associated with short sleep durations in children and adolescents. Flint and associates[9] confirmed by polysomnography (PSG) that insulin resistance was associated with short sleep duration, reduced percentage of rapid eye movement (REM) sleep time, and findings of obstructive sleep apnea (OSA) in 40 obese children. Javaheri and associates[10] found low sleep efficiency was associated with a higher systolic blood pressure (4 mm Hg) and a 3.5 times increased risk of prehypertension in 238 adolescents (findings not explained by obesity, sleep apnea, or socioeconomic status). In a study of 1024 middle-aged U.S. adults, Taheri and colleagues[11] found that getting less than 8 hours of sleep a night was associated with low leptin levels and elevated ghrelin levels, hormonal changes that are likely to increase appetite and may explain the increased BMI associated with short sleep duration in adults.

Many risk factors for insufficient sleep can be eliminated or reduced. A cross-sectional survey of a random representative sample of 20,778 Chinese children (ages 5-11 years) found that 28% slept less than 9 hours per day.[12] Multivariate logistic regression showed that the following factors were associated with short sleep duration: more time spent watching television or doing homework on weekdays, drinking caffeinated beverages after 6 PM, engaging in exciting activities before bedtime, and short sleep durations in the parents.

Studies confirm the benefits of sufficient sleep on children and adolescents. A study of 39 healthy children (ages 7-11 years) found longer habitual sleep duration was associated with better performance on measures of perceptual reasoning and overall IQ.[13] The average sleep duration reported was just over 10 hours, in good agreement with other studies.[2,14-16] Lemola and associates[17] evaluated the relationship between quantity and quality of sleep with positive attitudes in children. They found that sleep duration (confirmed by actigraphy for 7 nights) showed a nonlinear, reverse J-shaped relationship with optimism in 291 8-year-olds. Children with sleep duration in the middle of the distribution curve scored higher in optimism compared with children who slept less.

Given the relationships described here, it would appear that obtaining sufficient sleep is one element that may help to reduce obesity, prehypertension, and insulin resistance while at the same time improving mood in children and adolescents.

Treatment of Insufficient Sleep Syndrome in Children and Adolescents

Treatment of insufficient sleep syndrome in children and adolescents requires an appreciation of the range of their normal sleep needs and habits:

1. To recognize when a child's sleep/wake patterns and behaviors are abnormal, we must know what is normal.[15,18-23] Newborns at term typically sleep 16 to 18 hours per day. Sleep periods in infants during the first months of life typically last 50 to 300 minutes

519

followed by a 90- to 180-minute period of wakefulness. By 4 months of age, most infants consolidate their longest sleep time to the night. They normally wake about every 1.5 to 3 hours; most of these are brief, but one or two wakings typically last longer with infants "signaling" caregivers that they are wet or hungry. At this age infants typically take three naps, around midmorning, midafternoon, and early evening.

2. Infants 4 to 12 months usually sleep 9 to 10 hours at night and nap for 2 to 4.5 hours during the day. About 70% to 80% of infants sleep through the night by age 9 months. By 6 months the early evening nap is usually dropped. The 1- to 2-year-olds normally sleep 9 to 10 hours per night and take only a single nap, usually not over 2 hours. Twenty percent of toddlers and preschoolers awaken once each night, 50% wake at least one night per week.

Most children stop taking daytime naps between ages 3 to 5 years. Adolescents often sleep only 6.5 to 7.5 hours on school nights, then *crash and catch up* on weekends. Daytime napping often reappears in adolescents who curtail their sleep and accumulate sleep debt. A child who, on weekends, sleeps 2 hours more than during the week is providing strong evidence of weekday sleep deprivation.

At younger ages, children demonstrate greater variability in sleep needs and habits.[15,22] A longitudinal study by Iglowstein and associates[15] evaluated how nighttime, daytime, and total sleep duration changed with age in 463 children studied from age 1 month to 16 years. They found total sleep duration decreased from an average of 14.2 hours at 6 months of age to 8.1 hours at age 16. Of particular note, the range of "normal" (variance) was far greater at age 6 months (2.5 hours) than at age 16 (1 hour). The sleep schedule a child or adolescent prefers is often best identified during vacations. A *morningness* or *eveningness* preference (*lark* or *owl*) usually is clear by 3 to 4 years of age.[24]

CHILDHOOD OBESITY

The prevalence of obesity in the United States has doubled in the last two decades in younger children and tripled among adolescents.[25-27] OSA is significantly more common in obese or overweight children compared with nonobese children matched for age and gender.[28-30] Studies suggest obesity is an independent risk factor for OSA in children and adolescents[28,29,31,32] even after adjusting for race.[33]

Finding OSA on an overnight PSG is nearly 19 times more likely in an obese child compared to one of normal weight.[28] The severity of OSA on PSG is often worse in obese compared with nonobese children[29,33] even after adjusting for other confounding factors.[34-36] Obese children with OSA may be sleepier than nonobese children with a similar level of OSA severity.[37-39] In an obese child, even the presence of tonsillar hypertrophy alone or a narrow velopharyngeal space increases the risk for sleep-disordered breathing (SDB).[28,34,40-42]

Adenotonsillectomy (AT) is considered first-line treatment for significant symptomatic OSA in children with adenotonsillar enlargement. However, 76% of obese (vs. only 28% of nonobese) children had persistent OSA following AT; residual findings were only severe in the obese, occurring in 15%.[43] Other studies have confirmed that 45% to 56% of obese children are likely to have sufficient residual sleep apnea following AT to warrant use of positive airway pressure therapy, either continuous (CPAP) or bi-level (BiPAP).[44-47]

OSA also increases the likelihood that obese children will have systemic hypertension,[48-50] fatty liver disease,[51] and metabolic syndrome.[52,53] Obesity increased the risk of systemic hypertension 6.7 times, and 67% of obese children with an apnea-hypopnea index (AHI) greater than 5 had systemic hypertension compared with 23% of those with an AHI less than 5.[54] Redline and associates[52] found that obese adolescents with OSA had a 6.5-fold higher risk for metabolic syndrome compared with those without OSA (59% vs. 16%) even after adjusting for sex, age, race, and preterm status. The prevalence of hypertension was approximately 30% among children who had a BMI above the 95th percentile.[55,56] Thirty-two percent of 142 overweight or obese children had fatty liver disease, and 91% of these children had OSA on PSG; whereas only 3 of 376 nonobese subjects had fatty liver disease even though 66% had OSA on PSG.[51] They also found that the fatty liver disease improved after successful treatment of OSA in 32 of 42 obese children ($p < 0.0001$).

Diagnostic and Treatment Strategies for Childhood Obesity

Screening overweight or obese children for insulin resistance, hyperlipidemia, fatty liver disease,[57] hypothyroidism, and SDB should be routine; disorders such as Prader-Willi syndrome or hypothalamic or pituitary tumors should also be considered but are less common. Treatment strategies for pediatric obesity begin with lifestyle modification and behavior modification programs targeting the entire family and include dietary change, increased physical activity, treatment of co-morbidities, behavioral therapy, and for the morbidly obese adolescent, possible bariatric surgery.[58-62] Successful weight loss in the morbidly obese adolescents (BMI ≥ 40 kg/m^2) is associated with improvements in SDB.[63-66]

SYSTEMIC ARTERIAL HYPERTENSION

Childhood systemic hypertension (HTN) is often asymptomatic and is easily missed, even by health professionals.[67] Systemic hypertension in children and adolescents is defined as systolic blood pressure (SBP) or diastolic blood pressure (DBP) at or above the 95th percentile on *three* repeated measurements.[68] *Prehypertension* (an indication for recommending lifestyle changes) is defined as average SDB or DBP levels that are at or over the 90th but less than the 95th percentile for age and gender.[68] Adolescents with BP levels reaching 120/80 mm Hg or greater should be considered at least prehypertensive.[68]

OSA (AHI ≥ 5) was found to be an independent risk factor for elevated BP in 700 5- to 12-year-old randomly selected elementary school children in a prospective study.[69] In another study, SBP and DBP were significantly higher among 270 adolescents with AHI at or above 5, even after accounting for age, sex, and BMI percentile.[52] In a third study, 32% of 41 children with OSA, and 19% of 26 with primary snoring, had a blood pressure (BP) above the 95th percentile for age and sex compared with 2% to 5% in the general pediatric population.[50]

SDB in children who are otherwise healthy is independently associated with an increase in morning BP surge, BP load, 24-hour ambulatory BP values, and left ventricular remodeling (findings that, if left untreated, can increase cardiovascular morbidity).[70] Bixler and associates[69] found that even an AHI between 1 and 5 was associated with an approximately 2 mm Hg BP elevation in 25% of children studied (and even such modest BP elevations, over time, may predispose to metabolic syndrome).[71]

Ambulatory blood pressure monitoring is very useful for evaluating HTN in children and adolescents, often detecting the patterns of BP change seen in patients with SDB.[72-74] Isolated systolic HTN is the typical pattern of obesity-related primary HTN in children.[55,75] HTN in children with OSA is characterized by significantly greater variability of BP awake and asleep, higher night-to-day systolic BP differences, and a loss of *nocturnal dipping* (the normal 10-20% fall in the mean BP during sleep).[76] However, it remains to be shown that treatment of SDB in children and adolescents normalizes the associated BP abnormalities.

Treating Systemic Hypertension in Children and Adolescents

Treatment of HTN in children and adolescents begins with changes in lifestyle: healthy diet avoiding junk food and salt, weight loss, and exercise (40 minutes of aerobic-based exercise three to five times per week). Medications used to treat HTN in pediatric patients are similar to those in adults: angiotensin-converting enzyme inhibitors, angiotensin receptor antagonists, calcium antagonists, beta blockers, and (occasionally) diuretics and other antihypertensive agents.[67] BP control is often better if antihypertensive medications are dosed at bedtime especially among nondippers.[77] An AHI of 5 or greater on an overnight PSG in a child or adolescent warrants treatment for OSA.

BENIGN NEONATAL SLEEP MYOCLONUS

Benign neonatal sleep myoclonus (BNSM) is characterized by myoclonic jerks that occur during sleep but stop abruptly when the infant is aroused.[78-80] A recent retrospective review of 38 infants with BNSM found the limb jerks were first observed at a median age of 3 days (range 1-16 days) and spontaneously remitted between 2 weeks and 10 months (median 2 months).[80] The neurologic examinations of these infants are typically normal. The diagnosis is confirmed by video-electroencephalogram or video-PSG recording, showing a cluster of the typical limb movements not associated with ictal electroencephalogram (EEG) activity.[78]

BSNM limb jerks may occur during any stage of sleep,[78] but most commonly they occur at sleep onset (or sometimes they appear after the infant has been sleeping for more than 20 minutes or, even less commonly, shortly before awakening).[80] Video-PSG studies have shown that the limb movements of BNSM are typically bilateral and symmetrical, involve the arms and legs; and usually occur in clusters lasting only a few seconds (but occasionally can last up to 5 minutes). However, one video-EEG study of 18 infants found BNSM could occur unilaterally, involve the face or head, and could occur during the sleep-wake transition.[79] BNSM in another study consisted of brief salvos of four or five jerks recurring in clusters over 20 to 30 minutes during quiet (non–rapid eye movement [NREM]) sleep.[81]

BNSM can be provoked in some infants by rocking in a head-to-toe direction, or by exposure to repetitive sounds or loud noises.[80,82,83] A recent case-control study found BNSM in 67% of 78 infants of opioid-dependent mothers compared with 3% among the age-matched control subjects.[84] Familial cases of BNSM have been reported.[80,85,86] Reassurance is the best treatment approach to this benign transient condition.

INFANT COLIC

Infant colic (paroxysms of crying or fussing lasting 3 or more hours per day on 3 or more days per week for more than 3 weeks) usually first appears at age 2 to 3 weeks.[87] A prospective cohort study of 483 first-born infants found the prevalence of colic was 19% at 2 months and 13% at 4 months.[88] Periods of colic primarily occur in the evening, often start between 5 to 8 PM, typically last 1.75 to 2.75 hours, and usually end by midnight.[89] The majority of colic episodes begin when the infant is awake; only 8% start during sleep.[90]

Although the cause of colic is uncertain, recurrent abdominal pain is often suspected, particularly because passing flatus or feces sometimes provides relief.[91] A case-control study of 104 colicky infants found no medical cause in any. However, feeding problems (in 71%) and a history of pregnancy or birth complications (in 85%) were found about twice as often in sufferers than in thriving control subjects.[92] Some authors suggest colic may be caused by an imbalance in serotonin and melatonin secretion impacting on gastrointestinal smooth muscles,[93] by inadequate amounts of gastrointestinal lactobacillus and increased concentrations of coliform bacteria,[94] or by the absence of circadian rhythm of cortisol production in affected infants.[85] No significant differences in sleep architecture, arousals, or breathing patterns have been found between colicky infants and age-matched control subjects at 4.5 weeks and 6 months of age.[83,86,87] Infant colic is most likely *not* a sleep disorder.

A recently published double-blind, placebo-controlled study found infants fed formula enriched with lactalbumin and probiotics had fewer gastrointestinal symptoms but no less crying.[95] A recently published nested case-control study found no differences in fecal enzyme activities in 47 Turkish infants with colic and 142 control subjects.[96] Instead, they found much higher rates of impaired maternal-infant bonding and less education about parenting in the mothers of colicky infants.[96]

Nonpharmacologic interventions for infant colic include regular and uniform daily care, reduction in external stimuli, and swaddling when asleep.[97] Infant massage may reduce crying, improve sleep, aid relaxation, and help mother-infant interactions.[98] Providing the parents with educational materials, and reassuring them that colic usually ends by 3 to 4 months and does not predict long-term outcomes (sleep or otherwise) may be helpful.[88] Simply carrying or holding the infant, using sound machines, or treating with drugs aimed at gas reduction are not of benefit, and only 3% respond positively to rhythmic rocking. A few days of hospitalization may seem to lead to a breaking of the daily cycle of colic (raising interesting questions as to the possible cause).[97,99,100]

NOCTURNAL ASTHMA

An average of 1 out of every 10 school-aged children has asthma.[101,102] Prevalence rates for asthma are higher in children of African-American, Asian, and Native American ethnicities.[103] Thirteen million school days each year are missed in the United States because of asthma.[102] *Nocturnal asthma (NA)* is defined as asthma that occurs primarily at night, or at least is most severe at night. NA is associated with increased daytime symptoms, a need for more medication at night, and heightened airway reactivity and a worsening of lung function when sleeping.[104] The amplitude of the nocturnal decrease in peak expiratory flow rates, which exhibit circadian variation and are normally lowest around 4 AM, is increased in NA. Hypersensitivity responses to house dust allergens and inflammatory airway changes also show nocturnal increases. Box 41-1 summarizes factors that may contribute to nocturnal worsening of asthma.

Sleep/wake complaints are common in children with asthma. A 2006 case-control study found that 15% of asthmatic children have difficulty maintaining sleep, 15% had early morning awakening, 25% had daytime sleepiness, and 21% had daytime tiredness, far higher percentages than age-matched nonasthmatic control subjects.[105] One third of children with mild to moderate asthma awaken at least once per night, and 14% awaken three or more times per night.[106] Studies have shown that children with NA have less nighttime sleep, later bedtimes, and more daytime napping than healthy control subjects.[107] These children also have significantly less total sleep time (TST), increased wake after sleep onset (WASO), increased sleep-related arousals, and more motor restlessness;[108] they generate more calls to physicians, have more emergency department visits, and experience greater numbers of asthma-related deaths than do control subjects.[109,110] Children with asthma have their sleep disturbed by wheezing, coughing, and breathlessness, symptoms that may lead to tiredness, impaired activity, and increased absenteeism or tardy arrivals to school the following day.[111]

Braido and colleagues[112] found an inverse relationship between asthma control and the presence of sleep disturbances and recommended that a PSG be considered in asthmatic children who have sleep disturbances even when there is good control of their asthma and rhinitis. Children with a history of asthma were 3.8 times more likely to have obstructive sleep-disordered breathing (OSA) on a four-channel home PSG.[33] OSA and obesity are associated with asthma in children and adolescents.[113,114] Nearly half of 85 infants or young children with recurrent wheezing but *no* gastrointestinal symptoms had silent gastroesophageal reflux (GER) found by intraesophageal monitoring.[115]

Treating Nocturnal Asthma

Many of the medicines used to treat asthma are more effective and less toxic when taken at certain times of the day or on a certain schedule. This effect may reflect circadian rhythm function or pharmacokinetic properties. Fluticasone (an inhaled corticosteroid) more effectively reduces the nocturnal fall in peak expiratory flow (PEF) and postexercise forced expiratory volume in 1 second (FEV_1) than salmeterol (a long-acting β_2-agonist).[116] Salmeterol better improves asthma when used twice a day. Theophylline is effective in relieving nighttime asthma symptoms when taken once in the late afternoon. Prednisone decreases nocturnal airway inflammation and obstruction best when taken at 3 PM. Using a once-daily inhaler in the evening instead of in the morning can be very helpful especially if the asthma is worse or occurs only at night. However, administering aerosols by means of a pressurized metered-dose inhaler-spacer during sleep offers no advantage and was particularly poorly tolerated by young children.[117]

Creating an optimal sleeping environment often lessens the symptoms of NA, allergic rhinitis, and atopic dermatitis.[118-121] Methods to decrease NA symptoms are summarized in Table 41-1. Children with asthma exposed to environmental smoke were much more likely to report significant nocturnal symptoms and have lower morning and evening PEF values.[105] Airborne particle filters can help reduce symptoms of asthma and allergic rhinitis.[122,123] Education of middle and high school children about asthma physiology and self-management techniques has been shown to lead to significantly fewer days with activity limitations, fewer nights of sleep disturbance, and significantly fewer frequent emergency department visits and hospitalization.[124]

BOX 41-1 *Factors That May Contribute to Worsening of Asthma at Night*

- Peak expiratory flow rates lowest around 4 AM
- Hypersensitivity responses to house dust allergen and airway inflammation greater at night
- Greater nighttime activation of inflammatory cells and mediators
- Reduced mucociliary clearance and lung volume during sleep
- Increased pulmonary capillary blood volume, upper airway resistance, and intrapulmonary blood pooling during sleep
- Decreased effects of once-daily asthma medications by the early morning hours
- Bedroom exposure to bedroom dust mites or pet dander
- Slower clearing of gastroesophageal reflux events at night
- Bronchospasm induced by nocturnal fall in body temperature
- Nocturnal occurrence of sleep apnea, postnasal drip, or allergic rhinitis

---

TABLE 41-1

Creating the Optimal Sleep Environment to Lessen Symptoms of Nocturnal Asthma, Allergic Rhinitis, and Atopic Dermatitis

Items to Avoid	Items to Implement
Composite bedding	Wrap the mattress with a vinyl cover
Synthetic comforters	
Dust mite–laden bedding	Wash the top bedding cover with hot water (55° C) every 2 weeks
Foam bed pillows	
Recently painted bedrooms	
Carpeted bedrooms	Remove soft furniture from bedroom
Exposure to gas as a cooking fuel	
Exposure to tobacco smoke	Wet clean the bedroom floor every day
Presence of dog or cat in bedroom	Use airborne particle filters
	Be sure child obtains sufficient sleep
	Daily exercise for child
	Optimize child's body weight
	Patient and caregiver education

ALLERGIC RHINITIS

Allergic rhinitis (AR) is an inflammatory disease of the mucous membranes of the nose in which repeated exposure to environmental antigens results in vasomotor changes, hypersensitivity, inflammation, and mucus hypersecretion. Approximately 25% of children in the United States are affected by AR in one or more seasons of the year,[125] and AR is a major risk factor for the development of asthma in young children.[126] AR can be seasonal or perennial. Seasonal AR is often triggered by exposure to mold spores or tree, weed, or grass pollen, whereas in perennial AR nasal congestion is often the primary or sole symptom, and indoor allergens (dust mites, pet dander, mold, and cockroaches) may act as triggers. Perennial AR shows little or no seasonal variation in symptoms.

Symptoms of AR include nasal congestion, repetitive sneezing, watery nasal drainage, and itchy nose, ears, eyes, and throat; nasal symptoms may cause nose rubbing, and the child may exhibit dark circles beneath the eyes ("allergic shiners"). Prolonged exposure to an allergen in an atopic child can lead to allergen-specific IgE production. Reexposure triggers a cascade of events: episodes of sneezing, nasal itching, nasal congestion, and rhinorrhea. These symptoms occur within minutes of reexposure (early-phase response) followed 4 to 8 hours later by symptoms of nasal congestion, loss of smell, mucus hypersecretion, and nasal hyper-responsiveness to the same or even *other* allergens (late-phase response).[127]

AR predisposes children to adenoid hypertrophy, recurrent otitis media, and sinusitis, and is associated with learning and sleep problems.[127] Like asthma, the severity and symptoms of AR exhibit circadian variation; thus, symptoms are most often worse at night or early in the morning, which leads to compromise of nighttime sleep and results in decreased daytime QoL, irritability, moodiness, and poor academic achievement.[128]

Diagnosing and Treating Allergic Rhinitis

Allergy testing facilitates accurate diagnosis and the choice of specific treatments including allergen avoidance measures and immunotherapy.[127] Screening children with AR for OSA is warranted because children with self-reported hay fever (or sinus problems) are five times more likely to have PSG-confirmed OSA.[33]

AR is best treated by first reducing allergen triggers (see Table 41-1); then, if symptoms remain, the next steps involve adding medication and identifying and treating coexisting conditions (e.g., nocturnal GER disease and OSA).[129,130] Medication choices should be guided by the severity, seasonality, and persistence of the AR. In general, antihistamines are of limited benefit in AR caused by house dust mites and other perennial allergens, because symptoms are primarily nasal obstruction and not mediated by histamine.[130] In contrast, AR symptoms triggered by pollen (e.g., nasal itch, rhinorrhea, and sneezing) are often relieved by antihistamines.[130]

For *mild intermittent* AR symptoms, nonsedating oral antihistamines (most often H$_1$ receptor blockers such as cetirizine, fexofenadine, or loratadine) or decongestants (pseudoephedrine) may suffice. Oral nonsedating antihistamines may relieve runny nose, sneezing, or itching but may have little or no effect on nasal congestion. On the other hand, decongestants reduce nasal congestion and may lessen runny nose, but will not control sneezing or itching and may cause insomnia, irritability, and hyperactivity. Drugs which combine H$_1$ blockers with a decongestant are effective but approved by the Federal Drug Administration (FDA) only for children 12 years or older. Cromolyn nasal spray, available without a prescription, can be used shortly before exposure to an unavoidable predictable allergen.

Seasonal AR (hay fever) in a child may be controlled by intranasal corticosteroid spray every morning coupled with daily nasal saline sprays, gels, or irrigation. If symptoms persist after 1 to 2 weeks, a nonsedating H$_1$ receptor antagonist or nasal decongestant can be added as needed. Itchy eyes may be treated with eye drops (antihistamine with or without vasoconstrictor or topical mast cell stabilizer).

Moderately severe persistent AR is most effectively treated with topical nasal corticosteroids, which reduce mucosal inflammation and effectively treat sneezing, runny nose, itchy nose, and nasal stuffiness. Intranasal steroids are the treatment of choice for persistent moderately severe allergic rhinitis and are more effective than antihistamines for relief of nasal obstruction.[130] Many different formulations are available (fluticasone, triamcinolone, flunisolide, budesonide, beclomethasone); all work equally well, but some have particular odors or tastes that some patients may prefer or dislike. A large, well-designed study showed that triamcinolone aqueous nasal spray (110 μg once each morning) was effective in treating persistent perennial AR in children aged 2 to 5 years without suppressing their growth, increasing serum cortisol levels, or causing other unacceptable side effects.[131] A longer course of oral antihistamines and intranasal corticosteroids was as effective as a short course of an oral antibiotic coupled with oral corticosteroids in reducing adenoidal size and resolving all the symptoms of rhinosinusitis in 13 children, 7 of whom had extensive symptoms.[132]

Chronic obstructive nasal symptoms due to adenoidal hypertrophy were effectively controlled by intranasal corticosteroid therapy given for 4 to 28 months.[133] Failure to respond to intranasal medications is often due to poor compliance or inefficient use of nasal sprays.[130] Severe AR may require a short course (3-5 days) of oral corticosteroids. If these treatments are ineffective, allergy immunotherapy may be considered. Immunotherapy may be a useful but expensive treatment for AR, especially if the symptoms are triggered by specific pollens.[130] The benefits of immunotherapy in house dust mite–induced AR and asthma remain controversial.[130] A recently published double-blind, placebo-controlled study showed 30 weeks of sublingual immunotherapy with house dust extract was a safe and effective treatment for chronic AR related to house dust mites in 31 children (ages 7-15 years).[134]

Treating Allergic Rhinitis Can Improve Mild Obstructive Sleep Apnea in Children

Studies have shown that 6 to 12 weeks of morning intranasal corticosteroids can lessen mild OSA, improve both the quality of nocturnal sleep and daytime QoL, and reduce daytime sleepiness, fatigue, and inflammation.[135-139] Treating AR and adenoidal hypertrophy in children with mild OSA with 6 to 12 weeks of intranasal corticosteroids can lead to similar improvements.[135-139]

Significant improvements in sleep architecture and reductions in sleep-disordered breathing and adenoidal size were also observed in children with mild OSA treated for 6 weeks with intranasal budesonide at bedtime (32 μg on each side) in a double-blind, placebo-controlled, crossover study.[139] Oral montelukast (a leukotriene receptor antagonist) has been shown to reduce adenoid size, improve measures of OSA on PSG, and improve day and nighttime symptoms of AR in children whose OSA was too mild to readily justify treatment by adenotonsillectomy.[140,141] A 12-week trial of oral monelukast combined with intranasal budesonide significantly reduced AHI from a mean of 3.9 to 0.3 and lowered the respiratory arousal index from 4.6 to 0.8 per hour, changes not seen in the control group (children with similarly mild OSA who were not treated).[142]

SICKLE CELL DISEASE

Sickle cell disease (SCD) is an autosomal recessive disorder in which a substitution of valine for glutamic acid in the β-chain hemoglobin molecule[143] causes red blood cells to form sickle shapes and polymerize particularly when patients are exposed to hypoxemia or extremes of temperature or are dealing with infections.[144] SCD most often occurs in individuals of African descent, occurring in 1 in every 400 to 500 African Americans.[143] Individuals with sickle cell anemia (i.e., those who are homozygous for the abnormal hemoglobin S [HbS]) are most likely to exhibit severe clinical manifestations.[145]

Sleep disorders are common in children and adolescents with SCD. Not particularly surprising, Jacob and associates[146] found sleep/wake patterns were disrupted during painful crises. The parents of 54 SCD children (ages 4-10 years) reported that their children, even when their SCD was stable, still had significantly more nocturnal awakenings and sleep-disordered breathing than did healthy age-matched control subjects, as reported by parents.[147] The investigators found an increase of both parasomnias and sleep disordered breathing in three groups of SCD patients: those with nocturnal enuresis, those with higher frequencies of SCD complications, and those of lower socioeconomic status.

Children with SCD are at greater risk for adenotonsillar hypertrophy (ATH) because of compensatory lymphoid adenotonsillar hyperplasia following splenic infarction and repeated infections.[148-150] ATH, present in 55% of 85 SCD children, was associated with more episodes of tonsillitis, upper respiratory infections, and painful crises within 12 months, but only 11% had findings of OSA on overnight PSG (AHI > 1).[151] However, SCD children with OSA had lower mean Spo_2 values during REM sleep, higher respiratory disturbance index (RDI) values, lower Spo_2 nadirs, and a greater percentage of sleep time with Spo_2 less than 90% than those without OSA.[152]

The most common and distinctive pattern of sleep-disordered breathing in SCD is nocturnal oxygen desaturation (NOD), but most often this is *not related* to OSA.[153-157] A study of 20 SCD children found that 55% had NOD, but only 35% of these patients also had OSA, and most of the desaturations were unrelated to OSA events.[157] Another study found OSA on overnight PSG in 18% of 53 children with SCD with suspected sleep apnea; episodic NOD at 80% or less or low baseline Spo_2 during sleep was found in another 16%.[158]

SCD children whose baseline saturation when awake is at 94% or less are likely to have PSG-related abnormalities. Spivey and associates[157] found NOD (mean nocturnal Spo_2

88.9%) along with OSA on overnight PSG in 55% of 20 children with SCD. The average daytime Spo_2 correlated with nocturnal Spo_2, and children with the lower Spo_2 values awake had the greatest desaturations during sleep. Thirty-five percent also had OSA (mean RDI 14), but neither daytime nor nighttime pulse oximetry values alone predicted which child would have OSA on PSG. In children with SCD and a daytime Spo_2 of 94% or less, concomitant obstructive SDB was present in one third.

Nocturnal hypoxemia predisposes patients with SCD to painful vaso-occlusive crises[156,159,160] and central nervous system (CNS) events.[161] Approximately 11% of patients homozygous for HbS have a stroke by age 20.[162,163] Another recent study showed 28% of 96 children with SCD had "silent infarcts" on brain neuroimaging done before age 6 (for which lower hemoglobin levels were identified as a risk factor).[164] Stroke and silent infarctions in children with SCD are associated with lower hematocrit levels, cognitive impairment, and poor educational attainment.[165-169]

Hypoxemia in SCD is typically more common and more severe during sleep and can, if untreated, cause a hypercoagulable state that, in turn, could predispose to vaso-occlusive episodes, stroke, and seizures. SCD children with a mean overnight Spo_2 of 96% or less had a sixfold increased risk for developing a CNS event.[170] A mean nocturnal Spo_2 of 93% or less was associated with markers of white blood cell, platelet, and endothelial activation.[156] Hypoxemia, worse at night in SCD, may produce hypercoaguable states and lead to strokes, seizures, and silent infarcts. Heightened awareness of these associations is needed.

Diagnostic and Treatment Strategies for Sleep Disorders in Sickle Cell Disease

Identifying and aggressively managing nocturnal hypoxemia in children and adolescents with SCD is a cost-effective way of reducing the incidence of painful crises, CNS events, and pulmonary hypertension.[170] A daytime Spo_2 at or below 94% is a reasonable threshold to warrant pulmonary evaluation including an overnight PSG in children with SCD (because more than half have will have nocturnal hypoxemia and one third will have OSA).[157] Overnight home pulse oximetry may be a sufficient screening device to identify nocturnal hypoxemia in a child with SCD and a normal daytime Spo_2 who does not habitually snore and has no adenotonsillar hypertrophy. A history of frequent infections, painful crises, strokes, seizures, snoring, or poor sleep quality should prompt consideration of overnight PSG to evaluate for nocturnal hypoxemia and OSA.

Adenotonsillectomy (AT) benefits children with SCD most by reducing the number of subsequent infections.[149,153] The number of painful crises decreased following AT (done for recurrent tonsillitis, not for OSA), a finding attributed to reduced numbers of recurrent infections (suggesting that the real benefit, or least one of the real benefits, of AT for children with SCD is to reduce recurrent infections).[149,153] But surgery should be approached cautiously because individuals with SCD are at higher risk for postoperative complications, especially when the children are younger than 4 years, have a high preoperative HbS ratio, or also have OSA.[171] Giving SCD children transfusions to lower their HbS ratio below 40% (or achieve a hemoglobin level >100 g/L) coupled with aggressive intravenous (IV) hydration (1.5 times the maintenance fluid) 24 hours before surgery significantly reduced the incidence of postoperative complications in SCD children undergoing elective tonsillectomy.[171]

OSA unrelated to ATH in children or adolescents with SCD can be treated with CPAP or BiPAP. A small phase 1 trial showed treating OSA in children with SCD children with auto-adjusting continuous positive airway pressure (auto-PAP) improved their obstructive apnea-hypopnea index (OAHI), mean number of desaturations per hour of sleep (desaturation index), and mean nocturnal SpO_2, and resulted in improved daytime attention and processing speed.[172] In children with SCD, poor sleep quality was associated with increased daytime pain.[173] Strategies that encouraged good sleep hygiene, adequate pain control, and a positive attitude improved QoL for these children.[173,174]

Other treatment strategies to lessen painful crises in SCD include maintaining hydration and avoiding extremes of climate, physical exhaustion, and high altitudes without oxygen supplementation. Beginning at age 2 to 3 years, SCD patients should have yearly transcranial Doppler studies.[175-177] If they are found to have abnormally high arterial blood flow velocities (> 200 cm/second), exchange transfusion protocols should be started. If NOD or SDB is found, there should be, a diagnostic evaluation and aggressive management. Exchange transfusions (that decrease the percentage of HbS to values < 30% of the total hemoglobin) resulted in improvement and stabilization, have been shown to significantly decrease risk of stroke in SCD, and should also be started after a CNS event (stroke or seizure).[162,163]

Other important adjunct therapies for SCD are hydroxyurea and hydroxycarabamide. Hydroxyurea given prophylactically to children with SCD may reduce vaso-occlusion, hemolysis, and end-organ damage.[178-180] Hydroxyurea may preserve brain and spleen function and lower abnormally elevated transcranial Doppler velocities in children with SCD.[181-183] A case-control study found SCD children treated with hydroxyurea had significantly higher scores on various cognitive tests.[184] Hydroxyurea shortened hospitalization stay and reduced amount of opiates given for acute painful crises.[185] Hydroxycarbamide (an antimetabolic/cytotoxic agent that works by inhibiting ribonucleotide reductase, thereby blocking DNA synthesis and arresting cells in the sickle phase) promotes fetal hemoglobin (HbF) production, improves red blood cell hydration, acts as a nitric oxide donor, and reduces the frequency of painful crises and the overall mortality rate.[186,187]

NOCTURNAL GASTROESOPHAGEAL REFLUX DISEASE

Minor degrees of GER occur normally, particularly in children younger than 18 months of age.[188] Gastroesophageal reflux disease (GERD) is diagnosed when complications of significant and frequent reflux occur. The symptoms of GERD vary with age and are summarized in Table 41-2.[188] Approximately 2% of all children aged 7 to 16 years have symptoms of GERD, and the prevalence increases to 13% with obesity[189] and to 20% to 25% with asthma.[188] The risk of GERD is also higher among children with neurologic disorders or those treated with inhaled or oral corticosteroids, beta agonists,

TABLE 41-2

Symptoms of Gastroesophageal Reflux Disease by Age

Infants	Young Children	Older Children and Adolescents
Regurgitation	Abdominal pain	Recurrent abdominal pain
Recurrent vomiting	Recurrent vomiting	Heartburn
Irritability	Recurrent wheezing	Epigastric pain
Feeding resistance	Recurrent pneumonia	
Apnea	Heartburn	
Choking	Chronic cough	
Opisthotonic posturing during or after feeding	Hoarseness	
	Swallowing difficulty	
Excessive hiccups	Excessive eructation	
Failure to thrive and poor growth	Poor growth	
	Food refusal	
Recurrent pneumonia	Bad breath	
	Picky eater	

paracetamol, and antiepileptics.[190] Seventy percent of infants or young children with tracheomalacia or laryngomalacia have GERD.[191] Sleep-related GERD in infants and children may lead to esophagitis, stridor, recurrent cough, and wheezing. QoL in children with GERD is significantly lower than in children with chronic inflammatory disease or healthy age-matched control subjects.[192]

During sleep, gastric acid secretion peaks (between 10 PM and 2 AM),[193] the rate of swallowing decreases (from 25 to 5 times per hour), gastric emptying slows, and production of saliva nearly ceases. However, transient lower esophageal sphincter relaxations are actually suppressed in sleep and occur primarily during arousals. Probably for these reasons, the number of reflux events decreases in sleep, but the time to clear the gastric acid from the esophagus lengthens,[194] especially in the supine position.[195]

Diagnosing Gastroesophageal Reflux Disease

For an infant with typical reflux symptoms (regurgitation, vomiting, arching back, food refusal), a 2-week trial of a H_2-receptor blocker or a proton pump inhibitor (PPI) may be sufficient to empirically confirm the diagnosis.[188] Changing or thickening formulas in infants, and keeping the infant upright after feedings can be tried in infants younger than 3 months of age.

If symptoms persist, formal diagnostic testing should be considered. Intraesophageal pH monitoring can quantify the frequency and duration of acid reflux events, correlate the relationship between reflux and atypical symptoms (e.g., chronic cough, stridor, wheezing, irritability, or opisthotonic posturing), and assess treatment response.[196] Some specialists recommend recording an intraesophageal pH during a PSG in infants with unexplained SDB.[197] However, although infants with obstructive apnea often have GERD, episodes of apnea are seldom associated with a reflux event. When GER and obstructive apnea occur in close proximity, the obstructive apnea usually precedes the reflux.[198-201]

In one prospective study, 35 full-term infants with suspected OSA were recorded polysomnographically for two consecutive nights (one night with and one night without an intraesophageal probe, with order randomly assigned).[202] The authors found the presence of the pH probe significantly decreased both obstructive and central apneas present in 21 of 25 infants, prompting concerns that an esophageal pH probe in infants may compromise the diagnostic validity of the PSG. It is also known that some infants have nonacid reflux; although this would be undetected by esophageal pH monitoring, it can be diagnosed by impedance testing.[203]

Upper gastrointestinal series are neither sensitive nor specific for the diagnosis of GERD, but can be useful in identifying congenital abnormalities in infants. Esophagogastroduodenoscopy (EGD) with biopsy of the esophageal mucosa is indicated to further evaluate patients with GERD and recurrent abdominal pain, malabsorption, persistent vomiting, suspected erosive esophagitis, unexplained respiratory symptoms, or food allergies.[204-206] One should consider coupling these procedures with double fiberoptic airway bronchoscopy and bronchoalveolar lavage (BAL) under general anesthesia.[207] BAL can identify positive lipid-laden alveolar macrophages or neutrophilic inflammation. Children with medically refractory GERD or erosive esophagitis should be screened and (if indicated) treated for *Helicobacter pylori* infection, found in a third of such patients.[206,208]

Treating Gastroesophageal Reflux Disease in Children and Adolescents

Nonpharmacologic strategies to treat GERD can be effective. A 2-week trial of smaller, more frequent feedings with thickened formula, avoidance of supine sleep positions (if older than 6 months), and elimination of passive tobacco exposure significantly lessened symptoms of GERD in 59% of infants and normalized findings in 24%.[209] Modifying an infant's formula alone may reduce vomiting and irritability and improve quality of sleep in up to 25% of infants with GERD.[204,210] Using rice cereal to thicken an infant's formula decreases the volume and frequency of regurgitation but does not reduce esophageal acid exposure.[211] A prethickened formula with osmotic agents (Enfamil AR) significantly reduced GERD by the end of the first week and improved quality of sleep by 5 weeks in 104 infants with GERD.[210] A trial of a hypoallergenic infant formula may be useful because GERD apparently may be increased in some infants who are allergic to milk protein.[210,212] Passive tobacco exposure is a risk factor for esophagitis in infants and children.[213,214] And, adolescents who smoked tobacco had a 6.5 higher OR of reporting symptoms of GERD.[213] Nonpharmacologic strategies that may help lessen GERD in children and adolescents are listed in Box 41-2.

Pharmacologic treatments of GERD in children aim to increase the viscosity of the feedings or meals (by adding alginates); reduce gastric acid secretion and alter gastric pH (with antacids, histamine H_2 receptor antagonists [H_2 blockers], and PPIs); and improve gut motility (with prokinetic agents such as metoclopramide and domperidone).[215] H_2 blockers and, to a lesser extent, PPIs have been used extensively in infants and children with GERD and are considered safe.[215-221] Chronic antacid therapy is not recommended as treatment for children with GERD because it can lead to increased serum aluminum concentrations that could cause osteopenia and neurotoxicity.[200] Dosing guidelines, side effects, and efficacy

---

> **BOX 41-2** *Nonpharmacologic Treatment Strategies for Nocturnal Gastroesophageal Reflux Disease in Infants and Children*
>
> - Avoid eating 2 to 3 hours before bed
> - Provide frequent smaller meals
> - Elevate the head of the child's bed by 6 to 8 inches
> - Avoid caffeinated or carbonated beverages
> - Avoid foods containing acid, spice, or fats
> - Ensure daily physical exercise
> - Institute weight reduction measures (if patient is overweight)
> - Avoid passive or active exposure to tobacco

---

of drugs approved by the FDA for pediatric use are provided in Table 41-3.

Patients with chronic GERD refractory to medical treatments may require surgical procedures such as a Nissen fundoplication (whereby the upper part of the stomach is wrapped around the lower esophageal sphincter)[222] or insertion of a gastrojejunal feeding tube (to bypass the stomach); these two approaches have similar outcomes.[223,224] Young patients in particular with severe GERD or associated complications should be referred to a pediatric gastrointestinal specialist.

CYSTIC FIBROSIS

Cystic fibrosis (CF) is the most common inherited disease in patients of northern European heritage. CF is a chronic progressive disorder characterized by recurrent respiratory infections and gastrointestinal symptoms. Sleep in patients with CF is often fragmented, a finding attributed to nocturnal cough, hypoventilation, and hypoxemia.[225,226] Nocturnal coughing in CF patients is often maximal in the first hour of sleep, tends to be more severe in children with more advanced CF lung disease, and shows night-to-night variability.[227] Sixty-three percent of 123 children or young adults with CF complained that coughing always or sometimes interfered with their sleep. Although clinically significant OSA is present in less than 10% of young CF patients, a recent cross-sectional study of 63 CF children (aged 2-14 years) found that 56% had an obstructive apnea index at or above 1, and OSA was most common in those who had chronic rhinosinusitis, tonsillar hypertrophy, enlarged pharyngeal pillars, or specific orthodontic abnormalities (an overjet > 2 mm).[228]

Hypoxemia and hypercapnia are frequently present during sleep in patients with CF, especially during REM sleep.[229] Repeated episodes of nocturnal hypoxia can act as a stimulus for the development of pulmonary hypertension and right ventricular failure, complications that are associated with a poor prognosis in CF.[225] A prospective case-control study found 74% of 24 children with CF had excessive daytime sleepiness, 44% had difficulty falling asleep, 39% had trouble staying asleep, and 30% snored.[230] Overnight PSG confirmed reduced sleep efficiency, prolonged REM latency, and reduced percentage of REM sleep compared to age- and sex-matched healthy control subjects. Another study found 45 children with CF and stable pulmonary function also had significantly lower sleep efficiency compared to healthy control subjects.[231] Using multiple regression analyses, the authors found the

Pharmacologic Treatments for Gastroesophageal Reflux Approved by FDA for Oral Use in Infants and Children

Medication	Dose and Frequency	Common Side Effects	Treatment Role	Efficacy
HISTAMINE H_2 RECEPTOR AGONISTS (H_2RAS) THAT DECREASE GASTRIC ACID SECRETION				
Cimetidine	*Neonates:* 5-10 mg/kg/day divided q8-12h *Infants:* 10-20 mg/kg/day divided q6-12h *Children:* 20-40 mg/kg/day divided q6h	Headache, diarrhea, constipation, dizziness, muscle aches	Often first-line agent (8-12 weeks) for treatment of GERD in infants and children	Safe and effective in treating GERD in infants and children
Famotidine	*Infants < 3 mos old:* 0.5 mg/kg q24h; *Infants 3-12 months old:* 0.5 mg/kg q12h *Children (1-16 yrs):* 1mg/kg/day divided bid (80 mg/day max)			
Ranitidine	*Infants and Children (1 mo-16 yrs):* 5-10 mg/kg/day divided q12h			
PROTON PUMP INHIBITORS (PPIs)				
Omeprazole	10-20 kg: 0.7-3.5 mg/kg/day divided qd or bid; give before meals; available as oral suspension	Headache, diarrhea, abdominal pain, and constipation		
Lansoprazole	*Children < 30 kg:* 15 mg q24h *Children > 30 kg:* 30 mg q24h Capsules contents may be sprinkled on food or dissolved in apple juice			

FDA, U.S. Food and Drug Administration; *GERD,* gastroesophageal reflux disease.

FEV_1 values correlated positively with sleep duration and efficiency but negatively with the number and duration of nocturnal awakenings, age, and BMI. Other studies have shown that an FEV_1 of 64% or less predicted which children would have nocturnal hypoxemia (with 92% sensitivity but only 77% specificity),[232] and nocturnal hypoventilation with hypoxemia was also found to be more likely in CF patients whose resting Spo_2 (awake, sitting) was less than 94%.[233]

Sleep-Related Diagnostic and Treatment Strategies for Patients with Cystic Fibrosis

Diagnostic strategies for evaluating SDB in young CF patients begins with a comprehensive overnight PSG with carbon dioxide monitoring in those whose FEV_1 is 64% or less of predicted or who have a resting Spo_2 of less than 94%.[232,233] A single night of PSG will usually provide sufficient information to determine appropriate treatment of SDB in young patients.[234] The relevant treatment strategies include supplemental oxygen during sleep for sleep-related hypoxemia *unrelated* to either OSA or sleep-related hypoventilation,[235] BiPAP for those with nocturnal oxygen desaturation accompanied by sleep-related hypoventilation,[226] and AT or initiation of CPAP for those found to have significant OSA.[228] Supplemental oxygen during sleep may improve nocturnal symptoms in hypoxemic CF patients but does not improve long-term survival.[235] However, supplemental oxygen may lead to a worsening of sleep-related hypoventilation if present.[236-238]

Melatonin may be particularly beneficial for children with CF because of its antioxidant properties. Exogenous oral melatonin (3 mg or more) taken nightly for 3 weeks before bedtime was reported to improve sleep (and even reduce nitrite levels in exhaled breath condensates) in 20 older children with medically stable CF.[239] Complaints of sleep-disrupting coughing suggests the need to evaluate for nocturnal GERD and to manage CF respiratory disease aggressively.[227]

CHILDHOOD ATOPIC ECZEMA

Childhood atopic eczema (CAE), also known as *atopic dermatitis,* is a chronic skin condition characterized by pruritic red plaques that ooze when scratched. The dryness and itching of CAE may be associated with insomnia and sleep disruption.[240,241] CAE affects 5% to 20% of children in the United States and Britain and is associated with emotional distress, physical discomfort, reduced QoL, and sleeplessness.[240-242] Too often physicians underestimate the potential impact, but the effect on QoL of eczema in children is the same or greater than that observed in children with asthma or diabetes mellitus.[243]

Sixty percent of children with CAE report sleeplessness due to itching and soreness; this number increases to 83% during acute exacerbations.[244] The more scratching there is, the more likely are nighttime awakenings.[245] Frequent nocturnal awakenings (averaging 2.7 per night) were reported to occur in children with CAE when their eczema was flaring.[246] Sleep deprivation in CAE leads to daytime tiredness and impaired psychosocial and cognitive functioning, and it is more often reported during flares.[246] A recently published cross-sectional study of 13,318 children (ages 3-17 years) found ADHD was much more likely to be found in a child with CAE who specifically also had sleeping problems (OR 2.7).[247] Children with CAE also have an increased lifetime risks for asthma and allergic rhinitis.[248-253]

Children with an atopic parent are at greater risk for eczema, and exposure to certain environmental factors can modify the familial or genetic predispositions. Recent research has identified particular genotypes or gene mutations that increase the risk for CAE in an infant or child (filaggrin mutation,[254] CD14-159 C/T CC genotype, and IL-4Rα I75V single-nucleotide polymorphisms).[255] Infants or young children with genetic predispositions are far more likely to suffer CAE flares when exposed to a variety of allergens than CAE children without such predispositions.[254,256] Recent studies show that enhanced risk for CAE due to familial predisposition can be reduced by encouraging the use of hydrolyzed infant formulas[257] or breastfeeding for 4 months or more[258] and avoiding early exposure to dogs.[254,255]

Treating Chronic Atopic Eczema

Most patients with atopic eczema can be managed with emollients, moisturizers, and soap substitutes coupled with avoidance of environmental irritants.[259] Second-line treatments include elimination diets and topical corticosteroids or topical calcineurin inhibitors. Emollients are effective in healing the skin and preventing flares when applied daily in generous amounts over the entire body (500 g per week). Tar preparations are effective, but compliance is limited. Wet wrap dressings may be effective but increase the risk of skin infections.[260] Teaching caregivers about eczema[261] and about techniques for making their application of emollients "fun" for children can help.[262,263] It is important to encourage the child to assist in applying the skin creams.[262,263]

If emollients, moisturizers, and soap substitutes are not effective, other treatments for atopic eczema may be tried, including elimination diets and changes in infant formulas (to identify contributory food allergies),[260,264] topical antihistamines (to decrease itching),[265] topical corticosteroids,[266-268] topical calcineurin inhibitors,[266,269] and sublingual or subcutaneous immunotherapy.[270,271]

A strong association exists between atopic eczema and food allergy in infants: 90% of 51 infants (median age 34 weeks) with moderate atopic eczema seen in dermatology clinic were allergic to at least one food item (most often eggs, peanuts, or cow milk).[254] Choosing an extensively hydrolyzed casein formula in infancy can lessen the incidence of eczema in children as late as age 6 years, especially in those with a familial predisposition to allergy.[257] Given the likelihood of a food allergy in infants and young children, elimination diets should be tried, reintroducing one food at time.[260] Such screening in older children is less likely to be useful. Low zinc and copper levels are often found in children with CAE, but their significance is undetermined; nevertheless, supplementation is probably warranted.[272]

House dust mite (HDM) allergy, however, does play an important role in eczema in *older* children, and specific Immunoglobin E (IgE) assays for this allergy are available and should be conducted, particularly when the eczema is localized to exposed hands, feet, and neck. Pollen exposure may also exacerbate eczema, and therapy may need to be increased during hay fever season.[273] If the child fails to respond, search for an underlying immunodeficiency or chronic infection should be considered.[259] Also, environmental irritants should be identified and eliminated from the child's environment, and one should ensure that the treatments are being used as prescribed.[259] Sublingual immunotherapies have been shown to reduce symptoms and the need for other medications in CAE. A randomized, double-blind, placebo-controlled 18-month trial of sublingual immunotherapy in 56 CAE children sensitive to dust mites found this treatment effective in reducing symptoms in the children with mild to moderate (but not severe) disease.[271]

SLEEP DISORDERS IN CHILDREN WITH CANCER

Cancer occurs in 15 per 100,000 children.[274] Sleep problems are common in children with leukemia and brain tumors (cancers that account for approximately half of cancers in children).[275-281] Sleep problems in children with cancer vary and are often multifactorial.[282,283] Sleep, and respiratory patterns during sleep, may be impaired because of direct damage to the hypothalamus (the circadian pacemaker), the retinal hypothalamic tract (interrupting light input necessary to entrain circadian rhythms), and the brainstem respiratory control centers or cranial nerves (predisposing the child to obstructive or central sleep apnea). But sleep disorders in children with cancer may also be due to fear, sadness, depression, anxiety, worry, and nausea or other side effects of medication, chemotherapy, or radiotherapy. Still other factors, such as poor sleep/wake hygiene, exhausted parents reluctant to enforce appropriate limits, and disruption or regression of development, are often operative. The disruptive effects of pain on sleep in children with cancer are well known.[284-288]

Loss of undisturbed sleep and uninterrupted darkness may possibly contribute to cancer treatment failures, and improving the quality of nocturnal sleep in children with cancer may improve their response to cancer treatments.[289-293] Cancers are known to occur more frequently in blind individuals, shift workers, flight personnel, and Arctic residents; the common link between them, presumably, is disrupted coordination of their circadian rhythms for behavior, metabolism, endocrine function, and melatonin secretion, effects referred to by some as chronodisruption.[292,294] Sleep disturbances may lead to immune suppression and a shift to the predominance of cancer-stimulatory cytokines.[295]

The prevalence of insomnia is three times higher in patients undergoing cancer chemotherapy compared to the general population.[296] Rosen[275] and Rosen and Brand[282] found insomnia was the most common sleep complaint in children with leukemia referred to their pediatric sleep clinic, present in 39%. Medications (and medication schedules) also contribute to insomnia in children with cancer.[297-300] Corticosteroids, β-interferon, or asparaginase can be sedating, and cytarabine or vincristine cause either insomnia or sedation. Opiates may lead to daytime sedation and fatigue, cause respiratory depression, and exacerbate apnea during sleep.

Children with leukemia are often treated with monthly pulses of high-dose dexamethasone for 2.5 to 3 years, and a case series of children with leukemia treated with dexamethasone found that 56% complained of fatigue, 38% of insomnia, and 31% of hypersomnia.[277] Genes may influence which children with cancer are most susceptible to the effects of dexamethasone; thus, Vallance and associates[301] recently found that children on dexamethasone treatment, who had polymorphisms in three genes related to glucocorticoid metabolism (*AHSC, IL6, POLDIP3*) were most likely to experience sleep disruption.

Nocturnal sleep is often particularly disrupted in children with cancer during their frequent hospitalizations for cancer chemotherapy or procedures.[302,303] One study found that children with cancer receiving in-hospital chemotherapy had 20 or more awakenings per night.[303] In-hospital sleep for these children can be improved by treating their pain, creating a dark and quiet environment, and minimizing nocturnal interventions.[302,303]

Rosen and Brand[282] found excessive daytime sleepiness was the most common reason for referral to a pediatric sleep clinic in 70 children with cancer. This symptom was present in 60% of children with cancer and in 80% of children with CNS neoplasms involving the hypothalamus, thalamus, and brainstem. Children with brain tumors often had more than one sleep problem, most commonly excessive daytime sleepiness and SDB. SDB was found on overnight PSG in 40% overall and in 46% of those with brain tumors. Hypersomnia is very common in children receiving cranial radiation for brain tumors, leukemia, or lymphoma,[304] a condition often called the *radiation somnolence syndrome*.[304-309] It occurs in 40% to 71% of children treated with 2400 cGy cranial radiation, appearing 3 to 12 weeks after radiation and typically lasting 3 to 14 days.[305-307,310] Total sleep time increases both at night and during the day, and patients may become irritable with headaches, low-grade fevers, nausea, vomiting, decreased activity, dysphagia, and ataxia.[307] The radiation somnolence syndrome usually resolves spontaneously. Yet, Van Someren and colleagues[311] found that, 5 to 15 years following cranial radiation, 25 long-term survivors of childhood primary brain tumors had significantly longer sleep needs (8.7 hours vs. 7.7 hours in control subjects, confirmed by actigraphy), and were less tolerant of alterations in the timing of their sleep, than healthy control subjects.

Cancer-related fatigue (CRF) occurs in 70% to 80% of children or adolescents with cancer.[312-316] Often unrelenting, the CRF may prevent them from participating in physical, academic, and social activities, and effects may last for years following successful treatment.[317-319] Varying contributions of physical deconditioning, pain, poor nutrition, anemia, depression, anxiety, irregular sleep/wake schedules, poor sleep hygiene, opiate use, and organ system failure may contribute to it.[312-316] Neither rest nor sleep relieves CRF. CRF too often leads to the development or worsening of poor sleep hygiene (with excessive wake time spent in bed, and decreased daytime physical activity and light exposure), which may worsen the condition.[319-322]

Treatment strategies for CRF are summarized in Box 41-3.[283,314,323,324] Several recent studies examined the efficacy of modafinil for fatigue and attention problems in people with cancer.[325-328] A pilot study in adults found modafinil lessened CRF in 75% without adverse side effects.[329] A recently published multicenter double-blind, placebo-controlled trial of 631 adults with cancer found that 200 mg of modafinil significantly lessened CRF.[326] The use of modafinil to treat hypersomnia or CRF *in children* with cancer has not been studied. However, a small case series by Ivaneko and colleagues evaluated the efficacy and side effects of modafinil on 13 children (mean age 11 ± 5.3 years) with narcolepsy.[330] The mean dose was 346 ± 119 mg per day (available in 100- and 200-mg scored tablets). Modest lessening of excessive daytime sleepiness was observed. Exacerbation of seizures and psychotic reactions were observed in two children with preexisting conditions.

Craniopharyngiomas (CPs) are benign but locally aggressive neoplasms that most often present between ages 5 and 10 years and account for 9% of all pediatric brain tumors.[331] When CPs grow, they often encroach upon the hypothalamus, pituitary, and optic chiasm and then may cause narcolepsy-like symptoms, circadian dysrhythmicity, visual field deficits, insatiable appetite, rapid weight gain, obesity, hypersomnia, hypopituitarism, and headaches.[332-335] However, many of these symptoms develop or worsen after tumor resection and treatment. Reduced growth rates precede the diagnosis of CPs in children, whereas obesity more often develops after treatment.[336] Extreme obesity occurs in up to 40% after surgery.[337] Half of children and young adults remain obese following tumor resection primarily because of their inability to control their urge to eat, and hypersomnia persists in one third.[338] Insulin resistance may be the cause of their increased appetites.[339]

Subjective complaints of excessive daytime sleepiness were present in 30% of 115 childhood CP survivors.[333] Twenty-six percent of the cohort were obese, including 40% of those who complained of hypersomnia. Overnight PSG done on 10 obese sleepy patients revealed OSA in 2. Multiple sleep onset REM periods were observed on multiple sleep latency test (MSLT) in 4 of the 10 patients with obesity and hypersomnia, consistent with a diagnosis of secondary narcolepsy. Attempts to fully resect tumors involving the hypothalamus increased the likelihood of chronic hypersomnia, hyperphagia, and obesity,[340] whereas less extensive surgical resections led to more favorable long-term endocrine and quality of survival outcomes.[341-344]

Studies have found that CP survivors who become or remain excessively sleepy after treatment have low nocturnal serum melatonin levels,[338] and the melatonin levels correlated with BMI, obesity, and tumor involvement of the hypothalamus.[338] Chaotic circadian rhythms and hypersomnia in CP survivors may be helped by oral melatonin dosed nightly, strict sleep/wake schedules, weight management, and (if needed) adding CNS stimulants or wake-promoting agents during the day.[337,338,345-347] Bariatric surgery has been used to treat morbid obesity in survivors of CPs.[348]

Most sleep problems in children with cancer can be satisfactorily treated.[275,281] Treatments for insomnia in children with cancer begin with sleep hygiene and, if needed and appropriate, with sleep restriction, pain control, cognitive behavioral insomnia therapy, and sedative/hypnotics or melatonin.[282,283,322,349-352] The associated SDB, if present, is typically characterized by sleep-related hypoventilation with hypercapnia and hypoxemia, and can be treated by either BiPAP therapy (with a timed or backup rate, if necessary) or mechanical ventilation via a nasal mask or tracheotomy, in addition to the tumor therapy.[282]

CONGENITAL BLINDNESS

Light is the primary synchronizer of the endogenous circadian clock. More than half of blind individuals who completely lack light perception are unable to "entrain" their internal circadian clock, and their circadian rhythms *free run* on a cycle that is slightly longer than 24 hours. When their cycle slowly drifts later (usually about 30 minutes per day), their free-running rhythm passes out of phase with the desired time for sleep,

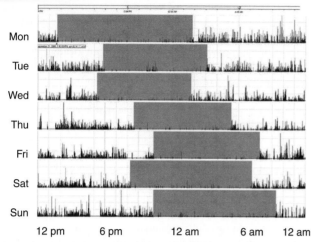

Figure 41-1 Actigraph of a congenitally blind adolescent with a free-running (non-24-hour) circadian rhythm disorder. More than half of blind individuals are unable to "entrain" their internal circadian clock; this failure allows their circadian clock to slowly drift later (usually about a half hour per day). As their free-rhythm passes out of phase with their desired time for sleep, nighttime insomnia and daytime sleepiness result. This 7-day actigraph tracing shows the characteristic progressive delay in sleep and wake times in an adolescent with congenital blindness and a non-24-hour, free-running circadian rhythm disorder. Grey areas are those with few movements and thus presumed sleep.

and nighttime insomnia and daytime sleepiness result. When desynchronized, blind individuals experience symptoms akin to jet lag (daytime sleepiness, early morning awakenings, poor night sleep, and reduced performance and alertness when awake). A non-24-hour free-running disorder is recognized by progressively delayed sleep times and periodic recurrent insomnia and is best diagnosed by having the patient or caregiver keep a 2- to 3-week record (sleep log or diary) of sleep/wake times coupled with actigraphy (Fig. 41-1).

Free-Running Sleep/Wake Disorder in Congenitally Blind Children

Treatment for a free-running (non-24-hour) sleep/wake disorder in blind persons begins by recommending regular bedtimes and awake times and absence of napping (for those past the age of napping). Low-dose oral melatonin (0.3-0.5 mg) taken 1 hour before the desired bedtime can help stabilize the endogenous melatonin, *phase-locking* the free-running rhythm to an approximately 24-hour period once it drifts to the desired bedtime.[353,354] Oral melatonin was effective in six of eight functionally blind intellectually disabled children and young adults with free-running disorders.[355] Some researchers advocate combination therapy using bright light exposure in the morning (for those children with some light perception) and melatonin at night; some also suggest adding vitamin B_{12} and hypnotics.[356-358]

IRON DEFICIENCY IN INFANCY

It is important to identify and aggressively treat iron deficiency with or without anemia in infants and children with excessive motor activity awake or asleep. Iron deficiency anemia (IDA) is the most common single nutrient deficiency, occurring in 20% to 25% of infants worldwide, with at least

as many having iron deficiency without anemia.[359] Sixty-nine percent of preschoolers and 35% of school-aged children had insufficient dietary iron intake. Iron deficiency in early life is associated with delayed development that persists to varying degrees after the iron deficiency has been satisfactorily treated.[360]

The peak period for IDA in children is 6 to 24 months, a crucial time for central nervous system development (including systems that control sleep). Impaired cognitive, emotional, and motor development in infants may result; the effects can linger even into adolescence despite correcting the deficiency.[359,361-368] A double-blind, controlled trial found that infants (aged 12-23 months) who were initially iron deficient had the lowest developmental scores 6 months following successful extended oral iron therapy.[369] Infant social-emotional behavior appears to be adversely affected by iron deficiency with or without anemia.[366] Infants with moderate to severe IDA were more wary, more fearful, less playful, and showed less pleasure than nonanemic infants.[368,369]

Short- and long-term changes in sleep architecture, sleep/wake patterns, and motor activity during sleep are seen in infants and toddlers with IDA.[359] Reduced numbers of sleep spindles (low spindle density), slower spindle frequencies (normally 14-16 Hz), and longer interspindle intervals were observed in infants with IDA at 6 months of age.[370] Six-month-old IDA infants also had (paradoxically) significantly *fewer* motor movements *awake* than did those without IDA, and the reduced motor activity awake was still present when they were retested at ages 12 and 18 months.[371] Iron-deficient infants were more restless when asleep, took longer daytime naps, and had more wake time at night and less nighttime NREM sleep than did control subjects.[372,373] Despite improvements in iron status with treatment, significant differences in sleep patterns persisted.[371] Risk factors for iron deficiency in infants and toddlers are summarized in Box 41-4.

Iron is an important cofactor in the metabolism of dopamine in the brain.[77] Ferritin (an iron-containing protein) carries iron across the blood-brain barrier. Dopamine plays important roles in regulating movement, motivation, cognition, sleep, and hormone release in the brain. Animal studies have shown that decreased availability of iron at crucial times in brain development leads to alterations in dopamine metabolism, myelination, and changes in dopamine-related behaviors, and some of these persist after repletion of brain iron stores.[360] Lower spontaneous eye blink rates (a noninvasive measure of dopamine function) were observed in 9- to 10-month-old iron-deficient infants compared with nonanemic control subjects (4.0 ± 1.9 vs. 5.3 ± 2.8 blinks per minute; $p = 0.02$).[364] After 12 months of iron therapy, the eye-blink rate had increased in the IDA infants by 2 beats per minute, but was unchanged in the nonanemic infants.

Iron deficiency may also contribute to symptoms of restless legs syndrome when awake, and to periodic limb movements, and excessive motor restlessness when sleeping. Cortese and associates[374] found that children with ADHD who had low serum ferritin levels (≤ 45 µg/L) were more likely reported to have sleep/wake transition disorders including abnormal movements during sleep. IDA and low serum ferritin levels have been found in as many as half of children with autism or Asperger syndrome.[374] An 8-week open-label pilot trial of oral iron supplementation in 33 children with autism spectrum disorder showed that restless sleep (present in 77% before treatment) improved significantly with iron repletion.[375] As opposed to enduring effects of iron deficiency on infants and toddlers, the clinical impact of IDA on older children and adolescents are reversed by iron repletion.

Infants, children, and adolescents with excessive motor restlessness or periodic limb movements when sleeping should be tested for iron depletion or deficiency by measuring serum ferritin, erythrocyte protoporphyrin, and hemoglobin levels. The earliest stage of iron deficiency in infants is evidenced by a low serum ferritin level of less than 10 µg/L (reflecting depletion of iron stores).[376] A transferrin saturation level of less than 10% reflects decreased iron transport (an intermediate stage of iron deficiency). A high erythrocyte protoporphyrin (≥ 35 µg/dL of whole blood) and a low hemoglobin (< 11 g/dL at sea level, < 10.7 g/dL for African-American infants) reflect decreased hemoglobin saturation. A low mean corpuscular volume less than 70 µm^3 is a late finding. Because a recent infection can depress hemoglobin in an infant, it is best to delay testing for 2 weeks in a recently ill infant or toddler.

Iron deficiency in an infant or toddler should be treated with oral elemental iron (3 mg/kg/day) once daily before breakfast (usually as ferrous sulfate syrup, which is 20% elemental iron).[376] Oral absorption of iron is improved by giving it with vitamin C (orange juice). Treat initially for 3 months, and check erythrocyte protoporphyrin and hemoglobin after the first month of treatment. Causes for iron deficiency and IDA should be explored.[377] Insufficient iron is the most common cause in children younger than 2 years, blood loss (gastrointestinal) in children 2 to 10 years, and menstrual loss in girls 10 years or older.[377] *Helicobacter pylori*-induced iron deficiency is most common in children 10 years or older.

Conclusion

Many medical disorders, particularly those present as chronic conditions, impair the restorative properties of sleep. These associated sleep disorders all too often go undiagnosed and undertreated and, in a reciprocal manner, may have a negative impact on these (and other) medical conditions. Chronically poor sleep quality, short sleep duration, and sleep-disordered breathing may predispose to the subsequent development of insulin resistance, systemic hypertension, metabolic syndrome, cancer, cardiovascular disorders, and fatty liver disease. Clinicians should search for complaints of disturbed sleep in children with chronic medical problems; treatment can potentially improve daytime functioning, behavior, academic performance, health, QoL, and longevity.

References

1. Bandla H, Splaingard M. Sleep problems in children with common medical disorders. *Pediatr Clin North Am.* 2004;51(1):203-227;viii.
2. Nixon GM, Thompson JM, Han DY, et al. Short sleep duration in middle childhood: Risk factors and consequences. *Sleep.* 2008;31(1):71-78.
3. Shi Z, Taylor AW, Gill TK, Tuckerman J, Adams R, Martin J. Short sleep duration and obesity among Australian children. *BMC Publ Health.* 2010;10:609.
4. Park S. Association between short sleep duration and obesity among South Korean adolescents. *West J Nurs Res.* 2011;33(2):207-223.
5. Taveras EM, Rifas-Shiman SL, Oken E, Gunderson EP, Gillman MW. Short sleep duration in infancy and risk of childhood overweight. *Arch Pediatr Adolesc Med.* 2008;162(4):305-311.
6. Beebe DW, Lewin D, Zeller M, et al. Sleep in overweight adolescents: Shorter sleep, poorer sleep quality, sleepiness, and sleep-disordered breathing. *J Pediatr Psychol.* 2007;32(1):69-79.
7. Tikotzky L, de Marcas G, Har-Toov J, Dollberg S, Bar-Haim Y, Sadeh A. Sleep and physical growth in infants during the first 6 months. *J Sleep Res.* 2010;19(1 Pt 1):103-110.
8. Seicean A, Redline S, Seicean S, et al. Association between short sleeping hours and overweight in adolescents: Results from a US suburban high school survey. *Sleep Breath.* 2007;11(4):285-293.
9. Flint J, Kothare SV, Zihlif M, et al. Association between inadequate sleep and insulin resistance in obese children. *J Pediatr.* 2007;150(4):364-369.
10. Javaheri S, Storfer-Isser A, Rosen CL, Redline S. Sleep quality and elevated blood pressure in adolescents. *Circulation.* 2008;118(10):1034-1040.
11. Taheri S, Lin L, Austin D, Young T, Mignot E. Short sleep duration is associated with reduced leptin, elevated ghrelin, and increased body mass index. *PLoS Med.* 2004;1(3):e62.
12. Li S, Zhu S, Jin X, et al. Risk factors associated with short sleep duration among Chinese school-aged children. *Sleep Med.* 2010;11(9):907-916.
13. Gruber R, Laviolette R, Deluca P, et al. Short sleep duration is associated with poor performance on IQ measures in healthy school-age children. *Sleep Med.* 2010;11(3):289-294.
14. Thorleifsdottir B, Bjornsson JK, Benediktsdottir B, et al. Sleep and sleep habits from childhood to young adulthood over a 10-year period. *J Psychosom Res.* 2002;53(1):529-537.
15. Iglowstein I, Jenni OG, Molinari L, Largo RH. Sleep duration from infancy to adolescence: Reference values and generational trends. *Pediatrics.* 2003;111(2):302-307.
16. Spruyt K, O'Brien LM, Cluydts R, Verleye GB, Ferri R. Odds, prevalence and predictors of sleep problems in school-age normal children. *J Sleep Res.* 2005;14(2):163-176.
17. Lemola S, Raikkonen K, Scheier MF, et al. Sleep quantity, quality and optimism in children. *J Sleep Res.* 2011;20(1 Pt 1):12-20.
18. McLaughlin Crabtree V, Williams NA. Normal sleep in children and adolescents. *Child Adolesc Psychiatr Clin North Am.* 2009;18(4):799-811.
19. Davis KF, Parker KP, Montgomery GL. Sleep in infants and young children: Part 1: Normal sleep. *J Pediatr Health Care.* 2004;18(2):65-71.
20. Quan SF, Goodwin JL, Babar SI, et al. Sleep architecture in normal Caucasian and Hispanic children aged 6-11 years recorded during unattended home polysomnography: Experience from the Tucson Children's Assessment of Sleep Apnea Study (TuCASA). *Sleep Med.* 2003;4(1):13-19.
21. Kahn A, Dan B, Groswasser J, Franco P, Sottiaux M. Normal sleep architecture in infants and children. *J Clin Neurophysiol.* 1996;13(3):184-197.
22. Iglowstein I, Latal Hajnal B, Molinari L, et al. Sleep behaviour in preterm children from birth to age 10 years: A longitudinal study. *Acta Paediatr.* 2006;95(12):1691-1693.
23. Grigg-Damberger M, Gozal D, Marcus CL, et al. The visual scoring of sleep and arousal in infants and children. *J Clin Sleep Med.* 2007;3(2):201-240.
24. Werner H, Lebourgeois MK, Geiger A, Jenni OG. Assessment of chronotype in four- to eleven-year-old children: Reliability and validity of the Children's Chronotype Questionnaire (CCTQ). *Chronobiol Int.* 2009;26(5):992-1014.
25. Hedley AA, Ogden CL, Johnson CL, et al. Prevalence of overweight and obesity among US children, adolescents, and adults, 1999-2002. *JAMA.* 2004;291:2847-2850.
26. Ogden CL, Carroll MD, Curtin LR, et al. Prevalence of overweight and obesity in the United States, 1999-2004. *JAMA.* 2006;295:1549-1555.
27. Ogden CL, Flegal KM, Carroll MD, Johnson CL. Prevalence and trends in overweight among US children and adolescents, 1999-2000. *JAMA.* 2002;288:1728-1732.

28. Xu Z, Jiaqing A, Yuchan L, Shen K. A case-control study of obstructive sleep apnea-hypopnea syndrome in obese and nonobese Chinese children. *Chest.* 2008;133(3):684-689.
29. Wing YK, Hui SH, Pak WM, et al. A controlled study of sleep related disordered breathing in obese children. *Arch Dis Child.* 2003;88(12):1043-1047.
30. Beebe DW, Lewin D, Zeller M, et al. Sleep in overweight adolescents: Shorter sleep, poorer sleep quality, sleepiness, and sleep-disordered breathing. *J Pediatr Psychol.* 2007;32:69-79.
31. Stepanski E, Zayyad A, Nigro C, Lopata M, Basner R. Sleep-disordered breathing in a predominantly African-American pediatric population. *J Sleep Res.* 1999;8(1):65-70.
32. Kohler M, Van den Heuvel C. Is there a clear link between overweight/obesity and sleep disordered breathing in children? *Sleep Med Rev.* 2008;12(5):347-361.
33. Redline S, Tishler P, Schluchter M, et al. Risk factors for sleep-disordered breathing in children. *Am J Respir Crit Care Med.* 1999;159:1527-1532.
34. Verhulst SL, Franckx H, Van Gaal L, De Backer WA, Desager KN. The effect of weight loss on sleep-disordered breathing in obese teenagers. *Obesity.* 2009;17:1178-1183.
35. Tauman R, O'Brien LM, Ivanenko A, Gozal D. Obesity rather than severity of sleep-disordered breathing as the major determinant of insulin resistance and altered lipidemia in snoring children. *Pediatrics.* 2005;116(1):e66-e73.
36. Marcus CL, Curtis S, Koerner CB, et al. Evaluation of pulmonary function and polysomnography in obese children and adolescents. *Pediatr Pulmonol.* 1996;21(3):176-183.
37. Gozal D, Kheirandish-Ghozal L. Obesity and excessive daytime sleepiness in prepubertal children with obstructive sleep apnea. *Pediatrics.* 2009;123(1):13-18.
38. Gozal D, Wang M, Pope Jr DW. Objective sleepiness measures in pediatric obstructive sleep apnea. *Pediatrics.* 2001;108(3):693-697.
39. Kalra M, Inge T, Garcia V, et al. Obstructive sleep apnea in extremely overweight adolescents undergoing bariatric surgery. *Obes Res.* 2005;13:1175-1179.
40. Chay OM, Goh A, Abisheganaden J, et al. Obstructive sleep apnea syndrome in obese Singapore children. *Pediatr Pulmonol.* 2000;29:284-290.
41. McKenzie SA, Bhattacharya A, Sureshkumar R, et al. Which obese children should have a sleep study? *Respir Med.* 2008;102(11):1581-1585.
42. Lam YY, Chan EYT, Ng DK, et al. The correlation among obesity, apnea-hypopnea index, and tonsil size in children. *Chest.* 2006;130:1751-1756.
43. Mitchell RB, Kelly J. Outcome of adenotonsillectomy for obstructive sleep apnea in obese and normal-weight children. *Otolaryngol Head Neck Surg.* 2007;137(1):43-48.
44. Morton S, Rosen C, Larkin E, Tishler P, Aylor J, Redline S. Predictors of sleep-disordered breathing in children with a history of tonsillectomy and/or adenoidectomy. *Sleep.* 2001;24(7):823-829.
45. O'Brien LM, Sitha S, Baur LA, Waters KA. Obesity increases the risk for persisting obstructive sleep apnea after treatment in children. *Int J Pediatr Otorhinolaryngol.* 2006;70(9):1555-1560.
46. Shine NP, Lannigan FJ, Coates HL, Wilson A. Adenotonsillectomy for obstructive sleep apnea in obese children: Effects on respiratory parameters and clinical outcome. *Arch Otolaryngol Head Neck Surg.* 2006;132(10):1123-1127.
47. Costa DJ, Mitchell R. Adenotonsillectomy for obstructive sleep apnea in obese children: A meta-analysis. *Otolaryngol Head Neck Surg.* 2009;140(4):455-460.
48. Reade EP, Whaley C, Lin JJ, et al. Hypopnea in pediatric patients with obesity hypertension. *Pediatr Nephrol.* 2004;19(9):1014-1020.
49. Leung LCK, Ng DK, Lau MW, et al. Twenty-four-hour ambulatory BP in snoring children with obstructive sleep apnea syndrome. *Chest.* 2006;130:1009-1017.
50. Marcus CL, Greene MG, Carroll JL. Blood pressure in children with obstructive sleep apnea. *Am J Respir Crit Care Med.* 1998;157(4 Pt 1):1098-1103.
51. Kheirandish-Ghozal L, Capdevila OS, Kheirandish E, Gozal D. Elevated serum aminotransferase levels in children at risk for obstructive sleep apnea. *Chest.* 2008;133:92-99.
52. Redline S, Storfer-Isser A, Rosen CL, et al. Association between metabolic syndrome and sleep-disordered breathing in adolescents. *Am J Respir Crit Care Med.* 2007;176(4):401-408.
53. Verhulst SL, Schrauwen N, Haentjens D, et al. Sleep-disordered breathing and the metabolic syndrome in overweight and obese children and adolescents. *J Pediatr.* 2007;150(6):608-612.
54. Leung LC, Ng DK, Lau MW, et al. Twenty-four-hour ambulatory BP in snoring children with obstructive sleep apnea syndrome. *Chest.* 2006;130(4):1009-1017.
55. Sorof JM, Poffenbarger T, Franco K, et al. Isolated systolic hypertension, obesity, and hyperkinetic hemodynamic states in children. *J Pediatr.* 2002;140(6):660-666.
56. Cook S, Weitzman M, Auinger P, et al. Prevalence of a metabolic syndrome phenotype in adolescents: Findings from the third National Health and Nutrition Examination Survey, 1988-1994. *Arch Pediatr Adolesc Med.* 2003;157(8):821-827.
57. Verhulst SL, Jacobs S, Aerts L, et al. Sleep-disordered breathing: A new risk factor of suspected fatty liver disease in overweight children and adolescents? *Sleep Breath.* 2009;13(2):207-210.
58. Steinbeck K. Childhood obesity. Treatment options. *Best Pract Res Clin Endocrinol Metab.* 2005;19(3):455-469.
59. Ford AL, Bergh C, Sodersten P, et al. Treatment of childhood obesity by retraining eating behaviour: Randomised controlled trial. *BMJ.* 2010;340:b5388.
60. Spivack JG, Bergh C, Sodersten P, et al. Primary care providers' knowledge, practices, and perceived barriers to the treatment and prevention of childhood obesity. *Obesity (Silver Spring).* 2010;18(7):1341-1347.
61. Hocevar SN, Key JD. Practice guidelines for the diagnosis, treatment and prevention of childhood and adolescent obesity. *J S C Med Assoc.* 2009;105(2):46-50.
62. Gronbaek HN, Madsen SA, Michaelsen KF. Family involvement in the treatment of childhood obesity: The Copenhagen approach. *Eur J Pediatr.* 2009;168(12):1437-1447.
63. Verhulst SL, Franckx H, Van Gaal L, De Backer W, Desager K. The effect of weight loss on sleep-disordered breathing in obese teenagers. *Obesity (Silver Spring).* 2009;17(6):1178-1183.
64. Kalra M, Inge T. Effect of bariatric surgery on obstructive sleep apnoea in adolescents. *Paediatr Respir Rev.* 2006;7(4):260-267.
65. Kalra M, Inge T, Garcia V, et al. Obstructive sleep apnea in extremely overweight adolescents undergoing bariatric surgery. *Obes Res.* 2005;13(7):1175-1179.
66. Scheuller M, Weider D. Bariatric surgery for treatment of sleep apnea syndrome in 15 morbidly obese patients: Long-term results. *Otolaryngol Head Neck Surg.* 2001;125(4):299-302.
67. Lurbe E, Alvarez J, Redon J. Diagnosis and treatment of hypertension in children. *Curr Hypertens Rep.* 2010;12(6):480-486.
68. National High Blood Pressure Education Program Working Group on High Blood Pressure in Children and Adolescents. The fourth report on the diagnosis, evaluation, and treatment of high blood pressure in children and adolescents. *Pediatrics.* 2004;114(2 Suppl):555-576.
69. Bixler EO, Vgontzas AN, Lin HM, et al. Blood pressure associated with sleep-disordered breathing in a population sample of children. *Hypertension.* 2008;52(5):841-846.
70. Amin R, Somers VK, McConnell K, et al. Activity-adjusted 24-hour ambulatory blood pressure and cardiac remodeling in children with sleep disordered breathing. *Hypertension.* 2008;51(1):84-91.
71. Srinivasan SR, Myers L, Berenson GS. Changes in metabolic syndrome variables since childhood in prehypertensive and hypertensive subjects: The Bogalusa Heart Study. *Hypertension.* 2006;48(1):33-39.
72. Sorof JM, Portman RJ. Ambulatory blood pressure measurements. *Curr Opin Pediatr.* 2001;13(2):133-137.
73. Simckes AM, Srivastava T, Alon US. Ambulatory blood pressure monitoring in children and adolescents. *Clin Pediatr (Phila).* 2002;41(8):549-564.
74. Lurbe E, Sorof JM, Daniels SR. Clinical and research aspects of ambulatory blood pressure monitoring in children. *J Pediatr.* 2004;144(1):7-16.
75. Flynn JT. Differentiation between primary and secondary hypertension in children using ambulatory blood pressure monitoring. *Pediatrics.* 2002;110(1 Pt 1):89-93.
76. Amin RS, Carroll JL, Jeffries JL, et al. Twenty-four-hour ambulatory blood pressure in children with sleep-disordered breathing. *Am J Respir Crit Care Med.* 2004;169(8):950-956.
77. Hermida RC, Ayala DE, Mojón A, Alonso I, Fernández JR. Reduction of morning blood pressure surge after treatment with nifedipine GITS at bedtime, but not upon awakening, in essential hypertension. *Blood Press Monit.* 2009;14(4):152-159.
78. Maurer VO, Rizzi M, Bianchetti MG, Ramelli GP. Benign neonatal sleep myoclonus: A review of the literature. *Pediatrics.* 2010;125(4):e919-e924.
79. Kaddurah AK, Holmes GL. Benign neonatal sleep myoclonus: History and semiology. *Pediatr Neurol.* 2009;40(5):343-346.

80. Paro-Panjan D, Neubauer D. Benign neonatal sleep myoclonus: Experience from the study of 38 infants. *Eur J Paediatr Neurol.* 2008;12(1):14-18.

81. Di Capua M, Fusco L, Ricci S, Vigevano F. Benign neonatal sleep myoclonus: Clinical features and video-polygraphic recordings. *Mov Disord.* 1993;8(2):191-194.

82. Alfonso I, Papazian O, Aicardi J, Jeffries HE. A simple maneuver to provoke benign neonatal sleep myoclonus. *Pediatrics.* 1995;96(6):1161-1163.

83. Coulter DL, Allen RJ. Benign neonatal sleep myoclonus. *Arch Neurol.* 1982;39(3):191-192.

84. Held-Egli K, Ruegger C, Das-Kundu S, Schmitt B, Bucher HU. Benign neonatal sleep myoclonus in newborn infants of opioid dependent mothers. *Acta Paediatr.* 2009;98(1):69-73.

85. Cohen R, Shuper A, Straussberg R. Familial benign neonatal sleep myoclonus. *Pediatr Neurol.* 2007;36(5):334-337.

86. Vaccario ML, Valenti MA, Carullo A, Di Bartolomeo R, Mazza S. Benign neonatal sleep myoclonus: Case report and follow-up of four members of an affected family. *Clin Electroencephalogr.* 2003;34(1):15-17.

87. Wessel MA, Cobb JC, Jackson EB, et al. Paroxysmal fussing in infancy, sometimes called colic. *Pediatrics.* 1954;14(5):421-435.

88. Wake M, Morton-Allen E, Poulakis Z, et al. Prevalence, stability, and outcomes of cry-fuss and sleep problems in the first 2 years of life: Prospective community-based study. *Pediatrics.* 2006;117(3):836-842.

89. Weissbluth M. Sleep and colic. In: Sheldon SH, Ferber R, Kryger MH, eds. *Principles and Practice of Pediatric Sleep Medicine.* Philadelphia: Elsevier Saunders; 2005:113-125.

90. Brazelton TB. Crying in infancy. *Pediatrics.* 1962;29:579-588.

91. Sadeh A, Sivan Y. Clinical practice: Sleep problems during infancy. *Eur J Pediatr.* 2009;168(10):1159-1164.

92. Zwart P, Vellema-Goud MG, Brand PL. Characteristics of infants admitted to hospital for persistent colic, and comparison with healthy infants. *Acta Paediatr.* 2007;96(3):401-405.

93. Weissbluth M, Weissbluth L. Colic, sleep inertia, melatonin and circannual rhythms. *Med Hypotheses.* 1992;38(3):224-228.

94. Savino F, Tarasco V. New treatments for infant colic. *Curr Opin Pediatr.* 2010;22(6):791-797.

95. Dupont C, Rivero M, Grillon C, et al. Alpha-lactalbumin-enriched and probiotic-supplemented infant formula in infants with colic: Growth and gastrointestinal tolerance. *Eur J Clin Nutr.* 2010;64(7):765-767.

96. Yalcin SS, Orun E, Mutlu B, et al. Why are they having infant colic? A nested case-control study. *Paediatr Perinat Epidemiol.* 2010;24(6):584-596.

97. Blom MA, van Sleuwen BE, de Vries H, et al. Health care interventions for excessive crying in infants: Regularity with and without swaddling. *J Child Health Care.* 2009;13(2):161-176.

98. Underdown A, Barlow J, Chung V, Stewart-Brown S. Massage intervention for promoting mental and physical health in infants aged under six months. *Cochrane Database Syst Rev.* 2006;(4):CD005038.

99. Don N, McMahon C, Rossiter C. Effectiveness of an individualized multidisciplinary programme for managing unsettled infants. *J Paediatr Child Health.* 2002;38(6):563-567.

100. Newnham CA, Milgrom J, Skouteris H. Effectiveness of a modified mother-infant transaction program on outcomes for preterm infants from 3 to 24 months of age. *Infant Behav Dev.* 2009;32(1):17-26.

101. American Lung Association. *Research and Program Services. Trends in Asthma Morbidity and Mortality.* Washington, DC: American Lung Association; November 2007.

102. Akinbami LJ. *The State of Childhood Asthma, United States, 1980–2005. Advance Data from Vital and Health Statistics.* Hyattsville, MD: National Center for Health Statistics; 2005.

103. Brim SN, Rudd RA, Funk RH, Callahan DB. Asthma prevalence among US children in underrepresented minority populations: American Indian/Alaska Native, Chinese, Filipino, and Asian Indian. *Pediatrics.* 2008;122(1):e217-e222.

104. Skloot GS. Nocturnal asthma: Mechanisms and management. *Mt Sinai J Med.* 2002;69(3):140-147.

105. Chugh IM, Khanna P, Shah A. Nocturnal symptoms and sleep disturbances in clinically stable asthmatic children. *Asian Pac J Allergy Immunol.* 2006;24(2-3):135-142.

106. Strunk RC, Sternberg AL, Bacharier LB, Szefler SJ. Nocturnal awakening caused by asthma in children with mild-to-moderate asthma in the childhood asthma management program. *J Allergy Clin Immunol.* 2002;110(3):395-403.

107. Kieckhefer GM, Ward TM, Tsai SY, Lentz MJ. Nighttime sleep and daytime nap patterns in school age children with and without asthma. *J Dev Behav Pediatr.* 2008;29(5):338-344.

108. Sadeh A, Horowitz I, Wolach-Benodis L, Wolach B. Sleep and pulmonary function in children with well-controlled, stable asthma. *Sleep.* 1998;21(4):379-384.

109. Horn CR, Clark TJ, Cochrane GM. Is there a circadian variation in respiratory morbidity? *Br J Dis Chest.* 1987;81(3):248-251.

110. Douglas NJ. Asthma at night. *Clin Chest Med.* 1985;6(4):663-674.

111. Lanier BQ, Nayak A. Prevalence and impact of nighttime symptoms in adults and children with asthma: A survey. *Postgrad Med.* 2008;120(4):58-66.

112. Braido F, Baiardini I, Ghiglione V, et al. Sleep disturbances and asthma control: A real life study. *Asian Pac J Allergy Immunol.* 2009;27(1):27-33.

113. Sulit LG, Storfer-Isser A, Rosen CL, Kirchner HL, Redline S. Associations of obesity, sleep-disordered breathing, and wheezing in children. *Am J Respir Crit Care Med.* 2005;171(6):659-664.

114. Chu YT, Chen WY, Wang TN, et al. Extreme BMI predicts higher asthma prevalence and is associated with lung function impairment in school-aged children. *Pediatr Pulmonol.* 2009;44(5):472-479.

115. Kang SK, Kim JK, Ahn SH, et al. Relationship between silent gastroesophageal reflux and food sensitization in infants and young children with recurrent wheezing. *J Korean Med Sci.* 2010;25(3):425-428.

116. Weersink EJ, Douma RR, Postma DS, Koeter GH. Fluticasone propionate, salmeterol xinafoate, and their combination in the treatment of nocturnal asthma. *Am J Respir Crit Care Med.* 1997;155(4):1241-1246.

117. Esposito-Festen J, Ijsselstijn H, Hop W, et al. Aerosol therapy by pressured metered-dose inhaler-spacer in sleeping young children: To do or not to do? *Chest.* 2006;130(2):487-492.

118. Ponsonby AL, Dwyer T, Trevillian L, et al. The bedding environment, sleep position, and frequent wheeze in childhood. *Pediatrics.* 2004;113(5):1216-1222.

119. Garner R, Kohen D. Changes in the prevalence of asthma among Canadian children. *Health Rep.* 2008;19(2):45-50.

120. Wong GW, Leung TF, Ma Y, et al. Symptoms of asthma and atopic disorders in preschool children: Prevalence and risk factors. *Clin Exp Allergy.* 2007;37(2):174-179.

121. Carter ER, Debley JS, Redding GR. Chronic productive cough in school children: Prevalence and associations with asthma and environmental tobacco smoke exposure. *Cough.* 2006;2:11.

122. Hacker DW, Sparrow EM. Use of air-cleaning devices to create airborne particle-free spaces intended to alleviate allergic rhinitis and asthma during sleep. *Indoor Air.* 2005;15(6):420-431.

123. Morris RJ, Helm TJ, Schmid W, Hacker D. A novel air filtration delivery system improves seasonal allergic rhinitis. *Allergy Asthma Proc.* 2006;27(1):63-67.

124. Magzamen S, Patel B, Davis A, Edelstein J, Tager IB. Kickin' asthma: School-based asthma education in an urban community. *J School Health.* 2008;78(12):655-665.

125. Smolensky MH, Lemmer B, Reinberg AE. Chronobiology and chronotherapy of allergic rhinitis and bronchial asthma. *Adv Drug Deliv Rev.* 2007;59(9-10):852-882.

126. Masuda S, Fujisawa T, Katsumata H, et al. High prevalence and young onset of allergic rhinitis in children with bronchial asthma. *Pediatr Allergy Immunol.* 2008;19(6):517-522.

127. Sih T, Mion O. Allergic rhinitis in the child and associated comorbidities. *Pediatr Allergy Immunol.* 2010;21(1):E107-E113.

128. Meltzer EO, Nathan R, Derebery J, et al. Sleep, quality of life, and productivity impact of nasal symptoms in the United States: Findings from the Burden of Rhinitis in America survey. *Allergy Asthma Proc.* 2009;30(3):244-254.

129. Muliol J, Maurer M, Bousquet J. Sleep and allergic rhinitis. *J Investig Allergol Clin Immunol.* 2008;18(6):415-419.

130. Turner PJ, Kemp AS. Allergic rhinitis in children. *J Paediatr Child Health.* 2010;Jun 27 [Epub ahead of print].

131. Weinstein S, Qaqundah P, Georges G, Nayak A. Efficacy and safety of triamcinolone acetonide aqueous nasal spray in children aged 2 to 5 years with perennial allergic rhinitis: A randomized, double-blind, placebo-controlled study with an open-label extension. *Ann Allergy Asthma Immunol.* 2009;102(4):339-347.

132. Georgalas C, Thomas K, Owens C, Abramovich S, Lack G. Medical treatment for rhinosinusitis associated with adenoidal hypertrophy in children: An evaluation of clinical response and changes on magnetic resonance imaging. *Ann Otol Rhinol Laryngol.* 2005;114(8):638-644.

133. Berlucchi M, Valetti L, Parrinello G, Nicolai P. Long-term follow-up of children undergoing topical intranasal steroid therapy for adenoidal hypertrophy. *Int J Pediatr Otorhinolaryngol.* 2008;72(8):1171-1175.

134. Yonekura S, Okamoto Y, Sakurai D, et al. Sublingual immunotherapy with house dust extract for house dust-mite allergic rhinitis in children. *Allergol Int.* 2010;59(4):381-388.

135. Storms W. Allergic rhinitis-induced nasal congestion: Its impact on sleep quality. *Prim Care Respir J.* 2008;17(1):7-18.

136. Lanier BQ. Use of intranasal corticosteroids in the management of congestion and sleep disturbance in pediatric patients with allergic rhinitis. *Clin Pediatr (Phila).* 2008;47(5):435-445.

137. Davies MJ, Fisher LH, Chegini S, Craig TJ. A practical approach to allergic rhinitis and sleep disturbance management. *Allergy Asthma Proc.* 2006;27(3):224-230.

138. Brouillette RT, Manoukian JJ, Ducharme FM, et al. Efficacy of fluticasone nasal spray for pediatric obstructive sleep apnea. *J Pediatr.* 2001;138(6):838-844.

139. Kheirandish-Gozal L, Gozal D. Intranasal budesonide treatment for children with mild obstructive sleep apnea syndrome. *Pediatrics.* 2008;122(1):e149-e155.

140. Santos CB, Hanks C, McCann J, et al. The role of montelukast on perennial allergic rhinitis and associated sleep disturbances and daytime somnolence. *Allergy Asthma Proc.* 2008;29(2):140-145.

141. Goldbart AD, Goldman JL, Veling MC, Gozal D. Leukotriene modifier therapy for mild sleep-disordered breathing in children. *Am J Respir Crit Care Med.* 2005;172(3):364-370.

142. Kheirandish L, Goldbart AD, Gozal D. Intranasal steroids and oral leukotriene modifier therapy in residual sleep-disordered breathing after tonsillectomy and adenoidectomy in children. *Pediatrics.* 2006;117(1):e61-e66.

143. Frenette PS, Atweh GF. Sickle cell disease: Old discoveries, new concepts, and future promise. *J Clin Invest.* 2007;117(4):850-858.

144. Roseff SD. Sickle cell disease: A review. *Immunohematology.* 2009;25(2):67-74.

145. Bender MA, Hobbs W. Sickle cell disease (Updated 2009 August 6). *GeneRev.* Accessed July 10, 2011. Last Revision: September 17, 2009. http://www.ncbi.nlm.nih.gov/books/NBK1377/. Bookshelf ID: NBK1377 PMID: HYPERLINK "/pubmed/20301551"20301551.

146. Jacob E, Miaskowski C, Savedra M, et al. Changes in sleep, food intake, and activity levels during acute painful episodes in children with sickle cell disease. *J Pediatr Nurs.* 2006;21(1):23-34.

147. Daniel LC, Grant M, Kothare SV, Dampier C, Barakat LP. Sleep patterns in pediatric sickle cell disease. *Pediatr Blood Cancer.* 2010;55(3):501-507.

148. Caboot JB, Allen JL. Pulmonary complications of sickle cell disease in children. *Curr Opin Pediatr.* 2008;20(3):279-287.

149. Ajulo SO. The significance of recurrent tonsillitis in sickle cell disease. *Clin Otolaryngol Allied Sci.* 1994;19(3):230-233.

150. Wittig RM, Roth T, Keenum AJ, Sarnaik S. Snoring, daytime sleepiness, and sickle cell anemia. *Am J Dis Child.* 1988;142(6):589.

151. Salles C, Ramos RT, Daltro C, et al. Association between adenotonsillar hypertrophy, tonsillitis and painful crises in sickle cell disease. *J Pediatr (Rio J).* 2009;85(3):249-253.

152. Souza LC, Viegas CA. Quality of sleep and pulmonary function in clinically stable adolescents with sickle cell anemia. *J Bras Pneumol.* 2007;33(3):275-281.

153. Hargrave DR, Wade A, Evans JP, Hewes DK, Kirkham FJ. Nocturnal oxygen saturation and painful sickle cell crises in children. *Blood.* 2003;101(3):846-848.

154. Kaleyias J, Mostofi N, Grant M, et al. Severity of obstructive sleep apnea in children with sickle cell disease. *J Pediatr Hematol Oncol.* 2008;30(9):659-665.

155. Raj AB, O'Brien LM, Bertolone SJ, et al. Cerebral oximetry improves detection of sickle cell patients at risk for nocturnal cerebral hypoxia. *Pediatr Pulmonol.* 2006;41(11):1088-1094.

156. Setty BN, Stuart MJ, Dampier C, Brodecki D, Allen JL. Hypoxaemia in sickle cell disease: Biomarker modulation and relevance to pathophysiology. *Lancet.* 2003;362(9394):1450-1455.

157. Spivey JF, Uong EC, Strunk R, et al. Low daytime pulse oximetry reading is associated with nocturnal desaturation and obstructive sleep apnea in children with sickle cell anemia. *Pediatr Blood Cancer.* 2008;50(2):359-362.

158. Samuels M, Stebbens VA, Davies SC, et al. Sleep related upper airway obstruction and hypoxaemia in sickle cell disease. *Arch Dis Child.* 1992;67:925-929.

159. Hargrave DR, Wade A, Evans JPM, Hewes DKM, Kirkham FJ. Nocturnal oxygen saturation and painful sickle cell crises in children. *Blood.* 2003;101(3):846-848.

160. Raj AB, O'Brien LM, Bertolone SJ, et al. Cerebral oximetry improves detection of sickle cell patients at risk for nocturnal cerebral hypoxia. *Pediatr Pulmonol.* 2006;41:1088-1094.

161. Kirkham FJ, Hewes DKM, Prengler M, Wade A, Lane R, Evans JPM. Nocturnal hypoxaemia and central-nervous-system events in sickle-cell disease. *Lancet.* 2001;357:1656-1659.

162. Wang WC. The pathophysiology, prevention, and treatment of stroke in sickle cell disease. *Curr Opin Hematol.* 2007;14(3):191-197.

163. Wang WC. Central nervous system complications of sickle cell disease in children: An overview. *Child Neuropsychol.* 2007;13(2):103-119.

164. Kwiatkowski JL, Zimmerman RA, Pollock AN, et al. Silent infarcts in young children with sickle cell disease. *Br J Haematol.* 2009;146(3):300-305.

165. Day S, Chismark E. The cognitive and academic impact of sickle cell disease. *J School Nurs.* 2006;22(6):330-335.

166. King AA, DeBaun MR, White DA. Need for cognitive rehabilitation for children with sickle cell disease and strokes. *Expert Rev Neurother.* 2008;8(2):291-296.

167. Schatz J, Buzan R. Decreased corpus callosum size in sickle cell disease: Relationship with cerebral infarcts and cognitive functioning. *J Int Neuropsychol Soc.* 2006;12(1):24-33.

168. Steen RG, Fineberg-Buchner C, Hankins G, et al. Cognitive deficits in children with sickle cell disease. *J Child Neurol.* 2005;20(2):102-107.

169. Steen RG, Miles MA, Helton KJ, et al. Cognitive impairment in children with hemoglobin SS sickle cell disease: Relationship to MR imaging findings and hematocrit. *AJNR Am J Neuroradiol.* 2003;24(3):382-389.

170. Kirkham FJ, Hewes DK, Prengler M, et al. Nocturnal hypoxaemia and central-nervous-system events in sickle-cell disease. *Lancet.* 2001;357(9269):1656-1659.

171. Halvorson DJ, McKie V, McKie K, Ashmore PE, Porubsky ES. Sickle cell disease and tonsillectomy. Preoperative management and postoperative complications. *Arch Otolaryngol Head Neck Surg.* 1997;123(7):689-692.

172. Marshall MJ, Bucks RS, Hogan AM, et al. Auto-adjusting positive airway pressure in children with sickle cell anemia: Results of a phase I randomized controlled trial. *Haematologica.* 2009;94(7):1006-1010.

173. Valrie CR, Gil KM, Redding-Lallinger R, Daeschner C. Brief report: Sleep in children with sickle cell disease: An analysis of daily diaries utilizing multilevel models. *J Pediatr Psychol.* 2007;32(7):857-861.

174. Valrie CR, Gil KM, Redding-Lallinger R, Daeschner C. Daily mood as a mediator or moderator of the pain-sleep relationship in children with sickle cell disease. *J Pediatr Psychol.* 2008;33(3):317-322.

175. Enninful-Eghan H, Moore RH, Ichord R, Smith-Whitley K, Kwiatkowski JL. Transcranial Doppler ultrasonography and prophylactic transfusion program is effective in preventing overt stroke in children with sickle cell disease. *J Pediatr.* 2010;157(3):479-484.

176. Suliman H, Wali Y, Al Saadoon M, et al. Hydroxyurea or chronic exchange transfusions in patients with sickle cell disease: Role of transcranial Doppler ultrasound in stroke prophylaxis. *J Pediatr Hematol Oncol.* 2009;31(1):42-44.

177. Mazumdar M, Heeney MM, Sox CM, Lieu TA. Preventing stroke among children with sickle cell anemia: An analysis of strategies that involve transcranial Doppler testing and chronic transfusion. *Pediatrics.* 2007;120(4):e1107-e1116.

178. Heeney MM, Ware RE. Hydroxyurea for children with sickle cell disease. *Hematol Oncol Clin North Am.* 2010;24(1):199-214.

179. Thornburg CD, Dixon N, Burgett S, et al. A pilot study of hydroxyurea to prevent chronic organ damage in young children with sickle cell anemia. *Pediatr Blood Cancer.* 2009;52(5):609-615.

180. Strouse JJ, Lanzkron S, Beach MC, et al. Hydroxyurea for sickle cell disease: A systematic review for efficacy and toxicity in children. *Pediatrics.* 2008;122(6):1332-1342.

181. Hankins JS, Helton KJ, McCarville MB, et al. Preservation of spleen and brain function in children with sickle cell anemia treated with hydroxyurea. *Pediatr Blood Cancer.* 2008;50(2):293-297.

182. Zimmerman SA, Schultz WH, Burgett S, et al. Hydroxyurea therapy lowers transcranial Doppler flow velocities in children with sickle cell anemia. *Blood.* 2007;110(3):1043-1047.

183. Kratovil T, Bulas D, Driscoll MC, et al. Hydroxyurea therapy lowers TCD velocities in children with sickle cell disease. *Pediatr Blood Cancer.* 2006;47(7):894-900.

184. Puffer E, Schatz J, Roberts CW. The association of oral hydroxyurea therapy with improved cognitive functioning in sickle cell disease. *Child Neuropsychol.* 2007;13(2):142-154.

185. Ballas SK, Bauserman RL, McCarthy WF, et al. Hydroxyurea and acute painful crises in sickle cell anemia: Effects on hospital length of stay and opioid utilization during hospitalization, outpatient acute care contacts, and at home. *J Pain Symptom Manage.* 2010;40(6):870-882.

186. Wiles N, Howard J. Role of hydroxycarbamide in prevention of complications in patients with sickle cell disease. *Ther Clin Risk Manag.* 2009;5:745-755.

187. Kumhaek C, Taylor JGt Zhu J, et al. Fetal haemoglobin response to hydroxycarbamide treatment and sar1a promoter polymorphisms in sickle cell anaemia. *Br J Haematol.* 2008;141(2):254-259.

188. Thakkar K, Boatright RO, Gilger MA, El-Serag HB. Gastroesophageal reflux and asthma in children: A systematic review. *Pediatrics.* 2010;125(4):e925-e930.

189. Pashankar DS, Corbin Z, Shah SK, Caprio S. Increased prevalence of gastroesophageal reflux symptoms in obese children evaluated in an academic medical center. *J Clin Gastroenterol.* 2009;43(5):410-413.

190. Ruigomez A, Wallander MA, Lundborg P, Johansson S, Rodriguez LA. Gastroesophageal reflux disease in children and adolescents in primary care. *Scand J Gastroenterol.* 2010;45(2):139-146.

191. Bibi H, Khvolis E, Shoseyov D, et al. The prevalence of gastroesophageal reflux in children with tracheomalacia and laryngomalacia. *Chest.* 2001;119(2):409-413.

192. Marlais M, Fishman JR, Koglmeier J, Fell JM, Rawat DJ. Reduced quality of life in children with gastro-oesophageal reflux disease. *Acta Paediatr.* 2010;99(3):418-421.

193. Moore JG. Circadian dynamics of gastric acid secretion and pharmacodynamics of H_2 receptor blockade. *Ann N Y Acad Sci.* 1991;618:150-158.

194. Kanaly T, Shaheen NJ, Vaughn BV. Gastrointestinal physiology and digestive disorders in sleep. *Curr Opin Pulm Med.* 2009;Sep 30 [Epub ahead of print].

195. Johnson LF, Demeester TR, Haggitt RC. Esophageal epithelial response to gastroesophageal reflux. A quantitative study. *Am J Dig Dis.* 1978;23(6):498-509.

196. Colletti RB, Christie DL, Orenstein SR. Statement of the North American Society for Pediatric Gastroenterology and Nutrition (NASPGN). Indications for pediatric esophageal pH monitoring. *J Pediatr Gastroenterol Nutr.* 1995;21(3):253-262.

197. Greenfeld M, Tauman R, Sivan Y. The yield of esophageal pH monitoring during polysomnography in infants with sleep-disordered breathing. *Clin Pediatr (Phila).* 2004;43(7):653-658.

198. Harris P, Munoz C, Mobarec S, Brockmann P, Mesa T, Sanchez I. Relevance of the pH probe in sleep study analysis in infants. *Child Care Health Dev.* 2004;30(4):337-344.

199. Rosen CL, Frost Jr JD, Harrison GM. Infant apnea: Polygraphic studies and follow-up monitoring. *Pediatrics.* 1983;71(5):731-736.

200. Tirosh E, Jaffe M. Apnea of infancy, seizures, and gastroesophageal reflux: An important but infrequent association. *J Child Neurol.* 1996;11(2):98-100.

201. Arad-Cohen N, Cohen A, Tirosh E. The relationship between gastroesophageal reflux and apnea in infants. *J Pediatr.* 2000;137:321-326.

202. Groswasser J, Scaillon M, Rebuffat E, et al. Naso-oesophageal probes decrease the frequency of sleep apnoeas in infants. *J Sleep Res.* 2000;9(2):193-196.

203. Francavilla R, Magista AM, Bucci N, et al. Comparison of esophageal pH and multichannel intraluminal impedance testing in pediatric patients with suspected gastroesophageal reflux. *J Pediatr Gastroenterol Nutr.* 2010;50(2):154-160.

204. Rudolph CD, Mazur LJ, Liptak GS, et al. Guidelines for evaluation and treatment of gastroesophageal reflux in infants and children: Recommendations of the North American Society for Pediatric Gastroenterology and Nutrition. *J Pediatr Gastroenterol Nutr.* 2001;32(Suppl 2):S1-S31.

205. Semeniuk J, Kaczmarski M, Uscinowicz M, Sobaniec-Lotowska M. Histological evaluation of esophageal mucosa in children with acid gastroesophageal reflux. *Folia Histochem Cytobiol.* 2009;47(2):297-306.

206. Moon A, Solomon A, Beneck D, Cunningham-Rundles S. Positive association between *Helicobacter pylori* and gastroesophageal reflux disease in children. *J Pediatr Gastroenterol Nutr.* 2009;49(3):283-288.

207. Ullmann N, Sacco O, Gandullia P, et al. Usefulness and safety of double endoscopy in children with gastroesophageal reflux and respiratory symptoms. *Respir Med.* 2010;104(4):593-599.

208. Emiroglu HH, Sokucu S, Suoglu OD, Gulluoglu M, Gokce S. Is there a relationship between *Helicobacter pylori* infection and erosive reflux disease in children? *Acta Paediatr.* 2010;99(1):121-125.

209. Orenstein SR, McGowan JD. Efficacy of conservative therapy as taught in the primary care setting for symptoms suggesting infant gastroesophageal reflux. *J Pediatr.* 2008;152(3):310-314.

210. Vanderhoof JA, Moran JR, Harris CL, Merkel KL, Orenstein SR. Efficacy of a pre-thickened infant formula: A multicenter, double-blind, randomized, placebo-controlled parallel group trial in 104 infants with symptomatic gastroesophageal reflux. *Clin Pediatr (Phila).* 2003;42(6):483-495.

211. Orenstein SR, Magill HL, Brooks P. Thickening of infant feedings for therapy of gastroesophageal reflux. *J Pediatr.* 1987;110(2):181-186.

212. Orenstein SR, Shalaby TM, Di Lorenzo C, et al. The spectrum of pediatric eosinophilic esophagitis beyond infancy: A clinical series of 30 children. *Am J Gastroenterol.* 2000;95(6):1422-1430.

213. Nelson SP, Chen EH, Syniar GM, Christoffel KK. Prevalence of symptoms of gastroesophageal reflux during childhood: A pediatric practice-based survey. Pediatric Practice Research Group. *Arch Pediatr Adolesc Med.* 2000;154(2):150-154.

214. Shabib SM, Cutz E, Sherman PM. Passive smoking is a risk factor for esophagitis in children. *J Pediatr.* 1995;127(3):435-437.

215. Tighe MP, Afzal NA, Bevan A, Beattie RM. Current pharmacological management of gastro-esophageal reflux in children: An evidence-based systematic review. *Paediatr Drugs.* 2009;11(3):185-202.

216. Tafuri G, Trotta F, Leufkens HG, et al. Off-label use of medicines in children: Can available evidence avoid useless paediatric trials? The case of proton pump inhibitors for the treatment of gastroesophageal reflux disease. *Eur J Clin Pharmacol.* 2009;65(2):209-216.

217. Sopo SM, Radzik D, Calvani M. Does treatment with proton pump inhibitors for gastroesophageal reflux disease (GERD) improve asthma symptoms in children with asthma and GERD? A systematic review. *J Investig Allergol Clin Immunol.* 2009;19(1):1-5.

218. Orenstein SR, Hassall E. Infants and proton pump inhibitors: Tribulations, no trials. *J Pediatr Gastroenterol Nutr.* 2007;45(4):395-398.

219. Gold BD, Freston JW. Gastroesophageal reflux in children: Pathogenesis, prevalence, diagnosis, and role of proton pump inhibitors in treatment. *Paediatr Drugs.* 2002;4(10):673-685.

220. Ward RM, Tammara B, Sullivan SE, et al. Single-dose, multiple-dose, and population pharmacokinetics of pantoprazole in neonates and preterm infants with a clinical diagnosis of gastroesophageal reflux disease (GERD). *Eur J Clin Pharmacol.* 2010;66(6):555-561.

221. Kierkus J, Furmaga-Jablonska W, Sullivan JE, et al. Pharmacodynamics and safety of pantoprazole in neonates, preterm infants, and infants aged 1 through 11 months with a clinical diagnosis of gastroesophageal reflux disease. *Dig Dis Sci.* 2011;56(2):425-434.

222. Frankel EA, Shalaby TM, Orenstein SR. Sandifer syndrome posturing: Relation to abdominal wall contractions, gastroesophageal reflux, and fundoplication. *Dig Dis Sci.* 2006;51(4):635-640.

223. Srivastava R, Berry JG, Hall M, et al. Reflux related hospital admissions after fundoplication in children with neurological impairment: Retrospective cohort study. *BMJ.* 2009;339:b4411.

224. Srivastava R, Downey EC, O'Gorman M, et al. Impact of fundoplication versus gastrojejunal feeding tubes on mortality and in preventing aspiration pneumonia in young children with neurologic impairment who have gastroesophageal reflux disease. *Pediatrics.* 2009;123(1):338-345.

225. Milross MA, Piper AJ, Dobbin CJ, Bye PT, Grunstein RR. Sleep disordered breathing in cystic fibrosis. *Sleep Med Rev.* 2004;8(4):295-308.

226. Yue HJ, Conrad D, Dimsdale JE. Sleep disruption in cystic fibrosis. *Med Hypotheses.* 2008;71(6):886-888.

227. van der Giessen L, Loeve M, de Jongste J, Hop W, Tiddens H. Nocturnal cough in children with stable cystic fibrosis. *Pediatr Pulmonol.* 2009;44(9):859-865.

228. Ramos RT, Salles C, Gregorio PB, et al. Evaluation of the upper airway in children and adolescents with cystic fibrosis and obstructive sleep apnea syndrome. *Int J Pediatr Otorhinolaryngol.* 2009;73(12):1780-1785.

229. Bradley S, Solin P, Wilson J, et al. Hypoxemia and hypercapnia during exercise and sleep in patients with cystic fibrosis. *Chest.* 1999;116:647-654.

230. Naqvi SK, Sotelo C, Murry L, Simakajornboon N. Sleep architecture in children and adolescents with cystic fibrosis and the association with severity of lung disease. *Sleep Breath.* 2008;12(1):77-83.

231. Amin R, Bean J, Burklow K, Jeffries J. The relationship between sleep disturbance and pulmonary function in stable pediatric cystic fibrosis patients. *Chest.* 2005;128(3):1357-1363.

232. de Castro-Silva C, de Bruin VM, Cavalcante AG, et al. Nocturnal hypoxia and sleep disturbances in cystic fibrosis. *Pediatr Pulmonol.* 2009;44(11):1143-1150.

233. Versteegh FG, Neijens HJ, Bogaard JM, et al. Relationship between pulmonary function, O_2 saturation during sleep and exercise, and exercise responses in children with cystic fibrosis. *Adv Cardiol.* 1986;35:151-155.

234. Milross MA, Piper AJ, Norman M, et al. Night-to-night variability in sleep in cystic fibrosis. *Sleep Med.* 2002;3(3):213-219.

235. Zinman R, Corey M, Coates AL, et al. Nocturnal home oxygen in the treatment of hypoxemic cystic fibrosis patients. *J Pediatr.* 1989;114(3):368-377.

236. Gozal D. Nocturnal ventilatory support in patients with cystic fibrosis: Comparison with supplemental oxygen. *Eur Respir J*. 1997;10:1999-2003.

237. Milross MA, Piper AJ, Norman M, et al. Low-flow oxygen and bilevel ventilatory support. *Am J Respir Crit Care Med*. 2001;163:129-134.

238. Regnis JA, Piper AJ, Henke KG, et al. Benefits of nocturnal nasal CPAP in patients with cystic fibrosis. *Chest*. 1994;106:1717-1724.

239. de Castro-Silva C, de Bruin VM, Cunha GM, et al. Melatonin improves sleep and reduces nitrite in the exhaled breath condensate in cystic fibrosis—A randomized, double-blind placebo-controlled study. *J Pineal Res*. 2010;48(1):65-71.

240. Carr JD. Evidence-based management of childhood atopic eczema. *Br J Nurs*. 2009;18(10):603-608.

241. Camfferman D, Kennedy JD, Gold M, Martin AJ, Lushington K. Eczema and sleep and its relationship to daytime functioning in children. *Sleep Med Rev*. 2010;14(6):359-369.

242. Ben-Gashir MA. Relationship between quality of life and disease severity in atopic dermatitis/eczema syndrome during childhood. *Curr Opin Allergy Clin Immunol*. 2003;3(5):369-373.

243. Lewis-Jones S. Quality of life and childhood atopic dermatitis: The misery of living with childhood eczema. *Int J Clin Pract*. 2006;60(8):984-992.

244. Camfferman D, Kennedy JD, Gold M, Martin AJ, Lushington K. Eczema and sleep and its relationship to daytime functioning in children. *Sleep Med Rev*. 2010;14(6):359-369.

245. Bartlet LB, Westbroek R, White JE. Sleep patterns in children with atopic eczema. *Acta Derm Venereol*. 1997;77(6):446-448.

246. Reid P, Lewis-Jones MS. Sleep difficulties and their management in preschoolers with atopic eczema. *Clin Exp Dermatol*. 1995;20(1):38-41.

247. Romanos M, Gerlach M, Warnke A, Schmitt J. Association of attention-deficit/hyperactivity disorder and atopic eczema modified by sleep disturbance in a large population-based sample. *J Epidemiol Community Health*. 2010;64(3):269-273.

248. Burgess JA, Dharmage SC, Byrnes GB, et al. Childhood eczema and asthma incidence and persistence: A cohort study from childhood to middle age. *J Allergy Clin Immunol*. 2008;122(2):280-285.

249. Foliaki S, Annesi-Maesano I, Tuuau-Potoi N, et al. Risk factors for symptoms of childhood asthma, allergic rhinoconjunctivitis and eczema in the Pacific: An ISAAC Phase III study. *Int J Tuberc Lung Dis*. 2008;12(7):799-806.

250. Brown SJ, Relton CL, Liao H, et al. Filaggrin null mutations and childhood atopic eczema: A population-based case-control study. *J Allergy Clin Immunol*. 2008;121(4):940-946.

251. Trakultivakorn M, Sangsupawanich P, Vichyanond P. Time trends of the prevalence of asthma, rhinitis and eczema in Thai children-ISAAC (International Study of Asthma and Allergies in Childhood) Phase Three. *J Asthma*. 2007;44(8):609-611.

252. Osman M, Tagiyeva N, Wassall HJ, et al. Changing trends in sex specific prevalence rates for childhood asthma, eczema, and hay fever. *Pediatr Pulmonol*. 2007;42(1):60-65.

253. Lima RG, Pastorino AC, Casagrande RR, et al. Prevalence of asthma, rhinitis and eczema in 6-7 years old students from the western districts of Sao Paulo City, using the standardized questionnaire of the "International Study of Asthma and Allergies in Childhood" (ISAAC), Phase IIIB. *Clinics (Sao Paulo)*. 2007;62(3):225-234.

254. Bisgaard H, Halkjaer LB, Hinge R, et al. Risk analysis of early childhood eczema. *J Allergy Clin Immunol*. 2009;123(6):1355-1360.

255. Biagini Myers JM, Wang N, LeMasters GK, et al. Genetic and environmental risk factors for childhood eczema development and allergic sensitization in the CCAAPS cohort. *J Invest Dermatol*. 2010;130(2):430-437.

256. Langan SM. Flares in childhood eczema. *Skin Therapy Lett*. 2009;14(8):4-5.

257. Berg AV, Kramer U, Link E, et al. Impact of early feeding on childhood eczema: Development after nutritional intervention compared with the natural course—The GINIplus study up to the age of 6 years. *Clin Exp Allergy*. 2010;40(4):627-636.

258. Kull I, Bohme M, Wahlgren CF, et al. Breast-feeding reduces the risk for childhood eczema. *J Allergy Clin Immunol*. 2005;116(3):657-661.

259. Hogan PA. Atopic eczema in children: What to do when treatment fails to work. *Australas J Dermatol*. 1996;37(3):119-122:quiz 123–124.

260. Yates JE, Phifer JB, Flake D. Clinical inquiries. Do nonmedicated topicals relieve childhood eczema? *J Fam Pract*. 2009;58(5):280-281.

261. Moore EJ, Williams A, Manias E, Varigos G, Donath S. Eczema workshops reduce severity of childhood atopic eczema. *Australas J Dermatol*. 2009;50(2):100-106.

262. Carr JD. Emollient treatment for childhood eczema: Involving children and parents. *J Fam Health Care*. 2006;16(4):105-107.

263. Robinson J. Managing atopic eczema in childhood: The health visitor and school nurse role. *Community Pract*. 2008;81(6):25-28.

264. Fiocchi A, Bouygue GR, Martelli A, Terracciano L, Sarratud T. Dietary treatment of childhood atopic eczema/dermatitis syndrome (AEDS). *Allergy*. 2004;59(Suppl 78):78-85.

265. Behrendt H, Ring J. Histamine, antihistamines and atopic eczema. *Clin Exp Allergy*. 1990;20(Suppl 4):25-30.

266. Schmitt J, Von Kobyletzki L, Svensson A, Apfelbacher C. Efficacy and tolerability of proactive treatment with topical corticosteroids and calcineurin inhibitors for atopic eczema: Systematic review and meta-analysis of randomized controlled trials. *Br J Dermatol*. 2011;164(2):415-428.

267. Green C, Colquitt JL, Kirby J, Davidson P. Topical corticosteroids for atopic eczema: Clinical and cost effectiveness of once-daily vs. more frequent use. *Br J Dermatol*. 2005;152(1):130-141.

268. Green C, Colquitt JL, Kirby J, Davidson P, Payne E. Clinical and cost-effectiveness of once-daily versus more frequent use of same potency topical corticosteroids for atopic eczema: A systematic review and economic evaluation. *Health Technol Assess*. 2004;8(47):1-120:iii, iv.

269. Anstey A. Management of atopic dermatitis: Nonadherence to topical therapies in treatment of skin disease and the use of calcineurin inhibitors in difficult eczema. *Br J Dermatol*. 2009;161(2):219-220.

270. Brunetti L, Francavilla R, Tesse R, et al. Effects of oral bacterial immunotherapy in children with atopic eczema/dermatitis syndrome: A pilot study. *BioDrugs*. 2005;19(6):393-399.

271. Pajno GB, Peroni DG, Barberio G, Boner AL. Efficacy of sublingual immunotherapy in asthma and eczema. *Chem Immunol Allergy*. 2003;82:77-88.

272. Hon KL, Wang SS, Hung EC, et al. Serum levels of heavy metals in childhood eczema and skin diseases: Friends or foes. *Pediatr Allergy Immunol*. 2010;21(5):831-836.

273. Kramer U, Weidinger S, Darsow U, et al. Seasonality in symptom severity influenced by temperature or grass pollen: Results of a panel study in children with eczema. *J Invest Dermatol*. 2005;124(3):514-523.

274. Reis L, Eisner M, Kosary C. *SEER Cancer Statistics Review*, 1975-2002. Bethesda, MD: National Cancer Institute; 2005.

275. Rosen GM. Sleep in children who have cancer. In: Carskadon, ed. *Sleep Medicine Clinics: Sleep in Children and Adolescents*. Philadelphia: Elsevier Saunders; 2007:491-500.

276. Hockenberry-Eaton M, Hinds PS. Fatigue in children and adolescents with cancer: Evolution of a program of study. *Semin Oncol Nurs*. 2000;16(4):261-272:discussion 272–278.

277. Harris JC, Carel CA, Rosenberg LA, Joshi P, Leventhal BG. Intermittent high dose corticosteroid treatment in childhood cancer: Behavioral and emotional consequences. *J Am Acad Child Psychiatry*. 1986;25(1):120-124.

278. Drigan R, Spirito A, Gelber RD. Behavioral effects of corticosteroids in children with acute lymphoblastic leukemia. *Med Pediatr Oncol*. 1992;20(1):13-21.

279. Meeske KA, Siegel SE, Globe DR, Mack WJ, Bernstein L. Prevalence and correlates of fatigue in long-term survivors of childhood leukemia. *J Clin Oncol*. 2005;23(24):5501-5510.

280. Nashed A, Al-Saleh S, Gibbons J, et al. Sleep-related breathing in children with mucopolysaccharidosis. *J Inherit Metab Dis*. 2009;32(4):544-550.

281. Rosen GM, Bendel AE, Neglia JP, Moertel CL, Mahowald M. Sleep in children with neoplasms of the central nervous system: Case review of 14 children. *Pediatrics*. 2003;112(1 Pt 1):e46-e54.

282. Rosen G, Brand SR. Sleep in children with cancer: Case review of 70 children evaluated in a comprehensive pediatric sleep center. *Support Care Cancer*. 2010;19(7):985-994.

283. Wright M. Children receiving treatment for cancer and their caregivers: A mixed methods study of their sleep characteristics. *Pediatr Blood Cancer*. 2011;56(4):638-645.

284. Miser AW, McCalla J, Dothage JA, Wesley M, Miser JS. Pain as a presenting symptom in children and young adults with newly diagnosed malignancy. *Pain*. 1987;29(1):85-90.

285. Ljungman G, Gordh T, Sorensen S, Kreuger A. Pain variations during cancer treatment in children: A descriptive survey. *Pediatr Hematol Oncol*. 2000;17(3):211-221.

286. Smith MT, Quartana PJ. The riddle of the sphinx: Sleep, pain, and depression. *Sleep Med*. 2010;11(8):745-746.

287. Smith MT, Haythornthwaite JA. How do sleep disturbance and chronic pain inter-relate? Insights from the longitudinal and cognitive-behavioral clinical trials literature. *Sleep Med Rev*. 2004;8(2):119-132.

288. Smith MT, Perlis ML, Smith MS, Giles DE, Carmody TP. Sleep quality and presleep arousal in chronic pain. *J Behav Med.* 2000;23(1):1-13.

289. Blask DE. Melatonin, sleep disturbance and cancer risk. *Sleep Med Rev.* 2009;13(4):257-264.

290. Erren TC, Reiter RJ. Axelrod, the pineal and the melatonin hypothesis: Lessons of 50 years to shape chronodisruption research. *Neuro Endocrinol Lett.* 2010;31(5):585-587.

291. Erren TC, Falaturi P, Reiter RJ. Research into the chronodisruption-cancer theory: The imperative for causal clarification and the danger of causal reductionism. *Neuro Endocrinol Lett.* 2010;31(1):1-3.

292. Erren TC, Reiter RJ. A generalized theory of carcinogenesis due to chronodisruption. *Neuro Endocrinol Lett.* 2008;29(6):815-821.

293. Reiter RJ, Tan DX, Korkmaz A, et al. Light at night, chronodisruption, melatonin suppression, and cancer risk: A review. *Crit Rev Oncog.* 2007;13(4):303-328.

294. Erren TC, Pape HG, Reiter RJ, Piekarski C. Chronodisruption and cancer. *Naturwissenschaften.* 2008;95(5):367-382.

295. Krueger JM, Majde JA, Rector DM. Cytokines in immune function and sleep regulation. *Handbook Clin Neurol.* 2011;98:229-240.

296. Palesh OG, Roscoe JA, Mustian KM, et al. Prevalence, demographics, and psychological associations of sleep disruption in patients with cancer: University of Rochester Cancer Center-Community Clinical Oncology Program. *J Clin Oncol.* 2010;28(2):292-298.

297. Conroy DA, Brower KJ. Alcohol, toxins, and medications as a cause of sleep dysfunction. *Handbook Clin Neurol.* 2011;98:587-612.

298. Meltzer LJ, Mindell JA, Owens JA, Byars KC. Use of sleep medications in hospitalized pediatric patients. *Pediatrics.* 2007;119(6):1047-1055.

299. Pagel JF. Medications and their effects on sleep. *Prim Care.* 2005;32(2):491-509.

300. Maddock C, Baita A, Orru MG, et al. Psychopharmacological treatment of depression, anxiety, irritability and insomnia in patients receiving interferon-alpha: A prospective case series and a discussion of biological mechanisms. *J Psychopharmacol.* 2004;18(1):41-46.

301. Vallance K, Liu W, Mandrell BN, et al. Mechanisms of dexamethasone-induced disturbed sleep and fatigue in paediatric patients receiving treatment for ALL. *Eur J Cancer.* 2010;46(10):1848-1855.

302. Jacob E, Hesselgrave J, Sambuco G, Hockenberry M. Variations in pain, sleep, and activity during hospitalization in children with cancer. *J Pediatr Oncol Nurs.* 2007;24(4):208-219.

303. Hinds PS, Hockenberry M, Rai SN, et al. Nocturnal awakenings, sleep environment interruptions, and fatigue in hospitalized children with cancer. *Oncol Nurs Forum.* 2007;34(2):393-402.

304. Kelsey CR, Marks LB. Somnolence syndrome after focal radiation therapy to the pineal region: Case report and review of the literature. *J Neurooncol.* 2006;78(2):153-156.

305. Vern TZ, Salvi S. Somnolence syndrome and fever in pediatric patients with cranial irradiation. *J Pediatr Hematol Oncol.* 2009;31(2):118-120.

306. Ryan J. Radiation somnolence syndrome. *J Pediatr Oncol Nurs.* 2000;17(1):50-53.

307. Uzal D, Ozyar E, Hayran M, Zorlu F, Atahan L, Yetkin S. Reduced incidence of the somnolence syndrome after prophylactic cranial irradiation in children with acute lymphoblastic leukemia. *Radiother Oncol.* 1998;48(1):29-32.

308. Faithfull S. Patients' experiences following cranial radiotherapy: A study of the somnolence syndrome. *J Adv Nurs.* 1991;16(8):939-946.

309. Littman P, Rosenstock J, Gale G, et al. The somnolence syndrome in leukemic children following reduced daily dose fractions of cranial radiation. *Int J Radiat Oncol Biol Phys.* 1984;10(10):1851-1853.

310. Jereczek-Fossa BA, Marsiglia HR, Orecchia R. Radiotherapy-related fatigue. *Crit Rev Oncol Hematol.* 2002;41(3):317-325.

311. Van Someren EJ, Swart-Heikens J, Endert E, et al. Long-term effects of cranial irradiation for childhood malignancy on sleep in adulthood. *Eur J Endocrinol.* 2004;150(4):503-510.

312. Ancoli-Israel S, Moore PJ, Jones V. The relationship between fatigue and sleep in cancer patients: A review. *Eur J Cancer Care (Engl).* 2001;10(4):245-255.

313. Cella D, Davis K, Breitbart W, Curt G. Cancer-related fatigue: Prevalence of proposed diagnostic criteria in a United States sample of cancer survivors. *J Clin Oncol.* 2001;19(14):3385-3391.

314. Morrow GR, Shelke AR, Roscoe JA, Hickok JT, Mustian K. Management of cancer-related fatigue. *Cancer Invest.* 2005;23(3):229-239.

315. Mock V. Evidence-based treatment for cancer-related fatigue. *Natl Cancer Inst Monogr.* 2004;32:112-118.

316. Kline N, DeSwarte J. Consensus statements, research on fatigue in children with cancer. *Semin Oncol Nurs.* 2000;16:277-278.

317. Wu M, Hsu L, Zhang B, Shen N, Lu H, Li S. The experiences of cancer-related fatigue among Chinese children with leukaemia: A phenomenological study. *Int J Nurs Stud.* 2010;47(1):49-59.

318. Chiang YC, Yeh CH, Wang KW, Yang CP. The experience of cancer-related fatigue in Taiwanese children. *Eur J Cancer Care (Engl).* 2009;18(1):43-49.

319. Clarke-Steffen L. Cancer-related fatigue in children. *J Pediatr Oncol Nurs.* 2001;18(2 Suppl 1):1-2.

320. Lee K, Cho M, Miaskowski C, Dodd M. Impaired sleep and rhythms in persons with cancer. *Sleep Med Rev.* 2004;8(3):199-212.

321. Moore P, Dimsdale JE. Opioids, sleep, and cancer-related fatigue. *Med Hypotheses.* 2002;58(1):77-82.

322. Walker AJ, Johnson KP, Miaskowski C, Lee KA, Gedaly-Duff V. Sleep quality and sleep hygiene behaviors of adolescents during chemotherapy. *J Clin Sleep Med.* 2010;6(5):439-444.

323. Berger AM, Mitchell SA. Modifying cancer-related fatigue by optimizing sleep quality. *J Natl Compr Cancer Netw.* 2008;6(1):3-13.

324. Young-McCaughan S, et al. Research and commentary: Change in exercise tolerance, activity and sleep patterns, and quality of life in patients with cancer participating in a structured exercise program. *Oncol Nurs Forum.* 2003;30(3):441-454:discussion 441-454.

325. Cooper MR, Bird HM, Steinberg M. Efficacy and safety of modafinil in the treatment of cancer-related fatigue. *Ann Pharmacother.* 2009;43(4):721-725.

326. Jean-Pierre P, Morrow GR, Roscoe JA, et al. A phase 3 randomized, placebo-controlled, double-blind, clinical trial of the effect of modafinil on cancer-related fatigue among 631 patients receiving chemotherapy: A University of Rochester Cancer Center Community Clinical Oncology Program Research base study. *Cancer.* 2010;116(14):3513-3520.

327. Lundorff LE, Jonsson BH, Sjogren P. Modafinil for attentional and psychomotor dysfunction in advanced cancer: A double-blind, randomised, cross-over trial. *Palliat Med.* 2009;23(8):731-738.

328. Wirz S, Nadstawek J, Kuhn KU, Vater S, Junker U, Wartenberg HC. [Modafinil for the treatment of cancer-related fatigue: An intervention study.] *Schmerz.* 2010;24(6):587-595.

329. Blackhall L, Petroni G, Shu J, Baum L, Farace E. A pilot study evaluating the safety and efficacy of modafinal for cancer-related fatigue. *J Palliat Med.* 2009;12(5):433-439.

330. Ivanenko A, Tauman R, Gozal D. Modafinil in the treatment of excessive daytime sleepiness in children. *Sleep Med.* 2003;4(6):579-582.

331. Zada G, Laws ER. Surgical management of craniopharyngiomas in the pediatric population. *Horm Res Paediatr.* 2010;74(1):62-66.

332. Marcus CL, Trescher WH, Halbower AC, Lutz J. Secondary narcolepsy in children with brain tumors. *Sleep.* 2002;25(4):435-439.

333. Muller HL, Muller-Stover S, Gebhardt U, et al. Secondary narcolepsy may be a causative factor of increased daytime sleepiness in obese childhood craniopharyngioma patients. *J Pediatr Endocrinol Metab.* 2006;19(Suppl 1):423-429.

334. Snow A, Gozal E, Malhotra A, et al. Severe hypersomnolence after pituitary/hypothalamic surgery in adolescents: Clinical characteristics and potential mechanisms. *Pediatrics.* 2002;110(6):e74.

335. Tachibana N, Taniike M, Okinaga T, et al. Hypersomnolence and increased REM sleep with low cerebrospinal fluid hypocretin level in a patient after removal of craniopharyngioma. *Sleep Med.* 2005;6(6):567-569.

336. Muller HL, Emser A, Faldum A, et al. Longitudinal study on growth and body mass index before and after diagnosis of childhood craniopharyngioma. *J Clin Endocrinol Metab.* 2004;89(7):3298-3305.

337. Muller HL. Childhood craniopharyngioma: Current controversies on management in diagnostics, treatment and follow-up. *Expert Rev Neurother.* 2010;10(4):515-524.

338. Muller HL, Handwerker G, Wollny B, Faldum A, Sorensen N. Melatonin secretion and increased daytime sleepiness in childhood craniopharyngioma patients. *J Clin Endocrinol Metab.* 2002;87(8):3993-3996.

339. Roth CL, Gebhardt U, Muller HL. Appetite-regulating hormone changes in patients with craniopharyngioma. *Obesity (Silver Spring).* 2011;19(1):36-42.

340. Kawamata T, Amano K, Aihara Y, Kubo O, Hori T. Optimal treatment strategy for craniopharyngiomas based on long-term functional outcomes of recent and past treatment modalities. *Neurosurg Rev.* 2010;33(1):71-81.

341. Schubert T, Trippel M, Tacke U, et al. Neurosurgical treatment strategies in childhood craniopharyngiomas: Is less more? *Childs Nerv Syst.* 2009;25(11):1419-1127.

342. Spoudeas HA, Saran F, Pizer B. A multimodality approach to the treatment of craniopharyngiomas avoiding hypothalamic morbidity: A UK perspective. *J Pediatr Endocrinol Metab.* 2006;19(Suppl 1):447-451.

343. Muller HL. More or less? Treatment strategies in childhood craniopharyngioma. *Childs Nerv Syst.* 2006;22(2):156-157.

344. Muller HL, Gebhardt U, Etavard-Gorris N, et al. Prognosis and sequela in patients with childhood craniopharyngioma—Results of HIT-ENDO and update on Kraniopharyngeom 2000. *Klin Padiatr.* 2004;216(6):343-348.

345. Lipton J, Megerian JT, Kothare SV, et al. Melatonin deficiency and disrupted circadian rhythms in pediatric survivors of craniopharyngioma. *Neurology.* 2009;73(4):323-325.

346. Muller HL, Handwerker G, Gebhardt U, et al. Melatonin treatment in obese patients with childhood craniopharyngioma and increased daytime sleepiness. *Cancer Causes Control.* 2006;17(4):583-589.

347. Muller HL. Childhood craniopharyngioma—Current concepts in diagnosis, therapy and follow-up. *Nat Rev Endocrinol.* 2010;6(11):609-618.

348. Muller HL, Gebhardt U, Wessel V, et al. First experiences with laparoscopic adjustable gastric banding (LAGB) in the treatment of patients with childhood craniopharyngioma and morbid obesity. *Klin Padiatr.* 2007;219(6):323-325.

349. Tang MF, Liou TH, Lin CC. Improving sleep quality for cancer patients: Benefits of a home-based exercise intervention. *Support Care Cancer.* 2010;18(10):1329-1339.

350. Barsevick A, Beck SL, Dudley WN, et al. Efficacy of an intervention for fatigue and sleep disturbance during cancer chemotherapy. *J Pain Symptom Manage.* 2010;40(2):200-216.

351. Kwekkeboom KL, Abbott-Anderson K, Wanta B. Feasibility of a patient-controlled cognitive-behavioral intervention for pain, fatigue, and sleep disturbance in cancer. *Oncol Nurs Forum.* 2010;37(3):E151-E159.

352. Kwekkeboom KL, Cherwin CH, Lee JW, Wanta B. Mind-body treatments for the pain-fatigue-sleep disturbance symptom cluster in persons with cancer. *J Pain Symptom Manage.* 2010;39(1):126-138.

353. Skene DJ, Arendt J. Circadian rhythm sleep disorders in the blind and their treatment with melatonin. *Sleep Med.* 2007;8(6):651-655.

354. Lewy AJ, Emens JS, Sack RL, Hasler BP, Bernert RA. Low, but not high, doses of melatonin entrained a free-running blind person with a long circadian period. *Chronobiol Int.* 2002;19(3):649-658.

355. Sack RL, Brandes RW, Kendall AR, Lewy AJ. Entrainment of free-running circadian rhythms by melatonin in blind people. *N Engl J Med.* 2000;343(15):1070-1077.

356. Pandi-Perumal SR, Trakht I, Spence DW, et al. The roles of melatonin and light in the pathophysiology and treatment of circadian rhythm sleep disorders. *Nat Clin Pract Neurol.* 2008;4(8):436-447.

357. Morgenthaler TI, Lee-Chiong T, Alessi C, et al. Practice parameters for the clinical evaluation and treatment of circadian rhythm sleep disorders. An American Academy of Sleep Medicine report. *Sleep.* 2007;30(11):1445-1159.

358. Yamadera H, Takahashi K, Okawa M. A multicenter study of sleep-wake rhythm disorders: Therapeutic effects of vitamin B_{12}, bright light therapy, chronotherapy and hypnotics. *Psychiatry Clin Neurosci.* 1996;50(4):203-209.

359. Peirano PD, Algarin CR, Chamorro RA, et al. Sleep alterations and iron deficiency anemia in infancy. *Sleep Med.* 2010;11(7):637-642.

360. Beard JL, Connor JR. Iron status and neural functioning. *Annu Rev Nutr.* 2003;23:41-58.

361. Carter RC, Jacobson JL, Burden MJ, et al. Iron deficiency anemia and cognitive function in infancy. *Pediatrics.* 2010;126(2):e427-e434.

362. Gupta SK, Bansal D, Malhi P, Das R. Developmental profile in children with iron deficiency anemia and its changes after therapeutic iron supplementation. *Indian J Pediatr.* 2010;77(4):375-379.

363. Herschman Z, Klapholz A. Aspirin to prevent pregnancy-induced hypertension. *N Engl J Med.* 1990;322(3):204-205.

364. Lozoff B, Armony-Sivan R, Kaciroti N, et al. Eye-blinking rates are slower in infants with iron-deficiency anemia than in nonanemic iron-deficient or iron-sufficient infants. *J Nutr.* 2010;140(5):1057-1061.

365. Shafir T, Angulo-Barroso R, Su J, Jacobson SW, Lozoff B. Iron deficiency anemia in infancy and reach and grasp development. *Infant Behav Dev.* 2009;32(4):366-375.

366. Lozoff B, Clark KM, Jing Y, et al. Dose-response relationships between iron deficiency with or without anemia and infant social-emotional behavior. *J Pediatr.* 2008;152(5):696-702.

367. Algarin C, Peirano P, Garrido M, Pizarro F, Lozoff B. Iron deficiency anemia in infancy: Long-lasting effects on auditory and visual system functioning. *Pediatr Res.* 2003;53(2):217-223.

368. Lozoff B, Klein NK, Nelson EC, McClish DK, Manuel M, Chacon ME. Behavior of infants with iron-deficiency anemia. *Child Dev.* 1998;69(1):24-36.

369. Lozoff B, Wolf AW, Jimenez E. Iron-deficiency anemia and infant development: Effects of extended oral iron therapy. *J Pediatr.* 1996;129(3):382-389.

370. Peirano P, Algarin C, Garrido M, Algarin D, Lozoff B. Iron-deficiency anemia is associated with altered characteristics of sleep spindles in NREM sleep in infancy. *Neurochem Res.* 2007;32(10):1665-1672.

371. Angulo-Kinzler RM, Peirano P, Lin E, Garrido M, Lozoff B. Spontaneous motor activity in human infants with iron-deficiency anemia. *Early Hum Dev.* 2002;66(2):67-79.

372. Angulo-Kinzler RM, Peirano P, Lin E, Algarin C, Garrido M, Lozoff B. Twenty-four-hour motor activity in human infants with and without iron deficiency anemia. *Early Hum Dev.* 2002;70(1-2):85-101.

373. Kordas K, Siegel EH, Olney DK, et al. Maternal reports of sleep in 6-18 month-old infants from Nepal and Zanzibar: Association with iron deficiency anemia and stunting. *Early Hum Dev.* 2008;84(6):389-398.

374. Cortese S, Konofal E, Bernardina BD, Mouren MC, Lecendreux M. Sleep disturbances and serum ferritin levels in children with attention-deficit/hyperactivity disorder. *Eur Child Adolesc Psychiatry.* 2009;18(7):393-399.

375. Dosman CF, Brian JA, Drmic IE, et al. Children with autism: Effect of iron supplementation on sleep and ferritin. *Pediatr Neurol.* 2007;36(3):152-158.

376. Kazal Jr LA. Prevention of iron deficiency in infants and toddlers. *Am Fam Physician.* 2002;66(7):1217-1224.

377. Huang SC, Yang YJ, Cheng CN, et al. The etiology and treatment outcome of iron deficiency and iron deficiency anemia in children. *J Pediatr Hematol Oncol.* 2010;32(4):282-285.

Sleep and Sleep Problems in Children with Psychiatric Disorders

Chapter 42

ANNA IVANENKO / VALERIE MCLAUGHLIN CRABTREE

Sleep complaints including sleep onset and maintenance insomnia, restless sleep, excessive daytime sleepiness, and bedtime fears and worries are seen frequently in children with psychiatric disorders. Nighttime awakenings are seen more frequently in children with mood and anxiety disorders than in children with other psychiatric disorders.[1] Children and adolescents with mood and anxiety disorders display both subjective and objective changes in their sleep patterns. Because of the substantial relationship between sleep disruptions and childhood psychiatric disorders, the need for treatment of the disrupted sleep is clear.

Dahl[2] has theorized a bidirectional relationship between mood and sleep disturbance in children. Dahl's theory is supported by a growing body of evidence that children with mood disorders have increased rates of sleep disturbance; while, conversely, children with sleep disturbance are significantly more likely to have psychiatric problems. Furthermore, even in children without mood disturbance, a stressful event may induce sleep disruption; and insufficient sleep in any child may directly lead to disruptive daytime behavior. In addition, children with sleep disorders and children with psychiatric disorders (particularly depression) may show similar symptoms. Finally, both sleep and mood regulation are supported by similar neurobehavioral systems.

SLEEP AND PEDIATRIC DEPRESSION

Subjective sleep disturbance is extremely common in pediatric depression. Sleep disturbances such as delayed sleep onset, nocturnal awakenings, shorter sleep duration, difficult morning awakening, and excessive daytime sleepiness have been associated with both depressed mood and co-morbid anxiety.[1,3,4] In particular, children with both hypersomnia and insomnia have increased rates of recurrent depression, longer episodes of depression, and more severe depressive symptoms.[3] The relationship between sleep disruption and depressive symptoms is very strong (Fig. 42-1): thus, the prevalence rate of sleep problems in depressed children and adolescents is very high, with nearly 75% of depressed children and adolescents reporting significant insomnia. Although insomnia is prevalent in both children and adolescents, subjective hypersomnia has been found to occur more frequently in depressed adolescents than in prepubertal children (34% vs. 16%).[5]

Sleep Complaints Predict Future Depression

Because of the common co-occurrence of sleep complaints and depressive symptoms, the role of sleep complaints in predicting future depression has been evaluated. Sleep complaints early in life have been theorized to be related to later development of depression and anxiety, and early depressive symptoms may also predict ongoing sleep difficulties. In a longitudinal study of sleep and depression in adolescents, 75% of adolescents initially reporting both sleep disturbances and symptoms of depression (but not meeting diagnostic criteria for major depressive disorder) met full criteria for major depressive disorder within 12 months.[6]

Ong and associates[7] examined the occurrence of sleep problems and the development of psychiatric symptoms over an extended period of time and found that young children described by their parents as having nonregular sleep habits prior to age 6 were significantly more likely to develop major depressive disorder or an anxiety disorder in adolescence. Several anxiety disorders (e.g., generalized anxiety disorder, obsessive-compulsive disorder, posttraumatic stress disorder [PTSD], panic disorder, agoraphobia, simple phobia, and social phobia) were associated with early sleep disturbances. Interestingly, none of the early childhood temperament domains were predictive of adult-onset mood disturbance.

Similarly, in a large longitudinal study of more than 2000 subjects, children who were rated by their parents as sleeping less, being overtired, and having difficulty sleeping were significantly more likely to report symptoms of anxiety and depression 14 years later than their peers who had no such earlier reports of sleep difficulties. In fact, in that study, parental reports of decreased sleep in childhood was the strongest predictor of future emotional difficulties.[8] In addition, adolescents with self-reports of insomnia had a significantly increased likelihood of exhibiting depressive symptoms 1 year later.[9] Further evidence that the existence of sleep difficulties early on is associated with future mood disturbance comes from a longitudinal study of twins. Sleep disturbances in these 8-year-old children predicted symptoms of depression at age 10; however, the reverse was not true, namely symptoms of depression at age 8 were not predictive of sleep problems at age 10.[10] Although depressive symptoms in childhood have not been shown to predict later sleep problems, some evidence in adolescents links depressive symptoms with persistent sleep problems. In a large sample of adolescents, those who had symptoms of depression at baseline but not 4 years later still had higher rates of sleep problems at the 4-year follow-up than did those who had not experienced depressive symptoms at baseline[11] (Fig. 42-2).

Circadian Rhythms in Adolescent Depression

Adolescent depression has been associated with disrupted circadian rhythm amplitude, particularly with *lower* amplitude circadian rhythms noted in depressed girls, even when

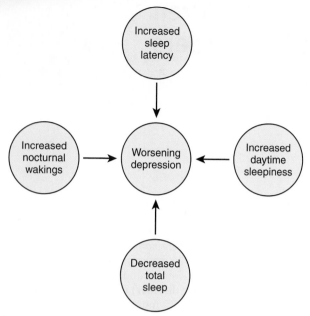

Figure 42-1 Hypothesized relationship between sleep and depression in childhood. The impact of changes in sleep on depression in childhood is shown schematically in this diagram; however, in fact, there are reciprocal relationships between depression and the sleep variables and among the sleep variables themselves.

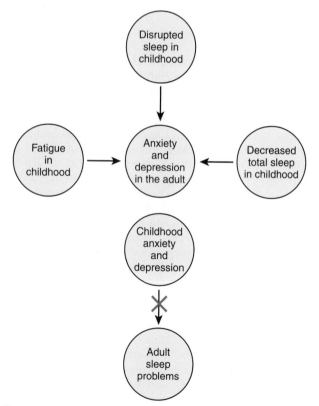

Figure 42-2 An association exists between sleep disturbances in the child and depression and anxiety in the adult; however, there is no similar association between depression and anxiety in the child and sleep problems in the adult.

controlling for total activity level. This may be related to poorer entrainment to the 24-hour day or decreased exposure to *zeitgebers* (time setters, such as light exposure). On the other hand, depressed adolescent boys showed *higher* circadian rhythm amplitude. Nevertheless, as a group the depressed adolescents exhibited decreased activity levels and lower light exposure than did their healthy peers, which may be hypothesized to be related to symptoms of anhedonia (the inability to experience pleasurable emotions from normally pleasurable events).[12]

Impact of Depression Treatment on Sleep Complaints

Relatively few studies have examined the effects on sleep complaints of treating coexisting depression in children. After undergoing 8 weeks of treatment, either with elective serotonin reuptake inhibitors (SSRIs) or cognitive behavior therapy (CBT), adolescents with major depressive disorder did not exhibit sleep improvements but did significantly reduce their caffeine intake.[4] Puig-Antich and associates found that 1 year after their depression had remitted, 90% of children no longer had symptoms of insomnia.[13] However, this improvement in sleep tended to apply more to subjective improvement rather than to documented changes in sleep. In particular, after treatment the children went to bed and fell asleep *later* than before, despite waking at the same time, and thus ended up actually sleeping 30 minutes less each night following their recovery than they did during the active depressive episode.[13]

SLEEP AND PEDIATRIC BIPOLAR DISORDER

Childhood bipolar disorder remains somewhat poorly understood. Symptoms present in children diagnosed with bipolar disorder often vary dramatically from those seen in adults with the same diagnosis. In particular, children tend to have mixed mania and depression with more rapid cycling of mood than is usually seen in adults.[14] Even though evidence for sleep disruption in pediatric depression and anxiety is mounting, few studies have examined sleep problems in children with bipolar disorder, most likely because of the difficulty in establishing this diagnosis in children and adolescents.

A primary feature of mania is a decreased need for sleep. This fact may represent one of the salient diagnostic features in pediatric bipolar disorder[15] with approximately 40% to 72% of children with this diagnosis reporting a significantly decreased need for sleep during a manic episode in comparison to only 6% of children with attention deficit hyperactivity disorder (ADHD) and 1% of healthy children.[16-18] As a result, decreased need for sleep may provide one of the best tools to differentiate between ADHD and bipolar disorder in children.[16,19]

During severe depressive episodes of bipolar disorder, 82% of children reported insomnia.[17] The vast majority of children with bipolar disorder have been reported to have moderate to severe sleep problems, most frequently bedtime resistance, difficulty initiating sleep, sleep-related anxiety, nocturnal awakenings, parasomnias, decreased sleep need, and excessive daytime sleepiness.[17,20] Based on family reports, sleep disruption is most frequently seen during mixed depressive-manic phases, occurring in 89% of affected children.[17]

SLEEP AND PEDIATRIC ANXIETY

Sleep is frequently inhibited in children with anxiety due to the hypervigilance and hyperarousability that frequently occur.[21] As in depression, a reciprocal relationship is theorized to occur between anxiety and sleep, with increased anxiety leading to disrupted sleep, which then exacerbates the anxiety, which then further disturbs sleep.[22] The majority of children with anxiety disorders evidence sleep disruption, with 83% to 92% of children reporting at least one sleep-related complaint.[22-24] The most common sleep complaints noted by parents of children with anxiety disorders include insomnia, refusal to sleep alone, nightmares, being overtired, general difficulty sleeping, and excessive sleeping.[22-24] Even among children without diagnosed anxiety disorders, those with symptoms of anxiety have been reported to have frequent nighttime awakenings, sleep with their lights on, sleep with a security object, have bedtime fears, require prolonged nighttime rituals, and have nightmares.[1]

Sleep Characteristics in Children with Post-Traumatic Stress Disorder

Because of the sleep-inhibiting effect of hypervigilance, sleep complaints are a hallmark feature of PTSD.[25] Children and adolescents with PTSD very often experience nightmares and nighttime anxiety, with both sleep initiation and sleep maintenance insomnia.[26-28] In children with a history of abuse, actigraphic evidence has demonstrated poorer sleep efficiency, increased nocturnal activity, and reduced quiet sleep in comparison to nonabused children and children with other psychiatric disorders.[29,30]

Sleep Complaints Predict Anxiety

Although there is significant overlap between depressive symptoms and sleep disruption, persistent sleep disruption in children may be even more strongly related to anxiety. In a large longitudinal study, children who had persistent sleep problems at ages 5, 7, and 9 years were significantly more likely to have anxiety at the ages of 21 and 26 years than those who had not experienced persistent sleep problems, even when controlling for gender, socioeconomic status, and childhood internalizing symptoms. While predictive of future anxiety, persistent sleep problems in childhood were not predictive of adult depression in this study.[31] In a separate, longitudinal study, children with sleep problems present at 4 years of age were significantly more likely to have symptoms of both anxiety and depression as adolescents. On the other hand, children with depression or anxiety in early childhood did not report future sleep problems in adolescence. As the children grew older, the co-occurrence of sleep problems and anxious/depressed symptoms grew stronger.[32]

SLEEP COMPLAINTS IN ATTENTION DEFICIT HYPERACTIVITY DISORDER

Children with ADHD have been noted to have significant night-to-night variability in their sleep patterns,[33] often making it difficult to find a consistent pattern of sleep in this population of children. Between 25% and 50% of parents report subjective sleep complaints in children and adolescents with ADHD,[34] including bedtime resistance, delayed sleep onset, nocturnal awakenings, difficulty with morning awakening, and excessive daytime sleepiness.[35] The consistent findings across objective studies include periodic limb movements, increased nighttime activity, sleep-disordered breathing, and decreased sleep efficiency.[35,36]

Although the relationship between sleep disturbance and ADHD has been shown to reflect confounding factors such as clinical co-morbidities and stimulant medication,[37] some evidence has shown that treatment of ADHD with stimulant medication makes little difference in the sleep disturbances,[38] either by subjective report or objective recording.[39] Furthermore, when psychiatric co-morbidities, including mood and anxiety disorders, conduct and oppositional-defiant disorders, and pharmacotherapy, were statistically controlled, children with ADHD did not show a frequency of sleep difficulties statistically different from those of normal control subjects.[40] (See Tsai and Huang[41] for a comprehensive review of sleep disturbance in children with ADHD.)

SLEEP COMPLAINTS IN CHILDREN WITH AUTISM SPECTRUM DISORDERS

Autism spectrum disorders (ASD) represent a common group of neurodevelopmental disabilities and, according to the DSM –IV[42] classification system, include the following categories: autistic disorder, Rett syndrome, childhood disintegrative disorder, Asperger's disorder, and pervasive developmental disorder not otherwise specified.

Autistic disorder is characterized by qualitative impairments in social interaction and communication with restricted, repetitive, and stereotyped patterns of behavior, interests, and activities. Delays or abnormal functioning in at least one of the afore mentioned areas have an onset prior to age 3 years.

Individuals with Asperger's syndrome have an intellectual capacity within the normal range but have a distinct profile of qualitative impairments in social interaction and restricted range of interest and activities apparent from early childhood. In Asperger's syndrome, the individual has deficits in the capacity to organize visual information or interpret visual cues (e.g., facial expressions and gestures) for use in interpreting the reactions and intentions of others.

Numerous research studies of sleep complaints in children and adolescents with ASD indicate a high prevalence of sleep onset and maintenance problems with night wakings, shortened night sleep, daytime napping, and parasomnias. ASD is discussed in Chapter 40. (See also Cortesi and associates[43] for a recent review.)

TREATMENT OF SLEEP DISTURBANCES IN CHILDREN WITH PSYCHIATRIC DISORDERS

Treating sleep disturbances in pediatric patients may not only serve to improve sleep and family functioning but may, in fact, provide a protective factor against future development of mood disturbance.[10] Unfortunately, despite a high prevalence of sleep complaints among children and adolescents with psychiatric morbidities, there are currently no well-designed, large-scale systematic studies on the effective treatments of sleep disturbances associated with early onset psychiatric disorders. Clinical research, however, indicates that successful treatment of primary psychiatric disorders results in significant improvement of sleep-related symptoms such as sleep initiation and maintenance insomnia, nocturnal fears, and nightmares.

Nonpharmacologic treatments have been shown to be effective for both primary and co-morbid insomnias in adults[44-46] and have been used for children with symptomatic insomnia related to mood and anxiety disorders. Adult research also suggests that concurrent treatment of insomnia and depressive disorders improves outcomes and may prevent further recurrence of major depression.[47,48] Furthermore, because of the disrupted circadian amplitude in adolescents with depression, increasing light exposure may be an appropriate intervention to improve the circadian rhythm and activity level of depressed pediatric patients.[12] This could be accomplished either through structured exposure to ambient lighting or with the use of a commercially available light therapy box.

Several multidisciplinary consensus groups have formulated a rational approach to pharmacologic treatment of pediatric insomnia, but they emphasize that nonpharmacologic treatment should be the first choice as intervention for children and adolescents with insomnia.[49,50] Sleep hygiene education stressing the importance of consistent age-appropriate bedtime and nighttime routines should be provided to every family seeking help for sleep-related problems in their children. Nighttime fears are commonly precipitated by watching frightening movies or TV programs; thus, avoiding exposure to television, computer games, and child-inappropriate websites close to bedtime, and creating soothing and safe environments for the child, may significantly reduce nocturnal anxiety. Other therapeutic interventions, such as systematic desensitization, exposure and response prevention with imagery exercises, and dream rehearsal techniques, have been shown to be effective in treating nightmares and bedtime fears in children.[51]

In one report, sleep problems significantly decreased in children with obsessive-compulsive disorders treated with family-based cognitive behavior therapy. This family-based treatment consisted of 14 90-minute sessions involving the child and at least one parent with focus on psycho-education, exposure with response prevention, cognitive therapy, and family interaction patterns. Significant improvements were noted in nightmares, complaints of being overtired, sleeping less or more than other children, difficulty sleeping, and requiring the presence of another person to sleep.[24]

Pharmacologic interventions may be warranted when the child does not adequately respond to behavioral interventions or when parents are unable to implement recommended behavioral interventions. Medication may be considered for the treatment of insomnia within the context of the comorbid psychiatric disorder. Once pharmacologic treatment for insomnia is chosen, it should be short-term, and clinicians should encourage regular and consistent follow-up visits with reevaluation of target insomnia symptoms and assessment of compliance. Rational selection of pharmacologic agents should be based on the presenting complaint, pharmacologic properties of the drug, drug-drug interactions, safety profile of the drug, potential side effects, and formulations available. Since a detailed description of pharmacotherapy of pediatric insomnia is beyond the scope of this chapter, the reader is referred to Chapter 36 and to a recent review by Owens and associates[50] for further details.

Interventions for Children with Depressive Disorders

Despite a high prevalence of sleep complaints in children and adolescents with depressive disorders, there are no strong evidence-based treatment recommendations available for insomnia in depressed youth. SSRIs emerged as effective pharmacologic agents for pediatric depression. However, little is known about how these agents affect children's sleep.

Fluoxetine has been shown to inhibit rapid eye movement (REM) sleep, increase the number of arousals and periodic limb movement in sleep, and cause oculomotor abnormalities in adults.[52] Similar changes in sleep characteristics, except for REM sleep suppression, were observed in a small group of children with major depression treated with fluoxetine.[53] Interestingly, most patients in this study reported poorer sleep quality when receiving the medication. On the other hand, children with anxiety disorders treated with fluvoxamine exhibited reductions in both anxiety and insomnia.[22]

One small retrospective study explored concomitant use of trazodone (a psychoactive compound with sedative and antidepressant properties) and the SSRI fluoxetine in a sample of adolescents with major depressive disorder. Two subgroups of patients were compared: those treated with combination of fluoxetine and trazodone and those treated with fluoxetine alone.[54] Based on self-reports, insomnia resolved sooner in adolescents treated with combination therapy. Changes in insomnia complaints were found to be *statistically* but not *clinically* significant.

Treatments in Children with Autism Spectrum Disorders

Behavioral Interventions

Few attempts have been made to investigate parental preference for behavioral and pharmacologic interventions among children with ASD. In one study, fewer than half of parents surveyed reported receiving any help for their children's sleep problems associated with developmental disabilities and ASD.[55] More recently, Williams and associates[56] conducted a study to determine the behavioral strategies and pharmacologic treatments most commonly prescribed by providers, and used by families, to promote sleep in children with ASD. Surveys asking about treatment modalities were completed by parents of children with ASD. The children were divided by intelligence quotient (IQ) into two groups: those less than 70 (mentally retarded) and those greater than 70 (not mentally retarded). Results of the survey indicated that behavioral interventions were tried far more frequently than medications. The behavioral interventions that were found most helpful included a regular bedtime, sleeping in parents' bed, wrapping the child in a blanket, using a noise masker, providing toys for bedtime, and using a darkened room. When survey results of children with ASD with mental retardation (MR) were compared with children with ASD without MR, similar effectiveness for behavioral interventions was noticed, except for use of a nightlight and reading, which were reported to be less effective for children with MR. In contrast, playing music at bedtime was found to be more helpful in the MR group.

Richdale and Wiggs[57] have written a comprehensive article on behavioral approaches to the treatment of sleep disorders in children with developmental disorders and autism that provides a systematic literature review of different behavioral interventions and their effectiveness in addressing sleep disturbances among children with developmental disabilities and ASD.

Nonpharmacologic interventions shown to be effective in children with ASD are listed in Table 42-1 and are discussed here.

TABLE 42-1

Nonpharmacologic Sleep Interventions Shown to Be Effective in Children with Autism Spectrum Disorders (ASDs)

Intervention	Description
Sleep hygiene	Establish an age-appropriate bedtime with consistent bedtime routine and elimination of sensory stimulation (TV, computers).
Positive bedtime routine	Promote positive interaction, relaxation, and self-soothing with reduced light exposure (dim light) and optimal temperature and noise control.
Faded bedtime	Start with bedtime late enough so that the child is able to fall asleep within 15 minutes; wake the child the next morning at a predetermined time. If the child is unable to fall asleep quickly at bedtime, he or she is then kept awake for an hour and put back to bed. The procedure can be repeated as often as necessary during the night and on successive nights until he or she falls asleep within 15 minutes and has no long wakings during the night. Once the sleep onset time is established, fading from the initial bedtime can be attempted by advancing bedtime by 30 minutes every night until the target bedtime is reached.[59]
Graduated behavioral approaches with social story	Graduated extinction is the progressive ignoring of undesired behaviors for increasing time periods, with periodic parental reassurance or with continuous parental presence. A social story (book with pictures illustrating bedtime routine) can be coupled with positive behavioral reinforcement and graduated extinction.[60]
Stimulus fading	A stimulus fading approach has been shown to be effective in addressing co-sleeping issues in patients with ASD.[61] Parents move a separate bed into their bedroom and place it right next to their own bed. The child is then encouraged to stay in his or her own bed while being able to communicate with the parents at bedtime. The child's bed is then gradually moved away from the parental bed (over 8 to 10 weeks). Once comfortable falling and staying asleep in his or her own bed, the child is moved to his own bedroom.
Sleep restriction	Parents obtain baseline sleep data by completing sleep logs for their child's sleep pattern for 1 to 2 weeks. Then they delay the child's initial bedtime to an hour later than the usual time of falling asleep; morning wake time, however, remains fixed. Once the sleep problems improve, parents gradually advance bedtime to one that is age-appropriate for the child.[62] (This is similar to the faded bedtime approach.)
Light therapy	Light therapy can be used in children with ASD who present with circadian sleep disorders such as irregular sleep-wake cycle and advanced or delayed sleep-phase syndrome.

Parental education about sleep and sleep hygiene are routinely recommended as part of the behavioral sleep program for children with ASD. Evening routines should promote relaxation, self-soothing with reduced light exposure (dim light) and an optimal temperature, and noise control. Dim light of approximately 15 watts helps to reduce nocturnal anxiety or separation anxiety and does not interfere with the endogenous melatonin secretion.

A visual schedule for bedtime routine has been proposed by Malow and McGrew[58] to train children with ASD to fall asleep on their own. Pictures of the bedtime routine include visual cues of using the bathroom, brushing teeth, getting a drink, reading a book, and getting in bed can be posted on the wall in the child's bedroom to communicate parental expectations.

Graduated behavioral approaches seem to be less stressful for the parents and the child.[59-62] Moore[60] reported a successful intervention for sleep onset and co-sleeping problems in a child with autism using social stories at bedtime. Social stories have been developed for children with autism to help them with understanding daily social situations that are difficult for them to comprehend because of their social communication deficits. A social story includes a book with pictures illustrating bedtime routine and is coupled with positive behavioral reinforcement and graduated extinction.

Co-sleeping and frequent night waking are commonly seen among children with ASD. Many of these children will seem to be unable fall or return to sleep without parental presence. An example of graduated extinction is verbal reassurances, by talking to the child from the hallway, standing outside the room, or using a baby monitor through which parents may speak to and comfort the child while he or she is trying to separate at bedtime and to fall asleep. We also successfully

have used tape or CD recorders with stories recorded by the parent; the child is taught to play them when the parent leaves the room.

Individually designed behavioral sleep interventions have been researched by Wiggs and Stores[63] in children with developmental disabilities including ASD. They have used individually written behavioral programs for sleep that included various interventions such as sleep hygiene, extinction, graduated extinction, and stimulus fading with positive reinforcement. A composite sleep index that included subjective and objective measures of sleep was used to measure the outcome in both an experimental (treatment) and control groups of children. Actigraphy was utilized to quantify sleep before and after treatment in mothers and children. Improvements in sleep were documented after intervention.

Piazza and associates[64] published a case report of a child with autism and severe intellectual disability whose disrupted sleep-wake pattern was treated by a gradual sleep phase delay until the desired bedtime was achieved.

Pharmacologic Interventions

Very limited evidence-based research is available on pharmacologic interventions for sleep disturbances in patients with ASD. According to surveys conducted among the physicians and parents of children with sleep disorders, a wide variety of medications have been prescribed to promote sleep in children with sleep initiation and maintenance problems, especially those who have neurodevelopmental disabilities including ASD.[56,65] Medications that were reported by the parents as most effective included clonidine, chloral hydrate, and hydroxyzine. Fifty percent of parents felt that zolpidem, amitriptyline, or diphenylhydramine was helpful in improving their child's sleep.[56] Alpha-agonists (clonidine, guanfacine) were prescribed by 67% of surveyed child psychiatrists for insomnia in children with mental retardation and developmental disabilities.[65]

Melatonin therapy has been shown to be effective in 70% to 90% of children with neurodevelopmental disorders (see review by Jan and associates[66]). A large retrospective study of over 100 children with ASD demonstrated improved quality of sleep in 85% of children with essentially no adverse reactions.[67] Other reports found melatonin supplementation (at doses ranging from 3-6 mg) effective in improving sleep in children with ASD.[68-70] In clinical practice, it may be appropriate to start treatment with melatonin at a lower dose (1 mg) and gradually increase the dose until clinical improvement is achieved. In most countries, melatonin is available over the counter without a prescription. Melatonin comes in sublingual tablets, liquid form, chewable tablets, tablets, and capsules and should be given approximately 30 minutes before bedtime. Immediate-release melatonin has a short half-life and is rapidly absorbed when given orally.

Controlled-release melatonin has been available for several years and was shown to be effective for sleep maintenance problems in children.[71] A recent controlled study using actigraphy demonstrated effectiveness of the controlled-release formulation of melatonin in children with ASD with increased sleep duration and reductions in sleep onset latency, night-to-night variability in bedtime, and wake time after sleep onset.[70]

The duration of melatonin therapy should depend on the child's response to both behavioral and pharmacologic treatment. To our knowledge there have not been studies investigating the optimal duration of treatment. However, several retrospective studies on the use of melatonin in pediatric patients have shown effectiveness of long-term use of melatonin for several years without evidence of tolerance or side effects.

Successful treatment of co-morbid psychiatric disorders such as ADHD, anxiety, and mood disorders is important in achieving improved sleep regulation in children with ASD.

Interventions in Children with Attention Deficit Hyperactivity Disorder

For children with ADHD, the initial primary focus of treatment should include management of daytime symptoms. A survey conducted among child psychiatrists revealed that alpha agonists (clonidine, guanfacine) were the most commonly prescribed medications for insomnia associated with ADHD.[65] For those with persistent sleep onset difficulty, melatonin has shown significant clinical benefit in both medicated (with other drugs) and unmedicated children.[72] In unmedicated children with rigorously diagnosed ADHD and insomnia, who are participating in a double-blind, placebo-controlled trial, a weight-based dosage (3 mg for children less than 40 kg, 6 mg for children at or above 40 kg) resulted in significantly decreased sleep onset latency and longer total sleep time.[73] Weiss and associates[74] demonstrated significant improvements in sleep onset latency in 20% of a sample of children with ADHD and sleep onset insomnia who were provided with sleep hygiene education (including establishment of regular bedtimes and rise times, with a target of 9.5 hours of sleep) and elimination of naps and caffeine. For those who did not initially respond to sleep hygiene instructions alone, 5 mg of melatonin was

> **BOX 42-1** *Key Facts in the Relationship between Sleep Disturbances and Psychiatric Disorders in Children*
>
> • Children with psychiatric disorders exhibit increased rates of sleep disturbances; children with sleep disturbances exhibit increased rates of psychiatric disorders.
> • A decreased need for sleep may provide one of the best tools to differentiate between ADHD and bipolar disorder in children.
> • As in depression, a reciprocal relationship is theorized to occur between anxiety and sleep: anxiety ⇒ disrupted sleep ⇒ exacerbation of the anxiety ⇒ further sleep disruption.
> • When psychiatric co-morbidity and pharmacotherapy are statistically controlled, children with ADHD do not show a frequency of sleep difficulties statistically different from that in normal control subjects.
> • Treating sleep disturbances in pediatric patients not only may serve to improve sleep and family functioning but in fact may be a protective factor for future development of mood disturbance.
>
> *ADHD*, attention deficit hyperactivity disorder.

added to the regimen 20 minutes before bedtime (as part of a double-blind, placebo-controlled crossover trial), and significant reductions in sleep onset latency were reported.

For a recent review of melatonin treatment for insomnia in children with ADHD, the reader is referred to the article by Bendz and Scates.[75]

CONCLUSION

In summary, sleep complaints are highly prevalent among children and adolescents with psychiatric disorders (Box 42-1). Sleep hygiene and cognitive behavior therapies for insomnia should be utilized first, prior to considering pharmacologic interventions, in children and adolescents with sleep problems associated with these disorders. No agents have been approved by the Food and Drug Administration (FDA) for the treatment of pediatric insomnia, and there is very limited evidence-based research available on the effective use of medications with sedative properties in the treatment of co-morbid insomnia in children with psychiatric disorders. Choosing a behavioral intervention and a pharmacologic agent should be individualized based on the type of sleep problem, primary psychiatric disorder, patient's individual characteristics, family dynamics, and the pharmacologic properties of currently available drugs.

REFERENCES

1. Ivanenko A, Crabtree VM, O'Brien LM, Gozal D. Sleep complaints and psychiatric symptoms in children evaluated at a pediatric mental health clinic. *J Clin Sleep Med.* 2006;15:42-48.
2. Dahl RE. The development and disorders of sleep. *Adv Pediatr.* 1998;45:73-90.
3. Liu X, Buysse DJ, Gentzler AL, Kiss E, Mayer L, et al. Insomnia and hypersomnia associated with depressive phenomenology and comorbidity in childhood depression. *Sleep.* 2007;30:83-90.
4. Whalen DJ, Silk JS, Semel M, Forbes EE, Ryan ND, et al. Caffeine consumption, sleep, and affect in the natural environments of depressed youth and healthy controls. *J Pediatr Psych.* 2008;33:358-367.

5. Ryan ND, Puig-Antich J, Ambrosini P, Rabinovich H, Robinson D, et al. The clinical picture of major depression in children and adolescents. *Arch Gen Psychiatry*. 1987;44:854-861.

6. Roberts RE, Lewinsohn PM, Seeley JR. Symptoms of DSM-III-R major depression in adolescence: Evidence from an epidemiological survey. *J Am Acad Child Adolesc Psychiatry*. 1995;34:1608-1617.

7. Ong SH, Wickramaratne P, Tang M, Weissman MM. Early childhood sleep and eating problems as predictors of adolescent and adult mood and anxiety disorders. *J Affect Disord*. 2006;96:1-8.

8. Gregory AM, Van der Ende J, Willis TA, Verhulst FC. Parent-reported sleep problems during development and self-reported anxiety/depression, attention problems, and aggressive behavior later in life. *Arch Pediatr Adolesc Med*. 2008;162:330-335.

9. Roberts RE, Roberts CR, Chen IG. Impact of insomnia on future functioning of adolescents. *J Psychosom Res*. 2002;53:561-569.

10. Gregory AM, Rijsdijk FV, Lau JYF, Dahl RE, Eley TC. The direction of longitudinal associations between sleep problems and depression symptoms: A study of twins aged 8 and 10 years. *Sleep*. 2009;32:189-199.

11. Patten CA, Choi WS, Gillin JC, Pierce JP. Depressive symptoms and cigarette smoking predict development and persistence of sleep problems in US adolescents. *Pediatrics*. 2000;106:E23.

12. Armitage R, Hoffmann R, Emslie G, Rintelmann J, Moore J, Lewis K. Rest-activity cycles in childhood and adolescent depression. *J Am Acad Child Adolesc Psychiatry*. 2004;43:761-769.

13. Puig-Antich J, Goetz R, Hanlon C, Tabrizi MA, Davies M, Weitzman ED. Sleep architecture and REM sleep measures in prepubertal major depressives. Studies during recovery from the depressive episode in a drug-free state. *Arch Gen Psychiatry*. 1983;40:187-192.

14. National Institute of Mental Health Research Roundtable on prepubertal bipolar disorder. *J Am Acad Child Adolesc Psychiatry*. 2001;40:871-878.

15. Geller B, Zimmerman B, Williams M, DelBello MP, Frazier J, Beringer L. Phenomenology of prepubertal and early adolescent bipolar disorder: Examples of elated mood, grandiose behaviors, decreased need for sleep, racing thoughts, and hypersexuality. *J Child Adolesc Psychopharmacol*. 2002;12:3-9.

16. Geller B, Zimmerman B, Williams M, DelBello MP, Bolhofner K, et al. DSM-IV mania symptoms in a prepubertal and early adolescent bipolar phenotype compared to attention-deficit hyperactive and normal controls. *J Child Adolesc Psychopharmacol*. 2002;12:11-25.

17. Lofthouse N, Fristad M, Splaingard M, Kelleher M. Parent and child reports of sleep problems associated with early-onset bipolar spectrum disorders. *J Fam Psychol*. 2007;21:114-123.

18. Kowatch RA, Youngstrom EA, Danielyan A, Findling RL. Review and meta-analysis of the phenomenology and clinical characteristics of mania in children and adolescents. *Bipolar Disord*. 2005;7:483-496.

19. Meyers OI, Youngstrom EA. A parent general behavior inventory subscale to measure sleep disturbance in pediatric bipolar disorder. *J Clin Psychiatry*. 2008;69:840-843.

20. Lofthouse N, Fristad M, Splaingard M, Kelleher K, Hayes J, Resko S. Web survey of sleep problems associated with early-onset bipolar spectrum disorders. *J Ped Psychol*. 2008;33:349-357.

21. Dahl RE. The regulation of sleep and arousal: Development and psychopathology. *Dev Psychopathol*. 1996;8:3-27.

22. Alfano CA, Ginsburg GS, Kingery JN. Sleep-related problems among children and adolescents with anxiety disorders. *J Am Acad Child Adolesc Psychiatry*. 2007;46:224-232.

23. Alfano CA, Beidel DC, Turner SM, Lewin DS. Preliminary evidence for sleep complaints among children referred for anxiety. *Sleep Med*. 2006;7:467-473.

24. Storch EA, Murphy TK, Lack CW, Geffken GR, Jacob ML, Goodman WK. Sleep-related problems in pediatric obsessive-compulsive disorder. *J Anxiety Disord*. 2008;22:877-885.

25. Sadeh A. Stress, trauma and sleep in children. *Child Adolesc Clin North Am*. 1996;5:685-700.

26. Pynoos RS, Frederick C, Nader K, Arroyo W, Steinberg A, et al. Life threat and posttraumatic stress in school-age children. *Arch Gen Psychiatry*. 1987;44:1057-1063.

27. Ross RJ, Ball WA, Sullivan KA, Caroff SN. Sleep disturbance as the hallmark of posttraumatic stress disorder. *Am J Psychiatry*. 1989;146:697-707.

28. Uhde TW. Anxiety disorders. In: Kryger MH, Roth T, Dement WC, eds. *Principles and Practice of Sleep Medicine*. 3rd ed. Philadelphia: WB Saunders; 2000:1123-1139.

29. Teicher MH, Glod CA, Harper D, Magnus E, Brasher C, et al. Locomotor activity in depressed children and adolescents: I. Circadian dysregulation. *J Am Acad Child Adolesc Psychiatry*. 1993;32:760-769.

30. Glod CA, Teicher MH, Hartman CR, Harakal T. Increased nocturnal activity and impaired sleep maintenance in abused children. *J Am Acad Child Adolesc Psychiatry*. 1997;36:1236-1243.

31. Gregory AM, Caspi A, Eley TC, Moffitt TE, O'Connor TG, Poulton R. Prospective longitudinal associations between persistent sleep problems in childhood and anxiety and depression disorders in adulthood. *J Abnorm Child Psych*. 2005;33:157-163.

32. Gregory AM, O'Connor TG. Sleep problems in childhood: A longitudinal study of developmental change and association with behavioral problems. *J Am Acad Child Adolesc Psychiatry*. 2002;41:964-971.

33. Crabtree VM, Ivanenko A, Gozal D. Clinical and parental assessment of sleep in children with attention-deficit/hyperactivity disorder (ADHD) referred to a pediatric sleep medicine center. *Clin Pediatr*. 2003;42:807-813.

34. Owens J. The ADHD and sleep conundrum: A review. *J Dev Behav Pediatr*. 2005;26:312-322.

35. Cortese S, Faraone S, Konofal E, Lecendreux M. Sleep in children with attention-deficit/hyperactivity disorder: Meta-analysis of subjective and objective studies. *J Am Acad Child Adolesc Psychiatry*. 2009;48:894-908.

36. Cohen-Zion M, Ancoli-Israel S. Sleep in children with attention-deficit hyperactivity disorder (ADHD): A review of naturalistic and stimulant intervention studies. *Sleep Med Rev*. 2004;8:379-402.

37. Corkum P, Moldofsky H, Hogg-Johnson S, Humphries T, Tannock R. Sleep problems in children with attention-deficit/hyperactivity disorder: Impact of subtype, comorbidity, and stimulant medication. *J Am Acad Child Adolesc Psychiatry*. 1999;38:1285-1293.

38. O'Brien LM, Ivanenko A, Crabtree VM, Holbrook CR, Bruner JL, et al. The effect of stimulants on sleep characteristics in children with attention deficit/hyperactivity disorder. *Sleep Med*. 2003;4:309-316.

39. Cockroft K, Ashwal J, Bentley A. Sleep and daytime sleepiness in methylphenidate medicated and un-medicated children with attention-deficit/hyperactivity disorder (ADHD). *Afr J Psychiatry*. 2009;12:275-279.

40. Mick E, Biederman J, Jetton J, Faraone SV. Sleep disturbances associated with attention deficit hyperactivity disorder: The impact of psychiatric comorbidity and pharmacotherapy. *J Child Adolesc Psychopharmacol*. 2000;10:223-231.

41. Tsai MH, Huang YS. Attention-deficit/hyperactivity disorder and sleep disorders in children. *Med Clin North Am*. 2010;94:615-632.

42. American Psychiatric Association. *Diagnostic and Statistical Manual of Mental Disorders*. 4th ed. Washington, DC: American Psychiatric Association; 2000.

43. Cortesi F, Giannotti F, Ivanenko A, Johnson K. Sleep in children with autistic spectrum disorder. *Sleep Med*. 2010;11(7):659-664.

44. Kupfer DJ, Reynolds 3rd CF. Management of insomnia. *N Engl J Med*. 1997;336(5):341-346.

45. Morin CM, Bootzin RR, Buysse DJ, et al. Psychological and behavioral treatment of insomnia: Update of the recent evidence (1998-2004). *Sleep*. 2006;29(11):1398-1414.

46. Bélanger L, Vallières A, Ivers H, Moreau V, Lavigne G, Morin CM. Meta-analysis of sleep changes in control groups of insomnia treatment trials. *J Sleep Res*. 2007;16(1):7-84.

47. Kupfer DJ. Pathophysiology and management of insomnia during depression. *Ann Clin Psychiatry*. 1999;11(4):267-276.

48. Ivanenko A. Sleep and mood disorders in children and adolescents. In: Ivanenko A, ed. *Sleep and Psychiatric Disorders in Children and Adolescents*. New York: Informa Healthcare; 2008:279-287.

49. Mindell JA, Emslie G, Blumer J, et al. Pharmacologic management of insomnia in children and adolescents: Consensus statement. *Pediatrics*. 2006;117(6):E1223-E1232.

50. Owens JA, Babcock D, Blumer J, et al. The use of pharmacotherapy in the treatment of pediatric insomnia in primary care: Rational approaches. A consensus meeting summary. *J Clin Sleep Med*. 2005;1(1):49-59.

51. Ollendick TH, Hagopian LP, Huntzinger RM. Cognitive-behavior therapy with nighttime fearful children. *J Behav Ther Exp Psychiatry*. 1991;22:113-121.

52. Dorsey CM, Lukas SE, Cunningham SL. Fluoxetine-induced sleep disturbance in depressed patients. *Neuropsychopharmacology*. 1996;14:437-442.

53. Armitage R, Emslie G, Rintelmann J. The effect of fluoxetine on sleep EEG in childhood depression: A preliminary report. *Neuropharmacology*. 1997;17:241-245.

54. Kallepalli BR, Bhatara VS, Fogas BS, et al. Trazodone is only slightly faster than fluoxetine in relieving insomnia in adolescents with depressive disorders. *J Child Adolesc Psychopharmacol*. 1997;7:97-107.

55. Wiggs L, Stores G. Severe sleep disturbance and daytime challenging behaviour in children with severe learning disabilities. *J Intell Disabil Res*. 1996;40(6):518-528.

56. Williams G, Sears L, Allard A. Parent perception of efficacy for strategies used to facilitate sleep in children with autism. *J Dev Phys Disabil.* 2006;18(1):25-33.

57. Richdale A, Wiggs L. Behavioral approaches to the treatment of sleep problems in children with developmental disorders: What is the state of the art?. *Int J Behav Consult Ther.* 2005;1(3):165-189.

58. Malow BA, McGrew SG. Sleep Interventions in children with autism spectrum disorders. In: Ivanenko A, ed. *Sleep and Psychiatric Disorders in Children and Adolescents.* New York: Informa Healthcare; 2008:339-349.

59. Piazza CC, Fisher W, Moser H. Behavioral treatment of sleep dysfunction in patients with the Rett syndrome. *Brain Dev.* 1991;13:232-237.

60. Moore PS. The use of social stories in a psychology service for children with learning disabilities: A case study of a sleep problem. *Br J Learn Disabil.* 2004;32:133-138.

61. Howlin P. A brief report on the elimination of long term sleeping problems in a 6-year-old autistic boy. *Behav Psychother.* 1984;12:257-260.

62. Christodulu KV, Durand MV. Reducing bedtime disturbance and night waking using positive bedtime routines and sleep restriction. *Focus Autism Other Dev Disabil.* 2004;19:130-139.

63. Wiggs L, Stores G. Behavioural treatment of sleep problems in children with severe learning disabilities and challenging daytime behaviour: Effect on sleep patterns of mother and child. *J Sleep Res.* 1998;7:119-126.

64. Piazza CC, Hagopian LP, Hughes CR, Fisher WW. Using chronotherapy to treat severe sleep problems. A case study. *Am J Ment Retard.* 1998;102:358-366.

65. Owens JA, Rosen CL, Mindell JA, Kirchner HL. Use of pharmacotherapy for insomnia in child psychiatry practice: A national survey. *Sleep Med.* 2010;11:692-700.

66. Jan JE, Wasdell MB, Reiter RJ, Weiss MD, et al. Melatonin therapy of pediatric sleep disorders: Recent advances, why it works, who are the candidates and how to treat. *Curr Pediatr Rev.* 2007;3:214-224.

67. Andersen IM, Kaczmarska J, McGrew SG, Malow BA. Melatonin for insomnia in children with autism spectrum disorders. *J Child Neurol.* 2008;23(5):482-485.

68. Paavonen EJ, Nieminen-von Wendt T, Vanhala R, Aronen ET, von Wendt L. Effectiveness of melatonin in the treatment of sleep disturbances in children with Asperger disorder. *J Child Adolesc Psychopharmacol.* 2003;13:83-95.

69. Garstang J, Wallis M. Randomized controlled trial of melatonin for children with autistic spectrum disorders and sleep problems. *Child Care Health Dev.* 2006;32(5):585-589.

70. Giannotti F, Cortesi F, Cerquiglini A, Sebastiani T, Vagnoni C, Bernabei P. The treatment of sleep disorders in childhood autism with melatonin or behavioral therapy: A randomized waiting list controlled study. *Sleep.* 2008(31):A58.

71. Jan JE, Hamilton D, Seward N, Fast DK, Freeman RD, Laudon M. Clinical trials of controlled-release melatonin in children with sleep-wake cycle disorders. *J Pineal Res.* 2000;29(1):34-39.

72. Bendz LM, Scates AC. Melatonin treatment for insomnia in pediatric patients with attention-deficit/hyperactivity disorder. *Ann Pharmacother.* 2010;44:185-191.

73. Van der Heijden KB, Smits MG, Van Someren EJ, Ridderinkhof KR, Gunning WB. Effect of melatonin on sleep, behavior, and cognition in ADHD and chronic sleep-onset insomnia. *J Am Acad Child Adolesc Psychiatry.* 2007;46:233-241.

74. Weiss MD, Wasdell MB, Bomben MM, Rea KJ, Freeman RD. Sleep hygiene and melatonin treatment for children and adolescents with ADHD and initial insomnia. *J Am Acad Child Adolesc Psychiatry.* 2006;45:512-519.

75. Bendz LM, Scates AC. Melatonin treatment for insomnia in pediatric patients with attention-deficit/hyperactivity disorder. *Ann Pharmacother.* 2010;44:185-191.

SECTION 10

Parasomnias
in Adults

REM Sleep Parasomnias in Adults:

REM SLEEP BEHAVIOR DISORDER, ISOLATED SLEEP PARALYSIS, AND NIGHTMARE DISORDERS

CARLOS H. SCHENCK / MARK W. MAHOWALD

Chapter
43

REM SLEEP BEHAVIOR DISORDER

…he was thrusting his sword in all directions, speaking out loud as if he were actually fighting a giant. And the strange thing was that he did not have his eyes open, because he was asleep and dreaming that he was battling the giant…. He had stabbed the wine skins so many times, believing that he was stabbing the giant, that the entire room was filled with wine….

MIGUEL DE CERVANTES, *Don Quijote de La Mancha* (1605), page 364, Editorial Juventud, S.A., Barcelona, 1995 edition (translation by CHS)

REM sleep behavior disorder (RBD) is a multifaceted motor, behavioral, and dream disorder of rapid eye movement (REM) sleep.[1,2] It is also a treatable disorder that predominantly affects middle-aged and older males who usually enact distinctly altered dreams that feature confrontation, aggression, and violence[1] (Box 43-1). The vigorous and violent behaviors of RBD commonly result in injury, which at times can be severe and even life-threatening[3,4] (Boxes 43-2 and 43-3). However, there is rarely a daytime tendency for irritability or displays of anger in patients with RBD. A controlled study found that although men with RBD had more aggressive (and less sexual) dreams than control subjects, they did not have an increased tendency for aggressiveness in their waking lives.[5] There has not been one reported case of marital separation or divorce related to RBD, and this finding probably reflects the many decades of marriage prior to the onset of RBD, so the wives of men with RBD understand that the violent dream-enacting behaviors are completely discordant from the usual pleasant waking personality. Nevertheless, RBD can pose serious risks to a marriage. A recently married, young adult Taiwanese woman with RBD attempted suicide because her husband would not sleep with her at night because her RBD disrupted his sleep excessively and compromised his work productivity.[6] Fortunately, once her RBD was diagnosed and effectively treated with clonazepam, the husband resumed sleeping in their conjugal bed, and their marriage was preserved. Some of the self-protection measures taken by the patients (e.g., tethering themselves to the bed, using sleeping bags or pillow barricades, or sleeping on a mattress in an empty room) reveal the recurrent and serious nature of these episodes. The potential for injury to one's self or bed partner raises important and challenging forensic medicine issues.[7] Recently there has been increased recognition of RBD in women, with a tendency for lesser severity, across a spectrum of clinical scenarios.[8]

RBD is the only parasomnia (i.e., sleep-related behavioral and experiential disorder) in the International Classification of Sleep Disorders, 2nd edition (ICSD-2), that requires polysomnographic (PSG) confirmation.[9] There are three reasons for this requirement:

1. The core electromyographic (EMG) abnormalities of RBD are present every night (given a sufficient amount of REM sleep).
2. RBD is not the only dream-enacting disorder in adults, and so objective confirmation is highly desirable.
3. There is a strong probability of future Parkinson's disease (PD) in males 50 years of age or older when initially diagnosed with idiopathic RBD; therefore, it is imperative to objectively diagnose RBD so that affected males (and their families) can be properly informed and be encouraged to plan for the future accordingly.

The core EMG abnormalities of RBD consist of intermittent or continuous loss of the usual skeletal muscle atonia of REM sleep (REM atonia), with increased muscle tone and excessive phasic muscle twitching associated with behavioral release[9] (Box 43-4), as shown in Figure 43-1. Periodic limb movements (PLMs) and nonperiodic twitching during non-REM (NREM) sleep are also common, indicating generalized REM/NREM sleep motor dyscontrol in RBD.[10]

RBD can present either acutely or as a chronic, progressive disorder. Acute RBD usually emerges in the context of alcohol/drug abuse and withdrawal, medication intoxication, other toxic-metabolic states, and acute relapsing multiple sclerosis.[10,11] A recently recognized cause of acute RBD (or acute onset RBD progressing to chronic RBD) involves the therapeutic use of psychotropic medications.[10] Also, excessive caffeine and chocolate ingestion have been implicated in the genesis or exacerbation of RBD.[10]

Chronic RBD may be preceded by a lengthy prodromal period with prominent limb and body movements during sleep and new onset sleep talking.[10] Idiopathic RBD is a chronic progressive disorder, with increasing complexity, intensity, and frequency of expressed behaviors. Although irregular jerking of the limbs may occur nightly (comprising the "minimal RBD syndrome"), the major behavioral episodes appear intermittently with a frequency minimum of usually once every 2 weeks to a maximum of four times nightly for 10 consecutive nights. Sleep talking runs the spectrum from short and garbled utterances to long-winded and clearly articulated speech. Angry speech with shouting and profanity, and also humorous speech with laughter, can emerge. Nonviolent activity involving sitting up, looking around, searching for objects, locomotion (usually running), and engaging in

549

BOX 43-1 *Altered Dream Content Typically Reported in REM Sleep Behavior Disorder*

- Dreams are described as vivid, intense, action-packed, unpleasant, and nightmarish.
- Dreams may involve being threatened or attacked by unfamiliar people, animals, or insects.
- Dreamer rarely is the primary aggressor.
- Dreamer often reports defending his wife (in the dream, whereas in reality he may actually be beating her in bed).

REM, rapid eye movement.

BOX 43-2 *Injuries to Patient and Bed Partner Resulting from REM Sleep Behavior Disorder*

- Bruises
- Subdural hematomas
- Lacerations (including arteries, nerves, tendons)
- Fractures (including high cervical fractures)
- Dislocations, sprains, abrasions, rug burns
- Tooth chipping, hair pulling

REM, rapid eye movement.

BOX 43-3 *Published Cases of REM Sleep Behavior Disorder Associated with Potentially Lethal Behaviors*

Choking/headlock	$N = 22\text{-}24$
Diving from bed	$N = 10$
Defenestration	$N = 7$
Punching a pregnant bed partner	$N = 2$

REM, rapid eye movement.
Data from Schenck CH, Lee SA, Cramer Bornemann MA, Mahowald MW. Potentially lethal behaviors associated with rapid eye movement sleep behavior disorder (RBD): Review of the literature and forensic implications. *J Forensic Sci.* 2009;54:6.

BOX 43-4 *Diagnostic Criteria for REM Sleep Behavior Disorder*

- Presence of REM sleep without atonia: excessive sustained or intermittent elevation of submental EMG tone or excessive phasic submental or (upper or lower) limb EMG twitching.
- Presence of at least one of the following:
  - Sleep-related injurious, potentially injurious, or disruptive behaviors by history
  - Abnormal REM sleep behaviors documented during polysomnographic monitoring
  - Absence of EEG epileptiform activity during REM sleep unless RBD can be clearly distinguished from any concurrent REM sleep-related seizure disorder
- The sleep disturbance is not better explained by another sleep disorder, medical or neurologic disorder, mental disorder, medication use, or substance use disorder.

EEG, electroencephalography; *EMG,* electromyography; *REM,* rapid eye movement.
Data from American Academy of Sleep Medicine. International Classification of Sleep Disorders, 2nd ed.: *Diagnostic and Coding Manual.* Westchester, IL: American Academy of Sleep Medicine; 2005.

---

various other activities can also occur[12] (Box 43-5). All categories of behaviors found in human RBD are mirrored in an experimental animal model of RBD produced by pontine tegmental lesions.[1]

Most patients with RBD who present for clinical evaluation complain of sleep injury and rarely of sleep disruption. They usually do not awaken from their own complex activity (unless stunned from an injury), but rather from the yelling of their wives who are being struck or choked. Two conclusions can be drawn from these observations: first, chronic RBD is primarily a motor-behavioral disorder and uncommonly also an arousal disorder; and, second, the very high arousal threshold in RBD constitutes another physiologic marker of REM sleep, which is known to have the highest threshold for arousal compared to NREM sleep.[10] In addition, the autonomic nervous system is generally not activated during episodes of vigorous or violent RBD activity, with a concurrent absence of tachycardia, as shown in Figure 43-1. For patients with RBD, arousal from a dream-enacting episode typically results in rapid alertness and orientation as well as detailed dream recall, all typical of most REM sleep awakenings, including those associated with nightmares. This type is very different from the confusional arousals from slow wave sleep found with sleepwalking and sleep terrors. After awakenings from RBD episodes, behavior and social interactions are appropriate, mitigating against either a NREM sleep phenomenon, delirious state, or ictal phenomenon.

Any patient suspected of having RBD should undergo a systematic evaluation consisting of the following:

1. Review of sleep/wake complaints (from patient and bed partner)
2. Neurologic and psychiatric examinations
3. A sleep laboratory study that includes continuous videotaping of behavior during standard PSG monitoring[13]

of the electro-oculogram (EOG), electroencephalogram (EEG), EMG (submental, lower/upper extremity muscles), electrocardiogram (ECG), oral-nasal airflow, respiratory effort along with written notations of observed behaviors by a certified technician.

Because of the association between RBD and narcolepsy, serious consideration should be given to administering a multiple sleep latency test (MSLT) the day following the overnight PSG study to document the presence or absence of objective hypersomnia and sleep onset REM episodes.

More extensive neurologic testing, including magnetic resonance brain imaging and comprehensive neuropsychological testing,[14] may also be warranted (Boxes 43-6 to 43-8).[15]

Parasomnia Overlap Disorder

A variant of RBD has been identified with PSG-documented overlapping parasomnias consisting of sleepwalking, sleep terrors, and RBD.[9,16] In addition to the RBD findings of absence of atonia in REM and (usually) the increased PLMs and nonperiodic limb movements during NREM sleep, these cases demonstrate additional motor-behavioral dyscontrol during NREM sleep. At least in these instances, the

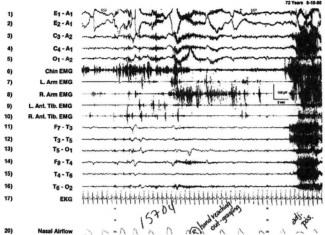

Figure 43-1 REM sleep polysomnogram of an older man with RBD and future PD. Intense, selective activation of the right arm EMG at 1:57:04 AM correlates with the observation, written down on the tracing by the attendant sleep technologist, of the "right hand reaching out-grasping." During this right arm EMG activation, there is pronounced suppression of the submental EMG tone (channel 6) that nearly restores the normal background "REM atonia." Preceding this activity, the submental EMG shows prominent, prolonged activation ("loss of REM atonia") unassociated with any behavioral release. The phasic and tonic motor activation seen in this tracing is not accompanied by any increased heart rate (channel 17), which is typical for RBD and is in stark contrast to the intense tachycardia found during sleep terrors arising from deep NREM sleep. The EEG (channels 3-5, 11-16) shows a typical REM sleep activation (low voltage, fast frequency) without any epileptiform activity. High-voltage rapid eye movement tracings (channels 1-2) are present in the first two thirds of this tracing and represent another form of phasic motor activation. EMG: channels 6-10; electro-oculogram: channels 1-2. *EEG,* electroencephalogram; *EMG,* electromyogram; *NREM,* non-REM; *RBD,* REM sleep behavior disorder; *REM,* rapid eye movement.

BOX 43-5 *Pleasant, Nonaggressive Behaviors Found in REM Sleep Behavior Disorder*

- Laughing, singing, giving speeches, whistling, dancing
- Clapping, "thumbs up" gesturing at someone
- Smoking a fictive cigarette, greeting someone
- Searching for a treasure
- Dealing textiles

REM, rapid eye movement.
 Data from Oudiette D, De Cock VC, Lavault S, Leu S, Vidailhet M, Arnulf I. Nonviolent elaborate behaviors may also occur in REM sleep behavior disorder. *Neurology.* 2009;72:551-557.

BOX 43-6 *Differential Diagnosis for Dream-Enacting Behaviors in Adults*

- REM sleep behavior disorder
- Sleepwalking and sleep terrors
- Obstructive sleep apnea ("OSA pseudo-RBD")[15]
- Nocturnal seizures (especially complex partial seizures)
- Malingering

RBD, REM sleep behavior disorder; *REM,* rapid eye movement.

BOX 43-7 *Etiologic Associations with Chronic REM Sleep Behavior Disorder*

- Idiopathic (cryptogenic?)
- Neurologic disorders
- Medication-induced
  - SSRIs, venlafaxine, mirtazapine, TCAs, MAOIs
  - Beta blockers (bisoprolol, atenolol)
  - Anticholinesterase inhibitors
  - Selegiline
- Caffeine, chocolate (when consumed in excess)

MAOIs, monoamine oxidase inhibitors; *REM,* rapid eye movement; *SSRIs,* selective serotonin reuptake inhibitors; *TCAs,* tricyclic antidepressants.

BOX 43-8 *Neurologic Disorders Most Commonly Linked with Chronic REM Sleep Behavior Disorder*

- Neurodegenerative disorders (especially parkinsonian disorders)
- Narcolepsy-cataplexy
- Cerebrovascular disorders

NOTE: Virtually all categories of neurologic disorders can trigger RBD, including toxic-metabolic, vascular, neoplastic, infectious, postinfectious, autoimmune, degenerative, developmental, congenital, and familial disorders.
 REM, rapid eye movement.

---

possibility of a unifying hypothesis for their disorders of arousal and RBD is suggested. The primary underlying feature is motor disinhibition during sleep—when it predominately occurs during NREM sleep, it manifests as a disorder of arousal, and when it predominately occurs during REM sleep, it manifests as RBD—with the parasomnia overlap disorder occupying an intermediate or mixed position, with features of both.

 In a series of 33 patients,[16] the mean age of parasomnia onset was 15 years (range: 1-66), and 70% ($N = 23$) were males. An idiopathic subgroup ($N = 22$) had a significantly earlier mean age of parasomnia onset (9 years; range: 1-28) than a symptomatic subgroup ($N = 11$) (27 years; range: 5-66), whose parasomnia began with a neurologic disorders ($N = 6$) (congenital Möbius syndrome; narcolepsy; multiple sclerosis; brain tumor [and treatment]; brain trauma; indeterminate disorder [exaggerated startle response/atypical cataplexy]); nocturnal paroxysmal atrial fibrillation ($N = 1$); post-traumatic stress disorder (PTSD)/major depression ($N = 1$); chronic ethanol/amphetamine abuse and withdrawal ($N = 1$); or mixed disorders (schizophrenia; brain trauma; substance abuse) ($N = 2$).

Epidemiology and Risk Factors

A phone survey of nearly 5000 individuals between the ages of 15 and 100 years of age indicated an overall prevalence of violent behaviors during sleep of 2%, one quarter of which were *likely* due to RBD, giving an estimated overall prevalence of RBD at 0.5%.[17] Another survey estimated the prevalence of RBD to be 0.38% in *elderly* individuals[18] (however, this is most likely an underestimate for this population, and the true prevalence of RBD in older adults may be > 1%).

As more patients with "idiopathic" RBD are carefully followed over time, it is becoming clear that the majority will eventually develop neurodegenerative disorders, most notably the synucleinopathies (PD, multiple system atrophy (MSA) including olivopontocerebellar degeneration and the Shy-Drager syndrome, dementia with Lewy body disease, or pure autonomic failure). RBD may be the first manifestation of these conditions and may precede any other manifestation of the underlying neurodegenerative process by more than 10 years—and for even as long as 50 years.[19-23]

Combined animal and human studies have identified physiologic and anatomic links between RBD and neurodegenerative disorders, leading to the proposal that neurodegeneration can begin in either the rostroventral midbrain or the ventral mesopontine junction and progressively extend to the rostral or caudal part of the brainstem. When the lesion starts in the ventral mesopontine region, RBD will develop first, but when the lesion initially involves the rostroventral midbrain, PD will be the initial manifestation.[24]

Systematic longitudinal study of patients with such neurologic syndromes indicates that RBD and REM sleep without atonia may be far more prevalent than previously suspected. Although the prevalence of RBD in PD is not definitively known, various subjective reports indicate that 25% of patients with PD have behaviors suggestive of RBD or sleep-related injurious behaviors, and PSG studies have found RBD in up to 47% of patients with PD with sleep complaints.[25-28] In one large series of patients with MSA, 90% were found to have REM sleep without atonia and 69% had clinical RBD.[29] The presentation of RBD with dementia so strongly suggests "dementia with Lewy bodies" that RBD has been proposed as one of the core diagnostic features of dementia with Lewy body disease.[30]

The link between PD and RBD is supported by the fact that impaired olfactory and color discrimination is common to both.[31,32] Also, the presence of cognitive deficits and slowing in the waking EEG in idiopathic RBD share common features with dementia with Lewy body disease.[23] The clinical features of RBD are identical in the idiopathic cases and in those with PD or MSA.[33] Interestingly, there is a striking male predominance in patients with PD who display RBD,[32] although somewhat less than the male predominance found in idiopathic RBD.

RBD and Narcolepsy

RBD is present in over half of patients with narcolepsy, and may be a presenting symptom in narcolepsy, including childhood narcolepsy.[34-37] Furthermore, tricyclic antidepressants, selective serotonin reuptake inhibitors (SSRIs), and venlafaxine, prescribed to treat cataplexy, can trigger or exacerbate RBD in narcoleptics.[10] The demographics (age and sex) of RBD in narcolepsy conform to those of narcolepsy (i.e., younger adults, and no gender predominance), indicating that RBD in these patients is yet another manifestation of state boundary dyscontrol (primarily REM sleep-wakefulness boundaries) seen in narcolepsy.[34] It is intriguing to note the

pathologic mirror images in motor dyscontrol involves sudden inappropriate atonia during wakefulness (in cataplexy) and inappropriately increased muscle tone during REM sleep (in RBD).

Pathophysiology

The generalized atonia of REM sleep results from active inhibition of motor activity by pontine centers of the peri-locus ceruleus region which exert an excitatory influence upon the reticularis magnocellularis nucleus of the medulla via the lateral tegmentoreticular tract. The reticularis magnocellularis nucleus, in turn, hyperpolarizes spinal motor neuron postsynaptic membranes via the ventrolateral reticulospinal tract.[1,38] Loss of muscle tone during REM sleep is very complex, and has been shown to be due to a combination of activation of brainstem motor inhibitory systems and deactivation of brainstem motor facilitatory systems. Normally the atonia of REM sleep is briefly interrupted by excitatory inputs, which produce the REMs and the muscle jerks and twitches characteristic of REM sleep.

Neuroimaging studies indicate dopaminergic abnormalities in RBD. Single photon emission computed tomography (SPECT) studies have found reduced striatal dopamine transporters, and decreased striatal dopaminergic innervation.[23,32] Positron emission tomography (PET) and SPECT studies have revealed decreased nigrostriatal dopaminergic projections in patients with MSA and RBD.[23,32] Impaired cortical activation as determined by EEG spectral analysis in patients with idiopathic RBD supports the relationship between RBD and neurodegenerative disorders.[39]

The overwhelming male predominance in RBD begs the question of hormonal influences, as suggested in male aggression studies in both animals and humans. However, serum sex hormone levels are normal in idiopathic RBD and in RBD associated with PD.[40,41] Another possible explanation for the male predominance is sex differences in brain development and aging.

Treatment of RBD

Ensuring the maximum safety of the sleeping environment should always be of paramount importance in conjunction with pharmacotherapy (or other somatic therapy) of RBD (Boxes 43-9 and 43-10). Clonazepam is the cornerstone for treating RBD in most cases, with the usual dose range being 0.25 mg to 2.0 mg at bedtime, extending up to 4 mg.[1] It was originally found to be effective in the first RBD patients identified in the index series at the Minnesota Regional Sleep Disorders Center.[1] These patients also had PLMs of NREM sleep, a PSG finding that in the 1980s was called "nocturnal myoclonus," that could be associated with the clinical complaint of sleep disruption. Case reports and case series in those years indicated that bedtime clonazepam was effective in controlling symptomatic "nocturnal myoclonus." Because our original RBD patients had PLMs of NREM sleep besides their RBD (a finding confirmed in over 60% of RBD patients subsequently reported in the worldwide literature), we decided to treat the RBD of our first patients with bedtime clonazepam in the hope that this medication would be successful in controlling a newly identified motor-behavioral disorder of REM sleep. We then realized that the clonazepam not only

BOX 43-9 *Treatment of REM Sleep Behavior Disorder: Initial Environmental Considerations*

To maximize the safety of the sleeping environment:
- Move bedside table and other hard objects away from the bed.
- Move bed away from the window.
- Place mattress on the floor.
- Have bed partner move to a separate bed or separate bedroom.

REM, rapid eye movement.

BOX 43-11 *Long-Term Benefits of Clonazepam in REM Sleep Behavior Disorder*[*]

• Initial nightly dose:	0.63 ± 0.40 mg
• Latest follow-up dose:	0.97 ± 0.89 mg
• Paired *t*-test:	No statistical difference
• Duration of treatment:	3.7 ± 2.3 years

[*]Without dosage tolerance (paired *t*-test) ($N = 49$).
 REM, rapid eye movement.
 Data from Schenck CH, Mahowald MW. Long-term, nightly benzodiazepine treatment of injurious parasomnias and other disorders of disrupted nocturnal sleep in 170 adults. *Am J Med.* 1996;100:333-337.

BOX 43-10 *Effective Pharmacologic Agents/Therapies for REM Sleep Behavior Disorder*

- Clonazepam
- Melatonin
- Pramipexole
- Levodopa
- Carbamazepine
- Clonidine
- Paroxetine
- Tricyclic antidepressants (desipramine, imipramine)
- Monoamine oxidase inhibitors
- Yi-gan san
- Zopiclone
- Temazepam
- Sodium oxybate
- Acetylcholinesterase inhibitors (donepezil, rivastigmine)
- Immunosuppressive therapy (in autoimmune limbic encephalitis)
- Pallidotomy (in RBD with PD)
- Customized bed alarm

REM, rapid eye movement.

controlled the abnormal behaviors of RBD, but also the disturbed dreaming that is almost as much the hallmark of RBD as the problematic behaviors. This linked benefit suggested a common pathophysiologic mechanism for generating the disturbed dreaming and abnormal behaviors of RBD, with a focus on brainstem motor pattern generators as encompassed by the "activation-synthesis" model of dream generation proposed by Hobson and McCarley[41a] (Bodkin and Schenck[8] discuss RBD, its dream disturbances, and this particular dream model).

A number of large case series totaling over 250 RBD patients have reported a response rate to clonazepam therapy of 87% to 90%.[1] Clonazepam is not usually associated with dosage tolerance (habituation effect), despite years of nightly therapy[42] (Box 43-11). The mechanism of action appears to be suppression of the excessive phasic motor-behavioral activity rather than restoration of REM atonia. Nevertheless, the literature is devoid of any double-blind, controlled, randomized trials of clonazepam therapy of RBD.[43,44] However, given the recurrent injuries usually associated with RBD (with major morbidity and potential lethality), it is doubtful that an ethical treatment trial can be devised with the approval of an

institutional review board. If such a trial could be devised and conducted in cases of milder RBD (i.e., not associated with violent behaviors), then the findings would not necessarily be considered generalizable to the more aggressive and violent cases of RBD.

Clonazepam side effects at times can occur with RBD, and include morning sedation, memory dysfunction, depression and personality changes (emerging at the outset of therapy), erectile dysfunction, hair loss, gastroesophageal reflux, and aggravation of obstructive sleep apnea (OSA). Underlying OSA should be ruled out before prescribing clonazepam.[45]

A recognized second-line (or co-first-line) therapy of RBD is bedtime melatonin at robust pharmacologic doses; doses ranging from 3 to 12 mg have been reported effective,[45-49a] and unpublished observations suggest that doses up to 15 mg may be useful. The mechanism of action appears to be partial restoration (up to 50%) of REM atonia. Therefore, combined melatonin-clonazepam therapy holds the appeal of utilizing complementary mechanisms of action on the tonic and phasic motor systems disturbed during REM sleep in RBD. Melatonin efficacy has been reported in four case series of idiopathic and symptomatic RBD totaling 43 patients,[46-49] and also in a case report of RBD with Alzheimer's disease.[50] Also, it was found in the first double-blind, placebo-controlled treatment study of RBD that melatonin (3 mg) was effective in seven of eight patients with idiopathic or symptomatic RBD.[49a] Side effects can include morning sedation and headaches.

Pramipexole, a dopamine receptor agonist, in two case series has been shown to be effective in 63% to 89% of patients with idiopathic RBD or RBD associated with mild cognitive impairment or mild PD.[51,52] On the other hand, a prospective study of patients with combined RBD-PD found no benefit when pramipexole was added to a stable levodopa regimen.[53] When used to treat RBD, the starting dose of pramipexole should be 0.125 mg at bedtime, with gradual increments by 0.125 mg up to a maximum of 2 to 4 mg at bedtime. Levodopa therapy for RBD has also been reported, but also with mixed results in patients with PD or dementia with Lewy bodies. A systematic study of 70 PD patients found that those with RBD generally used higher doses of levodopa than those without RBD in the context of comparable disease severity, suggesting a lack of substantial benefit of levodopa in treating RBD.[54] A perplexing contrast raised by these mixed therapeutic findings with pramipexole and levodopa therapy of RBD is that although these medications are usually successful in treating a major co-morbidity of RBD (i.e., PD), they are often considered third-line therapy of RBD.

Acetylcholinesterase inhibitors (AIs), which can also trigger RBD,[55] have been reported to be effective as therapy of idiopathic RBD. Donepezil has been reported in two case series of idiopathic RBD patients, with benefit identified in the 10- to 20-mg dose range.[56,57] Rivastigmine, in doses up to 6 mg at bedtime, was also reported to be effective. In these cases, it was proposed that enhancing central cholinergic neurotransmission with AI therapy could control RBD not associated with dementia.

Other therapies of RBD reported to be beneficial in case reports and small case series include clonidine (a potent suppressor of REM sleep),[58] desipramine/imipramine (tricyclic antidepressants that can also trigger or aggravate RBD),[1,8,59] paroxetine (in Japanese patients),[60,61] monoamine oxidase inhibitors,[62] carbamazepine,[63] gabapentin,[10] zopiclone,[64] temazepam,[64] and sodium oxybate (which is an effective anticataplectic agent).[65] The finding that paroxetine, an SSRI that can trigger or aggravate RBD in Caucasians[66]—along with fluoxetine[67] and other SSRIs[10]—was effective in controlling RBD in Japanese patients,[60,61] raises questions about racially mediated, divergent pharmacologic responses in RBD.

The herbal preparation *yi-gan san*, whose prescription is approved in Japan for treating insomnia, contains seven herbal ingredients, including *Angelicae redix* that has been reported to affect serotonin (5-HT$_2$) and γ-aminobutyric acid (GABA) receptors. Data on its use in RBD is limited to three cases from Japan, a 60-year-old man and 74- and 87-year-old women with aggressive dream-enactment, who reportedly responded to *yi-gan san* therapy taken at a dose of 2.5 g ($n = 1$) or 7.5 g ($n = 2$), with one patient also taking low-dose clonazepam (0.25 mg).[68]

Best practice guidelines for the pharmacotherapy of RBD have recently been published by the American Academy of Sleep Medicine.[69]

Immunosuppressive therapy (cycles of intravenous [IV] immunoglobulin and corticosteroids for more than 1 year) induced complete resolution of RBD in tandem with remission of autoimmune limbic encephalitis in three patients with potassium channel antibody-associated limbic encephalitis.[70] In contrast, RBD persisted in two patients with partial resolution of the limbic syndrome. (As an aside, these findings suggest that impairment of the limbic system may play a role in the pathogenesis of RBD, including the hyperemotional dream disturbances that are often enacted during RBD episodes.)

Pallidotomy has been effective in one case of RBD associated with PD,[71] whereas chronic bilateral subthalamic stimulation was not effective for RBD.[72,73] Interestingly, an isolated episode of RBD has been reported immediately following left subthalamic electrode implantation for the treatment of PD.[74] A novel nonpharmacologic therapy has been found to abort incipient RBD episodes involving a pressurized bed alarm system triggering a prerecorded calming message by the spouse or patient.[74a]

Finally, successful control of RBD with appropriate pharmacotherapy, or other somatic therapy, usually then also controls the "environmental sleep disorder,"[9] involving chronic, recurrent sleep disruption, in the spouse (typically the wife). This demonstrates how effective sleep therapy of one person can restore normal, uneventful sleep in the bed partner. These positive outcome scenarios, together with the stories shared by patients and spouses about the repeated hazards posed by chronic RBD (and various other parasomnias), are described in the DVD documentary film, "Sleep Runners: The Stories Behind Everyday Parasomnias."[74b]

RECURRENT ISOLATED SLEEP PARALYSIS

Sleep paralysis is essentially the atonia of REM sleep that has become dissociated and emerges inappropriately at times other than the typical periods of REM sleep during the night. It can either intrude into light NREM sleep at sleep onset or persist into awakening at the offset of REM or NREM sleep. In either case, its occurrence during sleep-wake transitions is often experienced as discomforting or frightening. It is typically found in association with narcolepsy, a disorder exhibiting multiple forms of REM sleep-wakefulness dissociations, but it is not specific to narcolepsy.[9] Sleep paralysis is similar to cataplexy, a state involving the intrusion of REM atonia during a period of full wakefulness. Unless the history includes hypersomnia or cataplexy, there is no need for a PSG evaluation of isolated sleep paralysis.[9]

Isolated sleep paralysis is characterized by an inability to perform voluntary movements at sleep onset, or upon awakening from sleep, in the absence of a diagnosis of narcolepsy[9] (Box 43-12). An episode is characterized by an inability to speak or to move the limbs, trunk, or head. The ability to breathe is usually not affected. Consciousness is preserved and full recall occurs. An episode of sleep paralysis can last from seconds to minutes. It usually resolves spontaneously, but can be aborted by sensory stimulation such as being touched or spoken to, or by the patient making a strong effort to move. The frequency of episodes varies greatly, from once in a lifetime to several times a year. During at least the initial episodes, intense anxiety is usually present, given the striking and novel experience of paralysis. Hallucinatory experiences may accompany the paralysis in about 25% to 75% of patients and may include auditory, visual, or tactile hallucinations or the sense of a presence in the room.

Sleep paralysis is known throughout the world, often with local expressions being used for this phenomenon, such as "kanashibari" in Japan, "ghost oppression" in China, and the "old hag" phenomenon in Newfoundland.

Most studies—usually of students under 30 years of age—from various countries suggest a 15% to 40% prevalence of at least one episode of sleep paralysis. No consistent gender differences have emerged from multiple studies. The mean age of onset is 14 to 17 years, although onset earlier and later in life

---

BOX 43-12 *Diagnostic Criteria for Isolated Sleep Paralysis*

- The patient complains of inability to move the trunk and all limbs at sleep onset or on waking from sleep.
- Each episode lasts seconds to a few minutes.
- Hallucinatory experiences may be present but are not essential to the diagnosis.
- Cataplexy is not present, and there are no other clinical or laboratory features suggesting a diagnosis of narcolepsy.
- Polysomnography, if performed, reveals the event to occur in a dissociated state with elements of REM sleep and wakefulness.

REM, rapid eye movement.
Data from American Academy of Sleep Medicine. International Classification of Sleep Disorders, 2nd ed. *Diagnostic and Coding Manual.* Westchester, IL: American Academy of Sleep Medicine; 2005.

has been reported. Most events appear to occur in the second and third decades, but may continue later in life. There are no known complications, apart from anxiety over the episodes.

Sleep deprivation and irregular sleep-wake schedules can precipitate episodes of sleep paralysis. Mental stress has been reported as a precipitating factor in some studies. Sleep paralysis appears more commonly with sleep in the supine position. Personality factors have usually not been shown to play a major role. Two families with apparent familial sleep paralysis occurring over three and four generations have been reported.[9] The authors postulate a maternal form of transmission.

Episodes of sleep paralysis elicited by awakening patients from sleep during the night tend to arise from REM sleep. The presence of early onset REM sleep after forced awakenings has been shown to predispose to sleep paralysis. It may be that subjects with less tolerance to sleep disruption are more likely to experience the phenomenon. Studies of sleep paralysis arising after forced awakenings during the night have shown onset chiefly from REM sleep. During the episodes, the PSG shows a dissociated state with either intrusion of alpha rhythm into REM sleep or persistence of REM atonia into wakefulness. The common feature is EMG atonia during the episode of paralysis.

The differential diagnosis of isolated sleep paralysis includes various conditions. Transient compression neuropathies may affect the radial, ulnar, median, or other nerves during the night and may be experienced by the individual as a form of paralysis or paresis. These neuropathies are usually unilateral and involve only a single limb. Paresthesias and numbness are usually present. Cataplexy produces similar generalized paralysis of skeletal muscles, but is a phenomenon of wakefulness precipitated by intense, abrupt emotional states. Atonic seizures occur during wakefulness. Nocturnal panic attacks are not usually associated with paralysis. Conversion disorders may mimic sleep paralysis, but the clinical features are usually sufficiently clear to make their distinction with ease. Familial periodic paralysis syndromes, especially hypokalemic periodic paralysis, may occur at rest and on awakening. However, the episodes usually last hours, may be associated with carbohydrate intake, and are usually accompanied by hypokalemia. There are also hyperkalemic and normokalemic periodic paralysis syndromes.

Treatment is usually unnecessary, apart from reassurance about the benign basis of the phenomenon, unless there is frequent recurrence, substantial sleep disruption, or excessive subjective distress. In such cases, REM suppressing agents, such as imipramine taken at bedtime (10-100 mg), or fluoxetine (10-20 mg) may be indicated.[75]

NIGHTMARE DISORDER

Nightmare disorder is characterized by recurrent nightmares, which are disturbing mental experiences that generally occur during REM sleep and result in awakening.[9] Nightmares are coherent dream sequences that seem real and become increasingly more disturbing as they unfold. Emotions usually involve anxiety, fear, or terror but frequently also anger, rage, embarrassment, disgust, and other negative feelings. Dream content most often focuses on imminent physical danger to the individual but may also involve other distressing themes. Nightmares should be distinguished from sleep terrors that arise abruptly from slow wave NREM sleep and are usually devoid of dream content, apart from some occasional fragmentary, frightening images that trigger (or are in response to) a "flight-or-fight response." The ability to detail the nightmare's contents upon awakening is common in nightmare disorder. Because nightmares typically arise during REM sleep, they may occur at any moment that REM propensity is high. Multiple nightmares within a single sleep episode may occur and may bear similar themes. Nightmares arising either immediately following a trauma (acute stress disorder ASD) or 1 month or more after a trauma (PTSD) can occur during NREM sleep, especially stage 2, as well as during REM sleep and at sleep onset. Post-traumatic nightmares may take the form of a realistic reliving of a traumatic event or depict only some of its elements. Postawakening anxiety and difficulty returning to sleep may be present (Box 43-13).

From 50% to 85% of adults report at least an occasional nightmare. Approximately 2% to 8% of the general population has a current problem with nightmares and this frequency is higher in clinical populations. Trauma-related nightmares are the most consistent problem reported by PTSD patients. Nightmares beginning within 3 months of a trauma are present in up to 80% of PTSD patients and predict delayed onset of PTSD. Although approximately 50% of PTSD cases resolve within 3 months, post-traumatic nightmares can persist throughout life. In adolescents and adults, women more frequently report nightmares and more readily discuss them.

Frequent nightmares are associated with enduring personality characteristics and psychopathologies, and they are inversely correlated with measures of well-being.[76,77] Associations with psychopathology have been detected for adults and adolescents. Measures of nightmare distress are much more robustly associated with psychopathology than are measures of nightmare frequency. Predisposing factors for ASD- and PTSD-associated nightmares include female gender, low socioeconomic and educational levels, and prior psychopathology. The severity, duration, and proximity of a traumatic event are the most important risk factors for PTSD. Social support, family history, childhood experiences, personality variables, and preexisting mental disorders may affect the development of ASD or PTSD. However, the disorder can develop in individuals without clear predisposing conditions, particularly if the stressor is extreme.

BOX 43-13 *Diagnostic Criteria for Nightmare Disorder*

- Recurrent episodes of awakenings from sleep with recall of intensely disturbing dream mentation, usually involving fear or anxiety but also anger, sadness, disgust and other dysphoric emotions.
- Recall of sleep mentation is immediate and clear.
- Alertness is full immediately on awakening, with little confusion or disorientation.
- Associated features include at least one of the following:
  - Return to sleep after the episodes is typically delayed and not rapid OR
  - Occurrence of episodes in the later half of the habitual sleep period

Data from American Academy of Sleep Medicine. International Classification of Sleep Disorders, 2nd ed. *Diagnostic and Coding Manual.* Westchester, IL: American Academy of Sleep Medicine; 2005.

The clinical use of pharmacologic agents affecting the neurotransmitters norepinephrine, serotonin, and dopamine are associated with the complaint of nightmares.[78] A majority of these agents are antidepressants, antihypertensives, and dopamine agonists. Agents affecting the neurotransmitters GABA, acetylcholine, and histamine as well as agents affecting the sleep-related immunologic response to infectious disease can be associated with the complaint of nightmares, including antiseizure, anesthetic, antibiotic, and antiviral medications.[78] Acute withdrawal from REM suppressing agents (e.g., tricyclic antidepressants, monoamine oxidase inhibitors, clonidine, alcohol, and amphetamines) may cause nightmares as a result of REM sleep rebound.

Nightmares generally diminish in frequency and intensity over the course of decades, but some patients at the age of 60 or 70 years still describe frequent episodes. Nightmare disorder can lead to sleep avoidance, sleep deprivation, and more intense nightmares, which can produce insomnia and daytime sleepiness. Nightmares associated with ASD and PTSD can develop at any age after physical or emotional trauma. Individuals with PTSD are at risk for depression and other mood disorders, adverse social and employment consequences, self-destructive and impulsive behavior, and substance abuse; it is not known to what extent the nightmares symptomatic of PTSD contribute to these complications.

If a nightmare disorder is apparently triggered by a particular medication, then a concerted effort should be attempted (including consulting with the prescribing physician) to discontinue that medication, if at all possible. Also, if a nightmare disorder is not associated with identified adverse affects on nocturnal or daytime functioning, then therapy may not be required apart from providing a diagnosis followed by reassurance. Adults with nightmares respond positively to the knowledge that non-trauma-associated nightmares do not necessarily indicate past or current trauma/abuse or psychiatric illness, and may be associated with creative personality characteristics. Recurrent nightmares often respond to behavioral approaches to therapy (e.g., desensitization and imagery rehearsal).[79] This approach deemphasizes discussion of any traumatic association of nightmares, emphasizing instead habitual pattern of recurrent nightmares. The nightmare sufferer is asked to change one of his nightmares "in any way you wish." They are then advised to rehearse the "new" dream while awake. Patients are taught to restructure the disturbing dream scenario into a more acceptable experience by rewriting the script as an exercise during wakefulness.[79] This therapeutic approach treats the nightmares as a sleep disturbance rather than a manifestation of specific psychopathology. Instruction in lucid dreaming as therapy of nightmares has also been cited in a case report.[80]

Pharmacotherapy, based largely on experience with PTSD, includes reported benefit with cyproheptadine and prazosin, guanfacine, clonidine, and other agents.[81-83] This approach can be coupled with cognitive therapy of insomnia that includes sleep hygiene, stimulus control, and sleep restriction.

SUMMARY

The main features of REM sleep are brain activation and dreaming along with tonic and phasic motor discharges that are largely suppressed due to generalized motor inhibition. Overactivation of some systems, insufficient suppression of others, or altered timing of activation and suppression, can lead to disorders associated with REM sleep, the so-called REM parasomnias. Overly intense dreaming leads to nightmares, overly active motor activity and/or insufficient motor suppression leads to RBD, and altered timing of motor inhibition leads to isolated sleep paralysis. The causes of these dysfunctions are many and include drug effects, neurodegenerative disease, and normal variation. Understanding their etiology is important to making proper diagnosis and designing proper care.

REFERENCES

1. Schenck CH, Mahowald MW. REM sleep behavior disorder: Clinical, developmental, and neuroscience perspectives 16 years after its formal identification in SLEEP. *Sleep*. 2002;25:120-138.
2. Mahowald MW, Schenck CH. The REM sleep behavior disorder odyssey [editorial]. *Sleep Med Rev*. 2009;13:381-384.
3. Schenck CH, Hurwitz TD, Bundlie SR, et al. Sleep-related injury in 100 adult patients: A polysomnographic and clinical report. *Am J Psychiatry*. 1989;146:1166-1173.
4. Schenck CH, Lee SA, Cramer Bornemann MA, Mahowald MW. Potentially lethal behaviors associated with rapid eye movement sleep behavior disorder (RBD): Review of the literature and forensic implications. *J Forensic Sci*. 2009;54:6.
5. Fantini ML, Corona A, Clerici S, et al. Increased aggressive dream content without increased daytime aggressiveness in REM sleep behavior disorder. *Neurology*. 2005;65:1010-1015.
6. Yeh S-B, Schenck CH. A case of marital discord and secondary depression with attempted suicide resulting from REM sleep behavior disorder in a 35-year-old woman. *Sleep Med*. 2004;5:151-154.
7. Cramer Bornemann MA, Mahowald MW, SchenckParasomnias CH. Clinical features and forensic implications. *Chest*. 2006;130:605-610.
8. Bodkin CL, Schenck CH. Rapid eye movement sleep behavior disorder affecting females: Relevance to general and specialty medical practice. *J Women's Health*. 2009;18:1955-1963.
9. American Academy of Sleep Medicine. International Classification of Sleep Disorders. *Diagnostic and Coding Manual*. Westchester, IL: American Academy of Sleep Medicine; 2005.
10. Mahowald MW, Schenck CH. REM sleep parasomnias. In: Kryger MH, Roth T, Dement WC, eds. *Principles and Practice of Sleep Medicine*. Philadelphia: Elsevier Saunders; 2011.
11. Tippmann-Peikert M, Boeve BF, Keegan BM. REM sleep behavior disorder initiated by acute brainstem multiple sclerosis. *Neurology*. 2006;66:1277-1278.
12. Oudiette D, De Cock VC, Lavault S, Leu S, Vidailhet M, Arnulf I. Nonviolent elaborate behaviors may also occur in REM sleep behavior disorder. *Neurology*. 2009;72:551-557.
13. Silber MH, Ancoli-Israel S, Bonnet MH. The visual scoring of sleep in adults. *J Clin Sleep Med*. 2007;3:121-131.
14. Ferini-Strambi L, Di Gioia MS, Castronovo V, et al. Neuropsychological assessment in idiopathic REM sleep behavior disorder (RBD). Does the idiopathic form of RBD really exist? *Neurology*. 2004;62:41-45.
15. Iranzo A, Santamaria J. Severe obstructive sleep apnea/hypopnea mimicking REM sleep behavior disorder. *Sleep*. 2005;28:203-206.
16. Schenck CH, Boyd JL, Mahowald MW. A parasomnia overlap disorder involving sleepwalking, sleep terrors, and REM sleep behavior disorder in 33 polysomnographically confirmed cases. *Sleep*. 1997;20:972-981.
17. Ohayon MM, Caulet M, Priest RG. Violent behavior during sleep. *J Clin Psychiatry*. 1997;58:369-376.
18. Chiu HF, Wing YK. REM sleep behaviour disorder: An overview. *Int J Clin Pract*. 1997;51:451-454.
19. Schenck CH, Bundlie SR, Mahowald MW. Delayed emergence of a parkinsonian disorder in 38% of 29 older males initially diagnosed with idiopathic REM sleep behavior disorder. *Neurology*. 1996;46:388-393.
20. Iranzo A, Molinuevo JL, Santamaria J, et al. Rapid-eye-movement sleep behaviour disorder as an early marker for a neurodegenerative disorder: A descriptive study. *Lancet Neurol*. 2006;5:572-577.
21. Postuma RB, Gagnon JF, Vendette M, Fantini ML, Massicotte-Marquez J, Montplaisir J. Quantifying the risk of neuro-degenerative disease in idiopathic REM sleep behavior disorder. *Neurology*. 2009;72:1296-1300.
22. Claassen DO, Josephs KA, Ahlskog JE, Silber MH, Tippmann-Peikert M, Boeve BF. REM sleep behavior disorder may precede other manifestations of synucleinopathies by up to half a century. *Neurology*. 2010;75(6):494-499.

23. Boeve BF. REM sleep behavior disorder: Updated review of the core features, the REM sleep behavior disorder-neurodegenerative disease connection, evolving concepts, controversies, and future directions. *Ann NY Acad Sci.* 2010;1184:17-56.

24. Lai Y-Y, Siegel JM. Physiological and anatomical link between Parkinson-like disease and REM sleep behavior disorder. *Molec Neurobiol.* 2003; 27:137-151.

25. Comella CL, Nardine TM, Diederich NJ, et al. Sleep-related violence, injury, and REM sleep behavior disorder in Parkinson's disease. *Neurology.* 1998;51:526-529.

26. Eisensehr I, Lindeiner H, Jager M, et al. REM sleep behavior disorder in sleep-disordered patients with versus without Parkinson's disease: Is there a need for polysomnography? *J Neurol Sci.* 2001;186:7-11.

27. Gagnon J-F, Bedard M-A, Fantini ML, et al. REM sleep behavior disorder and REM sleep without atonia in Parkinson's disease. *Neurology.* 2002;59:585-589.

28. Scaglione C, Vignatelli L, Plazzi G, et al. REM sleep behaviour disorder in Parkinson's disease: A questionnaire-based study. *Neurol Sci.* 2005; 25:316-321.

29. Plazzi G, Corsini R, Provini F, et al. REM sleep behavior disorders in multiple system atrophy. *Neurology.* 1997;48:1094-1097.

30. Ferman TJ, Boeve BF, Smith GE, et al. Dementia with Lewy bodies may present as dementia and REM sleep behavior disorder without parkinsonism or hallucinations. *J Int Neuropsych Soc.* 2002;8:904-914.

31. Postuma RB, Lang AE, Massicotte-Marquez J, et al. Potential early markers of Parkinson disease in idiopathic REM sleep behavior disorder. *Neurology.* 2006;66:845-851.

32. Iranzo A, Santamaria J, Tolosa E. The clinical and pathophysiological relevance of REM sleep behavior disorder in neurodegenerative diseases. *Sleep Med Rev.* 2009;13:385-401.

33. Iranzo A, Santamaria J, Rye DB, et al. Characteristics of idiopathic REM sleep behavior disorder and that associated with MSA and PD. *Neurology.* 2005;65:247-252.

34. Schenck CH, Mahowald MW. Motor dyscontrol in narcolepsy: Rapid-eye-movement (REM) sleep without atonia and REM sleep behavior disorder. *Ann Neurol.* 1992;32:3-10.

35. Bonakis A, Howard RS, Williams A, et al. Narcolepsy presenting as REM sleep behaviour disorder. *Clin Neurol Neurosurg.* 2008;110:518-520.

36. Nightingale S, Orgill JC, Ebrahim IO, et al. The association between narcolepsy and REM behavior disorder (RBD). *Sleep Med.* 2005;6:253-258.

37. Dauvilliers Y, Rompre S, Gagnon J-F, et al. REM sleep characteristics in narcolepsy and REM sleep behavior disorder. *Sleep.* 2007;30:844-849.

38. Boeve BF, Silber MH, Saper CB, et al. Pathophysiology of REM sleep behavior disorder and relevance to neurodegenerative disease. *Brain.* 2007;130:2770-2788.

39. Fantini ML, Gagnon J-F, Petit D, et al. Slowing of electroencephalogram in rapid eye movement sleep behavior disorder. *Ann Neurol.* 2003;53:774-780.

40. Iranzo A, Santamaria J, Vilaseca I, et al. Absence of alterations in serum sex hormone levels in idiopathic REM sleep behavior disorder. *Sleep.* 2007;30: 803-806.

41. Chou KL, Moro-de-Casillas ML, Amick MM, et al. Testosterone not associated with violent dreams or REM sleep behavior disorder in men with Parkinson's. *Mov Disord.* 2007;22:411-414.

41a. Hobson JA, McCarley R. The brain as a dream state generator: an activation-synthesis hypothesis of the dream process. *Am J Psychiatry.* 1977;134:1335-1348.

42. Schenck CH, Mahowald MW. Long-term, nightly benzodiazepine treatment of injurious parasomnias and other disorders of disrupted nocturnal sleep in 170 adults. *Am J Med.* 1996;100:333-337.

43. Gagnon JF, Postuma RB, Montplaisir J. Update on the pharmacology of REM sleep behavior disorder. *Neurology.* 2006;67:742-747.

44. Gugger JJ, Wagner ML. Rapid eye movement sleep behavior disorder. *Ann Pharmacother.* 2007;41:1833-1841.

45. Schuld A, Kraus T, Haack M, et al. Obstructive sleep apnea syndrome induced by clonazepam in a narcoleptic patient with REM-sleep-behavior disorder. *J Sleep Res.* 1999;8:321-322.

46. Kunz D, Bes F. Melatonin as a therapy in REM sleep behavior disorder patients: An open-labeled pilot study on the possible influence of melatonin on REM-sleep regulation. *Mov Disord.* 1999;14:507-511.

47. Takeuchi N, Uchimura N, Hashizume Y, et al. Melatonin therapy for REM sleep behavior disorder. *Psychiatry Clin Neurosci.* 2001;55:267-269.

48. Boeve BF, Silber MH, Ferman JT. Melatonin for treatment of REM sleep behavior disorder in neurologic disorders: Results in 14 patients. *Sleep Med.* 2003;4:281-284.

49. Kunz D, Mahlberg R. A two-part, double-blind, placebo-controlled trial of exogenous melatonin in REM sleep behaviour disorder. *J Sleep Res.* 2010;19(4):591-596.

49a. Kunz D, Mahlberg R. A two-part, double-blind, placebo-controlled trial of exogenous melatonin in REM sleep behavior disorder. *J Sleep Res.* 2010;19:S91-S96.

50. Anderson KN, Jamieson S, Graham AJ, et al. REM sleep behaviour disorder treated with melatonin in a patient with Alzheimer's disease. *Clin NeurolNeurosurg.* 2008;110:492-495.

51. Fantini ML, Gagno J-F, Filipini D, et al. The effects of pramipexole in REM sleep behavior disorder. *Neurology.* 2003;61:1418-1420.

52. Schmidt MH, Koshal VB, Schmidt HS. Use of pramipexole in REM sleep behavior disorder. *Sleep Med.* 2006;7:418-423.

53. Kumru H, Iranzo A, Carrasco E, et al. Lack of effects of pramipexole on REM sleep behavior disorder in Parkinson disease. *Sleep.* 2008;31:1418-1421.

54. Ozekmekci S, Apaydin H, Kilic E. Clinical features of 35 patients with Parkinson's disease displaying REM behavior disorder. *Clin Neurol Neurosurg.* 2005;107:306-309.

55. Yeh S-B, Yeh P-Y, Schenck CH. Rivastigmine-induced REM sleep behavior disorder (RBD) in an 88 year-old man with Alzheimer's disease. *J Clin Sleep Med.* 2010;6(2):192-195.

56. Ringman JM, Simmons JH. Treatment of REM sleep behavior disorder with donepezil: A report of three cases. *Neurology.* 2000;55:870-871.

57. Simmons J. Treatment of REM behavior disorder with acetylcholinesterase inhibitors. *Sleep.* 2009;32:A292.

58. Nash JR, Wilson SJ, Potokar JP, et al. Mirtazapine induces REM sleep behavior disorder (RBD) in parkinsonism. *Neurology.* 2003;61:1161: author reply.

59. Matsumoto M, Mutoh F, Naoe H, et al. The effects of imipramine on REM sleep behavior disorder in 3 cases. *Sleep Res.* 1991;20A:351.

60. Yamamoto K, Uchimura N, Habukawa M, et al. Evaluation of the effects of paroxetine in the treatment of REM sleep behavior disorder. *Sleep Biol Rhythms.* 2006;4:190-192.

61. Takahashi T, Mitsuya H, Murata T, et al. Opposite effect of SSRIs and tandospirone in the treatment of REM sleep behavior disorder. *Sleep Med.* 2008;9:317-319.

62. Mike ME, Kranz AJ. MAOI suppression of RBD refractory to clonazepam and other agents. *Sleep Res.* 1996;25:63.

63. Bamford C. Carbamazepine in REM sleep behavior disorder. *Sleep.* 1993;16:33-34.

64. Anderson KN, Shneerson JM. Drug treatment of REM sleep behavior disorder: The use of drug therapies other than clonazepam. *J Clin Sleep Med.* 2009;5:235-239.

65. Shneerson JM. Successful treatment of REM sleep behavior disorder with sodium oxybate. *Clin Neuropharmacol.* 2009;32:158-159.

66. Parish JM. Violent dreaming and antidepressant drugs: Or how paroxetine made me dream that I was fighting Saddam Hussein. *J Clin Sleep Med.* 2007;3:529-531.

67. Schenck CH, Mahowald MW, Kim SW, O'Connor KA, Hurwitz TD. Prominent eye movements during NREM sleep and REM sleep behavior disorder associated with fluoxetine treatment of depression and obsessive-compulsive disorder. *Sleep.* 1992;15:226-235.

68. Shinno H, Kamei M, Nakamura Y, Inami Y, Horiguchi J. Successful treatment with *yi-gan san* for rapid eye movement sleep behavior disorder. *Prog Neuro-Psychopharm Biol Psychiatry.* 2008;32:1749-1751.

69. Aurora RN, Zak RS, Maganti RK, et al. Best practice guide for the treatment of REM sleep behavior disorder (RBD). *J Clin Sleep Med.* 2010;6: 85-95.

70. Iranzo A, Graus F, Clover L, et al. Rapid eye movement sleep behavior disorder and potassium channel antibody-associated limbic encephalitis. *Ann Neurol.* 2005;59:178-182.

71. Rye DB, Dempsay J, Dihenia B, et al. REM-sleep dyscontrol in Parkinson's disease: Case report of effects of elective pallidotomy. *Sleep Res.* 1997;26:591.

72. Iranzo A, Valldeoriola F, Santamaria J, et al. Sleep symptoms and polysomnographic architecture in advanced Parkinson's disease after chronic bilateral subthalamic stimulation. *J Neurol Neurosurg Psychiatry.* 2002;72:661-664.

73. Arnulf I, Bejjani BP, Garma L, et al. Improvement of sleep architecture in PD with subthalamic stimulation. *Neurology.* 2000;55:1732-1734.

74. Piette T, Mescola P, Uytdenhoef P, et al. A unique episode of REM sleep behavior disorder triggered during surgery for Parkinson's disease. *J Neurol Sci.* 2007;253:73-76.

74a. Howell MJ, Arneson PA, Schenck CH. A novel therapy for REM sleep behavior disorder (RBD). *J Clin Sleep Med.* 2011 (in press).

74b. Slow-Wave Films, LLC, St. Paul, MN www.sleeprunners.com.

75. Koran L, Raghavan S. Fluoxetine for isolated sleep paralysis. *Psychosomatics.* 1993;34:184-187.

76. Ohayon M, Morselli P, Guilleminault C. Prevalence of nightmares and their relationship to psychopathology and daytime functioning in insomnia subjects. *Sleep*. 1997;20:340-348.

77. Zadra A, Donderi DC. Prevalence of nightmares and bad dreams and their relation to psychological well-being. *J Abnormal Psychol*. 2000;109:210-219.

78. Pagel JF. Helfter P. Drug induced nightmares—An etiology based review. *Hum Psychopharmacol*. 2003;18:59-67.

79. Krakow B, Zadra A. Clinical management of chronic nightmares: Imagery rehearsal therapy. *Behav Sleep Med*. 2006;4(1):45-70.

80. Abramovitch H. The nightmare of returning home: A case of acute onset nightmare disorder treated by lucid dreaming. *Israel J Psychiatry Rel Sci*. 1995;32(2):140-145.

81. Kinzie J, Fredrickson R, Ben R, Fleck J, Karls W. Posttraumatic stress disorder among survivors of Cambodian concentration camps. *Am J Psychiatry*. 1984;141(5):645-650.

82. Van Liempt S, et al. Pharmacotherapeutic treatment of nightmares and insomnia in posttraumatic stress disorder: An overview of the literature. *Ann NY Acad Sci*. 2006;1071:502-507.

83. Raskind M, Peskind E, Hoff D, et al. A parallel group placebo controlled study of prazosin for trauma nightmares and sleep disturbance in combat veterans with posttraumatic stress disorder. *Biol Psychiatry*. 2007;61(8):928-934.

NREM Sleep Parasomnias in Adults:

CONFUSIONAL AROUSALS, SLEEPWALKING, SLEEP TERRORS, AND SLEEP-RELATED EATING DISORDER

Chapter 44

MICHAEL J. HOWELL / CARLOS H. SCHENCK

Non–rapid eye movement (NREM) sleep parasomnias are characterized by abnormal nocturnal behavior, experiential phenomena, and autonomic nervous system activation due to incomplete or impaired arousal from (typically slow wave, stage N3) NREM sleep.[1] They have characteristic duration, complexity of behavior, autonomic nervous system activity, and degree of amnesia. *The International Classification of Sleep Disorders,* 2nd edition (ICSD-2), lists confusional arousals (CA), sleepwalking, sleep terrors, and sleep-related eating disorder as primary disorders of arousal from NREM sleep.[1] Sexsomnia is classified as a variant of confusional arousals[1] and will be covered in Chapter 45.

Managing these conditions effectively requires proper diagnosis made through obtaining a careful history and appropriate clinical investigations. These conditions can be associated with other sleep disorders, especially sleep-disordered breathing (SDB) and periodic leg movements (PLMs), which, if not appropriately identified and treated, may interfere with the treatment of the parasomnia. Furthermore, NREM parasomnias (particularly sleep-related eating disorder and sleepwalking) are increasingly being reported in association with commonly prescribed benzodiazepine receptor agonist (BZRA) sedative-hypnotic medications such as zolpidem, zaleplon, and zopiclone.[2]

The scientific understanding of NREM parasomnias therapy is still based on limited data. Most therapeutic studies consist of case reports or small noncontrolled case series. This chapter will review those reports and the few placebo-controlled studies. Future treatment strategies will require deeper insight into the mechanisms that underlie NREM parasomnias. This chapter will start by reviewing normal and abnormal arousal mechanisms as well as exploring the role of sleep inertia, genetic factors, and the effects of polyneuropharmacy.

GENERAL DESCRIPTIONS AND MECHANISMS

Confusional Arousals

Confusional arousals (CA) occur during an arousal from NREM sleep (Fig. 44-1) and are characterized by disoriented behavior (at times with aggressive, violent, or sexual manifestations), often with inappropriate vocalizations (Box 44-1). The episodes are poorly recalled the following day. Typically lasting less than 5 minutes (or even less than 1 minute), episodes occasionally last up to 40 minutes. These prolonged episodes are most commonly described in the setting of polyneuropharmacy. During these events, the patient's behavior is typically benign, although occasionally it can become aggressive and violent. A recognized

variant of confusional arousals in ICSD-2, namely severe morning sleep inertia, can have major adverse daytime consequences, such as being repeatedly tardy to work or school, and demonstrating recurrent, inappropriate behaviors at home.[1]

Precipitating factors for CA of any duration also include (in addition to untreated co-morbid sleep disorders and psychotropic medication) recovery from sleep deprivation and forced awakenings.[1]

Sleepwalking

Sleepwalking is the combination of ambulation with the persistence of impaired consciousness following an abrupt incomplete arousal from NREM sleep (Box 44-2). Amnesia for the sleepwalking is typical, and the behaviors are frequently described as routine but inappropriate (e.g., placing car keys in the refrigerator or rearranging furniture in a nonsensical manner). Attempting to arouse the patient during a sleepwalking episode is often difficult and may paradoxically worsen confusion and disorientation, possibly provoking an aggressive response.

The major predisposing factor for sleepwalking is heredity, with a positive family history being quite common. Other precipitating factors for sleepwalking include those noted earlier for CA.[1]

Occasionally NREM confusional or sleepwalking parasomnia behavior can become recurrent and persistent over time, as well as prolonged or dangerous. Alarming reports have described automobile driving, wielding of firearms, and sometimes the discharge of loaded firearms during a parasomnia episode. Recently, dangerous sleepwalking behaviors have been associated with sedative-hypnotic medications, in particular the BZRAs, as mentioned earlier.[2] Reports of repeated amnestic nocturnal eating and sexual activity have led to the creation of two new diagnostic categories in the ICSD-2: sleep-related eating disorder and sexsomnia.[1]

Sleep Terrors

Sleep terrors are episodes of intense fear beginning with a sudden cry or loud scream and accompanied by increased autonomic nervous system activity (Box 44-3). Adults having a sleep terror can impulsively bolt out of bed, without ability to properly judge what is happening, in response to an imagined threatening image or dream fragment. Severe injury or even death may result from running into furniture or walls, falling down stairs, or jumping through windows. Among all the NREM parasomnias, episodes of sleep terrors can be the most difficult to interrupt, and complete amnesia for the events is

559

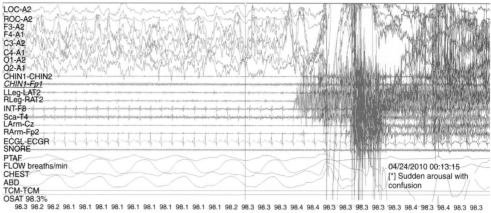

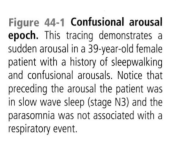

Figure 44-1 Confusional arousal epoch. This tracing demonstrates a sudden arousal in a 39-year-old female patient with a history of sleepwalking and confusional arousals. Notice that preceding the arousal the patient was in slow wave sleep (stage N3) and the parasomnia was not associated with a respiratory event.

BOX 44-1 *ICSD-2 Diagnostic Criteria for Confusional Arousals*

- Recurrent mental confusion or confusional behavior occurs during an arousal or awakening from nocturnal sleep or a daytime nap.
- The disturbance is not better explained by another sleep disorder, medical or neurologic disorder, mental disorder, medication use, or substance use disorder.

ICSD-2, International Classification of Sleep Disorders, Second Edition.

BOX 44-2 *ICSD-2 Diagnostic Criteria for Sleepwalking*

- Ambulation occurs during sleep.
- Persistence of sleep, an altered state of consciousness, or impaired judgment during ambulation is demonstrated by at least one of the following:
  1. Difficult arousability
  2. Mental confusion on being awakened from the episode
  3. Amnesia (complete or partial) for the episode
  4. Routine behaviors that occur at inappropriate times
  5. Inappropriate or nonsensical behaviors
  6. Dangerous or potentially dangerous behaviors
- The disturbance is not better explained by another sleep disorder, medical or neurologic disorder, mental disorder, or substance use disorder.

ICSD-2, International Classification of Sleep Disorders, Second Edition.

BOX 44-3 *ICSD-2 Diagnostic Criteria for Sleep Terrors*

- A sudden episode of terror occurs during sleep, usually initiated by a cry or loud scream that is accompanied by autonomic nervous system and behavioral manifestations of intense fear.
- At least one of the following associated features is present:
  1. Difficult arousability
  2. Mental confusion on being awakened from an episode
  3. Amnesia (complete or partial) for the episode
  4. Dangerous or potentially dangerous behaviors
- The disturbance is not better explained by another sleep disorder, medical or neurologic disorder, mental disorder, medication use, or substance use disorder.

ICSD-2, International Classification of Sleep Disorders, Second Edition.

EPIDEMIOLOGY AND CLINICAL ASSOCIATIONS

Although the incidence of NREM parasomnias peaks in childhood, these events are nevertheless not uncommon in adults with a prevalence range between 1% and 4%.[1,3-6] The majority of adult sleepwalkers report having been a sleepwalker as a child.[3]

NREM parasomnias have been associated with other sleep disorders. SDB, in particular obstructive sleep apnea (OSA), and PLMs (usually associated with restless legs syndrome [RLS]) are the most commonly identified precipitating factors during polysomnography (PSG) in adults and children with sleepwalking[7,8] (Box 44-4). In part, this apparent association is related to the high prevalence of OSA and PLMs. More importantly, these conditions may precipitate NREM parasomnias (at least in those who are otherwise predisposed) through repeated arousals and chronic sleep deprivation (caused by the frequent, recurrent sleep disruption). A telephone survey found several conditions to be independently associated with NREM parasomnias, including shift work, daytime sleepiness, smoking, and ethanol consumption at bedtime (in addition to OSA and other sleep disorders)[4] (Box 44-5). These conditions are all often characterized by nighttime sleep fragmentation.

Parasomnias among patients with mental illness are common, particularly in the setting of sedative-hypnotic medications. One group of investigators studying adult psychiatric

---

typical, albeit with notable exceptions in some adults. Sleep terrors can last for longer than 5 minutes, and attempts to abort an episode may result in even greater agitation. These behaviors often cause severe angst for cohabitants, whereas the patient usually does not appear to demonstrate any daytime consequences, apart from occasionally being physically or emotionally exhausted from a particularly intense or prolonged nocturnal episode.

As with sleepwalking, a positive family history is a common predisposing factor. Other factors that can precipitate and aggravate sleep terrors also include those already described for other disorders of arousal.[2]

BOX 44-4 *Disorders and Medications Associated with NREM Parasomnias*

CO-MORBID SLEEP DISORDERS
- Obstructive sleep apnea/other forms of sleep-disordered breathing
- Periodic limb movements
- Restless legs syndrome

MEDICAL DISORDERS
- Migraine
- Febrile illness
- Vitiligo
- Hyperthyroidism
- Encephalitis
- Stroke

MEDICATIONS
- Benzodiazepine receptor agonists: zolpidem, zaleplon
- Antidepressants: amitriptyline, bupropion, paroxetine, mirtazapine
- Mood stabilizer: lithium carbonate
- Antipsychotics: quetiapine, olanzapine
- Antihypertensive: metoprolol
- Anticonvulsant: topiramate
- Antibiotic: fluoroquinolone

OTHER ASSOCIATIONS
- Shift work
- Ethanol consumption at bedtime
- Smoking

NREM, non–rapid eye movement.

BOX 44-5 *Etiology of NREM Parasomnias*

- Conditions that deepen sleep and promote NREM parasomnias by impairing otherwise normal arousal mechanisms:
  - Sleep deprivation
  - Sedative-hypnotic medication
  - Ethanol intoxication
- Conditions that cause repeated cortical arousals and lead to NREM parasomnias through sleep fragmentation:
  - Obstructive sleep apnea
  - Periodic limb movement disorder
  - Narcolepsy
  - Disruptive sleeping environment
  - Ethanol withdrawal

NREM, non–rapid eye movement.

NREM parasomnias by impairing otherwise normal arousal mechanisms); and, second, those that cause repeated cortical arousals (leading to NREM parasomnias through sleep fragmentation).

These abnormal arousals are often associated with the normal alternating arousal microstructure of NREM sleep, the cyclic alternating pattern (CAP) (Fig. 44-2).[39] Abnormalities of the CAP may be used as a biomarker of treatment response and will be briefly mentioned later in the section on management. The complex behaviors that characterize these conditions are related to central pattern generators (CPGs). The isolated activation of CPGs at the same time as there is relatively little activity in brain regions that control executive function and memory accounts for the poor judgment and amnesia that characterize NREM parasomnias. (For a more thorough review of the CAP and CPGs in NREM parasomnias, see references 39-42 at the end of this chapter.)

Normal and Impaired Arousal Mechanisms

In the normal transition from light NREM sleep to wake, consciousness emerges quickly, typically within seconds. Stimuli of endogenous and exogenous origin activate neurons in the brainstem and the basal forebrain. These regions subsequently promote wakefulness both through direct activation of the cerebral cortex and by inhibiting thalamic reticular (sleep-promoting) neurons (thus blocking spindle oscillations).[43]

But the duration of a normal arousal transition depends upon an intricate combination of variables including duration of prior wakefulness, current sleep duration, circadian phase, effects of sedating or stimulating medications, and multiple genetic and behavioral factors; and, it depends on depth of NREM sleep: specifically, the speed of the conversion from NREM sleep to wakefulness depends upon the intensity of slow wave activity (SWA). Most arousals into wakefulness from NREM sleep are from the lighter stages (N1 or N2). In stages N1 and N2 there is minimal SWA and the threshold for stimulation to produce an awakening is low. By comparison, the threshold for an awakening from deep NREM sleep (N3), characterized by nearly continuous SWA, is high and the process of awakening is typically prolonged.[44] Subsequently, sleep inertia during N3 sleep arousals is strong and promotes a return to sleep.

outpatients reported a sleepwalking prevalence double that of the general population[9] and noted a high frequency of amnestic complex behaviors associated with ingestion of a BZRA medication.[10] These findings are consistent with other reports of abnormal nocturnal behavior induced by BZRAs, including prolonged complex behavior such as amnestic nocturnal eating, sexual activity, and operating a motor vehicle.[10-19] They frequently occurred in the setting of central nervous system polypharmacy or supratherapeutic doses.[2]

Sleepwalking has also been associated with a variety of other medications and medical conditions. Implicated medications have been reported in at least six classes: (1) the *antidepressants* amitriptyline,[20] bupropion,[21,22] paroxetine,[23] and mirtazapine;[24] (2) the *mood stabilizer* lithium;[25,26] (3) the *antipsychotics* quetiapine[27] and olanzapine;[28-30] (4) the *antihypertensive* metoprolol;[31] (5) the *antiseizure agent* topiramate;[32] and (6) the *antibiotic* fluoroquinolone.[33] Medical conditions reportedly associated with NREM parasomnias include migraine,[34,35] febrile illness,[36] vitiligo,[37] hyperthyroidism,[38] and encephalitis and stroke.[1]

PATHOPHYSIOLOGY

Sleepwalking and related NREM parasomnia disorders occur when there is an incomplete dissociation of NREM sleep from wakefulness, i.e., when the transition from NREM sleep to wakefulness is incomplete. Such abnormal partial arousals may reflect two interlinked sleep-related phenomena: first, those that deepen sleep and enhance sleep inertia (promoting

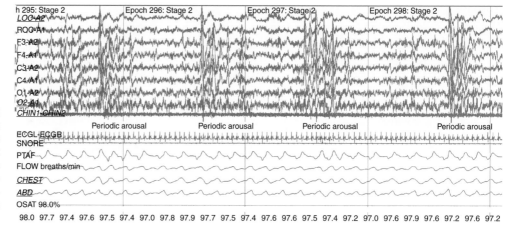

Figure 44-2 Cyclic alternating pattern. This graph demonstrates the microstructure of non–rapid eye movement (NREM) sleep by the cyclic alternating pattern (CAP). Notice the periodic arousals that recur every 30 to 40 seconds. Increased CAP rate, suggestive of NREM instability, has been associated with NREM parasomnias.

In NREM parasomnias, impaired arousal mechanisms and the persistence of sleep drive result in a failure of the brain to transition fully to wakefulness. Indeed, most sleepwalking and related disorders arise out of N3 sleep, and sleep-promoting factors (e.g., sleep deprivation and sedative-hypnotic medication) have been associated with these events.

Conversely, disorders that lead to fragmented NREM sleep promote sleepwalking and other disorders of arousal by increasing arousal frequency. OSA, PLMs, narcolepsy, and ethanol withdrawal all promote parasomnias by fragmenting NREM sleep. In fact, confusional arousals can often be precipitated in the sleep laboratory through sleep deprivation (which promotes SWA) combined with a sudden loud noise (see discussion under "Management").[45]

Some sleep disorders promote NREM parasomnias through both mechanisms working in parallel. In particular, OSA increases both sleep fragmentation and sleep inertia. OSA is typically characterized by repeated cortical arousals and, as a consequence, by an increased sleep drive (through chronic intermittent sleep deprivation). PLMs may do the same (although PLMs can occur in a more benign fashion, without cortical arousals).

Importantly, BZRA sedative-hypnotic medication may increase NREM parasomnia behaviors by further impairing the frontal lobe and hippocampal function. This occurs through enhancement of gamma-aminobutyric acid (GABA) inhibition upon cortical neurons and is related to dose and binding affinity. There has been an increase in sleep-associated amnestic complex behavior reported in parallel to the rise in use of sedative-hypnotic medication. These phenomena represent a distinct subset of adult onset NREM parasomnias. Thus, elaborate complicated behaviors develop as brain regions that encode motor behavior are activated during the episodes. Concurrently, owing to sedating medication, executive and memory function remain suppressed. These effects may produce behaviors that are more prolonged and inappropriate with persistent amnesia, including, for example, elaborate food preparation, sexual intercourse, and operation of a motor vehicle.[2,46]

Patients with combinations of predisposing conditions are at an increased risk for NREM parasomnias, for example, OSA patients prescribed BZRA sedative-hypnotic medication to assist continuous positive airway pressure (CPAP) therapy compliance or treat co-morbid insomnia. A similar situation applies to sleepwalking patients with RLS/PLM disorders misdiagnosed as insomnia and treated with sedative-hypnotic medication. This combination of a movement or sensory disorder inappropriately treated with medication for insomnia may lead (perhaps with considerable frequency) to sleepwalking and other complex amnestic behaviors.[2] This appears to be especially true among many cases of zolpidem-induced sleep-related eating disorder in which there is often underlying RLS.[47] Finally, the concurrent use of multiple psychotropic agents often provides the trigger for severe recurrent parasomnias. For instance, many of the cases of prolonged, complex amnestic behavior such as "sleep driving" have occurred with antidepressant medication used in combination with sedative-hypnotic medication.[2,48,49]

Intracranial monitoring and neuroimaging studies performed during NREM parasomnia events have demonstrated that during NREM parasomnias certain brain regions become more activated and *wake-like* while other regions continue to show slow, *sleep-like* activity (Box 44-6). One report captured a confusional arousal in a 20-year-old man who was undergoing intracerebral electroencephalographic (EEG) monitoring for refractory epilepsy. The cingulate and motor cortices demonstrated an arousal followed by brain waves consistent with wakefulness while, in parallel, the frontoparietal associative cortices had increased delta activity consistent with deep NREM sleep.[50] These findings were very similar to a sleepwalking event that was captured in a 16-year-old man with cranial single-photon emission computed tomography (SPECT). In this case, the parasomnia was characterized by activation (increased regional cerebral blood flow) of cingulate as well as motor coordination pathways with a relative paucity of activation in the frontal lobe.[51] This research is still in its early stages but further evaluations should provide greater insight into the regional nature of brain activation—and deactivation—in NREM sleep parasomnias.

An Alternative Proposed Mechanism for Sleep Terrors

Sleep terrors, while superficially similar to confusional arousals and sleepwalking (in regard to abrupt arousal from slow wave sleep), may nevertheless originate in part from a distinctive neurophysiologic mechanism[52] (Box 44-7). In particular, it has been suggested that instead of an overlap between NREM and wakefulness, as implicated in other NREM parasomnias, night terrors may represent a disorder of transition between NREM slow wave sleep and REM sleep.[52] This theory

---

BOX 44-6 *Dissociated Brain Activity during NREM Parasomnias*

- Intracranial EEG and functional neuroimaging reports suggest that dissociated brain activity occurs during NREM parasomnias.
- Motor regions become *awake-like,* whereas frontal (executive function) and medial temporal (memory) regions demonstrate *sleep-like* activity.
- These findings help explain the preservation of normal motor function with a relative paucity of judgment and memory functions.

EEG, electroencephalography; *NREM,* non–rapid eye movement.

BOX 44-7 *Possible Alternative Mechanism for Sleep Terrors*

Sleep terrors may represent an intrusion of REM sleep into NREM sleep. This mechanism is in contrast with that postulated for other NREM parasomnias, for which an overlap between features of NREM sleep and those of wakefulness is likely.

These findings help explain several unique features of sleep terrors compared with other NREM parasomnias:

- High level of autonomic activity (from REM sleep)
- Apparent vivid mentation (from REM sleep)
- Difficult arousability (from deep NREM [N3] sleep)
- Preponderance in childhood (greater proportion of both deep NREM [N3] sleep and REM sleep)
- Apparent clinical response to paroxetine (REM suppressor)

NREM, non–rapid eye movement; *REM,* rapid eye movement.

---

would explain several unique features of sleep terrors: the high autonomic activity and the apparent vivid mentation (both from REM) combined with very difficult arousability (from NREM slow wave sleep). Further, REM-NREM overlap may also explain the striking preponderance of night terrors in childhood because children have a greater proportion of both NREM slow wave sleep and REM sleep. Intriguingly, the antidepressant medication paroxetine, an agent reported to induce sleepwalking,[23] has conversely been reported to abolish sleep terrors[53] (see later discussion of treatment). The basis for this discrepancy is not known; however, paroxetine is a potent REM suppressor.[54] Thus, if night terrors were due to pathologic REM/NREM overlap, it would expected that paroxetine would block these phenomena. Conversely, paroxetine would not be expected to have a therapeutic effect on sleepwalking, a wake/NREM dissociative phenomenon. In fact, paroxetine has been demonstrated in certain cases to exacerbate sleepwalking (see later discussion of antidepressants).[23,55] Further neurophysiologic research is needed to distinguish the various pathophysiologic mechanisms of NREM parasomnias.

Genetics of NREM Parasomnias

Intrinsic factors predispose certain individuals to the impaired cortical arousal of NREM parasomnias. Sleepwalking and night terrors both often demonstrate familial patterns. In one study 80% of sleepwalkers and 96% of patients with night terrors could identify a family member who suffered from similar phenomena.[36] One group of investigators has followed parasomnias in a large group (*n* = 2944) of mono- and dizygotic twin pairs. Over a decade-long follow-up they report substantial genetic effects in sleepwalking among both children and adults.[3,56] Also, human leukocyte antigen (HLA) haplo typing has demonstrated that specific DQB1 alleles have been implicated among familial sleepwalking pedigrees.[57] Interestingly, similar findings regarding DQB1 alleles have been found among familial cases of narcolepsy and REM sleep behavior disorder.[58,59]

Conclusion

Sleepwalking and related disorders result from an incomplete dissociation of NREM sleep and wakefulness. Conditions promoting arousal or sleep may be implicated. Thus, both intrinsic and extrinsic conditions that provoke repeated cortical arousals may lead to parasomnias through sleep fragmentation. These abnormal arousals occur with isolated activation of motor regions with a relative paucity of activity in brain regions that control executive function and memory, thus accounting for the poor judgment and amnesia that characterize NREM parasomnias. Conversely, phenomena which lead to greater sleep inertia, such as sleep deprivation and sedating medications, promote NREM parasomnias by impairing otherwise normal arousal mechanisms.

MANAGEMENT

The first steps in management include assessment of the level of severity, consideration of eliminating presumed inducing agents, attention to maximizing environmental safety, and identification and treatment of any co-morbid sleep disorder(s). Most confusional arousals and many sleepwalking episodes are limited in duration and severity. Most patients may be given reassurance and advised to avoid sleep deprivation and any other identified presumed risk factor for that patient, such as the timing and extent of ethanol use. Situations that deserve more thorough investigation include violent and potentially injurious behavior, nonviolent but potentially dangerous behavior (e.g., leaving the house during the winter, walking into a lake during the summer, opening an upper floor window), and symptoms suggestive of another sleep disorder or neuropsychiatric condition[60] (Box 44-8).

When sleepwalking is associated with use of a sedative-hypnotic agent, it is of particular importance to carefully reconsider the diagnosis for which the medication was originally prescribed (Box 44-9). In these cases, patients may not have insomnia (for which the sedating agent was prescribed) but rather another disorder that leads to sleep initiation difficulties such as RLS or a delayed circadian rhythm.[2,61,62] Discontinuance of offending agents will typically resolve the abnormal nighttime behavior, particularly if another underlying condition is correctly identified and properly treated[2,62,63] (with, for example, dopamine agonists for RLS[64] or evening melatonin/morning light therapy for a delayed circadian rhythm).[65] Conversely, if a diagnosis of, say, psychophysiologic insomnia is correct, patients may still respond satisfactorily by decreasing the dose of the hypnotic agent or by switching to another agent. In fact, some cases of medication-induced

> ### BOX 44-8   *Situations That Warrant Polysomnographic Investigation of NREM Parasomnias*
>
> - History suggestive of a co-morbid sleep disorder or pertinent sleep finding (e.g., obstructive sleep apnea, periodic limb movements)
> - Violent or potentially injurious behavior
> - Repetitive and stereotyped behavior suggesting a possible epileptic etiology
>
> *NREM*, non–rapid eye movement.

> ### BOX 44-9   *Sedative-Hypnotic–Induced Parasomnia Behavior*
>
> - In the setting of sedative-hypnotic–induced parasomnia behavior, it is important to reconsider the diagnosis for which the sleeping agent was prescribed.
> - These insomnia medications may have been inappropriately prescribed for other disorders that lead to sleep initiation difficulties (e.g., circadian rhythm disorder, delayed sleep phase type; restless legs syndrome).

> ### BOX 44-10   *Polysomnographic Investigation of Presumed NREM Parasomnias*
>
> - PSG may demonstrate other sleep disorders in the setting of a presumed NREM parasomnia:
>   - Obstructive sleep apnea or upper airway resistance syndrome
>   - Periodic leg movements with frequent cortical arousal
>   - REM sleep behavior disorder (REM sleep without atonia on chin and limb EMG)
>   - Nocturnal seizure activity (requiring a seizure EEG montage for diagnosis)
> - Provoking an NREM parasomnia during PSG often requires the combination of sleep deprivation and sudden arousal from slow wave (N3) sleep.
>
> *EEG*, electroencephalography; *EMG*, electromyography; *NREM*, non–rapid eye movement; *PSG*, polysomnography; *REM*, rapid eye movement.

sleepwalking are related to patient self-administration of greater-than-recommended dosage.[2,12,16,46] When an alternative medication is needed, there is no consensus to guide decision making. Individual patients vary in their responsivity to different agents. Sometimes the same agent with a different formulation will resolve the nocturnal behavior; other patients require a switch in medication, whereas others need to discontinue sedative pharmacotherapy entirely.[2] Finally, patients with insomnia can also be successfully treated with cognitive behavioral therapy.[66]

Environmental safety is a critical component in treating all cases of potentially injurious sleepwalking behavior. The patient should be advised to remove any bedside object or furniture that could be injurious either to themselves or to a bed partner. Removal of firearms, knives, and other weapons is of paramount importance. Windows, and other exits that could result in a fall, should not be easily accessible to the sleepwalking patient. Automatically locking doors should be avoided as sleepwalkers may ambulate outside their residence without means of reentry. A housemate should conceal car keys; however, this is not an option for sleepwalkers who live alone. Furthermore, bedroom door alarms are helpful (and inexpensive) ways to fully awaken a sleepwalker (although it may paradoxically worsen the event in progress)[45] or at least to signal others that the sleepwalker has started to wander.

It has been demonstrated that in many violent parasomnia cases, injury to the victim is related to physical proximity to the sleeping person and could potentially be avoided. One report reviewed the nature of 32 medical and legal cases involving violent, sleep-related behavior. In the majority of the examples, the victim either was in passive close proximity to, or somehow provoked, the parasomniac subject (100% of confusional arousal cases, 81% of sleep terror cases, 40-90% of sleepwalking cases). The provocation was typically mild compared to the violent response and, importantly, the victims had not otherwise been sought out by the sleepwalker.[67] These results strongly suggest that patients with a history of violent

nocturnal behaviors should not sleep with a bed partner (at least until successful therapy has been achieved) and contact should be avoided during episodes.

PSG can sometimes be helpful in managing NREM parasomnias (Box 44-10); e.g., it may help facilitate diagnosis by ruling out other conditions predisposing to complex sleep-related behaviors, as well as helping identify reversible co-morbid conditions linked with a NREM parasomnia. PSG will often document multiple arousals from deep NREM sleep (N3); however, it does not routinely demonstrate abnormal nocturnal behavior.[1] This failing is likely due to the rarity of events as well as decreased depth of sleep during PSG testing secondary to inability to fully reproduce the natural sleep environment.[68]

Prior sleep deprivation combined with forced awakening during a PSG appears to be a useful tool in precipitating a NREM parasomnia episode in a known sleepwalker. One study of 10 sleepwalkers demonstrated increased likelihood of demonstrating complex behaviors arising from sleep after a night of sleep deprivation compared to baseline.[69] Another study of 10 patients reported that sleepwalkers had more frequent and complex somnambulistic episodes after sleep deprivation compared both to their own baseline sleep and to that of control subjects.[70]

Conversely, it has been noted that some sleepwalkers will paradoxically demonstrate an improvement in sleep study parameters after sleep deprivation. One group of investigators reported that despite 10 years of utilizing a standardized sleep deprivation protocol, no episode of sleepwalking was ever elicited in a laboratory setting.[71] These findings are not completely surprising as sleep deprivation promotes consolidation by decreasing arousals,[69] thus conceivably decreasing the probability for provoking an episode of NREM parasomnia.

Another possible explanation for the failure to trigger sleepwalking in the laboratory after sleep deprivation is the failure to reproduce normal nocturnal auditory stimuli during a PSG. Compared to the home, the laboratory environment is often acoustically sterile. At home, patients often sleep with the television or radio on and with noises from bed partners (snoring, mumbling, talking), any of which may be potential precipitants.

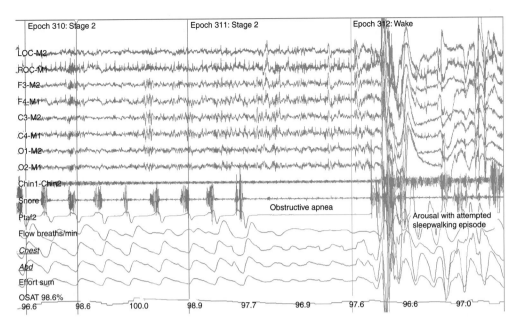

Figure 44-3 Obstructive sleep apnea with sleepwalking. This graph demonstrates an obstructive apnea that precedes an attempted sleepwalking episode in a 40-year-old male patient with a history of sleepwalking and symptoms concerning for sleep-disordered breathing.

This suggestion is consistent with the explanation that NREM parasomnias arise after a predisposed patient is primed (e.g., by sleep deprivation) and then induced by a precipitating factor.[45,72] There is evidence to support this explanation even for events during laboratory testing. In particular, one protocol recommended 25 hours of sleep deprivation leading up to a sleep laboratory study combined with an alarm awakening during SWS. Using these methods, investigators reported inducing somnambulistic events in 100% of patients with a history of sleepwalking compared to only 30% of patients who were not sleep deprived. Importantly, using this combined method of sleep deprivation and forced arousals, no control subject (i.e., without a history of sleepwalking) demonstrated somnambulistic events—a 100% sensitivity.[45]

In conclusion, it appears that sleep deprivation in itself is not an adequate method to induce NREM parasomnia episodes in the sleep laboratory, but the yield increases significantly when combined with a forced awakening protocol.

PSG recordings often demonstrate findings indicative of NREM instability and frequent cortical arousal. Immediately preceding the event there is often a 10-second buildup of hypersynchronous delta waves (see discussion on CAP earlier). Subsequently, postarousal EEG activity frequently shows slowed cortical activity, including delta waves in one or more EEG channels, with evolution either into a fully wakeful EEG activity or back to NREM sleep.[73]

The etiology of frequent cortical arousal in sleepwalkers is often related to other sleep disorders such as OSA (Fig. 44-3). Clinically symptomatic or severe co-morbid conditions (e.g., OSA and RLS) should always be treated. A pivotal report from 2005 studied 60 chronic sleepwalking patients with PSG and followed them prospectively for a year after diagnosis. Of the 60 sleepwalking patients, a high number ($n = 53$) were diagnosed as having SDB. In the majority of cases the SDB was mild, often not reaching criteria for OSA, but instead indicated upper airway resistance syndrome (UARS) and the majority of subjects did not demonstrate daytime sleepiness. Only three patients dropped out of the study, while of the remaining 50, all reported resolution of sleepwalking after treatment of SDB. Of those 50 patients, 42 patients reported

---

BOX 44-11 *Cyclic Alternating Pattern (CAP) and NREM Sleep*

- The CAP is an intrinsic oscillation between periods of cortical activity and inactivity during NREM sleep.
- The CAP oscillation typically occurs every 20 to 40 seconds and forms the scaffolding for various NREM normal and pathologic NREM phenomena:
  - K complexes
  - Slow wave activity
  - Epileptic activity
  - Confusional arousals
  - Sleepwalking episodes

NREM, non–rapid eye movement.

---

compliance with nasal CPAP while the remaining 8 patients described resolution of sleepwalking after upper airway surgical treatment. These dramatic results suggest that treatment of even mild, asymptomatic SDB may result in resolution of sleepwalking.[74] These findings have not yet been replicated in a separate study of sleepwalking patients; however, one review of sleep-related amnestic sexual activity reported four cases that resolved when concomitant OSA was treated with CPAP.[75]

The Cyclic Alternating Pattern as a Biomarker of Treatment Response

The CAP is an intrinsic oscillation throughout NREM sleep that cycles across periods of cortical arousal and quiescence (Box 44-11 and Fig. 44-2). This oscillation typically occurs every 20 to 40 seconds and provides the scaffolding for normal NREM phenomena (such as K complexes and delta bursts) as well as pathologic NREM phenomena (confusional arousals and sleepwalking events).[76] Interestingly, sleepwalking and sleep terror patients have an increased number of CAP cycles and a higher CAP rate, which is a measure of NREM

> **BOX 44-12** *Use of Abnormalities in the Cyclic Alternating Pattern (CAP) as Biophysiologic Markers of Treatment Response*
>
> - CAP abnormalities on EEG are relatively common in NREM parasomnias:
>   - Phase A1 activity (often referred to as *hypersynchronous delta activity*) often seen preceding parasomnia activity.
>   - Increased number of CAP oscillations
>   - Increased CAP rate
> - Resolution of CAP abnormalities identified during PSG correlates with the resolution of parasomnia behavior—this is particularly helpful because NREM parasomnia behavior may not occur frequently enough during overnight PSG to guide treatment.
>
> *EEG*, electroencephalogram; *NREM*, non–rapid eye movement; *PSG*, polysomnography.

> **BOX 44-13** *Treatment of NREM Parasomnias*
>
> - Several pharmacologic agents have been reported to have efficacy in treating NREM parasomnias:
>   - Diazepam
>   - Clonazepam
>   - Paroxetine (particularly for sleep terrors)
>   - Imipramine
>   - Trazodone
>   - *NOTE:* Agencies that regulate drug approval do not recognize NREM parasomnias as an indication for these agents, which therefore represents an "off-label" use.
> - Nonpharmacologic therapies that have been reported to have efficacy in treating NREM parasomnias include:
>   - Hypnotherapy
>   - Anticipatory (scheduled) awakenings
> - Studies investigating both pharmacologic and nonpharmacologic therapies typically have been noncontrolled case series or small clinical trials, and the findings occasionally have been contradictory.
>
> *NREM*, non–rapid eye movement.

instability.[77-80] Further, a subtype of cortical arousal in the CAP (phase A1) is characterized by hypersynchronous delta activity (HSD).[76] Interestingly, the majority of reports indicate that sleepwalking, sleep terrors, and confusional arousals are often preceded by a phase A1 run of HSD,[81] indicating that these events are linked to the CAP[81-82] (Box 44-12). Further, resolution of CAP abnormalities in patients who are being treated for sleep-disordered breathing is associated with a resolution of sleepwalking behaviors.[79] These insights suggest that treatment of NREM parasomnias should first be directed at resolving underlying sleep destabilizing processes and that the CAP changes (decrease in CAP rate and number of A1 events) may be used as a PSG marker of treatment response that can be correlated with the reported clinical response. These findings are particularly helpful as there is typically an absence of parasomnia behavior during PSG (see preceding discussion).[78,79,82] (For a more thorough review of the CAP and its role in NREM parasomnias, see references 71-79)

Types of Therapies

A variety of different therapies have been reported to treat NREM parasomnias. Pharmacologic interventions include a variety of benzodiazepine and antidepressant medications. Nonpharmacologic interventions include scheduled awakenings and hypnotherapy (Box 44-13).

Some agents demonstrate disparate efficacy depending upon which NREM parasomnia is being treated. In particular, it appears that antidepressants have a reported greater efficacy in the treatment of sleep terrors, whereas these agents have less benefit for sleepwalking and at times may, in fact, exacerbate sleepwalking. These findings suggest that sleepwalking and sleep terrors may arise, in part, from distinct mechanisms.

Importantly, the evidence for all therapies, pharmacologic and nonpharmacologic, is currently based on methodologically weak studies, typically case reports and case series. Only rarely have there been more rigorous clinical investigations, but sample size in these controlled studies typically has been small. Furthermore, as described here, some of the evidence is contradictory. Importantly, agencies that regulate drug approval do not recognize these treatments, and so the therapy of NREM parasomnias represents "off-label" use of

pharmacotherapy, which should be discussed with patients and their family.[83]

Benzodiazepines

The most commonly reported pharmacologic treatments for NREM parasomnias are various agents in the benzodiazepine (BZ) class of sedative-hypnotics. BZs act by increasing the chloride conductance through $GABA_A$ receptors.[84] BZs reported to be effective for NREM parasomnias are typically categorized as either intermediate- or long-acting agents. The use of BZs in the treatment of NREM parasomnias is seemingly paradoxical, as other sedative-hypnotics such as the BZRAs can induce amnestic nocturnal behavior.[2] The exact mechanism by which BZs suppress NREM parasomnias is uncertain; however, they may work through the suppression of cortical arousals.

Diazepam

One of the earliest reported pharmacologic studies, a double-blind crossover trial of diazepam, reported mixed results. In this investigation, five adults with chronic sleepwalking were given either 10 mg of diazepam or placebo. They reported that diazepam administration resulted in resolution of sleepwalking events in some, but not all, subjects. There was no significant difference between placebo and treatment groups; however, this was a small study and it is uncertain whether other sleep phenomena, such as subtle SDB, may have been present.[85]

Clonazepam

The most extensively studied agent in the treatment of NREM parasomnias is clonazepam. In 1989 a series was published of 61 patients with sleep-related injury who were treated with clonazepam;[86] 83.6% of patients had a "rapid and sustained" response to clonazepam. However, not all 61 patients treated with clonazepam had a NREM parasomnia. In fact, slightly more than half of patients ($n = 33$) had REM sleep behavior disorder, a condition whose first-line treatment is clonazepam,[87] and separate data for sleepwalking/night terrors were not reported.[86] Later, the same investigators reported on an expanded series of 170 patients with various sleep-disruptive disorders ($n = 69$ with sleepwalking/night terrors) who were treated with benzodiazepines, primarily clonazepam ($n = 136$).[88] The majority (86%) of these patients reported complete/nearly complete efficacy after a mean follow-up of 3.5 years. Importantly, the authors reported sustained efficacy with clonazepam with low risk of dosage tolerance.[88] In a separate small series, ten patients with a history of sleepwalking were followed after a variety of treatments were initiated. PSG was used to confirm the NREM parasomnia. Clonazepam was initiated in six patients, and sleepwalking being suppressed in five of them.[89] Conversely, a more recent report claims that clonazepam failed to demonstrate sustained efficacy in five sleepwalking patients. This investigation carefully excluded even subtle SDB or associated mental illness. After 1 year, all five of these patients treated with clonazepam reported persistence of sleepwalking and dropped out of the study.[74]

Antidepressant Medications

Reports have suggested that agents with serotoninergic activity (e.g., the commonly prescribed selective serotonin reuptake inhibitors [SSRI] antidepressants) are effective in the treatment of NREM parasomnias, in particular sleep terrors, in some patients.

The supposed mechanism by which these medications would resolve NREM parasomnias is derived from several features of serotoninergic neurons.[34,55] In particular, serotoninergic neurons can be activated by hypercapnic acidosis, which would be expected in the setting of SDB.[90,91] Further, serotoninergic neuronal activity activates spinal motor neurons,[92] and this effect can be dissociated from wakefulness.[55,93] Also, disorders associated with sleepwalking, such as migraine[34,35] and fever,[36] are often associated with surges of serotonin.[55] It has thus been suggested that because of impairment in serotonin regulation, serotoninergic neurons activated by nocturnal respiratory events trigger CPGs (for a review refer to references)[41,42] and produce sleep-related motor activity.[55]

Two early case reports provide some preliminary insight into the diversity of clinical effectiveness of antidepressant medication for NREM parasomnias. The first report described two patients with a history of sleep terrors and sleepwalking, both of whom failed diazepam therapy but responded well to imipramine, a tricyclic antidepressant with serotonin activity.[94] Later, a 7-year-old girl with sleep terrors who failed to respond to imipramine as well as to hydroxyzine (an antihistamine) or thioridazine (a dopamine blocking agent), was reported to have a compelling therapeutic response to trazodone, a phenylpiperazine antidepressant with strong effects on serotonin receptors.[95]

Paroxetine

There have been conflicting reports on the efficacy of paroxetine in NREM parasomnias. In 1994, a 30-year-old patient with a combination of sleep terrors and somnambulism was reported to be successfully treated with paroxetine.[96] Conversely, a letter in response to this report suggested that the nocturnal behavior was not actually sleepwalking but instead a nocturnal panic attack.[97] However, a later report noted either an elimination or reduction of night terrors in six patients treated with paroxetine[53] and concluded that SSRI's may be uniquely effective for night terrors through serotonin effects

on terror centers in the brainstem. In particular, the periaqueductal gray matter in the midbrain has been implicated. Finally, there has been a report of paroxetine inducing sleepwalking.[23] Clearly more research, in particular a randomized controlled trial, is needed.

The mechanism by which serotoninergic agents may potentially act on NREM parasomnias has not yet been fully elucidated. Any potential explanation should account for the apparent discrepancy in the effective treatment of some NREM parasomnias (sleep terrors, see later discussion) with some serotoninergic agents[53,94-96] and induction of other NREM parasomnias (sleepwalking) with others.[23,25,26] One plausible explanation for this inconsistency could be that sleep terrors arise from pathophysiologic mechanisms distinct (at least in part) from other NREM parasomnias (see "An Alternative Proposed Mechanism for Sleep Terrors," earlier).

Conversely, one series of sleepwalking patients, closely screened for underlying mood or anxiety disorders, included eight patients treated for these conditions with medications (SSRIs, trazodone, or anxiolytics) or by psychotherapy. After 1 year follow-up, all eight patients described a persistence of sleepwalking. These findings are in contrast to a dramatic elimination of sleepwalking behavior in patients who are effectively treated for SDB (see earlier discussion).[74]

Other Pharmacologic Treatments

There have been sporadic reports of successful resolution of NREM parasomnias with other BZs as well as other neuropsychiatric agents. These therapies were identified empirically through clinical practice and the studies were not blinded or placebo-controlled. In one series of PSG-confirmed NREM parasomnias, flurazepam resolved sleepwalking in two patients and a combination of clonazepam with phenytoin eliminated abnormal nocturnal behavior in another.[89] Another series reported 11 patients with either sleep terrors or sleepwalking who had a sustained response to alprazolam without significant dose escalation over a mean follow-up of 2.8 years.[88]

Psychotherapy and Hypnotherapy

Some reports suggest that psychotherapy may be helpful in the treatment of NREM parasomnias. In 1981, 11 sleepwalkers reported that hypnotherapy was helpful with lasting improvement after 1 year. However, close scrutiny of the blinded, crossover portion of this study reveals no difference between the active and suggestive treatment groups.[85] Later among 54 night terror/sleepwalking patients who presented with sleep-related injurious behavior, 22 were taught and treated with self-hypnosis. Of these 22, 14 (64%) reported substantial benefit. However, separate data for each of these two NREM parasomnias was not reported,[86] although often they coexist in the same patient. In another case series (involving some of the patients just described), 20 out of 23 sleepwalking patients who underwent self-hypnosis training described significant improvement after greater than 6 months of follow-up.[98] More recently, only 3 of 11 sleepwalkers treated with physician-administered hypnosis described significant improvement after 18 months follow-up.[99]

In cases in which psychotherapy is successful, it is uncertain whether this is an epiphenomenon, as controlled trials are lacking, or whether these treatments are addressing an underlying mental disorder which, once treated, helped eliminate the nocturnal behavior. Conversely, many patients with parasomnias are mislabeled as having underlying mental illness and have often undergone extensive psychotherapy with little resolution.[100] Thus, psychotherapy in the setting of parasomnias without other known mental illness is not supported by evidence. Nevertheless, in patients with episodes of NREM parasomnia that seem to be precipitated by stress, referral for stress-reduction psychotherapy could be considered.

Anticipatory Awakenings

Anticipatory awakening is a commonly used method, especially in childhood NREM parasomnias.[60] This technique involves purposefully arousing the parasomniac just prior to the onset of a typical episode, with the typical time of onset identified from repeated experience. Sustained positive results in four children have been reported;[101,102] however, there are negligible data in adults. This method appears to be a relatively low-risk therapy (unless the arousing stimulation triggers a major event); however, more investigations are needed.

Conclusion

In conclusion, while benzodiazepines, antidepressant medications, and hypnosis are commonly utilized to treat NREM parasomnias, their efficacy—though apparently substantial for the BZs—has not yet been convincingly proved in a methodologically rigorous manner (Box 44-14). Serotoninergic agents may have particular efficacy in the treatment of sleep terrors. However, as with other NREM parasomnias, adequately powered, randomized controlled trials are lacking. The absence of treatment data likely results from the diverse nature of these conditions, wide variations in episode frequency, their common co-morbidity with other sleep disorders, and concurrent polypharmacy. It is of paramount importance to identify and remove any inducing pharmacologic agents and treat any co-morbid sleep disorder. In particular, even subtle SDB should be considered as a potential target to resolve NREM parasomnias. Finally, if pharmacotherapy is utilized, patients should be made aware that these treatments are being used in an off-label—albeit presumably safe—manner, and they are apparently effective by suppressing the abnormal behavior on a night-to-night basis, but they are not curative of the NREM parasomnia.

SLEEP-RELATED EATING DISORDER

Sleep-related eating disorder (SRED) is characterized by a disruption of the nocturnal fast with episodes of feeding after an arousal from nighttime sleep (Box 44-15). The disorder resembles sleepwalking, especially in the setting of sedative-hypnotic medication-induced amnesia. The most commonly cited agents associated with SRED are the BZRAs, in particular zolpidem (Box 44-16). Like other NREM parasomnias, SRED is often associated with other sleep disorders, such as other NREM parasomnias, RLS, and SDB.[1,103]

SRED is common and has a diverse clinical presentation. A study of eating-disorder patients determined high prevalence rates in inpatients (17%), outpatients (9%), and an unselected group of college students (5%).[104] Adverse consequences include weight gain, ingestion of nonfood or toxic substances, and aggravation of associated medical conditions (e.g., diabetes mellitus, obesity).[104]

The etiology of SRED is unknown; however, the association with RLS may provide insight into pathophysiologic mechanisms. SRED is common among patients with RLS, and a substantial number of BZRA-associated cases of SRED occur in the setting of patients with RLS.[62,105-108] RLS is a condition distinct from, but often confused with, insomnia (which often responds to BZRA therapy). Difficulty initiating and maintaining sleep is a major presenting complaint in patients with RLS. Thus, the critical step in the pathogenesis of many amnestic SRED cases may in fact be an inaccurate diagnosis and treatment of RLS as insomnia.

Treatment

The first goal in treating dysfunctional nocturnal eating is to identify and correct any co-morbid sleep disorders (e.g., RLS and PLM) and eliminate suspected inducing agents. Discontinuing an offending medication is the best treatment for drug-induced SRED.[19,105-108] Rarely, patients who did not have nocturnal eating prior to exposure will have persisting episodes after cessation of the offending agent. It is not certain whether this is a temporary phenomenon or whether the offending agent is lowering a threshold in patients who were already predisposed to nocturnal eating.

Dopaminergics, opioids, and BZs are agents typically employed in the treatment of RLS and PLM. In the original case series of 38 SRED patients, combinations of these medications effectively eliminated nocturnal eating associated with RLS and PLM[109] (Box 44-17). Interestingly dopaminergic therapy also appears to often be helpful in the setting of SRED co-morbid with sleepwalking. In the original case series just described, eight sleepwalking patients with SRED were effectively treated with bromocriptine, levodopa, or clonazepam.[109] Interestingly, BZs, commonly employed in the treatment of other NREM parasomnias, are typically ineffective as monotherapy.[47] SRED associated with OSA may be effectively treated with CPAP. In two cases of SRED with OSA, CPAP eliminated the nocturnal eating.[109]

Two classes of pharmacotherapeutic agents have been studied and appear to be effective in treating nocturnal eating. In SRED, the anticonvulsant topiramate and the dopaminergics have both demonstrated promising results. However, research on the therapy of SRED is still in its infancy, and further investigations, in particular, randomized controlled trials, are necessary.

Dopaminergic Agents

Dopaminergic agents may be effective in the treatment of SRED. The original case series noted that either bedtime levodopa or bromocriptine was effective in eliminating nocturnal eating especially in patients with associated RLS.[109,110] Two follow-up reports from the same investigators also demonstrated improved control of nocturnal eating with dopaminergic and opioid therapy.[111,112] The mechanism by which dopamine agents may suppress nocturnal eating is unknown; their primary action may be through suppression of RLS (opioids also treat RLS) or conversely through appetite suppression. Recently, pramipexole, a dopamine receptor agonist, was investigated in a small double-blind, placebo-controlled crossover trial. Pramipexole was well tolerated in all patients, including those without known RLS or PLMD. On pramipexole subjects noted improved sleep, and reduced nighttime activity was documented with actigraphy. There was no improvement in the number or duration of awakenings.[113] The main side effects of dopamine agonists include sedation, orthostasis, nausea, manic episodes, paranoia, psychosis, and hallucinations.

Topiramate

Early studies indicate that the antiseizure medication topiramate may be an effective treatment for controlling abnormal nocturnal eating. An open-label trial of topiramate in four

patients with nocturnal eating demonstrated positive results. The agent was well tolerated, nocturnal eating diminished, and weight loss (mean of 11.1 kg) was noted in all four individuals over 8.5 months.[114] A case report with similar results was recently published. This 28-year-old obese man had a 10-year history of nocturnal eating episodes that were eliminated with topiramate. It was also reported that the agent was well tolerated over a 2-year follow-up.[115] In a case series published as an abstract, of 17 SRED patients treated with topiramate, 12 were treatment responsive. The agent was well tolerated, and over 1.8 years there was a mean weight loss of 9.2 kg among the treatment responders.[116] Another chart review of 25 follow-up SRED patients reported that 68% of SRED patients were treatment responders. However, over 1 year, only 28% of patients lost more than 10% of their body weight and 41% of patients discontinued the medication due to adverse effects.[117] The main side effects of topiramate are weight loss, paresthesias, renal calculus, cognitive dysfunction, and orthostasis.

Modulation of central nervous system serotonin may lead to effective treatment of nocturnal eating. Fluoxetine was reported to effectively resolve nocturnal eating in two of three SRED patients.[109] Further, other cases of nocturnal eating have also been responsive to serotoninergic medications. However, conclusions regarding SRED treatment are difficult to draw from these reports, as these subjects had diagnoses other than SRED, most commonly the night eating syndrome (NES).[118-120]

In conclusion, the clinical investigation of SRED patients should attempt to identify co-morbid sleep disorders and to eliminate inducing agents. In particular, sleepwalking, OSA, RLS, and PLM are treatable and commonly found in SRED patients. Attended PSG at a sleep laboratory is needed to identify and treat co-morbid sleep disorders. SRED is associated with psychotropic medications, most notably the BZRA zolpidem. Three types of pharmacotherapeutic agents have been studied as treatments for SRED and may be effective: dopaminergics, anticonvulsants (topiramate), and serotoninergics. Further research is needed.

A DVD documentary film, *Sleep Runners: The Stories Behind Everyday Parasomnias*, has been produced in which patients with sleepwalking, sleep terrors, SRED, and other parasomnias describe their personal experiences (along with their spouses and family) with these abnormal, recurrent nocturnal events, and the gratifying response to treatment.[121]

SUMMARY

Complex amnestic behaviors arise from NREM sleep due to a combination of impaired cortical arousal and inappropriate motor system activation. NREM sleep parasomnias include confusional arousals, sleepwalking, sleep terrors, and sleep-related eating disorder. There is often a genetic predisposition. Other predisposing factors include any process that increases the homeostatic sleep drive (such as sleep deprivation or sedative-hypnotic medications) or that precipitates arousal (such as SDB). In the sleep laboratory, the combination of sleep deprivation and sudden forced arousal during SWS is a useful diagnostic protocol for inducing a NREM parasomnia episode. Treatment should first focus upon addressing any underlying sleep disorders and conditions that inappropriately either enhance the sleep drive and deepen sleep, or precipitate sudden arousals. Various symptomatic therapies may need to be considered.

REFERENCES

1. American Academy of Sleep Medicine. *International Classification of Sleep Disorders: Diagnostic and Coding Manual*. 2nd ed. Westchester, IL: American Academy of Sleep Medicine; 2005.
2. Dolder CR, Nelson MH. Hypnosedative-induced complex behaviours: Incidence, mechanisms and management. *CNS Drugs*. 2008;22(12):1021-1036.
3. Hublin C, Kaprio J, Partinen M, Heikkila K, Koskenvuo M. Prevalence and genetics of sleepwalking: A population-based twin study. *Neurology*. 1997;48(1):177-181.
4. Ohayon MM, Guilleminault C, Priest RG. Night terrors, sleepwalking, and confusional arousals in the general population: Their frequency and relationship to other sleep and mental disorders. *J Clin Psychiatry*. 1999;60(4):268-276.
5. Pires ML, Benedito-Silva AA, Mello MT, Pompeia Sdel G, Tufik S. Sleep habits and complaints of adults in the city of Sao Paulo, Brazil, in 1987 and 1995. *Braz J Med Biol Res*. 2007;40(11):1505-1515.
6. Oluwole OS. Lifetime prevalence and incidence of parasomnias in a population of young adult Nigerians. *J Neurol*. 2010;257(7):1141-1147.
7. Espa F, Dauvilliers Y, Ondze B, Billiard M, Besset A. Arousal reactions in sleepwalking and night terrors in adults: The role of respiratory events. *Sleep*. 2002;25(8):871-875.
8. Guilleminault C, Palombini L, Pelayo R, Chervin RD. Sleepwalking and sleep terrors in prepubertal children: What triggers them? *Pediatrics*. 2003;111(1):e17-e25.
9. Lam SP, Fong SY, Ho CK, Yu MW, Wing YK. Parasomnia among psychiatric outpatients: A clinical, epidemiologic, cross-sectional study. *J Clin Psychiatry*. 2008;69(9):1374-1382.
10. Lam SP, Fong SY, Yu MW, Li SX, Wing YK. Sleepwalking in psychiatric patients: Comparison of childhood and adult onset. *Aust N Z J Psychiatry*. 2009;43(5):426-430.
11. Canaday BR. Amnesia possibly associated with zolpidem administration. *Pharmacotherapy*. 1996;16(4):687-689.
12. Fava GA. Amnestic syndrome induced by zopiclone. *Eur J Clin Pharmacol*. 1996;50(6):509.
13. Harazin J, Berigan TR. Zolpidem tartrate and somnambulism. *Milit Med*. 1999;164(9):669-670.
14. Morgenthaler TI, Silber MH. Amnestic sleep-related eating disorder associated with zolpidem. *Sleep Med*. 2002;3(4):323-327.
15. Sattar SP, Ramaswamy S, Bhatia SC, Petty F. Somnambulism due to probable interaction of valproic acid and zolpidem. *Ann Pharmacother*. 2003;37(10):1429-1433.
16. Liskow B, Pikalov A. Zaleplon overdose associated with sleepwalking and complex behavior. *J Am Acad Child Adolesc Psychiatry*. 2004;43(8):927-928.
17. Kintz P, Villain M, Dumestre-Toulet V, Ludes B. Drug-facilitated sexual assault and analytical toxicology: The role of LC-MS/MS: A case involving zolpidem. *J Clin Forensic Med*. 2005;12(1):36-41.
18. Yang W, Dollear M, Muthukrishnan SR. One rare side effect of zolpidem—Sleepwalking: A case report. *Arch Phys Med Rehabil*. 2005;86(6):1265-1266.
19. Tsai MJ, Tsai YH, Huang YB. Compulsive activity and anterograde amnesia after zolpidem use. *Clin Toxicol (Phila)*. 2007;45(2):179-181.
20. Ferrandiz-Santos JA, Mataix-Sanjuan AL. Amitriptyline and somnambulism. *Ann Pharmacother*. 2000;34(10):1208.
21. Khazaal Y, Krenz S, Zullino DF. Bupropion-induced somnambulism. *Addict Biol*. 2003;8(3):359-362.
22. Oulis P, Kokras N, Papadimitriou GN, Masdrakis VG. Bupropion-induced sleepwalking. *J Clin Psychopharmacol*. 2010;30(1):83-84.
23. Kawashima T, Yamada S. Paroxetine-induced somnambulism. *J Clin Psychiatry*. 2003;64(4):483.
24. Yeh YW, Chen CH, Feng HM, Wang SC, Kuo SC, Chen CK. New onset somnambulism associated with different dosage of mirtazapine: A case report. *Clin Neuropharmacol*. 2009;32(4):232-233.
25. Charney DS, Kales A, Soldatos CR, Nelson JC. Somnambulistic-like episodes secondary to combined lithium-neuroleptic treatment. *Br J Psychiatry*. 1979;135:418-424.
26. Landry P, Warnes H, Nielsen T, Montplaisir J. Somnambulistic-like behaviour in patients attending a lithium clinic. *Int Clin Psychopharmacol*. 1999;14(3):173-175.
27. Hafeez ZH, Kalinowski CM. Somnambulism induced by quetiapine: Two case reports and a review of the literature. *CNS Spectr*. 2007;12(12):910-912.
28. Kolivakis TT, Margolese HC, Beauclair L, Chouinard G. Olanzapine-induced somnambulism. *Am J Psychiatry*. 2001;158(7):1158.
29. Paquet V, Strul J, Servais L, Pelc I, Fossion P. Sleep-related eating disorder induced by olanzapine. *J Clin Psychiatry*. 2002;63(7):597.
30. Chiu YH, Chen CH, Shen WW. Somnambulism secondary to olanzapine treatment in one patient with bipolar disorder. *Prog Neuropsychopharmacol Biol Psychiatry*. 2008;32(2):581-582.
31. Hensel J, Pillmann F. Late-life somnambulism after therapy with metoprolol. *Clin Neuropharmacol*. 2008;31(4):248-250.
32. Varkey BM, Varkey LM. Topiramate induced somnabulism and automatic behaviour. *Indian J Med Sci*. 2003;57(11):508-510.
33. von Vigier RO, Vella S, Bianchetti MG. Agitated sleepwalking with fluoroquinolone therapy. *Pediatr Infect Dis J*. 1999;18(5):484-485.
34. Barabas G, Ferrari M, Matthews WS. Childhood migraine and somnambulism. *Neurology*. 1983;33(7):948-949.
35. Casez O, Dananchet Y, Besson G. Migraine and somnambulism. *Neurology*. 2005;65(8):1334-1335.
36. Kales JD, Kales A, Soldatos CR, Chamberlin K, Martin ED. Sleepwalking and night terrors related to febrile illness. *Am J Psychiatry*. 1979;136(9):1214-1215.
37. Mouzas O, Angelopoulos N, Papaliagka M, Tsogas P. Increased frequency of self-reported parasomnias in patients suffering from vitiligo. *Eur J Dermatol*. 2008;18(2):165-168.
38. Ajlouni KM, Ahmad AT, El-Zaheri MM, Ammari FL, Jarrah NS, et al. Sleepwalking associated with hyperthyroidism. *Endocr Pract*. 2005;11(1):5-10.
39. Guilleminault C, Kirisoglu C, da Rosa AC, Lopes C, Chan A. Sleepwalking, a disorder of NREM sleep instability. *Sleep Med*. 2006;7(2):163-170.
40. Guilleminault C, Lee JH, Chan A, Lopes MC, Huang YS, da Rosa A. Non-REM-sleep instability in recurrent sleepwalking in pre-pubertal children. *Sleep Med*. 2005;6(6):515-521.
41. Parrino L, Halasz P, Tassinari CA, Terzano MG. CAP, epilepsy and motor events during sleep: The unifying role of arousal. *Sleep Med Rev*. 2006;10(4):267-285.
42. Tassinari CA, Cantalupo G, Hogl B, Cortelli P, Tassi L, et al. Neuroethological approach to frontolimbic epileptic seizures and parasomnias: The same central pattern generators for the same behaviours. *Rev Neurol (Paris)*. 2009;165(10):762-768.

43. Steriade M, Llinas RR. The functional states of the thalamus and the associated neuronal interplay. *Physiol Rev.* 1988;68(3):649-742.

44. Neckelmann D, Ursin R. Sleep stages and EEG power spectrum in relation to acoustical stimulus arousal threshold in the rat. *Sleep.* 1993;16(5): 467-477.

45. Pilon M, Montplaisir J, Zadra A. Precipitating factors of somnambulism: Impact of sleep deprivation and forced arousals. *Neurology.* 2008;70(24):2284-2290.

46. Hwang TJ, Hsing-Chang N, Chen HC, Lin YT, Liao SC. Risk predictors for hypnosedative-related complex sleep behaviors: A pilot study. *J Clin Psychiatry.* 2010;71(10):1331-1335.

47. Howell MJ, Schenck CH. Treatment of nocturnal eating disorders. *Curr Treat Options Neurol.* 2009;11(5):333-339.

48. Mahowald MW, Schenck CH. Cramer Bornemann MA. Sleep-related violence. *Curr Neurol Neurosci Rep.* 2005;5(2):153-158.

49. Schenck CH, Connoy DA, Castellanos M, Johnson B, Wills L, et al. Zolpidem-induced sleep-related eating disorder (SRED) in 19 patients. *Sleep.* 2005;28(suppl):A259.

50. Terzaghi M, Sartori I, Tassi L, Didato G, Rustioni V, et al. Evidence of dissociated arousal states during NREM parasomnia from an intracerebral neurophysiological study. *Sleep.* 2009;32(3):409-412.

51. Bassetti C, Vella S, Donati F, Wielepp P, Weder B. SPECT during sleepwalking. *Lancet.* 2000;356(9228):484-485.

52. Arkin AM. Night-Terrors as anomalous REM sleep component manifestation in slow-wave sleep. *Waking-Sleeping.* 1978;(2):143-147.

53. Wilson SJ, Lillywhite AR, Potokar JP, Bell CJ, Nutt DJ. Adult night terrors and paroxetine. *Lancet.* 1997;350(9072):185.

54. Bell C, Wilson S, Rich A, Bailey J, Nutt D. Effects on sleep architecture of pindolol, paroxetine and their combination in healthy volunteers. *Psychopharmacology (Berl).* 2003;166(2):102-110.

55. Juszczak GR, Swiergiel AH. Serotonergic hypothesis of sleepwalking. *Med Hypotheses.* 2005;64(1):28-32.

56. Hublin C, Kaprio J, Partinen M, Koskenvu M. Parasomnias: Co-occurrence and genetics. *Psychiatr Genet.* 2001;11(2):65-70.

57. Lecendreux M, Bassetti C, Dauvilliers Y, Mayer G, Neidhart E, Tafti M. HLA and genetic susceptibility to sleepwalking. *Mol Psychiatry.* 2003;8(1):114-117.

58. Rogers AE, Meehan J, Guilleminault C, Grumet FC, Mignot E. HLA DR15 (DR2) and DQB1*0602 typing studies in 188 narcoleptic patients with cataplexy. *Neurology.* 1997;48(6):1550-1556.

59. Schenck CH, Garcia-Rill E, Segall M, Noreen H, Mahowald MW. HLA class II genes associated with REM sleep behavior disorder. *Ann Neurol.* 1996;39(2):261-263.

60. Wills L, Garcia J. Parasomnias: Epidemiology and management. *CNS Drugs.* 2002;16(12):803-810.

61. Provini F, Antelmi E, Vignatelli L, Zaniboni A, Naldi G, et al. Association of restless legs syndrome with nocturnal eating: A case-control study. *Mov Disord.* 2009;24(6):871-877.

62. Howell MJ, Schenck CH. Nocturnal eating and sleep related eating disorders are common in patients with restless legs syndrome. *Sleep.* 2010;11(6):583-585.

63. Schenck CH, Hurwitz TD, O'Connor KA, Mahowald MW. Additional categories of sleep-related eating disorders and the current status of treatment. *Sleep.* 1993;16(5):457-466.

64. Satija P, Ondo WG. Restless legs syndrome: Pathophysiology, diagnosis and treatment. *CNS Drugs.* 2008;22(6):497-518.

65. Barion A, Zee PC. A clinical approach to circadian rhythm sleep disorders. *Sleep Med.* 2007;8(6):566-577.

66. Sivertsen B, Omvik S, Pallesen S, Bjorvatn B, Havik OE, et al. Cognitive behavioral therapy vs. zopiclone for treatment of chronic primary insomnia in older adults: A randomized controlled trial. *JAMA.* 2006; 295(24):2851-2858.

67. Pressman MR. Disorders of arousal from sleep and violent behavior: The role of physical contact and proximity. *Sleep.* 2007;30(8):1039-1047.

68. Edinger JD, Fins AI, Sullivan Jr RJ, Marsh GR, Dailey DS, et al. Sleep in the laboratory and sleep at home: Comparisons of older insomniacs and normal sleepers. *Sleep.* 1997;20(12):1119-1126.

69. Mayer G, Neissner V, Schwarzmayr P, Meier-Ewert K. Sleep deprivation in somnambulism. Effect of arousal, deep sleep and sleep stage changes. *Nervenarzt.* 1998;69(6):495-501.

70. Joncas S, Zadra A, Paquet J, Montplaisir J. The value of sleep deprivation as a diagnostic tool in adult sleepwalkers. *Neurology.* 2002;58(6):936-940.

71. Guilleminault C. Hypersynchronous slow delta, cyclic alternating pattern and sleepwalking. *Sleep.* 2006;29(1):14-15.

72. Pressman MR. Factors that predispose, prime and precipitate NREM parasomnias in adults: Clinical and forensic implications. *Sleep Med Rev.* 2007;11:5-30.

73. Zadra A, Pilon M, Joncas S, Rompre S, Montplaisir J. Analysis of post-arousal EEG activity during somnambulistic episodes. *J Sleep Res.* 2004; 13(3):279-284.

74. Guilleminault C, Kirisoglu C, Bao G, Arias V, Chan A, Li KK. Adult chronic sleepwalking and its treatment based on polysomnography. *Brain.* 2005;128:1062-1069.

75. Schenck CH, Arnulf I, Mahowald MW. Sleep and sex: What can go wrong? A review of the literature on sleep related disorders and abnormal sexual behaviors and experiences. *Sleep.* 2007;30(6):683-702.

76. Terzano MG, Parrino L. Origin and significance of the cyclic alternating pattern (CAP). *Sleep Med Rev.* 2000;4(1):101-123.

77. Zucconi M, Oldani A, Ferini-Strambi L, Smirne S. Arousal fluctuations in non-rapid eye movement parasomnias: The role of cyclic alternating pattern as a measure of sleep instability. *J Clin Neurophysiol.* 1995; 12(2):147-154.

78. Guilleminault C, Lee JH, Chan A, Lopes MC, Huang YS, da Rosa A. Non-REM-sleep instability in recurrent sleepwalking in pre-pubertal children. *Sleep Med.* 2005;6(6):515-521.

79. Guilleminault C, Kirisoglu C, da Rosa AC, Lopes C, Chan A. Sleepwalking, a disorder of NREM sleep instability. *Sleep Med.* 2006;7(2):163-170.

80. Jacobson A, Kales A, Lehmann D, Zweizig JR. Somnambulism: All-night electroencephalographic studies. *Science.* 1965;148:975-977.

81. Espa F, Ondze B, Deglise P, Billiard M, Besset A. Sleep architecture, slow wave activity, and sleep spindles in adult patients with sleepwalking and sleep terrors. *Clin Neurophysiol.* 2000;111(5):929-939.

82. Guilleminault C, Poyares D, Aftab FA, Palombini L. Sleep and wakefulness in somnambulism: A spectral analysis study. *J Psychosom Res.* 2001; 51(2):411-416.

83. Harris M, Grunstein RR. Treatments for somnambulism in adults: Assessing the evidence. *Sleep Med Rev.* 2009;13(4):295-297.

84. Rudolph U, Mohler H. GABAA-based therapeutic approaches: GABAA receptor subtype functions. *Curr Opin Pharmacol.* 2006;6(1):18-23.

85. Reid WH, Haffke EA, Chu CC. Diazepam in intractable sleepwalking: A pilot study. *Hillside J Clin Psychiatry.* 1984;6(1):49-55.

86. Schenck CH, Milner DM, Hurwitz TD, Bundlie SR, Mahowald MW. A polysomnographic and clinical report on sleep-related injury in 100 adult patients. *Am J Psychiatry.* 1989;146(9):1166-1173.

87. Aurora RN, Zak RS, Maganti RK, Auerbach SH, Casey KR, et al. Best practice guide for the treatment of REM sleep behavior disorder (RBD). *J Clin Sleep Med.* 2010;6(1):85-95.

88. Schenck CH, Mahowald MW. Long-term, nightly benzodiazepine treatment of injurious parasomnias and other disorders of disrupted nocturnal sleep in 170 adults. *Am J Med.* 1996;100(3):333-337.

89. Kavey NB, Whyte J, Resor Jr SR, Gidro-Frank S. Somnambulism in adults. *Neurology.* 1990;40(5):749-752.

90. Richerson GB, Wang W, Tiwari J, Bradley SR. Chemosensitivity of serotonergic neurons in the rostral ventral medulla. *Respir Physiol.* 2001; 129(1-2):175-189.

91. Jacobs BL, Martin-Cora FJ, Fornal CA. Activity of medullary serotonergic neurons in freely moving animals. *Brain Res Brain Res Rev.* 2002; 40(1-3):45-52.

92. Rekling JC, Funk GD, Bayliss DA, Dong XW, Feldman JL. Synaptic control of motoneuronal excitability. *Physiol Rev.* 2000;80(2):767-852.

93. Steinfels GF, Heym J, Strecker RE, Jacobs BL. Behavioral correlates of dopaminergic unit activity in freely moving cats. *Brain Res.* 1983;258(2): 217-228.

94. Cooper AJ. Treatment of coexistent night-terrors and somnambulism in adults with imipramine and diazepam. *J Clin Psychiatry.* 1987;48(5): 209-210.

95. Balon R. Sleep terror disorder and insomnia treated with trazodone: A case report. *Ann Clin Psychiatry.* 1994;6(3):161-163.

96. Lillywhite AR, Wilson SJ, Nutt DJ. Successful treatment of night terrors and somnambulism with paroxetine. *Br J Psychiatry.* 1994;164(4):551-554.

97. van Sweden B, van Erp MG, Mesotten F, Peuskens J. Night terrors. *Br J Psychiatry.* 1994;165(6):834-835.

98. Hurwitz TD, Mahowald MW, Schenck CH, Schluter JL, Bundlie SR. A retrospective outcome study and review of hypnosis as treatment of adults with sleepwalking and sleep terror. *J Nerv Ment Dis.* 1991;179(4): 228-233.

99. Hauri PJ, Silber MH, Boeve BF. The treatment of parasomnias with hypnosis: A 5-year follow-up study. *J Clin Sleep Med.* 2007;3(4):369-373.

100. Mahowald MW, Schenck CH. Non-rapid eye movement sleep parasomnias. *Neurol Clin.* 2005;23(4):1077-1106:vii.

101. Tobin Jr JD. Treatment of somnambulism with anticipatory awakening. *J Pediatr.* 1993;122(3):426-427.

102. Frank NC, Spirito A, Stark L, Owens-Stively J. The use of scheduled awakenings to eliminate childhood sleepwalking. *J Pediatr Psychol.* 1997; 22(3):345-353.

103. Howell MJ, Schenck CH, Crow SJ. A review of nighttime eating disorders. *Sleep Med Rev.* 2009;13:23-34.

104. Winkelman JW, Herzog DB, Fava M. The prevalence of sleep-related eating disorder in psychiatric and non-psychiatric populations. *Psychol Med.* 1999;29(6):1461-1466.

105. Morgenthaler TI, Silber MH. Amnestic sleep-related eating disorder associated with zolpidem. *Sleep Med.* 2002;3(4):323-327.

106. Sansone RA, Sansone LA. Zolpidem, somnambulism, and nocturnal eating. *Gen Hosp Psychiatry.* 2008;30(1):90-91.

107. Chiang A, Krystal A. Report of two cases where sleep related eating behavior occurred with the extended-release formulation but not the immediate-release formulation of a sedative-hypnotic agent. *J Clin Sleep Med.* 2008;4(2):155-156.

108. Dang A, Garg G, Rataboli PV. Zolpidem induced nocturnal sleep-related eating disorder (NSRED) in a male patient. *Int J Eat Disord.* 2009;42:385-386.

109. Schenck CH, Hurwitz TD, O'Connor KA, Mahowald MW. Additional categories of sleep-related eating disorders and the current status of treatment. *Sleep.* 1993;16(5):457-466.

110. Schenck CH, Mahowald MW. Review of nocturnal sleep-related eating disorders. *Int J Eat Disord.* 1994;15(4):343-356.

111. Schenck CH, Mahowald MW. Combined buproprion-levodopa-trazadone therapy of sleep-related eating disorder and sleep disruption in two adults with chemical dependency. *Sleep.* 2000;23:587-588.

112. Schenck CH, Mahowald MW. Dopaminergic and opiate therapy of nocturnal sleep-related eating disorder associated with sleepwalking or unassociated with another nocturnal disorder. *Sleep.* 2002;25(suppl): A249-A250.

113. Provini F, Albani F, Vetrugno R, Vignatelli L, Lombardi C, et al. A pilot double-blind placebo-controlled trial of low-dose pramipexole in sleep-related eating disorder. *Eur J Neurol.* 2005;12(6):432-436.

114. Winkelman JW. Treatment of nocturnal eating syndrome and sleep-related eating disorder with topiramate. *Sleep Med.* 2003;4(3):243-246.

115. Martinez-Salio A, Soler-Algarra S, Calvo-Garcia I, Sanchez-Martin M. Nocturnal sleep-related eating disorder that responds to topiramate. *Rev Neurol.* 2007;45(5):276-279.

116. Schenck CH, Murakami MM. Topiramate therapy of sleep related eating disorder (SRED). *Sleep.* 2006;29:A268.

117. Winkelman JW. Efficacy and tolerability of open-label topiramate in the treatment of sleep-related eating disorder: A retrospective case series. *J Clin Psychiatry.* 2006;67:1729-1734.

118. Spaggiari MC, Granella F, Parrino L, Marchesi C, Melli I, Terzano MG. Nocturnal eating syndrome in adults. *Sleep.* 1994;17(4):339-344.

119. Miyaoka T, Yasukawa R, Tsubouchi K, Miura S, Shimizu Y, et al. Successful treatment of nocturnal eating/drinking syndrome with selective serotonin reuptake inhibitors. *Int Clin Psychopharmacol.* 2003;18(3): 175-177.

120. O'Reardon JP, Allison KC, Martino NS, et al. A randomized, placebo-controlled trial of sertraline in the treatment of night eating syndrome. *Am J Psychiatry.* 2006;163:893-898.

121. Sleep Runners. The Stories Behind Everyday Parasomnias (1 hour DVD documentary film). St. Paul, MN: Slow-Wave Films, LLC; 2004. *Deluxe Academic Edition.* 2007;www.sleeprunners.com.

Other Parasomnias in Adults:

SEXSOMNIA, SLEEP-RELATED DISSOCIATIVE DISORDER, CATATHRENIA, SLEEP-RELATED HALLUCINATIONS, AND SLEEP TALKING

Chapter
45

CARLOS H. SCHENCK / THOMAS D. HURWITZ

SEXSOMNIA

The first classification of sleep-related disorders associated with sexual behaviors and experiences has recently been published.[1] Several factors prompted the development of this classification. There has been growing awareness that abnormal sexual behaviors can emerge during sleep, described as "sleepsex," "atypical sexual behavior during sleep," and "sexsomnia."[2-4] In fact, *The International Classification of Sleep Disorders,* 2nd Edition (ICSD-2) in 2005 formally recognized this phenomenon by classifying it as a parasomnia, namely, a variant of confusional arousals (CA) and sleepwalking.[5] The cause of sleepsex can often be identified after clinical and polysomnography (PSG) evaluations, and then effectively treated. Furthermore, there is an expanding set of sleep disorders and other nocturnal disorders known to be associated with abnormal sexual behaviors and experiences, or the misperception of sexual behaviors and experiences. The forensic aspects of abnormal sleep-related sexual behavior have commanded increasing attention, and so a formal classification of the clinical features was desirable from this perspective as well. This section will focus on the clinical and therapeutic aspects of parasomnias with abnormal sleep-related sexual behaviors (sexsomnia) and sleep-related sexual seizures (epileptic sexsomnia) (Box 45-1).

Table 45-1 contains data on 31 published cases of parasomnias and seven published cases of epilepsy with abnormal sleep-related sexual behaviors and experiences that were reported in the aforementioned review.[1] The parasomnia group is strongly male predominant. Age of onset of sleepsex in both groups is during early adulthood. Sleepsex was a long-standing problem in eight parasomnia patients and in four epilepsy patients prior to clinical intervention.

Four categories of sleepsex behaviors were found in the parasomnia group, and five categories of sleepsex behaviors and experiences were found in the sleep epilepsy group. In the parasomnia group, females almost exclusively engaged in masturbation and sexual vocalizations, whereas males commonly engaged in sexual fondling and sexual intercourse with females. All 31 parasomnia patients had full amnesia for their sleepsex episodes, whereas there was recall of sleepsex episodes in five of seven patients with sleep-related seizures.

Aggressive and assaultive sleepsex behaviors, including sleepsex with minors—with subsequent legal consequences—affected a substantial number of parasomnia patients. Sleepsex was more frequently injurious to the bed partner than to the affected sexsomniac. Adverse psychosocial consequences were quite common in both the patients and their bed partners.

In the parasomnia group, histories of multiple non–rapid eye movement (NREM) sleep parasomnias were common, with CA being predominant. Sleepsex was rarely the only parasomnia behavior in the longitudinal histories of these patients. Two cases also involved sleepwalking with "sleep driving" and one case also involved sleep-related eating disorder. Besides a clinical evaluation, PSG monitoring (without penile tumescence monitoring) took place in the preponderance of cases. Obstructive sleep apnea (OSA) was present in three cases, possibly as a co-morbid feature that promoted sleepsex, with snoring during sleepsex being a prominent feature. Although 26 parasomnia patients with sexsomnia had PSG studies, sometimes on multiple nights, sexual behaviors during sleep rarely occurred, and usually it was sexual moaning arising from slow wave sleep. A total of eight patients had identified psychiatric disorders, but without any presumed link with the sexsomnia.

Parasomnias, OSA, and seizure-induced sleepsex appeared readily amenable to therapy. The benzodiazepine clonazepam was effective in almost all treated parasomnia cases. Continuous positive airway pressure (CPAP) was effective in all three treated OSA cases, and the mechanism of action presumably was suppression of OSA-induced CA that induced the sleepsex. Anticonvulsant medication was effective in all five treated seizure cases.

A variant of epileptic sexsomnia involves sleep-related hyperkinetic seizures with sexualized pelvic thrusting. Repetitive pelvic thrusting that often resembles sexual (coital) behavior is a prominent feature of sleep-related hyperkinetic seizures that are found most commonly in nocturnal frontal lobe epilepsy (NFLE), but also in nocturnal temporal lobe epilepsy (NTLE).[6-10] In a study of 442 surgically treated epileptic patients, 5.6% (*n* = 25) had exclusively sleep-related hyperkinetic seizures.[10] These 25 patients reported sensory-experiential (nonsexual) auras emerging from sleep that immediately preceded the hyperkinetic automatisms. These 25 patients, all resistant to drug treatment, underwent surgical resections of their epileptogenic zones; 18 of them were diagnosed with NFLE and 7 with NTLE. Sixteen of these patients had Taylor's dysplasia, as demonstrated by histopathologic findings, and were all free of their sleep-related seizures after 1 year; the status of the other 9 patients was not reported.

Physical and Psychosocial Consequences

In the parasomnia group, the bed partners often experienced physical injuries (ecchymoses, lacerations) from the sexual assaults and, to a lesser extent, the patients were also physically

573

injured (e.g., bruised penis or fractured digits). Moreover, both the patients and bed partners often experienced an array of adverse psychosocial consequences, mainly bewilderment, embarrassment, shame, and guilt. At times there was reactive emotional distancing that led to some marital discord. On the other hand, in four parasomnia cases, pleasurable aspects of the sleepsex were reported by the bed partners.

Likewise, in four epilepsy cases, pleasurable aspects of sleep-related sexual seizures were reported by three patients and one bed partner.

Finally, it should be emphasized that in the parasomnia and epilepsy cases just described, psychopathology was uncommonly present and was not an identified contributing factor to the abnormal sleep-related sexual behaviors and experiences. Furthermore, neither sexual deprivation/frustration nor a previous history of paraphilia or criminal sexual misconduct was reported.

Since the original sleep and sex review article was published in 2007, additional cases of sexsomnia were reported that have expanded awareness and raised intriguing questions

concerning contributing factors, co-morbidities, and therapeutic responsivities related to sexsomnia. One report from Italy involved three males (32, 42, and 46 years old) who were referred to a sleep disorders center because of sleep-related sexual episodes.[11] They had unremarkable medical, neurologic, and psychiatric histories. They each underwent PSG evaluation. A 42-year-old man had OSA (38.5 obstructions per hour), without any sexual or other parasomnia behavior during the PSG study. CPAP therapy controlled the OSA and induced a marked reduction of sexsomnia activity at home. A 32-year-old man had a prior sleepwalking (a NREM parasomnia) history. During his PSG evaluation, he had three minor (nonsexual) motor events from slow wave sleep. He was diagnosed to have a NREM parasomnia with sexsomnia; however, therapy was not mentioned. A 46-year-old man who reported sexsomnia without any history of childhood parasomnia or family history of parasomnia presented with a history, provided by his wife, of aggressive/violent sleep behaviors *and* sexual behaviors during sleep (involving full intercourse) that were at times associated with sexual dreams. These events occurred during the second half of the night and early morning hours, when rapid eye movement (REM) sleep is most predominant. PSG evaluation revealed REM sleep without atonia, although without any behaviors of REM sleep behavior disorder (RBD). He was, nevertheless, diagnosed to have RBD with sexsomnia; however, therapy with clonazepam (2 mg at bedtime) was not effective, nor were trials of dopamine agonists or carbamazepine.

Another report from France described two married women (36 and 40 years old) with sexsomnia.[12] Both patients had histories of traumatic and sexual psychological stress during childhood. They also both presented with amnestic sexsomnia manifesting as sexual moaning, "dirty talk," masturbation, sexual assault of the bed partner, and sexual intercourse with the bed partner. PSG evaluation identified multiple, abrupt, spontaneous arousals from slow wave sleep in both patients, without any associated unusual behaviors. Therefore, they were diagnosed with NREM parasomnias with sexsomnia. Therapy with the selective serotonin reuptake inhibitor (SSRI) escitalopram, 10 mg daily, induced complete control of the sexsomnia in both patients at least through the 9-month follow-up in one patient and the 2-year follow-up in the other (only one of these patients had a reported clinical depression). However, no rationale was given for the SSRI therapy of the sexsomnia. This issue is quite pertinent to opposite findings reported in another case. A 30-year-old man without a parasomnia history developed a *de novo* sexsomnia on a nightly basis for 3 weeks upon starting therapy of major depression with the same SSRI, escitalopram, also at 10 mg daily.[13] His sexsomnia involved full intercourse with his bed partner. The sexsomnia immediately ceased upon discontinuation of escitalopram. There was no recurrence of sexsomnia, or other parasomnia, when he was switched to duloxetine (a serotonin-norepinephrine reuptake inhibitor).

The Evaluation and Management of Sleep-Related Sexual Complaints

Increasingly, patients and their spouses are presenting to sleep disorders centers with a complaint of sexsomnia. A recent study from a sleep disorders center suggests that sexsomnia may be far more common than previously known—11% of

TABLE 45-1

Summary of Clinical Studies on Parasomnias and Epilepsy with Abnormal Sleep-Related Sexual Behaviors and Experiences*

Category	Parasomnias (n = 31)	Sleep-Related Epilepsy (n = 7)
Gender: %		
Male	80.6% (n = 25)	57.1% (n = 4)
Female	19.4% (n = 6)	42.9% (n = 3)
Age: years, mean ± SD		
TOTAL	31.9 ± 8.0 (n = 30)†	37.7 ± 8.5
Male	32.1 ± 8.5 (n = 24)	34.0 ± 3.5
Female	30.8 ± 6.4 (n = 6)	42.7 ± 11.6
Age at sleepsex onset: years, mean ± SD		
TOTAL	25.9 ± 8.7 (n = 17)‡	32.0 ± 9.6
Male	27.4 ± 7.9 (n = 15)	27.0 ± 9.1
Female	14.5 ± 3.5 (n = 2)	38.7 ± 5.6
Duration of sleepsex activity: years, mean ± SD		
TOTAL	9.5 ± 6.1 (n = 8)§	12-16 yr (n = 3), brief (n = 4)
Male	8.3 ± 6.5 (n = 6)	12 and 16 yr (n = 2)
Female	13.0 ± 4.2 (n = 2)	12 yr (n = 1)
Sleepsex behaviors: % of patients		
Masturbation	22.6% (n = 7) (4 male, 3 female)	14.3% (n = 1) (1 male)
Sexual vocalizations, talking, shouting	19.3% (n = 6) (2 moaning, 4 talking) (2 male, 4 female)	28.6% (n = 2) (1 moaning, 1 shouting) (2 male)
Fondling another person	45.2% (n = 14) (13 male, 1 female)	0
Sexual intercourse	41.9% (n = 13) (13 male, 0 female)	0
Sexual hyperarousal (experiential)	0%	28.6% (n = 2) (1 male, 1 female)
Ictal orgasm	N/A	42.9% (n = 3) (1 male, 2 female)
Ictal sexual automatisms	N/A	14.3% (n = 1) (1 male)
TOTAL sleepsex behaviors	n = 40	n = 9
Amnesia for sleepsex: %	100% (n = 31)	28.6% (n = 2)
Recall of sleepsex: %	0 (n = 0)	71.4% (n = 5)
Agitated/assaultive sleep-related sexual behaviors: %	45.2% (n = 14)	14.3% (n = 1)
Sleepsex with minors: %	29.0% (n = 9)	0%
Legal consequences from sleepsex: %	35.5% (n = 11) (2 with adults; 9 with minors‖)	0
Other consequences: %		
Adverse reports		
Physical		
Self	6.4% (n = 2)	71.4% (n = 5)
Other	61.3% (n = 19)	0.0
Psychosocial		
Self	67.7% (n = 21)	57.1% (n = 4)
Other	80.6% (n = 25)	14.3% (n = 1)
TOTAL	100.0% (n = 31)	100.0% (n = 7)
Positive reports		
Self/other—with or without adverse consequences	12.9% (n = 4)	57.1% (n = 4)
Sleep study: %		
Polysomnography (PSG)	83.9% (n = 26)	28.6% (n = 2)
Sleep EEG (without PSG)	0	14.3% (n = 1)
No PSG or sleep EEG	16.1% (n = 5)	57.1% (n = 4)
TOTAL parasomnias¶	71	N/A (not reported)
Mean number (± SD) per patient	2.2 ± 1.0 (range, 1-4)	

Continued

TABLE 45-1

Summary of Clinical Studies on Parasomnias and Epilepsy with Abnormal Sleep-Related Sexual Behaviors and Experiences*—cont'd

Category	Parasomnias (n = 31)	Sleep-Related Epilepsy (n = 7)
Final diagnosis—sleepsex etiology#: %		
DOA	90.3% (n = 28) (26 CA, 2 sleepwalking) (OSA co-morbidity with CA, 4)	N/A
RBD	9.7% (n = 3)	N/A
Sleep-related seizures	N/A	100% (n = 7)
Treatment efficacy**—control of sleepsex: %		
Clonazepam at bedtime	90.0% (9 of 10 patients): (6 of 7: DOA; 3 of 3: RBD)	
Nasal CPAP at bedtime	100.0% (3 of 3 patients: OSA)	N/A
Control of nocturnal seizures##	N/A	100% (n = 5)

*Data from 31 published cases of parasomnias and 7 published cases of epilepsy with abnormal sleep-related sexual behaviors and experiences.

[†]n = 1; age not reported.

[‡]Age at sleepsex onset was known in 54.8% of patients (17 of 31) and was unknown or not reported in 45.2% of patients (14 of 31).

[§]Duration of sleepsex was reported for n = 8 patients; 8 patients had only one reported episode of sleepsex and 1 had two reported episodes within 1 month, so duration is not applicable; n = 14, duration not known.

[‖]Adult males assaulted nine girls (8 to 15 years of age [n = 8] and a "teenage girl" [n = 1]).

[¶]CAs (n = 24); sleepwalking (n = 21); sleep talking and vocalizations, sexual and nonsexual (n = 15); sleep terrors (n = 7); RBD (n = 3); sleep-related eating disorder (n = 1). A history of enuresis was not included in these data.

[#]In all three patients with RBD, no behaviors (sexual or nonsexual) were documented in REM sleep.

**An additional patient with a DOA responded to clonazepam, but with remission maintained after clonazepam was discontinued. Another patient with a DOA did not respond to limited therapy consisting of low-dose (25 mg) clomipramine at bedtime. Therefore, findings in these two cases were kept separate from the treatment outcome data. For the remaining n = 17, treatment was not mentioned.

[##]Control of nocturnal seizures was achieved with anticonvulsant medications; n = 2. Treatment outcome was not mentioned.

CA, confusional arousals; *CPAP*, continuous positive airway pressure; *EEG*, electroencephalography; *OSA*, obstructive sleep apnea; *PSG*, polysomnography; *RBD*, REM sleep behavior disorder; *REM*, rapid eye movement; *DOA*, disorders of arousal.

From Schenck CH, Arnulf I, Mahowald MW. Sleep and sex: What can go wrong? A review of the literature on sleep related disorders and abnormal sexual behaviors and experiences. *Sleep*. 2007;30:683-702.

males and 4% of females of a consecutive series of all patients undergoing PSG evaluation.[14] Other patients with parasomnias, snoring, sleep-disordered breathing (SDB), or restless legs syndrome (RLS) complaints should be questioned a with their bed partners about any associated sleepsex (across a spectrum of activity, including vocalizations). For those patients having sleepsex, the frequency and severity, the longitudinal course, and any predisposing and precipitating factors (including prescription medication use) should be identified, along with any psychosocial and physical consequences. Covering the problematic sleepsex experiences identified by Mangan[15] can be useful in distinguishing between sleepsex initiator and recipient problems: the initiators often feel guilt, confusion, shame, disappointment, frustration, embarrassment, and self-incrimination, whereas the recipients often feel fear, lack of emotional intimacy, repulsion, sexual abandonment, annoyance, and suspicion. Screening psychological testing (e.g., the Minnesota Multiphasic Personality Inventory or the Beck Depression Inventory) should be administered, and formal psychiatric consultation should be considered on a case-by-case basis.

Time-synchronized video-PSG, with seizure-montage and upper/lower limb electromyographic (EMG) monitoring, are strongly recommended in evaluating the complaint of sleepsex. Although the yield in identifying parasomnia behaviors and confirming the diagnosis by video-PSG is substantial, sexual behaviors during sleep have rarely been documented (if there are any findings they are usually only sexual vocalizations).

Management of this problem can occur along two dimensions: (1) medical management, to treat any identified underlying sleep, medical, neurologic, or psychiatric disorder (including medication effects), which may be promoting the problematic sexuality; and (2) individual or couple psychotherapy to address the consequences of the problematic sexuality.

SLEEP-RELATED DISSOCIATIVE DISORDER

As a link with the previous section on sexsomnia, sexualized (repetitive behavior without affect) and frankly sexual behaviors (with affect) can emerge with sleep-related dissociative disorders. A particularly striking episode was demonstrated by video-PSG in a 22-year-old woman, with a duration of 7 minutes during well-defined EEG wakefulness.[15] She quietly lay awake in bed with eyes closed just prior to falling asleep. Then she gradually began jerking her head side-to-side, which proceeded to squirming in bed followed by a crescendo progression of pelvic thrusting, side-to-side movements, and other thrashing behaviors, along with moaning and groaning. Defensive, pained behaviors and moaning often accompanied the sexualized behaviors and were part of a reenactment of a past abuse scenario that she later believed she had been dreaming about, when in fact she had been awake and remembering in a dissociated state. In her "dream" that she was acting out in bed, her older sister was repeatedly shoving a ruler into her vagina, stomach, and legs that hurt her but sometimes

BOX 45-2 *Diagnostic Criteria for Sleep-Related Dissociative Disorders*

1. A dissociative disorder, fulfilling *DSM-IV* diagnostic criteria, is present and occurs in close association with the main sleep period AND
2. One of the following is present:
   - PSG demonstration of a dissociative episode or episodes that emerge during sustained EEG wakefulness, either in transition from wakefulness to sleep or after waking from NREM or REM sleep, OR
   - In the absence of a PSG-recorded episode of dissociation, there is a compelling history, provided by observers, for a sleep-related dissociative disorder, particularly if the sleep-related behaviors are similar to observed daytime dissociative behaviors, AND
   - The sleep disturbance is not better explained by another sleep disorder, medical or neurologic disorder, medication use, or substance use disorder.

EEG, electroencephalography; *NREM,* non–rapid eye movement; *PSG,* polysomnography; *REM,* rapid eye movement.
From American Academy of Sleep Medicine. International Classification of Sleep Disorders, 2nd ed. *Diagnostic and Coding Manual.* Westchester, IL: American Academy of Sleep Medicine; 2005.

BOX 45-3 *Differential Diagnosis for Sleep-Related Dissociative Disorders*

- NREM sleep parasomnias (sleepwalking, sleep terrors), RBD, and nocturnal seizures share some features with sleep-related dissociative disorders, but can usually be distinguished.
- NREM parasomnias and RBD usually have a shorter duration, and the observed behaviors are usually different from, those conditions and from seizures: behaviors present in dissociative disorders often suggest reenactments of past abuse and thus are quite inconsistent with usual parasomnia behaviors and ictal events.
- But there can be overlap: confusional arousals, sleepwalking, and postictal periods occasionally can be associated with confusional states lasting considerably longer than usual.
- NREM parasomnias emerge abruptly from (usually deep) NREM sleep. The behaviors of RBD occur within REM sleep and not after waking. Sleep-related dissociative disorders emerge gradually and from well-established wakefulness (after waking from any sleep stage or in the transition from the awake to the sleep state).
- Elaborate sleepwalking episodes usually are isolated events. Elaborate sleep-related dissociative disorders typically are recurrent.
- Abnormal toxic-metabolic states or medical disorders that can cause altered states of consciousness may mimic a dissociative disorder and must carefully be excluded.

NREM, non-REM; *PSG,* polysomnography; *RBD,* REM sleep behavior disorder; *REM,* rapid eye movement.

also sexually aroused her. Her case was one of a series of eight cases that first established, with PSG confirmation, the entity of sleep-related dissociative disorder, which is listed as a parasomnia in ICSD-2.[16]

The essential feature of a dissociative disorder (including sleep related dissociative disorder) is "disruption in the usually integrated functions of consciousness, memory, identity, or perception of the environment."[17] The disruption or disintegration of these basic functions results in a cognitive, emotional, behavioral, and perceptual separation—that is, a dissociation—from the overwhelming stress. Those afflicted with a dissociative disorder are prone to wandering around in a daze, sometimes for long distances, and may even end up in other cities before realizing where they are. This was the scenario for a 34-year-old woman who would repeatedly "just disappear out there" in the night after being subjected to overwhelming stress within a short time period.[15] She described "sleepwalking" when in fact she was "dissociating" after her brain awakened from sleep, but in an altered state of *wakeful* consciousness. She also described being typically "confused" when "snapping out" of her dissociated states (which to her seemed like sleepwalking episodes). This aspect of the nocturnal dissociative experience can be indistinguishable from the way many sleepwalking episodes terminate, with the person awakening in a confused state during an arousal from deep NREM sleep.

In the first case series reporting on nocturnal (sleep-related) dissociative disorders in 1989, it was emphasized that all eight cases had been referred to our sleep center with the provisional diagnosis of "injurious sleepwalking."[16] Whereas sleepwalking can usually be promptly controlled by means of applying proper sleep-wake habits, practicing relaxation techniques and self-hypnosis at bedtime, and bedtime pharmacotherapy with benzodiazepines, sleep-related dissociative disorders, in contrast, can be controlled only after the patient engages in long-term, specialized (inpatient and outpatient) psychiatric interventions. They are notoriously difficult conditions to treat.

As described in the ICSD-2, sleep-related dissociative disorders are dissociative disorders that can emerge throughout the usual sleep period but during well-established EEG wakefulness, either at the transition from wakefulness to sleep or within several minutes after an awakening from stage 1 or 2 NREM sleep or from REM sleep.[5] Furthermore, they are a sleep-related variant of dissociative disorders, which are defined in the Diagnostic and Statistical Manual of Mental Disorders, Fourth Edition (*DSM-IV*) as "…a disruption in the usually integrated functions of consciousness, memory, identity, or perception of the environment." Of the five listed diagnostic categories contained within the dissociative disorders section of the *DSM-IV,* three categories to date have been documented with nocturnal dissociative disorders: dissociative identity disorder (formerly called *multiple personality disorder*), dissociative fugue, and dissociative disorder not otherwise specified (Boxes 45-2 and 45-3). The similarity of the behaviors found with nocturnal dissociative disorders to the behaviors found with various parasomnias justifies their inclusion within the parasomnias section of *ICSD-2* and indicates how they are a distinct sleep-related variant of dissociative disorders.

Most patients with sleep-related dissociative disorders also have corresponding daytime dissociative disorders and have past or current histories of physical or sexual abuse. A variety of major psychiatric disorders is commonly present, including post-traumatic stress disorder (PTSD), major mood and anxiety disorders, self-mutilating behaviors, and suicide attempts, along with numerous psychiatric hospitalizations. Rarely, a sleep-related dissociative disorder can occur in isolation, without a daytime component and without a recalled or otherwise known history of physical or sexual abuse. During the sleep period, patients with sleep-related dissociative disorders can scream, walk, or run in a frenzied manner and engage in self-mutilating and other violent behaviors. The episodes, which can be elaborate and last several minutes to an hour or longer, often involve behaviors that represent reenactments of previous physical and sexual abuse situations. This activity may occur with

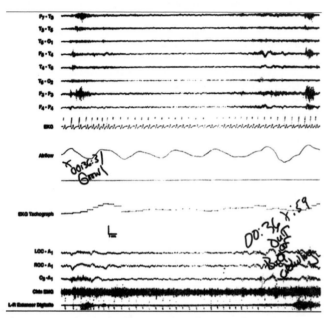

Figure 45-1 Nocturnal polysomnogram of an animalistic dissociative episode. Fifty-three minutes after sleep onset, a 19-year-old male suddenly begins to growl and then leave his bed and crawl away in the manner of a large jungle cat, as noted by the sleep laboratory technician. A 9-channel electroencephalograph (EEG) (the top 8 channels and C3-A1) indicates a corresponding wakeful state, characterized by desynchronized, low-voltage fast activity (activated EEG). The chin electromyogram (EMG) shows a moderate level of tone throughout the tracing, and there is intermittent twitching of the extensor digitorum and anterior tibialis EMGs. Minimal eye movements are present (LOC-A1; ROC-A1). (From Schenck CH, Milner DM, Hurwitz TD, Bundlie SR, Mahowald MW. Dissociative disorders presenting as somnambulism: Video and clinical documentation [8 cases]. *Dissociation.* 1989;2:194-204. Used with permission from the Ridgeview Institute.)

perceived dreaming, which is actually a dissociated wakeful memory of past abuse. Sexualized behavior can occur and can be paired with defensive behavior and with congruent verbalization. Other dissociative episodes may occur as confusional states, with or without elaborate behaviors, which are not associated with perceived dreaming. The individual is usually completely amnestic for the behaviors expressed during a nocturnal dissociative episode. A postassault headache can be reexperienced during nocturnal dissociation.[18] Nocturnal fugues,[16,19] with driving an automobile and flying on an airplane to another city, can also occur. Finally, eating uncooked foods[16] or binge eating high-calorie sweets[20] can occur during nocturnal dissociative episodes (at times representing behavior that emerges during the sleep period in a person with a nocturnal eating personality).

The prevalence is of sleep-related dissociative disorder is unknown. However, in a report on 100 consecutive patients who were referred to a multidisciplinary sleep disorders center and underwent clinical and PSG evaluations,[21] seven (7%) were diagnosed with a sleep-related dissociative disorder. Sleep related dissociative disorders occur predominantly in females. The age of onset ranges from childhood to middle adulthood.

Onset can be abrupt and fulminant, or it can be gradual and sporadic. The course is usually chronic and severe, with episodes often occurring several times weekly or multiple times nightly. Complications include repeated injuries to self or bed partner from the dissociative behaviors, including ecchymoses, fractures, lacerations, and burn wounds. Skin infections from self-mutilation can also occur. Additional perspectives are available for better understanding the phenomenon of nocturnal, sleep-related dissociation,[22] and nocturnal dissociative disorders.[23] Also, the 7-minute episode of nocturnal dissociation described earlier in a 22-year-old woman[16] is available as an educational resource, along with a catalogue of other parasomnia behaviors, for sleep physicians and fellows, sleep technologists, medical students, and physicians in postgraduate training.[24]

In video-PSG recordings of sleep-related dissociative episodes, EEG wakefulness has been present before, during, and after the episodes. An alpha EEG rhythm with abnormal behaviors emerging shortly after an arousal from NREM sleep is not necessarily diagnostic of a dissociative disorder, because disorders of arousal may also have an alpha rhythm. However, the lag time between EEG arousal and behavioral arousal can

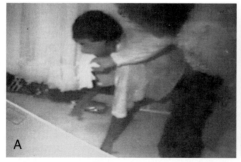
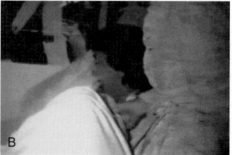

Figure 45-2 Video prints of a nocturnal dissociative episode. Still frames from a home movie record how a 19-year-old male crawls around his room while assuming the identity and behaviors of a large jungle cat. He is seen to clamp his teeth on a towel offered by his mother (**A**). He then drags a mattress across the room with his teeth as his mother attempts to intervene (**B**). Two identical episodes were documented to arise from electroencephalograph (EEG) wakefulness during overnight polysomnographic study with continuous audio-videotaping. (From Schenck CH, Milner DM, Hurwitz TD, Bundlie SR, Mahowald MW. Dissociative disorders presenting as somnambulism: Video and clinical documentation [8 cases]. *Dissociation.* 1989;2:194-204. Used with permission from the Ridgeview Institute.)

usually distinguish these two conditions. With disorders of arousal, the behaviors emerge almost immediately after the EEG arousal. With sleep-related dissociative disorders, there is often a lag time of 15 to 60 seconds between EEG arousal and behavioral activation. Finally, PSG monitoring may not capture a dissociative episode but is valuable in helping exclude other diagnostic possibilities. Figure 45-1 illustrates the PSG correlates of an episode of animalistic nocturnal dissociative disorder recorded in the sleep laboratory. Figure 45-2 shows video prints from a home movie recording another episode.

CATATHRENIA (SLEEP-RELATED GROANING)

Catathrenia is a rare, chronic disorder that usually emerges nightly and is characterized by expiratory groaning during sleep.[5] Although the initial reports emphasized that catathrenia was predominantly a REM sleep-related disorder emerging mainly during the second half of the night, and was not a treatable condition, more recent reports have expanded the database of this parasomnia/breathing disorder of sleep to now indicate that it can emerge throughout all stages of NREM and REM sleep during the course of the entire sleep period, and it can be treated (in many patients) with CPAP therapy. In fact, catathrenia can occur predominantly in NREM sleep in some patients, in contrast to other patients in whom it occurs mainly in REM sleep. This contrast raises provocative questions, as recently addressed in an editorial.[25] (Also, the pertinent literature will be described in the following paragraphs).

PSG evaluation with auditory monitoring reveals recurrent bradypneic episodes in which there is a deep inspiration is followed by protracted expiration when a monotonous vocalization is produced that closely resembles groaning. However, a variety of other abnormal expiratory sounds have been described, by history and during PSG monitoring, including "tremendous noises," "funny noises," "whining and squealing sounds," "high-pitched or cracking sounds," "loud humming sounds," "loud groans," loud roaring sounds, "groans with sexual connotation," and "mournful sounds" (in fact, the term *catathrenia* comes from the Greek words "kata," meaning "below," and "threnia," meaning "to lament"). The bradypneic episodes with groaning often recur in clusters and may be most abundant during the later REM sleep cycles. However, episodes can emerge during any stage of NREM sleep throughout the night. The groaning and other sounds are exclusively expiratory events and are not associated with any observed respiratory distress or anguished or emotional facial expression even though moaning and "mournful sounds" can occur. The expiratory sounds occur with the person lying in any position. These recurrent bradypneic episodes may closely resemble central sleep apneas, although there are usually distinguishable differences between the two conditions.

The affected person is usually unaware of the groaning, and it is the bed partner, roommate, or family member who is disturbed by it and urges clinical evaluation. The groaning and other sounds are usually loud, and are not associated with any abnormal motor activity, sleep talking, or dreaming. However, the groaning usually stops whenever the person changes position in bed, only to resume again later. General physical examinations and routine laboratory testing, along with neurologic and otorhinolaryngologic examinations, are unremarkable, even when including fibroscopy of the upper airways with static and dynamic vocal cord evaluations. The affected person

usually has no sleep-related complaint apart from occasional restless sleep and mild daytime fatigue—unless there is co-morbid OSA. Hoarseness in the morning has also been reported. No association with respiratory disorders or with psychological problems or psychiatric disorders has been found.

The onset appears to be insidious, but a nightly recurrence is quickly established. The course is chronic in all reported patients. However, it is unknown how many people have self-limited sleep-related groaning and do not seek medical attention. The main complication is interpersonal, as the bed partner or others in the same household have their sleep disrupted or become distressed from the groaning. The long-term consequences of this chronic disorder are unknown, but it appears to be a benign condition.

During PSG monitoring, a characteristic respiratory dysrhythmia with inter-groaning intervals during sleep has been detected. Monitoring respiratory sound signals during sleep is required for identifying vocalizations. Groaning and moaning sounds last from a few seconds to a minute, often repeat in clusters for 2 minutes to 1 hour, and may recur many times per night. The vocal sounds occur only during expiration, with respiratory signals being flat or prominently reduced during the protracted expiratory phase of a bradypnea. The bradypneas appear as a sudden change in respiratory rhythm lasting at least 2 seconds, with monotonous vocalization occurring only during a protracted expiratory phase of the bradypnea. These respiratory patterns often appear in clusters. During the groaning, the person remains still. EEG epileptiform activity does not precede or accompany the groaning. The groaning is associated with slightly decreased heart rate. Hemoglobin oxygen saturation remains normal, and there is no cardiac dysrhythmia. Groaning always ends with a sigh or grunt and is followed by a rebound in heart rate and arterial pressure. An EEG arousal, with or without a change in posture, often marks the end of groaning episodes. The sleep architecture is generally normal, with normal cycling across sleep stages. The presence of a preceding inspiration and of subsequent sound production is the key to the differentiation from true central apneas. There is typically considerable night-to-night consistency in these findings.

This respiratory dysrhythmia may bear close resemblance to that of postarousal central sleep apneas. The differential diagnosis also includes stridor, laryngospasm, snoring, nocturnal asthma, sleep talking, and moaning in epileptic seizures (including during REM sleep). Central sleep apnea may be confused with the bradypneic events, but the preceding deep inspiration and subsequent vocalizations (indicating ongoing breathing and not cessation of breathing) and lack of oxygen desaturation excludes this diagnostic possibility. Stridor can be either inspiratory or expiratory and may occur exclusively during sleep. Unlike sleep-related groaning, stridor may occur with every breath and not in clusters and tends not to occur as a prolonged expiration. In multiple system atrophy, however, stridor may occur in prolonged clusters (especially in REM sleep) that are interspersed with quiet breathing, but the stridor is always inspiratory. Sleep-related laryngospasm usually is accompanied by a sense of suffocation. Snoring is an inspiratory noise caused by vibrations of the soft parts of the oropharyngeal walls. Nocturnal asthma with bronchoconstriction is accompanied by wheezing. Sleep talking involves the production of words and speech (and not monotonous sounds). Moaning during epileptic seizures is usually accompanied by other epileptic behaviors.

Besides the two carefully documented initial case series describing catathrenia as a predominantly REM sleep–related condition,[26,27] and other similar case series, as critically reviewed,[25] the more recent literature has expanded awareness on catathrenia as also being a disorder of NREM sleep, with co-morbid OSA and upper airway resistance syndrome, and as being treatable with CPAP in a number of cases. In fact, a lively debate has been initiated as to whether catathrenia is a parasomnia, a breathing disorder of sleep, or both, and what the relationship is between the nocturnal groaning and sleep-disordered breathing.[25,28,29] Furthermore, a 2009 report called attention to the possibility of disturbed arousal mechanisms playing a role in the pathogenesis of nocturnal groaning—or at least in one subset of catathrenia.[30] In this study, eight patients with catathrenia (five males, three females, aged 11-32 years) underwent PSG and 76.5% of the groaning episodes were REM sleep related. Nearly two thirds of the groaning events emerged with arousals, and in virtually all of them the arousal occurred before or together with the onset of bradypnea. When considering the cumulative and ever-expanding literature on catathrenia, it is clear that various subtypes exist that need further elucidation in regard to pathogenesis, pathophysiology, and therapeutic interventions.

Regarding catathrenia responsive to CPAP therapy, in a case from Spain[31] a 62-year-old woman had a longstanding history of "producing tremendous noises during sleep" that was "very disturbing to her family." She had no subjective complaint concerning sleep except for a sporadic morning dry mouth. PSG monitoring revealed that these characteristic noises began a few minutes after falling asleep. An expiratory waxing and waning periodic groaning noise with an irregular movement of the abdominal wall was captured by video-PSG. These events occurred throughout the entire night and were independent of the sleep stage and body position. The PSG confirmed a respiratory dysrhythmia in all sleep stages, with frequent oxygen desaturations disproportionate to the expected values for a mild OSA disorder (16 events per hour; SaO_2 nadir of 79%). CPAP therapy (6 cm H_2O pressure) resulted in the noise disappearing almost completely. She tolerated the CPAP well. In another case from Turkey,[32] a 40-year-old woman had experienced a 33-year history of loud groaning while asleep, occurring in several periods every night, and a 3-year history, reported by her husband, of episodes where she "stops breathing and then gives a loud gasp or snort when aroused by the apnea." Her PSG test confirmed a diagnosis of moderate OSA. Groaning episodes started 3 minutes after falling asleep, with duration of about 2 to 10 seconds and a total number of 2 to 33 in every cluster; clusters lasted 2 to 8 minutes. The groaning occurred during expiration only and seven clusters of recurrent expiratory groaning were observed (three in N2 stage sleep, two in N3, and two in REM). Each event featured a deep inspiration followed by a short expiration, and then a prolonged period when the breathing signals were substantially reduced. During these noise-filled expiratory phases, decreased EMG activity in rectus abdominis and intercostalis muscles was detected. Body position had no influence on these events. During CPAP titration, the obstructive apnea was markedly reduced and the groaning sounds unexpectedly disappeared completely. At follow-up, the family reported the full control of the groaning with ongoing CPAP therapy, and the patient had less daytime subjective sleepiness.

Guilleminault and associates[33] reported a 100% (7/7) response to CPAP therapy in a group of exclusively premenopausal women 20 to 34 years old. "Distress from the social impact of their groaning, rather than a concern for their health, was the primary motivation for seeking treatment in each of our patients." One patient chose to continue with CPAP therapy for her catathrenia and upper airway resistance syndrome (UARS) for more than 3 years, because "her loud groaning had a conspicuous sexual connotation which was observed not only by her husband, but also her two daughters or anyone else that may be nearby." This case example demonstrates one form of adverse psychosocial impact that catathrenia can have on an individual and the household. Guilleminault,[33] in commenting on how their 100% response rate to CPAP therapy conflicted with some prior reports of poor response to CPAP therapy in catathrenia, made the following interesting and provocative statement:

> We have extensive experience treating women with UARS and we are aware that in pre-menopausal women nasal CPAP pressures well above 8 cm of water are often needed. The narrowest segment of the upper airway is typically behind the base of the tongue in these cases and is difficult to maintain patent at lower pressures. Our goal during CPAP titration was to achieve resolution of flow limitation which often arises from this stricture point…we were somewhat surprised at the amount of positive pressure needed to eliminate flow limitation…to find resolution of catathrenia.

Finally, the Mayo Clinic experience was recently reported in abstract form,[34] and the 11 reported cases were similar to the Guilleminault cases,[33] with groaning occurring in both NREM and REM sleep, and there was also associated sleep-disordered breathing. Therapy with CPAP was similarly successful.

On the other hand, cases of catathrenia not responsive to CPAP have been reported. As one example, in a case from Germany,[35] a 33-year-old man presented with whining and squealing sounds, but not groaning, during sleep that had an adverse impact on his wife. In fact, she had insisted on the consultation because of the utterance of a prolonged high-pitched whining and episodes of arrested breathing. He himself complained of nonrestorative sleep. PSG monitoring documented whining vocalizations in REM sleep during expirations after a deep inspiration.

Finally, catathrenia can be considered to be a cause of "environmental sleep disorder,"[5] with the bed partner or roommate having his or her sleep disturbed by the chronic, often nightly groaning. Therefore, strategies for assisting the person afflicted with the secondary sleep disruption should be offered, especially if there is no successful therapy of the catathrenia. The use of ear plugs, "white noise" generators (e.g., a fan), and similar measures should be discussed, and if all else fails, then sleeping in separate bedrooms may be the only realistic solution.

SLEEP-RELATED HALLUCINATIONS

This entity involves a sensory parasomnia that is not associated with the narcolepsy symptom complex. In other words, it is herein considered to be a separate entity, even though it can also be closely associated with narcolepsy. (An analogous situation exists for isolated sleep paralysis.) Sleep-related hallucinations are hallucinatory experiences, principally visual, that occur at sleep onset or on awakening from sleep.[5] Less commonly they are auditory, tactile, or kinetic phenomena. Hallucinations at sleep onset (hypnagogic hallucinations) may be difficult to differentiate from sleep-onset dreaming. Hallucinations on waking in the morning (hypnopompic hallucinations) may arise out of a period of REM sleep, and patients may also be uncertain whether they represent waking or dream-related experiences. Complex nocturnal visual hallucinations represent a distinct form of sleep-related hallucinations, and women are preferentially affected.[36] They typically occur following a sudden awakening, without recall of a preceding dream, and usually take the form of complex, vivid, relatively immobile, images of people or animals, sometimes distorted in shape or size. These hallucinations may remain present for many minutes but usually disappear if there is an increase in ambient light. Although patients are clearly awake, they often initially perceive the hallucinations as real and frightening. Patients with complex nocturnal visual hallucinations may jump out of the bed in terror, and on occasion have injured themselves. Some patients also may experience similar complex hallucinations during the day,[37] unassociated with napping or micro-sleep episodes.

Sleep-related hallucinations have been reported to occur with prevalence in large European population studies of 25% to 37% for hypnagogic hallucinations, while the equivalent reported prevalence for hypnopompic hallucinations is 7% to 13%.[38,39] Both hypnagogic and hypnopompic hallucinations are more common in younger persons and occur slightly more frequently in women than in men.

Sleep-related hallucinations appear to be most common in adolescence and early adulthood. In many patients, the frequency appears to decrease with age. The natural history of complex nocturnal visual hallucinations depends on the underlying cause.

Complex nocturnal visual hallucinations may in some cases be release phenomena in which loss of visual input or decreased reticular activating system activity results in the visual cortex generating aberrant images.

Sleep-related hallucinations appear to arise predominantly from REM periods. However, the very few reports of PSG in complex nocturnal visual hallucinations suggest an onset out of NREM sleep. Magnetic resonance imaging (MRI) scans of the brain, polysomnography, EEG testing, and neuropsychometric testing may help in the differential diagnosis and in identifying underlying disorders. Complex nocturnal visual hallucinations are a final common pathway with a number of possible causes. They may be seen in patients with narcolepsy,[5] Parkinson's disease,[40] dementia with Lewy bodies,[40] visual loss (Charles Bonnet hallucinations),[41] and midbrain and diencephalic pathology (peduncular hallucinosis),[41] as well as with the use of β-adrenergic receptor blocking medications. Anxiety disorders have been noted in some patients. A careful history and neurologic examination is needed to determine if any of these related conditions are present.

Most commonly the diagnosis of sleep-related hallucinations can be made clinically by careful attention to the history. However, if there is a question of seizures or another sleep disorder, then polysomnography may be indicated. This should be performed with additional EEG derivations and time-synchronized video recordings and should be interpreted by a reviewer experienced in the EEG appearance of seizures. In some patients, a normal daytime wake and sleep EEG may suffice to lower the probability of a seizure disorder without the need for polysomnography. The few descriptions of complex nocturnal visual hallucinations occurring during polysomnography suggest that they arise from NREM rather than REM sleep.

Differential diagnosis includes nightmares, exploding head syndrome, RBD, DOA from NREM sleep, nocturnal seizures, and migraines. Nightmares are frightening or otherwise disturbing dreams that awaken the patient from sleep.[5] They are clearly recognized as dreams and do not persist into wakefulness. Exploding head syndrome consists of a sudden sensation of an explosion in the head, usually at sleep onset and sometimes accompanied by a noise or flash of light.[5] It does not involve complex visual imagery and lasts seconds. In RBD, the patient acts out distinctly altered dreams during REM sleep, and so this is a combined sensory and motor parasomnia.[5] DOA from NREM sleep can be associated with dream mentation in adults,[42] but the patient subsequently recognizes that the dream occurred during sleep, and this is also an example of a combined sensory and motor parasomnia. Visual hallucinations can be due to epileptic seizures but are usually brief, stereotyped, and fragmentary in such cases. Complex visual hallucinations can be associated with migraines, but are usually followed by a headache.

Therapy usually entails reassuring the patient that the symptoms are benign, and often lessen with time. The lack of suspicion of a serious or progressive neurologic or psychiatric disorder being present should be communicated to the patient. Drug therapy is not usually beneficial.

SLEEP TALKING

Sleep talking (somniloquy) is not considered to be a disorder per se in the ICSD-2,[5] but it can be part of a symptom complex of a recognized disorder, such as sexsomnia (with "sleepsex talking"), RBD, sleepwalking sleep-related eating disorder, or nocturnal seizures (in which the vocalization tends to be stereotypic and recurrent). Sleep talking can also be the cause of an "environmental sleep disorder"[5] in the bed partner or roommate of the sleep talker, or in a group sleeping situation (e.g., college dormitory, military barracks, fire station, sleeping in a tent while camping). Sleep talking is highly prevalent, being reported in half of young children and in 5% of adults.[5] There is no apparent gender difference. Complications usually arise when sleep talking is very frequent or loud, or if the content is objectionable to others.

Therapy of sleep talking should be directed at any comorbid or underlying sleep disorder, as described earlier. Otherwise, therapy should be initiated for environmental sleep disorder for anyone bothered by the sleep talking. Also, if the content of the sleep talking brings up marital or relationship issues (e.g., sleep talking about a former spouse, girlfriend or boyfriend, or a current colleague or friend of the opposite gender), then referral to a marital or relationship therapist should be considered.

SUMMARY

The adult parasomnias discussed in this chapter exemplify how instinctual behaviors can be inappropriately released in sleep (e.g., sexsomnia), and they also illustrate how sleep-disordered breathing can promote parasomnias (e.g., OSA-induced CA with sexsomnia, or catathrenia with abnormal sound production during prolonged expirations).

The most common clinical scenarios for sexsomnia are in the context of a longstanding history of NREM sleep parasomnias, or in association with the recent onset of clinical OSA. Therapy of sexsomnia involves standard therapy for either of these two associated conditions (i.e., NREM parasomnias or OSA).

Sleep-related dissociative disorder is a psychiatric parasomnia promoted by a past and/or current history of emotional, physical, or sexual abuse, with the abnormal behaviors emerging during established EEG wakefulness during the sleep period. Therapy involves psychiatric management.

Sleep-related hallucinations are now known to encompass not only the classic hypnagogic/hypnopompic hallucinations commonly seen in narcolepsy but also more complex nocturnal visual hallucinations. Therapy is only sometimes necessary.

Finally, sleep talking can be a benign phenomenon, or it can be problematic by disrupting the sleep of the bed partner, and it may sometimes be a sign of a serious underlying parasomnia (e.g., RBD or NREM sleep parasomnia). Therapy is often not necessary, apart from treating an underlying parasomnia.

REFERENCES

1. Schenck CH, Arnulf I, Mahowald MW. Sleep and sex: What can go wrong? A review of the literature on sleep related disorders and abnormal sexual behaviors and experiences. *Sleep.* 2007;30:683-702.
2. Rosenfeld DS, Elhajjar AJ. Sleepsex: A variant of sleepwalking. *Arch Sex Behav.* 1998;27:269-278.
3. Guilleminault C, Moscovitch A, Yuen K, Poyares D. Atypical sexual behavior during sleep. *Psychosom Med.* 2002;64:328-336.
4. Shapiro CM, Trajanovic NN, Fedoroff JP. Sexsomnia—A new parasomnia? *Can J Psychiatry.* 2003;48:311-317.
5. American Academy of Sleep Medicine. International Classification of Sleep Disorders. *Diagnostic and Coding Manual.* 2nd ed. Westchester, IL: American Academy of Sleep Medicine; 2005.
6. Zucconi M, Oldani A, Ferini-Strambi L, Bizzozero D, Smirne S. Nocturnal paroxysmal arousals with motor behaviors during sleep: Frontal lobe epilepsy or parasomnia? *J Clin Neurophysiol.* 1997;14:513-522.
7. Provini F, Plazzi G, Tinuper P, Vandi S, Lugaresi E, Montagna P. Nocturnal frontal lobe epilepsy: A clinical and polygraphic overview of 100 consecutive cases. *Brain.* 1999;122:1017-1031.
8. Nobili L, Cossu M, Mai R, et al. Sleep-related hyperkinetic seizures of temporal lobe origin. *Neurology.* 2004;62:482-485.
9. Tinuper P, Provini F, Bisulli F, Lugaresi E. Hyperkinetic manifestations in nocturnal frontal lobe epilepsy: Semeiological features and physiopathological hypothesis. *Neurol Sci.* 2005;26:S210-S214.
10. Mai R, Sartori I, Francione S, et al. Sleep-related hyperkinetic seizures: Always a frontal onset? *Neurol Sci.* 2005;26:S220-S224.
11. Della Marca G, Dittoni S, Frusciante R, et al. Abnormal sexual behavior during sleep. *J Sex Med.* 2009;6(12):3490-3495.
12. Bejot Y, Juenet N, Garrouty R, et al. Sexsomnia: An uncommon variety of parasomnia. *Clin Neurol Neurosurg.* 2010;112:72-75.
13. Krol DGH. Sexsomnia during treatment with a selective serotonin reuptake blocker. *J Psychiatry (Netherlands).* 2008;50(11):735-739.
14. Chung SA, Yegneswaran B, Natarajan A, Trajanovic N, Shapiro CM. Frequency of sexsomnia in sleep clinic patients. *Sleep.* 2010;33:A226.
15. Mangan MA. A phenomenology of problematic sexual behavior occurring in sleep. *Arch Sex Behav.* 2004;33:287-293.
16. Schenck CH, Milner DM, Hurwitz TD, Bundlie SR, Mahowald MW. Dissociative disorders presenting as somnambulism: Video and clinical documentation (8 cases). *Dissociation.* 1989;2:194-204.
17. American Psychiatric Association. *Diagnostic and Statistical Manual of Mental Disorders.* 4th ed. Washington, DC: American Psychiatric Association; 1994.
18. Fleming J. Dissociative episodes presenting as somnambulism: A case report. *Sleep Res.* 1987;16:263.
19. Rice E, Fisher C. Fugue states in sleep and wakefulness: A psychophysiological study. *J Nerv Ment Dis.* 1976;163:79-87.
20. Coons P, Bowman E. Dissociation and eating. *Am J Psychiatry.* 1993;150:171-172.
21. Schenck C, Milner D, Hurwitz T, Bundlie S, Mahowald M. A polysomnographic and clinical report on sleep-related injury in 100 adult patients. *Am J Psychiatry.* 1989;146:1166-1173.
22. Mahowald M, Schenck C. Nocturnal dissociation—Awake? Asleep? Both? or Neither? *Sleep Hypnosis.* 2001;3:129-130.
23. Agargun M, Kara H, Ozer O, et al. Characteristics of patients with nocturnal dissociative disorders. *Sleep Hypnosis.* 2001;3:131-134.
24. Sleep Runners. The Stories Behind Everyday Parasomnias (1 hour DVD documentary film). St Paul: Slow-Wave Films, LLC; 2004(deluxe academic edition, 2007). Available at www.sleeprunners.com.
25. Ramar K, Gay P. Catathrenia: Getting the "cat" out of the bag. *Sleep Breath.* 2008;12:291-294.
26. Pevernagie D, Boon P, Mariman A, Verhaeghen D, Pauwels R. Vocalization during episodes of prolonged expiration: A parasomnia related to REM sleep. *Sleep Med.* 2001;2:9-30.
27. Vetrugno R, Provini F, Plazzi G, Vignatelli L, Lugaresi E, Montagna P. Catathrenia (nocturnal groaning): A new type of parasomnia. *Neurology.* 2001;56:681-683.
28. Vetrugno R, Lugaresi E, Ferini-Strambi L, Montagna P. Catathrenia (nocturnal groaning): What is it? *Sleep.* 2008;31:308-309.
29. Guilleminault C, Hagen CC, Khaja AM. Catathrenia is not expiratory snoring. *Sleep.* 2008;31:774-775.
30. Prihodova I, Sonka K, Kemlink D, Volna J, Nevsimalova S. Arousals in nocturnal groaning. *Sleep Med.* 2009;10:1051-1055.
31. Iriarte J, Alegre M, Urrestarazu E, Viteri C, Arocha J, Artieda J. Continuous positive airway pressure as treatment for catathrenia (nocturnal groaning). *Neurology.* 2006;66:609-610.
32. Songu M, Yilmaz H, Yuccturk AV, et al. Effect of CPAP on catathrenia and OSA: A case report and review of the literature. *Sleep Breath.* 2008;12:401-405.
33. Guilleminault C, Hagen CC, Khaja AM. Catathrenia: Parasomnia or uncommon feature of sleep disordered breathing? *Sleep.* 2008;31:132-139.
34. Abbasi A, Morgenthaler TI, Olson EJ, Tippman-Peikert M, Slocumb NL, Ramar K. Catathrena: A North American experience. *Sleep.* 2008;31:A263.
35. Steinig J, Lanz M, Krugel R, Happe S. Breath holding—A rapid eye movement (REM) sleep parasomnia (catathrenia or expiratory groaning). *Sleep Med.* 2008;9:455-456.
36. Silber MH, Hansen MR, Girish M. Complex nocturnal visual hallucinations. *Sleep Med.* 2005;6:363-366.
37. Manford M, Andermann F. Complex visual hallucinations. Clinical and neurobiological insights. *Brain.* 1998;121:1819-1840.
38. Ohayon M. Prevalence of hallucinations and their pathological associations in the general population. *Psychiatry Res.* 2000;97:153-164.
39. Ohayon M, Priest R, Caulet M, Guilleminault C. Hypnagogic and hypnopompic hallucinations: Pathological phenomena? *Br J Psychiatry.* 1996;169:459-467.
40. Barnes J, David AS. Visual hallucinations in Parkinson's disease: A review and phenomenological survey. *J Neurol Neurosurg Psychiatry.* 2001;70:727-733.
41. Mahowald M, Woods S, Schenck C. Sleeping dreams, waking hallucinations, and the central nervous system. *Dreaming.* 1998;8:89-102.
42. Kavey NB, Whyte J. Somnambulism associated with hallucinations. *Psychosomatics.* 1993;34:86-90.

Sleep-Related Medical Disorders

Sleep-Related Cardiac Disorders

RICHARD L. VERRIER / MURRAY A. MITTLEMAN

Sleep exerts a generally beneficial effect in healthy individuals. However, with development of cardiorespiratory disease, the sleep-induced surges in autonomic activity and disruptions in central control of sleep and airway function can predispose to cardiovascular events.

The annual toll of nocturnal, sleep-related cardiac events accounts for an estimated 20% of myocardial infarctions (or 250,000) and 15% of sudden cardiac deaths (or 48,750) in the United States.[1] Rapid eye movement (REM) sleep is characterized by surges in sympathetic and vagus nerve activity that are well tolerated in normal individuals but may provoke ventricular or atrial arrhythmias, myocardial ischemia, myocardial infarction, or worsening of heart failure symptoms in patients with heart disease. During non-REM (NREM) sleep, systemic blood pressure falls as a result of reduced cardiac metabolic demand,[2] potentially reducing flow through stenotic coronary vessels and precipitating myocardial ischemia or infarction. Sleep apnea reduces oxygen saturation with potential for arrhythmias, hypertension, and myocardial infarction. The major subgroups susceptible to adverse influences of surges in autonomic activity or depression of respiratory control during sleep are those with ischemic heart disease, heart failure, and channelopathies (Table 46-1).[3] In essence, sleep constitutes an autonomic stress test for the heart with unique autonomic, hemodynamic, and respiratory challenges.

CARDIAC EVENTS DURING SLEEP IN PATIENTS WITH CARDIOVASCULAR DISEASE

Nocturnal Ventricular Arrhythmias

A nocturnal trough in ventricular arrhythmias during sleep parallels the decreased nighttime incidence of myocardial infarction, sudden cardiac death, implantable cardioverter-defibrillator discharge, and myocardial ischemic events.[1,4,5] Physiologic triggering is suggested by the fact that the nighttime distribution of these events is not uniform (Fig. 46-1).[1]

Nocturnal ventricular arrhythmias and myocardial ischemia have been attributed to REM sleep–related surges in sympathetic nerve activity,[2,6,7] particularly in patients with endothelial dysfunction, coronary obstructive disease, or vasospasm. Concomitant direct and indirect effects of heart rate and arterial blood pressure are capable of accelerating cardiac electrical instability, intra-arterial platelet aggregation, and plaque disruption with release of proarrhythmic constituents. Sympathetic nerve activity remains elevated at night in patients with coronary artery disease,[5,8] myocardial infarction,[9,10] and

diabetes. Changes in cardiac substrate and mechanical function due to disease, hypoxia, sleep apnea, or aging can also amplify risk of nocturnal arrhythmias and ischemia. A nocturnal peak in sudden cardiac death and two- to fourfold increase in ventricular arrhythmia incidence have been documented in patients with sleep-disordered breathing.[11,12] A temporal association of nonsustained ventricular arrhythmias with apnea has been reported.[13] Frequent or complex arrhythmias are also characteristic of hypertensive patients who do not experience the typical nocturnal trough in blood pressure.[14] In patients who are predisposed to ventricular arrhythmias including torsades de pointes, nocturnal prolonged cycle lengths and asystolic events can facilitate the occurrence of early afterdepolarizations, which set the stage for these arrhythmias. Nocturnal heart rate pauses may be particularly arrhythmogenic in patients with the long QT 2 or 3 syndrome,[15] as lethal arrhythmias in these gene-based subtypes occur almost exclusively at rest or during sleep. (See later discussion under "Sudden Infant Death Syndrome.") A significant affective component of REM sleep dreams may be their vivid, bizarre, and emotionally intense nature and their capacity to generate anger and fear, emotions that have been linked in wakefulness to onset of myocardial infarction and sudden death.[16]

NREM sleep is generally salutary in its effects on ventricular arrhythmia vulnerability, due to increased vagus nerve activity. However, in some cases, arrhythmia frequency may be enhanced during NREM sleep, when latent slow rhythms are exposed by the generalized reduction in heart rate after withdrawal of overdrive suppression. Also, the relative hypotension of NREM sleep may exacerbate impaired coronary perfusion as a result of lowered blood pressure gradients in stenosed vessels with potential for ischemia-induced arrhythmia and myocardial infarction.[17]

Detection of Ventricular Arrhythmia Vulnerability

Quantification of risk for malignant ventricular arrhythmias constitutes an important frontier in cardiac care. T-wave alternans, a beat-to-beat fluctuation in the amplitude and shape of the T wave, has been demonstrated to serve as a marker of risk for life-threatening tachyarrhythmias.[18,19] A recent prospective study of patients with left ventricular dysfunction determined that this parameter monitored on ambulatory electrocardiograms (ECGs) identified patients' 1-year risk for cardiovascular death (primary endpoint) and sudden cardiac death (secondary endpoint) with odds ratios of 17.1 and 22.6, respectively.[20] A correlation between the severity of sleep apnea, indicated by oxygen desaturation and apnea-hypopnea index, with T-wave alternans magnitude in

TABLE 46-1

Patient Groups at Potentially Increased Risk for Nocturnal Cardiac Events

Condition (U.S. Patients/Year)	Possible Mechanism
Angina, MI, arrhythmias, ischemia, or cardiac arrest at night (20% of MIs [~250,000 cases/year] and 15% of sudden deaths [~48,750 cases/year] occur between midnight and 6 AM)	Disturbances in sleep, respiration, and autonomic balance may be factors in nocturnal arrhythmogenesis. The nocturnal pattern suggests a sleep state–dependent autonomic trigger or respiratory distress.
Unstable angina	Nondemand ischemia and angina peak between midnight and 6 AM.
Acute MI (1.5 million)	Nocturnal onset MI is more frequent in older and sicker patients and carries a higher risk of congestive heart failure.
Heart failure (5.3 million)	Sleep-related breathing disorders are pronounced in the setting of heart failure and may contribute to its progression and to mortality risk.
Spousal or family report of highly irregular breathing, excessive snoring, or apnea in patients with coronary disease (15 million U.S. patients with apnea)	Patients with hypertension or atrial or ventricular arrhythmias should be screened for the presence of sleep apnea.
Long QT syndrome	The profound cycle length changes associated with sleep may trigger pause-dependent torsades de pointes in these patients.
Near-miss or siblings of victims of SIDS (2500 total SIDS deaths annually in the United States or 1 death/2000 live births)	SIDS commonly occurs during sleep with characteristic cardiorespiratory symptoms.
Brugada syndrome in Western populations; Asians with warning signs of SUNDS	SUNDS is a sleep-related phenomenon and is genetically related to Brugada syndrome.
Atrial fibrillation (2.2 million)	Twenty-nine percent of episodes occur between midnight and 6 AM. Respiratory and autonomic mechanisms are suspected.

MI, myocardial infarction; *SIDS,* sudden infant death syndrome; *SUNDS,* sudden unexplained nocturnal death syndrome.
Adapted from Verrier RL, Mittleman MA. Sleep-related cardiac risk. In: Kryger MH, Roth T, Dement WC, eds. *Principles and Practice of Sleep Medicine,* 5th ed. Philadelphia: WB Saunders, 2011.

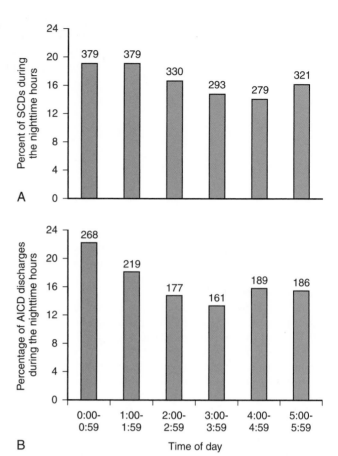

Figure 46-1 A, Hourly incidence of sudden cardiac death onset between midnight and 5:59 AM from 12 studies enrolling 1981 patients.[1] **B,** Hourly incidence of automatic implantable cardioverter defibrillator (ICD) discharge between midnight and 5:59 AM from 7 studies enrolling 1197 patients. The number of discharges observed each hour is indicated above each bar. (Redrawn from Lavery CE, Mittleman MA, Cohen MC, et al. Nonuniform nighttime distribution of acute cardiac events: A possible effect of sleep states. *Circulation.* 1997;96:3321-3327; used with permission from the American Heart Association.)

patients with congestive heart failure has also been reported.[21] Elevated T-wave alternans provoked by sleep apnea is illustrated as the difference in T-wave amplitude in a template of superimposed heart beats (Fig. 46-2).

Therapy

Similarly to treatment for daytime arrhythmias, antiarrhythmic therapy should address the electrically unstable myocardial substrate. Nocturnal β-adrenergic receptor blockade therapy may suppress marked surges in sympathetic nerve activity, but careful attention is required to avoid medications that disrupt sleep.[22] Caution with respect to dosing is also

advised for antihypertensive pharmacologic therapy, which may exacerbate the hypotensive effect of NREM sleep and introduce risk for transient myocardial ischemia and potential for myocardial infarction in patients with stenotic lesions.[17,23] Sleep-related cycle-length prolongation may be a risk factor in cardiac patients treated with class III antiarrhythmic agents (potassium channel blockers) or with diuretics, which also lower potassium. Thus, nocturnal monitoring for heart rate pauses is important in treating individuals for whom these medications are the primary treatment option. Despite associations of sleep-disordered breathing with nocturnal ventricular arrhythmias, evidence is lacking to support the efficacy of continuous positive airway pressure (CPAP) therapy for arrhythmia prevention or management.[24]

Nocturnal Asystole and QT Interval Changes

Benign asystoles are typical during sleep in normal individuals who are young or physically fit, such as athletes and heavy laborers. Sinus pauses less than 2 seconds, prolonged atrioventricular (AV) conduction, Wenckebach AV block, and bradycardia are attributed to effects of increased parasympathetic activity on AV node conduction. Periods of sinus

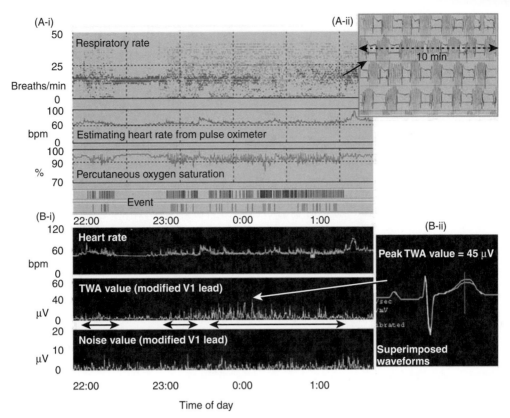

Figure 46-2 Results of overnight simplified respiratory polygraphy and continuous electrocardiography from a representative patient with sleep-disordered breathing[21] demonstrating increase in T-wave alternans levels during apneic events without elevation in noise level. In this patient, the apnoea–hypopnoea index was 35.5 events/hour, and 3% oxygen desaturation index was 33.8 events/hour. Sample simplified respiratory polygraphy is illustrated in (A-i). The first chart shows the time course of respiratory rate (breaths/min). The more dense series of dots was derived from nasal airflow and the more splayed dots from thoracic respiratory movements. A close-up illustration of the respiratory curve is presented in (A-ii). The time course of heart rates estimated from pulse oximeter signals (bpm) and percutaneous oxygen saturation (%) are shown in the second and third charts (A-i), respectively. The fourth chart shows events; the upper band indicates episodes of apnoea–hypopnoea and the lower band indicates periods of severe oxygen desaturation (SpO2, 90% for ≥10 s). Sample electrocardiogram (modified V1 lead) is illustrated (B-i). The time course of heart rate (bpm), T-wave alternans value (μV), and noise value (μV) are shown in the first, second, and third charts, respectively. Arrowed line indicates periods of apneic events. Template of superimposed electrocardiographic waveforms for peak T-wave alternans values during the night in the modified V1 lead (45 μV) are shown (B-ii). (Reprinted with permission from European Society of Cardiology.)

arrest 9 seconds or less during REM sleep in young adults with apparently normal cardiac function have been reported and attributed to exaggerated vagal tone.[25] However, in patients with coronary atherosclerosis and damaged endothelium, the acetylcholine released by surges in vagus nerve activity could provoke coronary vasoconstriction as a result of impaired release of endothelium-derived relaxing factor.[26] Reports vary of associations of apnea with nocturnal sinus pauses,[12] heart block,[27] or ventricular asystole or bradyarrhythmias.[28,29]

Therapy

CPAP therapy has been associated with reversal of sinus arrest and AV conduction block.[30]

Nocturnal Atrial Fibrillation

Atrial fibrillation afflicts 2.2 million people in the United States and 4.5 million in the European Union, in whom the arrhythmia is responsible for increased morbidity and mortality rates. It is likely that 10% to 25% of atrial arrhythmias are facilitated by vagal influences. Nocturnal atrial fibrillation provoked during periods of intense vagus nerve activity is termed "vagally mediated atrial fibrillation." Nocturnal

peaks in onset of atrial tachyarrhythmias and paroxysmal atrial fibrillation have been reported in patients younger than 61 years.[31] Atrial fibrillation during sleep may be evident in a rise in heart rate (Fig. 46-3).[32]

Risks of atrial fibrillation and its recurrence after cardioversion are increased two- to fourfold if breathing during sleep is disordered (Fig. 46-4).[12,13,33-36] Incidence of atrial fibrillation in apnea patients is strongly predicted by obesity and by nocturnal oxygen desaturation in subjects younger than 65 years old[36] and by heart failure in older patients. Mechanistic bases for apnea-induced atrial fibrillation include provocation of nocturnal hypoxemia, sympathetic nerve activity, and hemodynamic stress.

Therapy

At present there is no clear evidence for differentiating medical treatment for nighttime as compared with daytime atrial fibrillation. However, individuals with nocturnal onset of atrial fibrillation should be monitored for hypoxia and sleep-disordered breathing. The potential of CPAP as an adjunct therapy for prevention of atrial fibrillation is controversial.[24,33] Effectiveness of weight control when warranted has been documented.[37]

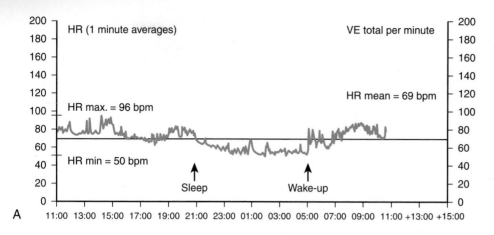

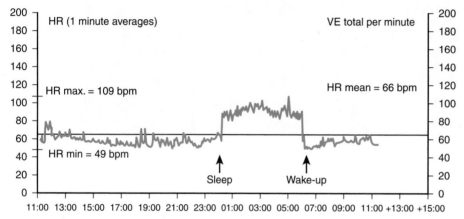

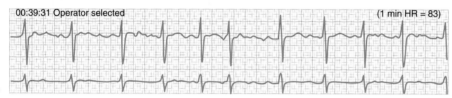

Figure 46-3 Heart rate trend from an ambulatory electrocardiogram (AECG) recording showing a normal circadian rhythm with a sleep-induced decrease in heart rate (**A**) as compared with a nocturnal increase in heart rate caused by paroxysmal atrial fibrillation at the onset of sleep and a drop in heart rate after awakening due to spontaneous conversion to sinus rhythm (**B**).[32] The AECG (at bottom) documents atrial fibrillation during the sleep period. (Redrawn from Singh J, Mela T, Ruskin J. Images in cardiovascular medicine. Sleep (vagal)-induced atrial fibrillation. *Circulation.* 2004;110:e32-33; used with permission from the American Heart Association.)

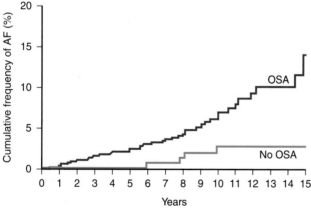

Figure 46-4 Incidence of atrial fibrillation based on presence or absence of obstructive sleep apnea (OSA).[36] Cumulative frequency curves for incident atrial fibrillation (AF) for subjects younger than 65 years of age with and without (OSA) during an average 4.7 years of follow-up (*P* = 0.002). (Redrawn from Gami AS, Hodge DO, Herges RM, et al. Obstructive sleep apnea, obesity, and the risk of incident atrial fibrillation. *J Am Coll Cardiol.* 2007;49:565-571; used with permission from American College of Cardiology.)

Nocturnal Myocardial Ischemia and Angina

Assessment and treatment of nocturnal angina has been a subject of concern for over 2 centuries. The renowned 20th century cardiologists Paul Dudley White and Samuel Levine remarked on the frequency of myocardial infarction and angina during sleep and suggested an association with dreaming. Nocturnal myocardial ischemia and angina are important prognostic markers of cardiovascular events and may occur during either REM or NREM sleep. In patients with stable coronary artery disease and preserved left ventricular function, nocturnal ischemic events occur primarily during REM sleep[6] and are attributed to increased sympathetic nerve activity and heart rate surges, and the resultant metabolic demands in a setting of flow-limited, stenotic coronary arteries.

Nighttime ischemic events remain, although less frequent, in cardiac patients receiving β-adrenergic receptor blockade therapy, which contains sympathetic nerve activity and demand-related myocardial ischemia. Non–demand-related nocturnal myocardial ischemia is prevalent among patients with more severe coronary disease, diabetes, acute coronary syndromes, and acute myocardial infarction, populations with significant endothelial and mechanical dysfunction. These nondemand nocturnal ischemic episodes may disclose a critical underlying coronary lesion, coronary vasospasm, or transient coronary artery stenosis. Mancia[17] hypothesized that the hypotension of NREM sleep "reduces the volume and velocity of blood flow, favoring the development of thrombi and embolic and ischemic phenomena before and after arousal." The nocturnal nadir in endogenous fibrinolytic activity may also play a role in nocturnal myocardial ischemia, with increased transient thrombus formation. Peaks in serum levels of plasminogen activator inhibitor and tissue plasminogen activator antigen increase blood viscosity or hypercoagulability at night and free radical generation. Patel and colleagues[8] documented a nocturnal peak in ischemic events in their study of 256 optimally medicated hospitalized patients with the acute coronary syndromes of unstable angina and non–Q-wave myocardial infarction. It is important to note, however, that the peak in out-of-hospital onset of these syndromes follows the usual circadian pattern.[38]

Therapy

Demand-related ischemic episodes can be effectively contained by β-adrenergic receptor blockade. Non–demand-related nocturnal myocardial ischemia is not reduced by antihypertensive treatment. Treatment of sleep apnea is capable of ameliorating angina in some patients.[39] The incidence of nocturnal ischemic activity in patients receiving optimal medical therapy[8] suggests that current approaches to management do not adequately address the factors involved.

Nocturnal Myocardial Infarction

REM-induced surges in autonomic nervous system activity both independent of and in association with sleep apnea are likely to constitute important triggers of the 20% of myocardial infarctions that occur at night by provoking tachycardia and hypertension. These phenomena may lead to coronary artery plaque rupture as well as to inappropriate decreases in the myocardial oxygen supply-demand relationship or to α-adrenergically mediated coronary vasoconstriction. Alternatively, the relative hypotension of slow wave sleep due to decreased cardiac metabolic demand may reduce coronary perfusion pressure through stenotic vessel segments, leading to malperfusion of the myocardium. Other factors known to contribute to myocardial infarction are operative during sleep, including increased ventricular diastolic pressures and volumes due to the fluid shifts resulting from the supine posture, unfavorable alterations in the balance of fibrinolytic and thrombotic factors, and chronic or episodic oxygen desaturation.

Specific patient groups experience an increased incidence of nighttime myocardial infarctions, particularly those with depressed ventricular function, advanced age, diabetes, or sleep apnea.[40] The risk for development of congestive heart failure is higher for nighttime than daytime myocardial infarctions, potentially as a result of either pathologic processes or a delay in obtaining high-quality care.[41]

Therapy

It is essential to avoid medications that enhance the hypotension of NREM sleep.[17] Antihypertensive treatment does not reduce the incidence of nocturnal myocardial infarction and myocardial ischemia.[23]

PATIENT GROUPS WITH ELEVATED RISK FOR NIGHTTIME CARDIOVASCULAR EVENTS

Patients with Hypertension

Patients whose nighttime arterial blood pressure declines less than 10% from day to night (referred to as "nondippers") are at increased risk of total and cardiovascular death, as well as all cardiovascular endpoints, frequent or complex ventricular arrhythmias, myocardial ischemia, cerebrovascular insult, and increased organ damage, including cardiac hypertrophy. Faulty baroreceptor reflex activation may account for the fact that arterial blood pressure during sleep remains significantly elevated in hypertensive patients with central hypersympathetic nerve activity, microarousals, reduced length and depth of NREM sleep, and shortened REM latency. Hypertension in sleep apnea patients has been attributed to impairment of resistance-vessel endothelium-dependent vasodilation.[42] Patients younger than 60 years old with uncontrolled hypertension should be monitored for the presence of sleep apnea.[43-45]

Therapy

CPAP has been found to reduce hypertension in patients with sleep-disordered breathing.[46-49]

Post-Myocardial Infarction Patients

During the first weeks after myocardial infarction, sleep is significantly disturbed.[9] Especially in patients with impaired left ventricular function, nocturnal oxygen desaturation may be generalized or episodic and may provoke ventricular tachycardia (Fig. 46-5), ventricular premature beats, and bouts of myocardial ischemia.[50] Heart rates remain elevated even during NREM sleep, and heart rate variability is depressed, indicating enhanced sympathetic nerve tone.[10] Nocturnal levels of norepinephrine are increased and nocturnal secretion of

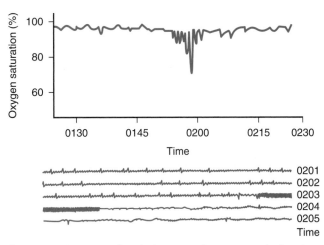

Figure 46-5 Importance of monitoring nocturnal oxygen saturation in patients who have sustained a myocardial infarction.[50] Nonsustained ventricular tachycardia (*lower panel*) and hypoxemia measured by pulse oximetry (*upper panel*) occurred simultaneously on the third night after infarction. The patient died on the following day of cardiogenic shock. (Redrawn from Galatius-Jensen S, Hansen J, Rasmussen V, et al. Nocturnal hypoxemia after myocardial infarction: Association with nocturnal myocardial ischaemia and arrhythmias. *Br Heart J.* 1994;72:23-30; used with permission from the British Medical Journal Publishing Group Ltd. and the British Cardiovascular Society.)

melatonin, an endogenous hormone that suppresses sympathetic nerve activity, is diminished. In patients with residual myocardial ischemia, both the duration and number of nighttime ischemic events are increased. These symptoms diminish across the first 6 months after myocardial infarction, after which ventricular tachycardia during sleep is relatively rare.

Heart Failure Patients

Sudden cardiac death in heart failure patients occurs at night in 20% of cases.[51] At least half of patients with congestive heart failure experience disturbed nighttime breathing. The apnea-hypopnea index is a powerful independent predictor of poor prognoses in clinically stable congestive heart failure patients.[52-54] These sleep-related nocturnal breathing disorders set in motion a cascade of arrhythmogenic factors that underlie an overall increase in mortality rate, particularly in patients with ischemic heart failure.[55] Nocturnal oxygen desaturations (Fig. 46-6),[56] elevated sympathetic nerve activity, ventricular stretch, remodeling of cardiac chambers, and left ventricular systolic dysfunction are implicated.[57] In patients with systolic heart failure, central sleep apnea, severe right ventricular systolic dysfunction, and low diastolic blood pressure are associated with increased mortality risks.[58]

Therapy

CPAP therapy reduces hypertension and improves left ventricular function in patients with obstructive[59,60] and central sleep apnea.[61-63] However, CPAP does not improve survival in heart failure patients with central sleep apnea.[62] An interventional trial is warranted to determine event-free survival of heart failure patients following CPAP.[64,65] Gottlieb and associates[56] have provided evidence suggesting that hypoxia rather than apnea frequency may be a more effective therapeutic target in heart failure patients.

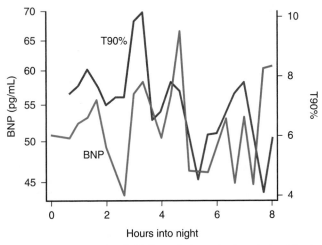

Figure 46-6 Mean BNP and t90. For each time point through the night, the mean brain (B-type) natriuretic peptide (BNP) of all patients (*blue line*) and the percentage of time with oxygen saturation less than 90% (t90) (*gray line*) are shown. Note that the BNP appears to fluctuate with the extent of hypoxemia. (Redrawn from Gottlieb JD, Schwartz AR, Marshall J, et al. Hypoxia, not the frequency of sleep apnea, induces acute hemodynamic stress in patients with chronic heart failure. *J Am Coll Cardiol.* 2009;54(18):1706-1712; used with permission from Journal of American College of Cardiology.)

Sudden Infant Death Syndrome

Sudden infant death syndrome (SIDS) is the leading cause of death in infants between 1 week and 1 year of age and typically occurs during sleep. The syndrome is diagnosed by exclusion criteria to include all causes that "remain unexplained after a thorough case investigation, including performance of a complete autopsy, examination of the death scene, and review of the clinical history." The toll of SIDS is approximately 1 death per 2000 live births or 2500 total SIDS deaths in the United States annually and may be attributable to a variety of causes that challenge the developing cardiorespiratory system.[66] Hypotension and bradycardia characterize the fatal event. In infants who later died of SIDS, heart rates were generally higher and exhibited a reduced range, normal breathing pauses were absent, variability in breathing was diminished, and respiration-induced heart rate variations were reduced, suggesting a defect in the normal reflex coordination of heart rate, arterial blood pressure, and respiration during sleep. Autonomic instability has also been documented in NREM sleep in infants with aborted SIDS events.[67]

Repolarization abnormalities and arrhythmias during sleep have been observed among SIDS victims with the long QT syndrome genotype linked to chromosome 3 (LQT3).[68] A 19-year, prospective, multicenter observational study of 34,442 infants determined that significant prolongation (35 msec or more) of the QT interval was typical of the 24 (0.07%) infants who died of SIDS within the first year of life.[69] T-wave alternans has been reported in infants who became SIDS victims or were successfully treated.[70,71]

Therapy

Straightforward opportunities for prevention of SIDS include placing infants in a supine (face-up) position for sleeping and avoidance of maternal smoking during gestation and passive smoking during the child's infancy. β-Adrenergic blockade is indicated[69,71] and diminishes T-wave alternans magnitude.[71]

The Brugada Syndrome and Sudden Unexplained Nocturnal Death

Sudden death during sleep due to ventricular arrhythmia has been reported in patients with the Brugada sybdrome or the sudden unexplained nocturnal death syndrome (SUNDS). These syndromes probably represent the same disorder, in which right precordial ST-segment elevation is diagnostic.[72,73]

The Brugada syndrome is responsible for 4% to 12% of all sudden cardiac deaths and for approximately 20% of deaths in patients with structurally normal hearts.[72] A single sodium channel mutation in the *SCN5A* gene, QT interval prolongation, and Brugada-like ECG are exhibited by 20% of Brugada patients; other gene mutations are suspected. Genetic defects in the sodium channel are associated with progressive conduction system disease and bradycardia.

Autopsies of SUNDS cases have established the absence of cardiovascular disease and developmental abnormalities in conduction pathways.

Therapy

Currently, implantation of cardioverter-defibrillators is indicated both for patients with Brugada syndrome[72] and those at risk for SUNDS.[73]

EFFECTS OF SLEEP-DISORDERED BREATHING ON CARDIAC EVENTS

Cardiac disease patients with obstructive or central sleep apnea experience a marked nocturnal peak in sudden death with close temporal association with onset of nonsustained ventricular tachycardia (Fig. 46-7).[11,12,74] This respiratory dysfunction affects 15 million Americans, or 4% to 9% of the adult U.S. population,[75] and constitutes an independent

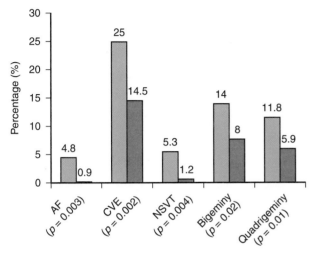

Figure 46-7 Arrhythmia prevalence (%) according to sleep-disordered breathing (SDB) status.[12] Blue bars, SDB; grey bars, non-SDB. *AF*, atrial fibrillation; *CVE*, complex ventricular ectopy; *NSVT*, nonsustained ventricular tachycardia. *N* = 228 with SDB; *N* = 338 without SDB. (Redrawn from Mehra R, Benjamin EJ, Shahar E, et al. Association of nocturnal arrhythmias with sleep-disordered breathing. The Sleep Heart Health Study. *Am J Respir Crit Care Med.* 2006;173: 910-916; used with permission from the American Thoracic Society.)

marker of ventricular arrhythmia risk.[52,53,76] Sleep apnea and hypoxia also potentiate the risk for daytime cardiovascular events, myocardial infarction,[77] stroke,[78-80] diabetes onset,[81] and death from any cause.[80] The postulated mechanism is the apnea-induced surge in arterial blood pressure and sympathetic nerve activity, which attain levels similar to waking at 249% to 299% above baseline and are not diminished during wakefulness (Fig. 46-8).[82,83] Apneic episodes provoke oxygen desaturation and hypoxia, which are highly conducive to nocturnal ischemia, bradyarrhythmia, and tachyarrhythmias in patients with coronary artery disease or heart failure[21,50,83-85] (see Fig. 46-2). Resistance-vessel endothelium-dependent vasodilation is impaired in patients with sleep apnea,[42] a potential factor in the development of hypertension and heart failure, and inflammatory processes are up-regulated, increasing cardiovascular morbidity.[86,87]

Therapy

Apnea treatment with CPAP, supplemental oxygen, or mechanical breathing-assist devices can improve exercise tolerance and lessen heart failure symptoms, but the efficacy of CPAP as an adjunct in prevention of cardiovascular events or arrhythmia management is controversial.[83,88-91] Weight control when indicated may ameliorate apnea and concomitant cardiovascular symptoms.[37,92]

SLEEP-DISRUPTING EFFECTS OF CARDIAC MEDICATIONS

Several widely employed cardiac medications have the potential to disrupt sleep, including antihypertensive agents and beta blockers, which reduce sudden death risk[93] but cross the blood-brain barrier.[22] The lipophilic beta blockers

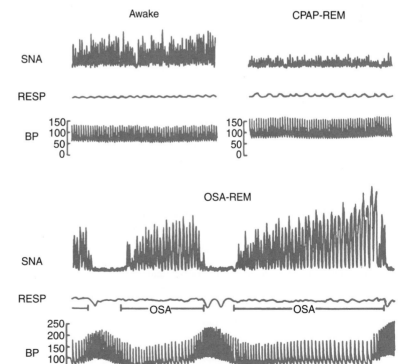

Figure 46-8 Recordings of sympathetic nerve activity (SNA), respiration (RESP), and intra-arterial blood pressure (BP) in the same subject when awake, with obstructive sleep apnea during rapid eye movement (REM) sleep, and with elimination of obstructive apnea by continuous positive airway pressure (CPAP) therapy during REM sleep.[82] SNA was very high during wakefulness but increased even further secondary to obstructive apnea during REM. BP increased from 130/65 mm Hg when awake to 256/110 mm Hg at the end of apnea. Elimination of apneas by CPAP resulted in decreased nerve activity and prevented BP surges during REM sleep. (Redrawn from Somers VK, Dyken ME, Clary MP, et al. Sympathetic neural mechanisms in obstructive sleep apnea. *J Clin Invest.* 1995;96:1897-1904; used with permission from The American Society for Clinical Investigation.)

propranolol and metoprolol increase the total number of awakenings and total wakefulness compared with placebo. These agents and the nonlipophilic atenolol are known to provoke nightmares. Blood-brain barrier penetration occurs with prolonged therapy. The mechanism of sleep disruption by beta-blocking agents may be depletion of endogenous melatonin, a key sleep-regulating hormone that affects sympathetic nervous system activity.[94] Sleep disturbance with neurologic side effects in 20% to 40% of patients have been reported in association with the widely prescribed antiarrhythmic agent amiodarone.

CONCLUSIONS AND IMPLICATIONS

Identification of the level of risk and determination of the particular pathophysiology provoking sleep-related cardiac events on an individual patient basis remain a frontier, requiring streamlined risk-assessment tools suitable for use in the routine flow of clinical evaluation. The needed technology will incorporate concurrent monitoring of ECG, blood pressure, oxygen desaturation, and respiratory variables to advance current understanding of causal links. Recent developments in ambulatory ECG-based technology for assessment of autonomic tone by heart rate turbulence[95] and of cardiac electrical instability by T-wave alternans[18-21] may be useful. Arrhythmia vulnerability is often compounded by disordered nighttime breathing, but whether sleep apnea treatment is capable of reducing risk for atrial fibrillation, myocardial infarction, and sudden death has not been established definitively and deserves intense investigation. Such multiparameter assessment could significantly improve diagnosis and therapy and reduce sleep-related cardiovascular events.

FUNDING SOURCES

HL-U34105277: A Planning Study: Sleep Apnea Intervention for Cardiovascular Disease Reduction.

DISCLOSURES

Dr. Richard L. Verrier is co-inventor of a patent for T-wave alternans measurement by the Modified Moving Average method, which was assigned to Beth Israel Deaconess Medical Center and licensed to GE Healthcare, Inc. and to Medtronic, Inc. He has received research equipment and honoraria from GE Healthcare and grant support from Medtronic, Inc. Dr. Murray A. Mittleman reports no conflicts of interest.

REFERENCES

1. Lavery CE, Mittleman MA, Cohen MC, et al. Nonuniform nighttime distribution of acute cardiac events: A possible effect of sleep states. *Circulation*. 1997;96:3321-3327.
2. Verrier RL, Harper RM. Central and autonomic mechanisms regulating cardiovascular function. In: Kryger MH, Roth T, Dement WC, eds. *Principles and Practice of Sleep Medicine*. Philadelphia: WB Saunders; 2011.
3. Verrier RL, Mittleman MA. Sleep-related cardiac risk. In: Kryger MH, Roth T, Dement WC, eds. *Principles and Practice of Sleep Medicine*. Philadelphia: WB Saunders; 2011.
4. Muller JE, Ludmer PL, Willich SN, et al. Circadian variation in the frequency of sudden cardiac death. *Circulation*. 1987;75:131-138.
5. Andrews TC, Fenton T, Toyosaki N, et al. for the Angina and Silent Ischemia Study Group (ASIS). Subsets of ambulatory myocardial ischemia based on heart rate activity: Circadian distribution and response to anti-ischemic medication. *Circulation*. 1993;98:92-100.
6. Nowlin JB, Troyer Jr WG, Collins WS, et al. The association of nocturnal angina pectoris with dreaming. *Ann Intern Med*. 1965;63:1040-1046.
7. Somers VK, Dyken ME, Mark AL, et al. Sympathetic nerve activity during sleep in normal subjects. *N Engl J Med*. 1993;328:303-307.
8. Patel DJ, Knight CJ, Holdright DR, et al. Pathophysiology of transient myocardial ischemia in acute coronary syndromes: Characterization by continuous ST-segment monitoring. *Circulation*. 1997;95:1185-1192.
9. Broughton R, Baron R. Sleep patterns in the intensive care unit and on the ward after acute myocardial infarction. *Electroencephalogr Clin Neurophysiol*. 1978;45:348-360.
10. Vanoli E, Adamson PB, Ba-Lin, et al. Heart rate variability during specific sleep stages: A comparison of healthy subjects with patients after myocardial infarction. *Circulation*. 1995;91:1918-1922.
11. Gami AS, Howard DE, Olson EJ, et al. Day-night pattern of sudden death in obstructive sleep apnea. *N Engl J Med*. 2005;352:1206-1214.
12. Mehra R, Benjamin EJ, Shahar E, et al. Association of nocturnal arrhythmias with sleep-disordered breathing. The Sleep Heart Health Study. *Am J Respir Crit Care Med*. 2006;173:910-916.
13. Monahan K, Storfer-Isser A, Mehra R, et al. Triggering of nocturnal arrhythmias by sleep-disordered breathing events. *J Am Coll Cardiol*. 2009;54(19):1797-1804.
14. Schillaci G, Verdecchia P, Borgioni C, et al. Association between persistent pressure overload and ventricular arrhythmias in essential hypertension. *Hypertension*. 1996;28:284-289.
15. Schwartz PJ, Priori SG, Spazzolini C, et al. Genotype-phenotype correlation in the long-QT syndrome: Gene-specific triggers for life-threatening arrhythmias. *Circulation*. 2001;103:89-95.
16. Mittleman MA, Maclure M, Sherwood JB, et al. Triggering of acute myocardial infarction onset by episodes of anger: Determinants of myocardial infarction onset study investigators. *Circulation*. 1995;92:1720-1725.
17. Mancia G. Autonomic modulation of the cardiovascular system during sleep. *N Engl J Med*. 1993;328:347-349.
18. Verrier RL, Kumar K, Nearing BD. Basis for sudden cardiac death prediction by T-wave alternans from an integrative physiology perspective. *Heart Rhythm*. 2009;6:416-422.
19. Nieminen T, Verrier RL. Usefulness of T-wave alternans in sudden death risk stratification and guiding medical therapy. *Ann Noninvasiv Electrocardiol*. 2010;15(3):276-288.
20. Sakaki K, Ikeda T, Miwa Y, et al. Time-domain T-wave alternans measured from Holter electrocardiograms predicts cardiac mortality in patients with left ventricular dysfunction: A prospective study. *Heart Rhythm*. 2009;6:332-337.
21. Takasugi N, Nishigaki K, Kubota T, et al. Sleep apnoea induces cardiac electrical instability assessed by T-wave alternans in patients with congestive heart failure. *Eur J Heart Fail*. 2009;11(11):1063-1070.
22. Kostis JB, Rosen RC. Central nervous system effects of beta-adrenergic blocking drugs: The role of ancillary properties. *Circulation*. 1987;75:204-212.
23. Floras JS. Antihypertensive treatment, myocardial infarction, and nocturnal myocardial ischaemia. *Lancet*. 1988;2:994-996.
24. Gami AS, Somers VK. Implications of obstructive sleep apnea for atrial fibrillation and sudden cardiac death. *J Cardiovasc Electrophysiol*. 2008;19:997-1003.
25. Guilleminault C, Pool P, Motta J, et al. Sinus arrest during REM sleep in young adults. *N Engl J Med*. 1984;311:1006-1010.
26. Ludmer PL, Selwyn AP, Shook TL, et al. Paradoxical vasoconstriction induced by acetylcholine in atherosclerotic coronary arteries. *N Engl J Med*. 1986;315:1046-1051.
27. Koehler U, Fus E, Grimm W, et al. Heart block in patients with obstructive sleep apnoea: Pathogenetic factors and effects of treatment. *Eur Respir J*. 1998;11:434-439.
28. Koehler U, Becker HF, Grimm W, et al. Relations among hypoxemia, sleep stage, and bradyarrhythmia during obstructive sleep apnea. *Am Heart J*. 2000;139(1 Pt 1):142-148.
29. Daccarett M, Segerson NM, Hamdan AL, et al. Relation of daytime bradyarrhythmias with high risk features of sleep apnea. *Am J Cardiol*. 2008;101(8):1147-1150.
30. Becker H, Brandenburg U, Peter JH, et al. Reversal of sinus arrest and atrioventricular conduction block in patients with sleep apnea during nasal continuous positive airway pressure. *Am J Respir Crit Care Med*. 1995;151:215-218.
31. Yamashita T, Murakawa Y, Hayami N, et al. Relation between aging and circadian variation of paroxysmal atrial fibrillation. *Am J Cardiol*. 1998;82:1364-1367.
32. Singh J, Mela T, Ruskin J. Images in cardiovascular medicine. Sleep (vagal)-induced atrial fibrillation. *Circulation*. 2004;110:e32-33.

33. Kanagala R, Murali NS, Friedman PA, et al. Obstructive sleep apnea and the recurrence of atrial fibrillation. *Circulation.* 2003;107:2589-2594.

34. Stevenson IH, Teichtahl H, Cunnington D, et al. Prevalence of sleep disordered breathing in paroxysmal and persistent atrial fibrillation patients with normal left ventricular function. *Eur Heart J.* 2008;29:1662-1669.

35. Konecny T, Brady PA, Orban M, et al. Interactions between sleep disordered breathing and atrial fibrillation in patients with hypertrophic cardiomyopathy. *Am J Cardiol.* 2010;105(11):1597-1602.

36. Gami AS, Hodge DO, Herges RM, et al. Obstructive sleep apnea, obesity, and the risk of incident atrial fibrillation. *J Am Coll Cardiol.* 2007;49:565-571.

37. Wang TJ, Parise H, Levy D, et al. Obesity and the risk of new-onset atrial fibrillation. *JAMA.* 2004;292:2471-2477.

38. Cannon CP, McCabe CH, Stone PH, et al. Circadian variation in the onset of unstable angina and non-Q-wave acute myocardial infarction (the TIMI Registry and TIMI III). *Am J Cardiol.* 1997;79:253-258.

39. Franklin KA, Nilsson JB, Sahlin C, et al. Sleep apnoea and nocturnal angina. *Lancet.* 1995;345(8957):1085-1087.

40. Kuniyoshi FH, Garcia-Touchard A, Gami AS, et al. Day-night variation of acute myocardial infarction in obstructive sleep apnea. *J Am Coll Cardiol.* 2008;52:343-346.

41. Mukamal KJ, Muller JE, Maclure M, et al. Increased risk of congestive heart failure among infarctions with nighttime onset. *Am Heart J.* 2000;140(3):438-442.

42. Kato M, Roberts-Thomson P, Phillips BG, et al. Impairment of endothelium-dependent vasodilation of resistance vessels in patients with obstructive sleep apnea. *Circulation.* 2000;102:2607-2610.

43. Nieto FJ, Young TB, Lind BK, et al. Association of sleep disordered breathing, sleep apnea, and hypertension in a large community-based study. Sleep Heart Health Study. *JAMA.* 2000;283(14):1829-1836.

44. Peppard PE, Young T, Palta M, et al. Prospective study of the association between sleep-disordered breathing and hypertension. *N Engl J Med.* 2000;342(19):1378-1384.

45. Haas DC, Foster GL, Nieto FJ, et al. Age-dependent associations between sleep-disordered breathing and hypertension: Importance of discriminating between systolic/diastolic hypertension and isolated systolic hypertension in the Sleep Heart Health Study. *Circulation.* 2005;111(5):614-621.

46. Becker HF, Jerrentrup A, Ploch T, et al. Effect of nasal continuous positive airway pressure treatment on blood pressure in patients with obstructive sleep apnea. *Circulation.* 2003;107(1):68-73.

47. Usui K, Bradley TD, Spaak J, et al. Inhibition of awake sympathetic nerve activity of heart failure patients with obstructive sleep apnea by nocturnal continuous positive airway pressure. *J Am Coll Cardiol.* 2005;45(12):2008-2011.

48. Arias MA, Garcia-Rio F, Alonso-Fernandez A, et al. Pulmonary hypertension in obstructive sleep apnea: Effects of continuous positive airway pressure: A randomized, controlled cross-over study. *Eur Heart J.* 2006;27(9):1106-1113.

49. Kapa S, Kuniyoshi FH, Somers VK. Sleep apnea and hypertension: Interactions and implications for management. *Hypertension.* 2008;51:605-608.

50. Galatius-Jensen S, Hansen J, Rasmussen V, et al. Nocturnal hypoxemia after myocardial infarction: Association with nocturnal myocardial ischaemia and arrhythmias. *Br Heart J.* 1994;72:23-30.

51. Carson PA, O'Connor CM, Miller AB, et al. Circadian rhythm and sudden death in heart failure: Results from prospective randomized amlodipine survival trial. *J Am Coll Cardiol.* 2000;36:541-546.

52. Bradley TD, Floras JS. Sleep apnea and heart failure: Part I: Obstructive sleep apnea. *Circulation.* 2003;107:1671-1678.

53. Bradley TD, Floras JS. Sleep apnea and heart failure: Part II: Central sleep apnea. *Circulation.* 2003;107:1822-1826.

54. Wang H, Parker JD, Newton GE, et al. Influence of obstructive sleep apnea on mortality in patients with heart failure. *J Am Coll Cardiol.* 2007;49:1625-1631.

55. Yumino D, Wang H, Floras JS, et al. Relationship between sleep apnoea and mortality in patients with ischaemic heart failure. *Heart.* 2009;95(10):819-824.

56. Gottlieb JD, Schwartz AR, Marshall J, et al. Hypoxia, not the frequency of sleep apnea, induces acute hemodynamic stress in patients with chronic heart failure. *J Am Coll Cardiol.* 2009;54(18):1706-1712.

57. Chami HA, Devereux RB, Gottdiener JS, et al. Left ventricular morphology and systolic function in sleep-disordered breathing: The Sleep Heart Health Study. *Circulation.* 2008;117(20):2599-2607.

58. Javaheri S, Shukla R, Zeigler H, et al. Central sleep apnea, right ventricular dysfunction and low diastolic blood pressure are predictors of mortality in systolic heart failure. *J Am Coll Cardiol.* 2007;49:2028-2034.

59. Kaneko Y, Floras JS, Usui K, et al. Cardiovascular effects of continuous positive airway pressure in patients with heart failure and obstructive sleep apnea. *N Engl J Med.* 2003;348(13):1233-1241.

60. Oliveira W, Campos O, Cintra F, et al. Impact of continuous positive airway pressure treatment on left atrial volume and function in patients with obstructive sleep apnea assessed by real-time three-dimensional echocardiography. *Heart.* 2009;95(22):1872-1878.

61. Sin DD, Logan AG, Fitzgerald FS, et al. Effects of continuous positive airway pressure on cardiovascular outcomes in heart failure patients with and without Cheyne-Stokes respiration. *Circulation.* 2000;102(1):61-66.

62. Bradley TD, Logan AG, Kimoff RJ, et al. Continuous positive airway pressure for central sleep apnea and heart failure. *N Engl J Med.* 2005;353(19):2025-2033.

63. Arzt M, Floras JS, Logan AG, et al. Suppression of central sleep apnea by continuous positive airway pressure and transplant-free survival in heart failure: A *post hoc* analysis of the Canadian Continuous Positive Airway Pressure for Patients with Central Sleep Apnea and Heart Failure Trial (CANPAP). *Circulation.* 2007;115(25):3173-3180.

64. Caples SM, Somers VK. CPAP treatment for obstructive sleep apnea in heart failure: Expectations unmet. *Eur Heart J.* 2007;28(10):1184-1186.

65. Floras JS. Should sleep apnea be a specific target of therapy in chronic heart failure? *Heart.* 2009;95(13):1041-1046.

66. Moon RY, Horne RS, Hauck FR. Sudden infant death syndrome. *Lancet.* 2007;370(9598):1578-1587.

67. Pincus SM, Cummins TR, Haddad GG. Heart rate control in normal and aborted-SIDS infants. *Am J Physiol.* 1993;264:R638-646.

68. Priori SG, Schwartz PJ, Napolitano C, et al. Risk stratification in the long-QT syndrome. *N Engl J Med.* 2003;348:1866-1874.

69. Schwartz PJ, Stramba-Badiale M, Segantini A, et al. Prolongation of the QT interval and the sudden infant death syndrome. *N Engl J Med.* 1998;338:1709-1714.

70. Weintraub RG, Gow RM, Wilkinson JL. The congenital long QT syndromes in childhood. *J Am Coll Cardiol.* 1990;16:674-680.

71. Mache CJ, Beitzke A, Haidvogl M, et al. Perinatal manifestations of idiopathic long QT syndrome. *Pediatr Cardiol.* 1996;17:118-121.

72. Antzelevitch C, Brugada P, Borggrefe M, et al. Brugada syndrome: Report of the second consensus conference: Endorsed by the Heart Rhythm Society and the European Heart Rhythm Association. *Circulation.* 2005;111:659-670.

73. Nademanee K, Veerakul G, Mower M, et al. Defibrillator Versus Beta-Blockers for Unexplained Death in Thailand (DEBUT): A randomized clinical trial. *Circulation.* 2003;107:2221-2226.

74. Lanfranchi PA, Somers VK, Braghiroli A, et al. Central sleep apnea in left ventricular dysfunction: Prevalence and implications for arrhythmic risk. *Circulation.* 2003;107:727-732.

75. Young T, Skatrud J, Peppard PE. Risk factors for obstructive sleep apnea in adults. *JAMA.* 2004;291(16):2013-2016.

76. Peker Y, Hedner J, Kraiczi H, et al. Respiratory disturbance index: An independent predictor of mortality in coronary artery disease. *Am J Respir Crit Care Med.* 2000;162:81-86.

77. Hung J, Whitford EG, Parsons RW, et al. Association of sleep apnea with myocardial infarction in men. *Lancet.* 1990;336:261-264.

78. Valham F, Mooe T, Rabben T, et al. Increased risk of stroke in patients with coronary artery disease and sleep apnea: A 10-year follow-up. *Circulation.* 2008;118(9):955-960.

79. Redline S, Yenokyan G, Gottlieb JD, et al. Obstructive sleep apnea-hypopnea and incident stroke: The Sleep Heart Health Study. *Am J Respir Crit Care Med.* 2010;182(2):269-277.

80. Yaggi HK, Concato J, Kernan WN, et al. Obstructive sleep apnea as a risk factor for stroke and death. *N Engl J Med.* 2005;353(19):2034-2041.

81. Seicean S, Kirchner HL, Gottlieb JD, et al. Sleep-disordered breathing and impaired glucose metabolism in normal-weight and overweight/obese individuals: The Sleep Heart Health Study. *Diabetes Care.* 2008;31:1001-1006.

82. Somers VK, Dyken ME, Clary MP, et al. Sympathetic neural mechanisms in obstructive sleep apnea. *J Clin Invest.* 1995;96:1897-1904.

83. Somers VK, White DP, Amin R, et al. Sleep apnea and cardiovascular disease: An American Heart Association/American College of Cardiology Foundation Scientific Statement from the American Heart Association Council for High Blood Pressure Research Professional Education Committee, Council on Clinical Cardiology, Stroke Council, and Council On Cardiovascular Nursing. In collaboration with the National Heart, Lung, and Blood Institute National Center on Sleep Disorders Research (National Institutes of Health). *Circulation.* 2008;118:1080-1111.

84. Davies SW, John LM, Wedzicha JA, et al. Overnight studies in severe chronic left heart failure: Arrhythmias and oxygen desaturation. *Br Heart J.* 1991;65:77-83.

85. Cripps T, Rocker G, Stradling J. Nocturnal hypoxia and arrhythmias in patients with impaired left ventricular function. *Br Heart J.* 1992;68:382-386.

86. Shamsuzzaman AS, Winnicki M, Lanfranchi P, et al. Elevated C-reactive protein in patients with obstructive sleep apnea. *Circulation.* 2002;105(21):2462-2464.

87. Jelic S, Lederer DJ, Adams T, et al. Vascular inflammation in obesity and sleep apnea. *Circulation.* 2010;121(8):1014-1021.

88. Milleron O, Pilliere R, Foucher A, et al. Benefits of obstructive sleep apnea treatment in coronary artery disease: A long-term follow-up study. *Eur Heart J.* 2004;25:728-734.

89. Marin JM, Carrizo SJ, Vicente E, et al. Long-term cardiovascular outcomes in men with obstructive sleep apnea-hypopnoea with or without treatment with continuous positive airway pressure: An observational study. *Lancet.* 2005;365:1046-1053.

90. Buchner NJ, Sanner BM, Borgel J, et al. Continuous positive airway pressure treatment of mild to moderate obstructive sleep apnea reduces cardiovascular risk. *Am J Respir Crit Care Med.* 2007;176:1274-1280.

91. Bradley TD, Floras JS. Obstructive sleep apnea and its cardiovascular consequences. *Lancet.* 2009;373:82-93.

92. Peppard PE, Young T, Palta M, et al. Longitudinal study of moderate weight change and sleep-disordered breathing. *JAMA.* 2000;284(23):3015-3021.

93. Olsson G, Wikstrand J, Warnold I, et al. Metoprolol-induced reduction in postinfarction mortality: Pooled results from five double-blind randomized trials. *Eur Heart J.* 1992;13(1):28-32.

94. Stoschitzky K, Sakotnik A, Lercher P, et al. Influence of beta-blockers on melatonin release. *Eur J Clin Pharmacol.* 1999;55(2):111-115.

95. Bauer A, Malik M, Schmidt G, et al. Heart rate turbulence: Standards of measurement, physiological interpretation, and clinical use: International Society for Holter and Noninvasive Electrophysiology Consensus. *J Am Coll Cardiol.* 2008;52:1353-1365.

Sleep, Chronic Pain, and Fatigue in Rheumatic Disorders

Chapter 47

CELESTE THIRLWELL / HARVEY MOLDOFSKY

Forty million people in the United States are impaired by rheumatic disorders, and by the year 2020 the number of patients affected by rheumatic disorders is projected to reach 59 million.[1] Pain, disordered sleep, and fatigue are among the common afflictions that affect people with rheumatic ailments.

The traditional model of medical practice holds that the rheumatic disorder itself is responsible for the pain and difficulties patients experience with sleep, psychological distress, and fatigue. By following this model, it is assumed that correct diagnosis and treatment of the rheumatologic disorder will cause the pain symptoms to improve, which in turn will cause sleep difficulties to improve, followed by decreased fatigue and improved overall well-being in the patient. This unidirectional approach does not hold because, even in the absence of objective evidence for active disease, patients with rheumatoid arthritis and systemic lupus erythematosus may complain of problems with pain, sleep, and fatigue.

There is mounting evidence, from human[2-4] and animal[2,5-7] experimental research studies, that there is a bidirectional relationship of disordered sleep to pain; thus the long-standing medical dictum of unidirectional diagnosis and treatment is no longer tenable.[2,8] These studies demonstrate that both disturbance of sleep and sleep restriction result in increased sensitivity to noxious stimuli and musculoskeletal pain symptoms. We suggest that not only is there a bidirectional relationship of disordered sleep to pain and fatigue but also other processes that impinge upon sleep and pain (i.e., immune function, systemic disturbances, and psychosocial distress) will impinge upon rheumatic ailments as well (Fig. 47-1).

This chapter will evaluate the nature of the interactions among rheumatologic disorders, chronic pain, fatigue, and sleep disturbances. Understanding and assessing these interrelated symptoms will aid the clinician in developing a comprehensive clinical assessment and management plan of rheumatologic patients.

GENERAL CLINICAL PRINCIPLES

The traditional history, physical examination, and specific laboratory tests remain invaluable in directing the physician to the diagnosis of the rheumatologic disorder and any co-morbid processes. Standardized screening inventories for sleep disorders, chronic fatigue and pain, and psychological functioning are invaluable. Adequate patient education and follow-up are needed to enhance treatment compliance.

Tiredness

Patients with rheumatic ailments will often report being tired. It is important to clarify what is meant by "tiredness." As previously outlined by Moldofsky,[9] tiredness can be classified into the categories of: cognitive fatigue, physical fatigue, or sleepiness. Patients with *cognitive fatigue* can present with problems with thinking, concentration, and memory. Multitasking becomes difficult and there may be a slowing in response times. *Physical fatigue* can present as overall physical exhaustion or reduced energy. Patients with *sleepiness* will describe an inability to remain alert or an inability to resist falling asleep. Sleepiness may occur in passive situations such as watching television, reading, or listening to a lecture. Sleepiness may also occur in active situations, such as being at work or driving a car.

Although sleepiness may be the result of insufficient sleep, daytime sleepiness may be the result of an unrecognized primary sleep disorder, such as obstructive sleep apnea, narcolepsy, or restless legs syndrome (RLS). The evaluation of *microsleep* has been developed to help assess subjective sleepiness.[10-14] Microsleep is an episode of sleep that may last from 3 to 30 seconds.[12,13] Clinical manifestations of microsleep include head nods, drooping eyelids, and lapses in focus and attention.[12,13] Microsleep episodes can become extremely dangerous in the context of activities that require continuous focused attention, such a driving or operating heavy machinery.[14]

Self-rating scales can be used to augment the clinical interview and can serve as standardized tools used to identify, differentiate, and track symptoms of tiredness (Box 47-1).[15-20]

Nonrestorative Sleep

Of special relevance in the rheumatologic patient is the concept of nonrestorative sleep. Quantity of sleep is not necessarily commensurate with quality of sleep. A brief nap can often leave a patient feeling refreshed and an 8-hour sleep, that is seemingly uninterrupted, can leave a patient feeling unrefreshed. Rheumatic patients who endorse unrefreshing or nonrestorative sleep, with or without pain, require polysomnographic (PSG) assessment for unrecognized primary sleep disorders, including the presence of *cyclic alternating pattern (CAP)* and *alpha electroencephalography (EEG) pattern*. CAP is a measure of sleep stability in non–rapid eye movement (NREM) sleep and is characterized by periodic episodes of aroused EEG activity followed by a period of more quiet sleep.[21,22] A high CAP rate has been found to correlate to severity of symptoms in fibro-myalgia syndrome (FMS).[23] The alpha EEG sleep pattern is often associated with light and unrefreshing sleep.[24] Three types of alpha EEG sleep patterns have been identified using detailed sleep EEG frequency analysis: tonic alpha EEG sleep (Fig. 47-2),[25] phasic alpha EEG sleep (Fig. 47-3),[26] and periodic K-alpha EEG sleep (Fig. 47-4).[27] Alpha EEG sleep patterns have been reported to occur in some patients with poor sleep quality in other rheumatic disorders including rheumatoid arthritis,[28-30] Sjögren's syndrome,[31] and systemic lupus erythematosus.[32,33]

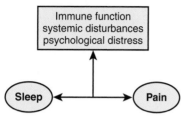

Figure 47-1 Bidirectional relationship of disordered sleep to pain and factors that impinge on this relationship in patients with rheumatic disorders.[8]

BOX 47-1 *Clinical Self-Rating Scales for the Assessment of Tiredness[15-20]*

FATIGUE
- Multidimentional Fatigue Inventory
- Fatigue Scale
- Fatigue Severity Scale

SLEEPINESS
- Stanford Sleepiness Scale
- Epworth Sleepiness Scale

Polysomnography

Other chapters in this volume will review the standard sleep assessment and treatment, including daily sleep diary, used in the evaluation of sleep hygiene; identification of substances or drugs that adversely affect sleep; qualitative and quantitative self-rating scales of sleep; and PSG studies used to identify sleep disorders.

Overnight polysomnography can be used in patients with rheumatologic disorders to diagnose suspected primary sleep disorders, identify any secondary sleep disorders, and provide objective evidence for nonrestorative sleep.

The multiple sleep latency test (MSLT) is a physiologic measure of sleepiness and can be used to identify co-morbid primary sleep disorders in rheumatologic patients such as narcolepsy[34,35] and hypersomnolence.[36] MSLT can also be used to identify episodes of microsleep and differentiate between the various forms of tiredness. Patients with cognitive or physical fatigue may not have a rapid onset of sleep during daytime naps. MSLT should follow overnight PSG to ensure the patient has not restricted his or her sleep.

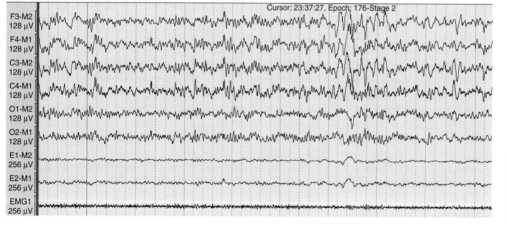

Figure 47-2 A 30-second epoch showing tonic alpha electroencephalography (EEG) using a standard bilateral 6 lead, frontal, central, and occipital EEG.

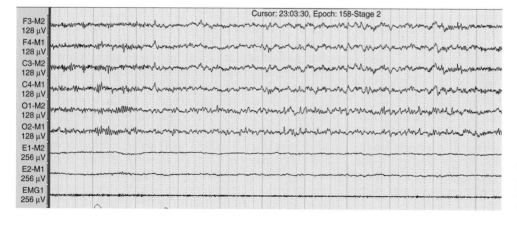

Figure 47-3 A 30-second epoch showing phasic alpha electroencephalography (EEG) using a standard bilateral 6 lead, frontal, central, and occipital EEG.

SPECIAL CONSIDERATIONS IN THE ASSESSMENT AND MANAGEMENT OF PATIENTS WITH RHEUMATOLOGIC DISORDERS

When assessing and managing patients with rheumatic disorders, certain special factors should be considered. Of particular relevance are the influence of sleep/wake-related immune functions on rheumatic disease; the influence of sleep disturbance on underlying co-morbid systemic disturbances; and the influence of psychosocial function in rheumatic patients.

Sleep/Wake-Related Immune Functions and Their Influence on Rheumatic Disease

Cytokines and immune functions directly affect the central nervous system (CNS) and are inextricably linked to the homeostatic regulation of sleep/waking brain and behavior.[37,38] For example, tumor necrosis factor-alpha (TNF-α) and interleukin 1β (IL-1β) modulate sleep/wake activity and are involved in a broad range of other biologic activities.[38] As well, systemic proinflammatory cytokine activity can clinically manifest as subjective symptoms of fatigue,[39] pain, and depression.[40] Traditionally, these subjective symptoms have been ignored by the rheumatologic literature, which has focused mainly on laboratory disease indices, joint pathology and function, and the adverse effects of disturbed cytokine-immune function on inflammatory rheumatic disorders.

Recently, rheumatologists acknowledge the relevance of assessing fatigue and disordered sleep. After examining outcome measures for assessing rheumatoid arthritis (RA) response to treatment, a combined committee of the European League Against Rheumatism (EULAR) and American College of Rheumatology (ACR) has recently released a consensus report recommending the study of disordered sleep and fatigue.[41]

The broadening of focus in rheumatic disorder management has been prompted by findings from studies involving disease-modifying antirheumatic drugs (DMARDs) in the management of patients with RA. Preliminary studies have shown the beneficial response of DMARDs on energy, sleep, and pain.[42-45] Long term outcome assessment of the response to treatment with the anti-TNF DMARD adalimumab demonstrates a clinically significant reduction in fatigue.[46] Immediate improvement in overnight sleep physiology and daytime alertness without any immediate changes in objective measures of disease activity were found in patients with RA receiving their first infusion of infliximab, a drug that neutralizes TNF-α.[47]

Sleep/Wake-Related Systemic Disturbances and Their Influence on Rheumatic Disorders

Commonly, patients with rheumatologic disorders develop other medical diseases that may impact on sleep/wake function and behavior. Limitation of mobility and decreased physical activity due to pain, sleep difficulty, and fatigue result in rheumatologic patients leading a sedentary life, predisposing them to become obese, possibly aggravating rheumatologic symptoms, such as osteoarthritis of the hips and knees. In rheumatologic patients with obesity, obstructive sleep apnea (OSA) may become an additional health burden. Co-morbidities associated with OSA include cardiovascular (e.g., nocturnal dysrhythmias, hypertension, congestive heart failure, myocardial infarction, and stroke) and metabolic (e.g., leptin resistance, insulin resistance, and obesity) complications.[48] Patients with systemic lupus erythematosus, who go on to develop end-stage renal disease may be predisposed to OSA, RLS, and sleep-related periodic limb movement disorder (PLMD).[32,33]

Psychosocial Distress in Rheumatic Patients with Disordered Sleep, Fatigue, and Pain

Inadequate sleep has a cumulative negative effect on mood, pain, and overall stress burden in patients with rheumatologic disorders. Patients may describe increased irritability and mood lability (i.e., "mood swings").[49] Sleep duration and sleep quality in 89 women with FMS are shown to be prospectively related to psychologic distress and fatigue.[50] A 1-year prospective study, using statistical path analysis techniques, demonstrated that 491 patients with FMS who complained of sleep problems were more likely to have increased pain symptoms on 1-year follow-up. Furthermore, increased pain predicted poorer physical functioning, which in turn predicted increased symptoms of depression.[51]

Depressive symptoms are seen in patients with rheumatic disorders. In RA patients, studies suggest that disturbed sleep may contribute to depression independent of pain and functional impairment.[52,53] Anxiety symptoms can also affect patients with rheumatologic disorders. In addition to difficulty with sleep and fatigue, patients with Sjögren's syndrome commonly have co-morbid anxiety and depression.

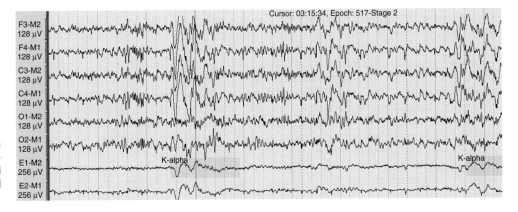

Figure 47-4 A 30-second epoch showing periodic K-alpha electroencephalography (EEG) using a standard bilateral 6 lead, frontal, central, and occipital EEG.

In a survey comparing 62 primary Sjögren's syndrome patients with healthy control subjects, 48% and 32% of patients had significantly higher scores for clinical anxiety and clinical depression, respectively.[54]

Maladaptive personality factors have been found to be associated with rheumatic disorders.[55,56] A patient's response to illness and ability to cope with stress can adversely be affected by the presence of a personality disorder.[57] In these patients it is possible that intrusive cognitions, such as maladaptive thought patterns and hypervigilance, may play a part in their sleep disturbance.[57]

Environmental and sociocultural variables must also be considered, as they can influence a patient's pain behavior, stress management, and treatment compliance (Box 47-2).[49,58,59] *Behavioral activation* and *motivational interviewing* are two evidence-based approaches that take into account a patient's subjective psychosocial experience and have been shown to improve outcomes in patients with psychologic distress.[60,61] Behavioral activation targets maladaptive depressive and avoidance behaviors, by scheduling activities and using graded task assignments to counteract inertia seen in patients with depression. By positively reinforcing the activities and tasks, patients become behaviorally activated and begin to engage in behaviors that are more adaptive and that promote health. Motivational interviewing is a nonjudgmental, nonconfrontational approach that attempts to increase a patient's awareness of problems caused by his or her behaviors. The aim of the therapy is to help patients think differently about their maladaptive behaviors and to consider what might be gained through changing to other behaviors that will positively influence their psychologic and physical health.

Operant conditioning and *cognitive behavioral therapy* have been shown to be of benefit with psychologic and environmental stressors in patients with FMS.[62-64] Operant conditioning involves effecting behavioral change by using positive reinforcement to cause adaptive behaviors to occur more frequently; negative reinforcement to cause maladaptive behaviors to occur less frequently; and extinction to reduce unwanted behaviors. In cognitive behavioral therapy, patients are taught to break down their reaction to stressors into three components: emotions, thoughts, and behaviors. They are taught to examine the interaction between these three components and learn new skills for solving their stress-related problems. *Mindfulness-based stress reduction (MBSR)* is an evidence-based approach that has shown to be effective in patients with chronic pain.[65-67] MBSR is an acceptance-based

approach that uses breathing exercises and meditation techniques to help patients cultivate moment-to-moment, nonjudgmental awareness of the events and experiences in their lives. This approach has also been successfully modified as treatment for mild to moderate depression and anxiety.[68,69] Further research needs to be conducted to evaluate whether MBSR has a direct treatment effect on disordered sleep.

A detailed explanation of the treatment pertaining to mood disorders, anxiety disorders, and personality disorders is beyond the scope of this chapter. However, the general principle of using treatments that do not further destabilize sleep or worsen sleep disorders is an important consideration. As well, appropriate chronotherapy should be followed.

CLINICAL FEATURES IN SPECIFIC RHEUMATOLOGIC DISORDERS

Inflammatory Arthritis

Inflammatory arthritis encompasses a wide spectrum of rheumatic diseases occurring mainly in the middle years of life. The hallmark of inflammatory joint disease is thickened synovium infiltrated with inflammatory cells lining the joint cavity. Activated cells release inflammatory cytokines that result in pain and tissue destruction. Some important proinflammatory cytokines are TNF-α and interleukin 1 (IL-1). There is currently no cure for inflammatory arthritis.[70] Although acute pain control is important, long-term disease control is the main objective.

RA is a systemic autoimmune disease characterized by inflammation most often in the hands and feet, resulting in pain, stiffness, swelling, deformity, and loss of function in the joints.[71] Approximately, 54% to 70% of adult RA patients endorse sleep problems and related daytime symptoms including: unrefreshing sleep, fatigue, headache, and sleepiness.[72-75] Subjective disturbed sleep in RA has been linked to pain, mood, and disease activity.[52-74]

Cervical spine disease may be seen in RA. The atlantoaxial joint refers to the articulation between C1, the atlas, and C2, the axis. Atlantoaxial joint subluxation is a complication seen in RA, anterior subluxations being the most common. As well, there may be atlantoaxial joint instability due to erosion of the odontoid process of C2 or of C1. With flexion, the atlantoaxial space should not increase significantly and any space larger than 2.5 or 3 mm is considered abnormal. In addition, there can be tenosynovitis of the transverse ligament of C1 and cervical myopathy due to erosion of the odontoid process and ligament laxity or rupture.[76-79] These abnormal atlantoaxial features may cause the cervical vertebrae to press against the upper airway, causing a narrowing of the lumen, and thus increasing the risk for restriction in airflow through the upper airway in sleep with consequent sleep apnea disorder. Case reports and small studies have identified OSA in fatigued individuals with RA.[29,74,80,81] In one small study, sleep-disordered breathing occurred frequently in nonobese patients with acquired retrognathia secondary to RA[82] (Box 47-3).

PSG in RA often reveals evidence of alpha EEG pattern and has been associated with the severity of morning joint pain and stiffness.[28,29] RLS and PLMD with arousals are also frequently seen in RA.[29,74,83]

BOX 47-3 *Risk Factors for Sleep-Disordered Breathing in Rheumatoid Arthritis[76-79] and Ankylosing Spondylitis[91-94]*

RHEUMATOID ARTHRITIS
- Retrognathia secondary to temporomandibular joint destruction
- Cervical spine disease leading to narrowing of upper airway
- Cervicle spine disease causing compression of the respiratory centers in the brainstem
- Atrophy of pharyngeal muscles due to steroid medication
- Weight gain

ANKYLOSING SPONDYLITIS
- Cervical ankylosis
- Limited chest expansion resulting in respiratory restriction
- Weight gain

BOX 47-4 *Medical Management of Osteoarthritis[95-98,161,162]*

- Anti-inflammatory drugs improve quality of sleep and relieve morning stiffness.
- Opiate pain medications can relieve hip and knee osteoarthritic pain; however, caution is required because of the respiratory depressant effect of opiates during sleep.
- Joint replacement surgery may relieve night pain and improve sleep and quality of life.
- Treatment of co-morbid primary sleep disorder (e.g., OSA, RLS, PLMD) also is indicated.

OSA, obstructive sleep apnea; *PLMD*, periodic limb movement disorder; *RLS*, restless legs syndrome.

Juvenile rheumatoid arthritis (JRA) is the most common type of arthritis that affects children. The few studies that have investigated sleep in children with JRA have shown evidence of sleep fragmentation, parasomnias, sleep-disordered breathing, daytime sleepiness, mood disturbances, and anxiety.[84-87] In children with JRA, a high CAP rate during NREM sleep has been noted to occur.[85]

As with RA, children with JRA are at potential risk for sleep apnea. A study of 85 children with JRA showed a 67% chance for retrognathia and a 52% chance for posterior rotation of the mandible, regardless of their temporal mandibular joint status.[86] Additional research is needed to determine the prevalence of sleep apnea and efficacy of response to DMARDs as to the impact on sleep apnea syndrome.

Ankylosing spondylitis is a chronic inflammatory disorder of the axial skeleton affecting the sacroiliac (SI) joint and the spine. The hallmark is bilateral sacroiliitis. The onset is in late adolescent and early adulthood. It has an insidious onset with back pain and tenderness in the bilateral SI joints and there is lumbar morning stiffness that improves with exercise. Ankylosing spondylitis has been associated with initial insomnia, unrefreshing sleep, morning stiffness, and fatigue.[88-90] The pathophysiology of the disease may predispose these patients to developing sleep-disordered breathing (see Box 47-3).[91-94]

Noninflammatory Disease

Osteoarthritis (OA) is a progressive disorder of the joints leading to deterioration of the articular cartilage and new bone formation at the joint surfaces and margins. OA is the most common arthritic disease affecting the older population and there is an increased incidence in occupations with repetitive trauma.[95] In obesity, OA of the knee is most common.[95] Clinical signs include dull aching pain, increased with activity and relieved by rest. However, as the disease progresses, pain occurs at rest as well. Joint stiffness upon awakening in the morning and after periods of inactivity during the day is common. Clinical symptoms include monoarticular involvement with no obvious joint pattern.

In the variant form of primary OA, *diffuse idiopathic skeletal hyperostosis (DISH)*, there is ossification of the anterior longitudinal ligament, which produces large osteophytes that extend to the length of the spine, leading to spinal fusion. The hallmark is ossification spanning three or more intervertebral disks. It is a multisystem disorder, associated with: diabetes mellitus, obesity, systemic hypertension, and coronary artery disease. There is stiffness in the morning and evening and dysphasia with cervical involvement. All of these systemic disturbances may be further adversely affected by sleep-disordered breathing and other underlying primary sleep disorders.[48,96]

Pain in OA is associated with light and restless sleep.[8,97,98] This poor-quality sleep has been shown to decrease pain thresholds and thus aggravate pain.[8,97] The prevalence of sleep apnea in OA is unknown, but both are common conditions in obese individuals and thus considerable overlap can be expected.[48]

Because disordered sleep is known to promote pain, the presence of a primary sleep disorder should be considered in the assessment and management of people with OA who complain of generalized musculoskeletal pain and morning stiffness (Box 47-4).

Connective Tissue Disease

Systemic lupus erythematosus (SLE) is a multisystemic autoimmune disease in which autoantibodies are directed against nuclear antigens. Its multiple clinical manifestations include rash, fever, thrombocytopenia, leukopenia, arthritis, nephritis, and neuropsychiatric disease.

Both fatigue and excessive daytime sleepiness have been reported in the literature.[33,99] Many studies rely only on subjective, self-report questionnaires and are not adequately designed to differentiate between fatigue and sleepiness. One study that was designed using a subjective measure (i.e., Epworth Sleepiness Scale score) and an objective measure (i.e., MSLT) found sleepiness in 51% of "fatigued" SLE test subjects. Their sleepiness could not be attributed to sleep restriction or to any primary sleep disorder other than narcolepsy.[33]

Fibromyalgia is a common co-morbidity in SLE.[100] As in RA and FMS, alpha EEG pattern is common in individuals with SLE.[32,33] Other primary sleep disorders that may occur in those with SLE are OSA and PLMD.[32,33]

Scleroderma is a progressive, chronic multisystem disease in which there are fibrosis-like changes in the skin and epithelial tissues of affected organs. Diffuse cutaneous scleroderma can affect the heart, lungs, gastrointestinal tract, and kidneys. Patients with scleroderma may suffer from dyspnea secondary to pulmonary fibrosis, gastroesophageal reflux, and

RLS, which may adversely affect sleep.[101] Primary sleep disorders associated with scleroderma include RLS and PLMD.[101] Exercise programs, which include maintaining range of motion and strengthening exercises, have been shown to be effective in improving well-being.[102]

Other Rheumatic Disorders

Behçet's disease involves vasculitis of small vessels, which commonly results in cutaneous lesions, ocular lesions, and aphthous ulcers of the genitalia and oral mucosa. In patient with Behçet's disease, fatigue is reported to be more common than insomnia, however, systematic PSG studies are lacking.[103] Case studies have shown an association of Behçet's disease with OSA, central sleep apnea, dyschronosis, and palatal myoclonus.[103-105]

Sjögren's syndrome (SS) is an autoimmune disorder characterized by autoantibodies targeting the exocrine glands that produce tears and saliva. Primary SS exists in the absence of another rheumatic disease. It is not uncommon for secondary SS to develop years after the onset of an associated rheumatic disorder such as RA, SLE, scleroderma, polymyositis, or dermatomyositis. Manifestations of SS include cutaneous vasculitis, sinusitis, ocular and oral dryness, and gastroesophageal reflux. It may affect other organs systems including kidneys, blood vessels, lungs, liver, pancreas, and peripheral nervous system and the brain.

In SS patients, sleep may be disturbed by pain, shortness of breath, sweating, restless legs symptoms, and PLMD.[31,106] These patients also suffer from difficulties with excessive daytime sleepiness, fatigue, depression, and anxiety.[31,54] An association with FMS and alpha EEG pattern has been reported.[31]

Sarcoidosis is a systemic, chronic granulomatous disease that can affect any organ system, characterized by abnormal collections of large numbers of activated macrophages and T lymphocytes. Clinical features include pulmonary infiltrates, bilateral hilar lymphadenopathy, fever, weight loss, fatigue, polyarthritis, and erythema nodosum. Pulmonary function tests are abnormal with either an obstructive or a restrictive pattern.

Sarcoidosis may be associated with complaints of excessive daytime sleepiness, fatigue, insomnia, and personality disturbances.[107] PSG studies show increased sleep fragmentation, sleep apnea, restless legs, and periodic leg movements of sleep.[108,109] Involvement of the tongue, tonsils, upper airway, and larynx can result in sleep apnea. In one case study, secondary narcolepsy due to neurosarcoidosis involving the diencephalon was reported and was successfully treated with irradiation of the brain.[107]

Nonarticular Rheumatism

Fibromyalgia syndrome (FMS) is characterized by chronic diffuse musculoskeletal pain and tenderness, physical discomfort, and fatigue. Patients with FMS may experience morning stiffness. There is no evidence of a pathologic process of the soft tissues. FMS pain symptoms reflect an overall reduced pain threshold.[110] In addition to the complaint of pain, patients may have a sleep disturbance, cognitive impairment, and hypersensitivity to outside stimuli such as sound, light, and odors.[110,111] There is an association with depression, panic disorder, generalized anxiety disorder, and post-traumatic stress

disorder (PTSD).[62-64,112-115] FMS often coexists with other rheumatologic disorders such as RA and SLE.[32,33,116,117] The presence of FMS has also been reported in hepatitis C infection, Lyme disease, endocrine disorder, and myxedema.[118-120]

Depending on the type of specialist seen by patients, not uncommonly patients with FMS may be labeled with diagnoses of other *central sensitivity syndromes (CSS)*, such as chronic fatigue syndrome, irritable bowel syndrome, chronic pelvic pain syndrome, temporomandibular joint pain, tension-type headaches, PTSD, multiple chemical sensitivities, and interstitial cystitis.[121] Bested and associates[122] published a book outlining therapeutic approaches to chronic fatigue syndrome and FMS. The treatment strategies include sleep hygiene, pacing and energy conservation, nutritional support, dietary supplements and herbs, complementary and pharmaceutical treatments, and legal support.

Research has shown that disturbances in the sleeping/waking brain play a role in the pathogenesis of FMS.[123-126] The studies support the hypothesis that disordered sleep may provoke the reduction of the normal physiologic inhibition to perception of noxious stimuli and thus result in central nervous system hypersensitivity or CSS.[110,121] Pain thresholds are shown to be reversibly reduced in subjects who have undergone 40 hours of sleep deprivation. Pain thresholds return to baseline after a slow wave sleep recovery period.[127] Noise used to disturb slow wave sleep in an experiment with healthy subjects artificially induces both musculoskeletal pain and fatigue.[128] Another study has shown that during partial sleep deprivation, young healthy women have a reduced ability to inhibit pain.[4]

The concept of FMS was characterized in 1975 by Moldofsky and associates[25] and subsequently modified in 1990 by Wolfe and associates,[129] where the prime criteria became chronic widespread body pain and the presence of tender points. Recently, researchers acknowledge that diagnosis of FMS rests on more than just body pain and merely testing for tender points.[58,62-64,110-115] These criteria do not adequately measure symptom severity or the effectiveness of new treatments.[130,131] Consequently, Wolfe and associates[132] have proposed a new set of diagnostic criteria, which would replace the tender point examination with a *widespread pain index (WPI)* and *symptom severity scale (SSS)*. Tender point testing would be replaced by identifying body areas in which the patient has experienced pain. In addition to *pain areas*, the new criteria would also include *fatigue, waking unrefreshed, cognitive symptoms, and somatic symptoms*. The WPI ranges from 0 to 19 and evaluates 19 possible body areas a patient has had pain over the last week. Body areas include the right and left shoulder girdles, right and left upper and lower arms, right and left hips, right and left upper and lower legs, right and left jaw, chest, abdomen, upper and lower back, and neck. A score of 1 is given for each body area in which pain has occurred. The SSS score is divided into two subsections. First, fatigue, waking unrefreshed, and cognitive symptoms are individually rated on a scale of 0 to 3, giving a possible subsection score ranging from 0 to 9. A score of 0 indicates no problem, a score of 1 indicates slight or mild problems, a score of 2 indicates moderate or considerable problems, and 3 indicates severe or life-disturbing problems. Second, the severity of generalized somatic symptoms is rated from 0 to 3. The list of possible somatic symptoms is extensive and ranges from dizziness, numbness, nausea, and irritable bowel syndrome to depression. A score of 0 indicates no somatic symptoms, a score of 1 indicates few somatic symptoms, a score of 2 indicates moderate somatic symptoms, and a score of 3 indicates a great deal of somatic symptoms. The two subsections of the SSS score are then added together to give a final score ranging from 0 to 12. For a patient to be diagnosed with FMS, he or she would have to have either a WPI of 7 or more *and* SSS of 5 or more *or* WPI 3 to 6 *and* SSS 9 or more, his or her symptoms would have been present for at least 3 months, and there would be an absence of any primary disorder that would otherwise explain the pain.

Nonrestorative sleep is common in FMS.[2,8,25,133] Patients with FMS may have co-morbid RLS and PLMD in sleep.[133,134] Moderate to severe sleep apnea has been shown to occur in a large-scale multicenter study.[135] Sleep instability, with frequent CAP and alpha EEG pattern, may be seen in patients with FMS.[24,136-139]

Other polysomnographic features of sleep disruption in patients diagnosed with FMS include: prolonged sleep latencies, decreased sleep efficiency, reduced sleep EEG spindles, reduced slow wave sleep, and rapid eye movement (REM) sleep.[136,137] There is also evidence of increased generalized restlessness and motor activity while sleeping.[136,140,141]

Some specific treatments have been shown to benefit some patients. Milnacipran, duloxetine, and pregabalin have been approved by the Food and Drug Administration (FDA) for treatment of FMS, but their effects on the sleep physiology in patients with FMS have not been systematically studied[114,115,142,143] (Table 47-1). Sodium oxybate has been found to reduce alpha sleep, increase delta sleep, improve fatigue symptoms, and decrease pain in patients with FMS.[144,145] These findings have been further substantiated by a recent double-blind, randomized, placebo-controlled study in which sodium oxybate was shown to be effective in improving sleep-related FMS symptoms and EEG sleep physiology.[135]

Current approaches to management are based on a biopsychosocial model of disease and combine both pharmacologic and nonpharmacologic approaches.[58,62-64,110,114,115,130] Nonpharmacologic approaches include cognitive, behavioral, and physical methods.[115,133] Complementary and alternative medicine approaches have also been used, but there

TABLE 47-1

FDA-Approved Medications for Treating Fibromyalgia[114,115,142,143]

Medication	Dose	Side Effects	Potential Complications
Milnacipran	*Starting dose*: 12.5 mg once daily *Days 2-3*: 12.5 bid *Days 4-7*: 25 mg bid *Day 8*: 50 mg bid *Maintenance dose*: 50 mg bid *Maximum dose*: 100 mg bid	*Gastrointestinal*: nausea, constipation, vomiting, dry mouth, abdominal pain, decreased appetite *Neurologic*: headache, dizziness, migraine, paresthesia, tremor, neuroleptic malignant syndrome, serotonin syndrome, parkinsonism *Cardiovascular*: hot flush, palpitations, tachycardia, hypertension; supraventricular tachycardia, hypertensive crisis *Dermatologic*: hyperhidrosis, rash, pruritus, night sweats, erythema multiforme, Stevens-Johnson syndrome *Genitourinary*: sexual dysfunction, prostatitis, urinary retention, cystitis, dysuria	• Caution in patients with renal impairment • Not recommended in patients with end-stage renal disease • Should be tapered and not abruptly discontinued after extended use
Duloxetine	*Starting dose*: 30 mg once daily for 1 week *Week 2*: 60 mg once daily *Maintenance dose*: 60 mg once daily	*Gastrointestinal*: nausea, constipation, vomiting, dry mouth, diarrhea, dyspepsia, gastritis *Neurologic*: somnolence, dizziness, headache, tremor, paraesthesia, dysgeusia, restless legs syndrome, seizures, reduction of REM sleep, increased REM sleep onset latency *Respiratory*: nasopharyngitis, cough, pharyngolaryngeal pain *Cardiovascular*: increase in blood pressure, increase in heart rate, palpitations, peripheral edema, phlebitis *Dermatologic*: hyperhidrosis, pruritus, night sweats, acne, alopecia, photosensitivity reaction *Genitourinary*: sexual dysfunction, pollakiuria, polyuria, dysuria, urinary retention	• Not recommended in patients with severe renal impairment and end-stage renal disease • Risk of elevation of serum transaminase • Reported seizures and tinnitus upon treatment discontinuation
Pregabalin	*Starting dose*: 75 mg bid for 1 week *Week 2*: 150 mg bid *Maintenance dose*: 300-450 mg/day *Maximum dose*: 225 mg bid	*Gastrointestinal*: nausea, constipation, dry mouth, increased appetite, vomiting, diarrhea, cholecystitis, cholelithiasis, *Neurologic*: dizziness, somnolence, ataxia, tremor, neuropathy, abnormal thinking, abnormal gait, myoclonus *Cardiovascular*: edema, thrombophlebitis, heart failure, hypotension, syncope, postural hypotension, depressed ST segment on ECG, ventricular fibrillation *Ocular*: reduced visual acuity, blurred vision, conjunctivitis, diplopia *Genitourinary*: sexual dysfunction, urinary incontinence *Dermatologic*: pruritus, alopecia, petechial rash, Stevens-Johnson syndrome	• Blurred vision resolved in a majority of cases with continued dosing • Risk of metabolic syndrome • Hypersensitivity side effects include skin redness, hives, rash, dyspnea, wheezing • Risk of arthralgia, leg cramps, myalgia, myasthenia

ECG, electrocardiogram; *REM*, rapid eye movement.

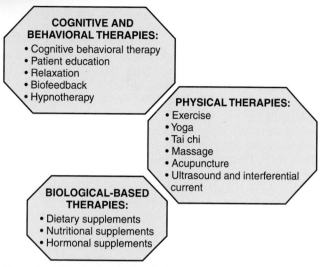

Figure 47-5 Nonpharmacologic methods that modulate symptoms of fibromyalgia syndrome: cognitive and behavioral therapies,[62-64,147-151] physical therapies,[146,150-157] and biologic therapies.[115,133,146]

is a lack of rigorous clinical trials for these modalities.[146] (Fig. 47-5)[62-64,115,133,146-157]

Patients with FMS are often exquisitely sensitive to pharmacologic agents.[110,114,115,133] Medications must be initiated at a fraction of the final dose and slowly increased to arrive at the lowest clinically effective dose with minimum adverse reactions. Triggers that may exacerbate FMS symptoms include strenuous physical activity, sleep disturbance, emotional stress, and a cold, damp, or humid environment.[110] Pain can be partially relieved by rest, warm baths, heat, and relaxation.[110] In patients with FMS, a graded, gentle aerobic fitness program during the part of the day in which the patient is experiencing the least pain and fatigue may improve sleep and symptoms of fibromyalgia.[150-152]

TREATMENT OF DISORDERED SLEEP IN PATIENTS WITH RHEUMATIC DISORDERS

For rheumatic patients with primary sleep disorders, such as narcolepsy, RLS, PLMD, or sleep apnea, the specific treatments for these sleep disorders that have been outlined in other chapters in this book should be instituted. Further systematic research needs to be conducted to evaluate the effects of treating these primary sleep disorders on the manifestations of the rheumatic disorders, fatigue, and chronic pain. There are generalized sleep management strategies and other more specific medication-based treatment approaches that are used in patients with rheumatic disorders.

Generalized Sleep Management

In patients with rheumatic disorders, there is often a dysregulation of sleep/wake, physiologic, and behavioral rhythms. Good sleep hygiene requires the elimination of daytime habits that adversely affect sleep. Stimulants, caffeine, nicotine, alcohol, or medications that destabilize sleep should be discontinued. Attention must also be paid to the sleep environment in order to minimize any environmental or psychologic stressors

that might interfere with sleep. Behaviors, disruptive thoughts, and worries that interfere with sleep can be addressed with cognitive behavioral therapy. In patients with chronic pain, cognitive behavioral therapy for insomnia, which addresses stress as well as maladaptive cognitive and behavioral patterns, has been shown to be effective.[115,158,159]

With respect to nighttime routine, faulty sleep habits such as variable bedtimes and restricted sleep times must be addressed. The sleep/wake cycle can be stabilized by following a routine of: regularly timed meals, daily aerobic exercise, and consistent sleep and wake times, and adequate duration of sleep.[160]

Heavy meals or vigorous exercise before bedtime can interfere with sleep. Specialized exercised programs geared to the abilities of the patient with rheumatic disease need to be developed by a physiotherapist. Where clinically indicated, an occupational therapist may be helpful to maximize mobility and home safety.

Specific Sleep Treatment Approaches

Specific treatment approaches should be individualized. When prescribing medication for the management in children, elderly, and medically ill patients with rheumatologic disorders, the general principle of starting pharmacologic agents at lower doses and titrating up slowly should be applied. This allows for finding the lowest effective tolerable dose and reduces the risk of adverse side effects. Iatrogenic toxicity and drug-drug interactions must also be monitored. The potential adverse effects on sleep of pain medication, over-the-counter sedatives, and herbal remedies needs to be considered. In particular, opioids should be used judiciously, as administration of high-potency opioids can cause central sleep apnea. Patients should be screened prior to the institution of opioid therapy for potentially hazardous sleep apnea disorder, which would be aggravated by opiates.[161,162]

As described above, DMARDs present a potential effective treatment for sleep disturbances in rheumatologic patients.[42,44,45] Pregabalin, duloxetine, and milnacipran have shown moderate effectiveness.[114,115,142,143] Sodium oxybate has been shown to improve sleep physiology and reduce pain and fatigue symptoms.[135,143-145]

Sedative-hypnotics, which include: barbiturates, chloral hydrate, benzodiazepines, and nonbenzodiazepine receptor agonists, do not have any long-term, specific benefit.[163,164] Barbiturates should not be used because they have a high risk of dependency and an increased risk of overdose.[163] Benzodiazepines decrease slow wave sleep as well as REM sleep and dependency may be a concern.[165] Intermittent use of nonbenzodiazepine benzodiazepine receptor agonists, such as zopiclone[166] and zolpidem,[167] can be of benefit for patients presenting with insomnia. These medications improve subjective sleep and daytime sleepiness but do not improve alpha EEG sleep or improve pain scores.[163,168]

Neuroleptics result in shortened sleep latency, increased sleep efficiency, decreased wake time after sleep onset, increased total sleep time, and decreased REM sleep.[168] In particular, chlorpromazine decreases pain scores, increases slow wave sleep, and reduces alpha EEG sleep. However, the long-term side effects, such as metabolic syndrome, potential development of tardive dyskinesia, and adverse extrapyramidal effects, have limited the clinical use of these drugs.[169]

Anticonvulsant agents such as gabapentin, pregabalin, and carbamazepine have antinociceptive properties and are sedating.[170] Their effects on sleep physiology have not been systematically studied.

Some antidepressants are sedating and improve sleep, but others can disrupt sleep and cause daytime fatigue and sleepiness.[168] Tricyclic antidepressants (TCAs), selective serotonin reuptake inhibitors (SSRIs), and serotonin-norepinephrine reuptake inhibitors (SNRIs) can precipitate or worsen PLMD, resulting in increased insomnia or daytime sleepiness.[171-173] Antidepressants from the SSRI class, such as fluoxetine, sertraline, and fluvoxamine, decrease REM sleep, increase REM latency, and fragment sleep.[171] One study showed that both amitriptyline and fluoxetine improve sleep in patients with FMS, and the combined effect is superior to either drug alone.[174] Further support for the potential benefit of using combination of medications requires study. Bupropion, a dopamine and norepinephrine reuptake inhibitor, decreases REM sleep latency, increases REM sleep, and has no effect on periodic leg movements in sleep.[175] Trazodone increases NREM stage N3 sleep, but does not alter sleep latency, sleep efficiency, or percentage wake time.[176] It also reduces alpha EEG sleep activity.[176] Mirtazapine, a serotonin and α_2-receptor blocker, promotes sleep by decreasing sleep latency, increasing sleep efficiency, and decreasing wake time after sleep onset with no significant changes in REM sleep.[171] Mirtazapine has been associated with an increased risk of RLS.[177] Amitriptyline and cyclobenzaprine, TCA agents, can have an initial beneficial effect on sleep, with amitriptyline having beneficial effects after 2 to 3 months.[178,179] However, neither of these medications reduces alpha EEG pattern.[180,181]

CONCLUSION

There is a need for well-designed studies that systematically evaluate the presence of sleep disorders and their treatment in a variety of rheumatologic disorders. As reviewed by Abad and associates,[182] there is a high prevalence of sleep disturbances in patients with rheumatic disorders. Unfortunately, researchers and clinicians outside the field of sleep medicine may not be aware of the bidirectional interaction between sleep and symptoms of patients with rheumatic disease. Furthermore, little attention is paid to other factors that impinge on sleep such as immune function, systemic disturbances, and psychosocial distress. This results in research design and clinical practice being based on the erroneous premise that rheumatologic disease unilaterally causes sleep problems, and there is a lack of attention paid to other associated factors.

Furthermore, there are inherent weaknesses in the brief self-rated questions about sleep used in large population surveys.[8] Often inquiries about sleep rely on overly simplified questions regarding sleep and lack the sensitivity and specificity to properly identify different types of disordered sleep. Papers continue to appear that do not investigate the potential adverse effects of a primary sleep disorder on the development and maintenance of a rheumatologic disorder. Without proper polysomnographic studies the actual prevalence of sleep disorders in specific rheumatologic patients cannot be ascertained. Patients are often unaware of the signs and symptoms of their primary sleep disorder. For example, patients who sleep alone might not be aware of snoring and patients are often unaware of their symptoms of RLS. As well, unrefreshing sleep, fatigue, and musculoskeletal symptoms may be masked by the features of the rheumatic disorder.

This highlights the importance of developing a research and clinical practice that employs validated behavioral and physiologic procedures (e.g., PSG and wrist actigraphy) in the determination of the specific nature of sleep/wake disturbance. Once identified, targeted treatment for the sleep disorder can be instituted and potential beneficial effects on the natural course of the rheumatologic disorder can be longitudinally evaluated.

Finally, further studies are needed to assess the efficacy of the combination of pharmacologic and nonpharmacologic strategies in the management of patients with rheumatic disorders, disordered sleep, chronic pain, and fatigue.

REFERENCES

1. National Institute of Arthritis and Musculoskeletal and Skin Diseases. National Institutes of Health, U.S. Department of Health and Human Services. Available at http://www.niams.nih.gov/.
2. Moldofsky H. The significance of the sleeping-waking brain for the understanding of widespread musculoskeletal pain and fatigue in fibromyalgia syndrome and allied syndromes. *J Joint Bone Spine.* 2008;7: 397-402.
3. Changani BS, Roehrs TA, Harris EJ, et al. Pain sensitivity in sleepy pain-free normals. *Sleep.* 2009;32:1011-1017.
4. Smith MT, Edwards RR, McCann UD, Haythornthwaite JA. The effects of sleep deprivation on pain inhibition and spontaneous pain in women. *Sleep.* 2007;30:494-505.
5. Silva A, Andersen ML, Tufik S. Sleep patterns in an experimental model of osteoarthritis. *Pain.* 2008;140:446-456.
6. Nascimento DC, Andersen ML, Hipolide JN, et al. Pain hypersensitivity induced by paradoxical sleep deprivation is not due to altered binding to the brain mu-opioid receptors. *Behav Brain Res.* 2007;178:216-220.
7. Wei H, Ma A, Wang YX, Pertovaara A. Role of spinal 5-HT receptors in cutaneous hypersensitivity induced by REM sleep deprivation. *Pharmacol Res.* 2008;57:469-475.
8. Moldofsky H. Rheumatic manifestations of sleep disorders. *Curr Opin Rheumatol.* 2010;22:59-63.
9. Moldofsky H. The contribution of sleep medicine to the assessment of the tired patient. *Can J Psychiatry.* 2000;45:798-802.
10. Tirunahari VL, Zaidi SA, Sharma R, et al. Microsleep and sleepiness: A comparison of multiple sleep latency test and scoring of microsleep as a diagnostic test for excessive daytime sleepiness. *Sleep Med.* 2003; 4:63-67.
11. Blaivas AJ, Patel R, Hom D, et al. Quantifying microsleep to help assess subjective sleepiness. *Sleep Med.* 2007;8:156-159.
12. Harrison Y, Horne JA. Occurrence of "microsleeps" during daytime sleep onset in normal subjects. *Electroencephalog Clin Neurophysiol.* 1996;98:411-416.
13. Vaughn BV, D'Cruz OF. Cardinal manifestations of sleep disorders. In: Kryger MH, Roth T, Dement WC, eds. *Principles and Practice of Sleep Medicine.* 4th ed. Philadelphia: Elsevier Saunders; 2005:594-601.
14. Drake C, Roehrs T, Breslau N, et al. The 10-year risk of verified motor vehicle crashes in relation to physiologic sleepiness. *Sleep.* 2010;33: 745-752.
15. Moldofsky H, MacFarlane JG. Fibromyalgia and chronic fatigue syndromes. In: Kryger MH, Roth T, Dement WC, eds. *Principles and Practice of Sleep Medicine.* 4th ed. Philadelphia: Elsevier Saunders; 2005:1225-1236.
16. Smets EM, Garseen B, Bonke B, et al. The Multidimensional Fatigue Inventory (MFI): Psychometric qualities of an instrument to assess fatigue. *J Psychosomat Res.* 1995;39:315-325.
17. Chalder T, Berelowitz G, Pawlikowska T, et al. Development of a fatigue scale. *J Psychosomat Med.* 1993;37:147-153.
18. Krupp LB, LaRocca NG, Muir-Nash J, et al. The fatigue severity scale: Application to patients with multiple sclerosis and systemic lupus erythematosus. *Arch Neurol.* 1989;46:1121-1123.
19. Hoddes E, Zarcone V, Smythe H, et al. Quantification of sleepiness: A new approach. *Psychophysiology.* 1973;10:431-436.
20. John MW. A new method for measuring daytime sleepiness: The Epworth Sleepiness Scale. *Sleep.* 1991;14:540-545.

21. Terzano MG, Parino L, Sherieri A, et al. Consensus report: Atlas, rules, and recording techniques for the scoring of cyclic alternating pattern (CAP) in human sleep. *Sleep Med.* 2002;3:187-199.

22. MacFarlane JG, Shahal B, Moldofsky H. Periodic K-alpha sleep EEG activity and periodic leg movements during sleep: Comparisons of clinical features and sleep parameters. *Sleep.* 1996;19:200-204.

23. Rizzi M, Sarzi-Puttini P, Atzeni F, et al. Cyclic alternating pattern: A new marker of sleep alteration in patients with fibromyalgia. *J Rheumatol.* 2004;31:1193-1199.

24. Benca R, Moldofsky H, Ancoli-Israel S. Special considerations in insomnia diagnosis and management: Depressed, elderly, and chronic pain populations. *J Clin Psychiatry.* 2004;65:26-35.

25. Moldofsky H, Scarisbrick P, England R, et al. Musculoskeletal symptoms and non-REM sleep disturbance in patients with "fibrositis syndrome" and healthy subjects. *Psychosomat Med.* 1975;37:341-351.

26. Anch AM, Lue FA, Maclean AW, et al. Sleep physiology and psychological aspects of the fibrositis (fibromyalgia) syndrome. *Can J Psychol.* 1991;45:178-184.

27. MacFarlane JG, Shahal B, Moldofsky H. Periodic K-alpha sleep EEG activity and periodic leg movements during sleep: Comparisons of clinical features and sleep parameters. *Sleep.* 1996;19:200-204.

28. Moldofsky H, Lue FA, Smythe HA. Alpha EEG sleep and morning symptoms in rheumatic arthritis. *J Rheumatol.* 1983;10:373-379.

29. Mahowald MW, Mahowald ML, Bundie SR, Ytterberg SR. Sleep fragmentation in rheumatoid arthritis. *Arthritis Rheum.* 1989;32:974-983.

30. Crosby LJ. Factors which contribute to fatigue associated with rheumatoid arthritis. *J Adv Nurs.* 1991;16:974-981.

31. Gudbjornsson B, Broman JE, Hetta J, Hallgren R. Sleep disturbances in patients with primary Sjogren's syndrome. *Br J Rheumatol.* 1993;32:1072-1076.

32. Valencia-Flores M, Resendiz M, Castano VA, et al. Objective and subjective sleep disturbances in patients with systemic lupus erythematosus. *Arthritis Rheum.* 1999;42:2189-2193.

33. Iaboni A, Gladman DD, Urowitz MB, Moldofsky H. Disordered sleep, sleepiness, and depression in chronically tired patients with systemic lupus erythematosus. *Sleep.* 2004;27:A327-A328.

34. Disdier P, Genton P, Harle JR, et al. Fibromyalgia and narcolepsy. *J Rheumatol.* 1993;20:888-889.

35. Disdier P, Genton P, Bolla G, et al. Clinical screening for narcolepsy/cataplexy in patients with fibromyalgia. *Clin Rheumatol.* 1994;13:132-134.

36. Sarzi-Puttini P, Rizzi M, Andreoli A, et al. Hypersomnolence in fibromyalgia syndrome. *Clin Exp Rheumatol.* 2002;20:69-72.

37. Moldofsky H, Dickstein J, Luk W- P. Sleep, health and immunocompetence. In: Berczi I, Gorczynski I, eds. *New Foundation of Biology (Neuroimmune Biology, vol. 1).* Amsterdam: Elsevier Science BV; 2001:255-268.

38. Kruger JM. The role of cytokines in sleep regulation. *Curr Pharm Des.* 2008;14:3408-3416.

39. Schafers M, Sommer C, Geis C, et al. Selective stimulation of either tumor necrosis factor receptor differentially induces pain behavior in vivo and ectopic activity in sensory neurons in vitro. *Neuroscience.* 2008;157:414-423.

40. Khairova RA, Machado-Vieira R, Du J, Manji HK. A potential role for pro-inflammatory cytokines in regulating synaptic plasticity in major depressive disorder. *Int J Neuropsychopharmacol.* 2009;12:561-578.

41. Aletaha D, Landewe R, Karonitsch T, et al. Reporting disease activity in clinical trials of patients with rheumatoid arthritis: EULAR/ARC collaborative recommendations. *Arthritis Rheum.* 2008;59:1371-1377.

42. Vgontzas AN, Zoumakis E, Lin HM, et al. Marked decrease in sleepiness in patients with sleep apnea by etanercept, a tumor necrosis factor-alpha antagonist. *J Clin Endocrinol Metab.* 2004;89:4409-4413.

43. Wolfe F, Michaud K, Li T. Sleep disturbance in patients with rheumatoid arthritis: Evaluation by medical outcomes study and visual analog sleep scales. *J Rheumatol.* 2006;33:1942-1951.

44. Genovese MC, Schiff M, Luggen M, et al. Efficacy and safety of the selective co-stimulation modulator abatacept following 2 years of treatment in patients with rheumatoid arthritis and an inadequate response to antitumour necrosis factor therapy. *Ann Rheum Dis.* 2008;67:547-554.

45. Wells G, Li T, Maxwell L, et al. Responsiveness of patient record outcomes including fatigue, sleep quality, activity limitation, and quality of life following treatment with abatacept for rheumatoid arthritis. *Ann Rheum Dis.* 2008;67:260-265.

46. Yount S, Sorensen MV, Cella D, et al. Adalimumab plus methotrexate or standard therapy is more effective than methotrexate or standard therapies alone in the treatment of fatigue in patients with active, inadequately treated rheumatoid arthritis. *Clin Exp Rheumatol.* 2007;25:838-846.

47. Zamarron C, Maceiras F, Mera A, Gomez-Reino JJ. Effect of the first infliximab infusion on sleep and alertness in patients with active rheumatoid arthritis. *Ann Rheum Dis.* 2004;63:88-90.

48. Iaboni A, Moldofsky H. Sleep and medical disorders. In: Smith HR, Comella CL, Hogl B, eds. *Sleep Medicine (Cambridge Clinical Guides).* Cambridge, United Kingdom: Cambridge University Press; 2008:186-207.

49. Winfield JB. Psychological determinants of fibromyalgia and related syndromes. *Curr Rev Pain.* 2000;4:276-286.

50. Hamilton NA, Affleck G, Tennen H, et al. Fibromyalgia: The role of sleep in affect and in negative event reactivity and recovery. *Health Psychol.* 2008;27:490-497.

51. Bigatti SM, Hernandez AM, Cronan TA, Rand KL. Sleep disturbances in fibromyalgia syndrome: Relationship to pain and depression. *Arthritis Care Res.* 2008;59:951-967.

52. Nicassio PM, Wallston KA. Longitudinal relationships among pain, sleep problems, and depression in rheumatoid arthritis. *J Abnorm Psychol.* 1992;101:514-520.

53. Cakirbay H, Bilici M, Kavakci O, et al. Sleep quality and immune functions in rheumatoid arthritis patients with and without major depression. *Int J Neurosci.* 2004;114:245-256.

54. Valtysdottir ST, Gudbjornsson Lindqvist U, et al. Anxiety and depression in patients with primary Sjogren's syndrome. *J Rheumatol.* 2000;27:165-169.

55. Cobb S. Contained hostility in rheumatoid arthritis. *Arthritis Rheum.* 1959;2:419-425.

56. Moos RH. Personality factors associated with rheumatoid arthritis: A review. *J Chron Dis.* 1964;17:41-55.

57. Leigh TJ. Sleep in rheumatic patients. *Scand J Rheumatol.* 1990;19:5-9.

58. Van Houdenhove B, Egle UT. Fibromyalgia: A stress disorder? Piecing the biopsychosocial puzzle together. *Psychother Psychosom.* 2004;73:267-275.

59. Turk DC, Monarch ES, Williams AD. Psychological evaluation of patients diagnosed with fibromyalgia syndrome: A comprehensive approach. *Rheum Dis Clin North Am.* 2002;28:219-233.

60. Hopko DR, Lejuez CW, Ruggiero KJ, et al. Contemporary behavioral activation treatments for depression: Procedures, principles, and progress. *Clin Psychol Rev.* 2003;23:699-717.

61. Lundahl B, Burke BL. The effectiveness and applicability of motivational interviewing: A practice-friendly review of four meta-analyses. *J Clin Psychol.* 2009;65:1233-1245.

62. Thieme K, Flor H, Turk DC. Psychological pain treatment in fibromyalgia syndrome: Efficacy of operant behavioural and cognitive behavioural treatments. *Arthritis Res Ther.* 2006;8:R121.

63. Thieme K, Turk DC, Flor H. Comorbid depression and anxiety in fibromyalgia syndrome: Relationship to somatic and psychosocial variables. *Psychosom Med.* 2004;66:837-844.

64. Turk DC, Monarch ES, Williams AD. Psychological evaluation of patients diagnosed with fibromyalgia syndrome: A comprehensive approach. *Rheum Dis Clin North Am.* 2002;28:219-233.

65. Carlson LE, Garland SN. Impact of mindfulness-based stress reduction (MBSR) on sleep, mood, stress and fatigue symptoms in cancer outpatients. *Int J Behav Med.* 2005;12:278-285.

66. Rosenweig S, Greeson JM, Reibel DK, et al. Mindfulness-based stress reduction for chronic pain conditions: Variation in treatment outcomes and role of home medication practice. *J Psychosom Res.* 2010;68:29-36.

67. Lush E, Salmon P, Floyd A, et al. Mindfulness meditation for symptom reduction in fibromyalgia: Psychophysiological correlates. *J Clin Psychol Med Settings.* 2009;16:200-207.

68. Tacon AM, McComb J, Caldera Y, et al. Mindfulness meditation, anxiety reduction, and heart disease: A pilot study. *Fam Commun Health.* 2003;26:25-33.

69. Williams JM, Russell I, Russell D. Mindfulness-based cognitive therapy: Further issues in current evidence and future research. *J Consult Clin Psychol.* 2008;76:524-529.

70. Sesin CA, Bingham CO. Remission in rheumatoid arthritis: Wishful thinking or clinical reality? *Semin Arthritis Rheum.* 2005;35:185-196.

71. Aletaha D, Neogi T, Silman AJ, et al. 2010 Rheumatoid arthritis classification criteria. An American College of Rheumatology/European League Against Rheumatism Collaborative Initiative. *Arthritis Rheum.* 2010;62:2569-2581.

72. Bourguignon C, Taibi D, Taylor AG. Sleep disturbances, fatigue, depression, and heart rate variability in menopausal women with and without RA. *Sleep.* 2005;28:302.

73. Drewes AM, Svendsen L, Taagholt SJ, et al. Sleep in rheumatoid arthritis: A comparison with healthy subjects and studies of sleep/wake interactions. *Br J Rheumatol.* 1998;37:71-81.

74. Hirsch M, Carlander B, Verge M, et al. Objective and subjective sleep disturbances in patients with rheumatoid arthritis: A reappraisal. *Arthritis Rheum.* 1994;37:41-49.
75. Walsh JK, Muelbach MJ, Lauter SA, et al. Effects of triazolam on sleep, daytime sleepiness, and morning stiffness in patients with rheumatoid arthritis. *J Rheumatol.* 1996;23:245-252.
76. Grob D. Principles of surgical treatment of cervical spine in rheumatoid arthritis. *Euro Spine J.* 1993;2:180-190.
77. Brasington Jr RD. Clinical features of rheumatoid arthritis. In: Hochberg MC, Silman AJ, Smolen JS, Weinblatt ME, Weisman MH, eds. *Rheumatology.* 4th ed. Spain: Mosby Elsevier; 2007:763-771.
78. Turesson C, Matteson EL. Extra-articular features of rheumatoid arthritis and systemic invoevment. In: Hochberg MC, Silman AJ, Smolen JS, Weinblatt ME, Weisman MH, eds. *Rheumatology.* 4th ed. Spain: Mosby Elsevier; 2007:773-783.
79. Hicks JE, Joe GO, Gerber LH. Rehabilitation of the patient with inflammatory arthritis and connective-tissue disease. In: DeLisa JA, Gans BM, Walsh NE, eds. *Physical Medicine and Rehabilitation: Principles and Practice.* 4th ed. Philadelphia: Lippincott Williams & Wilkins; 2005:721-763.
80. Redlund-Johnell I. Upper airway obstruction in patients with rheumatoid arthritis and temporomandibular joint destruction. *Scand J Rheumatol.* 1988;17:273-279.
81. Drossaers-Bakker KW, Hamburger HL, Bongartz EB, et al. Sleep apnoea caused by rheumatoid arthritis. *Br J Rheumatol.* 1998;37:889-894.
82. Alamondi OS. Sleep-disordered breathing in patients with acquired retrognathia secondary to rheumatoid arthritis. *Med Sci Monit.* 2006;12:CR530-CR534.
83. Gyori M, Sandra S, Szakacs Z, Koves P. Restless legs syndrome in rheumatoid arthritis. *Sleep.* 2004;27:A302.
84. Zamir G, Press J, Tal A, Tarasiuk A. Sleep fragmentation in children with juvenile rheumatoid arthritis. *J Rheumatol.* 1998;25:1191-1197.
85. Lopes MC, Guilleminault C, Rosa A, et al. Delta sleep instability in children with chronic arthritis. *Braz J Med Biol Res.* 2008;41:938-943.
86. Twilt M, Schulten AJ, Nicolaas P, et al. Facioskeletal changes in children with juvenile idiopathic arthritis. *Ann Rheum Dis.* 2006;65:823-825.
87. Bloom BJ, Owens JA, McGuinn M, et al. Sleep and its relationship to pain, dysfunction, and disease activity in juvenile rheumatoid arthritis. *J Rheumatol.* 2002;29:169-173.
88. Hultgren S, Broman JE, Gudbjornsson B, et al. Sleep disturbances in outpatients with ankylosing spondylitis: A questionnaire study with gender implications. *Scand J Rheumatol.* 2000;29:365-369.
89. Jamieson AH, Alford CA, Bird HA, et al. The effect of sleep and nocturnal movement on stiffness, pain and psychomotor performance in ankylosing spondylitis. *Clin Exp Rheumatol.* 1995;13:73-78.
90. Jones SD, Koh WH, Steiner A, et al. Fatigue in ankylosing spondylitis: Its prevalence and relationship to disease activity, sleep, and other factors. *J Rheumatol.* 1996;23:487-490.
91. Maksymowych WP. Etiology, pathogenesis and pathology of ankylosing spondylitis. In: Hochberg MC, Silman AJ, Smolen JS, Weinblatt ME, Weisman MH, eds. *Rheumatology.* 4th ed. Spain: Mosby Elsevier; 2007:1115-1130.
92. Defalque RJ, Hyder ML. Laryngeal mask airway in severe cervical ankylosis. *Can J Anaesth.* 1997;44:305-307.
93. Ortancil O, Sarikaya S, Sapmaz P, et al. The effect(s) of a six-week home-based exercise program on the respiratory muscle and functional status in ankylosing spondylitis. *J Clin Rheum.* 2009;15:68-70.
94. Solak O, Fidan F, Dunbar U, et al. The prevalence of obstructive sleep apnoea syndrome in ankylosing spondylitis patients. *Rhem.* 2009;48:433-435.
95. Stitik TP, Foye PM, Stskal D, et al. Osteoarthritis. In: DeLisa JA, Gans BM, Walsh NE, eds. *Physical Medicine and Rehabilitation: Principles and Practice.* 4th ed. Philadelphia: Lippincott Williams & Wilkins; 2005:765-786.
96. Mader R, Sarzi-Puttini P, Atzeni F. Extraspinal manifestations of diffuse idiopathic skeletal hypertosis. *Rheumatology.* 2009;48:1478-1481.
97. Moldofsky H, Lue FA, Saskin P. Sleep and morning pain in primary osteoarthritis. *J Rheum.* 1987;14:124-128.
98. Moldofsky H. Sleep influences on regional and diffuse pain syndromes associated with osteoarthritis. *Semin Arthritis Rheum.* 1989;18:18-21.
99. Tench CM, MMcCurdie I, White PD, D'Cruz DP. The prevalence and associations of fatigue in systemic lupus erythematosus. *Rheumatology (Oxford).* 2000;39:1249-1254.
100. Wolfe F, Petri M, Alarcon GS, et al. Fibromyalgia, systemic lupus erythematosus (SLE), and evaluation of SLE activity. *J Rheumatol.* 2009;36:82-88.
101. Prado GF, Allen RP, Trevisani VM, et al. Sleep disruption in systemic sclerosis (scleroderma) patients: Clinical and polysomnographic findings. *Sleep Med.* 2002;3:341-345.
102. Antonioli CM, Bua G, Frige A, et al. An individualized rehabilitation program in patients with systemic sclerosis may improve quality of life and hand mobility. *Clin Rheum.* 2009;28:159-165.
103. Hamuryudan V, Mat C, Saip S, et al. Thalidomide in the treatment of the mucocutaneous lesions of the Behcet syndrome. A randomized, double-blind, placebo-controlled trial. *Ann Intern Med.* 1998;128:443-450.
104. Yamada M, Kashiwamura K, Nakamura Y, et al. On psychiatric symptoms of neuro-Behcet's syndrome. *Folia Psychiatr Neurol Jpn.* 1978;32:191-197.
105. Sakurai N, Koike Y, Kaneoke Y, et al. Sleep apnea and palatal myoclonus in a patient with neuro-Behcet syndrome. *Intern Med.* 1993;32:336-339.
106. Tishler M, Barak Y, Paran D, Yaron M. Sleep disturbances, fibromyalgia and primary Sjogren's syndrome. *Clin Exp Rheumatol.* 1997;15:71-74.
107. Servan J, Marchand F, Garma L, et al. Narcolepsy disclosing neurosarchoidosis. *Rev Neurol (Paris).* 1995;151:281-283.
108. Turner GA, Lower EE, Corser BC, et al. Sleep apnea in sarcoidosis. *Sarcoidosis Vasc Diffuse Lung Dis.* 1997;14:61-64.
109. Verbraecken J, Hoitsma E, van der Grinten CP, et al. Sleep disturbances associated with periodic leg movements in chronic sarcoidosis. *Sarcoidosis Vasc Diffuse Lung Dis.* 2004;21:137-146.
110. Clauw DJ. Fibromyalgia. In: Hochberg MC, Silman AJ, Smolen JS, Weinblatt ME, Weisman MH, eds. *Rheumatology.* 4th ed. Spain: Mosby Elsevier; 2007:701-711.
111. Yunus MB. A comprehensive medical evaluation of patients with fibromyalgia syndrome. *Rheum Dis Clin North Am.* 2002;28:201-217.
112. Arnold LM, Hudson JI, Keck PE, et al. Comorbidity of fibromyalgia and psychiatric disorders. *J Clin Psychiatry.* 2006;76:1219-1225.
113. Buskila D, Cohen H. Comorbidity of fibromyalgia and psychiatric disorders. *Curr Pain Headache Rep.* 2007;11:333-338.
114. Hauser W, Thieme K, Turk DC. Guidelines on the management of fibromyalgia syndrome—A systematic review. *Euro J Pain.* 2010;14:5-10.
115. Arnold LM. Strategies for managing fibromyalgia. *Am J Med.* 2009;122:S31-S43.
116. Wolfe F, Cathey MA, Kleinheksel SM. Fibrositis (fibromyalgia) in rheumatoid arthritis. *J Rheumatol.* 1984;11:814-818.
117. Buskila D, Press J, Abu-Shakra M. Fibromyalgia in systemic lupus erythematosus: Prevalence and clinical implications. *Clin Rev Allergy Immunol.* 2003;25:25-28.
118. Thompson ME, Barkhuizen A. Fibromyalgia, hepatitis C infection and the cytokine connection. *Curr Pain Headache Rep.* 2003;7:342-347.
119. Golding DN. Hypothyroidism presenting with musculoskeletal symptoms. *Ann Rheum Dis.* 1970;29:10-14.
120. Bland JH, Frymoyer JW. Rheumatic syndromes of myxedema. *N Engl J Med.* 1970;282:1171-1174.
121. Yunus MB. Fibromyalgia and overlapping disorders: The unifying concept of central sensitivity syndromes. *Semin Arthritis Rheum.* 2007;36:339-356.
122. Bested AC, Logan AC, Howe R. Chronic fatigue syndrome and fibromyalgia. Nashville. *Cumberland House Pub.* 2006:1–254.
123. Paiva ES, Deodhar A, Jones KD, et al. Impaired growth hormone secretion in fibromyalgia patients: Evidence for augmented hypothalamic somatostatin. *Arthritis Rheum.* 2002;46:440-450.
124. Demitrack MA, Crofford LJ. Evidence for and pathophysiologic implications of the hypothalamic-pituitary-adrenal axis dysregulation in fibromyalgia and chronic fatigue syndrome. *Ann N Y Acad Sci.* 1998;840:684-697.
125. Klerman EB, Goldenberg DL, Brown EN, et al. Circadian rhythms of women with fibromyalgia. *J Clin Endocrin Metab.* 2001;86:1034-1039.
126. Pillemer SR, Bradley LA, Crofford LJ, et al. The neuroscience and endocrinology of fibromyalgia. *Arthritis Rheum.* 1997;40:1928-1939.
127. Onen SH, Alloui A, Gross A, et al. The effects of total sleep deprivation, selective sleep interruption and sleep recovery on pain tolerance thresholds in healthy subjects. *J Sleep Res.* 2001;10:35-42.
128. Lentz MJ, Landis CA, Rothermel J, et al. Effects of selective slow wave sleep disruption on musculoskeletal pain and fatigue in middle aged women. *J Rheumatol.* 1999;26:1586-1592.
129. Wolfe F, Smythe HA, Yunus MB, et al. The American College of Rheumatology 1990 criteria for the classification of fibromyalgia. Report of the Multicenter Criteria Committee. *Arthritis Rheum.* 1990;33:160-172.

130. Turk DC, Vierck CJ, Scarbrough E, et al. Fibromyalgia: Combining pharmacological and nonpharmacological approaches to treating the person, not just the pain. *J Pain.* 2008;9:99-104.
131. Clauw DJ. Fibromyalgia: Update on mechanisms and management. *J Clin Rheumatol.* 2007;13:102-109.
132. Wolfe F, Clauw DJ, Fitzcharles MA, et al. The American College of Rheumatology preliminary diagnostic criteria for fibromyalgia and measurement of symptom severity. *Arthritis Care Res.* 2010;62:600-610.
133. Moldofsky H, MacFarlane JG. Fibromyalgia and chronic fatigue syndromes. In: Kryger MH, Roth T, Dement WC, eds. *Principles and Practice of Sleep Medicine.* 4th ed. Philadelphia: Elsevier Saunders; 2005:1225-1236.
134. Stehlik R, Arvidsson L, Ulfberg J. Restless legs syndrome is common among female patients with fibromyalgia. *Euro Neurol.* 2009;61:107-111.
135. Moldofsky H, Inhaber NH, Guinta DR, Alvarez-Horine SB. Effects of sodium oxybate on sleep physiology and sleep/wake-related symptoms in patients with fibromyalgia syndrome: A double-blind, randomized, placebo-controlled study. *J Rheumatol.* 2010;37(10):2156-2166.
136. Branco J, Atalaia A, Paiva T. Sleep cycles and alpha-delta sleep in fibromyalgia syndrome. *J Rheumatol.* 1994;21:1113-1117.
137. Drewes AM, Nielsen KD, Taagholt SJ, et al. Sleep intensity in fibromyalgia: Focus on the microstructure of the sleep process. *Br J Rheumatol.* 1995;34:629-635.
138. Ware JC, Russell IJ, Campos E. Alpha intrusions into the sleep of depression and fibromyalgia syndrome (fibrositis) patients (abstract). *Sleep Res.* 1986;15:210.
139. Roizenblatt S, Moldofsky H, Benedito-Silva AA, Tufik S. Alpha sleep characteristics in fibromyalgia. *Arthritis Rheum.* 2001;44:222-230.
140. Shaver JL, Lentz M, Landis CA, et al. Sleep, psychological distress, and stress arousal in women with fibromyalgia. *Res Nurs Health.* 1997;20:247-257.
141. Wittig RM, Zorick FJ, Blumer D, et al. Disturbed sleep in patients complaining of chronic pain. *J Nerv Ment Dis.* 1982;70:429-431.
142. Moldofsky H. The significance of dysfunctions of the sleeping/waking brain to the pathogenesis and treatment of fibromyalgia. *Rheum Dis Clin North Am.* 2009;35:275-283.
143. Staud R. Pharmacological treatment of fibromyalgia syndrome: New developments. *Drugs.* 2010;70:1-4.
144. Scharf MB, Baumann M, Berkowitz DV. The effect of sodium oxybate on clinical symptoms and sleep patterns in patients with fibromyalgia. *J Rheumatol.* 2003;30:1070-1074.
145. Russell IJ, Bennett RM, Michalek JE. Oxybate SXB-26 Fibromyalgia Syndrome Study Group. Sodium oxybate relieves pain and improves function in fibromyalgia syndrome: A randomized, double-blind, placebo-controlled, multicenter clinical trial. *Arthritis Rheum.* 2009;60:299-309.
146. Holdcraft LC, Assefi N, Buchwald D. Complementary and alternative medicine in fibromyalgia and related syndromes. *Best Pract Res Clin Rheumatol.* 2003;17:667-683.
147. Haanen HC, Hoenderdos HT, Van Romunde LK, et al. Controlled trial of hypnotherapy in the treatment of refractory fibromyalgia. *J Rheumatol.* 1987;14:820-825.
148. Ferraccioli G, Ghirelli L, Scita F, et al. EMG biofeedback training in fibromyalgia syndrome. *J Rheumatol.* 1987;14:820-825.
149. Oliver K, Cronan TA, Walen HR, et al. Effects of social support and education on health care costs for patients with fibromyalgia. *J Rheumatol.* 2001;28:2711-2719.
150. Burckhardt CS, Mannerkorpi K, Hedenberg L, et al. A randomized, controlled clinical trial of education and physical training for women with fibromyalgia. *J Rheumatol.* 1994;21:714-720.
151. Rooks DS, Gautam S, Romelig M, et al. Group exercise, education, and combination self-management in women with fibromyalgia: A randomized trial. *Arch Intern Med.* 2007;167:2192-2200.
152. Busch AJ, Barber KA, Overend TJ, et al. Exercise for treating fibromyalgia syndrome. *Cochrane Database Syst Rev.* 2007;4:CD003786.
153. da Silva GD, Lorenzi-Filho G, Lage LV, et al. Effects of yoga and the addition of tui na in patients with fibromyalgia. *J Altern Complement Med.* 2007;13:1107-1113.
154. Taggart HM, Arslanian CL, Bae S, et al. Effects of tai chi exercise on fibromyalgia symptoms and health-related quality of life. *Orthop Nurs.* 2003;30:2257-2262.
155. Mayhew E, Ernst E. Acupuncture for fibromyalgia—A systemic review of randomized clinical trials. *Rheumatology (Oxford).* 2007;46:801-804.
156. Deluze C, Bosia L, Zirbs A, et al. Electroacupuncture in fibromyalgia: Results of a controlled trial. *BMJ.* 1992;14:820-825.
157. Almeida TF, Roizenblatt S, Benedito-Silva AA, et al. The effects of combined therapy (ultrasound and interferential current) on pain and sleep in fibromyalgia. *Pain.* 2003;104:665-672.
158. Jungquist CR, O'Brien C, Matteson-Rusby S, Smith MT, et al. The efficacy of cognitive-behavioral therapy for insomnia in patients with chronic pain. *Sleep Med.* 2010;11:302-309.
159. Krystal AD, Edinger JD. Sleep EEG predictors and correlates of the response to cognitive behavioral therapy for insomnia. *Sleep.* 2010;33:669-677.
160. Carskadon MA, Dement WC. Normal human sleep: An overview. In: Kryger MH, Roth T, Dement WC, eds. *Principles and Practice of Sleep Medicine.* 4th ed. Philadelphia: Elsevier Saunders; 2005:13-23.
161. Walker JM, Farney RJ, Rhondeau SM, et al. Chronic opioid use is a risk factor for the development of central sleep apnea and ataxic beathing. *J Clin Sleep Med.* 2007;3:455-461.
162. Alaltar MA, Scarf SM. Opioid-associated central sleep apnea: A case series. *Sleep Breath.* 2009;13:201-206.
163. Sweitzer PK. Drugs that disturb sleep and wakefulness. In: Kryger MH, Roth T, Dement WC, eds. *Principles and Practices of Sleep Medicine.* 3rd ed. Philadelphia: Saunders; 2000:441-461.
164. Gillin JC. The long and the short of sleeping pills. *N Engl J Med.* 1991;324:1735-1736.
165. Guilleminault C. Benzodiazepines, breathing and sleep. *Am J Med.* 1990;88:25S-28S.
166. Drewes AM, Andreasen A, Jennum P, et al. Zopiclone in the treatment of sleep abnormalitites in fibromyalgis. *Scand J Rheumatol.* 1991;20:288-293.
167. Moldofsky H, Lue FA, Mously C, et al. The effect of zolpidem in patients with fibromyalgia: A dose ranging, double blind, placebo controlled, modified crossover study. *J Rheumatol.* 1966;23:529-533.
168. Eisen J, Macfarlane J, Shapiro CM. Psychotropic drugs and sleep. ABC of sleep disorders. *BMJ.* 1993;306:1331-1334.
169. Moldofsky H, Lue FA. The relationship of alpha and delta EEG frequencies to pain and mood in "fibrositis" patients treated with chlorpromazine and L-tryptophan. *Electroencephalogr Clin Neurophysiol.* 1980;50:71-80.
170. Sammaritano M, Sherwin A. Effects of anticonvulsants on sleep. *Neurology.* 2000;54:S16-S24.
171. Sweitzer PK. Drugs that disturb sleep and wakefulness. In: Kryger MH, Roth T, Dement WC, eds. *Principles and Practice of Sleep Medicine.* 4th ed. Philadelphia: Elsevier Saunders; 2005:499-518.
172. Yang C, White DP, Winkelman JW. Antidepressants and periodic leg movements of sleep. *Biol Psychiatry.* 2005;58:510-514.
173. Nader P, Coralie L, Baleydier B, et al. Restless legs syndrome induced by citalopram: A psychiatric emergency? *Gen Hosp Psychiatry.* 3007;29:72-74.
174. Goldenberg D, Mayskiy M, Mossey C, et al. A randomized, double-blind crossover trial of fluoxetine and amitriptyline in the treatment of fibromyalgia. *Arthritis Rheum.* 1996;39:1852-1859.
175. Nofzinger EA, Fasiczka A, Berman S, et al. Buproprion SR reduces periodic limb movements associated with arousals from sleep in depressed patients with periodic limb movement disorder. *J Clin Psychiatry.* 2000;61:858-862.
176. Branco JC, Martini A, Palva T. Treatment of sleep abnormalities and clinical complaints in fibromyalgia with trazadone (abstract). *Arthritis Rheum.* 1996;39:591.
177. Kim SW, Shin IS, Kim JM, et al. Factors potentiating the risk of mirtazapine-associated restless legs syndrome. *Hum Psychopharmacol.* 2008;23:615-620.
178. Bennett RM, Gatter RA, Campbell SM, et al. A comparison of cyclobenzaprine and placebo in the management of fibrositis: A double blind controlled study. *Arthritis Rheum.* 1988;3:1535-1542.
179. Carette S, Bell MV, Reynolds WJ, et al. Comparison of amitriptyline, cyclobenzaprine and placebo in the treatment of fibromyalgia: A randomized double blind clinical trial. *Arthritis Rheum.* 1994;37:32-40.
180. Reynolds WJ, Moldofsky H, Saskin P, et al. The effects of cyclobenzaprine on sleep physiology and symptoms in patients with fibromyalgia. *J Rheumatol.* 1991;18:452-454.
181. Carette S, Oakson G, Guimont C, et al. Sleep electroencephalography and the clinical response to amitriptyline in patients with fibromyalgia. *Arthritis Rheum.* 1995;38:1211-1217.
182. Abad VC, Sarinas PSA, Guilleminault C. Sleep and rheumatologic disorders. *Sleep Med Rev.* 2008;12:211-228.

Inflammation and Sleep

MARK R. ZIELINSKI / JAMES M. KRUEGER

Chapter 48

Innate immunity involves cellular, inflammatory, behavioral, and other mechanisms to defend the host against exogenous pathogens and endogenous perturbations.[1] The other primary function of the innate immune system is to process antigens for the acquired immune system. The innate immune system and sleep are highly conserved among mammals, and homologous mediators are found in invertebrates such as fruit flies and worms (e.g., *Drosophila melanogaster* and *Caenorhabditis elegans*, respectively).[2] Importantly, the innate immune system is affected by sleep and sleep loss and alters sleep itself.[3] Moreover, the immune system and sleep interact to alter host defenses against pathogens. In addition, the immune system is involved with the pathology of various sleep-related disorders, and thus inflammatory mechanisms may be future targets for treatment.

INFLAMMATION

Mechanisms of Inflammation

Inflammation occurs in response to many stimuli, including pathogen exposure, cellular damage, irritants, cellular dysregulation, and waking activity.[1,3] As far back as the second century, in *De Medicina*, Aulus Cornelius Celsus described four classic signs of inflammation: rubor (redness), calor (increased temperature), tumor (swelling), and dolor (pain).[1] Soon after, Galen described a fifth inflammatory sign further described by Rudolf Virchow in the 19th century as laesa (loss of function). Inflammation is classified on the basis of its timing as acute or chronic. Acute inflammation occurs over seconds, minutes, hours, or days and allows the host to effectively heal damaged tissue and protect the body from disease. Some of the functions of the acute inflammatory response involve changing blood flow, activation/inhibition of cellular mediators, and the migration of cells such as neutrophils and macrophages. Chronic inflammation involves sustained inflammation and is associated with increased risk for cardiovascular disease,[4] type 2 diabetes,[5] inflammatory bowel disease,[6] asthma,[7] and colorectal cancer.[8] Sleep and prolonged wakefulness are strongly associated with altered acute and chronic inflammation, and short sleep duration is associated with the prevalence of many inflammatory diseases, such as type 2 diabetes,[9] cancer,[10] and cardiovascular disease.[11] Moreover, many sleep-related diseases including obstructive sleep apnea and insomnia have altered inflammation or inflammatory mechanism components.[12,13] Thus, it is plausible that inflammatory mechanisms are related to the pathology of sleep-related diseases.

Sleep Regulatory Substances

There is abundant evidence indicating that sleep regulatory substances such as interleukin 1β (IL-1β) or tumor necrosis factor-α (TNF-α) affect cognition,[14-16] memory,[17-19] performance,[17] pain,[20-22] depression,[23,24] sleepiness,[25-27] and fatigue.[28] IL-1β and TNF-α and other cytokines regulate the inflammatory response. Inflammation is associated with altering brain functions via the change in expression of several cytokines that are also linked to sleep. The first evidence that specific molecules in the body regulate sleep was inferred when Henri Pieron of France[29] and Kuniomi Ishimori of Japan[30] independently found that when cerebrospinal fluid from sleep-deprived dogs was transferred into dogs that slept *ad libitum,* the recipient dogs slept more. These findings started investigations of how molecules, now deemed sleep-regulatory substances, regulate sleep. Interestingly, these sleep regulatory substances are either inflammatory molecules or indirectly modulate inflammation.

Criteria for sleep regulatory substances are as follows. Sleep regulatory substances and their receptors fluctuate in the brain with sleep propensity. Sleep regulatory substances increase or inhibit sleep when injected systemically or locally into the central nervous systems (CNS). In addition, the removal of the sleep regulatory substances alters sleep. Sleep regulatory substances change during pathologic states associated with excessive sleepiness and alter duration of sleep.

Nearly 100 sleep regulatory substances have been identified, although only a few substances can be considered validated sleep regulatory substances.[3] IL-1β, TNF-α, and growth hormone–releasing hormone (GHRH) meet the sleep regulatory substance criteria for mediating non–rapid eye movement (NREM) sleep, while nitric oxide (NO) and prolactin meet the sleep regulatory substance criteria for mediating rapid eye movement (REM) sleep. However, many other inflammatory substances also have the capacity to alter sleep (Box 48-1). These substances have associated receptors, precursors, miRNAs, metabolites, and modulation of any of these associated substances has the potential to affect sleep as well.

Cytokines

Cytokines are protein, peptide, or glycoprotein signaling molecules acting as autocrines, paracrines, or endocrines.[1] Cytokines are produced by a variety of cells, including lymphocytes, neutrophils, myocytes, adipocytes, glia, and neurons, with the greatest production occurring in macrophages such as microglia in the CNS. The potency of cytokines is extremely

BOX 48-1 *Cytokines and Growth Factors Affecting Sleep*

Cytokine/Growth Factor	Effect on NREM Sleep
Interleukin 1α	↑
Interleukin 1β	↑
Interleukin 2	↑
Interleukin 4	↓
Interleukin 6	↑↓
Interleukin 8	↑
Interleukin 10	↓
Interleukin 12	↑
Interleukin 13	↓
Interleukin 15	↑
Interleukin 18	↑
Interleukin 1 receptor antagonist	↓
Epidermal growth factor	↑
Acidic fibroblast growth factor	↑
Erythropoietin	↑
Nerve growth factor	↑
Brain-derived neurotrophic factor	↑
Glia-derived neurotrophic factor	↑
Neurotrophin 3	↑
Neurotrophin 4	↑
Interferon-α	↑
Interferon-β	↑
Interferon-γ	↑↓
Tumor necrosis factor-α	↑
Tumor necrosis factor-β	↑
Granulocyte macrophage colony-stimulating factor	↑
Transforming growth factor-β	↓
Granulocyte colony-stimulating factor	↓
Insulin-like growth factor	↑
Soluble tumor necrosis factor receptor	↑↓
Soluble interleukin-1 receptor	↓

NREM, non–rapid eye movement.

high; for example, picomolar or femtomolar concentrations are often effective. Moreover, cytokines activate cells via their specific receptors to produce more cytokines resulting in rapid exponential activation of inflammatory or anti-inflammatory responses (Fig. 48-1). Cytokines are important for both innate and adaptive immune responses. The three key acute phase response cytokines—IL-1β, TNF-α, and IL-6—have been the most stringently investigated in regard to their actions on sleep.[3] In addition, IL-1β and TNF-α interfere with the expression of *Clock* genes by altering CLOCK-BMAL1-induced activation of E-box regulatory elements.[31,32] Thus, inflammatory mediators are a principal interceding component of the sleep homeostat (Fig. 48-2).

Interleukin 1 Superfamily

The interleukin 1 superfamily (IL1F) is composed of 11 members and their associated receptors. The best characterized form of the IL-1 family is IL-1β. IL-1β is produced by many cell types; for example, macrophages produce very high quantities of IL-1β.[33] IL-1α (IL1F1), IL-1β (IL1F2), and IL-18 (IL1F4) are agonists, and the interleukin 1 receptor antagonist (IL-1RA) (IL1F3) is an antagonist. There are additional IL-1 family members (i.e., IL1F5, IL1F6, IL1F7, IL1F8, IL1F9, and IL1F10) whose functions are currently not fully understood.

However, IL1F7 has recently been discovered to have anti-inflammatory regulatory functions modulating IL1F1, IL1F2, IL1F3, and IL1F4 and other pro- and anti-inflammatory cytokines. IL-1β was originally described as a pyrogenic molecule (i.e., an endogenous pyrogen).[34] However, its functions also include the regulation of inflammation, immune responses, hyperalgesia, hematopoiesis, and multiple CNS functions including sleep.[33] IL-1β has two receptor forms: the type 1 receptor, which is associated with inflammatory effects, and the type 2 receptor, which competitively inhibits IL-1β from binding to the type 1 receptor. The IL-1 type 2 receptor lacks an intracellular signaling domain and is often referred to as a decoy receptor. IL-1 regulates, or is regulated by, many inflammatory-regulating pathways including cyclooxygenase (COX), nuclear factor-kappa B (NF-κB), inducible nitric oxide synthase (iNOS), and prostaglandin E_2 (PGE$_2$).

IL-1α, IL-1β, IL-18 and IL-1RA all modulate sleep.[33] IL-1β was the first cytokine sleep regulatory substance identified.[35] IL-1β messenger ribonucleic acid (mRNA) levels in different brain regions fluctuate with the sleep/wake cycle and increase with sleep intensity.[3] Both central and systemic administrations of IL-1β enhance NREM sleep for hours and attenuate REM sleep in multiple species. Specifically, the duration of NREM sleep, electroencephalographic (EEG) delta power during NREM sleep (an indicator of increased sleep propensity), and sleepiness are all enhanced after IL-1β administration in mice, rats, rabbits, sheep, cats, monkeys, and humans. The increase in NREM sleep following exogenous IL-1β administration occurs at very low doses: in rats 400 femtomoles given intraventricularly enhance NREM sleep for hours. Mice that lack the IL-1 type 1 receptors have reduced NREM sleep and REM sleep compared to mice with intact receptors. These sleep deficits occur only during the night hours, suggesting an interaction with circadian regulatory events. However, inhibition of IL-1β pharmacologically or with antibodies attenuates spontaneous NREM sleep and the enhanced NREM sleep that follows sleep deprivation. In addition, the firing rate of hypothalamic sleep-active neurons is enhanced, but wake-active neurons are inhibited with exogenous IL-1β administration. Further, physiologic/pathologic increases in IL-1β associated with infection or increased food intake suggest that IL-1β from a variety of sources affects sleep.

The IL-1 receptor antagonist (IL-1RA) serves to inhibit IL-1β by competing with IL-1β for IL-1 binding sites on the IL-1 type 1 receptor.[33] Thus, IL-1RA mediates the inflammatory processes and modulates IL-1β to alter sleep. Indeed, the IL-1RA given intraperitoneally or intraventricularly inhibits IL-1β-induced NREM sleep in rabbits or rats.[3] Moreover, the IL-1RA attenuates the enhanced NREM sleep induced by bacterial cell wall components (e.g., muramyl dipeptide).[36]

IL-18 is a proinflammatory cytokine that binds to the IL-18 receptor, mediating acute and cell-mediated immune responses.[33] IL-18 binding protein (IL-18BP) binds to IL-18 with high affinity, preventing IL-18 from binding to the IL-18 receptor. IL-18 also mediates other proinflammatory cytokine production, including IL-1β and IL-12. However, IL-18 also mediates the production of the antisomnogenic cytokine IL-4 and the somnogenic cytokine interferon-γ (IFN-γ). IL-18 is involved in sleep regulation to the extent that its injection enhances duration of NREM sleep and IL-18 expression increases following sleep deprivation.[37] Moreover, an anti-IL-18 antibody attenuates muramyl dipeptide–induced sleep in rabbits.

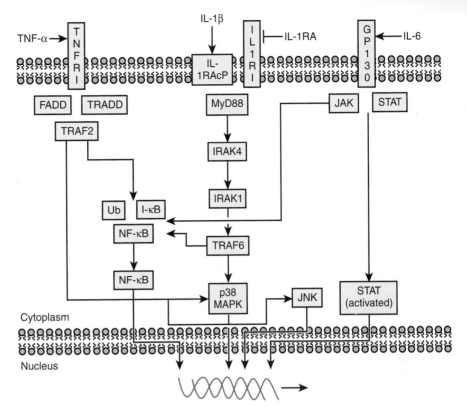

Figure 48-1 Extracellular sleep regulatory substances IL-1β, TNF-α, and IL-6 through their respective receptors, adaptor proteins, and intracellular signaling pathways influence gene expression. IL-1β binds to the type I IL-1 receptor (IL1RI) in conjunction with the IL-1 receptor accessory protein (IL-1RAcP) to signal MyD88. MyD88 activates IRAK4/IRAK1 to signal TNF receptor associated factor 6 (TRAF6). TRAF6 activates NF-κB, p38 MAPK, and c-Jun N-terminal kinase (JNK), and signaling transducers and activator of transcription (STAT). IL-6 binds to the gp130 component of the IL-6 receptor to activate JAK/STAT pathways that in turn activate NF-κB and STAT. Upon activation, NF-κB, p38 MAPK, JNK, and STAT traverse the nuclear membrane bind to DNA to influence transcription of multiple genes, some of which affect sleep. *IL,* interleukin; *MAPK,* mitogen-activated protein kinase; *MyD88,* myeloid differentiation primary response gene 88; *TNF,* tumor necrosis factor.

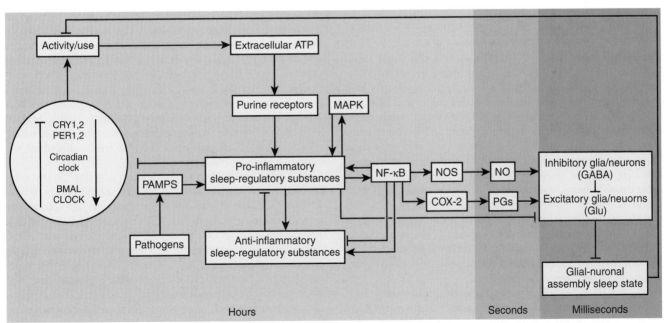

Figure 48-2 Local activity and pathogens such as LPS and influenza activate purine receptors and PAMPs, respectively. Proinflammatory sleep-regulatory substances such as IL-1β and TNF-α are activated through purine receptors and PAMPs. These substances induce their own production and interact with other sleep regulatory substances through the activation of NF-κB. The transcriptional and translational process involved take hours. These processes are mediated by MAPK. These processes alter the production of NOS and COX-2 to mediate the respective production of NO and PGs—that function over seconds. NO and PGs alter neurotransmission on a very rapid time scale of milliseconds. This occurs via receptors that alter postsynaptic glial/neuronal sensitivity such as α-amino-3-hydroxyl-5-methyl-4-isoxazole-propionate receptors. The end product is sleep, which inhibits glial/neural activity forming an inhibitory feedback loop. *COX,* cyclooxygenase; *IL,* interleukin; *LPS,* lipopolysaccharide; *MAPK,* mitogen-activated protein kinase; *NF-κB,* nuclear factor-kappa B; *NO,* nitric oxide; *NOS,* nitric oxide synthase; *PAMPs,* pathogen-associated molecular patterns; *PG,* prostaglandin; *TNF,* tumor necrosis factor.

Tumor Necrosis Factor Superfamily

The TNF family has two prototypic members—TNF-α and TNF-β[38]—although there are more than 40 unique ligand-receptor pairs currently recognized as belonging to this family. TNF-α mediates inflammation and the acute phase response. TNF-α also mediates apoptosis, tumorigenesis, septic shock, viral replication, fever, neuroprotection, neurotoxicity, and appetite. TNF-α and TNF-β are secreted by many types of cells, including T and B cells, macrophages, neurons, and glia. TNF-β shares some actions with TNF-α. The TNF receptor 1 (TNFR1) is expressed in most tissues, but the TNFR2 is found only on immunocytes, including microglia. Both receptors bind TNF-α and TNF-β. These TNF receptors activate multiple cellular pathways including NF-κB and mitogen-activated protein kinase (MAPK) pathways.

Brain TNF-α protein and mRNA levels increase during wakefulness.[3] As with IL-1β, systemic or CNS administration of TNF-α enhances NREM duration and EEG delta power in all species thus far examined. TNF-α suppresses REM sleep at high doses as found with IL-1β. TNF-α inhibitors inhibit spontaneous sleep and sleep following sleep loss. Furthermore, mice lacking TNFR1 fail to exhibit excess NREM sleep after TNF-α administration, although the mice respond to IL-1β. Further, the lack of the TNFR1 is associated with reduced durations of spontaneous NREM and REM sleep during the dark-light transition. In contrast, mice lacking both TNF receptors have less NREM sleep during dark hours and more REM sleep during daylight hours.[39] TNF-α also increases with various infectious diseases, including after bacterial and influenzavirus challenge.[36]

Interleukin-6 Superfamily

The members of the IL-6 cytokine superfamily share similar functions and a common signal transducer: gp130.[40] The proteotypic family member IL-6 is secreted by T cells and macrophages, myocytes, osteocytes, and microglia. IL-6 has both pro- and anti-inflammatory properties. IL-6 can be anti-inflammatory through its ability to inhibit TNF-α and activate the IL-1RA and IL-10.[41] IL-6 mediates fever and additional facets of the acute phase response. IL-6 binds to the type 1 cytokine receptor complex that has a ligand binding IL-6 receptor α chain and a signal transducing component gp130.[40] Upon activation, a signaling cascade occurs that leads to the activation of transcription factors, including janus kinases (JAKs), signal transducers and activators of transcription (STATS), and NF-κB. Although the differentiation and survival of neurons are influenced by the soluble IL-6 receptor, neurons can be unresponsive to IL-6.

Plasma IL-6 has a diurnal rhythm with peak values during sleep and nadirs during wakefulness.[42] Further, rat IL-6 protein levels in the cortex, hippocampus, and hypothalamus are higher during the beginning of the light period (i.e., when sleep propensity is the greatest) compared to the dark period.[43] Sleep deprivation increases IL-6 expression,[42] but IL-6 injections increase NREM sleep in rats and mice. In rats, recombinant IL-6 is also pyrogenic. Although pharmacologic inhibition of IL-6 alters sleep, IL-6 knockout mice have normal spontaneous NREM and REM sleep durations and body temperature. However, IL-6 knockout mice respond to sleep loss with longer sleep rebound responses compared to control mice, suggesting that IL-6 has a role in sleep regulation.

Circulating IL-6 increases during infections, and thereby modulates infection-altered sleep. IL-6 also mediates IL-1β and TNF-α production.

SLEEP-REGULATED INFLAMMATORY PATHWAYS

The most notable cellular pathways that mediate inflammation are the NF-κB, MAPK/extracellular receptor kinase (ERK), NO, and COX pathways (Fig. 48-3). There is much literature indicating that these pathways also modulate sleep regulatory substances, sleep, and sleep-related pathologies.

NF-κB Pathway

NF-κB is a transcription factor found in all nucleated cell types.[44] NF-κB has an important role in neuronal-glial function. It is present in neuronal tissue homogenates and is activated by neurotransmitters.[45] NF-κB is one of the key regulators of inflammatory immune responses and is involved with regulating cytokine production. NF-κB appears in multiple forms, with the most prevalent being inactive dimer combinations of its p50 and p65 subunits. NF-κB involves the rapid activation of primary transcription factors, including C-Jun and STATS, nuclear hormone receptors, and cytokines. NF-κB activation occurs after the stimulation of many cell-surface receptors. Activation results from a disinhibition of inhibitors of NF-κB called inhibitor of κBs (I-κBs). These I-κBs (including, I-κBα, I-κBβ, I-κBδ, I-κBε, and Bcl-3) are proteins that contain an ankyrin repeated sequence which mask the nuclear localization signal of NF-κB proteins and thereby keeps them in an inactivated state in the cytoplasm. Upon activation of I-κB kinase, the I-κB kinase phosphorylates two serine residues in one of the I-κB regulatory domains through ubiquitinations that lead I-κB to be degraded by proteosomes. Thereafter, the NF-κB complex translocates to the nucleus and activates genes with deoxyribonucleic acid (DNA) binding sites for NF-κB, such as proinflammatory cytokines, IL-1β, TNF-α, and IL-6. However, an auto-feedback loop occurs where translocated NF-κB transcribes I-κB to feedback and inhibit further NF-κB translocation.

NF-κB is involved in the regulation of sleep.[3] Many sleep regulatory substances activate NF-κB, including IL-1β and TNF-α. Additionally, many sleep regulatory substances are transcribed in response to NF-κB activation, including IL-1β, TNF-α, COX-2, iNOS, IL-2, and c-Fos. Conversely, many sleep regulatory substances that inhibit sleep also inhibit NF-κB activation, such as IL-4 and IL-10. There is a diurnal rhythm of cortical NF-κB levels with higher levels in the sleep period.[46] Further, the activation of cortical and lateral hypothalamic NF-κB expression increases following sleep deprivation. Peptide inhibition of NF-κB activation attenuates spontaneous sleep and IL-1β-enhanced sleep. In addition, NF-κB in cholinergic basal forebrain neurons may play a role in adenosine/sleep mechanisms. In contrast to the findings showing NF-κB activation-associated sleep enhancement, NF-κB p50 knockout mice have increased slow wave sleep and REM sleep.[47] These same mice have increased slow wave sleep and reduced REM sleep after lipopolysaccharide administration and more fragmented sleep after influenza administration, compared to control subjects administered identical pathogens.

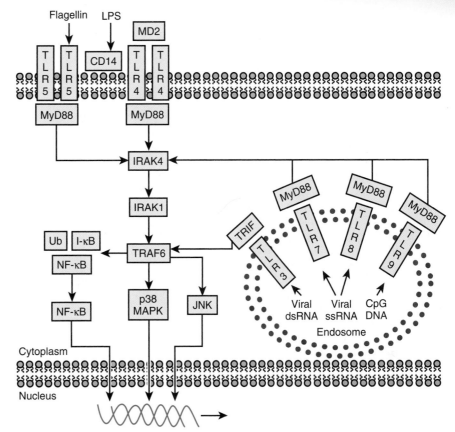

Figure 48-3 Toll-like receptors (TLRs) are pathogen recognition receptors (PRRs) that recognize bacterial and viral pathogens. The TLRs in turn activate pathways also activated by proinflammatory cytokines. The cell surface receptors TLR4 and TLR5 and the endosomal receptors TLR7, TLR8, and TLR9 signal through MyD88. MyD88 activates IRAK4/IRAK1 to signal TNF receptor associated factor 6 (TRAF6). The endosomal receptor TLR3 signals through the Toll/interleukin-1 receptor (TIR) domain containing adaptor-inducing interferon-β (TRIF) to signal TRAF6. TRAF6 activates NF-κB, p38 MAPK, and c-Jun N-terminal kinase (JNK). They in turn translocate to the nucleus and transcribe proinflammatory sleep regulatory substances such as IL-1β, TNF-α, and IL-6. *IL,* interleukin; *MAPK,* mitogen-activated protein kinase; *NF-κB,* nuclear factor-kappa B; *TNF,* tumor necrosis factor.

Mitogen-Activated Protein Kinase/ Extracellular Signal-Regulated Kinases Pathway

The MAPKs are extracellular signal-regulated protein kinases.[48] These enzymes mediate growth factor and cytokine receptor signaling. The MAPK/ERK pathway is activated by different heterotrimeric G proteins through scaffolds. In addition, G proteins modulate phospholipase C-beta to alter protein kinase C and calmodulin-dependent protein kinase II to stimulate or inhibit downstream mechanisms in the MAPK/ERK pathway. MAPKs are serine/threonine protein kinases that are activated by extracellular mitogens. Their cellular functions include cell survival/apoptosis, proliferation mitosis, and differentiation. MAPKs are stimulated by many growth factors including the sleep regulatory substances brain-derived neurotrophic factor (BDNF) and nerve growth factor (NGF). MAPKs also affect inflammation. In particular, p38 MAPK controls cellular responses to cytokines and stress.[49] Thus, MAPK p38 inhibitors inhibit the production of many proinflammatory cytokines, including IL-1β and TNF-α, and iNOS (discussed next).

There is currently little literature in the area of MAPKs and sleep. However, the fact that the MAPK/ERK pathway is involved in cytokine expression makes this link plausible. Further, MAPK p38 regulates certain aspects of circadian biology such as mediating TNFR1-induced increases in period 1 (Per1 mRNA).[32,50] The human immunodeficiency virus (HIV) gp120 component that activates the ERK pathway, increases calcium levels in rat brain cortical glia,[51] and increases NREM and REM sleep.[52] Further, c-Fos is affected by sleep loss, and

its stability is altered by MAPK.[53] Consequently, the MAPK/ERK pathway may be relevant to sleep and perhaps sleep disorders associated with pathologies.

Nitric Oxide

NO is involved in many physiologic and immunologic processes.[54,55] NO is synthesized from the terminal nitrogen of arginine in the presence of nicotinamide adenine dinucleotide phosphate (NADPH; reduced form) and dioxygen. This reaction is catalyzed by NOS. Different forms of NOS exist. Neuronal NOS (nNOS) is present in the central and peripheral nervous systems. Endothelial NOS (eNOS) is primarily found in blood vessels; NO is a vasodilator. iNOS modulates inflammation and immune functions and is produced by macrophages, monocytes, neutrophils, and microglia. Both nNOS and iNOS are implicated in sleep regulation.

Brain NO and iNOS increase during sleep deprivation.[56] The NO precursor, L-arginine, and other NO donors, including morpholinosydnonimine, or stress-activated protein kinase-interacting protein-1 (SIN-1), enhance NREM and REM sleep. Alternatively, iNOS inhibitors, including N-nitro-L-arginine-methyl-ester and 7-nitro-indazole inhibit sleep. In addition, mice lacking the iNOS gene have less NREM sleep and more REM sleep than control rats. NO production is influenced by multiple sleep regulatory substances including IL-1β, TNF-α, and GHRH. In addition, mice infected with influenza have marked increased NO levels in the lungs and iNOS and nNOS knockout mice have attenuated influenzavirus-induced sleep responses.[57] In summary, NO plays a role in sleep regulation in sickness and health.

Cyclooxygenase

COX is involved in the synthesis of prostanoids, such as prostaglandins, prostacyclin, and thromboxane.[58] COX converts arachidonic acid to prostaglandin H_2; this is the first step in prostanoid production and is the rate-limiting step in prostaglandin production. Three COX isoenzymes are currently known (COX-1, COX-2, and COX-3). COX-1 is constitutively expressed in most mammal cells, and COX-2 is inducible. COX-2 plays a role in inflammation; it is activated in macrophages by inflammatory signals. COX-3 is a splice variant of COX-1. Tissues including brain have various levels of endogenous COX-1 and COX-2.

Prostaglandin D_2 (PGD_2) seems to have a role in sleep regulation in mice, rats, monkeys, and humans.[59] For instance, COX-2 inhibition reduces spontaneous NREM sleep and TNF-α-induced sleep.[60] Lipopolysaccharide enhancement of PGD_2 and PGE_2 synthesis are both COX-2 dependent,[61,62] although PGE_2 inhibits sleep.[63] COX is induced by several sleep regulatory cytokines, including IL-1β and TNF-α.[58] In addition, the COX-2 inhibitor, diclofenac, inhibits TNF-α- and IL-1β-induced NREM sleep in rats.[64,65] Moreover, acetaminophen, a COX-1 and COX-2 inhibitor, inhibits sleep. The use of a selective COX-2 inhibitor (NS-398) requires a very high dose to inhibit spontaneous NREM sleep.[60] Although there is much evidence indicating the COX pathways mediate sleep, several issues remain to be resolved.

SLEEP AND PATHOGENS

For many millennia it has been recognized that good health is commonly associated with restful sleep. However, the mechanisms governing this association have been identified only in recent decades. One of the first endogenous sleep-promoting substances characterized was originally called *factor S*.[66] This substance was extracted and purified from human urine samples and rabbit brains and it was identified as a muramyl peptide similar in structure to monomeric muramyl peptides found in bacterial peptidoglycan.[67] That finding led to investigations on the effects of pathogens on sleep and the first description of changes in sleep over the course of an infection.[68] Those findings also led to the characterization of microbial component parts that are responsible for changing sleep.[36] Further investigations led to alterations in sleep as part of the acute phase response to infections (Box 48-2).

Bacteria are usually classified as being gram-negative or gram-positive.[1] Gram-negative bacteria, such as *Escherichia coli* and *Salmonella*, have cell walls containing peptidoglycan and lipopolysaccharide (LPS). Gram-negative bacteria and

> **BOX 48-2** *Characteristics of the Acute Phase Response*
>
> • Alterations in sleep
> • Fever (hypothermia in mice)
> • Reduced body weight
> • Leukocytosis
> • Increased cytokines, acute phase proteins, and complement proteins
> • Increased vascular permeability
> • Alterations in metabolism

LPS stimulate the innate immune system, in particular inflammation associated with enhanced proinflammatory cytokine activity. LPS binds to a receptor complex composed of Toll-like receptor 4 (TLR4), cluster of differentiation 14 (CD14), and myeloid differentiation 2 (MD2). When activated, this receptor complex stimulates proinflammatory cytokine pathways and consequent inflammation. In addition, LPS is pyrogenic and at high doses causes septic shock. These effects are mediated by the lipid A moiety of LPS that binds LPS to the bacterial membrane. LPS and its components, such as lipid A, are somnogenic in multiple species, including rabbits, rats, and mice.[36]

Gram-positive bacteria such as *Staphylococcus* and *Bacillus* contain larger amounts of the peptidoglycan in their cell wall and typically do not have LPS. Macrophages, including microglia, enzymatically degrade peptidoglycan to muramyl peptides.[1] Muramyl peptides in turn are recognized by nucleotide-binding oligomerization domain (NOD) proteins. Muramyl dipeptide, a substance initially isolated from the mycobacterial component of Freund's complete adjuvant, induces inflammatory cytokines including IL-1β, TNF-α, IL-6, and many others. Consequently, the sleep-promoting effects of muramyl dipeptide are due in part to enhanced proinflammatory cytokine release.

Alterations in sleep over the course of an infection were first experimentally studied in rabbits infected with gram-positive bacteria *Staphylococcus aureus*.[68] Within hours of infectious challenge NREM sleep is enhanced and REM sleep is inhibited. However, 20 hours following infection the animals have a prolonged reduction in NREM and REM sleep. The sleep effects occur concurrently with fever, fibrinogenemia, and neutrophilia. Other infectious agents, such as *Escherichia coli* and *Pasteurella multocida*, have similar effects, although the microbial species used, time of day, route of antigen entry, and prior sleep history influence the timing of the compensatory sleep responses.[36]

Influenza

Influenza is a negative sense RNA virus that affects many species.[69] Influenza induces an acute phase response characterized by fever (reduced body temperature in mice), airway inflammation and congestion, increased cytokine levels, headache, fatigue, gastrointestinal diarrhea or abdominal pain, and increased sleep.[36] Upon invasion of a cell, the positive RNA strand is synthesized and anneals with the negative sense viral RNA strand to form a double-stranded RNA (dsRNA). Viral dsRNA as well as synthetic dsRNAs, such as poly I:C, promote sleep. dsRNAs bind to the TLR3. Upon activation, the TLR3 induces multiple proinflammatory cytokines and chemokines, including IFN-α, IFN-β, IFN-γ, TNF-α, and IL-1β. Single-stranded RNA (ssRNA) and DNA bind to TLR7/8 and TLR9, respectively. The role of TLR7/8 and TLR9 in sleep remains uninvestigated, although ssRNA, whether viral or poly I or poly C, does not enhance sleep.

In humans, sleepiness and excessive sleep have been reported following influenza infection without altering other acute phase responses such as fever.[36] However, fever is a classic symptom associated with influenza infection in humans. In rabbits and mice, live influenzavirus, but not killed virus, increases sleep and fever (although mice exhibit reduced core body temperature). The exact brain mechanisms responsible for influenzavirus altered sleep remain incompletely understood. Viral RNA is found in the olfactory bulb shortly after intranasal challenge and enhanced olfactory bulb proinflammatory cytokine production occurs simultaneously.[70] If the olfactory tract is severed in mice, the onset of viral-induced hypothermia is delayed by about 15 hours, suggesting a role for olfactory bulb cytokines in influenza-induced hypothermia.[71] Although virus can locate to the olfactory bulb and induce inflammatory cytokines early after influenza infection,[70] other areas of the brain (e.g., the hypothalamus) are also likely involved in the sleep response to viral challenge. Regardless, the sleep-associated alterations from influenza manifest a few days after intranasal viral challenge in mice. These responses coincide with the time that the virus reaches the lungs. This suggests that sleep-inducing effects of influenza are not confined to the brain including the olfactory bulb, but also manifest via peripheral mechanisms such as the afferent vagal nerve input. Indeed, in rats, systemic cytokines, such as IL-1β, and LPS signal via the vagus nerve to induce cytokine production in the brain and enhance sleep.[72,73]

The magnitude and course of influenzavirus-induced sleep responses are dependent on endogenous sleep regulatory substances in the brain.[36] For instance, influenza-induced sleep changes are dependent on the expression of macrophage inflammatory protein 1α, suggesting the involvements of microglia in increasing sleep.[74] Mice that lack a functional GHRH receptor (i.e., lit/lit mice) have less spontaneous NREM and REM sleep compared to control mice.[75] In contrast to normal mice, influenza infection induces reduced NREM sleep in lit/lit mice.[76] Mice lacking the gene for nNOS have a greater suppression of REM sleep after influenza infection, but mice lacking the gene for iNOS have increased REM sleep and attenuated NREM sleep compared to control animals in response to viral challenge.[57] Further, mice lacking both TNF receptors have suppressed NREM sleep in response to influenza infection compared to control mice that have increased compensatory NREM sleep.[39] Consequently, the influenza-induced alterations in sleep are mediated by sleep regulatory substances and modulating these substances alters the acute phase response to influenza.

The immune-sleep interactions are complex when dealing with viruses. For instance, in humans, the level of antibodies generated from hepatitis A vaccine is attenuated following acute sleep deprivation.[77] A milder amount of sleep loss prior to influenza immunization attenuates anti-influenza IgG antibody titers 10 days after immunization.[78] However, the milder amount of sleep loss has no effect on influenza-induced antibody levels when the antibody titer is stabilized—approximately 3 weeks later. In mice, a bout of 7 hours of sleep deprivation has only minor effects on IgG catabolism.[79] It is noted, however, that the acute phase response effects occur through different mechanisms than those responsible for antibody production. Consequently, differences in sleep may not be predictors of individual immune parameters or the pathogenesis of influenza. In fact, sleep deprivation and influenza studies are inconsistent.[80-83] The discrepancies are likely due to differences in methodologies, such as length and type of sleep deprivation, time of day, viral preparation, and host immunologic status. Although speculative, the protective role of sleep deprivation on influenza might be attributed to the priming of the immune system by increasing proinflammatory cytokines and NF-κB. Enhanced cytokine levels, such as IL-1β, are associated with increased mortality and pathogenesis rates in response to influenza.[84] Moreover, certain other pathogenic challenges that follow sleep loss are protective. For instance, sleep restriction prior to B16 melanoma tumor cell implantation reduces metastasis in mice.[85] In addition, *D. melanogaster* that are sleep deprived prior to infection have enhanced resistance to bacteria mediated by NF-κB.[86]

Human Immunodeficiency Virus and Sleep

HIV is a retrovirus lentivirus. HIV infects humans and other primates, leading to acquired immunodeficiency syndrome (AIDS). The HIV infects immunogenic cells including CD4+ T helper cells, macrophages, and dendritic cells, thereby reducing their numbers and impairing the host's ability to combat pathogens.[87] The reduction in cell numbers occurs, in part, by the virus directly killing infected cells and increasing apoptosis, and by cytotoxic CD8+ T cells recognizing the infected cells and destroying them.

Individuals with HIV often have sleep complaints such as excessive daytime sleepiness, multiple awakenings during the night, and insomnia.[88] Adding to the complexity of this disease, many pharmaceuticals used in the treatment of HIV are associated with disturbances in sleep. Sleep disturbances tend to increase with the progression/severity of the disease. In asymptomatic patients with HIV-1 there are marked increases in slow wave sleep before the onset of AIDS.[89,90] Further, HIV is associated with decreased EEG slow wave activity.[91] Because individuals with HIV have impaired macrophage and glial cell functioning,[92] it is likely that these individuals cannot produce the typical cytokine responses necessary for normal sleep functioning. In support of this logic are the findings that individuals with HIV have impaired TNF-α release from macrophages.[87] Moreover, HIV infects microglia and when activated microglia secrete many substances involved in the regulation of sleep including IL-1β and TNF-α.[92]

PATHOGEN-ASSOCIATED MOLECULAR PATTERNS

Organisms rely on the innate immune system to recognize pathogen-associated molecular patterns (PAMPs).[93] PAMPs are conserved molecular constructs on pathogens. This recognition of pathogens is accomplished by pattern recognition receptors (PRRs) on certain cells. In the brain, glia are vital to pathogen recognition. Different types of PRRs lead to the activation of different intracellular molecular pathways including TLRs, retinoic acid–inducible gene-I-like receptors (RLRs), nucleotide-binding oligomerization domain-like receptors (NLRs), and DNA sensors. TLRs appear not to be able to recognize intracellular cytosolic pathogens and their components. However, viral ssRNA, dsRNA, and DNA, and derivatives of internalized or intracellular bacteria, are recognized by cytosolic PRRs including RLRs and NLRs. PRR activation by PAMPs results in proinflammatory and antimicrobial responses by activating multiple cellular pathways, including NF-κB, MAPK, and COX. Consequently, PAMPs activation of PRRs lead to the activation of many of the same molecules that alter sleep and inflammation, such as cytokines.

Toll-Like Receptors

TLRs are highly conserved among animals, from *D. melanogaster* to humans.[93] TLRs are integral glycoproteins with extracellular or luminal ligand binding domains with leucine-rich repeat motifs and a cytoplasmic signaling Toll/interleukin-1 receptor homology domain. Upon PAMP recognition, TLRs undergo receptor oligomerization to initiate intracellular signal transduction. A variety of cells, including macrophages, dendritic cells, B lymphocytes, and glia express TLRs on their cell surface or intracellularly within endosomal compartments. Currently, 11 TLRs are described in humans and 12 in mice. TLRs are classified by what they recognize; TLR1 (triacyl lipopeptides), TLR2 (glycolipids, lipopeptides, lipoproteins, lipoteichoic acid, HSP70, zymosan), TLR4 (LPS, certain heat shock proteins, fibrinogen), and TLR6 (diacyl lipopeptides) bind lipids, and TLR3 (dsRNA, poly I:C), TLR5 (flagellin), TLR8 (ssRNA), TLR9 (unmethylated CpG, oligodeoxynucleotide DNA), and TLR 11 (profilin) bind nucleic acids. The other TLR ligands have yet to be fully characterized. Upon activation of these TLRs the innate immune response initiates a large inflammatory response, which includes many sleep-regulatory substances such as IL-1β and TNF-α.

Nucleotide-Binding Oligomerization Domain-Like Receptor Family

NLRs are found in a variety of cells including glia. NOD1 and NOD2 detect bacterial components from the degradation of peptidoglycan. NOD1 senses diaminopimelic acid produced largely from gram-negative bacteria, and NOD2 recognizes muramyl dipeptide from both gram-positive and negative bacteria.[94] NOD1 and NOD2 activation leads to the activation of proinflammatory gene expression. NLRs induce a protein complex that catalyzes the cleavage of the IL-1 precursor, pro-IL-1, to IL-1.

Sleep and Pathogen-Associated Molecular Patterns

The role of PAMPs in sleep regulation is most notably demonstrated by muramyl dipeptides and LPS enhancing NREM sleep.[36] These pathogens are recognized by TLRs and activate cytokines including IL-1β and TNF-α to mediate sleep. Pathogenic viral dsRNAs and other dsRNAs that are also recognized as PAMPs by TLR3 are likely involved in the production of IL-1β and TNF-α as well as viral-induced interferons. Further, intracellular viral ssRNA and dsRNA activate the inflammation that induces cleavage of the pro-form of IL-1β into its mature active form.[95] In fact, mice lacking the TLR3, which recognizes dsRNA and activates cytokine synthesis, if infected with mouse-adapted influenzavirus have attenuated increases in NREM sleep, hypothermia, and body weight loss compared to the prototypical responses of normal mice infected with influenza.[96] Further, intracellular dsRNA that is produced during viral replication is also recognized by cytoplasmic PAMPs.[97] Thus, PAMPs play a crucial role in the recognition of pathogens that lead to the production of sleep regulatory cytokines and the acute phase response to infections.

INFLAMMATION AND SLEEP DISORDERS

Within the past few years our understanding of the causes and treatments of several sleep disorders has greatly improved. Recent findings indicate that certain sleep regulatory substances, such as cytokines, are associated with sleep-related disorders and may serve to help understand these disorders.[88]

In obstructive sleep apnea (OSA) the muscles of the soft palate encompassing the tongue and uvula relax and obstruct airway passage to temporarily stop breathing. This action disturbs sleep with brief arousals reducing EEG slow wave activity.[98] The hypoxia occurring in individuals with OSA is associated with inflammation. In addition, OSA is associated with cardiovascular disease, stroke, hypertension, obesity, and diabetes, all of which have chronic inflammation associated with them. These sleep-related disorders, such as OSA and insomnia, are linked to inflammation, but there remains a chicken-egg dilemma. Increased circulating inflammatory markers are associated with OSA, including C-reactive protein, TNF-α, IL-6, IL-8, and cellular adhesion molecules. Evidence also suggests that continuous positive airway pressure therapy reduces circulating TNF-α and IL-6 in patients with OSA.[99,100]

Individuals with insomnia have different EEG sleep patterns compared to noninsomniacs.[101] Notably, insomniacs have reduced EEG delta power at sleep onset,[102] and reduced theta and delta power during NREM and REM sleep compared to normal sleepers.[101] Further, many medical conditions are associated with insomnia and altered inflammation, including cardiovascular disease, gastrointestinal disorders, Parkinson's disease, asthma, and arthritis. In insomniacs, peak circulating IL-6 levels occur prior to sleep compared to normal sleepers; these changes might mediate the sleep pathogenesis. Also in humans, the peak in plasma TNF-α, which occurs close to waking in normal individuals, is absent in insomniacs, further indicating inflammatory cytokine disruption in this disease. Moreover, daytime plasma levels of IL-6 and TNF-α are elevated in insomniacs, and thereby might contribute to excess daytime sleepiness observed in these patients. There is also a correlation of insomnia with the removal of cytokines in patients undergoing chronic hemodialysis.[103] The cause of insomnia can vary greatly; however, stress is well known to induce insomnia and increase the sleep regulatory proinflammatory cytokines IL-1β, TNF-α, and IL-6.[23]

Sleep-regulatory inflammatory mediators likely play a role in the pathogenesis of sleep-related disorders. However, it is difficult to know if changes in plasma levels of inflammatory sleep regulatory substances are directly related to sleep disorders because sleep appears to be a fundamental property of local neuronal networks within the CNS. Nevertheless, it seems likely that changes in the array of circulating cytokines will provide useful clinical information because circulating cytokines affect the level of central cytokine expression. Further, there are transport mechanisms for cytokines from blood to brain. Thus, although currently speculative, assessing inflammatory sleep regulatory substances could be used in the future as an adjunct assessment of sleep-related disorders similar to current assessment of inflammatory biomarkers for diseases such as cancer. However, owing to the numerous diverse physiologic actions of cytokines their use for the treatment of sleep-related disorders seems unlikely at this time. Nonetheless, novel immunologic techniques for altering inflammatory molecules for many diseases are currently being investigated and show promise. Consequently, altering inflammatory sleep regulatory substances might play a vital role in future therapeutic interventions for certain sleep-related diseases.

CONCLUSION

Sleep and the immune system have a complex intertwining relationship. Many sleep regulatory substances are also mediators of inflammation. It is apparent that sleep has a host-defense function. Further, glial cells have a prominent role in modulating inflammation and interacting with neurons to regulate sleep. Sleep-related disorders have certain pathologies, some of which are associated with alterations in inflammation. Thus, targeting inflammatory and sleep regulatory substances or pathways may serve to aid in treating sleep-related disorders. Moreover, the treatment of sleep-related inflammatory pathways might serve to treat symptoms associated with certain pathogens or fight the pathogens themselves.

Acknowledgments

This work was supported in part by the National Institutes of Health, grant numbers NS25378, NS31453, and HD36520.

REFERENCES

1. Murphy KM, Travers P, Walport M. *Janeway's Immunobiology: The Immune System.* 7th ed. London: Garland Science; 2009.
2. Allada R, Siegel JM. Unearthing the phylogenetic roots of sleep. *Curr Biol.* 2008;18(15):R670-R679.
3. Krueger JM. The role of cytokines in sleep regulation. *Curr Pharm Des.* 2008;14(32):3408-3416.
4. Woollard KJ, Geissmann F. Monocytes in atherosclerosis: Subsets and functions. *Nat Rev Cardiol.* 2010;7(2):77-86.
5. Zeyda M, Stulnig TM. Obesity, inflammation, and insulin resistance—A mini-review. *Gerontology.* 2009;55(4):379-386.
6. Ye JH, Rajendran VM. Adenosine: An immune modulator of inflammatory bowel diseases. *World J Gastroenterol.* 2009;15(36):4491-4498.
7. Hamid Q, Tulic M. Immunobiology of asthma. *Annu Rev Physiol.* 2009;71:489-507.
8. Fantini MC, Pallone F. Cytokines: From gut inflammation to colorectal cancer. *Curr Drug Targets.* 2008;9(5):375-380.
9. Cappuccio FP, D'Elia L, Strazzullo P, et al. Quantity and quality of sleep and incidence of type 2 diabetes: A systematic review and meta-analysis. *Diabetes Care.* 2010;33(2):414-420.
10. Verkasalo PK, Lillberg K, Stevens RG, et al. Sleep duration and breast cancer: A prospective cohort study. *Cancer Res..* 2005;65(20):9595-9600.
11. Ayas NT, White DP, Manson JE, et al. A prospective study of sleep duration and coronary heart disease in women. *Arch Intern Med.* 2003;163(2):205-209.
12. Arnaud C, Dematteis M, Pepin JL, et al. Obstructive sleep apnea, immuno-inflammation, and atherosclerosis. *Semin Immunopathol.* 2009;31(1):113-125.
13. Kapsimalis F, Basta M, Varouchakis G, et al. Cytokines and pathological sleep. *Sleep Med.* 2008;9(6):603-614.
14. Trompet S, de Craen AJ, Slagboom P, et al. Genetic variation in the interleukin-1 beta-converting enzyme associates with cognitive function. The PROSPER study. *J Intern Med.* 2008;131(Pt 4):1069-1077.
15. Baune BT, Ponath G, Rothermundt M, et al. Association between genetic variants of IL-1beta, IL-6 and TNF-alpha cytokines and cognitive performance in the elderly general population of the MEMO-study. *Psychoneuroendocrinology.* 2008;33(1):68-76.
16. McAfoose J, Koerner H, Baune BT. The effects of TNF deficiency on age-related cognitive performance. *Psychoneuroendocrinology.* 2009;34(4):615-619.
17. Banks S, Dinges DF. Behavioral and physiological consequences of sleep restriction. *J Clin Sleep Med.* 2007;3(5):519-528.
18. Pickering M, O'Connor JJ. Pro-inflammatory cytokines and their effects in the dentate gyrus. *Prog Brain Res.* 2007;163:339-354.
19. Dantzer R. Cytokine-induced sickness behaviour: A neuroimmune response to activation of innate immunity. *Eur J Pharmacol.* 2004;500 (1-3):399-411.
20. Kundermann B, Hemmeter-Spernal J, Huber MT, et al. Effects of total sleep deprivation in major depression: Overnight improvement of mood is accompanied by increased pain sensitivity and augmented pain complaints. *Psychosom Med.* 2008;70(1):92-101.
21. Honore P, Donnelly-Roberts D, Namovic MT, et al. A-740003 [N-(1-{[(cyanoimino)(5-quinolinylamino) methyl]amino]-2,2-dimethylpropyl)-2-(3,4-dimethoxyphenyl)acetamide], a novel and selective P2X7 receptor antagonist, dose-dependently reduces neuropathic pain in the rat. *J Pharmacol Exp Ther.* 2006;319(3):1376-1385.
22. Kawasaki Y, Zhang L, Cheng JK, Ji RR. Cytokine mechanisms of central sensitization: Distinct and overlapping role of interleukin-1beta, interleukin-6, and tumor necrosis factor-alpha in regulating synaptic and neuronal activity in the superficial spinal cord. *J Neurosci.* 2008;28(20):5189-5194.
23. Anisman H, Merali Z. Cytokines, stress and depressive illness: Brain-immune interactions. *Ann Med.* 2003;35(1):2-11.
24. Vollmer-Conna U, Fazou C, Cameron B, et al. Production of pro-inflammatory cytokines correlates with the symptoms of acute sickness behavior in humans. *Psychol Med.* 2004;34:128–1297.
25. Obál Jr F, Krueger JM. Biochemical regulation of non–rapid-eye-movement sleep. *Frontiers Biosci.* 2003;8:520-550.
26. Moldofsky H. Sleep, neuroimmune and neuroendocrine functions in fibromyalgia and chronic fatigue syndrome. *Adv Neuroimmunol.* 1995;5(1):39-56.
27. Tringali G, Dello Russo C, Preziosi P, et al. Interleukin-1 in the central nervous system: From physiology to pathology. *Terapie.* 2000;55(1):171-175.
28. Omdal R, Gunnarsson R. The effect of interleukin-1 blockade on fatigue in rheumatoid arthritis—A pilot study. *Rheumatol Int.* 2005;25(6):481-484.
29. Legendre R, Pieron H. Recherches sur le besoin de sommeil consecutive a une veille prolongee. *Z Allg Physiol.* 1913;14:235-262.
30. Ishimori K. True causes of sleep—A hypnogenic substance as evidenced in the brain of sleep-deprived animals. *Tokyo Igakki Zasshi.* 1909;23:429-457.
31. Cavadini G, Petrzilka S, Kohler P, et al. TNF-alpha suppresses the expression of clock genes by interfering with E-box-mediated transcription. *Proc Natl Acad Sci.* 2007;104(31):12843-12848.
32. Petrzilka S, Taraborrelli C, Cavadini G, et al. Clock gene modulation by TNF-alpha depends on calcium and p38 MAP kinase signaling. *J Biol Rhythms.* 2009;24(4):283-294.
33. Dinarello CA. Immunological and inflammatory functions of the interleukin-1 family. *Annu Rev Immunol.* 2009;27:519-550.
34. Atkins E, Wood Jr WB. Studies on the pathogenesis of fever. I. The presence of transferable pyrogen in the blood stream following the injection of typhoid vaccine. *J Exp Med.* 1955;101(5):5519-5528.
35. Krueger JM, Walter J, Dinarello CA, et al. Sleep-promoting effects of endogenous pyrogen (interleukin-1). *Am J Physiol.* 1984;246(6 Pt 2): R994-R999.
36. Majde JA, Krueger JM. Links between the innate immune system and sleep. *J Allergy Clin Immunol.* 2005;116(6):1188-1198.
37. Kubota T, Fang J, Brown RA, et al. Interleukin-18 promotes sleep in rabbits and rats. *Am J Physiol Regul Integr Comp Physiol.* 2001;281(3):R828-R838.
38. Aggarwal BB. Signalling pathways of the TNF superfamily: A double-edged sword. *Nat Rev Immunol.* 2003;3(9):745-756.
39. Kapás L, Bohnet SG, Traynor TR, et al. Spontaneous and influenza virus-induced sleep are altered in TNF-alpha double-receptor deficient mice. *J Appl Physiol.* 2008;105(4):1187-1198.
40. Kishimoto T. Interleukin-6: From basic science to medicine—40 years in immunology. *Annu Rev Immunol.* 2005;23:1-21.
41. Xing Z, Gauldie J, Cox G, et al. IL-6 is an antiinflammatory cytokine required for controlling local or systemic acute inflammatory responses. *J Clin Invest.* 1998;101(2):311-320.
42. Opp MR. Cytokines and sleep. *Sleep Med Rev.* 2005;9(5):355-364.
43. Guan Z, Vgontzas AN, Omori T, et al. Interleukin-6 levels fluctuate with the light-dark cycle in the brain and peripheral tissues in rats. *Brain Behav Immun.* 2005;19(6):526-529.
44. Wang S, Liu Z, Wang L, et al. NF-kappaB signaling pathway, inflammation and colorectal cancer. *Cell Mol Immunol.* 2009;6(5):327-334.
45. O'Neill LA, Kaltschmidt C, NF-kappa B. A crucial transcription factor for glial and neuronal cell function. *Trends Neurosci.* 1997;20(6):252-258.
46. Chen Z, Gardi J, Kushikata T, et al. Nuclear factor-kappaB-like activity increases in murine cerebral cortex after sleep deprivation. *Am J Physiol.* 1999;276(6 Pt 2):R1812-R1818.
47. Jhaveri KA, Ramkumar V, Trammell RA, et al. Spontaneous, homeostatic, and inflammation-induced sleep in NF-kappaB p50 knockout mice. *Am J Physiol Regul Integr Comp Physiol.* 2006;291(5):R1516-R1526.
48. Anjum R, Blenis J. The RSK family of kinases: Emerging roles in cellular signaling. *Nat Rev Mol Cell Biol.* 2008;9(10):747-758.

49. Schieven GL. The p38alpha kinase plays a central role in inflammation. *Curr Top Med Chem.* 2009;9(11):1038-1048.

50. de Paula RM, Lamb TM, Bennett L, et al. A connection between MAPK pathways and circadian clocks. *Cell Cycle.* 2008;7(17):2630-2634.

51. Codazzi F, Menegon A, Zacchetti D, et al. HIV-1 gp120 glycoprotein induces [Ca^{2+}]i responses not only in type-2 but also type-1 astrocytes and oligodendrocytes of the rat cerebellum. *Eur J Neurosci.* 1995;7(6):1333-1341:1.

52. Opp MR, Rady PL, Hughes Jr TK, et al. Human immunodeficiency virus envelope glycoprotein 120 alters sleep and induces cytokine mRNA expression in rats. *Am J Physiol.* 1996;270(5 Pt 2):R963-R970.

53. Tanos T, Marinissen MJ, Leskow FC, et al. Phosphorylation of c-Fos by members of the p38 MAPK family. Role in the AP-1 response to UV light. *J Biol Chem.* 2005;280(19):18842-18852.

54. Murphy S, Gibson CL. Nitric oxide, ischaemia and brain inflammation. *Biochem Soc Trans.* 2007;35(Pt 5):1133-1137.

55. Brown GC, Bal-Price A. Inflammatory neurodegeneration mediated by nitric oxide, glutamate, and mitochondria. *Mol Neurobiol.* 2003;27(3):325-355.

56. Gautier-Sauvigné S, Colas D, Parmantier P, et al. Nitric oxide and sleep. *Sleep Med Rev.* 2005;9(2):101-113.

57. Chen L, Duricka D, Nelson S, et al. Influenza virus-induced sleep responses in mice with targeted disruptions in neuronal or inducible nitric oxide synthases. *J Appl Physiol.* 2004;97(1):17-28.

58. Choi SH, Aid S, Bosetti F. The distinct roles of cyclooxygenase-1 and -2 in neuroinflammation: Implications for translational research. *Trends Pharmacol Sci.* 2009;30(4):174-181.

59. Hayaishi O, Urade Y. Prostaglandin D2 in sleep-wake regulation: Recent progress and perspectives. *Neuroscientist.* 2002;8(1):12-15.

60. Yoshida H, Kubota T, Krueger JM. A cyclooxygenase-2 inhibitor attenuates spontaneous and TNF-alpha-induced non-rapid eye movement sleep in rabbits. *Am J Physiol Regul Integr Comp Physiol.* 2003;285(1):R99-109.

61. Hori M, Kita M, Torihashi S, et al. Upregulation of iNOS by COX-2 in muscularis resident macrophage of rat intestine stimulated with LPS. *Am J Physiol Gastrointest Liver Physiol.* 2001;280:G930-G938.

62. Rouzer CA, Jacobs AT, Nirodi CS, et al. RAW264.7 cells lack prostaglandin-dependent autoregulation of tumor necrosis factor-alpha secretion. *J Lipid Res.* 2005;46:1027-1037.

63. Masek K, Kadlecová O, Pöschlová N. Effect of intracisternal administration of prostaglandin E1 on waking and sleep in the rat. *Neuropharmacology.* 1976;15(8):491-494.

64. Terao A, Matsumura H, Yoneda H, et al. Enhancement of slow-wave sleep by tumor necrosis factor-alpha is mediated by cyclooxygenase-2 in rats. *Neuroreport.* 1998;9(17):3791-3796:1.

65. Terao A, Matsumura H, Saito M. Interleukin-1 induces slow-wave sleep at the prostaglandin D2-sensitive sleep-promoting zone in the rat brain. *J Neurosci.* 1998;18(16):6599-6607.

66. Pappenheimer JR, Koski G, Fencl V, et al. Extraction of sleep-promoting factor S from cerebrospinal fluid and from brains of sleep-deprived animals. *J Neurophysiol.* 1975;38(6):1299-1311.

67. Krueger JM, Pappenheimer JR, Karnovsky ML. Sleep-promoting effects of muramyl peptides. *Proc Natl Acad Sci U S A.* 1982;79(19):6102-6106.

68. Toth LA, Krueger JM. Alteration of sleep in rabbits by *Staphylococcus aureus* infection. *Infect Immun.* 1988;56(7):1785-1791.

69. Scholtissek C, Hinshaw VS, Olsen CW. Influenza in pigs and their role as the intermediate host. In: Nicholson KG, Webster RG, Hay A, eds. *Textbook of Influenza.* Oxford: Blackwell Healthcare; 1998.

70. Majde JA, Bohnet SG, Ellis GA, et al. Detection of mouse-adapted human influenza virus in the olfactory bulbs of mice within hours after intranasal infection. *J Neurovirol.* 2007;13(5):399-409.

71. Leyva-Grado VH, Churchill L, Harding J, et al. The olfactory nerve has a role in the body temperature and brain cytokine responses to influenza virus. *Brain Behav Immun.* 2010;24(2):281-288.

72. Hansen MK, Krueger JM. Subdiaphragmatic vagotomy blocks the sleep- and fever-promoting effects of interleukin-1beta. *Am J Physiol.* 1997;273(4 Pt 2):R1246-R1253.

73. Kapás L, Hansen MK, Chang HY, et al. Vagotomy attenuates but does not prevent the somnogenic and febrile effects of lipopolysaccharide in rats. *Am J Physiol.* 1998;274(2 Pt 2):R406-R411.

74. Toth LA, Hughes LF. Macrophage participation in influenza-induced sleep enhancement in C57BL/6J mice. *Brain Behav Immun.* 2004;18(4):375-389.

75. Obal Jr F, Alt J, Taishi P, et al. Sleep in mice with nonfunctional growth hormone-releasing hormone receptors. *Am J Physiol Regul Integr Comp Physiol.* 2003;284(1):R131-R139.

76. Alt JA, Obal Jr F, Traynor TR, et al. Alterations in EEG activity and sleep after influenza viral infection in GHRH receptor-deficient mice. *J Appl Physiol.* 2003;95(2):460-468.

77. Lange T, Perras B, Fehm HL, et al. Effect of sleep deprivation on response to immunization. *Psychosom Med.* 2003;65(5):831-835.

78. Spiegel K, Sheridan JF, Van Cauter E. Effect of sleep deprivation on response to immunization. *JAMA.* 2002;288(12):1471-1472.

79. Renegar KB, Floyd R, Krueger JM. Effect of sleep deprivation on serum influenza-specific IgG. *Sleep.* 1998;21(1):19-24.

80. Renegar KB, Floyd RA, Krueger JM. Effects of short-term sleep deprivation on murine immunity to influenza virus in young adult and senescent mice. *Sleep.* 1998;21(3):241-248.

81. Renegar KB, Crouse D, Floyd RA, et al. Progression of influenza viral infection through the murine respiratory tract: The protective role of sleep deprivation. *Sleep.* 2000;23(7):859-863.

82. Toth LA, Rehg JE. Effects of sleep deprivation and other stressors on the immune and inflammatory responses of influenza-infected mice. *Life Sci.* 1998;63(8):701-709.

83. Brown R, Pang G, Husband AJ, et al. Suppression of immunity to influenza virus infection in the respiratory tract following sleep disturbance. *Reg Immunol.* 1989;2(5):321-325.

84. Schmitz N, Kurrer M, Bachmann MF, et al. Interleukin-1 is responsible for acute lung immunopathology but increases survival of respiratory influenza virus infection. *J Virol.* 2005;79(10):6441-6448.

85. Zielinski MR, Davis JM, Wyatt Jr WC, et al. Effects of chronic sleep restriction and exercise training on metastasis. *Med Sci Sports Exerc.* 2007;39(Suppl 5):S62.

86. Williams JA, Sathyanarayanan S, Hendricks JC, et al. Interaction between sleep and the immune response in *Drosophila*: A role for the NFkappaB relish. *Sleep.* 2007;30(4):389-400.

87. Herbein G, Khan KA. Is HIV infection a TNF receptor signalling-driven disease? *Trends Immunol.* 2008;29(2):61-67.

88. Parish JM. Sleep-related problems in common medical conditions. *Chest.* 2009;135(2):563-572.

89. Norman SE, Chediak AD, Kiel M, et al. Sleep disturbances in HIV-infected homosexual men. *AIDS.* 1990;4(8):775-781.

90. Norman SE, Chediak AD, Freeman C, et al. Sleep disturbances in men with asymptomatic human immunodeficiency (HIV) infection. *Sleep.* 1992;15(2):150-155.

91. Darko DF, Mitler MM, White JL. Sleep disturbance in early HIV infection. *Focus.* 1995;10(11):5-6.

92. Persidsky Y, Poluektova L. Immune privilege and HIV-1 persistence in the CNS. *Immunol Rev.* 2006;213:180-194.

93. Mogensen TH. Pathogen recognition and inflammatory signaling in innate immune defenses. *Clin Microbiol Rev.* 2009;22(2):240-273.

94. Franchi L, Eigenbrod T, Muñoz-Planillo R, et al. The inflammasome: A caspase-1-activation platform that regulates immune responses and disease pathogenesis. *Nat Immunol.* 2009;10(3):241-247.

95. Allen IC, Scull MA, Moore CB, et al. The NLRP3 inflammasome mediates in vivo innate immunity to influenza A virus through recognition of viral RNA. *Immunity.* 2009;30(4):556-565.

96. Majde JA, Kapás L, Bohnet SG, et al. Attenuation of the influenza virus sickness behavior in mice deficient in Toll-like receptor 3. *Brain Behav Immun.* 2010;24(2):306-315.

97. Eisenacher K, Steinberg C, Reindl W, et al. The role of viral nucleic acid recognition in dendritic cells for innate and adaptive antiviral immunity. *Immunobiology.* 2008;212:701-714.

98. McNicholas WT. Chronic obstructive pulmonary disease and obstructive sleep apnea: Overlaps in pathophysiology, systemic inflammation, and cardiovascular disease. *Am J Respir Crit Care Med.* 2009;180(8):692-700:15.

99. Minoguchi K, Tazaki T, Yokoe T, et al. Elevated production of tumor necrosis factor-alpha by monocytes in patients with obstructive sleep apnea syndrome. *Chest.* 2004;126(5):1473-1479.

100. Yokoe T, Minoguchi K, Matsuo H, et al. Elevated levels of C-reactive protein and interleukin-6 in patients with obstructive sleep apnea syndrome are decreased by nasal continuous positive airway pressure. *Circulation.* 2003;107(8):1129-1134.

101. Basta M, Chrousos GP, Vela-Bueno A, et al. Chronic insomnia and stress system. *Sleep Med Clin.* 2007;2(2):279-291.

102. Merica H, Blois R, Gaillard JM. Spectral characteristics of sleep EEG in chronic insomnia. *Eur J Neurosci.* 1998;10(5):1826-1834.

103. Bornivelli C, Alivanis P, Giannikouris I, et al. Relation between insomnia mood disorders and clinical and biochemical parameters in patients undergoing chronic hemodialysis. *J Nephrol.* 2008;21(Suppl 13):S78-S83.

Sleep-Related Gastroesophageal Reflux Disease

SUSAN M. HARDING

Chapter 49

Gastroesophageal reflux disease (GERD) is characterized by the abnormal reflux of gastric contents into the esophagus and potentially to more proximal sites, including the pharynx and the lungs. Esophageal manifestations of GERD include heartburn, regurgitation, chest pain, dysphagia, esophageal stricture, and Barrett's esophagus, a predisposing condition to esophageal adenocarcinoma.[1] Symptoms and manifestations of GERD are not limited to the esophagus. Gastroesophageal reflux is a cause of cough, is a co-factor or trigger of asthma, and commonly coexists with and has impact upon idiopathic pulmonary fibrosis, chronic obstructive pulmonary disease (COPD), and bronchiolitis obliterans syndrome (BOS) in lung transplant recipients.[2]

Gastroesophageal reflux also occurs during sleep along with the potential for microaspiration and macroaspiration of gastric contents into the upper airway and lungs.[3] *Sleep-related GERD* is defined as GERD symptoms that are associated with sleep disturbances, arousals, early morning awakenings, unrefreshing sleep, daytime functioning difficulties, and excessive daytime sleepiness.[4,5] Furthermore, sleep-related laryngospasm is often caused by GERD, and GERD is prevalent in patients with obstructive sleep apnea (OSA).[6]

This chapter will review esophageal function during sleep and how sleep-related GERD presents, and then will discuss potential therapeutic options. Finally, disease states associated with sleep-related GERD will be discussed.

ESOPHAGEAL FUNCTION DURING SLEEP

Sleep influences esophageal function with physiologic changes noted during the transition from wake to sleep, with arousals, from one sleep stage to another, and from sleep to wake.[5] Box 49-1 reviews these changes.[7-15] The lower esophageal sphincter (LES) is the primary antireflux barrier and if the LES pressure is low, reflux events can occur.[16] Transient LES relaxations (TLESRs) are brief LES relaxations that are not associated with a swallow and are the primary reflux mechanism.[16] TLESRs occur during brief arousals and during wakefulness, so that reflux events during sleep occur primarily during arousals.[15] Delayed gastric emptying also predisposes to reflux.[8] The upper esophageal sphincter (UES) protects against aspiration, and UES pressure decreases during sleep.[10] Esophageal acid clearance depends on acid neutralization with saliva and swallowing, which triggers primary peristalsis.[13] Because sleep affects many of these mechanisms, sleep predisposes to GERD. Also, events causing arousals, including periodic limb movements and apneas, could trigger TLESRs and reflux events.[15] Medications that decrease the arousal response, such

as benzodiazepines, prolong esophageal refluxate clearance and may also predispose to aspiration.[17]

DIAGNOSING SLEEP-RELATED GERD

Sleep-related GERD is associated with prolonged reflux episodes, higher esophagitis grades, Barrett's esophagus, and esophageal adenocarcinoma.[18,19] Up to 75% of patients with GERD experience sleep-related GERD symptoms.[20] Symptoms of sleep-related GERD include multiple awakenings, substernal burning, heartburn, chest discomfort, sour or bitter taste in the mouth, regurgitation, water brash, coughing or choking, and excessive daytime sleepiness without a cause, even in the absence of esophageal symptoms.[21,22] Box 49-2 reviews findings associated with sleep-related GERD.[4,5]

Diagnostic testing is not required to make the diagnosis of sleep-related GERD.[4,6] However, esophageal pH testing, especially when combined with esophageal impedance monitoring, is very helpful in difficult or refractory cases. Esophageal pH monitoring is performed by placing pH probes intranasally, 5 cm above the LES. Probes may also be placed in other positions including near the UES and even in the pharynx. An acid reflux event is defined as an event when the pH dips below 4. It is usually performed for a 24-hour period with the patient recording mealtimes and symptoms. There is an event marker on the portable data acquisition device if a patient experiences symptoms during monitoring. Data is reported as the percentage of time when pH is less than 4. Normal value at the distal probe (5 cm above the LES) is a total less than 5.8%, upright value less than 8.2%, and supine (sleep time) value less than 3.5%. Proximal probe (just below the UES) normal value is a total time pH value less than 4 of 1.1%, upright value less than 1.7%, and supine (sleep time) value less than 0.6%.[23] Esophageal pH testing can be interpreted with polysomnography to assess the temporal relationship of reflux events with other sleep events.[24] Depending on the digital polysomnography (PSG) system, the pH data can be integrated directly onto a single montage. The signal from the data recorder will need to be split so that the pH data can be recorded both in the polysomnographic and in the pH system. If pH and PSG equipment are not fully compatible for data integration, the pH data can be time synchronized to polysomnography by hitting the event button on the pH data acquisition device to signal lights out or during a specific time during calibration. Catheter-free, wireless pH systems are also available and are deployed into the esophagus, usually by endoscopy.[25] Combined esophageal pH-impedance monitoring can assess both acid and nonacid reflux events.[26] Testing is recommended

---

BOX 49-1 *Events Affecting Reflux during Sleep*

- Basal gastric acid secretion peaks between 8 PM and 1 AM.[7]
- Sleep delays gastric emptying by disrupting gastromyoelectric function.[8]
- Saliva secretion ceases during sleep.[9]
- Swallowing does not occur during sleep and requires an arousal.[10]
- Sleep facilitates proximal refluxate migration.[11]
- Esophageal refluxate clearance is prolonged during sleep and requires an arousal.[12,13]
- Upper esophageal sphincter pressure decreases with sleep onset, predisposing to aspiration.[10]
- Reflux events tend to occur during the first two hours of sleep time.[14]
- Transient LES relaxations occur primarily during arousals.[15]

LES, lower esophageal sphincter.

BOX 49-2 *Associated Findings in Sleep-Related Gastroesophageal Reflux Disease*

- Sleep onset and sleep maintenance insomnia
- Poor daytime functioning
- Excessive daytime sleepiness
- Daytime fatigue
- Reduced work productivity
- Decreased health-related quality of life
- More health care provider visits
- Laryngospasm during sleep
- Asthma symptoms during sleep
- Obstructive sleep apnea

BOX 49-3 *Behavioral Approaches to Management of Sleep-Related Gastroesophageal Reflux Disease (GERD)*

- Weight loss if obese (BMI > 30)
- Sleeping in loose-fitting clothes
- No meals within 2 to 3 hours of bedtime
- Avoidance of foodstuffs that promote GERD
  - High fat-containing foods
  - Caffeine
  - Chocolate
  - Mint
  - Alcohol
  - Carbonated beverages (pH of 1.0 and CO_2 gas)
- Avoidance of acidic foods or those that precipitate GERD symptoms—for example:
  - Citrus fruits/citrus products
  - Tomato-based products
  - Spicy foods
  - Red wine
- Smoking cessation
- Positional therapy
  - Head of bed elevation
  - Left lateral decubitus sleeping position
- Treatment of primary sleep disorders that can disrupt sleep architecture
- Ensuring a sleep environment that is conducive to sleep
- Use of antacids and alginic acid with acute GERD symptoms

BMI, body mass index.

---

when patients have continued GERD symptoms despite GERD therapy.[24]

THERAPY OF SLEEP-RELATED GERD

Therapy of sleep-related GERD improves sleep quality, improves airway function in asthmatics with nocturnal asthma symptoms, reduces laryngospasm events during sleep, and reduces the apnea-hypopnea index (AHI) in some patients with OSA and GERD.[27-31] Furthermore, the interplay between OSA and GERD may be bidirectional so that the OSA events might influence GERD and GERD may influence OSA events.[31-33]

Therapy includes behavioral approaches, medications, endoscopic esophageal manipulations, surgical approaches, and nasal continuous positive airway pressure (CPAP). Although most of these therapies were not developed specifically for sleep-related GERD, careful attention to chronotherapeutic principles helps ensure adequate GERD control during sleep time.

Behavioral Approaches

Behavioral approaches are very important in the management of sleep-related GERD. Medications currently available in the United States for GERD suppress gastric acid secretion and

do not alter the motility disorder, the primary GERD mechanism.[34,35] Behavioral or lifestyle modification approaches should be integrated with medical and other therapies. Box 49-3 reviews these approaches.

Obesity is a risk factor for GERD development.[36] Abdominal fat increases intra-abdominal pressure, and thus gastric pressure, impeding the LES barrier. Although improvement in daytime GERD symptoms is noted with weight loss in obese patients, results vary. Nonetheless, weight loss should be recommended. Tight-fitting bed clothes can also impact LES function and should be avoided.[35]

Meal timing is important because gut motility is reduced during sleep.[8] Patients should avoid meals for at least 2 hours before bedtime. Small meals are preferable. In 261 asthmatic patients and 218 control subjects, Sontag and associates noted that 50% of the asthmatics had awakenings during sleep from heartburn and 33% of the asthmatics had suffocation, cough, or wheezing preceded by heartburn or regurgitation during sleep.[37] Sixty percent of these asthmatics ate right before bedtime and this timing was related to having reflux symptoms during sleep.[37]

Avoidance of foods that promote reflux is also important.[34,35] High-fat foods decrease gastric motility and emptying.[38] Caffeine lowers LES pressure and impairs adenosine-mediated sleep mechanisms.[39] Chocolate and mints, including peppermint, also lower LES pressure, as does alcohol.[40] Alcohol disrupts sleep and is associated with arousals that could trigger TLESRs and, thus, reflux events. Carbonated sodas have a pH of 1 and the release of CO_2 gas causes gastric distention that can trigger TLESRs.[41] Also important is avoidance of acidic foods or foods that are known to cause symptoms for the patient. These foods include citrus juices (orange juice has a pH of approximately 3), tomato-based products, red wine, and spicy foods. Unfortunately, avoidance of enjoyable foods is hard to do, so recommendations are to avoid these foods late in the day. Enjoy your chocolate with lunch instead of dinner!

Smoking worsens GERD. Nicotine lowers LES pressure and impacts sleep architecture.[42] Furthermore, smoking decreases salivation. Saliva contains bicarbonate and liquid. Swallowing initiates primary esophageal peristalsis that delivers saliva to the esophagus. Esophageal clearance occurs in two stages—volume clearance and acid neutralization. Most of the refluxate volume is cleared with the first two or three swallows, but a coating of acid material remains and subsequent swallows are required to deliver saliva for acid neutralization. If the patient is not open to smoking cessation, recommend smoking abstinence for an hour or more before bedtime.[43]

Positional therapy, including head of bed elevation and sleeping in the left lateral decubitus position, can reduce reflux. Head of bed elevation can be achieved by placing a wedge under the mattress or by placing 6- to 8-inch blocks under the legs at the head of the bed.[44] Pillows are not effective. A small study noted that reflux episodes were more frequent in the supine position and occurred less frequently in the left lateral decubitus position.[45]

Although these approaches have not been systematically evaluated in sleep-related GERD, a recent evidence-based review supported the effectiveness of weight loss and head of bed elevation.[46]

Finally, treatment of sleep disorders can decrease arousals and improve sleep-related symptoms. Also, ensure that the sleep environment is conducive to sleep. Animals and snoring bed partners can cause arousals!

Antacids

Current evidence-based guidelines developed by the American Gastroenterological Association Institute (AGAI) on the management of GERD include over-the-counter medications as part of behavioral therapy.[34,35] Acid secretion blockers will be discussed in the next section. Antacids provide acute symptom relief, but play no role in preventing sleep-related GERD. Alginates (alginic acid) may offer protection against the damaging effects of the refluxate.[47] Alginates (Gaviscon) have been available for more than 30 years and many formulations are available in different countries using various combinations of alginates and antacids. Gastric acid or other gelling agents such as aluminum hydroxide or bicarbonate combine with the alginates to form a raft or gel that floats on top of the gastric juice and forms a physical barrier.[48] Because many formulations contain aluminum, caution should be used in patients with kidney disease to avoid aluminum toxicity.[48] In experimental models, this alginate "raft" inhibited pepsin and the damaging effects of bile acids to the esophageal mucosa. Although alginates do not alter reflux itself, they may decrease the "toxicity" of the gastric refluxate to the esophagus and other sites, including extraesophageal sites. More investigation is needed in this area.

BOX 49-4 *Medications to Avoid with Sleep-Related Gastroesophageal Reflux Disease (GERD)*

MEDICATIONS THAT PROMOTE GERD
- Nitrates
- Calcium antagonists
- Benzodiazepines
- Tricyclic antidepressants
- Prostaglandins
- Bisphosphonates
- Progesterone
- Nicotine
- Oral corticosteroids (prednisone)
- Theophylline and aminophylline
- β_2-Adrenergic receptor agonists

MEDICATIONS THAT DECREASE SKELETAL MUSCLE TONE OR LOWER AROUSAL THRESHOLD DURING SLEEP
- Opioids
- Benzodiazepines
- Nonbenzodiazepine hypnotics
- Other sedatives and hypnotics

Avoidance of Medications That Can Potentiate GERD

Medications that potentiate GERD, lower skeletal muscle tone, or impair the arousal response during sleep should be reviewed to determine if the risk-benefit ratio indicates that it is best to discontinue the medication. Box 49-4 lists these medications. Medications can potentiate GERD by altering esophageal motility, lowering LES pressure, or increasing gastric acid secretion.[49] Intravenous (IV) and oral theophylline and aminophylline increase gastric acid secretion and decrease LES pressure.[50,51] Ekström and Tibbling[52] examined asthmatics with GERD while on and off their usual dose of oral slow-release theophylline and noted that GERD symptoms increased 170%, and that esophageal acid contact time increased 24%.[52] This effect was more pronounced in asthmatics with therapeutic theophylline levels. Although not used as commonly for treatment of nocturnal asthma and COPD, consider using lower doses of these medications if possible.

Oral or intravenous β_2-receptor agonists decrease LES pressure, but there are conflicting data concerning their impact on GERD.[53,54] Repeated doses of nebulized albuterol (β_2-receptor agonist) reduce LES pressure in a dose-dependent manner and decrease esophageal contraction amplitude.[55,56] This finding may have an impact on asthmatics, especially during exacerbations. No data are available on the long-acting inhaled β_2-receptor agonists frequently used today. The oral corticosteroid, prednisone, 60 mg for 7 days, increased esophageal acid contact times during sleep time and over the 24-hour period in asthmatics.[57]

Furthermore, medications that decrease skeletal muscle tone or reduce the arousal response should be avoided. The use of benzodiazepines was a predictor of heartburn during sleep in the more than 15,000 subjects of the Sleep Heart Health Study ($p < 0.0001$).[17] Also, zolpidem, the most commonly prescribed nonbenzodiazepine medication for sleep, decreases the arousal threshold.[58] Because the arousal response is vital for esophageal clearance of refluxate during sleep, it may impact sleep-related GERD. Gagliardi and associates[58] examined 16 GERD patients and 8 control subjects in a placebo-controlled, crossover study design using zolpidem 10 mg or placebo while performing esophageal pH testing combined with polysomnography. Zolpidem significantly increased esophageal acid contact times for individual reflux events compared with placebo during sleep ($p < 0.05$). Reflux events were associated with arousal or awakening 40% of the time with zolpidem compared to 89% with placebo ($p < 0.01$). The effect of zolpidem waned after the first 3 hours (elimination half-life of zolpidem is 2.5 hours). Because most GERD events occur during the first 2 hours of sleep, this finding may be significant.[14] Also, sleep-related GERD is a cause of insomnia and zolpidem is commonly prescribed, zolpidem may worsen GERD and thus the insomnia. Although more data are needed, this effect has the potential to extend to other medications in this class.

Medical Therapy of Sleep-Related GERD

Medications used to treat sleep-related GERD include acid-suppressive medications, prokinetic agents, and medications that inhibit TLESRs.[34,35]

Acid-Suppressive Medications

Acid-suppressive medications include H_2 receptor antagonists and proton pump inhibitors (PPIs). They suppress gastric acid secretion and reduce the acidity of the refluxate but *do not prevent reflux episodes*.[34,35] H_2 receptor antagonists were introduced in the 1970s. Box 49-5 lists H_2 receptor antagonists available. They have equal clinical efficacy if they are dosed correctly. Cimetidine has a higher potential for drug interactions, including clopidogrel. Dosing prior to bedtime suppresses gastric acid during the sleep period.

However, if symptoms are severe enough to cause sleep disruption, PPIs offer superior gastric acid suppression and should be considered first-line medical therapy. They were introduced in the late 1980s and have faster resolution rates for heartburn and esophagitis compared to H_2 receptor antagonists (H$_2$RAs).[34,35] They are most effective if the drug levels are high during meals when the gastric parietal cell is stimulated to secrete acid such that dosing of PPIs should be given 30 minutes *before* meals and not before bedtime. A formulation of dexlansoprazole does not require dosing before meals.[59] Box 49-5 reviews the PPIs currently available. Although many studies have compared PPIs to one another, and there are differences noted between PPIs, these differences are usually not clinically important in most patients.[60] Some patients may note a better response with a certain PPI compared to others. Currently, two PPIs (omeprazole and lansoprazole) are available for over-the-counter use in the United States. Omeprazole has the highest potential for drug interactions with digoxin, carbamepazine, warfarin, diazepam, phenytoin, and clopidogrel. Esomeprazole also has the potential for drug interactions, although to a lesser extent than omeprazole.[60] Omeprazole and esomeprazole inhibit the CYP2C19 enzyme, which converts clopidogrel into its active metabolite such that its antiplatelet activity is reduced, potentially placing patients at risk for myocardial infarction and stroke. The levels of CYP2C19 inhibition of the other PPIs vary. The Food and Drug Administration

---

BOX 49-5 *Potential Medications for Sleep-Related Gastroesophageal Reflux Disease (GERD)*

GASTRIC ACID SECRETION BLOCKERS
Histamine H_2 Receptor Antagonists
- Cimetidine, up to 800 mg twice a day, 400 mg four times a day
- Ranitidine, 150 mg twice a day
- Nizatidine, 150 mg twice a day
- Famotidine, 20 mg twice a day

Proton Pump Inhibitors
- Omeprazole, 20 mg daily or twice a day
- Esomeprazole, 20 mg or 40 mg daily or twice a day
- Lansoprazole, 30 mg daily or twice a day
- Dexlansoprazole, 30 mg or 60 mg daily
- Rabeprazole, 20 mg daily or twice a day
- Pantoprazole, 40 mg daily or twice a day

PROKINETIC AGENTS
Dopamine Receptor Antagonists
- Metaclopramide, 10 mg, four times a day
  FDA Black Box Warning (AGAI guidelines recommend not using this medication)
- Domperidone (non-USA) side effects related to hyperprolactinemia
- Itopride (non-USA)

Serotonergic Agents
- Mosapride (non-USA)

Motility Receptor Agonists
- Erythromycin
- Azithromycin
- Alemcinal (investigational)
- Mitemcinal (investigational)

Ghrelin Agonists (investigational)

ANTI-TLESR THERAPY
GABA-β Receptor Agonists
- Baclofen, 5 mg up to 20 mg, three times daily

Cholecystokinin Receptor Antagonists
- Loxiglumide (investigational)
- Mitemcinal (investigational)

Anticholinergics
- Atropine

Cannabinoid Receptor Agonists (investigational)

AGAI, American Gastroenterological Association Institute; *anti-TLESR*, anti–transient lower esophageal sphincter relaxation; *FDA*, U.S. Food and Drug Administration; *GABA-β*, gamma-aminobutyric acid-beta.

(FDA) issued a public health advisory stating that omeprazole and esomeprazole should not be taken with clopidogrel.[61] Cimetidine received the same FDA advisory (Food and Drug Administration, Nov. 17, 2009).[61] Lansoprazole and dexlansoprazole interact with theophylline. Pantoprazole has the lowest potential for drug interactions. Rabeprazole has a slightly faster onset of action. There is no need to decrease the dose of PPIs in patients with renal or hepatic disease.

Although nocturnal acid breakthrough (NAB) is noted during gastric pH monitoring in up to 70% of patients taking twice daily PPIs, there is no relationship between NAB and sleep-related GERD symptoms.[62] Early reports note that adding an H₂RA at bedtime controlled NAB; however, subsequent investigations note that a rapid tolerance develops after 1 week of therapy.[63,64]

In general, H₂RAs and PPIs are safe. Data suggest that their use increases the risk of community acquired pneumonia by 30%.[65] Long-term PPI therapy may decrease vitamin B_{12} absorption, so consider assessing vitamin B_{12} levels periodically.[66] Both H₂RA blockers and PPIs increase the risk of *Clostridium difficile* infection with the risk being higher with PPI use.[67] Data from the Women's Health Initiative notes that PPI use in postmenopausal women was modestly associated with spine, forearm or wrist, and total fractures, but use of PPIs was not associated with hip fractures. Use of PPIs was also associated with only a marginal effect on 3- to 4-year bone mineral density at the hip ($p = 0.05$), but not at other sites. The FDA issued a warning about this possible increased risk of bone fracture with the use of PPIs for a year or longer or at high doses.[68,69]

The use of acid suppressive therapy in pregnant women is not considered first-line therapy. More data are available with ranitidine and cimetidine, although PPIs have also been used.[70,71] Most H₂RAs and PPIs are classified as category B from the FDA for use during pregnancy.[71] The risk-benefit ratio to the individual needs to be carefully assessed before recommending their use during pregnancy.

Prokinetic Agents

Gastroesophageal reflux is a *motility disorder*, and *acid inhibitors do not impact reflux itself*—they just alter the pH of the refluxate. Unfortunately, prokinetic agents available for use in the United States that increase LES pressure, esophageal contractility and improve gastric motility are limited. The only medication available is metoclopramide, which now has an FDA black box warning.[72] Furthermore, evidence-based guidelines of the AGAI recommend *against* the use of metoclopramide.[34,35] Central nervous system (CNS) side effects, including drowsiness, irritability, and extra-pyramidal effects, are noted in 20% to 50% of patients taking metoclopramide. These side effects may not improve after discontinuing the drug.[73] Other prokinetic medications are outlined in Box 49-5. Hopefully, prokinetic agents that are currently being developed will show efficacy and be safe to use.

Inhibition of Transient Lower Esophageal Sphincter Relaxations

Since TLESRs are a major mechanism of reflux events, inhibition of TLESRs is a viable therapeutic option. Currently, only baclofen is available for clinical use. Baclofen reduces the frequency of TLESRs by approximately 50% and reflux events by 43%. Baclofen also increases LES pressure and gastric emptying rates.[74] However, baclofen crosses the blood-brain barrier and induces dizziness, lightheadedness, sleepiness, weakness, and trembling, thus limiting its current use to only refractory patients. Medications are currently being developed with better side effect profiles.

Endoscopic Therapies

Innovative endoscopic techniques are available as a potential alternative to medical and surgical GERD therapies.[75-82] One technique includes sewing stitches to form plications 1 cm below the Z-line (demarcating the squamocolumnar mucosal junction at the gastroesophageal junction) as well as at the 3, 6, and 9 o'clock positions for the circumferential position, and at 3, 2, and 1 cm below the Z-line for the linear configuration (Bard Endocinch).[76] The plication can also be formed by utilizing a suture-based implant device delivered just below the gastroesophageal junction (NDO plicator).[77,78] There are other proprietary devices available, some having more published experience analyzing outcomes than others.[77] Some endoscopic techniques were taken off the market because of safety concerns, including the Stretta procedure, which delivered radiofrequency energy to the LES.[79]

Despite advancements in techniques, none of these procedures are completely effective in controlling esophageal acid exposure, GERD symptoms, healing esophagitis, or freeing patients from having to take GERD medications.[80] Furthermore, the most recent AGAI Medical Position Statement on the Management of GERD gives grade insufficiency—that is, no recommendation is made because of insufficient evidence to recommend for or against its use.[34,35] There are no data examining outcomes in patients with sleep-related GERD. Be aware of these techniques because they are currently being marketed directly to consumers (Endogastric Solutions, EsophyX).[81] Future research may elicit their possible role.[80,82] At this time, there is insufficient evidence to recommend their use in treating sleep-related GERD.

Surgical Techniques for Sleep-Related GERD

Multiple funduscopic surgical techniques are available utilizing open or laparoscopic techniques for GERD therapy.[83] Specific operative techniques include the Nissen fundoplication, the Roselti-Nissen, the Toupet (a 270-degree wrap), the Hill gastropexy, and the Belsey Mark IV operation that uses a transthoracic approach.[84] The Roux-en-Y gastric bypass technique is used in bariatric surgery for morbidly obese patients who also have GERD.[85] Careful preoperative evaluation of potential surgical candidates is critical. Preoperative evaluation should include esophageal manometry, endoscopy, assessment of esophageal length, and objective GERD documentation. Surgical complications include vagal nerve injury, chest herniation, slipped fundoplication, dysphagia, and gas bloat symptoms.[84] Potential surgical indications include refractory GERD with symptoms despite medical therapy, esophagitis, and GERD associated with recurrent aspiration.[86]

In general, surgical success rates approach 90%. Long-term outcomes at 12-year follow-up comparing surgery versus omeprazole maintenance therapy for esophagitis show that 53% of patients in the surgically treated group remained in continuous remission versus 45% of patients in the omeprazole group that included dose adjustment ($p = 0.022$).[87] However, up to 62% of the surgically treated patients used GERD medications regularly at a median follow-up of 10 years in a prospective randomized trial comparing medical and surgical therapy, so surgery does not necessarily replace the need for GERD medications.[88] Success is improved by ensuring that the surgeon has good outcomes data and has adequate experience.[89] There is a learning curve, especially with laparoscopic techniques. There are minimal outcomes data in patients with sleep-related GERD, so careful selection of potential surgical candidates is essential, as well as careful evaluation by a gastroenterologist and a surgeon before recommending surgery.

Nasal Continuous Positive Airway Pressure

Nasal continuous positive airway pressure is a potential therapy for sleep-related GERD. It is especially useful in patients with OSA.[90] Green and associates[90] noted that OSA patients with sleep-related GERD who were compliant with CPAP therapy had a 48% reduction in sleep-related GERD symptoms ($p < 0.001$). There was also an association between higher CPAP pressures and GERD symptom improvement. Noncompliant CPAP patients had no improvement in their sleep-related GERD symptoms.[90] Ing and associates[91] noted that CPAP decreased esophageal acid contact times and the number of reflux episodes in 14 OSA patients and 8 control subjects. Tawk and associates[92] noted that 1 week of CPAP use in 16 OSA patients with an AHI greater than 20 and abnormal esophageal acid contact times decreased esophageal acid contact times during sleep from 16.3% ± 18.8% to 3.8% ± 7.6% with CPAP ($p < 0.01$).

Nasal CPAP improves LES barrier function.[93] Shepherd and associates[93] examined 10 healthy awake subjects in the supine position with and without 15 cm H_2O of nasal CPAP while monitoring esophageal and gastric manometry. Nasal CPAP increased intrathoracic pressure, which decreased the pressure gradient across the diaphragm. It also increased LES pressure, esophageal pressure, and gastric pressure, and decreased the duration of LES relaxation associated with swallows.[93]

Nasal CPAP also improves sleep-related esophageal symptoms associated with complicated esophageal diseases, including achalasia. Nasal CPAP can also be considered in patients without OSA who have uncontrolled sleep-related GERD despite aggressive behavioral and medical GERD therapy.[94]

SPECIFIC OUTCOMES IN DISEASE STATES ASSOCIATED WITH SLEEP-RELATED GERD

Reflux during sleep time can impair sleep, affect asthma during sleep, cause laryngospasm during sleep, and potentially affect OSA. Gastroesophageal reflux disease is a chronic disease that impacts around 7% of the adult population daily. Sleep-related GERD is more injurious than diurnal GERD. We previously reviewed symptoms of sleep-related GERD. Shaker and associates,[95] in a telephone-based survey by the Gallup Organization of 1000 persons experiencing heartburn at least once weekly, noted that 79% of the respondents reported heartburn during sleep and 75% of them reported that heartburn affected their sleep. Forty percent of respondents believed that this resulted in impairment of their daytime functioning.[95] Despite taking prescription GERD medication, only 49% reported adequate control of their sleep-related GERD symptoms.[95]

Medical GERD therapy improves sleep outcomes. For instance, Chand and colleagues[96] examined 18 consecutive patients without esophagitis and examined GERD symptoms, the Pittsburgh Sleep Quality Index (PSQI), and 48 hours of actigraphy at baseline and then at 1, 4, and 8 weeks of taking esomeprazole 40 mg 30 to 60 minutes before breakfast. The PSQI decreased from 8.5 to 4.5 at 4 weeks (> 5 indicates poor sleep). However, actigraphy did not change with treatment.[96] Johnson and associates[27] performed a large double-blind, placebo-controlled trial of 650 subjects with heartburn and sleep disturbance occurring 3 days a week with esomeprazole

20 mg, esomeprazole 40 mg, or placebo taken before breakfast. The primary outcome was relief of nighttime heartburn with secondary outcomes including PSQI, relief of the sleep disturbance, and work productivity.[27] Compared to placebo, both doses of esomeprazole improved sleep-related heartburn ($p < 0.0001$), increased the number of nights without GERD-related sleep disturbance ($p < 0.001$), and normalized sleep on the PSQI ($p < 0.001$).[27] DiMarino and associates[97] examined the effect of omeprazole on arousals, awakening, and sleep efficiency.[97] Omeprazole decreased the number of arousals from 11.6 ± 3.8 to 1.5 ± 0.8 ($p < 0.05$), the number of awakenings from 3.7 ± 0.9 to 1.3 ± 0.5 ($p < 0.05$), and increased sleep efficiency from 70.2% to 81.6% ($p < 0.05$). Thus, PPI therapy improves sleep-related GERD outcomes. No study thus far has addressed long-term therapy outcomes.

Sleep-Related GERD and Asthma

Nocturnal asthma or sleep-related asthma is characterized by an exaggeration of the normal circadian variation in lung function, airway inflammation, and heightened bronchial reactivity. Most asthma deaths occur between 6 PM and 3 AM. Gastroesophageal reflux is a potential asthma trigger.[98] Epidemiologic studies confirm the association of sleep-related GERD and asthma. Gislason and colleagues reviewed a subset of the European Community Respiratory Health Survey of 2661 participants. Asthma was more frequent in subjects with sleep-related GERD (9% vs. 4%).[99] Furthermore, sleep-related GERD was associated with wheeze (odds ratio [OR] 2.5, 95% confidence interval [CI] 1.6-3.9), sleep-related chest tightness (OR 2.3, 95% CI 1.4-3.8), cough during sleep time (OR 3.0, 95% CI 1.9-4.9), and asthma diagnosis (OR 2.2, 95% CI 1.0-4.7).[99] Gunnbjörnsdottir and associates[100] followed up the 16,191 participants of this same survey and noted that sleep-related GERD was independently related to asthma onset.

Sleep-related GERD also affects airway function. Cuttitta and associates[101] monitored esophageal pH and respiratory resistance in seven asthmatics with sleep-related GERD. During monitoring, 72 GERD episodes occurred lasting less than 5 minutes, and 29 lasted more than 5 minutes. Both long and short GERD episodes were associated with higher respiratory resistance compared to baseline. A significant correlation was also noted between respiratory resistance and GERD episode duration during sleep.[101]

Treatment of sleep-related GERD may improve asthma. In a multicenter, double-blind, placebo-controlled trial utilizing esomeprazole 40 mg twice daily for 16 weeks in 770 asthmatics, esomeprazole improved peak expiratory flow rates in asthmatics with sleep-related asthma and GERD symptoms.[28]

Sleep-Related GERD and Obstructive Sleep Apnea

Gastroesophageal reflux is prevalent in OSA patients.[31,102-108] Valipour examined 135 consecutive OSA patients and noted that 58% had "heartburn" or regurgitation.[102] The relationship between OSA and GERD is complex and may be bidirectional. For instance, Morse and colleagues noted no relationship between AHI and heartburn severity index in 136 subjects referred to the sleep laboratory; however, disturbed sleep quality was affected by GERD severity.[103] Also, a causal relationship between OSA and GERD was not found in a study by Kim and associates.[104] They examined 1023 consecutive patients referred for OSA. Utilizing a validated GERD questionnaire, gastroesophageal reflux symptoms did not correlate with OSA variables including apnea severity.[104] A temporal association between respiratory events and GERD events was present in approximately 70% of events. Furthermore, most GERD events occurred during stage N2 sleep (62%) followed by arousals (26%). They concluded that arousals may not be the primary cause of the GERD event.[104] Potentially a low basal LES pressure during sleep may be important in OSA patients with GERD and not TLESRs. This hypothesis is supported by Sabaté and associates[106] who noted similar findings in 68 obese subjects of whom 40% had both GERD and OSA. The presence of GERD correlated with low basal LES pressure ($p = 0.031$). They also found no relationship between esophageal pH data and AHI. Using state-of-the-art esophageal manometry during sleep, Kuribayashi and associates[107] that end-inspiratory UES and gastroesophageal junction pressure increases during obstructive sleep apnea events in OSA subjects without a hiatal hernia. Thus, these esophageal motor events actually augment the antireflux barrier during OSA events. More research is needed in this area.

Treatment of OSA with CPAP improves GERD symptoms and esophageal acid contact times as previously discussed. Surgical therapy for OSA also improved AHI and esophageal acid contact times.[108] Thirty-two OSA patients with abnormal esophageal acid contact times underwent uvulopharyngopalatoplasty, inferior turbinate reduction, and nasal septoplasty. At the 6-month follow-up, there was a notable reduction in the mean AHI from 51.2 ± 23.1 to 14.5 ± 10.0 and improvement in esophageal acid contact times (percentage of time pH < 4 dropped from 10.3% ± 5.2% to 4.5% ± 2.9%). A correlation was noted between AHI and arousal index and reduction in esophageal acid contact times ($r = 0.607, 0.730$; $p < 0.002$).[108] Furthermore, in a small trial without a placebo arm, 29 OSA patients treated with esomeprazole 40 mg daily for 2 to 6 months noted an improvement of the AHI from 37.9 ± 18.1 to 24.8 ± 11.5 ($p < 0.006$).[31] Epworth Sleepiness Scale improved from 14.2 ± 2.5 to 11.1 ± 2.4 ($p < 0.0001$).[31] Note that PPI therapy did not normalize the AHI or the Epworth Sleepiness Scale, so the clinical importance of this finding is limited. This does point out that the relationship between OSA and GERD may be a bidirectional one. Future research will further delineate how sleep-related GERD can affect OSA and vice-versa.

Sleep-Related GERD and Laryngospasm

Sleep-related laryngospasm presents as an abrupt awakening from sleep with an intense sensation of inability to breathe and stridor. The differential diagnosis includes OSA, epilepsy, panic disorder, sleep choking syndrome, sleep terrors, vocal cord dysfunction, sleep-related GERD without laryngospasm, and other upper airway pathologic processes. Thurnheer and associates[29] reported a case series of 10 patients and noted that patients reported abrupt interruptions of sleep accompanied by feelings of acute suffocation with an "apnea" period lasting 5 to 45 seconds, followed by stridor.[29] Nine of 10 patients had abnormal esophageal acid contact times by esophageal pH monitoring and six responded to medical GERD therapy.

COORDINATING THERAPY OF SLEEP-RELATED GERD

Because treatment of sleep-related GERD improves multiple outcomes, treatment should initially be aggressive, with a step-down approach in medication after there is adequate control of sleep-related GERD.

Education and implementation of behavioral therapy for sleep-related GERD should be carried out in all patients as outlined in Box 49-6. Furthermore, primary sleep disorders should be screened for, diagnosed, and treated, because arousals from these disorders could impact GERD by triggering TLESRs. Randomized, placebo-controlled trials evaluated sleep-related GERD with twice daily PPIs, which should be given 30 minutes *before* breakfast and dinner.[27] Because sleep-related GERD is associated with more severe esophagitis grade, Barrett's esophagus, and adenocarcinoma of the esophagus, consider referring the patient to a gastroenterologist for upper endoscopy, especially in the presence of dysphagia.[34,35]

Response to GERD therapy should be monitored with diaries. Potential outcomes to monitor include nocturnal awakenings, heartburn and regurgitation during sleep, and

---

BOX 49-6 *Therapy of Sleep-Related Gastroesophageal Reflux Disease (GERD)*

- **Educate and implement behavioral GERD therapy** (see Boxes 49-3 and 49-4).
- **Screen, diagnose, and treat primary sleep disorders that could cause arousals, including obstructive sleep apnea and periodic limb movement disorder.**
- **Begin twice-daily PPI therapy, 30 minutes before breakfast and dinner.**
- **Consider referral to gastroenterologist for endoscopy if dysphagia is present or as outlined by AGAI guidelines.[34,35]**
- **At 2-month follow-up, has sleep-related GERD improved?**
  If yes: Consider stepdown therapy:
  - **Once-daily PPI therapy, 30 minutes before dinner.**
  - **Consider changing PPI to H$_2$RA at bedtime.**
  - **Continue behavioral GERD therapy.**
  - **Selected patients may desire surgical fundoplication (refer to AGAI guidelines).[34,35]**
  If no: Consider combined esophageal pH impedance monitoring while patient is on sleep-related GERD therapy:
  GERD not controlled:
  - **Refer to gastroenterologist.**
  - **Consider the addition of CPAP during sleep or prokinetic agents at bedtime (if non-USA*) along with referral to gastroenterologist for further evaluation of treatment options for refractory GERD.**
  GERD controlled:
  - **Symptoms may not be GERD-related. Consider repeating combined esophageal pH impedance monitoring after discontinuing PPI therapy for 7 days.**
  - **Refer to gastroenterologist.**

*The only prokinetic agent available in the United States is metoclopramide, which has severe nervous system side effects and is not recommended for use.

AGAI, American Gastroenterological Association Institute; CPAP, continuous positive airway pressure; H$_2$RA, histamine H$_2$ receptor antagonist; PPI, proton pump inhibitor.

the Epworth Sleepiness Scale. If symptoms markedly improve after 2 months of medical GERD therapy, then step-down therapy can be implemented as outlined in Box 49-6. If symptoms return after implementing step-down therapy, then stepping back up to the previous PPI dosing is indicated.

If outcomes are not improved after 2 months of therapy, then evaluation of GERD is indicated. Optimal investigation should include combined esophageal pH-impedance monitoring done while the patient remains on medical GERD therapy. Referral to a gastroenterologist for endoscopy should be considered if not done so already. If no significant reflux is present and symptoms continue, consider other diagnoses that could be causing symptoms. Next, consider discontinuing medical GERD therapy for 7 days and repeat esophageal pH-impedance monitoring.

Although not evaluated in controlled trials, if significant GERD is still present on esophageal testing while on medical GERD therapy, then consider adding a prokinetic medication (outside the United States). Unfortunately, metoclopramide is the only prokinetic agent available in the United States, and its use is associated with potentially nonreversible neurologic sequelae, including tardive dyskinesia, so its use is not recommended. Other prokinetic agents are approved for GERD outside the United States that are not available in the United States. Adding nasal CPAP therapy or surgical fundoplication can also be considered. A careful evaluation by a gastroenterologist is recommended for refractory sleep-related GERD.

SUMMARY

Sleep-related GERD disrupts sleep, causes arousals, leads to excessive daytime sleepiness, impairs daytime functioning, and is associated with esophagitis and Barrett's esophagus. Sleep-related GERD can impact airflow obstruction in asthmatics, cause laryngospasm during sleep, and is often present in OSA patients. Management of sleep-related GERD includes behavioral, medical, and surgical interventions. No long-term data are available to determine the best long-term therapeutic options. Nasal CPAP therapy improves sleep-related GERD and is especially useful in patients with OSA; however, it can also be used in patients with refractory sleep-related GERD. Esophageal testing is recommended in those patients who do not improve with behavioral therapy and twice daily PPIs. Surgical fundoplication can improve sleep-related GERD in selected patients. Treatment of sleep-related GERD improves multiple outcomes including the number of awakenings from sleep, daytime functioning, and Epworth Sleepiness Scale. Hopefully, prokinetic medications will be developed to better address GERD. Future research will determine optimal long-term therapeutic options for sleep-related GERD.

REFERENCES

1. Richter JE. The many manifestations of gastroesophageal reflux disease: Presentation, evaluation, and treatment. *Gastroenterol Clin North Am.* 2007;36(3):577-599.
2. Fass R, Achem SR, Harding S, et al. Supra-oesophageal manifestations of gastro-oesophageal reflux disease (GERD) and the role of nighttime gastro-oesophageal reflux. *Aliment Pharmacol Therapeut.* 2004;20(suppl 9):26-38.
3. Highland KB, Harding SM. GERD-related lung disease. GERD in the 21st century, Series #15. *Pract Gastroenterol.* 2005;29(10):74-80.
4. Gerson LB, Fass R. A systematic review of the definitions, prevalence, and response to treatment of nocturnal gastroesophageal reflux disease. *Clin Gastroenterol Hepatol.* 2009;7(4):372-378.
5. Harding SM. Sleep-related gastroesophageal reflux: Evidence is mounting. *Clin Gastroenterol Hepatol.* 2009;7(9):919-920.
6. Harding SM. Gastroesophageal reflux during sleep. *Sleep Med Clin.* 2007;2(1):41-50.
7. Moore JG. Circadian dynamics of gastric acid secretion and pharmacodynamics of H_2 receptor blockade. *Ann N Y Acad Sci.* 1991;618:150-158.
8. Elsenbruch S, Orr WC, Harnish MJ, et al. Disruption of normal gastric myoelectric functioning by sleep. *Sleep.* 1999;22(4):453-458.
9. Schneyer LH, Pigman W, Hanahan L, et al. Rate of flow of human parotid, sublingual, and submaxillary secretion during sleep. *J Dent Res.* 1956;35(1):109-114.
10. Kahrilas PJ, Dodds WJ, Dent J, et al. Effect of sleep, spontaneous gastroesophageal reflux, and a meal on upper esophageal sphincter pressure in normal human volunteers. *Gastroenterology.* 1987;92(2):466-471.
11. Orr WC, Elsenbruch S, Harnish MJ, et al. Proximal migration of esophageal acid perfusions during waking and sleep. *Am J Gastroenterol.* 2000;95(1):37-42.
12. Orr WC, Johnson LF, Robinson MG. The effect of sleep on swallowing, esophageal peristalsis, and acid clearance. *Gastroenterology.* 1984;86(5 Pt 1):814-819.
13. Orr WC, Johnson LF. Responses to different levels of esophageal acidification during waking and sleep. *Dig Dis Sci.* 1998;43(2):241-245.
14. Hila A, Castell DO. Nighttime reflux is primarily an early event. *J Clin Gastroenterol.* 2005;39(7):579-583.
15. Freidin N, Fisher MJ, Taylor W, et al. Sleep and nocturnal acid reflux in normal subjects and patients with reflux oesophagitis. *Gut.* 1991;32(11):1275-1279.
16. Mittal RK, Balaban DH. The esophagogastric junction. *N Engl J Med.* 1997;336(13):924-932.
17. Fass R, Quan SF, O'Connor GT, et al. Predictors of heartburn during sleep in a large prospective cohort study. *Chest.* 2005;127(5):1654-1666.
18. Adachi K, Fujishiro H, Katsube T, et al. Predominant nocturnal acid reflux in patients with Los Angeles grade C and D reflux esophagitis. *J Gastroenterol Hepatol.* 2001;16(11):1191-1196.
19. Dickman R, Parthasarathy S, Malagon IB, et al. Comparisons of the distribution of oesophageal acid exposure throughout the sleep period among the different gastro-oesophageal reflux diseases groups. *Aliment Pharmacol Ther.* 2007;26(1):41-48.
20. Farup C, Kleinman L, Sloan S, et al. The impact of nocturnal symptoms associated with gastroesophageal reflux disease on health-related quality of life. *Arch Intern Med.* 2001;161(1):45-52.
21. Mody R, Bolge SC, Kannan H, et al. Effects of gastroesophageal reflux disease on sleep and outcomes. *Clin Gastroenterol Hepatol.* 2009;7(9):953-959.
22. Jansson C, Nordenstedt H, Wallander MA, et al. A population-based study showing an association between gastroesophageal reflux disease and sleep problems. *Clin Gastroenterol Hepatol.* 2009;7(9):960-965.
23. Harding SM, Richter JE, Guzzo MR, et al. Asthma and gastroesophageal reflux: Acid suppressive therapy improves asthma outcomes. *Am J Med.* 1996;100(4):398-405.
24. Sexton MW, Harding SM. Sleep-related reflux: A unique clinical challenge. *J Resp Dis.* 2003;24(9):398-406.
25. Ayazi S, Lipham JC, Portale G, et al. Bravo catheter-free pH monitoring: Normal values, concordance, optimal diagnostic thresholds, and accuracy. *Clin Gastroenterol Hepatol.* 2009;7(1):60-67.
26. Mainie I, Tutuian R, Shay S, et al. Acid and non-acid reflux in patients with persistent symptoms despite acid suppressive therapy: A multicenter study using combined ambulatory impedance pH monitoring. *Gut.* 2006;55(10):1398-1402.
27. Johnson DA, Orr WC, Crawley JA, et al. Effect of esomeprazole on nighttime heartburn and sleep quality in patients with GERD: A randomized placebo-controlled trial. *Am J Gastroenterol.* 2005;100(9):1914-1922.
28. Kiljander TO, Harding SM, Field SK, et al. Effects of esomeprazole 40 mg twice daily on asthma therapy: A randomized, placebo-controlled trial. *Am J Respir Crit Care Med.* 2005;173(9):1090-1097.
29. Thurnheer R, Henz S, Knoblauch A. Sleep-related laryngospasm. *Eur Respir J.* 1997;10(9):2084-2086.
30. Senior BA, Khan M, Schwimmer C, et al. Gastroesophageal reflux and obstructive sleep apnea. *Laryngoscope.* 2001;111(12):2144-2146.
31. Friedman M, Gurpinar B, Lin HC, et al. Impact of treatment of gastroesophageal reflux on obstructive sleep apnea-hypopnea syndrome. *Ann Otol Rhinol Laryngol.* 2007;116(11):805-811.
32. Lipan MJ, Reidenberg JS, Laitman JT. Anatomy of reflux: A growing health problem affecting structures of the head and neck. *Anat Rec B New Anat.* 2006;289(6):261-270.

33. Nguyen AT, Jobin V, Payne R, et al. Laryngeal and velopharyngeal sensory impairment in obstructive sleep apnea. *Sleep*. 2005;28(5):585-593.
34. Kahrilas PJ, Shaheen NJ, Vaezi MF. American Gastroenterological Association Institute; Clinical Practice and Quality Management Committee. American Gastroenterological Association Institute technical review on the management of gastroesophageal reflux disease. *Gastroenterology*. 2008;135(4):1392-1413.
35. Kahrilas PJ, Shaheen NJ, Vaezi MF, et al. American Gastroenterological Association. American Gastroenterological Association Medical Position Statement on the management of gastroesophageal reflux disease. *Gastroenterology*. 2008;135(4):1383-1391.
36. Hampel M, Abraham NS, El-Serag HB. Meta-analysis: Obesity and the risk for gastroesophageal reflux disease and its complications. *Ann Intern Med*. 2005;143:199-211.
37. Sontag SJ, O'Connell S, Miller TQ, et al. Asthmatics have more nocturnal gasping and reflux symptoms than nonasthmatics, and they are related to bedtime eating. *Am J Gastroenterol*. 2004;99(5):789-796.
38. Becker DJ, Sinclair J, Castell DO, et al. A comparison of high and low fat meals on postprandial esophageal acid exposure. *Am J Gastroenterol*. 1989;84(7):782-786.
39. Pehl C, Pfeiffer A, Wendl B, et al. The effect of decaffeination of coffee on gastro-oesophageal reflux in patients with reflux disease. *Aliment Pharmacol Ther*. 1997;11(3):483-486.
40. Vitale GC, Cheadle WG, Patel B, et al. The effect of alcohol on nocturnal gastroesophageal reflux. *JAMA*. 1987;258(15):2077-2079.
41. Holloway RH, Hongo M, Berger K, et al. Gastric distention: A mechanism for postprandial gastroesophageal reflux. *Gastroenterology*. 1985;89(4):779-784.
42. Kahrilas PJ, Gupta RR. Mechanisms of acid reflux associated with cigarette smoking. *Gut*. 1990;31:4-10.
43. Waring JP, Eastwood TF, Austin JM, Sanowski RA. The immediate effects of cessation of cigarette smoking on gastroesophageal reflux. *Am J Gastroenterol*. 1989;84(9):1076-1078.
44. Hamilton JW, Boisen RJ, Yamamoto DT, et al. Sleeping on a wedge diminishes exposure of the esophagus to refluxed acid. *Dig Dis Sci*. 1998;33(5):518-522.
45. Khoury RM, Camacho-Lobato L, Katz PO, et al. Influence of spontaneous sleep positions on nighttime recumbent reflux in patients with gastroesophageal reflux disease. *Am J Gastroenterol*. 1999;94(8):2069-2073.
46. Kaltenbach T, Crockett S, Gerson LB. Are lifestyle measures effective in patients with gastroesophageal reflux? An evidence-based approach. *Arch Intern Med*. 2006;166(9):965-971.
47. Strugala V, Avis J, Joliffe IG, et al. The role of an alginate suspension on pepsin and bile acids—key aggressors in the gastric refluxate. Does this have implications for the treatment of gastro-oesophageal reflux disease? *J Pharm Pharmacol*. 2009;61(8):1021-1028.
48. Dettmar PW, Hampson VC, Taubel J, et al. The suppression of gastro-oesophageal reflux by alginates. *Int J Clin Pract*. 2007;61(10):1654-1662.
49. Lagergren J, Bergström R, Adami HO, et al. Association between medications that relax the lower esophageal sphincter and risk for esophageal adenocarcinoma. *Ann Intern Med*. 2000;133(3):165-175.
50. Johannesson N, Andersson KE, Joelsson B, et al. Relaxation of lower esophageal sphincter and stimulation of gastric secretion and diuresis by antiasthmatic xanthines. Role of adenosine antagonism. *Am Rev Respir Dis*. 1985;131(1):26-30.
51. Stein MR, Towner TG, Weber TW, et al. The effect of theophylline on the lower esophageal sphincter pressure. *Ann Allergy*. 1980;45(4):238-241.
52. Ekström T, Tibbling L. Influence of theophylline on gastro-oesophageal reflux and asthma. *Eur J Clin Pharmacol*. 1988;35(4):353-356.
53. DiMarino AJ, Cohen S, et al. Effect of an oral beta$_2$-adrenergic agonist on lower esophageal sphincter pressure in normals and in patients with achalasia. *Dig Dis Sci*. 1982;27(12):1063-1066.
54. Michoud MC, Leduc T, Proulx F, et al. Effect of salbutamol on gastroesophageal reflux in healthy volunteers and patients with asthma. *J Allergy Clin Immunol*. 1991;87(4):762-767.
55. Crowell MS, Zayat EN, Lacy BE, et al. The effects of an inhaled beta$_2$-adrenergic agonist on lower esophageal function: A dose-response study. *Chest*. 2001;120(4):1184-1189.
56. Lacy BE, Mathis C, DesBiens J, et al. The effects of nebulized albuterol on esophageal function in asthmatic patients. *Dig Dis Sci*. 2008;53(10):2627-2633.
57. Lazenby JP, Guzzo MR, Harding SM, et al. Oral corticosteroids increase esophageal acid contact times in patients with stable asthma. *Chest*. 2002;121(2):625-634.
58. Gagliardi GS, Shah AP, Goldstein M, et al. The effect of zolpidem on the sleep arousal response to nocturnal acid exposure. *Clin Gastroenterol Hepatol*. 2009;7(9):948-952.
59. Metz DC, Vakily M, Dixit T, et al. Dual delayed release formulation of dexlansoprazole MR; a novel approach to overcome the limitations of conventional single release proton pump inhibitor therapy. *Aliment Pharmacol Ther*. 2009;29(9):928-937.
60. Wolfe MM. Overview and comparison of the proton pump inhibitors for the treatment of acid-related disorders. Available online at http://www.uptodateonline.com/online/content/topic.do?topicKey=acidpep/10094&:view=print. Accessed March 1, 2010.
61. Omeprazole FDA. Health Advisory. Nov. 17, 2009. Available at http://www.fda.gov/Drugs/DrugSafety/PublicHealthAdvisories/ucm190825.htm; accessed Feb. 17, 2010.
62. Peghini PL, Katz PO, Bracy NA, Castell DO. Nocturnal recovery of gastric acid section with twice-daily dosing of proton pump inhibitors. *Am J Gastroenterol*. 1998;93(5):753-757.
63. Peghini PL, Katz PO, Castell DO. Ranitidine controls nocturnal acid breakthrough on omeprazole: A controlled study in normal subjects. *Gastroenterology*. 1998;115(6):1335-1339.
64. Fackler WK, Ours TM, Vaezi MF, Richter JE. Long-term effect of H$_2$RA therapy on nocturnal acid breakthrough. *Gastroenterology*. 2002;122(3):625-632.
65. Herzig SJ, Howell MD, Ngo LH, Marcantonio ER. Acid-suppressive medication use and the risk for hospital-acquired pneumonia. *JAMA*. 2009;30(20):2120-2128.
66. Laine L, Ahnen D, McClain C, et al. Potential gastrointestinal effects of long-term acid suppression with proton pump inhibitors. *Aliment Pharmacol Ther*. 2000;14(6):651-668.
67. Leonard J, Marshall JK, Moayyedi P. Systematic review of the risk of enteric infection in patients taking acid suppression. *Am J Gastroenterol*. 2007;102(9):2047-2056.
68. FDA News Release. May 25, 2010. Possible fracture risk with high dose, long-term use of proton pump inhibitors. Available at www.fda.gov/NewsEvents/Newsroom/Pressannouncements/ucm213377.htm?sms_22=email. Accessed June 2, 2010.
69. Gray SL, LaCroix AZ, Larson J, et al. Proton pump inhibitor use, hip fracture, and change in bone mineral density in postmenopausal women: Results from the Women's Health Initiative. *Arch Intern Med*. 2010;170(9):765-771.
70. Larson JD, Patatanian E, Miner Jr PB, et al. Double-blind, placebo-controlled study of ranitidine for gastroesophageal reflux symptoms during pregnancy. *Obstet Gynecol*. 1997;90(1):83-87.
71. Gill SK, O'Brien L, Einarson TR, Koren G. The safety of proton pump inhibitors (PPIs) in pregnancy: A meta-analysis. *Am J Gastroenterol*. 2009;104(6):1541-1545.
72. Bernstein R. Warnings on metaclopramide treatment. *Clin Gastroenterol Hepatol*. 2009;7(10):1138-1139.
73. Kenney C, Hunter C, Davidson A, Jankovic J. Metoclopramide, an increasingly recognized cause of tardive dyskinesia. *J Clin Pharmacol*. 2008;48(3):379-384.
74. Zhang Q, Lehmann A, Rigda R, et al. Control of transient lower esophageal sphincter relaxations and reflux by the GABA (B) agonist baclofen in patients with gastroesophageal reflux disease. *Gut*. 2002;50(1):19-24.
75. Schwartz MP, Wellink H, Gooszen HG, et al. Endoscopic gastroplication for the treatment of gastroesophageal-oesophageal reflux disease: A randomised, sham-controlled trial. *Gut*. 2007;56(1):20-28.
76. Mahmood Z, McMahon BP, Arfin Q, et al. Endocinch therapy for gastroesophageal reflux disease: A one year prospective follow up. *Gut*. 2003;52(1):34-39.
77. Rothstein R, Filipi C, Caca K, et al. Endoscopic full-thickness plication for the treatment of gastroesophageal reflux disease: A randomized, sham-controlled trial. *Gastroenterology*. 2006;131(3):704-712.
78. Cadière GB, Rajan A, Germay O, Himpens J. Endoluminal fundoplication by a transoral device for the treatment of GERD: A feasibility study. *Surg Endosc*. 2008;22(2):333-342.
79. Meier PN. Efficacy of endoscopic antireflux procedures: At least durability for radiofrequency energy delivery. *Gastrointest Endosc*. 2007;65(3):375-376.
80. Fry CL, Mönkemüller K, Malfertheiner P, et al. Systematic review: Endoluminal therapy for gastro-oesophageal reflux disease: Evidence from clinical trials. *Eur J Gastroenterol Hepatol*. 2007;19(12):1125-1139.
81. Spirit Magazine. Southwest Airlines, Jan. 2010, p 43 (advertisement).

82. Cadière GB, Van Sante N, Graves JE, et al. Two-year results of a feasibility study on antireflux transoral incisionless fundoplication (TIF) using EsophyX. *Surg Endosc.* 2009;23(5):957-964.

83. Salminen PT, Hiekkanen HI, Rantala AP, Ovaska JT. Comparison of long-term outcome of laparoscopic and conventional Nissen fundoplication: A prospective randomized study with an 11-year follow up. *Ann Surg.* 2007;246(2):201-206.

84. Granderath FA, Kamolz T, Granderath UM, Pointner R. Gas-related symptoms after laparoscopic 360 degrees Nissen or 270 degrees Toupet fundoplication in gastroesophageal reflux disease patients with aerophagia as comobidity. *Dig Liver Dis.* 2007;39(4):312-318.

85. Houghton SG, Romero Y, Sarr MG. Effect of Roux-en-Y gastric bypass in obese patients with Barrett's esophagus; attempts to eliminate duodenogastric reflux. *Surg Obes Relat Dis.* 2008;4(1):1-4.

86. Johnson WE, Hagen JA, DeMeester TR, et al. Outcome of respiratory symptoms after antireflux surgery on patients with gastroesophageal reflux disease. *Arch Surg.* 1996;131(5):489-492.

87. Lundell L, Miettinen P, Myrvold HE, et al. Comparison of outcomes twelve years after antireflux surgery or omeprazole maintenance therapy for reflux esophagitis. *Clin Gastroenterol Hepatol.* 2009;7(12):1292-1298.

88. Spechler SJ, Lee E, Ahnen D, et al. Long-term outcomes of medical and surgical therapies for gastroesophageal reflux disease: Follow up of a randomized controlled trial. *JAMA.* 2001;285(18):2331-2338.

89. Dassinger MS, Torquati A, Houston HL, et al. Laparoscopic fundoplication: 5-year follow-up. *Am Surg.* 2004;70(8):694-695.

90. Green BT, Broughton WA, O'Connor JB, et al. Marked improvement in nocturnal gastroesophageal reflux in a large cohort of patients with obstructive sleep apnea treated with continuous positive airway pressure. *Arch Intern Med.* 2003;163(1):41-45.

91. Ing AJ, Ngu MC, Breslin AB. Obstructive sleep apnea and gastroesophageal reflux. *Am J Med.* 2000;108(suppl 4a):S120-S125.

92. Tawk M, Goodrich S, Kinasewitz G, et al. The effect of 1 week of continuous positive airway pressure treatment in obstructive sleep apnea patients with concomitant gastroesophageal reflux. *Chest.* 2006;130(4):1003-1008.

93. Shepherd KL, Holloway AH, Hillman DR, Eastwood PR. The impact of continuous positive airway pressure on the lower esophageal sphincter. *Am J Physiol Gastrointest Liver Physiol.* 2007;292(5):G1200-G1205.

94. Kerr P, Shoenut JP, Steens RD, et al. Nasal continuous positive airway pressure. A new treatment for nocturnal gastroesophageal reflux? *J Clin Gastroenterol.* 1993;17(4):276-278.

95. Shaker R, Castell DO, Schoenfeld PS, et al. Nighttime heartburn is an under-appreciated clinical problem that impacts sleep and daytime function: The results of a Gallup survey conducted on behalf of the American Gastroenterological Association. *Am J Gastroenterol.* 2003;98(7):1487-1493.

96. Chand N, Johnson DA, Tabangin M, Ware JC. Sleep dysfunction in patients with gastro-oesophageal reflux disease: Prevalence and response to GERD therapy, a pilot study. *Aliment Pharmacol Ther.* 2004;20(9):969-974.

97. DiMarino Jr JA, Banwait KS, Eschinger E, et al. The effect of gastro-oesophageal reflux and omeprazole on key sleep parameters. *Aliment Pharmacol Ther.* 2005;22(4):325-329.

98. Harding SM. Nocturnal asthma: Role of nocturnal gastroesophageal reflux. *Chronobiol Int.* 1999;16(5):641-662.

99. Gislason T, Janson C, Vermeire P, et al. Respiratory symptoms and nocturnal gastroesophageal reflux: A population-based study of young adults in three European countries. *Chest.* 2002;121(1):158-163.

100. Gunnbjörnsdottir MF, Omenaas E, Gislason T, et al. Obesity and nocturnal gastro-esophageal reflux are related to onset of asthma and respiratory syndrome. *Eur Respir J.* 2004;24(1):116-121.

101. Cuttitta G, Cibella F, Visconti A. Spontaneous gastroesophageal reflux and airway patency during the night in adult asthmatics. *Am J Respir Crit Care Med.* 2000;161(1):177-181.

102. Valipour A, Makker HK, Hardy R, et al. Symptomatic gastroesophageal reflux in subjects with a breathing sleep disorder. *Chest.* 2002;121(6):1748-1753.

103. Morse CA, Quan SF, Mays MZ, et al. Is there a relationship between obstructive sleep apnea and gastroesophageal reflux disease? *Clin Gastroenterol Hepatol.* 2004;2(9):761-768.

104. Kim HN, Vorona RD, Winn MP, et al. Symptoms of gastro-oesophageal reflux disease and the severity of obstructive sleep apnoea syndrome are not related in sleep disorders center patients. *Aliment Pharmacol Ther.* 2005;21(9):1127-1133:1.

105. Ozturk O, Ozturk L, Ozdogan A, et al. Variables affecting the occurrence of gastroesophageal reflux in obstructive sleep apnea patients. *Eur Arch Otorhinolaryngol.* 2004;261(4):229-232.

106. Sabaté JM, Jouët P, Merrouche M, et al. Gastroesophageal reflux in patients with morbid obesity: A role of obstructive sleep apnea syndrome? *Obes Surg.* 2008;18(11):1479-1484.

107. Kuribayashi S, Massey BT, Hafeezullah M, et al. Upper esophageal sphincter and gastroesophageal junction pressure changes act to prevent gastroesophageal reflux and esophagolaryngeal reflux during apneic episodes in patients with obstructive sleep apnea. *Chest.* 2010;137(4):769-776.

108. Wang L, Liu JX, Qin YX, et al. [Research on the relationship between obstructive sleep apnea hypopnea syndrome and gastroesophageal reflux.]. *Zhonghua Er Bi Yan Hou Tou Jing Wai Ke Za Zi.* 2009;44(1):26-30.

Neurologic Disorders and Sleep

Approach to Sleep-Related Seizure Identification and Management

Chapter 50

JENNIFER L. DeWOLFE / BETH ANN MALOW

Sleep and epilepsy are dynamically interrelated; understanding these relationships can provide insight into identifying and managing seizures in the sleep laboratory. This chapter will review seizure definitions, seizure classification, differential diagnoses of sleep-related seizures, identification of seizures during polysomnography (PSG), neurophysiologic techniques, and management of seizures during PSG monitoring with an emphasis on current evidence-based information.

DEFINITIONS

Clinical Definitions

An *epileptic seizure* is the manifestation of excessive or hypersynchronous activity of cerebral neurons and is usually self-limited.[1] *Epilepsy* is a chronic neurologic condition characterized by recurrent unprovoked epileptic seizures. *Ictal* is defined as the period of a seizure and *interictal* refers to the period between seizures.[2] An *aura* is the subjective ictal onset that may precede observable ictal phenomena. If an aura does not progress, it is known as a sensory seizure. Seizure *semiology* refers to the signs and symptoms of the ictal event. *Postictal* state is the transient clinically abnormal central nervous system (CNS) function after the clinical seizure has ended.[1] *Status epilepticus* is continuous clinical and electrographic seizure activity or recurrent epileptic seizures without return to consciousness between seizures for longer than 30 minutes.[3]

Electroencephalography Definitions

The electroencephalogram (EEG) records the electrical activity of the cerebral cortex as measured by electrodes on the scalp. Each *channel* or *derivation* is generated by two electrode inputs into a differential amplifier. The output of the amplifier represents the algebraic sum of the potential difference between the two electrodes. *Polarity* refers to the positivity or negativity of the activity recorded at the first electrode input compared to the second, recorded as a downward or upward graphical deflection, respectively. *Montage* is the organization of PSG channels in an EEG recording or *tracing*. EEG epochs are typically reviewed in 10 seconds per page (vs. 30 seconds in typical PSG scoring) (see later discussion under "Neurophysiologic Recording Techniques").

Epileptiform Discharges

The term *epileptiform* refers to the characteristic morphology of an abnormal discharge (graphical deflection) detected on scalp electrodes when neurons over at least several square centimeters fire synchronously. Epileptiform discharges indicate underlying cortical irritability and may be associated with epileptic seizures. *Ictal epileptiform discharges* occur as rhythmic patterns associated with epileptic seizures with clinical manifestations or without clinical manifestations (*electrographic epileptic seizures*). *Interictal epileptiform discharges (IEDs)* occur in between epileptic seizures and are suggestive of underlying cortical tissue that is potentially *epileptogenic* (i.e., able to generate epileptic seizures).[4]

There are several types of interictal epileptiform patterns: individual spikes or sharp waves, spike and slow wave or sharp and slow wave complexes, multiple spike complexes (polyspikes), and multiple spike and slow wave complexes (polyspikes and waves). There are four key characteristics of epileptiform discharges: (1) they stand out from the background (paroxysmal), (2) they show abrupt change in polarity, (3) they have individual spikes or a sharp wave component (e.g., of spike or sharp and slow wave discharges) with a duration of less than 200 ms (< 70 ms = spike; 70-200 ms = sharp wave), and (4) they involve a physiologic field (a voltage gradient across the scalp as measured by at least two electrodes). Spikes and sharp waves are commonly followed by a slow wave lasting 150 to 350 ms. IEDs tend to have a negative polarity, and may correlate with location of seizure onset.[5] Localization-related (partial onset) IEDs have an electrical field that is limited to one electrode location and its immediate adjacent electrodes[6] (Figs. 50-1 to 50-3). Generalized IEDs have an electrical field that is bilateral and extends to include electrode locations both anterior and posterior to the vertex (excluding focal vertex discharges)[6] (Figs. 50-4 and 50-5).

SLEEP-RELATED EPILEPSIES

Generalized Epilepsies

Generalized interictal epileptiform discharges suggest primary generalized epilepsy. In some primary generalized epilepsies, IEDs are increased in non–rapid eye movement (NREM) sleep, especially NREM stage 1 (N1) and NREM stage 2 (N2) sleep.[5,7-9]

Juvenile myoclonic epilepsy is a common primary generalized epilepsy syndrome characterized by clinical myoclonic, absence (brief unresponsive staring), and generalized tonic-clonic seizures typically 1 to 2 hours after awakening. The EEG demonstrates 4- to 6-Hz generalized spike and wave and polyspike and wave discharges that increase at sleep onset and on awakening and considerably decrease during NREM and rapid eye movement (REM) sleep and wakefulness.[8]

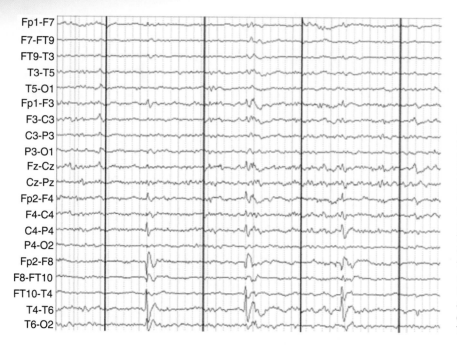

Figure 50-1 Right temporal lobe interictal epileptiform discharges (phase reversal FT10), anterior to posterior bipolar montage, 10-second epoch. Interictal epileptiform discharge (IED) characteristics: (1) stands out from the background, (2) abrupt change in polarity, (3) spike or sharp wave component (e.g., of spike or sharp and slow wave discharge) duration less than 200 ms, (4) involves a physiologic field. There are three interictal epileptiform discharges (IEDs) lateralized to the right hemisphere, localized to the right anterior temporal region. There is a phase reversal at FT10 with a field involving FP2, F4, C4, F8, FT10, T4, T6, and O2. See Figure 50-2 for average referential montage and Figure 50-3 for Pz referential montage. See Neurophysiologic Recording Techniques.

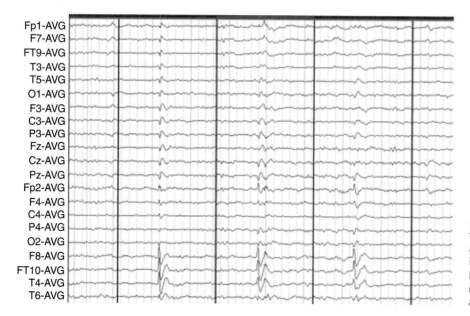

Figure 50-2 Right temporal lobe interictal epileptiform discharges (F8, FT10, T4 > Fp2, T6 > F4, C4), average referential montage, 10-second epoch. The interictal epileptiform discharges (IEDs) seen in Figure 50-1 are present on this average referential montage and demonstrate typical spikes with an aftergoing slow wave.

Childhood absence epilepsy, Lennox-Gastaut syndrome, and West syndrome are primary generalized epilepsy syndromes with clinical seizures manifesting mostly during wakefulness and have increased IEDs and polyspikes during N1 and N2 sleep. In childhood absence epilepsy while awake, IEDs have a characteristic 3-Hz generalized spike and wave pattern and become less well formed and may appear to be focal with a shifting fragmentation during slow wave sleep.[5,8,10] Lennox-Gastaut syndrome is a heterogeneous generalized epilepsy syndrome typically characterized by mental retardation, intractable multiple seizure types, and slow 1.5- to 2.5-Hz generalized spike and wave discharges on a slow electrographic background. West syndrome is characterized by infantile spasms, psychomotor retardation, and hypsarrhythmia on EEG. Hypsarrhythmia is an electrographic pattern manifesting as a disorganized background

with high amplitude slowing and multifocal spikes. Lennox-Gastaut and West syndromes may demonstrate relative burst-suppression (periods of high-amplitude EEG activity interrupted by periods of low-amplitude or suppressed EEG activity) patterns during sleep.[8,11] In REM sleep, generalized IEDs and hypsarrhythmia are decreased, often with a restricted field[8,12] (Table 50-1).

Localization-Related (Partial) Epilepsies

Localization-related epilepsies are characterized by partial seizures arising from one part of the brain. Seizure semiology correlates with initial activation of only part of one cerebral hemisphere and categorized by cerebral lobe of seizure onset (Figs. 50-6 to 50-9). Multifocal seizures have more than one independent seizure onset focus.[1] During partial seizures,

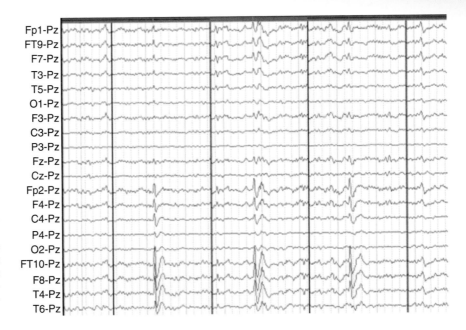

Figure 50-3 Right temporal lobe interictal epileptiform discharges (FT10, F8, T4 > Fp2 > T6, F4, C4, P4), Pz referential montage, 10-second epoch. The IEDs from Figures 50-1 and 50-2 are still present on this Pz referential montage. Interictal epileptiform discharges (IEDs) should maintain typical epileptiform characteristics in multiple montages. See Neurophysiologic Recording Techniques.

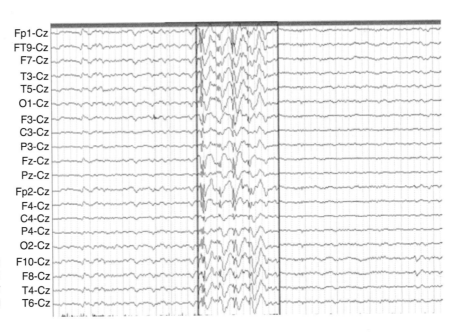

Figure 50-4 Generalized 2.5-Hz spike and wave and polyspike and wave discharges, Cz referential montage, 10-second epoch. See Figure 50-5 for 30-second epoch. See Neurophysiologic Recording Techniques.

consciousness and awareness may be maintained (i.e., simple partial seizures) or impaired (e.g., complex partial seizures). Cerebral location of epileptiform activity, slow frequencies, and cortical and subcortical networking areas involved determine the impact on consciousness or awareness.[13] Partial onset seizures may spread to adjacent cerebral cortex. Simple partial seizures may progress to complex partial seizures. Clinical generalized tonic-clonic convulsions may develop if epileptiform activity spreads diffusely to both cerebral hemispheres (i.e., secondary generalization).

Temporal Lobe

Temporal lobe epilepsy is the most common epilepsy in adults.[14] Temporal lobe IEDs are increased during NREM sleep and decreased during REM sleep.[8,15,16] Temporal lobe seizures are more frequent while awake than asleep, with a peak between 11 AM and 5 PM in patients undergoing scalp video-EEG on the seizure monitoring unit and in patients undergoing intracranial video-EEG recordings.[15,17,18] About one quarter of temporal lobe seizures occur during sleep and, if so, happen more frequently in N1 or N2 sleep and are more likely to secondarily generalize than seizures that occur while awake.[19,20] Partial seizures are common in temporal lobe epilepsy and may present clinically with an aura (i.e., simple partial seizure) that may then progress to a complex partial seizure with loss of awareness accompanied by a blank stare, decreased responsiveness, and automatic behaviors (e.g., oral and manual automatisms). Complex partial seizures typically resolve spontaneously in less than 2 minutes based on extra- and intracranial seizure monitoring unit studies.[21-23] Postictal confusion is usually not prolonged. Placing additional EEG electrodes over the anterior temporal region can increase

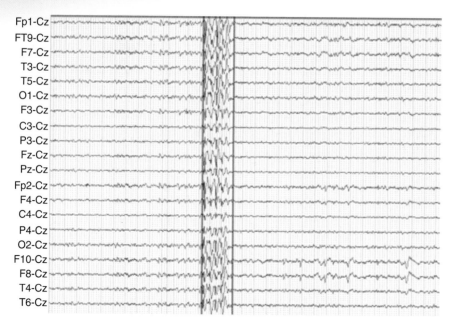

Figure 50-5 Generalized 2.5-Hz spike and wave and polyspike and wave discharges, Cz referential montage, 30-second epoch. Interictal epileptiform discharges (IEDs) from Figure 50-4 are present on this 30-second epoch. See Neurophysiologic Recording Techniques.

TABLE 50-1

Timing of Seizures and Interictal Epileptiform Discharges in Generalized Epilepsies

Form of Epilepsy	Morphology of IEDs	NREM	SWS	REM	Wake	Sleep Onset	Upon Awakening
Primary generalized epilepsy	Generalized	↑		↓	+		
Juvenile myoclonic epilepsy	4- to 6-Hz gen. polyspike waves	↓	↓	↓	↓	↑	↑
Childhood absence epilepsy	3-Hz gen. spike waves	↑ IEDs	↓ less well-formed IEDs	↓ IEDs	+		
Lennox-Gastaut	Slow 2.5-Hz gen. spike wave; BS in sleep	↑ IEDs	↓ IEDs	↓ IEDs	+		
West syndrome	Hypsarrhythmia; BS in sleep	↑ IEDs	↓ IEDs	↓ IEDs	+		

BS, burst suppression; *gen.,* generalized; *IEDs,* interictal epileptiform discharges; *NREM,* non–rapid eye movement sleep; *REM,* rapid eye movement sleep; *SWS,* slow wave sleep; ↑, increased frequency; ↓, decreased frequency; +, present.

recording of interictal and ictal epileptiform activity in temporal lobe epilepsies.[24]

Benign focal epilepsy of childhood (benign epilepsy with centrotemporal spikes [BECTS], rolandic epilepsy) is the most common epilepsy syndrome in children.[25] Typically, BECTS is associated with centrotemporal IEDs, mostly during sleep.[26,27] More than 50% of these seizures occur during sleep and are characterized by stereotyped unilateral face and arm clonic activity with frequent secondary generalization.[8,28,29]

Frontal Lobe

Frontal lobe seizures occur frequently during sleep (30-60%)[19] with a peak occurring between 11 PM and 5 AM.[18] They secondarily generalize equally in sleep and wake.[19] Frontal lobe seizures are typically stereotyped, short, and frequent; may cluster; and have a very brief to no detectable postictal state. Some frontal lobe seizures may be associated with affective manifestations, such as fear. Motor manifestations are common and correlate to cortical location of epileptiform activity (e.g., clonic activity associated with primary motor cortex or fencing posture with supplementary sensorimotor cortex).

Movements may be complex and bizarre (e.g., hypermotor activity) and can have associated vocalizations. Ictal EEG and IEDs may be nonlocalized (e.g., diffuse and bilateral), absent, or unilateral.[20] Ictal EEG may not demonstrate epileptiform activity, especially if the seizure focus is deep midline in the brain.

Supplementary sensorimotor seizures are localized to the mesial superior frontal gyrus, are associated with IEDs in the vertex, typically arise from sleep, and may cluster (several seizures in one night).[30,31] Seizure semiology consists of stereotyped brief asymmetrical tonic "fencing posture" with one shoulder extended, other upper extremity flexed at the elbow, and head deviated toward extended arm.[32] Ictal EEG is best viewed in a transverse bipolar montage and may display no epileptiform activity or a high-amplitude slow transient at the vertex followed by low-amplitude fast beta activity (i.e., electrodecremental response) focally at the vertex or more diffusely.

Autosomal dominant nocturnal frontal lobe epilepsy is an inherited localization-related epilepsy associated with mutations in the genes coding for the α_4, α_2, and β_2 subunits of

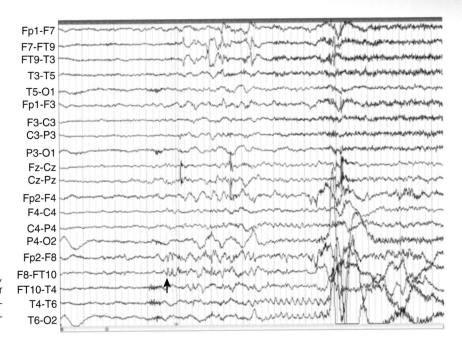

Figure 50-6 Right temporal lobe seizure onset, 5.5-Hz rhythmic theta, anterior to posterior bipolar montage, 10-second epoch. Arrow indicates electroencephalogram (EEG) onset of right temporal lobe seizure. Note the phase reversal pattern localized to F8.

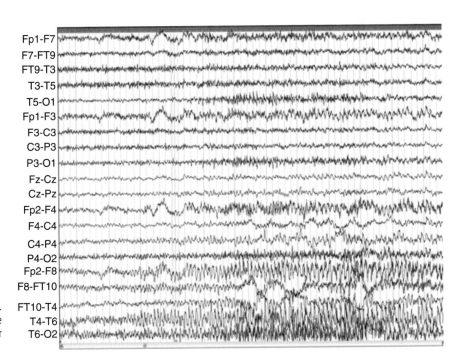

Figure 50-7 Right temporal lobe seizure continued. Ictal pattern evolves into rhythmic spikes over the right frontotemporal region, anterior to posterior bipolar montage, 10-second epoch.

the ligand-gated neuronal acetylcholine receptor. Seizures are activated by sleep, occur soon after sleep onset or in the early hours of the morning, consist of stereotyped brief motor activity ranging from simple repetitive motor manifestations to hypermotor thrashing movements, and may have associated vocalizations.[33] Seizures tend to cluster with multiple seizures in a night. Seizure semiology may vary within a family.

Other Epilepsies

Electroconvulsive status epilepticus in sleep (ESES) is an EEG pattern of almost continuous 2.5-Hz (or slower) generalized slow spike waves during NREM sleep associated with several epileptic syndromes, namely, two childhood clinical syndromes: continuous spike waves in slow wave sleep (CSWS) and Landau-Kleffner syndrome.[8,34,35] CSWS is associated with global cognitive regression, motor impairment, and partial onset (usually frontotemporal or frontocentral foci) and generalized seizures. Landau-Kleffner syndrome, also known as *acquired epileptic aphasia*, is associated with subacute language difficulty, focal central or posterior temporal IEDs that progress to ESES during NREM sleep, and rare seizures. In both these conditions, seizures and ESES usually resolve in midadolescence. Neuropsychological status will not improve in the presence of ESES. However, neurologic dysfunction

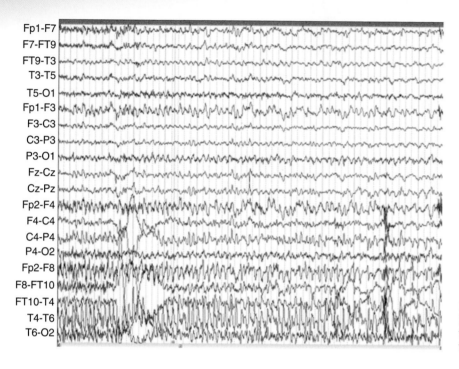

Figure 50-8 Right temporal lobe seizure continued. Ictal pattern slows to spike waves over the right frontotemporal region, anterior to posterior bipolar montage, 10-second epoch.

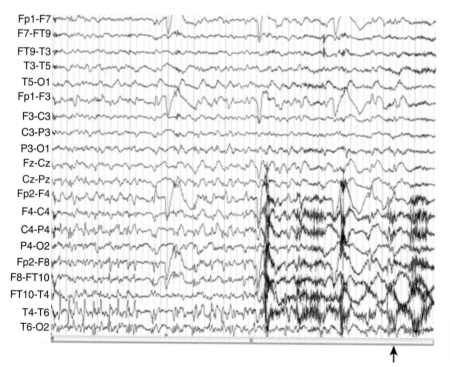

Figure 50-9 Right temporal lobe seizure termination. Spike waves stop. *Arrow* indicates electrographic seizure offset, anterior to posterior bipolar montage, 10-second epoch.

may persist after resolution of ESES and longer duration of ESES is associated with poorer long-term prognosis[8,35-38] (Table 50-2).

INTERRELATION OF SLEEP AND EPILEPSY

Sleep stages can affect IEDs and seizures. People with epilepsy (PWE) may have disrupted sleep architecture and poor quality sleep. Poor quality sleep and sleep deprivation can have potential effects on seizures. Seizures, IEDs, and epilepsy treatments can, in turn, affect sleep.

Effects on Sleep Architecture

It is clear that the sleep state modulates the expression of epilepsy. Epilepsy itself can also modify sleep. PWE have known changes in sleep architecture including prolonged sleep onset and REM latency; increased N2 sleep, sleep fragmentation, and wake time; and reduced REM and slow wave sleep.[39-42] Seizures during sleep increase N1 sleep and reduce REM sleep and daytime alertness. Seizures during the day reduce REM sleep the following night. This sleep instability can lead to sleep deprivation.[39,42,43]

TABLE 50-2

Timing of Seizures and Interictal Epileptiform Discharges in Localization-Related and Other Epilepsies

Epilepsy	Timing/Morphology	Localization	NREM	REM	Wake
Temporal	Peak between 11 PM and 5 AM		↑ IEDs	↓ IED/SZs	↑ SZs
BECTS	NREM	Centrotemporal	↑ IEDs/SZs	↓ IED/SZs	+ IED/SZs
Frontal	Peak between 11 PM and 5 AM		↑ IEDs/SZs	↓ IED/SZs	+ IED/SZs
SSMA	More common during sleep	Vertex	↑ IEDs/SZs	↓ IED/SZs	+ IED/SZs
ADNFLE	Soon after sleep onset, early morning	Frontal	↑ IEDs/SZs	↓ IED/SZs	Usually no IED/SZs
ESES	Almost continuous rhythmic slow ≤ 2.5-Hz spike waves in NREM	Generalized	↑ IEDs/SZs	↓ IED/SZs	No IED/SZs
Landau-Kleffner	Almost continuous rhythmic slow ≤ 2.5-Hz spike waves in NREM	Centrotemporal progress to ESES	↑ IEDs/SZs	↓ IED/SZs	+ IED/SZs

ADNFLE, autosomal dominant nocturnal frontal lobe epilepsy; *BECTS,* benign epilepsy with centrotemporal spikes; *ESES,* electroconvulsive status epilepticus in slow wave sleep; *IEDs,* interictal epileptiform discharges; *NREM,* non–rapid eye movement sleep; *REM,* rapid eye movement sleep; *SSMA,* supplementary sensorimotor area seizures; *SZs,* seizures; ↑, increased frequency; ↓, decreased frequency; +, present

Sleep Deprivation and Sleep Hygiene

Sleep deprivation may increase cortical excitability and the risk of seizures in some PWE, especially in those with idiopathic generalized epilepsy.[43-46] Although sleep deprivation may increase cortical excitability in patients with localization-related epilepsies,[47] this may not result in increased seizures.[48,49]

Inadequate sleep hygiene can be associated with daytime sleepiness and insomnia.[50] Although inadequate sleep hygiene is not uncommon, studies in PWE demonstrate that the majority of patients do not have multiple poor sleep behaviors. PWE tend to have fewer poor sleep behaviors than people without epilepsy. PWE with poor sleep are less likely to be seizure free.[50-54]

Epilepsy Treatment

Antiepileptic Drugs

Selection of antiepileptic drugs (AEDs) can be difficult, and thus, referral to a neurologist or epileptologist for seizure management is recommended. AEDs are selected based on multiple factors including but not limited to seizure type (Table 50-3), ease of use, efficacy, co-morbid conditions, potential interactions with concurrent medications, known allergy to medication class/ingredient, and other potential side effects/benefits. AEDs can have indirect and direct effects on sleep.

AEDs can affect sleep indirectly via alterations in weight. Weight gain may increase risk of developing primary sleep disorders such as obstructive sleep apnea (OSA). Benzodiazepines, carbamazepine (CBZ), gabapentin (GBP), phenobarbital (PB), pregabalin (PRG), primidone (PRM), and valproic acid (VPA) can cause weight gain.[55-59] Weight neutral AEDs include lamotrigine (LTG), levetiracetam (LEV), phenytoin (PHT), and tiagabine (TGB),[57,60] and felbamate (FBM), topiramate (TPM), and zonisamide (ZNS) have been associated with weight loss.[57,61,62]

Direct effects of AEDs on sleep include somnolence, insomnia, and sleep architecture modulation. Most AEDs are associated with somnolence; however, FBM and LTG are also linked with insomnia.[42,56,58,59,61,63-73]

Potentially beneficial effects on sleep architecture include decreased sleep onset latency (benzodiazepines, CBZ, PB, PHT, PRM),[50,65,74-76] increased slow wave (N3) sleep (CBZ, GBP, PRG, PRM),[50,77,78] increased REM sleep (GBP, LTG,

TABLE 50-3

Antiepileptic Drugs Indicated for Generalized or Partial Seizures

Generalized Seizures	Partial Seizures
Carbamazepine (not absence seizures)	Carbamazepine
Ethosuximide (absence, petit mal only)	Felbamate (with and without secondary generalization)
Lamotrigine	Gabapentin (with and without secondary generalization)
Levetiracetam	Lacosamide
Phenobarbital	Lamotrigine
Phenytoin	Levetiracetam
Primidone	Oxcarbazepine
Topiramate	Phenobarbital
Valproic acid	Phenytoin
	Pregabalin
	Primidone
	Tiagabine
	Topiramate
	Valproic acid
	Zonisamide

PRG),[42,50,59,79,80] increased sleep efficiency (CBZ, LEV, PB), and increased total sleep time (CBZ and LEV).[50,75,81-85]

Potentially disruptive effects on sleep architecture include decreased slow wave sleep (benzodiazepines, ethosuximide [ESX], LTG), decreased REM (benzodiazepines, CBZ, PB, PRM), and increased N1 and N2 sleep (benzodiazepines, ESX, LTG, LEV, PB). Benzodiazepines and barbiturates can increase spindle activity[42,50,65,74-78,81-88] (Table 50-4).

Vagal Nerve Stimulators and Cortical Resective Surgery

Vagal nerve stimulators (VNS) and epilepsy cortical resective surgery can affect sleep. VNS have been shown to cause significant OSA, especially at higher stimulus frequencies. Continuous positive airway pressure and reducing stimulus frequency has successfully improved VNS-induced obstructive apneas.[89-91] VNS can improve daytime sleepiness but increase daytime REM sleep, as demonstrated by increased number of sleep onset REM periods during multiple sleep latency tests.[92]

A recent report demonstrated resolution of significant OSA following cortical resective surgery for medically intractable

TABLE 50-4

Direct and Indirect Effects of Antiepileptic Drugs on Sleep

AED	Somnolence	Weight	Sleep Latency	REM Latency	N1	N2	SWS	REM	Sleep Efficiency	TST	Misc
BZ	+	↑	↓	↑		↑	↓	↓			↑ spindles
CBZ	+	+/- ↑	↓				↑	↓	↑	↓	
ESX					↑		↓				
FMB	±, insomnia	↓									
GBP	+	↑					↑	↑			
LTG	±, insomnia	N				↑		↑			
LEV	+	N				↑			↑	↑	
OXC	+										
PB	+	↑	↓	↑		↑		↓	↑		↑ spindles
PHT	+	N	↓								
PRG	+	↑					↑	↑↓			
PRM	+	↑	↓								↑ spindles
TGB	+	N					↑				
TPM	+	↓									
VPA	+	↑					↑				
ZNS	+	↓									

AED, antiepileptic drug; *BZ,* benzodiazepines; *CBZ,* carbamazepine; *ESX,* ethosuximide; *FBM,* felbamate; *GBP,* gabapentin; *LTG,* lamotrigine; *LEV,* levetiracetam; *Misc,* miscellaneous; *N,* neutral; *N1,* non–rapid eye movement (NREM) stage 1 sleep; *N2,* NREM stage 2 sleep; *OXC,* oxcarbazepine; *PB,* phenobarbital; *PHT,* phenytoin; *PRG,* pregabalin; *PRM,* primidone; *REM,* rapid eye movement sleep; *SWS,* slow wave sleep; *TGB,* tiagabine; *TPM,* topiramate; *TST,* total sleep time; *VPA,* valproic acid; *ZNS,* zonisamide; +, present; ↑, increased; ↓, decreased, ±, some reports positive.

Adapted from Foldvary-Schaefer N, Grigg-Damberger M. Sleep and epilepsy. *Semin Neurol.* 2009;29(4):419-428.

epilepsy.[93] The full effects of epilepsy surgery on primary sleep disorders, such as OSA, are unknown and require further evaluation.

DIFFERENTIAL DIAGNOSIS OF SLEEP-RELATED SEIZURES

Sleep-related epileptic seizures can occur throughout the night, are less common during REM sleep, are stereotyped, and can occur at any age. In particular, frontal lobe seizures are usually brief, lack a prolonged postictal state, and may cluster in a given night. However, all nocturnal behaviors are not epileptic seizures. Other disorders may have sleep-related manifestations including parasomnias, sleep-related movement disorders, primary sleep disorders, and psychogenic events (Table 50-5).

Parasomnias

Parasomnias are "unpleasant or undesirable behavioral or experiential phenomena that occur predominantly or exclusively during the sleep period" as defined by the International Classification of Sleep Disorders.[94,95] Parasomnias may occur during wake-sleep transitions, NREM sleep, or REM sleep (see Section 10, "Adult Parasomnias").

NREM Arousal Parasomnias

NREM arousal parasomnias are the most common parasomnias, and occur most frequently out of slow wave sleep (N3 sleep) during the first third of the night, although they may occur during N2 sleep. These patients typically show impaired awareness and amnesia for the event, although some may have partial recollection or associated dream mentation.[96] The spectrum of NREM arousal parasomnias includes confusional arousals, somnambulism, and sleep terrors. During events, EEG findings suggest incomplete awakening with slower mixed alpha and theta frequencies. Arousal parasomnias are common in young children and infrequently may persist into adulthood. Individuals may have more than one arousal parasomnia and co-morbid primary sleep disorders, such as OSA. Obstructive apneas may trigger a NREM arousal parasomnia episode.[94] Atypical presentations of NREM arousal parasomnias such as stereotyped behaviors, adult onset, or event clustering should be studied with video extended EEG monitoring in addition to standard polysomnography monitoring to characterize the event, define sleep stage during which events arise, and evaluate for lack of associated possible epileptiform activity to help distinguish from nocturnal epileptic seizures.[97]

Confusional Arousals. Confusional arousals manifest as sudden arousal presenting with confusion and disorientation with variable associated semipurposeful movements, vocalizations (e.g., unintelligible gibberish to clear speech), and agitation. Duration ranges from 1 to 2 minutes up to 10 minutes or longer. Arousal threshold increases during episodes and if attempts are made to awaken the patient, he or she may become agitated. Triggers include stress, febrile illness, sleep deprivation, and erratic sleep schedule.[94,98]

Somnambulism. Somnambulism, or sleep walking, is associated with a sudden arousal from sleep with abrupt simple to complex semipurposeful to goal-oriented motor behaviors. People may abruptly get out of bed and leave the bedroom or house. Some complex behaviors include talking, sleep-related eating, driving, and dressing, and can be sexual or violent.[96] Events can last several minutes up to a half hour. Sometimes

TABLE 50-5

Differential Diagnosis of Sleep-Related Nocturnal Behaviors

Disorder	Sleep Stage/ Timing	Semiology	Event Amnesia	Dream Recall	Onset Age	Recommended Test
Catathrenia	N2 > REM	Variable, multiple, may be prolonged	Yes	No	Any	VPSG
Confusional arousals	N3, 1st 3rd	Variable, brief to prolonged	Typical	±	Any, common childhood	None; if stereotyped, then vEEG-PSG or LTMvEEG
Nocturnal epileptic seizures	NREM > REM	Stereotypical, brief, may cluster or 2nd gen.	±	No	Any	vEEG-PSG or LTMvEEG
Hypnic jerks	Sleep onset	Stereotypical, brief	No	±	Any	None
Nocturnal panic attacks	N2-3	Variable, brief to prolonged, ~1/night	No	No	Any	vEEG-PSG vs. LTMvEEG
Obstructive sleep apnea	N1-3, REM	Variable	±	±	Any	VPSG
Periodic limb movements in sleep	NREM > REM	Stereotypical, periodic	Yes	No	Any, ↑ with age	None
Psychogenic nonepileptic events	Wake	Variable, brief to prolonged	±	No	Any	vEEG-PSG vs. LTMvEEG
REM behavior disorder	REM, last 3rd	Variable, brief to prolonged	±	Yes, if woken	Adult	vEEG-PSG
Sleep-related bruxism	N2	Stereotypical, brief	±	No	Any, ↓ with age	Usually none
Sleep-related rhythmic movement disorder	Sleep onset, N1-2 > N3, REM	Stereotypical, brief to prolonged	±	No	Usually <5 y/o	vEEG-PSG vs. LTMvEEG
Sleep terrors	N3, 1st 3rd	Variable, prolonged	Yes	±	Usually childhood	None; if stereotypical, then vEEG-PSG or LTMvEEG
Somnambulism	N3, 1st 3rd	Variable, brief to 30 minutes	Typical	±	Usually childhood	None; if stereotypical, then vEEG-PSG or LTMvEEG
Somniloquy	NREM > REM	Variable	±	No	Any, common childhood	Usually none

EEG, electroencephalogram; *LTMvEEG*, long-term monitoring video electroencephalogram; *N1*, non–rapid eye movement (NREM) stage 1 sleep; *N2*, NREM stage 2 sleep; *N3*, NREM stage 3 sleep; *REM*, rapid eye movement sleep; *PSG*, polysomnography; *vEEG-PSG*, video polysomnography with extended EEG; ↑, increases; ↓, decreases; *1st 3rd*, first third of sleep period; *2nd gen*, secondarily generalized seizure; *last 3rd*, last third of sleep period; ±, yes and no.

people may be directed back to bed and often return to sleep after the event.[94] Inadvertent self-injuries and even death have been attributed to somnambulism.[99,100]

Sleep Terrors. Sleep terrors are characterized by abrupt arousal associated with autonomic and emotional symptoms, commonly including tachycardia, fear, and agitation. Individuals are often inconsolable during the episode and may try to get out of the room as if trying to get away from something. Vocalizations may be present and range from incoherent mumblings to blood-curdling screams. Event duration is variable and patients are typically amnestic for the events. Episodes usually occur during childhood, but infrequently they persist into adulthood.[94,101]

REM Parasomnias

REM Behavior Disorder. REM behavior disorder (RBD) is a parasomnia arising out of REM sleep with variable simple to complex nocturnal behaviors associated with loss of normal muscle atonia and impaired suppression of movement generators during REM sleep.[102] Behaviors may be violent including punching, grabbing, fighting, or kicking. Injuries to self and others have been attributed to RBD.[103] Violence is usually not manifested when patients are awake.[99] Patients may report detailed dream recall or be amnestic for the dream and motoric events after awakening from a night with RBD symptoms. Often, if woken during the spell, the patient can report dream content correlating with observed movements. Vocalizations may be present. RBD tends to occur in older adults and may be the harbinger of neurodegenerative disorders. RBD can be induced with excessive alcohol use[104] or withdrawal or other medications (e.g., certain antidepressants).[105,106] PSG findings demonstrate REM without atonia in the electromyographic (EMG) channels of the chin or limbs without epileptiform activity on EEG.[103] PSG is required for definitive diagnosis.[107]

Sleep Paralysis. Sleep paralysis is a REM parasomnia associated with voluntary muscle paralysis, sparing extraocular muscles and diaphragmatic muscles, and retained awareness; it can be hypnagogic or hypnopompic. Duration of events is usually brief, but rarely may be prolonged. Episodes resolve spontaneously, although they may may be broken if the patient is touched (sensory trick). Manifestations are attributed to intrusion of REM into wakefulness.[98] Triggers include altered sleep schedule, disrupted sleep, and REM-influencing medications such as antidepressants. Sleep paralysis may be isolated or can be associated with narcolepsy. Diagnostic procedures are not indicated unless narcolepsy is suspected.[98,108]

Sleep-Related Movement Disorders

Hypnic Jerks

Hypnic jerks, or sleep starts, are common simple movement disorders occurring at sleep onset and consisting of one to two whole body jerks. They may be associated with a sense of falling, hypnagogic dream, or sensory flash. Patients are aware of events and have no associated amnesia.[95,109]

Periodic Limb Movements in Sleep

Periodic limb movements in sleep (PLMS) (see Chapter 24) are stereotyped repetitive movements of the limbs, typically legs, during sleep. Movements are unilateral or bilateral, usually involve the first toe, and ankle dorsiflexion and may also involve flexion of knee and hip (triple flexion). PLMS begin at any age and become more common with increased age.[94] On PSG, duration of 0.5 to 10 seconds, a minimum 8 μV increase in voltage above resting EMG tone, and four consecutive periodic to semiperiodic events are required.[95] PLMS can disrupt sleep, potentially trigger NREM arousal parasomnias,[94] are more frequent in PWE,[110] and may lead to daytime sleepiness.

Sleep-Related Rhythmic Movement Disorder

Sleep-related rhythmic movement disorder (SRMD)[95] is typically reported at sleep onset, but may occur during any sleep stage (see Chapter 27). It is characterized by stereotyped, rhythmic movements of large muscle groups in variable body locations (e.g., body rocking, head banging), and occurs most frequently in children younger than 5 years of age. Persistence of SRMD into adulthood is unusual and is associated with mental retardation, although it has been reported in normal adults.[111,112] SRMD may be associated with rhythmic movement artifact, but not epileptiform discharges, on EEG.

Sleep-Related Bruxism

Sleep-related bruxism (tooth grinding or clenching), is a sleep-related movement disorder[95] that manifests as simple stereotyped movements of the face and jaw. Episodes typically arise from N2 sleep and may or may not have associated awareness of events.[94] Bruxism can occur at any age, although it is less common with increasing age[113-115] and may lead to dental damage or temporomandibular joint dysfunction.[109] Bruxism can be diagnosed by history and, potentially, clinical examination (enamel wear) and is frequently noted by patients' dentists. Complex partial seizures can be associated with oral automatisms such as lip smacking and chewing. Although sleep-related bruxism is not usually confused with epileptic seizures, if it is accompanied by other nocturnal behaviors, further evaluation with video-PSG with extended EEG monitoring to rule out epileptic seizures or other parasomnias should be considered.

Primary Sleep Disorders

Obstructive Sleep Apnea

It is well known that OSA can disrupt sleep and that apneas are associated with arousals. Patients are usually not aware of apneas. They may manifest dream enacting behaviors during apnea-related arousals that may resemble RBD.[116] Untreated OSA may trigger parasomnias and exacerbate seizures.[93,117] Video with PSG can record obstructive apneas and allow characterization of postarousal behaviors.

Co-morbid OSA in PWE is common. In one study on PWE without OSA undergoing PSG prior to epilepsy surgery, significant OSA was diagnosed in one third of patients.[118] OSA has been associated with worsening seizure control in children and elderly PWE.[117,119] Continuous positive airway pressure and oral appliances improve OSA and seizure control in pilot studies on PWE with OSA (whether it was known or previously undiagnosed). Comprehensive trials are needed to further investigate the impact of OSA treatment on seizure control in people with epilepsy.[120,121]

Gastroesophageal Reflux Disease

Sleep-related gastroesophageal reflux disease may disrupt sleep and cause arousals, potentially triggering an arousal parasomnia. Arousals induced by gastroesophageal reflux may be accompanied by epigastric pain, crying, vomiting, and respiratory problems (see Chapter 49).[122,123]

Psychogenic Disorders

Psychogenic Nonepileptic Spells

Psychogenic nonepileptic spells (PNES), or dissociative episodes, arise from wakefulness and are rare from 12 AM to 5 AM. Clinically, patients can appear to be asleep and may actually believe they are asleep.[19,124] Movements are typically variable, range from minimal to bizarre violent thrashing, may start and stop several times, and can have a brief to prolonged (> 10 minutes) duration. Awareness during events may be altered, and event recall is variable. Associated EEG demonstrates normal waking background, at times with movement artifact, and no epileptiform activity.[19] Long-term video-EEG monitoring is useful to help distinguish PNES from epileptic seizures.[125]

Nocturnal Panic Attacks

Nocturnal panic attacks arise from NREM sleep, most frequently at the transition from stage N2 to slow wave sleep.[126] Usually only one event occurs in a given night. Symptoms include sudden arousal with a sense of fear, palpitations, and possible hyperventilation. Patients are intensely aware of the event, may take up to 2 hours to fall back to sleep after the event, and retain vivid event recall the following morning.[94,127]

Other Paroxysmal Nocturnal Events

Catathrenia

Catathrenia manifests as nocturnal moaning or groaning that may cluster throughout sleep and usually arises from stage N2, although it may occur during REM sleep as well. Amnesia of episodes is typical.[94,128]

Somniloquy

Somniloquy (sleep talking), typically arises from light NREM sleep, but it may occur during REM sleep. Speech ranges from single words to short sentences without evident emotion. Somniloquy is common, especially in children, and co-morbid parasomnias may be present. Unless associated with another primary sleep disorder, arousal parasomnia, or RBD, diagnostic studies are not indicated.[94]

Neurophysiologic Recording Techniques

Proficient knowledge of EEG recording and interpretation is required for physicians and technologists utilizing EEG monitoring techniques.[97] The International 10-20 System of Electrode Placement is typically used for electrode placement. The 10 and 20 refer to percentage of distance from standard cerebral landmarks[129] (see Fig. 50-10). Electrode names have a letter corresponding to the underlying cerebral region: Fp, frontopolar; F, frontal; T, temporal; C, central; P, parietal; O, occipital; and z, midline. Numbers correspond to electrode locations overlying specific cerebral regions, with odd numbers indicating the left hemispheric positions and even numbers indicating right hemispheric positions (e.g., T6 represents an electrode over the right posterior temporal lobe).

Montages

In a *bipolar montage*, channels are generated by adjacent pairs of electrodes, typically arranged in chains.[130] The second input of the first channel will then be the first input of the next channel (e.g., channel 1: Fp1-F7; channel 2: F7-T3; channel 3: T3-T5; channel 4: T5-O1). Anterior to posterior montages can be arranged from left to right (double banana) (e.g., left lateral chain, left parasagittal chain, central chain, right parasagittal chain, right lateral chain) or alternating left and right chains (left lateral chain, right lateral chain, left parasagittal chain, right parasagittal chain, central chain). Coronal (transverse) montages begin on the left and progress to the right in chains starting anteriorly and ending posteriorly.[6] Montages may be modified and personalized for optimal review.

In a *referential montage*, the first electrode input is compared to a standard number of electrodes in the second input.

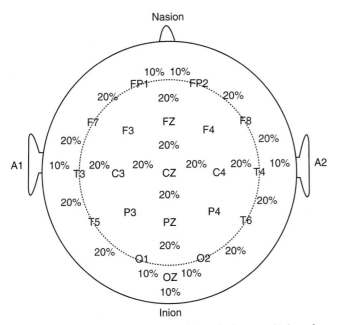

Figure 50-10 10/20 international system of electrode placement. (Redrawn from Gandhi Pangrahi BK, Bhatia M, Anand S. Expert model for detection of epileptic activity in EEG signature. *Expert Systems with Applications.* 2010;37(4):3513-3520.)

Common reference: all channels have the same second input of the electrode pair. In a *Cz referential montage* the second input in all channels on the polygraph is Cz (e.g., channel 1: Fp1-Cz; channel 2: F7-Cz; channel 3: T3-Cz; channel 4: T5-Cz; channel 5: O1-Cz). In a *combined ear referential montage* the second input in all channels is A1 and A2, linked together (M1 and M2, mastoids linked, in PSG). *Average referential montage*: the second input in all channels is the combination of all scalp electrodes (usually excluding A1, A2, Fp1, Fp2 due to frequency of artifacts in these electrodes).[6] Recordings are usually acquired referentially and then remontaged for optimal viewing. Analysis of the same cerebral activity with different montages aids in the localization and characterization of abnormal electrical activity.

By convention, when reviewing EEGs in bipolar montage, downward deflections are positive and upward deflections are negative. Downward deflections occur when the first electrode in a channel becomes more positive or the second electrode in a channel becomes more negative. Upward deflections occur with the first electrode has greater negativity or the second electrode has greater positivity. For referential montages, the same principle holds: a downward deflection occurs when the first electrode is more positive than the reference (deflects upward when it is more negative).

Epileptiform discharges are typically associated with negative electrophysiologic deflections. For bipolar montages, a *phase reversal* occurs in the channels over the epileptogenic source in partial epilepsies. For example, an epileptogenic source localized to T4 will have a downward (positive) deflection in F8-T4 channel (relatively more positive first electrode minus a negative second electrode results in a positive deflection) and an upward (negative) deflection in T4-T6 channel (negative first electrode minus a relatively more positive second electrode results in a negative deflection). For epileptiform discharges with a phase reversal in bipolar montages, identifying the common electrode in adjacent channels can localize the epileptogenic source (e.g., T4 in the previous example). In average or common referential montages, the channel with the highest amplitude of the epileptiform discharge indicates the epileptogenic source. Using our earlier example in both average and Pz common referential montages, channels with T4 will have the highest negative (upward) amplitude. The immediate adjacent channels within the epileptogenic field (i.e., F8, T6) will also demonstrate negative deflections, but will have decreased amplitudes compared to channels containing T4 (see Figs. 50-1 to 50-3).

For anterior to posterior bipolar montages, channels with an occipital electrode in the second input may appear to have reversed polarity (i.e., positive discharges may be upward) as in upward deflections associated with positive occipital sharp transients of sleep (POSTS), a common normal physiologic variant in light NREM sleep[6] (see Fig. 50-13 later in the chapter). Further details regarding EEG techniques and conventions can be found in a standard EEG reference.[131]

Video Electroencephalography and Polysomnography

Video and extended EEG monitoring can be combined with standard PSG physiologic recordings (vEEG-PSG) on analog or digital systems. Analog EEG-PSG signal may be stored directly onto a videotape with video signal and encoded data and time permitting synchronous review on paper and video. Playback speeds may be adjusted to allow characterization of sleep or EEG features. Digital recordings can be stored on magnetic or optical media with synchronized video.[97] Split-screen mode or two synchronized monitors can be used to view EEG-PSG and video simultaneously.[132]

Computerized digital vEEG-PSG systems offer advantages over conventional analog systems due to data acquisition versatility, customizable analysis, video synchronization, and increased storage capacity.[133,134] Reviewers may easily modify postacquisition data and adjust display settings (e.g., filters and sensitivities), change montages (including specific channels), adjust temporal resolution (paper speed), and correlate with synchronized video and technologist annotations for specific events or epochs of interest to help distinguish artifact from normal variant or epileptiform activity. Certain montages allow organization of EEG derivations to help distinguish evolving rhythmic epileptiform patterns from synchronous delta and theta frequencies in NREM sleep.[97] IEDs should maintain epileptiform morphology in alternate montages. Thus, reviewing suspicious EEG findings in an alternate montage can increase the diagnostic yield of the study.[134] Supplemental spike and seizure detection software, which is available in many digital video EEG-PSG systems, can automatically detect epileptiform abnormalities.[97]

According to the 2007 American Academy Sleep Medicine Manual for the Scoring of Sleep and Associated Events, a minimum of three EEG derivations (F4-M1, C4-M1, O2-M1) with an additional three contralateral derivations for backup (F3-M2, C3-M2, O1-M2) are recommended to sample activity from the frontal, central, and occipital regions referenced to a mastoid (M) electrode.[107] Limited EEG monitoring during PSG (four channels or less) is not sufficient to distinguish epileptic seizures from nonepileptic events. Additionally, limited EEG is inadequate for localizing seizures. In one study, extended EEG monitoring with 7 or 18 channels increased seizure localization and identification.[135] Placing additional anterior temporal electrodes (i.e., FT9 and FT10) increases identification of epileptiform activity over the temporal lobes.[24]

The history may provide enough information to diagnose epileptic seizures (e.g., reliable witnessed generalized tonic-clonic). However, for recurrent frequent violent sleep-related behaviors, combining vEEG-PSG can help characterize sleep-related behaviors associated with complex movements and provide a definitive diagnosis and guide appropriate management. The differential diagnosis for sleep-related events includes nocturnal epileptic seizures, NREM arousal disorders, rhythmic movement disorders, RBD, panic disorder, or psychogenic nonepileptic events. Reviewing synchronous video, EEG, and PSG data allows for staging sleep prior to and during events, determining event onset in relation to sleep onset, and correlating EEG abnormalities. Interictal electrographic EEG findings also may help identify predisposition toward epileptic seizures.[97]

Video review in real time or slower speeds may help define the event. Nighttime recordings may be enhanced with infrared recording. Mounted cameras with ability to pan, tilt, and zoom to allow for close-ups or full body view may be used alone or for simultaneous view with double mounted cameras.[97]

There are no guidelines for diagnostic tests indicated for specific disorders and specific EEG montages to use for diagnosis of sleep-related behaviors; although in 2006, the

---

TABLE 50-6

Proposed Electroencephalography Montages for Video with Extended Electroencephalography-Polysomnography*

Channel Number	16-Channel A-P Bipolar	18-Channel A-P Bipolar	16-Channel Transverse Bipolar	18-Channel Transverse Bipolar	16-Channel Referential	18-Channel Referential
1	Fp1-F7	Fp1-F7	F7-Fp1	F7-Fp1	F7-A1	F7-A1
2	F7-T3	F7-T3	Fp1-Fp2	Fp1-Fp2	T3-A1	T3-A1
3	T3-T5	T3-T5	Fp2-F8	Fp2-F8	T5-A1	T5-A1
4	T5-O1	T5-O1	F7-F3	F7-F3	Fp1-A1	Fp1-A1
5	FP1-F3	FP1-F3	F3-Fz	F3-Fz	F3-A1	F3-A1
6	F3-C3	F3-C3	Fz-F4	Fz-F4	C3-A1	C3-A1
7	C3-P3	C3-P3	F4-F8	F4-F8	P3-A1	P3-A1
8	P3-O1	P3-O1	T3-C3	T3-C3	O1-A1	O1-A1
9	Fp2-F4	Fz-Cz	C3-Cz	C3-Cz	Fp2-A2	Fz-A1
10	F4-C4	Cz-Pz	Cz-C4	Cz-C4	F4-A2	Pz-A2
11	C4-P4	Fp2-F4	C4-T4	C4-T4	C4-A2	Fp2-A2
12	P4-O2	F4-C4	T5-P3	T5-P3	P4-A2	F4-A2
13	Fp2-F8	C4-P4	P3-Pz	P3-Pz	O2-A2	C4-A2
14	F8-T4	P4-O2	Pz-P4	Pz-P4	F8-A2	P4-A2
15	T4-T6	Fp2-F8	P4-T6	P4-T6	T4-A2	O2-A2
16	T6-O2	F8-T4	O1-O2	T5-O1	T6-A2	F8-A2
17		T4-T6		O1-O2		T4-A2
18		T6-O2		O2-T6		T6-A2

*Based on International 10- to 20-electrode placement.
A, ear or mastoid; A-P, anterior to posterior; Avg, average; C, central; F, frontal; Fp, frontopolar; O, occipital; P, parietal; T, temporal; z, midline. Additional anterior temporal electrodes (FT9, FT10) may be considered. Any electrodes may be used for input 2 on the referential montage (e.g., Cz, average of all of the electrodes excluding Fp1, Fp2, A1, A2).
Adapted from Guideline 6: A proposal for standard montages to be used in clinical EEG. *J Clin Neurophysiol.* 2006;23(2):111-117.

American Clinical Neurophysiology Society proposed guidelines for standard EEG montages for evaluation of epileptic seizures.[23] vEEG-PSG increases correct diagnostic interpretations over standard PSG.[97] Accurate diagnosis is helpful to avoid unnecessary treatment with AEDs in patients misdiagnosed with epileptic seizures or to initiate AEDs in patients misdiagnosed with nonepileptic events.[125]

For suspected complex partial seizures, increased EEG coverage over the temporal lobes may increase EEG yield (e.g., F7, FT9, T3, T5, F8, FT10, T4, T6). In children with suspected BECTS, include electrodes over the centrotemporal parasagittal regions (C3, C4). Montages depend on EEG channel availability.[97] The American Clinical Neurophysiology Society recommends no fewer than 16 channels of simultaneous EEG channels and utilization of bipolar and referential montages for suspected epileptic seizures. Table 50-6 shows suggested montages.[23] A 16-channel anterior to posterior bipolar montage provides widespread coverage to sample interictal and ictal activity during sleep. Additional anterior temporal electrodes, FT9 and FT10, are commonly utilized to capture temporal lobe epileptiform activity.[97]

Clinical Case

A 31-year-old man with a history of febrile seizures as a child developed almost nightly nocturnal spells. His wife reported that within 1 hour of falling asleep he aroused, looked scared, then fumbled with the bed sheets and moved his jaw repeatedly, had a blank stare, and then returned to sleep. He did not respond to her during the spell. The spells were all the same with duration of fewer than 90 seconds. Afterward, he responded almost immediately and was unable to recall the event.

Differential Diagnosis

Differential diagnosis includes NREM arousal parasomnia, epileptic seizures, and psychogenic spells. RBD is possible, but unlikely because of stereotyped clinical manifestations and young age. Event amnesia makes nocturnal panic disorder improbable. Bruxism is not associated with the other manifestations, although it may precipitate an arousal parasomnia. History of febrile illness predisposes to development of epilepsy; however, the history is not sufficient to establish a definitive diagnosis.

Because of the frequency of his sleep-related events, vEEG-PSG was performed. Several typical events were recorded, arising from all stages of NREM sleep. Associated EEG demonstrated evolving rhythmic theta pattern over the right temporal lobe that increased in frequency and became more sharply contoured, progressing to rhythmic spikes. IEDs were noted over the same distribution in stages N2 and N3 sleep. He was diagnosed with complex partial seizures and treated with carbamazepine and became seizure free. Long-term video-EEG in an epilepsy monitoring unit may have been considered for less frequent events (e.g., once weekly).[97]

Suspected NREM Arousal Disorders. NREM arousal parasomnias, confusional arousals, somnambulism, and sleep terrors may be diagnosed by history alone. Consider vEEG-PSG if events are stereotyped, begin in adulthood, occur multiple times a night, are atypical, or do not respond to trial of medications. vEEG-PSG allows event characterization by video review, identifying sleep staging preceding and during spells, and extended EEG monitoring to evaluate for the absence of ictal and interictal epileptiform activity. EEG patterns correlating with arousal parasomnias include diffuse rhythmic synchronous delta, intermixed alpha, theta, and delta, stage N1 sleep pattern, nonreactive alpha activity, or low-voltage delta and beta activity.[94,97,136]

Suspected REM Behavior Disorder. RBD may be suspected by history; however, definitive diagnosis requires video recording or PSG demonstrating REM without atonia in chin or limb EMG, with or without behaviors, and the absence of epileptiform activity on EEG. vEEG-PSG allows simultaneous sleep staging, video to characterize behaviors and review of extended EEG for the absence of ictal epileptiform patterns.[95,97,107]

Suspected Psychogenic Disorder. PNES and other psychogenic spells occur while awake, even if the patient appears to be asleep.[19] Behaviors of PNES may be complex, peculiar, and potentially violent including flailing, alternating limb movements, pelvic thrusting, and side-to-side head movements. Events may be prolonged, start and stop numerous times, and have a variable presentation event to event. PNES may be suspected by history; however, recording spells on vEEG-PSG enables the physician to characterize the behaviors and correlate normal waking EEG immediately preceding and during spells with absence of interictal and ictal epileptiform activity.[97]

Disadvantages and Limitations of Video-EEG-PSG

The major disadvantages of vEEG-PSG evaluations for suspected epileptic seizures, parasomnias, and psychogenic events are increased time and relative expense.[101] Extra time is necessary to place additional EEG electrodes for extended EEG monitoring, monitor sleep-related behaviors, and vEEG-PSG documentation. Physicians must dedicate more time to review spells and interpret correlating EEG. Equipment must allow for additional EEG inputs, storage capacity, and means to modify speed of EEG review (10 seconds per page or 30 mm/second). Most digital PSG systems allow for review modifications.[97,134]

vEEG-PSG has limitations. Patients may not have a typical spell on the night of study. The patient's typical clinical event may manifest atypical signs, which may not be easily categorized. The EEG may be obscured by extracranial artifact and clear epileptiform activity may not be evident.[20] Some epileptic seizures do not have an epileptiform correlate on scalp EEG. Thus, the absence of well-defined ictal EEG patterns may not rule out epileptic seizures. Ictal epileptiform patterns may have a diffuse bilateral onset or evolve into rhythmic theta and delta frequencies misinterpreted as synchronous delta associated with NREM arousal parasomnias. NREM arousal parasomnias may have diffuse alpha frequencies on correlating EEG. An additional consecutive night of vEEG-PSG may increase the yield of capturing events; however, this will increase the overall cost.[125]

Artifacts and Pitfalls

Artifacts are common during sleep-related events during PSG and vEEG-PSG studies and can obscure the recording, potentially reducing the diagnostic yield. Commonly encountered

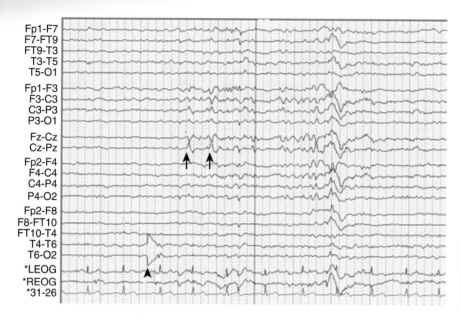

Figure 50-11 Vertex sharp waves, normal physiologic variant, electrode pop artifact, anterior to posterior bipolar montage, 10-second epoch. Vertex sharp waves (normal variant) with phase reversal at Cz (*arrows*). Electrode pop artifact in T6 (*arrowhead*).

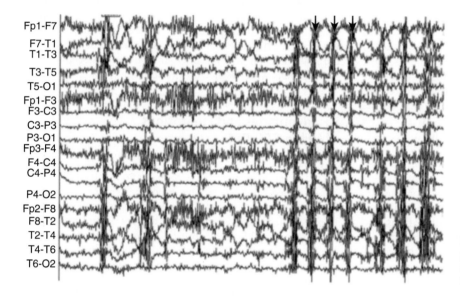

Figure 50-12 Sleep-related bruxism, anterior to posterior bipolar montage, 10-second epoch. Note the rhythmic myogenic artifact associated with jaw movements (*arrows*).

artifacts include eye movements, eyelid blinks, and electrode pops (Fig. 50-11). Familiarity with artifacts may help reduce misinterpretation as parasomnia-associated EEG changes or epileptiform activity.[97]

Some artifacts may be diagnostic, including characteristic rhythmic myogenic artifact associated with bruxism (Fig. 50-12) or body rocking artifact in rhythmic movement disorders.[97]

Pitfalls in vEEG-PSG interpretation by inexperienced reviewers include misinterpreting sharply contoured and rhythmic normal variants or artifacts as epileptiform activity or EEG characteristic of parasomnias. EEG interpretation may be aided by review of synchronous video.[137] Sharply contoured artifacts include movement artifact and electrode pops (see Fig. 50-11). Sharply contoured normal variants include vertex sharp waves (see Fig. 50-11), small sharp spikes, sawtooth waves, wicket spikes, and positive occipital sharp transients of sleep (Fig. 50-13). Rhythmic artifacts may be attributed to movements. Rhythmic normal physiologic variants include hypersynchronous theta of drowsiness and rhythmic midtemporal theta of drowsiness. If interpretation is uncertain, a trained electroencephalographer should be consulted.[97,125]

POLYSOMNOGRAPHY TECHNOLOGIST ROLE

There are no standard protocols for PSG technologist role during nocturnal behaviors in the sleep laboratory. The following recommendations are based on experience of the authors and others.

The role of the polysomnography technologist (PSGT) is crucial when performing vEEG-PSG to capture sleep-related events. PSGTs should be aware of vEEG-PSG studies prior to the date of study. Laboratory specific routine and emergency protocols should be reviewed and readily available in case needed. The PSGT can help maintain patient and equipment safety, document behaviors, annotate the record, and communicate with the sleep physician (Box 50-1).

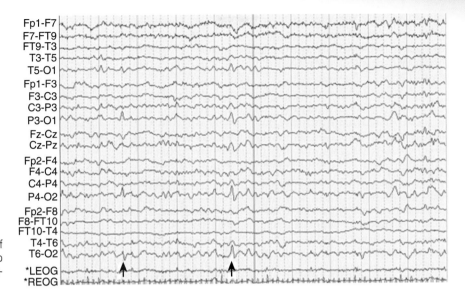

Figure 50-13 Positive occipital sharp transients of sleep (POSTS), normal physiologic variant, anterior to posterior bipolar montage, 10-second epoch. Symmetrical POSTS in the occipital channels (*arrows*).

BOX 50-1 *Recommended Responsibilities of the Polysomnographic Technologist in the Management of the Patient with Abnormal Nocturnal Behaviors in the Sleep Laboratory*

Identify patient charts with vEEG-PSG orders before sleep study:
- Flag charts.
- Review event semiology.
- Review event-related medications (if applicable).
- Review laboratory emergency protocols.

Contact patient before study:
- Remind him/her to bring medications.
- Establish emergency contact.

Hook-up process:
- Confirm event semiology.
- Confirm patient took event medications (if applicable).
- Ensure patient brought rescue medications (if applicable).
- Confirm emergency contact information.

Nocturnal behaviors during study:
- Ensure patient safety.
- Interact with patient to determine:
  - Level of consciousness
  - Ability to follow commands
  - Memory, dream recall
- Do not forcefully wake patient.
  - If out of bed, gently guide him/her back to bed.
- If generalized convulsion lasts > 5 minutes, initiate emergency protocol.
  - Administer rescue medications (if applicable).
- Ensure equipment safety.
- Document behaviors and patient response on study.
- Notify sleep physician and emergency contact if necessary.

With suspicious EEG findings during study:
- Review suspect EEG pattern in alternate montage.
- Document any correlating clinical manifestations.
- Document on study.

EEG, electroencephalogram; *vEEG-PSG*, video polysomnography with extended EEG.

Preparing the Charts

Consider flagging patient charts with orders for vEEG-PSG. The PSGT should review the chart for nocturnal behavior semiology including frequency and duration of events and occurrence during sleep. Do events stop spontaneously? Does the patient return to baseline after the event? Patients should be reminded to bring all of their home medications, including seizure medications if applicable. Does the patient take "rescue medications" (i.e., medications to abort seizures or to reduce the risk of recurrent seizures after the event)? Determine the patient's emergency contact including a working phone number and establish when to call the contact prior to the study.

Responsibilities During Polysomnography

PSGTs and physicians should be very familiar with the protocols regarding seizures and other nocturnal behaviors that occur in the sleep laboratory. PSGTs should confirm event semiology during the hookup process and ensure that the patient brought his or her medications. Emergency contact information should be confirmed.

If the patient manifests abnormal nocturnal behaviors during the PSG, the PSGT should interact with the patient to determine level of consciousness, response to verbal stimulus, and ability to follow commands (e.g., "stick out your tongue" or "raise your right thumb"). Memory testing can be done by giving the patient a few key words to remember (e.g., "remember blue wagon"). The PSGT should ensure that the patient is safe and that nothing can fall on him. If the patient attempts to get out of bed, try to gently guide him back. Do not attempt to awaken the patient forcefully. Patients may unknowingly become agitated and combative both during and after the event if attempts are made to awaken him forcefully. If patient is awake after the event, ask him to recall the key words given during the event and inquire if he recalls the spells or associated dreams. After completion of the study, again ask if the patient recalls behaviors.

After attending to the patient, ensure the sleep equipment is secured. PSGT should document all nocturnal behaviors on the vEEG-PSG for the physician to review. A clear description of clinical manifestations and response to PSGT should be recorded.

In the case of convulsive activity, have another technician help roll the patient to the lateral position to prevent aspiration and place supplemental oxygen via nasal cannula. If convulsive activity persists longer than 5 minutes, initiate emergency protocol (e.g., call a code, call 911). If applicable and PSGT is trained to do so, administer prescribed rescue medications to the patient (e.g., oral lorazepam, rectal diazepam).

PSGT should annotate the vEEG-PSG for suspicious EEG activity and any associated clinical manifestations for the physician review. The suspicious EEG should be viewed in alternate montages to assess if the morphology remains suspicious. For example, if sharply contoured activity is present over the right temporal region (i.e., T4-M2, T6-M2), then reference to an alternate second input (e.g., T4-M1, T6-M1). If the sharply contoured morphology does not persist on alternate montages/derivations, then it is unlikely to be epileptiform. Annotating suspicious EEG activity along with any associated clinical manifestations or lack thereof is important to highlight epochs in question for more detailed review by the sleep physician.

After patient and equipment safety is addressed, the sleep physician should be notified immediately of recurrent partial seizures, generalized convulsions, or any patient-related emergencies. If indicated, the patient's emergency contact should be notified as well.

Patient Referral

Patients with (1) interictal epileptiform activity, (2) clear electrographic ictal epileptiform activity associated with clinical events, or (3) recurrent stereotyped events without definite associated electrographic epileptiform discharges on vEEG-PSG, especially if atypical for sleep disorders, should be referred to an epileptologist or neurologist for further outpatient evaluation and management. Patients with a history of epilepsy, epilepsy risk factors, or central nervous system disease who manifest unusual nocturnal behaviors or movements not captured by vEEG-PSG should be referred as well. Printouts of the electrographic abnormalities and, if possible, video with EEG-PSG findings on disk should be forwarded.

If appropriate, admission to an epilepsy monitoring unit (EMU) may increase the diagnostic yield. Advantages of EMU evaluations include secured (i.e., glued) electrodes allowing for longer recording duration maintained continuously over several days instead of just overnight, thus possibly increasing the yield of capturing events. Equipment may be able to accommodate extra EEG electrode coverage, especially over the temporal lobes.[97] Activation procedures that may induce events include controlled weaning of antiepileptic medications, sleep deprivation, photic stimulation, and hyperventilation. Long-term video-EEG monitoring can classify seizure types, distinguish nonepileptic events, quantify seizures and IEDs, and establish seizure localization during presurgical evaluation for epilepsy surgery.[125] Establishing a definitive diagnosis can change management and allow for correct appropriate treatment.

Disadvantages of EMU admission include cost, limited availability, and time commitment. Some EMUs may not have additional equipment to simultaneously stage sleep or evaluate other primary sleep disorders. The addition of electro-oculogram (EOG) electrodes and EMG electrodes in an EMU may enhance diagnostic yield by helping determine the sleep stage preceding the clinical event.[97] The disadvantages should be weighed against the financial and social costs, both to the patient and society, of misdiagnosed and uncontrolled seizures.[101]

REFERENCES

1. Blume W, Luders HO, Mizrahi E, Tassinari C, Boas WVE, Engel J. Glossary of Descriptive Terminology for Ictal Semiology. *ILAE Epilepsy Classification and Terminology.* 1997 [cited Aug. 10, 2009]. Available from http://www.ilae-epilepsy.org/ctf/over_frame.html.
2. *McGraw-Hill Concise Dictionary of Modern Medicine.* New York: McGraw-Hill; 2002.
3. Treiman DM. Generalized convulsive status epilepticus in the adult. *Epilepsia.* 1993;34(suppl 1):S2-S11.
4. Nair D, Burgess R, McINtyre CC, Luders H. Chronic subdural electrodes in the management of epilepsy. *Clin Neurophysiol.* 2008;119(1):11-28.
5. Walczak T, Jayakar P, Mizrahi EM. Interictal electroencephalography. In: Engel J, Pedley TA, eds. *Epilepsy: A Comprehensive Textbook.* 2nd ed. Lippincott Williams & Wilkins; 2007:809-821.
6. Stern J, Engel J. How to use this book. In: Engel J, ed. *Atlas of EEG Patterns.* Lippincott Williams & Wilkins; 2004:3-12.
7. Niedermeyer E. Sleep electroencephalograms in petit mal. *Arch Neurol.* 1965;12:625-630.
8. Dinner DS. Effect of sleep on epilepsy. *J Clin Neurophysiol.* 2002;19(6):504-513.
9. Broughton R. *Epilepsy and sleep: A synopsis and prospectus.* Amsterdam: Elsevier Science Publishers; 1984.
10. Ross J, Johnson LC, Walter RD. Spike and wave discharges during stages of sleep. *Ann Neurol.* 1966;14:399-407.
11. Passouant P, Besset A, Carrier A, et al. *Night Sleep and Generalized Epilepsies.* Basel: Karger; 1974.
12. Jeavons PM, Bower BD. The natural history of infantile spasms. *Arch Dis Child.* 1961;36:17-21.
13. Englot DJ, Blumenfeld H. Consciousness and epilepsy: Why are complex-partial seizures complex? *Prog Brain Res.* 2009;177:147-170.
14. Engel J. Mesial temporal lobe epilepsy: What have we learned? *Neuroscientist.* 2001;7:340-352.
15. Crespel A, Baldy-Moulinier M, Coubes P. The relationship between sleep and epilepsy in frontal and temporal lobe epilepsies: Practical and physiopathologic considerations. *Epilepsia.* 1998;39:150-157.
16. Quigg M, Staume M, Menaker M, Bertram EH. Temporal distribution of partial 8 seizures: Comparison of an animal model with human partial epilepsy. *Ann Neurol.* 1998;43:748-755.
17. Hofstra WA, Grootemarsink BE, Dieker R, van der Palen J, de Weerd AW. Temporal distribution of clinical seizures over the 24-h day: A retrospective observational study in a tertiary epilepsy clinic. *Epilepsia.* 2009;50(9):2019-2026.
18. Hofstra WA, Spetgens WP, Leijten FS, van Rijen PC, Gosselaar P, et al. Diurnal rhythms in seizures detected by intracranial electrocorticographic monitoring: An observational study. *Epilepsy Behav.* 2009;14(4):617-621.
19. Bazil CW, Walczak TS. Effects of sleep and sleep stage on epileptic and nonepileptic seizures. *Epilepsia.* 1997;38(1):56-62.
20. Lawson JA, Cook MJ, Vogrin S, Litewka L, Strong D, et al. Clinical, EEG, and quantitative MRI differences in pediatric frontal and temporal lobe epilepsy. *Neurology.* 2002;58(5):723-729.
21. Afra P, Jouny CC, Bergey GK. Duration of complex partial seizures: An intracranial EEG study. *Epilepsia.* 2008;49(4):677-684.
22. Pellock JM. Overview: Definitions and classifications of seizure emergencies. *J Child Neurol.* 2007;22(5 suppl):13S.
23. Jenssen S, Gracely EJ, Sperling MR. How long do most seizures last? A systematic comparison of seizures recorded in the epilepsy monitoring unit. *Epilepsia.* 2006;47(9):1499-1503.
24. Sadle R, Goodwin J. Multiple electrodes for detecting spikes in partial complex seizures. *Can J Neurol Sci.* 1989;16(3):326-329.
25. Lerman P, Kivity S. Benign focal epilepsy in childhood. *Arch Neurol.* 1975;32:261-264.
26. Lerman P, Kivity-Ephraim S. Carbamazepine sole anticonvulsant for focal epilepsy in childhood. *Epilepsia.* 1974;15:229-234.
27. Nayrac P. Les pointes-ondes prerolandiques: Expression EEG tres particuliere: Etude electroclinique de 21 cas. *Rev Neurol.* 1957;99:201-206.
28. Gregory DL, Wong PK. Topographical analysis of the centrotemporal discharges in benign rolandic epilepsy in childhood. *Epilepsia.* 1984;25:705-711.
29. Beaussart M. Benign epilepsy of children with rolandic (centrotemporal) paroxysmal foci—A clinical entity: Study of 221 cases. *Epilepsia.* 1972;13:795-811.

30. Anand I, Dinner DS. Relation of supplementary motor area epilepsy and sleep. *Epilepsia.* 1997;38(suppl 8):48-49.

31. King DW, Smith JR. Supplementary sensorimotor area epilepsy in adults. *Adv Neurol.* 1996;70:285-291.

32. Penfield W, Jasper H. *Epilepsy and the Functional Anatomy of the Human Brain.* Boston: Little, Brown; 1954.

33. Marini C, Guerrini R. The role of the nicotinic acetylcholine receptors in sleep-related epilepsy. *Biochem Pharmacol.* 2007;74(8):1308-1314.

34. Jayakar PB, Seshia SS. Electrical status epilepticus during slow-wave sleep: A review. *J Clin Neurophysiol.* 1991;8:299-311.

35. Nickels K, Wirrell E. Electrical status epilepticus in sleep. *Semin Pediatr Neurol.* 2008;15(2):50-60.

36. Landau WM, Kleffner FR. Syndrome of acquired aphasia with convulsive disorder in children. *Neurology.* 1957;7:523-530.

37. Tassinari C, Buereau M, Dravet C, Dalla Bernardina B, Roger J. *Epilepsy with Continuous Spikes and Waves during Slow Sleep, Otherwise Described As ESES (Epilepsy with Electrical Status Epilepticus during Slow Sleep).* 2nd ed. London: John Libbey; 1992.

38. Mascetti L, Foret A, Bonjean M, Matarazzo L, Dang-Vu T, Maquet P. Some facts about sleep relevant for Landau-Kleffner syndrome. *Epilepsia.* 2009;50(suppl 7):43-46.

39. Bazil CW, Castro LH, Walczak TS. Reduction of rapid eye movement sleep by diurnal and nocturnal seizures in temporal lobe epilepsy. *Arch Neurol.* 2000;57(3):363-368.

40. Mendez M, Radtke RA. Interactions between sleep and epilepsy. *J Clin Neurophysiol.* 2001;18(2):106-127.

41. Touchon J, Baldy-Moulinier M, Billiard M, Besset A, Cadilhac J. Sleep organization and epilepsy. *Epilepsy Res Suppl.* 1991;2:73-81.

42. Foldvary N, Perry M, Lee J, Dinner D, Morris HH. The effects of lamotrigine on sleep in patients with epilepsy. *Epilepsia.* 2001;42(12):1569-1573.

43. Foldvary-Schaefer N, Grigg-Damberger M. Sleep and epilepsy. *Semin Neurol.* 2009;29(4):419-428.

44. Shahar E, Genizi J, Ravid S, Schif A. The complementary value of sleep-deprived EEG in childhood onset epilepsy. *Eur J Paediatr Neurol.* 2010;14(4):308-312.

45. Pinikahana J, Dono J. The lived experience of initial symptoms of and factors triggering epileptic seizures. *Epilepsy Behav.* 2009;15(4):513-520.

46. Scalise A, Desiato MT, Gigli GL, Romigi A, Tombini M, et al. Increasing cortical excitability: A possible explanation for the proconvulsant role of sleep deprivation. *Sleep.* 2006;29(12):1595-1598.

47. Badawy RA, Curatolo JM, Newton M, Berkovic SF, Macdonell RA. Sleep deprivation increases cortical excitability in epilepsy: Syndrome-specific effects. *Neurology.* 2006;67(6):1018-1022.

48. Rocamora R, Sanchez-Alvarez JC, Salas-Puig J. The relationship between sleep and epilepsy. *Neurologist.* 2008;14(6) (suppl 1):S35-S43.

49. Malow BA, Passaro E, Milling C, Minecan DN, Levy K. Sleep deprivation does not affect seizure frequency during inpatient video-EEG monitoring. *Neurology.* 2002;59(9):1371-1374.

50. Foldvary-Schaefer N. Sleep complaints and epilepsy: The role of seizures, antiepileptic drugs and sleep disorders. *J Clin Neurophysiol.* 2002;19(6):514-521.

51. Herman ST. Epilepsy and sleep. *Curr Treat Options Neurol.* 2006;8(4):271-279.

52. Lannon SL. Sleep hygiene in people with epilepsy [abstract]. *Epilepsia.* 1997;38:227.

53. Manni R, Politini L, Ratti MT, Marchioni E, Sartori I, et al. Sleep hygiene in adult epilepsy patients: A questionnaire-based survey. *Acta Neurol Scand.* 2000;101(5):301-304.

54. Thomas S, DeWolfe J. Sleep behaviors in a population of subjects with epilepsy (abstract). *Epilepsia Suppl.* 2008;1(suppl O):156.

55. Perucca E. Pharmacological and therapeutic properties of valproate: A summary after 35 years of clinical experience. *CNS Drugs.* 2002;16(10):695-714.

56. Ketter T, Post R, Theodore W. Positive and negative psychiatric effects of antiepileptic drugs in patients with seizure disorders. *Neurology.* 1999;53(suppl 2):S53-S67.

57. Ben-Menachem E. Weight issues for people with epilepsy—A review. *Epilepsia.* 2007;48(suppl 9):42-45.

58. Morris G. Gabapentin. *Epilepsia.* 1999;40(suppl 5):S63-S70.

59. Arain AM. Pregabalin in the management of partial epilepsy. *Neuropsychiatr Dis Treat.* 2009;5:407-413.

60. Walia K, Khan E, Ko D, Raza S, Khan Y. Side effects of antiepileptics—A review. *Pain Pract.* 2004;4(3):194-203.

61. Ben-Menachem E, Sander J, Stefan H, Schwalen S, Schauble B. Topiramate monotherapy in the treatment of newly or recently diagnosed epilepsy. *Clin Ther.* 2008;30(7):1180-1195.

62. Wellmer J, Wellmer S, Bauer J. The impact of zonisamide on weight. A clinical study in 103 patients with epilepsy. *Acta Neurol Scand.* 2009;119(4):233-238.

63. Nieto-Barrera M, Brozmanova M, Capovilla G, Christe W, Pedersen B, et al. A comparison of monotherapy with lamotrigine or carbamazepine in patients with newly diagnosed partial epilepsy. *Epilepsy Res.* 2001;46(2):145-155.

64. Wagner M. Felbamate: A new antiepileptic drug. *Am J Hosp Pharm.* 1994;51(13):1657-1666.

65. Placidi F, Scalise A, Marciani M, Romigi A, Diomedi M, Gigli G. Effect of antiepileptic drugs on sleep. *Clin Neurophysiol.* 2000;111(suppl 2):S115-S119.

66. Sadler M. Lamotrigine associated with insomnia. *Epilepsia.* 1999;40(3):322-325.

67. Abou-Khalil B. Levetiracetam in the treatment of epilepsy. *Neuropsychiatr Dis Treat.* 2008;4(3):507-523.

68. Martinez W, Ingenito A, Blakeslee M, Barkley G, McCague K, D'Souza J. Efficacy, safety, and tolerability of oxcarbazepine monotherapy. *Epilepsy Behav.* 2006;9(3):448-456.

69. Iivanainen M, Savolainen H. Side effects of phenobarbital and phenytoin during long-term treatment of epilepsy. *Acta Neurol Scand Suppl.* 1983;97:49-67.

70. Mattson R, Cramer J, Collins J, Smith D, Delgado-Escueta A, et al. Comparison of carbamazepine, phenobarbital, phenytoin, and primidone in partial and secondarily generalized tonic-clonic seizures. *N Engl J Med.* 1985;313(3):145-151.

71. Bauer J, Cooper-Mahkorn D. Tiagabine: Efficacy and safety in partial seizures—Current status. *Neuropsychiatr Dis Treat.* 2008;4(4):731-736.

72. DeWolfe JL, Knowlton RC, Beasley MT, Cofield S, Faught E, Limdi NA. Hyperammonemia following intravenous valproate loading. *Epilepsy Res.* 2009;85(1):65-71.

73. Brodie M, Duncan R, Vespignani H, Solyom A, Bitenskyy V, Lucas C. Dose-dependent safety and efficacy of zonisamide: A randomized, double-blind, placebo-controlled study in patients with refractory partial seizures. *Epilepsia.* 2005;46(1):31-41.

74. Ballenger JC, Post RM. Carbamazepine in manic-depressive illness: A new treatment. *Am J Psychiatry.* 1980;137(7):782-790.

75. Manni R, Ratti MT, Galimberti CA, Morini R, Perucca E, Tartara A. Daytime sleepiness in epileptic patients on long-term monotherapy: MSLT, clinical and psychometric assessment. *Neurophysiol Clin.* 1993;23(1):71-76.

76. Wolf P, Roder-Wanner UU, Brede M. Influence of therapeutic phenobarbital and phenytoin medication on the polygraphic sleep of patients with epilepsy. *Epilepsia.* 1984;25(4):467-475.

77. Yang JD, Elphick M, Sharpley AL, Cowen PJ. Effects of carbamazepine on sleep in healthy volunteers. *Biol Psychiatry.* 1989;26(3):324-328.

78. Gann H, Riemann D, Hohagen F, Muller WE, Berger M. The influence of carbamazepine on sleep-EEG and the clonidine test in healthy subjects: Results of a preliminary study. *Biol Psychiatry.* 1994;35(11):893-896.

79. Placidi F, Diomedi M, Scalise A, Marciani MG, Romigi A, Gigli GL. Effect of anticonvulsants on nocturnal sleep in epilepsy. *Neurology.* 2000;54(5) (suppl 1):S25-S32.

80. Rao ML, Clarenbach P, Vahlensieck M, Kratzschmar S. Gabapentin augments whole blood serotonin in healthy young men. *J Neural Transm.* 1988;73(2):129-134.

81. Karacan I, Orr W, Roth T, Kramer M, Thornby J, et al. Dose-related effects of phenobarbitone on human sleep-waking patterns. *Br J Clin Pharmacol.* 1981;12(3):303-313.

82. Bell C, Vanderlinden H, Hiersemenzel R, Otoul C, Nutt D, Wilson S. The effects of levetiracetam on objective and subjective sleep parameters in healthy volunteers and patients with partial epilepsy. *J Sleep Res.* 2002;11(3):255-263.

83. Cicolin A, Magliola U, Giordano A, Terreni A, Bucca C, Mutani R. Effects of levetiracetam on nocturnal sleep and daytime vigilance in healthy volunteers. *Epilepsia.* 2006;47(1):82-85.

84. Bazil C, Battista J, Basner R. Effects of levetiracetam on sleep in normal volunteers. *Epilepsy Behav.* 2005;7(3):539-542.

85. Manni R, Ratti MT, Perucca E, Galimberti CA, Tartara A. A multiparametric investigation of daytime sleepiness and psychomotor functions in epileptic patients treated with phenobarbital and sodium valproate: A comparative controlled study. *Electroencephalogr Clin Neurophysiol.* 1993;86(5):322-328.

86. Röder-Wanner U, Wolf P. Effects of treatment with dipropylacetate and ethosuximide on sleep organization in epileptic patients. In: Dam M, Gram L, Penry JK, eds. *Advances in Epileptology: XIIth Epilepsy International Symposium.* New York: Raven Press; 1981:145-157.

87. Maxion H, Jacobi P, Schneider E, Kohler M. *Effect of the Anticonvulsant Drugs Primidone and Diphenylhydantoin on Night Sleep in Healthy Volunteers and Epileptic Patients.* Basel: Karger; 1975.

88. Legros B, Bazil C. Effects of antiepileptic drugs on sleep architecture: A pilot study. *Sleep Med.* 2003;4(1):51-55.

89. Marzec M, Edwards J, Sagher O, Fromes G, Malow BA. Effects of vagus nerve stimulation on sleep-related breathing in epilepsy patients. *Epilepsia.* 2003;44(7):930-935.

90. Hsieh T, Chen M, McAfee A, Kifle Y. Sleep-related breathing disorder in children with vagal nerve stimulators. *Pediatr Neurol.* 2008;38(2):99-103.

91. Malow BA, Edwards J, Marzec M, Sagher O, Fromes G. Effects of vagus nerve stimulation on respiration during sleep: A pilot study. *Neurology.* 2000;55(10):1450-1454.

92. Malow B, Edwards J, Marzec M, Sagher O, Ross D, Fromes G. Vagus nerve stimulation reduces daytime sleepiness in epilepsy patients. *Neurology.* 2001;57(5):879-884.

93. Foldvary-Schaefer N, Stephenson L, Bingaman W. Resolution of obstructive sleep apnea with epilepsy surgery? Expanding the relationship between sleep and epilepsy. *Epilepsia.* 2008;49(8):1457-1459.

94. Derry CP, Duncan JS, Berkovic SF. Paroxysmal motor disorders of sleep: The clinical spectrum and differentiation from epilepsy. *Epilepsia.* 2006;47(11):1775-1791.

95. International Classification of Sleep Disorders. *Diagnostic and Coding Manual.* 2nd ed. Westchester, IL: American Academy of Sleep Medicine; 2005.

96. Aldrich M, ed. *Parasomnias.* Oxford, England: Oxford University Press; 1999.

97. Malow BA. Neurological monitoring techniques. In: Kryger M, Roth T, Dement W, eds. *Principles and Practice of Sleep Medicine.* 4th ed. St. Louis: Elsevier; 2005:1422-1433.

98. Sheldon S, ed. *Disorders of development and maturation of sleep, and sleep disorders of infancy, childhood, and cerebral palsy.* New York: Marcel Dekker; 2000.

99. Mahowald MW, Schenck CH, Rosen GM, Hurwitz TD. The role of a sleep disorder center in evaluating sleep violence. *Arch Neurol.* 1992;49(6):604-607.

100. Mahowald MW, Schenck CH, Goldner M, Bachelder V, Cramer-Borneman M. Parasomnia pseudo-suicide. *J Forensic Sci.* 2003;48(5):1158-1162.

101. Yogarajah M, Powell HW, Heaney D, Smith SJ, Duncan JS, Sisodiya SM. Long term monitoring in refractory epilepsy: The Gowers Unit experience. *J Neurol Neurosurg Psychiatry.* 2009;80(3):305-310.

102. Trotti LM. REM sleep behaviour disorder in older individuals: Epidemiology, pathophysiology and management. *Drugs Aging.* 2010;27(6):457-470.

103. Schenck C, Bundlie S, Ettinger M, Mahowald MW. Chronic behavioural disorders of REM sleep: A new category of parasomnia. *Sleep.* 1986;9:293-308.

104. Hoque R, Chesson Jr AL. Pharmacologically induced/exacerbated restless legs syndrome, periodic limb movements of sleep, and REM behavior disorder/REM sleep without atonia: Literature review, qualitative scoring, and comparative analysis. *J Clin Sleep Med.* 2010;6(1):79-83.

105. Schenck CH, Hurwitz TD, Mahowald MW. REM sleep behaviour disorder: An update on a series of 96 pateints and a review of the world literature. *J Sleep Res.* 1993;2:224-231.

106. Boeve BF, Silber MH, Saper CB, Ferman TJ, Dickson DW, et al. Pathophysiology of REM sleep behaviour disorder and relevance to neurodegenerative disease. *Brain.* 2007;130(Pt 11):2770-2788.

107. Iber C, Ancoli-Israel S, Chesson A, Quan S. *The AASM Manual for the Scoring of Sleep and Associated Events: Rules, Terminology and Technical Specifications.* Westchester, IL: American Academy of Sleep Medicine; 2007.

108. Takeuchi T, Miyasita A, Sasaki Y, Inugami M, Fukuda K. Isolated sleep paralysis elicited by sleep interruption. *Sleep.* 1992;15(3):217-225.

109. Walters AS. Clinical identification of the simple sleep-related movement disorders. *Chest.* 2007;131(4):1260-1266.

110. Khatami R, Zutter D, Siegel A, Mathis J, Donati F, Bassetti CL. Sleep-wake habits and disorders in a series of 100 adult epilepsy patients—A prospective study. *Seizure.* 2006;15(5):299-306.

111. Newell KM, Incledon T, Bodfish JW, Sprague RL. Variability of stereotypic body-rocking in adults with mental retardation. *Am J Ment Retard.* 1999;104(3):279-288.

112. Mayer G, Wilde-Frenz J, Kurella B. Sleep related rhythmic movement disorder revisited. *J Sleep Res.* 2007;16(1):110-116.

113. Laberge L, Tremblay RE, Vitaro F, Montplaisir J. Development of parasomnias from childhood to early adolescence. *Pediatrics.* 2000;106:67-74.

114. Lavigne G, Montplaisir J. Restless legs syndrome and sleep bruxism: Prevalence and association among Canadians. *Sleep.* 1994;17:739-743.

115. Saletu A, Parapatics S, Anderer P, Matejka M, Saletu B. Controlled clinical, polysomnographic and psychometric studies on differences between sleep bruxers and controls and acute effects of clonazepam as compared with placebo. *Eur Arch Psychiatry Clin Neurosci.* 2010;260(2):163-174.

116. Iranzo A, Santamaria J. Severe obstructive sleep apnea/hypopnea mimicking REM sleep behavior disorder. *Sleep.* 2005;28(2):203-206.

117. Miano S, Paolino MC, Peraita-Adrados R, Montesano M, Barberi S, Villa MP. Prevalence of EEG paroxysmal activity in a population of children with obstructive sleep apnea syndrome. *Sleep.* 2009;32(4):522-529.

118. Malow BA, Levy K, Maturen K, Bowes R. Obstructive sleep apnea is common in medically refractory epilepsy patients. *Neurology.* 2000;55(7):1002-1007.

119. Chihorek AM, Abou-Khalil B, Malow BA. Obstructive sleep apnea is associated with seizure occurrence in older adults with epilepsy. *Neurology.* 2007;69(19):1823-1827.

120. Malow BA, Weatherwax KJ, Chervin RD, Hoban TF, Marzec ML, et al. Identification and treatment of obstructive sleep apnea in adults and children with epilepsy: A prospective pilot study. *Sleep Med.* 2003;4(6):509-515.

121. Malow BA, Foldvary-Schaefer N, Vaughn BV, Selwa LM, Chervin RD, et al. Treating obstructive sleep apnea in adults with epilepsy: A randomized pilot trial. *Neurology.* 2008;71(8):572-577.

122. Wise M, ed. *Sleep and Epilepsy: The Clinical Spectrum.* Amsterdam: Elsevier Science; 2002.

123. Sheikh S, Stephen T, Sisson B. Prevalence of gastroesophageal reflux in infants with brief apneic episodes. *Can Respir J.* 1999;6:401-404.

124. Thacker K, Devinsky O, Perrine K, Alper K, Luciano D. Nonepileptic seizures during apparent sleep. *Ann Neurol.* 1993;33(4):414-418.

125. Cascino GD. Clinical indications and diagnostic yield of video-electroencephalographic monitoring in patients with seizures and spells. *Mayo Clin Proc.* 2002;77(10):1111-1120.

126. Mellman T, Uhde T. Electroencephalographic sleep in panic disorder. *Arch Gen Psychiatry.* 1989;46:178-184.

127. Hauri P, Friedman M, Ravaris C. Sleep in patients with spontaneous panic attacks. *Sleep.* 1989;12:323-337.

128. Vetrugno R, Provini F, Plazzi G, Vignatelli L, Lugaresi E, Montagna P. Catathrenia (nocturnal groaning): A new type of parasomnia. *Neurology.* 2001;56:681-683.

129. Jasper H. The 10-20 electrode system of the Internation Federation. *Electroencephalogr Clin Neurophysiol.* 1958;10:370-375.

130. Guideline 6. A proposal for standard montages to be used in clinical EEG. *J Clin Neurophysiol.* 2006;23(2):111-117.

131. Daly D, Pedley T. *Practice of Clinical Electroencephalography.* New York: Raven Press; 2002.

132. Tinuper P, Grassi C, Bisulli F, Provini F, Plazzi G, et al. Split-screen synchronized display. A useful video-EEG technique for studying paroxysmal phenomena. *Epileptic Disord.* 2004;6(1):27-30.

133. Penzel T, Hirshkowitz M, Harsh J, Chervin RD, Butkov N, et al. Digital analysis and technical specifications. *J Clin Sleep Med.* 2007;3(2):109-120.

134. Lagerlund TD, Cascino GD, Cicora KM, Sharbrough FW. Long-term electroencephalographic monitoring for diagnosis and management of seizures. *Mayo Clin Proc.* 1996;71(10):1000-1006.

135. Foldvary-Schaefer N, De Ocampo J, Mascha E, Burgess R, Dinner D, Morris H. Accuracy of seizure detection using abbreviated EEG during polysomnography. *J Clin Neurophysiol.* 2006;23(1):68-71.

136. Zadra A, Pilon M, Joncas S, Rompre S, Montplaisir J. Analysis of postarousal EEG activity during somnambulistic episodes. *J Sleep Res.* 2004;13(3):279-284.

137. DeWolfe JL. Utilization of video in routine EEG. *Epilepsia.* 2009;3 (suppl O):207:(abstract).

Sleep-Disordered Breathing and Cerebrovascular Disease

Chapter
51

H. KLAR YAGGI / PAUL DIEFFENBACH

When considered separately from cardiovascular disease, stroke is the third leading cause of death in the United States and ranks as the leading cause of long-term disability.[1] Patients with minor stroke and transient ischemic attack (TIA) are also at high risk for poor outcomes despite current prevention strategies. Twenty-five percent of patients with TIA will have a completed stroke, experience a cardiovascular event, or die within 90 days. Therefore, understanding underlying pathophysiology, developing novel therapeutic approaches, and reducing recurrent vascular events after TIA are of crucial importance.

The treatment of obstructive sleep apnea (OSA) may provide a novel therapeutic target to improve outcomes among patients after cerebrovascular events. Sleep apnea is highly prevalent in patients after stroke and TIA[2-6] and has been found to be associated with poor outcomes after stroke.[7] Moreover, in prospective studies sleep apnea independently increases the risk of incident ischemic stroke,[8] as well as composite risk of stroke, TIA, and death.[9] These independent risks are likely mediated through a variety of mechanisms including intermittent hypoxia,[10] nocturnal sympathetic activation,[11] systemic hypertension,[12] cardiac dysrhythmias,[13] negative intrathoracic pressure swings,[14] paradoxical embolization,[15] metabolic dysregulation,[16] and snoring-induced carotid vibratory trauma.[17] Continuous positive airway pressure (CPAP) safely and effectively treats sleep apnea,[18] attenuates the physiologic sequelae of sleep apnea,[19] and may ultimately help to improve outcomes among patients with stroke and TIA.[20] This chapter will review evidence of the association between sleep apnea and stroke, mechanisms by which sleep-disordered breathing might predispose to increased cerebrovascular risk, and recent literature regarding the impact of CPAP therapy on cerebrovascular outcomes.

AUTONOMIC CHANGES IN THE CARDIOVASCULAR SYSTEM DURING SLEEP, AND THE CIRCADIAN OCCURRENCE OF SUDDEN DEATH EVENTS

Studies in normal humans using microneurography, which allows for direct recording of peripheral sympathetic nerve traffic, suggest that the cardiovascular influence of sleep is more complex than a generalized inhibition of the sympathetic nervous system.[11] The most striking example is rapid eye movement (REM) sleep, which replaces non-REM (NREM) sleep for several minutes at regular intervals and is accompanied by skeletal muscle atonia, bursts of REMs, and muscle twitches. During REM sleep, sympathetic nerve activity increases significantly and blood pressure and heart rate return to levels

similar to those during wakefulness. Conversely, there are marked reductions in blood pressure ("nocturnal dipping"), heart rate, and sympathetic activity during NREM sleep, which accounts for most of sleep time. These changes become more marked at deeper stages of NREM (i.e. slow wave sleep).[11] These observations might explain the reason myocardial ischemia, infarction, and stroke are less common during the night than during daytime periods of similar duration, particularly the morning hours[21] (Fig. 51-1). In contrast, this observed morning circadian pattern of adverse cardiovascular events appears to be inverted among patients with OSA, in whom the peak circadian time for sudden death occurs during the sleeping hours between midnight and 6 AM.[22] These sudden death events likely consist at least in part of acute strokes, as evidenced by epidemiologic data showing a 20% incidence of acute stroke as a cause of sudden death.[23]

OBSTRUCTIVE SLEEP APNEA AND CEREBROVASCULAR OUTCOMES

Overnight polysomnography is considered the gold standard diagnostic test to evaluate the presence of sleep apnea. A number of cross-sectional and case-control studies have used overnight polysomnography in order to evaluate the association between sleep apnea and cerebrovascular disease. In a recent meta-analysis pooling results from this literature, Johnson and Johnson[2] estimated a 72% prevalence of sleep apnea among poststroke and post-TIA patients, with over half of these patients having moderate-severe disease (Table 51-1). One significant limitation of these case-control and cross-sectional studies, however, is their inability to establish the temporal course in a cause-and-effect relationship. Such study designs might reflect reverse causal pathways whereby sleep-disordered breathing has been the consequence rather than the cause of cerebrovascular disease. For example, several case reports of sleep apnea after bulbar stroke have been reported in the literature.[24,25] Therefore, it is difficult to be certain whether sleep apnea is a cause or consequence of the cerebrovascular outcome. The direction of this arrow of causation can ultimately only be definitively determined by analysis of incident cerebrovascular disease events.

Several recent prospective observational cohort studies have helped to clarify this temporal relationship and have demonstrated that sleep apnea increases the risk for stroke,[26,27] stroke and all-cause death,[28,29] and fatal and nonfatal cardiovascular events (including stroke).[19] In one study, after excluding prevalent stroke and adjusting for traditional cerbrovascular

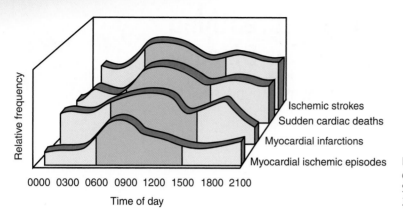

Figure 51-1 Circadian variation in ischemic stroke and cardiovascular events in the general population. (Redrawn from Mohsenin V. Sleep-related breathing disorders and risk of stroke. *Stroke.* 2001;32:1271, used with permission.)

TABLE 51-1

Prevalence of Sleep Apnea in Stroke or Transient Ischemic Attack, Stratified by Apnea-Hypopnea Index (AHI)*

Cutpoint	No. of Studies (No. of Patients)	Prevalence (%)† (95% CI)
AHI > 5	9 (908)	72 (60-81)
AHI > 10	24 (1980)	63 (58-68)
AHI > 20	15 (1405)	38 (31-46)
AHI > 30	10 (865)	29 (21-37)
AHI > 40	3 (318)	14 (7-25)
Central*	17 (1286)	7 (5-12)

*AHI = (number of apneas + number of hypopneas)/duration of sleep (hours).
†Percentage of patients who had primarily central apnea.
Adapted with permission from Johnson K, Johnson D. Frequency of sleep apnea in stroke and TIA: A meta-analysis. *J Clin Sleep Med.* 2010;6(2):131-137.

TABLE 51-2

Proposed Mechanisms Causally Linking Sleep-Disordered Breathing to Incident Stroke

Mechanism	Consequence
Intermittent hypoxia-induced activation of vascular inflammatory pathways	Impaired endothelial function, accelerated atherogenesis, thrombosis
Autonomic-mediated increases in circulating catecholamines	Hypertension, increased intracranial pressure
Negative intrathoracic pressure created from inspiratory effort against closed airway	Impaired autoregulation, decreased stroke volume, alterations in cerebral blood flow
Predisposition to cardiac arrhythmias	Atrial fibrillation, increased embolic stroke risk
Right-to-left shunting through a patent foramen ovale	Paradoxical embolism
Metabolic dysregulation	Metabolic syndrome, diabetes, vascular inflammation, and worsened atherogenesis
Snoring-induced mechanical carotid trauma	Increased carotid plaque burden

---

risk factors (including hypertension), sleep apnea was associated with a twofold increased risk for TIA, stroke, or all-cause death.[9] In a trend analysis, increasing severity of sleep apnea at baseline was associated with an increased risk for the development of the composite endpoint ($P = 0.005$).[9] Those patients in the highest severity quartile of the cohort (apnea-hypopnea index [AHI] > 36) had a greater than threefold increased risk for the development of stroke or death. A similar magnitude of risk was observed in a longitudinal examination of the Wisconsin sleep cohort, but the odds ratio (OR) was no longer statistically significant after adjustments for confounders.[26] Recently published data from the Sleep Heart Health Study demonstrated a statistically significant OR of 2.86 for incident stroke in men with moderate-severe sleep apnea (AHI ≥ 20), and a 6% increase per AHI unit increase in male patients with mild-moderate disease (5 ≤ AHI < 25).[8] Interestingly, a significant association between AHI and incident stroke was observed only in the most severely affected women (AHI > 25). The associations seen in these studies strongly imply that there are mechanisms specific to sleep apnea that confer a risk for the development of cerebrovascular disease.

Pathophysiologic Mechanisms of Cerebrovascular Disease in Sleep Apnea

Patients with sleep apnea have recurrent "cycles" of sleep, airway obstruction, arousal, and resumption of ventilation. Several physiologic stresses arise from this intermittent airway occlusion during sleep including: intermittent hypoxia of varying duration and severity, the generation of strenuous respiratory efforts and severely negative intrathoracic pressures, increased right-sided heart pressures, sympathetic activation, reduced total sleep time, and snoring with vibratory injury (Table 51-2). These stresses, unique to sleep-disordered breathing, serve as potential mechanisms for the increased risk of adverse cerebrovascular events and are discussed in further detail in the next paragraphs.

Intermittent Hypoxia and Inflammation

Systemic inflammation plays an important role in the development of atherosclerosis. The pathogenesis of inflammation and atherosclerosis in sleep apnea has not been entirely elucidated; however, intermittent hypoxia followed by reoxygenation (common to sleep apnea) appears to play a key role. Repetitive episodes of hypoxia may selectively activate vascular inflammatory pathways.[10,30] A higher frequency of repetitive oxygen desaturations has been correlated with increasing severity of atherosclerosis.[31] It has been suggested that hypoxia-reoxygenation cycles that occur in OSA patients may trigger formation of reactive oxygen species and facilitate oxidative stress in a manner similar to ischemia-reperfusion injury.[32] Two- to threefold increases in basal and stimulated levels of superoxide production have been found in the leukocytes of subjects with OSA compared to non-weight-matched control subjects.[33,34] Accelerated free radical formation and oxidative stress correlate with increased levels of oxidized lipids,[35-37] prostaglandins,[38] protein,[39] and DNA[40] seen in patients with OSA. This increased stress can have deleterious effects on leukocytes and platelets, inducing the expression of adhesion molecules and proinflammatory cytokines, which in turn may lead to endothelial dysfunction and consequently to atherosclerosis.[34,36,41-44] Notably, markers of oxidative stress in OSA, including lipid peroxidation, enhanced leukocyte free radical formation, and the decline in nitric oxide (NO) bioavailability, have been shown to regress or partially reverse after CPAP therapy.[33,38,45,46]

Nocturnal Sympathetic Activation

Sympathetic overactivity in the pathogenesis of cerebrovascular complications in OSA has been suggested for several years, and evidence continues to accumulate. Early reports found increased plasma and urinary catecholamine levels in patients with sleep apnea and a fall in these levels after treatment with tracheostomy.[47] Others employed more direct measures of sympathetic nerve activity through the use of a tungsten microelectrode in the peroneal nerve.[48] This methodology demonstrated increased muscle sympathetic nerve activity following acute apneic events. Superimposed on these bursts of sympathetic activation are "surges" of blood pressure of up to levels of 240 mm Hg at apnea termination. These acute blood pressure elevations during apnea appear to be driven by changes in baroreceptor sensitivity during sleep and chemoreceptor responses to progressive hypoxia.[49] Considering that humans typically spend one third of their lives sleeping, these nocturnal increases in blood pressure might in themselves contribute to hypertensive cardiovascular and cerebrovascular consequences. Indeed, patients with sleep apnea commonly do not have the normal nocturnal fall or "dipping" in blood pressure.[50] Among patients with hypertension, those who exhibit a diminished nocturnal decline in blood pressure, "nondippers,"[51] have been reported to have more cardiovascular target organ damage than "dippers"[52,53] including silent cerebrovascular damage.[54] Three longitudinal studies conducted in patients with hypertension have confirmed that a diminished nocturnal decline in blood pressure predicted cardiovascular events[55,56] including worsened stroke prognosis.[57] Moreover, diminished nocturnal decline of blood pressure is a risk factor for cardiovascular death independent of overall blood pressure load during a 24-hour period, with 5% decrease in nocturnal dipping associated with a 20% increase in cardiovascular death.[58]

Sleep Apnea and Daytime Hypertension

In addition to acute blood pressure swings at night, evidence supports that sustained *diurnal* hypertension can arise from obstructive apnea. This appears to be in part related to a "carryover" phenomenon of heightened sympathetic activity.[48] In the Sleep Heart Health Study,[59] sleep apnea was associated with prevalent hypertension even after controlling for potential confounders such as age, gender, body mass index (BMI and other measures of adiposity), alcohol, and smoking. Overall, the odds of hypertension appeared to increase with increases in respiratory disturbance index (RDI) in a dose-responsive fashion. From prospective results of the Wisconsin Sleep Cohort, the presence of sleep apnea at baseline was accompanied by a substantially increased risk for future hypertension at 4-year follow-up.[60] Even after adjusting for baseline hypertension status, age, gender, BMI, waist and neck circumference, and weekly alcohol and cigarette use, the risk for hypertension remained elevated (two- to threefold). The Seventh Report of the Joint Committee on Prevention, Detection, Evaluation, and Treatment of High Blood Pressure (JCN 7) recognizes the etiologic role of sleep apnea as an identifiable cause of hypertension.[61]

Cardiac Arrhythmia

Sleep apnea is associated with cardiac arrhythmias, including both conduction abnormalities such as second-degree atrioventricular block[62] and potentially life-threatening arrhythmias such as ventricular tachycardia.[63] Sleep apnea has also been specifically associated with atrial fibrillation.[64-66] In a recent analysis of participants from the Sleep Heart Health Study, individuals with severe sleep-disordered breathing had two to four times the odds of complex arrhythmia (atrial fibrillation, non-sustained ventricular tachycardia, and complex ventricular ectopy) compared to patients without sleep-disordered breathing even after adjustment for potential confounders.[13] The association between sleep apnea and atrial fibrillation provides an indirect mechanism for stroke via embolic phenomenon.

Mechanical Load

Large negative intrapleural pressures are generated as a result of attempting inspiration against an obstructed upper airway. This large negative intrapleural pressure results in elevated cardiac transmural pressure, or afterload, because of the high pressure differential between the inraventricular and intrapleural spaces.[67] These increases in afterload and corresponding decreases in cardiac output, combined with surges in systemic blood pressure in relation to individual obstructive apneic events, predispose to significant swings in cerebral blood flow during apneic episodes (Fig. 51-2).[68] Such large variations in cerebral blood flow are hypothesized to predispose the cerebrovascular system to increased sheering stress, ischemia, and acute cerebrovascular events.[69]

Paradoxical Embolism

A patent foramen ovale (PFO) is a defect in the interatrial septum that normally allows right-to-left shunting in the fetal circulation, but persists after birth in an estimated 27% of the general population.[70] Younger adult patients with cryptogenic stroke have three to six times increased prevalence of PFO compared to other stroke patients,[71] suggesting a high rate of stroke via paradoxical embolization in this patient subset. OSA may increase the risk of stroke by being provocative of right-to-left shunting through a patent foramen ovale.[15] The increased right-sided heart pressures associated with apneic events may serve to increase the exposure time of right-to-left shunting through a patent foramen ovale, which increases the risk of paradoxical embolism. In one study of OSA patients with PFO, Beelke and associates[15] found right-to-left shunting on transcranial Doppler study during nocturnal sleep in 9 out of 10 patients, but only during OSA episodes lasting more than 17 seconds. Patients with sleep apnea have also been shown

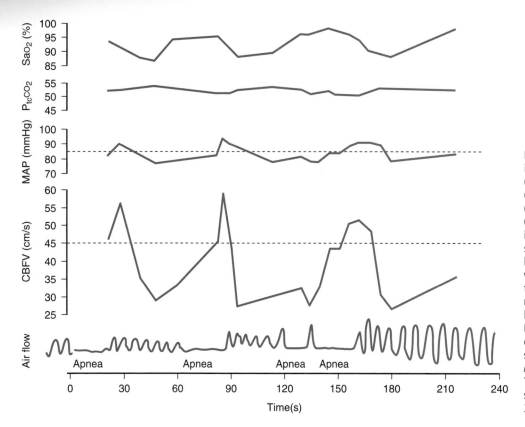

Figure 51-2 Simultaneous recordings of arterial oxygen saturation (SaO$_2$), transcutaneous arterial PCO$_2$ (PtcCO$_2$), mean arterial blood pressure (MAP), cerebral blood flow velocity (CBFV), and respiratory airflow during sleep in a patient with obstructive sleep apnea. The recording shows long periods of low CBFV compared with baseline (*dashed line*) during the obstructive apnea with a steep rise at the end of the apnea parallel to rises in MAP. (Adapted from Balfors E, Franklin K. Impairment in cerebral perfusion during obstructive sleep apneas. *Am J Respir Crit Care Med.* 1994;150:1587-1591, and from Yaggi H, Mohsenin V. Obstructive sleep apnoea and stroke. *Lancet Neurol.* 2004;3(6):333-342.)

to have greatly increased prevalence of patent foramen ovale by both transcranial Doppler[72] and transesophageal echocardiography[73] detection methods compared to age-matched control populations, indirectly implicating the pathophysiology of OSA in the recurrence of detectable PFO in adults.

Short Sleep Duration and Metabolic Dysregulation

There is significant overlap between sleep apnea and the cluster of cardiovascular risk factors that constitutes the "metabolic syndrome." In fact, there is accumulating evidence to suggest that sleep restriction may worsen these metabolic abnormalities. In the Sleep Heart Health Study cohort, sleep durations of 6 hours or less were associated with an increased prevalence of diabetes mellitus and impaired glucose tolerance by oral glucose tolerance test with 1.5-fold to 2.5-fold risk after adjustment for age, sex, and body habitus.[16] Moreover, a twofold increased incidence of diabetes was observed in Massachusetts Male Aging Study participant with short sleep duration even after adjustment for age, self-rated health status, and waist circumference.[74] Recently, sleep duration has also been linked to the development of incident coronary artery calcification, with longer sleep duration demonstrating a clear protective effect.[75] Several studies have also demonstrated an independent association between sleep-disordered breathing and increased risk for glucose intolerance,[76] insulin resistance,[77,78] and even overt clinical diabetes.[79,80]

Snoring and Carotid Atherosclerosis

A novel mechanism has recently emerged linking sleep apnea to stroke via a direct pathogenic relationship between snoring and carotid atherosclerosis. Snores originate from the upper airway during sleep and are a result of vibrations of the

pharyngeal wall and associated structures. It has been hypothesized that oscillatory pressure waves/vibrations originating in the upper airway during snoring may be transmitted through the surrounding tissue to the carotid artery wall. The proximity of the carotid artery bifurcation to the lateral pharyngeal wall is such that it is likely exposed to these vibrations and may cause pathologic damage to the arterial wall endothelium, triggering an inflammatory cascade leading to early atherosclerosis or embolic phenomenon. In this context, a recent cross-sectional study[17] was conducted on 110 patients who underwent overnight polysomnography with quantification of snoring, carotid artery ultrasound, and simultaneous quantification of femoral artery atherosclerosis as a distant (from the upper airway) control artery. A significant association was observed (in a dose-response fashion) between percentage of time snoring and the prevalence of carotid artery atherosclerosis (but not femoral atherosclerosis) even after adjustment for confounding variables. Of note, early epidemiologic studies linking sleep-disordered breathing to stroke used snoring as a "proxy measure" for sleep-disordered breathing;[4,81-86] however, these new data suggest a more direct pathogenic relationship attributable to snoring.

Therapy for Sleep Apnea and Impact on Cerebrovascular Risk

Compared to control groups, CPAP (the main medical therapy for sleep apnea) shows significant improvements in objective and subjective measures of sleepiness, quality of life, and cognitive function.[87] CPAP has also been demonstrated to improve left ventricular function in patients with congestive heart failure and sleep apnea[88-91] and to decrease automobile accidents.[92] To date no published *long-term* prospective randomized controlled trials have demonstrated that the treatment of sleep apnea decreases the risk of cerebrovascular events in terms of either primary or secondary prevention. However, long-term longitudinal observational cohort studies have evaluated the impact of CPAP therapy on cardiovascular outcomes, and short-term randomized controlled trials have evaluated the impact of CPAP on hypertension and intermediate cerebrovascular endpoints in patients with sleep apnea.

Long-Term Observational Studies

One early investigation that gives some insight into the impact of sleep apnea treatment on the risk of stroke (and myocardial infarction) was a retrospective cohort study of patients who were diagnosed with sleep apnea in the 1970s using polysomnography.[93] This study was conducted prior to the availability of CPAP, when the only known definitive therapy for sleep apnea consisted of tracheostomy. Here, 7 years of follow-up was provided on 198 patients, of which 71 patients received tracheostomy (considered "effective treatment") and 127 received "conservative treatment" consisting of recommended weight loss (the only alternative). Any new hypertension, myocardial infarction, or stroke occurring since the original polysomnography was considered the main vascular morbidity outcome. Despite the fact that at study entry the tracheostomy group included more patients with a history of hypertension, myocardial infarction, or stroke, it was the conservatively treated group who developed considerably more vascular events.

Over the past decade, prospective observational cohort studies designed to examine the impact of treatment efficacy on long-term cardiovascular outcomes in patients with sleep apnea have demonstrated that CPAP therapy may reduce mortality rate in severe sleep apnea[94] and protect against death from cardiovascular disease.[95] In a study conducted by Marin and associates[19] the incidence of both fatal and nonfatal cardiovascular events (including stroke) was highest in patients with severe untreated sleep apnea. Patients who received and complied with CPAP (who largely had severe sleep apnea) had a significantly reduced cardiovascular risk, suggesting that long-term therapy with CPAP may reduce risk for cardiovascular events. In another study, CPAP compliance in patients found to have OSA after stroke or TIA has been similarly associated with reduced rates of recurrent cardiovascular events (predominantly recurrent stroke).[96]

Until very recently, most other observational studies or controlled trials on CPAP use after ischemic stroke were small investigations that examined short-term proxy outcomes including subjective well-being,[97] depressive symptoms,[98] and Barthel activities of daily living index.[98,99] Although these studies were able to show a correlation between CPAP use and improved sense of well-being[97] and fewer depressive symptoms,[98] many of them were plagued by very poor CPAP tolerance and compliance.[99-101]

A recent 5-year observational study by Martinez-Garcia and associates[20] has demonstrated a highly significant protective effect of CPAP on cardiovascular morbidity and mortality rates after cerebrovascular events. Out of 166 patients with acute ischemic stroke who underwent polysomnography, those who had an AHI greater than 20 and did not tolerate CPAP had an increased risk of mortality compared to CPAP-tolerant patients, those with mild sleep apnea, and those without sleep apnea (Fig. 51-3). In a linear regression model, intolerance to CPAP in moderate-severe OSA showed a hazard

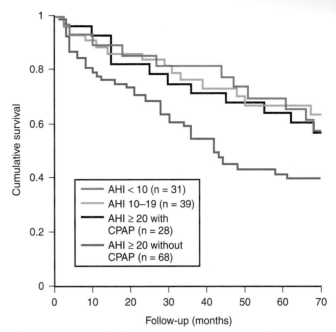

Figure 51-3 Accumulated survival curve for study groups of patients with stroke, by apnea-hypopnea index (AHI) cutoff point and continuous positive airway pressure (CPAP) tolerance. (Redrawn from Martinez-Garcia MA, Soler-Cataluna JJ, Ejarque-Martinez L, et al. Continuous positive airway pressure treatment reduces mortality in patients with ischemic stroke and obstructive sleep apnea: A 5-year follow-up study. *Am J Respir Crit Care Med.* 2009;180(1): 36-41, used with permission.)

ratio of 1.58 for mortality risk in this population after adjustment for age, sex, Barthel index, AHI, CPAP treatment groups, previous stroke or TIA, diabetes, hypercholesterolemia, body mass index, current smoking, arterial hypertension, atrial fibrillation, significant carotid stenosis, and fibrinogen levels. Furthermore, patients who did not tolerate CPAP specifically showed a statistically significant increase in deaths due to ischemic stroke (25% vs. 10-12% in the other groups, $p = 0.03$).

A criticism of these observational studies has been that the lack of treatment group randomization allows for bias from unaccounted differences between CPAP users and nonusers, especially regarding compliance with other medical co-therapy (e.g., medications, lifestyle adjustments). However, in methodologic work in which both observational studies examining treatment efficacy and randomized trials existed on a variety of clinical topics, the results of well-designed observational studies did not systematically overestimate the magnitude of the effects of treatment as compared with those in randomized, controlled trials on the same topic.[102] Whether the preceding observational findings are ultimately confirmed by longer-term randomized, controlled trials remains to be seen, and a significant international effort is underway to conduct such trials. Early published efforts (largely short-term studies) in the conduct of randomized controlled trials examining the impact of CPAP on blood pressure and other intermediate measures of cerebrovascular risk are discussed next.

Short-term Randomized Controlled Trials with CPAP Therapy: Effect on Blood Pressure

Short-term (up to 3 months) randomized controlled trials of CPAP therapy have been published looking at arterial blood pressure as the primary outcome. Though the studies vary with respect to the magnitude of blood pressure reduction, overall there appears to be significant reduction in both 24-hour systolic and diastolic pressures following CPAP treatment. The characteristics of the patients selected for these trials give clues to those most likely to gain any blood pressure–lowering benefits. In general, those more likely to experience benefit have more severe and symptomatic sleep apnea, are hypertensive or on hypertensive therapy at baseline, receive more effective therapy for sleep apnea (longer use), and have more frequent oxygen desaturations.[89-91] Those less likely to experience benefit are normotensive at baseline, are asymptomatic, and have milder sleep apnea.[103,104] A systematic literature review conducted by the Cochrane Collaboration[87] found that mean 24-hour systolic and diastolic pressures were significantly lower on CPAP (−7.24 mm Hg systolic, −3.07 mm Hg diastolic). Other meta-analyses have indicated that magnitude of the blood pressure reduction increases significantly with more severe sleep apnea and longer effective nighttime use of CPAP.[105] A recent large randomized controlled trial investigating this question found a small (−2.1 mm Hg systolic, −1.3 mm Hg diastolic), but highly statistically significant, effect of CPAP use versus sham-CPAP in a population of recently diagnosed patients with untreated hypertension and an AHI greater than 15, with a somewhat larger effect seen in those with more severe hypertension and with greater CPAP compliance.[106] Although the magnitude of the blood pressure changes with CPAP therapy remains somewhat controversial, when extrapolated to antihypertensive epidemiologic data, even relatively modest blood pressure reductions would be predicted to significantly reduce stroke and coronary heart disease event risk.[107,108]

CPAP Treatment and Intermediate Cerebrovascular Endpoints

In addition to reduction of blood pressure, CPAP therapy has been demonstrated to improve a number of "intermediate" cerebrovascular endpoints. Effective CPAP therapy eliminates cyclic hypoxia, decreases inflammatory markers of atherosclerosis,[34] reduces sympathetic activity and catecholamines,[90] reduces recurrent atrial fibrillation,[109] and improves left ventricular function.[88] Recently, a short-term randomized controlled trial demonstrated that CPAP also significantly decreases early signs of atherosclerosis as measured by carotid intima media thickness and arterial stiffness.[110] Based on these results, the potential cerebrovascular event risk reduction of CPAP therapy may be more than that conferred just by its blood pressure–lowering effects. This question awaits the results of future longer-term randomized controlled trials.

Acute TIA/Minor Stroke as a Therapeutic Target for Secondary Prophylaxis

Patients with TIA/minor stroke are ideal candidates for the prevention of recurrent vascular events. Over 300,000 TIAs occur annually in the United States.[111] Despite current prevention strategies, patients with TIAs are at high risk for recurrent vascular events with 25% of patients developing completed stroke, myocardial infarction, congestive heart failure hospitalization, or death within 90 days after initial TIA presentation.[112] Importantly, half of these events occur within the first 72 hours. New approaches to reduce this recurrent vascular event rate are needed (particularly in the acute post-TIA period). Recent work has demonstrated that sleep apnea

is common among TIA patients (60%) and that it is feasible to initiate CPAP in the acute TIA setting using autotitrating CPAP devices.[113] Using a protocol for rapid administration of autotitrating CPAP immediately after TIA, acute TIA patients showed a 90-day compliance rate comparable to non-TIA patients and with greater compliance than stroke patients.[99] Moreover, data from this feasibility trial, combined with other published data on cardiovascular outcomes in patients with stroke or TIA,[96] support the hypothesis that CPAP therapy may help to reduce recurrent vascular events after TIA.

SUMMARY/PUBLIC HEALTH IMPLICATIONS

Multiple prospective observational cohort studies have demonstrated that OSA significantly increases the risk of stroke independent of potential confounding risk factors. This implies that there are mechanisms mediated by sleep apnea that confer vascular risk. The current literature suggests that such mechanisms include intermittent hypoxia, systemic inflammation, and athersclerosis; nocturnal sympathetic activation; diurnal hypertension; cardiac arrythmias (including atrial fibrillation); mechanical load; paradoxical embolism, metabolic dysregulation; and snoring-induced vibratory injury.

The increasing prevalence of sleep-disordered breathing in the population suggests that the population attributable risk percent (the percentage of the total risk for cerebrovascular disease due to sleep apnea) is high, making the identification of sleep apnea an important public health issue. This is particularly true given that sleep apnea is a potentially modifiable risk factor. Indeed, guidelines from the American Heart Association/American Stroke Association Stroke Council regarding the primary prevention of ischemic stroke recommend "questioning bed partners and patients, particularly those with abdominal obesity and hypertension, about symptoms of sleep-disordered breathing and referring to a sleep specialist as appropriate."[114]

Short-term randomized, controlled trials of CPAP investigating hypertension and other intermediate cardiovascular endpoints, as well as long-term observational cohort studies with follow-up of cerebrovascular and cardiovascular outcomes, together suggest a clinically significant risk reduction associated with the use of CPAP. However, there are currently no published long-term randomized studies demonstrating the efficacy of treating sleep apnea in reducing stroke risk. Such studies are critical prior to instituting large-scale sleep apnea screening guidelines. In the meantime, clinicians should have a low threshold for polysomnographic evaluation in patients with symptoms of sleep-disordered breathing.

REFERENCES

1. American Heart Association. *2005 Heart and Stroke Statistical Update.* Dallas: American Heart Association; 2005.
2. Johnson KG, Johnson DC. Frequency of sleep apnea in stroke and TIA patients: A meta-analysis. *J Clin Sleep Med.* 2010;6(2):131-137.
3. Bassetti C, Aldrich M. Sleep apnea in acute cerebrovascular diseases: Final report on 128 patients. *Sleep.* 1999;22:217-223.
4. Dyken M, Somers V, Yamada T, Ren Z, Zimmerman M. Investigating the relationship between stroke and obstructive sleep apnea. *Stroke.* 1996;27:401-407.
5. Mohsenin V, Valor R. Sleep apnea in patients with hemispheric stroke. *Arch Phys Med Rehabil.* 1995;76:71-76.
6. Parra O. Sleep-disordered breathing and stroke: Is there a rationale for treatment? [letter; comment]. *Eur Respir J.* 2001;18(4):619-622.

7. Sahlin C, Sandberg O, Gustafson Y, et al. Obstructive sleep apnea is a risk factor for death in patients with stroke: A 10-year follow-up. *Arch Intern Med.* 2008;168(3):297-301.

8. Redline S, Yenokyan G, Gottlieb DJ, et al. Obstructive sleep apnea-hypopnea and incident stroke: The Sleep Heart Health Study. *Am J Respir Crit Care Med.* 2010;182(2):269-277.

9. Yaggi HK, Concato J, Kernan WN, Lichtman JH, Brass LM, Mohsenin V. Obstructive sleep apnea as a risk factor for stroke and death. *N Engl J Med.* 2005;353(19):2034-2041.

10. Ryan S, Taylor CT, McNicholas WT. Selective activation of inflammatory pathways by intermittent hypoxia in obstructive sleep apnea syndrome. *Circulation.* 2005;112(17):2660-2667.

11. Somers VK, Dyken ME, Mark AL, Abboud FM. Sympathetic-nerve activity during sleep in normal subjects. *N Engl J Med.* 1993;328(5):303-307.

12. Peppard PE, Young T, Palta M, Skatrud J. Prospective study of the association between sleep-disordered breathing and hypertension. *N Engl J Med.* 2000;342(19):1378-1384.

13. Mehra R, Benjamin EJ, Shahar E, et al. Association of nocturnal arrhythmias with sleep-disordered breathing: The Sleep Heart Health Study. *Am J Respir Crit Care Med.* 2006;173(8):910-916.

14. Balfors EM, Franklin KA. Impairment of cerebral perfusion during obstructive sleep apneas. *Am J Respir Crit Care Med.* 1994;150(6 Pt 1):1587-1591.

15. Beelke M, Angeli S, Del Sette M, et al. Obstructive sleep apnea can be provocative for right-to-left shunting through a patent foramen ovale. *Sleep.* 2002;25(8):856-862.

16. Gottlieb DJ, Punjabi NM, Newman AB, et al. Association of sleep time with diabetes mellitus and impaired glucose tolerance. *Arch Intern Med.* 2005;165(8):863-867.

17. Lee SA, Amis TC, Byth K, et al. Heavy snoring as a cause of carotid artery atherosclerosis. *Sleep.* 2008;31(9):1207-1213.

18. Guest JF, Helter MT, Morga A, Stradling JR. Cost-effectiveness of using continuous positive airway pressure in the treatment of severe obstructive sleep apnea/hypopnea syndrome in the UK. *Thorax.* 2008;63(10):860-865.

19. Marin JM, Carrizo SJ, Vicente E, Agusti AG. Long-term cardiovascular outcomes in men with obstructive sleep apnea-hypopnea with or without treatment with continuous positive airway pressure: An observational study. *Lancet.* 2005;365(9464):1046-1053.

20. Martinez-Garcia MA, Soler-Cataluna JJ, Ejarque-Martinez L, et al. Continuous positive airway pressure treatment reduces mortality in patients with ischemic stroke and obstructive sleep apnea: A 5-year follow-up study. *Am J Respir Crit Care Med.* 2009;180(1):36-41.

21. Marler JR, Price TR, Clark GL, et al. Morning increase in onset of ischemic stroke. *Stroke.* 1989;20(4):473-476.

22. Gami AS, Howard DE, Olson EJ, Somers VK. Day-night pattern of sudden death in obstructive sleep apnea. *N Engl J Med.* 2005;352(12):1206-1214.

23. Tokashiki T, Muratani A, Kimura Y, Muratani H, Fukiyama K. Sudden death in the general population in Okinawa: Incidence and causes of death. *Jpn Circ J.* 1999;63(1):37-42.

24. Chaudhary BA, Elguindi AS, King DW. Obstructive sleep apnea after lateral medullary syndrome. *South Med J.* 1982;75(1):65-67.

25. Askenasy JJ, Goldhammer I. Sleep apnea as a feature of bulbar stroke. *Stroke.* 1988;19(5):637-639.

26. Arzt M, Young T, Finn L, Skatrud JB, Bradley TD. Association of sleep-disordered breathing and the occurrence of stroke. *Am J Respir Crit Care Med.* 2005;172(11):1447-1451.

27. Munoz R, Duran-Cantolla J, Martinez-Vila E, et al. severe sleep apnea and risk of ischemic stroke in the elderly. *Stroke.* 2006;37(9):2317-2321.

28. Marshall NS, Wong KK, Liu PY, Cullen SR, Knuiman MW, Grunstein RR. Sleep apnea as an independent risk factor for all-cause mortality: The Busselton Health Study. *Sleep.* 2008;31(8):1079-1085.

29. Young T, Finn L, Peppard PE, et al. Sleep disordered breathing and mortality: Eighteen-year follow-up of the Wisconsin sleep cohort. *Sleep.* 2008;31(8):1071-1078.

30. Savransky V, Nanayakkara A, Li J, et al. Chronic intermittent hypoxia induces atherosclerosis. *Am J Respir Crit Care Med.* 2007;175(12):1290-1297.

31. Hayashi M, Fujimoto K, Urushibata K, Uchikawa S, Imamura H, Kubo K. Nocturnal oxygen desaturation correlates with the severity of coronary atherosclerosis in coronary artery disease. *Chest.* 2003;124:936-941.

32. Lavie L. Obstructive sleep apnoea syndrome—An oxidative stress disorder. *Sleep Med Rev.* 2003;7(1):35-51.

33. Schulz R, Mahmoudi S, Hattar K, et al. Enhanced release of superoxide from polymorphonuclear neutrophils in obstructive sleep apnea. Impact of continuous positive airway pressure therapy. *Am J Respir Crit Care Med.* 2000;162(2 Pt 1):566-570.

34. Dyugovskaya L, Lavie P, Lavie L. Increased adhesion molecules expression and production of reactive oxygen species in leukocytes of sleep apnea patients. *Am J Respir Crit Care Med.* 2002;165(7):934-939.

35. Barcelo A, Miralles C, Barbe F, Vila M, Pons S, Agusti AG. Abnormal lipid peroxidation in patients with sleep apnoea. *Eur Respir J.* 2000;16(4):644-647.

36. Lavie L, Vishnevsky A, Lavie P. Evidence for lipid peroxidation in obstructive sleep apnea. *Sleep.* 2004;27(1):123-128.

37. Saarelainen S, Lehtimaki T, Jaak-kola O, et al. Autoantibodies against oxidised low-density lipoprotein in patients with obstructive sleep apnoea. *Clin Chem Lab Med.* 1999;37(5):517-520.

38. Carpagnano GE, Kharitonov SA, Resta O, Foschino-Barbaro MP, Gramiccioni E, Barnes PJ. 8-Isoprostane, a marker of oxidative stress, is increased in exhaled breath condensate of patients with obstructive sleep apnea after night and is reduced by continuous positive airway pressure therapy. *Chest.* 2003;124(4):1386-1392.

39. Vatansever E, Surmen-Gur E, Ursavas A, Karadag M. Obstructive sleep apnea causes oxidative damage to plasma lipids and proteins and decreases adiponectin levels. *Sleep Breath.* Berlin/Heidelberg: Springer; 2010:1-8. Available at http://dx.doi.org/10.1007/s11325-010-0378-8.

40. Yamauchi M, Nakano H, Maekawa J, et al. Oxidative stress in obstructive sleep apnea. *Chest.* 2005;127(5):1674-1679.

41. El-Solh A, Mador M, Sikka P, Dhillon R, Amsterdahm D, Grant B. Adhesion molecules in patients with coronary artery disease and moderate-to-severe obstructive sleep apnea. *Chest.* 2002;121:1541-1547.

42. Ohga E, Nagase T, Tomita T, et al. Increased levels of circulating I-CAM-1, VCAM-1, and L-selectin in obstructive sleep apnea syndrome. *J Appl Physiol.* 1999;87:10-14.

43. Lavie L, Dyugovskaya L, Lavie P. Sleep-apnea-related intermittent hypoxia and atherogenesis: Adhesion molecules and monocytes/endothelial cells interactions. *Atherosclerosis.* 2005;183(1):183-184.

44. Lavie L. Sleep-disordered breathing and cerebrovascular disease: A mechanistic approach. *Neurol Clin.* 2005;23(4):1059-1075.

45. Ip MS, Lam B, Chan LY, et al. Circulating nitric oxide is suppressed in obstructive sleep apnea and is reversed by nasal continuous positive airway pressure. *Am J Respir Crit Care Med.* 2000;162(6):2166-2171.

46. Lavie L, Hefetz A, Luboshitzky R, Lavie P. Plasma levels of nitric oxide and L-arginine in sleep apnea patients: Effects of nCPAP treatment. *J Mol Neurosci.* 2003;21(1):57-63.

47. Fletcher E, Miller J, Schaaf J. Urinary catecholamines before and after tracheostomy in patients with obstructive sleep apnea and hypertension. *Sleep.* 1987;10:35-44.

48. Somers V, Dyken M, Clary M, Abboud F. Sympathetic neural mechanisms in obstructive sleep apnea. *J Clin Invest.* 1995;96:1897-1904.

49. O'Donnell C, King E, Schwartz A, Robatham J, Smith P. Relationship between blood pressure and airway obstruction during sleep in the dog. *J Appl Physiol.* 1994;77:1819-1828.

50. Hla KM, Young T, Finn L, Peppard PE, Szklo-Coxe M, Stubbs M. Longitudinal association of sleep-disordered breathing and nondipping of nocturnal blood pressure in the Wisconsin Sleep Cohort Study. *Sleep.* 2008;31(6):795-800.

51. O'Brien E, Sheridan J, O'Malley K. Dippers and non-dippers. *Lancet.* 1988;2(8607):397.

52. Bianchi S, Bigazzi R, Baldari G, Sgherri G, Campese VM. Diurnal variations of blood pressure and microalbuminuria in essential hypertension. *Am J Hypertens.* 1994;7(1):23-29.

53. Verdecchia P, Schillaci G, Guerrieri M. Circadian blood pressure changes and left ventricular hypertrophy. *Circulation.* 1990;81:528-536.

54. Shimada K, Kawamoto A, Matsubayashi K, Ozawa T. Silent cerebrovascular disease in the elderly. Correlation with ambulatory pressure. *Hypertension.* 1990;16(6):692-699.

55. Verdecchia P, Porcellati C, Schillaci G, et al. Ambulatory blood pressure. An independent predictor of prognosis in essential hypertension. *Hypertension.* 1994;24(6):793-801.

56. Staessen JA, Thijs L, Fagard R, et al. Predicting cardiovascular risk using conventional vs. ambulatory blood pressure in older patients with systolic hypertension. Systolic Hypertension in Europe Trial Investigators. *JAMA.* 1999;282(6):539-546.

57. Kario K, Pickering TG, Matsuo T, Hoshide S, Schwartz JE, Shimada K. Stroke prognosis and abnormal nocturnal blood pressure falls in older hypertensives. *Hypertension.* 2001;38(4):852-857.

58. Ohkubo T, Hozawa A, Yamaguchi J, et al. Prognostic significance of the nocturnal decline in blood pressure in individuals with and without high 24-h blood pressure: The Ohasama study. *J Hypertens.* 2002;20(11):2183-2189.

59. Neito F, Young T, Lind B, et al. Association of sleep-disordered breathing, sleep apnea, and hypertension in a large community based study. *JAMA.* 2000;283:1829-1836.

60. Peppard P, Young T, Palta M, Skatrud J. Prospective study of the association between sleep-disordered breathing and hypertension. *N Engl J Med.* 2000;342:1378-1384.

61. Chobanian AV, Bakris GL, Black HR, et al. The Seventh Report of the Joint National Committee on Prevention, Detection, Evaluation, and Treatment of High Blood Pressure: The JNC 7 report. *JAMA.* 2003;289(19):2560-2572.

62. Zwillich C, Devlin T, White D, Douglas N, Weil J, Martin R. Bradycardia during sleep apnea. Characteristics and mechanism. *J Clin Invest.* 1982;69:1286-1292.

63. Fichter J, Bauer D, Arampatzis S, Fries R, Heisel A, Sybrecht G. Sleep-related breathing disorders are associated with ventricular arrhythmias in patients with an implantable cardioverter defibrillator. *Chest.* 2002;122:558-561.

64. Javaheri S, Parker T, Liming J, et al. Sleep apnea in 81 ambulatory male patients with stable heart failure: Types and their prevalences, consequences, and presentations. *Circulation.* 1998;97:2154-2159.

65. Kanagala R, Murali N, Friedman P, et al. Obstructive sleep apnea and the recurrence of atrial fibrillation. *Circulation.* 2003;107:2589-2594.

66. Gami AS, Pressman G, Caples SM, et al. Association of atrial fibrillation and obstructive sleep apnea. *Circulation.* 2004;110(4):364-367.

67. Bradley T. Right and left ventricular functional impairment and sleep apnea. *Clin Chest Med.* 1992;13:459-479.

68. Balfors E, Franklin K. Impairment of cerebral perfusion during obstructive sleep apneas. *Am J Respir Crit Care Med.* 1994;150:1587-1591.

69. Franklin KA. Cerebral haemodynamics in obstructive sleep apnoea and Cheyne-Stokes respiration. *Sleep Med Rev.* 2002;6(6):429-441.

70. Hagen PT, Scholz DG, Edwards WD. Incidence and size of patent foramen ovale during the first 10 decades of life: An autopsy study of 965 normal hearts. *Mayo Clin Proc.* 1984;59(1):17-20.

71. Overell JR, Bone I, Lees KR. Interatrial septal abnormalities and stroke: A meta-analysis of case-control studies. *Neurology.* 2000;55(8):1172-1179.

72. Beelke M, Angeli S, Del Sette M, et al. Prevalence of patent foramen ovale in subjects with obstructive sleep apnea: A transcranial Doppler ultrasound study. *Sleep Med.* 2003;4(3):219-223.

73. Shanoudy H, Soliman A, Raggi P, Liu JW, Russell DC, Jarmukli NF. Prevalence of patent foramen ovale and its contribution to hypoxemia in patients with obstructive sleep apnea. *Chest.* 1998;113(1):91-96.

74. Yaggi HK, Araujo AB, McKinlay JB. Sleep duration as a risk factor for the development of type 2 diabetes. *Diabetes Care.* 2006;29(3):657-661.

75. King CR, Knutson KL, Rathouz PJ, Sidney S, Liu K, Lauderdale DS. Short sleep duration and incident coronary artery calcification. *JAMA.* 2008;300(24):2859-2866.

76. Sulit L, Storfer-Isser A, Kirchner HL, Redline S. Differences in polysomnography predictors for hypertension and impaired glucose tolerance. *Sleep.* 2006;29(6):777-783.

77. Ip MS, Lam B, Ng MM, Lam WK, Tsang KW, Lam KS. Obstructive sleep apnea is independently associated with insulin resistance. *Am J Respir Crit Care Med.* 2002;165(5):670-676.

78. Punjabi N, Sorkin J, Katzel L, Goldberg A, Schwartz A, Smith P. Sleep-disordered breathing and insulin resistance in middle-aged and overweight men. *Am J Respir Crit Care Med.* 2002;165:677-682.

79. Reichmuth KJ, Austin D, Skatrud JB, Young T. Association of sleep apnea and type II diabetes: A population-based study. *Am J Respir Crit Care Med.* 2005;172(12):1590-1595.

80. Botros N, Concato J, Mohsenin V, Selim B, Doctor K, Yaggi HK. Obstructive sleep apnea as a risk factor for type 2 diabetes. *Am J Med.* 2009;122(12):1122-1127.

81. Bassetti C. Habitual snoring, sleep apnoea, and stroke prevention. *J Neurol Neurosurg Psychiatry.* 1997;62(3):303.

82. Jennum P, Schultz-Larsen K, Davidsen M, Christensen NJ. Snoring and risk of stroke and ischaemic heart disease in a 70 year old population. A 6-year follow-up study. *Int J Epidemiol.* 1994;23(6):1159-1164.

83. Koskenvuo M, Kaprio J, Telakivi T, Partinen M, Heikkila K, Sarna S. Snoring as a risk factor for ischaemic heart disease and stroke in men. *Br Med J (Clin Res Educ).* 1987;294:16-19.

84. Neau J, Meurice J, Paquereau J, Chavagnat J, Ingrand P, Gil R. Habitual snoring as a risk factor for brain infarction. *Acta Neurol Scand.* 1995;92:63-68.

85. Palomaki H. Snoring and the risk of ischemic brain infarction. *Stroke.* 1991;22:1021-1025.

86. Spriggs D, French J, Murdy J, Curless R, Bates D, James O. Snoring increases the risk of stroke and adversely affects prognosis. *Q J Med.* 1992;83:555-562.

87. Giles T, Lasserson T, Smith B, White J, Wright J, Cates C. Continuous positive airways pressure for obstructive sleep apnea in adults. *Cochrane Database Syst Rev.* 2006;3:CD001106.

88. Kaneko Y, Floras J, Usui K, et al. Cardiovascular effects of continuous positive airway pressure in patients with heart failure and obstructive sleep apnea. *N Engl J Med.* 2003;348:1233-1241.

89. Becker H, Jerrentrup A, Ploch T, et al. Effect of nasal continuous positive airway pressure treatment on blood pressure in patients with obstructive sleep apnea. *Circulation.* 2003;107:68-73.

90. Faccenda J, Mackay T, Boon N, Douglas N. Randomized placebo-controlled trial of continuous positive airway pressure on blood pressure in the sleep apnea-hypopnea syndrome. *Am J Respir Crit Care Med.* 2001;163:344-348.

91. Pepperell J, Ramdassingh-Dow S, Crosthwaite N, et al. Ambulatory blood pressure after therapeutic and subtherapeutic nasal continuous positive airway pressure for obstructive sleep apnea: A randomised parallel trial. *Lancet.* 2002;359:204-210.

92. Findley L, Smith C, Hooper J, Dineen M, Suratt P. Treatment with nasal CPAP decreases automobile accidents in patients with sleep apnea. *Am J Respir Crit Care Med.* 2000;161:857-859.

93. Partinen M, Guilleminault C. Daytime sleepiness and vascular morbidity at seven-year follow-up in obstructive sleep apnea patients. *Chest.* 1990;97:27-32.

94. Marti S, Sampol G, Munoz X, et al. Mortality in severe sleep apnoea/hypopnoea syndrome patients: Impact of treatment. *Eur Respir J.* 2002;20:1511-1518.

95. Doherty LS, Kiely JL, Swan V, McNicholas WT. Long-term effects of nasal continuous positive airway pressure therapy on cardiovascular outcomes in sleep apnea syndrome. *Chest.* 2005;127(6):2076-2084.

96. Martinez-Garcia MA, Galiano-Blancart R, Roman-Sanchez P, Soler-Cataluna JJ, Cabero-Salt L, Salcedo-Maiques E. Continuous positive airway pressure treatment in sleep apnea prevents new vascular events after ischemic stroke. *Chest.* 2005;128(4):2123-2129.

97. Wessendorf TE, Wang YM, Thilmann AF, Sorgenfrei U, Konietzko N, Teschler H. Treatment of obstructive sleep apnoea with nasal continuous positive airway pressure in stroke. *Eur Respir J.* 2001;18(4):623-629.

98. Sandberg O, Franklin KA, Bucht G, Eriksson S, Gustafson Y. Nasal continuous positive airway pressure in stroke patients with sleep apnoea: A randomized treatment study. *Eur Respir J.* 2001;18(4):630-634.

99. Hsu CY, Vennelle M, Li HY, Engleman HM, Dennis MS, Douglas NJ. Sleep-disordered breathing after stroke: A randomised controlled trial of continuous positive airway pressure. *J Neurol Neurosurg Psychiatry.* 2006;77(10):1143-1149.

100. Hui DS, Choy DK, Wong LK, et al. Prevalence of sleep-disordered breathing and continuous positive airway pressure compliance: Results in Chinese patients with first-ever ischemic stroke. *Chest.* 2002;122(3):852-860.

101. Bassetti CL, Milanova M, Gugger M. Sleep-disordered breathing and acute ischemic stroke: Diagnosis, risk factors, treatment, evolution, and long-term clinical outcome. *Stroke.* 2006;37(4):967-972.

102. Concato J, Shah N, Horwitz RI. Randomized, controlled trials, observational studies, and the hierarchy of research designs. *N Engl J Med.* 2000;342(25):1887-1892.

103. Barbe F, Mayoralas LR, Duran J, et al. Treatment with continuous positive airway pressure is not effective in patients with sleep apnea but no daytime sleepiness. A randomized, controlled trial. *Ann Intern Med.* 2001;134(11):1015-1023.

104. Monasterio C, Vidal S, Duran J, et al. Effectiveness of continuous positive airway pressure in mild sleep apnea-hypopnea syndrome. *Am J Respir Crit Care Med.* 2001;164(6):939-943.

105. Haentjens P, Van Meerhaeghe A, Moscariello A, et al. The impact of continuous positive airway pressure on blood pressure in patients with obstructive sleep apnea syndrome: Evidence from a meta-analysis of placebo-controlled randomized trials. *Arch Intern Med.* 2007;167(8):757-764.

106. Duran-Cantolla J, Aizpuru F, Montserrat JM, et al. Continuous positive airway pressure as treatment for systemic hypertension in people with obstructive sleep apnoea: Randomised controlled trial. *BMJ.* 2010;341:c5991.

107. MacMahon S, Peto R, Cutler J, et al. Blood pressure, stroke, and coronary heart disease. Part 1, Prolonged differences in blood pressure: Prospective observational studies corrected for the regression dilution bias. *Lancet.* 1990;335(8692):765-774.

108. Turnbull F. Effects of different blood-pressure-lowering regimens on major cardiovascular events: Results of prospectively-designed overviews of randomised trials. *Lancet*. 2003;362(9395):1527-1535.

109. Kanagala R, Murali N, Friedman P, et al. Obstructive sleep apnea and the recurrence of atrial fibrillaiton. *Circulation*. 2003;107(20):2589-2594.

110. Drager LF, Bortolotto LA, Figueiredo AC, Krieger EM, Lorenzi GF. Effects of continuous positive airway pressure on early signs of atherosclerosis in obstructive sleep apnea. *Am J Respir Crit Care Med*. 2007;176(7):706-712.

111. Johnston SC. Clinical practice. Transient ischemic attack. *N Engl J Med*. 2002;347(21):1687-1692.

112. Johnston SC, Gress DR, Browner WS, Sidney S. Short-term prognosis after emergency department diagnosis of TIA. *JAMA*. 2000;284(22):2901-2906.

113. Bravata DM, Concato J, Fried T, et al. Autotitrating CPAP for patients with acute transient ischemic attack: A randomized feasibility trial. *Stroke*. 2010;41(7):1464-1470.

114. Goldstein LB, Adams R, Alberts MJ, et al. Primary prevention of ischemic stroke: A guideline from the American Heart Association/American Stroke Association Stroke Council: cosponsored by the Atherosclerotic Peripheral Vascular Disease Interdisciplinary Working Group; Cardiovascular Nursing Council; Clinical Cardiology Council; Nutrition, Physical Activity, and Metabolism Council; and the Quality of Care and Outcomes Research Interdisciplinary Working Group. *Circulation*. 2006;113(24):E873-E923.

Chapter 52

Sleep Disorders Associated with Dementia

DANIEL A. COHEN

Dementia is a clinical syndrome defined by cognitive impairment to a degree that is severe enough to interfere with previously attained levels of occupational and social functioning.[1] The term is generally used in the context of a progressive course and reflects a deviation from normal aging. Memory is most commonly affected, but patients may also have problems with other cognitive processes, including concentration, reasoning, planning, problem solving, language, tool use, and navigating directions. They may also experience other personality and behavioral changes. After diagnosis of the specific dementia syndrome, the goals of care may be broadly defined as: (1) instituting specific disease-modifying therapies to minimize progression (when possible), (2) maintaining safety in the care environment, and (3) providing symptomatic treatments to enhance cognitive and behavioral function. There are theoretical, empirical, and practical reasons why addressing sleep disorders in this population can contribute to meeting these goals of care (Fig. 52-1). This chapter will present a framework for understanding the relationship of sleep disorders and dementia, provide an overview of sleep disturbances found in the major dementia syndromes, and review the evidence-based approach to treatment of sleep disorders in dementia.

RELATIONSHIP OF SLEEP DISORDERS AND DEMENTIA

Mechanisms of Sleep Disorders in Dementia

The prevalence of sleep abnormalities in dementia tends to increase with the severity of cognitive impairment,[2,3] suggesting that pathophysiology associated with dementia can affect the fundamental mechanisms of sleep-wake regulation. The ability to sustain stable sleep and wakefulness is governed by a functional switch that arises from the mutually inhibitory connections between specific arousal and sleep-promoting neural circuits.[4] The state of the switch predominantly depends on interactions between processes of sleep homeostasis, which is an accumulated drive for sleep from recent waking activity, and the phase of the endogenous circadian rhythm generated by pacemaker activity in the hypothalamic suprachiasmatic nuclei (SCN).[5] Abnormalities in homeostatic mechanisms, circadian rhythm generation or expression, and fundamental components of the sleep-wake circuitry are all potential causes of sleep-wake disorders in dementia.

Sleep homeostasis reflects the drive for sleep as a function of the sleep-wake history. Over the course of hours spent awake, extracellular adenosine accumulates in the basal forebrain and other regions, and this product of energy metabolism increases sleepiness in a negative-feedback manner.[6-12] A marker of this homeostatic sleep pressure is the amount of slow wave sleep (SWS) or slow wave activity (SWA; spectral power in the frequency range of approximately 0.5-4.5 Hz) during sleep.[13] SWS/SWA increases with the prior duration of waking and also shows a rebound increase during recovery following SWS deprivation.[14-17] Rather than simply being a marker of homeostatic sleep pressure, the ability to generate adequate SWS/SWA appears to be necessary for the homeostatic recovery function of sleep.[18,19] In response to sleep deprivation, patients with Alzheimer's disease (AD) had blunted SWS rebound during recovery sleep compared to elderly control subjects,[20] suggesting that homeostatic mechanisms may be impaired by neurodegenerative diseases. The effect of dementia on homeostatic sleep regulation is currently an understudied area of research.

Circadian phase and amplitude abnormalities have been demonstrated in the setting of dementia,[21-24] and dementia patients make up a significant proportion of patients diagnosed with the circadian rhythm sleep disorder called irregular sleep-wake rhythm.[25] Primary degeneration of the SCN and progressive reduction of SCN melatonin receptor expression has been demonstrated,[26-29] possibly explaining why circadian abnormalities tend to worsen with disease progression.[22,23,30,31] In addition, a functional disconnection has been proposed between SCN pacemaker activity and the rhythmic expression of clock genes in peripheral targets[32] or possibly the disruption of the underlying molecular mechanisms regulating the SCN circadian pacemaker activity.[33] A genetic susceptibility to specific polymorphisms of monoamine oxidase A (MAO-A) and up-regulation of MAO-A levels in dementia may reduce the conversion of serotonin to melatonin and cause sleep-wake rhythm disruption.[34,35] Finally, patients with dementia are at a higher risk of reduced exposure to environmental time cues, such as light, that would normally entrain the circadian system.[36] These circadian abnormalities have been proposed as a significant cause of the sundowning syndrome, with confusion and agitation in the evening.[37,38]

The sleep-wake circuitry itself may be damaged in the setting of dementia. For example, cell loss in brainstem components of the arousal system have been demonstrated in AD including up to 40% neuron loss of dorsal raphe serotoninergic neurons, noradrenergic locus ceruleus cell loss, and neuropathologic changes to the cholinergic pedunculopontine neurons.[39-41] Neuropathology may also affect the orexin/hypocretin neurons,[42] the cell population lost in narcolepsy that is postulated to stabilize the sleep-wake circuitry to prevent rapid state changes.[4] Degeneration of the brainstem

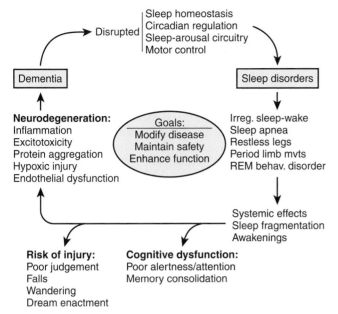

Figure 52-1 **Framework for understanding the relationship between sleep disorders and dementia.** Neuropathology causing dementia syndromes increases the prevalence of sleep disorders. Sleep disorders, in turn, can further impair cognitive function and increase safety hazards during unsupervised awakenings. In addition, sleep disorders may cause cellular, metabolic, immunologic, and vascular changes that may further exacerbate underlying neuropathology. Therefore, treating sleep disorders can substantially assist with meeting the goals of care for patients with dementia.

circuits that regulate the physiologic components of rapid eye movement (REM) sleep can lead to the loss of the normal skeletal muscle atonia of REM sleep and cause the dream-enacting behaviors of REM behavioral disorder (RBD).[43]

Contribution of Sleep Disorders to Neuropathologic Changes

Sleep serves a homeostatic function to promote recovery from waking activity.[44] For example, with increasing hours awake, cortical neuronal excitability and firing rates progressively increase, which are both metabolically demanding and carry the potential for excitotoxicity and seizures;[45] cortical firing rates are restored to a lower, more sustainable level following sleep. Conceivably, disrupted sleep may therefore exacerbate neuropathologic changes in the setting of dementia. Recent evidence suggests several mechanisms in which sleep disorders may cause neuronal injury: inflammatory processes appear to be a common mechanism in many neurodegenerative causes of dementia,[46] and chronic sleep restriction causes an increase in proinflammatory cytokines;[47] abnormal folding and aggregation of proteins within distinct neural networks are found in neurodegenerative disease,[48] and disrupted sleep may interfere with the processing of these disease-related proteins. For example, chronic sleep restriction causes the accumulation of toxic extracellular amyloid-β, which is implicated in the pathogenesis of AD;[49] intermittent hypoxia as a consequence of obstructive sleep apnea (OSA) leads to neuronal apoptosis, glial scar formation, and altered morphology and connectivity of neurons;[50,51] and finally, alterations in glucose regulation, endothelial function, sympathetic nervous system tone, and other systemic changes result from insufficient sleep and sleep

disorders such as OSA, increasing the risk for atherosclerosis and a vascular contribution to dementia.[52-58] Therefore, it is possible that treatment of sleep disorders early in the course of dementia can serve a neuroprotective role, but this hypothesis has only recently received preliminary testing.[59]

Implications of Sleep Disorders on Safety

Disturbed nocturnal sleep in patients with dementia makes them more vulnerable to falls, wandering, and other safety hazards if they are unsupervised.[60] As such, tending to these individuals through the night causes caregivers' sleep quality to be reduced, leading to significant emotional distress and daytime sleepiness.[2,60,61] Even on nights in which they do not have to awaken to provide care and supervision, caregiver sleep may be lighter and poorer quality as they may maintain some degree of continuous vigilance for sounds that indicate the patient with dementia has gotten out of bed.[62] The logistical difficulties of continually maintaining a safe environment for these patients likely explains why sleep disruption is a primary factor in the decision for placement in a long-term care facility.[63,64] Improvements in bed, window, and door alarms could potentially alleviate some of the caregiver difficulties and delay institutionalization.[62]

Influence of Sleep Disorders on Cognitive Functioning

Treatment of sleep disorders in dementia may provide a symptomatic benefit to improve cognitive functioning.[65] Sleep loss is associated with difficultly sustaining alertness, concentration, and performance in a variety of cognitive tasks.[66-69] The effects of chronic sleep loss can accumulate over weeks, increasing the rate at which performance deteriorates over consecutive hours awake.[70] In the setting of dementia, a condition in which there is low cognitive reserve, the impact of chronic sleep loss on cognition and daily functioning may be particularly pronounced.[71] In addition, the dissipation of sleep inertia upon awakening, which reflects the intrusion of sleep maintenance mechanisms into the waking state,[72] may be more pronounced in the setting of a sleep disorder and dementia. For example, sleep apnea can increase morning confusion in patients with AD.[73] Therefore, a sleep disorder may render individuals with baseline cognitive impairment much more vulnerable to substantial variability in their cognitive abilities over a 24-hour period. Treatment of a sleep disorder can improve alertness and attention,[74] and this improvement in vigilance state could improve performance in many cognitive domains. In addition, sleep has been implicated in the strengthening of synaptic connectivity and memory storage,[75] suggesting that treating sleep disorders has the potential to enhance memory capabilities beyond the effects of improved alertness and attention alone.

SLEEP DISORDERS IN SPECIFIC DEMENTIA SYNDROMES

Alzheimer's Disease

AD is the most common cause of dementia, and the prevalence increases exponentially with age.[76] The medial temporal lobes are particularly affected, causing a primary memory storage deficit and accelerated forgetting of salient facts and events.

Language and visuospatial deficits are also common, but social comportment tends to be preserved until later stages of the illness. Sleep complaints are two to three times more common in those with AD compared to elderly control subjects and can be found in up to half of the individuals in this population.[35,77-80] The prevalence estimates of sleep symptoms vary depending on the severity of disease, living situation in the home versus an institution, and co-morbid medical conditions. Total sleep time tends to reduce with healthy aging.[81] In contrast, sleeping more than usual was the most common reported sleep symptom in a community-based sample of 205 AD patients,[2] and daytime napping is three times more common in AD compared to elderly control subjects.[82] AD may cause a mild increase in the apnea-hypopnea index (AHI),[83,84] although not all studies agree.[73,85] Fundamental changes in neurophysiologic features of sleep have been documented, including slowing of the posterior dominant rhythm and a reduction in stage N3 sleep, fast spindle activity, and stage REM.[86-89] There are also increases in delta and theta power spectra in waking and sleep.[87,88] These changes can make sleep stage scoring challenging. Circadian abnormalities include lower amplitude, more variable, or disorganized circadian rhythms; reduced cerebrospinal fluid (CSF) melatonin concentrations; and circadian misalignment including circadian phase delay.[21-24,31,90,91] Sleep-wake rhythm disruption has been demonstrated in the face of normal circadian patterns of cortisol secretion, suggesting that disruption of SCN output pathways may be more significant than primary degeneration of the SCN itself, at least in earlier stages of the disease.[31] Overt clinical manifestations of RBD are rare in AD, although the presence of excessive muscle activity during REM sleep may be a more common finding.[92]

Vascular Dementia

Vascular dementia (VaD) is the second most common type of dementia, commonly caused by small vessel cerebrovascular disease and subcortical ischemia.[93] There is generally a slowing of cognitive processing speed and poor executive control. These patients tend to be forgetful, but recall improves with the aid of cues, and recognition memory for salient facts and events is relatively preserved.[93] The burden of subcortical white matter pathologic change appears to be an important factor in the degree of sleep-wake disruption in this population.[94] Patients with VaD were shown to have greater degrees of sleep disruption compared to those with AD,[95,96] but a more recent study found the opposite result.[97] Patients with VaD appear to have lower amplitude and less organized circadian temperature rhythms compared to AD patients, possibly from subcortical lesions disconnecting SCN output pathways.[98] However, these patients may be more responsive to circadian interventions such as light (see later discussion), possibly because the SCN may be relatively intact. Given the strong association of sleep-disordered breathing and stroke,[99-101] treatment of sleep apnea may be a particularly important aspect of minimizing the development or progression of VaD.[58]

Parkinson's Disease and Dementia with Lewy Bodies

Parkinson's disease (PD) with dementia and dementia with Lewy bodies (DLB) are related conditions associated with the abnormal accumulation of alpha synuclein protein that forms neuronal inclusions called *Lewy bodies.* These conditions may be considered along a spectrum, and the time course of the motor (tremor, rigidity, bradykinesia, impaired postural reflexes) and nonmotor symptoms (cognitive impairment, autonomic dysfunction, sleep disturbances) correlates with the distribution of Lewy bodies in the brainstem, limbic regions, and neocortical structures.[102-104] Problems with visuospatial and executive functioning are prominent, and there are significant fluctuations within and across days in alertness, arousal, and awareness of the environmental context.[104] Prominent cognitive fluctuations are considered a reliable distinguishing feature between the dementia of DLB versus AD,[105] although a primary sleep disorder such as sleep apnea in AD may also cause substantial fluctuations. Visual hallucinations, which may be mediated, at least in part, by dysregulated REM, are considered a core feature of DLB.[106-108] Up to 80% of patients with DLB will have RBD,[43] and RBD supports the diagnosis of DLB over other causes of dementia.[104] For the purpose of this chapter, sleep disturbances in PD and DLB will be discussed together.

Sleep complaints are twice as common in PD compared to age-matched control subjects, and insomnia and excessive daytime sleepiness occur in up to 50% of patients.[109-111] A narcolepsy phenotype has been reported, likely related to the loss of orexin neurons in the hypothalamus.[42,111] Poor sleep quality and daytime sleepiness are more frequent in Lewy body diseases than in AD.[112-114] Sleep-disordered breathing was shown to be worse in PD compared to age-matched control subjects, with a mean AHI of 12.2 compared to 5.7 and with a 3% to 4% lower oxygen nadir.[115] However, not all studies find an increase in sleep-disordered breathing in this population.[116] The prevalence of restless legs syndrome is roughly six times greater in PD, and there are three times as many periodic limb movements of sleep compared to control subjects.[117,118] Dopaminergic therapies used for the motor symptoms in these disorders may be an additional source of daytime sleepiness.[119]

Disorders of Tau Accumulation

Disorders of abnormal tau accumulation include progressive supranuclear palsy (PSP), frontotemporal dementia (FTD), and corticobasal degeneration (CBD). PSP is characterized by impaired voluntary eye movements, axial rigidity, and impaired postural reflexes with falls relatively early in the course. PSP appears to be associated with a greater degree of insomnia than AD or PD, and the number of nighttime awakenings correlates with the severity of impaired motor function.[120] The degree of nocturnal sleep disruption does not appear to be explained by significant sleep-disordered breathing or periodic limb movement disorder. A recent study confirmed the greater number of arousals, increased stage N1 sleep, and increased wake after sleep onset in PSP compared to PD, yet with similar degrees of daytime sleepiness measured by the multiple sleep latency test (MSLT).[121] In addition, REM sleep without atonia was found in 27% with polysomnographic evidence of RBD in 13%,[121] but others suggest that the prevalence of RBD is likely to be lower in this population.[43] Other findings in PSP include reduced sleep spindles, lower percentage of stage REM sleep, and slowing of the wake electroencephalographic (EEG) frequencies in the frontal regions.[122]

FTD is characterized by prominent problems with social conduct early in the course of the illness (behavioral variant

FTD), executive dysfunction, and in some patients a progressive aphasia. Sleep diary combined with actigraphy demonstrated disrupted sleep and rest-activity patterns in FTD, and these disturbances may occur relatively early in the disease course.[123] Another study demonstrated a highly fragmented and phase advanced activity rhythm that was apparently desynchronized from the body temperature rhythm.[124] This pattern suggests that the SCN may be intact, but output pathways may be disrupted and cause abnormal expression of some behavioral rhythms.

CBD, a relatively rare disorder, may have less frequent sleep symptoms compared to other neurodegenerative conditions.[125]

Huntington's Disease

Huntington's disease (HD) is an autosomal dominant disorder characterized by a hyperkinetic state and involuntary choreoathetoid movements that generally subside during sleep. Sleep EEG findings have demonstrated increased sleep onset latency, reduced sleep efficiency, frequent nocturnal awakenings, more time spent awake, and less SWS, with some relationship to disease severity.[126] HD is associated with an increase in spindle density in stage N2 sleep, although the clinical significance of this finding is uncertain.[126,127] There does not appear to be a significant increase in SDB in HD.[128]

Prion Diseases

Prion diseases, including fatal familial insomnia, sporadic fatal insomnia, and sporadic Creutzfeldt-Jakob disease produce the most profound changes in sleep-wake organization, with diffuse theta during wakefulness, remarkably disturbed sleep efficiency, and behavioral and polysomnographic difficulty distinguishing wakefulness, non-REM (NREM) sleep, and REM sleep.[129] These conditions are also associated with a relatively rapidly deteriorating course compared to other neurodegenerative conditions.

TREATMENT OF SPECIFIC SLEEP DISORDERS

Irregular Sleep-Wake Rhythm

Light Therapy

Because impaired circadian regulation of sleep-wake cycles is considered a predominant mechanism of sleep disruption in dementia, there has been significant interest in the use of light therapy as a method to either entrain the circadian pacemaker or strengthen the amplitude the circadian rhythm. In addition, bright light can directly improve subjective and objective measures of alertness and attention.[130] Therefore, light therapy may help sleep-wake organization by directly increasing alertness, reducing naps, and thereby increasing homeostatic pressure to sleep at night. Light studies in this population have generally been small, often included a mixture of dementia types, and were conducted mostly with institutionalized patients, and many have lacked a control condition, suggesting that social interaction or other aspects of the treatment may have played a part. Virtually all the studies in this population used sleep logs, nurse reports, or more commonly actigraphy and not polysomnographically measured sleep.

(Table 52-1 provides a summary of 14 light studies reporting sleep-wake, or rest-activity, effects of light.) Taken collectively, light therapy appears to have substantial promise in promoting a better diurnal sleep-wake rhythm in patients with dementia. However, the optimal dose, timing, and method of delivery have not been fully determined in this population. For example, there has been a recent increase in the use of blue wavelength light technology given the spectral sensitivity of the circadian system and the alerting effects of short-wavelength light,[131] but these light boxes have not yet been studied in dementia patients. Bright light exposure in dementia has also been shown to reduce restlessness, sundowning, and agitation behavior,[132-137] although light therapy also has the potential to increase agitation in some individuals.[138]

Melatonin

Melatonin has also been used to improve the circadian regulation of sleep-wake states in dementia. In a small ($n = 20$), 4-week, double-blind, placebo-controlled trial in patients with moderate AD, melatonin 3 mg increased nocturnal sleep duration by approximately 100 minutes, with small improvements in tests of cognitive function.[139] However, a multicenter randomized, placebo-controlled trial of 157 patients with moderate AD compared two dose formulations of melatonin (2.5 mg slow release or 10 mg immediate release) to placebo and found no significant differences across groups; there was a nonsignificant trend for a 30-minute increase in nocturnal sleep time in the 10 mg melatonin group.[140] There were no significant adverse events compared to placebo. A randomized, double-blind, crossover trial in moderate AD using 6 mg slow-release melatonin also failed to demonstrate a beneficial effect on sleep, although this study may have been underpowered because only 25 participants completed the protocol.[141] A study in 41 nursing home patients with severe AD failed to find a benefit of melatonin 10 mg (8.5 mg immediate, 1.5 mg sustained release) on sleep, circadian rest-activity patterns, or agitation compared to placebo.[142] In combination with morning light therapy, melatonin 5 mg (versus placebo) reduced daytime sleep time in nursing home patients with AD, but there was no improvement in nighttime sleep.[143] Finally, in a long-term study (for an average of 15 months) of 189 dementia patients living in Dutch assisted living centers, patients were randomized in a "2 × 2" design to (1) melatonin 2.5 mg versus placebo; and (2) common area ceiling lighting greater than 1000 lux versus standard intensity overhead lighting.[144] Melatonin alone was associated with a 27-minute increase in total sleep time at night. However, caregiver ratings of withdrawn behavior increased, an effect that was ameliorated by the combination of light and melatonin. These authors therefore suggested that melatonin only be used in combination with light treatment.

Structured Behavioral Activities

In an uncontrolled intervention study in institutionalized patients with an irregular sleep-wake rhythm, the sleep pattern and behavioral symptoms of wandering, agitation, and confusion simultaneously improved in 8 of 24 patients by structured daily activities for 3 hours each day (9-11 AM and 2-3 PM).[91] In a controlled trial with 147 nursing home patients with dementia, 2 hours of individualized activities per day for 3 weeks did not significantly increase nighttime sleep duration.[145] However, the intervention reduced daytime sleep

TABLE 52-1

Summary of Light Studies for Sleep in Patients with Dementia

Study	No. of Patients	Population	Design	Intervention	Timing	Finding(s)
Satlin et al, 1992[132]	10	AD, severe sundowning	Open label	1500-2000 lux	7-9 PM	Improved circadian rest-activity pattern
Colenda et al, 1997[161]	4	AD, community dwelling	Open label	2000 lux (visor)	2 hr, morning	Phase advance activity rhythm, no consistent sleep benefit; improved stability of day-to-day activity rhythm[162]
Okumoto, 1998[162]	1	VaD, nursing home	Open, repeated challenge	4000 lux	9:30-11:30 AM	Sleep much more consolidated at night during 34-46 daylight exposure periods compared with 2 baseline periods (44-54 days)
Van Someren et al, 1997[163]	29	Severe dementia, geriatrics ward	Open label	Common area overhead lighting 1100 lux	Ad libitum	Reduced fragmentation of the rest-activity rhythm
Yamadera, 2000[162a]	29	AD, inpatient setting	Open label	3000 lux	9-11 AM	5% increase in sleep efficiency, decreased awakenings
Mishima et al, 1998[164]	22	AD and VaD, chronic care	Crossover	5000-8000 lux	9-11 AM	Decreased nighttime activity in VaD (not AD)
Lyketsos et al, 1999[165]	15	Dementia, chronic care	Crossover	10,000 lux	Morning, 1 hr	Increase nighttime sleep by 1.7 hr
Fontana Gasio et al, 2003[166]	17	Dementia, nursing homes	Parallel (*n* = 4 control subjects)	Dawn-dusk simulation	Dawn 34 min, dusk 30 min	Phase advance sleep-wake rhythm, trend for increased sleep time (~26 min)
Fetveit et al, 2003[167]	11	Dementia, nursing home	Open label	6000-8000 lux	Morning, 2 hr, within 8-11 AM	13% increase in sleep efficiency
Ancoli-Israel et al, 2003[168]	92	Severe AD, nursing home	Parallel	2500 lux	9:30-11:30 AM *or* 5:30-7:30 PM	Lengthened maximum sleep bout, a measure of sleep consolidation
Skjerve et al, 2004[137]	10	Severe VaD or AD, chronic care	Open label	5000-8000 lux	Morning, 45 min	Decreased behavioral symptoms but no effect on sleep-wake variables
Dowling et al, 2005,[169] 2007[136]	70	Severe AD, long-term care	Parallel	2500 lux	9:30-10:30 AM *or* 3:30-4:30 PM	No benefit of bright light therapy on sleep, but small improvements in agitation
Sloane et al, 2007[170] Barrick et al, 2010[138]	66*	Dementia, residential care and inpatient ward	Parallel	Common area overhead lighting 2500 lux	7-11 AM 4-8 PM 7-11 AM	Morning and all-day light increased nocturnal sleep by approximately 11 min; however, agitation was increased
Riemersma-van der Lek et al, 2008[144]	189	Moderate AD, assisted Living	Parallel	Common area overhead lighting > 1000 lux	10 AM-6 PM	10-min increase in nighttime sleep

*Separate analyses published on a single experiment.
NOTE: Parallel and crossover designs include an experimental control condition such as standard lighting or predominantly red wavelength light.
AD, Alzheimer's disease; *VaD,* vascular dementia.

by 35%, suggesting that increasing daytime activity can influence either homeostatic or circadian mechanisms to enhance daytime alertness.

Multicomponent Therapy

Two recent studies in nursing homes used multicomponent interventions in the attempt to improve sleep-wake patterns.[146,147] The interventions consisted of: scheduled daytime activity; bright light exposure through outdoor sun exposure or a light box; structured bedtime routines; and reduced ambient noise at night. Patients randomized to the interventions had some benefit on reducing daytime sleep but did not achieve more nighttime sleep. However, one study demonstrated that this approach may have some efficacy for patients who are still capable of living at home.[148] In that study of 36 dementia patients, those randomized to a similar multicomponent intervention including a suggested 30-minute daily walk showed a 36-minute average reduction in the time spent awake at night. The benefits of the intervention remained during a 6-month follow-up interval, and this study provided preliminary evidence that such a program may delay the timing of institutionalization.

Hypnotics, Stimulants, and Other Agents

Many different classes of sedating medications are routinely used in patients with dementia, including antipsychotics, sedating antidepressants, anxiolytics, and sedative/hypnotics.[2] However, use of these agents for insomnia in the setting of dementia usually arises from clinical opinion, case reports, and open label trials, with little to no data documenting the safety and efficacy of these medications in placebo-controlled trials. A large meta-analysis of hynotic use (benzodiazepines and benzodiazepine receptor agonists) in the elderly concluded that the modest improvement in sleep quality is generally outweighed by a higher incidence of adverse events, including falls and cognitive decline.[149] It is possible that the risk of confusion and serious falls may be even higher in patients with dementia, but clinical trials with hypnotic agents have generally excluded this population. Medications with anticholinergic properties, including over-the counter diphenhydramine-containing products, can trigger episodes of delirium in this population. Although antipsychotics such as quetiapine may improve nocturnal sleep consolidation in patients with dementia,[150] antipsychotics have been shown to increase the mortality rate in these patients.[151] Agents such as trazodone, mirtazipine, and rameleteon are often used to treat insomnia in patients with dementia owing to clinicians' perception that adverse cognitive effects are unlikely, but clinical trials are needed.

The sleep-wake state influences the circadian pacemaker,[152] and pharmacologic agents that influence the sleep-wake cycle may help facilitate circadian entrainment.[153] Therefore, it is possible that medications to improve wakefulness during the day may help entrain the circadian system and promote nocturnal sleep. For example, a 78-year-old patient with Alzheimer's disease and severe insomnia showed a remarkable improvement in nocturnal sleep with methylphenidate 10 mg twice a day; the insomnia returned with drug withdrawal and the medication effect was confirmed by restarting therapy.[154] In an open label trial of modafinil up to 200 mg per day, five of eight patients with dementia improved, including two patients who had a substantial improvement in the actigraphy measured daytime:nighttime activity ratio.[155] These preliminary reports suggest that enhancing wakefulness can lead to improved nocturnal sleep in patients with dementia, opening the door to future clinical trials.

REM Sleep Behavior Disorder

RBD (see Chapter 43) is strongly associated with α-synuclein-related neurodegenerative diseases, including PD, DLB, and multisystem atrophy.[43] Sleep-related injury to the patient or bed partner is common in RBD, occurring in 33% to 65% of patients.[156] The first step in managing this condition involves assuring safety of the patient and the bed partner in the bedroom environment. This action includes placing a mattress on the floor next to the bed and soft padding over bedside furniture; removing sharp objects or weapons from the bedroom; securing windows; and sleeping in a separate bedroom from the partner.[156] The Standards of Practice Committee of the American Academy of Sleep Medicine reviewed the evidence-based treatment approach to this disorder,[156] and all evidence was considered weak at level 4. Clonazepam (usual recommended dose 0.5-2.0 mg, maximum dose 4 mg) is generally considered the most effective agent,[43,156] but it should be used cautiously in those with gait impairment or cognitive dysfunction.[156] Melatonin (at doses 3-12 mg) has demonstrated efficacy as well.[43,156] Given the potential for clonezepam to worsen cognitive function, melatonin is emerging as a first-line treatment for RBD in the setting of dementia.[156] Serotoninergic medications may induce RBD and should be minimized when possible, although REM suppression from these medications can improve RBD symptoms in some individuals.[156] Other agents, such as acetylcholinesterase inhibitors used for cognitive symptoms in dementia, have also been reported to either improve[156] or exacerbate[157] RBD.

Obstructive Sleep Apnea

In a 6-week, sham controlled study in community-dwelling individuals with mild-moderate AD, continuous positive airway pressure (CPAP) use was associated with a reduction of the Epworth Sleepiness Scale (ESS) score of approximately 3 points as well as a small benefit in composite neuropsychological functioning compared to baseline.[158,159] In these patients, all with a reliable live-in caregiver, the average usage of CPAP therapy was 4.8 hours per night, comparable to other OSA populations.[160] In a follow-up study, the authors compared five patients who decided to continue CPAP therapy to five patients who decided not to continue treatment after the trial; with a mean follow-up of 13 months, the CPAP treated group showed less deterioration in performance on measures of global cognition and executive functioning.[59] This preliminary evidence suggests the possibility that CPAP use for OSA can serve a neuroprotective role in slowing the decline of dementia.

SUMMARY AND RECOMMENDATIONS

Sleep disorders in dementia are common, compromise patient safety, decrease cognitive functioning, increase caregiver burden, and may exacerbate underlying neuropathologic changes. Different dementia syndromes may have differential predilection for various types of sleep-wake abnormalities and responses to treatment, but substantial overlap exists: further research is needed to elucidate unique mechanisms and treatment targets for sleep disorders among different dementia phenotypes. Treatment studies are often limited to institutionalized patients, limiting generalizability to individuals with dementia who remain in the community, a group that represents the majority of patients with dementia. Light therapy appears to have significant promise, but the optimal dose, timing, and method of delivery remains to be determined. Table 52-1 summarizes the findings of several light studies for sleep disorders in patients with dementia.[161-170] Melatonin treatment responses have generally been disappointing when used alone, including one study showing an adverse effect of withdrawn behavior, but the efficacy and side effects may be more favorable when combined with light therapy. Clinical trials are long overdue to determine the safety and efficacy of the Food and Drug Administration (FDA)-approved hynotics, sedating antidepressants such as trazodone and mirtazapine, and wake-promoting agents such as modafinil in improving sleep-wake behavior of these patients. Positive airway pressure appears to be reasonably tolerated in mild-moderate dementia patients living at home with a reliable caregiver, and some preliminary data suggest the exciting possibility that treatment of

BOX 52-1 *Approach to Sleep Disruption in Dementia*

- Screen for intrinsic sleep disorders (consider PSG).
- Assess for conditions causing pain.
- Minimize caffeine, alcohol, nicotine use/intake.
- Assess adequacy of overnight supervision/alarms.
- Dim night-light with blue wavelength filtered out may be helpful.
- Establish consistent bed and wake times and routines.
- Minimize fluids within 2 hours of bedtime.
- Replace napping with structured, enjoyable activities.
- Encourage a regimen of 30 minutes of walking per day if possible.
- Outdoor sun exposure for 1 to 2 hours (with use of sunscreen) can help entrain the circadian system.
- Daytime activities should be performed near a window or lightbox.
- Evening bright light is recommended only with phase-advanced disruption.
- Melatonin 3 mg 30 to 60 minutes can be taken before bed.
- Consider bedtime trazodone or mirtazapine (Remeron) if patient is depressed.
- Consider modafinil for daytime sleepiness.

PSG, polysomnography.

sleep apnea (or perhaps other sleep disorders) can have a neuroprotective role. With an aging population and an increasing prevalence of dementia, it will become more and more critical to develop safe and effective therapies for sleep disorders in dementia. Box 52-1 outlines a reasonable approach to addressing sleep-wake disruption in patients with dementia based on the current literature.

REFERENCES

1. Doody RS, Stevens JC, Beck C, et al. Practice parameter: Management of dementia (an evidence-based review). Report of the Quality Standards Subcommittee of the American Academy of Neurology. *Neurology*. 2001;56:1154-1166.
2. McCurry SM, Logsdon RG, Teri L, et al. Characteristics of sleep disturbance in community-dwelling Alzheimer's disease patients. *J Geriatr Psychiatry Neurol*. 1999;12:53-59.
3. Moe KE, Vitiello MV, Larsen LH, Prinz PN. Symposium: Cognitive processes and sleep disturbances: Sleep/wake patterns in Alzheimer's disease: Relationships with cognition and function. *J Sleep Res*. 1995;4:15-20.
4. Saper CB, Scammell TE, Lu J. Hypothalamic regulation of sleep and circadian rhythms. *Nature*. 2005;437:1257-1263.
5. Reppert SM, Weaver DR. Coordination of circadian timing in mammals. *Nature*. 2002;418:935-941.
6. Benington JH, Kodali SK, Heller HC. Stimulation of A1 adenosine receptors mimics the electroencephalographic effects of sleep deprivation. *Brain Res*. 1995;692:79-85.
7. Benington JH, Heller HC. Restoration of brain energy metabolism as the function of sleep. *Prog Neurobiol*. 1995;45:347-360.
8. Christie MA, Bolortuya Y, Chen LC, McKenna JT, McCarley RW, Strecker RE. Microdialysis elevation of adenosine in the basal forebrain produces vigilance impairments in the rat psychomotor vigilance task. *Sleep*. 2008;31:1393-1398.
9. Landolt HP. Sleep homeostasis: A role for adenosine in humans? *Biochem Pharmacol*. 2008;75:2070-2079.
10. Porkka-Heiskanen T. Adenosine in sleep and wakefulness. *Ann Med*. 1999;31:125-129.
11. Portas CM, Thakkar M, Rainnie DG, Greene RW, McCarley RW. Role of adenosine in behavioral state modulation: A microdialysis study in the freely moving cat. *Neuroscience*. 1997;79:225-235.
12. Basheer R, Porkka-Heiskanen T, Stenberg D, McCarley RW. Adenosine and behavioral state control: Adenosine increases c-Fos protein and AP1 binding in basal forebrain of rats. *Brain Res Mol Brain Res*. 1999;73:1-10.
13. Borbely AA. From slow waves to sleep homeostasis: New perspectives. *Arch Ital Biol*. 2001;139:53-61.
14. Borbely AA, Baumann F, Brandeis D, Strauch I, Lehmann D. Sleep deprivation: Effect on sleep stages and EEG power density in man. *Electroencephalogr Clin Neurophysiol*. 1981;51:483-495.
15. Dijk DJ, Brunner DP, Beersma DG, Borbely AA. Electroencephalogram power density and slow wave sleep as a function of prior waking and circadian phase. *Sleep*. 1990;13:430-440.
16. Dijk DJ, Beersma DG. Effects of SWS deprivation on subsequent EEG power density and spontaneous sleep duration. *Electroencephalogr Clin Neurophysiol*. 1989;72:312-320.
17. Ferrara M, De Gennaro L, Bertini M. Selective slow-wave sleep (SWS) deprivation and SWS rebound: Do we need a fixed SWS amount per night? *Sleep Res Online*. 1999;2:15-19.
18. Bjorness TE, Kelly CL, Gao T, Poffenberger V, Greene RW. Control and function of the homeostatic sleep response by adenosine A1 receptors. *J Neurosci*. 2009;29:1267-1276.
19. Walsh JK, Randazzo AC, Stone K, et al. Tiagabine is associated with sustained attention during sleep restriction: Evidence for the value of slow-wave sleep enhancement? *Sleep*. 2006;29:433-443.
20. Reynolds III CF, Kupfer DJ, Hoch CC, et al. Sleep deprivation as a probe in the elderly. *Arch Gen Psychiatry*. 1987;44:982-990.
21. Mishima K, Tozawa T, Satoh K, Matsumoto Y, Hishikawa Y, Okawa M. Melatonin secretion rhythm disorders in patients with senile dementia of Alzheimer's type with disturbed sleep-waking. *Biol Psychiatry*. 1999;45:417-421.
22. Harper DG, Volicer L, Stopa EG, McKee AC, Nitta M, Satlin A. Disturbance of endogenous circadian rhythm in aging and Alzheimer disease. *Am J Geriatr Psychiatry*. 2005;13:359-368.
23. Harper DG, Stopa EG, McKee AC, Satlin A, Fish D, Volicer L. Dementia severity and Lewy bodies affect circadian rhythms in Alzheimer disease. *Neurobiol Aging*. 2004;25:771-781.
24. Lee JH, Friedland R, Whitehouse PJ, Woo JI. Twenty-four-hour rhythms of sleep-wake cycle and temperature in Alzheimer's disease. *J Neuropsychiatry Clin Neurosci*. 2004;16:192-198.
25. Sack RL, Auckley D, Auger RR, et al. Circadian rhythm sleep disorders: Part II, advanced sleep phase disorder, delayed sleep phase disorder, free-running disorder, and irregular sleep-wake rhythm. An American Academy of Sleep Medicine review. *Sleep*. 2007;30:1484-1501.
26. Stopa EG, Volicer L, Kuo-Leblanc V, et al. Pathologic evaluation of the human suprachiasmatic nucleus in severe dementia. *J Neuropathol Exp Neurol*. 1999;58:29-39.
27. Wu YH, Swaab DF. The human pineal gland and melatonin in aging and Alzheimer's disease. *J Pineal Res*. 2005;38:145-152.
28. Harper DG, Stopa EG, Kuo-Leblanc V, et al. Dorsomedial SCN neuronal subpopulations subserve different functions in human dementia. *Brain*. 2008;131:1609-1617.
29. Wu YH, Zhou JN, Van Heerikhuize J, Jockers R, Swaab DF. Decreased MT1 melatonin receptor expression in the suprachiasmatic nucleus in aging and Alzheimer's disease. *Neurobiol Aging*. 2007;28:1239-1247.
30. Werth E, Savaskan E, Knoblauch V, et al. Decline in long-term circadian rest-activity cycle organization in a patient with dementia. *J Geriatr Psychiatry Neurol*. 2002;15:55-59.
31. Hatfield CF, Herbert J, van Someren EJ, Hodges JR, Hastings MH. Disrupted daily activity/rest cycles in relation to daily cortisol rhythms of home-dwelling patients with early Alzheimer's dementia. *Brain*. 2004;127:1061-1074.
32. Wu YH, Fischer DF, Kalsbeek A, et al. Pineal clock gene oscillation is disturbed in Alzheimer's disease, due to functional disconnection from the "master clock." *FASEB J*. 2006;20:1874-1876.
33. Morton AJ, Wood NI, Hastings MH, Hurelbrink C, Barker RA, Maywood ES. Disintegration of the sleep-wake cycle and circadian timing in Huntington's disease. *J Neurosci*. 2005;25:157-163.
34. Wu YH, Feenstra MG, Zhou JN, et al. Molecular changes underlying reduced pineal melatonin levels in Alzheimer disease: Alterations in preclinical and clinical stages. *J Clin Endocrinol Metab*. 2003;88:5898-5906.
35. Craig D, Hart DJ, Passmore AP. Genetically increased risk of sleep disruption in Alzheimer's disease. *Sleep*. 2006;29:1003-1007.
36. Campbell SS, Kripke DF, Gillin JC, Hrubovcak JC. Exposure to light in healthy elderly subjects and Alzheimer's patients. *Physiol Behav*. 1988;42:141-144.

37. Martin J, Marler M, Shochat T, Ancoli-Israel S. Circadian rhythms of agitation in institutionalized patients with Alzheimer's disease. *Chronobiol Int.* 2000;17:405-418.

38. Volicer L, Harper DG, Manning BC, Goldstein R, Satlin A. Sundowning and circadian rhythms in Alzheimer's disease. *Am J Psychiatry.* 2001;158:704-711.

39. Aletrino MA, Vogels OJ, Van Domburg PH, Ten Donkelaar HJ. Cell loss in the nucleus raphes dorsalis in Alzheimer's disease. *Neurobiol Aging.* 1992;13:461-468.

40. Chan-Palay V. Neuronal communication breakdown in neurotransmitter systems in Alzheimer's and Parkinson's dementias. *J Neurocytol.* 1990;19:802-806.

41. Mufson EJ, Mash DC, Hersh LB. Neurofibrillary tangles in cholinergic pedunculopontine neurons in Alzheimer's disease. *Ann Neurol.* 1988;24:623-629.

42. Fronczek R, Overeem S, Lee SY, et al. Hypocretin (orexin) loss in Parkinson's disease. *Brain.* 2007;130:1577-1585.

43. Boeve BF, Silber MH, Saper CB, et al. Pathophysiology of REM sleep behaviour disorder and relevance to neurodegenerative disease. *Brain.* 2007;130:2770-2788.

44. Savage VM, West GB. A quantitative, theoretical framework for understanding mammalian sleep. *Proc Natl Acad Sci U S A.* 2007;104: 1051-1056.

45. Vyazovskiy VV, Olcese U, Lazimy YM, et al. Cortical firing and sleep homeostasis. *Neuron.* 2009;63:865-878.

46. Brown GC, Neher JJ. Inflammatory neurodegeneration and mechanisms of microglial killing of neurons. *Mol Neurobiol.* 2010;41:242-247.

47. Vgontzas AN, Zoumakis E, Bixler EO, et al. Adverse effects of modest sleep restriction on sleepiness, performance, and inflammatory cytokines. *J Clin Endocrinol Metab.* 2004;89:2119-2126.

48. Seeley WW, Crawford RK, Zhou J, Miller BL, Greicius MD. Neurodegenerative diseases target large-scale human brain networks. *Neuron.* 2009;62:42-52.

49. Kang JE, Lim MM, Bateman RJ, et al. Amyloid-beta dynamics are regulated by orexin and the sleep-wake cycle. *Science.* 2009;326(5955):1005-1007.

50. Aviles-Reyes RX, Angelo MF, Villarreal A, Rios H, Lazarowski A, Ramos AJ. Intermittent hypoxia during sleep induces reactive gliosis and limited neuronal death in rats: Implications for sleep apnea. *J Neurochem.* 2010;112:854-869.

51. Zeng YM, Cai KJ, Chen XY, Wu MX, Lin X. Effect of chronic intermittent hypoxia on the expression of Nip3, cell apoptosis, beta-amyloid protein deposit in mice brain cortex. *Chin Med J (Engl).* 2009;122:68-73.

52. Arzt M, Young T, Finn L, Skatrud JB, Bradley TD. Association of sleep-disordered breathing and the occurrence of stroke. *Am J Respir Crit Care Med.* 2005;172:1447-1451.

53. Young T, Peppard P, Palta M, et al. Population-based study of sleep-disordered breathing as a risk factor for hypertension. *Arch Intern Med.* 1997;157:1746-1752.

54. Silvestrini M, Rizzato B, Placidi F, Baruffaldi R, Bianconi A, Diomedi M. Carotid artery wall thickness in patients with obstructive sleep apnea syndrome. *Stroke.* 2002;33:1782-1785.

55. Gottlieb DJ, Redline S, Nieto FJ, et al. Association of usual sleep duration with hypertension: The Sleep Heart Health Study. *Sleep.* 2006;29: 1009-1014.

56. Punjabi NM, Shahar E, Redline S, Gottlieb DJ, Givelber R, Resnick HE. Sleep-disordered breathing, glucose intolerance, and insulin resistance: The Sleep Heart Health Study. *Am J Epidemiol.* 2004;160:521-530.

57. Ikehara S, Iso H, Date C, et al. Association of sleep duration with mortality from cardiovascular disease and other causes for Japanese men and women: The JACC Study. *Sleep.* 2009;32:295-301.

58. Roman GC. Facts, myths, and controversies in vascular dementia. *J Neurol Sci.* 2004;226:49-52.

59. Cooke JR, Ayalon L, Palmer BW, et al. Sustained use of CPAP slows deterioration of cognition, sleep, and mood in patients with Alzheimer's disease and obstructive sleep apnea: A preliminary study. *J Clin Sleep Med.* 2009;5:305-309.

60. Rowe MA, McCrae CS, Campbell JM, Benito AP, Cheng J. Sleep pattern differences between older adult dementia caregivers and older adult noncaregivers using objective and subjective measures. *J Clin Sleep Med.* 2008;4:362-369.

61. Simpson C, Carter PA. Pilot study of a brief behavioral sleep intervention for caregivers of individuals with dementia. *Res Gerontol Nurs.* 2010;3:19-29.

62. Rowe M, Lane S, Phipps C. CareWatch: A home monitoring system for use in homes of persons with cognitive impairment. *Top Geriatr Rehabil.* 2007;23:3-8.

63. Hope T, Keene J, Gedling K, Fairburn CG, Jacoby R. Predictors of institutionalization for people with dementia living at home with a carer. *Int J Geriatr Psychiatry.* 1998;13:682-690.

64. Bianchetti A, Scuratti A, Zanetti O, et al. Predictors of mortality and institutionalization in Alzheimer disease patients 1 year after discharge from an Alzheimer dementia unit. *Dementia.* 1995;6:108-112.

65. Pallier PN, Morton AJ. Management of sleep/wake cycles improves cognitive function in a transgenic mouse model of Huntington's disease. *Brain Res.* 2009;1279:90-98.

66. Dawson D, Reid K. Fatigue, alcohol and performance impairment. *Nature.* 1997;388:235.

67. Van Dongen HP, Maislin G, Mullington JM, Dinges DF. The cumulative cost of additional wakefulness: Dose-response effects on neurobehavioral functions and sleep physiology from chronic sleep restriction and total sleep deprivation. *Sleep.* 2003;26:117-126.

68. Belenky G, Wesensten NJ, Thorne DR, et al. Patterns of performance degradation and restoration during sleep restriction and subsequent recovery: A sleep dose-response study. *J Sleep Res.* 2003;12:1-12.

69. McCauley P, Kalachev LV, Smith AD, Belenky G, Dinges DF, Van Dongen HP. A new mathematical model for the homeostatic effects of sleep loss on neurobehavioral performance. *J Theor Biol.* 2009;256:227-239.

70. Cohen DA, Wang W, Wyatt JK, et al. Uncovering residual effects of chronic sleep loss on human performance. *Sci Transl Med.* 2010;2:14ra3.

71. Lee JH, Bliwise DL, Ansari FP, et al. Daytime sleepiness and functional impairment in Alzheimer disease. *Am J Geriatr Psychiatry.* 2007;15:620-626.

72. Balkin TJ, Braun AR, Wesensten NJ, et al. The process of awakening: A PET study of regional brain activity patterns mediating the reestablishment of alertness and consciousness. *Brain.* 2002;125:2308-2319.

73. Bliwise DL, Yesavage JA, Tinklenberg JR, Dement WC. Sleep apnea in Alzheimer's disease. *Neurobiol Aging.* 1989;10:343-346.

74. Huang YS, Guilleminault C, Li HY, Yang CM, Wu YY, Chen NH. Attention-deficit/hyperactivity disorder with obstructive sleep apnea: A treatment outcome study. *Sleep Med.* 2007;8:18-30.

75. Maquet P. The role of sleep in learning and memory. *Science.* 2001;294:1048-1052.

76. Rocca WA, Hofman A, Brayne C, et al. Frequency and distribution of Alzheimer's disease in Europe: A collaborative study of 1980-1990 prevalence findings. The EURODEM-Prevalence Research Group. *Ann Neurol.* 1991;30:381-390.

77. Lyketsos CG, Lopez O, Jones B, Fitzpatrick AL, Breitner J, DeKosky S. Prevalence of neuropsychiatric symptoms in dementia and mild cognitive impairment: Results from the cardiovascular health study. *JAMA.* 2002;288:1475-1483.

78. Tractenberg RE, Singer CM, Kaye JA. Symptoms of sleep disturbance in persons with Alzheimer's disease and normal elderly. *J Sleep Res.* 2005;14:177-185.

79. Chen JC, Borson S, Scanlan JM. Stage-specific prevalence of behavioral symptoms in Alzheimer's disease in a multi-ethnic community sample. *Am J Geriatr Psychiatry.* 2000;8:123-133.

80. Hart DJ, Craig D, Compton SA, et al. A retrospective study of the behavioural and psychological symptoms of mid and late phase Alzheimer's disease. *Int J Geriatr Psychiatry.* 2003;18:1037-1042.

81. Klerman EB, Dijk DJ. Age-related reduction in the maximal capacity for sleep—Implications for insomnia. *Curr Biol.* 2008;18:1118-1123.

82. Ohadinia S, Noroozian M, Shahsavand S, Saghafi S. Evaluation of insomnia and daytime napping in Iranian Alzheimer disease patients: Relationship with severity of dementia and comparison with normal adults. *Am J Geriatr Psychiatry.* 2004;12:517-522.

83. Hoch CC, Reynolds III CF, Nebes RD, Kupfer DJ, Berman SR, Campbell D. Clinical significance of sleep-disordered breathing in Alzheimer's disease. Preliminary data. *J Am Geriatr Soc.* 1989;37:138-144.

84. Erkinjuntti T, Partinen M, Sulkava R, Telakivi T, Salmi T, Tilvis R. Sleep apnea in multiinfarct dementia and Alzheimer's disease. *Sleep.* 1987;10:419-425.

85. Smallwood RG, Vitiello MV, Giblin EC, Prinz PN. Sleep apnea: Relationship to age, sex, and Alzheimer's dementia. *Sleep.* 1983;6:16-22.

86. Prinz PN, Vitaliano PP, Vitiello MV, et al. Sleep, EEG and mental function changes in senile dementia of the Alzheimer's type. *Neurobiol Aging.* 1982;3:361-370.

87. Montplaisir J, Petit D, Gauthier S, Gaudreau H, Decary A. Sleep disturbances and EEG slowing in Alzheimer's disease. *Sleep Res Online.* 1998;1:147-151.

88. Montplaisir J, Petit D, Lorrain D, Gauthier S, Nielsen T. Sleep in Alzheimer's disease: Further considerations on the role of brainstem and forebrain cholinergic populations in sleep-wake mechanisms. *Sleep.* 1995;18:145-148.

89. Rauchs G, Schabus M, Parapatics S, et al. Is there a link between sleep changes and memory in Alzheimer's disease? *Neuroreport.* 2008;19: 1159-1162.

90. Liu RY, Zhou JN, van Heerikhuize J, Hofman MA, Swaab DF. Decreased melatonin levels in postmortem cerebrospinal fluid in relation to aging, Alzheimer's disease, and apolipoprotein E-epsilon 4/4 genotype. *J Clin Endocrinol Metab.* 1999;84:323-327.

91. Okawa M, Mishima K, Hishikawa Y, Hozumi S, Hori H, Takahashi K. Circadian rhythm disorders in sleep-waking and body temperature in elderly patients with dementia and their treatment. *Sleep.* 1991;14: 478-485.

92. Gagnon JF, Petit D, Fantini ML, et al. REM sleep behavior disorder and REM sleep without atonia in probable Alzheimer disease. *Sleep.* 2006;29:1321-1325.

93. Roman GC, Erkinjuntti T, Wallin A, Pantoni L, Chui HC. Subcortical ischaemic vascular dementia. *Lancet Neurol.* 2002;1:426-436.

94. Meguro K, Ueda M, Kobayashi I, et al. Sleep disturbance in elderly patients with cognitive impairment, decreased daily activity and periventricular white matter lesions. *Sleep.* 1995;18:109-114.

95. Aharon-Peretz J, Masiah A, Pillar T, Epstein R, Tzischinsky O, Lavie P. Sleep-wake cycles in multi-infarct dementia and dementia of the Alzheimer type. *Neurology.* 1991;41:1616-1619.

96. Fuh JL, Wang SJ, Cummings JL. Neuropsychiatric profiles in patients with Alzheimer's disease and vascular dementia. *J Neurol Neurosurg Psychiatry.* 2005;76:1337-1341.

97. Fernandez-Martinez M, Castro J, Molano A, Zarranz JJ, Rodrigo RM, Ortega R. Prevalence of neuropsychiatric symptoms in Alzheimer's disease and vascular dementia. *Curr Alzheimer Res.* 2008;5:61-69.

98. Mishima K, Okawa M, Satoh K, Shimizu T, Hozumi S, Hishikawa Y. Different manifestations of circadian rhythms in senile dementia of Alzheimer's type and multi-infarct dementia. *Neurobiol Aging.* 1997;18:105-109.

99. Partinen M, Palomaki H. Snoring and cerebral infarction. *Lancet.* 1985;2:1325-1326.

100. Dyken ME, Somers VK, Yamada T, Ren ZY, Zimmerman MB. Investigating the relationship between stroke and obstructive sleep apnea. *Stroke.* 1996;27:401-407.

101. Bassetti C, Aldrich MS, Chervin RD, Quint D. Sleep apnea in patients with transient ischemic attack and stroke: A prospective study of 59 patients. *Neurology.* 1996;47:1167-1173.

102. Press DZ. Parkinson's disease dementia—A first step? *N Engl J Med.* 2004;351:2547-2549.

103. Alafuzoff I, Ince PG, Arzberger T, et al. Staging/typing of Lewy body related alpha-synuclein pathology: A study of the BrainNet Europe Consortium. *Acta Neuropathol.* 2009;117:635-652.

104. McKeith IG, Dickson DW, Lowe J, et al. Diagnosis and management of dementia with Lewy bodies: Third report of the DLB Consortium. *Neurology.* 2005;65:1863-1872.

105. Ferman TJ, Smith GE, Boeve BF, et al. DLB fluctuations: Specific features that reliably differentiate DLB from AD and normal aging. *Neurology.* 2004;62:181-187.

106. Manni R, Pacchetti C, Terzaghi M, Sartori I, Mancini F, Nappi G. Hallucinations and sleep-wake cycle in PD: A 24-hour continuous polysomnographic study. *Neurology.* 2002;59:1979-1981.

107. Whitehead DL, Davies AD, Playfer JR, Turnbull CJ. Circadian rest-activity rhythm is altered in Parkinson's disease patients with hallucinations. *Mov Disord.* 2008;23:1137-1145.

108. Sinforiani E, Terzaghi M, Pasotti C, Zucchella C, Zambrelli E, Manni R. Hallucinations and sleep-wake cycle in Alzheimer's disease: A questionnaire-based study in 218 patients. *Neurol Sci.* 2007;28:96-99.

109. Tandberg E, Larsen JP, Karlsen K. A community-based study of sleep disorders in patients with Parkinson's disease. *Mov Disord.* 1998;13: 895-899.

110. Gjerstad MD, Wentzel-Larsen T, Aarsland D, Larsen JP. Insomnia in Parkinson's disease: Frequency and progression over time. *J Neurol Neurosurg Psychiatry.* 2007;78:476-479.

111. Baumann C, Ferini-Strambi L, Waldvogel D, Werth E, Bassetti CL. Parkinsonism with excessive daytime sleepiness—A narcolepsy-like disorder? *J Neurol.* 2005;252:139-145.

112. Boddy F, Rowan EN, Lett D, O'Brien JT, McKeith IG, Burn DJ. Subjectively reported sleep quality and excessive daytime somnolence in Parkinson's disease with and without dementia, dementia with Lewy bodies and Alzheimer's disease. *Int J Geriatr Psychiatry.* 2007;22:529-535.

113. Grace JB, Walker MP, McKeith IG. A comparison of sleep profiles in patients with dementia with Lewy bodies and Alzheimer's disease. *Int J Geriatr Psychiatry.* 2000;15:1028-1033.

114. Rongve A, Boeve BF, Aarsland D. Frequency and correlates of caregiver-reported sleep disturbances in a sample of persons with early dementia. *J Am Geriatr Soc.* 2010;58:480-486.

115. Maria B, Sophia S, Michalis M, et al. Sleep breathing disorders in patients with idiopathic Parkinson's disease. *Respir Med.* 2003;97: 1151-1157.

116. Cochen De Cock V, Abouda M, Leu S, et al. Is obstructive sleep apnea a problem in Parkinson's disease? *Sleep Med.* 2010;11(3):247-252.

117. Loo HV, Tan EK. Case-control study of restless legs syndrome and quality of sleep in Parkinson's disease. *J Neurol Sci.* 2008;266:145-149.

118. Diederich NJ, Vaillant M, Leischen M, et al. Sleep apnea syndrome in Parkinson's disease. A case-control study in 49 patients. *Mov Disord.* 2005;20:1413-1418.

119. Micallef J, Rey M, Eusebio A, et al. Antiparkinsonian drug-induced sleepiness: A double-blind placebo-controlled study of l-dopa, bromocriptine and pramipexole in healthy subjects. *Br J Clin Pharmacol.* 2009;67:333-340.

120. Aldrich MS, Foster NL, White RF, Bluemlein L, Prokopowicz G. Sleep abnormalities in progressive supranuclear palsy. *Ann Neurol.* 1989;25:577-581.

121. Arnulf I, Merino-Andreu M, Bloch F, et al. REM sleep behavior disorder and REM sleep without atonia in patients with progressive supranuclear palsy. *Sleep.* 2005;28:349-354.

122. Montplaisir J, Petit D, Decary A, et al. Sleep and quantitative EEG in patients with progressive supranuclear palsy. *Neurology.* 1997;49: 999-1003.

123. Anderson KN, Hatfield C, Kipps C, Hastings M, Hodges JR. Disrupted sleep and circadian patterns in frontotemporal dementia. *Eur J Neurol.* 2009;16:317-323.

124. Harper DG, Stopa EG, McKee AC, et al. Differential circadian rhythm disturbances in men with Alzheimer disease and frontotemporal degeneration. *Arch Gen Psychiatry.* 2001;58:353-360.

125. Colosimo C, Morgante L, Antonini A, et al. Non-motor symptoms in atypical and secondary parkinsonism: The PRIAMO study. *J Neurol.* 2010;257(1):5-14.

126. Wiegand M, Moller AA, Lauer CJ, et al. Nocturnal sleep in Huntington's disease. *J Neurol.* 1991;238:203-208.

127. Emser W, Brenner M, Stober T, Schimrigk K. Changes in nocturnal sleep in Huntington's and Parkinson's disease. *J Neurol.* 1988;235: 177-179.

128. Bollen EL, Den Heijer JC, Ponsioen C, et al. Respiration during sleep in Huntington's chorea. *J Neurol Sci.* 1988;84:63-68.

129. Landolt HP, Glatzel M, Blattler T, et al. Sleep-wake disturbances in sporadic Creutzfeldt-Jakob disease. *Neurology.* 2006;66:1418-1424.

130. Phipps-Nelson J, Redman JR, Dijk DJ, Rajaratnam SM. Daytime exposure to bright light, as compared to dim light, decreases sleepiness and improves psychomotor vigilance performance. *Sleep.* 2003;26:695-700.

131. Lockley SW, Evans EE, Scheer FA, Brainard GC, Czeisler CA, Aeschbach D. Short-wavelength sensitivity for the direct effects of light on alertness, vigilance, and the waking electroencephalogram in humans. *Sleep.* 2006;29:161-168.

132. Satlin A, Volicer L, Ross V, Herz L, Campbell S. Bright light treatment of behavioral and sleep disturbances in patients with Alzheimer's disease. *Am J Psychiatry.* 1992;149:1028-1032.

133. Lovell BB, Ancoli-Israel S, Gevirtz R. Effect of bright light treatment on agitated behavior in institutionalized elderly subjects. *Psychiatry Res.* 1995;57:7-12.

134. Koyama E, Matsubara H, Nakano T. Bright light treatment for sleep-wake disturbances in aged individuals with dementia. *Psychiatry Clin Neurosci.* 1999;53:227-229.

135. Haffmans PM, Sival RC, Lucius SA, Cats Q, van Gelder L. Bright light therapy and melatonin in motor restless behaviour in dementia: A placebo-controlled study. *Int J Geriatr Psychiatry.* 2001;16:106-110.

136. Dowling GA, Graf CL, Hubbard EM, Luxenberg JS. Light treatment for neuropsychiatric behaviors in Alzheimer's disease. *West J Nurs Res.* 2007;29:961-975.

137. Skjerve A, Holsten F, Aarsland D, Bjorvatn B, Nygaard HA, Johansen IM. Improvement in behavioral symptoms and advance of activity acrophase after short-term bright light treatment in severe dementia. *Psychiatry Clin Neurosci.* 2004;58:343-347.

138. Barrick AL, Sloane PD, Williams CS, et al. Impact of ambient bright light on agitation in dementia. *Int J Geriatr Psychiatry.* 2010;25(10):1013-1021.

139. Asayama K, Yamadera H, Ito T, Suzuki H, Kudo Y, Endo S. Double blind study of melatonin effects on the sleep-wake rhythm, cognitive and non-cognitive functions in Alzheimer type dementia. *J Nippon Med Sch.* 2003;70:334-341.

140. Singer C, Tractenberg RE, Kaye J, et al. A multicenter, placebo-controlled trial of melatonin for sleep disturbance in Alzheimer's disease. *Sleep.* 2003;26:893-901.

141. Serfaty M, Kennell-Webb S, Warner J, Blizard R, Raven P. Double blind randomised placebo controlled trial of low dose melatonin for sleep disorders in dementia. *Int J Geriatr Psychiatry.* 2002;17:1120-1127.

142. Gehrman PR, Connor DJ, Martin JL, Shochat T, Corey-Bloom J, Ancoli-Israel S. Melatonin fails to improve sleep or agitation in double-blind randomized placebo-controlled trial of institutionalized patients with Alzheimer disease. *Am J Geriatr Psychiatry.* 2009;17:166-169.

143. Dowling GA, Burr RL, Van Someren EJ, et al. Melatonin and bright-light treatment for rest-activity disruption in institutionalized patients with Alzheimer's disease. *J Am Geriatr Soc.* 2008;56:239-246.

144. Riemersma-van der Lek RF, Swaab DF, Twisk J, Hol EM, Hoogendijk WJ, Van Someren EJ. Effect of bright light and melatonin on cognitive and noncognitive function in elderly residents of group care facilities: A randomized controlled trial. *JAMA.* 2008;299:2642-2655.

145. Richards KC, Beck C, O'Sullivan PS, Shue VM. Effect of individualized social activity on sleep in nursing home residents with dementia. *J Am Geriatr Soc.* 2005;53:1510-1517.

146. Alessi CA, Martin JL, Webber AP. Cynthia Kim E, Harker JO, Josephson KR. Randomized, controlled trial of a nonpharmacological intervention to improve abnormal sleep/wake patterns in nursing home residents. *J Am Geriatr Soc.* 2005;53:803-810.

147. Ouslander JG, Connell BR, Bliwise DL, Endeshaw Y, Griffiths P, Schnelle JF. A nonpharmacological intervention to improve sleep in nursing home patients: Results of a controlled clinical trial. *J Am Geriatr Soc.* 2006;54:38-47.

148. McCurry SM, Gibbons LE, Logsdon RG, Vitiello MV, Teri L. Nighttime insomnia treatment and education for Alzheimer's disease: A randomized, controlled trial. *J Am Geriatr Soc.* 2005;53:793-802.

149. Glass J, Lanctot KL, Herrmann N, Sproule BA, Busto UE. Sedative hypnotics in older people with insomnia: Meta-analysis of risks and benefits. *BMJ.* 2005;331:1169.

150. Savaskan E, Schnitzler C, Schroder C, Cajochen C, Muller-Spahn F, Wirz-Justice A. Treatment of behavioural, cognitive and circadian rest-activity cycle disturbances in Alzheimer's disease: Haloperidol vs. quetiapine. *Int J Neuropsychopharmacol.* 2006;9:507-516.

151. Liperoti R, Onder G, Landi F, et al. All-cause mortality associated with atypical and conventional antipsychotics among nursing home residents with dementia: A retrospective cohort study. *J Clin Psychiatry.* 2009;70:1340-1347.

152. Webb IC, Patton DF, Landry GJ, Mistlberger RE. Circadian clock resetting by behavioral arousal: Neural correlates in the midbrain raphe nuclei and locus coeruleus. *Neuroscience.* 2010;166:739-751.

153. Buxton OM, Copinschi G, Van Onderbergen A, Karrison TG, Van Cauter E. A benzodiazepine hypnotic facilitates adaptation of circadian rhythms and sleep-wake homeostasis to an eight hour delay shift simulating westward jet lag. *Sleep.* 2000;23:915-927.

154. Kittur S, Hauser P. Improvement of sleep and behavior by methylphenidate in Alzheimer's disease. *Am J Psychiatry.* 1999;156:1116-1117.

155. Howcroft DJ, Jones RW. Does modafinil have the potential to improve disrupted sleep patterns in patients with dementia? *Int J Geriatr Psychiatry.* 2005;20:492-495.

156. Aurora RN, Zak RS, Maganti RK, et al. Best practice guide for the treatment of REM sleep behavior disorder (RBD). *J Clin Sleep Med.* 2010;6:85-95.

157. Yeh SB, Yeh PY, Schenck CH. Rivastigmine-induced REM sleep behavior disorder (RBD) in an 88-year-old man with Alzheimer's disease. *J Clin Sleep Med.* 2010;6:192-195.

158. Chong MS, Ayalon L, Marler M, et al. Continuous positive airway pressure reduces subjective daytime sleepiness in patients with mild to moderate Alzheimer's disease with sleep disordered breathing. *J Am Geriatr Soc.* 2006;54:777-781.

159. Ancoli-Israel S, Palmer BW, Cooke JR, et al. Cognitive effects of treating obstructive sleep apnea in Alzheimer's disease: A randomized controlled study. *J Am Geriatr Soc.* 2008;56:2076-2081.

160. Ayalon L, Ancoli-Israel S, Stepnowsky C, et al. Adherence to continuous positive airway pressure treatment in patients with Alzheimer's disease and obstructive sleep apnea. *Am J Geriatr Psychiatry.* 2006;14:176-180.

161. Colenda CC, Cohen W, McCall WV, Rosenquist PB. Phototherapy for patients with Alzheimer's disease with disturbed sleep patterns: Results of a community-based pilot study. *Alzheimer Dis Assoc Disord.* 1997;11:175-178.

162. Okumoto Y, Koyama E, Matsubara H, Nakano T, Nakamura R. Sleep improvement by light in a demented aged individual. *Psychiatry Clin Neurosci.* 1998;52(2):194-196.

162a. Yamadera H, Ito T, Suzuki H, Asayama K, Ito R, Endo S. Effects of bright light on cognitive and sleep–wake (circadian) rhythm disturbances in Alzheimer-type dementia. *Psychiatry and Clinical Neurosciences.* 2000;54:352-353.

163. Van Someren EJ, Kessler A, Mirmiran M, Swaab DF. Indirect bright light improves circadian rest-activity rhythm disturbances in demented patients. *Biol Psychiatry.* 1997;41:955-963.

164. Mishima K, Hishikawa Y, Okawa M. Randomized, dim light controlled, crossover test of morning bright light therapy for rest-activity rhythm disorders in patients with vascular dementia and dementia of Alzheimer's type. *Chronobiol Int.* 1998;15:647-654.

165. Lyketsos CG, Lindell Veiel L, Baker A, Steele C. A randomized, controlled trial of bright light therapy for agitated behaviors in dementia patients residing in long-term care. *Int J Geriatr Psychiatry.* 1999;14:520-525.

166. Fontana Gasio P, Krauchi K, Cajochen C, et al. Dawn-dusk simulation light therapy of disturbed circadian rest-activity cycles in demented elderly. *Exp Gerontol.* 2003;38:207-216.

167. Fetveit A, Skjerve A, Bjorvatn B. Bright light treatment improves sleep in institutionalised elderly—An open trial. *Int J Geriatr Psychiatry.* 2003;18:520-526.

168. Ancoli-Israel S, Gehrman P, Martin JL, et al. Increased light exposure consolidates sleep and strengthens circadian rhythms in severe Alzheimer's disease patients. *Behav Sleep Med.* 2003;1:22-36.

169. Dowling GA, Mastick J, Hubbard EM, Luxenberg JS, Burr RL. Effect of timed bright light treatment for rest-activity disruption in institutionalized patients with Alzheimer's disease. *Int J Geriatr Psychiatry.* 2005;20:738-743.

170. Sloane PD, Williams CS, Mitchell CM, et al. High-intensity environmental light in dementia: Effect on sleep and activity. *J Am Geriatr Soc.* 2007;55:1524-1533.

Chapter 53

Sleep Disturbances and Disorders and Their Treatment in Multiple Sclerosis

RAJINDER SINGH / HRAYR ATTARIAN

Sleep disturbances in multiple sclerosis (MS) are well known; however, there is very little written on the treatment. This chapter summarizes the sleep disorders associated with MS, their impact on the primary illness, and their treatment options.

The limited literature that exists about poor sleep in MS patients is divided into three broad categories: prevalence of sleep disturbances in MS, the relationship of sleep disturbances with fatigue, and the distinct sleep disorders co-morbid with MS. The discussion will concentrate on the treatment options available for the last two categories.

Early recognition and treatment of sleep disturbances in MS patients can translate into improved quality of life and less disability, as sleep issues have been shown to be independent predictors for both reduced quality of life and for mental and physical status.[1,2]

NONSPECIFIC SLEEP DISTURBANCES AND FATIGUE IN MULTIPLE SCLEROSIS

Although not a sleep complaint per se, daytime fatigue overlaps with the symptom of daytime sleepiness and is one of the most common symptoms of MS. *The Multiple Sclerosis Council for Clinical Practice Guidelines* defines *fatigue* as "a subjective lack of physical and/or mental energy that is perceived by the individual or caregiver to interfere with usual and desired activities."[3] It is distinguished from excessive daytime sleepiness (EDS) by the absence of episodes of inappropriate sleep during the day. A variety of subjective rating scales exist including the Fatigue Severity Scale (FSS),[4] Fatigue Impact Scale (FIS),[5] Fatigue Descriptive Scale,[6] and Modified Fatigue Impact Scale[7] (MFIS), among others. In contrast, EDS has subjective measures including the Epworth Sleepiness Scale (ESS)[8] and objective measures including the multiple sleep latency test (MSLT).[9]

There are robust data to suggest a strong correlation between sleep problems and fatigue in MS.[10-12] Data on the prevalence of EDS in MS are limited (see later discussion). In studies in which both fatigue and sleepiness have been measured, the two symptoms frequently occur together but are not the same.[13] It is likely that in both clinical practice and clinical studies the distinction is imprecise.

Lobentanz and associates[2] reported on a series of 504 patients in which fatigue, as measured by the FSS score, was an independent predictor of decreased occupational functioning as measured by the Quality of Life Index (QLI).[14] In this group, more than 60% reported that fatigue was one of the three most troubling symptoms of

their disease. Therefore, fatigue control could be key in improving the MS patient's quality of life and sense of independence.[15]

Fatigue has been described by MS patients even in the absence of obvious causes such as motor weakness, cognitive deficits, and mood disorders.[15] The cause of fatigue in MS patients, however, seems to be multifactorial. One theory is that fatigue is a result of demyelination or the inflammatory process itself.[16] Heesen and associates[17] demonstrated elevations of inflammatory cytokines (tumor necrosis factor [TNF-α] and interferon [IFN-γ]) in MS patients which correlated with scores on the MFIS. Studies utilizing either functional imaging or electroencephalogram (EEG) have shown that a larger cortical area is activated in a fatigued MS patient than in a nonfatigued patient while performing the same task.[16,18] Moreover, functional magnetic resonance imaging (MRI) studies during tasks designed to induce cognitive and motor fatigue in MS and normal control subjects have shown increased cortical activation in multiple cortical and subcortical areas compared to normal subjects, suggesting that MS fatigue could be in part secondary to a need to recruit compensatory neural circuits.[18] These observations could be consistent with the hypothesis that lesion load may correlate with fatigue.[16,19] However, that hypothesis was not confirmed by Codella and associates,[20] who compared magnetization transfer and diffusion transfer MRI scans of 14 MS patients with fatigue and 14 MS patients without fatigue and did not find a difference in lesion load between the two groups.

The prevalence of sleep disturbances in MS patients has led some to explore the potential link between fatigue and disordered sleep. Possible etiologies of sleep disturbance include spasticity, lack of sphincter control, immobility, motor weakness, pain, periodic leg movements (PLM), restless legs syndrome (RLS), abnormal sleep-wake cycles, sleep-disordered breathing, narcolepsy, rapid eye movement (REM) sleep behavior disorder, and depression. Iatrogenic causes include medications such as benzodiazepines and antispasticity drugs, which can induce daytime hypersomnolence, and corticosteroids, which may result in insomnia and even hynagogic hallucinations[21] (Table 53-1). In a cross-sectional survey of 1063 patients with MS, Bamer and associates[22] found that 51% patients with MS had moderate to severe subjective sleep problems, with women at higher risk than men. Merlino and associates[1] found a strong relationship between immobility, pain, and social isolation and poor sleep in patients with MS. Using actigraphs and sleep logs, Attarian and associates[10] compared three groups of 15 subjects each: a MS group with fatigue, an age- and sex-matched MS group without fatigue, and an age- and sex-matched healthy control group. In this study 13 of 15 patients in the fatigued group experienced disrupted sleep, but only 2 of 15 in the group without fatigue had sleep disturbances and only one patient in the healthy control group had subjective but no actigraphically documented sleep problems. Kaynak and associates[11] further confirmed these findings by using polysomnography. In comparing 27 MS patients with fatigue, 10 MS patients without fatigue, and 13 control subjects they demonstrated a higher prevalence of nonspecific polysomnographic sleep disruptions in the MS with fatigue group as measured by the total arousal index.

Vetrugno and associates,[23] on the other hand, did not find an association, in their group of relapsing remitting MS patients, between fatigue and sleep disturbances. Attarian and associates[24] randomized 30 subjects with relapsing remitting MS and sleep disturbance in a double-blind controlled fashion to either placebo or eszopiclone. This study found a significant improvement in sleep continuity in subjects who took eszopiclone versus placebo, but there was no significant difference in the degree of improvement in fatigue between those who took active medication and those who took placebo. Therefore, the relationship between fatigue and nonspecific sleep disturbance remains unclear.

Most medications that have been studied in the treatment of MS fatigue are those with some degree of impact on sleep-wake patterns. These drugs include the antiviral amantadine that has CNS stimulant activity,[25] the stimulant pemoline[26,27] (now unavailable in the United States because of liver toxicity), aminopyridines,[28] selective serotonin reuptake inhibitors,[29] and modafinil. None has shown robust efficacy.[25,27-29] The newest medication for this indication is the wake-promoting agent modafinil. There are many anecdotal case reports of its efficacy, but it is uncertain whether these findings are due to a placebo effect.[30]

Fatigue and Modafinil

Modafinil (see Chapter 6) is a wake-promoting drug that is approved by the Food and Drug Administration (FDA) as therapy for narcolepsy with and without cataplexy, residual EDS in treated obstructive sleep apnea syndrome, and shift work disorder. Despite a paucity of evidence regarding the utility of modafinil in controlling symptoms of fatigue in MS patients, it is widely used.[30]

Rammohan and associates[15] conducted a single-blind crossover study of 72 patients and found a significant reduction compared to placebo in three fatigue scales (MFIS, FSS, and a visual analog scale) and the ESS, with modafinil 200 mg when compared to placebo. However, a randomized, double-blind, placebo-controlled, parallel group 35-day study of 115 patients by Stankoff and associates[13] showed no significant difference between the treatment and placebo groups using the MFIS as the primary measure of efficacy. In a *post hoc* analysis of these data, the authors reported that modafinil "tended to provide more benefit than placebo" among those patients who also reported EDS.[13] A retrospective analysis of 39 patients treated for fatigue with modafinil in an MS clinic for a median of 1.25 years (range 1 month to 5 years) showed a higher percentage of responders in patients who also reported EDS as compared to those with the complaint of fatigue without EDS.[31]

These results suggest that MS fatigue could be linked to EDS and that the impact of modafinil on fatigue may be due to its efficacy in the treatment of EDS,[13,31] but the data are weak.

Excessive Daytime Sleepiness

EDS refers to the abnormal tendency to fall asleep during the day. The prevalence of EDS in MS has been measured with both subjective and objective measures in several studies with inconsistent results. Knudsen and associates[32] compared 48 MS patients either in active disease or in remission and found that the mean ESS score was within normal limits with no difference between groups. Six patients, three in each group, showed an ESS of 10 or greater (normal scores are <10). Attarian and associates[24] reported normal ESS scores in 14 of 15 fatigued MS patients. Taphoorn and associates[33] found normal latencies on the MSLT in 60 MS patients who presented with fatigue and sleep disturbance. Frausher and colleagues[34] also found no evidence of sleepiness on both objective and subjective measures in 61 MS patients. On the other hand, ESS of 10 or greater was reported[12] in 19 of 59 MS clinic patients (32%) surveyed by questionnaire and 58 of 110 patients (60%) in Standkoff's series.[13]

Like fatigue, EDS in MS may be caused by factors related to the inflammatory or demyelinating aspects of the disorder. Heesen and associates[17] reported that in MS patients levels of TNF-α showed a significant ($p = 0.0001$) positive correlation with the ESS.[17] A small number of patients have shown unequivocal evidence of "symptomatic narcolepsy" secondary to demyelinating lesions of the hypothalamus as described later in the chapter.[35] Other specific sleep disorders implicated in both fatigue and/or EDS may emerge secondary to the pathology of MS and are discussed later.

SPECIFIC SLEEP DISORDERS AND MULTIPLE SCLEROSIS

Sleep-Disordered Breathing

Demyelinating lesions, especially those involving the brainstem, may directly influence respiratory function at multiple anatomic levels. Auer and associates[36] described two nocturnal deaths associated with MS plaque involving the medullary respiratory centers at postmortem examination; in one of these patients, sleep studies had shown nocturnal hypoventilation with hypercarbia and hypoxia. A variety of abnormal respiratory patterns including paroxysmal hyperventilation, central apneas, and apneustic breathing have also been described.[37,38] Respiratory muscle weakness of both bulbar and diaphragmatic muscles can contribute to sleep-disordered breathing. However, an increased prevalence of obstructive sleep apnea in MS is not established. Several small studies have shown no increased prevalence or only a few cases.[11,21]

The clinician should remain alert to the possibility of significant respiratory dysfunction during sleep, especially hypoventilation in patients with prominent weakness or brainstem dysfunction. Treatment of nocturnal respiratory hypoventilation with noninvasive positive pressure ventilation (NIPPV) or other forms of respiratory support may be necessary (see Chapter 20).

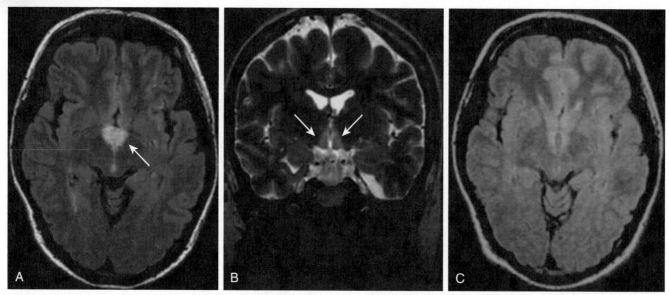

Figure 53-1 A patient with multiple sclerosis, excessive daytime sleepiness, and SOREMPs with low hypocretin (<40 pg/mL). A 22-year-old female patient with bilateral hypothalamic lesions of multiple sclerosis (originally reported by Iseki and associates[61] and Oka and associates[52]). Her nocturnal sleep time was 15 hours, sleep latency by MSLT was 2.8 minutes, and REM latency was 4.7 minutes with 5 SOREMPs. Her HLA was DR2 negative and an MRI scan revealed FLAIR hyperintensity in the hypothalamus bilaterally. **A,** Axial section of FLAIR image. **B,** Coronal section of T_2-weighted image. Bilateral hypothalamic plaque is demonstrated as a median high-intensity area (*arrow*). **C,** The plaque disappeared 1 month later with steroid treatments. *FLAIR,* fluid-attenuated inversion recovery; *MRI,* magnetic resonance imaging; *MSLT,* multiple sleep latency test; *REM,* rapid eye movement; *SOREMPs,* sleep onset REM periods. (From Nishino S, Kanbayashi T. Symptomatic narcolepsy, cataplexy and hypersomnia, and their implications in the hypothalamic hypocretin/orexin system. *Sleep Med Rev.* 2005;9[4]:287.)

Restless Legs Syndrome and Periodic Limb Movement Disorder

An established factor contributing to poor sleep in MS patients is RLS (see Chapter 24). RLS is described as an unpleasant feeling or an irresistible urge to move the legs that occurs at rest primarily in the evening or at bedtime. Patients report temporary relief of symptoms with movement. The prevalence of RLS in the general population in North America and Western Europe is estimated to be around 5%.[39] In the MS population, however, it has been reported to be over 30%.[39,40] A prospective case control study of 861 patients and 649 control subjects in Italy found the risk of RLS in MS to be 5.4 times that of control subjects.[39] In this MS population the significant risk factors for RLS were older age, longer MS duration, primary progressive form, higher global pyramidal and sensory disability, and the presence of leg jerks before sleep. Measures of iron storage (a risk factor for RLS; see Chapter 24) did not differ between the groups. Clinical evidence of RLS followed the onset of MS by a mean period of 5 years. MS/RLS(+) patients reported a significantly higher frequency of insomnia, longer sleep latency, shorter total sleep time, EDS, snoring, and hypnotic use. In another study, Moreira and associates,[41] also found MS patients with RLS had increased sleep latency, as well as decreased sleep duration and sleep efficiency as measured by the Pittsburgh Sleep Quality Index (PSQI).[42] MS patients with fatigue were shown to have a higher rate of RLS than MS patients without fatigue, 40.7% and 30% respectively, but the difference was not statistically significant.[11] However, in a study of MS patients with and without RLS, a higher prevalence of fatigue was found in the RLS patients, and this finding correlated with clinical disability and sleep quality.[41] Therefore, given that RLS has a significantly higher prevalence in MS and appears to contribute to fatigue and poor sleep, timely recognition and treatment may prove to be useful in improving quality of life in these patients. However, no clinical trials have directly studied the impact of treatment of RLS in this population. The treatment of RLS in MS is approached as it is for RLS in other conditions, but has not been specifically studied in this population (see Chapter 24).

Periodic limb movement disorder (PLMD) (see Chapter 24) is another disorder that may contribute to poor sleep and fatigue in MS patients, but the evidence remains equivocal. PLMD is commonly associated with RLS but is not the same entity. PLMD is the clinical sleep disturbance caused by repetitive stereotypic limb movements during sleep (PLMS) most frequently involving the lower extremities. Movements occur about every 20 to 40 seconds and typically involve extension of the big toe with some degree of flexion of the ankle, knee, and hip. PLMD is considered a sleep disorder because the movements often cause arousal and lead to nonrestorative sleep. Kaynak and associates,[11] using polysomnography, showed that MS patients with fatigue had higher rates of periodic leg movements per hour with and without arousal, more wake time after sleep onset, and an increased total arousal index as compared to normal control subjects without MS. Although the total arousal index was significantly higher in the fatigued MS group as compared to the nonfatigued MS group, PLMS with and without arousal were not significantly different between the two patient groups.

PLMD may be treated with the same medications as used in the treatment of RLS; in addition, PLMD has been reported to respond to physical therapy[43] and electrical stimulation.[44] Whether treatment of PLMD improves sleep quality in MS is unknown.

Circadian Rhythm Disorders

Early on there was some evidence that because of the presence of pineal calcification in patients with MS and fatigue there was a possibility of increased prevalence of circadian rhythm

TABLE 53-1

Select Medications Used in the Treatment of Multiple Sclerosis with Potential Effects on Sleep and Wake

Medication*	Indication in MS	Side Effect(s)	PSG Data	Mechanism of Action
Interferon-β[62,63]	Disease-modifying therapy	Fatigue, hypersomnolence and insomnia	?	Reduced antigen presentation and T cell proliferation. Altered cytokine expression
Methylprednisolone[64,65]	Treatment of acute relapse	Insomnia	Decrease in REM sleep	Decreased cytokine cascade. Decreased activation of T cells. Decreased ability of immune cells to penetrate the CNS
Modafinil[66]	MS fatigue	Insomnia	Reduction in mean sleep latency	Unknown
Methylphenidate[67]	MS fatigue	Insomnia	Suppressed REM sleep	Increased catecholamine release and inhibition of reuptake
Amantadine[64]	MS fatigue	Insomnia	?	Presynaptic dopamine-releasing agent
4-Aminopyridine[68]	MS fatigue	Insomnia	?	Blockade of potassium channels in neurons
Baclofen[69,70]	Spasticity	Sedation	Total sleep time increased. Wake after sleep onset reduced.	GABA$_B$ receptor agonist
Clonazepam[71]	Spasticity/anxiety	Somnolence	Total sleep time increased. Sleep latency and wake after sleep onset reduced. Spindle activity increased. REM sleep reduced.	GABA$_A$ receptor agonist
Tizanidine[72]	Spasticity	Daytime drowsiness	Improvement in sleep induction and maintenance	Central α$_2$-adrenoreceptor agonist
Selective serotonin reuptake inhibitors[73]	Depression/anxiety	Insomnia or sedation	Decreased total sleep time. Increased Stage 1 sleep. Decreased REM. Increase sleep latency. "Prozac eyes". Periodic limb movements	5-HT reuptake inhibition
Gabapentin[74]	Pain/seizures	Sleepiness	Decreased stage 1 sleep. Increased stage 3 sleep. Reduced periodic limb movements. Increased REM sleep	May promote formation of GABA in the CNS
Oxybutinin[75]	Urinary frequency	Sedation	Decreased REM sleep. Increased REM latency	Anticholinergic agent

*Data from cited references.
CNS, central nervous system; GABA, γ-aminobutyric acid; 5-HT, 5-hydroxytryptamine; MS, multiple sclerosis; PSG, polysomnography; REM, rapid eye movement.
Modified from Brass SD, Duquette P, Proulx-Therrien J, Auerbach S. Sleep disorders in patients with multiple sclerosis. *Sleep Med Rev.* 2010;14(2):121-129.[60]

disorders in MS patients.[45,46] Cortical and subcortical pathways affected in MS also play a role in sleep-wake cycles and control of body core temperature (BCT).[23] The suprachiasmatic nucleus (SCN) plays an important role in regulation of the 24-hour cycle based on light exposure (see Section 8, "Circadian Rhythm Disorders"). This signal is carried via the retinohypothalamic input through the optic nerve. Because the optic nerve is commonly affected in MS patients, it is plausible that a lesion of the optic nerve could cause circadian rhythm disturbances.

A relationship between fatigue and sleep-wake cycles or BCT has been evaluated in a variety of study designs with conflicting results. For example, Attarian and associates[10] found support for a possible relationship between fatigue and abnormal sleep-wake cycles measured actigraphically in patients with relapsing remitting and progressive types of MS who were takings immunomodulators at the time of the study. Taphoorn and associates[33] studied 16 MS patients selected for both fatigue and sleep complaints including 13 with optic nerve lesions and did not find actigraphic evidence of

abnormal 24-hour sleep-wake cycling. A study by Vetrugno and associates[23] of six MS patients with fatigue, in which only one patient had visual dysfunction and five patients had corticospinal tract or brainstem dysfunction, found normal BCT rhythmicity as compared to normal control subjects during polysomnographic analysis. Such observations need further validation.

No published data exist on the treatment of circadian rhythm disorders in MS using either light therapy, chronotherapy, or melatonin.

Narcolepsy

The association of narcolepsy and MS has been suggested for decades. This idea was originally based on case reports of MS patients with concomitant narcolepsy[47,48] and has been strengthened by the association of both disorders with the DQB10602 allele of the HLA-DR2 serotype and increasing evidence that narcolepsy, like MS, may be an autoimmune disorder (see Chapter 22). Poirier and associates[49] reported a greater frequency of sleep attacks, cataplexy, and sleep paralysis as assessed by questionnaire and clinical interview in 70 MS patients. There was no difference in frequency of symptoms between DR2 positive and negative patients. A subset of DR2 positive patients with a clinical history consistent with cataplexy were studied polysomnographically, and none fulfilled neurophysiologic criteria for narcolepsy. An early small study exploring the possible relationship of the HLA-DR2 antigen and sleep latency on the MSLT showed no difference in latencies between MS patients positive for HLA-DR2 and those who were negative; none of the patients showed sleep onset REM.[50]

There are reports of "symptomatic narcolepsy" (see Chapter 22) in MS attributed to lesions of the hypothalamus accompanied by low cerebrospinal fluid (CSF) hypocretin (orexin) during attacks.[35,51-53] Improvement in EDS and normalization of CSF hypocretin followed immunosuppressive treatment in patients with acute and subacute hypothalamic lesions.[35,54] A study of 48 MS patients without hypothalamic lesions did not show abnormalities of CSF hypocretin or a higher prevalence of EDS[32] either during acute attacks or during periods of remission. It is likely that most cases of MS-associated narcolepsy are secondary to hypothalamic lesions affecting the hypocretin (orexin) system.[32,35]

The treatment of narcoleptic symptoms in MS should be the same as that in idiopathic narcolepsy (see Chapter 22) with additional attention to the possibility that immunotherapy of the demyelinating disease has been reported to result in remission of symptoms in patients with hypothalamic lesions[35,53,54] (Fig. 53-1).

Parasomnias

There have been rare case reports of REM sleep behavior disorder (RBD)[55,56] (see Chapter 43) attributed to MS plaque involving the pons. In a consecutive series of 135 MS patients, three patients met all of the clinical criteria for RBD, compared to no subjects in the control population.[57] Of the three MS RBD patients, only one demonstrated a pontine plaque and the remaining two were treated with selective serotonin reuptake inhibitors, medications known to precipitate RBD.[58] RBD in the MS patient should be treated as one would treat idiopathic RBD. The role of antidepressants in exacerbating or precipitating RBD may be particularly important in MS because many of these patients are treated pharmacologically for depression.[59]

CONCLUSION

In summary, despite their prevalence, sleep disturbances in MS are still poorly understood and infrequently studied. Their treatment also remains unexplored. Most therapies are symptomatic and target the individual complaints rather than the underlying cause.

REFERENCES

1. Merlino G, Fratticci L, Lenchig C, Valente M, Cargnelutti D, et al. Prevalence of "poor sleep" among patients with multiple sclerosis: An independent predictor of mental and physical status. *Sleep Med.* 2009;10(1):26-34.
2. Lobentanz IS, Asenbaum S, Vass K, Sauter C, Klosch G, et al. Factors influencing quality of life in multiple sclerosis patients: Disability, depressive mood, fatigue and sleep quality. *Acta Neurol Scand.* 2004;110(1):6-13.
3. Fatigue Guidelines Development Panel of the Multiple Sclerosis Council for Clinical Practice Guidelines. *Fatigue and Multiple Sclerosis. Evidence-Based Management Strategies for Fatigue in Multiple Sclerosis.* Washington, DC: Paralyzed Veterans of America; 1998.
4. Krupp LB, LaRocca NG, Muir-Nash J, Steinberg AD. The fatigue severity scale. Application to patients with multiple sclerosis and systemic lupus erythematosus. *Arch Neurol.* 1989;46(10):1121-1123.
5. Fisk JD, Pontefract A, Ritvo PG, Archibald CJ, Murray TJ. The impact of fatigue on patients with multiple sclerosis. *Can J Neurol Sci.* 1994;21(1):9-14.
6. Iriarte J, Katsamakis G, de Castro P. The Fatigue Descriptive Scale (FDS): A useful tool to evaluate fatigue in multiple sclerosis. *Mult Scler.* 1999;5(1):10-16.
7. Tellez N, Rio J, Tintore M, Nos C, Galan I, Montalban X. Does the Modified Fatigue Impact Scale offer a more comprehensive assessment of fatigue in MS? *Mult Scler.* 2005;11(2):198-202.
8. Johns MW. A new method for measuring daytime sleepiness: The Epworth Sleepiness Scale. *Sleep.* 1991;14(6):540-545.
9. Arand D, Bonnet M, Hurwitz T, Mitler M, Rosa R, Sangal RB. The clinical use of the MSLT and MWT. *Sleep.* 2005;28(1):123-144.
10. Attarian HP, Brown KM, Duntley SP, Carter JD, Cross AH. The relationship of sleep disturbances and fatigue in multiple sclerosis. *Arch Neurol.* 2004;61(4):525-528.
11. Kaynak H, Altintas A, Kaynak CD, Uyanik O, Saip S, et al. Fatigue and sleep disturbance in multiple sclerosis. *Eur J Neurol.* 2006;13(12):1333-1339.
12. Stanton BR, Barnes F, Silber E. Sleep and fatigue in multiple sclerosis. *Mult Scler.* 2006;12(4):481-486.
13. Stankoff B, Waubant E, Confavreux C, Edan G, Debouverie M, et al. Modafinil for fatigue in MS: A randomized placebo-controlled double-blind study. *Neurology.* 2005;64(7):1139-1143.
14. Mezzich JE, Ruiperez MA, Yoon G, Liu J, Zapata-Vega MI. Measuring cultural identity: Validation of a modified Cortes, Rogler and Malgady Bicultural Scale in three ethnic groups in New York. *Cult Med Psychiatry.* 2009;33(3):451-472.
15. Rammohan KW, Rosenberg JH, Lynn DJ, Blumenfeld AM, Pollak CP, Nagaraja HN. Efficacy and safety of modafinil (Provigil) for the treatment of fatigue in multiple sclerosis: A two centre phase 2 study. *J Neurol Neurosurg Psychiatry.* 2002;72(2):179-183.
16. Leocani L, Colombo B, Comi G. Physiopathology of fatigue in multiple sclerosis. *Neurol Sci.* 2008;29(suppl 2):S241-S243.
17. Heesen C, Nawrath L, Reich C, Bauer N, Schulz KH, Gold SM. Fatigue in multiple sclerosis: An example of cytokine mediated sickness behaviour? *J Neurol Neurosurg Psychiatry.* 2006;77(1):34-39.
18. DeLuca J, Genova HM, Capili EJ, Wylie GR. Functional neuroimaging of fatigue. *Phys Med Rehab Clin North Am.* 2009;20(2):325-337.
19. Tedeschi G, Dinacci D, Lavorgna L, Prinster A, Savettieri G, et al. Correlation between fatigue and brain atrophy and lesion load in multiple sclerosis patients independent of disability. *J Neurol Sci.* 2007;263(1-2):15-19.
20. Codella M, Rocca MA, Colombo B, Rossi P, Comi G, Filippi M. A preliminary study of magnetization transfer and diffusion tensor MRI of multiple sclerosis patients with fatigue. *J Neurol.* 2002;249(5):535-537.
21. Tachibana N, Howard RS, Hirsch NP, Miller DH, Moseley IF, Fish D. Sleep problems in multiple sclerosis. *Eur Neurol.* 1994;34(6):320-323.
22. Bamer AM, Johnson KL, Amtmann D, Kraft GH. Prevalence of sleep problems in individuals with multiple sclerosis. *Mult Scler.* 2008;14(8):1127-1130.
23. Vetrugno R, Stecchi S, Scandellari C, Pierangeli G, Sabattini L, et al. Sleep-wake and body core temperature rhythms in multiple sclerosis with fatigue. *Clin Neurophysiol.* 2007;118(1):228-234.
24. Attarian HP, Applebee G, Applebee A, Wang B, Clark M, et al. Eszopiclone for improving sleep continuity in MS patients with sleep disturbances and its impact on daytime fatigue. *Int J Mult Scler Care.* 2011;13(2):84-90.
25. Taus C, Giuliani G, Pucci E, D'Amico R, Solari A. Amantadine for fatigue in multiple sclerosis. *Cochrane Database Syst Rev.* 2003(2):CD002818.
26. Weinshenker BG, Penman M, Bass B, Ebers GC, Rice GP. A double-blind, randomized, crossover trial of pemoline in fatigue associated with multiple sclerosis. *Neurology.* 1992;42(8):1468-1471.
27. Bakshi R. Fatigue associated with multiple sclerosis: Diagnosis, impact and management. *Mult Scler.* 2003;9(3):219-227.
28. Solari A, Uitdehaag B, Giuliani G, Pucci E, Taus C. Aminopyridines for symptomatic treatment in multiple sclerosis. *Cochrane Database Syst Rev.* 2001(4):CD001330.
29. Tremlett HL, Luscombe DK, Wiles CM. Prescribing for multiple sclerosis patients in general practice: A case-control study. *J Clin Pharm Ther.* 2001;26(6):437-444.

30. Kumar R. Approved and investigational uses of modafinil: An evidence-based review. *Drugs*. 2008;68(13):1803-1839.

31. Littleton ET, Hobart JC, Palace J. Modafinil for multiple sclerosis fatigue: Does it work? *Clin Neurol Neurosurg*. 2010;112(1):29-31.

32. Knudsen S, Jennum PJ, Korsholm K, Sheikh SP, Gammeltoft S, Frederiksen JL. Normal levels of cerebrospinal fluid hypocretin-1 and daytime sleepiness during attacks of relapsing-remitting multiple sclerosis and monosymptomatic optic neuritis. *Mult Scler*. 2008;14(6):734-738.

33. Taphoorn MJ, van Someren E, Snoek FJ, Strijers RL, Swaab DF, et al. Fatigue, sleep disturbances and circadian rhythm in multiple sclerosis. *J Neurol*. 1993;240(7):446-448.

34. Frauscher B, Egg R, Brandauer E, Ulmer H, Berger T, et al. Daytime sleepiness is not increased in mild to moderate multiple sclerosis: A pupillographic study. *Sleep Med*. 2005;6(6):543-547.

35. Kanbayashi T, Shimohata T, Nakashima I, Yaguchi H, Yabe I, et al. Symptomatic narcolepsy in patients with neuromyelitis optica and multiple sclerosis: New neurochemical and immunological implications. *Arch Neurol*. 2009;66(12):1563-1566.

36. Auer RN, Rowlands CG, Perry SF, Remmers JE. Multiple sclerosis with medullary plaques and fatal sleep apnea (Ondine's curse). *Clin Neuropathol*. 1996;15(2):101-105.

37. Howard RS, Wiles CM, Hirsch NP, Loh L, Spencer GT, Newsom-Davis J. Respiratory involvement in multiple sclerosis. *Brain*. 1992;115(Pt 2):479-494.

38. Ferini-Strambi L, Filippi M, Martinelli V, Oldani A, Rovaris M, et al. Nocturnal sleep study in multiple sclerosis: Correlations with clinical and brain magnetic resonance imaging findings. *J Neurol Sci*. 1994;125(2):194-197.

39. Manconi M, Ferini-Strambi L, Filippi M, Bonanni E, Iudice A, et al. Multicenter case-control study on restless legs syndrome in multiple sclerosis: The REMS study. *Sleep*. 2008;31(7):944-952.

40. Manconi M, Fabbrini M, Bonanni E, Filippi M, Rocca M, et al. High prevalence of restless legs syndrome in multiple sclerosis. *Eur J Neurol*. 2007;14(5):534-539.

41. Moreira NC, Damasceno RS, Medeiros CA, Bruin PF, Teixeira CA, et al. Restless leg syndrome, sleep quality and fatigue in multiple sclerosis patients. *Braz J Med Biol Res*. 2008;41(10):932-937.

42. Buysse DJ, Reynolds III CF, Monk TH, Berman SR, Kupfer DJ. The Pittsburgh Sleep Quality Index: A new instrument for psychiatric practice and research. *Psychiatry Res*. 1989;28(2):193-213.

43. De Mello MT, Esteves AM, Tufik S. Comparison between dopaminergic agents and physical exercise as treatment for periodic limb movements in patients with spinal cord injury. *Spinal Cord*. 2004;42(4):218-221.

44. Kovacevic-Ristanovic R, Cartwright RD, Lloyd S. Nonpharmacologic treatment of periodic leg movements in sleep. *Arch Phys Med Rehab*. 1991;72(6):385-389.

45. Sandyk R, Awerbuch GI. Relationship of nocturnal melatonin levels to duration and course of multiple sclerosis. *Int J Neurosci*. 1994;75(3-4):229-237.

46. Sandyk R, Awerbuch GI. Pineal calcification and its relationship to the fatigue of multiple sclerosis. *Int J Neurosci*. 1994;74(1-4):95-103.

47. Berg O, Hanley J. Narcolepsy in two cases of multiple sclerosis. *Acta Neurol Scand*. 1963;39:252-256.

48. Schrader H, Gotlibsen OB, Skomedal GN. Multiple sclerosis and narcolepsy/cataplexy in a monozygotic twin. *Neurology*. 1980;30(1):105-108.

49. Poirier G, Montplaisir J, Dumont M, Duquette P, Decary F, et al. Clinical and sleep laboratory study of narcoleptic symptoms in multiple sclerosis. *Neurology*. 1987;37(4):693-695.

50. Rumbach L, Tongio MM, Warter JM, Collard M, Kurtz D. Multiple sclerosis, sleep latencies and HLA antigens. *J Neurol*. 1989;236(5):309-310.

51. Kato T, Kanbayashi T, Yamamoto K, Nakano T, Shimizu T, et al. Hypersomnia and low CSF hypocretin-1 (orexin-A) concentration in a patient with multiple sclerosis showing bilateral hypothalamic lesions. *Intern Med*. 2003;42(8):743-745.

52. Oka Y, Kanbayashi T, Mezaki T, Iseki K, Matsubayashi J, et al. Low CSF hypocretin-1/orexin-A associated with hypersomnia secondary to hypothalamic lesion in a case of multiple sclerosis. *J Neurol*. 2004;251(7):885-886.

53. Vetrugno R, Stecchi S, Plazzi G, Lodi R, D'Angelo R, et al. Narcolepsy-like syndrome in multiple sclerosis. *Sleep Med*. 2009;10(3):389-391.

54. Nishino S, Kanbayashi T. Symptomatic narcolepsy, cataplexy and hypersomnia, and their implications in the hypothalamic hypocretin/orexin system. *Sleep Med Rev*. 2005;9(4):269-310.

55. Tippmann-Peikert M, Boeve BF, Keegan BM. REM sleep behavior disorder initiated by acute brainstem multiple sclerosis. *Neurology*. 2006;66(8):1277-1279.

56. Plazzi G, Montagna P. Remitting REM sleep behavior disorder as the initial sign of multiple sclerosis. *Sleep Med*. 2002;3(5):437-439.

57. Gomez-Choco MJ, Iranzo A, Blanco Y, Graus F, Santamaria J, Saiz A. Prevalence of restless legs syndrome and REM sleep behavior disorder in multiple sclerosis. *Mult Scler*. 2007;13(6):805-808.

58. Mahowald M, Schenck C. Principles and practice of sleep medicine. In: Kryger MH, Roth T, Dement WC, eds. *Principles and Practice of Sleep Medicine*. 5th ed. Philadelphia: Saunders/Elsevier; 2011:1085.

59. Ferini-Strambi L. Sleep disorders in multiple sclerosis. *Handb Clin Neurol*. 2011;99:1139-1146.

60. Brass SD, Duquette P, Proulx-Therrien J, Auerbach S. Sleep disorders in patients with multiple sclerosis. *Sleep Med Rev*. 2010;14(2):121-129.

61. Iseki K, Mezaki T, Oka Y, Terada K, Tomimoto H, et al. Hypersomnia in MS. *Neurology*. 2002;59(12):2006-2007.

62. Culebras A. Other neurological disorders. In: Kryger MH, Roth T, Dement WC, eds. *Principles and Practice of Sleep Medicine*. 4th ed. Philadelphia: WB Saunders; 2005:883.

63. Markowitz CE. Interferon-beta: Mechanism of action and dosing issues. *Neurology*. 2007;68:S8-S11.

64. Schweitzer PK. Drugs that disturb sleep. In: Kryger MH, Roth T, Dement WC, eds. *Principles and Practice of Sleep Medicine*. 4th ed. Philadelphia: WB Saunders; 2005:509-511. Also available at www.sleepmedtext.com.

65. Sioka JS. The mechanism of action of methylprednisolone in the treatment of multiple sclerosis. *Mult Scler*. 2005;11(4):425-432.

66. Mitler MM, O'Malley MB. Wake-promoting medications: Efficacy and adverse effects. In: Kryger MH, Roth T, Dement WC, eds. *Principles and Practice of Sleep Medicine*. 4th ed. Philadelphia: WB Saunders; 2005:488-489. Available at www.sleepmedtext.com.

67. Nishino S, Mignot E. Wake-promoting medications: Basic mechanisms and pharmacology. In: Kryger MH, Roth T, Dement WC, eds. *Principles and Practice of Sleep Medicine*. 4th ed. Philadelphia: WB Saunders; 2005:468-476. Available at www.sleepmedtext.com.

68. Korenke AR. Sustained-release fampridine for symptomatic treatment of multiple sclerosis. *Ann Pharmacother*. 2008;42(10):1458-1465.

69. Mignot E. Narcolepsy: Pharmacology, pathophysiology, and genetics. In: Kryger MH, Roth T, Dement WC, eds. *Principles and Practice of Sleep Medicine*. 4th ed. Philadelphia: WB Saunders; 2005:763-765. Available at www.sleepmedtext.com.

70. Finnimore AJ, Roebuck M, Sajkov D, McEvoy RD. The effects of the GABA agonist, baclofen, on sleep and breathing. *Eur Respir J*. 1995;8:230-234.

71. Mendelson WB. Hypnotic medications: Mechanisms of action and pharmacology effects. In: Kryger MH, Roth T, Dement WC, eds. *Principles and Practice of Sleep Medicine*. 4th ed. Philadelphia: WB Saunders; 2005:449-451. Available at www.sleepmedtext.com.

72. Tanaka H, Fukuda I, Miyamoto A, Oka R, Cho K, Fujieda K. Effects of tizanidine for refractory sleep disturbance in disabled children with spastic quadriplegia. *No To Hattatsu*. 2004;36(6):455-460.

73. Schweitzer PK. Drugs that disturb sleep. In: Kryger MH, Roth T, Dement WC, eds. *Principles and Practice of Sleep Medicine*. 4th ed. Philadelphia: WB Saunders; 2005:499-504. Available at www.sleepmedtext.com.

74. Buysse DJ, Schweitzer PK, Moul DE. Clinical pharmacology of other drugs used as hypnotics. In: Kryger MH, Roth T, Dement WC, eds. *Principles and Practice of Sleep Medicine*. 4th ed. Philadelphia: WB Saunders; 2005:459-464. Available at www.sleepmedtext.com.

75. Diefenbach K, Donath F, Maurer A, et al. Randomised, double blind study of the effects of oxybutynin, toiterodine, trospium chloride and placebo on sleep in healthy young volunteers. *Clin Drug Invest*. 2003;23(6):395-404.

Therapy of Sleep Disturbances Associated with Psychiatric Disorders

Sleep in Mood Disorders

ANDREW D. KRYSTAL

Sleep and mood disorders are related in important and complex ways. Mood disorders are, in fact, so strongly associated with changes in sleep that alterations in sleep are among the defining features of these conditions. As such, it is not surprising that sleep problems are highly prevalent among individuals with mood disorders. For many years the predominant view was that these sleep problems were symptoms of the associated mood disorders; however, research studies that speak to this question suggest otherwise. These studies suggest that the relationship between sleep and mood disorders is complex and bidirectional. There is evidence that sleep problems, rather than being simply symptoms of mood disorders, may be predictors for the subsequent onset of mood disorders and may have important effects on their course and treatment response. Contrary to the symptom model, wherein sleep-specific therapy is superfluous to mood disorder therapy and not indicated, there is reason to believe that sleep disorders occurring in those with mood disorders merit specific therapeutic attention.

The relationship of sleep and mood disorders becomes further complicated when attributes of the treatments for mood disorders are considered. Most treatments for mood disorders have effects on sleep. Some are therapeutic, some problematic, and some of uncertain significance. Further, depriving patients with mood disorders of sleep in research settings may be therapeutic for major depression, but may trigger or exacerbate mania.[1]

This chapter reviews the data relevant to sleep in patients with mood disorders and discusses how the data suggest that the relationship of sleep and mood disorders is complex, bidirectional, and of clinical importance. The mood disorders comprise a number of conditions, which include a set of depressive disorders and a set of bipolar spectrum disorders.[2] This chapter addresses the prototypical conditions for each of these disorder subtypes: major depressive disorder (MDD) and bipolar I disorder (BPD). These conditions are of particular interest because both include a disturbance of sleep among their core features and, among the various mood disorders, they have been the subject of the most sleep-related research by far. Through reviewing the data on sleep in MDD and BPD and considering the implications for both research and clinical practice this chapter makes the case that in order to understand mood disorders and to optimally treat patients with mood disorders it is necessary to take sleep into account.

MAJOR DEPRESSIVE DISORDER

MDD is a common condition that occurs roughly twice as frequently in women than men. It is estimated that the lifetime prevalence in women is 10% to 25% compared with

5% to 12% in men.[2] The onset of MDD occurs on average around 25 years of age, but individuals may experience their first episode of depression at any age. The course of MDD varies considerably among affected individuals. Some experience a single episode, whereas in others, it is a highly recurrent condition. The diagnostic criteria for MDD are listed in Box 54-1.[2]

Given that sleep difficulty (either insomnia or hypersomnia) is among the diagnostic criteria for MDD, it is not surprising that sleep problems are nearly universal in MDD patients, reportedly occurring in up to 90%.[3] The particular type of sleep disturbance varies among those with MDD, who may report difficulty with sleep onset, problems staying asleep, waking too early in the morning without being able to return to sleep, diminished sleep quality, nightmares, and excessive daytime sleepiness.

MDD has also been associated with a particular set of alterations in sleep that are evident in the polysomnogram (PSG) (Table 54-1). PSG evidence of sleep disturbance includes prolonged sleep onset latency, increased wake time after sleep onset, decreased sleep efficiency (sleep time divided by time in bed), and increased number of awakenings throughout the night and in the early morning.[4-7] Studies of PSG data have also observed alterations in the timing, characteristics, and amount of sleep stages in MDD patients compared with normal control subjects. These alterations include a shortening of the time until the onset of the first period of rapid eye movement (REM) sleep (REM latency),[5,8-15] an increase in the number of eye movements occurring per minute during REM sleep (REM density),[6,16-18] an increase in the percentage of sleep composed of REM sleep,[6,7,12] a longer lasting first REM period of the night,[7,19,20] and a decrease in the relative amount of slow wave sleep.[5-7,19]

The significance of these alterations in the sleep stage data has been the subject of considerable debate. In terms of their implications for understanding the pathophysiology of MDD, the question has been raised about whether these sleep stage alterations are trait markers (identifiers of those individuals predisposed to the development of MDD who are not experiencing a current MDD episode) or state markers (indicators of changes in the brain occurring in association with an episode of MDD). Some polysomnographic characteristics of MDD patients are more evident during acute episodes of depression, including REM density and decreased sleep efficiency, suggesting that they might be state markers, at least to a degree.[21-23] Other PSG features of MDD, such as shortened REM latency and decreased amount of slow wave sleep, appear to be more akin to trait markers because they are present in those predisposed to developing depression even when they are not having episodes.[23-27] Shortened REM latency and reduced slow-wave

BOX 54-1 *Diagnostic Criteria for Major Depressive Episode*

- Five of the following nine symptoms must be present over a period of at least 2 weeks.
- One of the five symptoms has to be either depressed mood or loss of interest or pleasure.
  1. Depressed mood, present most of the day, every day, as noted by subjective report or objectively
  2. Loss of interest or pleasure in all or almost all activities, most of the day, nearly every day
  3. Significant change in appetite nearly every day or significant change in weight (5% of body weight over a 1-month period)
  4. Insomnia or hypersomnia nearly every day
  5. Observable psychomotor agitation or retardation present nearly every day
  6. Fatigue or lack of energy nearly every day
  7. Feelings of worthlessness or excessive guilt nearly every day
  8. Indecisiveness, diminished ability to concentrate, nearly every day
  9. Recurrent thoughts of death (not just fear of dying), recurrent suicidal ideation with or without intent or plan

TABLE 54-1

Polysomnographic Alterations in Major Depressive Disorder

Variable	Change
Sleep onset latency	↑
Wake after sleep onset	↑
Sleep efficiency	↓
Number of awakenings	↑
REM latency	↓
REM density	↑
Proportion of REM sleep	↑
Duration of the first REM period	↑
Proportion of slow wave sleep	↓

↑, increase; ↓, decrease; *REM*, rapid eye movement.

sleep are also present in the first-degree relatives of those with MDD. These abnormalities may therefore represent biomarkers of a familial predisposition to MDD.[24,28]

A factor limiting the value of these PSG features of MDD for understanding the pathophysiology of this condition and limiting their clinical utility is the finding that these changes in sleep are not specific to those with MDD.[10] These markers reliably distinguish those with MDD from healthy control subjects but may also occur in those with other psychiatric disorders.[10] In this regard, in a large meta-analysis comparing PSG data across different groups of patients with psychiatric disorders, all of the patient groups studied had more sleep abnormalities than healthy control subjects, though it should be noted that the most severe disturbance was seen in those with MDD.[10] Diminished slow wave sleep and shortened REM latency were not found to distinguish MDD patients from other groups of psychiatric patients.[10] Indeed, shortened REM latency compared with healthy control subjects has been reported for patients with alcoholism,[29] post-traumatic stress disorder,[30,31] schizophrenia,[32,33] panic disorder,[34,35] and eating disorders.[36,37] Some have speculated that this finding reflects a high rate of co-morbid depression in these conditions; however, some studies have controlled for the degree of co-morbid depression and still noted shorter REM latency in those with psychiatric disorders compared with healthy control subjects.[38] Of the characteristic polysomnographic findings in MDD, increased REM density and total amount of REM sleep, so far, appear to be the most specific for those with MDD.[10] Nevertheless, the relationship between these PSG characteristics and the predisposition to developing depression, and the neurophysiologic mechanisms that occur acutely during episodes of depression that underlie these changes, remain largely unknown. In addition, the clinical utility of these markers remains limited.

Although disturbances of sleep may not be specific to MDD, there is increasing evidence that sleep disturbance may have important effects on the course of MDD and response to treatment. This view runs contrary to what has long been the prevailing opinion regarding the relationship of sleep disturbance and MDD. Insomnia has generally been considered to be a "symptom" of MDD that did not have independent importance and, like the other symptoms of MDD, was expected to resolve with antidepressant therapy.[39] As such, targeting treatment specifically to insomnia when it occurred with MDD was viewed as superfluous.[39] However, the available evidence suggests that this symptom model of the relationship of insomnia to MDD is incorrect.

Contrary to the traditional view, there is evidence that insomnia is a risk factor for the development of future depression.[40-43] Further, disturbed sleep fails to resolve in 44% to 53% of these patients despite the administration of appropriate antidepressant therapy,[44-45] and this persistent disturbance of sleep is correlated with an increased risk of relapse of MDD, impairment in concentration, daytime sleepiness, and impairment in the ability to perform daily activities.[46-47] Although a causal link between insomnia and MDD has not been proved, there is a compelling body of literature demonstrating that disturbed sleep is correlated with either suicidal ideation or completed suicide.[48-61]

A number of studies also suggest that sleep disturbance affects the response to antidepressant treatment. MDD patients with a greater degree of sleep disturbance have a slower response to antidepressant therapy and a lower depression remission rate.[62-66] Further, several studies suggest that targeting treatment specifically to the sleep disturbance in those with MDD may result in a faster and more robust response to antidepressant therapy. In one study, patients with insomnia and depression received antidepressant treatment with either nortriptyline or maprotiline and in addition received insomnia-specific therapy with either the benzodiazepines lormetazepam or flunitrazepam, or with placebo.[66] Those subjects treated with lormetazepam improved in their depression severity to a greater degree than those subjects receiving placebo. In another study, in patients with MDD and co-morbid insomnia, all subjects received fluoxetine treatment for their MDD and in addition received either eszopiclone 3 mg or placebo.[67,68] Eszopiclone treatment of insomnia not only led to improvement in sleep compared with placebo but also was associated with a more rapid antidepressant response, a greater improvement in depression severity, and a greater percentage of depression responders and remitters. Similar findings emerged from a study where cognitive behavioral therapy for insomnia was compared with a control behavioral intervention as add-on therapy to escitalopram in depressed patients with insomnia.[69] The subjects receiving the cognitive behavioral therapy for insomnia had a 62% rate of depression remission compared with 33% among subjects receiving the control behavioral intervention. These studies suggest that improving sleep in those with depression and co-morbid insomnia may improve depression outcome. However, there is one study that suggests otherwise. In this study, zolpidem extended release was compared with placebo as adjunctive insomnia therapy given along with selective serotonin reuptake inhibitor antidepressant therapy and, although zolpidem extended release led to significant improvement in sleep and daytime function compared with placebo, no effect on the depression response was observed.[70] Further work will be needed to reconcile this observation with those of prior studies. It is possible that the other therapies evaluated have antidepressant effects themselves that were unrecognized, or that zolpidem extended release somehow prevents the improvement in depression that would otherwise accompany improvement in sleep in those with depression and co-morbid insomnia. Another unresolved issue is whether treating insomnia decreases the risk for suicide and for relapse. Nonetheless, all studies carried out to date suggest that targeting treatment specifically to insomnia that occurs with MDD improves outcome, at least in terms of sleep and possibly in terms of speed and degree of antidepressant response. On this basis, it is hard to avoid the conclusion that targeting treatment to insomnia in this setting should be the standard of care.

Another important sleep-related consideration in MDD that has implications for clinical practice and how we understand MDD are the sleep effects of antidepressant therapies. A number of antidepressants have sleep-enhancing effects, which may have a therapeutic impact on sleep disturbance but may lead to daytime sleepiness. Others increase the risks of experiencing disturbed sleep. Antidepressants that have been found to have a therapeutic effect on difficulties falling asleep or staying asleep in controlled trials in those with MDD, primary insomnia, or healthy control subjects include doxepin, mirtazapine, amitriptyline, and trimipramine.[71-79] Trazodone has also been found to have a therapeutic effect on sleep when administered as add-on therapy to ongoing antidepressant treatment.[80] (See Chapter 8, "Pharmacology of Psychotropic Drugs," for a detailed description of the effects of these agents and other antidepressants on sleep.) Based on these sleep effects these agents are often used "off-label" as insomnia therapies.[81] They are also the antidepressants most likely to be associated with daytime sedation. It is important to note that the studies in which therapeutic effects on sleep were observed with these agents generally employed dosages below those used to treat depression. There are, as of yet, no studies evaluating the effects of monotherapy with a sedating antidepressant in which a single agent was used to target insomnia as well as depression. However, we can infer that the agents that have been found to have therapeutic effects on sleep at low dosages are likely to do so at higher dosages as well, but this remains to be determined, and there is some reason to believe that for some agents, such as mirtazapine, higher dosages may actually be associated with less sleep-enhancing effects than lower dosages.[82]

The sleep-wake effects of the selective serotonin reuptake inhibitors (SSRIs) and serotonin-norepinephrine reuptake inhibitors (SNRIs) are more complex. Data on these effects largely derive from adverse effects rates in clinical trials in depressed patients: For SSRIs the rate of insomnia is 7% to 22% compared with 4% to 11% for placebo; at the same time, the rate of daytime somnolence with the SSRIs is 4% to 24% versus 4% to 11% for placebo.[83] For SNRIs the rate of insomnia is 4% to 23% versus 2% to 10% and the rate of daytime somnolence is 5% to 23% versus 3% to 10% for placebo.[83] Bupropion, on the other hand, does not appear to be associated with daytime somnolence to any significant degree but is associated with a rate of insomnia that is comparable to that of the SSRIs and SNRIs (insomnia rate of 5-20% vs. 2-8% for placebo).[83]

The reason for the relatively increased risk of both disturbed sleep and daytime sleepiness with SSRIs and SNRIs is unknown. One possibility is that the sleep-wake effects of these agents varies among individuals. Another possibility is that this may reflect the tendency of these medications to cause or exacerbate restless legs syndrome and periodic movements of sleep, which can be associated with either sleep disturbance, daytime sleepiness, or both.[84] Along with mirtazapine, the SSRIs and SNRIs appear to be the antidepressant medications most strongly associated with these sleep conditions.[84,85]

Antidepressant medications also have effects on sleep architecture, which may not be of clinical relevance but have been of interest with respect to the pathophysiology of major depression. Of these effects the one that has received the most attention is the suppression of REM sleep, which has been noted with a large number of antidepressant therapies including use of monoamine oxidase inhibitors, tricyclic antidepressants, electroconvulsive therapy, SSRIs, and SNRIs.[10,86-92] The REM suppression observed with antidepressant therapies has been interpreted as further evidence for the hypothesis that an increase in REM intensity underlies or is a central feature of MDD; this hypothesis is based on evidence for shortened REM latency and an increase in the percentage and density of REM sleep in MDD. It has further been hypothesized on this basis that suppression of REM sleep may be necessary if an antidepressant effect is to be achieved. This hypothesis, however, is contradicted by antidepressant agents that have demonstrated efficacy in the treatment of MDD in placebo-controlled trials but do not consistently suppress REM sleep, including bupropion, nefazodone, mirtazapine, and trazodone.[83] Thus, the suppression of REM sleep that occurs with the majority of antidepressants is currently of uncertain significance, as is the increase in the amount of slow wave sleep and increase in electroencephalographic (EEG) slow wave activity during non-REM (NREM) sleep which have been observed with nefazodone, trazodone, and mirtazapine.[79,93-96]

Among the more interesting observations related to sleep and MDD are the antidepressant effects of sleep deprivation. Studies of this phenomenon report that a single night of sleep deprivation is associated with a 50% or greater response rate.[97-99] Interestingly, however, the therapeutic effects are lost when sleep occurs following the period of sleep deprivation, even if the duration of that sleep is brief.[97,100] Attempts have been made to prolong the therapeutic effects of sleep deprivation by various means, including advancing the sleep phase, but none of these efforts have been successful.[101,102] As a result, sleep deprivation remains of high interest but limited clinical utility.

In summary, sleep and MDD are related in important and complex ways. The longstanding model in which sleep disturbance is a symptom of MDD without independent importance is contradicted by a growing body of research. This literature suggests that the relationship is complex and bidirectional and suggests that sleep disturbance may have important effects on the course and treatment response in MDD. How changes in sleep might play a mechanistic role in the development or perpetuation or recurrence of MDD remains unknown, as is the mechanism by which sleep disturbance might increase suicidality and impede the antidepressant response. Further studies will be needed in order to shed light on these issues. Additional treatment studies are needed to resolve whether improvement in sleep may speed and enhance the antidepressant response, and studies are needed to determine if effectively addressing sleep problems decreases the rate of relapse. Yet, the available literature is clear that optimal clinical management of MDD should include an assessment for sleep problems and the implementation of effective therapy for disturbed sleep if found in patients with depression.

BIPOLAR I DISORDER

BPD, with a prevalence of 0.4% to 1.6%, is significantly less prevalent than MDD and, unlike MDD, is equally likely in both genders.[2] BPD, however, tends to be a more recurrent disorder than MDD, with affected individuals experiencing a higher number of lifetime episodes. The diagnostic criteria for BPD are summarized in Box 54-2.[2]

Among the criteria for mania is a "decreased need for sleep," which although easily confused with insomnia is altogether a different phenomenon.[103] It differs from insomnia in terms of the associated impairment. Although manic patients and those with insomnia may be unable to sleep when given the opportunity to do so, insomnia patients would be expected to

experience impairment in function or quality of life as a result, whereas manic patients would not, as their difficulty sleeping may not cause them to sleep less than needed.[2]

In light of the antidepressant effects of sleep deprivation, the fact that a decrease in the amount of sleep occurs with mania has been interpreted as evidence that loss of sleep might play a role in the development of mania. According to this hypothesis, sleep loss and mania are mutually reinforcing such that decreased sleep predisposes toward the development of mania, which further decreases sleep, thereby further promoting the development of mania, and so on.[103] There is relatively little experimental support for this hypothesis other than several studies suggesting that sleep deprivation tends to trigger mania in those with BPD.[103-105] The mechanisms by which this might occur have not been determined; however, this model has been accepted by many practitioners as a basis for the need to administer treatments that increase sleep time when treating manic patients even though no studies have been carried out that demonstrate the antimanic utility of sedation. Yet, the primary treatments for mania—lithium, valproic acid, and carbamazepine—are generally believed to have significant sleep-enhancing effects; however, few studies of their sleep effects have been carried out. In addition, a number of antipsychotic agents are used to treat mania and there is reason to believe that many of these agents can increase sleep time, though this has not been systematically studied in manic patients.[106]

In contrast to mania, the depressed phase of BPD is reportedly often associated with hypersomnia; at least hypersomnia occurs more commonly than in those with unipolar depression.[107] Notably, objective testing of BPD patients with depression using the multiple sleep latency test have not identified objective evidence of daytime sleepiness in this population.[107] Whether the experience of hypersomnolence has therapeutic implications for those with bipolar depression has yet to be determined.

Though less well investigated in BPD patients than in MDD patients, some studies have evaluated the PSG sleep architectural profile of manic patients. The findings indicate that manic patients have shortened REM latency, much as is seen in those with MDD.[108,109] In terms of the effects of antimanic treatments on REM sleep, one study that was carried out with lithium identified that this medication suppressed REM sleep and increased the amount of slow wave sleep.[110] Studies with the antipsychotic agents often used to treat mania suggest that REM suppression occurs with risperidone, ziprasidone, and quetiapine.[106] Thus, the extent to which suppression of REM sleep might be important for antimanic therapies remains undetermined. Given the lack of specificity of this finding, in that it occurs in those who do not have mood disorders, it seems unlikely that suppression of REM sleep is necessary for the treatment of mania.[10]

In summary, alterations in sleep are characteristic of both mania and depression in BPD patients. In mania, there appears to be a decreased need for sleep, whereas those with depression experience hypersomnia. It has been hypothesized but not established that decreased sleep might play a role in the evolution of mania and, although it is standard practice to administer sleep-enhancing agents to treat mania, studies demonstrating a link between enhancement of sleep and a therapeutic antimanic effect are lacking. A small amount of research has been carried out on sleep architecture in mania

---

BOX 54-2 *Bipolar Disorder*

- A *bipolar I disorder* is diagnosed when the patient has experienced at least one manic episode, with or without previous history of depressive episodes. A *manic episode* is a period of abnormally and persistently elevated, expansive, or irritable mood, lasting at least 1 week or of any duration if hospitalization is necessary.
- During the period of mood disturbance, three (or more) of the following symptoms are present to a significant degree (four symptoms if the mood is irritable):
  1. Grandiosity or inflated self-esteem
  2. Decreased need for sleep
  3. Pressure to keep talking or being more talkative than usual
  4. Flight of ideas or a subjective feeling that thoughts are racing
  5. Distractibility (attention too easily drawn to irrelevant or unimportant external stimuli)
  6. Psychomotor agitation or an increase in goal-directed activity (work, social, or sexual)
  7. Impulsivity with increased involvement in high-risk, high-reward activities with potential for painful consequences (e.g., expensive shopping sprees or sexual indiscretions)

and on the sleep architectural effects of antimanic therapies, but this work has not appeared to influence how we understand mania or its treatment. Finally, the sleep of BPD patients in the depressed phase has been relatively less characterized, and it has not been determined whether there are treatment or pathophysiologic implications to the apparent increase in the experience of hypersomnolence in this group.

CONCLUSION

Important relationships exist between sleep and mood disorders. This chapter focused on two mood disorders, MDD and BPD, which are prototypical for the major classes of mood disorders. The relationships with sleep have been much better characterized for MDD than for BPD. For MDD a growing literature suggests that these relationships are complex, bidirectional, and have clear treatment implications: there is a need to identify and treat sleep disturbance in those with MDD. For those with BPD, sleep appears to play an important role and the loss of sleep is often addressed by practitioners, but the research base related to this issue is more limited. However, the literature that does exist suggests that, like with MDD, alterations in sleep appear to have a major impact on the course of those with MDD and are likely to be important treatment considerations.

Sleep architectural changes for understanding pathophysiology and for treatment remains unresolved. For example, this is one of a number of unresolved issues related to the relationships of sleep and mood disorders. For example, although there are data suggesting that the treatment of insomnia enhances the antidepressant response in those with insomnia co-morbid with depression, further work is needed to confirm this understanding. Another example is that data suggest that residual insomnia following antidepressant therapy increases the risk of relapse; however, it remains unknown if treating this residual insomnia decreases the relapse risk. Similarly, insomnia is correlated with increased suicidality among MDD patients, but it remains unknown whether treating sleep disturbance decreases the risk of suicidality. Carrying out the work needed to address these issues promises to improve our understanding of mood disorders and the mechanisms by which they are affected by sleep and also has the potential to improve the treatment of the many individuals who suffer with mood disorders.

REFERENCES

1. Giedke H, Schwarzler F. Therapeutic use of sleep deprivation in depression. *Sleep Med Rev.* 2002;6:361-377.
2. American Psychiatric Association. *Diagnostic and Statistical Manual of Mental Disorders.* 4th ed. Washington, DC: American Psychiatric Association; 2000.
3. Thase ME. Antidepressant treatment of the depressed patient with insomnia. *J Clin Psychiatry.* 1999;60(suppl 17):28-31.
4. Gillin JC, Duncan WC, Pettigrew KD, et al. Successful separation of depressed, normal and insomniac subjects by EEG sleep data. *Arch Gen Psychiatry.* 1979;36:85-90.
5. Kupfer DJ, Ulrich RF, Coble PA, et al. Electroencephalographic sleep of younger depressives. *Arch Gen Psychiatry.* 1985;42:806-810.
6. Waller DA, Hardy BW, Pole R, et al. Sleep EEG in bulimic, depressed and normal subjects. *Biol Psychiatry.* 1989;25:661-664.
7. Berger M, Doerr P, Lund RD, et al. Neuroendocrinological and neurophysiological studies in major depressive disorders: Are there biological markers for the endogenous subtype? *Biol Psychiatry.* 1982;17:1217-1242.
8. Kupfer DJ, Foster FG. Interval between onset of sleep and rapid-eye-movement sleep as an indicator of depression. *Lancet.* 1972;2:684-686.
9. Kupfer DJ, Reynolds III CF, Ehlers CL. Comparison of EEG sleep measures among depressive subtypes and controls in older individuals. *Psychiatry Res.* 1989;27:13-21.
10. Benca RM, Obermeyer WH, Thisted RA, et al. Sleep and psychiatric disorders: A meta-analysis. *Arch Gen Psychiatry.* 1992;49:651-668.
11. Akiskal HS, Lemmi H, Yerevanian B, King D, Belluomini J. The utility of the REM latency test in psychiatric diagnosis: A study of 81 depressed outpatients. *Psychiatry Res.* 1982;7(1):101-110.
12. Emslie GJ, Rush AJ, Weinberg WA, et al. Children with major depression show reduced rapid eye movement latencies. *Arch Gen Psychiatry.* 1990;47:119-124.
13. Gillin JC, Duncan W, Pettigrew KD, Frankel BL, Snyder F. Successful separation of depressed, normal, and insomniac subjects by EEG sleep data. *Arch Gen Psychiatry.* 1979;36(1):85-90.
14. Hartmann E, Verdone P, Snyder F. Longitudinal studies of sleep and dreaming patterns in psychiatric patients. *J Nerv Ment Disord.* 1966;142:117-126.
15. Mendels J, Hawkins DR. Sleep and depression: A controlled EEG study. *Arch Gen Psychiatry.* 1967;16:344-354.
16. Kupfer DJ, Targ E, Stack J. Electroencephalographic sleep in unipolar depressive subtypes: Support for a biological and familial classification. *J Nerv Ment Disord.* 1982;170(8):494-498.
17. Jones DA, Kelwala S, Bell J, et al. Cholinergic REM sleep induction response correlation with endogenous depressive subtype. *Psychiatry Res.* 1985;14:99-110.
18. Foster FG, Kupfer DJ, Coble PA, et al. Rapid eye movement sleep density. An objective indicator in severe medial-depressive syndromes. *Arch Gen Psychiatry.* 1976;33:1119-1123.
19. Borbely AA, Tobler I, Loepfe M, et al. All night spectral analysis of the sleep EEG in untreated depressives and normal controls. *Psychiatry Res.* 1984;12:27-33.
20. Feinberg M, Gillin JC, Carroll BJ, et al. EEG studies of sleep in the diagnosis of depression. *Biol Psychiatry.* 1982;17:305-316.
21. Kerkhofs M, Hoffman G, De Martelaere V, et al. Sleep EEG recordings in depressive disorders. *J Affect Disord.* 1985;9:47-53.
22. Schulz H, Lund RD, Cording C, et al. Bimodal distribution of REM sleep latencies in depression. *Biol Psychiatry.* 1979;14:595-600.
23. Thase ME, Fasiczka AL, Berman SR, et al. Electroencephalographic sleep profiles before and after cognitive behavioral therapy of depression. *Arch Gen Psychiatry.* 1998;55:138-144.
24. Giles DE, Etzel BA, Reynolds III CF, et al. Stability of polysomnographic parameters in unipolar depression: A cross-sectional report. *Biol Psychiatry.* 1989;25:807-810.
25. Hauri PJ, Chernic D, Hawkins DR, et al. Sleep of depressed patients in remission. *Arch Gen Psychiatry.* 1974;31:386-391.
26. Rush AJ, Erman MK, Giles DE, et al. Polysomnographic findings in recently drug-free and clinically remitted depressed patients. *Arch Gen Psychiatry.* 1986;43:878-884.
27. Lee JH, Reynolds III CF, Hoch CC, et al. Electroencephalographic sleep in recently remitted, elderly depressed patients in double-blind placebo maintenance therapy. *Neuropsychopharmacology.* 1993;8:143-150.
28. Giles DE, Kupfer DJ, Rush AJ, et al. Controlled comparison of electroencephalographic sleep in families of probands with unipolar depression. *Am J Psychiatry.* 1998;155:192-199.
29. Gillin JC, Smith TL, Irwin M, Kripke DF, Brown S, Schuckit M. Short REM latency in primary alcoholic patients with secondary depression. *Am J Psychiatry.* 1990;147(1):106-109.
30. Kauffman CD, Reist C, Djenderedjian A, et al. Biological markers of affective disorders and post-traumatic stress disorder: A pilot study with desipramine. *J Clin Psychiatry.* 1987;48:366-367.
31. Greenberg R, Pearlman CA, Gampel D. War neuroses and the adaptive function of REM sleep. *Br J Med Psychol.* 1972;45:27-33.
32. Hiatt JF, Floyd TC, Katz PH, et al. Further evidence of abnormal non-rapid-eye-movement sleep in schizophrenia. *Arch Gen Psychiatry.* 1985;42:797-802.
33. Zarcone VP, Benson KL, Berger PA. Abnormal rapid eye movement latencies in schizophrenia. *Arch Gen Psychiatry.* 1987;44:45-48.
34. Lauer CJ, Garcia D, Pollmacher T, et al. All-night EEG sleep in anxiety disorders and major depression. In: Horne J, ed. *Sleep '90; Bochum.* Germany: Pontenagel Press; 1991.
35. Uhde TW, Roy-Byrne P, Gillin JC, et al. The sleep of patients with panic disorder: A preliminary report. *Psychiatry Res.* 1985;12:251-259.
36. Katz JL, Kuperberg A, Pollack CP, et al. Is there a relationship between eating disorder and affective disorder? New evidence from sleep recordings. *Am J Psychiatry.* 1984;141:753-759.

37. Neil JF, Merikangas JR, Foster FG, et al. Waking and all-night sleep EEGs in anorexia nervosa. *Clin Electroencephalogr.* 1980;11:9-15.

38. Zarcone VP, Benson KL. BPRS symptom factors and sleep variables in schizophrenia. *Psychiatry Res.* 1997;66:111-120.

39. NIH Consensus Conference. Drugs and insomnia. The use of medications to promote sleep. *JAMA.* 1984;11(251):2410-2414.

40. Breslau N, Roth T, Rosenthal L, et al. Sleep disturbance and psychiatric disorders: A longitudinal epidemiologic study of young adults. *Biol Psychiatry.* 1996;39:411-418.

41. Chang PP, Ford DE, Mead LA, et al. Insomnia in young men and subsequent depression. *Am J Epidemiol.* 1997;146:105-114.

42. Ford DE, Kamerow DB. Epidemiologic study of sleep disturbance and psychiatric disorders: An opportunity for prevention? *JAMA.* 1989;262:1479-1484.

43. Livingston G, Blizard B, Mann A. Does sleep disturbance predict depression in elderly people? A study in inner London. *Br J Gen Pract.* 1993;43:445-448.

44. Carney CE, Segal ZV, Edinger JD, Krystal AD. A comparison of rates of residual insomnia symptoms following pharmacotherapy or cognitive-behavioral therapy for major depressive disorder. *J Clin Psychiatry.* 2007;68(2):254-260.

45. Nierenberg AA, Keefe BR, Leslie VC, et al. Residual symptoms in depressed patients who respond acutely to fluoxetine. *J Clin Psychiatry.* 1999;60:221-225.

46. Asnis GM, Chakrabartty A, DuBoff EA, et al. Zolpidem for persistent insomnia in SSRI-treated depressed patients. *J Clin Psychiatry.* 1999;60:668-676.

47. Reynolds III CF, Frank E, Houck PR, et al. Which elderly patients with remitted depression remain well with continued interpersonal psychotherapy after discontinuation of antidepressant medication? *Am J Psychiatry.* 1997;154:958-962.

48. Choquet M, Menke H. Suicidal thoughts during early adolescence: Prevalence, associated troubles and help-seeking behavior. *Acta Psychiatr Scand.* 1989;81:170-177.

49. Choquet M, Kovess V. Suicidal thoughts among adolescents: An intercultural approach. *Adolescence.* 1993;28(111):649-661.

50. Agargun MY, Kara H, Solmaz M. Sleep disturbances and suicidal behavior in patients with major depression. *J Clin Psychiatry.* 1997;58:249-251.

51. Agargun MY, Kara H, Solmaz M. Subjective sleep quality and suicidality in patients with major depression. *J Psychiatr Res.* 1997;31(3):377-381.

52. Agargun MY, Cilli A, Kara H, Tarhan N, Kincir F, Oz H. Repetitive and frightening dreams and suicidal behavior in patients with major depression. *Compr Psychiatry.* 1998;39(4):198-202.

53. Agargun MY, Besiroglu L, Cilli A, et al. Nightmares, suicide attempts, and melancholic features in patients with unipolar major depression. *J Affect Disord.* 2007;98:267-270.

54. Chellappa S, Araujo JF. Sleep disorders and suicidal ideation in patients with depressive disorder. *Psychiatry Res.* 2007;153:131-136.

55. Bernert R, Joiner T, Cukrowicz K, Schmidt N, Krakow B. Suicidality and sleep disturbances. *Sleep.* 2005;28(9):1135-1141.

56. Fawcett J, Scheftner WA, Fogg L, et al. Time-related predictors of suicide in major affective disorder. *Am J Psychiatry.* 1990;147:1189-1194.

57. Smith M, Perlis M, Haythornthwaite J. Suicidal ideation in outpatients with chronic musculoskeletal pain. *Clin J Pain.* 2004;20(2):111-118.

58. Roberts R, Roberts C, Chen I. Functioning of adolescents with symptoms of disturbed sleep. *J Youth Adolesc.* 2001;30(1):1-18.

59. Tanskanen A, Tuomilehto J, Vinamaki H, Vartiainene E, Lehtonen J, Puska P. Nightmares are predictors of suicide. *Sleep.* 2001;24(7):844-847.

60. Turvey CL, Conwell Y, Jones MP, et al. Risk factors for late-life suicide: A prospective, community-based study. *Am J Geriatr Psychiatry.* 2002;10:398-406.

61. Vignau J, Bailly D, Duhamel A, Vervaecke P, Beuscart R, Collinet C. Epidemiologic study of sleep quality and troubles in French secondary school adolescents. *J Adolesc Health.* 1997;21:343-350.

62. Winokur A, Reynolds CF. The effects of antidepressants and anxiolitics on sleep physiology. *Prim Psychiatry.* 1994;1:22-27.

63. Buysse D, Reynolds CF, Houck PR, et al. Does lorazepam impair the antidepressant response to nortriptyline and psychotherapy? *J Clin Psych.* 1997;58(10):426-432.

64. Dew M, Reynolds CF, Houck PR, et al. Temporal profiles of the course of depression during treatment. Predictors of pathways toward recovery in the elderly. *Arch Gen Psychiatry.* 1997;54(11):1016-1024.

65. Thase M, Buysse DJ, Frank E, et al. Which depressed patients will respond to interpersonal psychotherapy? The role of abnormal EEG sleep profiles. *Am J Psychiatry.* 1997;154(4):502-509.

66. Nolen WA, Haffmans PM, Bouvy PF, et al. Hypnotics as concurrent medication in depression. A placebo-controlled, double-blind comparison of flunitrazepam and lormetazepam in patients with major depression, treated with a (tri)cyclic antidepressant. *J Affect Disord.* 1993;28:179-188.

67. Fava M, McCall WV, Krystal A, Wessel T, Rubens R, et al. Eszopiclone co-administered with fluoxetine in patients with insomnia coexisting with major depressive disorder. *Biol Psychiatry.* 2006;59(11):1052-1060.

68. Krystal A, Fava M, Rubens R, Wessel T, Caron J, et al. Evaluation of eszopiclone discontinuation after cotherapy with fluoxetine for insomnia with coexisting depression. *J Clin Sleep Med.* 2007;3(1):48-55.

69. Manber R, Edinger JD, Gress JL, San Pedro-Salcedo MG, Kuo TF, Kalista T. Cognitive behavioral therapy for insomnia enhances depression outcome in patients with comorbid major depressive disorder and insomnia. *Sleep.* 2008;31(4):489-495.

70. Fava M, Asnis G, Shrivastava R, Lydiard RB, Bastani B, et al. Improved insomnia symptoms and daily functioning in patients with comorbid major depressive disorder and insomnia following zolpidem extended-release 12.5 mg and escitalopram co-treatment. *Sleep.* 2008;31:A324.

71. Krystal AD, Durrence H, Scharf M, Jochelson P, Rogowski R, et al. Long-term efficacy and safety of doxepin 1 mg and 3 mg in a 12-week sleep laboratory and outpatient trial of elderly subjects with chronic primary insomnia. *Sleep.* 2010;33(11):1553-1561.

72. Roth T, Rogowski R, Hull S, et al. Efficacy and safety of doxepin 1, 3 and 6 mg in adults with primary insomnia. *Sleep.* 2007;30:1555-1561.

73. Roth T, Zorick F, Wittig R, McLenaghan A, Roehrs T. The effects of doxepin HCl on sleep and depression. *J Clin Psychiatry.* 1982;43:366-368.

74. Ruigt GS, Kemp B, Groenhout CM, Kamphuisen HA. Effect of the antidepressant Org 3770 on human sleep. *Eur J Clin Pharmacol.* 1990;38:551-554.

75. Feuillade P, Pringuey D, Belugou JL, Robert P, Darcourt G. Trimipramine: Acute and lasting effects on sleep in healthy and major depressive subjects. *J Affect Disord.* 1992;24:135-145.

76. Hajak G, Rodenbeck A, Voderholzer U, Riemann D, Cohrs S, et al. Doxepin in the treatment of primary insomnia: A placebo-controlled, double-blind, polysomnographic study. *J Clin Psych.* 2001;62(6):453-463.

77. Hohagen F, Montero RF, Weiss E. Treatment of primary insomnia with trimipramine: an alternative to benzodiazepine hypnotics? *Eur Arch Psychiatry Clin Neurosci.* 1994;244(2):65-72.

78. Riemann D, Voderholzer U, Cohrs S, Rodenbeck A, Hajak G, et al. Trimipramine in primary insomnia: Results of a polysomnographic double-blind controlled study. *Pharmacopsychiatry.* 2002;35(5):165-174.

79. Winokur A, Sateia MJ, Hayes JB, Bayles-Dazet W, MacDonald MM, Gary KA. Acute effects of mirtazapine on sleep continuity and sleep architecture in depressed patients: A pilot study. *Biol Psychiatry.* 2000;48(1):75-78.

80. Nierenberg AA, Adler LA, Peselow E, et al. Trazodone for antidepressant-associated insomnia. *Am J Psychiatry.* 1994;151:1069-1072.

81. Krystal AD. A compendium of placebo-controlled trials of the risks/benefits of pharmacological treatments for insomnia: The empirical basis for U.S. clinical practice. *Sleep Med Rev.* 2009;13(4):265-274.

82. Fawcett J, Barkin RL. Review of the results from clinical studies on the efficacy, safety and tolerability of mirtazapine for the treatment of patients with major depression. *J Affect Disord.* 1998;51(3):267-285.

83. Krystal AD, Thase ME, Tucker VL, Goodale EP. Bupropion HCl and sleep in patients with depression. *Clin Psych Rev.* 2007;3:123-128.

84. Hoque R, Chesson Jr AL. Pharmacologically induced/exacerbated restless legs syndrome, periodic limb movements of sleep, and REM behavior disorder/REM sleep without atonia: Literature review, qualitative scoring, and comparative analysis. *J Clin Sleep Med.* 2010;6(1):79-83.

85. Yang C, White DP, Winkelman JW. Antidepressants and periodic leg movements of sleep. *Biol Psychiatry.* 2005;58:510-514.

86. Bowers M, Kupfer DJ. Central monoamine oxidase inhibition and REM sleep. *Brain Res.* 1971;35:561-564.

87. Wyatt RJ, Fram DH, Buchbinder R, et al. Treatment of intractable narcolepsy with a monoamine oxidase inhibitor. *N Eng J Med.* 1971;285:987-991.

88. Wyatt RJ, Fram DH, Kupfer DJ, et al. Total prolonged drug-induced REM sleep suppression in anxious-depressed patients. *Arch Gen Psychiatry.* 1971;24:145-155.

89. Gillin JC, Wyatt RJ, Fram D, Shyder F. The relationship between changes in REM sleep and clinical improvement in depressed patients treated with amitriptyline. *Psychopharmacolgy (Berl).* 1978;59:267-272.

90. Mayers AG, Baldwin DS. Antidepressants and their effect on sleep. *Hum Psychopharmacol.* 2005;20:533-559.

91. Kupfer DJ, Spiker DG, Coble PA, Neil JF, Ulrich R, Shaw DH. Sleep and treatment prediction in endogenous depression. *Am J Psychiatry.* 1981;138:429-434.

92. Thase ME. Depression and sleep: Pathophysiology and treatment. *Dialogues Clin Neurosci.* 2006;8:217-226.

93. Winokur A, DeMartinis 3rd NA, McNally DP, Gary EM, Cormier JL, Gary KA. Comparative effects of mirtazapine and fluoxetine on sleep physiology measures in patients with major depression and insomnia. *J Clin Psych.* 2003;64(10):1224-1229.

94. Ware JC, Pittard JT. Increased deep sleep after trazodone use: A double-blind placebo-controlled study in healthy young adults. *J Clin Psychiatry.* 1990;51(suppl):18-22.

95. Scharf MB, Sachais BA. Sleep laboratory evaluation of the effects and efficacy of trazodone in depressed insomniac patients. *J Clin Psychiatry.* 1990;51:13-17.

96. Mouret J, Lemoine P, Minuit MP, Benkelfat C, Renardet M. Effects of trazodone on the sleep of depressed subjects—A polygraphic study. *Psychopharmacology.* 1988;95:37-43.

97. Van den Burg W, Van den Hoofdakker RH. Total sleep deprivation on endogenous depression. *Arch Gen Psychiatry.* 1975;32:1121-1125.

98. Pflug B, Tolle R. Disturbance of the 24-hour rhythm in endogenous depression by sleep deprivation. *Int Pharmacopsychiatry.* 1971;6:187-196.

99. Post RM, Kotin J, Goodwin FK. Effects of sleep deprivation on mood and central amine metabolism in depressed patients. *Arch Gen Psychiatry.* 1976;33:627-632.

100. Weigand M, Berger M, Zulley J, et al. The influence of daytime naps on the therapeutic effect of sleep deprivation. *Biol Psychiatry.* 1987;22:386-389.

101. Sack DA, Dancan W, Rosenthal NE, et al. The timing and duration of sleep in partial sleep deprivation therapy of depression. *Acta Psychiatr Scand.* 1988;77:219-224.

102. Berger M, Vollmann J, Hohagen F, et al. Sleep deprivation combined with consecutive sleep phase advance as a fast-acting therapy in depression: An open pilot trial in medicated and unmedicated patients. *Am J Psychiatry.* 1997;154:870-872.

103. Wehr TA, Sack DA, Rosenthal NE. Sleep reduction as a final common pathway in the genesis of mania. *Am J Psychiatry.* 1987;144:201-204.

104. Wehr TA. Sleep loss as a possible mediator of diverse causes of mania. *Br J Psychiatry.* 1991;159:576-578.

105. Zimanova J, Vojtechovsky M. Sleep deprivation as a potentiation of antidepressant pharmacotherapy. *Act Nerv Super (Praha).* 1974;16:188-189.

106. Krystal AD, Goforth H, Roth T. Effects of antipsychotic medications on sleep in schizophrenia. *Int Clin Psychopharm.* 2008;23:150-160.

107. Nofzinger EA, Thase ME, Reynolds III CF, et al. Hypersomnia in bipolar depression: A comparison with narcolepsy using the multiple sleep latency test. *Am J Psychiatry.* 1991;148:1177-1181.

108. Hudson JI, Lipinski JF, Frankenburg FR, et al. Electroencephalographic sleep in mania. *Arch Gen Psychiatry.* 1988;45:267-273.

109. Linkowski P, Kerkhofs M, Rielaert C, et al. Sleep during mania in manic-depressive males. *Eur Arch Psychiatry Neurol Sci.* 1986;235:339-341.

110. Kupfer DJ, Reynolds III CF, Weiss BL, et al. Lithium carbonate and sleep in affective disorders: Further considerations. *Arch Gen Psychiatry.* 1974;30:79-84.

Chapter 55

Sleep in Anxiety Disorders

CONSTANCE GUILLE / BERNADETTE M. CORTESE /
THOMAS W. UHDE

Epidemiologic studies demonstrate that one in four persons meet diagnostic criteria for at least one anxiety disorder during their lifetime,[1] making the anxiety disorders one of the most prevalent psychiatric disorders. Women are more likely than men to develop an anxiety disorder (lifetime rate: 30.5% vs. 19.2%), and the severity of these disorders can result in significant impairment, morbidity, and mortality.[1]

Sleep disturbances are common in anxiety disorders and patients may present with a range of complaints such as difficulty falling asleep, inability to sleep through the night, early morning awakening, apprehension about getting sufficient sleep, lack of restful sleep, nightmares, sleep panic attacks, or restless broken sleep. Many of these sleep problems are collectively referred to as "insomnia" by patients with anxiety disorders.

The high prevalence of subjective insomnia in anxiety disorders contributes to the impression among clinicians that the treatment of core anxiety symptoms will be associated with parallel improvement in sleep quality. Whether this impression plays out in reality, however, requires more systematic study under controlled conditions. In fact, there is a growing belief among anxiety experts that sleep problems may need to be selectively targeted, independently of anxiety symptoms, in order achieve a full remission of both anxiety and sleep problems.

The high prevalence of co-morbid insomnia in primary anxiety disorders and co-morbid anxiety symptoms in primary insomnia suggests an important underlying relationship between these clinical entities. The exact nature of this relationship remains unclear, but emergent advances in our knowledge may lead in the near future to more targeted or "evidence-based" interventions in the management of patients who suffer from co-morbid anxiety and insomnia.[2]

In the anxiety disorders, the most extensive sleep research has been conducted in panic disorder (PD), post-traumatic stress disorder (PTSD), generalized anxiety disorder (GAD), and to a lesser extent, obsessive-compulsive disorder (OCD).[3-11] Although all of these disorders are associated with "insomnia," there are also some qualitative and objective electroencephalographic (EEG) differences. Nightmares, which frequently replicate in exact detail recent (and sometimes distant) traumatic events, are a common feature of acute stress and post-traumatic stress disorders. Patients with GAD and PD, especially those patients with sleep panic attacks,[12-16] share particularly poignant characteristics with primary insomnia in terms of symptomatology, co-morbidity, pharmacologic treatment response, and sleep EEG measures. In contrast to GAD and PD, social anxiety disorder[17] can be easily distinguished from primary insomnia on a number of clinical and physiologic criteria,[11]

largely based on the absence of either impressive clinical or EEG findings.

This chapter provides an overview of the epidemiology and phenomenology of GAD, PTSD, PD, and OCD, each manifesting sleep disturbances as a facet of illness. For the reader's convenience, pharmacologic and nonpharmacologic treatments are discussed separately, although in real-world practice of psychiatry these modalities are often used in combination or provided in a sequential fashion. We highlight current knowledge regarding sleep problems and their treatment *within these anxiety disorders*. Given that little research has been undertaken to specifically study the treatment of insomnia or syndrome-specific sleep problems (e.g., sleep panic attacks) in patients with primary anxiety disorders, we highlight the sleep effects of drugs that are most commonly used to treat GAD, PTSD, PD, and OCD.

GENERALIZED ANXIETY DISORDER

Epidemiology and Phenomenology

GAD is a common condition affecting 3% to 8% of the general population during a given year. The lifetime prevalence of GAD is 5% to 8%. Women are more likely than men to be affected (2:1). The age of onset is in the late teenage years or early adulthood and GAD often presents with other co-morbid psychiatric conditions including panic disorder, depression, and substance abuse.[18]

GAD is characterized by chronic, excessive worry for most days during at least a 6-month period. Worrying occupies much of the individual's time and results in significant impairment (e.g., occupation, relationships, school). The "worry" is difficult to control and distressing and is accompanied by somatic symptoms including *sleep disturbance*, muscle tension, irritability, and restlessness.

In people reporting insomnia and co-morbid anxiety, GAD is often the co-morbid anxiety condition (55.6% of the cases).[19] Of interest, primary insomnia and GAD are individual disorders, which when occurring alone, are each typically associated with physiologic hyperarousal and increased vigilance ("feeling keyed up") as part of their syndromes. Intermittent fatigue and disturbances in concentration and memory are also features of both conditions. Likewise, symptoms of "worry," difficulty concentrating, feelings of jitteriness, agitation, and muscle tension are almost universally reported in part or whole by patients with GAD and primary insomnia. The subjective sleep complaints, including problems falling or maintaining sleep, and worrying about obtaining good quality or sufficient amounts of sleep, are nearly identical in both patients diagnosed with GAD and patients diagnosed with primary insomnia. For reasons that remain unclear, however, patients with primary insomnia experience their symptoms exclusively within the context of a sleep problem while those with GAD experience symptoms in a wider range of contexts and situations. Whether primary insomnia and GAD represent distinctly different neurobiologic disorders remains to be determined in future research.

Objective Evidence of Sleep Dysfunction

The objective evidence of sleep disturbance in GAD is consistent with the subjective reports of insomnia in these individuals. Decreased total sleep time and sleep efficiency, increased wake within total sleep time, and greater early morning awakenings (late insomnia) have all been reported in adult outpatients diagnosed with nonorganic insomnia related to GAD.[20,21] Monti and Monti[22] compiled the data from six different polysomnography (PSG) studies in patients with GAD and found that wake time after sleep onset was significantly increased in patients versus control subjects in four out of the six studies (mean increase: 32.8 minutes; range: 14.8-49.0 minutes), and total sleep time was significantly reduced in five of the six studies (mean decrease: 54.8 minutes; range 27.0-101.4 minutes). After a review of all sleep variables assessed in these six studies, the authors concluded that GAD is related to sleep maintenance insomnia and, to a lesser degree, sleep onset insomnia. Although other GAD-related PSG findings have been reported, including significant decreases in slow wave sleep[23] and increases in stage N1 sleep,[24] these findings are much more inconsistent and need further investigation before a consensus on their role in GAD-related insomnia can be made.[6,11]

Pharmacologic Treatment

The four major drug classes to be considered for the treatment of GAD include selective serotonin reuptake inhibitors (SSRIs) (escitalopram), serotonin-norepinephrine reuptake inhibitors (SNRIs) (venlafaxine), benzodiazepines, and buspirone. Other medications that may be useful are the tricyclic antidepressants (TCAs; imipramine), antihistamines, and β-adrenergic antagonists (propranolol), but there is less empirical support for the use of these medications and they should be employed only when conventional pharmacologic approaches are ineffective or only partially effective. Of the evidence-based treatment choices, many have dual indications; thus, treatment decisions are often guided by co-morbid conditions as well as patient preference (Table 55-1).

Even though escitalopram is the only SSRI approved by the Food and Drug Administration (FDA) for the treatment of GAD, in practice, many of the SSRIs are used for this indication. SSRIs are a particularly good choice for patients who have co-morbid GAD and depression. The main disadvantages of these medications however, include the potential to transiently increase anxiety and/or *insomnia*, as well as the time it could take (4-6 weeks or more) to reach maximum effect. Starting these medications at a very low dose and increasing slowly can reduce the chances of developing medication-induced anxiety or *insomnia*.[18] It is also reasonable to start an SSRI with a benzodiazepine with plans to taper the benzodiazepine in

4 to 6 weeks when the SSRI has taken effect. Alternatively, if insomnia is the only activating effect of the SSRI, the addition of low-dose trazodone (50-100 mg) at bedtime is widely used to *improve sleep* in those with antidepressant-induced insomnia.[25]

If the GAD patient is already taking an SSRI for a mood or other anxiety disorder, the dose of the SSRI can first be increased to a higher but therapeutic range as long as the patient is not experiencing untoward side effects.[18] If remission is not achieved after at least a 6-week trial of the medication, or the patient cannot tolerate the medication, another SSRI may be tried. Although all the SSRIs have similar mechanism of actions and adverse events, a patient failing to achieve therapeutic benefit from one SSRI may respond to another.

There are limited data regarding the secondary improvement in insomnia following the targeted treatment of GAD. Some SSRIs may actually *induce insomnia* in patients with anxiety or primary insomnia as well as healthy subjects.[26,27] SSRIs have other effects on sleep and have been shown to decrease rapid eye movement (REM) sleep as well as to produce oculomotor abnormalities in stages 2, 3, and 4 of non-REM (NREM) sleep.[28,29] The latter effects on increased eye movements and arousals theoretically might be linked to complaints of insomnia reported by some depressed patients treated with fluoxetine.[30]

On the other hand, there is also some evidence that older patients with anxiety disorders (> 60 years of age with mainly GAD) may show decreased scores on the Pittsburgh Sleep Quality Index (PSQI) suggesting that *quality of sleep may improve* after the targeted treatment of anxiety in elderly patients.[31]

The extended-release formulation of venlafaxine is an FDA-approved medication for the treatment of GAD and is a potent inhibitor of serotonin and norepinephrine reuptake and a weak inhibitor of dopamine reuptake. Venlafaxine appears to be a good choice for patients with GAD and *insomnia* as well as patients with GAD and depression. In clinical trials, dosages of 75 to 225 mg per day were shown to *reduce insomnia* as well as poor concentration, restlessness, irritability, and excessive muscle tension associated with GAD.[32] Further, venlafaxine is used for the treatment of depression and would be beneficial for those with this co-morbid diagnosis. Precautions should be taken with patients with preexisting hypertension, as doses 300 mg or more per day of venlafaxine have been shown to increase diastolic blood pressure. Abrupt discontinuation of venlafaxine may produce a discontinuation syndrome consisting of nausea, *somnolence*, or *insomnia*. Therefore, when discontinuing venlafaxine, it should be tapered gradually over at least 2 to 4 weeks.

Benzodiazepines administered to GAD patients, with insomnia as target symptoms, have been shown to reduce insomnia.[33] The decision to initiate a benzodiazepine as a monotreatment or in combination with other medications for GAD should be weighed carefully. Although benzodiazepines are *sedating* and can immediately relieve anxiety symptoms and insomnia, patients may be less motivated to employ behavioral and cognitive strategies to address their anxiety or sleep difficulties.[34]

Buspirone, a 5-HT$_{1A}$ (serotonin) receptor partial agonist, is a FDA approved medication for the treatment of GAD. Although studies have shown that buspirone is effective in 60% to 80% of patients with GAD, data also suggest that buspirone is more effective in reducing the cognitive symptoms

TABLE 55-1

Pharmacologic Treatment for Generalized Anxiety Disorder (GAD)

Medication (Class)	Treatment of Co-Morbid Conditions	Precautions
FIRST-LINE AGENTS		
*Venlafaxine (SNRI)	Depression Panic with/without Agoraphobia Social phobia Menopausal symptoms Obsessive compulsive disorder PTSD Premenstrual dysphoric disorder Attention deficit hyperactivity disorder	*Preexisting hypertension:* monitor BP at baseline and each visit *Withdrawal/discontinuation syndrome:* taper medication slowly when discontinuing
*Duloxetine (SNRI)	Depression Fibromyalgia Peripheral neuropathy	*Withdrawal/discontinuation syndrome:* taper medication slowly when discontinuing
*Escitalopram (SSRI)	Depression Depression prophylaxis in CVA Obsessive compulsive disorder Panic disorder Trichotillomania	*Serotonin syndrome:* do not combine with other serotoninergic medications Drug-drug interactions—inhibitor of P-450 2D6: e.g., increase TCAs, atomoxetine, risperdal
*Paroxetine (SSRI)	Depression Obsessive compulsive disorder Panic disorder PTSD Premenstrual dysphoric disorder social phobia	*Serotonin syndrome:* do not combine with other serotoninergic medications Anticholinergic effects Drug-drug interactions—inhibitor of P-450 2D6: e.g., increase TCAs, atomoxetine, risperdal
*Buspirone (partial agonist of 5-HT$_{1A}$)	Depression Nicotine dependence	*Not pharmacologically related to benzodiazepines:* do not use for benzodiazepine withdrawal
Benzodiazepines	Panic disorder (alprazolam) Muscle relaxant Seizures Alcohol withdrawal	*Tolerance/dependence:* use only for short duration/fixed amount of time *Withdrawal:* taper with long-acting benzodiazepine to decrease chance of symptomatic withdrawal *Lethal in combination with alcohol:* avoid use in patients with alcohol abuse or dependence or at high risk for overdose
SECOND-LINE AGENTS		
Imipramine (TCA)	Depression Nocturnal enuresis Cataplexy Diabetic neuropathy Panic disorder	*Anticholinergic effects:* delirium and confusion in the elderly; precipitate narrow-angle glaucoma; bethanechol to treat urinary retention *Cardiac—prolonged QRS complex:* do not use in patients with history of arrhythmia, or potential for overdose *Drug-drug interactions*—TCAs Substrate of P-450 2D6 enzymes: increase TCAs with SSRIs and decrease with dexamethasone Monitor TCA level Monitor ECG for QRS prolongation
Propranolol (β-adrenergic antagonists)	Hypertension Essential tremor Migraine prophylaxis Performance anxiety	*Cardiovascular disease:* can cause bradycardia and hypotension
Diphenhydramine (antihistamines)	Allergic rhinitis Insomnia	*Anticholinergic effects:* can cause delirium and confusion in the elderly

*FDA-approved medications for the treatment of GAD. Medications listed in the first column are not necessarily FDA-approved for the co-morbid conditions listed in the second column.

BP, blood pressure; *ECG,* electrocardiogram; *FDA,* U.S. Food and Drug Administration; *5-HT$_{1A}$,* 5-hydroxytryptamine (serotonin) receptor 1A; *PTSD,* post-traumatic stress disorder; *SNRI,* serotonin-norepinephrine reuptake inhibitor; *SSRI,* selective serotonin reuptake inhibitor; *TCA,* tricyclic antidepressant.

of GAD (e.g., worry, distress, difficulty concentrating) compared to reducing somatic symptoms (e.g., insomnia, muscle tension, restlessness).[35] Thus, buspirone would not be the first choice of medication for those with GAD and a *prominent sleep disturbance* and somatic symptoms. Further, data also indicate that patients who have previously undergone treatment with a benzodiazepine for GAD are less likely to respond to monotherapy with buspirone. Some studies,

however, have reported benefit of combined treatment with benzodiazepine and buspirone, possibly owing to the immediate, muscle relaxant, sedative, and anxiolytic effects of benzodiazepines and cognitive effects of buspirone.[36] The major disadvantage of buspirone is that it takes at least 2 to 3 weeks for the anxiolytic effects to become evident. One approach to this limitation is to initiate buspirone treatment with a benzodiazepine and then taper the benzodiazepine in 3 to 4 weeks, at which point the buspirone should have reached its maximum effects.

Nonpharmacologic Treatment

Cognitive behavioral therapy (CBT) has demonstrated effectiveness as a nonpharmacologic intervention for GAD,[37] primary insomnia,[38] and co-morbid GAD and insomnia.[39] Although Stanley and associates[39] employed a CBT intervention that addressed both GAD and sleep management and demonstrated clinical efficacy on anxiety and depression measures in their co-morbid GAD and insomnia patients, sleep was not reported as a specific outcome measure. The evidence base regarding whether GAD-targeted treatment improves sleep (or sleep-targeted treatment improves GAD) is very limited. One might predict, however, that CBT specifically designed to target the cognitive distortions of worry would be useful in treating both GAD and insomnia. In an important preliminary investigation, Bélanger and associates[40] treated patients with co-morbid GAD and insomnia with a CBT intervention targeting the GAD-related worries[41] but not sleep complaints. In this study, 86.5% reported that they had never experienced insomnia without worry and the majority reported difficulties maintaining sleep; indeed, 25% reported suffering from all phases of insomnia (i.e., early, middle, and late). Although sleep dysfunction was not directly addressed in the treatment, a significant post-treatment improvement on the Insomnia Severity Index[42] was demonstrated. The authors concluded that even though a specific treatment for sleep was not utilized, the CBT specific for GAD had a significant positive impact on sleep dysfunction.[40]

POST-TRAUMATIC STRESS DISORDER

Epidemiology and Phenomenology

The lifetime prevalence of PTSD is estimated to be 8% to 13% of the general population. Among groups exposed to significant trauma, rates of PTSD vary substantially (e.g., 15% Vietnam veterans; 24% urban youth; 39% traffic accident victims). Women are at greater risk for developing PTSD during their lifetime compared to men (10-12% vs. 5-6%) and PTSD is most prevalent in young adults owing to their propensity to exposure to traumatic events. PTSD however, can appear at any age including childhood.[18]

PTSD is a syndrome that develops after a person has witnessed or experienced a traumatic event that involved actual or threatened death or serious injury and resulted in intense fear, helplessness, or horror. Subsequently the person persistently re-experiences the event in the form of intrusive thoughts, nightmares, or flashbacks and desperately tries to avoid being reminded of the event. In addition, the person typically reports symptoms of physiologic hyperarousal including insomnia, exaggerated startle response, and increased vigilance. This constellation of symptoms can begin immediately following the stressor (termed *acute stress disorder*), but symptoms persisting longer than 1 month warrant a diagnosis of PTSD. Patients can also be asymptomatic immediately following or even years after a trauma, and later may present with symptoms consistent with the diagnosis of PTSD.[43]

Sleep disturbance, including nightmares and insomnia, is so common in PTSD that it has been considered the hallmark feature.[44] Prevalence of nightmares in people with PTSD is estimated to reach up to 70%, and rates for insomnia are as great as 50%. Recurrent PTSD-related nightmares typically contain features of the original traumatic event, allowing for the trauma to be repeatedly experienced or "relived" during sleep. The re-experiencing aspect of trauma-related nightmares is one of the main characteristics that set these sleep events apart from sleep panic attacks or sleep paralysis experiences. Compared to night terrors, a person experiencing PTSD-related nightmares, a syndrome-specific sleep problem, becomes alert quickly after awakening and is not as confused upon awakening. In contrast to REM sleep behavior disorder, complex body movements while asleep are uncommon in those with PTSD. Given the sleep disturbances associated with PTSD, including a question about trauma in the overall evaluation of the patient with sleep difficulties may be helpful in discerning the etiology of sleep disruption and facilitate appropriate therapy.

People with trauma exposure(s) have greater numbers of medical problems, somatic complaints, and prescription drugs compared to age-matched control subjects, all of which can negatively influence sleep quality.[45] The evaluation of sleep problems is further compounded by the high rates of co-morbid psychiatric illnesses in PTSD. For example, two thirds of patients with PTSD have at least two other psychiatric diagnoses, including depressive disorders, bipolar disorders, substance-abuse related disorders, and other anxiety disorders.[43] Thus, documentation of co-morbid conditions is an important part of the sleep evaluation given that neuropsychiatric and substance-related disorders, as well as the medications used to treat these problems, have their own effects on sleep and wakefulness.

Objective Evidence of Sleep Dysfunction

Despite the dominance of sleep complaints in PTSD, the objective evidence of PTSD-related sleep disturbance is less coherent. Studies utilizing PSG have revealed sleep abnormalities in people who develop PTSD after a variety of traumas including, but not limited to, military combat,[4,46] serious accidents,[47] domestic violence,[48] and other violent crimes.[49] These studies frequently report PTSD-related changes in REM sleep. The specific nature of these findings, however, varies from study to study. For example, increased REM latency, REM percentage, REM density, and REM fragmentation have been widely reported,[4,8,46,50] but not in all studies.[5] Similarly, variable findings are evident with studies that assessed PSG measured decreases in sleep efficiency.[8,46] A confound and potential source of variance underlying these inconsistent findings is the lack of control for length of illness and associated secondary disorders, including depression or substance abuse/dependence. In fact, a recent meta-analysis of 20 PSG studies concluded that PTSD-related sleep dysfunction (i.e., increased stage 1 sleep, reduced slow wave sleep, and greater REM sleep density) was mediated by such variables as age, sex, and co-morbid depression.[51] Several more recent investigations attempted to control for such factors as duration of illness, co-morbidity, or use of hypnotic medication. Yet these studies also failed to provide a clear picture. For example, Habukawa and associates[47] reported reduced sleep efficiency due to increased wake time after sleep onset and increased REM interruption in a homogeneous group of young adults with PTSD, whereas Klein and associates[52] reported no PSG-measured sleep disturbance in a well-controlled sample of recent motor vehicle accident survivors with PTSD. Future research using newer assessment tools (e.g., combining neuroimaging strategies with EEG recordings) may be necessary to identify reliable sleep disturbances in PTSD.

Pharmacologic Treatment

Sertraline (Zoloft) and paroxetine (Paxil) are FDA-approved SSRIs and are considered first-line treatments for PTSD owing to their efficacy, tolerability, and safety. SSRIs can potentially reduce symptom clusters of PTSD including re-experiencing of the trauma, avoidance, and emotional numbing as well as hyperarousal. Although SSRIs are considered a "first-line" pharmacologic treatment of PTSD, studies have shown SSRIs to induce insomnia in these patients.[26,27] When sleep problems are a core feature of PTSD, starting an SSRI at a very low dose and increasing slowly is one approach to decrease the chances of developing medication-induced anxiety or insomnia. Treatment with an SSRI, however, can result in incomplete remission of PTSD, and many patients continue to experience debilitating symptoms including trauma-related nightmares and sleep disturbances (Table 55-2).

Preclinical data provide a rationale for the specific involvement of the postsynaptic α_1-adrenoreceptor in the pathophysiologic process of nightmares and disrupted sleep associated with PTSD.[53,54] Prazosin, an α_1-adrenoreceptor antagonist that easily crosses the blood-brain barrier, is being investigated for the treatment of sleep dysfunction in PTSD. Prazosin has been shown to substantially reduce PTSD-associated trauma nightmares and sleep disturbances,[55] as well as to significantly increase total sleep time, REM sleep time, and mean REM period duration[56] in combat veterans with chronic PTSD. Although the sleep-related improvements of prazosin are notable, it remains unclear to what extent other features of PTSD might improve with prazosin treatment;[55] also, there may be a reappearance of nightmares once prazosin is discontinued.[57] Prazosin has also been reported to worsen cataplexy[58] and, therefore, should only be used with great caution and under special circumstances in patients with narcolepsy. Other medications that also target the noradrenergic system include clonidine (Catapres) and guanfacine, which have shown some utility in the treatment of PTSD as an adjunct or monotherapy. A recent study, however, showed no benefit of guanfacine for the treatment of PTSD.[59]

There are numerous "off-label" treatment options for those with PTSD based on small or open-label studies as well as a few controlled studies and include drug classes such as the SNRIs (venlafaxine, duloxetine, and desvenlafaxine), TCAs (imipramine, amitriptyline), monoamine oxidase inhibitors (MAO-Is) (phenelzine), anticonvulsants (valproic acid, lamotrigine, topiramate, gabapentin), and second generation antipsychotics (risperidone, olanzapine, quetiapine). These agents should be employed only after attempting to further titrate an SSRI, or switching to a different SSRI. If, given an adequate dose and duration (at least 6 weeks), the SSRI has failed to induce remission or treatment response is inadequate, other "off-label" medication trials are warranted. Treatment choices for patients who are refractory to SSRIs should preferably include a pharmacologic agent that can also target a co-morbid condition or residual symptoms. For example, venlafaxine would be a good choice for a patient with major depression and treatment refractory PTSD or amitriptyline or gabapentin for a patient with co-morbid neuropathic pain. Other examples include valproate for those with co-morbid seizure disorder or risperidone for those with prominent flashbacks or dissociation associated with treatment refractory PTSD.

Nonpharmacologic Treatment

Cognitive behavioral therapy in the treatment of co-morbid PTSD and insomnia has also been investigated. The available literature suggests that although many symptoms of PTSD, along with some symptoms of sleep disturbance such as nightmares,[60,61] improve with CBT for PTSD, insomnia is often resistant to behavioral treatments that target the other core features of this disorder. It may be necessary, therefore, for patients to undergo *insomnia-targeted CBT* to achieve a more complete response. For example, DeViva and colleagues[62] administered a five-session CBT for insomnia in a group of PTSD patients who had previously responded well to CBT for their PTSD symptoms but still reported significant insomnia. In this small sample of treated PTSD patients, additional behavioral treatment targeting insomnia improved self-reported sleep time, sleep onset latency, wake time after sleep onset, sleep efficiency, sleep quality, impairment resulting from sleep difficulty, and maladaptive sleep-related cognitions. In another small preliminary investigation, Germain and associates[63] demonstrated that a very brief behavioral intervention (90-minute session), targeting PTSD-related nightmares and insomnia, not only significantly improved self-report sleep quality and sleep disturbances, but also overall daytime PTSD symptom severity and individual PTSD symptom clusters. Taken together, these studies underscore the importance of targeting sleep dysfunction in the behavioral treatment of PTSD.

PANIC DISORDER

Epidemiology and Phenomenology

Epidemiologic studies demonstrate that the lifetime prevalence of PD is 4%. Women are two to three times more likely to report symptoms consistent with PD compared to men. The average age of onset of the disorder is in late adolescence or early adulthood, although the onset can occur during childhood.[18] New onset PD is uncommon in midadulthood and in older people and should prompt a thorough medical workup. For those with onsets during later years of life, a careful medical evaluation should include a complete blood count; metabolic panel; fasting glucose; liver, renal, and thyroid panels; urinalysis including drug screen; and electrocardiogram (ECG). If a patient is presenting to an emergency room or with chest pain, especially with cardiac risk factors, cardiac tests, including ECG and cardiac enzymes are warranted. Atypical neurologic signs or symptoms may also warrant obtaining further studies including an electroencephalogram or a magnetic resonance imaging (MRI) scan. Suspicion of the rare possibility of carcinoid syndrome or pheochromocytoma can be evaluated by testing a 24-hour urine sample for serotonin metabolites and catecholamines.[64]

Panic attacks are self-characterized as events of profound and sudden, "out-of-the-blue" anxiety that achieve peak intensity over a short period of time, usually within 3 to

TABLE 55-2

Pharmacologic Treatment for Post-traumatic Stress Disorder (PTSD)

Medication (Class)	Treatment of Co-Morbid Conditions	Precautions
FIRST-LINE AGENTS		
*Sertraline (SSRI)	Depression Premenstrual dysphoric disorder Panic disorder Obsessive compulsive disorder Social phobia	*Serotonin syndrome:* do not combine with other serotoninergic medications Drug-drug interactions—inhibitor of P-450 2D6: e.g., increase TCAs, atomoxetine, risperdal
*Paroxetine (SSRI)	GAD Depression Obsessive compulsive disorder Panic disorder PTSD Premenstrual dysphoric disorder Social phobia	*Serotonin syndrome:* do not combine with other serotoninergic medications Anticholinergic effects Drug-drug interactions—inhibitor of P-450 2D6: e.g., increase TCAs, atomoxetine, risperdal
Prazosin (α_1-adrenoreceptor antagonist)	Hypertension PTSD nightmares and sleep disruption Benign prostatic hyplasia	*Cardiovascular effects:* hypotension, tachycardia, syncope
Clonidine, (α_2-adrenergic agonist)	PTSD nightmares and sleep disruption Hypertension Opiate withdrawal	*Cardiovascular effects:* hypotension Depression
SECOND-LINE AGENTS		
Desvenlafaxine (SNRI)	Depression Menopausal symptoms	*Preexisting hypertension:* monitor BP at baseline and each visit *Withdrawal/discontinuation syndrome:* taper medication slowly when discontinuing
Duloxetine (SNRI)	See Table 55-1 for GAD	
Venlafaxine (SNRI)	See Table 55-1 for GAD	
Imipramine (TCA)	See Table 55-1 for GAD	

Amitriptyline (TCA)	Depression
	Peripheral neuropathy
	Migraine prophylaxis
	Postherpetic neuralgia
		Anticholinergic effects: greatest effect compared with other TCAs; delirium and confusion in the elderly; precipitate narrow-angle glaucoma; bethanechol to treat urinary retention
		Cardiac—prolonged QRS complex: do not use in patients with history of arrhythmia, or potential for overdose
		Drug-drug interactions—TCAs
		    Substrate of P-450 2D6 enzymes: increase TCAs with SSRIs and decrease with dexamethasone
		    Monitor TCA level
		    Monitor ECG for QRS prolongation

Risperidone (antipsychotic)	Prominent flashbacks or dissociation Bipolar disorder Schizophrenia Autistic–irritability	*Metabolic syndrome:* monitor weight, BP, lipid profile
Lamotrigine	Bipolar disorder Seizure disorder	*Stevens-Johnson syndrome:* monitor for rash; start at low dose and titrate slowly to decrease risk of rash
Valproic acid	Bipolar disorder Migraine prophylaxis Seizure disorder	*Hepatotoxicity:* baseline and monitor liver function tests *Thrombocytopenia:* baseline and monitor complete blood count *Polycystic ovary (PCO) disease:* monitor for menstrual irregularity, signs/symptoms of PCO

*FDA-approved medications for the treatment of post-traumatic stress disorder. Medications listed in the first column are not necessarily FDA-approved for the co-morbid conditions listed in the second column.
BP, blood pressure; *ECG,* electrocardiogram; *FDA,* U.S. Food and Drug Administration; *GAD,* generalized anxiety disorder; *SNRI,* serotonin-norepinephrine reuptake inhibitor; *SSRI,* selective serotonin reuptake inhibitor; *TCA,* tricyclic antidepressant.

10 minutes. Associated cognitions usually involve fears of serious medical diseases or, sometimes, mental illnesses. Often, there is a fear of imminent death or impending doom. During panic attacks patients may report trouble concentrating and often experience a range of psychosensory disturbances, primarily depersonalization (the feeling that they are not real) or derealization (the events around them are not real).[18] The

physical symptoms include, but are not limited to, tachycardia, palpitations, dyspnea, and sweating. After achieving peak intensity, the "attack" will typically gradually dissipate over the following 15 to 30 minutes, and it does not usually last for more than 1 hour. Between panic attacks patients are concerned about having another attack, or worry about the implication of the attack ("I'm having a heart attack" or "I'm going crazy)."[65] As a result of the attacks, patients begin to change their behavior to prevent future attacks.[66] The majority of patients with panic attacks, particularly if the panic attacks remain untreated, begin to avoid situations (e.g., being alone outside their home, being in a crowd, on a bridge, in a car) where help would not be immediately available in case of sudden incapacitation. These individuals develop secondary fears and avoid an increasingly large array of situations and circumstances (i.e., they avoid situations and conditions they associate with prior "spontaneous" panic attacks). These avoidance behaviors are referred to as "agoraphobia." In our clinical experience, agoraphobia always develops in these individuals as a secondary complication of the panic attacks.

Patients with PD often experience sleep disturbances such as frequent awakenings, restless broken sleep, and nonrestorative sleep.[67-69] Approximately 65% to 70% of PD patients report lifetime sleep panic attacks and 30% to 45% have recurrent sleep panic attacks.[15,16,70-72] There are panic disorder patients who experience sleep panic attacks as their predominant symptom.[11] Sleep panic attacks are similar in quality and duration to wake panic attacks: there is an abrupt arousal from sleep with a sense of impending doom, fear, palpitations, shortness of breath, chest discomfort, feelings of unreality, and hot or cold flashes. In several studies involving small sample sizes, PD patients with sleep panic attacks reported higher rates of insomnia, especially nonrestorative sleep and frequent awakenings.[15,16,73] Singareddy and Uhde[14] found that depression is more common in PD patients with sleep panic attacks. In this study, 78.5% of PD patients with sleep panic reported difficulty sleeping, and 91% of PD patients with a history of both sleep panic and depression reported sleep problems. In addition, PD patients with sleep panic or sleep panic plus depression self-reported particularly severe sleep restriction (i.e., sleep duration of ≤ 5 hours per night) compared to PD patients who exclusively panic during wakefulness. In the same study a separate group of PD patients with hypersomnia (i.e., patients sleeping 9 or more hours per sleeping period) were identified.[14] Historically, hypersomnia has been associated with primary dysthymia or "atypical" depressions.[74] Interestingly, Matza and associates,[75] who compared atypical versus nonatypical depression in the National Comorbidity Survey, found a higher rate of PD in the depressed individuals with atypical features (i.e., hypersomnia). These studies suggest that in addition to insomnia, hypersomnia should be assessed in the clinical workup and management of sleep dysfunction associated with PD.

Objective Evidence of Sleep Dysfunction

Although some studies have provided objective evidence of sleep disturbance (i.e., increased sleep latency, decreased total sleep time, and sleep efficiency) that is consistent with the self-report of insomnia in panic patients,[15,16,76,77] the sleep architecture of PD has been found to be remarkably normal.[11,78-80]

Panic patients who suffer from sleep panic attacks, however, may be particularly vulnerable to sleep dysfunction (e.g., insomnia) caused by an acquired fear of sleep and the sleep environment.[11,81,82] Although sleep EEG studies reveal that these fearful sleep arousals occur during the first third of the sleep period (i.e., first or second NREM sleep cycle), during stage N2 sleep, or within the first few minutes of stage N3 sleep, and typically during transition from stage N2 to stage

N3 sleep,[16,68,80] sleep architecture is otherwise unimpressive.[16,82] For example, using a 2 night PSG protocol, Landry and associates[80] failed to find any differences in sleep measures of medication-free sleep panic patients compared to normal control subjects.

Pharmacologic Treatment

Although paroxetine (Paxil) is the only FDA-approved SSRI for the treatment of PD, in practice, all SSRIs (fluoxetine, fluvoxamine, paroxetine, sertraline, citalopram, escitalopram) are likely effective and can be employed as a first-line treatment.[83] If the first SSRI employed is ineffective or intolerable, it is quite reasonable to switch to another SSRI. Although all the SSRIs have similar mechanism of actions, a patient failing to achieve therapeutic benefit from one SSRI may respond to another.[84] Anecdotal evidence suggests that PD patients are particularly sensitive to the activating effects (e.g., insomnia, agitation, and jitteriness) of some SSRIs (e.g., fluoxetine [Prozac]). Paroxetine is a particularly good choice for such jitteriness-prone patients owing to its sedating effects. Most of the troublesome effects of SSRIs may be diminished by starting with very low doses and gradually titrating to therapeutic levels. Given that a 6-week trial is usually necessary for the medication to take full effect, short-term use of a benzodiazepine is reasonable while titrating the SSRI (Table 55-3).[83]

Alprazolam (Xanax) is the only benzodiazepine that is FDA approved for the treatment of PD, but controlled trials have also demonstrated the efficacy of lorazepam (Ativan) and clonazepam (Klonopin).[83] In practical reality, some patients require long-term treatment with benzodiazepines in order to achieve and sustain a complete blockade of panic attacks. Other patients, however, after experiencing first-hand that benzodiazepines can block panic attacks and reduce generalized anxiety, develop the strategy of simply ensuring access to 1 or 2 tablets of a benzodiazepine (e.g., alprazolam) on their person at all times, yet never use the medication for years. In such patients, perception of self-control (PSC) via immediate access to an antianxiety agent itself appears to be therapeutic. Theoretically, either long-term benzodiazepine or PSC approaches offer potential advantages over taking benzodiazepines immediately after a spontaneous (i.e., out-of-the-blue) panic attack or just prior to known stressful events. These latter methods are tricky because spontaneous panic attacks are not prevented (i.e., patients continue to experience unprovoked panic attacks) and patients fail to learn or fully apply cognitive or behavioral skills that are known to be effective in the treatment of anxiety.[64]

When a benzodiazepine is selected, a longer acting benzodiazepine (e.g., Klonopin) is ideal to prevent spontaneous, uncued panic attacks. Benzodiazepines may also be useful in treating sleep panic attacks. The muscle relaxant and sedative properties of benzodiazepines theoretically should increase sleep panic attacks in patients who report relaxation-induced anxiety.[11] Despite this theory, our clinical experience suggests that benzodiazepines can be helpful in some patients suffering from sleep panic attacks. Thus, until further research is conducted to identify predictors of benzodiazepine response, the use and benefit of this class of medication in treating sleep panic attacks must be assessed on a case-by-case basis.[84]

TCAs can be effective in PD but have more adverse side effects and are less well-tolerated than SSRIs. Of the TCAs, clomipramine and imipramine have been shown to be effective for the

TABLE 55-3

Pharmacologic Treatment for Panic Disorder

Medication (Class)	Treatment of Co-Morbid Conditions	Precautions
FIRST-LINE AGENTS		
*Paroxetine (SSRI) All SSRIs are used in practice	Depression Social phobia Post-traumatic stress disorder Sleep panic attacks	Sedating *Serotonin syndrome:* do not combine with other serotoninergic medications *Withdrawal syndrome:* taper gradually when discontinuing
*Alprazolam (benzodiazepines)	Muscle relaxant Seizure Alcohol withdrawal	*Short-acting:* potential for rebound anxiety *Tolerance/dependence/withdrawal:* taper with long-acting benzodiazepine to decrease chance of symptomatic withdrawal *Lethal in combination with alcohol:* avoid use in patients with alcohol abuse or dependence or at high risk for overdose
SECOND-LINE AGENTS		
Venlafaxine, desvenlafaxine, and duloxetine (SNRIs)	See Table 55-1 for GAD and Table 55-2 for PTSD	
Amitriptyline, imipramine (TCAs)	See Table 55-1 for GAD and Table 55-2 for PTSD	
Doxepine (TCA)	Depression Insomnia Alcohol abuse/dependence	*Sedation:* greatest histamine blockade
Nortriptyline (TCA)	Depression	Orthostatic hypotension *Anticholinergic effects:* fewer anticholinergic effects compared to other TCAs

*FDA-approved medications for the treatment of panic disorder. Medications listed in the first column are not necessarily FDA-approved for the co-morbid conditions listed in the second column.
FDA, U.S. Food and Drug Administration; *GAD,* generalized anxiety disorder; *SNRI,* serotonin-norepinephrine reuptake inhibitor; *SSRI,* selective serotonin reuptake inhibitor; *TCA,* tricyclic antidepressant.

treatment of PD, but full clinical benefit is not usually reached until 8 to 12 weeks and use is often limited by anticholinergic side effects. Imipramine has also shown efficacy in a small (n = 7) open-label investigation of sleep panic attacks.[85] Another study reported that nortriptyline fully remitted sleep panic attacks in three patients.[86] The MAOIs phenelzine (Nardil) and tranylcypromine (Parnate) are similarly effective for the treatment of PD but require at least 8 to 12 weeks of therapy to achieve maximum efficacy. Use is limited by the need for dietary restriction (e.g., tyramine-free diet). Even though the sedating effects of both MAOIs and TCAs can be beneficial for the treatment of insomnia, both classes of medication reduce REM sleep.

Nonpharmacologic Treatment

CBT is an effective treatment for PD and involves educating the patient about increased perception of physiologic sensations and addressing maladaptive patterns of thinking including catastrophic thinking. The major focus of cognitive therapy is to target the patients' false beliefs about panic attacks. For example, patients with PD misinterpret bodily sensations associated with panic attacks. An individual with panic attacks may experience depersonalization or derealization and, based on this perceptual disturbance, believes she/he is "going crazy" or may experience a pounding heart beat and believe he or she is having an impending myocardial infarction. By eliciting the patient's beliefs about the symptoms, the beliefs can be challenged, thus helping the individual understand that panic attacks are time limited and not life threatening.

Although cognitive influences are minimal during sleep, patients with sleep panic attacks also express significant catastrophic thinking in regard to the consequences of sleep panic attacks. In fact, maladaptive cognitive thinking can play a critical role in secondary impairment in sleep and the worsening of sleep panic attacks. For example, sleep panic patients may develop maladaptive sleep habits, such as having the TV or lights on while sleeping, delaying sleep onset time, and so on. Although these habits appear to emerge as a consequence of, rather than a cause for, sleep panic attacks, recent data, demonstrating that sleep deprivation can potentiate anxiety and fear responding during a biologic challenge of panic,[87] suggest that poor sleep may also promote sleep panic attacks.

To date, Craske and associates[88] have the only published randomized, controlled trial to investigate CBT for sleep panic attacks. In this study, 43 panic disorder patients with sleep panic attacks (average of at least six sleep panic attacks over the past 6 months) were assigned to either CBT or a wait-list control group. The CBT intervention consisted of 11 60-minute sessions conducted over 10 weeks that included education about common misappraisals of arousal sensations, cognitive structuring regarding the benign nature of these sensations, breathing retraining, interoceptive exposure, deep relaxation, and finally modification of maladaptive sleep habits. A significant reduction in the frequency of sleep panic attacks (and daytime panic attacks) in the CBT group compared to the wait-list control group was demonstrated. Moreover, efficacy was maintained at the 9-month follow-up visit. This study highlights an important issue in targeting sleep hygiene in the treatment of sleep panic. Although a high priority is placed on the establishment of healthy sleep hygiene by most sleep experts and sleep treatment manuals, these measures are likely to be ineffective for sleep panic patients until other pharmacologic or CBT interventions (e.g., education, exposure, relaxation) have been instituted. Sleep panic patients are likely to be noncompliant with sleep hygiene measures until they are confident that they will not die of a medical event during their sleep. A higher priority is given, therefore, to educating the patient about sleep panic attacks (and PD) and managing the sleep panic attacks prior to initiating sleep hygiene measures in the treatment of PD.

OBSESSIVE COMPULSIVE DISORDER

Epidemiology and Phenomenology

The lifetime prevalence of OCD is 2% to 3%. Unlike most anxiety disorders, adult men and women are equally affected and in adolescents, boys are more likely to develop OCD compared to girls. Although the average age of onset of OCD is 20 years old, there appears to be a bimodal distribution; approximately two thirds of cases develop prior to age 25, and a third of cases develop after age 35.[18] Co-morbid psychiatric diagnoses are common in those with OCD. Approximately 67% of patients have been found to have a co-occurring diagnosis of depression and 25% have a diagnosis of social phobia. OCD and Tourette's syndrome are thought to share genetic underpinnings with about 5% to 7% of patients with OCD presenting with Tourette's syndrome and 25% to 30% presenting with a tic disorder.[89,90]

Patients with OCD can have obsessions or compulsions, but the majority of patients (up to 75%) will present with both obsessions and compulsions.[18] Given that obsessions and compulsions share many clinical features, it is easiest to conceptualize obsessions as thoughts and compulsions as behaviors. These thoughts or behaviors are intrusive, experienced as foreign to the person's sense of self, and produce anxiety and distress, which result in the person taking countermeasures against the initial idea or impulse. The most common patterns of obsessions are "contamination" fears. For example, a sponge is viewed with marked anxiety and distress because it is carrying germs. The thought or perceived contact with a sponge (obsession) results in great distress and is followed by a need to wash excessively (compulsion) to counteract or alleviate the initial anxiety. The obsessions or compulsions or both are time consuming (take at least 1 hour per day), or are disruptive and interfere with social, occupational, or academic functioning. In addition to "contamination" fears, obsessions can be categorized as "pathologic doubt" (e.g., fear that the stove was left on, or the home was not locked), "intrusive thoughts" (e.g., a repetitious thought usually of a sexual or violent content that is reprehensible to the individual), and "symmetry" (e.g., excessive need for order and precision).[65]

Sleep disturbances associated with OCD have been found to be the result of the total symptom burden of the disorder, rather than the disorder itself.[91] Sleep disturbances can result from heightened levels of OCD-related anxiety and engagement in rituals before or during the bedtime routine that interferes with sleep onset. For example, those with pathologic doubt may need to continuously check the door to assure themselves its locked before falling asleep, or an intrusive thought may persist, causing arousal and resulting in the need to repeat a mental or behavioral routine. Further, obsessive concerns about contamination or symmetry obviously need to be quieted before falling asleep. Some patients can develop obsessions around sleep itself.

For example, a patient becomes fixated on needing to get a certain amount of sleep and becomes anxious when unable to fall asleep or unable to fall back asleep if awakened in the middle of the night. The excessive worry or obsession is often built around the potential for negative repercussions of suboptimal sleep.

Evidence of Objective Sleep Dysfunction

Despite the fact that some patients with OCD report significant disruption or distress surrounding sleep,[91] objective PSG measures have been shown to be normal in patients with pure OCD.[92,93]

Pharmacologic Treatment

SSRIs are effective medications for the treatment of OCD and are also useful in treating the common co-morbid conditions associated with OCD, including depression, social phobia, and other anxiety disorders (Table 55-4). The majority of the SSRIs including fluoxetine, fluvoxamine, paroxetine, and sertraline are FDA approved, but citalopram and escitalopram are used "off label" based on favorable placebo-controlled studies. Although some therapeutic benefit can be seen with these medications in the first 4 weeks, 8 to 16 weeks of treatment is often needed to reach maximum benefit. Further, higher doses of the SSRIs are often required to obtain maximal benefit in patients with OCD compared to patients with depression or other anxiety disorders (e.g., fluoxetine 40-80 mg/day, fluvoxamine 200-300 mg/day, paroxetine 40-80 mg/day, and sertraline 100-200 mg/day).[18,83] As reviewed in the section on panic disorder, initiation of SSRIs may induce insomnia and restlessness as well as other side effects (e.g., nausea, diarrhea, and headache). The severity of these side effects can be decreased by starting at a low dose and increasing as tolerated. Most side effects are transient and will subside within 2 weeks. In clinical practice, it appears that short-term use of a benzodiazepine can also decrease the activating effects of SSRIs and can subsequently be tapered once the SSRI has been titrated to a therapeutic dose.

Clomipramine is also FDA approved for the treatment of OCD. Of the TCAs, clomipramine has the greatest serotoninergic action. And in relation to SSRIs, its serotonin reuptake potency is exceeded only by paroxetine and sertraline.[83] Despite its efficacy in the treatment of OCD, it is often employed only after an SSRI has failed owing to its unfavorable side effect profile, particularly at the higher doses often required to treat OCD. These side effects, largely related to anticholinergic properties, include dry mouth, constipation, urinary hesitancy, and potential for confusion or delirium in the elderly. Clinically, clomipramine's sedative effects, however, can be a favorable asset for those with sleep difficulties.

If an adequate trial of SSRI monotherapy or clomipramine is ineffective, then combining medications can be helpful. However, there is potential for a drug-drug interaction with SSRIs (especially fluvoxamine, fluoxetine, paroxetine, and sertraline) inhibiting cytochrome P-450 2D6 enzymes, resulting in potentially toxic levels of clomipramine. If this strategy is employed, using lower doses of clomipramine (75-150 mg/day) is likely to decrease the risk of toxicity. Clomipramine and desmethylclomipramine levels should be monitored as well as

TABLE 55-4

Pharmacologic Treatment for Obsessive Compulsive Disorder

Medication (Class)	Treatment of Co-Morbid Conditions	Precautions
FIRST-LINE AGENTS		
*Paroxetine (SSRIs) *Fluoxetine *Fluvoxamine *Sertraline All SSRIs are used in practice	See Table 55-1 for GAD and Table 55-2 for PTSD	*Serotonin syndrome:* do not combine with other serotoninergic medications *Withdrawal syndrome:* taper gradually when discontinuing Drug-drug interactions—inhibitor of P-450 2D6: e.g., increase TCAs, atomoxetine, risperdal

*Clomipramine (TCA)	Cataplexy
	Depression
		Anticholinergic effects: delirium and confusion in the elderly; precipitate narrow-angle glaucoma; bethanechol to treat urinary retention
		Cardiac—prolonged QRS complex: do not use in patients with history of arrhythmia, or potential for overdose
		Drug-drug interactions—TCAs
		   Substrate of P-450 2D6 enzymes: increase TCAs with SSRIs and decrease with dexamethasone
		   Monitor TCA level
		   Monitor ECG for QRS prolongation

SECOND-LINE AGENTS		
Haloperidol	Tourette's syndrome Psychotic disorder Schizophrenia Tic disorder Delirium	*Cardiac—torsades de pointes:* baseline ECG, and 1 month, caution when combined with other medications that prolong QT interval *Acute dystonia/dyskinesias:* monitor throughout treatment *Tardive dyskinesia:* monitor throughout treatment
Pimozide	Tourette's syndrome Schizophrenia Tic disorder	*Cardiac—torsades de pointes:* baseline ECG, then at 1 month; caution when combined with other medications that prolong QT interval *Acute dystonia/dyskinesias:* monitor throughout treatment *Tardive dyskinesia:* monitor throughout treatment
Venlafaxine, desvenlafaxine, and duloxetine (SNRIs)	See Table 55-1 for GAD and Table 55-2 for PTSD	

*FDA-approved medications for the treatment of obsessive compulsive disorder. Medications listed in the first column are not necessarily FDA-approved for the co-morbid conditions listed in the second column.

ECG, electrocardiogram; *FDA,* U.S. Food and Drug Administration; *GAD,* generalized anxiety disorder; *PTSD,* post-traumatic stress disorder; *SNRI,* serotonin-norepinephrine reuptake inhibitor; *SSRI,* selective serotonin reuptake inhibitor; *TCA,* tricyclic antidepressant.

periodic ECGs because high levels of TCAs can prolong the QRS interval and increase the risk of an arrhythmia.[18]

There are several strategies to augment the effect of SSRIs and they include buspirone, clonazepam, trazodone, venlafaxine, lithium, typical and atypical antipsychotics, and anticonvulsants. Evidence for augmentation comes primarily from open-label or uncontrolled trials with small sample sizes.[83] Augmentation choices for those that are refractory to SSRIs include a pharmacologic agent that targets a co-morbid or residual problem. For example, haloperidol would be a reasonable choice for a patient with OCD and co-morbid Tourette's disorder or a tic disorder, or venlafaxine for a patient with co-morbid depression. Other examples include using a sedating medication in the evening (i.e., trazodone) for those with prominent sleep disturbances and OCD.

Nonpharmacologic Treatment

There are no studies to date employing cognitive or behavioral therapy for the treatment of sleep problems associated with OCD; however, several lines of evidence seem to suggest that sleep problems are related to the total symptom burden of OCD,[91] underscoring the need for adequate treatment of the disorder. Behavioral therapy is the most well studied nonpharmacologic intervention for OCD, and well-controlled studies have found that medication, behavioral therapy, or a combination of both is effective at significantly reducing symptoms of OCD.[94] The principle of behavioral therapy is exposure and response prevention. Patient and therapist create a list of feared exposures or anxiety-provoking thoughts and order these stimuli from most anxiety inducing to least anxiety provoking. The patient and therapist begin with the least anxiety producing thought or situation and gradually expose the patient (either in the imagination or in real life) to the stimulus. The patient is prohibited from completing the compensatory action or thought associated with the stimulus. With repeated exposures, anxiety is decreased by habituation to the stimulus resulting in a decreased need to perform the compensatory behavior.

While patients with OCD may develop maladaptive sleep habits that ostensibly should be treated with sleep hygiene intervention, physicians are likely to have greater success in reducing maladaptive sleep patterns by targeting OCD symptoms, rather than sleep hygiene alone. In patients whose obsessions revolve around sleep itself (e.g., a patient fixates on the amount of sleep and fears negative repercussions of suboptimal sleep), cognitive behavioral strategies may be effective. Helping these patients understand how their obsessive thought actually leads to worsening of their sleep and ways to challenge the validity of their obsession or belief might be helpful in reducing their sleep difficulties.

DISCUSSION

Myriad challenges confront the clinician who must treat the patient with coexisting anxiety and sleep problems. Do we use pharmacologic versus psychosocial treatments? Do we use sequential or combination treatments? A review of empirical data indicates that there are many unknowns and few answers to these questions.[95]

For example, there is no information on the relative value of targeting the treatment of syndrome-specific sleep problems (e.g., sleep panic attacks in panic disorder patients) and coexisting insomnia versus just the standard treatment of the anxiety disorder (e.g., PD) . Does it make a difference? There are theoretical reasons to believe that patients with coexisting disturbed sleep should receive focused and specific treatment of the sleep problem (e.g., sleep panic attacks in panic disorder or trauma-related nightmares in PTSD), but we lack sufficient research data to convincingly justify this approach. Such research is necessary if we are to move toward a more personalized approach to the care of patients with co-morbid anxiety and sleep problems.

Beyond the syndrome-specific sleep problems associated with some anxiety disorders (e.g., sleep panic attacks in panic disorder, trauma-related nightmares in PTSD), insomnia is a prevalent complaint in GAD, PD, and PTSD. Untreated insomnia is a condition with serious medical consequences and is estimated to cost the United States between $92 billion and $107 billion in combined direct and indirect costs each year.[96] The anxiety disorders are highly associated with insomnia. Yet, there are few guidelines and virtually no empirical data on how to best treat patients with coexisting anxiety disorders and insomnia. The *traditional model* is to view insomnia as a secondary complication of the underlying anxiety disorder. The implication of this traditional model is that the successful treatment of the primary anxiety disorder will lead to an automatic remission in insomnia. Beyond the lack of empirical data to support this notion, a potential negative outcome of this belief is that patients will receive only partial treatment for their overall impairments. For example, when a person has been experiencing extreme distress and impairment for many years as a consequence of his coexisting anxiety and insomnia, it is understandable that clinicians and patients alike might be quite pleased with 50% to 70% improvement. Under such circumstances, it is easy to overlook the degree to which there might be significant residual problems (an incomplete response), especially if the theoretical view is that any "secondary" problems, such as insomnia, will eventually improve over time. Thus, our theoretical models have practical repercussions. In the aforementioned illustration, the patient might both achieve a reduction in anxiety yet continue to suffer from a condition (i.e., insomnia), which itself has significant morbidity and negative health consequences.

Of course, the traditional model might be correct and in such cases the insomnia would likely improve with the sustained successful treatment of the core anxiety condition. The challenge is how to make such decisions in the absence of objective information from well-controlled clinical trials.

We need to know when the exclusive treatment of the anxiety symptoms is sufficient and when it is necessary to simultaneously treat both the anxiety and sleep problems. And, to complicate this task, it is likely that the preferable approach (i.e., treating "core" anxiety symptoms alone

versus the independent treatment of the anxiety syndrome and sleep problems as separate disorders) might be different across different anxiety disorders. For example, it is probable that the standard treatment of OCD would be adequate to eliminate the relentless worrying about "getting just the right amount of sleep," which characterizes some patients with OCD. In contrast, it is unlikely that the blockade of wake panic attacks alone will be sufficient to effectively treat the insomnia, sleep loss, and fear of sleeping in patients with PD and sleep panic attacks.

Until empirically driven decision trees have been established, clinicians should recognize the importance of evaluating and tracking the course of syndrome-specific sleep problems, insomnia, and hypersomnia in all patients with primary anxiety disorders. Sleep complaints must be taken into account when assessing treatment response. By employing life-charting methods to plot sleep factors (i.e., syndrome-specific sleep problems, insomnia, and hypersomnia), the physician-patient team will be much more likely to achieve a full remission in patients with primary anxiety disorders.

REFERENCES

1. Kessler RC, Berglund P, Demler O, Jin R, Merikangas KR, Walters EE. Lifetime prevalence and age-of-onset distributions of DSM-IV disorders in the National Comorbidity Survey Replication. *Arch Gen Psychiatry.* 2005;62(6):593-602.
2. Uhde TW, Cortese BM. Anxiety and insomnia. In: Stein DJ, Hollander E, Rothbaum B, eds. *Textbook of Anxiety Disorders.* 2nd ed. Washington, DC: American Psychiatric Publishing; 2009:699-714.
3. Dow BM, Kelsoe Jr JR, Gillin JC. Sleep and dreams in Vietnam PTSD and depression. *Biol Psychiatry.* 1996;39:42-50.
4. Engdahl BE, Eberly RE, Hurwitz TD, Mahowald MW, Blake J. Sleep in a community sample of elderly war veterans with and without posttraumatic stress disorder. *Biol Psychiatry.* 2000;47:520-525.
5. Hurwitz TD, Mahowald MS, Kuskowski M, Engdahl BE. Polysomnographic sleep is not clinically impaired in Vietnam combat veterans with chronic posttraumatic stress disorder. *Biol Psychiatry.* 1998;44:1066-1073.
6. Papadimitriou GN, Linikowski P. Sleep disturbance in anxiety disorders. *Int Rev Psychiatry.* 2005;17:229-236.
7. Mellman TA. Psychobiology of sleep disturbance in posttraumatic stress disorder. *Ann NY Acad Sci.* 1997;821:142-149.
8. Ross RJ, Ball WA, Dinges DF, Kribbs NB, Morrison AR, et al. Rapid eye movement sleep disturbance in posttraumatic stress disorder. *Biol Psychiatry.* 1994;35:195-202.
9. Sheikh JI, Woodward SH, Leskin GA. Sleep in post-traumatic stress disorder: Convergence and divergence. *Depress Anxiety.* 2003;18:187-197.
10. Uhde TW, Roy-Byrne PP, Gillin JC, Mendelson WD, Boulenger J-P, et al. The sleep of patients with panic disorder: A preliminary report. *Psychiatry Res.* 1984;12:251-259.
11. Uhde TW. The anxiety disorders. In: Kryger MH, Roth T, Dement W, eds. *Principles and Practice in Sleep Medicine.* 3rd ed. Philadelphia: WB Saunders; 2000:1123-1139.
12. Craske MG, Tsao JC. Assessment and treatment of nocturnal panic attacks. *Sleep Med Rev.* 2005;9:173-184.
13. Cortese BM, Uhde TW. Immobilization panic. *Am J Psychiatry.* 2006;163:1453-1454.
14. Singareddy R, Uhde TW. Nocturnal sleep panic and depression: Relationship to subjective sleep in panic disorder. *J Affect Disord.* 2009;112:262-266.
15. Mellman TA, Uhde TW. Sleep panic attacks: New clinical findings and theoretical implications. *Am J Psychiatry.* 1989;146:1204-1207.
16. Mellman TA, Uhde TW. Electroencephalographic sleep in panic disorder. A focus on sleep-related panic attacks. *Arch Gen Psychiatry.* 1989;46:178-184.
17. Brown TM, Black B, Uhde TW. Sleep architecture in social phobia. *Biol Psychiatry.* 1994;35:420.
18. Sadock JB, Sadock VA. *Kaplan and Sadock's Synopsis of Psychiatry: Behavioral Sciences and Clinical Psychiatry.* 9th ed. Philadelphia: Lippincott Williams & Wilkins; 2003.
19. Ohayon MM, Caulet M, Lemoine P. Comorbidity of mental and insomnia disorders in the general population. *Compr Psychiatry.* 1998;39:185-197.

20. Saletu B, Saletu-Zyhlarz G, Anderer P, Brandstätter N, Frey R, et al. Non-organic insomnia in generalized anxiety disorder. 2. Comparative studies on sleep, awakening, daytime vigilance and anxiety under lorazepam plus diphenhydramine (Somnium) versus lorazepam alone, utilizing clinical, polysomnographic and EEG mapping methods. *Neuropsychobiology*. 1997;36:130-152.

21. Saletu B, Saletu-Zyhlarz G, Anderer P, Brandstater N, Frey R, et al. Non-organic insomnia in generalized anxiety disorder: Controlled studies on sleep. Awakening and daytime vigilance utilizing polysomnography and EEG mapping. *Neuropsychobiology*. 1997;36:117-129.

22. Monti JM, Monti D. Sleep disturbance in generalized anxiety disorder and its treatment. *Sleep Med Rev*. 2000;4:263-276.

23. Arriaga F, Paiva T. Clinical and EEG sleep changes in primary dysthymia and generalized anxiety: A comparison with normal controls. *Neuropsychobiology*. 1991;24(3):109-114.

24. Fuller KH, Waters WF, Binks PG, Anderson T. Generalized anxiety and sleep architecture: A polysomnographic investigation. *Sleep*. 1997;20(5):370-376.

25. Nierenberg AA, Adler LA, Peselow E, Zornberg G, Rosenthal M. Trazodone for antidepressant-associated insomnia. *Am J Psychiatry*. 1994;151(7):1069-1072.

26. Davis LL, Frazier EC, Williford RB, Newell JM. Long-term pharmacotherapy for post-traumatic stress disorder. *CNS Drugs*. 2006;20(6):465-476.

27. Winokur A, Gary KA, Rodner S, Rae-Red C, Fernando AT, Szuba MP. Depression, sleep physiology, and antidepressant drugs. *Depress Anxiety*. 2001;14:19-28.

28. Schenck CH, Mahowald MW, Kim SW, O'Connor KA, Hurwitz TD. Prominent eye movements during NREM sleep and REM sleep behavior disorder associated with fluoxetine treatment of depression and obsessive-compulsive disorder. *Sleep*. 1992;15(3):226-235.

29. Armitage R, Trivedi M, Rush AJ. Fluoxetine and oculomotor activity during sleep in depressed patients. *Neuropsychopharmacology*. 1995;12(2):159-165.

30. Dorsey CM, Lukas SE, Cunningham SL. Fluoxetine-induced sleep disturbance in depressed patients. *Neuropsychopharmacology*. 1996;14(6):437-442.

31. Blank S, Lenze E, Mulsant BH, Dew MA, Karp JF, et al. Outcomes of late-life anxiety disorders during 32 weeks of citalopram treatment. *J Clin Psychiatry*. 2006;67:468-472.

32. Stahl SM, Ahmed S, Haudiquet V. Analysis of the rate of improvement of specific psychic and somatic symptoms of general anxiety disorder during long-term treatment with venlafaxine ER. *CNS Spectr*. 2007;12(9):703-711.

33. Fontaine R, Beaudry P, Le Morvan P, Beauclair L, Chouinard G. Zopiclone and triazolam in insomnia associated with generalized anxiety disorder: A placebo-controlled evaluation of efficacy and daytime anxiety. *Int Clin Psychopharmacol*. 1990;5:173-183.

34. Westra HA, Stewart SH. Cognitive behavioural therapy and pharmacotherapy: Complementary or contradictory approaches to the treatment of anxiety? *Clin Psychol Rev*. 1998;18(3):307-340.

35. Thayer JF, Friedman BH, Borkovec TD. Autonomic characteristics of generalized anxiety disorder and worry. *Biol Psychiatry*. 1996;39:255.

36. Rapee RM, Barlow DH. Generalized anxiety disorders, panic disorders and phobias. In: Sutker PB, Adams, eds. *Comprehensive Handbook of Psychopathology*. 3rd ed. New York: Kluwer Academic; 2001:131.

37. Newman MG, Borkovec TD. Cognitive-behavioral treatment of generalized anxiety disorder. *Clin Psychol*. 1995;48:5-7.

38. Morin CM, Hauri PJ, Espie CA, Spielman AJ, Buysse DJ, Bootzin RR. Nonpharmacologic treatment of chronic insomnia. An American Academy of Sleep Medicine review. *Sleep*. 1999;22:1134-1156.

39. Stanley MA, Wilson NL, Novy DM, Rhoades HM, Wagener PD, et al. Cognitive behavior therapy for generalized anxiety disorder among older adults in primary care: A randomized clinical trial. *JAMA*. 2009;301(14):1460-1467.

40. Bélanger L, Morin CM, Langlois F, Ladouceur R. Insomnia and generalized anxiety disorder: Effects of cognitive behavior therapy for gad on insomnia symptoms. *J Anxiety Disord*. 2004;18:561-571.

41. Dugas MJ, Ladouceur R. Treatment of GAD: Targeting intolerance of uncertainty in two types of worry. *Behav Modif*. 2000;24:635-657.

42. Morin CM. *Insomnia: Psychological Assessment and Management*. New York: Guilford Press; 1993.

43. Perkonigg A, Kessler RC, Storz S, Wittchen HU. Traumatic events and posttraumatic stress disorder in the community: Prevalence, risk factors and comorbidity. *Acta Psychiatr Scand*. 2000;101:46.

44. Ross RJ, Ball WA, Sullivan KA, Caroff SN. Sleep disturbance as the hallmark of posttraumatic stress disorder. *Am J Psychiatry*. 1989;146(6):697-707.

45. Meltzer-Brody S, Hidalgo R, Connor KM, Davidson JRT. Posttraumatic stress disorder: Prevalence, health care use and costs, and pharmacologic considerations. *Psychiatr Scand*. 2000;30:722.

46. Mellman TA, Nolan B, Hebding J, Kulick-Bell R, Dominguez R. A polysomnographic comparison of veterans with combat-related PTSD, depressed men, and non-ill controls. *Sleep*. 1997;20(1):46-51.

47. Habukawa M, Uchimura N, Maeda M, Kotorii N, Maeda H. Sleep findings in young adult patients with posttraumatic stress disorder. *Biol Psychiatry*. 2007;62(10):1179-1182.

48. Humphreys J, Lee K. Sleep disturbance in battered women living in transitional housing. *Issues Ment Health Nurs*. 2005;26(7):771-780.

49. Germain A, Hall M, Katherine Shear M, Nofzinger EA, Buysse DJ. Ecological study of sleep disruption in PTSD: A pilot study. *Ann N Y Acad Sci*. 2006;1071:438-441.

50. Woodward SH, Murburg MM, Bliwise DL. PTSD-related hyperarousal assessed during sleep. *Physiol Behav*. 2000;70(1-2):197-203.

51. Kobayashi I, Boarts JM, Delahanty DL. Polysomnographically measured sleep abnormalities in PTSD: A meta-analytic review. *Psychophysiology*. 2007;44(4):660-669.

52. Klein E, Koren D, Arnon I, Lavie P. No evidence of sleep disturbance in post-traumatic stress disorder: A polysomnographic study in injured victims of traffic accidents. *Isr J Psychiatry Relat Sci*. 2002;39(1):3-10.

53. Pickworth WB, Sharpe LG, Nozaki M, Martin WR. Sleep suppression induced by intravenous and intraventricular infusions of methoxamine in the dog. *Exp Neurol*. 1977;57(3):999-1011.

54. Birnbaum S, Gobeske KT, Auerbach J, Taylor JR, Arnsten AF. A role for norepinephrine in stress-induced cognitive deficits: Alpha-1-adrenoceptor mediation in the prefrontal cortex. *Biol Psychiatry*. 1999;46(9):1266-1274.

55. Raskind MA, Peskind ER, Hoff DJ, Hart KL, Holmes HA, et al. A parallel group placebo controlled study of prazosin for trauma nightmares and sleep disturbance in combat veterans with post-traumatic stress disorder. *Biol Psychiatry*. 2007;61(8):928-934.

56. Taylor FB, Martin P, Thompson C, Williams J, Mellman TA, et al. Prazosin effects on objective sleep measures and clinical symptoms in civilian trauma posttraumatic stress disorder: A placebo-controlled study. *Biol Psychiatry*. 2008;63(6):629-632.

57. Peskind ER, Bonner LT, Hoff DJ, Raskind MA. Prazosin reduces trauma-related nightmares in older men with chronic posttraumatic stress disorder. *J Geriatr Psychiatry Neurol*. 2003;16:165-171.

58. Aldrich MS, Rogers AE. Exacerbation of human cataplexy by prazosin. *Sleep*. 1989;12(3):254-256.

59. Neylan TC, Lenoci M, Samuelson KW, Metzler TJ, Henn-Haase C, et al. No improvement of posttraumatic stress disorder symptoms with guanfacine treatment. *Am J Psychiatry*. 2006;163(12):2186-2188.

60. Cooper NA, Clum GA. Imaginal flooding as a supplementary treatment for PTSD in combat veterans: A controlled study. *Behav Ther*. 1989;20:381-391.

61. Keane TM, Fairbank JA, Caddell JM, Zimering RT. Implosive (flooding) therapy reduces symptoms of PTSD in Vietnam combat veterans. *Behav Ther*. 1989;20:245-260.

62. DeViva JC, Zayfert C, Pigeon WR, Mellman TA. Treatment of residual insomnia after CBT for PTSD: Case studies. *J Trauma Stress*. 2005;18:155-159.

63. Germain A, Shear MK, Hall M, Buysse DJ. Effects of a brief behavioral treatment for PTSD-related sleep disturbances: A pilot study. *Behav Res Ther*. 2007;45(3):627-632.

64. Simon NM, Pollock HM. The current status of the treatment of panic disorder: Pharmacology and cognitive behavioral therapy. *Psychiatr Ann*. 2000;30(11):689.

65. American Psychiatric Association. *Diagnostic and Statistical Manual of Mental Health Disorders*. 4th ed. Washington, DC: American Psychiatric Association; 2000.

66. Keller MB, Hanks DL. Course and outcome in panic disorder. *Prog Neuropsychopharmacol Biol Psychiatry*. 1993;17:551.

67. Arriaga F, Paiva T, Matos-Pires A, Cavaglia F, Lara E, Bastos L. The sleep of non-depressed patients with panic disorder: A comparison with normal controls. *Acta Psychiatr Scand*. 1996;93(3):191-194.

68. Hauri PJ, Friedman M, Ravaris CL. Sleep in patients with spontaneous panic attacks. *Sleep*. 1989;12(4):323-337.

69. Uhde TW, Singareddy R. Biological research in anxiety disorders. In: Maj M, ed. *Psychiatry as a Neuroscience*. New York: John Wiley & Sons; 2002:237-285.

70. Roy-Byrne PP, Mellman TA, Uhde TW. Biologic findings in panic disorder. *J Anxiety Disord*. 1988;2:17-29.

71. Uhde TW, Mellman TA. Commentary on "Relaxation-induced panic (RIP): When resting isn't peaceful." *Integr Psychiatry*. 1988;6:147-149.

72. Singareddy R, Uhde TW. Sleep panic arousals. In: Thorpy MJ, Plazzi G, eds. *The Parasomnias and Other Sleep-Related Movement Disorders.* New York: Cambridge University Press; 2010:278-289.

73. Crake MG, Barlow DH. Nocturnal panic. *J Nerv Ment Dis.* 1989;177:160-168.

74. Akiskal HS, Lemmi H, Dickson H, King D, Yerevanian B. Van Valkenburg, C. Chronic depressions. Part 2. Sleep EEG differentiation of primary dysthymic disorders from anxious depressions. *J Affect Disord.* 1984;6:287-295.

75. Matza LS, Revicki DA, Davidson JR, Stewart JW. Depression with atypical features in the National Comorbidity Survey: Classification, description, and consequences. *Arch Gen Psychiatry.* 2003;60:817-826.

76. Lydiard RB, Zealberg J, Laraia MT, Fossey M, Prockow V, et al. Electroencephalography during sleep of patients with panic disorder. *J Neuropsychiatry Clin Neurosci.* 1989;1:372-376.

77. Sloan EP, Natarajan M, Baker B, Dorian P, Mironov D, et al. Nocturnal and daytime panic attacks—Comparison of sleep architecture, heart rate variability, and response to sodium lactate challenge. *Biol Psychiatry.* 1999;45:1313-1320.

78. Stein MB, Enns MW, Kryger MH. Sleep in nondepressed patients with panic disorder: II. Polysomnographic assessment of sleep architecture and sleep continuity. *J Affect Disord.* 1993;28(1):1-6.

79. Stein MB, Uhde TW. Infrequent occurrence of EEG abnormalities in panic disorder. *Am J Psychiatry.* 1989;146:517-520.

80. Landry P, Marchand L, Mainguy N, Marchand A, Montplaisir J. Electroencephalography during sleep of patients with nocturnal panic disorder. *J Nerv Ment Dis.* 2002;190:559-562.

81. Krystal JH, Woods SW, Hill CL, Charney DS. Characteristics of panic attack subtypes: Assessment of spontaneous panic, situational panic, sleep panic, and limited symptom attacks. *Compr Psychiatry.* 1991;32(6):474-480.

82. Craske MG, Lang AJ, Mystkowski JL, Zucker BG, Bystritsky A, Yan-Go F. Does nocturnal panic represent a more severe form of panic disorder? *J Nerv Ment Dis.* 2002;190(9):611-618.

83. Labbate L, Fava M, Rosenbaum JF, Arana GW. *Handbook of Psychiatric Drug Therapy.* 6th ed. 2010:182.

84. Pigott HE, Leventhal AM, Alter GS, Boren JJ. Efficacy and effectiveness of antidepressants: Current status of research. *Psychother Psychosom.* 2010;79(5):267-279.

85. Mellman TA, Uhde TW. Patients with frequent sleep panic: Clinical findings and response to medication treatment. *J Clin Psychiatry.* 1990;51:513-516.

86. Lopes FL, Nardi AE, Nascimento I, Valenca AM, Zin WA. Nocturnal panic attacks. *Arq Neuropsiquiatr.* 2002;60(3-B):717-720.

87. Babson KA, Feldner MT, Trainor CD, Smith RC. An experimental investigation of the effects of acute sleep deprivation on panic-relevant biological challenge responding. *Behav Ther.* 2009;40(3):239-250.

88. Craske MG, Lang AJ, Aikins D, Mystokowski JL. Cognitive behavioral therapy for nocturnal panic. *Behav Ther.* 2005;36:43-54.

89. Nelson E, Rice J. Stability of diagnosis of obsessive compulsive disorder in the epidemiologic catchment area study. *Am J Psychiatry.* 1997;154:826.

90. Wolff M, Alsobrook JP, Pauls DL. Genetic aspects of obsessive compulsive disorder. *Psychiatr Clin North Am.* 2000;23(3):535.

91. Ivarsson T, Larsson B. Sleep problems as reported by parents in Swedish children and adolescents with obsessive-compulsive disorder (OCD), child psychiatric outpatients and school children. *Nord J Psychiatry.* 2009;63(6):480-484.

92. Robinson D, Walsleben J, Pollack S, Lerner G. Nocturnal polysomnography in obsessive-compulsive disorder. *Psychiatry Res.* 1998;80(3):257-263.

93. Hohagen F, Lis S, Krieger S, Winkelmann G, Riemann D, et al. Sleep EEG of patients with obsessive-compulsive disorder. *Eur Arch Psychiatry Clin Neurosci.* 1994;243(5):273-278.

94. Anthony MM, Swinson RP. Comparative and combined treatments for obsessive compulsive disorder. In: Sammons MT, Schmidt NB, eds. *Combined Treatment for Mental Disorders; A Guide to Psychological and Pharmacological Interventions.* Washington, DC: American Psychological Association; 2001:53.

95. National Institutes of Health. NIH State-of-the-Science Conference Statement on manifestations and management of chronic insomnia in adults. *NIH Consens State Sci Statements.* 2005;22(2):1-30.

96. Rosekind MR, Gregory KB. Insomnia risks and costs: Health, safety, and quality of life. *Am J Manag Care.* 2010;16(8):617-626.

Seasonal Affective Disorder

BRENDA BYRNE / GEORGE BRAINARD

Seasonal affective disorder (SAD), a depressive disorder associated with fall/winter decrements in functioning and spring/summer remission, was introduced to psychiatry's *Diagnostic and Statistical Manual* (DSM) in the early 1980s. An early research report had described the suppression of melatonin secretion from the pineal gland by bright artificial light presented to the eyes, suggesting that the human brain shared with other animals specific responses to light.[1] A report of successful therapy with bright light of a seasonal manic-depressive disorder[2] was followed by a description of the syndrome of seasonal affective disorder and a report of the treatment of 29 fall/winter SAD sufferers by bright artificial light.[3]

At present, SAD is represented in the DSM-IV-TR as a "seasonal pattern specifier" that may be appended to diagnoses of major depressive disorder in bipolar I, bipolar II, or recurrent forms, summarized in Box 56-1.[4]

Rosenthal[5] has argued that accumulation of evidence presents a strong case for construct validity of SAD and that SAD should be defined as a specific disorder in DSM-V instead of remaining a modifier of other mood disorders.

SYMPTOMS OF SAD AND SUBSYNDROMAL SAD

Although meeting criteria for major depression or bipolar disorder, SAD sufferers generally have much in common with an "atypical" depressive pattern, that is, increased appetite, especially for carbohydrates, weight gain, and hypersomnia. Hypersomnia generally refers to long periods of sleep and excessive daytime sleepiness with daytime napping.[6,7] Increased awakenings and reduced sleep efficiency, and similar elements of restless sleep are also commonly reported by SAD sufferers.[3] Many SAD sufferers report a general sentiment of "don't want to be bothered" and cognitive difficulties. Box 56-2 lists the authors' clinical impressions of some of the more commonly encountered symptoms of SAD.

A minority of SAD sufferers present with more typical depressive complaints of poor appetite, weight loss, and insomnia. It is thought that this symptom picture predicts a less successful outcome for light therapy.[3,8]

The earliest description of depressive symptoms in 29 SAD sufferers reported that 100% of these patients reported sadness, a decrease in physical activity, and interpersonal difficulties, 97% reported work difficulties, 90% reported irritability, 79% reported carbohydrate cravings, 76% reported weight increase, 71% of female subjects reported difficulties around menses, 97% reported increased sleep time, and 90% reported interrupted, unrefreshing sleep.[3]

A more recent assessment of 454 SAD patients in Vancouver, BC yielded similar prevalence rates for several SAD symptoms, summarized in Box 56-3.[8]

At least half of women with SAD report intensified premenstrual mood symptoms in the fall and winter.[9] The first author of this chapter has observed that many SAD sufferers report cold intolerance and avoid being out of doors in the winter.

The earliest studies of SAD identified it as a predominantly bipolar disorder; 76% of the first cohort of 29 SAD patients treated with light had been diagnosed as bipolar II (a history of recurrent major depressive episodes alternating with hypomanic episodes).[3] Over a longer period of time, however, bipolar subjects in SAD studies have made up only between 11% and 50% of study cohorts.[8]

Many people experiencing decrements in fall/winter functioning do not meet criteria for major affective (unipolar or bipolar) disorder and so do not have a diagnosis to which DSM-IV-TR permits appending a seasonal pattern specifier. Researchers have termed this group *subsyndromal SAD (S-SAD)*. Compared to SAD sufferers, who make up 0.8% to 2.2% of North American populations, S-SAD sufferers are more numerous—11% to 25% among various studies—and generally reports less seasonal impairment in mood, energy, or productivity. S-SAD symptoms can significantly degrade overall well-being, however.[9]

SAD or S-SAD symptoms may develop in any season, given exposure to several days of dark weather or prolonged indoor environments. Mood and energy generally recover with exposure to bright—and preferably warm—environments, a notable benefit of winter vacations in tropical climates. Typically the establishment of spring weather brings complete remission of symptoms.

BOX 56-1 *Criteria for Seasonal Pattern Specifier*

- Regular onset in fall or winter of major depressive episodes in major depressive disorder, bipolar I or bipolar II disorders, or recurrent forms. (Disregard cases in which a recurrent seasonal stressor has an obvious psychosocial impact.)
- Full remission or a shift to mania or hypomania in the spring.
- This pattern of fall/winter depression and spring remission is reported for the past 2 years and no nonseasonal major depression episodes are reported during this period.
- Lifetime seasonal major depressive disorder episodes outnumber lifetime nonseasonal major depressive disorder episodes.

BOX 56-2 *Common Signs and Symptoms of Seasonal Affective Disorder*

- Fatigue, loss of energy
- Hypersomnia: prolonged sleep periods and excessive daytime sleepiness, often associated with reduced sleep efficiency
- Carbohydrate craving and increased eating
- Weight gain
- Cognitive problems: concentration, information processing
- Depressed mood: sadness, irritability, despair, loss of interest and pleasure, low self-esteem, extreme guilt
- Social withdrawal

BOX 56-3 *Frequency (%) of Clinical Signs and Symptoms of Seasonal Affective Disorder (SAD)**

Hypersomnia	68
Insomnia	24
Appetite	
Increased	55
Decreased	27
Carbohydrate craving	77
Weight	
Gain	51
Loss	14
Anxiety	87
Suicidal ideation	45

*In a series of 454 patients with SAD in Vancouver, British Columbia, Canada.

PREVALENCE AND NATURAL HISTORY OF SAD

Estimates of the prevalence of SAD have varied widely, depending on whether method of estimation was based on screening instruments or clinical interviews. An early study using the the Seasonal Pattern Assessment Questionnaire (SPAQ)[10] at four latitudes in the United States yielded prevalence rates ranging from 1.4% for winter SAD in Sarasota, FL (27°N latitude) to 9.7% in Nashua, NH (42.5°N latitude). Prevalence rates for S-SAD were higher: 2.6% in Sarasota and 11% in Nashua.[11] Studies using more stringent DSM diagnostic criteria have reported lower estimates of SAD prevalence, between 0.8% and 2.2% in North America and between 1.7% and 2.2% in Canada.[12]

A review of the literature of SAD and latitude supports the conclusion that, except for studies of North American populations, the correlation between latitude and SAD prevalence is weak. Factors of climate assume more importance in some areas; for example, summer SAD is reported more commonly in hot and humid climates such as in Japan and China,[13] and weather may account for significant degrees of SAD. Genetic vulnerability and sociocultural factors also may play more important roles in emergence of SAD than does latitude alone. For instance, reported prevalence of SAD among residents of Reykjavik, Iceland (latitude of 64°N) is 3.8% compared to a SAD prevalence of 13.7% among residents of Tromsö, Norway (latitude of 69°N).[12,13]

SAD affects people of all ages but is most prevalent among women of childbearing years, with a ratio of females to males within this age group at about 1.6 to 1.[9] In older populations, men and women are more equally afflicted but at lower rates overall. Though a recurrent disorder, SAD may have a limited course in the life of an individual. In a follow-up study of the first 59 patients treated with light for SAD at the National Institute of Mental Health (NIMH), 42% of subjects continued to report SAD symptoms, and 41% of these continued to use light therapy after a mean interval of 8.8 years. Full remission of symptoms was reported in 14% of the subjects, and 44% were experiencing nonseasonal depression.[14]

PATHOGENESIS

The composite of physiologic and mood disturbances in SAD permit a range of clinical presentations. An effort to account for these variations is offered in the "dual vulnerability hypothesis."[15] According to this understanding, separate factors of seasonality and mood disturbance account, respectively, for seasonal fall/winter appetite, weight, sleep, and energy changes and for unipolar and bipolar mood changes. Seasonality alone may be activated without a significant affective component, resulting in S-SAD. Mood factors alone may predominate, resulting in nonseasonal depressive disorders. When these two factors coexist, clinical pictures of SAD or of winter depression with incomplete summer remission emerge.

Early observations of SAD prompted interest in possible causal factors. Major hypotheses focused on factors of day length (photoperiod), hours of sunshine, and temperature.[3] Early SAD therapy applied light in morning and evening hours to extend the subjective photoperiod of subjects. Studies at the NIMH demonstrated that healthy humans retain responses to day length, and researchers in Chicago demonstrated that, compared to other environmental variables, photoperiod accounted for 26% of the total variance in the weekly risk of fall-onset SAD symptoms.[16]

The effects of morning light therapy have been shown in a number of studies to be superior to those of light at evening[17,18] or later morning hours.[19] This finding and other lines of investigation have focused attention on the possible role of circadian rhythm disturbances in the genesis of SAD.

Alignment of internal rhythms with the 24-hour day is effected by endogenous (internal) pacemakers, primarily those of the suprachiasmatic nuclei (SCN) of the hypothalamus. Cycles of light and darkness form the primary environmental influence, which continually entrains the endogenous pacemaker to the 24-hour light/dark cycle of the external world. Applied to SAD, a phase-shift hypothesis proposes that SAD sufferers, with their tendency to oversleep in fall/winter, have intrinsic circadian rhythms that are phase-delayed (that is, occurring later than normal relative to external clock time). Using a "constant routine" protocol that minimizes environmental influences on intrinsic circadian rhythms, Lewy and associates[20] noted that, based on levels of the circadian hormone melatonin detected in saliva, the timing of sleep of 71% of SAD subjects studied ($N = 68$) was phase-delayed relative to the timing of sleep of normal control subjects, whereas the timing of sleep in 29% was phase-advanced relative to that of control subjects. The phase shift theory would predict that morning bright light therapy would be more efficacious than light therapy at other times during the day, because morning therapy is most likely to produce a phase advance of circadian rhythms, presumably rectifying the underlying abnormality. Nevertheless, research support for this theory has been mixed, as some SAD subjects have responded to evening light therapy and to midday natural light[21,22] as well as, or in preference to, morning light. In addition, in other SAD studies the degree of phase advance resulting from light therapy has not been found to reliably correlate with clinical improvement.[23,24]

Overall, accumulated evidence suggests that circadian misalignment may be an important factor in the development of SAD, that phase delays are more common than phase advances, and that morning light therapy provides more benefit than evening light therapy.[19] The best outcomes may likely result from matching timing of light therapy to the phase-delayed or phase-advanced state of the patient.[25] Light therapy, correctly timed, can correct circadian misalignments and relieve SAD symptoms. Despite the current dominance of the phase shift hypothesis, however, a substantial minority of SAD patients may not have advanced or delayed circadian phases and may respond to light or to other treatment approaches for other reasons.

ASSESSING SAD

Assessment of seasonality, as it requires retrospective accounts of symptoms over 2 or more years, must be based on patients' subjective reports or the reports of close observers. Inquiry into seasonal symptoms should take into account that light therapy has been effective not only for classic SAD but also for the milder symptoms of S-SAD[26] and for symptom pictures that combine seasonal and nonseasonal complaints. Presence of the "atypical" depressive symptoms of hyperphagia, weight gain, and hypersomnia, which are typical for SAD, predict efficacy of light therapy.[9] A history of seasonal stressors (anniversaries of severe losses, seasonal job layoffs, or seasonal exacerbations of family difficulties) should be considered as alternative causes of depression, fatigue, and dissatisfaction. Elements of inquiry in assessing SAD are noted in Box 56-4.

The presence of depression in SAD deserves careful assessment, because suicide is a risk of depression whether seasonal or nonseasonal in character. In two studies, SAD outpatients had more severe psychopathology scores than those of nonseasonal major depression sufferers,[27] including scores of nonseasonal mood sufferers who had attempted suicide.[28]

Instruments and inventories may be helpful to establish the diagnosis and confirm seasonality (Box 56-5). Seasonality can be established by utilizing the SPAQ a self-report instrument allowing persons to note how moods and behaviors change across months and seasons of the year (Fig. 56-1).[10] A "global seasonality score"(GSS) can be derived from a subset of questions in the SPAQ which ask to what degree changes are experienced in sleep length, social activity, mood (overall feeling of well-being), weight, appetite, and energy level. Each is rated on a 5-point scale from "no change" to "extremely marked change," so that responses yield a GSS score from 0 to 24.

The SPAQ, including the GSS, is suitable for initial screening but not adequate for diagnosis[9] or for the assessment of treatment effects. Seasonal depression can be established by the Structured Interview Guide for the Hamilton Depression Scale—Seasonal Affective Disorder Version (SIGH-SAD),[29]

> **BOX 56-4** *Elements of Inquiry in Assessing for Seasonal Affective Disorder (SAD)*
>
> SAD more likely:
> - Seasonal onset and offset of mood, cognitive and vegetative symptoms
> - Evidence of spring/summer-associated hypomania or mania
> - Presence of combined hyperphagia, weight gain, and hypersomnia
> - Anticipatory anxiety about fall and winter
> - Symptom relief from travel to warm sunny climates in winter
> - Cold intolerance
> - Family history of affective disorders and of alcoholism
>
> Nonseasonal depression more likely:
> - Skipped winters or year-round depressions
> - Annual conditions or anniversary reactions that might provoke fall or winter symptoms

---

> **BOX 56-5** *Seasonal Affective Disorder (SAD) Assessment Tools*
>
> - **Seasonal Pattern Assessment Questionnaire (SPAQ)**[13]: A six-item instrument to assess how a subject's mood and behavior change over months and seasons. Useful in initial assessment for suspected SAD. This questionnaire, which is in the public domain, can be copied freely.[13]
> - **Structured Interview Guide for the Hamilton Depression Rating Scale–Seasonal Affective Disorder Version (SIGH-SAD)**[30]: A 10-page structured interview guide, scorable to obtain a 21-item Hamilton depression score, an 8-item atypical symptoms score, a 29-item total score indicating severity of SAD, and an atypical balance score indicating what percentage of the total depression score is composed of atypical symptoms. Frequently used in SAD research studies to track symptoms over time, typically administered weekly.
> - **Beck Depression Inventory II (BDI-II)**[29]: A 21-item multiple-choice instrument for assessing severity of depression over the previous 2 weeks. Can be quickly completed by patients and used to track symptoms over time.

---

an interview instrument that is commonly utilized in SAD treatment studies. It yields a 29-item Total score, a 21-item Hamilton score, an 8-item Atypical symptoms score and—based on the 8-item divided by the 29-item scores—an Atypical Balance score. The Atypical Balance score represents the proportion of symptoms in the Total score which are considered "atypical" in major depression and which occur commonly in SAD: carbohydrate craving, increased eating and weight, hypersomnia and difficulty rising in the morning. The SIGH-SAD is also available in a self-report form.[30] The presence, and severity, of the depressive component of SAD can be assessed by the Beck Depression Inventory II (BDI-II).[31] The BDI-II and SIGH-SAD are suitable for repeated assessments to track changes in the severity of the disorder over time. The Fatigue Severity Scale is a self-administered inventory that tracks a common complaint in SAD; it may also be useful in assessing treatment progress.[32] Estimates of the optimal

To what degree do the following change <u>with the seasons</u>?
(CHECK ONE LINE ONLY FOR EACH QUESTION.)

	0 No change	1 Slight change	2 Moderate change	3 Marked change	4 Extremely marked change
A. Sleep length	—	—	—	—	—
B. Social activity	—	—	—	—	—
C. Mood (overall feeling of well-being)	—	—	—	—	—
D. Weight	—	—	—	—	—
E. Appetite	—	—	—	—	—
F. Energy level	—	—	—	—	—

Overall seasonality score: _____

7 points or less:	Seasonal problems unlikely
8-10 points:	"Winter blues" (S-SAD) likely
11 points or more:	SAD likely

Figure 56-1 Scoring for global seasonality scale. (From Rosenthal NE, Bradt GH, Wehr TA. *Seasonal Pattern Assessment Questionnaire.* Bethesda, MD: National Institute of Mental Health; 1987.)

time to schedule daily light therapy can be obtained with the Morningness-Eveningness Questionnaire.[33]

Summer SAD

Seasonal patterns of summer depression and winter remission have been identified, but summer SAD is less well studied than its winter counterpart. No diagnostic criteria for summer SAD are included in the DSM-IV-TR. An NIMH survey of seasonal changes in Maryland identified a 5:1 ratio of winter SAD to summer SAD.[34] Summer SAD is found more commonly in the southern United States and in other warm and humid climates than in temperate climates. In contrast to winter SAD, summer SAD sufferers report more typical depressive symptoms of appetite and sleep loss. The disorder may be triggered or worsened by heat and humidity or by exposure to intense light. It can be usefully treated with antidepressant medications, and some SAD sufferers respond well to travel to cold environments.[13,35]

MANAGEMENT

Bright Light Therapy

Bright light therapy has proved to be useful in treating SAD, S-SAD, and nonseasonal depression with winter exacerbation,[9] although more research is clearly needed to establish its efficacy in these conditions. Bright light therapy may be more helpful for the seasonal component of SAD than for the depressive component, but its use as adjunctive therapy in nonseasonal depressions has also been suggested.[36] In the case of SAD, well over 60 studies have examined its efficacy over placebo, including two quantitative meta-analyses of fluorescent light box studies and two large-sample studies.[18,19,37] Methodologic limitations, including the lack of a convincing control condition, affect many studies. Nevertheless, the response rate to bright light in SAD is generally considered to be about 65%.[9]

Initial descriptions of bright light therapy utilized various configurations of fluorescent white light tubes installed in a box behind a diffusing screen (Fig. 56-2). Intensity, or

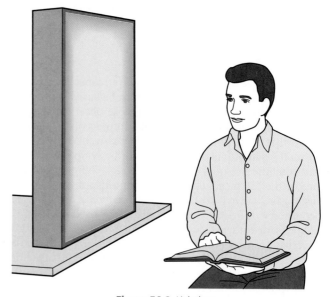

Figure 56-2 Light box.

illuminance, of visible light is measured in lux units, and the original light boxes emitted 2500 lux. In early SAD studies, subjects sat at a prescribed distance from a light box for 2 to 6 hours per day, usually in divided morning and evening doses. Treatment regimens were greatly modified with the findings that duration could be shortened as light illuminance was increased[38] and that morning light had benefits superior to evening light.[18] By the late 1980s it was also determined that filtering out ultraviolet wavelengths to reduce possible risks to retina and skin did not reduce the efficacy of white light therapy.[39] A typical current starting dose for light therapy is 30 minutes exposure to broadband white light (minus ultraviolet wavelengths) at 10,000 lux in the early morning. Such intensity appears very bright, compared to ordinary room light, but is considerably dimmer than natural outdoor illumination.[22] Lux measurements are a function of distance between the light source and the eye, and manufacturers of light units typically specify distances required to obtain

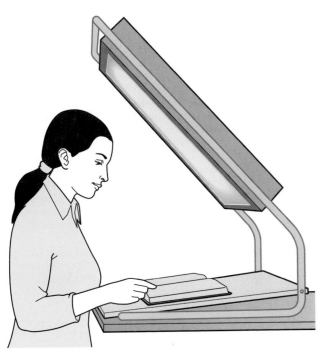

Figure 56-3 Work station light unit. (Adapted from the original artwork of Joan Krecjar and the Light Research Program of Thomas Jefferson University.)

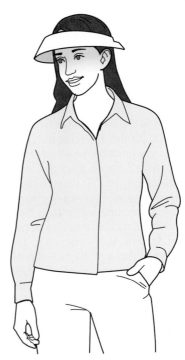

Figure 56-4 Light visor. (Adapted from the original artwork of Joan Krecjar and the Light Research Program of Thomas Jefferson University.)

ranges of illuminance of up to 10,000 lux. Though 30 minutes is a typical starting duration of light therapy, some patients achieve benefit with durations closer to 15 minutes while others may require durations of 45 or 60 minutes or longer.

Since early development of the "light box," alternate light fixture designs have been developed to illuminate a desk or table top with reflected light (Fig. 56-3), to provide smaller and more portable light units, including head-mounted light visors (Fig. 56-4), and to offer light sources with restricted bandwidths.

Light therapy has also been presented in "dawn simulation," or exposure to gradually increasing light beginning prior to wake time, sending a "dawn signal" to the brain even through closed eyelids (Fig. 56-5). Though somewhat more challenging to configure, dawn simulation outcomes have equaled or exceeded standard light therapy in at least two studies.[19,40]

Preliminary studies suggested the possibility that different portions of the visible spectrum may have different potency for treating SAD,[41,42] yet such a relationship has not been conclusively demonstrated. Rather, studies have focused on the effects of different wavelengths of light on levels of melatonin; the extent of melatonin suppression has not, however, been shown to be related to the extent of improvement in clinical SAD symptoms. Since the development of light-emitting diodes (LEDs), which can emit narrower bandwidths of light, studies of light wavelengths in SAD have become more feasible and more precise. Extensive studies have identified wavelengths in the blue part of the spectrum, between 446 to 477 nm, as most potent for suppressing melatonin in healthy humans.[43] Further, in healthy humans monochromatic blue light with a peak of 460 nm has been shown to have twice the potency in suppressing melatonin, inducing a circadian phase delay, and promoting alertness, performance and attention compared to monochromatic green light with a peak of 555 nm.[44,45]

Narrowband blue light also has shown promise in correcting SAD symptoms, based on a comparison with a dim red

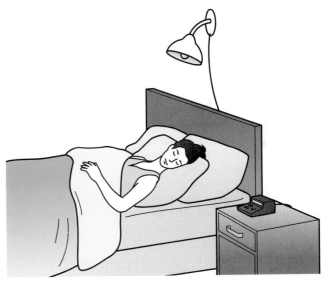

Figure 56-5 Dawn simulator. (Adapted from the original artwork of Joan Krecjar and the Light Research Program of Thomas Jefferson University.)

light placebo condition,[46] on a comparison with red light of similar visual intensity[47] and in comparison to an equal photon dose of broad bandwidth white light.[48] To date, however, broadband white light remains the most tested and most well established type of bright light therapy for SAD.

Bright light therapy is thought to be effective as well for the milder symptoms of S-SAD.[9] An uncontrolled study of 29 SAD subjects and 15 S-SAD subjects found similar response rates—64% to 69% for SAD and 40% to 67% for S-SAD—after 2 weeks of light therapy.[26]

A wide variety of light units have come onto the market, and patients may need some assistance sorting through alternative designs, prices, and claims for efficacy. A reliable nonprofit source of information for clinicians and the public includes the website for the Society of Light Treatment and Biological Rhythms (www.sltbr.org),[49] which lists a number of "corporate members" offering light units (though without specific endorsement from SLTBR). Ideally, white light units have adjustments for intensity and specify what distances between the light and the eye would produce intensities ranging from 2500 to 10,000 lux when the unit is set at maximum brightness. Some light units can be adjusted to aim light either directly at the patient's eye or toward a work surface, thus helpfully providing treatment via reflected light.

Patients may have to schedule an earlier than usual rising time to allow for a morning bright light treatment prior to their usual daily activities. This may also be beneficial for correcting phase delays in the sleep/wake cycle. Terman and associates[50,51] recommend that light therapy should begin no later than 8.5 hours after evening melatonin onset, which is impractical to determine in most treatment settings, or 2.5 hours from the midpoint of the sleep period, and they offer the Morningness-Eveningness Questionnaire as a tool for estimating the ideal light therapy start time, based on the patient's habitual retiring and rising times.[33] Patients should be reminded to stay at the recommended distance from the light source during the treatment period and glance at it frequently for a few seconds or, when the light is aimed at a work surface, to look more steadily toward this reflected light. Some patients will benefit from evening bright light therapy. Guidance about a schedule of evening light exposure can be based on convenience, as long as bright light therapy does not adversely affect nighttime sleep; some trial and error may be necessary to establish the ideal time for evening light therapy in individual cases.

Bright light therapy is generally continued on a daily basis until the springtime. Some patients find that they can skip one or more light treatment days with no relapse. Given a good response to light therapy, it can usefully be started in the early fall in subsequent years so that SAD symptoms can be forestalled. This is ideal for patients who can predict with some confidence when they will begin to feel seasonal depression or for whom SAD symptoms are particularly severe. Alternatively, patients who notice onset of symptoms only gradually can begin light therapy after the earliest symptoms of SAD have appeared. Bright light therapy procedures are summarized in Box 56-6.

Side Effects and Risks of Bright Light Therapy

Bright light therapy is relatively very safe. In a study in 1995, ophthalmologic examinations of SAD patients before and after short-term treatment and after 3 to 6 years of light therapy each fall and winter revealed no ocular abnormalities.[34] Subsequent years have not provided evidence of ocular risk to SAD patients using bright light therapy. Side effects of light therapy are rare and, if they occur, are mild and subside within a few days or, if necessary, with reductions in treatment times or light intensities. They are listed in Box 56-7.

Bright light therapy units generally filter out ultraviolet ranges of the light spectrum, thus reducing the risk of skin and retinal damage. Bright light therapy undertaken even over years appears to pose no risk to patients in good ocular health.[52] Nevertheless, caution and ophthalmologic consultation is advised in ocular conditions whose ocular manifestations can be exacerbated by bright light, including macular

---

BOX 56-6 *Bright Light Therapy Procedure*

- Determine if patient is using photosensitizing medications, has preexisting eye problems, or has a history of bipolar disorder. Consult prescribing physicians, ophthalmologist, or mental health provider if indicated.
- Prescribe 30 minutes of exposure to light at 10,000 lux, with no ultraviolet wavelengths, as close as possible to time of awakening, or have patient complete "Morningness Eveningness Questionnaire"[53] to determine a recommended light therapy start time. Patient's eyes should remain open but not staring fixedly at the light source.
- Monitor for early side effects; if present and persisting for more than 2 to 3 days, shorten duration of light therapy or reduce light intensity by dialing it down or increasing distance between patient and light unit.
- Hold treatment schedule steady for 1 week and assess for changes. If some improvement is noted, continue schedule. If no improvement is noted, increase time of exposure to 45 minutes or longer, in 15-minute increments.
- Continue to follow for 3 to 4 weeks.
    If good response, patient can continue with daily program until springtime.
    If no response, consider:
    - Increasing duration of exposure to 45 and then 60 minutes; or
    - Adding a period of evening light therapy; or
    - Switching to evening light therapy for 1 or more weeks
    - If patient reports too much advance of sleep phase, shorten duration of light therapy.
- Advise patient to begin light therapy in the following fall before the typical onset of symptoms, possibly for shorter periods at first.
- For patients unable or unwilling to schedule daily light therapy, consider dawn simulation or high-density negative ion treatment.
- If inadequate response to light therapy is noted, consider adding or altering antidepressant medication regimen.

BOX 56-7 *Side Effects of Bright Light Therapy for Seasonal Affective Disorder (SAD)**

Reported by 19% to 21% of subjects:
- Headache
- Eye or vision problem

Reported by 6% to 7% of subjects:
- Nausea or vomiting
- Hypomania or agitation
- Sedation

Reported by 1% to 3% of subjects:
- Dizziness
- Anxiety ("feeling wired")
- Irritability
- Tightness in chest

*In a series of 70 patients exposed to 10,000 lux 30 minutes per day for 5 days.

Data from Kogan AO, Guilford PM. Side effects of short-term 10,000-lux light therapy. Am J Psychiatry. 1998;155:293-294.

BOX 56-8 *Common Photosensitizing Medications*

- Lithium
- Phenothiazines (antipsychotics, antiemetics)
- Chloroquine (antimalarial drug)
- Hematoporphyrins (uses in treatment of cancer)
- 8-Methoxypsoralen (used in ultraviolet treatment for psoriasis)
- Melatonin
- Hypericum (St. John's wort)

Data from Lam RW, Levitt AJ, eds. *Canadian Consensus Guidelines for the Treatment of Seasonal Affective Disorder.* Vancouver, BC: Clinical and Academic Publishing; 1999.

---

degeneration, retinitis pigmentosa, glaucoma, diabetes mellitus, and systemic lupus erythematosus, and in patients who have recently undergone cataract surgery and lens removal. Light, especially that of the ultraviolet spectrum, can interact with photosensitizing medications and cause ocular injury; a partial list of these medications appears in Box 56-8.[9,11]

Full-blown manic episodes and hypomania have been reported in SAD patients treated with bright light, however.[53] As a result patients with bipolar disorder, especially those not well controlled by medication, and patients with or without bipolar disorder who report springtime episodes of mania or hypomania, should be closely followed, preferably by a psychiatrist, during initial periods of light therapy or at any time that manic or hypomanic symptoms emerge. Patients who seem at risk for being overenergized by light should be cautioned not to prolong treatment periods beyond what has been recommended and to report feeling overenergized, euphoric, excessively irritable, or sleepless immediately. In the event of such symptoms, diminishing exposure time or moving light therapy to the evening hours may be useful, and in extreme cases light therapy may have to be paused, discontinued, or supplemented with medication.

Case 1: Successful Treatment of SAD with Bright Light Therapy

"Emily" is a 50-year-old divorced woman who lives with her grown child and works as a store manager. She presents as a volunteer for a research study comparing bright blue light to dim red light in the treatment of SAD. She consents to the research study. She has a multiyear history of seasonal symptoms including irritability, feeling "down," depression, and anxiety. She also complains of fatigue and diminished motivation. Although she works full time, she spends much of her free time sleeping, stating that "I can't get anything done." Symptoms are seasonal, beginning in December, becoming most intense in January, and resolving in the spring. She has a history of depression, and about 10 years ago was treated with citalopram and fluoxetine, each for about 2 months, but both were discontinued because of side effects. She is currently free of psychiatric and other medical conditions and is on no medications.

Her global assessment of functioning (GAF) score for the worst week of the previous month is 53, suggesting moderately impairing mental health symptoms. Based on the Structured Clinical Interview for DSM Disorders (SCID) she meets criteria for major depressive disorder, melancholic, recurrent with seasonal pattern, of moderate severity. Her global seasonality score (GSS) on the SPAQ is 20 (on a scale of 0 to 24), with items endorsing "extremely marked change" on sleep length, mood (overall feeling of well-being), and weight; "marked change" on appetite and energy level; and "moderate change" on social activity.

By random selection she is assigned to therapy with narrowband bright blue light from an array of light-emitting diodes behind a diffusing screen. She is instructed to sit about 50 cm in front of the light unit for 45 minutes between 6 AM and 8 AM each morning for 3 weeks. The SIGH-SAD questionnaire is administered at baseline and at the end of each of the 3 treatment weeks.

These scores make clear her successful response to light, from points of view both of response and of remission. Response, defined as a final SIGH-SAD score of less than 50% of baseline, was achieved by the end of week 1. In addition, remission, defined as a final SIGH-SAD score of less than 8, was achieved by the end of week 2. The proportion of atypical symptoms remained unchanged by the end of week 3.

Emily's scores:

	Total SIGH-SAD score:		Atypical Balance score:	
Baseline:		31		58.1%
Week 1:		15		40.0%
Week 2:		6		83.3%
Week 3:		4		50.0%

Following study termination, she continues light therapy, using standard bright white light.

In a follow-up phone call made to her 6 years after her participation in the study, Emily states that she began taking Zoloft, 2 weeks on and 2 weeks off, for premenstrual dysphoric disorder (PMDD). She continues to find light "mandatory" to her well-being, however, and uses her light unit whenever her access to natural outdoor light is reduced.

This case and its follow-up illustrate the rapid response possible with light therapy, the efficacy of narrowband blue light in symptom reduction, the extended utility of bright white light therapy in successive years, and the therapeutic impact of natural outdoor light for people willing to spend time out of doors in the fall and winter.[54]

Medication Management

Psychopharmacology

Open-label trials of desipramine, tranylcypromine, reboxetine, and bupropion showed improvement with the drug therapy.[55] An open-label trial of escitalopram for SAD patients ($N = 20$) over 8 weeks produced a response rate of 95% (SIGH-SAD < 50% of baseline value) and a remission rate (SIGH-SAD score < 8) of 85%.[56] In an open-label trial of duloxetine, a serotinin-norepinephrine reuptake inhibitor, response rates were 80.8% and remission rates were 76.9% ($N = 26$).[57] Agomelatine, a novel antidepressant on the market so far only in Europe, acts as a melatonergic (MT$_1$ and MT$_2$) receptor agonist and a serotonin 5-HT$_{2C}$ receptor antagonist. In an uncontrolled study of 37 SAD patients over 14 weeks its use yielded a response rate in SAD sufferers of 75.7% and a remission rate of 70.3%. Progressive decrease of symptoms was noted during the second week onward, and only one adverse event (of mild fatigue) was noted.[58]

In various studies, fluoxetine has equaled or significantly outperformed placebo[59] in reducing SAD symptoms. Sertraline has also outperformed placebo in reducing depression scores and in response rates.[55,60] Citalopram significantly outperformed placebo in preventing recurrence of some depressive symptoms after a 1-week period of successful light therapy.[61]

In a multicenter SAD prevention study ($N = 1042$), bupropion XL significantly outperformed placebo in preventing development of symptoms from early autumn through the winter; recurrence rates were 15.7% in the bupropion group and 28% in the placebo group.[62]

Psychopharmacology versus Light Therapy

A multicenter double-blind, randomized, controlled trial over three winters in Canada compared light therapy 30 minutes per day to fluoxetine 20 mg per day for SAD sufferers ($N = 96$) over an 8-week period. Therapeutic effects of light therapy compared to fluoxetine were significantly greater at the end of week 1 but not at later points of comparison. Light therapy resulted in a significantly lower incidence of treatment-emergent adverse events of agitation and sleep disturbance. Both treatments were considered to be well tolerated, and similar percentages of patients reported at least one adverse event self-rated as severe: 33.3% of light-treated patients and 35.4% of fluoxetine-treated patients. Overall, both treatments showed symptom reduction over time, with each condition showing a 67% response rate. Differences in rates of remission were also nonsignificant; 50% of light-treated patients and 54% of fluoxetine-treated patients reached remission.[61]

A number of factors are generally considered in the choice of light therapy versus medication versus a combination treatment or novel treatment for SAD. The Canadian Consensus Guidelines[11] recommend that the decision for a first-line treatment consider factors such as severity of depression, anticipated side effects of treatment, safety, patient preference, patient compliance, and cost. One treatment regimen at a time should be used initially. Light therapy usually is effective in a shorter period of time than antidepressants, is inexpensive after an initial purchase of a light therapy unit, is simple to initiate and then taper off season after season, and appeals to patients who wish a more "natural" remedy. Light therapy and antidepressants may usefully be combined when a patient has had a partial response to either approach or when depression is severe, treatment-resistant, and associated with prolonged dysfunction.

Case 2: Combination Approach in Management of SAD

"Alice" is a 32-year-old married woman who presents in February with 3 years of "horrible" winter depression symptoms including low mood, poor concentration, lack of enjoyment or libido, social withdrawal, and poor self-image. She also complains of morning awakening, appetite decrease, and weight loss, also occurring during the winter months. Poor concentration, low energy, and deficits in memory and task prioritization make full-time work difficult for her. She denies suicidal ideation. She invariably feels well in spring and summer.

Her first depressive episode occurred in November 1998, 2 months after moving into a darker house. She tried light

therapy 1 year ago and noticed a slight improvement in symptoms. Her psychiatrist also treated her with sertraline, which was not effective, and was in the process of tapering it in preparation for a trial of bupropion at the time of presentation. She reports no depressive episodes prior to 3 years ago and denies a history of manic or hypomanic symptoms.

She is mildly overweight, yet denies a history of medical or other psychiatric conditions. She denies substance abuse but describes her father as an alcoholic. Alice agreed to begin 30 minutes of morning bright light therapy at 10,000 lux. After 10 days of no improvement she increases morning light to 45 minutes and adds 30 minutes of evening bright light, again with no benefit. Bupropion 150 mg twice a day is initiated after 1 month of ineffective bright light therapy, and she begins to feel better about 3 weeks later. This improved mood occurs in late March, several weeks earlier than the onset of improvement in the previous 2 years. The combined use of bright light therapy and an antidepressant makes uncertain the relative effectiveness of each form of treatment.

Following spring and summer remission, Alice discontinues bupropion in early July and resumes bright light therapy in September. However, in early October SAD symptoms return and persist despite increasing her exposure to daylight once or twice a day and the addition of evening bright light therapy and institution of cognitive behavior therapy. A cognitive behavior focus increases her awareness of automatic negative thoughts about the fall and winter, and she begins to resist inaction and to pursue personal goals. Bupropion, 400 mg per day, is added without improvement, yet symptoms resolve following a vacation to Florida. Nevertheless, she relapses quickly upon her return, prompting the addition of citalopram up to 80 mg per day with slight relief by late January and complete relief by early March.

This case illustrates the often persistent nature of SAD, its sometimes nonclassic symptom picture, the importance of persisting in efforts to maximize medication benefits, and the contribution of psychotherapy and a cognitive behavioral approach to ongoing treatment. As this case makes evident, light therapy sometimes fails; the subject's complaints of more typical nonseasonal symptoms of poor appetite and disturbed sleep may have predicted a less successful outcome of light therapy in her case. Light therapy predictably is more successful in patients presenting a classic SAD picture of carbohydrate craving, weight gain, and hypersomnia.

Negative Ion Therapy

An unanticipated treatment for SAD emerged from light therapy studies in which negative ion generators used as placebos appeared to have a therapeutic effect. Negative ions are molecules in the air which, because they contain an extra electron, are negatively charged. They are found in nature in association with sun, wind, and moving water, and they are a feature of some manufactured air purifiers. A SAD study employing negative ion generators as treatment devices found that high-density negative ions were superior to low-density negative ions. Percentage improvement in SIGH-SAD scores for the high-density negative ion group was 47.9% compared to 22.7% for the low-density negative ion group. Percentage improvement for the bright light treatment group was 57.1%.[63] Side effects of treatment with high-density ions (93 minutes per day for 3 weeks) was low, with 14.3% of subjects reporting drowsiness and appetite increase and 19% of subjects reporting weight gain. Given its status as a yet minor tool of SAD treatment, no rigorous effort to document treatment emergent side effects for air ionization treatment has been undertaken. An earlier study had shown that both bright light and high-density negative ion treatments appeared to act as specific antidepressants in SAD patients and reported that a careful monitoring of potential side effects of treatment with negative air ionization found no differences between high- and low-density groups.[37] Though having an apparent antidepressant effect, no optimum timing or dose of air ionization has been established, nor is the mechanism of action known. Along with dawn simulation and antidepressant medication, high-density ionization has been recommended as a treatment alternative when bright light treatment is impractical, ineffective, or not well tolerated.[63]

Cognitive Behavior Therapy

Rohan and associates,[64] in a series of studies, developed a psychotherapeutic approach to SAD treatment using strategies of cognitive behavior therapy (CBT).[64] CBT has been used effectively to treat nonseasonal depression.[65] It is typically a time-limited approach aiming to provide patients with awareness and skills that produce enduring results. Rohan developed a CBT protocol to offer to SAD subjects in groups during the winter season. Subjects ($N = 69$) were randomly assigned to this CBT program, to light therapy, to a combination treatment (CBT + light therapy), and to a minimum-contact control group. Treatments were held concurrently during a 6-week period. On the outcome measures of the SIGH-SAD and the Beck Depression Inventory-II (BDI-II), the scores of all three active treatments groups but not the control group, showed significant reduction in symptoms between pre- and post-treatment. Although the results of CBT alone were impressive, especially because subject expectations were lowest for CBT, the authors reported that only the combined CBT plus light therapy treatment resulted in a statistically larger proportion of SIGH-SAD remissions compared to the control group. For practitioners wishing to incorporate CBT into SAD treatment, therapist and participant guides based on this CBT program are available.[66]

Although the results of Rohan's group CBT for SAD patients are impressive, the effort to recruit, screen, and admit patients to groups may not be practical for many locales or provider practices. Even so, the CBT focus on practicing self-awareness and actively coping with seasonal symptoms may be usefully incorporated into the care of individual SAD patients whether light, medication or a combination or novel treatment is delivered.

Finally, Box 56-9 lists additional information and resources regarding SAD.

SUMMARY

Seasonal affective disorder, though a relative newcomer to psychiatric nosology, is related to observations about human responses to light and to seasons and was described at least as early as the age of Hippocrates.[5] Light is the basic empowering force of life for diverse species, ranging from the simplest single-celled plankton to highly complex organisms. Light therapy, at proper illuminances and at correct circadian timing, has been demonstrated to be corrective for SAD. Further work is needed to identify the most effective wavelengths of light for reversing SAD symptoms. Multiple studies reveal that SAD is multidimensional, having both common elements and divergent aspects in its clinical presentations. At this stage of our understanding, treatment planning can best proceed by considering the likely impact of light therapy along with the therapeutic alternatives of medication, negative ion treatment, and psychotherapy.

Acknowledgments

The authors gratefully acknowledge John Kemp for his able assistance in obtaining reference materials, Benjamin Warfield, MFA, for assistance in obtaining elements of the figure, and John Kemp and Melissa Ayer, MS, for carefully editing the final draft.

Both authors are supported by the National Space Biomedical Research Institute under NASA NCC 9-58 and NASA Grant #NNX09AM68G. GCB is also supported by the Institute of Integrative Medicine Scholars Program. We acknowledge with gratitude the SAD patients who generously consented to having their case studies presented here.

BOX 56-9 *Seasonal Affective Disorder (SAD) Information and Treatment Resources*

- **Society for Light Treatment and Biological Rhythms: www.sltbr.org**
- **Center for Environmental Therapeutics: www.cet.org**
- **Lam RW, Levitt AJ, eds.** *Canadian Consensus Guidelines for the Treatment of Seasonal Affective Disorder.* **Vancouver, BC: Clinical and Academic Publishing; 1999.**
- **Rosenthal NE.** *Winter blues: Everything You Need to Know to Beat Seasonal Affective Disorder.* **New York: Guilford Press; 2006**

Data from Rohan KJ. *Coping with the Seasons: A Cognitive-Behavioral Approach to Seasonal Affective Disorder. Therapist Guide and Participant Workbook.* Oxford, England: Oxford University Press; 2009.

REFERENCES

1. Lewy AJ, Wehr TA, Goodwin FK, et al. Light suppresses melatonin secretion in humans. *Science.* 1980;210(4475):1267-1269.
2. Lewy AJ, Kern HE, Rosenthal NE, et al. Bright artificial light treatment of a manic-depressive patient with a seasonal mood cycle. *Am J Psychiatry.* 1982;139(11):1496-1498.
3. Rosenthal NE, Sack DA, Gillin JC, et al. Seasonal affective disorder. A description of the syndrome and preliminary findings with light therapy. *Arch Gen Psychiatry.* 1984;41(1):72-80.
4. American Psychiatric Association. *Diagnostic and Statistical Manual of Mental Disorders.* 4th ed. Washington, DC: American Psychiatric Association; 2000.
5. Rosenthal NE. Issues for DSM-V: Seasonal affective disorder and seasonality (editorial). *Am J Psychiatry.* 2009;166(8):852.
6. Kaplan KA, Harvey AG. Hypersomnia across mood disorders: A review and synthesis. *Sleep Med Rev.* 2009;13:275-285.
7. American Academy of Sleep Medicine. *International Classification of Sleep Disorders: Diagnostic and Coding Manual.* 2nd ed. Westchester, IL: American Academy of Sleep Medicine; 2005.
8. Sohn CH, Lam RW. Treatment of seasonal affective disorder: Unipolar versus bipolar differences. *Curr Psychiatry Rep.* 2004;6(6):478-485.
9. Lam RW, Levitt AJ, eds. *Canadian Consensus Guidelines for the Treatment of Seasonal Affective Disorder.* Vancouver, BC: Clinical and Academic Publishing; 1999.
10. Rosenthal NE, Bradt GH, Wehr TA. *Seasonal Pattern Assessment Questionnaire.* Bethesda, MD: National Institute of Mental Health; 1987.
11. Rosen LN, Targum SD, Terman M, et al. Prevalence of seasonal affective disorder at four latitudes. *Psychiatry Res.* 1990;31:131-144.
12. Mersch PPA, Middendorp HM, Bouhuys AL, et al. Seasonal affective disorder and latitude: A review of the literature. *J Affect Disord.* 1999;53:35-48.

13. Rosenthal NE. *Winter Blues: Everything You Need to Know to Beat Seasonal Affective Disorder.* New York: The Guilford Press; 2006.

14. Schwartz PJ, Brown C, Wehr TA, et al. Winter seasonal affective disorder: A follow-up study of the first 59 patients of the National Institute of Mental Health Seasonal Studies Program. *Am J Psychiatry.* 1996;153(8):1028-1036.

15. Lam RW, Tam EM, Yatham LN, et al. Seasonal depression: The dual vulnerability hypothesis revisited. *J Affect Disord.* 2001;63(1-3):123-132.

16. Young MA, Meaden PM, Fogg LF, et al. Which environmental variables are related to the onset of seasonal affective disorder? *J Abnorm Psychol.* 1997;106(4):554-562.

17. Eastman CI, Young MA, Fogg LF, et al. Bright light treatment of winter depression: A placebo-controlled trial. *Arch Gen Psychiatry.* 1998;55(10):883-889.

18. Lewy AJ, Bauer VK, Cutler NL, et al. Morning vs. evening light treatment of patients with winter depression. *Arch Gen Psychiatry.* 1998;55(10):890-896.

19. Terman JS, Terman M, Lo ES, et al. Circadian time of morning light administration and therapeutic response in winter depression. *Arch Gen Psychiatry.* 2001;58:69-75.

20. Lewy AJ, Lefler BJ, Emens JS, et al. The circadian basis of winter depression. *Proc Natl Acad Sci U S A.* 2006;103:7414-7419.

21. Doghramji K, Gaddy JR, Stewart KT, et al. 2- versus 4-hour evening phototherapy of seasonal affective disorder. *J Clin Psychiatry.* 1991;52(5):213-216.

22. Wirz-Justice A, Graw P, Krauchi K, et al. "Natural" light treatment of seasonal affective disorder. *J Affect Disord.* 1996;27(2-3):109-120.

23. Murray G, Michalak EE, Levitt AJ, et al. Therapeutic mechanism in seasonal affective disorder: Do fluoxetine and light operate through advancing circadian phase? *Chronobiol Int.* 2005;22(5):937-943.

24. Sohn CH, Lam RW. Update on the biology of seasonal affective disorder. *CNS Spectr.* 2005;10(8):635-646.

25. Levitan RD. The chronobiology and neurobiology of winter seasonal affective disorder. *Dialogues Clin Neurosci.* 2007;9(3):315-324. Available at http://www.dialogues-cns.org.

26. Levitt AJ, Lam RW, Levitan R. A comparison of open treatment of seasonal major and minor depression with light therapy. *J Affect Disord.* 2002;71(1-3):243-248.

27. Sullivan B, Payne TW. Affective disorders and cognitive failures: A comparison of seasonal and nonseasonal depression. *Am J Psychiatry.* 2007;164:1663-1667.

28. Pendse BP, Engstrom G, Traskman-Bendz L. Psychopathology of seasonal affective disorder patients in comparison with major depression patients who have attempted suicide. *J Clin Psychiatry.* 2004;65:322-327.

29. Williams JBW, Link MJ, Rosenthal NE, et al. *Structured Interview Guide for the Hamilton Depression Rating Scale. Seasonal Affective Disorder Version (SIGH-SAD),* New York: State Psychiatric Institute; 2002.

30. Williams JBW, Link MJ, Terman M. *Seasonal Affective Disorder Version—Self-Rating Version (SIGH-SAD-SR). Structured Interview Guide for the Hamilton Depression Rating Scale.* New York: State Psychiatric Institute; 1998.

31. Beck AT, Steer RA, Brown GK. Beck Depression Inventory II. Upper Saddle River, NJ: Pearson Education, Inc; 1996. Available at www.pearson assessments.com.

32. Krupps LB. *Fatigue severity scale. National Women's Health Resource Center.* 2010. Available at http://www.healthywomen.org/content/article/fatigue-severity-scale-fss.

33. Center for Environmental Therapeutics. Available at www.cet.org. Assessed Sept. 2010;12.

34. Kasper S, Wehr TA, Bartko JJ, et al. Epidemiological findings of seasonal changes in mood and behavior. A telephone survey of Montgomery County. *Maryland. Arch Gen Psychiatry.* 1989;46(9):823-833.

35. Wehr TA, Sack DA, Rosenthal NE. Seasonal affective disorder with summer depression and winter hypomania. *Am J Psychiatry.* 1987;144(12):1602-1603.

36. Martiny K. Adjunctive bright light in non-seasonal major depression. *Acta Psychiat Scand Suppl.* 2004;425:7-28.

37. Terman M, Terman JS, Ross DC. A controlled trial of timed bright light and negative air ionization for treatment of winter depression. *Arch Gen Psychiatry.* 1998;55(10):875-882.

38. Terman JS, Terman M, Schlager D, et al. Efficacy of brief, intense light exposure for treatment of winter depression. *Psychopharmacol Bull.* 1990;26:3-11.

39. Lam RW, Buchanan A, et al. The effects of ultraviolet-A wavelengths in light therapy for seasonal depression. *J Affect Disord.* 1992;24(4):237-243.

40. Avery DH, Eder DN, Bolte MA, et al. Dawn simulation and bright light in the treatment of SAD: A controlled study. *Biol Psychiatry.* 2001;50(3):205-216.

41. Brainard GC, Sherry D, Skwerer RG, Waxler M, Kelly K, Rosenthal NE. Effects of different wavelengths in seasonal affective disorder. *J Affect Disord.* 1990;20(4):209-216.

42. Oren DA, Brainard GC, Johnston SH, Joseph-Vanderpool JR, Sorek E, Rosenthal NE. Treatment of seasonal affective disorder with green light and red light. *Am J Psychiatry.* 1991;148(4):509-511.

43. Brainard CG, Hanifin JP, Greeson JM, et al. Action spectrum for melatonin regulation in humans: Evidence for a novel circadian photoreceptor. *J Neurosci.* 2001;21:6405-6412.

44. Lockley SW, Brainard GC, Czeisler CA. High sensitivity of the human circadian melatonin rhythm to resetting by short wavelength light. *J Clin Endocrinol Metab.* 2003;88(9):4502-4505.

45. Lockley SW, Evans EE, Scheer F, et al. Short-wavelength sensitivity for the direct effects of light on alertness, vigilance, and the waking electroencephalogram in humans. *Sleep.* 2006;29(2):161-168.

46. Glickman G, Byrne B, Pineda C, et al. Light therapy for seasonal affective disorder with blue arrow-band light-emitting diodes (LED). *Biol Psychiatry.* 2006;59(6):502-507.

47. Strong RE, Marchant BK, Reimherr FW, et al. Narrow-band blue-light treatment of seasonal affective disorder in adults and the influence of additional nonseasonal symptoms. *Depress Anxiety.* 2009;26:273-278.

48. Anderson JL, Glod CA, Dai J, et al. Lux vs. wavelength in light treatment of seasonal affective disorder. *Acta Psychiatr Scand.* 2009;120(3):203-212.

49. Society for Light Treatment and Biological Rhythms. Available at: www.sltbr.org. Accessed April 11, 2010.

50. Terman JS, Terman M, Lo ES, et al. Circadian time of morning light administration and therapeutic response in winter depression. *Arch Gen Psychiatry.* 2001;58(1):69-75.

51. Terman M, White TM, Jacob J. Automated Morningness-Eveningness Questionnaire. New York: State Psychiatric Institute; 2002. Available at: www.cet.org. Accessed April 11, 2010.

52. Gallin PF, Terman M, Reme CE, et al. Ophthalmologic examination of patients with seasonal affective disorder, before and after bright light therapy. *Am J Ophthalmol.* 1995;119:202-210.

53. Chan KY, Lam RW, Perry KF. Mania precipitated by light therapy for patients with SAD. *J Clin Psychiatry.* 1994;55:454.

54. Wirz-Justice A, Graw P, Krauchi K, et al. "Natural" light treatment of seasonal affective disorder. *J Affect Disord.* 1996;27:109-120.

55. Westrin A, Lam RW. Seasonal affective disorder: A clinical update. *Ann Clin Psychiatry.* 2007;19(4):239-246.

56. Pjrek E, Winkler D, Stastny J, et al. Escitalopram in seasonal affective disorder: Results of an open trial. *Pharmacopsychiatry.* 2007;40(1):20-24.

57. Pjrek E, Winkler D, Praschak-Rieder N, et al. Treatment of seasonal affective disorder with duloxetine: An open-label study. *Pharmacopsychiatry.* 2008;41:100-105.

58. Pjrek E, Winkler D, Konstantinidis A, et al. Agomelatine in the treatment of seasonal affective disorder. *Psychopharmacology.* 2007;190(4):575-579.

59. Lam RW, Gorman CP, Michalon M, et al. Multicenter, placebo-controlled study of fluoxetine in seasonal affective disorder. *Am J Psychiatry.* 1995;152:1765-1770.

60. Lam RW, Levitt AJ, Levitan AJ, et al. The Can-SAD study: A randomized controlled trial of the effectiveness of light therapy and fluoxetine in patients with winter seasonal affective disorder. *Am J Psychiatry.* 2006;163:805-812.

61. Martiny K, Lunde M, Simonsen C, et al. Relapse prevention by citalopram in SAD patients responding to 1 week of light therapy. A placebo-controlled study. *Acta Psychiatr Scand.* 2004;109:230-234.

62. Modell JG, Rosenthal NE, Harriett AE, et al. Seasonal affective disorder and its prevention by anticipatory treatment with bupropion XL. *Biol Psychiatry.* 2005;58:658-667.

63. Terman M, Terman J. Controlled trial of naturalistic dawn simulation and negative air ionization for seasonal affective disorder. *Am J Psychiatry.* 2006;163:2126-2133.

64. Rohan KJ, Roecklein KA, Lacy TJ, et al. Winter depression recurrence one year after cognitive-behavioral therapy, light therapy, or combination treatment. *Behav Ther.* 2009;40:225-238.

65. Beck AT, Rush JA, Shaw BF, et al. *Cognitive Therapy of Depression.* New York: Guilford Press; 1979.

66. Rohan KJ. *Coping with the Seasons: A Cognitive-Behavioral Approach to Seasonal Affective Disorder.* Oxford: Oxford University Press; 2009.

Schizophrenia and Its Associated Sleep Disorders

Chapter 57

KATHLEEN L. BENSON

EPIDEMIOLOGIC OVERVIEW

Schizophrenia is one of the most devastating and costly mental disorders. Although recent decades have seen advancements in pharmacologic treatment, schizophrenia is still neither preventable nor curable. Schizophrenia has an early onset and patients can anticipate lifelong mental disability and suffering as well as social and economic marginalization. In addition to the immense human cost, schizophrenia is also associated with costs of higher morbidity and mortality rates. Epidemiologic studies of schizophrenia suggest estimates of both prevalence and incidence.[1] Mean lifetime prevalence has been estimated at 5.5 cases per 1000 population. Incidence, or annual new case appearance, has been estimated at 15.9 cases per 100,000 population. Incidence estimates broadly taken suggest that schizophrenia is more common in males than females, with a male-to-female ratio of 1.4, or three men for every two women affected. Finally, all-cause mortality estimates suggest that schizophrenics have a two- to threefold increased risk of dying, with a large portion of this increased mortality rate due to suicide.

DIAGNOSIS

Popular culture frequently misconstrues *schizophrenia* as "split personality" or "multiple personality." In actuality, the term *schizophrenia* represents the splitting or disintegration of normal thought processes such that cognitive impairment or formal thought disorder is believed to be the fundamental or defining symptom of the illness. The American Psychiatric Association is the recognized source of the current clinical criteria used to diagnose schizophrenia. These criteria listed in the *Diagnostic and Statistical Manual of Mental Disorder*, Fourth Edition (DSM-IV)[2] are presented in Box 57-1. The characteristic or defining symptoms of the illness are defined within Criterion A and encompass two main categories: positive symptoms and negative symptoms. Positive symptoms reflect a "psychotic dimension" that includes hallucinations and delusions and a "disorganization dimension" that includes disorganized speech and catatonic behavior. Negative symptoms include affective flattening ("restrictions in the range and intensity of emotional expression"), avolition ("restrictions in the initiation of goal-directed behavior"), and poverty of speech ("restrictions in the fluency and productivity of thought and speech"). Diagnostic Criterion B specifies an overlapping marked deterioration in occupational and social functioning. Schizophrenia is also a diagnosis of exclusion because psychotic disturbances attributable to a variety of medical, psychiatric and substance abuse disorders must be eliminated.

COURSE AND OUTCOME

The course and outcome of schizophrenia as presented here have been synthesized and summarized from a variety of sources.[3-6] The onset of schizophrenia typically occurs in the late teens through the middle thirties. The onset may be abrupt or can begin with a slowly developing prodromal phase associated with subtle changes in behavior, mild thought disorder, and social withdrawal. The active phase may ensue with the presentation of positive symptoms such as hallucinations and delusions. Although active symptoms may recur episodically (relapse or acute exacerbation), some amount of psychoticism usually persists during the waning or residual phase of the illness. In the long run, positive symptoms may decline, but negative symptoms such as affective flattening and avolition may increase with the progression of the disease.

Although it is commonly assumed that the diagnosis of schizophrenia is synonymous with a negative outcome, for most patients advances in pharmacologic treatment have resulted in fewer and briefer hospitalizations. Overviews of long-term studies[4-6] suggest that 18% to 27% of patients may even have a full recovery, while another 20% may remain seriously impaired or require long-term institutionalization. About 50% to 60% may recover to levels at which they can function occupationally and socially but may require outpatient interventions or rehospitalization with any subsequent relapse.

Prognostic indicators of better outcome include more acute onset, episodic course, female sex, and lack of family history of schizophrenia. Poorer outcomes have been linked to poor premorbid functioning, baseline negative symptoms, longer duration of no treatment, as well as the presence at onset of neurologic soft signs.[4-6]

ETIOLOGIC FACTORS

Although the etiology of schizophrenia remains unknown, risk factors associated with the development of the disease include both genetic and environmental factors. Schizophrenia is clearly familial. Family, twin, and adoption studies provide strong evidence that schizophrenia is highly heritable. Meta-analysis of twin studies has examined the impact of genes and environment on liability to schizophrenia and estimated genetic heritability to be 81% and shared environmental influences to be 11%.[7] Genome-wide association studies suggest that the genetic architecture of schizophrenia may include multiple common variants, each of small effect but acting together to increase the risk of developing the disease; genetic

> **BOX 57-1** *DSM-IV Diagnostic Criteria for Schizophrenia*

A. *Characteristic symptoms:* Two (or more) of the following, each present for a significant portion of time during a 1-month period (or less if successfully treated):
1. Delusions
2. Hallucinations
3. Disorganized speech (e.g., frequent derailment or incoherence)
4. Grossly disorganized or catatonic behavior
5. Negative symptoms (i.e., affective flattening, alogia, or avolition)

NOTE: Only one Criterion A symptom is required if delusions are bizarre or hallucinations consist of a voice keeping up a running commentary on the person's behavior or thoughts, or two or more voices conversing with each other.

B. *Social/occupational dysfunction:* For a significant portion of the time since the onset of the disturbance, one or more major areas of functioning such as work, interpersonal relations, or self-care are markedly below the level achieved before the onset (or when the onset is in childhood or adolescence, failure to achieve expected level of interpersonal, academic, or occupational achievement).

C. *Duration:* Continuous signs of the disturbance persist for at least 6 months. This 6-month period must include at least 1 month of symptoms (or less if successfully treated) that meet Criterion A (i.e., active-phase symptoms) and may include periods of prodromal or residual symptoms. During these prodromal or residual symptom periods, the signs of the disturbance may be manifested by only negative symptoms or two or more symptoms listed in Criterion A presented in an attenuated form (e.g., odd beliefs, unusual perceptual experiences).

D. *Schizoaffective disorder/mood disorder exclusion:* Schizoaffective disorder and mood disorder with psychotic features have been ruled out because either (1) no major depressive, manic, or mixed episodes have occurred concurrently with the active-phase symptoms; or (2) if mood episodes have occurred during active-phase symptoms, their total duration has been brief relative to the duration of the active and residual symptom periods.

E. *Substance/general medical condition exclusion:* The disturbance is not due to the direct physiologic effects of a substance (e.g., a drug of abuse, a medication) or a general medical condition.

F. *Relationship to a pervasive developmental disorder:* If there is a history of autistic disorder or another pervasive developmental disorder, the additional diagnosis of schizophrenia is made only if prominent delusions or hallucinations are also present for at least 1 month (or less if successfully treated).

DSM-IV, Diagnostic and Statistical Manual of Mental Disorders, 4th ed. Modified with permission from the American Psychiatric Association: Diagnostic and Statistical Manual of Mental Disorders, 4th ed. Washington, DC, American Psychiatric Press, 2000.

Environmental factors that might play a role in the etiology of schizophrenia include obstetric complications (e.g., premature birth, low birth weight, preeclampsia, and hypoxia) as well as prenatal or gestational exposure to infection. Seasonality of birth, with winter-spring births as a risk factor for schizophrenia, suggests that maternal influenza infection during pregnancy might compromise fetal brain development. Exposure to other microbial infections (e.g., toxoplasmosis and genitourinary diseases) during the gestational period might also compromise neurodevelopment. Although infections might have direct effects on the fetus, it is more likely that the mother's immune response to the infection (production of serum antibodies and cytokines) might contribute even more directly to developmental brain damage.[9] Although family history and environmental factors may be viewed as separate but contributory risk factors, there is strong evidence that genetic risk and prenatal exposure to infection might interact synergistically to elevate the risk of developing schizophrenia.[10] Both etiologic factors—genetic risk and environmental exposure to prenatal infection—are consistent with the prevailing model, which views schizophrenia as a neurodevelopmental disorder.[11,12]

PATHOPHYSIOLOGY

Although decades of study have revealed a wide range of pathology, there is no *specific* laboratory finding diagnostic of schizophrenia. Documented abnormalities[2,5,6,13,14] include a wide range of neuropsychologic and cognitive deficits in such areas as attention, memory, and psychomotor abilities; neurophysiologic deficits in perception and processing of sensory stimuli such as abnormalities in smooth pursuit eye movements and evoked potentials; brain structural abnormalities such as ventricular enlargement, decreased volumes of gray and white matter, decreased thalamic volume, and focal abnormalities of temporal lobe regions; functional brain abnormalities such as reduced metabolic activity of the prefrontal region (hypofrontality); and widespread abnormalities of neuronal synchrony and circuitry.

Documented abnormalities of several neurotransmitter systems have also been published, but investigations of the dopamine (DA) system have been the most extensive. Such investigations were driven by two early observations: first, the potency of antipsychotic (AP) medication correlates with their degree of DA D_2 receptor blockade; and second, DA-enhancing drugs such as amphetamines can mimic paranoid schizophrenia. Broadly speaking, the DA hypothesis, as currently conceptualized, attributes schizophrenia to an imbalance between subcortical and cortical DA systems with hyperstimulation of subcortical mesolimbic DA D_2 receptors associated with positive symptoms and understimulation of prefrontal cortex DA D_1 receptors associated with negative symptoms and cognitive impairment.[15]

CHARACTERISTIC SLEEP PATTERNS

Abnormal sleep patterns also rank as one of the major pathophysiologic findings in schizophrenia. Typically, marked sleep disruption accompanies the presence of psychotic symptoms with psychotic agitation being associated with periods of total sleeplessness. When psychotic symptoms are less severe, sleep patterns are frequently characterized by a pronounced insomnia—long sleep onset latencies, reduced total sleep time

architecture may also include highly penetrant, individually rare variants.[8] Because the concordance rate for monozygotic twins only approaches 50%, genetic makeup alone is not sufficient for the development of schizophrenia, and nongenetic or sporadic forms of the disorder must exist.

(TST), and sleep fragmented by episodes of waking. Furthermore, the onset of relapse is often signaled by an increasing insomnia.[16] In addition, clinically stable, medicated patients subjectively report sleep disturbance, notably early and middle insomnia.[17] Often schizophrenics sleep during the day and remain awake at night; these sleep-wake reversals correlate with subjective complaints of poor sleep quality.[18] Poor sleep quality is also related to a higher incidence of nightmares.[19] Co-morbid alcohol and substance abuse, not uncommon in schizophrenia, also disturb sleep and may precipitate relapse.

In contrast to subjective reports, objective assessments of sleep patterns have been derived from overnight in-laboratory polysomnographic (PSG) study. Although these PSG studies have differed in many respects such as protocol design, patient characteristics (e.g., age, medication status and history, as well as clinical features and history), type of control group, sample size and related statistical power, and algorithms to quantify sleep parameters, they have revealed a wide range of dyssomnias that are consistent with subjective complaints. In the next section, the discussion highlights some of the major PSG findings and refers the reader to more comprehensive reviews.[20-22]

Measures of Sleep Maintenance

- *Poor sleep efficiency* is defined as a reduction in TST relative to time in bed.[21]
- Early, middle, and late insomnia is seen, with sleep onset insomnia being the most typically reported.[17,21]
- Residual insomnia has been reported in patients maintained on antipsychotic medication.[17,21]
- A resurgence of more severe insomnia is one of the prodromal signs of impeding psychotic relapse and is frequently the result of the discontinuation of antipsychotic medication.[16]

Abnormalities of NREM Sleep

- Slow wave sleep (SWS) is that portion of non–rapid eye movement (NREM) sleep characterized by high-amplitude, low-frequency brain waves.
- SWS deficits are frequently, but not consistently, observed in PSG recordings of schizophrenic patients.[22]
- Although prior exposure to, or withdrawal from, AP medications has been advanced to explain these inconsistencies, SWS deficits have been observed in first episode, AP-naive patients with schizophrenia.[23]
- Studies of total sleep deprivation in healthy subjects have shown that SWS increases in proportion to the amount of prior waking.[24]
- The homeostatic model of SWS was advanced by Feinberg[25] in 1974 and maintains that a homeostatic drive builds up during waking and dissipates in SWS across successive NREM sleep cycles. Thus, the SWS homeostatic response might serve a restorative role in the central nervous system.
- SWS deficits might mean that the integrity of homeostatic regulatory mechanism and its related restorative functions are impaired in schizophrenia.
- On a theoretical level, SWS deficits may be associated with possible microstructural brain abnormalities. Consistent with schizophrenia as neurodevelopmental disorder, Feinberg[26] has proposed that schizophrenia

may result from excess synaptic pruning, that is, a malfunction in the normal maturational process of synaptic elimination during the second decade of life. Excess synaptic pruning would result in less capability for synchronous electroencephalographic (EEG) slow wave activity and a resulting SWS deficit.[26]

REM Sleep Onset Latency

- *Rapid eye movement (REM) sleep onset latency* is defined as the elapsed time between sleep onset and the onset of the first REM sleep period, alternatively viewed as the length of the first NREM sleep period.
- Significantly shortened REM latencies have been observed in approximately one half of studies comparing the sleep of unmedicated patients with schizophrenia to that of nonpsychiatric and psychiatric control subjects.[22]
- Shortened REM latencies may be the result of an active advance of REM sleep mechanisms.[22]
- Shortened REM latencies may also reflect the passive advance of the first REM sleep period due to SWS deficits in the first NREM period.[27]

REM Sleep Time and REM Sleep Eye Movement Activity

- Relative to nonpsychiatric control subjects, REM sleep time in patients with schizophrenia is neither significantly augmented nor reduced.[20,21]
- Both visual and computer-automated scoring of REM sleep eye movements have shown no differences in REM sleep eye movement density between schizophrenics, nonpsychiatric control subjects, and patients with major depressive disorder, a psychiatric control group.[28,29]

PHARMACOLOGIC TREATMENT

Broadly stated, most patients diagnosed with schizophrenia are treated with one or more AP agents (Box 57-2). An expansive review of these agents is beyond the scope of this chapter; however, the reader is referred to other sources such as Miyamoto and associates[30] to explicate their chemical designs and receptor binding profiles, which in turn are associated with differential side effects and clinical outcome.

First-Generation Antipsychotics

First-generation antipsychotics (FGAs) came into use in the 1950s with the introduction of chlorpromazine, the first recognized AP agent. This introduction not only shifted treatment regimens from practices such as electroconvulsive therapy and psychosurgery to psychopharmacology, but also made possible the large-scale deinstitutionalization of patients with schizophrenia. Following the release of chlorpromazine, other FGAs were approved for the treatment of schizophrenia.

What the FGAs have in common is a high affinity for binding to the DA D_2 postsynaptic receptor. DA receptor occupancy by FGAs not only predicts their therapeutic response, but also predicts their adverse effects. These effects include extrapyramidal side effects (EPS) such as akathisia, dystonia,

BOX 57-2 *First- and Second-Generation Antipsychotics*

Agent	Usual Adult Daily Maintenance Dose (mg)	Elimination Half-Life (hr)
First-Generation Antipsychotics		
Chlorpromazine (Thorazine)	50-400	16-30
Fluphenazine (Prolixin)	1-15	15-30
Haloperidol (Haldol)	1-15	12-36
Perphenazine (Trilafon)	8-24	8-20
Thioridazine (Mellaril)	50-400	7-20
Thiothixene (Navrane)	6-30	10-20
Trifluoperazine (Stelazine)	4-30	10-20
Second-Generation Antipsychotics		
Aripiprazole (Abilify)	10-30	75
Clozapine (Clozaril)	200-600	6-26
Olanzapine (Zyprexa)	5-20	21-54
Paliperidone (Invega)	6-12	23
Quetiapine (Seroquel)	150-750	6
Risperidone (Risperdal)	2-8	3-20
Ziprasidone (Geodon)	80-160	4-10

and parkinsonism. A more damaging side effect linked to D_2 receptor blockade is tardive dyskinesia (TD). The FGAs may also be associated with a rare but potentially fatal side effect called the neuroleptic malignant syndrome. Furthermore, the FGAs are associated to varying degrees with cholinergic side effects, including sedation, changes in blood pressure and myocardial conduction, sexual dysfunction, and weight gain. These FGA-associated side effects are one of the principal reasons for treatment noncompliance. Finally, the mechanism of action of FGAs needs further explication because the gradual onset of their therapeutic efficacy is not consistent with their rapid blockade of DA D_2 receptors.

Second-Generation Antipsychotics

The development of the second-generation antipsychotics (SGAs) was motivated by several factors: (a) many patients with chronic schizophrenia had an inadequate response to traditional FGA treatment; (b) although FGAs were successful in treating positive symptoms, they appeared less successful in treating negative symptoms; and (c) FGA-associated side effects such as EPS and TD were, as mentioned previously, a source of noncompliance and difficult management issues. Between 1989 and 2006, seven SGAs were approved by the FDA for the treatment of schizophrenia. In contrast to the FGAs, the SGAs have a broader spectrum of activity with differential effects on DA, serotonin (5-HT), and α-adrenergic, cholinergic, and histaminic receptors, as well as the various subtypes of the aforementioned neurotransmitters. Relative to the FGAs, the SGAs are characterized by weaker affinity for the DA D_2 receptor and stronger affinity for 5-HT receptors, particularly the $5-HT_{2A}$ receptor. For this reason, the SGAs, as a group, are known as "atypical" APs. Although the SGAs appear to have some advantage over the FGAs in the treatment of negative symptoms, cognitive dysfunction, and relapse prevention, the pharmacologic mechanisms responsible for their therapeutic properties have not been definitively identified. Furthermore, the

differential receptor profile of the SGAs relative to the FGAs is associated with another set of serious side effects. Patients taking clozapine may be at risk of agranulocytosis or of seizures at higher doses. More commonly, the SGAs are associated with weight gain, dyslipidemias, and impaired glucose regulation including type 2 diabetes mellitus. Weight gain may be particularly striking and puts the patient at increased risk of developing sleep-related breathing disorders and other obesity-related morbidities. Relative to the FGAs, the incidence of EPS and TD in SGA-treated schizophrenics is reduced, but EPS and TD are not uncommon with SGAs at higher doses.

On a final note, there is pressing need for more head-to-head comparisons of FGAs and SGAs in terms of their efficacy, side effects, and cost. The National Institute of Mental Health-sponsored Clinical Antipsychotic Trials of Intervention Effectiveness (CATIE) study[31] compared one FGA to several SGAs in terms of efficacy and side effects. The CATIE study found no significant difference in efficacy between the FGA perphenazine and three SGAs (risperidone, quetiapine, and ziprasidone). Although olanzapine was more effective than perphenazine, it was associated with greater weight gain and metabolic morbidity. At present (circa 2010), SGAs are considered first-line treatment for schizophrenia. Relative to FGAs, they appear to offer better compliance and fewer hospitalizations.

New Directions in Antipsychotic Drug Development

Although the last 50 years have witnessed major advances in the pharmacologic treatment of schizophrenia, limitations of efficacy as well as the morbidities of adverse effects have motivated the development of more novel medications covering a wide range of neurobiologic systems. It has been suggested that aripiprazole, although classed with the SGAs in Box 57-2, actually represents the next generation of APs because it is a partial dopamine agonist and, as distinct from the other SGAs, has an affinity for DA D_2 receptors far in excess of serotonin receptors. In addition to DA, the role of the excitatory neurotransmitter glutamate in the pathophysiology of schizophrenia is being widely examined.[32]

Treating Co-Morbid Psychiatric Illness

As mentioned previously, SGAs are currently first-line treatment for patients with schizophrenia; however, optimization of therapeutic response may require augmentation with additional AP agents. For many patients with schizophrenia, the efficacy of APs to treat negative symptoms and cognitive dysfunction is limited; consequently, adjunct psychoactive agents may also be prescribed. Also, other psychoactive agents may be enlisted to treat co-morbid psychiatric illness. For example, adjunct mood stabilizers such as valproate may be prescribed for schizophrenics with problems of impulse control and those with schizoaffective disorder. Patients with schizophrenia are also at high risk for suicidal behavior and co-morbid depression; for these patients adjunct antidepressants may be prescribed. Finally, it is not uncommon for schizophrenics to also be enrolled in dual diagnosis programs to treat co-morbid problems of alcohol and substance abuse.

BOX 57-3 *Effect of First- and Second-Generation Antipsychotics on Major Polysomnographic Sleep Variables*

Agent	SL	TST	SLP%	WASO	#Wakes	S1	S2	SWS	RL	REM
First-Generation Antipsychotics										
Chlorpromazine	↓	↑		↓			ns	↑	↑	ns
Thiothixene or Haloperidol	↓↓	↑ ns	↑↑	ns ns	ns ns	ns ns	ns ns	↑ ns	↑↑	ns
Flupentixol or Haloperidol	↓	↑	↑	ns		↑	ns	ns	ns	ns
Haloperidol	↓	↑	ns	ns	ns	↑	↓	ns	↑	ns
Second-Generation Antipsychotics										
Clozapine	↓	↑↑↑	↑↑↑	↓↓			↑↑↑	↓		
Olanzapine		↑	↑	↓		↓	↑	↑↑	↑	↑
Paliperidone	↓	↑	↑	ns	↓	↓	↑	ns	ns	↑
Quetiapine*	↓	↑	↑	↓	ns	ns	↑	ns	ns	↓
Risperidone†	ns	ns	ns	ns	ns	ns	ns	↑	ns	ns
Ziprasidone*	ns	↑	↑	↓	↓	↓	↑	↑	↑	↓

*Studied only nonpsychiatric control subjects.
†Risperidone relative only to haloperidol.
　NREM, non-REM sleep; *ns*, no significant change in mean value relative to a baseline or placebo condition; *REM*, rapid eye movement sleep time; *RL*, REM latency; *S1*, NREM sleep stage 1; *S2*, NREM sleep stage 2; *SL*, sleep onset latency; *SLP%*, percentage of time asleep relative to time in bed; *SWS*, NREM slow wave sleep; *TST*, total sleep time; *#Wakes*, number of awakenings; *WASO*, waking minutes after sleep onset.

EFFECTS OF ANTIPSYCHOTICS ON SLEEP PATTERNS

Objective Findings

Although the clinical efficacy of FGAs and SGAs has been amply documented, objective evidence that these agents counteract the insomnia and other sleep abnormalities associated with schizophrenia is particularly sketchy. The 13 available studies are summarized in Box 57-3. Arrows indicate significant increases or decreases in mean values; "ns" indicates no significant change in mean value relative to a baseline or placebo condition. The reader is encouraged to view this summary with caution. Double-blind, placebo-controlled studies are rare, sample sizes are small, and head-to-head comparisons of different APs have rarely been undertaken. Not all studies have utilized subjects as their own control group (longitudinal protocol); instead, most have utilized cross-sectional comparison groups. Note also that quetiapine and ziprasidone were studied only in nonpsychiatric control subjects; as yet, aripiprazole has undergone no PSG evaluation in schizophrenics or control subjects.

In general terms, FGAs appear to improve measures of sleep maintenance by increasing TST and sleep efficiency (SE) and by reducing both sleep latency (SL) and the amount of time waking after sleep onset.[33-37] The FGAs may also increase REM latency. The sole study of chlorpromazine suggested an ability to increase SWS time.[33]

Broadly stated, SGAs also appear to have sedating properties. From among the SGAs, the effect of clozapine on the sleep of patients with schizophrenia has been the most widely studied.[36,38,39] Clozapine appears to have a strong consolidating effect on sleep, with three studies documenting increases in TST, SE, and NREM stage N2. Clozapine may also decrease both SL and wake time after sleep onset. Olanzapine has also been shown to be a sleep-promoting agent with increases in TST, SE, and SWS.[40,41] In the only head-to-head comparison of two AP agents, a significant enhancement of SWS was observed in schizophrenics treated with risperidone relative to those treated with haloperidol; significant differences in other sleep variables were not observed.[42] PSG studies of paliperidone's effects on the sleep patterns in patients with schizophrenia revealed increased TST, SE, NREM stage 2, and REM sleep minutes; also observed were decreased SL, number of awakenings, and NREM stage 1.[43] PSG studies of quetiapine, ziprasidone, and aripiprazole have not been evaluated in patients with schizophrenia. However, in PSG studies of healthy control subjects, quetiapine and ziprasidone have augmented TST, SE, and NREM stage 2 and decreased the amount of wake time after sleep onset.[44,45] Such effects suggest that improvements in both sleep induction and consolidation might be expected in patients with schizophrenia.

Subjective Complaints

Residual Insomnia

As previously noted, insomnia is one of the cardinal features of schizophrenia. Difficulty falling asleep is the most frequent complaint, but restless sleep and increased bouts of waking after sleep onset are often described. These indices of hyperarousal have been associated with clinical measures of psychosis.[46,47] Commonly the mental health practitioner must balance clinical efficacy of an AP agent against a range of potential adverse effects and thus will prescribe a maintenance dose that is the lowest clinically effective dose. As a result, some degree of untreated hyperarousal and associated insomnia may be present in schizophrenics on maintenance doses of APs. The CATIE study[31] reported that rates of insomnia in AP-treated schizophrenics ranged from 16% to 30%. Although some residual hyperarousal may contribute to these insomnia rates, some APs (e.g., aripiprazole) may themselves may have associated side effects of insomnia, disturbed sleep, and anxiety.[48]

Clinicians may take one or more approaches to treat co-morbid insomnia: (a) change the dose of the treating AP agent; (b) switch to a different, more sedating AP agent; or (c) prescribe a low dose of an adjunct, more sedating AP. Head-to-head objective data on the sedative properties of currently approved APs are not available; however, patient reports as well as receptor-binding profiles (antihistaminergic and anti-α_1-adrenergic properties) suggest that chlorpromazine, clozapine, olanzapine, and quetiapine are among the more sedating AP agents.[30,48]

Clinicians might also consider adjunct use of an anxiolytic or a sedative hypnotic.[49] Note that these agents should be prescribed cautiously, particularly for those schizophrenics with a sleep-related breathing disorder or a history of alcohol or drug abuse. In addition, investigational studies suggest that melatonin might serve as an adjunct treatment for residual insomnia. Melatonin is the principal hormonal product of the pineal gland. Abnormal nocturnal secretory patterns of melatonin have been associated with insomnia. Consequently, abnormal patterns of melatonin secretion might also occur in schizophrenia. This hypothesis prompted study of nocturnal melatonin production in schizophrenics; these studies observed that the nighttime peak in melatonin secretion was blunted, and that normalization of melatonin production levels did not occur following clinical improvement with AP treatment.[50,51] In two studies, exogenous melatonin was used as an adjunct treatment for residual insomnia in AP-treated schizophrenics; these studies reported that melatonin replacement was associated with improved sleep maintenance as measured by actigraphy[52] and by self-report.[53]

Sedation as a Side Effect of Antipsychotic Drug Treatment

Rates of AP-related somnolence in patients with schizophrenia were also reported in the CATIE study; these rates ranged from 24% to 31%.[31] Although somnolence may be symptomatic of an underlying sleep disorder, sedation in AP-treated schizophrenics may be a direct side effect of AP treatment. As mentioned in the previous section, the SGAs clozapine, olanzapine, and quetiapine are recognized sedating medications. The remaining SGAs are associated with lower rates of somnolence. Sedation as a side effect of FGA treatment is associated with high-milligram, low-potency agents such as chlorpromazine and thioridazine. In contrast, the low-milligram, high-potency FGAs such as haloperidol are associated with less somnolence. It is important to note that levels of somnolence are also affected by the half-life of the agent, amount of drug, and dosing schedule. Somnolence secondary to AP treatment is usually addressed by changing AP medication or reducing its dosage. Case studies suggest that aripiprazole when added to ongoing clozapine therapy may improve psychotic symptoms while decreasing clozapine-associated sedation.[54]

Modafinil is a wakefulness-promoting agent that has been approved by the FDA to treat the daytime sleepiness associated with narcolepsy. Because modafinil might also improve daytime sleepiness in an off-label condition such as AP-associated somnolence, research protocols have been designed to study the effect of modafinil as an adjunct to AP treatment. Modafinil was shown to increase wake time, reduce TST, and reduce fatigue in case studies[55] and in an open-label pilot study[56] of AP-treated schizophrenics. In contrast, a double-blind, placebo-controlled trial of modafinil as an adjunct to AP treatment only observed a nonsignificant trend toward less nighttime and daytime total sleep.[57] Although these studies

suggest that modafinil might be beneficial in offsetting the sedative effects of some APs, the use of modafinil as an adjunct to AP treatment in schizophrenia is not FDA approved and its use demands further study given that stimulant drugs might exacerbate psychosis in patients with schizophrenia.[58]

CO-MORBID SLEEP DISORDERS

The previous sections discussed both insomnia and sedation as effects of AP treatment in schizophrenia. But patients with schizophrenia may also suffer from a range of additional co-morbid sleep disorders. These co-morbid conditions may encompass sleep-related movement disorders, sleep-related breathing disorders, parasomnias, and sleep disorders associated with poor sleep hygiene, alcohol/substance abuse, and circadian rhythm disorders (Box 57-4). Baseline prevalence rates of these sleep disorders in schizophrenics who are naïve to AP treatment have never been established; however, it is clear that many of these co-morbid sleep disorders have been induced by or exacerbated by AP treatment.

Sleep-Related Movement Disorders

Both restless legs syndrome (RLS) and periodic limb movement disorder (PLMD) are sleep-related movement disorders associated with sleep disturbance.

RLS is characterized by an urge to move the legs and is often associated with unpleasant sensations in the legs. RLS occurs or worsens when the patients is at rest. It is immediately but temporarily relieved by activity such as walking or moving the legs. It has a circadian component with worsening in the evening and night. As such, RLS is associated with sleep onset insomnia because it profoundly interferes with the ability to attain a state of persistent sleep. About 80% to 90% of patients with RLS also experience periodic limb movements (PLMs). PLMs are periodic episodes of repetitive limb movement (usually the lower extremities) occurring most typically during NREM sleep. The disorder, PLMD, may be associated with autonomic or cortical arousals or outright awakenings. Consequently, PLMs can be associated with complaints of restless or unrefreshing sleep.

For many years, the pathophysiology of schizophrenia has centered on the dopamine hypothesis of schizophrenia owing primarily to the relationship between the clinical potency of AP agents and the blockade of the DA D_2 receptor.

BOX 57-4 *Sleep Disorders Associated with Schizophrenia*

Direct effects of antipsychotic treatment
- Residual insomnia or untreated hyperarousal
- Sedation as a side effect of antipsychotic drug treatment

Sleep-related movement disorders
- Restless legs syndrome
- Periodic limb movement disorder

Sleep-disordered breathing

Parasomnias
- Somnambulism
- Sleep-related eating disorder

Poor sleep hygiene

In this context, psychoticism has been attributed to pathologic hyperstimulation of subcortical mesolimbic DA D_2 receptors. In contrast, because RLS and PLMD respond to DA agonists, the pathophysiology of RLS and PLMD may reflect a DA *deficiency*.[59] It is not surprising then that D_2 receptor blockade associated with AP agents might induce RLS and PLMD in AP-treated schizophrenics.

In confirmation, studies have determined that the prevalence rates of RLS in AP-treated schizophrenics are more than twice that of healthy control subjects.[60] Prevalence rates of PLMD in schizophrenics are not as well known because the diagnosis of PLMD requires overnight PSG study. In contrast, the diagnosis of RLS is made by clinical interview. Two published reports suggest that prevalence rates of PLMD in schizophrenics treated with FGAs are in the range of 13% to 14%.[61,62]

Recent studies have reported the development of RLS and PLMD in patients taking SGAs such as risperidone,[63] olanzapine,[64-67] quetiapine,[68] and clozapine.[69] Olanzapine has also been associated with the induction of restless arms syndrome.[70] The standard treatment for RLS and PLMD are DA agonists such as ropinirole and pramipexole; however, for patients with schizophrenia, DA agonists are not first-line choices. In schizophrenic patients who develop RLS and PLMD following AP management, clinicians might consider a reduction in AP dose or a change to a different AP agent. Adjunct treatments such as clonazapam might also be considered. Patients should also be evaluated for possible iron deficiency, a known risk factor for the development of RLS,[71] and be encouraged to limit use of substances such as caffeine that might worsen sleep-related movements. Although DA agonists such as ropinirole and pramipexole should not be the first choice of treatment for patients with schizophrenia who develop RLS or PLMD, it is possible that such agents might be necessary when their benefits outweigh the risk.

Finally, akathisia is a common side effect of many AP agents. Akathisia is characterized by generalized inner disquiet and motor restlessness evidenced by fidgeting and pacing; it can induce significant sleep disruption. RLS can be distinguished from akathisia because RLS is associated with symptomatic relief by movement, and unlike akathisia, it is associated with a circadian worsening of symptoms in the evening or at night. Pharmacologic treatment of AP-induced akathisia may include anticholinergic agents (e.g., benztropine), β-adrenergic antagonists (e.g., propranolol), and benzodiazepines (e.g., clonazepam).[72]

Somnolence Associated with Sleep-Related Breathing Disorder

Increased somnolence associated with the receptor binding profile of certain APs was addressed in a previous section. However, somnolence in AP-treated schizophrenics may also indicate the presence of a sleep-related breathing disorder (SBD) that has been exacerbated or induced by an AP agent. A common adverse effect of AP treatment is the emergence of obstructive sleep apnea syndrome (OSAS). Prevalence rates of OSAS in schizophrenics never exposed to AP agents are unknown. However, a wide range of high prevalence rates for OSAS have been reported in studies that enrolled patients with schizophrenia in research protocols (rates of 17%,[61] 19%,[73] and 48%[62]). In a study of schizophrenic patients referred to a sleep clinic for a suspected sleep disorder, more than 46% had a respiratory disturbance index (RDI) greater than 10 events per hour of sleep; the mean RDI was 64.8 events per hour of sleep, and the best predictor of RDI was obesity.[74]

One of the adverse side effects of AP treatment is weight gain, which can occur following the use of certain FGAs and SGAs such as clozapine, olanzapine, thioridazine, chlorpromazine, and risperidone.[75] More recent data suggest that quetiapine should be added to this list.[76] Clozapine and risperidone have been associated not only with significant morbid obesity but also with the development of moderate to severe SBD.[77] Weight gain is one of a constellation of factors associated with insulin resistance and known as the *metabolic syndrome*. The *metabolic syndrome* increases not only the risk of obesity and SBD but also the risks of impaired glucose tolerance, type 2 diabetes, and coronary heart disease. These AP-related adverse effects are consistent with the heightened mortality rate associated with schizophrenia. Published reports found significant weight loss and improved metabolic measures when aripiprazole was substituted for olanzapine[78] or when aripiprazole was added as an adjunct to olanzapine.[79]

Although daytime sleepiness is a relatively frequent side effect seen in schizophrenics treated with APs, clinicians must consider the differential diagnosis of co-morbid OSAS for those patients who are obese by history or who have gained weight during the course of AP treatment. OSAS in patients with schizophrenia has been treated effectively with nasal continuous positive airway pressure (CPAP); these patients have shown relatively good compliance and significant clinical improvement.[80,81]

Parasomnias

Somnambulism is associated with a partial arousal from SWS. Psychotropic agents that increase SWS may predispose schizophrenics to somnambulistic behaviors. Somnambulism has been reported to occur following the addition of lithium to FGAs[82] and following treatment with olanzapine.[83] Both lithium and olanzapine have also been credited with SWS enhancement. Clonazepam has been reported to ameliorate AP-induced somnambulism,[84] but hypnotics should be prescribed with caution if there is co-morbid SBD. Another parasomnia, sleep-related eating disorder, may be induced by APs such as haloperidol,[85] olanzapine,[86] and risperidone.[87] Treatment options for sleep-related eating disorders might include topiramate or a sedative agent.

Poor Sleep Hygiene

Many schizophrenics exhibit sleep-wake reversals, sleeping during the day and remaining active at night. Others may exhibit polyphasic sleep patterns with extended periods of daytime napping that interfere with subsequent consolidation of nocturnal sleep. Although daytime napping might indicate AP-associated sedation or somnolence associated with a sleep disorder such as OSAS, many schizophrenic patients lack daytime structure and may prefer to avoid social interactions. As a result, they may develop bad habits in relation to daytime napping and the circadian assignment of their major sleep period. Excess caffeine intake and the use of alcohol or psychoactive drugs such as cannabis and cocaine can further erode good sleep hygiene. Both mental health and sleep medicine specialists should be cognizant of the fact that most patients with schizophrenia can benefit from sleep hygiene counseling.

CONCLUSION

Schizophrenia is an illness with great personal and societal costs. Prior to treatment, most schizophrenics experience moderate to severe sleep disruption. These abnormalities often include a marked difficulty in attaining persistent sleep, reduced sleep time with sleep punctuated by restless bouts of wakefulness, and a loss of the deeper stages of SWS. A broad array of AP agents has been developed with differential receptor binding profiles. Although APs are efficacious agents, their effects on negative symptoms and cognitive dysfunction have been more limited. Their range of associated adverse side effects has likewise proved problematic. Nevertheless, most FGAs and SGAs improve sleep maintenance and structure, and this normalization of sleep may contribute to their clinical efficacy and to their tolerance.

Mental health specialists should explicitly incorporate in their treatment plans strategies to deal aggressively with complaints of poor sleep quality in patients with schizophrenia. They should be sensitive to any resurgence of severe insomnia as it may indicate pending relapse; they should also be sensitive to the emergence or exacerbation of sleep disorders associated with AP treatment. Untreated sleep disorders in patients with schizophrenia may undermine the recuperative value of sleep and can adversely affect both treatment compliance and clinical outcome.

REFERENCES

1. McGrath J, Saha S, Chant D, Welham J. Schizophrenia: A concise overview of incidence, prevalence, and mortality. *Epidemiol Rev.* 2008;30:67-76.
2. American Psychiatric Association. *Diagnostic and Statistical Manual of Mental Disorders.* 4th ed. Washington, DC: American Psychiatric Press; 2000:297-317.
3. Van Os J, Kapur S. Schizophrenia. *Lancet.* 2009;374(9690):635-645.
4. White C, Stirling J, Hopkins R, Morris J, Montague L, et al. Predictors of 10-year outcome of first-episode psychosis. *Psychol Med.* 2009;39:1447-1456.
5. Black DW, Andreasen NC. Schizophrenia, schizophreniform disorder, and delusional (paranoid) disorders. In: Hales RE, Yudofsky SC, Talbott JA, eds. *Textbook of Psychiatry.* 3rd ed. Washington, DC: American Psychiatric Press; 1999:425-477.
6. Tsuang MT, Faraone SV, Green AI. Schizophrenia and other psychotic disorders. In: Nicholi AM, ed. *The Harvard Guide to Psychiatry.* 3rd ed. Cambridge, MA: Belknap Press of Harvard University Press; 1999:240-280.
7. Sullivan PF, Kendler KS, Neale MC. Schizophrenia as a complex trait. *Arch Gen Psychiatry.* 2003;60:1187-1192.
8. Wray NR, Visscher PM. Narrowing the boundaries of the genetic architecture of schizophrenia. *Schiz Bull.* 2010;36:14-23.
9. Brown AS, Derkits EJ. Prenatal infection and schizophrenia: A review of epidemiologic and translational studies. *Am J Psychiatry.* 2010;167:261-280.
10. Clarke MC, Tanskanen A, Huttunen M, Whittaker JC, Cannon M. Evidence for an interaction between familial liability and prenatal exposure to infection in the causation of schizophrenia. *Am J Psychiatry.* 2009;166:1025-1030.
11. Lewis DA, Levitt P. Schizophrenia as a disorder of neurodevelopment. *Annu Rev Neurosci.* 2002;25:409-432.
12. Rapoport JL, Addington AM, Frangou S, et al. The neurodevelopmental model of schizophrenia: Update 2005. *Mol Psychiatry.* 2005;10:434-449.
13. Uhlhaas PJ, Singer W. Abnormal neural oscillations and synchrony in schizophrenia. *Nat Rev Neurosci.* 2010;11(2):100-113.
14. Feinberg I, Guazzelli M. Schizophrenia: A disorder of the corollary discharge systems that integrate the motor systems of thought with the sensory systems of consciousness. *Br J Psychiatry.* 1999;174:196-204.

15. Guillin O, Abi-Dargham A, Laruelle M. Neurobiology of dopamine in schizophrenia. *Int Rev Neurobiol.* 2007;78:1-39.
16. Chemerinski E, Ho B, Flaum M, et al. Insomnia as a predictor for symptom worsening following antipsychotic withdrawal in schizophrenia. *Compr Psychiatry.* 2002;43:393-396.
17. Haffmans PM, Hoencamp E, Knegtering HJ, et al. Sleep disturbance in schizophrenia. *Br J Psychiatry.* 1994;165:697-698.
18. Hofstetter JR, Mayeda AR, Happel CG, et al. Sleep and daily activity preferences in schizophrenia: Associations with neurocognition and symptoms. *J Nerv Ment Dis.* 2003;191(6):408-410.
19. Lusignan F-A, Zadra A, Dubuc M-J, et al. Dream content in chronically-treated persons with schizophrenia. *Schiz Res.* 2009;112:164-173.
20. Benca RM, Obermeyer WH, Thisted RA, et al. Sleep and psychiatric disorders: A meta-analysis. *Arch Gen Psychiatry.* 1992;49:651-668.
21. Chouinard S, Poulin J, Stip E, et al. Sleep in untreated patients with schizophrenia: A meta-analysis. *Schiz Bull.* 2004;30(4):957-967.
22. Benson KL, Feinberg I. Schizophrenia. In: Kryger MH, Roth T, Dement WC, eds. *Principles and Practice of Sleep Medicine.* 5rd ed. Philadelphia: Elsevier Saunders; 2011:1501-1511.
23. Poulin J, Daoust A, Forest G, et al. Sleep architecture and its clinical correlates in first episode and neuroleptic-naive patients with schizophrenia. *Schiz Res.* 2003;62:147-153.
24. Webb WB, Agnew HW. Stage 4 sleep: Influence of time course variables. *Science.* 1971;174:1354-1356.
25. Feinberg I. Changes in sleep cycle patterns with age. *J Psychiatr Res.* 1974;10:283-306.
26. Feinberg I. Schizophrenia: Caused by a fault in programmed synaptic elimination during adolescence? *J Psychiatr Res.* 1983;17:319-334.
27. Feinberg I, Braum N, Koresko RL, et al. Stage 4 sleep in schizophrenia. *Arch Gen Psychiatry.* 1969;21:262-266.
28. Lauer CJ, Schreiber W, Pollmächer T, et al. Sleep in schizophrenia: A polysomnographic study on drug-naive patients. *Neuropsychopharm.* 1997;16:51-60.
29. Benson KL, Zarcone VP. REM sleep eye movement activity in schizophrenia and depression. *Arch Gen Psychiatry.* 1993;50:472-474.
30. Miyamoto S, Duncan GE, Marx CE, Lieberman JA. Treatments for schizophrenia: A critical review of pharmacology and mechanisms of action of antipsychotic drugs. *Mol Psychiatry.* 2005;10:79-104.
31. Lieberman JA, Stroup TS, McEvoy JP, et al. Effectiveness of antipsychotic drugs in patients with chronic schizophrenia. *N Engl J Med.* 2005;353(12):1209-1223.
32. Goff DC, Coyle JT. The emerging role of glutamate in the pathophysiology and treatment of schizophrenia. *Am J Psychiatry.* 2001;158:1367-1377.
33. Kaplan J, Dawson S, Vaughan T, et al. Effect of prolonged chlorpromazine administration on the sleep of chronic schizophrenics. *Arch Gen Psychiatry.* 1974;31:62-66.
34. Maixner S, Tandon R, Eiser A, et al. Effects of antipsychotic treatment on polysomnographic measures in schizophrenia: A replication and extension. *Am J Psychiatry.* 1998;155:1600-1602.
35. Taylor SF, Tandon R, Shipley JE, et al. Effect of neuroleptic treatment on polysomnographic measures in schizophrenia. *Biol Psychiatry.* 1991;30:904-912.
36. Wetter TC, Lauer CJ, Gillich G, et al. The electroencephalographic sleep pattern in schizophrenic patients treated with clozapine or classical antipsychotic drugs. *J Psychiatr Res.* 1996;30:411-419.
37. Nofzinger EA, van Kammen DP, Gilbertson MW, et al. Electroencephalographic sleep in clinically stable schizophrenic patients: Two-weeks versus six-weeks neuroleptic free. *Biol Psychiatry.* 1993;33:829-835.
38. Hinze-Selch D, Mullington J, Orth A, et al. Effects of clozapine on sleep: A longitudinal study. *Biol Psychiatry.* 1997;42:260-266.
39. Lee JH, Woo JI, Meltzer HY. Effects of clozapine on sleep measures and sleep-associated changes in growth hormone and cortisol in patients with schizophrenia. *Psychiatry Res.* 2001;103:157-166.
40. Salin-Pascual RJ, Herrera-Estrella M, Galicia-Polo L, et al. Olanzapine acute administration in schizophrenic patients increases delta sleep and sleep efficiency. *Biol Psychiatry.* 1999;46:141-143.
41. Müller MJ, Rossbach W, Mann K, et al. Subchronic effects of olanzapine on sleep EEG in schizophrenic patients with predominantly negative symptoms. *Pharmacopsychiatry.* 2004;37(4):157-162.
42. Yamashita H, Morinobu S, Yamawaki S, et al. Effect of risperidone on sleep in schizophrenia: A comparison with haloperidol. *Psychiatry Res.* 2002;109:137-142.
43. Luthringer R, Staner L, Noel N, et al. A double-blind, placebo controlled, randomized study evaluating the effect of paliperidone extended-release tablets on sleep architecture in patients with schizophrenia. *Int Clin Psychopharmacol.* 2007;22:299-308.

44. Cohrs S, Rodenbeck A, Guan Z, et al. Sleep-promoting properties of quetiapine in healthy subjects. *Psychopharmacology*. 2004;174(3):421-429.

45. Cohrs S, Meier A, Neumann A-C, et al. Improved sleep continuity and increased slow wave sleep and REM latency during ziprasidone treatment: A randomized, controlled, crossover trial of 12 healthy male subjects. *J Clin Psychiatry*. 2005;66(8):989-996.

46. Neylan TC, van Kammen DP, Kelley ME, et al. Sleep in schizophrenic patients on and off haloperidol therapy. *Arch Gen Psychiatry*. 1992;49:643-649.

47. Zarcone VP, Benson KL. BPRS symptom factors and sleep variables in schizophrenia. *Psychiatry Res*. 1997;66:111-120.

48. Krystal AD, Goforth HW, Roth T. Effects of antipsychotic medications on sleep in schizophrenia. *Int Clin Psychopharmacol*. 2008;23:150-160.

49. Kane JM, Sharif ZA. Atypical antipsychotics: Sedation versus efficacy. *J Clin Psychiatry*. 2008;69(suppl 1):18-31.

50. Robinson S, Rosca P, Durst R, et al. Serum melatonin levels in schizophrenic and schizoaffective hospitalized patients. *Acta Psychiatr Scand*. 1991;84(3):221-224.

51. Monteleone P, Natale M, LaRocca A, et al. Decreased nocturnal secretion of melatonin in drug-free schizophrenics: No change after subchronic treatment with antipsychotics. *Neuropsychobiology*. 1997;36:159-163.

52. Shamir E, Laudon M, Barak Y, et al. Melatonin improves sleep quality of patients with chronic schizophrenia. *J Clin Psychiatry*. 2000;61:373-377.

53. Kumar PNS, Andrade C, Bhakta SG, et al. Melatonin in schizophrenic outpatients with insomnia: A double-blind, placebo-controlled study. *J Clin Psychiatry*. 2007;68(2):237-241.

54. Rocha FL, Hara C. Benefits of combining aripiprazole to clozapine: Three case reports. *Prog Neuro Psychopharm Biol Psychiatry*. 2006;30:1167-1169.

55. Makela EH, Miller K, Cutlip WD. Three case reports of modafinil use in treating sedation induced by antipsychotic medications. *J Clin Psychiatry*. 2003;64(4):485-486.

56. Rosenthal MH, Bryant SL. Benefits of adjunct modafinil in an open-label, pilot study in patients with schizophrenia. *Clin Neuropharmacol*. 2004;27(1):38-43.

57. Pierre JM, Peloian JH, Wirshing DA, et al. A randomized, double-blind, placebo-controlled trial of modafinil for negative symptoms in schizophrenia. *J Clin Psychiatry*. 2007;68:705-710.

58. Narendran R, Young CM, Valenti AM, et al. Is psychosis exacerbated by modafinil?. *Arch Gen Psychiatry*. 2002;59:292-293.

59. Allen RP, Earley CJ. Restless legs syndrome: A review of clinical and pathophysiologic features. *J Clin Neurophysiol*. 2001;18:128-147.

60. Kang SG, Lee HJ, Jung SW, et al. Characteristics and clinical correlates of restless legs syndrome in schizophrenia. *Prog Neuro Psychopharmacol Biol Psychiatry*. 2007;31:1078-1083.

61. Benson KL, Zarcone VP. Sleep abnormalities in schizophrenia and other psychotic disorders. *Rev Psychiatry*. 1994;13:677-705.

62. Ancoli-Israel S, Martin J, Jones DW, et al. Sleep disordered breathing and periodic limb movements in sleep in older patients with schizophrenia. *Biol Psychiatry*. 1999;45:1426-1432.

63. Wetter TC, Brunner J, Bronisch T. Restless legs syndrome probably induced by risperidone treatment. *Pharmacopsychiatry*. 2002;35:109-111.

64. Kraus T, Schuld A, Pollmächer T. Periodic leg movements in sleep and restless legs syndrome probably caused by olanzapine. *J Clin Psychopharmacol*. 1999;19:478-479.

65. Khalid I, Rana L, Khalid TJ, Roehrs T. Refractory restless legs syndrome likely caused by olanzapine. *J Clin Sleep Med*. 2009;5(1):68-69.

66. Kang SG, Lee HJ, Kim L. Restless legs syndrome and periodic limb movements during sleep probably associated with olanzapine. *J Psychopharmacol*. 2009;23(5):597-601.

67. Aggarwal S, Dodd S, Berk M. Restless leg syndrome associated with olanzapine: A case series. *Curr Drug Saf*. 2010;5(2):129-131.

68. Pinninti NR, Mago R, Townsend J, et al. Periodic restless legs syndrome associated with quetiapine. *J Clin Psychopharmacol*. 2005;25:617-618.

69. Duggal HS, Mendhekar DN. Clozapine-associated restless les syndrome. *J Clin Psychopharmacol*. 2007;27:89-90.

70. Konstantakopoulos G, Oulis P, Michalopoulou PG, et al. Olanzapine-induced "restless arms syndrome." *J Clin Psychophamacol*. 2009;29:89-90.

71. Allen R. Dopamine and iron in the pathophysiology of restless legs syndrome (RLS). *Sleep Med*. 2004;5:385-391.

72. Fleischhacker WW, Roth SD, Kane JM. The pharmacologic treatment of neuroleptic-induced akathisia. *J Clin Psychopharmacol*. 1990;10:12-21.

73. Takahashi KI, Shimizu T, Sugita T, et al. Prevalence of sleep-related respiratory disorders in 101 schizophrenic patients. *Psychiatry Clin Neurosci*. 1998;52:229-231.

74. Winkelman JW. Schizophrenia, obesity, and obstructive sleep apnea. *J Clin Psychiatry*. 2001;62:8-11.

75. Allison DB, Mentore JL, Heo M, et al. Antipsychotic-induced weight gain: A comprehensive research synthesis. *Am J Psychiatry*. 1999;156:1686-1696.

76. Williams SG, Alinejad NA, Williams JA, Cruess DF. Statistically significant increase in weight caused by low-dose quetiapine. *Pharmacotherapy*. 2010;30:1011-1015.

77. Wirshing DA, Pierre JM, Wirshing WC. Sleep apnea associated with antipsychotic-induced obesity. *J Clin Psychiatry*. 2002;63:369-370.

78. Newcomer JW, Campos JA, Marcus RN, et al. A multicenter, randomized, double-blind study of the effects of aripiprazole in overweight subjects with schizophrenia or schizoaffective disorder switched from olanzapine. *J Clin Psychiatry*. 2008;69:1046-1056.

79. Henderson DC, Fan X, Copeland PM. Aripiprazole added to overweight and obese olanzapine-treated schizophrenic patients. *J Clin Psychopharmacol*. 2009;29(2):165-169.

80. Boufidis S, Kosmidis MH, Bozikas VP, et al. Treatment outcome of obstructive sleep apnea syndrome in a patient with schizophrenia: A case report. *Int J Psychiatry Med*. 2003;33:305-310.

81. Karanti A, Landén M. Treatment refractory psychosis remitted upon treatment with continuous positive airway pressure: A case report. *Psychopharmacol Bull*. 2007;40(1):113-117.

82. Charney DS, Kales A, Soldatos CR, Nelson JC. Somnambulistic-like episodes secondary to combined lithium-neuroleptic treatment. *Br J Psychiatry*. 1979;135:418-424.

83. Kolivakis TT, Margolese HC, Beauclair L, et al. Olanzapine-induced somnambulism. *Am J Psychiatry*. 2001;158:1158.

84. Goldbloom D, Chouinard G. Clonazepam in the treatment of neuroleptic-induced somnambulism. *Am J Psychiatry*. 1984;141:1486.

85. Horiguchi J, Yamashita H, Mizuno S, et al. Nocturnal eating/drinking syndrome and neuroleptic-induced restless legs syndrome. *Int Clin Psychopharmacol*. 1999;14:33-36.

86. Paquet V, Strul J, Servais L, et al. Sleep-related eating disorder induced by olanzapine. *J Clin Psychiatry*. 2002;63:597.

87. Lu M-L, Shen WW. Sleep-related eating disorder induced by risperidone. *J Clin Psychiatry*. 2004;65(2):273.

SECTION **14**

Special Situations and the Future

Sleep in Women

GRACE W. PIEN / BARBARA A. PHILLIPS / NANCY A. COLLOP

Chapter 58

Historically, women have been both underdiagnosed with sleep disorders and under represented in sleep research compared to men. Over the past several decades, this imbalance has started to shift. Nevertheless, the substantial gender differences that can exist in the prevalence, clinical manifestations, responses to treatment, and other characteristics of specific sleep disorders remain underappreciated and often unexplored. Pregnancy and menopause, conditions that are unique to women, also often affect normal sleep and may increase the risk for certain sleep disorders.

This chapter will review gender differences in common sleep disorders including insomnia, obstructive sleep apnea (OSA), restless legs syndrome (RLS), and narcolepsy and will discuss features of these conditions that are specific to understanding and caring for affected women. The changes in sleep that occur during pregnancy and the menopausal transition will be reviewed, along with evaluation and treatment of sleep complaints in these populations and the effect of these conditions on specific sleep disorders. Finally, nighttime eating disorders will be considered, as they are generally more likely to affect women than men.

INSOMNIA IN WOMEN

Epidemiology

Among the most prevalent and distressing sleep problems faced by women (and physicians caring for them) is insomnia.[1] Beginning at approximately the time of menarche, women are more likely to report sleep complaints than men, and this gap widens with age.[1-3] On average, the frequency of sleep complaints in women is about twice that of men.[4] One of the conundrums in this area is that although women are more likely than men to complain about their sleep, they actually appear to sleep better. Most population-based studies indicate that sleep is better preserved in women than men with aging. Between the ages of 30 and 40, differences in sleep structure begin to emerge, with better sleep efficiency, more slow wave sleep, and shorter sleep latencies in women compared to men.[5-9] This apparent contradiction is largely unexplained, but may result at least in part because of the subjective nature of insomnia identification and the increased vigilance of women.[10]

Definition and Diagnosis

One of the problems with assessing the prevalence and impact of insomnia in women (or anyone) is its definition. *Insomnia* has many definitions. In 2005, a National Institutes of Health

(NIH) Consensus Conference[10] defined insomnia as any of the following: difficulty going to sleep; difficulty staying asleep; waking up too early, being unable to return to sleep; and perhaps, nonrestorative sleep. *The International Classification of Sleep Disorders,* 2nd edition (ICSD-II), defines *insomnia* as a complaint of difficulty initiating sleep, difficulty maintaining sleep, or waking up too early *or* sleep that is chronically nonrestorative or poor in quality; "the above sleep difficulty occurs despite adequate opportunity and circumstances for sleep" and the nighttime sleep difficulty includes the presence of daytime consequences.[11] *The Diagnostic and Statistical Manual of Mental Disorders (DSM-IV)* criteria include complaints of sleep problems three times a week for a month, but also daytime consequences.[12] The Research Diagnostic Criteria for Insomnia Disorder include sleep complaints, nonrestorative sleep, and daytime impairment in the definition, but do not have duration, severity, or frequency criteria.[13] The obvious problem with most of these definitions is their subjectivity; one person's "difficulty falling asleep" might be described by another as "this is to be expected after such a hectic day." The subjective uncertainty about the definition of insomnia is reflected in the NIH Consensus Conference report: "Although chronic insomnia is considered to be common....Conclusive evidence from epidemiologic studies has been limited by their different definitions of chronic insomnia and by the lack of standardized...screening methods. Population-based studies suggest that about 30 percent of the general population has complaints of sleep disruption, while approximately 10 percent has associated symptoms of daytime functional impairment....Not surprisingly, prevalence appears to be greater in clinical practices, where about one-half of respondents report symptoms of sleep disruption."[10]

In an attempt to address the subjective nature of insomnia, research investigators have somewhat arbitrarily chosen criteria so that numerical data could be collected and analyzed. One commonly used set of criteria is as follows: (1) difficulties initiating or maintaining sleep, defined as a sleep onset latency or wake after sleep onset greater than 30 minutes, with a corresponding sleep time of less than 6.5 hours at least three nights per week (as measured by daily sleep diaries); (2) insomnia duration longer than 6 months; and (3) significant distress or impairment of daytime functioning (usually assessed by a questionnaire).[14]

Another problem in defining *insomnia* is its overlap with sleep deprivation. Investigators, the press, and well-meaning organizations sometimes blur the line between insomnia and sleep deprivation. The diagnosis of insomnia assumes adequate opportunity to sleep, coupled with inadequate ability to fall and stay asleep. Sleep deprivation occurs when there is adequate ability to sleep, but inadequate opportunity. The stressed-out 28-year-old graduate student with a husband, two children, and a part-time job may find only 6 hours to sleep in a 24-hour period but sleeps pretty well when she gets a chance. She has sleep deprivation. The 49-year-old perimenopausal woman whose primary daytime activities are church and watching television, and who goes to bed at 10 PM, falls asleep at midnight, wakes at 4 AM, falls back asleep again at 6 AM, and finally gets out of bed at 8 AM also gets only 6 hours of sleep. She has insomnia. Although the consequences of sleep deprivation appear to be significant,[15] it is not at all clear that the consequences of insomnia are the same. Yet the public is bombarded with "health messages" that lump insomnia and sleep deprivation together.

Thus, the true prevalence and outcomes of insomnia are unknown, because in clinical practice and in most large population-based studies or surveys, insomnia is very much in the mind of the beholder. Many studies and clinicians allow self-definition of insomnia (e.g., "Do you have insomnia?") in assessing its impact, response to treatment, and prevalence. The subjective nature of insomnia is likely to account for some of the difference in the prevalence of insomnia between men and women. Women are more likely than men to report and seek treatment for most symptoms and medical conditions,[16] and sleep disturbances are no exception.

Other potential explanations for the increased prevalence of insomnia in women exist. Mood disturbances, particularly anxiety, dysthymia, and depression, are much more prevalent in women than in men.[17,18] These disorders are commonly associated with insomnia.[19,20] Indeed, the NIH Consensus Conference Report noted, "Insomnia usually appears in the presence of at least one other disorder. Particularly common comorbidities are major depression, generalized anxiety, substance abuse, dementia, and a variety of physical problems."[10]

Another likely explanation for women's increased risk of insomnia is the association between pain and sleep disturbance. Women are more likely than men to report pain and to be diagnosed with pain disorders. This relationship is likely bidirectional, with pain causing sleep disturbances and sleep disturbances lowering the pain threshold, resulting in a downward spiral of increasing pain and worsening sleep. One laboratory-controlled study has shown that reductions in total sleep time significantly increase pain sensitivity, even in healthy disease-free individuals.[21]

Pathophysiology

Insomnia is thought to be a disorder of hyperarousal. Indeed, there is evidence that insomnia is associated with an overall increase of adrenocorticotropic hormone (ACTH) and cortisol secretion, which supports this idea.[22] However, the situation is likely to be much more complex than that, and data are not always consistent. The current understanding of the theoretical basis of insomnia has been recently reviewed.[23]

Consequences

Women who report insomnia may overemphasize the role of sleep in their lives. They may report that their sleep disturbance causes problems with performance, relationships, and mood. It has been difficult to document these findings with objective testing. In particular, although individuals with insomnia may report fatigue, they generally score low on subjective tests of sleepiness and are not generally objectively sleepy with multiple sleep latency testing (MSLT) or maintenance of wakefulness testing (MWT). Cross-sectional studies suggest that individuals with insomnia fare poorly in many domains, but such studies typically do not control well for mood disturbance, medication use, and other lifestyle factors.[24]

The NIH Consensus Conference noted that "it is difficult to separate the effects of insomnia from the effects of comorbid conditions."[10] Insomnia complaints have been associated with many adverse outcomes, but prospective studies controlling for confounders are not available for most of the putative sequelae of insomnia, with the notable exception of depression. Numerous prospective studies have demonstrated that self-reported insomnia precedes depression,[19,25] and this has generally been taken to demonstrate that insomnia causes depression. An alternative hypothesis, however, is simply that insomnia is the earliest or most sensitive marker of depression. As the NIH Consensus Conference notes, "The research diagnostic criteria for insomnia recently developed by the American Academy of Sleep Medicine…share many of the criteria of major depressive disorder."[10]

Clinicians caring for women with insomnia may find themselves confronted by concerned, anxious individuals who are convinced that sleep difficulties are literally going to kill them. Several investigators have demonstrated that insomnia is not associated with an increased risk of death.[26,27] Based on data gathered by telephone survey of more than 1 million American Cancer Society volunteers, Kripke and associates[26] reported that reporting insomnia was associated with reduced mortality rate at 7-year follow-up. In that study, participants were asked, "On average, how many times a month do you have insomnia?" and hazard ratios were calculated with "never" having insomnia being assigned a hazard ratio of 1. Compared with "never," any reported frequency of insomnia was associated with a statistically reduced risk of death 7 years later. Using a more precise (but still subjective) definition of insomnia, we confirmed that insomnia does not appear to confer an increased risk of death after controlling for confounders.[27]

There are conflicting reports about the association between insomnia and hypertension or heart disease, with some data suggesting an increased risk with insomnia,[28,29] but other data finding a reduced risk, at least in men.[30] It is also possible that the effects of insomnia are different for women than for men.

Treatment and Natural History

Data are accumulating that cognitive-behavioral therapies (CBT) are as effective as pharmacologic therapies for treatment of insomnia. The NIH Consensus Conference report on chronic insomnia noted, "Behavioral and cognitive-behavioral therapies (CBTs) have demonstrated efficacy in [randomized controlled trials]….When these cognitive methods have been added to the behavioral methods to compose a cognitive-behavioral treatment package, [they have] been found to be as effective as prescription medications are for brief treatment of chronic insomnia. Moreover, there are indications that the beneficial effects of CBT, in contrast to those produced by medications, may last well beyond the termination of treatment."[10] These findings have been bolstered by recent work by Morin and associates.[14]

Although hypnotic use may be a useful adjunct in the acute management of insomnia, particularly in combination with CBT, chronic hypnotic use is suboptimal treatment and may actually reduce the effectiveness of CBT.[14] A recent comprehensive review noted, "[Benzodiazepine receptor agonists, BZRAs] and psychological and behavioral methods are effective to treat insomnia in the short-term and the latter have significantly more durable effects when active treatment is discontinued; there is only very limited evidence that BZRAs retain their efficacy during long-term treatment."[31]

The shifting emphasis to CBT is being driven not only by growing evidence of its efficacy, but also by recent reports of adverse effects of hypnotic use, particularly chronic hypnotic use. Kripke and associates[32,33] first sounded the alarm, but subsequent credible reports have demonstrated an increased mortality risk with chronic hypnotic use.[34,35] Associations between chronic hypnotic use and increased risks for motor vehicle crashes[36] and skin cancers[37] have also been reported.

Furthermore, a recent 3-year observational study of individuals with insomnia showed that approximately two thirds of those who met diagnostic criteria for insomnia at baseline still reported problems 3 years later,[38] independently of whether pharmacologic treatment was initiated.

Insomnia is a prevalent and distressing problem for women. It is often chronic and difficult to treat, and CBT is likely to be the safest, most effective long-term treatment.

SLEEP IN PREGNANT WOMEN

Changes in Normal Sleep with Pregnancy

During pregnancy, most women report alterations in their sleep.[39-47] Sleep complaints and changes in sleep patterns start occurring in the first trimester.[44,46,47] Sleep patterns are likely to be influenced by some of the dramatic changes in reproductive hormone levels that accompany pregnancy: levels of estrogens and progesterone rise throughout the gestational period and peak at term, falling rapidly after delivery.[48]

Sleepiness is a common first-trimester complaint.[13] Increases in first-trimester total sleep time of more than 30 minutes have been observed compared to the prepregnancy period in surveys[49] and home sleep studies,[44] though sleep efficiency and the percentage of slow wave sleep fall.[44] Total nocturnal sleep time decreases by late in the second trimester.[44] Although the percentage of slow wave sleep increases compared to the first trimester,[40] complaints of restless sleep also increase.[46]

During the third trimester, more than 98% of women experience nocturnal awakenings.[49] Declines in slow wave[42,44,50] and rapid eye movement (REM) sleep[39-41,44] are observed and are offset by more stage 1 sleep.[41] Despite less nocturnal sleep time compared to the first two trimesters,[39,44] total sleep time approximates prepregnancy sleep time,[44,49] perhaps because the majority of pregnant women take daytime naps.[43,45] In the final trimester, common complaints causing sleep disruption include general discomfort, urinary frequency, spontaneous awakenings, and restless sleep. Fetal movement, heartburn, leg discomfort, fatigue, and difficulty falling asleep or maintaining sleep are also frequently reported.[41,43,46,51]

Following delivery, maternal sleep is most disturbed in the first month,[44] with mean 24-hour total sleep time at 2 weeks postpartum less than 6 hours, including naps.[52] Maternal sleep time and sleep efficiency increase as the infant's circadian rhythm matures, with a transition to uninterrupted sleep generally occurring around the twelfth week postpartum.[53] Dramatically higher percentages of slow wave sleep have been observed in breastfeeding women compared to bottle-feeding women and nongravid control subjects, and have been attributed to high levels of circulating prolactin in lactating women.[54]

Characteristics associated with poor sleep among pregnant women include age over 30[49] and in the postpartum period, primiparity.[55] Sleep quality has also been reported to be impaired among preeclamptic women.[56] Women with affective disorders can experience sleep disruption earlier in pregnancy than other women, but have been observed to be otherwise similar compared to control subjects.[57]

Management of Difficulty Sleeping During Pregnancy

Despite moderate to high levels of fatigue[43] and the high prevalence of disturbed sleep among pregnant women, they generally do not report complaints to their physicians.[47,58] However, despite speculation about potential associations between postpartum sleep disruption and mood disorders ranging from postpartum depression to overt psychosis,[59-62] little is known about the effects of sleep restriction and sleep disturbance on either pregnant or postpartum women.[43]

For pregnant women with general sleep complaints, sleep hygiene techniques and therapies targeted at pregnancy-associated complaints can be beneficial after excluding specific sleep disorders through history and, if necessary, additional testing. Less commonly, pregnant women may experience severe, persistent insomnia. Although behavioral therapies should be attempted, medication (Table 58-1) can be considered for use in refractory cases after discussion of potential risks and benefits. Two hypnotic agents are designated as class B in pregnancy (i.e., fetal harm possible but unlikely[63]): (1) zolpidem, a nonbenzodiazepine hypnotic;[64] and (2) diphenhydramine, a sedating antihistamine.[64] Zolpidem is preferable, given its shorter duration of action and lack of anticholinergic effects. Zaleplon, another shorter-acting agent, is class C (possible adverse fetal effects based on animal studies, no evidence of adverse fetal effects in humans[63]) in pregnancy.[65] Most of the other sedative-hypnotics (see Table 58-1) should be avoided as they are pregnancy class D (human data shows risk, though benefits may outweigh these) or X (benefit unlikely to outweigh clear evidence of increased human or animal risk).[63,64]

SLEEP AND THE MENOPAUSAL TRANSITION

Problems with sleep are widely reported among middle-aged women and have commonly been attributed to the menopausal transition or cited as a symptom of menopause.[66-72] In fact, a recent NIH panel on menopausal symptoms concluded that sleep disturbance is an important problem in women during the perimenopausal and early postmenopausal periods.[73] Nevertheless, whether difficulty sleeping increases among women in the late reproductive years and results from symptoms of the menopausal transition, particularly hot flashes and night sweats, or whether the aging process itself causes an increase in sleep problems that is incorrectly attributed to menopause is not well understood. Studies measuring subjective sleep

TABLE 58-1

Pregnancy Safety Classifications of Common Medications for Sleep Disorders

Drug	Drug Class	Pregnancy Category*	Comments†
INSOMNIA			
Diphenhydramine	Antihistamine	B	No evidence of fetal harm in animal studies
Zolpidem	Imidazopyridine	C	No evidence of fetal harm in animal studies
Amitriptyline	Tricyclic antidepressant	C	Animal teratogen at high doses; insufficient human data
Doxepin	Tricyclic antidepressant	C	Possible association with major birth defects, polydactyly
Eszopiclone	Nonbenzodiazepine hypnotic	C	No evidence of animal teratogenicity even at high doses but decreased weight and survival of pups; insufficient human data
Ramelteon	Melatonin receptor agonist	C	Fetal structural abnormalities, growth and developmental retardation in some animal studies; insufficient human data
Trazodone	Antidepressant	C	Fetal toxicity and teratogenicity in animals at high doses
Zaleplon	Nonbenzodiazepine hypnotic	C	Increased stillbirths in animal studies; insufficient human data
Lorazepam	Benzodiazepine	D	"Floppy infant syndrome," respiratory depression, possible association with anal atresia
Estazolam	Benzodiazepine	X	May have adverse effects similar to those of other benzodiazepines
Flurazepam	Benzodiazepine	X	No reported major adverse effects in animals or humans, but known adverse effects of other benzodiazepines
Quazepam	Benzodiazepine	X	May have adverse effects similar to those of other benzodiazepines
Temazepam	Benzodiazepine	X	Potential interaction with diphenhydramine, causing stillbirth in animals and one human case
Triazolam	Benzodiazepine	X	May have adverse effects similar to those of other benzodiazepines
RESTLESS LEGS SYNDROME			
Oxycodone	Opioid	B	No evidence of teratogenic effects in animal studies; potential neonatal respiratory depression, withdrawal symptoms
Pergolide	Dopamine agonist	B	No evidence of fetal harm in animal studies
Carbidopa-levodopa	Dopaminergic	C	Teratogenicity and toxicity in animals, limited human data showing no adverse effects
Gabapentin	Anticonvulsant	C	Some fetal toxicity in animals, limited human data
Levodopa	Dopaminergic	C	See entry for carbidopa-levodopa
Pramipexole	Dopamine agonist	C	Pregnancy disruption and early embryonic loss in animals, insufficient human data
Ropinirole	Dopamine agonist	C	Teratogenicity and toxicity in animals at high doses, insufficient human data
Codeine	Opioid	C/D	Neonatal respiratory depression, neonatal withdrawal symptoms
Hydrocodone	Opioid	C/D	Teratogenicity in animals, possible association with human fetal malformations
Propoxyphene HCl	Opioid	C/D	Neonatal withdrawal symptoms
Carbamazepine	Anticonvulsant	D	Increased incidence of major and minor malformations, including spina bifida
Clonazepam	Benzodiazepine	D	Neonatal respiratory depression
NARCOLEPSY			
Excessive somnolence			
Pemoline	CNS stimulant	B	No evidence of teratogenicity, but increased stillbirths in animal studies; limited human data
Armodafinil	Wake-promoting agent	C	Increased incidence of fetal visceral and skeletal variations at intermediate and high doses in animals; inadequate human data
Dextroamphetamine	Amphetamine	C	Increased risk of premature delivery and low birth weight, neonatal withdrawal symptoms
Methylphenidate	CNS stimulant	C	Teratogen in animals at high doses; inadequate human data
Metamphetamine	Amphetamine	C	See entry for dextroamphetamine
Modafinil	Wake-promoting agent	C	Fetal toxicity in animals at high doses in some but not all studies; inadequate human data
Cataplexy, other REM-related symptoms			
Sodium oxybate	CNS depressant	B	No evidence of teratogenicity in animal studies

quality have observed that peri- and postmenopausal women generally report worse sleep quality compared to premenopausal women.[67,69,70,74] In several large, cross-sectional, community-based surveys, higher rates of self-reported difficulty sleeping have been observed among peri- and postmenopausal compared to premenopausal women.[67,69,71,72,75] For instance, in a survey of nearly 1500 Scottish women aged 45 to 54, the prevalence of sleep problems among peri- and postmenopausal women was 40% and 35%, respectively, compared to 22% among premenopausal women.[71]

Role of Vasomotor Symptoms

The role of vasomotor symptoms (i.e., hot flashes) in menopausal sleep disturbances remains unclear.[73] Hot flashes (also known as *hot flushes, vasomotor symptoms, night sweats)* are reported by 75% of women during the menopausal transition and are the most common symptom of menopause.[76] Hot flashes are a transient but sudden sensation of intense heat, occurring in the upper body in association with vasodilation and sweating, and resulting in heat loss.[77] Hot flashes often cause physical and emotional distress and can interfere with daytime activities or disrupt sleep.[78] Many women report that hot flashes persist for 4 to 5 years during the menopausal transition, and are most prevalent in the late peri- and early postmenopausal periods.[79] Variations in prevalence of hot flashes between ethnicities and races have been reported in some studies: in the multiethnic, community-based Study of Women's Health Across the Nation (SWAN), African-American women were most likely and Asian women least likely to report hot flashes. Similarly, in the Penn Ovarian Aging Study, African-American women were nearly twice as likely as white women to report hot flashes.[80] Although hot flashes can occur at any time throughout the day and night, the majority of women have more symptoms from late afternoon until the early morning, including during sleep.[81]

Although population-based surveys have generally demonstrated an association between menopausal status and subjective sleep problems, some of these studies failed to control for vasomotor symptoms. Even among studies taking vasomotor symptoms into account, the findings are conflicting. In the SWAN study, both vasomotor symptoms and menopausal status were independently associated with sleep difficulties;[67] women in late perimenopause were at greatest risk for difficulty sleeping. In a recent survey of midlife women from California, the prevalence of chronic insomnia was also highest among perimenopausal women, compared to pre- and postmenopausal participants.[1] After adjustment for hot flashes, however, symptoms of insomnia were not consistently more common among peri- and postmenopausal women: although advancing menopausal status was associated with difficulty maintaining sleep, global sleep dissatisfaction was *least* prevalent among perimenopausal women after adjusting for hot flashes and other variables. Similarly, in the Penn Ovarian Aging Study, sleep quality did not worsen with advancing menopausal status after accounting for reproductive hormone levels, hot flashes, and other symptoms associated with the transition.[82] These study results imply that menopausal status may be less important to sleep quality than the degree to which women are symptomatic with vasomotor symptoms.

Studies of the relationship between menopausal status, vasomotor symptoms, and *objective* measurements of sleep are also limited and contradictory. Perimenopausal women were observed to have longer and more numerous awakenings from sleep than premenopausal women in a study utilizing actigraphy.[83] However, investigators have failed to find significant differences in polysomnographic sleep measures among pre-, peri-, and postmenopausal women.[84] Furthermore, polysomnographic measures from 589 women participating in the Wisconsin Sleep Cohort Study demonstrated that although postmenopausal women reported significantly more dissatisfaction with sleep, they spent more time in bed asleep, slept for longer periods, and had a greater proportion of slow wave sleep compared to premenopausal women.[75] Women in this study who experienced nocturnal hot flashes were more likely to report dissatisfaction with sleep, but differences in objectively measured sleep parameters between women with and without hot flashes were not observed.[75]

It is generally believed that hot flashes cause arousals and awakenings from sleep, leading in turn to daytime fatigue, yet in only a few studies have simultaneous physiologic recordings of hot flashes and sleep measures been made. In 1981, Erlik and associates[85] recorded sleep electroencephalography and skin conductance (a method for detecting hot flashes) in 9 postmenopausal women with frequent, severe hot flashes. They found that 45 of 47 hot flashes recorded in these women were associated with a waking episode within 5 minutes before or after the onset of the hot flash. Nevertheless, not all hot flashes were associated with awakenings from sleep. Similarly, a subsequent study in which sleep and sternal skin conductance were recorded in postmenopausal women found that women with hot flashes had lower sleep efficiency, awoke more often, and had more changes in sleep stages than women without hot flashes.[86]

More recently, sleep electroencephalogram and sternal skin conductance recordings were used to examine whether hot flashes were associated with increased arousal and awakening frequency in 31 cycling and postmenopausal women.[87] The investigators failed to find significant differences between women with and without hot flashes. Given large differences in some of the raw data measurements in this study, however, insufficient sample size may have contributed to the lack of detected differences.

Reproductive Hormones and Sleep in Menopausal Women

Few studies have examined whether levels of reproductive hormones predict difficulty sleeping or other symptoms of the menopausal transition.[68,82,88,89] Among African-American and white women in the Penn Ovarian Aging Study, lower mean levels of estradiol initially predicted difficulty sleeping among the oldest subjects, who were 45 to 49 years of age at the time and still premenopausal.[89] Analyses performed in the same cohort after 8 years used a more in-depth measure of sleep quality, at which time many subjects had reached the late transition and postmenopausal stages: these results demonstrated that lower levels of inhibin B, a marker of the early menopausal transition, were a strong predictor of poorer self-reported sleep quality.[82] Higher follicle-stimulating hormone (FSH) levels were also associated with poorer sleep in some analyses in this study.

When levels of reproductive hormones were measured in a subset of women participating in the SWAN study, higher mean urinary log FSH levels were also associated with poor sleep in premenopausal women.[68] Since FSH stimulates the gonadal production of inhibin B, with inhibin B suppressing pituitary FSH secretion as part of a closed-loop feedback system, higher FSH levels are likely to result from a fall in inhibin B levels.[90] More rapid changes in serum levels of FSH over time were also associated in the SWAN study with less favorable self-reported sleep quality.[91] Thus, findings from both the Penn Ovarian Aging Study and SWAN investigators suggest that changes in hormone levels along the FSH axis are likely to affect sleep quality.

Evaluation of Sleep Complaints in Menopausal Women

Sleep complaints in midlife women should not be automatically attributed to perimenopausal symptoms. Clinical evaluation should include a detailed sleep history, with an assessment of the adequacy of total sleep time, possible mood disorders, and medical conditions or medications that may cause sleep disruption. Common sleep disorders should be ruled out. Symptoms of sleep-disordered breathing should prompt further evaluation for OSA, as the prevalence of this condition increases approximately threefold in postmenopausal compared to premenopausal women. Because many individuals with difficulty sleeping experience symptoms of anxiety and depression, in some cases it may be important to consider referral for further mental health evaluation and treatment.

Given the association between vasomotor symptoms and sleep complaints, one focus of treatment for menopause-associated sleep problems has been on the use of hormone replacement therapy to reduce hot flashes. The Women's Health Initiative and other studies have observed that hormonal therapy increases breast cancer risk and fails to confer long-term cardiovascular benefits,[92] and therefore, current recommendations are for use of the lowest effective dose when needed for brief periods of time following menopause.[93] Estrogen replacement has been demonstrated to decrease sleep disruption due to vasomotor symptoms,[85,94] and it can improve both subjective and objective sleep quality in postmenopausal women without vasomotor symptoms exposed to external stimuli.[95] The latter data suggest that estrogen may improve sleep in part by preventing arousals rather than by reducing vasomotor symptoms. Nevertheless, studies of estrogen replacement do not uniformly demonstrate benefit.[96] Progestins also relieve hot flashes at higher doses.[97] Side effects are frequent, however, and although progestins are used in combination with estrogen in women with a uterus, because of the increased risk of uterine hyperplasia and cancer conferred by unopposed estrogen use, this combination may also exacerbate the overall risk of adverse events compared to estrogen.[98-100]

Aside from hormone replacement therapy, the most widely studied medications for vasomotor symptoms have been the selective serotonin-reuptake inhibitors (SSRIs) and serotonin-norepinephrine reuptake inhibitors (SNRIs). Venlafaxine has been examined in several studies and has been demonstrated to reduce hot flashes by 51% to 65%.[101] Paroxetine also reduced hot flash frequency by 25% over placebo in a trial of women who were mildly symptomatic with hot flashes.[102] However, because venlafaxine and paroxetine are both alerting and can cause sleep disruption and insomnia,[103,104] these medications may have limited utility for treating menopausal sleep disturbances. Conflicting results have been observed with fluoxetine,[105,106] which has more sedating qualities.

There are limited data regarding the effectiveness of centrally acting nonhormonal medications such as gabapentin and clonidine for treating sleep disturbances related to vasomotor symptoms.[107,108] During menopause, the thermoregulatory center of the hypothalamus appears to lower and narrow the range within which core body temperature can fluctuate without provoking the sweating and vasodilation that characterize hot flashes: the thermoneutral zone. These medications are thought to widen the thermoneutral zone.[109]

A number of alternative and complementary therapies have been evaluated for treating vasomotor symptoms. Black cohosh is the best studied and has been demonstrated to have a moderate effect on hot flashes;[110] soy isoflavone products, which contain phytoestrogens, have shown conflicting results.[111,112] Studies of vitamin E, dong quai (*Angelica sinensis*) root, and red clover and most other biologically based, nonhormonal compounds have failed to demonstrate efficacy.[111,112]

Behavioral treatments may also have a role in treating vasomotor symptoms and improving sleep. In a small study of 19 women in the menopausal transition, cognitive behavioral therapy (adapted for the treatment of menopausal hot flashes) was moderately successful at reducing the frequency of vasomotor symptoms.[113] Paced respiration, a slow, controlled diaphragmatic breathing technique that is thought to decrease sympathetic activity,[114] may also reduce hot flashes by as much as 50%.[115] However, additional studies of these promising preliminary therapies are needed before they can be recommended and adopted for widespread use.

OBSTRUCTIVE SLEEP APNEA IN WOMEN

OSA is characterized by repetitive partial or complete collapse of the upper airway during sleep that often results in sleep disruption and complaints of excessive daytime sleepiness. Early studies of patients presenting to clinics declared the disease a male-dominant disorder, with an estimated male:female ratio of 10:1.[116] However, more recent epidemiologic studies show the true male:female ratio of OSA to be close to 3:1 to 2:1, much less lopsided than what was noted in clinical settings.[117,118] It is now thought that women with OSA often have clinical presentations that may delay or obscure their diagnoses, and that women have unique therapeutic considerations and perhaps different prognoses compared to men.

Symptoms

The classic symptoms associated with OSA include snoring, daytime hypersomnolence, and witnessed apneas during sleep. However, studies suggest that women are *more likely* to present with depression or hypothyroidism without sleep complaints, and *less likely* to have witnessed apneas.[119-121] Women may have more insomnia, nightmares, and restless legs complaints than men.[122] Women are also more likely to come to their clinic appointments unaccompanied, meaning that supplemental information from bed partners is less likely to be obtained.[118]

To summarize, women with sleep-disordered breathing frequently do not have "classic symptoms," may not have as "attentive" a bed partner, and are not usually thought of by physicians as being likely to have OSA—all possible reasons why they are relatively underdiagnosed.

Polysomnography

Polysomnographic (PSG) indices for OSA have also been observed to be different between genders. Women tend to have fewer apneas than hypopneas, and their events are shorter.[123,124] Women are also more likely to have a mild form of sleep-disordered breathing that is often termed the upper airway resistance syndrome.[125]

Positional and REM-related sleep apnea are two common forms of OSA. Men are more likely to be diagnosed with supine position-dependent OSA, and women are more likely to experience obstructive events predominantly during REM sleep.[126] REM-related OSA is twice as common in women and is not modified by position, although it is more common when women are younger.[127]

Anatomic Factors

Body Mass Index and Body Habitus

In middle-aged men and women with OSA with similar apnea-hypopnea indices (AHIs), women tend to have a higher body mass index (BMI).[128,129] In addition to BMI, the distribution of total body fat is relevant to the risk of OSA.[130] When comparing men and women with comparable body mass indices and waist circumferences, men exhibit greater upper body obesity, with smaller hip circumferences and greater subscapular skinfold thickness.[131] The finding that compared to men, women with a similar severity of OSA have a higher body mass index may therefore be explained by differences in distribution of body weight by gender.

Upper Airway Anatomy

Upper airway caliber, a major determinant of OSA, is determined by parapharyngeal tissue fat distribution, craniofacial dimensions that affect airway size, and the size of the surrounding tissues (lateral pharyngeal walls and tongue).[132] In normal individuals, total neck soft tissue volume is greater in men than in women, and men have larger soft palates and upper tongue volume than women.[133] Controversy exists as to whether there is a difference by gender in the prevalence of craniofacial abnormalities.[134,135] It has also been suggested that a descended larynx, which evolved to accommodate speech in humans, may place men at a higher risk for sleep-disordered breathing. The male larynx is lower to allow for the deeper male voice and this increases the collapsibility of the upper airway.[136] Interestingly, awake upper airway diameter has been shown to be *greater* in men than in women,[132,137] but narrows more with recumbency[138] and changes in lung volume.[137] Actual upper airway size is a better predictor of clinical severity of OSA in men than in women.[139]

Upper Airway Compliance

Upper airway compliance, or its propensity for collapse, is determined by: tonic and phasic upper airway muscle activation; its biomechanical properties (e.g., connective tissue composition, surface tension); and its responsiveness to change in position. Techniques have shown that men have increased upper airway compliance (more collapsibility) with increasing neck size.[140]

Physiologic Factors

Neuromuscular Reflexes

The neuromuscular reflexes of the upper airway are key to maintaining patency. Both mechanoreceptors and chemoreceptors are utilized to activate the pharyngeal dilator muscles, which are the tensor palatini and genioglossus muscles.

In patients with OSA, it does not appear that upper airway dilator muscles differ by gender in responsiveness. Therefore, it is unlikely that muscle tone per se explains gender differences in OSA.[141-143]

Central Ventilatory Control

Differential responses of ventilatory drive to hypoxia and hypercapnia likely play a role in gender differences regarding OSA. Men have a greater awake ventilatory response to hypoxia and hypercarbia; however, with sleep onset, ventilatory responses to hypoxia are similar.[144-146] This difference results in a greater reduction in ventilation in men compared to women during the wake-sleep transition, and is a stimulus for ventilatory instability in men. In addition, women have a lower apnea threshold (i.e., they tolerate a lower arterial partial pressure of carbon dioxide (Pco_2) before developing apnea) during non-REM (NREM) sleep and are less likely to develop ventilatory instability during sleep.[147] Women are, however, much more likely to respond to flow limitation with increasing respiratory effort and rate, whereas men respond with near-apneic inspiratory flow reduction.[141,148] These differences are likely to play a role in both the development of and response to airway obstruction.

Hormonal Effects

It has been postulated that the gender differences in OSA are related to levels of sex hormones. In one female cohort, those with OSA had lower levels of 17-hydroxyprogesterone, progesterone, and estradiol.[149] It is well know that progesterone levels are related to ventilatory chemoresponsiveness and may influence upper airway dilator muscle activity.[150-152] Testosterone has also been shown to precipitate or worsen OSA,[153,154] and is potentially important in women with polycystic ovary syndrome, a condition of testosterone excess with a high prevalence of OSA.[155]

Leptin is associated with both obesity and ventilatory control and women have higher circulating levels of leptin. Like progesterone, leptin stimulates breathing, which may serve to preserve ventilation in the face of increased work of breathing due to obesity.[156] In obese mice, leptin has been shown to have a greater role in ventilatory control in females compared to males during both wakefulness and NREM sleep.[157] Thus, differences between men and women in leptin levels and function may explain gender differences in the ventilatory response to upper airway obstruction.

Arousal from Sleep

Arousals from sleep result in sleep fragmentation and unrefreshing sleep. In the setting of sleep apnea, arousals from sleep are primarily triggered by increased inspiratory effort. Women are more likely to experience arousals from sleep with increasing inspiratory effort, which may prevent them from developing hypoxia during obstructive events.[158-162] In addition, responses following arousals vary by gender, with increased minute ventilation during the first breath after an arousal in men compared to women.[163]

Sleep-Disordered Breathing and Pregnancy

Obstructive sleep-disordered breathing is uncommon in premenopausal women. However, pregnancy alters hormonal balance, body habitus, and pulmonary function, and thus changes the risk for developing OSA. Increased levels of estrogen and placental growth hormones result in upper airway mucosal edema, which can decrease upper airway size and increase resistance.[164-166] Progesterone, as previously noted, increases ventilation. Uterine enlargement, diaphragmatic elevation, and relaxation of the costochondral ligaments during

pregnancy change the shape and dimensions of the thorax,[167] leading to decreases in functional residual capacity and oxygen reserve.[167] These physical changes during pregnancy, with abdominal distention and weight gain, may precipitate or worsen preexisting sleep apnea.[168] Finally, in late pregnancy, airway closure can occur above functional residual capacity, leading to ventilation-perfusion mismatch[167] and magnifying the adverse consequences of abnormal breathing events.

Several recent studies have established that symptoms of sleep-disordered breathing are common among pregnant women. The prevalence of self-reported snoring in pregnancy has been estimated to be between 14% and 46%, with snoring being more common with advancing gestation.[169,170] Furthermore, many pregnant women also develop other symptoms of sleep-disordered breathing, such as snorting and gasping.[171,172] Nevertheless, only small increases in the number of apneas and hypopneas have been observed during pregnancy,[173,174] raising the question of whether other parameters such as flow limitation may be relevant.

This issue is important because sleep-disordered breathing has been proposed as a risk factor for adverse maternal-fetal outcomes, including preeclampsia and small-for-gestational age births. Several observational studies have reached different conclusions.[49,169,170] Two studies focusing primarily on infant outcomes (birth weight, Apgar scores) failed to find significant differences between infants born to snorers and nonsnorers.[49,170] In contrast, other studies have observed higher rates of gestational hypertension, preeclampsia[169,175] and delivery of small-for-gestational age infants[169] among habitual snorers compared to nonsnorers.[169]

In the general population, CPAP therapy has been shown to lower blood pressure in patients with OSA.[176] The use of nasal CPAP in the hypertensive conditions of pregnancy has been examined in only a small, uncontrolled trial.[177] In this investigation, when autotitrating nasal CPAP was administered to 11 women with severe preeclampsia, mean nocturnal blood pressure was significantly reduced.[177] These results should be interpreted cautiously, given the lack of a control group and other study limitations.

Sleep Apnea and Menopause

The prevalence and clinical severity of OSA in women increases dramatically after menopause, with postmenopausal women having approximately three times the rate of OSA observed in premenopausal women, as previously noted.[178-180] The increase in OSA prevalence with menopause has been attributed to hormonal status, changes in body habitus, and overall fat distribution. In one study of 133 obese females (BMI ≥ 30 kg/m^2), postmenopausal women exhibited larger neck circumferences and higher waist-to-hip circumference ratios.[181] In addition, menopause results in increased abdominal adiposity, suggesting that changes in fat distribution after menopause play an important role.[182]

The role of hormones is clearly an important aspect of the postmenopausal development of OSA. It has been shown that combination estrogen and progesterone replacement reduces apnea and hypopneas[183-185] and that postmenopausal women on hormone replacement therapy have a similar prevalence of OSA as premenopausal women.[178] It is possible that the effect of hormone replacement therapy on sleep-disordered breathing may require an extended duration of therapy to show a protective effect, as existing trials have generally been only 2 to 3 months in duration. Progesterone therapy in males with OSA has not proved to be effective,[186,187] suggesting that progesterone alone does not relieve OSA, but that the progesterone-deficient state may predispose to the development of OSA.

Treatment

Treatment considerations for OSA should be tailored to individual patients, and gender differences should be factored into this decision. Young and Finn demonstrated a significant mortality rate difference in women diagnosed with OSA, compared to men, despite comparable disease severity and treatment options;[188] however, more recent analyses from the Sleep Heart Health Study suggest otherwise.[189] In the latter study, although there was an impressive linear relationship with hazard ratios based on AHI in women, it was suggested that perhaps because women tended to have less severe disease, the female groups with severe OSA may have been underpowered. Further work with prospective studies is needed in this area.

Continuous Positive Airway Pressure Therapy

Nasal continuous positive airway pressure (CPAP) is the therapy of choice for OSA. Results of studies examining the role of gender in predicting adherence to CPAP are conflicting, with men more likely to use CPAP therapy in some studies,[190,191] and women more or similarly likely to be adherent in others.[192,193] The benefits of CPAP may be different between genders because (as already outlined) the symptom complex is different. Similarly, measures to improve adherence may need to be different between genders.

Oral Appliance Therapy

Oral appliances (OAs) are an accepted therapy for OSA in patients with mild to moderate disease. Oral appliances typically come in two forms, mandibular advancement devices and tongue retention devices, both of which increase posterior pharyngeal space and relieve upper airway obstruction. In one study, women with OSA were more likely to have treatment success with OA than men, particularly those with milder forms of OSA.[194] However, another study came to the opposite conclusion.[195] To date, no studies have shown a significant gender difference in adherence to OA therapy.[196]

Upper Airway Surgery

Upper airway surgery for treatment of OSA includes a vast array of techniques and very few randomized controlled trials.[197] Overall, upper airway surgery is not considered a first-line treatment for OSA in adults. Gender differences regarding the outcome of upper airway surgery have not been examined.

Weight Loss

Despite the fact that women with OSA are generally heavier than their male counterparts, weight loss was found to be a more effective treatment strategy for men.[198] It is possible that this is explained by the gender differences in body fat distribution.

Bariatric surgery has become a very popular treatment for morbid obesity and has been shown to reduce the AHI.[199] Because the vast majority of patients who undergo bariatric surgery are female, this clearly has gender implications.

It should be noted that men have been shown to have a higher mortality rate with this surgery[200] and that OSA may persist even after substantial weight loss, suggesting the need for long-term follow-up.[201,202]

RESTLESS LEGS SYNDROME AND PERIODIC LIMB MOVEMENT DISORDER

Restless Legs Syndrome

RLS is a sleep-related movement disorder whose primary feature is unpleasant leg sensations in the evening that interfere with sleep.[203] These sensations are most typically described as restlessness or a need to move, although such terms as "creepy-crawling," "burning," or "itching" have all been used. The discomfort is rarely described as painful, and the use of such a descriptor should prompt consideration of an alternative diagnosis, such as neuropathy. The distressing sensations generally involve the legs, but can also occur in the arms. RLS symptoms are most intense at night, typically between 10 PM and 2 AM. Symptoms are worse at rest and improve with movement or stimulation, including walking, rubbing, or stretching. Because of the nature and timing of RLS symptoms, patients with RLS often complain of insomnia.

The diagnosis of RLS is made by history and physical examination. PSG is not routinely necessary to establish the diagnosis.[204,205] Box 58-1 includes the historical diagnostic criteria. The specificity of these criteria is not ideal, and there is no objective gold standard. However, careful assessment of the four cardinal features, accompanied by a physical examination, has been determined to be approximately 84% specific for RLS, with cramps, positional discomfort, and local leg disease being the most common mimickers.[206] Benes and associates[207] have reported that three of the four essential criteria (urge to move the legs, made worse by rest and worse in the evening) almost completely determine the correlation

---

BOX 58-1 *ICSD-2 Diagnostic Criteria for Restless Legs Syndrome (RLS) in Adults*

- The patient reports an urge to move the legs, usually accompanied or caused by uncomfortable and unpleasant sensations in the legs.
- The urge to move or the unpleasant sensations begin or worsen during periods of rest or inactivity such as lying down or sitting.
- The urge to move or the unpleasant sensations are partially or totally relieved by movement, such as walking or stretching, or at least as long as the activity continues.
- The urge to move or the unpleasant sensations are worse, or only occur, in the evening or at night.
- The condition is not better explained by another current sleep disorder, medical or neurologic disorder, mental disorder, medication use, or substance use disorder.

From American Academy of Sleep Medicine (AASM). *The International Classification of Sleep Disorders: Diagnostic and Coding Manual,* 2nd ed. Westchester, IL: American Academy of Sleep Medicine; 2005.

with expert diagnosis. Adding response to dopaminergic medication to the essential criteria improves the diagnostic accuracy.

The prevalence of any degree of RLS symptoms is estimated to be somewhere in the 10% to 15% range for all adults, with lower rates in the young and higher rates in the elderly.[203] Because the diagnosis of RLS is based on symptom report, prevalence rates vary with different criteria for frequency and severity. For example, in the RLS Epidemiology, Symptoms and Treatment (REST) study, RLS symptoms were endorsed by 7.2% of the survey population. However, symptoms occurring at least twice per week were reported by only 5% of the subjects, and were moderately or severely distressing in only 2.7%.[208]

After the third decade, women are twice as likely as men are to endorse RLS symptoms, which may be related to parity. Pregnancy is an important risk factor for RLS, both during pregnancy and in subsequent years,[209-211] and pregnancy-related RLS is discussed in detail here. Approximately a fourth of pregnant women experience RLS symptoms, which typically peak in severity in the third trimester and resolve promptly after delivery. Lower hemoglobin, mean corpuscular volumes, and serum folate levels appear to be risk factors for RLS in pregnancy.[210,211] In the years after pregnancy, the risk of RLS is associated with bearing children in a dose-dependent way. In one study, nulliparous women had the same risk for RLS as did men up to age 64. However, for women who had borne children, the risk of RLS increased with the number of children. A woman with one child had twice the risk of RLS as a nulliparous woman and the risk increased with additional children.[209]

The rate of RLS has been observed to be lower in Asian than in European populations,[212] but the prevalence in African Americans is similar to that of Caucasians.[213]

There is clearly a familial tendency for the development of both RLS and periodic limb movements. Two recent genome-wide association studies have reported positive association with sequence variants in or around specific genes on chromosomes 6p, 2p, and 15q. The molecular findings, together with the variable expressivity of the phenotype, suggest a substantial clinical and genetic heterogeneity of RLS.[214,215] In an Icelandic cohort of patients with RLS and periodic limb movements of sleep, Stefansson and associates[215] observed a common variant on chromosome 6p21.2, which was replicated in a U.S. sample. These investigators found an association between the variant and periodic limb movements (PLMs) in sleep without RLS (and the absence of such an association for RLS without PLMS) and suggested that they had identified a genetic determinant of periodic limb movements in sleep (PLMS). They also observed that serum ferritin levels were decreased in those with the genetic variant and noted that these findings bolster the hypothesis that iron depletion is involved in the pathogenesis of the disease.

Understanding the pathophysiology of RLS is currently an active area of research, and dysfunction of both iron and dopamine have been implicated. There appear to be contributions from the spinal cord, peripheral nerves, and central dopamine receptors.[216,217] The impairment of dopamine transport or function in the central nervous system (CNS) due to reduced iron levels appears to play a critical role in most patients with this disorder.[217]

When RLS appears without a known predisposing or exacerbating condition, it is considered "primary." Primary RLS is more likely to have earlier age of onset and to be familial. RLS can also be "secondary" to another condition, especially iron deficiency, pregnancy, and renal failure. One study of the age at onset of RLS demonstrated a bimodal distribution, with the largest peak of RLS symptom onset occurring at 20 years of age, and a smaller peak in the mid-40s. Age at onset is different between patients with primary RLS (early onset) and those with secondary RLS,[218] with the cut-off between early and late onset RLS at approximately 36 years of age.

Individuals with RLS have been well documented to have an increased likelihood of mood disturbance.[219-221] Studies demonstrating this relationship have been cross-sectional, so causality (whether RLS causes depression or vice versa) is not established. Indeed, because of the cross-sectional nature of most studies of RLS and associated conditions, the impact of RLS is not well delineated. For example, RLS symptoms have been reported to be associated with daytime sleepiness and objectively disturbed sleep,[222] but have also been shown not to impair daytime alertness.[223] A large group of conditions has now been reported to be associated with RLS[224-232] (Box 58-2). Many of these conditions and disorders also lack objective diagnostic criteria, such as attention deficit hyperactivity disorder (ADHD), depression, and fibromyalgia. However, RLS appears to be associated with many significant medical conditions, and may be a marker for poor overall health. Indeed, one study has reported an increased risk of death in individuals with RLS.[233]

Several medications have been linked to both RLS and periodic limb movements, including tricyclic antidepressants, lithium, selective serotonin reuptake inhibitors, and dopamine antagonists (including some antipsychotics and antiemetics).[234] The data are particularly strong for the association between RLS and antidepressants; one study of patients recorded RLS as a side effect in 9% of new antidepressant users. The likelihood of RLS symptoms was especially high for those taking mirtazapine.[234] Lifestyle may also contribute to RLS symptoms. Higher body mass index, caffeine intake, sedentary lifestyle, smoking, earning a lower income, and reduced alcohol consumption have all been associated with an increased likelihood of reporting RLS symptoms.[203]

The evaluation of the RLS patient with new or exacerbated symptoms should include questions pertaining to the preceding factors as well as a thorough neurologic examination (primarily to rule out neuropathy, which may be confused with RLS) and testing for iron deficiency with a serum ferritin level.

BOX 58-2 *Conditions Associated with Restless Legs Syndrome*

- Attention deficit hyperactivity disorder[226]
- Chronic obstructive pulmonary disease[229]
- Depression and panic disorder[275]
- Fibromyalgia[227]
- Migraine[231]
- Medication use[276]
- Multiple sclerosis[224,277]
- Neuropathy[228]
- Parkinson's disease treatment[278]
- Pulmonary hypertension[230]

The treatment for RLS in patients who have frequent or intense symptoms includes both nonpharmacologic and pharmacologic modalities. Nonpharmacologic measures include education, moderate exercise,[235] smoking cessation, alcohol avoidance, caffeine reduction or elimination, and discontinuation of offending medications if it is safe to do so. Some have found that working at night and sleeping during the day has helped. Iron supplementation should be prescribed for those who are iron deficient. Recently, pneumatic compression devices have been shown to relieve symptoms in a randomized, double-blinded sham-controlled trial.[236]

In terms of pharmacologic treatment, dopamine receptor agonists are first-line treatment. The dopamine receptor agonists ropinirole and pramipexole are both approved by the Food and Drug Administration (FDA) and recommended for this purpose.[237,238] In April 2011, the FDA also approved gabapentin enacarbil extended-release tablets, 600 mg at 5 PM.

One consideration in the pharmacologic treatment of RLS is the large placebo effect; in a meta-analysis of 24 trials, Fulda and Wetter reported that the pooled placebo effect was about 40%.[239] The placebo effect appeared to be largest when assessed using the International Restless Legs Severity Scale (IRLSS), moderate for daytime functioning, small to moderate for subjective and objective sleep parameters, very small for PLMS and absent for sleep efficiency.

Another consideration in the pharmacologic management of RLS is the appearance of augmentation. The International Restless Legs Study Group has established diagnostic standards for the dopaminergic augmentation of RLS, based on usual time of RLS symptom onset each day, number of body parts with RLS symptoms, latency to symptoms at rest, severity of the symptoms when they occur, and effects of dopaminergic medication on symptoms. Either a 4-hour advance in usual starting time for RLS symptoms or a combination of the occurrence of other features indicates augmentation, according to these recommendations.[240]

Periodic Limb Movements of Sleep

Much confusion exists about the presentation and overlap of RLS and PLMS. PLMS, originally called *nocturnal myoclonus,* and sometimes periodic leg movements (PLMs), consist of rhythmic extensions of the big toe and dorsiflexions of the ankle with occasional flexions of the knee and hip. These movements usually occur during the first part of the night and increase in frequency with age. Each movement lasts approximately 2 to 4 seconds with a frequency of one every 20 to 40 seconds.[11] During an overnight sleep study, PLMs are scored if they are part of a series of four or more consecutive movements lasting 0.5 to 5.0 seconds, with an intermovement interval of 4 to 90 seconds. A PLMS index of greater than 15 (movements per hour of sleep) is generally considered elevated in adults (Box 58-3).

PLMS are most commonly identified in association with other sleep disorders. The most notable association is the occurrence of PLMS in the overwhelming majority (> 80%) of RLS patients, suggesting a like pathophysiology. PLMS has also been described in the obstructive sleep apnea-hypopnea syndrome, the upper airway resistance syndrome, narcolepsy, and REM sleep behavior disorder.[241,242] PLMS are also frequently observed in patients taking antidepressants and probably represent a serotoninergic phenomenon.[243] When

individuals with complaints of insomnia or hypersomnia have PLMS and no other sleep disorder is present, they are referred to as having periodic limb movement disorder (PLMD). Such patients are probably rare. Patients with PLMS associated with RLS are treated like any other RLS patient. If PLMs are noted on PSG but symptoms of RLS are not present, there is no evidence to support treatment, especially pharmacologic, to suppress PLMS/PLMD, even in the face of insomnia or hypersomnia.[242] Indeed, there is no FDA-approved agent to treat PLMS or PLMD. The revised diagnostic criteria for PLMD take into account the coexistence of leg jerks with many medical conditions and medications, and also raise the threshold for an "abnormal" number of periodic limb movements of sleep from 5 to 15 for adults (see Box 58-3).

Restless Legs Syndrome and Periodic Limb Movements of Sleep in Pregnancy

Although RLS is infrequently recognized by physicians taking care of pregnant patients,[58] the prevalence of RLS has been observed to increase during pregnancy[49,211,244] and to resolve rapidly post partum.[58] In a large cross-sectional study of approximately 16,000 pregnant women in Japan, Suzuki and associates[244] observed that 15% of subjects reported RLS symptoms at 3 to 4 months of gestation, increasing to 23% at term. Women with RLS reported significantly lower average sleep time, more difficulty in initiating and maintaining sleep, more early morning awakenings, and more excessive daytime somnolence than women without RLS.[244] Risk factors for RLS may include primiparity, advancing pregnancy, less than 7 hours of sleep, lack of daytime napping, smoking, and use of medication or alcohol.[244]

BOX 58-3 *ICSD-2 Diagnostic Criteria for Periodic Limb Movement Disorder (PLMD)*

- Polysomnography demonstrates repetitive, highly stereotypical limb movements that are
  - 0.5 to 5 seconds in duration
  - Of amplitude less than or equal to 25% of toe dorsiflexion during calibration
  - In a sequence of four or more movements
  - Separated by an interval of more than 5 seconds (from limb movement onset) and less than 90 seconds (typically an interval of 20 to 40 seconds)
- The periodic limb movements of sleep index exceeds 5 per hour in children and 15 per hour in most adult cases.
- There is clinical sleep disturbance or a complaint of daytime fatigue.
- The periodic limb movements are not better explained by another current sleep disorder, medical or neurologic disorder, mental disorder, medication use, or substance use disorder.

NOTE: If periodic limb movements of sleep are present without clinical sleep disturbance, they can be noted as a polysomnographic finding, but criteria are not met for a diagnosis of PLMD.

From American Academy of Sleep Medicine (AASM). *The International Classification of Sleep Disorders: Diagnostic and Coding Manual,* 2nd ed. Westchester, IL: American Academy of Sleep Medicine; 2005.

Although PLMs are common in individuals with RLS,[245] whether they contribute significantly to sleep disruption during pregnancy is just beginning to be studied. When assessed in a series of 10 women with multiple gestations in the third trimester of pregnancy, periodic limb movements were present in all subjects (mean 21.7 events/hour).[246] Only four subjects reported symptoms of RLS associated with the pregnancy,[246] suggesting that PLMS may be present in the absence of RLS. However, the frequency of arousals due to PLMS was not reported.

Reduced serum ferritin levels, the most specific marker for iron deficiency,[247] have been demonstrated in pregnant women with RLS.[211] However, pregnant women without RLS symptoms have similar reductions in ferritin, an observation attributed to the normal hemodilution that accompanies pregnancy.[211] In contrast, although serum folate levels remain within the normal range in pregnant women with RLS, levels are consistently lower than in control subjects.[211]

Treatment of Restless Legs Syndrome in Pregnancy

For pregnant women who develop RLS, evaluation for iron deficiency with a serum ferritin level and a trial of folate supplementation are a reasonable approach. Folic acid has been reported to improve symptoms in pregnant patients with RLS who are folate deficient.[248] Iron replacement reduces or eliminates symptoms in patients with serum ferritin levels below 45 µg/L.[249] Conservative treatments (walking, stretching, massage of the affected limbs, application of heat, and relaxation techniques) may also be helpful. Abstinence from tobacco and alcohol should be reinforced, and adequate time should be set aside for sleep.[244]

None of the medications commonly used to treat RLS is entirely safe in pregnancy. Nevertheless, for women with severe symptoms, standard pharmacologic therapies for idiopathic RLS, such as dopaminergic agents, opiates, and benzodiazepine medications, can be considered.[250] There are no controlled clinical trials upon which to base treatment recommendations. For short-term use, oxycodone and pergolide are currently classified as class B in pregnancy; however, pergolide use has been reported in association with valvular heart anomalies in nongravid individuals.[251] Most benzodiazepines, anticonvulsants, other opioids, and dopamine agonists have been classified as class C, D, or X in pregnancy (see Table 58-1).

By 10 days after delivery, the majority of patients with pregnancy-associated RLS report symptom resolution.[58] In a few women, symptoms persist beyond the month following delivery.[58,211] These cases can be managed using standard therapies, although consideration should be given to the excretion of opioids, benzodiazepines, and anticonvulsant medications in breast milk, and to the possibility that lactation may be diminished by the use of dopaminergic medications.[205]

NARCOLEPSY

Differences Between Women and Men

Few studies have examined whether gender differences exist in the epidemiology, clinical presentation, and response to treatment of women and men with narcolepsy. A slight male predominance in the prevalence of narcolepsy has been observed.[252-255] These studies include one of the earliest case series of patients with narcolepsy,[255] as well as studies in French and French-Canadian populations[254] and Olmstead County in Minnesota.[253] Among individuals with narcolepsy with cataplexy, the higher prevalence among males may be less pronounced,[252,253] having been estimated at 1.4 males to each female, compared to 1.8 males to each female when considering narcolepsy patients with or without cataplexy.[253] In the community-based Wisconsin Sleep Cohort Study,[252] 5.9% of males had a mean sleep onset latency of 8 minutes or less and at least two sleep onset REM sleep periods on multiple sleep latency testing (consistent with the diagnosis of narcolepsy) without cataplexy, compared to 1.1% of females, suggesting a high rate of narcolepsy without cataplexy with a distinct male preponderance. However, a study from an ethnically and racially diverse community, King County in Washington State, described more females than males in a registry of narcolepsy patients.[256]

With regard to the clinical presentation of narcolepsy, the median age of onset was not significantly different by sex among subjects in the Olmstead County or French and French-Canadian populations,[253,254] nor have differences in Epworth Sleepiness Scale scores or HLA type been reported.[254] Although observations of greater objective sleepiness (i.e., shorter mean latency to sleep onset on the MSLT) were made among female French Canadians with narcolepsy compared to their male counterparts, this finding was not replicated in a comparison group from France in the same study.[254] Sex differences were not observed in the ability to remain awake, as assessed by the maintenance of wakefulness test, in a large sample of patients with narcolepsy who were free of medication when tested.[257] The rate of episodes of cataplexy has been observed both to be similar between women and men[254] and higher among men.[258] A small study of plasma orexin A levels in 12 men and women with narcolepsy did not show significant differences between groups.[259] Sex differences in the clinical course of narcolepsy or response to pharmacologic or other treatments have not been described.

Narcolepsy and Pregnancy

Little information exists about how pregnancy affects the course of narcolepsy.[260] The clinical presentation of narcolepsy usually occurs during adolescence or young adulthood,[261] and symptoms may be exacerbated by the sleep disturbance associated with pregnancy. Individuals with narcolepsy often require medication for excessive daytime somnolence (e.g., modafinil, methylphenidate, amphetamines) or REM-related symptoms including cataplexy (e.g., tricyclic agents, SSRI agents, sodium oxybate). However, prematurity, low birth weight and withdrawal symptoms have been reported in infants born to women taking amphetamines[262] and many of these drugs are designated class C in pregnancy (see Table 58-1). Similarly, the widely used wakefulness-promoting agents modafinil, armodafinil, and methylphenidate have been labeled class C.[263] Pemoline, a CNS stimulant with a chemical structure dissimilar to the amphetamines, is class B in pregnancy[64] but has been associated rarely with liver failure (nonpregnant individuals);[264] because of its potential toxicity, it is rarely indicated in the treatment of narcolepsy.[262] Selegiline, which has both alerting and anticataplectic effects, and fluoxetine, which has anti-REM effects, are also class C.[265]

Given the limited treatment options, the reduction or discontinuation of stimulant drugs has been advised for women attempting to conceive and for pregnant women, except in cases in which potential benefits to the patient clearly outweigh risks to the fetus.[265] Whenever possible, narcolepsy should be managed during pregnancy by maintenance of adequate sleep time, scheduled naps, and if necessary, a reduction in work and family responsibilities. Women with disabling cataplectic episodes or who must maintain daytime alertness (e.g., who must drive) may continue to require medication.

NIGHTTIME EATING DISORDERS

Eating during usual sleep hours is well described in the sleep medicine literature. Nighttime eating can be divided into that done during wakefulness (night eating) and that done during sleep (sleep-related eating disorder, SRED). The latter is involuntary and beyond the individual's control. SRED occurs more often in females, with some case series noting a female predominance as high as 80%. SRED tends to occur in younger age groups and has been associated with childhood sleepwalking. Patients with SRED may eat bizarre foods (e.g., raw bacon or cat food) with variable recall of the event ranging from none to substantial.[11]

The precipitation of SRED has been associated with use of several different medications, including hypnotics such as zolpidem and triazolam, as well as psychiatric medications such as olanzapine and resperidone.[266,267] It appears to be more common in patients with eating disorders and dissociative disorders. Patients can have many adverse consequences from SRED including weight gain, ingestion of poisonous or allergic substances, poor dentition, lacerations or burns from food preparation, household fires, and secondary depression.[268] Treatment of SRED can be problematic, with most experts suggesting that benzodiazepines alone are less effective than topiramate, or dopaminergic or serotonin modulating therapies.[269,270]

Night eating is the conscious consumption of food after the last meal and prior to desired time to get out of bed. In contrast to SRED, the patient is aware of eating and will consume "standard" foods, albeit ones often high in calories and fat. These patients exhibit anorexia in the morning and may ingest more than 50% of their total caloric intake at night.[271] It is less clear whether there is a gender preference with night eating, but it has been associated with eating disorders, which are more common in females. Studies of treatment suggest sertraline and topiramate are effective. Use of hypnotics and sedating drugs have not been shown to be of benefit.[272,273]

CONCLUSION

Much has been learned about both normal and disordered sleep in women over the past decades. We have come to recognize how conditions specific to women such as pregnancy and menopause can affect normal sleep, and how women's risk for sleep problems such as sleep-disordered breathing and restless legs syndrome may be impacted by changes in the hormonal milieu. Differences between women and men in the prevalence, clinical characteristics, and perhaps even the pathophysiology of some sleep disorders such as obstructive sleep apnea have emerged and inform our clinical practice and care of patients. Nevertheless, we are still learning about both gender differences in sleep disorders and about how reproductive status and specific hormones influence sleep and sleep quality across all stages of women's lives and especially those during which substantial changes in hormonal levels occur. Future studies that not only recognize but leverage these differences to ascertain the efficacy and effectiveness of various treatments for specific sleep disorders depending on patient gender have the potential to improve the health of both women and men. Finally, improved dissemination to both health care providers and patients themselves of existing and new insights that affect women's sleep is imperative for improving recognition and treatment of sleep disorders in female patients.

REFERENCES

1. Ohayon MM. Severe hot flashes are associated with chronic insomnia. *Arch Intern Med.* 2006;166:1262-1268.
2. Camhi SL, Morgan WJ, Pernisco N, Quan SF. Factors affecting sleep disturbances in children and adolescents. *Sleep Med.* 2000;1:117-123.
3. Ohayon MM, Caulet M, Guilleminault C. How a general population perceives its sleep and how this relates to the complaint of insomnia. *Sleep.* 1997;20:715-723.
4. Zhang B, Wing YK. Sex differences in insomnia: A meta-analysis. *Sleep.* 2006;29:85-93.
5. Van Cauter E, Leproult R, Plat L. Age-related changes in slow wave sleep and REM sleep and relationship with growth hormone and cortisol levels in healthy men. *JAMA.* 2000;284:861-868.
6. Latta F, Leproult R, Tasali E, Hofmann E, L'Hermite-Baleriaux M, et al. Sex differences in nocturnal growth hormone and prolactin secretion in healthy older adults: Relationships with sleep EEG variables. *Sleep.* 2005;28:1519-1524.
7. Redline S, Kirchner HL, Quan SF, Gottlieb DJ, Kapur V, Newman A. The effects of age, sex, ethnicity, and sleep-disordered breathing on sleep architecture. *Arch Intern Med.* 2004;164:406-418.
8. Latta F, Leproult R, Tasali E, Hofmann E, Van Cauter E. Sex differences in delta and alpha EEG activities in healthy older adults. *Sleep.* 2005;28:1525-1534.
9. Lauderdale DS, Knutson KL, Yan LL, Rathouz PJ, Hulley SB, et al. Objectively measured sleep characteristics among early-middle-aged adults: The CARDIA study. *Am J Epidemiol.* 2006;164:5-16.
10. National Institutes of Health. NIH State of the Science Conference Statement on Manifestations and Management of Chronic Insomnia in Adults. *J Clin Sleep Med.* 2005;1:412-421.
11. American Academy of Sleep Medicine (AASM). *The International Classification of Sleep Disorders: Diagnostic and Coding Manual.* 2nd ed. Westchester, IL: American Academy of Sleep Medicine; 2005.
12. American Psychiatric Association. *Diagnostic and Statistical Manual of Mental Disorders.* Washington, DC: American Psychiatric Association; 1994.
13. American Academy of Sleep Medicine. *International Classification of Sleep Disorders, Revised Edition: Diagnostic and Coding Manual.* Rochester, MN: American Academy of Sleep Medicine; 2000:114–117.
14. Morin CM, Vallieres A, Guay B, Ivers H, Savard J, et al. Cognitive behavioral therapy, singly and combined with medication, for persistent insomnia: A randomized controlled trial. *JAMA.* 2009;301:2005-2015.
15. Dinges D, Rogers N, Baynard M. Chronic sleep deprivation. In: Kryger M, Roth T, Dement W, eds. *Principles and Practice of Sleep Medicine.* 4th ed. Philadelphia: Elsevier Saunders; 2005:67-76.
16. Owens GM. Gender differences in health care expenditures, resource utilization, and quality of care. *J Manag Care Pharm.* 2008;14:2-6.
17. Grigoriadis S, Robinson GE. Gender issues in depression. *Ann Clin Psychiatry.* 2007;19:247-255.
18. Bekker MH, van Mens-Verhulst J. Anxiety disorders: Sex differences in prevalence, degree, and background, but gender-neutral treatment. *Gend Med.* 2007;4(Suppl B):S178-S193.
19. Ford DE, Kamerow DB. Epidemiologic study of sleep disturbances and psychiatric disorders. An opportunity for prevention? *JAMA.* 1989;262:1479-1484.
20. Phillips B, Mannino D. Correlates of sleep complaints in adults: The ARIC study. *J Clin Sleep Med.* 2005;1:277-283.
21. Roehrs T, Hyde M, Blaisdell B, Greenwald M, Roth T. Sleep loss and REM sleep loss are hyperalgesic. *Sleep.* 2006;29:145-151.
22. Vgontzas AN, Bixler EO, Lin HM, Prolo P, Mastorakos G, et al. Chronic insomnia is associated with nyctohemeral activation of the hypothalamic-pituitary-adrenal axis: Clinical implications. *J Clin Endocrinol Metab.* 2001; 86:3787-3794.

23. Perlis M, Smith M, Pigeon W. Etiology and pathophysiology of insomnia. In: Kryger M, Roth T, Dement W, eds. *Principles and Practice of Sleep Medicine.* 4th ed. Philadelphia: Elsevier Saunders; 2005:714-725.
24. Daley M, Morin CM, LeBlanc M, Gregoire JP, Savard J, Baillargeon L. Insomnia and its relationship to health-care utilization, work absenteeism, productivity and accidents. *Sleep Med.* 2009;10:427-438.
25. Dodge R, Cline MG, Quan SF. The natural history of insomnia and its relationship to respiratory symptoms. *Arch Intern Med.* 1995;155:1797-1800.
26. Kripke DF, Garfinkel L, Wingard DL, Klauber MR, Marler MR. Mortality associated with sleep duration and insomnia. *Arch Gen Psychiatry.* 2002;59:131-136.
27. Phillips B, Mannino DM. Does insomnia kill? *Sleep.* 2005;28:965-971.
28. Vgontzas AN, Liao D, Bixler EO, Chrousos GP, Vela-Bueno A. Insomnia with objective short sleep duration is associated with a high risk for hypertension. *Sleep.* 2009;32:491-497.
29. Phillips B, Mannino DM. Do insomnia complaints cause hypertension or cardiovascular disease? *J Clin Sleep Med.* 2007;3:489-494.
30. Phillips B, Buzkova P, Enright P. Cardiovascular Health Study Research G. Insomnia did not predict incident hypertension in older adults in the cardiovascular health study. *Sleep.* 2009;32:65-72.
31. Riemann D, Perlis ML. The treatments of chronic insomnia: A review of benzodiazepine receptor agonists and psychological and behavioral therapies. *Sleep Med Rev.* 2009;13:205-214.
32. Kripke DF, Simons RN, Garfinkel L, Hammond EC. Short and long sleep and sleeping pills. Is increased mortality associated? *Arch Gen Psychiatry.* 1979;36:103-116.
33. Kripke DF, Klauber MR, Wingard DL, Fell RL, Assmus JD, Garfinkel L. Mortality hazard associated with prescription hypnotics. *Biol Psychiatry.* 1998;43:687-693.
34. Mallon L, Broman JE, Hetta J. Is usage of hypnotics associated with mortality? *Sleep Med.* 2009;10:279-286.
35. Hublin C, Partinen M, Koskenvuo M, Kaprio J. Sleep and mortality: A population-based 22-year follow-up study. *Sleep.* 2007;30:1245-1253.
36. Gustavsen I, Bramness JG, Skurtveit S, Engeland A, Neutel I, Morland J. Road traffic accident risk related to prescriptions of the hypnotics zopiclone, zolpidem, flunitrazepam and nitrazepam. *Sleep Med.* 2008;9:818-822.
37. Kripke DF. Possibility that certain hypnotics might cause cancer in skin. *J Sleep Res.* 2008;17:245-250.
38. Morin CM, Belanger L, LeBlanc M, Ivers H, Savard J, et al. The natural history of insomnia: A population-based 3-year longitudinal study. *Arch Intern Med.* 2009;169:447-453.
39. Brunner DP, Munch M, Biedermann K, Huch R, Huch A, Borbely AA. Changes in sleep and sleep electroencephalogram during pregnancy. *Sleep.* 1994;17:576-582.
40. Driver HS, Shapiro CM. A longitudinal study of sleep stages in young women during pregnancy and postpartum. *Sleep.* 1992;15:449-453.
41. Hertz G, Fast A, Feinsilver SH, Albertario CL, Schulman H, Fein AM. Sleep in normal late pregnancy. *Sleep.* 1992;15:246-251.
42. Karacan I, Heine W, Agnew H, Williams RL, Webb WB, Ross JJ. Characteristics of sleep patterns during late pregnancy and post partum periods. *Am J Obstet Gynecol.* 1968;101:579-586.
43. Lee KA, DeJoseph JF. Sleep disturbances, vitality, and fatigue among a select group of employed childbearing women. *Birth.* 1992;19:208-213.
44. Lee KA, Zaffke ME, McEnany G. Parity and sleep patterns during and after pregnancy. *Obstet Gynecol.* 2000;95:14-18.
45. Mindell JA, Jacobson BJ. Sleep disturbances during pregnancy. *JOGNN: J Obstet Gynecol Neonat Nurs.* 2000;29:590-597.
46. Schweiger MS. Sleep disturbance in pregnancy. A subjective survey. *Am J Obstet Gynecol.* 1972;114:879-882.
47. Suzuki S, Dennerstein L, Greenwood KM, Armstrong SM, Satohisa E. Sleeping patterns during pregnancy in Japanese women. *J Psychosom Obstet Gynecol.* 1994;15:19-26.
48. Liu JH, Rebar RW. Endocrinology of pregnancy. In: Creasy RK, Resnik R, eds. *Maternal-Fetal Medicine.* 4th ed. Philadelphia: Saunders; 1999:379-391.
49. Hedman C, Pohjasvaara T, Tolonen U, Suhonen-Malm AS, Myllyla VV. Effects of pregnancy on mothers' sleep. *Sleep Med.* 2002;3:37-42.
50. Hoppenbrouwers T, Hodgman JE, Berntsen I, Sterman MB, Harper RM. Sleep in women during the last trimester of pregnancy. *Sleep Res.* 1979;8:150.
51. Baratte-Beebe KR, Lee K. Sources of midsleep awakenings in childbearing women. *Clin Nurs Res.* 1999;8:386-397.
52. Shinkoda H, Matsumoto K, Park YM. Changes in sleep-wake cycle during the period from late pregnancy to puerperium identified through the wrist actigraph and sleep logs. *Psychiatry Clin Neurosci.* 1999;53:133-135.
53. Horiuchi S, Nishihara K. Analyses of mothers' sleep logs in postpartum periods. *Psychiatry Clin Neurosci.* 1999;53:137-139.
54. Blyton DM, Sullivan CE, Edwards N. Lactation is associated with an increase in slow-wave sleep in women. *J Sleep Res.* 2002;11:297-303.
55. Waters MA, Lee KA. Differences between primigravidae and multigravidae mothers in sleep disturbances, fatigue, and functional status. *J Nurse-Midwifery.* 1996;41:364-367.
56. Ekholm EM, Polo O, Rauhala ER, Ekblad UU. Sleep quality in preeclampsia. *Am J Obstet Gynecol.* 1992;167:1262-1266.
57. Coble PA, Reynolds III CF, Kupfer DJ, Houck PR, Day NL, Giles DE. Childbearing in women with and without a history of affective disorder. II. Electroencephalographic sleep. *Comp Psychiatry.* 1994;35:215-224.
58. Goodman JD, Brodie C, Ayida GA. Restless leg syndrome in pregnancy. *BMJ.* 1988;297:1101-1102.
59. Karacan I, Williams RL, Hursch CJ, McCaulley M, Heine MW. Some implications of the sleep patterns of pregnancy for postpartum emotional disturbances. *Br J Psychiatry.* 1969;115:929-935.
60. Errante J. Sleep deprivation or postpartum blues? *Topics Clin Nurs.* 1985;6:9-18.
61. Kennedy HP, Beck CT, Driscoll JW. A light in the fog: Caring for women with postpartum depression. *J Midwifery Women's Health.* 2002;47:318-330.
62. Sharma V, Mazmanian D. Sleep loss and postpartum psychosis. *Bipolar Disord.* 2003;5:98-105.
63. Food and Drug Administration. Labeling and prescription drug advertising; content and format for labeling for human prescription drugs. *Fed Reg.* 1979;44:37434-37467.
64. Briggs GG, Freeman RK, Yaffe SJ. *Drugs in Pregnancy and Lactation.* Philadelphia: Lippincott, Williams & Wilkins; 2002.
65. *Physicians' Desk Reference.* Montvale, NJ: Thomson; 2003.
66. Baker A, Simpson S, Dawson D. Sleep disruption and mood changes associated with menopause. *J Psychosom Res.* 1997;43:359-369.
67. Kravitz HM, Ganz PA, Bromberger J, Powell LH, Sutton-Tyrrell K, Meyer PM. Sleep difficulty in women at midlife: A community survey of sleep and the menopausal transition. *Menopause.* 2003;10:19-28.
68. Kravitz HM, Janssen I, Santoro N, Bromberger JT, Schocken M, et al. Relationship of day-to-day reproductive hormone levels to sleep in midlife women. *Arch Intern Med.* 2005;165:2370-2376.
69. Kuh DL, Wadsworth M, Hardy R. Women's health in midlife: The influence of the menopause, social factors and health in earlier life. *Br J Obstet Gynaecol.* 1997;104:923-933.
70. Owens JF, Matthews KA. Sleep disturbance in healthy middle-aged women. *Maturitas.* 1998;30:41-50.
71. Porter M, Penney GC, Russell D, Russell E, Templeton A. A population based survey of women's experience of the menopause. *Br J Obstet Gynaecol.* 1996;103:1025-1028.
72. Shin C, Lee S, Lee T, Shin K, Yi H, Kimm K, Cho N. Prevalence of insomnia and its relationship to menopausal status in middle-aged Korean women. *Psychiatry Clin Neurosci.* 2005;59:395-402.
73. National Institutes of Health. NIH State-of-the-Science Conference Statement on Management of Menopause-Related Symptoms. *NIH Consensus & State of the Science Statements.* 2005;22:1-38.
74. Dennerstein L, Dudley EC, Hopper JL, Guthrie JR, Burger HG. A prospective population-based study of menopausal symptoms. *Obstet Gynecol.* 2000;96:351-358.
75. Young T, Rabago D, Zgierska A, Austin D, Laurel F. Objective and subjective sleep quality in premenopausal, perimenopausal, and postmenopausal women in the Wisconsin Sleep Cohort Study. *Sleep.* 2003;26:667-672.
76. Avis NE, Crawford SL, McKinlay SM. Psychosocial, behavioral, and health factors related to menopause symptomatology. *Women's Health.* 1997;3:103-120.
77. Freedman RR. Physiology of hot flashes. *Am J Hum Biol.* 2001;13:453-464.
78. Utian WH. Psychosocial and socioeconomic burden of vasomotor symptoms in menopause: A comprehensive review. *Health Qual Life Outcomes.* 2005;3:47.
79. Kronenberg F. Hot flashes: Epidemiology and physiology. *Ann N Y Acad Sci.* 1990;592:52-86.

80. Freeman EW, Sammel MD, Lin H, Gracia CR, Pien GW, et al. Symptoms associated with menopausal transition and reproductive hormones in midlife women [see comment]. *Obstet Gynecol.* 2007;110:230-240.

81. Albright DL, Voda AM, Smolensky MH, Hsi B, Decker M. Circadian rhythms in hot flashes in natural and surgically-induced menopause. *Chronobiol Int.* 1989;6:279-284.

82. Pien GW, Sammel MD, Freeman EW, Lin H, DeBlasis TL. Predictors of sleep quality in women in the menopausal transition. *Sleep.* 2008;31:991-999.

83. Baker A, Simpson S, Dawson D. Sleep disruption and mood changes associated with menopause. *J Psychosom Res.* 1997;43:359-369.

84. Shaver J, Giblin E, Lentz M, Lee K. Sleep patterns and stability in perimenopausal women. *Sleep.* 1988;11:556-561.

85. Erlik Y, Tataryn IV, Meldrum DR, Lomax P, Bajorek JG, Judd HL. Association of waking episodes with menopausal hot flushes. *JAMA.* 1981;245:1741-1744.

86. Woodward S, Freedman RR. The thermoregulatory effects of menopausal hot flashes on sleep. *Sleep.* 1994;17:497-501.

87. Freedman RR, Roehrs TA. Lack of sleep disturbance from menopausal hot flashes. *Fertil Steril.* 2004;82:138-144.

88. Freeman EW, Sammel MD, Liu L, Gracia CR, Nelson DB, Hollander L. Hormones and menopausal status as predictors of depression in women in transition to menopause. *Arch Gen Psychiatry.* 2004;61:62-70.

89. Hollander LE, Freeman EW, Sammel MD, Berlin JA, Grisso JA, Battistini M. Sleep quality, estradiol levels, and behavioral factors in late reproductive age women. *Obstet Gynecol.* 2001;98:391-397.

90. Stenchever MA. Reproductive endocrinology. In: Stenchever MA, Droegemueller W, Herbst AL, et al. eds. *Comprehensive Gynecology.* 4th ed. St. Louis: Mosby; 2001:71-124.

91. Sowers MF, Zheng H, Kravitz HM, Matthews K, Bromberger JT, et al. Sex steroid hormone profiles are related to sleep measures from polysomnography and the Pittsburgh Sleep Quality Index. *Sleep.* 2008;31:1339-1349.

92. Rossouw JE, Anderson GL, Prentice RL, LaCroix AZ, Kooperberg C, et al. Risks and benefits of estrogen plus progestin in healthy postmenopausal women: Principal results from the Women's Health Initiative randomized controlled trial. *JAMA.* 2002;288:321-333.

93. Stephenson J. FDA orders estrogen safety warnings: Agency offers guidance for HRT use. *JAMA.* 2003;289:537-538.

94. Polo-Kantola P, Erkkola R, Helenius H, Irjala K, Polo O, et al. When does estrogen replacement therapy improve sleep quality? *Am J Obstet Gynecol.* 1998;178:1002-1009.

95. Moe KE, Larsen LH, Vitiello MV, Prinz PN. Estrogen replacement therapy moderates the sleep disruption associated with nocturnal blood sampling. *Sleep.* 2001;24:886-894.

96. Thomson J, Oswald I. Effect of oestrogen on the sleep, mood, and anxiety of menopausal women. *Br Med J.* 1977;2:1317-1319.

97. Bertelli G, Venturini M, Del Mastro L, Bergaglio M, Sismondi P, et al. Intramuscular depot medroxyprogesterone versus oral megestrol for the control of postmenopausal hot flashes in breast cancer patients: A randomized study. *Ann Oncol.* 2002;13:883-888.

98. Grady D. Clinical practice. Management of menopausal symptoms. *N Engl J Med.* 2006;355:2338-2347.

99. Loprinzi CL, Michalak JC, Quella SK, O'Fallon JR, Hatfield AK, et al. Megestrol acetate for the prevention of hot flashes. *N Engl J Med.* 1994;331:347-352.

100. Schiff I, Tulchinsky D, Cramer D, Ryan KJ. Oral medroxyprogesterone in the treatment of postmenopausal symptoms. *JAMA.* 1980;244:1443-1445.

101. Loprinzi CL, Kugler JW, Sloan JA, Mailliard JA, LaVasseur BI, et al. Venlafaxine in management of hot flashes in survivors of breast cancer: A randomised controlled trial. *Lancet.* 2000;356:2059-2063.

102. Stearns V, Slack R, Greep N, Henry-Tilman R, Osborne M, et al. Paroxetine is an effective treatment for hot flashes: Results from a prospective randomized clinical trial. *J Clin Oncol.* 2005;23:6919-6930.

103. Rudolph RL, Derivan AT. The safety and tolerability of venlafaxine hydrochloride: Analysis of the clinical trials database. *J Clin Psychopharmacol.* 1996;16:S54-S59:discussion S59-S61.

104. Stearns V, Beebe KL, Iyengar M, Dube E. Paroxetine controlled release in the treatment of menopausal hot flashes: A randomized controlled trial. *JAMA.* 2003;289:2827-2834.

105. Loprinzi CL, Sloan JA, Perez EA, Quella SK, Stella PJ, et al. Phase III evaluation of fluoxetine for treatment of hot flashes. *J Clin Oncol.* 2002;20:1578-1583.

106. Suvanto-Luukkonen E, Koivunen R, Sundstrom H, Bloigu R, Karjalainen E, et al. Citalopram and fluoxetine in the treatment of postmenopausal symptoms: A prospective, randomized, 9-month, placebo-controlled, double-blind study. *Menopause.* 2005;12:18-26.

107. Goldberg RM, Loprinzi CL, O'Fallon JR, Veeder MH, Miser AW, et al. Transdermal clonidine for ameliorating tamoxifen-induced hot flashes. *J Clin Oncol.* 1994;12:155-158.

108. Guttuso Jr T, Kurlan R, McDermott MP, Kieburtz K. Gabapentin's effects on hot flashes in postmenopausal women: A randomized controlled trial. *Obstet Gynecol.* 2003;101:337-345.

109. Freedman RR. Hot flashes: Behavioral treatments, mechanisms, and relation to sleep. *Am J Med.* 2005;118:124-130.

110. Osmers R, Friede M, Liske E, Schnitker J, Freudenstein J, Henneicke-von Zepelin HH. Efficacy and safety of isopropanolic black cohosh extract for climacteric symptoms. *Obstet Gynecol.* 2005;105:1074-1083.

111. Nedrow A, Miller J, Walker M, Nygren P, Huffman LH, Nelson HD. Complementary and alternative therapies for the management of menopause-related symptoms: A systematic evidence review. *Arch Intern Med.* 2006;166:1453-1465.

112. Nelson HD, Vesco KK, Haney E, Fu R, Nedrow A, et al. Nonhormonal therapies for menopausal hot flashes: Systematic review and meta-analysis. *JAMA.* 2006;295:2057-2071.

113. Keefer L, Blanchard EB. A behavioral group treatment program for menopausal hot flashes: Results of a pilot study. *Appl Psychophysiol Biofeedback.* 2005;30:21-30.

114. Freedman RR. Management of hot flashes. In: Liu JH, Gass MLS, eds. *Management of the Perimenopause.* New York: McGraw Hill; 2006:38-55.

115. Freedman RR, Woodward S, Brown B, et al. Biochemical and thermoregulatory effects of behavioral treatment for menopausal hot flashes. *Menopause.* 1995;2:211-218.

116. Chaudhary BA, Speir Jr WA. Sleep apnea syndromes. *South Med J.* 1982;75:39-45.

117. Young T, Palta M, Dempsey J, Skatrud J, Weber S, Badr S. The occurrence of sleep-disordered breathing among middle-aged adults. *N Engl J Med.* 1993;328:1230-1235.

118. Quintana-Gallego E, Carmona-Bernal C, Capote F, Sanchez-Armengol A, Botebol-Benhamou G, et al. Gender differences in obstructive sleep apnea syndrome: A clinical study of 1166 patients. *Respir Med.* 2004;98:984-989.

119. Shepertycky MR, Banno K, Kryger MH. Differences between men and women in the clinical presentation of patients diagnosed with obstructive sleep apnea syndrome. *Sleep.* 2005;28:309-314.

120. Young T, Hutton R, Finn L, Badr S, Palta M. The gender bias in sleep apnea diagnosis. Are women missed because they have different symptoms? *Arch Intern Med.* 1996;156:2445-2451.

121. Ambrogetti A, Olson LG, Saunders NA. Differences in the symptoms of men and women with obstructive sleep apnoea. *Aust N Z J Med.* 1991;21:863-866.

122. Valipour A, Lothaller H, Rauscher H, Zwick H, Burghuber OC, Lavie P. Gender-related differences in symptoms of patients with suspected breathing disorders in sleep: A clinical population study using the sleep disorders questionnaire. *Sleep.* 2007;30:312-319.

123. Leech JA, Onal E, Dulberg C, Lopata MA. A comparison of men and women with occlusive sleep apnea syndrome. *Chest.* 1988;94:983-988.

124. Ware JC, McBrayer RH, Scott JA. Influence of sex and age on duration and frequency of sleep apnea events. *Sleep.* 2000;23:165-170.

125. Exar EN, Collop NA. The upper airway resistance syndrome. *Chest.* 1999;115:1127-1139.

126. O'Connor C, Thornley KS, Hanly PJ. Gender differences in the polysomnographic features of obstructive sleep apnea. *Am J Respir Crit Care Med.* 2000;161:1465-1472.

127. Koo BB, Patel SR, Strohl K, Hoffstein V. Rapid eye movement-related sleep-disordered breathing: Influence of age and gender. *Chest.* 2008;134:1156-1161.

128. Guilleminault C, Quera-Salva MA, Partinen M, Jamieson A. Women and the obstructive sleep apnea syndrome. *Chest.* 1988;93:104-109.

129. Redline S, Kump K, Tishler PV, Browner I, Ferrette V. Gender differences in sleep disordered breathing in a community-based sample. *Am J Respir Crit Care Med.* 1994;149:722-726.

130. Trinder J, Kay A, Kleiman J, Dunai J. Gender differences in airway resistance during sleep. *J Appl Physiol.* 1997;83:1986-1997.

131. Millman RP, Carlisle CC, McGarvey ST, Eveloff SE, Levinson PD. Body fat distribution and sleep apnea severity in women. *Chest*. 1995;107: 362-366.

132. Schwab RJ. Genetic determinants of upper airway structures that predispose to obstructive sleep apnea. *Respir Physiol Neurobiol*. 2005;147: 289-298.

133. Whittle AT, Marshall I, Mortimore IL, Wraith PK, Sellar RJ, Douglas NJ. Neck soft tissue and fat distribution: Comparison between normal men and women by magnetic resonance imaging. *Thorax*. 1999;54: 323-328.

134. Ferguson KA, Ono T, Lowe AA, Ryan CF, Fleetham JA. The relationship between obesity and craniofacial structure in obstructive sleep apnea. *Chest*. 1995;108:375-381.

135. Riha RL, Brander P, Vennelle M, Douglas NJ. A cephalometric comparison of patients with the sleep apnea/hypopnea syndrome and their siblings. *Sleep*. 2005;28:315-320.

136. Lin CM, Davidson TM, Ancoli-Israel S. Gender differences in obstructive sleep apnea and treatment implications. *Sleep Med Rev*. 2008;12: 481-496.

137. Brooks LJ, Strohl KP. Size and mechanical properties of the pharynx in healthy men and women. *Am Rev Respir Dis*. 1992;146:1394-1397.

138. Martin SE, Mathur R, Marshall I, Douglas NJ. The effect of age, sex, obesity and posture on upper airway size. *Eur Respir J*. 1997;10:2087-2090.

139. Mohsenin V. Gender differences in the expression of sleep-disordered breathing: Role of upper airway dimensions. *Chest*. 2001;120: 1442-1447.

140. Mohsenin V. Effects of gender on upper airway collapsibility and severity of obstructive sleep apnea. *Sleep Med*. 2003;4:523-529.

141. Pillar G, Malhotra A, Fogel R, Beauregard J, Schnall R, White DP. Airway mechanics and ventilation in response to resistive loading during sleep: Influence of gender. *Am J Respir Crit Care Med*. 2000;162: 1627-1632.

142. Jordan AS, Catcheside PG, O'Donoghue FJ, Saunders NA, McEvoy RD. Genioglossus muscle activity at rest and in response to brief hypoxia in healthy men and women. *J Appl Physiol*. 2002;92:410-417.

143. Eckert DJ, Malhotra A, Lo YL, White DP, Jordan AS. The influence of obstructive sleep apnea and gender on genioglossus activity during rapid eye movement sleep. *Chest*. 2009;135:957-964.

144. White DP, Douglas NJ, Pickett CK, Weil JV, Zwillich CW. Sexual influence on the control of breathing. *J Appl Physiol*. 1983;54:874-879.

145. White DP, Douglas NJ, Pickett CK, Weil JV, Zwillich CW. Hypoxic ventilatory response during sleep in normal premenopausal women. *Am Rev Respir Dis*. 1982;126:530-533.

146. White DP, Schneider BK, Santen RJ, McDermott M, Pickett CK, et al. Influence of testosterone on ventilation and chemosensitivity in male subjects. *J Appl Physiol*. 1985;59:1452-1457.

147. Zhou XS, Shahabuddin S, Zahn BR, Babcock MA, Badr MS. Effect of gender on the development of hypocapnic apnea/hypopnea during NREM sleep. *J Appl Physiol*. 2000;89:192-199.

148. Schneider H, Krishnan V, Pichard LE, Patil SP, Smith PL, Schwartz AR. Inspiratory duty cycle responses to flow limitation predict nocturnal hypoventilation. *Eur Respir J*. 2009;33:1068-1076.

149. Netzer NC, Eliasson AH, Strohl KP. Women with sleep apnea have lower levels of sex hormones. *Sleep Breath*. 2003;7:25-29.

150. Zwillich CW, Natalino MR, Sutton FD, Weil JV. Effects of progesterone on chemosensitivity in normal men. *J Lab Clin Med*. 1978;92:262-269.

151. Regensteiner JG, Woodard WD, Hagerman DD, Weil JV, Pickett CK, et al. Combined effects of female hormones and metabolic rate on ventilatory drives in women. *J Appl Physiol*. 1989;66:808-813.

152. Popovic RM, White DP. Upper airway muscle activity in normal women: Influence of hormonal status. *J Appl Physiol*. 1998;84: 1055-1062.

153. Schneider BK, Pickett CK, Zwillich CW, Weil JV, McDermott MT, et al. Influence of testosterone on breathing during sleep. *J Appl Physiol*. 1986;61:618-623.

154. Johnson MW, Anch AM, Remmers JE. Induction of the obstructive sleep apnea syndrome in a woman by exogenous androgen administration. *Am Rev Respir Dis*. 1984;129:1023-1025.

155. Fogel RB, Malhotra A, Pillar G, Pittman SD, Dunaif A, White DP. Increased prevalence of obstructive sleep apnea syndrome in obese women with polycystic ovary syndrome. *J Clin Endocrinol Metab*. 2001;86:1175-1180.

156. O'Donnell CP, Tankersley CG, Polotsky VP, Schwartz AR, Smith PL. Leptin, obesity, and respiratory function. *Respir Physiol*. 2000;119: 163-170.

157. Polotsky VY, Wilson JA, Smaldone MC, Haines AS, Hurn PD, et al. Female gender exacerbates respiratory depression in leptin-deficient obesity. *Am J Respir Crit Care Med*. 2001;164:1470-1475.

158. Berry RB, Gleeson K. Respiratory arousal from sleep: Mechanisms and significance. *Sleep*. 1997;20:654-675.

159. Gleeson K, Zwillich CW, White DP. The influence of increasing ventilatory effort on arousal from sleep. *Am Rev Respir Dis*. 1990;142:295-300.

160. Berry RB, Light RW. Effect of hyperoxia on the arousal response to airway occlusion during sleep in normal subjects. *Am Rev Respir Dis*. 1992;146:330-334.

161. Vincken W, Guilleminault C, Silvestri L, Cosio M, Grassino A. Inspiratory muscle activity as a trigger causing the airways to open in obstructive sleep apnea. *Am Rev Respir Dis*. 1987;135:372-377.

162. Berry RB, Mahutte CK, Light RW. Effect of hypercapnia on the arousal response to airway occlusion during sleep in normal subjects. *J Appl Physiol*. 1993;74:2269-2275.

163. Jordan AS, McEvoy RD, Edwards JK, Schory K, Yang CK, et al. The influence of gender and upper airway resistance on the ventilatory response to arousal in obstructive sleep apnoea in humans. *J Physiol*. 2004;558:993-1004.

164. Mabry RL. Rhinitis of pregnancy. *South Med J*. 1986;79:965-971.

165. Driver HS, McLean H, Kumar DV, Farr N, Day AG, Fitzpatrick MF. The influence of the menstrual cycle on upper airway resistance and breathing during sleep. *Sleep*. 2005;28:449-456.

166. Pilkington S, Carli F, Dakin MJ, Romney M, De Witt KA, et al. Increase in Mallampati score during pregnancy. *Br J Anaesth*. 1995;74:638-642.

167. Popovich JJ. The lungs in pregnancy. In: Fishman AP, Elias JA, Fishman JA, Grippi MA, Kaiser LR, Senior RM, eds. *Fishman's Pulmonary Diseases and Disorders*. New York: McGraw-Hill; 1998:243-250.

168. Pien GW, Schwab RJ. Sleep disorders during pregnancy. *Sleep*. 2004;27:1405-1417.

169. Franklin KA, Holmgren PA, Jonsson F, Poromaa N, Stenlund H, Svanborg E. Snoring, pregnancy-induced hypertension, and growth retardation of the fetus. *Chest*. 2000;117:137-141.

170. Loube DI, Poceta JS, Morales MC, Peacock MD, Mitler MM. Self-reported snoring in pregnancy. Association with fetal outcome. *Chest*. 1996;109:885-889.

171. Pien GW, Fife D, Pack AI, Nkwuo JE, Schwab RJ. Changes in symptoms of sleep-disordered breathing during pregnancy. *Sleep*. 2005;28: 1299-1305.

172. Calaora-Tournadre D, Ragot S, Meurice JC, Pourrat O, D'Halluin G, et al. Obstructive sleep apnea syndrome during pregnancy: Prevalence of main symptoms and relationship with pregnancy induced-hypertension and intra-uterine growth retardation. *Rev Med Intern*. 2006;27: 291-295.

173. Guilleminault C, Palombini L, Poyares D, Takaoka S, Huynh NT, El-Sayed Y. Pre-eclampsia and nasal CPAP: Part 1. Early intervention with nasal CPAP in pregnant women with risk-factors for pre-eclampsia: Preliminary findings. *Sleep Med*. 2007;9:9-14.

174. Maasilta P, Bachour A, Teramo K, Polo O, Laitinen LA. Sleep-related disordered breathing during pregnancy in obese women. *Chest*. 2001;120:1448-1454.

175. Perez-Chada D, Videla AJ, O'Flaherty ME, Majul C, Catalini AM, et al. Snoring, witnessed sleep apnoeas and pregnancy-induced hypertension. *Acta Obstet Gynecol Scand*. 2007;86:788-792.

176. Pepperell JC, Ramdassingh-Dow S, Crosthwaite N, Mullins R, Jenkinson C, et al. Ambulatory blood pressure after therapeutic and subtherapeutic nasal continuous positive airway pressure for obstructive sleep apnoea: A randomised parallel trial. *Lancet*. 2002;359:204-210.

177. Edwards N, Blyton DM, Kirjavainen T, Kesby GJ, Sullivan CE. Nasal continuous positive airway pressure reduces sleep-induced blood pressure increments in preeclampsia. *Am J Respir Crit Care Med*. 2000;162:252-257.

178. Bixler EO, Vgontzas AN, Lin HM, Ten Have T, Rein J, et al. Prevalence of sleep-disordered breathing in women: Effects of gender. *Am J Respir Crit Care Med*. 2001;163:608-613.

179. Dancey DR, Hanly PJ, Soong C, Lee B, Hoffstein V. Impact of menopause on the prevalence and severity of sleep apnea. *Chest*. 2001;120: 151-155.

180. Young T, Finn L, Austin D, Peterson A. Menopausal status and sleep-disordered breathing in the Wisconsin Sleep Cohort Study. *Am J Respir Crit Care Med*. 2003;167:1181-1185.

181. Tremollieres FA, Pouilles JM, Ribot CA. Relative influence of age and menopause on total and regional body composition changes in postmenopausal women. *Am J Obstet Gynecol*. 1996;175:1594-1600.

182. Toth MJ, Tchernof A, Sites CK, Poehlman ET. Effect of menopausal status on body composition and abdominal fat distribution. *Int J Obes Relat Metab Disord.* 2000;24:226-231.
183. Keefe DL, Watson R, Naftolin F. Hormone replacement therapy may alleviate sleep apnea in menopausal women: A pilot study. *Menopause.* 1999;6:196-200.
184. Pickett CK, Regensteiner JG, Woodard WD, Hagerman DD, Weil JV, Moore LG. Progestin and estrogen reduce sleep-disordered breathing in postmenopausal women. *J Appl Physiol.* 1989;66:1656-1661.
185. Cistulli PA, Barnes DJ, Grunstein RR, Sullivan CE. Effect of short-term hormone replacement in the treatment of obstructive sleep apnoea in postmenopausal women. *Thorax.* 1994;49:699-702.
186. Cook WR, Benich JJ, Wooten SA. Indices of severity of obstructive sleep apnea syndrome do not change during medroxyprogesterone acetate therapy. *Chest.* 1989;96:262-266.
187. Rajagopal KR, Abbrecht PH, Jabbari B. Effects of medroxyprogesterone acetate in obstructive sleep apnea. *Chest.* 1986;90:815-821.
188. Young T, Finn L. Epidemiological insights into the public health burden of sleep disordered breathing: Sex differences in survival among sleep clinic patients. *Thorax.* 1998;53(Suppl 3):S16-S19.
189. Punjabi NM, Caffo BS, Goodwin JL, Gottlieb DJ, Newman AB, et al. Sleep-disordered breathing and mortality: A prospective cohort study. *PLoS Med.* 2009;6:E1000132.
190. McArdle N, Devereux G, Heidarnejad H, Engleman HM, Mackay TW, Douglas NJ. Long-term use of CPAP therapy for sleep apnea/hypopnea syndrome. *Am J Respir Crit Care Med.* 1999;159:1108-1114.
191. Pelletier-Fleury N, Rakotonanahary D, Fleury B. The age and other factors in the evaluation of compliance with nasal continuous positive airway pressure for obstructive sleep apnea syndrome. A Cox's proportional hazard analysis. *Sleep Med.* 2001;2:225-232.
192. Sin DD, Mayers I, Man GC, Pawluk L. Long-term compliance rates to continuous positive airway pressure in obstructive sleep apnea: A population-based study. *Chest.* 2002;121:430-435.
193. Anttalainen U, Saaresranta T, Kalleinen N, Aittokallio J, Vahlberg T, Polo O. CPAP adherence and partial upper airway obstruction during sleep. *Sleep Breath.* 2007;11:171-176.
194. Marklund M, Stenlund H, Franklin KA. Mandibular advancement devices in 630 men and women with obstructive sleep apnea and snoring: Tolerability and predictors of treatment success. *Chest.* 2004;125:1270-1278.
195. Krishnan V, Collop NA, Scherr SC. An evaluation of a titration strategy for prescription of oral appliances for obstructive sleep apnea. *Chest.* 2008;133:1135-1141.
196. McGown AD, Makker HK, Battagel JM, L'Estrange PR, Grant HR, Spiro SG. Long-term use of mandibular advancement splints for snoring and obstructive sleep apnoea: A questionnaire survey. *Eur Respir J.* 2001;17:462-466.
197. Franklin KA, Anttila H, Axelsson S, Gislason T, Maasilta P, et al. Effects and side-effects of surgery for snoring and obstructive sleep apnea—A systematic review. *Sleep.* 2009;32:27-36.
198. Newman AB, Foster G, Givelber R, Nieto FJ, Redline S, Young T. Progression and regression of sleep-disordered breathing with changes in weight: The Sleep Heart Health Study. *Arch Intern Med.* 2005;165:2408-2413.
199. Rasheid S, Banasiak M, Gallagher SF, Lipska A, Kaba S, et al. Gastric bypass is an effective treatment for obstructive sleep apnea in patients with clinically significant obesity. *Obes Surg.* 2003;13:58-61.
200. Livingston EH, Huerta S, Arthur D, Lee S, De Shields S, Heber D. Male gender is a predictor of morbidity and age a predictor of mortality for patients undergoing gastric bypass surgery. *Ann Surg.* 2002;236:576-582.
201. Pillar G, Peled R, Lavie P. Recurrence of sleep apnea without concomitant weight increase 7.5 years after weight reduction surgery. *Chest.* 1994;106:1702-1704.
202. Lettieri CJ, Eliasson AH, Greenburg DL. Persistence of obstructive sleep apnea after surgical weight loss. *J Clin Sleep Med.* 2008;4:333-338.
203. Phillips B, Young T, Finn L, Asher K, Hening WA, Purvis C. Epidemiology of restless legs symptoms in adults. *Arch Intern Med.* 2000;160:2137-2141.
204. National Heart, Lung, and Blood Institute. Restless legs syndrome: Detection and management in primary care. National Heart, Lung, and Blood Institute Working Group on Restless Legs Syndrome. *Am Fam Physician.* 2000;62:108-114.
205. Chesson Jr AL, Wise M, Davila D, Johnson S, Littner M, et al. Practice parameters for the treatment of restless legs syndrome and periodic limb movement disorder. An American Academy of Sleep Medicine Report. Standards of Practice Committee of the American Academy of Sleep Medicine. *Sleep.* 1999;22:961-968.
206. Hening WA, Allen RP, Washburn M, Lesage SR, Earley CJ. The four diagnostic criteria for restless legs syndrome are unable to exclude confounding conditions ("mimics"). *Sleep Med.* 2009;10:976-981.
207. Benes H, von Eye A, Kohnen R. Empirical evaluation of the accuracy of diagnostic criteria for restless legs syndrome. *Sleep Med.* 2009;10:524-530.
208. Allen RP, Walters AS, Montplaisir J, Hening W, Myers A, et al. Restless legs syndrome prevalence and impact: REST general population study. *Arch Intern Med.* 2005;165:1286-1292.
209. Berger K, Luedemann J, Trenkwalder C, John U, Kessler C. Sex and the risk of restless legs syndrome in the general population. *Arch Intern Med.* 2004;164:196-202.
210. Manconi M, Govoni V, De Vito A, Economou NT, Cesnik E, et al. Restless legs syndrome and pregnancy. *Neurology.* 2004;63:1065-1069.
211. Lee KA, Zaffke ME, Baratte-Beebe K. Restless legs syndrome and sleep disturbance during pregnancy: The role of folate and iron. *J Women's Health Gender-Based Med.* 2001;10:335-341.
212. Tan EK, Seah A, See SJ, Lim E, Wong MC, Koh KK. Restless legs syndrome in an Asian population: A study in Singapore. *Mov Disord.* 2001;16:577-579.
213. Lee HB, Hening WA, Allen RP, Earley CJ, Eaton WW, Lyketsos CG. Race and restless legs syndrome symptoms in an adult community sample in east Baltimore. *Sleep Med.* 2006;7:642-645.
214. Pichler I, Hicks AA, Pramstaller PP. Restless legs syndrome: An update on genetics and future perspectives. *Clin Genet.* 2008;73:297-305.
215. Stefansson H, Rye DB, Hicks A, Petursson H, Ingason A, et al. A genetic risk factor for periodic limb movements in sleep. *N Engl J Med.* 2007;357:639-647.
216. Montplaisir J, Michaud M, Denesle R, Gosselin A. Periodic leg movements are not more prevalent in insomnia or hypersomnia but are specifically associated with sleep disorders involving a dopaminergic impairment. *Sleep Med.* 2000;1:163-167.
217. Connor JR, Boyer PJ, Menzies SL, Dellinger B, Allen RP, et al. Neuropathological examination suggests impaired brain iron acquisition in restless legs syndrome. *Neurology.* 2003;61:304-309.
218. Whittom S, Dauvilliers Y, Pennestri MH, Vercauteren F, Molinari N, et al. Age-at-onset in restless legs syndrome: A clinical and polysomnographic study. *Sleep Med.* 2007;9:54-59.
219. Phillips B, Hening W, Britz P, Mannino D. Prevalence and correlates of restless legs syndrome: Results from the 2005 National Sleep Foundation Poll. *Chest.* 2006;129:76-80.
220. Picchietti D, Winkelman JW. Restless legs syndrome, periodic limb movements in sleep, and depression. *Sleep.* 2005;28:891-898.
221. Lee HB, Hening WA, Allen RP, Kalaydjian AE, Earley CJ, et al. Restless legs syndrome is associated with DSM-IV major depressive disorder and panic disorder in the community. *J Neuropsychiatry Clin Neurosci.* 2008;20:101-105.
222. Hornyak M, Feige B, Voderholzer U, Philipsen A, Riemann D. Polysomnography findings in patients with restless legs syndrome and in healthy controls: A comparative observational study. *Sleep.* 2007;30:861-865.
223. Gamaldo C, Benbrook AR, Allen RP, Oguntimein O, Earley CJ. Evaluating daytime alertness in individuals with restless legs syndrome (RLS) compared to sleep restricted controls. *Sleep Med.* 2009;10:134-138.
224. Deriu M, Cossu G, Molari A, Murgia D, Mereu A, et al. Restless legs syndrome in multiple sclerosis: A case-control study. *Mov Disord.* 2009;24:697-701.
225. Italian RSG, Manconi M, Ferini-Strambi L, Filippi M, Bonanni E, et al. Multicenter case-control study on restless legs syndrome in multiple sclerosis: The REMS study. *Sleep.* 2008;31:944-952.
226. Walters AS, Silvestri R, Zucconi M, Chandrashekariah R, Konofal E. Review of the possible relationship and hypothetical links between attention deficit hyperactivity disorder (ADHD) and the simple sleep related movement disorders, parasomnias, hypersomnias, and circadian rhythm disorders. *J Clin Sleep Med.* 2008;4:591-600.
227. Stehlik R, Arvidsson L, Ulfberg J. Restless legs syndrome is common among female patients with fibromyalgia. *Eur Neurol.* 2009;61:107-111.
228. Hattan E, Chalk C, Postuma RB. Is there a higher risk of restless legs syndrome in peripheral neuropathy? *Neurology.* 2009;72:955-960.
229. Lo Coco D, Mattaliano A, Lo Coco A, Randisi B. Increased frequency of restless legs syndrome in chronic obstructive pulmonary disease patients. *Sleep Med.* 2009;10:572-576.
230. Minai OA, Malik N, Foldvary N, Bair N, Golish JA. Prevalence and characteristics of restless legs syndrome in patients with pulmonary hypertension. *J Heart Lung Transplant.* 2008;27:335-340.

231. Rhode AM, Hosing VG, Happe S, Biehl K, Young P, Evers S. Comorbidity of migraine and restless legs syndrome—A case-control study. *Cephalalgia*. 2007;27:1255-1260.

232. Lee JE, Shin HW, Kim KS, Sohn YH. Factors contributing to the development of restless legs syndrome in patients with Parkinson disease. *Mov Disord*. 2009;24:579-582.

233. Mallon L, Broman JE, Hetta J. Restless legs symptoms with sleepiness in relation to mortality: 20-year follow-up study of a middle-aged Swedish population. *Psychiatry Clin Neurosci*. 2008;62:457-463.

234. Rottach KG, Schaner BM, Kirch MH, Zivotofsky AZ, Teufel LM, et al. Restless legs syndrome as side effect of second generation antidepressants. *J Psychiatr Res*. 2008;43:70-75.

235. Aukerman MM, Aukerman D, Bayard M, Tudiver F, Thorp L, Bailey B. Exercise and restless legs syndrome: A randomized controlled trial. *J Am Board Fam Med*. 2006;19:487-493.

236. Lettieri CJ, Eliasson AH. Pneumatic compression devices are an effective therapy for restless legs syndrome: A prospective, randomized, double-blinded, sham-controlled trial. *Chest*. 2009;135:74-80.

237. Littner MR, Kushida C, Anderson WM, Bailey D, Berry RB, et al. Practice parameters for the dopaminergic treatment of restless legs syndrome and periodic limb movement disorder. *Sleep*. 2004;27:557-559.

238. Silber MH, Girish M, Izurieta R. Pramipexole in the management of restless legs syndrome: An extended study. *Sleep*. 2003;26:819-821.

239. Fulda S, Wetter TC. Where dopamine meets opioids: A meta-analysis of the placebo effect in restless legs syndrome treatment studies. *Brain*. 2008;131:902-917.

240. Garcia-Borreguero D, Allen RP, Kohnen R, Hogl B, Trenkwalder C, et al. Diagnostic standards for dopaminergic augmentation of restless legs syndrome: Report from a World Association of Sleep Medicine-International Restless Legs Syndrome Study Group consensus conference at the Max Planck Institute. *Sleep Med*. 2007;8:520-530.

241. Exar EN, Collop NA. The association of upper airway resistance with periodic limb movements. *Sleep*. 2001;24:188-192.

242. Chervin RD. Periodic leg movements and sleepiness in patients evaluated for sleep-disordered breathing. *Am J Respir Crit Care Med*. 2001;164:1454-1458.

243. Yang C, White DP, Winkelman JW. Antidepressants and periodic leg movements of sleep. *Biol Psychiatry*. 2005;58:510-514.

244. Suzuki K, Ohida T, Sone R, Takemua S, Miyake T, et al. The prevalence of restless legs syndrome among pregnant women in Japan and the relationship between restless legs syndrome and sleep problems. *Sleep*. 2003;26:673-677.

245. Allen RP, Earley CJ. Restless legs syndrome: A review of clinical and pathophysiologic features. *J Clin Neurophysiol*. 2001;18:128-147.

246. Nikkola E, Ekblad U, Ekholm E, Mikola H, Polo O. Sleep in multiple pregnancy: Breathing patterns, oxygenation, and periodic leg movements. *Am J Obstet Gynecol*. 1996;174:1622-1625.

247. Beutler E. The common anemias. *JAMA*. 1988;259:2433-2437.

248. Botez MI, Lambert B. Folate deficiency and restless legs syndrome in pregnancy. *N Engl J Med*. 1977;297:670.

249. Sun ER, Chen CA, Ho G, Earley CJ, Allen RP. Iron and the restless legs syndrome. *Sleep*. 1998;21:371-377.

250. Earley CJ. Clinical practice. Restless legs syndrome. *N Engl J Med*. 2003;348:2103-2109.

251. Pritchett AM, Morrison JF, Edwards WD, Schaff HV, Connolly HM, Espinosa RE. Valvular heart disease in patients taking pergolide. *Mayo Clin Proc*. 2002;77:1280-1286.

252. Mignot E, Lin L, Finn L, Lopes C, Pluff K, et al. Correlates of sleep-onset REM periods during the multiple sleep latency test in community adults. *Brain*. 2006;129:1609-1623.

253. Silber MH, Krahn LE, Olson EJ, Pankratz VS. The epidemiology of narcolepsy in Olmsted County, Minnesota: A population-based study. *Sleep*. 2002;25:197-202.

254. Dauvilliers Y, Montplaisir J, Molinari N, Carlander B, Ondze B, et al. Age at onset of narcolepsy in two large populations of patients in France and Quebec. *Neurology*. 2001;57:2029-2033.

255. Daniels LE. Narcolepsy. *Medicine*. 1934;13:1–122.

256. Longstreth Jr WT, Ton TG, Koepsell T, Gersuk VH, Hendrickson A, et al. Prevalence of narcolepsy in King County, Washington, USA. *Sleep Med*. 2009;10:422-426.

257. Mitler MM, Walsleben J, Sangal RB, Hirshkowitz M. Sleep latency on the maintenance of wakefulness test (MWT) for 530 patients with narcolepsy while free of psychoactive drugs. *Electroencephalogr Clin Neurophysiol*. 1998;107:33-38.

258. Mattarozzi K, Bellucci C, Campi C, Cipolli C, Ferri R, et al. Clinical, behavioural and polysomnographic correlates of cataplexy in patients with narcolepsy/cataplexy. *Sleep Med*. 2008;9:425-433.

259. Higuchi S, Usui A, Murasaki M, Matsushita S, Nishioka N, et al. Plasma orexin-A is lower in patients with narcolepsy. *Neurosci Lett*. 2002;318:61-64.

260. Hoover-Stevens S, Kovacevic-Ristanovic R. Management of narcolepsy in pregnancy. *Clin Neuropharmacol*. 2000;23:175-181.

261. Guilleminault C, Anagnos A. Narcolepsy. In: Kryger MH, Roth T, Dement WC, eds. *Principles and Practices of Sleep Medicine*. 4th ed. Philadelphia: W.B. Saunders Company; 2005:780-790.

262. Littner M, Johnson SF, McCall WV, Anderson WM, Davila D, et al. Practice parameters for the treatment of narcolepsy: an update for 2000. *Sleep*. 2001;24:451-466.

263. Physicians' Desk Reference. Montvale, NJ: Thomson; 2010.

264. Shevell M. Pemoline associated hepatic failure: A critical analysis of the literature. *Pediatric Neurology*. 1997;16:353.

265. Practice parameters for the use of stimulants in the treatment of narcolepsy. Standards of Practice Committee of the American Sleep Disorders Association. *Sleep*. 1994;17:348-351.

266. Morgenthaler TI, Silber MH. Amnestic sleep-related eating disorder associated with zolpidem. *Sleep Med*. 2002;3:323-327.

267. Paquet V, Strul J, Servais L, Pelc I, Fossion P. Sleep-related eating disorder induced by olanzapine. *J Clin Psychiatry*. 2002;63:597.

268. Winkelman JW. Clinical and polysomnographic features of sleep-related eating disorder. *J Clin Psychiatry*. 1998;59:14-19.

269. Winkelman JW. Efficacy and tolerability of open-label topiramate in the treatment of sleep-related eating disorder: A retrospective case series. *J Clin Psychiatry*. 2006;67:1729-1734.

270. Provini F, Albani F, Vetrugno R, Vignatelli L, Lombardi C, et al. A pilot double-blind placebo-controlled trial of low-dose pramipexole in sleep-related eating disorder. *Eur J Neurol*. 2005;12:432-436.

271. Howell MJ, Schenck CH, Crow SJ. A review of nighttime eating disorders. *Sleep Med Rev*. 2009;13:23-34.

272. Winkelman JW. Treatment of nocturnal eating syndrome and sleep-related eating disorder with topiramate. *Sleep Med*. 2003;4:243-246.

273. O'Reardon JP, Allison KC, Martino NS, Lundgren JD, Heo M, Stunkard AJ. A randomized, placebo-controlled trial of sertraline in the treatment of night eating syndrome. *Am J Psychiatry*. 2006;163:893-898.

274. Briggs GG, Freeman RK, Yaffe SJ. *Drugs in Pregnancy and Lactation*. Philadelphia: Lippincott, Williams & Wilkins; 2008.

275. Lee HB, Hening WA, Allen RP, Kalaydjian AE, Earley CJ, et al. Restless legs syndrome is associated with DSM-IV major depressive disorder and panic disorder in the community. *J Neuropsychiatry Clin Neurosci*. 2008;20:101-105.

276. Pearson VE, Gamaldo CE, Allen RP, Lesage S, Hening WA, Earley CJ. Medication use in patients with restless legs syndrome compared with a control population. *Eur J Neurol*. 2008;15:16-21.

277. Manconi M, Ferini-Strambi L, Filippi M, Bonanni E, Iudice A, et al. Multicenter case-control study on restless legs syndrome in multiple sclerosis: The REMS study. *Sleep*. 2008;31:944-952.

278. Lee JE, Shin HW, Kim KS, Sohn YH. Factors contributing to the development of restless legs syndrome in patients with Parkinson disease. *Mov Disord*. 2009;24:579-582.

Sleep Disorders in Geriatric Patients

KENDRA BECKER / CHARLES POON / JENNIFER L. MARTIN

Chapter
59

SLEEP AND THE GERIATRIC PATIENT

Studies estimate that about half of American adults older than age 65 report at least one chronic sleep complaint.[1] Common complaints include difficulty falling asleep, trouble staying asleep, early morning awakenings, and excessive daytime sleepiness and fatigue. As one ages, there are changes to the architecture of sleep as measured with polysomnography (PSG). There is an increased percentage of time spent in stage N1 sleep and decreased time in stage N3 (i.e., slow wave) sleep. There is decreased sleep efficiency, increased number of arousals per hour slept, and increased sleep latency. Interrupted and fragmented nighttime sleep can then lead to increased daytime sleepiness, inadvertent dozing, and compensatory naps. Age-related changes in circadian rhythms also play a role. Older adults may experience sleepiness earlier in the evening and concomitant early morning awakenings. Daytime napping may compound the problem by reducing the drive for sleep at the usual bedtime hour, thereby delaying sleep onset at night without delaying the undesirable early morning awakenings. Given increased co-morbidities among older adults, contributory factors for sleep difficulties include acute and chronic medical illnesses, medication effects, psychiatric disorders, primary sleep disorders, social changes, poor sleep habits, and circadian rhythm shifts.

There are significant consequences of poor sleep. Poor sleep or chronic use of sedating medications for sleep may lead to falls and accidents.[2,3] Sleep-disordered breathing, restless legs syndrome (RLS), and rapid eye movement (REM) sleep behavior disorder, which are more common in older adults relative to younger adults, may contribute to serious cardiovascular, pulmonary, or neurologic complications and memory impairment. Sleep disturbance is also associated with risk of depression among older adults.[4]

Special considerations in the evaluation and treatment of sleep complaints of older patients include presentation of insomnia that is typically co-morbid with one or more medical or psychiatric conditions, plus thoughtful management of sleep disorders such as sleep apnea, RLS, periodic limb movement disorder (PLMD), and REM sleep behavior disorder. Each of these issues will be discussed in this chapter with special emphasis on age-related concerns.

INSOMNIA

Insomnia is defined by ongoing difficulty with sleep initiation, duration, consolidation, or quality that occurs despite adequate time and opportunity for sleep and results in daytime impairment.[5] Some patients complain of trouble falling asleep (sleep onset insomnia), others complain of difficulty staying asleep (sleep maintenance insomnia), and some suffer from both difficulties of falling and staying asleep. Among older adults, it is more common for patients to report awakenings in the early morning hours, sometimes with an inability to return to sleep. This is often a result of an age-related advance (i.e., shift earlier) of circadian rhythms in combination with insomnia. In the absence of a contributing cause, these complaints are referred to as "primary insomnia." Among older adults, insomnia is more typically co-morbid with another condition. This co-morbid condition may actually cause the insomnia or may exacerbate the severity of the insomnia. Medical co-morbidities that can contribute to insomnia include frequent urination (commonly caused by benign prostatic hypertrophy, timing of diuretic use, fluid intake prior to bed, or poorly controlled diabetes in older adults), musculoskeletal pain, cardiovascular disease, gastroesophageal reflux, malignancy, renal disease, chronic obstructive pulmonary disease, congestive heart failure, and neurologic disorders. Polypharmacy in geriatric patients can also contribute to insomnia, as many medications can increase daytime sleepiness or nighttime wakefulness. Insomnia due to a mental disorder, such as depression and anxiety, is also common among older adults.

Pathophysiology

The pathophysiology of primary insomnia is largely unknown. It is postulated that insomnia is related to a state of hyperarousal, including physiologic and cognitive arousal. Insomniacs may have an increased physiologic arousal that is incompatible with the initiation or maintenance of sleep and is manifested by increased respiration, heart rate, and metabolic rate.[6,7] Insomnia is also associated with cognitive arousal that involves worry and rumination brought on by acute stressors or genetic predisposition that leads to long-term nighttime cognitive arousal. Poor behavioral sleep practices are involved in the maintenance of insomnia over time, and are the focus of behavioral treatments.[8] Many age-related changes in behavior, such as increased daytime napping, reduced daytime physical activity, and variable sleep schedules contribute directly to the maintenance of insomnia problems.

As mentioned previously, co-morbid conditions and symptoms may play a key role in the onset and maintenance of insomnia. For example, studies suggest that treating insomnia can improve both sleep and pain symptoms among older patients with osteoarthritis.[9] Anxiety and depression, which are common in older adults, can also contribute to the development and maintenance of insomnia.[4,10]

Prevalence

In a large study of adults in six European countries, 16% met diagnostic criteria for insomnia.[11,12] Studies show that difficulty in initiating and maintaining sleep affects nearly half of adults older than the age of 65, representing an increased prevalence in older versus younger patients.[13] Older women tend to report more sleep disturbance compared with older men.[14] One study found that 36% of men and 54% of women older than age 65 living in the community reported insomnia symptoms.[15]

Clinical Consequences

The clinical consequences of insomnia can be numerous. Insomnia impacts daytime function, results in loss of productivity, and impairs neurocognitive function. A recent study of insomniacs with short sleep duration showed poorer neuropsychologic performance in processing speed, set-switching attention, and visual memory, which are key components of executive control of attention.[16] Among older adults, these consequences may be especially problematic. Napping can be both a cause and a consequence of insomnia, and some studies suggest napping may be one of the key symptoms of sleep fragmentation among older adults.[17]

Evaluation

A diagnostic workup of insomnia should include the elucidation of the patient's sleep-related habits, including the sleep environment, circadian tendencies, and use of prescription drugs, caffeine, and alcohol plus a review of medical conditions and psychiatric symptoms likely to impact sleep. Specific concerns among older patients are (1) improper sleep scheduling with frequent napping, variable bedtimes or rise times, and excessive time in bed; (2) routine use of products containing alcohol, nicotine, or caffeine, especially near bedtime; (3) engagement in mentally stimulating, physically activating, or emotionally upsetting activities close to bedtime; (4) use of the bed for activities other than sleep; and (5) failure to maintain a comfortable sleep environment.

PSG is not routinely indicated for the workup of insomnia, but may be helpful if other sleep disorders are suspected or if the patient has not benefited from insomnia treatment. It is appropriate to have patients maintain a sleep diary for a week or more, particularly when the patient reports an irregular sleep schedule, or in preparation for behavioral therapies. This can be done in conjunction with wrist actigraphy to provide objective data when self-report data may be unreliable, for example, among patients with cognitive impairment. When comparing actigraphy's ability to assess sleep parameters to PSG in a study of older women, actigraphy had excellent concordance in total sleep time measurement compared to PSG among older adults.[18]

Treatment

There are two general approaches to the treatment of insomnia: pharmacologic treatments and nonpharmacologic treatments. Treatment selection should be individualized based on the patient's wishes and considering the risk/benefit ratio of each. Major concerns of pharmacotherapy of insomnia with older patients are interactions with other medications, gait/balance problems that can increase fall risk, and adverse cognitive effects of sedatives. The limitations of behavioral treatments include availability of skilled providers, greater time commitment on the part of both patient and provider, and the need for multiple appointments to address the insomnia problem.

Although several drug classes are used in clinical practice (Table 59-1), sedative-hypnotics are considered the first-line drugs used for insomnia. The longer acting medications, such as diazepam, are typically not recommended in older adults, and caution must be used with all benzodiazepines in older adults as they may increase the risk of falls and confusion and may worsen upper airway resistance in patients with sleep apnea.[19-22] Newer selective benzodiazepine receptor agonists, including zolpidem, zaleplon, and eszopiclone, have less deleterious effects on sleep architecture and more agreeable side effect profiles compared to benzodiazepines.[23] Ramelteon, a melatonin receptor agonist approved for treatment of insomnia, has been shown to reduce sleep latency in older adults with insomnia without next-morning residual effects.[24,25] In addition, one study found ramelteon was not associated with impaired balance during the night, suggesting this medication may not increase risk for nighttime falls compared to other sedating medications.[26] Medications are typically considered a short-term treatment for insomnia, and this is particularly true of benzodiazepine hypnotics. Newer medications, such as ramelteon and zaleplon, are increasingly being considered for longer-term use.[27,28] An open-label trial of long-term hypnotic treatment with zaleplon for 6 to 12 months demonstrates safe and effective treatment for insomnia in older adults.[28] Additional research is needed on the long-term use of medications for sleep in older adults. Data are not available to guide clinicians about when to discontinue medications if medical status changes or frailty increases, potentially making a sedative-hypnotic inappropriate.

When medication therapy is considered, it is important to concurrently target underlying causes for the insomnia. Table 59-1 lists currently approved medications for insomnia and other commonly used medications (used off-label), noting considerations for their use in older adults related to half-life and side effects. For example, an older patient with neuropathic pain and insomnia may benefit from gabapentin, which enhances slow wave sleep, improves sleep efficiency, and decreases spontaneous arousals in patients with insomnia.[29] Risk of depression increases with age and as depression and insomnia may overlap, sedating antidepressants such as mirtazapine, trazodone, or doxepin can be considered. However, these medications must be used with caution because of anticholinergic side effects and the relative lack of available research literature on their use for insomnia in the absence of depression.[23] Recent literature suggests that doxepin at a low dose is efficacious in improving sleep with older patients with primary insomnia without reported anticholinergic side effects or memory impairment.[30,31] Antihistamines (contained in over-the-counter sleep aids) should be avoided in older adults because they can lead to excessive somnolence and confusion.[32]

There is strong evidence to support the use of nonpharmacologic interventions for insomnia among older adults, including two recent meta-analytic reviews showing that behavioral treatments lead to significant improvements.[33,34]

TABLE 59-1

Medications for Insomnia That Have Been Tested for Use in Older Patients

Medication Class	Agent	Dosing*	Half-life (hr)	Additional Considerations
BENZODIAZEPINES				
Short-acting	Triazolam[129]	0.125-0.25 mg	1.6-5.4	Tested only for short-term use (< 1 month) in older adults with evidence of withdrawal insomnia.[131]
Intermediate-acting	Temazepam[130]	7.5-15 mg	10-20	Potentially serious side effects include impaired cognitive performance[132] and increased fall risk.[133]
Selective benzodiazepine receptor agonists	Zaleplon[28,134]	5-10 mg	0.9-1.1	Improved side effect profile over that of traditional benzodiazepines, but evidence of postural instability remains.
	Zolpidem[135]	5 mg	1.4-4.5	Evaluated for longer-term use (up to 1 year) in older adults.[28]
	Eszopiclone[136]	1-2 mg	6	
ANTIDEPRESSANTS				
Tricyclics†	Amitriptyline	25-100 mg	10-26	May alleviate co-morbid depressive symptoms.
	Nortriptyline	25-100 mg	18-44	Except doxepin, not evaluated for primary insomnia in older patients.
	Doxepin[30]	1-3 mg	6-8	Cardiac and anticholinergic side effects may make use of these agents inappropriate in older patients.
Alpha-2 agonist†	Mirtazapine	15 mg initially ≤ 30 mg	20-40	May alleviate co-morbid depressive symptoms. Hepatic impairment may be a significant concern for older patients.
Serotonin antagonist and reuptake inhibitor†	Trazodone[137]	25-50 mg	*1st Phase:* 3-6 *2nd Phase:* 5-9	May alleviate co-morbid depressive symptoms. Not tested for long-term treatment of insomnia in older adults. Some side effects, including orthostatic hypotension, constipation, and urinary retention, may be of concern.
Melatonin receptor agonist	Ramelteon[138,139]	8 mg	1-3	No impact on postural stability at night in older adults,[26] suggesting lower fall risk. Tested for longer-term use in older adults.[138] Hepatic impairment may be a significant concern for older patients.

*Start with lowest dose and increase gradually.
†Off-label use.
Superscript numbers refer to references listed at the end of this chapter.

Importantly, these improvements are likely to be maintained after the termination of therapy for up to 2 years and the benefits are superior to medications when treatments are compared head to head.[35-37] An outline of cognitive behavioral therapy for insomnia is shown in Table 59-2. These treatments are most typically provided by psychologists with expertise in behavioral sleep medicine;[38] however, similar interventions provided by nurse practitioners, physicians, and other health professionals may be beneficial as well.

SLEEP-DISORDERED BREATHING

Obstructive Sleep Apnea

Obstructive sleep apnea (OSA) is a disorder of at least five obstructed breathing events (including apneas and hypopneas) per hour of sleep with coexistent daytime somnolence. *Apneas* are defined as breathing pauses of 10 seconds or more, whereas hypopneas are reductions in breathing amplitude. OSA is a common disorder that often requires lifelong care and can result in significant morbidity and even death if left untreated.

Pathophysiology

Although the pathophysiology of OSA is not age-specific, some age-related changes to airway anatomy and body composition are relevant considerations. OSA patients typically have reduced upper airway size owing to excess surrounding soft tissue and reduced neural output to the upper airway muscles during sleep that results in partial or complete upper airway closure.[39] The loss of lean muscle mass and increase in

body fat with aging (particularly among women after menopause) is one factor that may place older adults at higher risk for OSA. The primary defect therefore results in an inability to oppose negative pressure within the airway during inspiration leading to airway collapse.[39] Apneas and hypopneas typically terminate when the patient arouses briefly from sleep. The arousals may not be noticed by the patient but may manifest as increased heart rate, elevated blood pressure, or raised sympathetic tone. Arousals are protective in ending apneas and hypopneas because they resume upper airway muscle tone and airway patency; however, they disrupt sleep architecture and may result in daytime symptoms, particularly in older adults. As older adults may often sleep alone, they may report only midsleep awakenings without awareness of the apneic events that precipitate the awakenings.

Prevalence in Older Adults

Studies suggest that OSA is a relatively common condition, with as much as 20% of the adult population having an apnea-hypopnea index (AHI) of 5 or higher.[40] OSA prevalence particularly increases in early adulthood (age 18 to 45 years) and begins to plateau around 55 to 65 years of age.[41] This plateau may be related to increased mortality rate after age 65 among those with OSA, although support for this assumption is sparse. Comparatively, the prevalence of OSA in patients age 65 and older is two- to threefold higher compared to those who are 30 to 64 years old.[41] In an early study of sleep-disordered breathing in older adults, 70% of men and 56% of women aged 65 to 99 years had at least 10 respiratory events (apneas plus hypopneas) per hour of sleep.[42] Subsequent studies

TABLE 59-2

Cognitive Behavioral Therapy for Insomnia in Older Adults

Treatment Component or Approach	Related Considerations
Sleep education is provided to outline the rationale for recommendations.	Education should be provided about age-related changes in sleep and impact of co-morbid conditions on sleep.
Sleep restriction is used to improve sleep continuity by regulating time spent in bed.	Sleep efficiency of 85% is used as the "cutoff" for good sleep. Daytime activities the patient might engage in to avoid napping should be considered. If naps are needed, a brief (30-minute) nap is sometimes allowed.
Stimulus control is used to change the association between the bed/bedroom and wakefulness to an association with sleep. Patients are instructed to get out of bed if not asleep within 15-30 minutes.	Patients must be reminded to use assistive devices (e.g., cane, walker, eyeglasses) if out of bed at night. If fall risk is a concern, patient may instead sit on edge of bed or in a chair near bed for safety.
Sleep hygiene education is provided to address daytime habits and improve the sleep environment.	Review liquids consumed with evening medications, and consider whether some may be taken before bedtime (e.g., with dinner) to reduce fluid intake near bedtime.
Cognitive therapy is used to challenge the patient's dysfunctional beliefs and misconceptions about sleep and insomnia.	Age-related misperceptions about sleep are common. Realistic expectations must be discussed when co-morbid conditions may limit progress. Patients with mild cognitive problems may still benefit from behavioral aspects of treatment.
Relaxation training is sometimes recommended to reduce arousal at bedtime. Techniques can include progressive muscle relaxation, meditation, yoga, biofeedback, or imagery.	Consider patient preferences in choosing an approach, and incorporate relaxing activities the patient already uses when possible.

confirm that sleep-disordered breathing is highly prevalent in older individuals.[43]

Clinical Consequences

The manifestations of OSA in adults commonly include snoring, daytime somnolence, poor concentration, and awakening with a sense of choking or gasping for air. Older adults may also experience additional symptoms, such as sleep maintenance insomnia, nonrestorative sleep, or even depression, mood changes, and irritability. Patients with mild OSA (i.e., an AHI of 5-15) may experience passive daytime sleepiness as their primary symptom, that is, their somnolence becomes apparent when they are unstimulated or sedentary. Patients with moderate to severe OSA (AHI of 15 or greater) may have daytime somnolence that limits daytime activities and can increase risk for motor vehicle violations or accidents.[44]

Primarily in severe cases, OSA has also been associated with diabetes, hypertension, coronary artery disease, congestive heart failure, and stroke, all of which are common in older patients. It remains unclear, however, if these associations are due to common factors that lead to both OSA and the co-morbid conditions, or if OSA plays a role in the etiology and worsening of these disorders. At least one longitudinal population study showed that patients with OSA had three times the adjusted odds of developing hypertension compared to patients without OSA.[45] OSA is also particularly common in patients with resistant hypertension and should be regularly screened by primary care providers in such patients.[46] OSA has also been associated with insulin resistance and other factors related to the metabolic syndrome.[47] Studies show that OSA is associated with elevations in C-reactive protein,[48] which is reduced when OSA is treated with continuous positive airway pressure (CPAP) therapy.[49]

Overall, patients with severe OSA have increased mortality rate.[50-52] This may be attributed to co-morbid disorders associated with OSA including pulmonary hypertension, systemic hypertension, diabetes, obesity, myocardial infarction, cerebrovascular disease, and cardiac arrhythmias. Also, OSA induces excessive daytime sleepiness, inattention, and fatigue,

which may contribute to cognitive deficits. In-hospital morbidity and mortality rates tend to be higher for patients with OSA, particularly in the perioperative period.[53,54] Stroke patients with untreated OSA show attenuated functional improvement with stroke rehabilitation as well.[55]

Evaluation

Diagnosis of OSA initially depends on obtaining a good sleep history from the patient and a bed partner when possible. Physical examination should assess for obesity, narrow oropharyngeal airway, high blood pressure, and abnormal jaw structure. Overnight polysonography (PSG) is needed to evaluate respiration, thoracoabdominal movement, and oxygenation patterns during sleep and is considered the gold standard for diagnosis of OSA.[56]

Treatment

Treatment of OSA is particularly important for older patients with cardiac disorders and stroke. Patients treated for OSA show a significant increase in ejection fraction and an improvement in systolic blood pressure and heart rate after only 1 month of treatment.

For clinically significant and symptomatic OSA, the most common therapy is positive airway pressure (PAP) delivered by CPAP, bilevel positive airway pressure (BiPAP), or autotitrating positive airway pressure (APAP).[56] PAP acts as a pneumatic splint that reduces obstruction and maintains patency of the pharyngeal airway. Symptomatic patients benefit most significantly and typically report improved sleep quality, daytime alertness, and energy.[57] In general, adherence is best when a nurse or technician spends time teaching optimal use and ensuring optimal comfort of the mask during initiation of therapy. Cost of PAP therapy may be another limiting factor as many older patients may have a fixed income and lack funds to sustain their treatment.

Surgical options generally are not recommended for older patients, primarily due to increased risk of complications and the limited efficacy of surgical interventions. Uvulopalatopharyngoplasty (UPPP) theoretically opens the airway and tightens tissues in the throat and palate to decrease upper airway obstruction. Laser-assisted uvulopalatoplasty is a technique whereby a carbon dioxide laser is used to reshape and reduce the size of the uvula and superficial palate. Other surgical options may include treatment of anatomic abnormalities such as a deviated septum, enlarged tonsils, or nasal polyps. These options can improve OSA and snoring in some patients,[56] however, studies have failed to show consistent clinical utility of these surgical procedures compared to conservative therapy,[58] and these procedures may involve considerable perioperative morbidity in older patients. Examples of surgical complications include palatal mucosal breakdown, transient neuralgias, tongue base abscess formation, and airway compromise due to edema.[59,60]

Oral appliances may improve symptoms of OSA by holding the tongue and mandible in a more anterior position. These devices have shown efficacy in improving the frequency of respiratory events, arousals, snoring, and oxyhemoglobin desaturation.[61-63] Some (but not all) studies suggest resolution of OSA is most likely in patients with only mild to moderate OSA.[62,64] Oral appliances may be difficult for older patients to tolerate[65] and some studies suggest long-term relapse of OSA may be significant due to nonadherance, appliance failure due to wear and tear, or weight gain.[66,67] Edentulous older patients generally cannot use oral appliance therapy.

Although behavioral recommendations are seldom sufficient to treat sleep apnea among older adults, patients should be encouraged to abstain from drinking alcohol and smoking, and overweight patients should be encouraged to lose weight. Sleeping on the side rather than in the supine position may improve the frequency of obstructive events for patients with OSA primarily in the supine position. In addition, maintaining patency of the nasal passages by use of a humidifier or decongestants may be helpful in some cases.

Central Sleep Apnea

Central sleep apnea (CSA) describes a form of abnormal respiratory pauses caused by a lack of respiratory effort. *The International Classification of Sleep Disorders* (ICSD-2) describes several subtypes of CSA including Cheyne-Stokes breathing, high altitude periodic breathing, CSA due to a medical condition, and CSA due to a drug or substance. Spontaneous CSA is rare and is subdivided by the arterial carbon dioxide level ($Paco_2$). Hypercapnic CSA occurs secondary to insufficient ventilator drive (e.g., in *congenital central alveolar hypoventilation syndrome,* formerly known as *Ondine's curse*). Patients with normocapnic spontaneous CSA have normal $Paco_2$ levels during wakefulness but breathe at a serum $Paco_2$ near or below the apneic threshold during sleep leading to cycles of hyperventilation and hypocapnia causing arousals. CSA is especially important in geriatric populations as it appears to increase with age and co-morbid conditions.

Pathophysiology

Normal respiration functions to regulate levels of arterial oxygen (Pao_2) and $Paco_2$ at a homeostatic level. Several feedback loops involving chemoreceptors, intrapulmonary vagal receptors, respiratory control centers in the brainstem, and respiratory muscles work to maintain a balance in serum chemistry. Cortical brain areas influence respiration during wakefulness in a process termed behavioral control. Awake stimulation

and pulmonary mechanoreceptors affect behavioral control to maintain respiration. During sleep, behavioral control is lost and chemical control predominantly regulates ventilation. The greatest stimulus affecting chemical control is serum $Paco_2$. CSA occurs when respiratory instability lowers $Paco_2$ near a specific value. This value where apnea begins to occur is commonly termed the apneic threshold. The apneic threshold typically increases when a person goes from wake to sleep. In normal individuals, the increase in apneic threshold is accompanied by an increase in the serum $Paco_2$ during sleep. However, co-morbid conditions such as heart failure, high altitude, or central nervous system (CNS) disturbances may increase the respiratory rate and decrease the difference between serum $Paco_2$ and the apneic threshold. As a result, periods of apnea are more likely to occur as a result of hyperventilation that causes a reduction in $Paco_2$ below the apneic threshold. CSA can also occur as a result of CNS disease (encephalitis), neuromuscular disease (e.g., post-polio syndrome), abnormal ventilator mechanics (e.g., kyphoscoliosis), or blunted chemoreceptor responsiveness (e.g., narcotics), which can all diminish respiratory muscle activity. Although respiratory abnormalities may not be apparent during wakefulness, they may be evident during sleep when behavioral control of respiration decreases. Patients with any of the disorders mentioned above should undergo a thorough evaluation to screen for CNS.

Prevalence in Older Adults

The estimated prevalence of CSA is 4% (women 0.4%, men 7.8%)[68] based on a prospective study of adults randomly selected from the general population. CSA appears to increase in prevalence particularly in individuals older than 60 years of age.[33] It remains unclear whether this rise is directly linked to advanced age or merely associated with a higher prevalence of co-morbid disease. Undoubtedly, CSA occurs at a higher rate with the presence of certain other risk factors. Cheyne-Stokes breathing has been reported in 15% to 55% of patients with heart failure and up to 26% of patients who have recently had a stroke.[69-71] Narcotics (e.g., methadone) also increase the rate of CSA as high as 30% in methadone-treated patients.[72] Primary CSA appears to affect mostly middle- or older-aged individuals. Cheyne-Stokes breathing increases in prevalence among individuals older than 60 years.[43]

Clinical Consequences

Similar to OSA patients, CSA patients may present with symptoms of excessive somnolence, nighttime awakenings, and hypoxia.[73] Patients may report unrefreshing sleep or choking and shortness of breath upon awakening. Overall, somnolence tends to be less severe than in OSA Concomitant insomnia may result from and worsen CSA in older patients, as the recurrent sleep-wake transition may worsen respiratory instability. Patients with heart failure, arrhythmias such as atrial fibrillation,[74] and stroke may also be at higher risk for CSA. Unlike OSA, however, CSA has no known predictive physical examination findings. These patients may have a normal body habitus, and a high index of suspicion must be sought based on the patient's clinical history.

The long-term clinical effects of CSA are unknown. Most data on morbidity and mortality stem from studies of patients with medically optimized heart failure and CSA, particularly Cheyne-Stokes breathing. One study showed a significantly worsened 2-year survival rate for patients with heart failure and Cheyne-Stokes breathing (56%) compared to patients with heart failure alone (86%).[75] This lower survival rate has been attributed to various etiologies including increased sympathetic tone, increased pulmonary artery pressure, and prolonged circulation time. Unfortunately, data regarding the long-term effects of other forms of CSA is lacking.

Evaluation

Patients with suspected CSA should undergo nocturnal PSG. An apnea is scored when there is a drop in peak thermal sensor excursion by more than 90% from baseline for at least 10 seconds. An apnea is classified as central when it is associated with lack of inspiratory effort. Effort is usually measured during PSG by thoracoabdominal movement. Additional methods to measure respiratory muscle effort can include esophageal manometry and respiratory muscle electromyography (EMG), which are less commonly employed techniques.[76,77]

Treatment

Treatment of CSA is generally recommended for all symptomatic patients, but the decision should be made on an individual basis. Evidence suggests that up to 20% of CSA cases resolve spontaneously, depending on the underlying cause. There are no agreed-upon clinical guidelines for the treatment for CSA; however, several approaches may be considered.

If an underlying disorder is present, its treatment should be considered first-line therapy. For example, patients with Cheyne-Stokes breathing who have heart failure should receive optimized medical therapy for heart failure. For these patients, medical therapy, atrial overdrive pacing, and resynchronization therapy appear to improve CSA in small studies, presumably by improving cardiac function.[78-80] Supplemental oxygen has also been effective at improving nocturnal hypoxia and sleep architecture, New York Heart Association activity class, and ejection fraction for patients with heart failure and Cheyne-Stokes breathing.[81]

Positive airway pressure, however, has been a mainstay treatment for CSA. CPAP has been shown to improve the AHI for patients with CSA.[82,83] In the Canadian Positive Airway Pressure Trial (CANPAP), 258 patients with CSA and heart failure were randomly assigned to receive either CPAP or no CPAP for 2 years.[84] The study did not show an improvement in mortality or transplant-free survival rate with CPAP, and there was an early increase in adverse events favoring the control group that was likely secondary to decreased cardiac output in patients who received CPAP and were preload dependent (e.g., patients with atrial fibrillation or hypovolemia). There were, however, significant improvements in the 6-minute walk tests, CSA index, nocturnal oxygen, and ejection fraction with CPAP. Post-hoc analysis of the CANPAP trial showed a slight benefit from patients who achieved an AHI lower than 15 on CPAP.[85] Although its effect on survival remains questionable, CPAP can be used to improve nocturnal and daytime symptoms in patients with CSA.

BiPAP is effective for treating patients with hypercapnic CSA associated with hypoventilation. Examples of such patients include those with neuromuscular disease, chest wall disease, or central nervous system disease. A high inspiratory-to-expiratory PAP ratio provides support to improve ventilation. This feature may be particularly helpful for patients with prolonged apneas; however, some studies suggest that the use of BiPAP for CSA without a backup rate may actually worsen the AHI.[86] Possible explanations for this may include an exacerbation of hyperventilation, hypocapnia, and lowering serum bicarbonate levels near the apneic threshold. However, studies using BiPAP with a backup rate have shown at least a similar improvement in apneas and hypopneas when compared to CPAP. This has been especially studied in patients with heart failure and Cheyne-Stokes breathing.[87,88] Adaptive servoventilation has recently been suggested as a strategy for treating CSA, particularly Cheyne-Stokes breathing. The device provides a fixed end-expiratory pressure while varying inspiratory pressure to compensate for decreases in inspiratory flow. In small, short-term trials the device has been found to be more effective than conventional PAP for controlling CSA, improving sleep architecture, and decreasing daytime somnolence.[89,90] Long-term outcome studies are still needed.

Finally, certain medications have been explored to treat CSA in limited studies. The carbonic anhydrase inhibitor, acetazolamide, theoretically produces a serum metabolic acidosis that stimulates the central respiratory drive, decreasing the likelihood of hypoventilation with varying levels of carbon dioxide. One small study of six patients with Cheyne-Stokes breathing found a significant improvement after 1 week of treatment with acetazolamide.[91] Another drug that has been prescribed in the setting of heart failure and Cheyne-Stokes breathing is theophylline. Theophylline inhibits phosphodiesterase-5, which stimulates respiration and theoretically improves central chemosensitivity to carbon dioxide and reduces the likelihood of apneas;[92] however, the drug has the potential to cause tachyarrhythmias and other cardiac events and this effect has limited its use.

RESTLESS LEGS SYNDROME

RLS is a sleep movement disorder in which there is an urge or need to move the legs to stop the unpleasant sensations. All of the following symptoms must be endorsed to diagnose RLS: (1) involuntary urge to move, with uncomfortable sensations in the legs (paresthesias); (2) increasing at rest or inactivity; (3) relieved by movement or stretching, and (4) worsening at night. Patients often describe symptoms as "creepy-crawly," jittery, internal itch, shock-like, or painful sensation. Other body parts may be involved including the arms.

Pathophysiology

RLS appears to have a strong genetic component, with 50% of patients reporting a family history and a greater than sixfold chance of RLS among first-degree relatives of RLS patients. Genetic studies have revealed links to the RLS susceptibility gene on chromosome 12q and 14q. RLS appears to have central dopamine involvement, which is suggested by the therapeutic reduction of RLS symptoms with the use of a dopamine agonist.

One common cause of RLS is iron deficiency anemia. Older patients are particularly at risk for anemia or low iron stores in the absence of anemia, which can result from nutritional deficiencies, gastrointestinal disorders, or malignancies. Iron is a cofactor at the rate-limiting step in the production of dopamine. Inadequate iron stores may decrease dopamine production in the brain and contribute to primary RLS.

RLS is related to many medical conditions that are also more common in older adults, such as rheumatoid arthritis, uremia (15-40% of patients on hemodialysis have RLS), diabetes, hypothyroidism, and peripheral neuropathy. Use of specific medications (e.g., selective serotonin reuptake inhibitors [SSRIs]) is also implicated. In one study of older adults, a higher incidence of RLS was reported in patients with anxiety, those with depression, and those with lower cognitive performance.[93]

Prevalence

The prevalence of RLS is 2% to 15% and is likely higher among older adults.[94] One study of RLS in an older French population (mean age 68.6 years) found that RLS was present in 24.2% of 318 participants, with higher rates in women (29.7%) than men (12.1%).[93] Another study reported a prevalence of 9.8% among 369 subjects in a German population age 65 to 83 years old, which was higher in women (13.9%) compared to men (6.1%).[95]

Clinical Consequences

Concomitant with RLS symptoms, patients may complain of delayed sleep onset, daytime sleepiness, and sometimes depression. RLS severity, sleep disturbances, and depressive symptoms are interrelated in some research. Hornyak and associates[96] found that RLS patients endorsed somatic symptoms of depression (especially sleep disturbances), but not cognitive symptoms of depression. Given that both RLS and depression increase with age, there may be a higher correlation between these disorders among older adults.

Evaluation

Workup of RLS should include a history, physical examination, and routine laboratory tests. Thyroid function should be checked to assess for hypothyroidism, a basic metabolic panel to assess for kidney function and diabetes plus a complete serum iron panel to evaluate for clinically significant abnormalities in iron levels or binding.

RLS is a clinical diagnosis made by interviewing the patient to determine whether diagnostic criteria are met, and PSG is not routinely indicated for a diagnosis. At times, however, PSG is used to evaluate for co-morbid PLMD if suspected (see later discussion).

Treatment

Treatment of RLS should target underlying causes of the disorder if identified. Table 59-3 outlines medications used for the treatment of RLS, noting specific considerations for older patients. Iron repletion should be used when ferritin levels

---

TABLE 59-3

Pharmacologic Treatments for Restless Legs Syndrome (RLS), with Special Considerations for Use in Older Patients

Agent	Dosing for Older Patients	Half-life (hr)	Additional Considerations
DOPAMINE AGONIST			
Carbidopa/levodopa (Sinemet)[98]	25/100-50/200 mg PO qhs	0.75-1.5	Patients with occasional symptoms can use prn, which may reduce side effect risk. Strong empirical support exists for RLS treatment. Concerns remain about augmentation; see Chapter 24 for discussion of RLS.
Nonergot (D_2/D_3) dopamine agonist[98]	1-3 hr before bedtime as dose titration		Strong empirical support exists for treatment of moderate to severe primary RLS. Orthostatic hypotension may be a concern with older patients.
Pramipexole	0.125-0.5 mg qhs	8	
Ropinirole	0.25-3 mg	6	
Gabapentin	100-1200 mg	5-7	May be most useful for older patients with secondary RLS from peripheral neuropathy. Daytime sedation may be problematic in older patients. Dosing is dependent on creatinine clearance.
OPIATES			
Codeine	15 mg PO qhs	2.5-4	Consider only for older patients with co-morbid pain. Significant side effects (dizziness, nausea, exacerbation of sleep apnea) may make this medication inappropriate for many older patients. Significant rebound RLS may occur when drug is discontinued.
BENZODIAZEPINES			
Clonazepam	0.25 mg PO qhs	≤ 60	Long half-life may cause drug accumulation.
Other benzodiazepines	See Table 59-1	See Table 59-1	Consider for some patients with co-morbid insomnia who are not at risk for adverse events. Potentially serious side effects include impaired cognitive performance[132] and increased fall risk.[133]
Iron (ferrous sulfate)	Replace deficiency with 325 mg tid; improved absorption with vitamin C	6	Suggested for patients with ferritin <20 ng/mL and on case-by-case basis for patients with ferritin levels 20-50 ng/mL. Constipation is common; stool softener may be needed.

qhs, at bedtime; *tid,* three times a day.
Superscripts refer to references listed at the end of this chapter.

are below 20 ng/mL and may be used when ferritin levels are between 20 and 50 ng/mL.[97] Few treatments have been systematically evaluated for safety and efficacy in the management of RLS among older patients specifically. Because a number of the conditions that may contribute to RLS are more common with advanced age, addressing such conditions (e.g., diabetic peripheral neuropathy) is likely to be a key focus of RLS management. There is the greatest evidence for direct pharmacologic treatment of RLS with agents that targets dopamine. Although not specific to older patients, two meta-analyses showed that dopamine agonists were significantly more efficacious in the treatment of RLS than placebo, and that pramipexole may be more efficacious and better tolerated than ropinirole.[98,99] Alternative pharmacologic treatments for RLS include other dopaminergic agents, gabapentin, opiates, and benzodiazepines, which should be used with caution in older patients (see Table 59-3). Nonpharmaceutical management includes massage, hot baths, avoidance of sleep deprivation, and good sleep hygiene,[100] which may be appropriate for older adults given the low risk for adverse consequences from these behavioral recommendations.

PERIODIC LIMB MOVEMENT DISORDER

PLMD, also called *nocturnal myoclonus,* is a similar and sometimes overlapping disorder with RLS. It is a diagnosis made with overnight PSG which shows evidence of limb movements in combination with a sleep complaint or daytime fatigue. A limb movement is described as rhythmic extensions of the big toe and dorsiflexion of the ankle with occasional flexions of the knee or hip. A periodic limb movement (PLM) event is scored on a sleep study as movements that last 0.5 to 10 seconds, in a sequence of four or more, separated by an interval of 5 to 90 seconds, with an amplitude change of 8 μV above baseline. As many as 90% of patients with RLS have periodic limb movements during sleep (PLMS), but PLMD independent of RLS is rare. In contrast to RLS, PLMD occurs during sleep and requires PSG evidence in combination with a sleep-related complaint for diagnosis. A diagnosis

of PLMD also requires the clinician to establish that the condition is not caused by another medical or sleep disorder. Figure 59-1 shows a sample PSG recording of PLMS. One study found that PLMS can be exacerbated by the use of medications suggesting PLMS are likely the result of enhanced serotoninergic availability and secondarily decreased dopaminergic effects.[101]

REM BEHAVIOR DISORDER

REM sleep behavior disorder (RBD) is a parasomnia that occurs most commonly in older persons. Underlying this disorder is disinhibition of the process that normally prevents transmission of muscle activity during dreaming. Thus, the patient may thrash about in bed, sometimes falling or leaping from the bed and incurring significant injury during REM sleep. Patients often describe vivid and violent dreams. The bed partner often complains that the patient is punching or kicking, fighting in a dream, and sleep talking. In one study, 32% of RBD patients had injured themselves and 64% had assaulted their spouses.[102]

The minimal diagnostic criteria for RBD are (1) presence of REM sleep without atonia, defined as sustained or intermittent elevation of submental EMG tone or excessive phasic muscle activity in the limb EMG; (2) sleep-related injurious or potentially injurious disruptive behaviors by history or abnormal REM behaviors on PSG; (3) absence of electroencephalograph (EEG) epileptiform activity during REM sleep unless RBD can be clearly distinguished from concurrent REM sleep-related seizure disorder; and (4) sleep disturbance that is not better explained by another sleep, medical, mental, or neurologic disorder, medications, or substance use disorder.[77,103]

Pathophysiology

The pathophysiology and anatomical substrates of RBD are unknown but are presumed to involve the regulation of both brainstem mechanisms that control REM sleep atonia

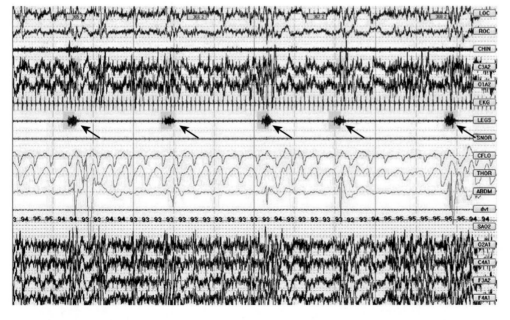

Figure 59-1 Sample polysomnography (PSG) recording from a 73-year-old patient with periodic limb movements in sleep. Episodes of limb movements are highlighted. Periodic movements in the leg electromyograph are shown in the recording of this 120-second epoch.

and as yet undefined locomotor centers. In cases in which structural lesions were identified by neuroimaging, the midbrain and dorsal pons were involved.[104] Medications can also induce RBD, particularly antidepressant medications. Given the high prevalence of depression in older adults, medication-induced RBD should be considered a potential cause of RBD. Recently, a literature search was conducted on 15 articles that demonstrated clomipramine, selegiline, and phenelzine had the strongest evidence for drug-induced RBD.[105]

RBD may also be associated with other sleep disorders, particularly OSA. Arousals that occur from respiratory events during REM due to OSA can lead to dream-enacting behaviors and mimic RBD. One study found that abnormal behaviors and unpleasant dreams (presenting as RBD-like symptoms) resolved in OSA patients when the OSA was treated with CPAP therapy.[106] This suggests that RBD-like symptoms may be caused by the disruption of REM sleep caused by OSA in some patients. PSG should therefore be performed in patients with suspected RBD because OSA can imitate RBD and treatment of the OSA may eliminate RBD-like symptoms. If OSA is diagnosed in a patient with suspected RBD, the OSA should first be treated.

Prevalence

The estimated prevalence of RBD in the general population has been reported as high as 0.5%. A recent study of sleep disorders patients found rates of RBD of approximately 5%.[107] It is more common in males and with increasing age. The mean age of RBD patients has been reported to be 52 to 61 years of age.[107,108] One study of adults age 70 or older found that 0.8% reported history of sleep-related injury, with 0.4% of individuals having confirmed RBD. In a population of patients with RBD presenting to a regional sleep laboratory, nearly two thirds of patients were older than age 50 at diagnosis.[109]

RBD may be idiopathic or secondary to a neurodegenerative disease.[104] A study of 93 RBD patients found neurologic disorders were present in 57% of patients.[107] RBD often predates neurodegenerative disease diagnosis by years. In a study of Parkinson's disease, RBD developed before parkinsonism in 52% of the patients.[107]

Evaluation

The diagnosis of suspected RBD is confirmed by PSG with video monitoring. First, other sleep disorders (especially sleep apnea) need to be ruled out. In the absence of such disorders, and the presence of REM sleep, the patient will be monitored acting out dreams and display REM atonia (REM sleep on EEG and electro-oculogram with activity in the EMG) (Fig. 59-2).

Treatment

The main goal of treatment is the prevention of harm to the patient and family by creating a safe sleep environment and having the bed partner sleep in a different bed until symptoms are controlled. The aim of medication treatment is a reduction in dream enactment behavior. The 2010 Best Practice Guidelines for the treatment of RBD suggest clonazepam to decrease the occurrence of sleep-related injury caused by RBD in patients for whom pharmacologic therapy is necessary.[110] A review of the literature identified 22 studies of the treatment of RBD using clonazepam, with 90% of patients positively responding to treatment.[110] Other benzodiazepines are also used, but as mentioned earlier, caution is warranted among older adults as benzodiazepines increase risk of falls and memory impairment, and can worsen dementia or sleep apnea.[19-22] Melatonin has been shown to effectively treat motor atonia in patients with RBD and has fewer side effects than benzodiazepines[19-22] although less research is available. Of six studies reviewed, 31 out of 38 patients experienced improvement in RBD with melatonin.[110] Melatonin leads to a reduction of muscle tone in REM[111] in contrast to the persistence of tonic muscle tone with clonazepam treatment.

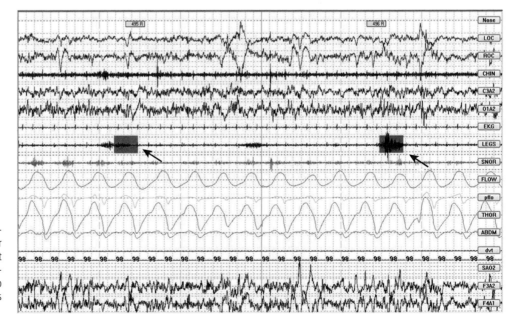

Figure 59-2 Sample polysomnography (PSG) recording from an older patient with rapid eye movement (REM) sleep behavior disorder. Electromyography activity during REM sleep without atonia are highlighted in this 120-second epoch.

CIRCADIAN RHYTHM SLEEP DISORDERS

Circadian rhythms describe 24-hour physiologic patterns of events. Circadian rhythm sleep disorders (CRSD) are characterized by chronic or recurrent sleep disturbance resulting from misalignment between the environment and an individual's sleep-wake cycle.

There are several distinct circadian rhythm sleep disorders.[112] Of particular relevance to older adults, advanced sleep phase disorder (ASPD) describes a condition in which sleep begins and ends earlier than the desired time for sleep. Random, short bouts of sleep with overall preserved total sleep time describes irregular sleep-wake phase disorder. Individuals with a sleep schedule that gradually delays and is unaffected by time cues (e.g., enucleated blind individuals) may have a free-running rhythm. Generally, circadian rhythm sleep disorders are due to an alteration of the internal timekeeping system that regulates sleep or to a change in environmental time cues. This alteration can result from a mixture of exogenous and endogenous factors that affect normal waking function.

Pathophysiology

Studies of mammalian physiology have discovered that sleep, alertness, core body temperature, and the secretion of hormones such as melatonin and cortisol vary consistently across the day with a schedule slightly longer than 24 hours.[113] As a result, diurnal variation is constantly affected by environmental cues such as activity, scheduled sleep, and solar light/dark cycles. Absence of these time cues may lead to development of circadian abnormalities.

Circadian rhythms are especially responsive to light and dark signals. Timing of environmental light is important in training the normal circadian rhythm.[114-116] It remains less clear whether wavelength or intensity of light may cause different changes in the circadian system. Recently, non-rod and non-cone ganglion cells have been discovered that continue to entrain circadian rhythms even in blind individuals.[117] These photoreceptors contain melanopsin, which is most sensitive to blue wavelength light. Other cues such as sleep schedules and daily activity play a less certain role in regulating circadian rhythms. Burgess and Eastman[118] showed that manipulation of wake time causes shifts in the normal secretion of melatonin; however, this effect may be a reflection of light exposure due to the change in morning rise time.

Prevalence

Prevalence studies of CRSD are limited. An advance in the timing of sleep is common with age,[119,120] and as a result, older adults are at elevated risk for ASPD. To date, there are no true prevalence data for circadian rhythm sleep disorders available for older adults specifically; however, some data suggest rates of approximately 1% in middle-age to

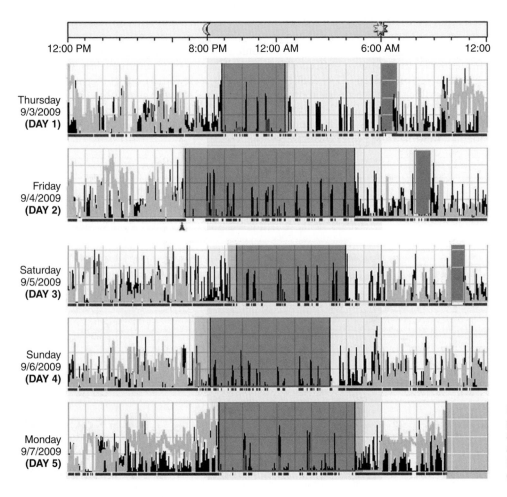

Figure 59-3 Sample wrist actigraphy record from an older patient with advanced sleep phase syndrome. Shaded areas indicate periods in bed. Note the irregular schedule and daytime naps co-occurring with the advanced phase.

older adults.[112] In addition, a telephone survey found that ASPD symptoms were twice as common as delayed sleep phase disorder (DSPD) symptoms among adults aged 40 to 64 years.[121] Among older adults with dementia and those in nursing home settings, circadian abnormalities are nearly ubiquitous.[122,123]

Clinical Consequences

Among older patients, a presentation of insomnia characterized with early morning awakenings and evening sleepiness indicates a high likelihood of ASPD. Common symptoms of circadian rhythm disorders are fatigue and functional limitation. Older adults appear particularly prone to an advanced sleep schedule. A study of healthy adults aged 20 to 59 showed a relationship between older age and earlier bedtime and wake time. In addition, older age was associated with less time in bed overall and better mood and increased alertness in the mornings.[124]

Assessment

The diagnosis of circadian rhythm disorder often depends on the clinical history. Other methods of assessing sleep cycle abnormalities include sleep diaries, actigraphy[77,112] and questionnaires. In research settings, salivary dim light melatonin onset is also used, though this is not widely available in clinical settings. Figure 59-3 shows a sample actigraphic recording of an older patient with ASPD.

Treatment

Treatment of CRSD requires interventions that target underlying circadian timing. Chronotherapy involves a process of delaying bedtime gradually around the 24-hour clock until the desired schedule is obtained.[125] This treatment is typically used for DSPD and has not been formally studied with older adults or with ASPD.

Circadian phase shifting involves using environmental time cues (especially light) to resynchronize the circadian rhythm. In the case of advanced sleep phase syndrome, evening light exposure is used to delay the onset of sleep. In the case of irregular sleep-wake patterns such as those observed in residents of long-term care facilities, the important factor may be increasing daytime light exposure in general.[126]

Melatonin has been used to entrain irregular circadian rhythms in patients with free-running sleep disorders.[127] Melatonin administration in the morning shifts sleep later, while administration in the evening advances the circadian rhythm.[128] Thus, melatonin performs opposite to phototherapy on the sleep-wake schedule. In the treatment of ASPD, the response to melatonin supplements suggests it should be taken in the morning; however, questions remain about the safety of administration of melatonin in the morning because of sleepiness that is experienced by some patients. Unfortunately, there are no clear guidelines regarding optimal dosage of the drug. Doses between 0.5 and 5 mg have been used in most studies, and the threshold for effect occurs at the physiologic serum levels near 50 pg/mL. A specific melatonin receptor agonist, ramelteon, has been licensed as an effective hypnotic in the United States, and this drug may have clinical effectiveness on promoting sleep in circadian rhythm disorders.

SUMMARY AND CONCLUSIONS

In summary, sleep complaints are common among geriatric patients. A key consideration in the evaluation and treatment of sleep complaints among older adults is that insomnia is typically co-morbid with one or more medical or psychiatric conditions. Management of other sleep disorders such as sleep apnea, RLS, periodic limb movement disorder, REM sleep behavior disorder and addressing circadian rhythm shifts are often an important focus of a comprehensive treatment plan. Sleep disorders are worthy of treatment because effective interventions can improve health and quality of life and reduce mortality risk among older adults.

Acknowledgments

This work is supported by grants NIH/NIA K23 AG028452 (Martin), VA RR&D IIR 1RX000135, Cedars Sinai Sleep Medicine Fellowship Program and the VA Greater Los Angeles Healthcare System, Geriatric Research, Education and Clinical Center.

REFERENCES

1. Foley DJ, Monjan AA, Brown SL, Simonsick EM, Wallace RB, Blazer DG. Sleep complaints among elderly persons: An epidemiologic study of three communities. *Sleep*. 1995;18:425-432.
2. Stone KL, Ancoli-Israel S, Blackwell T, et al. Actigraphy-measured sleep characteristics and risk of falls in older women. *Arch Intern Med*. 2008;168:1768-1775.
3. Le Couteur DG, Latimer Hill E, Cumming RG, Lewis R, Carrington S. Sleep disturbances and falls in older people. *J Gerontol: Med Sci*. 2007;62A:62-66.
4. Martin JL, Fiorentino L, Jouldjian S, Josephson KR, Alessi CA. Sleep quality among residents of assisted living facilities: Impact on quality of life, functional status and depression. *J Am Geriatr Soc*. 2010;58: 829-836.
5. American Academy of Sleep Medicine. *I. Insomnia. The International Classification of Sleep Disorders*. 2nd ed. Westchester, IL: American Academy of Sleep Medicine; 2005:1–31.
6. Bonnet MH, Arand DL. Heart rate variability in insomniacs and matched normal sleepers. *Psychosom Med*. 1998;60:610-615.
7. Bonnet MH, Arand DL. 24-Hour metabolic rate in insomniacs and matched normal sleepers. *Sleep*. 1995;18:581-588.
8. Spielman A, Glovinsky PB. The varied nature of insomnia. In: Hauri PJ, ed. *Case Studies in Insomnia*. New York: Plenum Press; 1991.
9. Vitiello MV, Rybarczyk B, VonKorff M, Stepanski EJ. Cognitive behavioral therapy for insomnia improves sleep and decreases pain in older adults with co-morbid insomnia and osteoarthritis. *J Clin Sleep Med*. 2009;5:355-362.
10. Birrer RB, Vemuri SP. Depression in later life: A diagnostic and therapeutic challenge. *Am Fam Physician*. 2004;69:2375-2382.
11. American Psychiatric Association. *Diagnostic and Statistical Manual of Mental Disorders: DSM-IV*. 4th ed. Washington, DC: American Psychiatric Association Press; 1994.
12. Ohayon MM, Roth T. What are the contributing factors for insomnia in the general population? *J Psychosom Res*. 2001;51:745-755.
13. Monane M. Insomnia in the elderly. *J Clin Psychiatry*. 1992;53:23-28.
14. Su TP, Huang SR, Chou P. Prevalence and risk factors of insomnia in community-dwelling Chinese elderly: A Taiwanese urban area survey. *Aust N Z J Psychiatry*. 2004;38:706-713.
15. Maggi S, Langlois JA, Minicuci N, et al. Sleep complaints in community-dwelling older persons: Prevalence, associated factors, and reported causes. *J Am Geriatr Soc*. 1998;46:161-168.
16. Fernandez-Mendoza J, Calhoun S, Bixler EO, et al. Insomnia with objective short sleep duration is associated with deficits in neuropsychological performance: A general population study. *Sleep*. 2010;33:459-465.
17. Goldman SE, Hall M, Boudreau R, et al. Association between nighttime sleep and napping in older adults. *Sleep*. 2008;31:733-740.
18. Blackwell T, Redline S, Ancoli-Israel S, et al. Comparison of sleep parameters from actigraphy and polysomnography in older women: The SOF Study. *Sleep*. 2008;31:283-291.
19. Ray WA, Thapa PB, Gideon P. Benzodiazepines and the risk of falls in nursing home residents. *J Am Geriatr Soc*. 2000;48:682-685.

20. Mendelson WB, Garnett D, Gillin JC. Single case study: Flurazepam-induced sleep apnea syndrome in a patient with insomnia and mild sleep-related respiratory changes. *J Nerv Ment Dis.* 1981;169:261-264.

21. Wagner J, Wagner ML. Non-benzodiazepines for the treatment of insomnia. *Sleep Med Rev.* 2000;4:551-581.

22. Mitler MM. Nonselective and selective benzodiazepine receptor agonists—Where are we today? *Sleep.* 2000;23:S39-S47.

23. National Institutes of Health. Manifestations and management of chronic insomnia in adults. *Sleep.* 2005;28:1049-1057.

24. Roth T, Seiden D, Zee P, Sainati S, Weigand S, Zhang J. Phase III outpatient trail of ramelteon for the treatment of chronic insomnia in elderly patients. *J Am Geriatr Soc.* 2005;53:S25-S26.

25. Roth T, Seiden D, Sainati S, Wang-Weigand S, Zhang J, Zee PC. Effects of ramelteon on patient-reported sleep latency in older adults with chronic insomnia. *Sleep Med.* 2006;7:312-318.

26. Zammit G, Wang-Weigand S, Rosenthal R, Peng X. Effect of ramelteon on middle-of-the-night balance in older adults with chronic insomnia. *J Clin Sleep Med.* 2009;5:34-40.

27. Mayer G, Wang-Weigand S, Roth-Schechter B, Lehmann R, Staner C, Partinen M. Efficacy and safety of 6-month nightly ramelteon administration in adults with chronic primary insomnia. *Sleep.* 2009;32: 351-360.

28. Ancoli-Israel S, Richardson GS, Mangano RM, Jenkins L, Hall P, Jones WS. Long-term use of sedative hypnotics in older patients with insomnia. *Sleep Med.* 2005;6:107-113.

29. Lo HS, Yang CM, Lo HG, Lee CY, Ting H, Tzang BS. Treatment effects of gabapentin for primary insomnia. *Clin Neuropharmacol.* 2010;33: 84-90.

30. Krystal AD, Durrence HH, Scharf M, et al. Efficacy and safety of doxepin 1 mg and 3 mg in a 12-week sleep laboratory and outpatient trial of elderly subjects with chronic primary insomnia. *Sleep.* 2010;33: 1553-1561.

31. Roth T, Rogowski R, Hull S, et al. Efficacy and safety of doxepin 1 mg, 3 mg, and 6 mg in adults with primary insomnia. *Sleep.* 2010;30: 1555-1561.

32. Basu R, Dodge H, Stoehr GP, Ganguli M. Sedative-hypnotic use of diphenhydramine in a rural, older adult, community-based cohort: Effects on cognition. *Am J Geriatr Psychiatry.* 2003;11:205-213.

33. Irwin MR, Cole JL, Nicassio PM. Comparative meta-analysis of behavioral interventions for insomnia and their efficacy in middle-aged adults and in older adults 55+ years of age. *Health Psychol.* 2006;25:3-14.

34. Pallesen S, Nordhus IH, Kvale G. Nonpharmacological interventions for insomnia in older adults: A meta-analysis of treatment efficacy. *Psychotherapy.* 1998;35:472-482.

35. Sivertsen B, Omvik S, Pallesen S, et al. Cognitive behavioral therapy vs. zopiclone for treatment of chronic primary insomnia in older adults. *JAMA.* 2006;295:2851-2858.

36. Vallieres A, Morin CM, Guay B. Sequential combinations of drug and cognitive behavioral therapy for chronic insomnia: An exploratory study. *Behav Res Ther.* 2005;43:1611-1630.

37. Jacobs GD, Pace-Schott EF, Stickgold R, Otto MW. Cognitive behavioral therapy and pharmacotherapy for insomnia: A randomized controlled trial and direct comparison. *Arch Intern Med.* 2004;164:1888-1896.

38. Stepanski EJ, Perlis ML. Behavioral sleep medicine—An emerging subspecialty in health psychology and sleep medicine. *J Psychosom Res.* 2000;49:343-347.

39. White DP. Pathogenesis of obstructive and central sleep apnea. *Am J Respir Crit Care Med.* 2005;172:1363-1370.

40. Young T, Palta M, Dempsey J, Skatrud J, Weber S, Badr S. The occurrence of sleep disordered breathing among middle-aged adults. *N Engl J Med.* 1993;328:1230-1235.

41. Jennum P, Riha RL. Epidemiology of sleep apnoea/hypopnoea syndrome and sleep disordered breathing. *Eur Respir J.* 2009;33:907-914.

42. Ancoli-Israel S, Kripke DF, Klauber MR, Mason WJ, Fell R, Kaplan O. Sleep disordered breathing in community-dwelling elderly. *Sleep.* 1991;14:486-495.

43. Johansson P, Alehagen U, Svanborg E, Dahlstrom U, Brostrom A. Sleep disordered breathing in an elderly community-living population: Relationship to cardiac function, insomnia symptoms and daytime sleepiness. *Sleep Med.* 2009;10:1005-1011.

44. George CF. Sleep apnea, alertness and motor vehicle crashes. *Am J Respir Crit Care Med.* 2007;176:954-956.

45. Peppard PE, Young T, Palta M, Skatrud J. Prospective study of the association between sleep-disordered breathing and hypertension. *N Engl J Med.* 2000;342:1378-1384.

46. Logan AG, Perlikowski SM, Mente A, et al. High prevalence of unrecognized sleep apnoea in drug-resistant hypertension. *J Hyperten.* 2001;19:2271-2277.

47. Punjabi NM, Sorkin JD, Katzel LI, Goldberg AP, Schwartz AR, Smith PL. Sleep-disordered breathing and insulin resistance in middle-aged and overweight men. *Am J Respir Crit Care Med.* 2002;165:677-682.

48. Steiropoulos P, Tsara V, Nena E, et al. Effect of continuous positive airway pressure treatment on serum cardiovascular risk factors in patients with obstructive sleep apnea-hypopnea syndrome. *Chest.* 2007;132: 834-851.

49. Ishida K, Kato M, Kato Y, et al. Appropriate use of nasal continuous positive airway pressure decreases elevated C-reactive protein in patients with obstructive sleep apnea. *Chest.* 2009;2009:1-125.

50. Marshall NS, Wong KK, Liu PY, Cullen SR, Knuiman MW, Grunstein RR. Sleep apnea as an independent risk factor for all-cause mortality: The Busselton Health Study. *Sleep.* 2008;31:1079-1085.

51. Young T, Finn L, Peppard PE, et al. Sleep disordered breathing and mortality: Eighteen-year follow-up of the Wisconsin sleep cohort. *Sleep.* 2008;31:1071-1078.

52. Punjabi NM, Caffo BS, Goodwin JL, et al. Sleep-disordered breathing and mortality: A prospective cohort study. *PLoS Med.* 2009;6(8):e1000132.

53. Mickelson SA. Preoperative and postoperative management of obstructive sleep apnea patients. *Otolaryngol Clin North Am.* 2007;40:877-889.

54. Somers VK, White DP, Amin R, et al. Sleep apnea and cardiovascular disease: An American Heart Association/American College of Cardiology Foundation Scientific Statement from the American Heart Association Council for High Blood Pressure Research Professional Education Committee, Council on Clinical Cardiology, Stroke Council, and Council on Cardiovascular Nursing. In collaboration with the National Heart, Lung, and Blood Institute National Center on Sleep Disorders Research (National Institutes of Health). *Circulation.* 2008;118:1080-1111.

55. Kaneko Y, Hajek VE, Zivanovic V, Raboud J, Bradley D. Relationship of sleep apnea to functional capacity and length of hospitalization following stroke. *Sleep.* 2003;26:293-297.

56. Epstein LJ, Kristo D, Strollo PJ, et al. Clinical guideline for the evaluation, management and long-term care of obstructive sleep apnea in adults. *J Clin Sleep Med.* 2009;5:263-276.

57. Montserrat JM, Ferrer M, Hernandez L, et al. Effectiveness of CPAP treatment in daytime function in sleep apnea syndrome: A randomized controlled study with an optimized placebo. *Am J Respir Crit Care Med.* 2001;164:608-613.

58. Sundaram S, Bridgman SA, Lim J, Lasserson TJ. Surgery for obstructive sleep apnoea. *Cochrane Database Syst Rev.* 2005;4:CD001004.

59. Terris DJ, Chen V. Occult mucosal injuries with radiofrequency ablation of the palate. *Otolaryngol Head Neck Surg.* 2001;125:468-472.

60. Pazos G, Mair EA. Complications of radiofrequency ablation in the treatment of sleep-disordered breathing. *Otolaryngol Head Neck Surg.* 2001;125:462-467.

61. Mehta A, Qian J, Petocz P, Darendelier MA, Cistulli PA. A randomized, controlled study of a mandibular advancement splint for obstructive sleep apnea. *Am J Respir Crit Care Med.* 2001;163:1457-1461.

62. Cistulli PA, Gotsopoulos H, Marklund M, Lowe AA. Treatment of snoring and obstructive sleep apnea with mandibular repositioning appliances. *Sleep Med Rev.* 2004;8:443-457.

63. Gotsopoulos H, Chen C, Qian J, Cistulli PA. Oral appliance therapy improves symptoms in obstructive sleep apnea: A randomized, controlled trial. *Am J Respir Crit Care Med.* 2002;166:743-748.

64. Kushida CA, Morgenthaler TI, Littner MR, et al. Practice parameters for the treatment of snoring and obstructive sleep apnea with oral appliances: An update for 2005. *Sleep.* 2010;29:240-243.

65. Mohsenin N, Mostofi MT, Mohsenin V. The role of oral appliances in treating obstructive sleep apnea. *J Am Dent Assoc.* 2003;134:442-449.

66. Marklund M, Sahlin C, Stenlund H, Persson M, Franklin KA. Mandibular advancement device in patients with obstructive sleep apnea: Long-term effects on apnea and sleep. *Chest.* 2001;120:162-169.

67. Marklund M, Stenlund H, Franklin KA. Mandibular advancement devices in 630 men and women with obstructive sleep apnea and snoring: Tolerability and predictors of treatment success. *Chest.* 2004;125: 1270-1278.

68. Bixler EO, Vgontzas AN, Lin HM, et al. Prevalence of sleep-disordered breathing in women: Effects of gender. *Am J Respir Crit Care Med.* 2001;163:608-613.

69. Lanfranchi P, Somers VK, Braghiroli A, Corra U, Eleuteri E, Giannuzzi P. Central sleep apnea in left ventricular dysfunction: Prevalence and implications for arrhythmic risk. *Circulation.* 2003;107:727-732.

70. Sin DD, Fitzgerald F, Parker JD, Newton G, Floras JS, Bradley TD. Risk factors for central and obstructive sleep apnea in 450 men and women with congestive heart failure. *Am J Respir Crit Care Med.* 1999;160:1101-1106.

71. Javaheri S, Parker TJ, Liming JD, et al. Sleep apnea in 81 ambulatory male patients with stable heart failure types and their prevalences, consequences, and presentations. *Circulation.* 1998;97:2154-2159.

72. Wang D, Teichtahl H, Drummer O, et al. Central sleep apnea in stable methadone maintenance treatment patients. *Chest.* 2005;128:1348-1356.

73. Eckert DJ, Jordan AS, Merchia P, Malhotra A. Central sleep apnea: Pathophysiology and treatment. *Chest.* 2007;131:595-607.

74. Leung RS, Huber MA, Rogge T, Maimon N, Chiu KL, Bradley TD. Association between atrial fibrillation and central sleep apnea. *Sleep.* 2005;28:1543-1546.

75. Hanly PJ, Zuberi-Khokhar NS. Increased mortality associated with Cheyne-Stokes respiration in patients with congestive heart failure. *Am J Respir Crit Care Med.* 1996;153:272-276.

76. American Academy of Sleep Medicine. *II. Sleep Related Breathing Disorders. The International Classification of Sleep Disorders.* 2nd ed. Westchester, IL: American Academy of Sleep Medicine; 2005:33–77.

77. American Academy of Sleep Medicine. *The International Classification of Sleep Disorders.* 2nd ed. Westchester, IL: American Academy of Sleep Medicine; 2005.

78. Luthje L, Renner B, Kessels R, et al. Cardiac resynchronization therapy and atrial overdrive pacing for the treatment of central sleep apnoea. *Eur J Heart Fail.* 2009;11:273-280.

79. Baylor P, Tayloe D, Owen D, Sanders C. Cardiac failure presenting as sleep apnea. *Chest.* 1988;94(6):1298-1300.

80. Garrigue S, Bordier P, Jais P, et al. Benefit of atrial pacing in sleep apnea syndrome. *N Engl J Med.* 2002;346:404-412.

81. Sasayama S, Izumi T, Matsuzaki M, et al. Improvement of quality of life with nocturnal oxygen therapy in heart failure patients with central sleep apnea. *Circ J.* 2009;73:1255-1262.

82. Naughton MT, Benard DC, Liu PP, Rutherford R, Rankin F, Bradley TD. Effects of nasal CPAP on sympathetic activity in patients with heart failure and central sleep apnea. *Am J Respir Crit Care Med.* 1995;152:473-479.

83. Naughton MT, Liu PP, Benard DC, Goldstein RS, Bradley TD. Treatment of congestive heart failure and Cheyne-Strokes respiration during sleep by continuous positive airway pressure. *Am J Respir Crit Care Med.* 1995;151:92-97.

84. Bradley TD, Logan AG, Kimoff RJ, et al. Continuous positive airway pressure for central sleep apnea and heart failure. *N Engl J Med.* 2005;353:2025-2033.

85. Arzt M, Floras JS, Logan AG, et al. Suppression of central sleep apnea by continuous positive airway pressure and transplant-free survival in heart failure: A post hoc analysis of the Canadian Continuous Positive Airway Pressure for Patients with Central Sleep Apnea and Heart Failure Trial (CANPAP). *Circulation.* 2007;115:3173-3180.

86. Johnson KG, Johnson DC. Bilevel positive airway pressure worsens central apneas during sleep. *Chest.* 2005;128:2141-2150.

87. Kohnlein T, Welte T, Tan LB, Elliott MW. Assisted ventilation for heart failure patients with Cheyne-Stokes respiration. *Eur Respir J.* 2002;20:934-941.

88. Willson GN, Wilcox I, Piper AJ, et al. Noninvasive pressure preset ventilation for the treatment of Cheyne-Stokes respiration during sleep. *Eur Respir J.* 2001;17:1250-1257.

89. Philippe C, Stoica-Herman M, Drouot X, et al. Compliance with and effectiveness of adaptive servoventilation versus continuous positive airway pressure in the treatment of Cheyne-Stokes respiration in heart failure over a six-month period. *Heart.* 2006;92:337-342.

90. Allam JS, Olson EJ, Gay PC, Morgenthaler TI. Efficacy of adaptive servoventilation in treatment of complex and central sleep apnea syndromes. *Chest.* 2007;132:1839-1846.

91. Javaheri S. Acetazolamide improves central sleep apnea in heart failure: A double-blind, prospective study. *Am J Respir Crit Care Med.* 2006;173:234-237.

92. Javaheri S, Parker TJ, Wexler L, Liming JD, Lindower P, Roselle GA. Effect of theophylline on sleep-disordered breathing in heart failure. *N Engl J Med.* 1996;335:562-567.

93. Celle S, Roche F, Kerleroux J, et al. Prevalence and clinical correlates of restless legs syndrome in an elderly French population: The synapse study. *J Gerontol Biol Sci.* 2010;65:167-173.

94. Natarajan R. Review of periodic limb movement and restless leg syndrome. *J Postgrad Med.* 2010;56:157-162.

95. Rothdach AJ, Trenkwalder C, Haberstock J, Keil U, Berger K. Prevalence and risk factors of RLS in an elderly population: The MEMO study: Memory and Morbidity in Augsburg Elderly. *Neurology.* 2000;54:1064-1068.

96. Hornyak M, Kobasz M, Berger M, Reimann D, Voderholzer U. Impact of sleep-related complaints on depressive symptoms in patients with restless legs syndrome. *J Clin Psychiatry.* 2005;66:1139-1145.

97. Silber MH, Ehrenberg BL, Allen RM, et al. An algorithm for the management of restless legs syndrome. *Mayo Clin Proc.* 2004;79:916-922.

98. Zintzaras E, Kitsios GD, Papathanasiou AA, et al. Randomized trials of dopamine agonists in restless legs syndrome: A systematic review, quality assessment, and meta-analysis. *Clin Ther.* 2010;32:221-237.

99. Quilici S, Abrams KR, Nicolas A, et al. Meta-analysis of the efficacy and tolerability of pramipexole versus ropinirole in the treatment of restless legs syndrome. *Sleep Med.* 2008;9:715-726.

100. Edinger JD, Fins AI, Sullivan RJ, Marsh GR, Dailey DS, Young M. Comparison of cognitive-behavioral therapy and clonazepam for treating periodic limb movement disorder. *Sleep.* 1996;19:442-444.

101. Yang C, White DP, Winkelman JW. Antidepressants and periodic leg movements of sleep. *Biol Psychiatry.* 2005;58:510-514.

102. Olson EJ, Boeve BF, Silber MH. Rapid eye movement sleep behaviour disorder: Demographic, clinical and laboratory findings in 93 cases. *Brain.* 2000;123:331-339.

103. American Academy of Sleep Medicine. *V. Parasomnias. The International Classification of Sleep Disorders.* 2nd ed. Westchester, IL: American Academy of Sleep Medicine; 2005:137–176.

104. Boeve BF, Silber MH, Saper CB, et al. Pathophysiology of REM sleep behaviour disorder and relevance to neurodegenerative disease. *Brain.* 2007;130:2770-2788.

105. Hoque R, Chesson Jr AL. Pharmacologically induced/exacerbated restless legs syndrome, periodic limb movements of sleep, and REM behavior disorder/REM sleep without atonia: Literature review, qualitative scoring, and comparative analysis. *J Clin Sleep Med.* 2010;6:79-83.

106. Iranzo A, Santamaria J. Severe obstructive sleep apnea/hypopnea mimicking REM sleep behavior disorder. *Sleep.* 2005;28:203-206.

107. Olson EJ, Boeve BF, Silber MH. Rapid eye movement sleep behaviour disorder: Demographic, clinical and laboratory findings in 93 cases. *Brain.* 2000;123:331-339.

108. Schenck CH, Hurwitz TD, Mahowald MW. Symposium: Normal and abnormal REM sleep regulation: REM sleep behaviour disorder: An update on a series of 96 patients and a review of the world literature. *J Sleep Res.* 1993;2:224-231.

109. Bonakis A, Howard RS, Ebrahim IO, Merritt S, Williams A. REM sleep behaviour disorder (RBD) and its associations in young patients. *Sleep Med.* 2009;10:641-645.

110. Aurora RN, Zak RS, Maganti RK, et al. Best practice guide for the treatment of REM sleep behavior disorder (RBD). *J Clin Sleep Med.* 2010;6:85-95.

111. Kunz D, Bes F. Melatonin as a therapy in REM sleep behavior disorder patients: An open-labeled pilot study on the possible influence of melatonin on REM-sleep regulation. *Mov Disord.* 1999;14:507-511.

112. American Academy of Sleep Medicine. *IV. Circadian Rhythm Sleep Disorders. The International Classification of Sleep Disorders.* 2nd ed. Westchester, IL: American Academy of Sleep Medicine; 2005:117–136.

113. Dijk DJ, Lockley SW. Integration of human sleep-wake regulation and circadian rhythmicity. *J Appl Physiol.* 2002;92:852-862.

114. Czeisler CA, Duffy JF, Shanahan TL, et al. Stability, precision, and near-24-hour period of the human circadian pacemaker. *Science.* 1999;284:2177-2181.

115. Czeisler CA, Allan JS, Strogatz SH, et al. Bright light resets the human circadian pacemaker independent of the timing of the sleep-wake cycle. *Science.* 1986;223:667-671.

116. Duffy JF, Wright KP. Entrainment of the human circadian system by light. *J Biol Rhythms.* 2005;20:326-338.

117. Lockley SW, Brainard GC, Czeisler CA. High sensitivity of the human circadian melatonin rhythm to resetting by short wavelength light. *J Clin Endocrinol Metab.* 2003;88:4502-4505.

118. Burgess HJ, Eastman CI. A late wake time phase delays the human dim light melatonin rhythm. *Neurosci Lett.* 2006;395:191-195.

119. Carrier J, Monk TH, Reynolds CF, Buysse DJ, Kupfer DJ. Are age differences in sleep due to phase differences in the output of the circadian timing system? *Chronobiol Int.* 1999;16:79-91.

120. Duffy JF, Zeitzer JM, Rimmer DW, Klerman EB, Dijk DJ, Czeisler CA. Peak of circadian melatonin rhythm occurs later within the sleep of older subjects. *Am J Physiol Endocrinol Metab.* 2002;282:E297-E303.

121. Ando K, Kripke ZD, Ancoli-Israel S. Delayed and advanced sleep phase symptoms. *Isr J Psychiatry*. 2002;39:81-90.

122. Martin JL, Webber AP, Alam T, Harker JO, Josephson KR, Alessi CA. Daytime sleeping, sleep disturbance and circadian rhythms in nursing home residents. *Am J Geriatr Psychiatry*. 2006;14:121-129.

123. Ancoli-Israel S, Klauber MR, Jones DW, et al. Variations in circadian rhythms of activity, sleep and light exposure related to dementia in nursing home patients. *Sleep*. 1997;20:18-23.

124. Carrier J, Monk TH, Buysse DJ, Kupfer DJ. Sleep and morningness-eveningness in the "middle" years of life (20-59 y). *J Sleep Res*. 1997;6:230-237.

125. Sack RL, Auckley D, Auger RR, et al. Circadian rhythm sleep disorders Part I, Basic principles, shift work and jet lag disorders An American Academy of Sleep Medicine Review. *Sleep*. 2007;30:1460-1483.

126. Shochat T, Martin J, Marler M, Ancoli-Israel S. Illumination levels in nursing home patients: Effects on sleep and activity rhythms. *J Sleep Res*. 2000;9:373-380.

127. Redman JR, Armstrong SML, Ng KT. Free-running activity in the rat: Entrainment by melatonin. *Science*. 1983;219:1089-1091.

128. Lewy AJ, Bauer VK, Ahmed S, et al. The human phase response curve (PRC) to melatonin is about 12 hours out of phase with the PRC to light. *Chronobiol Int*. 1998;15:71-83.

129. Elie R, Frenay M, LeMorvan P, Bourgouin J. Efficacy and safety of zopiclone and triazolam in the treatment of geriatric insomnia. *Int Clin Psycholpharmacol*. 1990;5(Suppl 2):39-46.

130. Glass JR, Sproule BA, Herrmann N, Busto UE. Effects of 2-week treatment with temazepam and diphenhydramine in elderly insomniacs: A randomized, placebo-controlled trial. *J Clin Pharmacol*. 2008;28:182-188.

131. Linnoila M, Viukari M, Lamminsivu U, Auvinen J. Efficacy and side effects of lorazepam, oxazepam and temazepam as sleeping aids in psychogeriatric inpatients. *Int Pharmacopsychiat*. 1980;15:129-135.

132. Nakra BR, Gfeller JD, Hassan R. A double-blind comparison of the effects of temazepam and triazolam on residual, daytime performance in elderly insomniacs. *Int Psychoger*. 1992;4:45-53.

133. Morin CM, Bastien CH, Brink D, Brown TR. Adverse effects of temazepam in older adults with chronic insomnia. *Hum Psychopharm*. 2003;18:75-82.

134. Hedner J, Yaeche R, Emilien G, Farr I, Salinas E. Zaleplon shortens subjective sleep latency and improves subjective sleep quality in elderly patients with insomnia. The Zaleplon Clinical Investigator Study Group. *Int J Geriatr Psych*. 2000;15:704-712.

135. Roger M, Attali P, Coquelin JP. Multicenter, double-blind, controlled comparison of zolpidem and triazolam in elderly patients with insomnia. *Clin Ther*. 1993;15(1):127-136.

136. Ancoli-Israel S, Krystal AD, McCall WV, et al. A 12-week, randomized, double-blind, placebo-controlled study evaluating the effect of eszopiclone 2 mg on sleep/wake function in older adults with primary and comorbid insomnia. *Sleep*. 2010;33:225-234.

137. Schwartz T, Nihalani N, Virk S, et al. A comparison of the effectiveness of two hypnotic agents for the treatment of insomnia. *Int J Psychiatr Nurs Res*. 2004;10:1146-1150.

138. Richardson GS, Zammit G, Wang-Weigand S, Zhang J. Safety and subjective sleep effects of ramelteon administration in adults and older adults with chronic primary insomnia: A 1-year, open-label study. *J Clin Psychiatry*. 2009;70:467-476.

139. Mini LJ, Wang-Weigand S, Zhang J. Self-reported efficacy and tolerability of ramelteon 8 mg in older adults experiencing severe sleep-onset difficulty. *Am J Geriatr Psychother*. 2007;5:177-184.

Drug Abuse, Dependency, and Withdrawal

Chapter 60

ABIGAIL L. KAY / KRYSTAL R. STOBER / RONALD SEROTA / STEPHEN P. WEINSTEIN

One of the many challenges faced by the sleep specialist is determining the cause(s) of a patient's sleep difficulties. As the use of alcohol, and most illicit substances, can result in sleep disturbances,[1] it is important that all patients who present with sleep difficulties be screened for drug and alcohol use, abuse, or dependence. Patients with sleep difficulties demonstrate an increased use of drugs and alcohol when compared to the general public. It has also been reported that patients who have been abstinent from drug use may continue to have sleep problems long after the discontinuation of the drug.[1]

A detailed substance abuse history is often not obtained before initiating care, although it is essential for accurate diagnosis and safe treatment. There are many reasons, including the physician's attitudes toward patients who misuse substances, the physician's inability to treat the disorder, lack of time, or the physician's belief in the lack of efficacy of treatment.[2] Validated self-administered questionnaires (addressed later in this chapter) sent to the patients' homes before the first appointment provide clinicians with a time-saving, yet effective means of collecting a thorough drug and alcohol history. Regardless of the reasons why substance abuse disorders are not directly assessed, the necessity has been demonstrated in the connection between sleep difficulties and substance use. For this reason, if substance abuse is suspected, a referral and collaboration with an addiction specialist is essential and can lead to a more successful outcome or, in some circumstances, can be lifesaving.

Physician education in basic addiction treatment is necessary so that the physician can then assuage his or her own concerns about treatment efficacy and can then instill hope in patients about recovery. For many drugs of abuse (e.g., alcohol, opiates, tobacco) there are Food and Drug Administration (FDA)–approved medications to help patients achieve remission. For other drugs (e.g., cocaine) some non-FDA-approved medications may help the patient attain remission. For all substance-abusing patients, counseling, family therapy and 12-step programs are also helpful in achieving and maintaining remission.

This chapter will discuss (1) factors that place someone at an increased risk for addiction; (2) how to obtain a drug and alcohol history; (3) sleep issues related to commonly abused substances; (4) addiction issues related to commonly prescribed medications for sleep disorders; and (5) possible alternative medication options. It is hoped that this chapter will help the sleep specialist achieve more successful outcomes with this patient population.

DEFINITIONS

There are multiple ways to define *substance misuse*. This chapter will use the criteria as defined in the *Diagnostic and Statistical Manual of Mental Disorders,* Fourth Edition, text

revised (DSM-IV-TR),[3] for substance abuse and substance dependence, which are summarized in Table 60-1.

Tolerance and withdrawal are often confused with *substance dependence* (as defined by the DSM-IV-TR) when they are in fact not synonymous. First, a person's body being physiologically dependent on a substance (i.e., tolerance and withdrawal) is not required for someone to meet DSM-IV-TR criteria for substance dependence. It is common for a patient to be physiologically dependent on a given medication without feeling out of control, distressed, or motivated to use despite negative consequences (e.g., treatment with antidepressants and beta blockers).[4] *Substance dependence,* known more commonly outside the field as "addiction," is in contrast a psychological phenomenon involving a sense of distress in response to substance use, as well as a loss of control over use or continued use despite negative consequences.

Pseudoaddiction

The concept of pseudoaddiction was introduced in 1989. It was a term developed to describe behaviors seen in patients with inadequately treated pain. In their attempt to receive appropriate pain management, these patients may act in ways which are perceived by their treatment team as drug seeking behavior. For example, they act in ways to show the doctor how much pain they are in, or they request medication before it is due. When the patient's pain is adequately treated these behaviors resolve, in contrast to the patient with a substance abuse disorder who may continue to seek additional opiates.[5]

It is extremely important to differentiate pseudoaddiction from substance dependence or abuse, and may require a consult from an addiction specialist in some cases. All patients must be reminded routinely that they are expected to take medication as prescribed as part of a mutually agreed upon contract and should not increase the dose without consulting with the prescriber and receiving approval first.

NEUROBIOLOGY OF ADDICTION

Genetic Predisposition

It has been demonstrated in numerous studies over many decades that there is a genetic predisposition toward different addictions and that as much as 40% to 60% of this predisposition may be ascribed to genetics.[6-8] Adoption and twin studies have been an important part of determining the genetic predisposition for drug addiction. In one study it was shown that sons who had alcoholic fathers, but who were raised from

TABLE 60-1

DSM-IV-TR Definitions of Substance Abuse and Substance Dependence

Substance Abuse	Substance Dependence
A. Within a 12-month period, the person's use of substances indicates a maladaptive pattern that is causing clinically significant levels of impairment or distress. At least one of the following criteria must be met:	Within a 12-month period, the person's use of substances indicates a maladaptive pattern that is causing clinically significant levels of impairment or distress. At least three of the following criteria must be met:

(1) The patterned use leads to inability to carry out primary employment, educational, or home responsibilities.	(1) Physiologic tolerance, involving either:
	  (a) needing increasing quantities of a substance in order to feel intoxicated or before achieving desired effect OR
	  (b) after continued use of the substance, becoming increasingly less intoxicated by the same quantity

(2) The patterned use leads to situations in which the safety or well-being of the patient or another person is affected (e.g., driving under the influence).	(2) Physiologic withdrawal, as indicated by either:
	  (a) meeting criteria for withdrawal syndrome consistent with the substance of use OR
	  (b) replacement of the substance with a similar substance in an effort to avoid or mitigate withdrawal symptoms

(3) Legal problems occur in relation to substance use.	(3) The person is using increasingly larger quantities over longer periods of time than intended.
(4) The substance use persists despite interpersonal difficulties caused or worsened by the substance use.	(4) The person reports repeated desire to control or decrease substance use, or has failed at attempts to do so.
B. The person does not meet criteria for dependence on this substance.	(5) The person has spent a significant amount of time using, pursuing, or recuperating from the effects of the substance.
	(6) As a result of substance use the person has reduced or discontinued involvement in important activities related to work, education, recreation, or interpersonal life.
	(7) The substance use persists despite known negative physical or psychological symptoms caused or worsened by the substance use.
	Specify if with physiologic dependence (meeting criteria for tolerance or withdrawal) or without physiologic dependence (not meeting criteria for tolerance or withdrawal)

DSM-IV-TR, Diagnostic and Statistical Manual of Mental Disorders, Fourth Edition.

birth by nonalcoholic parents, were at higher risk of becoming alcoholics.[7] In other studies, which looked at monozygotic twins, dizygotic twins, and nontwin siblings, increased rates of substance dependence was demonstrated in twins, more so in the monozygotic twins, as compared to the nontwins.[8] This does not mean that those with a genetic predisposition toward addiction are the only people who are at risk for becoming addicted to a substance. Genetic predisposition is related to the initiation and continuation of substance use; this means that a predisposed person is more likely to have a highly positive physiologic response upon exposure to the substance, thus increasing likelihood of addiction and continued use.[8,9]

Initiation of Substance Use

Substance dependence is one of few chronic illnesses in which there is a behavioral choice involved in the initiation of the disorder; in other words, a person must first choose to expose himself or herself to a substance before becoming addicted to it. This can often lead to a series of moral and character judgments about substance users from society, from their families, and most importantly, from their health care providers. For this reason it is important for professionals to consider the vulnerabilities that are often associated with substance use and the development of an addiction.

During adolescence the prefrontal cortex, a region which is central in executive decision making as well as behavioral inhibition, is still in the process of developing. This leads to adolescents being a particularly at-risk subgroup of the population. Adolescents are more susceptible to peer pressure and

more likely to engage in risk-taking behaviors and experimentation with substance use.[10] Unfortunately, the age of first use can be extremely important, as there is evidence that those who start using a given substance in their early teens can be at increased risk of later developing substance dependence. For example, those who initiate drinking at the age of 14 have four times the risk of becoming dependent on alcohol when compared to those who initiated drinking at age 20 or older.[11]

In addition to underdeveloped prefrontal cortices, there are additional potential problems facing the already at-risk adolescent population. Teens are at an increased risk for depression compared to other age groups, which is concerning, as depression is also a risk factor involved in the initiation of drug use.[10] Additionally, studies indicate that those who have used nicotine in their adolescence may be at higher risk for addiction than those who initiate use as an adult.[12,13]

Finally, there are the issues surrounding sleep disturbances in teens. Research has found that approximately 10% of adolescents within the general population report experiencing insomnia,[14,15] which does not take into account the other sleep disturbances that may also impact adolescents. Multiple studies support the conclusion that sleep problems, substance use, and psychiatric problems are frequently experienced simultaneously by adolescents.[16,17] This is most significant to sleep experts (as well as substance abuse specialists) because researchers have determined that sleep problems among adolescents can serve as an early indicator of an increased risk of substance use or abuse.[15] It also appears that the high correlation between sleep disturbance and adolescent substance use may be bidirectional, meaning that sleep problems could lead to self-medicating with abusable substances, which often leads to further sleep disturbance (due to the effects of the substance), which can then trigger even further substance use.[18,19]

Sleep specialists, and other physicians who encounter adolescents with sleep disturbances, may have the opportunity to intervene at a key time in these patients' development. Potentially, in addressing the sleep disturbance they may circumvent adolescent patients experimenting with substances in an effort to self-medicate. If this is already an ongoing issue with a patient, it is advised that physicians work with the patients and their families to get specialized care in addressing the issue proactively, before it becomes a longer term, adult problem with substances.

Psychiatric Disorders

The co-morbidity found between severe mental illness (e.g., bipolar disorder and schizophrenia) and substance abuse disorders is very high, with a lifelong incidence of approximately 50%,[20] a rate that is well over twice that of the general public.[21] Additionally, patients with co-morbid substance abuse and psychiatric illness have a poor prognosis when untreated.[20]

Chronic Illness Model

As noted earlier, patients who suffer from substance dependence are commonly blamed for their illness,[9] with the reasoning that they chose to expose themselves to a substance to which they could become addicted. It is important to note, however, that there are other chronic illnesses besides addiction, such as diabetes mellitus and hypertension (see later discussion), for which this is true. In fact, when addiction is viewed through this lens, researchers have found many similarities between the course of substance dependence and that of other chronic illnesses, which have both genetic and environmental contributions.

In their 2005 paper, Dackis and O'Brien[9] note that "Addiction is best conceptualized as a disease of brain reward centers that ensure the survival of organisms and species. By activating and dysregulating endogenous reward centers, addictive drugs essentially hijack brain circuits that exert considerable dominance over rational thought, leading to progressive loss of control over drug intake in the face of medical, interpersonal, occupational and legal hazard." In other words, the poor judgment and "noncompliance" frequently observed in the addicted patient (e.g., risky behavior, missing appointments, medication noncompliance, continuing substance use despite physician warnings) can be a symptom of a chronic brain illness rather than intentionally disruptive or actively chosen self-harmful behavior.

Addictions research leaders McLellan and associates[8] advocate that health care experts approach substance abusing patients as they would patients with other chronic illnesses; they, too, as noted earlier, draw a parallel to other diseases, reminding us that poor treatment compliance rates exist for other chronic medical illnesses. They specifically refer to research that finds high noncompliance rates in the medication regimens and treatment of adult patients with type 1 diabetes,[22] hypertension,[23] and asthma.[24] When we compare the compliance rates for diabetes and hypertension to those of substance abuse disorders, we find that the psychosocial statistics and the compliance and relapse rates are strikingly similar.[8,25]

McLellan's group encourages health professionals to shift perspectives and recognize that low compliance and high relapse rates, as in these other illnesses, should not indicate hopelessness in treating the illness. Instead, these researchers support the use of the chronic disease model and serve as proof of the need for long-term care and disease management for addiction.[8]

Once seen from a medical rather than moral perspective, perhaps treating an addicted patient may seem less daunting. Practitioners can take into account the psychosocial issues that contribute to poor compliance with these illnesses (e.g., poor support from family members, low socioeconomic status, and co-morbid psychiatric illness[25]) and when possible can refer patients to resources and specialists that can help to address these issues. At the same time researchers would be encouraged to seek physiologic and neurologic explanations for some of the actions that characterize addictions and other chronic diseases.

Brain Circuitry: Pathways of Addiction and Relapse

The reward pathway in the brain, and its dysregulation to addiction, has been studied extensively. If looked at from the point of view of survival, it is adaptive that food, water, and sex activate the reward pathway[7] and thus drive humans and animals to repeat the behavior. Dopamine appears to be a key neurotransmitter with respect to addiction. Unlike natural adaptive rewards, substances with potential for abuse have the ability to increase the dopamine to considerably higher levels and thus provide a significantly greater reward value ("high"). Either directly or indirectly, most substances with potential for abuse affect dopamine levels. It is known that substances that result in increased levels of dopamine in the brain (most notably those that do so in the nucleus accumbens, a central component of the reward pathway) have the potential to result in abuse.[26] The mesolimbic dopamine pathway is central in the reward pathway.[27] This pathway begins in the ventral tegmental area and projects to multiple areas in the limbic system, including the nucleus accumbens, amygdala, hippocampus, and the prefrontal cortex. Gamma-aminobutyric acid (GABA) neurons in the mesolimbic and mesocortical dopaminergic pathways are able to work both in conjunction with and parallel to one another.[7]

These increased dopamine levels also strengthen conditioned learning such that cues associated with the drug then result in increased dopamine levels, which lead to an increased craving for the drug.[6] In substance abuse treatment a relevant adage is often used: "Avoid people, places, and things." This guidance of staying away from stimuli associated with old patterns of substance abuse is used to help those in recovery avoid the cravings elicited by the increased dopamine level that is triggered by the learned conditioned response.

OBTAINING A DRUG AND ALCOHOL HISTORY

The National Institute on Alcohol Abuse and Alcoholism notes that self-report measures are tools that are fairly accurate, inexpensive, and noninvasive. Teplin and associates[1] recommend that basic screening questionnaires become part of every patient's initial evaluation. Unfortunately, most doctors do not screen for drug and alcohol use, or they may merely limit screening to tobacco and alcohol use rather than elicit a full substance use history. There are many questionnaires from which to choose. Two questionnaires that these authors recommend include the Michigan Alcohol Screening Test (MAST) and the Drug Abuse Screening Test (DAST). These screening tools, as well as information pertaining to their validity and other screening tools may be accessed at the URLs listed at the end of this chapter under "Additional Resources."

If the screening tools suggest there is any evidence of substance abuse, additional information from Table 60-2 should be gathered.

A thorough history can be a significant aid to the sleep specialist and help prevent unknowingly prescribing the exact medication which a patient abuses.

SPECIFIC SLEEP ISSUES FOR PATIENTS ABUSING SUBSTANCES

For all patients with a substance abuse disorder, it is important to treat the disorder as well as any co-morbid medical or psychiatric issues, because almost all substances of abuse may be associated with a sleep disturbance that can be compounded by a sleep

disturbance to a psychiatric or medical illness.[1,28] One study found a much higher rate of sleep problems in patients with addiction problems compared to the general public.[29] As with all patients with sleep disturbances, it is important to evaluate their sleep habits as a possible cause or as a contributor to their sleep disturbance,[28] especially considering the physical impact of substance use and resulting potential for disrupting sleep schedules. Table 60-3 presents a brief summary of the more commonly abused substances and their subsequent effects on sleep.

Sleep Disorders as a Risk for Relapse

Sleep disruption, whether insomnia, hypersomnia, increased arousals from sleep, or vivid dreams, is often seen in either acute intoxication or withdrawal from most drugs of abuse. It has been hypothesized that sleep difficulties in patients with a substance abuse disorder are a risk factor for relapse. Although the acute withdrawal period tends to be short for most drugs of abuse, the term "protracted withdrawal" has been developed for the symptoms (e.g., a sleep disturbance) that may continue for a significant amount of time even after the substance has been discontinued. At this time it has not been scientifically demonstrated that improved sleep will prevent relapse,[30] but it is clear that disrupted sleep is a risk for relapse.

COMMON SUBSTANCES OF ABUSE

Alcohol

There are multiple studies that show that up to 20% of the general population has used alcohol to help them sleep.[30] Although alcohol *acutely* decreases sleep latency, it has been shown that tolerance to this effect develops quickly such that after three nights it is no longer effective.[31] This rapid tolerance can often result in confusion in the effects of alcohol on sleep, as the effects seen before the development of tolerance can be the opposite of those seen after. Unlike the decrease in sleep latency seen prior to the development of tolerance, there is an increase in sleep latency as well as increased rapid eye movement (REM) sleep in patients in early cessation of chronic use, and both are predictors of relapse in patients with substance abuse disorders.[30]

Unfortunately alcohol also results in an increase in the time spent awake during the second half of the night and, even in low doses, leads to increased sleep fragmentation and an increase in the number of awakenings.[32] Alcohol's disrupting effects on sleep during the second half of the night are thought to be secondary to a "rebound" effect that occurs once the

---

TABLE 60-2

Additional Information to Be Gathered in Cases with Evidence of Substance Abuse

Potential Substances of Abuse	Required Information*
Alcohol	Age at first use
Tobacco	Date of most recent use
Cocaine	Frequency and quantity of substance use (per day/week/month/year)
Stimulants	
Hallucinogens	Route of self-administration (IV, PO, smoked, snorted, inhaled)
Opiates	
Sedative-hypnotics	Effects of intoxication and of withdrawal of the substance on the patient
"Club drugs"	
	For a substance prescribed by a physician: history of perceived need for more than prescribed dose to produce desired effect; note additional amount required
	History of attempts, successful or not, to obtain a prescription drug from a nonphysician
	History of inpatient or outpatient treatment for substance abuse
	Family history of substance abuse

*All elements of assessment are to be determined for each suspected substance of abuse.
IV, intravenous; *PO*, per os (oral).

TABLE 60-3

Summary of Effects of Commonly Abused Substances on Sleep

Substance	Sleep Latency	NREM	REM	Unique Issue(s)
Alcohol	↓ (use < 3 days) ↑ (use > 3 days)		↓	↑ sleep disruption in 2nd half of night
Opiates		↓ N3 sleep ↑ N2 sleep		Chronic use associated with sleep-related periodic breathing and central sleep apnea
Stimulants	↑		Suppression	↓ total sleep time
Marijuana		↑	↓	

NREM, non–rapid eye movement; *REM*, rapid eye movement.

alcohol has been metabolized by the body.[31] One study noted that those who had persistent insomnia from baseline to 1 year had more than double the risk of developing alcohol abuse a year later when compared to those without insomnia.[19] Studies have shown that insomnia is seen almost twice as frequently in patients with alcoholism.[28,33] Disruptions in sleep may be seen even after the patient has been abstinent from alcohol for years. In patients who are currently drinking, as well as those up to 8 weeks after withdrawal, an increase in sleep latency is also seen (recall the rapid development of tolerance to the initial decrease in sleep latency), and there is a decrease in the time spent asleep. Additionally it has been found that there is an increase in slow wave sleep during periods of drinking but a decrease during withdrawal as well as a suppression of REM sleep when drinking and a REM rebound during withdrawal. Furthermore, alcohol can increase upper airway resistance as well as result in an increased risk for sleep apnea.[33]

Patients with insomnia may use alcohol as a "sleep aid," but in one study it was noted that patients with a history of alcoholism only felt their sleep was improved during the first week they returned to drinking. It was hypothesized that their subsequent increase in alcohol intake may have been a response to the resulting tolerance to the sedating effect, but the overall effect was a return to their uncontrolled use. It is also important to recall that although sedative-hypnotic agents are normally considered safe, they can be lethal when mixed with alcohol,[33] and this effect cautions their use in this population.

Interestingly, alcohol may mimic an augmentation of restless legs syndrome (RLS) in a patient with this diagnosis.[34] There are multiple studies with seemingly conflicting results, reporting either increasing or a masking of periodic limb movements (PLMs) with the use of alcohol.[32,35] Despite these conflicting results of the effects of alcohol on periodic limb movements, as with other substances of abuse, it is important that patients are not actively self-medicating with alcohol while in treatment for their sleep disorder, as this will make an accurate diagnosis and successful treatment extremely difficult.

Cocaine and Amphetamine

Cocaine and amphetamine use results chemically in increased levels of dopamine and physically in feelings of euphoria and alertness.[36] Although many studies have been done to evaluate the effects of cocaine withdrawal on sleep, the results are conflicting. One theory for this is that the conditioned cues, to which a patient is normally exposed, are not experienced in the controlled research setting. Another theory hypothesizes these differences may result from the different methods used in various studies, as some studies were retrospective while others prospective, and some were inpatient while others were outpatient.[37] Studies have reported subjective complaints of difficulty falling asleep, increased sleep latency, hypersomnolence, increased sleep/rebound hypersomnia, decrease in REM sleep, and decrease in total sleep time during subacute and acute withdrawal.[37-39] Interestingly enough, patients may not feel that their sleep is in fact worse during this time.[36]

Ecstasy

Ecstasy (3,4-methylenedioxymethamphetamine [MDMA]) has become an increasingly popular recreational drug. MDMA shares a chemical similarity to the stimulant amphetamine and the hallucinogen mescaline. It causes a large release of serotonin and dopamine, resulting in the user experiencing powerful feelings of empathy and closeness to others, combined with the sensation of both a stimulant and a psychedelic drug. MDMA also inhibits the reuptake of serotonin from the synaptic gap.[40]

The damage to brain serotonin neurons (5-HT neurotoxicity) may lead to chronic alterations in sleep and circadian rhythms.[41] There has been evidence for some time that chronic, heavy recreational use of MDMA is associated with sleep disorders as well as a range of other psychological problems.[42,43] Allen and associates (1993),[44] in an age- and gender-matched control group study found that heavy recreational users of MDMA had less total sleep and less non-REM (NREM) sleep than did their matched control subjects. Clearly, MDMA is a potent neurotoxin with both short- and long-term effects on sleep.

Marijuana: *Cannabis sativa* or Tetrahydrocannabinol

Like other substances of abuse, marijuana use affects sleep. There are multiple studies with mixed results on the effects of marijuana on sleep, but common findings include a subjective feeling of sedation, reports of decreased sleep quality, an increase in NREM sleep, and a decrease in REM sleep.[36,45] The opposite of these effects are seen during withdrawal.[35] Withdrawal from marijuana often results in complaints of sleep difficulty and "strange dreams," which may be the result of increased REM sleep; this may continue for close to 2 months after cessation and can interfere with attempts to abstain.[36,45]

ABUSE PROBLEMS IN PRESCRIPTION MEDICATIONS

Sedative-Hypnotic Agents

Barbiturates, benzodiazepines, and nonbenzodiazepine hypnotic agents all share the common feature of acting at the $GABA_A$ receptor sites. It appears that the α_1 subunit of this receptor, which is thought to be involved in the sedative effects of benzodiazepines, may also be involved in its ability to result in physical dependence. Unfortunately, this class of medication is also known for its potential for abuse.[46]

Studies have looked at patients in the general population who were chronically using this class of drugs. These individuals were found to get less sleep as compared to patients with insomnia who were not receiving hypnotics. On the other hand, other studies demonstrated an increase of at most 45 minutes total sleep time with the use of these medications.[47] These conflicting results combined with the increased risk of using sedative-hypnotics in patients with a history of drug or alcohol misuse makes use of this class of medications in this population very concerning. In one review article the authors stated "…all benzodiazepine receptor agonists…should be used with caution, if at all, in substance-abusing or substance-dependent patients."[28] The authors of this chapter are in strong agreement with this statement.

Barbiturates

Barbiturates (phenobarbital, secobarbital, pentobarbital, etc.) deserve at least a mention among the sedative-hypnotics that were used to treat sleep disorders but were found to have a very high abuse potential. Because long-term barbiturate use led to dependence and a severe, potentially life-threatening withdrawal syndrome when abruptly stopped (including delirium and grand mal seizures),[48] alternative medications were sought by the medical world. In the 1960s barbiturates were, for the most part, replaced by benzodiazepines, which at that time were seen as a safer, less abusable alternative.[49] Although perhaps safer, the abuse potential of benzodiazepines has since become an issue as well (see following discussion).

Anxiolytics: Benzodiazepines

Although clinically effective in helping to address anxiety and sleep difficulties, abuse of benzodiazepines is on the rise,[46] thus presenting a challenge for the sleep specialist. Studies have generally shown that benzodiazepine use is more reinforcing for patients who have a history of moderate alcohol intake (12 or more drinks per week), substance abuse, anxiety, or insomnia. Patients who are currently misusing substances, those with a current or past history of alcoholism[50,51] and the elderly are all at an increased risk for using benzodiazepines inappropriately,[46] reinforcing the importance of obtaining a thorough history of current and past substance use in all patients. The past is often the best predictor of the future, and studies have demonstrated that individuals with a history of misuse of sedatives are at increased risk of misusing them again.[50] Therefore, the sleep specialist must carefully evaluate if the benefit of prescribing them to address a sleep problem outweighs the risk of the patient worsening any current substance abuse or restarting a pattern of misuse (cost-benefit ratio).

Yet another challenge with using benzodiazepines as a sleep agent, in patients with or without a history of addiction, is the rapid adaptation to their sedative effect. Increasing doses may be required to gain the same effect,[46] which limits their long-term use as a sleeping aid. There is a significant subset of patients who are in opiate replacement treatments (methadone, buprenorphine) or who are prescribed opiates for a legitimate purpose (e.g., severe chronic pain) who combine benzodiazepines with their prescribed opiates in order to experience a "high."[46] This effect does not occur with opiate replacement therapy (methadone, buprenorphine) when prescribed alone, at an appropriate dose.[52]

In some circumstances, after the physician has taken into account the patient's likelihood of abuse and failure to respond to other medication options, the physician may determine that there is a true need to treat with a benzodiazepine. As the benzodiazepine chosen for abuse is not random, but based on multiple characteristics of a given drug, specifically its rate of onset and half-life (prolonged in the older patient), the clinician must take these characteristics into consideration when choosing a medication. Those which have a fast rate of onset create more of a high, and those with a fast offset (i.e., end of perceived high) require repeated use to maintain the high. Each of these factors must be taken into account as a medication like diazepam has a long half-life, generally associated with being less rewarding, but its rapid onset actually results in its increased abuse potential.[50,53]

An additional challenge is rebound insomnia that may occur upon discontinuation of the hypnotic agent. The patient may fear this result[54] and may attempt to obtain the medication from other sources, legal or illegal. For patients with a substance abuse disorder, a discontinuation syndrome may result in patient distress, which in turn can lead to resuming use of the hypnotic agent, with or without a prescription. Additionally, there is a subset of patients who may seek sedative-hypnotic agents to help treat symptoms of withdrawal from other substances (e.g., stimulant abuse).[55]

Nonbenzodiazepine Hypnotics

The nonbenzodiazepine hypnotics ("Z-drug" hypnotics) are known to be extremely useful in the treatment of insomnia, owing to their quick onset and short duration of action.[46] Like their benzodiazepine counterparts, they too act at the $GABA_A$ receptor.[56] In studies that looked at zolpidem use in both human and animal models, there was less risk of physical dependence than seen with benzodiazepines. However, other animal studies demonstrated withdrawal symptoms which are comparable to those seen with chronic benzodiazepine treatment.[46] Further case series have presented examples of patients who demonstrated zolpidem abuse and dependence.[57,58] Many of these patients escalated the dose of the medication and reported reinforcing and paradoxical effects from the medication. Frequently these patients had current or past psychiatric or addiction histories. One small study of the abuse potential of zaleplon versus triazolam found that patients ranked them similarly in terms of liking the drug and its possible street value.[59] Interestingly one animal study demonstrated that zolpidem appeared to be more reinforcing than midazolam.[46] In each of the manufacturer's drug information guides, there are warnings to use caution when prescribing these medications to patients with a history of drug or alcohol abuse. Although this class of drug may have a lower liability for abuse,[28] it is still extremely important to be careful prescribing them to patients with a history of drug or alcohol problems.

Sodium Oxybate

Gamma-hydroxybutyrate (GHB) was initially a dietary supplement that was considered to be useful for sleep and weight loss, and was used by bodybuilders who thought its use led to an increased release of growth hormone. GHB is also a popular "club drug," which is used at "raves" (dance parties that last all night and promote use of mind-altering substances) as it increased sexual arousal and provided an alcohol-like euphoria without the subsequent hangover. It was later dubbed the "date-rape" drug owing to the anterograde amnesia it produced in the victim, especially when mixed with alcohol.[60]

Its use for the treatment of cataplexy in patients with narcolepsy is strongly regulated to prevent diversion and misuse. There have been few studies on its abuse potential, although there has been an increase in emergency room visits of patients presenting after having overdosed on GHB. One study looked at its abuse potential and found that it was comparable to that of triazolam and pentobarbital, but noted that there may be an increased risk of accidental overdose.[61] As with any medication with the potential for abuse, it is recommended that the sleep specialist discuss the risks and benefits of the medication with the patient, using strong caution in patients with a history of substance abuse.

Opiates

With a sharp increase in prescription methadone (824%) and oxycodone (660%) seen from 1997 to 2003, it is extremely important that sleep specialists are aware of the sleep ramifications of this class of medication. In a study of people without a history of drug abuse, researchers found that even low-dose opioids decreased stage N3 sleep, by 30% to 50%, and also increased stage N2 sleep.[62] Another small study looked at healthy patients' sleep architecture after intravenous morphine and found they had a decrease in slow wave sleep without an increase in arousals or awakenings.[62]

Multiple studies have examined the effects of more chronic opiate use patterns on sleep. Several studies have concluded that central sleep apneas and ataxic breathing may result from chronic use of opiates.[62-64] It was determined that the impact of chronic opioid use is dose-related, with higher doses having more of an impact on irregular breathing with central apneas and hypopneas.[63] Other studies of patients on methadone found that these patients actually have increased arousals from sleep.[65]

Additionally, patients in methadone treatment often have co-morbid disorders such as psychiatric or alcohol use disorders, which are independently known to be associated with sleep disorders. One study, based on self-report, looked at 225 patients on methadone maintenance and found that 84% met criteria for clinically significant sleep disturbances. Unfortunately, patients in methadone treatment sometimes abuse sedative-hypnotics in an effort to achieve intoxication when combined with methadone. Under these circumstances prescribing this medication for insomnia creates a risk for abuse. Hence, it is important to use nonaddictive sleep medications in this population when possible and evaluate and treat any co-morbid disorders that may affect sleep.[65]

Stimulants

As with opiates, prescriptions for stimulants have been increasing since 1990 with the production quota for methylphenidate increasing from 1768 kg to 14,957 kg between 1990 and 2000.[66]

Dextroamphetamine and Methylphenidate

Methamphetamine, D-amphetamine sulfate, and methylphenidate hydrochloride have been used in the past in the treatment of excessive daytime sleepiness, as seen in the case of narcolepsy, but each has potential for abuse. Secondary to their high water solubility they can all be misused by intravenous (IV) injection.[67] Methylphenidate can also be misused by smoking. One study, which looked at data from 2002, suggested that diversion is indicated in more recent stimulant abuse and that "an estimated 21 million persons aged 12 years or older were found to have misused at least one prescription stimulant at least once in their lifetimes."[66] Additional risk factors for misuse of stimulants include being in treatment for a psychiatric disorder and use of illegal drugs.[68] Another study looked at patients on 120% or more of the maximum stimulant dose, as recommended by the American Academy of Sleep Medicine Standards of Practice Committee, and found that

this group of patients "...demonstrated a significantly higher prevalence of psychosis, substance abuse, and psychiatric hospitalizations compared to the standard-dose group."[69] They additionally noted that patients who are at risk of developing a given psychiatric disorder may "request or require higher doses of stimulants."

Available research indicates a low risk of addiction to stimulants for patients with narcolepsy,[67,70] but this conclusion is based either on anecdotal evidence[71] or, in other instances, specifically excluded patients with psychiatric disorders, including alcoholism.[72] Unfortunately there do not appear to be studies to support or refute the addiction potential of stimulants for patients with narcolepsy who also have a personal or a family history of addiction. Thus, at this time we strongly urge extreme caution with the use of this class of medication in patients with any history of drug or alcohol abuse or dependence, seeing that their relative safety in this population is unclear.

Modafinil

There is significantly less information available on the abuse potential of modafinil as compared to the stimulants discussed previously.[73] Unlike stimulants, which cause an increase in dopamine, modafinil does not seem to have a similar mechanism of action and thus is thought to have a lower risk of potential for abuse.[67] Chemically it is not likely to be abused in IV form or by smoking.[67] Postmarketing surveillance indicated that the abuse/misuse of modafinil is low; however, animal studies have demonstrated both positive and negative results[73] with respect to its addiction potential. New research demonstrates that dopamine may be involved in modafinil's mechanism of action, with one study noting that mice that lack dopamine transporters or that lack D_1 or D_2 receptors do not get the wake-promoting effect from modafinil.[26] One study in humans showed some results that might indicate abuse potential in subjects who had a history of stimulant abuse,[73,74] but another group of researchers did not generate the same findings.[75,76] One small study demonstrated its reinforcing effects were influenced by the task at hand and concluded that modafinil has "some, albeit limited, abuse potential."[73] An additional factor, which may be in part why modafinil is of lower risk than amphetamines, is the fact that amphetamines has a defined, unpleasant, withdrawal,[67] which might lead to further use in an attempt to ameliorate the withdrawal process.

Animal studies indicate that modafinil may be useful in the treatment of stimulant abuse.[77] Most recent clinical studies focus on modafinil's usefulness in the treatment of cocaine dependence. It is thought that modafinil's glutamate-enhancing properties might be helpful in the cocaine-dependent patient, as continued use of cocaine results in depleted extracellular glutamate levels. Another study demonstrated that modafinil was safe when used with IV cocaine and significantly decreased the cocaine-induced euphoria. In a double-blind, placebo-controlled study it was found that patients in the treatment group (400 mg modafinil total in a single daily dose) had a significantly greater proportion of negative urine drug screens as compared to the placebo group during the 8-week study.[78] Given the known abuse potential of stimulants and the potential for modafinil to be a treatment for cocaine abuse, these authors feel that modafinil appears to be a safer choice for the treatment of excessive daytime sedation and narcolepsy in the patient with a history of substance abuse. However, it is important to discuss the risk, no matter how small, with your patients and have them inform you if they feel the medication has any reinforcing effects.

APPROACHING THE SUBSTANCE ABUSING PATIENT

Substance-abusing patients have long been a challenging population for health care professionals to treat, as discussed earlier, owing to treatment noncompliance issues and complications accompanying excessive substance use. In response to the need for skills to help manage resistant and difficult patients, research clinicians Miller and Rollnick[79] developed motivational interviewing (MI). MI is a patient-centered, evidence-based practice designed to reduce patients' resistance, help them recognize discrepancies between their current circumstances and where they would like to be, increase self-efficacy and confidence in their ability to change, and increase intrinsic motivation. Research has begun to focus on incorporating MI skills into medical college curricula in an effort to teach medical students basic motivational interviewing skills; results indicate that MI skills assist medical students in achieving behavioral change and managing resistant behaviors with patients.[80-82] It offers an effective means of initiating treatment and it is highly recommended that physicians familiarize themselves with at least basic MI skills to better equip them in approaching substance-abusing patients.

SUBSTANCE ABUSE TREATMENT

If history, physical examination, laboratory studies, or standardized questionnaires indicate the possibility of adverse consequences of drug or alcohol involvement, it is helpful for the nonaddiction specialist to have some familiarity with evidence-based practices/treatment. This section will briefly summarize some of the evidence-based practices (EBPs), both nonpharmacologic and pharmacologic, that are utilized in drug and alcohol treatment settings. The sleep specialist should be aware of these EBPs but is not necessarily expected to provide care under these models. The following discussion will present a concise description of each approach and offer some suggested articles should the reader be interested in further exploration.

Cognitive Behavioral Therapy

Cognitive behavioral strategies are based on models that focus on learning processes that play a major role in the development of maladaptive behaviors. Initially cognitive behavior therapy (CBT) was brought into substance abuse treatment as a method to prevent relapse in alcohol treatment and was subsequently applied to cocaine treatment. CBT focuses on teaching people to recognize dysfunctional thought processes and cope with or stop distressing thoughts that frequently lead to destructive behaviors (i.e., substance abuse). Specific techniques involve self-monitoring, cognitive restructuring, recognizing behavioral cues, identifying and developing strategies to avoid and cope with high-risk situations, and building problem-solving skills.[83-85] CBT can

be utilized in outpatient or inpatient care and in individual or group therapy formats.

Matrix Model

In an intensive outpatient treatment setting, the matrix model is an evidence-based approach for stimulant abuse and dependence. The 16-week intervention consists of therapy group work focusing on relapse prevention, education (e.g., addiction, relapse, coping), and support from peers, while individual therapy simultaneously addresses personal issues that arise during group therapy.[86-89] Additional aspects include family member education, reinforcing positive behavior change, and promotion of the patient's self-esteem and self-worth.

Supportive-Expressive Psychotherapy

There is also research to support the more analytically oriented supportive-expressive psychotherapy (SEP). SEP is time-limited and adapted for use with primarily heroin- and cocaine-dependent individuals. The supportive techniques are designed to create comfort and rapport while the patient shares feelings and thoughts about personal experiences; the primary goal is to bolster self-esteem and self-efficacy.[90-94] Expressive techniques focus on the patient learning to verbally explore and process his or her substance use patterns and problematic relationship patterns, so that he or she may understand the meanings attached to the substance use and instead learn to cope with relationship problems more directly. This therapy is conducted in individual therapy settings, both inpatient and outpatient.

Other Strategies

Other evidence-based strategies include the following:
  Relapse prevention: intended to enhance self-control, learning to anticipate problems, and developing effective coping strategies[95]
  Community reinforcement approach plus vouchers: an intensive outpatient approach (24 weeks, twice a week) designed to engage and retain patients in treatment by utilizing vouchers scaled to reflect increased treatment involvement and drug abstinence[96]
  Contingency management interventions: an effective prize-based model allowing patients in outpatient care to earn a chance to "win" low cost incentives for providing drug-free urine test results[97]
  12-Step facilitation: designed to promote abstinence by actively engaging patients toward becoming affiliated with 12-step groups in their community[98]

Treating Substance Abusers with Insomnia

With all of the literature on the abuse or addiction potential of many frequently used medications, there is often hesitation and the need for guidance in how physicians *should* proceed in treating sleeping difficulties. Next are some alternative means of treating the addicted patient with insomnia.

Alternative Medications

For the patient with current alcohol dependence there are multiple medications, without FDA approval, which have been suggested for the treatment of insomnia. Trazodone is one option, but like the sedative-hypnotics, it can be lethal if mixed with alcohol and the risk for priapism limits its use in men.[18] One author noted that he had found mirtazapine useful for his patients with alcoholism and insomnia; however, this was not based on a control group design[18] and studies have not been done in patients with substance abuse disorders.[28]

There are some studies that show gabapentin is useful in treating insomnia in the patient with alcoholism.[18] Gabapentin has the advantage that it is not metabolized through the liver and is overall a safe medication to use in a patient who is drinking alchohol.[18,28] It is important to note that in one controlled study gabapentin was not found to differ, as a sleep aid, from placebo in the recovering alcohol-dependent patient.[28]

In one study quetiapine, a sedating second-generation antipsychotic, was shown to be beneficial for reduction of alcohol use in patients with alcohol dependence and sleep disturbances. The authors of this small study ($n = 30$) noted that, although there is evidence for this class of drugs reducing the craving for alcohol, it is also important to consider that it may have been the improved sleep, rather than the drug, which accounted for the decrease in drinking.[99] Another quetiapine study looked specifically at the treatment of alcoholism in type B alcoholics: those with an earlier age of onset, worse level of dependence and use of other drugs, increased psychopathology, and poor prognosis after treatment for alcohol dependence. This study concluded that quetiapine helped increase the number of days of abstinence and decrease the number of days of heavy drinking in patients who also received weekly medical management-based counseling.[100] When prescribing any sedating atypical antipsychotic for the use of sleep it is extremely important that the physician weigh the extreme risks of this class of medications with any potential benefit on sleep. This medication puts the patient at risk for tardive dyskinesia (a potentially permanent movement disorder), neuroleptic malignant syndrome (which has a potential to result in death), diabetes mellitus, metabolic syndrome, and other complications.[56]

Ramelteon may be a good option for patients with a history of substance abuse as it does not have potential for abuse; however, studies looking at its use in the substance-abusing patient are lacking.[28] Additionally there is some evidence that melatonin levels are lowered in patients with alcohol dependence,[101] which would make ramelteon a good option for these patients; again, however, studies are needed to properly demonstrate this effect.

Hydroxyzine, an antihistamine with mild anxiolytic properties, does not appear to have potential for dependence[56] and thus may be a useful sleep agent in patients with a current or past history of substance abuse.

Nonpharmacologic Treatments

As with non-substance-abusing patients, nonpharmacologic treatments of insomnia have also been shown to be beneficial with substance-abusing patients. In patients with a substance abuse disorder these authors feel nonpharmacologic approaches should be the first-line treatment or, at the least, should be included with any pharmacologic approach in an effort to empower patients and help them to rely less on medication in order to affect change in their lives.

Progressive muscle relaxation is a technique for relaxation involving alternately tensing and relaxing muscles in the body. In one study, behavioral therapy involving progressive muscle relaxation was used with patients receiving 1 month of inpatient treatment for their alcoholism; patients reported improvement in their sleep as compared to the group who did not receive this intervention.[18]

Cognitive behavioral techniques have been found to be extremely helpful for patients without medical or psychiatric causes for their insomnia.[59] One study's results indicated that CBT techniques were superior to pharmacotherapy alone.[102] Another study, which examined the usefulness of CBT for recovering alcoholics with at least 1 month of sobriety, found that the participants had better sleep outcomes with cognitive behavioral interventions, which included sleep hygiene education.[103]

In light of the high level of psychological dependence on substances to alter physical and mental states, the authors of this chapter strongly suggest that all patients with substance abuse problems should be educated about proper sleeping habits (e.g., maintaining consistent sleep schedules, timing of caffeine and nicotine use, healthy sleeping environments), offered cognitive behavioral therapy (e.g., to teach thought-stopping techniques and other cognitive skills that promote sleep), and trained in progressive muscle relaxation.

CONCLUSION

Although the sleep specialist is presented with many challenges when treating the patient with a sleep problem as well as a current or past history of substance abuse, their knowledge of this area will help them work more effectively with this population. Obtaining a thorough substance abuse history on each patient will allow the sleep specialist to quickly determine if the past or present use or misuse of a substance is contributing to the patient's sleep complaint. Additionally, it will help them to avoid prescribing the very drug to which a patient is or has been addicted or a drug that may interact with whatever the patient already has on board. In addition, basic training in motivational interviewing for the sleep specialist will provide physicians with the skills needed to approach even the most challenging addicted patients in a way that can facilitate their working relationship and help to promote behavior change and reduce resistance.

As can be seen from the material presented here, there are many different pharmacologic and nonpharmacologic approaches in the treatment of sleep disorders in patients with a substance abuse disorder. When treating sleep difficulties, it is suggested that treatment initiation should start with a strategy that involves utilizing the least addictive approach first. For example, with little risk, nonpharmacologic approaches can be initiated, with cognitive behavioral therapy delivered by a trained professional in conjunction with basic proper sleeping habits and monitoring by the sleep specialist. Should that effort fail, medication with the least abuse potential can be initiated (e.g., ramelteon or hydroxyzine). The patient's provider needs to monitor self-reports of sleep improvement, as well as side effects, blood drug levels, and behavioral changes until the patient reports sleep improvement, all the while being mindful of the possibility and risk of misuse.

Although sleep specialists are presented with many challenges when treating patients with a current or past history of substance abuse, their knowledge of this area will allow them to treat these patients' sleep problems in a safer way, and thus allow them to play a key role in each patient's path toward recovery.

ADDITIONAL RESOURCES

These authors recommend further resources for the reader interested in more information on drug abuse, dependency, and withdrawal:

Ries RK, Fiellin DA, Miller SC, Saitz R. *Principles of Addiction Medicine.* 4th ed. Philadelphia: Lippincott Williams & Wilkins; 2009.

Galanter M, Kleber HD, eds. *The American Psychiatric Publishing Textbook of Substance Abuse Treatment.* 4th ed. Washington, DC: American Psychiatric Pub; 2008.

The Substance Abuse and Mental Health Services Administration (SAMHSA) provides free online book downloads of their Treatment Improvement Protocols (TIPs). You can obtain more information at their website: http://www.samhsa.gov/

The National Institute on Drug Abuse has excellent online screening tools and advice on how to evaluate a patient for addiction, including CPT billing code information at their website:

http://www.drugabuse.gov/NIDAMED/screening/

MAST information can be accessed online:

http://pathwayscourses.samhsa.gov/aaap/aaap_4_pg15_pop2.htm

http://pubs.niaaa.nih.gov/publications/Assesing%20Alcohol/Instrument PDFs/42_MAST.pdf

DAST information can be accessed online:

http://www.emcdda.europa.eu/html.cfm/index3618EN.html

http://www.emcdda.europa.eu/attachements.cfm/att_4092_EN_DA ST%202008.pdf

REFERENCES

1. Teplin D, Raz B, Daiter J, et al. Screening for substance use patterns among patients referred for a variety of sleep complaints. *Am J Drug Alcohol Abuse.* 2006;32:111-120.
2. Friedmann PD, McCullough D, Chin MH, et al. Screening and intervention for alcohol problems: A national survey of primary care physicians and psychiatrists. *J Gen Intern Med.* 2000;15:84-91.
3. American Psychiatric Association. *Substance Use Disorders — Quick Reference to the Diagnostic and Statistical Manual of Mental Disorders.* 4th ed. (DSM-IV-TR) Washington, DC: American Psychiatric Association Publication; 2000:110-115.
4. Koob GF, Kandel D, Volkow ND. Pathophysiology of addiction. In: Tasman A, Kay J, Lieberman JA, eds. *Psychiatry.* 3rd ed. Vol 1. London: John Wiley & Sons; 2008:354-378.
5. Weissman DE. Pseudoaddiction #69. *J Pal Med.* 2005;8(6):1283-1284.
6. Volkow ND, Li T. Drug addiction: The neurobiology of behavior gone awry. *Nat Rev Neurosci.* 2004;5:963-970.
7. Cami J, Farre M. Mechanisms of disease drug addiction. *N Engl J Med.* 2003;349(10):975-986.
8. McLellan AT, Lewis D, O'Brien CP, Kleber HD. Drug dependence, a chronic medical illness implications for treatment, insurance, and outcomes evaluation. *JAMA.* 2000;284(13):1689-1695.
9. Dackis C, O'Brien CP. Neurobiology of addiction: Treatment and public policy ramifications. *Nat Neurosci.* 2005;8(11):1431-1436.
10. Kelley AE, Schochet T, Landry CF, et al. Risk taking and novelty seeking in adolescence: Introduction to part I. *Acad Sci.* 2004;1021:27-32.
11. Grant BF. The impact of a family history of alcoholism on the relationship between age at the onset of alcohol use and DSM-IV alcohol dependence: Results from the National Longitudinal Alcohol Epidemiologic Survey. Alcohol Health & Research World NIAAA's Epidemiologic Bulletin No. 39, 1998.
12. Pahl K, Brook DW, Morojele NJ, et al. Nicotine dependence and problem behaviors among urban South African adolescents. *J Behav Med.* 2010;33(2):101-109.
13. Adriani W, Spijker S, Deroche-Gamonet V, et al. Evidence for enhanced neurobehavioral vulnerability to nicotine during preadolescence in rats. *J Neurosci.* 2003;23(11):4712-4716.
14. Johnson EO, Roth T, Schultz L, Breslau N. Epidemiology of DSM-IV insomnia in adolescence: Lifetime prevalence, chronicity, and an emergent gender difference. *Pediatrics.* 2006;117:247-256.
15. Roane BM, Taylor DJ. Adolescent insomnia as a risk factor for early adult depression and substance abuse. *Sleep.* 2008;31(10):1351-1356.
16. Johnson EO, Breslau N. Sleep problems and substance use in adolescence. *Drug Alcohol Dependence.* 2001;64:1-7.
17. Breslau N, Roth T, Rosenthal L, et al. Sleep disturbance and psychiatric disorders: A longitudinal epidemiological study of young adults. *Biol Psychiatry.* 1996;39(6):411-418.
18. Brower KJ. Alcohol's effects on sleep in alcoholics. *Alcohol Res Health.* 2001;25:110-125.
19. Wong MW, Brower KJ, Fitzgerald HE, et al. Sleep problems in early childhood and early onset of alcohol and other drug use in adolescence. *Alcohol Clin Exp Res..* 2004;28(4):578-587.
20. Rach Beisel J, Scott J, Dixon L. Co-occurring severe mental illness and substance use disorders: A review of recent research. *Psychiatr Serv.* 1999;50:11.
21. Brook JS, Pahl K, Rubenstone E. Epidemiology of addiction. In: Galanter M, Kleber HD, eds. *Textbook of Substance Abuse Treatment.* 4th ed. Washington, DC: American Psychiatric Pub; 2008.
22. Graber AL, Davidson P, Brown A, et al. Dropout and relapse during diabetes care. *Diabetes Care.* 1992;15:1477-1483.
23. Clark LT. Improving compliance and increasing control of hypertension: Needs of special hypertensive populations. *Am Heart J.* 1991;121:664-669.
24. Dekker FW, Dieleman FE, Kaptein AA, Mulder JD. Compliance with pulmonary medication in general practice. *Eur Respir J.* 1993;6:886-890.
25. O'Brien CP, McLellan AT. Myths about the treatment of addiction. *Lancet.* 1996;347:237-240.
26. Volkow ND, Fowler JS, Logan J, et al. Effects of modafinil on dopamine and dopamine transporters in the male human brain. *JAMA.* 2009;30(11):1148-1154.
27. Koob GF. The neurobiology of addiction: A neuroadaptational view relevant for diagnosis. *Addiction.* 2006;101(suppl 1):23-30.
28. Conroy D, Arndt JT, Brower KJ. Insomnia in patients with addictions: A safer way to break the cycle. *Curr Psychiatry.* 2008;7(5):97-109.
29. Teplin D, Raz B, Daiter J, et al. Screening for substance use patterns among patients referred for a variety of sleep complaints. *The American Journal of Drug and Alcohol Abuse.* 2006;32:111-120
30. Brower KJ, Perron BE. Sleep disturbance as a universal risk factor for relapse in addiction to psychoactive substances. *Med Hypotheses.* 2010;74:928-933.
31. Roehrs T, Roth T. Sleep, sleepiness, and alcohol use. *Alcohol Res Health.* 2001;25(2):101-109.
32. Aldrich MS, Shipley JE. Alcohol use and periodic limb movements of sleep. *Alcohol Clin Exp Res.* 1993;17(1):192-196.
33. Brower KJ. Insomnia, alcoholism and relapse. *Sleep Med Rev.* 2003;7(6):523-539.
34. Allen RP, Picchietti D, Hening WA, et al. Restless legs syndrome: Diagnostic criteria, special considerations, and epidemiology. A report from the restless legs syndrome diagnosis and epidemiology workshop at the National Institutes of Health. *Sleep Med.* 2003;4:101-119.
35. Cohen-Zion M, Drummond SPA, Padula CB, et al. Sleep architecture in adolescent marijuana and alcohol users during acute and extended abstinence. *Addiction Behav.* 2009;34:976-979.
36. Schierenbeck T, Riemann D, Berger M, et al. Effect of illicit recreational drugs upon sleep: Cocaine, ecstasy and marijuana. *Sleep Med Rev.* 2008;12:381-389.
37. Coffey SF, Dansky BS, Carrigan MH, et al. Acute and protracted cocaine abstinence in an outpatient population: A prospective study of mood, sleep and withdrawal symptoms. *Drug Alcohol Dependence.* 2000;59: 277-286.
38. Thompson PM, Gillin CJ, Golshan S, et al. Polygraphic sleep measures differentiate alcoholics and stimulant abusers during short-term abstinence. *Biol Psychiatry.* 1995;38:831-836.
39. Pace-Scott EF, Stickgold AM, Wigren PE, et al. Sleep quality deteriorates over a binge-abstinence cycle in chronic smoked cocaine users. *Psychopharmacolgy.* 2005;179:873-883.
40. Koesters SC, Rogers PD. Rajasingham, CR. MDMA ("ecstasy") and other "club drugs": The new epidemic. *Pediatr Clin North Am.* 2002;49(2):415-433.
41. McCann U, Ricaurte GA. Effects of 3,4-methylenedioxymethamphetamine (MDMA) on sleep and circadian rhythms. *Sci World J.* 2007;7(2):231-238.
42. Morgan JA. Ecstasy (MDMA): A review of its possible persistent psychological effects. *Psychopharmacology.* 2000;152:230-248.
43. Montoya AG, Sorrentino R, Lukas SE, et al. Long-term neuropsychiatric consequences of "ecstasy" (MDMA): A review. *Harvard Rev Psychiatry.* 2002;10(4):212-220.
44. Allen RP, McCann UD, Ricaurte GA. Persistent effects of 3,4-methylen edioxymethamphetamine (MDMA, "Ecstasy") on human sleep. *Sleep.* 1993;16:560-564.
45. Bolla KI, Lesage SR, Gamaldo CE, et al. Sleep disturbance in heavy marijuana users. *Sleep.* 2008;31(6):901-908.
46. Licata SC, Rowlett JK. Abuse and dependence liability of benzodiazepine-type drugs: $GABA_A$ receptor modulation and beyond. *Pharmacol Biochem Behav.* 2008;90:74-89.

47. Kripke DF. Chronic hypnotic use: Deadly risks, doubtful benefit. *Sleep Med Rev.* 2000;4(1):5-20.

48. Morgan WW. Abuse liability of barbiturates and other sedative hypnotics. *Adv Alcohol Substance Abuse.* 1990;9(1-2):67-82.

49. Ator NA. Contributions of GABA A receptor subtypeselectivity to abuse liabilityand dependence potential of pharmacological treatments for anxiety and sleep disorders. *CNS Spectrum.* 2005;10(1):31-39.

50. Griffiths RR, Weerts EM. Benzodiazepine self-administration in humans and laboratory animals—Implications for problems of long-term use and abuse. *Psychopharmacology.* 1997;134:1-37.

51. Ciraulo DA, Nace EP. Benzodiazepine treatment of anxiety or insomnia in substance abuse patients. *Am J Addictions.* 2000;9:276-284.

52. IDU HIV. *Prevention Methadone Maintenance Treatment.* Feb. 2002. Available at http://www.cdc.gov/idu/facts/MethadoneFin.pdf. Accessed Sept. 11, 2010.

53. O'Brien CP. Benzodiazepine use, abuse, and dependence. *J Clin Psychiatry.* 2005;66(suppl 2):28-33.

54. Griffiths RR, Johnson MW. Relative abuse liability of hypnotic drugs: A conceptual framework and algorithm for differentiating among compounds. *J Clin Psychiatry.* 2005;66(9):21-38.

55. Salzman C. Addiction to benzodiazepines. *Psychiatr Quart.* 1998;69(4):251-261.

56. Albers LJ, Hahn RK, Reist C, eds. *Handbook of Psychiatric Drugs,* 2011 Edition. Blue Jay, CA: Current Clinical Strategies Publishing; 2008.

57. Liappas IA, Malitas PN, Dimopoulos NP, et al. Zolpidem dependence case series: Possible neurobiological mechanisms and clinical management. *J Psychopharmacol.* 2003;17(1):131-135.

58. Victorri-Vigneau C, Kailly E, Veyrac G, et al. Evidence of zolpidem abuse and dependence: Results of the French Centre for Evaluation and Information on Pharcacodependence (CEIP) network survey. *Br J Clin Pharmacol.* 2007;64(2):198-209.

59. Wagner J, Wagner ML. Non-benzodiazepines for the treatment of insomnia. *Sleep Med Rev..* 2000;4(6):551-581.

60. Fuller DE, Hornfeldt. From club drug to orphan drug: Sodium Oxybate (Xyrem) for the treatment of cataplexy. *Pharmacotherapy.* 2003;23(9):1205-1209.

61. Carter LP, Richards BD, Minstzer MZ, et al. Relative abuse liability of GHB in humans: A comparison of psychomotor, subjective, and cognitive effects of supratherapeutic doses of Triazolam, Pentobarbital, and GHB. *Neuropsychopharmacology.* 2006;31:2537-2551.

62. Dimsdale JE, Nomran D, DeJardin D, et al. The effect of opioids on sleep architecture. *J Clin Sleep Med.* 2007;3(1):33-36.

63. Walker JM, Farney RJ, Rhondeau SM, et al. Chronic opioid use is a risk factor for the development of central sleep apnea and ataxic breathing. *J Clin Sleep Med.* 2007;3(5):455-462.

64. Walker JM, Farney RJ. Are opioids associated with sleep apnea? A review of the evidence. *Curr Pain Headache Rep.* 2009;13:120-126.

65. Stein MD, Herman DS, Bishop S, et al. Sleep disturbances among methadone maintained patients. *J Substance Abuse Treat.* 2004;26:175-180.

66. Kroutil LA, Van Brunt DL, Herman-Stahl MA, et al. Nonmedical use of prescription stimulants in the United States. *Drug Alcohol Dependence.* 2006;84:135-143.

67. Jasinski DR, Kovacevic-Ristanovic R. Evaluation of the abuse liability of modafinil and other drugs for excessive daytime sleepiness associated with narcolepsy. *Clin Neuropharmacol.* 2000;23(3):149-156.

68. Herman-Stahl MA, Krebs CP, Kroutil LA, et al. Risk and protective factors for nonmedical use of prescription stimulants and methamphetamine among adolescents. *J Adolesc Health.* 2006;39:374-380.

69. Auger RR, Goodman SH, Silber MH, et al. Risks of high-dose stimulants in the treatment of disorders of excessive somnolence: A case-control study. *Sleep.* 2005;28(6):667-672.

70. Billiard M. Narcolepsy: Current treatment options and future approaches. *Neuropsychiatric Dis Treat.* 2008;4(3):557–566.

71. Guillerminault C. Amphetamines and narcolepsy: Use of the Stanford Database. *Sleep.* 1993;16(3):199-201.

72. Rogers AE, Aldrich MS, Berrios AM, et al. Compliance with stimulant medications in patients with narcolepsy. *Sleep.* 1997;20(1):28-33.

73. Stoops WW, Lile JA, Fillmore MT, et al. Reinforcing effects of modafinil: Influence of dose and behavioral demands following drug administration. *Psychopharmacology.* 2005;182:186-193.

74. Jasinski DR. An evaluation of the abuse potential of modafinil using methylphenidate as a reference. *J Psychopharmacol.* 2000;14:53-60.

75. Rush CR, Kelly TH, Hays LR, et al. Acute behavioral and physiological effects of modafinil in drug abusers. *Behav Pharmacol.* 2002;133:105-116.

76. Rush CR, Kelly TH, Hays LR, et al. Discriminative-stimulus effects of modafinil in cocaine-trained humans. *Drug Alcohol Dependence.* 2002;67:311-322.

77. Reichel CM, See RE. Modafinil effects on reinstatement of methamphetamine seeking in a rat model of relapse. *Psychopharmacology.* 2010; 210:337-346.

78. Dackis CA, Kampman KM, Lynch KG, et al. A double-blind, placebo-controlled trial of modafinil for cocaine dependence. *Neuropsychpharmacology.* 2005;30:205-211.

79. Miller WR, Rollnick S. *Motivational Interviewing: Preparing People for Change.* 2nd ed. New York: Gilford Press; 2002.

80. Bell K, Cole BA. Improving medical students' success in promoting health behavior change: A curriculum evaluation. *J Gen Intern Med.* 2008;23:1503-1506.

81. Martino S, Haeseler F, Belitsky R, et al. Teaching brief motivational interviewing to year three medical students. *Med Educ.* 2007;41: 160-167.

82. Haesler F, Fortin AH, Pfeiffer C, et al. Assessment of a motivational interviewing curriculum for year 3 medical students using a standardized patient case. *Patient Educ Counseling.* 2011;84(7):27-30.

83. Carroll K, Rounsaville B, Keller D. Relapse prevention strategies for the treatment of cocaine abuse. *Am J Drug Alcohol Abuse.* 1991;17(3): 249-265.

84. Barlow DH. *Clinical Handbook of Psychological Disorders.* New York,: Guilford Press; 2001.

85. McHugh RK, Hearon BA, Otto MW. Cognitive behavioral therapy for substance use disorders. *Psychiatr Clin North Am.* 2010;33(3):511-525.

86. Huber A, Ling W, Shoptaw S. Integrating treatments for methamphetamine abuse: A psychosocial perspective. *J Addictive Dis.* 1997;16:41-50.

87. Rawson RA, Marinelli-Casey P, Anglin MD, et al. A multi-site comparison of psychosocial approaches for the treatment of methamphetamine dependence. *Addiction.* 2004;99:708-717.

88. Rawson RA, Obert JL, McCann MJ, et al. Psychological approaches to the treatment of cocaine dependence: A neurobehavioral approach. *J Addictive Dis.* 1991;11:97-119.

89. Rawson RA, Obert JL, McCann MJ, et al. Cocaine treatment outcome: Cocaine use following inpatient, outpatient, and no treatment. In: Harris LS, ed. *Problems of Drug Dependence: Proceedings of the 47th Annual Scientific Meeting.* No. 67. NIDA Research Monograph Series; 1986:271-277.

90. Luborsky L, McLellan AT, Woody GE, et al. Therapist success and its determinants. *Arch Gen Psychiatry.* 1985;42(6):602-611.

91. Woody GE, Luborsky L, McLellan AT, et al. Psychotherapy for opiate addicts: Does it help? *Arch Gen Psychiatry.* 1983;40(6):639-645.

92. Woody GE, McLellan AT, Luborsky L, et al. Twelve-month follow-up of psychotherapy for opiate dependence. *Am J Psychiatry.* 1987;144(5): 590-596.

93. Woody GE, McLellan AT, Luborsky L, et al. Psychotherapy in community methadone programs: A validation study. *Am J Psychiatry.* 1995;152(9):1302-1308.

94. Woody GE. Research findings on psychotherapy of addictive disorders. *Am J Addictions.* 2003;12(2):S19-S26.

95. Marlatt G, Gordon JR, eds. *Relapse Prevention: Maintenance Strategies in the Treatment of Addictive Behaviors.* New York: Guilford Press; 1985.

96. Higgins ST, Wong CJ, Badger GJ, et al. Contingent reinforcement increases cocaine abstinence during outpatient treatment and 1 year of follow-up. *Consult Clin Psychol.* 2000;68:64-72.

97. Petry NM, Martin B. Low-cost contingency management for treating cocaine and opioid abusing methadone patients. *J Consult Clin Psychol.* 2002;70:398-405.

98. Donovan DM, Wells EA. "Tweaking 12-step": The potential role of 12-step self-help group involvement in methamphetamine recovery. *Addiction.* 2007;102(1):121-129.

99. Monnelly EP, Ciraulo DA, Knapp C, et al. Quetiapine for treatment of alcohol depedence. *J Clin Psychopharmacol.* 2004;24(5):532-535.

100. Kampman KM, Pettinati HM, Lynch KG, et al. A double-blind, placebo-controlled pilot trial of quetiapine for the treatment of type A and type B alcholism. *J Clin Psychopharmacol.* 2007;27(4):344-351.

101. Arnedt JT, Conroy DA, Brower KJ. Treatment options for sleep disturbances during alcohol recovery. *J Addictive Dis.* 2007;26(4):41-54.

102. Jacobs GD, Pace-Schott EF, Stickgold R, et al. Cognitive behavior therapy and pharmacotherapy for insomnia: A randomized controlled trial and direct comparison. *Arch Intern Med.* 2004;164:1888-1896.

103. Currie SR, Clark S, Hodgins DC, et al. Randomized controlled trial of briefcognitive-behavioralinterventionsforinsomniainrecoveringalcoholics. *Addiction.* 2004;99:1121-1132.

Effects of Drugs on Sleep

PAULA K. SCHWEITZER / EHREN R. DODSON

INTRODUCTION

A number of drugs can affect the architecture of sleep and lead to changes in the durations of various sleeps stages or the frequency of stage transitions. The best available polysomnographic (PSG) data describing these architectural changes are presented in the table below (Table A-1). Drugs that affect PSG-recorded total sleep time (TST), total wake time (TWT), wake after sleep onset (WASO), or the number of awakenings are said to affect sleep continuity (with improved sleep continuity leading to increased TST and decreased TWT, WASO, and number of awakenings).

The long-term significance of drug effects on rapid eye movement (REM) sleep and slow wave sleep (SWS) is uncertain because the precise functions of these sleep stages remain unknown. However, certain short-term effects have been recognized (for example, an increase in REM sleep—REM rebound—with bothersome nightmares or vivid dreaming after discontinuation of a REM-suppressing agent).

PSG data from well-designed, placebo-controlled studies exist for the majority of drugs that have been evaluated as hypnotics; however, similar information is limited for most other drugs. Although objective measures of sleepiness—such as multiple sleep latency (MSLT) and daytime performance testing—exist and have been reported for some drugs, the majority of the data are subjective. Furthermore, conclusions from both objective and subjective data may be limited by factors such as the specific population studied, lack of placebo control, particular dosage and duration of drug treatment, concomitant medication usage, and effects of underlying disease. Interpretation of the following data should be understood within the context of these limitations.

TABLE A-1

Effects of Drugs on Sleep and Wake

Drug Class/Drug	Mechanism of Action and Other Receptor Pharmacology	Effect on Sleep Architecture				Subjective Effect(s)	Comment(s)
		Sleep Latency	Sleep Continuity	SWS	REM Sleep		
Alcohol	Multiple receptor effects including GABA$_A$ agonism						
Acute ingestion		↓	↑	↑	↓	Sedating	Impairs performance
Withdrawal			↓	↓	↑	Fragments sleep; nightmares	
ANTIEPILEPTICS							
Established drugs						Sedating	Most impair performance
Barbiturates	GABA agonism via increased duration of chloride channel opening; enzyme induction	↓	↑	↔↓	↓	Very sedating	High doses have direct action on chloride channel; ↑ spindle density
Benzodiazepines	GABA$_A$ agonism	↓	↑	↓	↓	Sedating	↑ spindle density
Carbamazepine	NE agonism; partial adenosine agonism; enzyme induction	↓	↑	↑	↓	Sedating	↓ MSLT latency
Ethosuximide	Selective reduction of T-type calcium channel currents		↓	↓	↔↑	May be less sedating than other drugs	
Phenytoin	Decreased sodium flux; enzyme induction	↓	↓	↑	↓	Sedating	↑ drowsiness on wake maintenance test
Valproic acid	GABA potentiation		?↑	↔	↔	May be less sedating than other drugs	

Continued

TABLE A-1

Effects of Drugs on Sleep and Wake—cont'd

Drug Class/Drug	Mechanism of Action and Other Receptor Pharmacology	Effect on Sleep Architecture				Subjective Effect(s)	Comment(s)
		Sleep Latency	Sleep Continuity	SWS	REM Sleep		
Newer drugs						Sedating	
Felbamate	Unknown; glycine blockade; GABA potentiation					Insomnia, fatigue	Interactions with other anticonvulsants, theophylline, warfarin
Gabapentin	Binds with high affinity to the alpha$_2$-delta site (an auxiliary subunit of voltage-gated calcium channels)	↔	↑	↑	↔↑	Sedating	FDA indications include seizures, postherpetic neuralgia; evaluated for multiple disorders
Lacosamide	Sodium channel inactivation; collapsin-response mediator protein-2 affinity					Fatigue, insomnia	
Lamotrigine	Unknown; sodium channel inhibition			↔↓	↔↑	Mildly sedating	FDA indications include seizures, bipolar disorder
Levetiracetam	Unknown; no affinity for GABA	↔	↑	↑	↓	Mildly sedating	No change in MSLT latency
Pregabalin	Unknown; binds with high affinity to the alpha$_2$-delta subunit of voltage-gated calcium channels	↓	↑	↑	↓	Sedating	FDA indications include seizures, neuropathic pain, postherpetic neuralgia, fibromyalgia; evaluated for multiple disorders
Rufinamide	Unknown; sodium channel modulation					Sedating, fatigue	
Tiagabine	GABA reuptake inhibition	↔↓	↑	↑	↔	Sedating	Evaluated for anxiety, insomnia, pain
Topiramate	Unknown; excitatory amino acid receptor blockade; GABA potentiation					Sedating	FDA indications include seizures, migraine; evaluated for multiple disorders; some cognitive impairments noted
Vigabatrin	GABA analog; inhibits GABA transaminase	↔	↔	↔	↔	Moderately sedating	Associated with specific adverse event of peripheral visual field defect
Zonisamide	Unknown; sodium and calcium channel inhibition					Mildly sedating	
ANTIHISTAMINES							
First-generation H$_1$ antagonists	H$_1$ antagonism; significant CNS penetration; also mACh, alpha, 5-HT antagonism					Sedating	↓ MSLT latency; impair performance; possible tolerance to sedation
Chlorpheniramine	H$_1$, mACh, alpha, 5-HT antagonism	↔↓	↔↑		↔↓	Sedating	
Clemastine	H$_1$, mACh, alpha, 5-HT antagonism					Sedating	
Cyproheptadine	H$_1$, mACh, alpha, 5-HT antagonism					Sedating	
Diphenhydramine	H$_1$, mACh, alpha, 5-HT antagonism	↔↓	↔↑		↔↓	Sedating	Primary ingredient in most over-the-counter sleep aids
Doxylamine	H$_1$, mACh, alpha, 5-HT antagonism	↔↓	↔↑		↔↓	Sedating	
Hydroxyzine	H$_1$, mACh, alpha, 5-HT antagonism	↔↓	↔↑		↔↓	Sedating	
Second-generation H$_1$ antagonists	H$_1$ antagonism but little CNS penetration					Nonsedating	
Cetirizine	H$_1$ antagonism					More sedating than other second-generation drugs, particularly at higher doses	Nonsedating per MSLT; performance impairment at higher doses

TABLE A-1

Effects of Drugs on Sleep and Wake—cont'd

Drug Class/Drug	Mechanism of Action and Other Receptor Pharmacology	Effect on Sleep Architecture				Subjective Effect(s)	Comment(s)
		Sleep Latency	Sleep Continuity	SWS	REM Sleep		
Desloratadine	H_1 antagonism					Nonsedating	No performance impairment
Fexofenadine	H_1 antagonism					Nonsedating	No performance impairment even at higher doses
Levocetirizine	H_1 antagonism					Nonsedating	No performance impairment
Loratadine	H_1 antagonism					Nonsedating	Nonsedating per MSLT; performance impairment at higher doses
H_2 antagonists	H_2 antagonism						Sedation may occur with dose increases or drug interactions
Cimetidine	H_2 antagonism	↔	↔	↑?	↔	Nonsedating	
Famotidine	H_2 antagonism	↓?	↔	↔	↔	Nonsedating	
Ranitidine	H_2 antagonism	↔	↔	↔	↔	Nonsedating	
ANTIHYPERTENSIVE DRUGS							
Alpha$_1$ antagonists							
Prazosin	Alpha$_1$ antagonism		↑		↑	Transient sedation	Used to treat nightmares in PTSD
Terazosin	Alpha$_1$ antagonism					Transient sedation	
Alpha$_2$ agonists							
Clonidine	Alpha$_2$ agonism		↔↑	↑	↓	Sedation, nightmares, insomnia	Performance impairment
Methyldopa	Alpha$_2$ agonism; NE depletion		↑	↓	?	Sedation, nightmares	Performance impairment
ACE inhibitors Enalapril, captopril, lisinopril, others	ACE inhibition	↔	↔	↔	↔	Rare fatigue, insomnia, nightmares	Dry irritating cough may disturb sleep
Beta antagonists	Beta-adrenergic receptor blockade						fatigue, insomnia, nightmares
Acebutolol	Selective beta$_1$ antagonism						
Atenolol	Selective beta$_1$ antagonism		↔↓		↓		Insomnia less likely than with other beta antagonists
Bisoprolol	Selective beta$_1$ antagonism						
Carvedilol	Selective beta$_1$ antagonism; alpha$_1$ antagonism					Fatigue, insomnia	
Metoprolol	Selective beta$_1$ antagonism		↓		↓	Fatigue, insomnia, nightmares	
Nadolol	Nonselective beta antagonism						
Pindolol	Nonselective beta antagonism		↓		↓	Fatigue, insomnia, nightmares	
Propranolol	Nonselective beta antagonism		↓		↓	Fatigue, insomnia, nightmares	More disruptive of sleep than other beta antagonists
Sotalol	Nonselective beta antagonism						Insomnia less likely than with other beta antagonists
Timolol	Nonselective beta antagonism						
Calcium channel blockers Nifedipine, verapamil, others	Calcium ion influx inhibition					Rare fatigue, rare sleep disturbance	No deficits in alertness or performance
Other							
Reserpine	NE uptake inhibition		↓	↓	↑	Sedation, nightmares	

Continued

Effects of Drugs on Sleep and Wake—cont'd

Drug Class/Drug	Mechanism of Action and Other Receptor Pharmacology	Effect on Sleep Architecture				Subjective Effect(s)	Comment(s)
		Sleep Latency	Sleep Continuity	SWS	REM Sleep		
DOPAMINE AGONISTS							
Amantadine	Dopamine reuptake inhibition					Insomnia	Also used as an antiviral agent
Apomorphine	D_4, D_2, D_3 agonism					Sedating	
Benztropine	mACh, H_1 antagonism		↔↓	↔↑	↓		Cognitive impairment
Bromocriptine	D_2 agonism; D_1 antagonism; ergot-derived					Sedating	
Hyoscyamine	mACh antagonism		↔↓	↔↑	↓		Cognitive impairment
Levodopa	Precursor of dopamine and NE		↓	↔↑	↔↓	Improved sleep at low doses; insomnia, nightmares at higher doses	↑ REM density at high doses; ↑ spindles; cognitive impairment
Pergolide	D_1, D_2 agonism; ergot-derived	↓	↑			Sedating	Decreases PLMs
Pramipexole	D_2, D_3 agonism; non–ergot-derived			?↑	↓	Sedating; vivid dreams	Decreases PLMs; ↓ MSLT latency
Ropinirole	D_2, D_3 agonism; non–ergot-derived	↓	↑	↔	↔	Sedating	Decreases PLMs; ↓ MSLT latency
Selegiline	Selective MAO-B inhibition; partial metabolism to amphetamine		↓		↓	Insomnia	↓ SL in patient population; transdermal formulation used for depression
HYPNOTICS							
Benzodiazepine receptor agonists	$GABA_A$ agonism					Sedating	May ↑ spindles
Estazolam	$GABA_A$ agonism	↓	↑	↓	↓	Sedating	
Eszopiclone	$GABA_A$ agonism	↓	↑	↔	↔	Sedating	No residual sedation
Flurazepam	$GABA_A$ agonism	↓	↑	↓	↓	Sedating	Residual sedation likely
Quazepam	$GABA_A$ agonism	↓	↑	↓	↓	Sedating	
Temazepam	$GABA_A$ agonism	↓	↑	↓	↓	Sedating	
Triazolam	$GABA_A$ agonism	↓	↑	↓	↓	Sedating	No residual sedation
Zaleplon	$GABA_A$ agonism (selective alpha$_1$ subunit–binding)	↓	↔	↔	↔	Sedating	No residual sedation
Zolpidem, zolpidem controlled-release	$GABA_A$ agonism (selective alpha$_1$ subunit–binding)	↓	↑	↔	↓	Sedating	No residual sedation
Other							
Doxepin	H_1 antagonism	↓	↑	↔	↔	Sedating	FDA indication for insomnia at doses of 3-6 mg
Ramelteon	Melatonin receptor agonism	↓	↔	↔	↔	Sedating	May affect circadian phase
HYPOLIPIDEMIC DRUGS							
Atorvastatin, lovastatin, simvastatin, rosuvastatin	HMG-CoA reductase inhibition	↔	↔			Insomnia?	Limited data, variable effects on sleep and performance
Gemfibrozil, ezetimibe	Varies						
PSYCHOTHERAPEUTIC DRUGS							
Antidepressants							
Tricyclics	5-HT, NE reuptake inhibition; strong alpha$_1$, mACh, H_1 antagonism	↓	↑	↔	↓	Tertiary more sedating than secondary; may increase PLMs	↑ SWS during the first NREM sleep period but not overall; may impair performance; may ↑ PLMs
Amitryptiline	5-HT, NE reuptake inhibition; alpha$_1$, mACh, H_1, $5-HT_2$ antagonism	↓	↑	↔	↓	Very sedating	↑ REM density
Clomipramine	5-HT, NE reuptake inhibition; alpha$_1$, mACh, H_1, $5-HT_2$ antagonism	↓	↑	↔	↓↓	Not as sedating as other tertiary amines	↑ eye movements in NREM sleep

TABLE A-1

Effects of Drugs on Sleep and Wake—cont'd

Drug Class/Drug	Mechanism of Action and Other Receptor Pharmacology	Effect on Sleep Architecture				Subjective Effect(s)	Comment(s)
		Sleep Latency	Sleep Continuity	SWS	REM Sleep		
Desipramine	NE, 5-HT reuptake inhibition; mACh antagonism	↔			↓	Less sedating than tertiary amines	
Doxepin	NE, 5-HT reuptake inhibition; alpha$_1$, mACh, H$_1$ antagonism	↓	↑	↔	↓	Sedating	↑ REM density
Imipramine	5-HT, NE reuptake inhibition; alpha$_1$, mACh, H$_1$ antagonism	↓	↑	↔	↓	Very sedating	
Nortriptyline	NE, 5-HT reuptake inhibition; alpha$_1$, mACh, H$_1$ antagonism		↔		↓	Less sedating than tertiary amines	
Protriptyline	NE, 5-HT reuptake inhibition	↔	↔			Less sedating than tertiary amines	
Trimipramine	5-HT reuptake inhibition; alpha$_1$, mACh, H$_1$ antagonism	↓	↑	↔	↔	Sedating	Variable effects on REM
SSRIs	Primarily 5-HT reuptake inhibition					Insomnia more likely than sedation	Sleep continuity may improve with long-term use; may ↑ PLMs and slow eye movements
Citalopram	Exclusive 5-HT reuptake inhibition		↔		↓		
Escitalopram	Exclusive 5-HT reuptake inhibition						
Fluoxetine	Primarily 5-HT reuptake inhibition		↓	↓	↓	Vivid dreams	
Fluvoxamine	Exclusive 5-HT reuptake inhibition		↓	↓	↓	Vivid dreams	
Paroxetine	Primarily 5-HT reuptake inhibition	↑	↓		↓		May be more sedating than other SSRIs
Sertraline	Primarily 5-HT reuptake inhibition	↑	↓		↓	Vivid dreams	
SNRIs	5-HT, NE reuptake inhibition					Insomnia more likely than sedation	May ↑ PLMs
Desvenlafaxine	5-HT, NE reuptake inhibition					Insomnia, somnolence	
Duloxetine	5-HT, NE reuptake inhibition; weak dopamine reuptake inhibition		↓		↓	Fatigue, insomnia, somnolence	FDA indications include depression, anxiety, neuropathic pain, fibromyalgia
Milnacipran	5-HT, NE reuptake inhibition	?↓	?↑				FDA indication for fibromyalgia
Venlafaxine	5-HT, NE reuptake inhibition; weak dopamine reuptake inhibition		↓	↓	↓	Insomnia, somnolence	
MAOIs							
Isocarboxazid	MAO-A, MAO-B inhibition					Insomnia	
Moclobemide	Selective inhibition of MAO-A		↓		↔	Rare insomnia	Minimal effect on sleep; not available in USA
Phenelzine	MAO-A, MAO-B inhibition		↓		↓↓	Insomnia	Rare report of daytime somnolence at high dose
Selegiline transdermal	Selective inhibition of MAO-B; less selective at higher doses				?↓	Insomnia	Oral formulation used in Parkinson's disease treatment
Tranylcypromine	MAO-A, MAO-B inhibition		↓		↓↓	Insomnia	Rare report of daytime somnolence at high dose
Other							
Bupropion	NE, dopamine reuptake inhibition				↑	Insomnia, nightmares	Limited data, may ↓ PLMs

Continued

TABLE A-1

Effects of Drugs on Sleep and Wake—cont'd

Drug Class/Drug	Mechanism of Action and Other Receptor Pharmacology	Effect on Sleep Architecture				Subjective Effect(s)	Comment(s)
		Sleep Latency	Sleep Continuity	SWS	REM Sleep		
Lithium	Unknown; 5-HT potentiation; 5-HT_{1B} partial agonism		↑	↔↑	↔↓	Sedating	May impair performance
Mirtazapine	Alpha_2, 5-HT_2, H_1, alpha_1 antagonism	↓	↑	↔	↔	Sedating	
Nefazodone	5-HT reuptake inhibition; 5-HT_2 antagonism; weak alpha_1 antagonism		↑	↔	↔	Sedating	
Trazodone	5-HT reuptake inhibition; alpha_1, H_1, 5-HT_2 antagonism, 5-HT agonism	↓	↔↑	↑	↔↓	Very sedating	May impair performance
Antipsychotics							
Traditional drugs							
Chlorpromazine	D_2, 5-HT_2, alpha_1, H_1, mACh antagonism		↑	?	?	Moderately sedating	May impair performance
Haloperidol	D_2, 5-HT_2, alpha_1 antagonism		↑	?	?	Mildly sedating	
Thioridazine	D_2, 5-HT_2, alpha_1, D_1, H_1, mACh antagonism		↑	?	?	Very sedating	May impair performance
Newer drugs							
Aripiprazole	D_2, 5-HT_{1A} partial agonism; 5-HT_{2A} antagonism					Insomnia	Unlikely to impair performance
Clozapine	5-HT_2, alpha_1, H_1, cholinergic, D_1, D_2 blockade	↓	↑	↓?	↔↓	Markedly sedating	↑ REM density
Iloperidone	D_2, 5-HT_2 antagonism					Sedating	
Lamotrigine	Unknown; sodium channel inhibition, weak 5-HT_3 inhibition			↓?		Mildly sedating	Less likely to impair performance
Loxapine	Dopamine, 5-HT_2 antagonism	↓	↑		?↑	Mildly sedating	
Olanzapine	D_2, 5-HT_{2A}, mACh, H_1, alpha_1, D_1 antagonism	↔↓	↑	↑	↔↓	Markedly sedating	May impair performance; used off-label as hypnotic
Quetiapine	H_1, alpha_1, alpha_2, 5-HT_{2A}, D_2 antagonism		↑	↔	↓	Moderately sedating	May impair performance; used off-label as hypnotic
Risperidone	D_2, 5-HT_2, alpha_1 antagonism		↑	↑	↓	Mildly sedating	
Sertindole	5-HT_2, alpha_1, D_2 antagonism					Mildly sedating	Less sedating than others in this class
Ziprasidone	D_2, 5-HT_2, alpha_1, D_1 antagonism		↑			Mildly sedating	
Anxiolytics							
Alprazolam, chlordiazepoxide, diazepam, lorazepam	GABA_A agonism	↓	↑	↓	↓	Sedating	Performance impairment
Buspirone	5-HT_{1A} partial agonism; D_2 antagonism	↔	↔	↔	↔	Nonsedating	No effect on MSLT
STIMULANTS							
Amphetamine, methamphetamine	Dopamine, NE (also 5-HT at higher doses) release and reuptake inhibition	↑	↓	↔↓	↓	Increased alertness, insomnia	↑ MSLT latency
Armodafinil	Unknown; dopamine reuptake inhibition					Increased alertness	↑ MSLT latency
Caffeine	Adenosine receptor antagonism	↑	↓	↓		Increased alertness, insomnia	↑ MSLT latency
Lisdexamfetamine	Prodrug of dextroamphetamine						
Methylphenidate, dexmethylphenidate	Dopamine, NE release and reuptake inhibition	↑	↓	↔↓	↓	Increased alertness, insomnia	↑ MSLT latency; extended release formulas available

TABLE A-1

Effects of Drugs on Sleep and Wake—cont'd

Drug Class/Drug	Mechanism of Action and Other Receptor Pharmacology	Effect on Sleep Architecture				Subjective Effect(s)	Comment(s)
		Sleep Latency	Sleep Continuity	SWS	REM Sleep		
Modafinil	Unknown; dopamine reuptake inhibition	↔↑	?	↔		Increased alertness	↑ MSLT latency
Nicotine	Cholinergic agonism	↑	↓		↓	Insomnia	Insomnia on withdrawal
Pemoline	Unknown	↑	↓			Mildly increased alertness	No longer available in USA (hepatic failure)
Theophylline	Phosphodiesterase inhibition; adenosine receptor antagonism		↓	↓		Insomnia	Symptom relief may result in improved sleep
PAIN MEDICATIONS							
NSAIDs	Prostaglandin inhibition						
Acetaminophen							
Aspirin			↓	↓	↔	No effect	
Ibuprofen			↓	↓	↔	No effect	
Opioids							Respiratory depression, central sleep apnea, performance impairment
Fentanyl, hydrocodone, hydromorphone, oxycodone	Opioid agonism		↔↓	↓	↔↓	Sedating	
Methadone	Opioid agonism; NMDA antagonism					Sedating	
Morphine	Opioid agonism	↔↓	↓	↓	↓	Acutely sedating, insomnia with chronic use	↑ sleep disturbance on withdrawal
Tramadol	Opioid agonism; weak reuptake inhibition of NE, 5-HT			↓	↓	Sedating	
Skeletal muscle relaxants							
Baclofen	Unknown; GABA$_B$ agonism					Sedating	Interacts with alcohol and other CNS depressants
Cyclobenzaprine	mACh, 5-HT$_2$ antagonism; NE agonism					Sedating	Long half-life
Orphenadrine	mACh, H$_1$, NMDA antagonism					Sedating	
Tizanidine	Alpha$_2$ agonism					Sedating	
Other							
Triptans	Selective 5-HT$_2$ receptors					Sedating	
RESPIRATORY DRUGS							
Bronchodilators							
Fomoterol, salmeterol, terbutaline	Beta$_2$ agonism						Restlessness, particularly with long-acting drugs; improved sleep with improved symptoms
Ipratropium, tiotropium	ACh antagonism					Improved sleep with disease treatment	Improved Sao$_2$ with disease treatment
Corticosteroids			↓	↔↓	↓	Insomnia	Results inconsistent
Dexamethasone	Glucocorticoid agonist						
Hydrocortisone	Glucocorticoid agonist						
Prednisone	Glucocorticoid agonist					Case reports: insomnia	
Leukotriene modifiers							
Montelukast, zafirlukast, zileuton	Leukotriene antagonism					Case reports of insomnia, restlessness, dream abnormalities, somnambulism	Improved sleep quality, sleepiness, and performance accompany symptom improvement
Other							
Phenylpropanolamine	Alpha agonism					Insomnia	
Pseudoephedrine	Alpha agonism		↓			Insomnia	

Continued

TABLE A-1

Effects of Drugs on Sleep and Wake—cont'd

Drug Class/Drug	Mechanism of Action and Other Receptor Pharmacology	Effect on Sleep Architecture				Subjective Effect(s)	Comment(s)
		Sleep Latency	Sleep Continuity	SWS	REM Sleep		
Theophylline	Phosphodiesterase inhibition; adenosine receptor antagonism		↓	↓		Insomnia	Symptom relief may result in improved sleep
OTHER DRUGS							
Melatonin	Melatonin receptor agonism	↓	↔↑	↔	↔↓		May affect circadian phase
Sodium oxybate (gamma-hydroxybutyrate [GHB])	Unknown; possibly a direct neurotransmitter; GABA$_B$ modulation	↓	↑	↑	↔↓	Sedating	FDA indication for sleepiness and cataplexy in narcolepsy
Valerian	Unknown; may inhibit GABA, affect 5-HT, inhibit adenosine	↔↓	↔↑	↑	↔↑	Sedating	

ACE, angiotensin-converting enzyme; *ACh,* acetylcholine; *CNS,* central nervous system; *D_1 to D_4,* dopamine receptor types 1 to 4; *FDA,* U.S. Food and Drug Administration; *GABA,* γ-aminobutyric acid; *H_1,* histamine receptor type 1; *HMG-CoA,* 3-hydroxy-3-methylglutaryl–coenzyme A; *5-HT,* 5-hydroxytryptamine (serotonin); *mACh,* muscarinic acetylcholinergic; *MAOI,* monoamine oxidase inhibitor; *MSLT,* multiple sleep latency test; *NE,* norepinephrine; *NMDA, N*-methyl-D-aspartate; *NREM,* non-*REM; NSAIDs,* nonsteroidal anti-inflammatory drugs; *PLM,* period limb movement; *PTSD,* post-traumatic stress disorder; *REM,* rapid eye movement; *SNRI,* serotonin-norepinephrine reuptake inhibitor; *SSRI,* selective serotonin reuptake inhibitor; *SWS,* slow wave sleep; ↑, increase; ↓, decrease; ↔, no change; ?, mixed results.

From Avidan A, Barkoukis TJ: *Review of Sleep Medicine*, 3rd ed. Philadelphia: Elsevier; 2011.

TABLE A-2

Drugs Reported to Cause Vivid Dreams or Nightmares in Clinical Studies or Case Reports

Drug Class	Example(s)	Possible Mechanism for Inducing Nightmares	Comments
Alcohol		REM rebound	With acute use and withdrawal
Amphetamine		Norepinephrine, dopamine	With chronic use and withdrawal
Antibiotics/antivirals	Amantadine	Sleep-related immunologic response?	
	Ciprofloxacin		
	Erythromycin		
	Ganciclovir		
Antidepressants			
Tricyclics	Amitriptyline	Norepinephrine, serotonin	With use and withdrawal
	Clomipramine		
	Desipramine		
	Doxepin		
	Imipramine		
	Nortriptyline		
SSRIs	Escitalopram	Serotonin	Suppressed dream recall frequency but increased dream intensity and bizarreness
	Fluoxetine		
	Fluvoxamine		
	Paroxetine		Nightmares possibly more common than with other SSRIs
	Sertraline		
Other	Bupropion	Dopamine	Nightmares more common than with other antidepressants
	Nefazodone	Serotonin	
	Venlafaxine	Norepinephrine, serotonin	
Antiepileptics	Ethosuximide		
	Gabapentin	GABA	
	Lamotrigine		
	Tiagabine	GABA	
	Valproic acid	GABA	
	Zonisamide		
Antihypertensives			
ACE inhibitors	Captopril	Norepinephrine?	
	Enalapril		
	Losartan		
	Quinapril		
Beta antagonists	Atenolol	Norepinephrine	Nightmares common in this class of drugs
	Labetolol		
	Metoprolol		
	Propranolol		
Other	Clonidine	Norepinephrine	
	Digoxin	Unknown	
	Methyldopa	Norepinephrine	
Antipsychotics	Chlorpromazine	Unknown	
	Clozapine		
	Risperidone		
	Thioridazine		
	Thiothixene		
Barbiturates		REM rebound	Upon withdrawal
Benzodiazepines	Triazolam	GABA, REM rebound	Upon withdrawal
Cholinergic agonists	Rivastigmine	Acetylcholine	
	Tacrine		
Dopamine agonists	Amantadine	Dopamine	With chronic use
	Levodopa		
	Ropinirol		
	Selegiline		
Other	Chlorpheniramine	Histamine?	
	GHB	GABA	
	Naproxen	Unknown	
	Tramadol	Unknown	
	Zopiclone	GABA	

ACE, angiotensin-converting enzyme; GABA, γ-aminobutyric acid; GHB, gamma-hydroxybutyrate; REM, rapid eye movement; SSRIs, selective serotonin reuptake inhibitors.
From Avidan A, Barkoukis TJ: *Review of Sleep Medicine,* 3rd ed. Philadelphia: Elsevier; 2011.

TABLE A-3

Characteristics of Drugs Used for the Treatment of Insomnia

Drug	Drug Type	Half-life (hours)*	Dose (mg)	FDA Indication
DRUGS WITH FDA INDICATION FOR INSOMNIA				
Doxepin†	Histamine antagonist	10-30	3-6	Insomnia
Estazolam	Benzodiazepine receptor agonist	10-24	1-2	Insomnia
Eszopiclone	Benzodiazepine receptor agonist	5-6	1-3	Insomnia
Flurazepam	Benzodiazepine receptor agonist	48-120	15-30	Insomnia
Quazepam	Benzodiazepine receptor agonist	39-73	7.5-15	Insomnia
Ramelteon	Melatonin receptor agonist	1-2.6	8	Insomnia
Temazepam	Benzodiazepine receptor agonist	8-20	15-30	Insomnia
Triazolam	Benzodiazepine receptor agonist	1.5-5	0.125-0.25	Insomnia
Zaleplon	Selective benzodiazepine receptor agonist	1	5-20	Insomnia
Zolpidem	Selective benzodiazepine receptor agonist	1.5-2.4	5-10	Insomnia
Zolpidem extended-release	Selective benzodiazepine receptor agonist	1.6-4.5	6.25-12.5	Insomnia
OTHER DRUGS USED TO TREAT INSOMNIA				
Amitriptyline	Tricyclic antidepressant	5-45	25-150‡	Depression
Chloral hydrate	Two-carbon molecule	5-10	500-1000	Preoperative sedation
Chlordiazepoxide	Benzodiazepine receptor agonist	36-120	5-25	Anxiety
Clonazepam	Benzodiazepine receptor agonist	24-56	0.5-4	Anxiety, panic disorder, seizures
Diazepam	Benzodiazepine receptor agonist	36-100	2-10	Anxiety, panic disorder
Diphenhydramine	Histamine antagonist	4-8	25-50	Allergy symptoms
Doxepin†	Tricyclic antidepressant	10-30	25-150‡	Depression, anxiety
Doxylamine	Histamine antagonist	10	6.25-25	Allergy symptoms
Gabapentin	Anticonvulsant	5-9	300+	Postherpetic neuralgia, epilepsy
Lorazepam	Benzodiazepine receptor agonist	12-16	0.5-2	anxiety
Melatonin	Melatonin agonist	0.6-1		Not regulated; dietary supplement
Mirtazapine	Antidepressant	13-40	15-30‡	Depression
Nefazodone	Antidepressant	2-18	50-150‡	Depression
Olanzapine	Antipsychotic	20-54	5-20	Schizophrenia, bipolar disorder
Trimipramine	Antidepressant	15-40	25-150‡	Depression
Trazodone	Antidepressant	3-14	25-150‡	Depression

*Half-life includes active metabolites.
†Doxepin is available in low doses (3-6 mg) for the treatment of insomnia (FDA indication). It is also formulated in much higher doses (100-300 mg) for the treatment of depression.
‡This is the dose range used clinically off-label for treatment of insomnia. However, no dose range studies have been published for insomnia. Recommended doses for treatment of depression are higher.
FDA, U.S. Food and Drug Administration.
From Avidan A, Barkoukis TJ: *Review of Sleep Medicine,* 3rd ed. Philadelphia: Elsevier; 2011.

INDEX

A

Accreditation Council for Graduate Medical Education (ACGME), 6–7
Accreditation of Sleep Disorders Centers (ASDC), 7
Acetazolamide, impact, 248–249
Acetylcholine (ACh), 63
    clinical correlations, 67
    neurotransmitter signaling, 65–67
    overview, 65–66
    sleep-wake regulation, 66–67
Acetylcholinesterase (AChE), enzymatic breakdown, 65–66
Acetylcholinesterase inhibitors (AChEi), blockade, 66f
Acetyl-serotonin O-methyltransferase (ASMT), 500
Achondroplasia (AC), 507–508
    SDB predisposition, 507b
    treatment strategies, 507–508
Acid inhibitors, impact, 621
Acid-suppressive medications, 620–621
Acid suppressive therapy, usage, 621
Acrylic occlusal splints, usage, 327f
Actigraphy, 24, 38–39
    basis, 470–471
    data, example, 405f
    indications, 38–39
    interpretation, 39
    movement recordation, 28
    procedures, 39
    usage, 357, 403–404
Acupressure, 133
    application, 133
    meridians, stimulation, 133
Acupuncture, 133
    safety profile, 133
    side effects, 133
Acute exercise, effects, 157
Acute insomnia (adjustment insomnia), 144–145
    causes, 145b
Acute phase response, characteristics, 612b
Acute serotonin syndrome, 131–132
Acute sleep deprivation, 381
Acute TIA, therapeutic target, 652
Adaptive seroventilation (ASV), 25, 210, 249–252
    diagnostic features, 403b
    efficacy, 200
Adapt SV, 250
Addiction
    chronic illness model, 751
    genetic predisposition, 749–750
    neurobiology, 749–751
    pathways, 751
    psychiatric disorders, 751
    relapse, 751
    substance use, initiation, 750–751
Adenoidal size, improvement, 523–524
Adenosine, 74–75
    clinical correlations, 75
    distribution, 51

Adenosine (Continued)
    extracellular levels, 53
    GPCR subtypes, brain expression, 74–75
    overview, 74–75
    receptors, blockade, 52–53
    role, endogenous sleep-promoting factor, 52–53
    sleep drive, relationship, 51–53
    sleep-promoting substance, 95
    sleep-wake regulation, 75
Adenosine triphosphate (ATP) hydrolysis, 51–52
Adenotonsillar hypertrophy (ATH), 506
    obstructive sleep apnea (OSA), impact, 525
    risk, 524
Adenotonsillectomy (AT), 428–429
    decisions, 428
    nonrespiratory outcomes, benefit data, 428
    scheduling, 428–429
    treatment, usage, 494
Adenylate cyclase (AC), involvement, 64
Adjunctive insomnia, 676–677
Adolescents
    congenital blindness, actigraph, 530f
    depression, circadian rhythms, 539–540
    GERD, treatment, 526
    insomnia, point-prevalence rates, 453
    insufficient sleep syndrome, treatment, 519–520
    prefrontal cortex, development, 750
    sleep disorders, commonness, 524
    systemic hypertension, treatment, 521
    treatment, discussion, 471
Adrenergic receptor subtypes, NE interaction, 70–71
Adults
    achondroplasia (AC), 507
    co-morbid insomnias, nonpharmacologic treatments (effectiveness), 541–542
    dream-enacting behaviors, differential diagnosis, 551b
    excessive daytime sleepiness (EDS), 448
    overweight treatment selection guidelines, 199
    positive airway pressure titration, steps, 211t
    primary insomnias, nonpharmacologic treatments (effectiveness), 541–542
    restless legs syndrome (RLS), 479
        diagnostic criteria, 482t
        ICSD-2 diagnostic criteria, 725b
    sleep architecture, studies, 271t
    sleep medicine diagnostics, introduction, 28
    sleep-related breathing disorders (SRBDs), 448
Advanced sleep phase
    circadian misalignment, 466f
    syndrome, 38–39
    types, 403b
Advanced sleep phase disorder (ASPD), 370, 402, 472
    actigraphy, usage, 403–404
    chronotherapy, 408
    chronotype, 405
    clinical diagnosis, 402–405
    conceptualization, 402
    diagnosis, 403–404

Advanced sleep phase disorder (ASPD) (Continued)
    diagnostic tools, 402–405
    DMLO, usage, 404–405
    genetic factors, 405
    melatonin, usage, 409
    nondiagnostic associated clinical features, 405–406
    phase angle disorders, 405–406
    phototherapy, 408–409
    polysomnography, usage, 405
    sleep diaries, 402–403
    treatment, 408–409
Affinity, 67b
Age, effects, 270
Aggressive sleepsex behaviors, 573
Agonists, 67b
Airflow, creation, 206
Airway patency, pressure requirements, 210
Airways, classification, 218–219
Akathisia
    characterization, 711
    medications, impact, 355b
Alcohol
    avoidance, 153–154, 157
    history, obtaining, 751–752
    sleep hygiene, relationship, 199
    substance abuse, 752–753
    use, Quetiapine (impact), 757
Allergic rhinitis (AR), 523–524
    chronic obstructive nasal symptoms, 523
    diagnosis, 523
    mild intermittent symptoms, 523
    moderately severe persistence, 523
    seasonal AR (hay fever), control, 523
    symptoms, 523
        lessening, optimal sleep environment (creation), 522t
    treatment, 523–524
Allostatic loads, 57
Alpha agonists, usage, 462
Alpha-amino-3-hydroxy-5-methyl-4-isoxazole proprionate (AMPA), ion channel classification, 71–72
Alpha EEG, 595–596
Alpha intrusions, 33–34
Alprazolam (Xanax)
    comparison, 103
    usage, 688
Altered dream content, 550b
Altered sleep homeostasis, 161
Alternating leg muscle activation (ALMA), 347
    differential diagnosis, 347
    pattern, PSG recording, 347
Alternative medical systems, 133–134
Alveolar hypoventilation, 255–256
Alzheimer's disease (AD), 418–420
    clinical diagnostic criteria, 418
    clinical treatments, 419–420
    combination therapy, 420
    definitions, 418

Page numbers followed by *b,* indicate box; *f,* figure; *t,* table.

Alzheimer's disease (AD) (Continued)
 description, 418
 endogenous circadian markers, measurements, 418
 light therapy, 419–420
 pharmacologic treatment, 420
 progressive neurodegenerative disorder, 418
 sleep-disordered breathing (SDB), prevalence, 418
 sleep disorders, 657–658
 sleep disturbances, 418
 sleep-wake disturbances, wrist actigraphy (basis), 418
 SWS rebound, 656
AM Aligner (Airway Management), 239f
 fitting, patient mouth, 239f
Amantadine, usage, 334
Ambulatory blood pressure monitoring, usefulness, 521
Ambulatory electrocardiogram (AECG) recording, 588f
American Academy of Dental Sleep Medicine (AADSM), 6
American Academy of Sleep Medicine (AASM)
 criteria, 23–24
 formation, 5
 hypopnea definition, 207
 PAP criteria, 207
 practice guidelines, standards, 28
American Association of Sleep Technologists, 6
American Board of Internal Medicine, examination administration, 7
American Board of Sleep Medicine (ABSM), 7
American Sleep Disorders Association (ASDA), formation, 5
Amnestic parasomnia episodes, 106
Amnestic SRED, medications, 569b
Amphetamine derivatives
 co-administration, 93
 effects, 91f
 pharmacologic effects, 87
Amphetamine-like compounds, 85–93
 historical perspective/limitations, 85–87
 structure, comparison, 87
Amphetamine-like stimulants
 alternative, 94
 chemical structures, 87f
 effects, 90f
 usage, 96
Amphetamines, 85–93
 absorption, 88
 abuse, 753
 action, molecular targets, 88
 adverse effects, 298–299
 chemical entities, 87–88
 DA/NE release, 92
 drug-drug interactions, 93
 effectiveness, 85–86
 historical perspective/limitations, 85–87
 idiopathic hypersomnia usage, 298–299
 pregnancy risk, 299
 schematic representation, 89f
 side effects, 92
 stimulants, abuse/misuse, 93
 structure, 87
 structure-activity relationships, 87–88
 synthesis, 85
 toxicity, 92
 use, 92, 753
Amyotrophic lateral sclerosis (ALS), 259
Anastomotic leak, 197
Angelman syndrome, 497
Angina, nocturnal myocardial ischemia (relationship), 588–589
Animalistic dissociative episode, nocturnal polysomnogram, 578f

Ankylosing spondylitis, 599
 sleep-disordered breathing, risk factors, 599b
Antacids, usage, 619
Antagonists, 67b
Anterior bipolar montages, 639
Anticholinergics
 treatment-related side effects, 340
 usage, 334
Anticipatory awakenings, 568
 scheduled awakening, 478
Anticyclic modulating ventilation, 250–251
Antidepressants, 109–116, 462
 abuse, potential, 115–116
 basic pharmacology, 112
 clinical management, 115–116
 clinical pharmacology, 112
 initiation, 115–116
 maintenance, 115–116
 medications
  impact, 112t
  usage, 567
 patient initiation, 115–116
 precautions, 115–116
 treatment, discontinuation, 115
 treatment-related side effects, 340
 usage, 114–115
Antidiuretic hormone, 76
Antiepileptic drugs (AEDs), 635
 direct effects, 635, 636t
 impact, 635
 indirect effects, 636t
 selection, difficulty, 635
Antiepileptics, 119–121
 abuse, potential, 120–121
 basic pharmacology, 119
 clinical management, 120–121
 clinical pharmacology, 119
 double-blind crossover study, 119
 impact, 119–120
 initiation, 120–121
 maintenance, 120–121
 off-label usage, 120–121
 precautions, 120–121
Antihistamines, 121–122
 abuse, potential, 122
 adverse events, 122
 basic pharmacology, 121
 clinical management, 122
 clinical pharmacology, 121
 impact, 121
 initiation, 122
 maintenance, 122
 precautions, 122
 sleep disorder efficacy, clinical evidence, 121–122
Anti-Ma2 antibodies, 487
Antipsychotic drugs, 116–118
 abuse, potential, 118
 basic pharmacology, 116
 clinical application, 116
 clinical management, 118
 clinical pharmacology, 116
 development, 708
 5-HT$_2$ receptor mediation, 118
 grouping, 116
 initiation, 118
 maintenance, 118
 precautions, 118
 sedation, side effect, 710
 sleep disorder efficacy, clinical evidence, 118
Antipsychotic medications, 462
Anxiety
 issues, 471
 prediction, sleep complaints (impact), 541
 response, initiation, 163
 symptoms, 339
 valerian, impact, 130–131

Anxiety disorder
 diagnostic criteria, 682
 insomnia, relationship, 146
 sleep disturbances, commonness, 682
 subjective insomnia, prevalence, 682
Anxiolytics, abuse problems, 754
Apnea-hypopnea index (AHI), 35
 change, 196f
 cutoff point, 651f
 fenfluramine, impact, 195–196
 improvement, 196
 increase, 657–658
  absence, 273
 reduction, 618
 stratification, 648t
 wedge pressure, correlation, 246–247
 Zaleplon, impact, 200
Apnea of prematurity (AOP), 436–437
 frequency, 436–437
 observation, 437
Apnea Positive Pressure Long-term Efficacy Study (APPLES), 4
Apnea threshold, 246
 partial pressure of carbon dioxide in arterial blood (PaCO$_2$), representation, 246f
Apneustic breathing, 435
Apparent life-threatening event (ALTE), 437
 differential diagnosis, 437b
 management/workup, 437
Arginine vasopressin (AVP), 76
Armodafinil, 93–94
 action, mechanism, 94
 chemical structure, 87f
 clinical observations, 94
 FDA approval, 93
 idiopathic hypersomnia usage, 299
 Modafinil, contrast, 202t
 pharmacokinetics, 93
 side effects, 93–94
 structure, 93
 uses, 93
 wake-promoting agent usage, 202
Arousal parasomnias, 476–478
 comparison, 476t
 differential diagnosis, 477
 nocturnal seizures, contrast, 477t
Arousals
 dopamine, impact, 333
 mechanisms, 561–562
 reaction, importance, 247
 transition, duration, 561
Arousal side, ARAS node representation, 48–49
Arrhythmia prevalence, 591f
Arterial oxygen saturation (SaO$_2$), 272–273
 ILD, relationship, 282–283
 maintenance, 280
 recordings, 650f
Artifacts, 641–642
Ascending arousal system
 components, 46f
 evidence, discovery, 45f
Ascending reticular activating system (ARAS), 43–44
 cessation, 48
 origin, 45
 ventral branch, 45–46
 VLPO, interaction, 48–49
Aserinsky, Eugene, 4
Asian Sleep Research Society, 6
Asperger's syndrome, social interaction impairments, 541
Assaultive sleepsex behaviors, 573
Assist-control ventilation (spontaneous-timed ventilation mode), 260
Assist ventilation mode (spontaneous ventilation mode), 260

Associated Professional Sleep Societies (APSS), 5–6, 28
Associated sleep apnea, treatment, 294
Association for the Psychological Study of Sleep (APSS), 28
  formation, 5
Association of Polysomnographic Technologists (APT)
  federation formation, 5–6
  formation, 6
Association of Professional Sleep Societies (APSS), formation, 5–6
Association of Sleep Disorders Center (ASDC), formation, 5
Asthma, 275–278
  control, sleep disturbance (inverse relationship), 522
  diagnosis, 275
  inflammatory cells, involvement, 275
  management, 276
  mechanisms, 275
  OSA, relationship, 276–277
  severity, classification, 276
  sleep disturbance/architecture, 276
  sleep-related GERD, relationship, 622
  step-up/step-down pharmacotherapy, 276
  transient worsening, 275
  treatment, 277
  worsening, factors, 522b
Asthmatic patient, OSA (prevalence), 276–277
Atherosclerosis (development), systemic inflammation (impact), 648–649
Atomoxetine, 95
  usage, 86–87
Atonia, 49–50
Atopic dermatitis, 527
  symptom (lessening), optimal sleep environment (creation), 522t
Atopic eczema, food allergy (association), 528
Atopic parent, eczema risk, 527–528
Atrial fibrillation
  incidence, 588f
  risks, 587
Attended laboratory clinical polysomnography (sleep study), 28
Attention deficit hyperactivity disorder (ADHD), 85–86
  atomoxetine, usage, 86–87
  interventions, 544
  sleep complaints, 541
Augmentation Severity Rating Scale (ASRS), 23
Aura, 629
Australasian Sleep Society, 6
Autism spectrum disorders (ASDs), 499–502
  behavioral insomnia, treatment strategies, 501b
  behavioral interventions, 542–543
  co-sleep/night waking, commonness, 543
  diagnostic sleep studies, 500
  nonpharmacologic sleep interventions, effectiveness, 543t
  oral melatonin, prescribing, 501b
  pharmacologic interventions, 543–544
  sleep complaints, 541
  sleep problems, risk factors, 499b
  symptoms, 502
  treatments, 542–544
    medications, usage, 501–502
Autocrine signaling, 67b
Autoreceptors, 67b
Autosomal dominant nocturnal frontal lobe epilepsy, 632–633
Autotitrating positive airway pressure (APAP), 209–210
  titration, 210
  usage, AASM standard operating procedure guidelines, 209b

AveoTSD, 235–237
  health professional fitting kit, 237f
  sample, 237f
Average referential montage, 639
Average volume-assured pressure support (AVAPS), 260, 264
Awakenings
  nightmares, relationship, 186
  number, increase, 33
Ayurvedic medicine, 133–134
  safety profile, 134
  side effects, 134

B

Bacteria, classification, 612
Bad sleepers, 278
Balenotherapy, 135
Ballismus, 352
Barbiturates, abuse problems, 754
Bariatric surgery, 226–227
  goal, 226–227
Bariatric weight loss surgery
  prospective studies, summary, 197t
  studies, 196–197
Basal forebrain (BF)
  cholinergic neurons
    impact, 66–67
    lesions, 45–46
  neurons, role, 47
Basal ganglia, wake-promoting role, 47–48
Baseline diagnostic polysomnography, 29–36
  indications, 29
  interpretation, 30–36
  movement, detection/measurement, 30
  procedures, 29–30
Beck Depression Inventory Second Edition (BDI-II), 14, 697b
Bed Partner Questionnaire, 231–232
  completion, 237
  usage, 232b
Bedroom clock, elimination, 153, 156
Bedroom comfort, 152–153, 155
Bedroom noise, elimination, 152, 155
Bedroom temperature, regulation, 152, 155
Bedtime pass, 450–451
Bedtimes
  decrease, 156
  liquids, limitation, 154, 157
  regularity, 153, 156
  relaxing activities, 157
  rules, 153
  snack, consumption, 154, 157
Behavioral activation, 598
Behavioral arousal, EEG (relationship), 43–48
Behavioral disorders, 11b–12b
Behavioral insomnia
  diagnosis/treatment, 500–501
  treatment strategies, 501b
Behavioral interventions, 195–200
Behavioral states
  temporal regulation, SCN (impact), 54
  transitions, 48–49
Behavioral therapeutics, developments, 169–170
Behavioral treatments, AASM endorsement, 163t
Behavioral variant FTD, 658–659
Behçet's disease, 600
Benign epilepsy with centrotemporal spikes (BECTS), 632
Benign focal epilepsy, 632
Benign neonatal sleep myoclonus (BNSM), 478, 521
  limb jerks, occurrence, 521
  provocation, 521
Benign sleep myoclonus, 348–349
  pathogenesis, 348–349

Benzodiazepine hypnotics, 174
Benzodiazepine receptor agonists (BZRAs), 99, 178–179
  amnestic effects, 104
  amnestic parasomnia episodes, 106
  cognitive effects, 104–105
  daytime function, 103–104
  dependence liability, 105–106
  discontinuation effects, 105
  drug abuse, 105
  drugs, metabolism, 104
  falls, 104–105
    risk, increase, 104
  half-lives, 100
  long-term BZRA use, 105
  metabolism, 100–101
    reduction, CYP3A4 inhibitors (impact), 101
  mortality risk, elevation, 105
  pharmacodynamic drug-drug interactions, 101
  pharmacokinetics, 100–102
  plasma concentration, 105f
  receptor subtype affinity, dependence liability (relationship), 106
  residual effects, 104
  safety, 104–106
  sedative/amnestic activities, 99
  tolerance, development, 102
Benzodiazepine receptor agonists (BZRAs)
  hypnotics, 173–175
  administration, 178
  approval, 178
  availability, 177–178
  efficacy, 102–104
    assessments, PSG usage, 102
  indication, 102
  indication, absence, 103
  list, 174t
  nonbenzodiazepines, 175t
  pharmacokinetic properties, 174
  positive allosteric modulators, 174
  usage, 173
Benzodiazepines, 34
  abuse problems, 754
  administration, 683
  CNS depressant, 200
  usage, 458–460, 566, 683
Berlin Questionnaire (BQ), 19
  screening tool, usefulness, 231
Bilevel positive airway pressure (BiPAP), 25, 209
  Auto SV (ASV), 250
  CPAP, contrast, 263–264
  NIPPV modality, 259
Biocalibrations, 37
Bi-occipital spike-wave discharges, runs, 503f
Biofeedback
  physiologic signals, monitoring, 165
  relaxation, relationship, 165
Biologic compounds, 127–133
Bio/neurofeedback, evaluation, 165
Biot's breathing, 435
Bipolar disorders (depressive episodes), 678b
  insomnia, report, 540
Bipolar I disorders (BPD), 678–679
  depressed phase, 678
  mania/depression, sleep alterations, 678–679
  prevalence, 678
Bipolar montage, 639
  EEG review, 639
Blind, non-24-hour sleep-wake syndrome (melatonin treatment), 416f
Blindness, role, 365
Blindness-related dyssomnia, 38–39
Blood pressure, 213
  CPAP therapy, impact, 651–652
  dippers/nondippers, 649

Blood pressure (Continued)
  PAP therapy, impact, 213
  reduction
      CPAP treatment, 652
      nocturnal dipping, 647
  surges, 649
Blood tests, 24
Board of Registered Polysomnographic
    Technologists (BRPT), operation, 7
Body habitus, women, 723
Body mass index (BMI)
  elevation, 196–197
  OSA, association, 18
  women, 723
Body movements, 354–356
Bona fide cataplexy, 486–487
Bone damage, 325
Brain
  activation, stimulation, 181
  activity, 30–34
  arousals, reactions, 247
  circuitry, 751
  information, chemical transfer, 65
  response, impairment, 52f
  sleep-wake behavior, active role, 45f
Brain-derived neurotrophic factor (BDNF),
    77–78
Brain nitric oxide, increase, 611
Brainstem
  ascending reticular activating system, 43–46
  cholinergic activating system, location, 48f
  disorders, 25
  systems, projections, 49f
  tumor, 444f
Brain TNF-α protein levels, increase, 610
Breathalyzer, usage, 382
Breathing disturbances, 247
Bremer, Frederic, 43–44, 45f
Bright light therapy, 453, 698–701
  continuation, 700
  descriptions, 698–699
  procedure, 700b
  risks, 700–701
  safety, 700
  side effects, 700–701, 700b
Bronchodilators, reversibility (absence), 271
Brugada syndrome, 590
  therapy, 590
Bruxism, 324
  identification, 326f
  medications, impact, 356b
  neurologic diseases, reports, 326
  scoring, events, 326b
BTBD9, RLS sensory symptoms (relationship),
    309
Bupropion, 95
  action mechanism, 114
  DA uptake inhibitor, 88–90
Burst mode, 47
Buspirone
  GAD treatment, FDA approval, 683–685
  usage, 683
Butyrophenones, 116

C
Caffeine, 95
  absorption, 95
  effects, 53f
  intake, impact, 14
  limitation/avoidance, 153, 157
  metabolism, 95
  products, 101–102
  responses (mediation), adenosine receptors
      (impact), 53
  scheduled naps, combination, 384–385

Cambridge-Hopkins RLS questionnaire
    (CH-RLSq), 23
Canadian Sleep Society, 6
Cancer
  shift work, relationship, 371–372
  sleep disorders, 528–529
Cancer-related fatigue (CRF)
  occurrence, 529
  treatment strategies, 529, 529b
Cannabinoids, 77
CANPAP nonresponders, comparison, 249
Carbachol, injection, 50–51
Carbamazepine, sleep-enhancing effects, 678
Carbon dioxide (CO_2)
  stimulation, 249
  therapeutic application, 248
Cardiac abnormalities, 440
Cardiac arrhythmia, 649
Cardiac drugs, effect, 248
Cardiac events, 35
  sleep-disordered breathing, effects, 591
  therapy, 591
Cardiac medications, sleep-disrupting effects,
    591–592
Cardiac resynchronization (CRT) therapy, 248
Cardiometabolic disease, shift work
    (relationship), 371
Cardiopulmonary measures, 30, 34–35
Cardiovascular disease
  cardiac events, 585–589
  OSA risk factor, 4
Cardiovascular disorders
  OSA predisposition, 10
  prevalence, 251f
Cardiovascular events, circadian variation, 648f
Cardiovascular morbidity/mortality rates, CPAP
    (impact), 651
Cardiovascular system, autonomic changes, 647
Carotid atherosclerosis, snoring (relationship),
    650
Carskadon, Mary, 4–5
Cataplexy, 289, 485
  attacks, frequency (variation), 289
  diagnostic categories, ICSD-2, 487
  improvement, 292
  Orexin, presence, 49f
  pediatric narcolepsy, pharmacologic
      treatment, 490t
  treatment, 293, 491
      antidepressant drugs, usage, 114–115
      pharmacotherapy, 488
Cataplexy Hypnagogic hallucinations Excessive
    daytime sleepiness Sleep attacks Sleep
    paralysis (CHESS), 486b
Catathrenia (sleep-related groaning), 579–580
  CPAP therapy, response, 580
  night-to-night consistency, 579
  onset, insidiousness, 579
  paroxysmal nocturnal event, 638
  PSG evaluation, auditory monitoring, 579
  respiratory dysrhythmia, 579
Catechol-O-methyltransferase (COMT)
  impact, 70
  inhibitors, 354
Catechol-O-methyltransferase (COMT)
    Inhibitors, usage, 334
Caudate dopamine, effects, 91f
Center for Medicare and Medicaid Services
    (CMS)
  enrollment form (CMS-855S), 234
  hypopnea definition, 207
  PAP criteria, 207
Central adrenal insufficiency, 496
Central apnea, 208t, 434–438
  conditions, 444
  conventional events, 435–436

Central apnea (Continued)
  definition, 434–435
  extreme events, 435–436
  genetics, 438–439
  normative data, 436
  term, usage, 434–435
  ventilation, sleep (impact), 434
Central breathing disturbances
  normalization, inability, 250
  therapeutic approach, 248f
Central chemoreceptors, CSA role, 247
Central nervous system (CNS)
  arousal, 33–34
      illustration, 33f
  depressants, impact, 195
  GHB depressant effects, 490
  penetration, increase, 87
  stimulant
      definition, 85
      usage, 85
Central pattern generators (CPGs)
  activation, 475, 479–480
  schematic, 476f
Central sensitivity syndromes (CSS), 600
Central sleep apnea (CSA), 209
  OA, comparison, 243f–245f
  pathophysiology, 246–247
      central chemoreceptors, role, 247
      factors, 246b
  syndromes, defining, 245
  treatment, 247–252
      options, 247b
Central ventilatory control, women, 724
Cerebellar tremor, 352
Cerebral blood flow velocity (CBFV),
    recordings, 650f
Cerebral palsy (CP), 502–503
  incidental spike-wave discharges, 503–504
  sleep-disordered breathing, treatment, 503
Cerebrovascular complications, pathogenesis
    (sympathetic overactivity), 649
Cerebrovascular disease, 25
  pathophysiologic mechanisms, 648–650
Cerebrovascular disorders, OSA predisposition,
    10
Cerebrovascular outcomes, OSA (relationship),
    647–652
Cerebrovascular risk, sleep apnea (impact),
    650–652
Cervical-medullary compression, clinical
    symptoms, 505b
Cervical pillows, studies, 198
Cervical spine disease, presence, 598
Chamomile, 132
  safety profile, 132
  side effects, 132
Channel, term (usage), 629
Chemical signing mechanisms, membrane
    proteins (impact), 78
Chest wall deformities, 255–256, 267
Cheyne-Stokes pattern, 200
Cheyne-Stokes respiration (CSR), 245
  characterization, 245
  importance, 248
Chiari 1 malformations (CM1), 506
Chiari 2 malformations (CM2), 506
Chiari malformations (CMs), 25, 443–444,
    505–506
  characterization, 443
  medical therapies, selection, 444
  obstructive sleep apnea (OSA), presence, 506
  respiratory complications, 444b
  sleep-disordered breathing, treatment, 506
  sleep-related breathing disorders, diagnostic
      approach, 506
Childhood, benign focal epilepsy, 632

Childhood absence epilepsy, 630
Childhood atopic eczema (CAE), 527–528
    sleeplessness, 527
Childhood CP survivors, excessive daytime
        sleepiness (subjective complaints), 529
Childhood history, 18
Childhood obesity, 520
    diagnostic strategies, 520
    risk, increase, 428
    treatment strategies, 520
Childhood obstructive sleep apnea (OSA)
    adjunctive therapies, 432
    CPAP indications, 429b
    leukotriene receptor antagonist montelukast,
        effectiveness, 431
    management, AAP guidelines, 427b
    nasal steroids, 431
    pharmacologic treatments, 431
    research areas, 432b
    treatment, tracheostomy (clinical indications),
        431b
    weight loss, 431–432
Childhood RLS, diagnostic criteria, 482b
Childhood sleep-related breathing disorders
    dental/orthodontic therapies, 431
    oral appliances, 431
Childhood systemic hypertension (HTN), 520
Children
    abnormal craniofacial anatomy, 430
    achondroplasia (AC), 507
        cervicomedullary compression, risk, 507
    adjunctive supportive care, 431–432
    Angelman syndrome (AS), 497
    anxiety, issues, 471
    atopic parent, eczema risk, 527–528
    attention deficit hyperactivity disorder
        (ADHD), interventions, 544
    autism spectrum disorders (ASDs)
        behavioral interventions, 542–543
        nonpharmacologic sleep interventions, 543t
        pharmacologic interventions, 543–544
        sleep complaints, 541
        treatments, 542–544
    bariatric surgery, 431
    bedtime, 471
        pass, 450–451
    behavioral extinction, 449
    behavioral insomnia, diagnosis/treatment,
        500–501
    behavioral interventions, 449b
    brainstem tumor, 444f
    cancer
        sleep disorders, 528–529
        sleep problems, 529
    cancer-related fatigue, treatment strategies,
        529b
    cardiac abnormalities, 440
    CCHS
        acute respiratory failure, vulnerability, 440
        therapy, 439
    central adrenal insufficiency, 496
    central apnea, 434–438
        normative data, 436
        term, usage, 434–435
    central sleep apnea, conditions, 435b
    cerebral palsy, SDB (treatment), 503
    cervical-medullary compression, 505b
    chronic snoring, 431
    circadian rhythm disorders
        background, 465–466
        evaluation, sleep history (usage), 468b
        treatment, 469
    circadian rhythms, disturbances, 500
    clinical history, usage, 469
    cognitive behavioral insomnia (CBI)
        treatments, 501

Children (Continued)
    complex patients, surgical therapies, 430–431
    continuous positive airway pressure (CPAP),
        429–430
    CPAP adherence data, absence, 429
    CPAP initiation/treatment, 429
    craniofacial procedures, 430
    daytime ventilation, 439–440
    delayed sleep phase, treatment guidelines, 473f
    diagnostic sleep studies, 500
    Down Syndrome (DS)
        sleep-disordered breathing, risk factors,
            494b
        sleep problems, 493
    eczema, house dust mite (HDM) allergy
        (impact), 528
    epileptic parasomnias, diagnostic issue, 504
    extinction with parental presence (E/PP), 450
    fragile X syndrome (FXS), 498–499
        clinical features, 498b
        sleep problems, 499
    gastroesophageal reflux, oral use
        pharmacologic treatments (FDA
        approval), 527t
    gastroesophageal reflux disease (GERD),
        pharmacologic treatments, 526
    GERD, treatment, 526
    graduated extinction (GE), 450
    growth hormone (GH), trials, 442
    insomnia
        absence/presence, parental practices, 449b
        parent education/problem prevention, 449
        presentation, 448
        treatment, Rett syndrome (inclusion), 497
    inspiratory vital capacity (IVC), 508
    insufficient sleep syndrome, treatment,
        519–520
    leukemia, dexamethasone (treatment), 528
    long-acting stimulant medication, 471
    medical disorders, sleep insufficiency/short
        sleep duration (impact), 519–520
    melatonin, secretion, 498
    narcolepsy, sleep medicine (therapy), 475–479
    nasal insufflation, 430
    neural crest abnormalities, 440
    neurodevelopmental disorders, 493–502
        melatonin therapy, effectiveness, 544
    neuromotor tone, 430
    neuromuscular disease (NMD), 508
        polysomnographic findings, 509
        sleep-disordered breathing, prediction,
            508–509
    nocturnal GERD, nonpharmacologic
        treatment strategies, 526b
    nonepileptic parasomnias, diagnostic issues,
        504
    obesity, odds ratio, 519
    obsessive-compulsive disorders, sleep
        problems (decrease), 542
    obstructive sleep apnea (OSA)
        commonness, 493
        improvement, allergic rhinitis (treatment),
            523–524
        perioperative complications/postoperative
            complications, risk factors, 429b
        persistence, 494
    PAP interface, 430
    polysomnographic findings, 509
    postoperative respiratory complications, risk
        factors, 428
    post-traumatic stress disorder (PTSD), sleep
        characteristics, 541
    Prader-Willi syndrome (PWS), 494–496
        central hypersomnia, 495
        exogenous growth hormone, risks/benefits,
            495–496

Children (Continued)
    sudden/premature death, risk (increase), 496
    psychiatric disorders
        pharmacologic interventions, 542
        sleep disturbances, relationship, 544b
    psychiatric disorders, sleep disturbances
        (treatment), 541–544
    respiratory abnormalities, 439–440
    respiratory control, 434
        anatomy/physiology, 434
    respiratory support therapies, 430
    Rett syndrome (RS), 496–497
        symptomatic/supportive treatments, 497b
    ROHHAD, 440–441
    scheduled awakenings, 451
    secondary obesity, PWS (impact), 494
    sleep complaints, 541
    sleep-disordered breathing (SDB), 520–521
    sleep disorders, commonness, 524
    sleep disturbances, psychiatric disorders
        (relationship), 544b
    sleep problems, decrease, 542
    sleep/wake patterns/behaviors, 519–520
    Smith-Magenis syndrome (SMS), 497–498
    soft tissue reduction surgery, 430
    systemic hypertension, treatment, 521
    total sleep duration, population-based
        epidemiologic study, 467f
    tracheostomy, 430
    treatment, success, 472
    wake maintenance zone, 466
    Williams syndrome (WS), 498
Children, autism spectrum disorders (ASDs),
        499–502
    behavioral insomnia, diagnosis/treatment,
        500–501
    diagnostic sleep studies, 500
    oral melatonin, prescribing, 501b
    risk factors, 499b
Children, epilepsy
    cervical-medullary compression, clinical
        symptoms, 505b
    insomnia (treatment), oral melatonin (usage),
        505
    sleep disorders, treatment, 504–505
Children, sleep
    actigraphy, usage, 500–501
    delay, 471
    disturbance, extinction, 449–450
    experience, 467
    graduated extinction, 450
    homeostatic drive, 465
    problems
        clinical evaluations, 468–469
        commonness, 499
        problems, evaluation, 467
    process, 448
    psychosocial/developmental issues, 467–468
    regulation, opponent-process model, 466f
Chinese medicine, 133
Chloral hydrate, 462
Chlorpheniramine, REM latency (relationship),
        121
Chokroverty, Sudhansu, 6
Cholecystokinin (CCK), 76
Cholinergic nucleus basalis of Meynert,
        degeneration, 333
Chorea, 352
    medications, impact, 355b
Chronic atopic eczema, treatment, 528
Chronic hypercapnia
    cause, 254
    treatment, absence, 257
Chronic hypoventilation, 254–258
    causes, 254f
    mechanisms, 254–257

Chronic illness model, 751
Chronic insomnia, 161, 172
  Morin's model, 184f
  unregulated pharmacologic approaches,
    172–173
Chronic invasive ventilation, spirometric results,
  256f
Chronic obstructive nasal symptoms, 523
Chronic obstructive pulmonary disorder
    (COPD), 177–178, 209, 255, 270–275
  acute exacerbations, 255
  co-morbid conditions, 272
  etiology/pathophysiology, 271–272
  overlap syndrome, relationship, 266–267
  PAP therapy, usage (contrast), 266
  placebo-controlled, crossover study, 272
  prevalence, estimation, 270
  risk factors, 274
  treatment, 274–275
Chronic pain, clinical principles, 595–596
Chronic primary insomnia, physiologic
    activation (relationship), 144
Chronic pulmonary disease
  etiology/pathophysiology, 271–272
  inclusion, 270
Chronic RBD
  etiologic associations, 551b
  neurologic disorders, 551b
  prodromal period, 549–550
Chronic respiratory failure (treatment), PAP/
    oxygen (usage), 275t
Chronic sleep deficiency, 381
Chronotherapy, 406, 408
  delayed sleep phase intervention, 472
  treatment, failure, 408
Chronotype, 405
Circadian amplitude, measurement, 363–364
Circadian clock
  adaptation, 391
  advancement, 392–396
  delay, 397–398
  flight, examples, 393f, 395f, 397f–398f
  gene, identification, 4
  landing, delay, 393–394
  light boxes, availability, 399
  light/melatonin, phase-shifting effect, 392f
  melatonin, availability, 399
  phase delay, usage, 397–398
  preflight advancement, 397
  problem, 394
  reset, light/melatonin (usage), 391
  short trips, coping, 399
  sleep, advancement, 397
  sleep/wake schedule, misalignment, 390
  synchronization, environmental stimulus, 391
Circadian disruption, 379–381
Circadian misalignment, effects, 372f, 697
Circadian pacemaker, sleep-wake state (impact),
  661
Circadian parameters, alterations, 161
Circadian period, measurement, 364
Circadian phase, 379–381
  abnormalities, 656
  hormonal markers, 374f
  light, intensity, 367
  measurement, 363–364
    DLMO, usage, 373
  outpatient circadian phase assessment, 374
Circadian phase resetting
  duration/pattern, 367
  light, properties, 365–367
  photic history, 367
  timing, 365–367
Circadian photic resetting, light (properties),
  366f

Circadian rhythm, 365–367
  abnormalities, 656
  amplitude, reduction, 416–417
  blindness, role, 365
  defining, 363–365
  disorder, nonentrained type, 370–371
  disruptions, 390
    anatomic basis, 417f
  disturbances, 500
  establishment, 465
  evening type clock, 369
  homeostatic drive, counterweight, 465
  impact, 368f
  measurement, 364f
    usage, 372–375
  morning type clock, 369
  persistence, 363
  reset ability, 364–365
Circadian rhythm disorders, 129
  evaluation
    issues, 467–469
    sleep history, usage, 468b
  melatonin, impact, 130
  sleep disorder, 668–669
  treatment, 469–474
    issues, 467–469
Circadian rhythm sleep disorders (CRSDs), 14,
    369–372
  Alzheimer's disease, impact, 418–420
  circadian phase, 369f
  clinical diagnostic criteria, 420–421
  clinical sleep disorders, percentage, 363
  clinical treatments, 421
  diagnosis
    circadian rhythms, measurement, 372–375
    clinical criteria, problems, 372
  diagnostic criteria, 364b, 403b
    irregular sleep-wake type, 416b
    medical condition, 419b
    nonentrained type, 412b
  light therapy, 419–421
  medical condition, impact, 418–421
  neurodevelopmental disorders (NDDs), 420
  neurologic disorders, 420–421
  pharmacologic treatment, 421
  shift work type, ICSD-2 diagnostic criteria,
    378b
  sleep, timing, 369f
  sleep disorder category, 11b–12b
  sleep patterns, 55f
  treatment, clinical criteria (problems), 372
Circadian sleep disorders, SCN dysfunction
    (impact), 55
Circadian sleep-wake cycle (alteration),
    melatonin (usage), 458
Circadian system, 363–365
Circadian timing system, temporal organization,
  54f
Circulation time (prolongation), left ventricular
    failure (impact), 247
Clinical Antipsychotic Trials of Intervention
    Effectiveness (CATIE), 708
Clinical sleep medicine/research, international
    training (support), 6
Clinical sleep professional societies, evolution, 5
Clock genes, anomalies, 500
Clomipramine, FDA approval, 690
Clonazepam
  long-term benefits, 553b
  NREM parasomnia treatment, FDA approval,
    187
  side effects, 553
  usage, 566–567
Cocaine, use/abuse, 753
Coffin-Lowry syndrome, 487

Cognitive behavioral insomnia (CBI) treatments,
  501
Cognitive behavioral therapy (CBT), 598
  effectiveness, 685, 689
Cognitive-behavioral therapy for insomnia
    (CBTi), 453
  approaches, 453
Cognitive behavior principles, 162–169
Cognitive behavior therapy (CBT), 185, 703
  impact, 14
  integrated psychological therapy, 167–169
  pharmacotherapy, comparison, 169
  studies, 188–189
Cognitive behavior therapy for insomnia
    (CBT-I), 151, 172
  comparison, 154
Cognitive behavior therapy-I (CBT-I), evidence
    base, 169
Cognitive control, 166
  instructions, 168b
Cognitive distortions, 189
Cognitive function, assessment, 19
Cognitive functioning, sleep disorders (impact),
  657
Cognitive model, 162
Cognitive symptoms, 600–601
Cognitive therapeutics, developments, 169–170
Cognitive therapy, 453
  focus, 454
  goals, 454b
Cognitive treatments, AASM endorsement, 163t
Coincidence detectors, 71–72
Coleman, Richard, 30
Colic, cause, 521
Combined ear referential montage, 639
Co-morbid insomnias
  nonpharmacologic treatments, effectiveness,
    541–542
  prevalence, 682
Co-morbid OSAS, differential diagnosis, 711
Co-morbid primary sleep disorders, usage, 596
Co-morbid psychiatric illness, 708
Co-morbid sleep conditions, 278
Co-morbid sleep disorders, 710–712
Complementary and alternative medicine
    (CAM)
  biologic compounds, usage, 128f
  female use, 127f
  NCCAM definition, 126
  prevalence, 127f
  research, 127f
  therapies, 126
  use, medical treatment, 126
Complex nocturnal visual hallucinations, 581
Complex partial seizures, 641
Complex sleep apnea, 251
Computerized digital vEEG-PSG systems,
    advantages, 640
Concentration-response curves (CRCs), 67b
Confusion, episodes, 17
Confusional arousals, 476–478, 559
  dominance, 573
  epoch, 560f
  ICSD-2 diagnostic criteria, 560b
  manifestation, 636
Congenital alveolar hypoventilation syndrome
    (CCHS)
  acute respiratory failure, vulnerability, 440
  cardiac abnormalities, 440
  clinical features, 438b
  diagnosis, 439
  genetics, 438–439
  individual education program (IEP), 440
  neural crest abnormalities, 440
  presentation, 439

Congenital alveolar hypoventilation syndrome (CCHS) *(Continued)*
respiratory abnormalities, 439–440
testing, 24
therapy, 439
Congenital blindness, 529–530
adolescent, actigraph, 530f
Congenital central hypoventilation syndrome (CCHS), 438–440
Congenitally blind children, free-running sleep/wake disorder, 530
Congestive heart failure (CHF), 209
Conjugate saccades, presence, 44f
Connective tissue disease, 599–600
Contamination fears, 690
Continuous positive airway pressure (CPAP), 208–209, 429–430
application, 249
BiPAP, contrast, 263–264
clinical outcomes, 231t
CPAP-related blood pressure changes, randomized controlled trials (meta-analysis), 213
cutoff point, 651f
device, usage, 233
effects, 249f
efficacy, 251f
impact, 4, 249
therapy
short-term randomized controlled trials, 651–652
usage, 218
titration, quality (improvement), 200
tolerance, 25
treatment, cerebrovascular endpoints, 652
usage, 197
cessation, 196–197
success, 230
Continuous spike waves in slow wave sleep (CSWS), 633–634
Control ventilation mode (timed ventilation mode), 260
Convulsive activity, technician (assistance), 644
Core insomnia symptoms, improvement, 165
Cortex norepinephrine, effects, 91f
Cortical arousal
EEG, impact, 48f
etiology, 565
Cortical EEG, changes, 43
Cortical myoclonus, 348
Cortical resective surgery, 635–636
Corticobasal degeneration (CBD), 330–331
Corticoganglionic degeneration (CBGD), 353
Corticotropin-releasing hormone (CRH), action, 75
Cortisol rhythms
salivary melatonin, relationship, 373
urinary melatonin, relationship, 373–375
Cortistatin, 76
Craniocervical junction (CCJ), 505
compression
clinical symptom, 506
disorders, risk, 506
Craniomandibular complex, 233
Craniopharyngiomas (CPs), benign characteristic, 529
Critical care ventilators, portable ventilators (contrast), 260
Culture (shape), sleep (impact), 3
Cyclic adenosine monophosphate (cAMP), formation (catalysis), 64
Cyclic alternating pattern (CAP), 561
biomarker, 565–566
biophysiologic markers, 566b
composition, 34
graph, 562f

Cyclic alternating pattern (CAP) *(Continued)*
illustration, 34f
NREM sleep, relationship, 563b
periodic EEG events, 476–477
presence, 595–596
types, 34
Cycloxygenase (COX), 612
CYP3A4 inhibitors, impact, 101
Cystic fibrosis (CF), 278–280, 526–527
episodic nocturnal desaturations, cause, 279–280
gas exchange, 278–280
hypoxemia/hypercapnia, presence, 526–527
melatonin, impact, 527
NIPPV, usage, 280
nocturnal hypopneas, impact, 279
nocturnal low flow oxygen, impact, 280
pathophysiology, 278
sleep
architecture, 278–280
characteristics, 279
sleepers, category, 278
sleep-related diagnostic/treatment strategies, 527
studies, 279t
treatment, 280
Cytochrome P-450 (CYP) 2D6, metabolism, 93
Cytochrome P-450 (CYP) hepatic enzymes, antidepressant effects, 115
Cytokines, 77–78
manipulation, 78
sleep promotion, 77
usage, 607–610
Cytosine-thymine-guanine (CTG) trinucleotide repeat, 24
Czeisler, Charles, 4
Cz referential montage, 639

D

D-amphetamine, DAT binding affinity, 90–91
Dawn simulator, 699f
Daytime clenching, damage, 324
Daytime dissociative disorders, sleep-related dissociative disorders (correspondence), 577–578
Daytime function, disruptions, 390
Daytime hypertension, sleep apnea (relationship), 649
Daytime hypoventilation, 262–263
Daytime impairment, types, 143b
Daytime QOL, improvement, 523
Daytime sleepiness
excess, 14–16, 294
GHB, usage, 489–491
Methylphenidate, usage, 488
Modafinil, usage, 488–489
orexin/hypocretin system, impact, 333
sodium oxybate, usage, 489–491
symptomatic treatment, 340
treatment, 488–491
pharmacotherapy, 488
Dead space to tidal volume ratio (VD/VT), 256
Deafferentation theory, 43–44
Deep brain stimulation (DBS), 334
treatment-related side effects, 340
Deep sleep, 43
Delayed sleep phase
circadian misalignment, 466f
intervention, chronotherapy (usage), 472
treatment
guidelines, 473f
sleep scheduling, usage, 470, 470f
types, 403b
Delayed sleep phase disorder (DSPD), 370, 402
actigraphy, example, 405f
chronotherapy, 406

Delayed sleep phase disorder (DSPD) *(Continued)*
free-running disorder, development, 406
treatment, failure, 408
chronotype, 405
clinical diagnosis, 402–405
combination treatments, 408
conceptualization, 402
diagnosis, 403
diagnostic features, 403b
entrainment, range, 406
genetic factors, 405
melatonin, 407–408
treatment, 407–408
nondiagnostic associated clinical features, 405–406
phase angle disorders, 405–406
phototherapy, 406–407
treatment, testing, 407
teenager problem, 465
treatment, 406–408
vitamin B$_{12}$, usage, 408
Delayed sleep phase syndrome (DSPS), 38–39, 453, 470–472
correction, 471
treatment, 471
Delta activity, low level, 187
Delta waves, 43
De Medicina (Aulus Cornelius Celsus), 607
Dement, William, 4–5, 7–8
Dementia
amplitude abnormalities, 656
circadian phase abnormalities, 656
definition, 656
patients, ISWR (light treatment), 419f
sleep, light studies, 660t
sleep disorders
mechanisms, 656–657
relationship, 656–657
relationship, framework, 657f
treatment, 657
sleep disruption, approach, 662b
sleep-wake states, circadian regulation (improvement), 659
syndromes, sleep disorders, 657–659
Dementia, frequency, 335
Dementia with Lewy bodies (DLB), 330–331
inclusion, sleep disorders, 658
Dental damage, 324–325
Dental evaluation/prognosis, 230–232
Depolarized plateau, production, 47
Depression
circadian rhythms, 540
commonness, 335
development, insomnia (risk factor), 676
diagnosis, 146
DSM4R basis, 146
prediction, sleep complaints (impact), 539
remission rate, 676–677
severity, dream recall (correlation), 185
sleep, hypothesis, 540f
sleep alterations, 678–679
symptoms, 339
Depressive disorder (treatment) Trazodone/Fluoxetine (combination usage), 542
Depressive symptoms, 597–598
Derivation, term (usage), 629
Desensitization, 67b
Desipramine, 88–90
Dextroamphetamine, abuse problems, 755
Diacylglycerol (DAG), conversion, 64
Diazepam, usage, 566
Dickens, Charles (sleep description), 3
Dietary Supplemental and Education Act (1994), 127
Differential diagnosis, usage, 641

Diffuse idiopathic skeletal hyperostosis (DISH), 599

Diffuse Lewy body disease (DLBD)
  dementia, inclusion, 353–354
  etiology, 353
  pathologic findings, 353
  treatment, 354

Digit symbol substitution test (DSST), 122

Dim light cortisol onset (DLCO), 373
  melatonin, administration, 407

Dim light melatonin onset (DLMO), 24
  circadian phase measurement, 373
  delay, 404–405
  usage, 404–405

Diphenhydramine
  efficacy, 122
  pediatric use, 122

Directional asymmetry, 391–392

Disease states, NIPPV usage, 262–267

Disordered sleep
  bidirectional relationship, 596f
  clinical presentation/manifestation, 448
  psychosocial distress, 597–598
  treatment, 602–603

Disorders of tau accumulation, 658–659

Dissociated brain activity, 563b

Dissociative disorder, feature, 577

Disturbed nocturnal sleep, 290, 293
  treatment options, 293

Diurnal involuntary movement disorders, 349–352

Diurnal NIPPV, 267

Doctoral level nonphysician clinicians, clinical training (history), 7

Dopamine (DA), 73–74
  biogenic monoamine transporter, 85
  clinical correlations, 73–74
  D_1/D_2 receptor sites, 116
  D_2 receptors, blockade, 116
  metabolism, iron (cofactor), 530–531
  movement, 88
  overview, 73
  receptors, 116
  reuptake inhibitors, schematic representations, 89f
  sleep-wake regulation, 73
  uptake inhibitors, effects, 90f

Dopamine agonists (DAs), impact, 333–334

Dopamine beta-hydroxylase (DBH), impact, 70

Dopaminergic agonists, treatment-related side effects, 340

Dopaminergic system, presynaptic modulation, 88–92

Dopaminergic terminal neurotransmission, schematic representations, 89f

Dopamine transporter (DAT), 70
  binding affinity, 90–91
  cloning, 88
  synaptic dopamine clearance, 73

Dorsal raphe (DR), serotonin (impact), 62

Dorsal raphe neurons (DRNs), 48
  noradrenergic/serotoninergic neurons, REMS-off neurons, 51

Dorso-medial hypothalamic (DMH) nucleus, SCN/SPZ projection, 55–56

Down Syndrome (DS), 493–494
  adenotonsillectomy (AT), treatment, 494
  sleep-disordered breathing, risk factors, 494b
  sleep problems, 493

Doxepin, examination, 114

Dream content, 183
  alteration, 550b

Dream-enacting behaviors, differential diagnosis, 551b

Dreaming, characteristics, 182

Dreams
  abnormalities, diagnostic implications, 183t
  change, steps, 184–185
  components, 182
  construction, tonic phasic hypothesis, 181
  content, examination, 183
  correlates, 182–183
  disorders, psychology (role), 183–187
  enactment behavior, 50
  focus, reasons, 189
  function, hypotheses, 181–182
  recall, depression (correlation), 185
  Recognize, Identify, Stop, Change (RISC) method, 184
  scenarios, change, 184–185
  sensory images, 182
  story, emotional component, 182
  studies, 181
  vividness, drugs (impact), 769t

Driving risks, 382–383

Drowsy driving, 382

Drug abuse
  definitions, 749
  DSM-IV definitions, 750t

Drug Abuse Screening Test (DAST), 751–752

Drug dependence
  definitions, 749
  DSM-IV definitions, 750t

Drug history, obtaining, 751–752

Drug-induced movement disorders, 354

Drug withdrawal
  definitions, 749
  tolerance, confusion, 749

Duchenne muscular dystrophy (DMD), 508
  expiratory muscles, weakness, 509
  respiratory care, 509

Durable medical equipment, prosthetics, orthotics, and supplies (DMEPOS) codes, 234

Dysfunctional Beliefs and Attitudes Sleep (DBAS) Scale, 23, 25, 166f–167f

Dystonia, 352
  medications, impact, 355b

E

Early childhood, insomnia (absence/presence), 449b

Edison, Thomas (light bulb invention), 3

Efficacy, 67b

Electroconvulsive status epilepticus in sleep (ESES), 633–634

Electroencephalogram (EEG), 29–30
  activity, 29
  alpha intrusions, 33–34
  arousal effects, 88–92
  behavioral arousal, relationship, 43–48
  beta, excess, 34
  beta activity, increase, 34
  coverage, 641
  invention, 4
  sleep spindle activity, excess, 34
  theta rhythms, 33

Electroencephalography (EEG), 25
  waveforms, 32f

Electrographic epileptic seizures, 629

Electromyogram (EMG), 29–30

Electromyography (EMG), 25

Electro-oculogram (EOG), 29–30
  waveforms, 32f

Encephale isole, 43–44

Endogenous circadian markers, measurements, 418

Endogenous circadian pacemaker, location, 379

Endothelial nitric oxide synthase (eNOS), 611

Endothelium-dependent flow-mediated dilation (E-DFMD), 213–214

Endothelium-independent nitroglycerin-induced dilation (E-INTGD), 213–214

Endotoxin (lipopolysaccharide), 77

End-tidal CO_2 measurement, usefulness, 30

Epilepsy, 503–505, 633–634
  chronic neurologic condition, 629
  clinical features, 504
  excessive daytime sleepiness (EDS), 505
  in-laboratory video-PSG (V-PSG), recommendation, 504
  interictal epileptiform discharges, 635t
  obstructive sleep apnea (OSA), 504
  seizures
    relationship, 505
    timing, 635t
  sleep, interrelation, 634–636
  sleep disorders, 505
    treatment, 504–505
  sleep problems, 504
  treatment, 635–636
  vagal nerve stimulation, 504

Epileptic parasomnias, diagnostic issues, 504

Epileptic seizure, 629

Epileptic sexsomnia, sleep-related hyperkinetic seizures (involvement), 573

Epileptiform discharges, 629

Epileptogenic, term (usage), 629

Episodic hyperventilation, breath holding, 496

Episodic nocturnal desaturations, impact, 279–280

Epworth Sleepiness Scale (ESS), 19, 23f
  basis, 281
  breathing disorders, 231
  score, baseline, 196–197
  usage, 237

Erythrocyte growth factor (EGF), 77–78

Escitalopram, usage, 683

Essential tremor (ET), 352
  Propranolol, usage, 352

Eszopiclone (Lunesta), usage, 460

European Sleep Research Society, 6

Evening type clock, 369

Exaggerated physiologic tremor, 352

Excessive daytime sleepiness (EDS), 14–16, 289
  bedtimes, 16
    shortness, impact, 16
  commonness, 335
  consequences, 14–16
  fatigue, contrast, 14
  improvement, 292
  multiple sclerosis, relationship, 667
  napping, 16
  parasomnias, 17
  pediatric narcolepsy, pharmacologic treatment, 489t
  pharmacologic compounds, usage, 86t
  Prader-Willi syndrome relationship, 441
  recommendations, 302
  RLS, impact, 17
  sleep disruption, impact, 337
  sleep patterns, 16
  stimulants, usage, 292
  subjective complaints, 529
  treatment, 292–293

Excessive fragmentary myoclonus (EFM), 349
  differential diagnosis, 349
  EMG pattern, 349

Excessive motor restlessness, iron deficiency (impact), 531

Exchange diffusion, 88

Excitatory amino acid transporter (EAAT), 71b

Exercise, impact, 156–157

Exogenous leptin, impact, 76–77

Exogenous melatonin
    efficacy, 128
    relationship, 129
    side effect, 396
Expiratory muscles, weakness, 509
Expiratory positive airway pressure (EPAP), 259
Expiratory pressure, 250
    titration, 250
Extended EEG monitoring, 639–640
Extended EEG-polysomnography, 640t
Extinction-based sleep treatments, response, 450
Extinction with parental presence (E/PP), 450
Extracellular receptor kinase (ERK), 610
Extracellular signal-regulated kinases pathway, 611
Extracellular sleep regulatory substances,
    pathways, 609f
Extraoral evaluation, 233
Extrapyramidal motor symptoms (EPS),
    production (risk), 118
Extrasynaptic receptor signaling, 65
Extrinsic PEEP, 255
Eye movement desensitization and reprocessing
    (EMDR), 186
Eye movement detection, 29

F
Facial dyskinesias, medications (impact), 356b
Factor S, 57–58
Faded bedtime with/without response cost
    (FB/RC), 451–452
Family history, 18
Fatal familial insomnia (FFI), 356–357
    sleep disorders, 659
Fatigue, 600–601, 666–667
    clinical principles, 595–596
    description, 666
    excessive daytime sleepiness, contrast, 14–16
    Modafinil, relationship, 667
    polysomnography, 596
    psychosocial distress, 597–598
    scales (reduction), Modafinil (usage), 667
    shift work, relationship, 382
    sleep-wake cycles, relationship, 669
Fatigue Impact Scale (FIS), 666
Fatigue-related crashes, ATSB operational
    definition, 382
Fatigue Severity Scale (FSS), 666
    basis, 281
Fatty acid amide hydrolase (FAAH), 77
Fatty acid amides, 77
Federation of Latin American Sleep Societies, 6
Fellowship Training Committee (ASDA), 6
Fencamfamin, structure (similarity), 87
Fenfluramine, impact, 195–196
Fibroblast growth factor (FGF), 77–78
Fibromyalgia
    balenotherapy, impact, 135
    massage, impact, 135
    SLE co-morbidity, 599
    traditional Chinese medicine, impact, 133
    treatment
        antidepressant drugs, usage, 114
        FDA-approved medications, 601t
Fibromyalgia syndrome (FMS), 600
    concept, characterization, 600–601
    nonrestorative sleep, commonness, 601
    symptoms, modulation (nonpharmacologic
        methods), 602f
First-generation antipsychotics (FGAs)
    sleep maintenance improvement, 709
    usage, 707–708, 708b
First night effect, 31–33
5-hydroxytryptamine (5-HT), 63, 85
    monoamine neurotransmitter, 200

5-hydroxytryptophan, 131
Flashbacks, 186
Flip-flop switches, formation, 62
Flow generator
    airflow creation, 206
    tubing, connection, 207
Fluoxetine
    PSG studies, 113
    Trazodone, combination usage, 542
Flyover night, 155
Follicle-stimulating hormone (FSH), melatonin
    (impact), 129–130
Foods
    allergy, atopic eczema (association), 528
    avoidance, 618–619
Forced desynchrony protocol, 368–369
Forced expiratory volume in 1 second (FEV$_1$),
    reduction, 273, 278
Forebrain arousal system, 46–48
Fragile X mental retardation 1 (FMR1) gene, 498
Fragile X mental retardation 1 protein (FMRP),
    498
Fragile X syndrome (FXS), 498–499
    clinical features, 498b
Fragmentary myoclonus, excess, 349
Fragmented sleep, all-night histogram, 274f
Free-running circadian rhythm disorder,
    congenitally blind adolescent (actigraph),
    530f
Free-running disorder, development, 406
Free-running sleep-wake cycle, 414
Free-running type, 411
    circadian rhythm disorder, 370–371
Friedman anatomic staging system, 219t
Friedman tongue position (FTP), 219f
    description, 218–219
Friedman tonsil classification system, 219f
Frontal Assessment Battery (FAB), 19
Frontal lobe epilepsy, 25
Frontal Lobe Epilepsy and Parasomnias (FLEP)
    scale, 23
Frontal lobe seizures, occurrence, 632
Frontotemporal dementia, characterization,
    658–659
Full face mask, 206–207
    oronasal mask, 261f
Functional magnetic resonance imaging (fMRI),
    25
Functional Outcomes in Sleep Questionnaire
    (FOSQ), basis, 281
Functional residual capacity (FRC), decrease,
    279–280

G
Gabapentin, double-blind crossover study, 119
Galanin, 75
Gamma-aminobutyric acid (GABA), 34, 72–73
    alpha subtypes, differential brain distribution,
        99–100
    benzodiazepine receptors, impact, 99
    BZRA hypnotics, 174
    clinical correlations, 73
    GABAergic interactions, 50
    GABAergic transmission, enhancement, 73
    impact, 46–47
    overview, 72
    receptor subtypes, 99
    sleep-wake control, 99
    sleep-wake regulation, 72–73
    synaptic vesicle release, 62
Gamma-aminobutyric acid A (GABA$_A$) receptor,
    100f
    complex, 99–100
    subtypes, alpha subunit basis, 100t

Gamma-aminobutyric acid class A (GABA$_A$)
    receptor
    ligand-gated ion channel, 72f
    synaptic signaling importance, 72
Gamma-hydroxybutyrate (GHB), 75
    central nervous system depressant effects, 490
    narcolepsy treatment, 462
    synthesis, 72
    usage, 489–491
Gap junctions, 78
Gastric banding, 196–197
Gastric bypass, effectiveness, 227
Gastric refluxate, toxicity, 619
Gastroesophageal reflux
    occurrence, 617
    pharmacologic treatments, FDA approval,
        527t
Gastroesophageal reflux disease (GERD)
    behavioral approaches, 618–619
    characterization, 617
    development, obesity (risk factor), 618
    diagnosis, 525–526
        upper gastrointestinal series, impact, 526
    endoscopic therapies, 621
    pharmacologic treatments, 526
    positional therapy, 619
    potentiation, medications (avoidance),
        619–620
    primary sleep disorder, 638
    sleep complaints, 272
    smoking, impact, 619
    symptoms, 525t
    treatment, 277, 526
    worsening, 525
GBR12909, DA uptake inhibitor, 88–90
Generalized 2.5-Hx spike/wave/polyspike/wave
    discharges, 631f–632f
Generalized anxiety disorder (GAD), 188–189,
    682–685
    benzodiazepines, usage, 683
    buspirone, usage, 683
    characterization, 682
    cognitive behavioral therapy (CBT),
        effectiveness, 685
    epidemiology, 682–683
    Escitalopram, usage, 683
    nonpharmacologic treatment, 685
    pharmacologic treatment, 683–685
        list, 684t
    phenomenology, 682–683
    Pregabalin, impact, 119–120
    research, 682
    sleep dysfunction, objective evidence, 683
    Venlafaxine, usage, 683
Generalized Anxiety Disorder (GAD-7)
    Assessment, 14, 16f
Generalized epilepsies, 629–630
    interictal epileptiform discharges, 632t
    seizures, timing, 632t
Generalized seizures, antiepileptic drugs
    (impact), 635t
Generalized sleep management, 602
Genetic testing, 24
George Gauge
    components, 235f
    placement, 235
    record, 235, 235f
Geriatric patient, central sleep apnea, 739–740
    bilevel positive airway pressure, effectiveness, 740
    clinical consequences, 739–740
    evaluation, 740
    pathophysiology, 739
    positive airway pressure, 740
    prevalence, 739
    treatment, 740

Geriatric patient, circadian rhythm sleep disorders, 744–745
  assessment, 745
  clinical consequences, 745
  light/dark signals, response, 744
  pathophysiology, 744
  prevalence, 744–745
  treatment, 745
  wrist actigraphy record, 744f
Geriatric patient, insomnia (cognitive behavioral therapy), 738t
Geriatric patient, obstructive sleep apnea, 737–739
  clinical consequences, 738
  evaluation, 738
  pathophysiology, 737
  prevalence, 737–738
  symptoms (improvement), oral appliances (usage), 739
  treatment, 738–739
Geriatric patient, periodic limb movement disorder, 742
Geriatric patient, REM behavior disorder, 742–743
  diagnostic criteria, 742
  evaluation, 743
  pathophysiology, 742–743
  polysomnography (PSG) recording, 742f
  prevalence, 743
  treatment, 743
Geriatric patient, restless legs syndrome, 740–742
  clinical consequences, 741
  evaluation, 741
  pathophysiology, 740–741
  pharmacologic treatments, 741t
  prevalence, 741
  treatment, 741–742
Geriatric patient, sleep, 735
  clinical consequences, 736
  evaluation, 736
  insomnia medications, 737t
  medication therapy, 736
  pathophysiology, 735–736
  prevalence, 736
  treatment, 736–737
Geriatric patient, sleep-disordered breathing, 737–740
Ghost oppression (sleep paralysis), 554
Ghrelin, 76–77
Girls, Rett Syndrome (symptomatic/supportive treatments), 497b
Glial-derived neurotrophic factor (GDNF), 77–78
Glial EAAT, 71–72
Global Initiative for Chronic Obstructive Lung Disease (GOLD) criteria, 270
Global seasonality score (GSS), 697
  scoring, 698f
Glutamate, 71–72
  clinical correlations, 72
  overview, 71–72
  sleep-wake regulation, 72
Glutamatergic compounds, 96
Glycine, 74
Goldman equation, 71b
Good sleepers, 278
G protein-coupled receptors (GPCRs), 63–64
  impact, 78
  signaling, details, 64
Graduated extinction (GE), 450
Gram-positive bacteria, peptidoglycan (presence), 612
Growth factors, impact, 608b
Growth hormone (GH), 76
  impact, 442–443
  trials, demonstration, 442

Growth hormone-releasing hormone (GHRH), 76
  impact, 607
Guanasine triphosphate (GTP), circulation, 64
Guillain-Mollaret triangle, involvement, 350

H

H_1 antagonists, use, 122
H_2 receptor antagonists
  impact, 620
  safety, 621
Haemophilus influenzae, 278
Hallucinations, commonness, 335
Hard palate shortening (transpalatal advancement pharyngoplasty), 221–222
Hatfield, Mark, 7–8
Hay fever (seasonal AR), control, 523
Head, sagittal MRI, 237f
Healthcare Common Procedures Coding System (HCPCS), 234
Heart, CPAP (effects), 249f
Heart failure (HF)
  improvement, CRT therapy (usage), 248
  patients, 590
    differences, 247
  sudden cardiac death, 590
  therapy, 590
Heart rate trend, AECG recording, 588f
Hemifacial spasm, 351
  treatment, 351
Heteroreceptors, 67b
High dopa dyskinesias (HDD), occurrence, 354
Histamine, 73
  clinical correlations, 73
  overview, 73
  sleep-wake regulation, 73
Histamine H_1 receptor antagonists, 179
Histaminergic H3 antagonists, 96
HLA DQB1*0602 test, 24
Home noninvasive nocturnal ventilation, impact, 509
Homeostatic mechanisms, abnormalities, 656
Homeostatic sleep drive, impact, 55f
Home sleep testing (HST), 28–29, 39–40
  classification, 39t
  indications, 39
  interpretation, 40
  procedures, 39–40
Hops (humulus lupulus), 132–133
  active ingredient, 132–133
  safety profile, 133
  side effects, 133
Horne and Ostberg Questionnaire (HOQ), 23
Hot baths
  impact, 153
  usage, 157, 184
House dust mite (HDM) allergy, 528
Human immunodeficiency virus (HIV), sleep (relationship), 613
Human sleep, staging (AASM rules update), 43
Humoral sleep factors, research, 58
Humoral somnogens, impact, 62
Huntington's disease (HD), sleep disorders, 659
Hydroxytryptophan, 131–132
  safety profile, 131–132
  side effects, 131–132
Hyoid expansion, 224–225
  Repose screws, insertion, 224f
Hyoid suspension, 224
  nonabsorbable sutures, usage, 224f
Hyomandibular suspension, 224–225
  hyoid expansion, combination, 225
  Repose screws, insertion, 224f
Hyperarousal, pattern, 104

Hypercapnia
  importance (absence), PAP therapy (impact), 264
  presence, 526–527
  ventilation, responses, 255f
Hypercapnic ventilatory response, 247
Hyperekplexia, 348, 351
  classification, 351b
  treatment, 351
Hyperphagia, atypical depressive symptoms, 697
Hypersomnias
  conditions (ICSD-2), 297
  sleep disorder category, 11b–12b
Hypersomnolence, demonstration, 43–44
Hypertension (HTN), 589
  incidence, 213
  therapy, 589
  treatment, 521
Hyperventilation, hypercarbia (association), 441
Hypervigilance, 186
Hypnagogic foot tremor, 347
Hypnagogic hallucinations (HHs), 289, 485–486, 580–581
  treatment, 293
Hypnic jerks, 349, 638
Hypnic starts, 475
Hypnopompic hallucinations, 580–581
Hypnotic agents, usage, 214
Hypnotic BZRAs
  FDA approval, 101t
  half-lives, 100
Hypnotic medication, dependence, 105–106
Hypnotic response, assessment, 128
Hypnotics
  indications, 102
  interaction, agents (impact), 101b
  self-administration, 106
Hypocarbia, hyperventilation (association), 441
Hypocretin-1 measurement, narcolepsy analysis, 291b
Hypocretin-based therapies, 95–96
Hypocretin deficiency, biochemical implications, 290
Hypocretin neurons
  impact, 290f
  loss, 290–291
  transplantation, 295
Hypocretin/Orexin, discovery, 487
Hypocretin receptor function, 96
Hypocretin system (Orexin system), impact, 290
Hypomania, reports, 701
Hypopharyngeal obstruction (correction), surgery (usage), 220
Hypopnea, 34–35
  AASM definition, 207, 208t
  CMS definition, 207
Hypothalamic SCN, pacemaker activity, 656
Hypoventilation syndromes, 209
Hypoxemia
  presence, 526–527
  treatment, PAP/oxygen (usage), 275t
Hypoxemic CF patients, arterial oxygen saturation (maintenance), 280
Hypoxia
  episodes, repetition, 648–649
  ventilation, responses, 255f
Hypoxic ventilatory response, 247

I

Ictal EEG, demonstration, 632
Ictal epileptiform discharges, occurrence, 629
Idiopathic hypersomnia (IH), 16, 297–300
  amphetamines, usage, 298–299
  Armodafinil, usage, 299

Idiopathic hypersomnia (IH) *(Continued)*
  behavioral treatment, 299
  characteristics, 298b
  definition, 297–298
  epidemiologic study, absence, 297
  long sleep time, inclusion, 297
  management, 298–299
  melatonin, usage, 299
  methylphenidate, usage, 299
  Modafinil, usage, 299
  pathophysiology, 297–298
  pharmacologic treatment, 298–299
  prevalence, 297–298
  treatment, 299
Idiopathic pulmonary fibrosis (IPF), 281
  ILD variation, 282
  pulmonary hypertension, occurrence, 281
Idiopathic RBD, 552
Imagery rehearsal therapy (IRT), 186
  program, execution (method), 186
Immobilization test, 28, 38
Immune signals, 77–78
Immune-sleep interactions, complexity, 613
Impulse control disorders (ICDs), impact, 316
Incandescent light bulb, invention (Edison), 3
Incident stroke, SDB linkage (mechanisms), 648t
Inducible NOS (iNOS), 611
  impact, 75
Infants
  achondroplasia (AC), 507
    cervicomedullary compression risk, 507
  apparent life-threatening events, 437–438
    differential diagnosis, 437b
  atopic eczema, food allergy (association), 528
  bedtime pass, 450–451
  benign sleep myoclonus, 348–349
  central apnea
    normative data, 435–436
    term, usage, 434–435
  Chiari type I malformation, 443f
  colic, 521
    cause, 521
    nonpharmacologic interventions, 521
  extinction with parental presence (E/PP), 450
  faded bedtime, response cost (inclusion/
    exclusion), 451–452
  gastroesophageal reflux, oral use
    pharmacologic treatments (FDA
    approval), 527t
  graduated extinction (GE), 450
  insomnia, 448–452
  iron deficiency, 530–531
    risk factors, 530b
  iron deficiency anemia (IDA), 530
  napping, 520
  nocturnal GERD, nonpharmacologic
    treatment strategies, 526b
  oxygen saturation, acute decreases, 436
  periodic breathing, 435f, 438
  positive routines (PRs), 451
  respiratory abnormalities, 439–440
  rhythmic movements, 476
  Standard Treatments, 452
Inflammation, 607–610
  impact, 648–649
  mechanisms, 607
  occurrence, 607
  sleep disorders, relationship, 614–615
Inflammatory arthritis, 598–599
Inflammatory mediators, manipulation, 78
Influenza, 612–613
Influenzavirus-induced sleep responses
  attenuation, 611
  magnitude/course, 613
Information, chemical transfer, 65

Inhibitory postsynaptic potential (IPSP), impact, 99
Innate immunity, 607
Inositol triphosphate (IP$_3$), conversion, 64
Inputs, collective synaptic potentials, 48f
Insomnia, 13–14, 128–129
  acupuncture, impact, 133
  adolescence, 452–454
  ancillary tests, 24–25
  anxiety disorder, relationship, 146
  balneotherapy, impact, 135
  behavioral conditioning, inappropriateness,
    145–146
  behavioral extinction, 449
  cause, SSRIs (impact), 502
  classification, 144–148
  clinical consequences, 736
  cognitive approaches, 165–169
  cognitive control, 166
  cognitive model, 162
  complaints, 13, 421
  daytime/evening behaviors, assessment, 13–14
  daytime habits/behaviors, 13–14
  daytime symptoms, 13–14
  defining, problems, 717–718
  definition, 143
  development, 145–146
    factors, 162f
  diagnosis, 143b
  differential diagnosis, 13b, 144–148
  disorders, differential diagnosis, 145b
  dreams, content, 183
  dysfunctional beliefs, 165
  EEG sleep patterns, 614
  efficacy, BZRA dose range, 103
  exercise, impact, 156–157
  extinction, 449–450
  features, 161
  hydroxytryptophan, impact, 131
  impairments, 143–144
  investigational compounds, 178–179
  investigations, 23–25
  massage, impact, 135
  medical conditions, 146–147
  medical issues, 146–148
  medical problems
    association, 144
    prevalence, 147t
  medications, 457–462, 737t
  middle childhood, 452
  models, 161–162
  napping, 14
  neurocognitive model, 161–162
  oral melatonin, usage, 505
  paradoxical intention, 164–165
  patient health questionnaire (PHQ9), 14
  performance, 144
  pharmacologic agents, approval (absence), 470
  physiologic effects, 144
  Predisposing, Precipitating, Perpetuating (3P)
    model, 161
  prescribing guidelines, 176–178
  prevalence, 143
    increase, 143
  psychiatric illnesses, relationship, 146
  psychobiologic inhibition/attention-intention-
    effort model, 162
  psychological management, 162–169
  psychological/psychiatric effects, 14
  psychology, role, 183–185
  residual insomnia, 709–710
  sleep deprivation, contrast, 143
  sleep disorders
    category, 11b–12b
    relationship, 147–148
  sleep history, elements, 148–149

Insomnia *(Continued)*
  sleep restriction therapy, 163–164
  St. John's wort, impact, 132
  stimulus control treatment, 163
  subclassifications, 144b
  subjective nature, 717
  substance use/abuse/withdrawal, impact, 147
  symptoms, 458
    improvement, 165
  term, misuses, 448
  treatment, 184–185, 273–274
    antidepressant drugs, usage, 114
    CAM biologic compounds, usage, 128f
    cognitive therapy, goals, 454b
    drugs, usage characteristics, 770t
    response, 144
    sleep hygiene therapy, evidence, 154–155
    valerian, impact, 130–131
    yi-gan san, usage, 554
  valerian, impact, 130–131
Insomnia medications
  considerations, 177
  FDA approval, 173–176, 175t
  selection, 178
  usage, 147, 176–177
Insomnia Severity Index (ISI), 19, 22f
Inspiratory positive airway pressure (IPAP), 209,
    259
Instrumental conditioning, 161
Intellectual disability (ID), 493, 502
Intensified hypnic jerks, 348
Intensive care unit (ICU) management, 264–266
Intensive sleep retraining (ISR), 169
Intercollicular transections, 43–44
Inter-groaning intervals, 579
Interictal, term (usage), 629
Interictal epileptiform discharges (IEDs)
  impact, 634
  occurrence, 629
Interleukin 1 (IL-1), 77
  IL-1B, extracellular sleep regulatory
    substances, 609f
  IL-1RA, impact, 608
  IL-18, impact, 608
  impact, 607
  superfamily, 608
Interleukin 6 (IL-6) superfamily, 610
Intermaxillary fixation (IMF), 225–226
Intermediate cerebrovascular endpoints, CPAP
    treatment, 652
Intermediolateral (IML) cell column,
    projections, 56
Intermittent hypoxia, impact, 648–649
Internal globus pallidus (GPi), stimulation, 334
International 10-20 System of Electrode
    Placement, 639
International Classification of Sleep Disorders
    (ICSD)
  ICSD-2 sleep disorder categories, 11b–12b
  publication, 10
International normalized ratio (INR) elevation,
    melatonin (usage), 78
International RLS Severity (IRLS) Rating, 23
Interpersonal therapy (IPT), 185
Interstitial lung disease (ILD), 281–283
  arterial oxygen saturation, 282–283
  clinical presentation, 281
    variation, 281
  co-morbid sleep conditions, 281
  contributing conditions, 281
  OSA, impact, 281
  pathophysiology, 281
  sleep architecture, 282–283
    studies, 282t
  treatment, steroids (usage), 283

Intra-arterial blood pressure, recordings, 591f
Intracellular G proteins, usage, 64f
Intracranial EEG study, usage, 25
Intraoral evaluation, 233
Intravenous immunoglobulin (IVIG) therapy, 487
Intrinsic positive end-expiratory pressure (iPEEP), 255
Intrusive thoughts, 690
Invasive mechanical ventilation, 259
    challenge, increase, 267
Invasive ventilation, 258–259
Inventories, usage, 19–23
Inverse agonists, 67b
Involuntary movement disorders, 349–350
    persistence, 350–351
Involuntary movements, persistence, 351–352
Ion channel
    classification, 71–72
    gating, 71b
Ionotropic receptors, 64f
    cell surface proteins, 63
Iron deficiency, 5
    risk factors, 530b
Iron deficiency anemia (IDA), 530
    peak period, 530
Iron lung ventilators, usage, 258–259
Irregular sleep-wake rhythm (ISWR), 370–371, 415–418, 472–474
    characterization, 415–416
    circadian rhythms
        amplitude, reduction, 416–417
        disruption, anatomic basis, 417f
    clinical diagnostic criteria, 417
    clinical treatments, 418
    definitions, 415–417
    demographics, 418
    description, 415–417
    hypnotics, usage, 661
    light therapy, 659
    light treatment, 419f
    melatonin, usage, 659
    multicomponent therapy, 660
    multiphasic sleep, 371
    sleep, anatomic basis, 417f
    stimulants, usage, 661
    structured behavioral activities, impact, 659–660
    treatment, 659–661
        steps, 473
Ischemic stroke, circadian variation, 648f
Isolated sleep paralysis (ISP), 475–476
    characterization, 554
    diagnostic criteria, 554b
    differential diagnosis, 555
    recurrence, 554–555
Isolated sleep-related motor symptoms, 347–349

J
Janus kinases (JAKs), 610
Jet lag, 38–39, 148
    age, effects, 392
    cause, 390
    circadian clock/sleep-wake schedule, misalignment, 390
    defining, 390
    directional asymmetry, 391–392
    disorder, 369–370
    duration, 390
    exogenous melatonin, side effect, 396
    flight, examples, 393f, 395f, 397f–398f
    length, determination (factors), 391–392
    light boxes, availability, 399
    management, approaches, 392

Jet lag (Continued)
    melatonin
        availability, 399
        usage, 398–399
    occurrence, 390
    phase delay, usage, 397–398
    preflight interventions, testing, 396–397
    preflight schedules, melatonin (recommendation), 396
    reduction, methods, 398–399
    risks, 378–379
    short trips, coping, 399
    sleep, advancement, 397
    sleeping pills, usage, 399
    stimulants, usage, 399
Juvenile myoclonic epilepsy, 629
Juvenile rheumatoid arthritis (JRA), 599

K
Kainate subtypes, ion channel classification, 71–72
Kales, Anthony, 4
Kanashiban (sleep paralysis), 554
Karolinska Sleepiness Scale (KSS), 19, 23b
K complexes, 30–31
Klearway Oral Appliance, 236f
    engagement, 236f
Kleine-Levin syndrome, 301
    compulsive eating, absence, 301–302
        treatment (effect), pharmacologic agents (usage), 302t
    pharmacologic treatments, 300–301
    prophylactic treatment, 301
    symptomatic treatment, 301
    treatment (effect), pharmacologic agents (usage), 301t
Kleitman, Nathaniel, 4
Knockin mice, 71b
Knockout mice, 71b
    absence, 85
Kyphoscoliosis, 258

L
Laboratory clinical polysomnography, 28
Laboratory tests, classification, 39t
Landau-Kleffner syndrome, 633–634
Laryngospasm, sleep-related GERD (relationship), 623
Latency, sleep measure, 74
Latency to persistent sleep, 30
Lateral hypothalamus (LH), neurons, 46f
Lateral pontine tegmentum (LPT), REMS-off neurons (location), 50
Laterodorsal tegmental (LDT)
    brainstem cholinergic activating system location, 48f
    LDT/PPT REMS-on neurons, 51
    nuclei, 45
Learned insomnia, symptoms, 146b
Left eye EOG, 37
Left ventricular ejection fraction (LVEF), 248
Left ventricular function (reduction), CPAP (impact), 249
Leg movements
    durations, range, 38
    events, 36f
Leg muscle activation, alternation, 347
Lennox-Gastaut syndrome, 630
Leptin, 76–77
Leukemia, dexamethasone (treatment), 528
Levodopa (L-dopa) (LD)
    LD-induced nighttime myoclonus, 354
    LD-related abnormal movements, occurrence, 354
    treatment-related side effects, 340

Lewy body dementia (LBD), 50
Ligand-gated ion channel, 72f
Light
    alerting effects, 399
    box, 698f
        availability, 399
    bulb, invention (Edison), 3
    delay regions, timing, 391
    exposure, 470
    information, capture, 365
    intensity, 367
    phase advance, timing, 391
    phase-shifting effect, 392f
    rhythms, 365–367
    therapy, 412–413, 419–420, 659
        dawn simulation, 699
    visor, 699f
Light-dark cycle, melatonin (impact), 367
Limb jerks, 521
Lipid rafts, 65
Lipopolysaccharide (LPS), 609f
    endotoxin, 77
Lithium, sleep-enhancing effects, 678
Localization-related epilepsies
    interictal epileptiform discharges, 635t
    partial epilepsies, 630–633
    seizures, timing, 635t
Locus ceruleus (LC)
    lesions, 45–46
    neurons (innervation), hypocretin neurons (impact), 290f
    nonadrenergic neurons, 46f
    noradrenergic/serotoninergic neurons, REMS-off neurons, 51
Long-acting agents, usage, 292
Long-term health risks, 383–384
Long-term hypocretin deficiency, 96
Long-term NIPPV, 258
Long-term nocturnal NIPPV, consideration, 259
Long-term nocturnal ventilation, 258
Long-term oxygen therapy (LTOT), 274
    usage, 266
Loop gain, 246
Low calorie diet (LCD), 195
Low dopa dyskinesias (LDD), initiation, 354
Low-dose doxepin, availability, 177–178
Lower esophageal sphincter (LES)
    pressure (reduction)
        oral/intravenous β2-receptor agonists, impact, 619
    pressure (reduction), nicotine (impact), 619
Lower esophageal sphincter (LES), antireflux barrier, 617
Lower teeth, acrylic occlusal splints, 327f
Lumbar puncture, 24
Luteotropic hormone (LH), melatonin (impact), 129–130

M
Maintenance insomnia, 539
Maintenance of Wakefulness Test (MWT), 24, 37–38
    indications, 37
    principles, usage, 37–38
    procedures, 37–38
Major affective disorder, criteria, 695
Major depressive disorder (MDD), 112, 675–678
    antidepressant treatment, sleep disturbance (impact), 676–677
    development, insomnia (risk factor), 676
    diagnosis, 113
    diagnostic criteria, 676b
    occurrence, 675
    polysomnographic alterations, 676t

Major depressive disorder (MDD) (*Continued*)
  polysomnographic features, limitations, 676
  sleep alterations, association, 675
  sleep deprivation, antidepressant effects, 677
  sleep difficulty, diagnostic criteria, 675
  sleep disturbance, symptom, 678
  sleep-related consideration, 677
  SSRIs/SNRIs, sleep-wake effects, 677
Major mood disorder (MMD), 188–189
Malignant ventricular arrhythmias, risk
    (quantification), 585–586
Mallampati classification, 218–219
Mallampati score, 18
Mallampati scoring system, 282f
Mandible
  advancement, 238f
  forward titration, 237
Mandibular advancement appliance (MAA),
    usage, 326
Mania
  feature, 540
  primary treatments, 678
  sleep alterations, 678–679
Manic episodes, reports, 701
Manipulation treatments, 135
Manual tracking test (MTT), 122
Marijuana (*Cannabis sativa*/
    tetrahydrocannabinol), 753
Mask interfaces, 261f
Mask leaks, minimization, 261
Massage, 135
Maxillomandibular advancement (MMA),
    225–226
Maximal inspiratory pressure, 250
Mazindol, 94–95
  schedule IV controlled drug, 94–95
m-chlorophenylpiperazine (mCPP), action, 115
Meal, timing, 618
Mean arterial blood pressure (MAP), recordings,
    650f
Mean basal forebrain extracellular adenosine
    values, 52f
Mean BNP, 590f
Mechanical load, 649
Medial pontine reticular formation (mPRF),
    carbachol (injection), 50–51
Median preoptic nucleus (MnPO), sleep-active
    neurons (location), 48
Medical disorders, sleep insufficiency/short sleep
    duration (impact), 519–520
Medical GERD therapy, impact, 622
Medical history, 18
Medical Outcomes Study Short Form (SF-36), 143
Medical reports, examination, 19
Medicare, level II coding system, 234
Medication, impact, 18
Medications
  sedative-hypnotic properties, 462
Meditation, 134
Melancholia, description, 109
Melanin-concentrating hormone (MCH), 76
  lateral hypothalamic orexin neurons,
      combination, 46–47
  neurons, 46f
Melanopsin, sensitivity, 365
Melatonin, 74, 367
  administration, higher doses (impact), 396
  age-related insomnia, link, 128
  availability, 399
  biologic compound, 127–130
  clinical correlations, 74
  effects, 129
  efficacy, assessment, 398–399
  endogenous role, 56–57
  hormonal measures, 373

Melatonin (*Continued*)
  idiopathic hypersomnia usage, 299
  impact, 56–57, 129–130
  oral melatonin, prescribing, 501b
  overview, 74
  phase-shifting effect, 392f
  pineal gland production, 56
  pineal gland secretion, 384
  preflight schedules, recommendation, 396
  production, SCN (temporal relationship), 367
  prolonged-release formulations, 129
  research studies, summary, 128t
  safety profile, 129–130
  salivary melatonin, 373
  secretion, inversion, 498
  side effects, 129–130
  sleep-wake regulation, 74
  test dose, 399
  urinary melatonin, 373–375
  urine, collection, 374
  usage, 398–399, 409
    effectiveness, 399
Melatonin receptor agonists, 179, 458
Membrane receptors, neurotransmitter response,
    63
Memory
  consolidation, 181–182
    hypothesis, prediction, 182
  formation, synaptic (Hebbian) theories, 71–72
  testing, 643
Meningomyelocele, 505–506
  sleep-disordered breathing, treatment, 506
Menopausal status, vasomotor symptoms
    (relationship), 721
Menopausal transition
  sleep, 719–723
  vasomotor symptoms
    population-based surveys, 721
    role, 721–722
Menopausal women
  reproductive hormones, sleep (association), 722
  sleep complaints, evaluation, 722–723
Menopause, sleep apnea (relationship), 724–725
Menstruation-related hypersomnia, 302
  treatment (effect), pharmacologic agents
    (usage), 302t
Mental disorders, 146
Mental status examination, 19
Mesopontine cholinergic REMS hypothesis,
    49–50
Mesopontine tegmentum, LDT nuclei, 45
Metabolic dysregulation, short sleep duration
    (relationship), 650
Metabolic syndrome, 650, 711
Metabolism, circadian misalignment (effects),
    372f
Metabotropic glutamate receptor 5 system
    (mGluR5), 498
Metabotropic glutamate receptor family, 72
Metabotropic receptors, 64f
  extracellular signal response, 63–64
  signaling, intracellular G proteins (usage), 64f
Methylenedioxyamphetamine (MDA) (Love),
    impact, 87
Methylphenidate
  abuse problems, 755
  adverse effects, 299
  idiopathic hypersomnia usage, 299
  side effect profile, 92
  side effects, 488
  structure, similarity, 87
  sustained release formulations, usage, 292
  usage, 488
Michigan Alcohol Screening Test (MAST),
    751–752

Midbrain junction, postmortem brain analysis,
    43–44
Middle childhood, 452
Mind-body treatments, 134
Mindfulness-based stress reduction (MBSR)
  evidence-based approach, 598
  therapy, 453
Mindfulness-based therapy, 169
Mindfulness training, cognitive behavioral
    therapy (combination), 134
Minimal inspiratory pressure, 250
Minimally invasive tongue base stabilization,
    223–224
Minor stroke, therapeutic target, 652
Mirtazapine
  administration, 114
  usage, 462
Mitogen-activated protein kinase (MAPK), 611
  extracellular signal-regulated protein kinases,
      611
  pathways, 610
Mixed apnea, 208t, 435
Modafinil, 93–94
  abuse problems, 755–756
  action
    mechanism, 94
    mode, 96
  Armodafinil, contrast, 202t
  Armodafinil, *R*-enantiomer, 488
  chemical structure, 87f
  clinical observations, 94
  idiopathic hypersomnia usage, 299
  pharmacokinetics, 93
  side effects, 93–94
  structure, 93
  SWD usage, 384
  uses, 86–87, 93
Modified Fatigue Impact Scale (MFIS), 666
Modified Mallampati classification system,
    218–219
Modified Mallampati system, usage, 218–219
Monoamine oxidase A (MAO-A),
    polymorphism, 656
Monoamine oxidase B (MAO-B) inhibition, 95
Monoamine oxidase B (MAO-B) inhibitors,
    usage, 334
Monoamine oxidase inhibitors (MAOIs), 86, 112
  acute serotonin syndrome, 131–132
  co-administration, 93
  usage, 113
Monoaminergic activity, reduction (permissive
    role), 51
Montage, 639
  term, usage, 629
Montefiore Sleep Questionnaire, 19, 20f–22f
Mood disorders, 185–186
  remission, predictor, 185
  sleep disorders, relationship, 675
  treatment, 185–186
Mood regulatory hypothesis, 181–182
Mood swings, 597
Morbidity, sleep disorders (impact), 281
Morbidity/mortality rates, 257–258
Morningness-Eveningness Questionnaire
    (MEQ), 405
Morning type clock, 369
Mortality rate, 212–213
Motility disorder, 621
Motivational interviewing, 598
Motor activity
  classification, 346b
  reduction, 43
Motor parasomnias, 345
Motor stereotypes, 308–309
Motor vehicle collision risk, factors, 382–383

Mournful sounds, 579
Movement, detection/measurement, 30, 36
Movement disorders
  clinical approach, 357
  therapy, general approach, 357–358
Movement Disorders Society (MDS) task force,
    RLS medication identification, 315
mRNA levels, increase, 610
Multiple sclerosis (MS)
  bilateral hypothalamic lesions, 668f
  excessive daytime sleepiness (EDS),
    prevalence, 667
  fatigue, 666–667
    description, 666
  narcolepsy, association, 669–670
  narcoleptic symptoms, treatment, 670
  nonspecific sleep disturbances, 666–667
  periodic limb movement disorder, 668
  restless legs syndrome, 668
  sleep disorders, 667–670
  sleep disturbances, 666
    prevalence, 666–667
  treatment, medications (usage), 669t
Multiple Sleep Latency Test (MSLT), 4–5, 24, 36–37
  daytime alertness measurement, 102–103
  ease, 156
  indications, 36
  interpretation, 37
  measure, 201
  narcolepsy analysis, 291b
  occurrence, 106
  procedures, 28, 36–37
  usage, 36, 53f, 335
Multiple system atrophy (MSA), 50, 330–331
  neurodegenerative disease, 352–353
  onset, median age, 353
  treatment, 353
Muscarinic cholinergic/histamine H_1 receptors,
    risperidone (affinity), 117
Muscle
  damage, 325
  fatigue, 255–256
  tension (reduction), hot baths (usage), 184
Myelomeningocele
  respiratory complications, 444b
  shunt malfunction, 443–444
Myocardial infarction, risk, 651
Myoclonic jerks, occurrence, 348
Myoclonus (cause/exacerbation), medications
    (usage), 354b

N
Napping, 14, 16
  curtailment/elimination, 153, 156
  excess, 16
Naps
  caffeine, combination, 384–385
  opportunities, 37
  recommendations, 156
Narcolepsy, 485–491
  amphetamines, usage, 85
  Armodafinil, usage, 292
  autoimmune hypothesis, genome-wide
    association studies (impact), 291
  behavioral modification, 291–292
  clinical characteristics, 485–486
  co-morbid conditions, 290
  diagnosis, 291
    hypocretin-1 measurement criteria, 291b
    MSLT, usage, 291b
  diagnostic categories, ICSD-2, 487
  disorders, 294
  epidemiology, 486
  excessive weight gain, 486

Narcolepsy (Continued)
  features, 290
  future treatment, 294–295
  genetic/immunologic aspects, 290–291
  genetic testing, 487
  human leukocyte antigen (HLA) allele
    DQB1*0602, relationship, 485
  hypocretin deficiency, biochemical
    implications, 290
  hypocretin (orexin) system, impact, 290
  investigational agents, 491
  likelihood, positive HLA DQB1*0602 test
    result, 24
  long-acting agents, usage, 292
  management, 291–295
  microdialysis experiments, 91–92
  Modafinil, usage, 292
  modafinil, usage, 86–87
  nonpharmacologic considerations, 294–295
  Orexin, presence, 49f
  overnight polysomnogram, 486
  Paraxanthine, usage, 295
  pathophysiology, 290–291
  pharmacologic treatment, 292–295
    initiation, recommendations, 294
  pregnancy, relationship, 728–729
  prevalence, 289, 486
  RBD, relationship, 552
  recommendations, 302
  selegiline, impact, 95
  sleep disorder, 669–670
  sleep medicine, therapy, 485
  sodium oxybate (SXB), usage, 292
  symptoms, 289–290
  thyrotropin-releasing hormone (TRH), usage,
    295
  treatment, 5, 291–295
    initiation, algorithm, 294f
    strategies, 487–491
  women/men, contrast, 728
Narcolepsy-cataplexy
  diagnosis, 486–487
    establishment, genetic testing, 487
  syndrome, cardinal symptoms, 486b
Narcolepsy-cataplexy
  clinical difference, 291
  inclusion, 289
Nasal airway obstruction
  commonness, 225
  surgery, 225
Nasal continuous positive airway pressure (nasal
    CPAP), 622
Nasal insufflation, 430
  therapy, 201
Nasal mask, 261f
Nasal patency medical therapy, 202
Nasal pillows, 261f
Nasal pressure channel, 34–35
Nasal pressure signal amplitude, 34–35
Nasal valve
  cross-sectional area (increase), corrective
    procedures (usage), 225
  repair, 225
    orbital rim, drill hole, 226f
  suspension, performing, 225
National Center for Sleep Disorders Research
    (NCSDR), 7–8
National Health Interview Survey (NHIS)
  dataset, analysis, 126
National Sleep Foundation (NSF), formation, 8
National Supplier Clearinghouse, application
    review, 234
Necrosis factor (NF-κB)
  impact, 610
  pathway, 610

Nefazodone, 113
Negative ion therapy, 702–703
Neimann-Pick type C disease, 487
Neocortical EEG activation, 49–50
Nernst equation, 71b
Nerve conduction velocity (NCV) tests, 25
Nerve growth factor (NGF), 77–78
Neural crest abnormalities, 440
Neurocognitive model, 161–162
Neurodegenerative disorders, 332
Neurodevelopmental disorders (NDDs), 420,
    493–502
Neurohormones, 74–78
Neuroimaging, 25
Neuroleptics, avoidance, 339–340
Neurologic examination, components, 18–19
Neurologic history, 18
Neuromuscular disease (NMD), 256–257, 267
  mechanism, understanding, 256
  polysomnographic findings, 509
  respiratory failure, 267
  sleep-related hypoventilation, management, 509
  survival, home noninvasive nocturnal
    ventilation (impact), 509
  treatment, absence, 258
Neuromuscular disorders, 508–510
Neuromuscular reflexes, women, 723
Neuronal nicotinic acetylcholine (nACh)
    channels, expression, 65–66
Neuronal NOS (nNOS), 611
  impact, 75
Neurons
  intrinsic excitability, 78
Neuropathologic changes, sleep disorders
    (contribution), 657
Neuropeptides, 74–78
  signaling mechanisms, 65f
Neuropeptide S (NPS), 75
Neuropeptide Y (NPY), 77
Neurophysiologic recording techniques, 639–642
Neurotransmitters
  receptor signaling mechanisms, 66t
  receptor subtypes, 69f–70f
  signaling, 65–74
    mechanisms, 65f
  synthesis pathways, 68f
Nicotinamide adenine dinucleotide phosphate
    (NADPH), 611
Nightmares, 186–187, 478
  disorder, 555–556
    diagnostic criteria, 555b
  dysphoric emotion, 17
  frequency, 555
    reduction, 556
  history, 188
  pharmacologic agents, clinical use, 556
  subclassification, 186
  treatment, 186–187
  vividness, drugs (impact), 769t
Nighttime bruxism, damage, 324
Nighttime cardiovascular events, risk (increase),
    589–590
Nighttime eating disorders, 729
Nighttime ischemic events, 588–589
Nisoxetine, 88–90
Nitric oxide (NO), 75, 611
  impact, 607
Nitric oxide synthase (NOS), impact, 75
N-methyl-D-aspartate (NMDA), ion channel
    classification, 71–72
Nocturia, presence, 335
Nocturnal acid breakthrough (NAB), 620–621
Nocturnal angina, assessment/treatment, 588
Nocturnal arousal, obstructive sleep apnea
    (impact), 326

Nocturnal arterial hemoglobin saturation, NREM/REM sleep (effect), 272f
Nocturnal asthma (NA), 521–522
  sleep architecture, studies, 277t
  sleeping environment, creation, 522
  sleep/wake complaints, 522
  symptoms (lessening), optimal sleep environment (creation), 522t
  treatment, 522
Nocturnal asystole
  QT interval changes, 586–587
  therapy, 587
Nocturnal atrial fibrillation, 587
  therapy, 587
Nocturnal cardiac events, risk (increase), 586t
Nocturnal complaints, improvement, 277
Nocturnal dipping, 521
  blood pressure, reduction, 647
Nocturnal dissociative episode, video prints, 578f
Nocturnal frontal lobe epilepsy (NFLE), 17
  cause, 477
Nocturnal GERD, 525–526
  nonpharmacologic treatment strategies, 526b
Nocturnal hypopneas, impact, 279
Nocturnal hypoventilation, ICSD-2 definition, 508
Nocturnal hypoxemia
  documentation, 274
  SCD predisposition, 524
Nocturnal jerks, 354–356
Nocturnal leg cramps, 346–347
  clinical diagnosis, 347
  differential diagnosis, 347
  etiology, 347
  treatment, 347
Nocturnal low flow oxygen, impact, 280
Nocturnal motor hyperactivity, 354–357
Nocturnal myocardial infarction, 589
  therapy, 589
Nocturnal myocardial ischemia
  angina, relationship, 588–589
  therapy, 589
Nocturnal NIPPV
  BiPAP, combination, 274–275
  initiation, 267
  usage, 266
Nocturnal oxygen desaturation (NOD), 524
Nocturnal oxygen saturation, monitoring (importance), 589f
Nocturnal panic attacks, 638
  differential diagnosis, 356
Nocturnal polysomnogram, usage, 479f
Nocturnal polysomnography, 23–24
  usage, 4–5
Nocturnal seizures, arousal parasomnias (contrast), 477t
Nocturnal sleep
  disruption, 528
  disturbance, 290
  QOL, improvement, 523
Nocturnal sympathetic activation, 649
Nocturnal ventilation, serial adjustments, 510
Nocturnal ventricular arrhythmias, 585–586
  therapy, 586
Non-24-hour circadian rhythm disorder, congenitally blind adolescent (actigraph), 530f
Non-24-hour sleep-wake syndrome (N24HSWS), 38–39, 370–371, 411–413
  adolescent onset, 411
  benzodiazepines, impact, 413
  circadian period, 413
  circadian rhythm disruption, anatomic basis, 417f
  clinical definition, 413

Non-24-hour sleep-wake syndrome (N24HSWS) (Continued)
  clinical diagnostic criteria, 411
  clinical treatments, 412–413
  definitions, 411
  demographics, 411–412
  description, 411
  hypnotic medications, impact, 413
  light therapy, 412–413
  melatonin treatment, 413
  pharmacologic treatment, 413
  phase jumps, 411
  phase response curve (PRC), 412
  risk groups, 371
  scalloping pattern, 411
  sighted patients example, 412f
  sleep, anatomic basis, 417f
  totally blind patient impact, 413–415
Nonarticular rheumatism, 600–602
Nonbenzodiazepine benzodiazepine receptor agonists, 460
Nonbenzodiazepine hypnotics, 174–175
  abuse problems, 754
  characteristics, 176t
  usage, 200
Nonbenzodiazepine RAs, impact, 103
Nonbenzodiazepines, 175t
Nondipping, 213
Nondopaminergic pathways, degeneration, 333
Nonentrained sleep/wake rhythm, 472
Nonepileptic parasomnias, diagnostic issues, 504
Noninflammatory disease, 599
Noninvasive positive pressure ventilation (NIPPV), 258–259
  complications, 261–262
  critical care ventilators, portable ventilators (contrast), 260
  efficacy, 261–262
  equipment, introduction, 260–262
  evolution, 259
  failure, 265–266
  impact, 509
  initiation, 262–263, 265–266
  inspired gas, humidification (absence), 262
  interfaces, 261
    advantages/disadvantages, 262t
  modality, 259
  nocturnal use, 259
  oxygen supplementation, 262
  titration, 264
  triggering, 261
  usage, 262–267
Noninvasive ventilation, action (mechanism), 259
Nonphysician certification, 7
Non-Rapid Eye Movement (NREM) arousal disorders, 641
  parasomnias, 636–637
Non-Rapid Eye Movement (NREM) parasomnias, 187, 476–478
  antidepressant medications, usage, 567
  Benzodiazepines, usage, 566
  CAP usage, biophysiologic markers (abnormalities), 566b
  Clonazepam, usage, 566–567
    FDA approval, 187
  Diazepam, usage, 566
  disorders, association, 561b
  dissociated brain activity, 563b
  dysfunctional behaviors, psychological basis, 187
  etiology, 561b
  genetics, 563
  hypnotherapy, 567–568
  increase, BZRA sedative-hypnotic medication (impact), 562

Non-Rapid Eye Movement (NREM) parasomnias (Continued)
  intracranial monitoring/neuroimaging studies, 562
  management, 477–478
  medications, association, 561b
  Paroxetine, usage, 567
  pathophysiology, 476–477
  pharmacologic treatments, 567
  polysomnographic investigation, 564b
  psychotherapy, 567–568
  therapies, types, 566–567
  treatment, 187, 566b, 568b
Non-Rapid Eye Movement Sleep (NREMS)
  abnormalities, 707
  architecture, maturation (delay), 493
  arousal mechanisms, 561–562
  cyclic alternating pattern (CAP), relationship, 565b
  description, 4
  management, 563–568
  mediation, 607
  microstructure, demonstration, 562f
  onset, 43
  parasomnias
    characterization, 559
    descriptions/mechanisms, 559–560
    epidemiology/clinical associations, 560–561
  pathophysiology, 561–563
  profile, fragmentation, 562
  reports, 183
  stages, 43
  treatment response, CAP biomarker, 565–566
Nonrestorative sleep, 595–596, 601
Nonseasonal depression, bright light therapy (usage), 698
Non-shift workers, comparison, 383t
Nonspecific sleep disturbances, 666–667
Noradrenergic neurons
  degeneration, 333
  REMS-off neurons, 51
Norepinephrine (NE), 70–71
  biogenic monoamine transporter, 85
  clinical correlations, 71
  movement, 88
  overview, 70–71
  sleep-wake regulation, 71
  uptake inhibitors, effects, 90f
Norepinephrine transporter (NET), 88
  inhibition, 70
NREM sleep, burst mode, 47
Nucleotide-binding oligomerization domain (NOD), 614
Nucleotide-binding oligomerization domain-like receptor family, 614
Nucleus tractus solitarius (NTS), 434
Number of awakenings (NAWK), parameters, 169
Numbing, 186

O
Obesity
  adults, treatment selection guidelines, 199t
  antiobesity medication, 195–196
  co-morbid condition, 226
  odds ratio, 519
  OSA risk factor, 195
  prevalence, 520
  severity, 196
  systemic hypertension (increase), OSA (impact), 520
  treatment algorithm, 198f

Obesity hypoventilation syndrome (OHS), 254–255, 263–266
  case series, 255f
  death, risk (increase), 258
  diagnosis, 257–258
  hypercapnia, presence, 254–255
  ICU management, 264–266
  management, 265f
  morbidity/mortality rates, 257–258
  pathogenesis, mechanisms, 256f
  prevalence, 257, 257f, 257t
  untreated OHS, survival curves, 258f
Objective sleep dysfunction, evidence, 690
Obsessive-compulsive disorder (OCD), 690–691
  Clomipramine, FDA approval, 690
  epidemiology, 690
  nonpharmacologic treatment, 691
  objective sleep dysfunction, evidence, 690
  pharmacologic treatment, 690–691
    list, 691t
  phenomenology, 690
  prevalence, 690
  research, 682
  sleep disturbances, 690
  sleep problems, decrease, 542
Obstructive apnea, 208t
Obstructive lung disease, pulmonary function (measures), 271t
Obstructive sleep apnea (OSA), 273
  alleviation, 195
  asthma, relationship, 276–277
  BMI, association, 18
  cerebrovascular complications, pathogenesis (sympathetic overactivity), 649
  cerebrovascular outcomes, relationship, 647–652
  classes, 18
  description (Dickens), 3
  disorder predisposition, 10
  hypnotics, impact, 199–200
  insurance/billing, 234
  nasal insufflation therapy, 201
  nasal patency medical therapy, 202
  occurrence, 273
  opioids, impact, 200
  oxygen therapy, 201
  pharmacologic interventions, 200–202
  polysomnographic characteristics, 338
  positive airway pressure therapy, overview, 206–207
  preoperative screening/management, 197
  prevalence, 276–277
  primary sleep disorder, 638
  REMS suppressant therapy, 201
  risk factors, 4, 232t
  sedatives, impact, 199–200
  serotoninergic agents, impact, 200–201
  sleep complaints, 272
  sleep-related GERD, relationship, 622–623
  sleepwalking, relationship, 565f
  soft palate muscles, relationship, 614
  supplemental oxygen, usage (problems), 201
  support treatment options, evidence levels, 427
  surgical treatment, 428
  syndrome, historical accounts review, 3
  treatment, 647, 661
    CPAP, usage, 623
    options, efficacy/acceptability matrix, 231f
    oral appliance, usage (clinical/cephalometric positive predictors), 233b
    tracheostomy, introduction, 5
  ventilatory stimulants, 201
  wake-promoting agents, 201–202

Obstructive sleep apnea/hypopnea syndrome (OSAHS), 218
  clinical assessment, 218–219
  CPAP therapy, first-line treatment, 218
  Friedman anatomic staging system, 219t
  postoperative follow-up, 227–228
  preoperative considerations, 220
  surgery, approach, 218
  treatment, nasal surgery (usage), 225
Obstructive sleep apnea syndrome (OSAS), 93
  characterization, 243–245
  nocturnal jerks/body movements, 354–356
Obstructive sleep-disordered breathing events, 208f
Occipital electroencephalographic derivations, 38
Occupational history, 18
Occupational performance/safety, 382
Occupational safety/health risks, 381–384
Olanzapine, structure (similarity), 117
Oleamide, 77
Open eyes, light exposure, 470
Operant conditioning, 598
Opiates, 77
  abuse problems, 755
Oral appliances (OAs)
  clinical outcomes, 231t
  complications, 239
  components, 237
  delivery/recall, 237
  dental codes, 234
  fabrication, clinical procedures, 234–235
  medical codes, 234
  retention, 230
  selection, 235–237
  SOAP format, 232
  solutions, 239
  therapeutic effect, 233
  therapy
    function, 230
    sleep-related breathing disorder screening/treatment protocol, 232f
  titratable OA, incremental advancement, 238
  titration, 237–239
  usage
    clinical/cephalometric positive predictors, 233b
    initiation, follow-up evaluation, 238t
    success, 230
Oral dyskinesias, medications (impact), 356b
Oral melatonin, prescribing, 501b
Orexin (ORX), 75
  antagonists, 179
  impact, 62
  presence, 49f
  system, impact, 290
Orexin-A, 46–47
Orexin-B, 46–47
Orexinergic neurons, degeneration, 333
Orexin neurons, 46f
Organized sleep medicine, 5–6
Orlistat, antiobesity medication, 195–196
Oronasal mask (full face mask), 261f
Oropharyngeal narrowing, degree, 282f
OSLER test, 250
Osteoarthritis (OA), 599
  medical management, 599b
  pain, 599
Outpatient circadian phase assessment, 374
Overlap syndrome, 272
  COPD, relationship, 266–267
  prevalence, 257
Overnight PSG
  diagnostic test, gold standard, 647
  obstructive sleep apnea, location, 520
  usage, 262–263

Overnight simplified respiratory polygraphy/continuous electrocardiography, results, 587f
Oversedation, development, 220
Overweight adults, treatment selection guidelines, 199t
Oxygen
  desaturation, predisposition, 266–267
  provision, 254
  saturation
    continuous monitoring, 40
    decrease, 34–35
  supplementation, 248, 262
  therapy, 201
  usage, 275t

P
Pain
  behavior, environmental/sociocultural variables, 598b
  disordered sleep, bidirectional relationship, 596f
  psychosocial distress, 597–598
Painful legs and moving toes (PLMT), 308
Palatal myoclonus (palatal tremor), 349–350
  Guillain-Mollaret triangle, involvement, 350
  surgical treatment, 350
  treatment, 350
Palatal obstruction (correction), surgery (usage), 220
Palatal stiffening, 220
  efficacy, 220
Panic attacks, 686–688
Panic disorder (PD), 686–690
  Alprazolam (Xanax), usage, 688
  benzodiazepines, selection, 688
  cognitive behavioral therapy (CBT), effectiveness, 689
  cognitive influences, 689
  epidemiology, 686–688
  nonpharmacologic treatment, 689–690
  Paroxetine (Paxil), treatment (FDA approval), 688
  pharmacologic treatment, 688–689
    list, 689t
  phenomenology, 686–688
  research, 682
  sleep disturbances, 688
  sleep dysfunction, objective evidence, 688
  treatment, 356
Paracrine, 67b
Paradoxical embolism, 649–650
Paradoxical insomnia, 148
Paradoxical intention (PI), 164–165
Paraneoplastic syndrome, 487
Parasomnia-like behaviors, case reports, 106
Parasomnias, 17, 475–479, 636–638
  commonness, 560–561
  definition, 475
  hypnic starts, 475
  ICSD-2 polysomnographic confirmation, 549
  isolated sleep paralysis, 475–476
  laboratory assessment, 357
  management, 478t
  occurrence, 475–476
  overlap disorder, 550–551
  pathophysiology, 475
  presence, 50
  prevalence, 475
  rhythmic movement disorder, 476
  sleep disorder category, 11b–12b
Paraxanthine, usage, 295
Parkinsonian syndromes, list, 331t
Parkinsonian tremor (rest tremor), 351–352

Parkinsonism
  advancement, hypnograms, 332f
  chromosome 17 (FTDP-17), linkage, 332
  treatment, amphetamines (usage), 85
Parkinson plus syndromes (P+), 330–332
Parkinson's disease (PD)
  Amantadine, usage, 334
  anticholinergics
    treatment-related side effects, 340
    usage, 334
  antidepressants, treatment-related side effects, 340
  anxiety, symptoms, 339
  Carbidopa, usage, 333
  Catechol-O-methyltransferase (COMT)
    Inhibitors, usage, 334
  classical pathophysiology, 333
  co-morbid nonmotor symptoms, 335, 339–340
  daytime sleepiness, orexin/hypocretin system (impact), 333
  deep brain stimulation, 334
    treatment-related side effects, 340
  definitions, 330–332
  dementia, frequency, 335
  depression
    commonness, 335
    symptoms, 339
  dopamine agonists (DAs), impact, 333–334
  dopaminergic agonists, treatment-related side effects, 340
  early morning awakening, 335
  epidemiology, 332
  excessive daytime sleepiness (EDS), commonness, 335
  hallucinations, commonness, 335
  impact, 330
  laboratory assessment, 357
  Levodopa (L-dopa)
    abnormal movements, 354
    arms, kicking/flailing, 354
    treatment-related side effects, 340
    usage, 333
  manifestations, 331b
  medications, usage, 339t
  monoamine oxidase B inhibitors (MAO-B), usage, 334
  motor symptoms, 334–335, 338
  neurodegenerative disorders, 332
  neuroleptics, avoidance, 339–340
  nocturia, presence, 335
  nonmotor symptoms (NMS), 335
  objective measures, 338
  pathophysiology, 333
  polysomnogram, example, 336f
  polysomnography, usage, 338
  premotor symptoms, 18
  primary sleep disorders, 336–337, 340–341
  progressiveness, 330
  RBD, relationship, 333, 552
  REM sleep polysomnogram, 551f
  selegiline, treatment-related side effects, 340
  sleep complaints, 332–333
  sleep-disordered breathing, prevalence, 337
  sleep disorders, 658
    classification, 334–337
    pathophysiology, 333
  sleep fragmentation, reports, 332
  sleepiness (measurement), MSLT (usage), 335
  sleep problems
    diagnosis, 337–338
    history, 337
    treatment, 338–341
  subjective measures, 337–338
  syndromes, 332–333

Parkinson's disease (PD) (Continued)
  treatment, 333–334
    medications, usage, 339t
    treatment-related side effects, 336, 340
    tremor, disappearance, 335
    Unified Parkinson's Disease Rating Scale, 337
Parkinson's Disease Sleep Scale (PDSS), 23
Parkinson's plus syndrome, sleep dysfunction, 352–354
Paroxetine (Paxil)
  characteristics, 112
  PD usage, FDA approval, 688
  usage, 567, 686
Paroxysmal nocturnal events, 638–639
Partial epilepsies (localization-related epilepsies), 630–633
Partial implant extrusion, complication, 220
Partial pressure of carbon dioxide in arterial blood (PaCO$_2$)
  interspace, 246
Partial seizures
  antiepileptic drugs, impact, 635t
  commonness, 631–632
Passive deafferentation theory, 43–44
Patent foramen ovale (PFO), defect, 649–650
Pathogen-associated molecular patterns (PAMPs), 613–614
  recognition, 613–614
  sleep, relationship, 614
Pathologic doubt, 690
Patient health questionnaire (PHQ9), 14
  Depression Scale, 15f
Patient injury, RBD (impact), 550b
Patient referral, 644
Pattern recognition receptors (PRRs), usage, 613–614
Pediatric anxiety, sleep (relationship), 540–541
Pediatric bipolar disorder, sleep (relationship), 540
Pediatric depression, sleep (contrast), 539–540
Pediatric insomnia
  alpha agonists, 462
  antidepressants, 462
  antihistamines, 460
    recommendation, 460
  antipsychotic medications, 462
  benzodiazepines, usage, 458–460
  chloral hydrate, 462
  Eszopiclone (Lunesta), usage, 460
  herbal preparations, pharmacology/clinical properties, 463t
  hypnotic medications, development/testing, 457
  medications, 457
    clinical properties, 461t
    pharmacology, 459t
  melatonin, usage, 458
  Mirtazapine, usage, 462
  nonbenzodiazepine benzodiazepine receptor agonists, 460
  pharmacologic agents, approval (absence), 470
  pharmacologic treatment, approach, 542
  Ramelteon, usage, 458
  research directions, 462–463
  sedative-hypnotics
    properties, 461t
    usage, 458–460
  sodium oxybate (Xyrem), usage, 462
  Trazodone, usage, 462
  Zaleplon (Sonata), usage, 460
  Zolpidem (Ambien), usage, 460
Pediatric insomnia, treatment, 449
Pediatric narcolepsy
  cataplexy, pharmacologic treatment, 490t
  excessive daytime sleepiness, pharmacologic treatment, 489t
  sleepiness, behavioral management, 488b

Pediatric neurologic disorders, 502–510
Pediatric obstructive sleep apnea (OSA)
  conventional treatments, 428–430
  nasal insufflation, 430
  oxygen, usage, 430
  rapid maxillary expansion, treatment, 431
  respiratory support therapies, 430
  surgical therapies, 430–431
  treatment options, 427b
Pediatrics, medications (off-label use), 457
Pedunculopontine nucleus (PPN), degeneration, 333
Pedunculopontine tegmental (PPT)
  brainstem cholinergic activating system location, 48f
  cholinergic neurons, presence, 45
Pemoline, structure (similarity), 87
People with epilepsy (PWE), 634
Peptide pro-opio-melanocortin (POMC), expression, 77
per (circadian clock gene), 4
Perception of self-control (PSC), 688
Perfectionism, 183
Peri-intubation complications, risk (increase), 266
Periodic breathing, 435, 438
Periodic K-alpha electroencephalography, 30-second epoch, 597f
Periodic leg movements (PLMs), 308–309
  basal ganglia, impact, 311
  diet, impact, 312
  dopamine alterations, 311–312
  functional anatomy, 310–311
  iron alterations, 311–312
  lifestyle, effects, 312
  measurement, 308
  movements, 310
  nonspecificity, 308
  occurrence, 308–309
  prevalence estimates, 308
  SSRI/SNRI, impact, 312
  thalamocortical pathways, impact, 311
Periodic leg movements in sleep (PLMS), medications (impact), 356b
Periodic limb movement disorder (PLMD), 308
  definition, 479
  diagnosis, 480
  ICSD-2 diagnostic criteria, 727b
  impact, 668
  iron/dopamine deficiency, role, 481
  movement, 148
  pathophysiology, 479–480
  prevalence, 479
  sleep disorder, 668
Periodic limb movement index (PLMI), 479
Periodic limb movements (PLMs), 479–482
  definition, 479
  diagnosis, 480
  iron deficiency, impact, 531
  pathophysiology, 479–480
  prevalence, 479
  spontaneous flexor-withdrawal, 309
  treatment, 481
Periodic limb movements in sleep (PLMS), 307, 638
  genetic predisposition, 480
  iron deficiency, association, 480
  occurrence, night-to-night variability, 479
  treatment, 481
Periodic limb movements in sleep index (PLMI), 308
Periodic limb movements of sleep (PLMS), 307
  exacerbation, 118
  increase, 113
  women, 727

Periodic limb movement with cortical arousals (PLMA), 480
Periodontal damage, 325
Peripheral nerves, RLS involvement, 310
Persistent sleep, latency, 30
Personality types, research, 186
Pharmacodynamics, 67b
Pharmacokinetics, 67b
Pharmacologic interventions, 195
Pharyngeal airway
    narrowing, supine sleeping (risk factor), 197
    obstruction, forced inspiration (usage), 225
Phase advance shift rotation, diagrammatic representation, 379f
Phase delay/phase advance, 466–467
Phase delay shift rotation, diagrammatic representation, 379f
Phase response curve (PRC), 412
Phase reversal, occurrence, 639
Phasic alpha electroencephalography, 30-second epoch, 596f
Phenothiazines, 116
Phosphatidylinositol-4,5-bisphosphate (PIP$_2$), conversion, 64
Phospholipase C (PLC), stimulation, 64
Photic history, 367
Photosensitizing medications, 701b
Phototherapy, 406–409
    treatment, 407
Physical activity, impact, 14
Physical examination, 18–19
Physiologic arousal, reduction, 184
Physiologic hypnic fragmentary myoclonus (PHM), 349
Physiologic hypnic jerks, 348
Physiologic signals, monitoring, 165
Physiologic tremor, exaggeration, 352
Pickwickian syndrome, 4
Pittsburgh Sleep Quality Index (PSQI), 19, 668
    basis, 281
    correlation, 281
    increase, 278
    usage, 337–338
Plasma concentration, 105f
Polarity, term (usage), 629
Poliomyelitis, 259
Polycythemia, complete blood count (usage), 271–272
Polysomnogram, 28, 181
    all-night histogram, 274f
    performing, 262–263
Polysomnographic (PSG) criteria, 325–326
Polysomnographic (PSG) estimates, 102
Polysomnographic (PSG) laboratory techniques, 113
Polysomnographic (PSG) reevaluation, 25
Polysomnographic (PSG) sleep variables, FGAs/SGAs (effects), 709b
Polysomnographic (PSG) techniques, 116
Polysomnographic technologist, responsibilities, 643b
Polysomnographic (PSG) technologists
    impact, 5
    training, 7
Polysomnography, 639–641
    clinical indications, 29
    recording montage, 29t
    usage, 405
Polysomnography technologist (PSGT)
    responsibilities, 643–644
    role, 641
    vEEG-PSG annotation, 644
Ponto-geniculo-occipital (PGO) spikes, 181
Ponto-geniculo-occipital (PGO) waves, 49–50
Poor sleep hygiene, symptoms, 146b

Portable ventilators, critical care ventilators (contrast), 260
Positional therapy, 197–199
    strategies, 197–198
Positive airway pressure (PAP)
    adherence, education (role), 214–215
    blood pressure, 213
    determination, 210
    devices, function, 206
    endothelial function, 213–214
    heart function, 213
    humidification, effect, 214
    hypnotic agents, usage, 214
    inflammation, 213
    interfaces, 207f
    machines, 209f
    mask, construction, 206–207
    Medicare qualification, 40
    modalities, 208–210
    moods, impact, 214
    mortality rate, 212–213
    neurocognition, impact, 214
    success, 200
    titration
        algorithms, 264
        grading system, 212t
        success, steps, 211t
    treatment, 249
        modality, 23–24
    usage, 275t
Positive airway pressure (PAP) therapy, 195, 200, 263–264
    acceptance, problems, 215
    adherence, 214–215, 264
    adverse effects, 214
    benefits, 210–214
    COPD, contrast, 266
    impact, 213
    indications, 207
    outcome studies, 210–211
    prevalence, 214
Positive HLA DQB1*0602 test result, 24
Positive occipital sharp transients of sleep (POSTS), 643f
Positive pressure ventilation, 258–259
Positron emission tomography (PET), 25
Postarousal central sleep apneas, respiratory dysrhythmia (resemblance), 579
Posterior bipolar montages, 639
Posterior fossa decompression, 506
Posterior hypothalamus, orexin (impact), 62
Posterior-lateral hypothalamic (PLH) region, wake-promoting neurons (existence), 46–47
Postictal, term (usage), 629
Post-myocardial infarction patients, 589–590
Post-traumatic stress disorders (PTSDs), 186–187, 357, 685–686
    development, 685
    diagnosis, 188
    epidemiology, 685
    nonpharmacologic treatment, 686
    off-label treatment options, 686
    Paroxetine (Paxil), usage, 686
    pharmacologic treatment, 686
        list, 687t
    phenomenology, 685
    prevalence, 685
    research, 682
    Sertraline (Zoloft), usage, 686
    sleep characteristics, 541
    sleep disturbance, 685
    sleep dysfunction, objective evidence, 685–686
    trauma exposure, medical problems, 685
    treatment, 357
Post-tuberculosis, 259

Prader-Willi syndrome (PWS), 441–443, 494–496
    central hypersomnia, 495
    clinical features, 495b
    excessive daytime sleepiness, 441
    exogenous growth hormone, risks/benefits, 495–496
    genetic basis, 494
    premature death, risk (increase), 496
    sleep-disordered breathing (SDB), 441–442
        commonness, 495
    sleep hypoventilation, 495
    sudden death
        cases, 442–443
        risk, increase, 496
    treatment, success, 442
Pramipexole, usage, 553
Predisposing, Precipitating, Perpetuating (3P) model, 161
Pregabalin, effects, 119–120
Pregnancy
    acid suppressive therapy, usage, 621
    narcolepsy, 728–729
    periodic limb movements of sleep, 727–728
    restless legs syndrome, 727–728
        treatment, 728
    RLS commonness, 317
    safety classifications, sleep disorder medications, 720t–721t
    sleep
        changes, 719
        management, difficulty, 719
    sleep-disordered breathing, relationship, 724
Pregnant women, sleep, 719
    characteristics, 719
Prematurity, apnea, 436–437
Preoptic area (POA), sleep-promoting nuclei, 62
Preschoolers
    bedtime pass, 450–451
    extinction with parental presence (E/PP), 450
    faded bedtime, response cost (inclusion/exclusion), 451–452
    graduated extinction (GE), 450
    insomnia, 448–452
    positive routines (PRs), 451
    scheduled awakenings (SAs), 451
    Standard Treatments, 452
Prescription medications, abuse problems, 753–756
Pressure-cycled ventilators, 260
Pressure-preset machines, pressure delivery, 260
Pressure-preset ventilation, volume-preset ventilation (contrast), 260
Presynaptic EAAT, 71–72
Presynaptic receptors, importance, 65
Presynaptic terminal, receptors (involvement), 67b
Pretrigeminal cat preparation, 49–50
Primary anxiety disorders, co-morbid insomnia (prevalence), 682
Primary insomnia, 148, 735
    physiologic problem, 148
    sleep efficiency, 129
Primary insomnias
    nonpharmacologic treatments, effectiveness, 541–542
Primary signaling mechanisms, 65f
Primary sleep disorders, 340–341, 638
    gastroesophageal reflux disease, 638
    obstructive sleep apnea, 638
Prion diseases, sleep disorders, 659
Probable RSL, 481
Process S, homeostatic sleep drive (impact), 55f
Profile of Mood States (POMS) test, usage, 183–184

Progressive muscle relaxation (PMR), 453
  therapy, 454
Progressive supranuclear palsy (PSP), 330–332, 353
  neurodegenerative disease, 353
  treatment, 353
Prokinetic agents, 621
Prolactin (PRL), 76
Prolonged expiratory apnea, cyanosis
  (inclusion), 435
Propriospinal myoclonus (PSM), 347–348
  diagnosis, 348
  differential diagnosis, 348
  EEG/EMG correlation study, 348
  occurrence, 348
  treatment, 348
Propriospinal psychogenic myoclonus, 348
Prostaglandin D_2 (PGD$_2$), sleep regulation role,
  612
Prostaglandins (PGs), 77
Protein kinase C (PKC), DAG activation, 64
Proton pump inhibitor (PPI)
  acid-suppressive medication, 620
  safety, 621
  usage, 277
Protriptyline, usage, 201
Pseudoaddiction, 749
Pseudomonas aeruginosa (mucoid type), impact, 278
Psychiatric disorders, 11b–12b
  pharmacologic interventions, 542
  sleep disturbances
    relationship, 544b
    treatment, 541–544
Psychobiologic inhibition/attention-intention-
  effort model, 162
Psychodynamic psychotherapy (PPT), 181, 185
  practice, 188
  revision, 188–189
Psychogenic disorders, 638
  suspicion, 641
Psychogenic nonepileptic spells (PNES), 638
  dissociative episodes, 638
  occurrence, 641
Psychologic arousal, 183
Psychology, role, 183–187
Psychomotor vigilance test (PVT), 24
Psychopharmacologic revolution, 109
Psychophysiologic insomnia, 13
Psychotropic medication, characteristics, 110t–111t
PTPRD (chromosome 9), 309
Pulmonary function impairment, combination, 274
Pulmonary function test (PFT), 264
Pulmonary hypertension, occurrence, 281
Pure autonomic failure, 50
Pyramidal cells, collective synaptic potentials, 48f

Q
QRS duration, level, 35
QT interval changes, 586–587
Quality of life (QOL), 143
  improvement, 523, 525
Quality of Life Index (QLI), 666
Quan, Stuart, 5
Questionnaires, usage, 19–23
Quetiapine
  importance, 117
  treatment usage, clinical reports, 118
Quite wake EEG, 44f

R
Racemic modafinil, development, 93
Radiofrequency tongue base reduction (RFBOT),
  221–222
  radiofrequency energy, delivery, 222f

Ramelteon
  melatonin receptor agonist, 179
  nonsedating medication, 176
  usage, 458
Rapid eye movement (REM), 17
  abnormalities, diagnostic implications, 183t
  correlates, 182–183
  density, 493
  description, 4
  duration, reduction, 119–120
  parasomnias, 637–638
  periods, interruption, 188
  rebound, 115–116
  REM-off switch, 50f
  REM-on switch, 50f
  sleep (decrease), TCAs (impact), 200–201
  waking, impact, 182f
Rapid eye movement behavior disorder (RBD),
  637, 641
  suspicion, 641
Rapid eye movement sleep (REMS)
  activity (generation), monoaminergic activity
    (reduction), 51
  behavior disorder, 30, 479
  behavioral disorder, 549–554
  behavioral state, 43
    description, 49
  discovery, 181
  eye movement activity, 707
  flip-flop switch model, 50f
  fragments, intrusion, 48–49
  generalized atonia, 552
  inhibition, Fluoxetine (impact), 542
  latency, 31–33
  management, 479
  nocturnal polysomnogram, 479f
  onset latency, 707
  parasomnias, 478–479
    management, 478–479
  patterns, abnormality, 31
  polysomnogram, 551f
  promotion, PPN (impact), 333
  REMS-off neurons, 49–50
  suppressant therapy, 201
  time, 707
  total sleep, proportion, 182
  transmission mode, 47
  W/REMS, 50–51
Rapid eye movement sleep behavior disorder
  (RBD), 17, 330, 345
  acetylcholinesterase inhibitors (AIs), usage,
    554
  altered dream content, 550b
  bed partner injuries, 550b
  bedtime melatonin, second-line therapy, 553
  characteristics/treatability, 549
  chronic RBD
    etiologic associations, 551b
    neurologic disorders, 551b
    prodromal period, 549–550
  Clonazepam, long-term benefits, 553b
  development, 18–19
  diagnostic criteria, 550b
  EMG abnormalities, 549
  epidemiology, 551–552
  evaluation, 550
  idiopathic RBD, 552
  lethal behaviors, association, 550b
  narcolepsy, relationship, 552
  nonaggressive behaviors, 551b
  pallidotomy, usage, 554
  parasomnia, 50
  Parkinson's disease, relationship, 333, 552
  pathophysiology, 552
  patient injury, 550b

Rapid eye movement sleep behavior disorder
    (RBD) (Continued)
  pharmacologic agents/therapies, 553b
  Pramipexole, usage, 553
  presentation, 549
  REM sleep polysomnogram, 551f
  risk factors, 551–552
  treatment, 552–554, 661
    environmental considerations, 553b
Rapid eye movement sleep (REMS) regulation,
    46–47
  circuitry, impact, 49–51
  mesopontine cholinergic hypothesis, 49–50
  pathways/transmitter systems, 49–50
  reciprocal interaction model, proposal, 49–50
Rapid-onset obesity with hypothalamic
    dysfunction, hypoventilation, and
    autonomic dysregulation (ROHHAD),
    440–441
  treatment considerations, 441
  tumors, neural crest origin, 440
Reality testing, loss, 182
Reboxetine, 95
Receptors
  overview, 63–64
  pharmacology, terminology, 67b
  signaling, complexity, 64–65
Rechtschaffen, Alan, 4
Recognize, Identify, Stop, Change (RISC)
    method, 184
Recurrent hypersomnia, 300–302
  characterization, 300
  definitions, 300
  management, 300–302
  manifestations, 300t
  pathophysiology, 300
  prevalence, 300
  prophylactic treatment, 301
  symptomatic treatment, 301
  treatment, types, 301
Recurrent isolated sleep paralysis, 554–555
Referential montage, 639
Reflux
  events, 618b
  promotion, foods (avoidance), 618–619
Relaxation
  biofeedback, relationship, 165
  hot baths, impact, 153
  techniques, 165
Repetitive oxygen desaturations, frequency
    (increase), 648–649
Reproductive hormones, sleep (association), 722
Residual insomnia, 709–710
Respiration (RESP), recordings, 591f
Respiratory airflow, recordings, 650f
Respiratory control, 434
  anatomy/physiology, 434
  system, instability, 247
Respiratory depression, development, 220
Respiratory disturbance index (RDI), 35
  apnea episodes, relationship, 207
  change, 196f
  increase, absence, 273
  reduction, 222
Respiratory dysrhythmia
  inter-groaning intervals, 579
  postarousal central sleep apneas, resemblance,
    579
Respiratory effort-related arousal (RERA), 34–35
  CNS arousal, relationship, 207
  definition, 208t
Respiratory events, detection (scoring
    technique), 40
Respiratory muscle weakness, 267
Respiratory pause, 434–435

Restless leg syndrome (RLS), 131, 307–308, 479, 481–483
  assessment, 312–317
  augmentation, 316
  basal ganglia, impact, 311
  Cabergoline, usage, 314–315
  clinical features, 482
  commonness, pregnancy, 317
  co-morbid gastrointestinal disorders, 312
  complaint, 148
  conditions, 726b
  consensus criteria, self-administered
      questionnaires, 308
  definition, 481
  diagnosis, 307–309, 482–483
  diagnostic criteria, 482b
  diet, impact, 312
  discomfort, sensation, 482
  dopamine agonist, selection, 314
  dopamine alterations, 311–312
  dopaminergic systems, dysfunction, 337
  dopaminergic treatment, levodopa (usage), 315
  EDS symptom, 17
  epidemiology, 307
  exacerbation, 118
  expressivity, enhancement (factors), 314b
  frequency, conditions, 317b
  functional anatomy, 310–311
  genetics, 309–310
      underpinnings, 309
  heme iron formulations, usage, 313–314
  history, 481
  impulse control disorders, impact, 316
  intravenous iron, usage (clinical practice
      guidelines), 314
  iron alterations, 311–312
  iron deficiency, 5, 312
      impact, 531
  iron supplementation
      implementation, 312–313
      objective data, 312
  lifestyle, effects, 312
  maintenance difficulty, 482
  management, 483
  medications
      impact, 356b
      usage, MDS task force identification, 315
  motor stereotypes, 308–309
  natural history, 307
  neurobehavioral disturbance, 482
  nonheme iron formulations, usage, 313–314
  nonrestorative sleep, 482
  off-label treatment, 315
  pathophysiology, 309–312, 481–482
  peripheral nerves, involvement, 310
  pharmacologic intervention, 314
  pharmacologic treatment, 741t
  PLMs, demonstration, 308
  prevalence, 307, 481
  sensory discomfort, 481–482
  sensory symptoms, BTBD9 (relationship), 309
  severity scale value, 482
  sleep disorder, 668
  sleep initiation, 482
  spinal cord, involvement, 310
  SSRI/SNRI, impact, 312
  supraspinal networks, involvement, 310–311
  symptoms
      control, peripheral nervous system
          (impact), 310
      mimicking, 18–19
  thalamocortical pathways, impact, 311
  treatment, 312–317, 727
      complications, 316
      flowchart, 313f

Restless leg syndrome (RLS) (Continued)
      ICD/compulsive behaviors, association, 316
      pharmacologic agents, usage, 315b
      special clinical situations, 316–317
Restrictive lung disease, pulmonary function
      (measures), 271t
Restrictive-malabsorptive procedures, 227
Rest tremors (Parkinsonian tremors), 351–352
Retinohypothalamic tract (RHT), impact, 365
Retroglossal obstruction, soft tissue reduction
      surgery, 430
Retrolingual obstruction, surgery, 222–225
Rett syndrome (RS), 441
      development, 496
      dysrhythmic breathing patterns, 441b
      symptomatic/supportive treatments, 497b
      wakefulness data, 442f
Rheumatic disease, sleep/wake-related immune
      functions (impact), 597
Rheumatic disorders, 600
      clinical principles, 595–596
      disordered sleep, treatment, 602–603
      maladaptive personality factors, 598
      polysomnography, 596
      sleep/wake-related systemic disturbances,
          impact, 597
Rheumatic patients, psychosocial distress,
      597–598
Rheumatoid arthritis (RA), 598
      cervical spine disease, presence, 598
      polysomnography, 598
      sleep-disordered breathing, risk factors, 599b
Rheumatoid disease, pain behavior/stress
      management/treatment compliance
      (environmental/sociocultural variables),
      598b
Rheumatologic disorders
      assessment/management, 597–598
      clinical features, 598–602
Rhythmic masticatory muscle activity (RMMA),
      17, 325–326
Rhythmic movement disorders, 345–346, 476
      differential diagnosis, 345
      treatment, 346
Right eye EOG, 37
Right temporal lobe interictal epileptiform
      discharges, 630f–631f
Right temporal lobe seizure onset, 633f–634f
Right temporal lobe seizure termination, 634f
Riluzole, glutamate antagonist, 72
Rise time, 261
Risperidone, affinity, 117
Rolandic epilepsy, 632
Roux-en-Y gastric bypass (RYGB), 196–197, 227
R sleep, increase, 278

S

Salivary cortisol, usage, 373
Salivary melatonin, cortisol rhythms
      (relationship), 373
Sarcoidosis, 600
Scheduled awakening (SAs), 451
      anticipatory awakening, 478
      polysomnographic sleep variables, FGAs/SGAs
          (effects), 709b
      sleep patterns, antipsychotic drugs (effects),
          709–710
Scheduled naps, caffeine (combination), 384–385
Schizophrenia
      antipsychotic drugs
          development, 708
          treatment, sedation (side effect), 710
      Clinical Antipsychotic Trials of Intervention
          Effectiveness (CATIE), 708

Schizophrenia (Continued)
      co-morbid psychiatric illness, treatment, 708
      co-morbid sleep disorders, 710–712
      course/outcome, 705
      diagnosis, 705
      DSM-IV diagnostic criteria, 706b
      environmental factors, 706
      epidemiologic overview, 705
      etiologic factors, 705–706
      first-generation antipsychotics (FGAs), usage,
          707–708, 708b
      multiple personality, contrast, 705
      NREM sleep, abnormalities, 707
      parasomnias, 711
      pathophysiology, 706
      periodic limb movement disorder (PLMD),
          710–711
      personal/societal costs, 712
      pharmacologic treatment, 707–708
      polysomnographic (PSG) sleep variables,
          FGAs/SGAs (effects), 709b
      prognostic indicators, 705
      REM sleep onset latency, 707
      REM sleep time/eye movement activity, 707
      restless legs syndrome (RLS), 710
      second-generation antipsychotics (SGAs),
          usage, 708, 708b
      sleep disorders, association, 710b
      sleep hygiene, problems, 711–712
      sleep maintenance, measures, 707
      sleep patterns, 706–707
          objective assessments, 707
          subjective complaints, 709–710
      sleep-related movement disorders, 710–711
      somnolence, sleep-related breathing disorder
          (association), 711
      split personality, contrast, 705
      symptoms, 705
Scleroderma, 599–600
Scotoperiod, 56
Seasonal affective disorder (SAD), 695
      assessment, 697–698
          inquiry, elements, 697b
          tools, 697b
      Beck Depression Inventory Second Edition
          (BDI-II), 697–698, 697b
      bright light therapy, 698–701
          continuation, 700
          procedure, 700b
          risks, 700–701
          side effects, 700–701, 700b
      circadian misalignment, impact, 697
      clinical signs/symptoms, 696b
      cognitive behavior therapy (CBT), 703
      constant routine protocol, 696–697
      correction, narrowband blue light (usage), 699
      dawn simulator, 699f
      depression, presence, 697
      depressive complaints, 695
          description, 695
      global seasonality score (GSS), 697
          scoring, 698f
      hypomania, reports, 701
      impact, 696
      internal rhythms, alignment, 696–697
      light box, 698f
      light-emitting diodes (LEDs), usage, 699
      light therapy
          dawn simulation, 699
          psychopharmacology, contrast, 702
      light visor, 699f
      major affective disorder criteria, 695
      management, 698–703
          combination approach, case study, 702
      manic episodes, reports, 701

Seasonal affective disorder (SAD) *(Continued)*
  medication management, 701–702
  morning light therapy, effects, 696
  natural history, 696
  negative ion therapy, 702–703
  pathogenesis, 696–697
  photosensitizing medications, 701b
  physiologic/mood disturbances, composite, 696
  prevalence, 696
  psychopharmacology, 701–702
    light therapy, contrast, 702
  Seasonal Pattern Assessment Questionnaire (SPAQ), 697–698, 697b
  signs, 696b
  Structured Interview Guide for the Hamilton Depression Rating Scale-Seasonal Affective Disorder Version (SIGH-SAD), 697–698, 697b
  symptoms, 695, 696b
    development, 695
  treatment, case study, 701
  work station light unit, 699f
Seasonal AR (hay fever), control, 523
Seasonality, assessment, 697
Seasonal Pattern Assessment Questionnaire (SPAQ), 697b
Seasonal pattern specifier (DSM-IV-TR), 695
  criteria, 695b
Secondary obesity, PWS (impact), 494
Secondary prophylaxis, acute TIA/minor stroke (therapeutic target), 652
Second-generation antidepressant drugs, impact, 112
Second-generation antipsychotics (SGAs)
  sedating properties, 709
  usage, 708, 708b
Sedative-hypnotic agents, abuse problems, 753–754
Sedative-hypnotic-induced parasomnia behavior, 564b
Sedative-hypnotics, usage, 458–460
Seizures
  postmarketing observation, 120
  semiology, 629
  timing, 632t
Selective histamine H_1 receptor antagonist, 176
Selective melatonin receptor agonists, 175–176
Selective serotonin reuptake inhibitors (SSRIs), 71b, 112
  acute serotonin syndrome, 131–132
  blockade, 66f
  impact, 68
  marketing, 113
  sleep-wake effects, 677
Selegiline, 95
  treatment-related side effects, 340
Sensorimotor rhythm (SMR), real-time viewing, 165
Sensory parasomnia, 580–581
Septoplasty, 225
Serotonin (SERT) (5-HT), 68–70
  biogenic monoamine transporter, 85
  clinical correlations, 68–70
  impact, 62
  modulation, 569
  overview, 68
  receptors, 200t
  release, increase, 88
  sleep-wake regulation, 68
  subtypes, 200t
Serotonin 5-HT$_{2A}$ receptor antagonists, 179
Serotoninergic neurons
  degeneration, 333
  REMS-off neurons, 51

Serotoninergic system, difficulty, 200
Serotonin-norepinephrine reuptake inhibitors (SNRIs), 71b, 112
  impact, 68
  marketing, 113
  sleep-wake effects, 677
Sertraline (Zoloft), usage, 686
Sexsomnia, 573–576
  evaluation/diagnosis, 574b
  physical/psychosocial consequences, 573–574
  traumatic/sexual psychological stress, histories, 574
Shakespeare, William (sleep description), 3
Shift rotation, impact, 379
Shift systems, difference, 378–379
Shift work, 378–379
  cancer, relationship, 371–372
  cardiometabolic disease, relationship, 371
  CRSD shift work type, ICSD-2 diagnostic criteria, 378b
  driving risks, 382–383
  drowsy driving, 382
  long-term health risks, 383–384
  nonstandard working hours, 378
  occupational safety/health risks, 381–384
  prevalence, 378
Shift work disorder (SWD), 369–370
  CRSD, impact, 378
  description, 378
  management, treatments/countermeasures, 384–385
  Modafinil (Provigil)
    effects (assessment), efficacy measures (improvement), 385f
    usage, 384
Shift workers
  cardiovascular disease, 383–384
  comparison, 383t
  disease contribution, mechanisms (model), 384f
  wakefulness/acute sleep deprivation, 381
Shift-work sleep disorder (SWSD), 38–39, 93
Short sleep duration, metabolic dysregulation (relationship), 650
Short-term nocturnal ventilation, 267
Short-term RDI, reduction, 222
Shoulder-head elevation pillow (SHEP), design, 199
Sibutramine, efficacy, 195–196
Sibutramine Cardiovascular Outcomes (SCOUT) trial, 195–196
Sickle cell disease (SCD), 524–525
  adenotonsillectomy (AT), impact, 524–525
  adjunct therapies, 525
  autosomal recessive disorder, 524
  children, baseline saturation, 524
  hypoxemia, 524
  sleep disorders, diagnostic/treatment strategies, 524–525
Siffre, Michel, 4
Signaling molecules, 74–78
Signal transducers and activators of transcriptions (STATS), 610
Silent Night, 235
Silent Nite
  oral appliance, 236f
  snoring appliance, 236f
Single nucleotide polymorphism (SNP) markers, 480
Single photon emission computed tomography (SPECT), 25
Sjögren's syndrome (SS), 600
  co-morbid anxiety/depression, 597–598
Sleep
  abnormal events, 13b, 16–17
  advancement, 397

Sleep *(Continued)*
  AEDs, direct effects, 635
  alterations, 612
  anatomic basis, 417f
  antiepileptic drugs, direct/indirect effects, 636t
  arousal, women, 724
  arousal levels, psychological experience, 182t
  attacks, 485
  attitudes, change (cognitive strategies), 168b
  Bed Partner Questionnaire, usage, 232b
  behaviors, problems, 29–30
  beliefs, change (cognitive strategies), 168b
  caffeine intake, impact, 14
  cardiac events, 585–589
  cardiovascular system, autonomic changes, 647
  circadian regulation, 53–57
  consolidation, 53–56
    melatonin, impact, 56–57
    SCN, impact, 55–56
  continuity measures, increase, 113
  control
    GABA, impact, 99
    neuronal circuitry, 52f
  cytokines, impact, 608b
  deficiency, 383
  depression, relationship, 540f
  descriptions, 3
  diagnostic studies, 500
  diaries, 402–403
    documents, usage, 23
    sample, 404f
  difficulties, hypnotics (impact), 332–333
  dopamine, impact, 333
  drives, 57
    adenosine, relationship, 51–53
  drug-induced movement disorders, 354
  drugs, effects, 761t–768t
  dysfunction, 352–354
    objective evidence, 683, 685–686, 688
  electrophysiologic recordings, making (ability), 4
  enhancement, substances (usage), 172
  environment, review, 152–153
  epilepsy, interrelation, 634–636
  epochs, classification, 30–31
  esophageal function, 617
  evaluation questions, 13b
  evening activites, impact, 153
  expectations, abnormality, 14
  factor, research, 58
  fragmentation, 332f
    reports, 332
  function
    disruptions, 390
    unified theory, elusiveness, 51
  gate, opening, 368–369
  growth factors, impact, 608b
  health, promotion, 6
  histograms, 32f
  history, 3
    usage, 468b
  HIV, relationship, 613
  homeostasis, 656
    alteration, 161
  homeostatic drive, 465
  homeostatic regulation, 51–53
  humoral regulation, 57–58
  hypoventilation, 495
  impact, 8
  importance (Hippocrates), 3
  improvement
    antidepressants, impact, 603
    exercise, impact, 156–157
  inertia, 381

Sleep (*Continued*)
  initiation, 482
  involuntary movement disorders, 349–350
    persistence, 350–351
  involuntary movements, persistence, 351–352
  laboratory, nocturnal behaviors, 643b
  light studies, 660t
  macroarchitecture, 30–33
    change, 33
  maintenance
    improvement, FGAs, impact, 709
    measures, 707
  menopausal transition, 719–723
  menopausal women, reproductive hormones
    (association), 722
  microarchitecture, 33–34
    waveforms/events, comparison, 33
  modulation, interleukin (usage), 608
  motor activities, classification, 346b
  movement disorders, 345
    clinical approach, 357
    therapy, general approach, 357–358
  MS medications, effects, 669t
  neuropharmacology
    alternative therapies, 78
    historical background, 62–63
  NREM, description, 4
  occupational safety/health risks, 381–384
  onset, 539
    enhancement, alcohol (impact), 14
  organizations, 8
  outcomes (improvement), medical GERD
    therapy (impact), 622
  panic attacks, 688
  parameters, amphetamine derivatives (effects),
    91f
  pathogen-associated molecular patterns,
    relationship, 614
  pathogens, impact, 612–613
  pediatric anxiety, relationship, 540–541
  pediatric bipolar disorder, relationship, 540
  pediatric depression, relationship, 539–540
  periodic limb movement disorder, 479–481
  periodic limb movements, 479–481
  personification, 3
  perspective (early civilization), 3
  pharmacology
    considerations, 63f
    variability, 62–63
  phenomenology, 43
  physical activity, impact, 14
  pregabalin, effects, 119–120
  problems, occurrence, 539
  promotion
    IL-1β, usage, 77
    VLPO, usage, 75
  propensity, circadian rhythm (impact), 368f
  proposal (Aristotle), 3
  purpose, analysis, 3
  quality, impaired/daytime symptoms, 272
  reflux, events, 618b
  research, importance, 6
  respiratory airflow, recordings, 650f
  restriction, therapy, 163–164
    example, 168–169
    guidelines, 164b
  schedules, delay, 398
  scheduling, 166, 470f
  science, 4–5
  scientific observations, 4
  scoring, AASM Manual, 326b
  spindles, 30–31
  stages, 31f
    amount/sequence/pattern, 31
  staging, BZRA (impact), 102–103

Sleep (*Continued*)
  study, 233
    attended laboratory clinical
      polysomnography, 28
  substance abuse, impact, 752t
  supine position, risk factor, 197
  switches, 48–49
    identification, 4
  talking, 581
  threshold time, 163
  timing, 53–56, 369f
    SCN, impact, 55–56
  training, 449
  treatment, 277
    approaches, 602–603
    iatrogenic toxicity/drug-drug interactions,
      monitoring, 602
  trying, avoidance, 154
  wakefulness, differentiation, 30
Sleep, geriatric patient, 735
SLEEP (journal), publication, 5–6
Sleep-active neurons, location, 48
Sleep apnea
  cerebrovascular disease, pathophysiological
    mechanisms, 648–650
  daytime hypertension, relationship, 649
  episode, 34–35
  growth hormone, influence, 442–443
  impact, 650–652
  menopause, relationship, 724–725
  oral appliances
    FDA approval, 240t–241t
    usage, medical codes, 234
  pathophysiology, 246
  therapy, 650–652
  treatment, 294
    impact, 651
Sleep architecture, 272–273
  age, effects, 270
  amphetamine derivatives, effects, 91f
  antidepressant medications, effects, 677
  antiepileptics, effects, 119–120
  antihistamines, effects, 121
  antipsychotic drugs, impact, 116–118
  COPD, inclusion (studies), 273t
  cystic fibrosis, 278–280
    studies, 279t
  effects, 634
  impact, 112–114
  improvement, 523–524
  studies, 271t, 273, 277t
Sleep complaints, 10, 539
  attention deficit hyperactivity disorder
    (ADHD), relationship, 541
  depressive symptoms, co-occurrence, 539
  differential diagnosis, 13b
  history, 13–17
  impact, 541
  treatment, absence, 10
  vasomotor symptoms, association, 722
Sleep deprivation
  antidepressant effects, 677–678
  brain response, impairment, 52f
  forced awakening, combination, 564
  insomnia, contrast, 143
  sleep hygiene, relationship, 635
Sleep-disordered breathing (SDB), 34
  development, 200
  event definitions, 207, 208t
  geriatric patient, 737–740
  impact, 591
  improvement, 523–524
  incident stroke, linking (mechanisms), 648t
  multiple sclerosis, relationship, 667
  occurrence, 505

Sleep-disordered breathing (SDB) (*Continued*)
  Prader-Will syndrome, relationship, 441–442
  prediction, 508–509
  predisposition, 507b
  pregnancy, relationship, 724
  prevalence, 337, 418
    increase, 652
  problems, 496
  risk factors, 599b
  snoring, proxy measure, 650
  status, 591f
  treatment, 503
  ventilation, 258–259
Sleep disorders
  antihistamine efficacy, clinical evidence, 121–122
  antipsychotic drug efficacy, clinical evidence,
    118
  cancer, 528–529
  classification, 10
  commonness, 524
  consequences, 10
  contribution, 657
  CPAP, impact, 4
  dementia, relationship, 656–657
    framework, 657f
  diagnostic/treatment strategies, 524–525
  differential diagnosis, 11b–12b
  dream correlates, 182–183
  efficacy, clinical evidence, 114–115
  factors, 10–13
  follow-up, 25
  impact, 6, 657
  inflammation, relationship, 614–615
  insomnia, relationship, 147–148
  mechanisms, 656–657
  medications, pregnancy safety classifications,
    720t–721t
  mood disorders, relationship, 675
  NREM parasomnias, association, 560
  occurrence, 519
  pathophysiology, 333
  patient assessment, 19b
  presentation, 10
  prevalence, 10
  PSG, usage, 338
  psychodynamic treatments, 188
  psychological treatments, 188–189
  psychology, role, 183–187
  psychotherapy treatments, 188–189
  reevaluation, 25
  REM correlates, 182–183
  role, examples, 3
  schizophrenia, association, 710b
  symptoms, 10–13
  treatment, 5, 657, 659–661
Sleep disruption, 379–381
  approach, 662b
  polysomnographic features, 601
  shift work, relationship, 382
Sleep disturbances
  antidepressant drugs, off-label usage, 115
  impact, 676–677
  prevalence, 666–667
  psychiatric disorders, relationship, 544b
  treatment, 541–544
Sleep duration, 53–56
  chronic sleep deficiency, 381
  circadian rhythm, impact, 368f
  shortness, insulin resistance/systemic arterial
    hypertension, 519
Sleep efficiency (SE), parameters, 169
Sleep Heart Health Study, initiation, 4
Sleep hygiene (SH), 453
  advice, difference, 151
  alcohol, impact, 199

Sleep hygiene (SH) (*Continued*)
  deprivation, relationship, 635
  discussions, usefulness, 154
  focus, 454
  instructions, 158
  problems, 711–712
    symptoms, 146b
  rules, 151–154
    evidence, 155–158
    identification, 152
    publication results, 152t
  smoking cessation, impact, 199
  therapy, effectiveness, 154–155
Sleepiness
  behavioral management, 488b
  cause, SSRIs (impact), 502
  excess, 13b
  levels, improvement, 384
  measurement, MSLT (usage), 335
  MSLT measure, 596
  physiologic determinants, data, 380f
  risk factors, comparison, 382f
  symptom, development, 485
Sleepiness-related collisions, incidence, 383
Sleepiness-related crashes, ATSB operational
    definition, 382
Sleeping pills, usage, 399
Sleeping/waking brain play, disturbances, 600
Sleep latency
  improvement, 384
  measurement, 30
  reduction
    BZRA hypnotics, impact, 102
    neuroleptics, impact, 602
Sleep logs
  basis, 470–471
  example, 469f
  usage, 23, 469
Sleep maintenance insomnia, 735
Sleep medicine, 4–5
  board certification, 7
  clinical procedures, 38–39
  emergence, 8
  history, 181
  modified Mallampati system, adoption, 218–219
  organization, 5–6
  therapy, 485
  U.S. clinical training, 6–7
Sleep medicine diagnostics
  home testing procedures, 28–29
  laboratory procedures, 28
  overview, 28
  procedures, descriptions, 28–29
Sleep onset insomnia, 143, 183, 735
Sleep onset latency (SOL)
  decrease, melatonin (usage), 128
  impact, 115
  parameter, 169
  reduction, 113
Sleep onset REM periods (SOREMPs), 297
  addition, 486
Sleep paralysis, 289–290, 485–486
  isolation, 475–476
  recurrence, 554–555
  REM parasomnia, association, 637–638
  sleep deprivation/irregular sleep-wake
    schedules, impact, 555
  terms, 554
  treatment, 293
Sleep patterns, 16, 55f
  antipsychotic drugs, effects, 709–710
    objective findings, 709
  resetting, 164
  schizophrenia, impact, 706–707
  subjective complaints, 709–710

Sleep phase syndrome, advance/delay, 38–39
Sleep physiology
  antidepressant medication, impact, 112t
  antiepileptic medication, impact, 120t
  antiepileptics, effects, 119–120
  antihistamines, effects, 121
  antipsychotic drugs, impact, 116–118
  antipsychotic medication, impact, 117t
  impact, 112–114
Sleep problems
  diagnosis, 337–338
  history, 337
  treatment, quetiapine (usage), 118
Sleep-promoting circuitry, 48
Sleep-promoting factor, 57–58
Sleep-regulated inflammatory pathways,
    610–612
Sleep regulation
  NF-κB, involvement, 610
  opponent-process model, 466f
  process model, 4
  two-process model, 54–55
Sleep-regulatory inflammatory mediators, role,
    614–615
Sleep regulatory substances, 607
Sleep-related breathing disorders (SRBDs)
  clinical examination, 232–234
  complexity, 243–245
  diagnosis, 23–24
  diagnostic approach, 506
  events, 35f
  oral appliance, usage, 233
  polysomnographic patterns, 243f–245f
  retention, 233
  screening/treatment protocol, 232f
  sleep disorder category, 11b–12b
  somnolence, association, 711
  split-night sleep study procedures, 210
  stability, 233
  therapeutic algorithm, 251f
  tolerance, 233
Sleep-related bruxism (tooth grinding) (SB), 638
  anterior-to-posterior bipolar montage, 642f
  arousals, relationship, 326
  behavioral therapies, 328
  bone damage, 325
  clinical diagnosis, 325
  demographics, 324
  dental damage, 324–325
  dental pathophysiology, 324–325
  diagnosis, 325–326
  etiology, 326
  muscle damage, 325
  nonfunctional oral activity, 324
  occlusal interventions, 327–328
  oral appliances, usage, 327–328
  periodontal damage, 325
  permanent interventions, 327
  pharmacologic interventions, 328
  risk factors, 326
  signs/symptoms, 325b
  teeth, wearing (photograph), 325f
  temporomandibular joint damage, 325
  treatment, 327–328
    modalities, 327
Sleep-related cardiac events, 585
Sleep-related daytime, improvement, 277
Sleep-related disorder
  classification, 573
  history, 232–233
Sleep-related dissociative disorder, 576–579
  daytime dissociated disorders,
    correspondence, 577–578
  diagnostic criteria, 577b
  differential diagnosis, 577b

Sleep-related dissociative disorder (*Continued*)
  ICSD-2 description, 577
  prevalence, 578
Sleep-related dissociative episodes, video-PSG
    recordings, 578–579
Sleep-related eating, case reports, 106
Sleep-related eating disorder (SRED), 568–570
  amnestic SRED, medications, 569b
  dopaminergic agents, usage, 569
  etiology, 568
  ICSD-2 diagnostic criteria, 568b
  pharmacologic treatment, 569b
  Topiramate, usage, 569–570
  treatment, 568–570
Sleep-related epilepsies, 629–634
Sleep-related esophageal symptoms
    (improvement), nasal CPAP (usage), 622
Sleep-related events, artifacts, 641–642
Sleep-related GERD
  associated findings, 618b
  asthma, relationship, 622
  diagnosis, 617–618
  impact, 638
  laryngospasm, relationship, 623
  management, behavioral approaches, 618b
  medical therapy, 620–621
  medications, 620b
    avoidance, 619b
  obstructive sleep apnea, relationship, 622–623
  outcomes, 622–623
  surgical techniques, 621
  therapy, 618–622, 623b
    coordination, 623–624
  treatment, 622
Sleep-related groaning (catathrenia), 579–580
Sleep-related hallucinations, 580–581
  appearance, 581
  differential diagnosis, 581
  occurrence, 581
Sleep-related hyperkinetic seizures, involvement,
    573
Sleep-related hypoventilation, 262–263
  ICSD-2 definition, 508
  management, 509
  symptoms, 508
  treatment, nocturnal ventilation (serial
    adjustments), 510
Sleep-related leg cramps, 17
Sleep-related movement disorders, 17, 345–347,
    638
  polysomnographic criteria, 36
  rhythmic movement activity, occurrence, 17
  schizophrenia, relationship, 710–711
  sleep disorder category, 11b–12b
Sleep-related nocturnal behaviors, differential
    diagnosis, 637t
Sleep-related panic attacks, 356
Sleep-related rhythmic movement disorder
    (SRMD), 638
Sleep-related seizure
  clinical definitions, 629
  definitions, 629
  differential diagnosis, 636–639
  electroencephalography definitions, 629
  epileptiform discharges, 629
Sleep-related sexual behaviors, parasomnias/
    epilepsy (clinical studies), 575t–576t
Sleep-related sexual complaints, evaluation/
    management, 574–576
Sleep Research Society (SRS), 5
Sleep restriction therapy (SRT), 453–454
Sleepsex, 573
  categories, 573
  complaint, evaluation, 576
  management, 576

Sleep talking (somniloquy), paroxysmal nocturnal event, 638–639
Sleep terrors, 187, 476–478, 559–560
characterization, 637
ICSD-2 diagnostic criteria, 560b
mechanism, alternative, 562–563, 563b
Sleep-wake behavior, brain (role), 45f
Sleep-wake circuitry, damage, 656–657
Sleep-wake consolidation, enhancement, 371
Sleep-wake cycles
circadian regulation, 56f
regulation, 367–369
Sleep-wake disturbances, wrist actigraphy basis, 418
Sleep-wake features, 13
Sleep-wake modulation, therapeutic mechanisms, 78
Sleep-wake neurochemistry, overview, 62
Sleep-wake regulation, 66–67
melatonin, endogenous role, 56–57
Sleep/wake-related immune functions, 597
Sleep/wake-related systemic disturbances, 597
Sleep-wake schedule, 13, 37
Sleep/wake schedule, circadian clock (misalignment), 390
Sleep-wake state modulation, endogenous substances (impact), 62
Sleep-wake syndrome, 38–39
Sleepwalking, 187, 476–478, 559
cortical arousal, etiology, 565
description, 577
environmental safety, 564
ICSD-2 diagnostic criteria, 560b
medications/medical conditions, association, 561
obstructive sleep apnea, relationship, 565f
parasomnia behavior, 559
personality case studies, 187
sedative-hypnotic agent, association, 563–564
somnambulism, 636–637
spectral analysis scoring method, 187
Slow wave, 30–31
Slow wave activity (SWA), increase, 656
Slow wave sleep (SWS)
amount, 656
increase, 711
Tiagabine, impact, 119
Smith-Magenis syndrome (SMS), 497–498
Smoking
cessation, sleep hygiene (relationship), 199
decrease/avoidance, 154, 157
prevalence, 199
Snoring
carotid atherosclerosis, relationship, 650
odds ratio (OR), 276–277
oral appliances
dental codes, 234
FDA approval, 240t–241t
risk factors, 232t
Social history, 18
Sodium oxybate (SXB) (Xyrem), 293–294, 462
abuse problems, 754–755
anticataplectic drug usage, 293
dosing/titration, 293
usage, 72, 292, 489–491
warning, 292–293
Somatic symptoms, 600–601
Somatostatin (SS), 76
Somnambulism
medications, impact, 356b
sudden arousal, association, 636–637
zolpidem/zaleplon, impact, 106
Somniloquy (sleep talking), paroxysmal nocturnal event, 638–639

Somnogen
impact, 62
production, 57–58
Somnolence, sleep-related breathing disorder (association), 711
Spectral analysis scoring method, 187
Spina bifida, 505–506
Spinal cord
glycine, inhibitory signal, 74
IML cell column projection, 56
restless legs syndrome, 310
Spinal myoclonus, 350
Spinal segmental myoclonus, 348
Spindle activity, increase, 34
Spirometry, usage, 270
Split-night diagnostic-titration
sleep histogram, 212f
study, 36–37
Split-night titration, 210
Spontaneous awakening, occurrence, 466
Spontaneous-timed (ST) ventilation mode, 260–261
Sporadic Creutzfeldt-Jakob disease, sleep disorders, 659
Sporadic fatal insomnia, sleep disorders, 659
St. John's wort, 132
impact, 132
safety profile, 132
side effects, 132
Stage 1 sleep, elevation, 103
Stage 3-4 sleep
nonbenzodiazepine RAs, impact, 103
reduction, BZRA (impact), 102–103
Stanford Center for Narcolepsy, 486
Stanford Sleepiness Scale, 19
Staphylococcus aureus, 278
State-Trait Anxiety Inventory (STAI), 14
Status cataplecticus, 289
Status epilepticus, 629
Status post-uvulopalatopharyngoplasty (UPPP), 210
Stepanski, Edward, 7
Step-up/step-down pharmacotherapy, 276
Steroids, usage, 283
Stimulants
abuse problems, 755–756
side effects, 292
tolerance, 292
treatments, 95–96
usage, 399
Stimulus control
rules, 155
treatment, 163
Stimulus control therapy (SCT), 167–168, 453–454
components, 163b
instructions, 454, 454b
Stimulus dyscontrol, 161
STOP-BANG, 19
Stress
central adrenal insufficiency, 496
management, 598b
Stress axis hormones, 75
Stroke
accumulated survival curve, 651f
death, ranking, 647
long-term observational studies, 651
risk, 651
increase, OSA (impact), 652
sleep apnea, prevalence, 648t
Structured behavioral activities, 659–660
Structured Interview Guide for the Hamilton Depression Rating Scale-Seasonal Affective Disorder Version (SIGH-SAD), 697b
Study of Women's Health Across the Nation (SWAN), 721

Subjective, Objective, Assessment, and Plan (SOAP) format, 232–234
Subjective insomnia, prevalence, 682
Subjective sleep disturbance, 539
Sublaterodorsal nucleus (SLD)
REMS-on neurons, location, 50
SLD-PC REMS-on neurons, GABAergic interactions, 50
spinally projecting neurons, 50
Submucosal minimally invasive lingual excision (SMILE), 221–222
lingual arteries, identification, 223f
Subparaventricular zone (SPZ), projection, 55–56
Substance abuse
abusers, insomnia treatment, 756–757
alternative medications, impact, 756–757
cognitive behavioral therapy (CBT), usage, 756
components, 752–753
contingency management interventions, 756
DSM-IV definitions, 750t
evidence/information, 752t
impact, 752t
matrix model, 756
patient, approach, 756
Ramelteon, impact, 757
relapse prevention, 756
sleep disorders, relapse risk, 752
sleep issues, 752
supportive-expressive psychotherapy, 756
treatment, 756–757
community reinforcement, 756
strategies, 756
twelve-step facilitation, 756
Substance dependence, DSM-IV definitions, 750t
Substances, impact, 18
Substance use, initiation, 750–751
Substantia nigra, dopaminergic circuits, 73
Subsyndromal SAD (S-SAD)
bright light therapy, 698
effectiveness, 699
signs, 696b
symptoms, 695, 696b
development, 695
Subthalamic nucleus (STN), stimulation, 334
Sudden death, 10
events, circadian occurrence, 647
Sudden infant death syndrome (SIDS), 590
therapy, 590
Sudden unexplained nocturnal death (SUND), 590
therapy, 590
Sudden unexplained nocturnal death syndrome (SUNDS), 590
autopsies, 590
Suggested immobilization test (SIT), 28, 38
indications, 38
interpretation, 38
laboratory procedure, 38
procedures, 38
recordings, 38
Summer SAD, 698
Supplementary sensorimotor seizures, localization, 632
Supportive-expressive psychotherapy (SEP), 756
Suprachiasmatic nucleus (SCN), 4, 71b
biologic clock, role, 54f
dysfunction, impact, 55
endogenous circadian pacemaker, location, 379
impact, 54
light input, indirect assessment, 367
melatonin production, temporal relationship, 367
near-24-hour rhythms, generation, 363
projection, 55–56

Supraspinal networks, RLS (involvement), 310–311
Sympathetic nerve activity (SNA), recordings, 591f
Symptomatic cervicomedullary decompression, suboccipital craniectomy (usage), 507
Symptomatic narcolepsy, 670
Symptomatic obstructive sleep apnea, adenotonsillectomy (AT) treatment, 520
Symptom severity scale (SSS), 600–601
Synaptic GABA$_A$ receptor-mediated tonic inhibition, increase, 119
Synaptic transmission, regulation, 66f
Synaptic vesicle release, 62
Synucleinopathies, 50
Systemic arterial hypertension, 520–521
  co-morbidity, fibromyalgia, 599
Systemic hypertension, treatment, 521
Systemic inflammation, impact, 648–649
Systemic lupus erythematosus (SLE), 599

T

Tai chi, 134
  safety profile, 134
  side effects, 134
Talk therapy, 188
Tap III oral appliance, 236f
  device, usage, 239
Tau accumulation, disorders (sleep disorders), 658–659
Teenagers, DSPS (problem), 465
Temazepam, efficacy, 122
Temporal lobe epilepsy, 631–632
Temporomandibular damage, 325
Tetrahydrocannabinol, 753
Thalamic relay nuclei, 47
Thalamocortical (TC) neurons, firing modes, 47
Thalamocortical (TC) sensory transmission, inhibition, 47
Thalamus, functional integrity, 47
Therapeutic alliance, 189
Therapeutics, 149
Theta rhythms, 33
Thioxanthines, 116
Third wave psychological therapy, 169
Thyroid hormones, melatonin (impact), 129–130
Thyrotropin-releasing hormone (TRH), 96
Thyrotropin-releasing hormone (TRH), usage, 295
Tiagabine, impact, 119
Tics, 350–351
  medications, impact, 355b
Time zones, flying, 392
Tiredness, 595
  assessment, clinical self-rating scales, 596b
Titratable OA, incremental advancement, 238
Toddlers
  bedtime pass, 450–451
  extinction with parental presence (E/PP), 450
  faded bedtime, response cost (inclusion/exclusion), 451–452
  graduated extinction (GE), 450
  insomnia, 448–452
  iron deficiency anemia (IDA), 530
  positive routines (PRs), 451
  rhythmic movements, 476
  scheduled awakenings (SA), 451
  Standard Treatments, 452
Toll-like receptors (TLRs), 611f, 614
Tongue base
  radiofrequency reduction, 222
  stabilization, 223f
Tonic alpha electroencephalography, 30-second epoch, 596f

Tonic phasic hypothesis, 181
Topiramate, usage, 569–570
Total lung capacity (TLC), reduction, 281
  free-running sleep-wake cycle, 414
Totally blind patients, non-24-hour sleep-wake syndrome, 413–415
  clinical definition, 413
  clinical diagnostic criteria, 413–415
  clinical treatments, 415
  definitions, 413
  demographics, 415
  description, 413
  example, 414f
  onset, occurrence, 415
  pharmacologic treatment, 415
Total sleep duration, population-based epidemiologic study, 467f
Total sleep time (TST)
  decrease, 33
  increase, 121–122
  measure, 113
Tourette's syndrome, tics, 350–351
  treatment, 350–351
Tracheostomy, 227, 430
  introduction, 5
Tracing, term (usage), 629
Traditional Chinese medicine, 133
Transcutaneous arterial PCO_2 ($PtCCO_2$), recordings, 650f
Transient ischemic attack (TIA), 647
  sleep apnea, prevalence, 648t
Transient LES relaxations (TLESRs), 617
  inhibition, 620
Transient LES sphincter relaxations, inhibition, 621
Transmission mode, 47
Transpalatal advancement pharyngoplasty (hard palate shortening), 221–222
Transporter, 71b
Trauma exposure, medical problems, 685
Traumatic brain injury (TBI), 421
Trazodone, 113
  add-on therapy, 677
  Fluoxetine, combination usage, 542
  side effects, 462
  usage, 462
Tremors, 351–352
  medications, impact, 355b
Tricyclic antidepressants (TCAs), 112
  impact, 70, 200–201
  pharmacologic effects, 112
  sleep architecture/physiology effects, 112–113
  therapy, combination, 86
Triggering, 261
Tuberomammillary nucleus (TMN)
  brain histamine source, 73
  histamine, impact, 62
  lesion, 45–46
  neurons, GABA (presence), 46–47
Tumor necrosis factor alpha (TNF-α), 77, 607
  impact, 607
  sleep-promoting cytokine, classification, 77
Tumors, neural crest origin, 440
Turbinate reduction, 225

U

Ullanlinna Narcolepsy Scale (UNS), 23
Undisturbed sleep, loss, 528
Unified Parkinson's Disease Rating Scale, 337
Uninterrupted darkness, loss, 528
United States, sleep medicine (clinical training), 6–7
Untreated OHS, survival curves, 258f

Upper airway (UA)
  anatomy, women, 723
  collapsibility, posture (impact), 198–199
  compliance, women, 723
  investigations, 24
  surgeries, 195
  women, 725
Upper esophageal sphincter (UES), protection, 617
Upper teeth, acrylic occlusal splints, 327f
Urinary melatonin, cortisol rhythms (relationship), 373–375
Urine tests, 24
Uvulopalatatopharyngoplasty (UPPP), 220–221, 430
  efficacy, 220
  goal, 220
  tonsils, removal, 221f

V

Vagal nerve stimulation, 504
Vagal nerve stimulators (VNS), 635–636
Valerian, 130–131
  action, mechanisms, 130t
  components, 130
  depressant effect, 131
  pharmacodynamic interactions, 131
  safety profile, 131
  side effect, 131
  species, 130
  usage, 130
Valerianaceae, species, 130b
Valeriana officinalis, remedies, 172–173
Valproic acid, sleep-enhancing effects, 678
Valvular regurgitation, fenfluramine side effect, 195–196
Vascular dementia (VaD), sleep disorders, 658
Vasoactive intestinal peptide (VIP), 76
Vasomotor symptoms
  role, 721–722
  sleep complaints, association, 722
Vaso-occlusive crises, 524
Venlafaxine
  extended-release formulation, 683
  usage, 683
Ventilation
  method, 260
  modes, 260–261
  responses, 255f
Ventilation/perfusion mismatch, 279–280
Ventilators
  classification, 260
  rise time, 261
  strategy, mode (determination), 267
  synchronization, 261
Ventilatory control system (interference), drugs (impact), 248–249
Ventilatory stimulants, 201
Ventral intermediate (VIM) thalamic nucleus, stimulation, 334
Ventral tegmental area (VTA), 92
Ventral tegmentum, dopaminergic circuit, 73
Ventricular arrhythmia
  NREM sleep, impact, 585
  vulnerability, detection, 585–586
Ventro-lateral periaqueductal gray (vlPAG)
  GABAergic interactions, 50
  REMS-off neurons, location, 50
Ventrolateral preoptic (VLPO)
  ARAS, interaction, 48–49
  nucleus, neurons (presence), 49f
  sleep promotion, 75
  sleep switch identification, 4
Vertex sharp waves, 642f

Very low calorie diet (VLCD), 195
Video EEG-PSG
  disadvantages/limitations, 641–642
  interpretation, 642
  PSGT annotation, 644
Video electroencephalography (EEG), 639–641
  monitoring, 639–640
  montages, 640t
Video review, real time speed, 640
Vigilance, states, 43
Visual analog scale (VAS), 19
Vitamin B_{12}, usage, 408
Voltage-gated ion channels, 78
Volume-cycled ventilators, 260
Volume-preset ventilation, 260
  pressure-preset ventilation, contrast, 260
von Economo, Baron Constantine, 43–44, 45f

W
Wake
  drugs, effects, 761t–768t
  maintenance zone, 466
  MS medications, effects, 669t
  periodic limb movements, spontaneous
    flexor-withdrawal, 309
  times, rules, 153
Wake after sleep onset (WASO), 102
  decrease, 116–117
  increase, 33
  parameters, 169
  reduction, 113
  tiagabine, impact, 119
Wake control
  GABA, impact, 99
  neuronal circuitry, 52f
Wakefulness
  dopaminergic effects, anatomic target
    mediation, 92
  duration, acute sleep deprivation, 381
  sleep, differentiation, 30
  test, maintenance, 37–38
  testing, maintenance, 24
    procedures, 28
Wakefulness/REMS (W/REMS), 45
Wake maintenance zone (WMZ),
  368–369
Wake-promoting agents, usage, 201–202
Wake-promoting circuitry, 43–44
Wake-promoting forebrain arousal systems,
  rostral, 47
Wake-up time, phase advancing, 471
Waking
  arousal levels, psychological experience,
    182t
  impact, 182f
  state, EEG characterization, 44f

Waking unrefreshed, 600–601
Wedge pressure, AHI (correlation), 246–247
Weight loss, 195–197
Weight reaccumulation, occurrence, 196
Weight reduction, exercise (impact), 195
West syndrome, 630
White, David, 5
Widespread pain index (WPI), 600–601
Williams syndrome (WS), 498
Women, insomnia, 717–719
  CBT, emphasis, 719
  definition/diagnosis, 717–718
  epidemiology, 717
  hyperarousal disorder, 718
  natural history, 718–719
  outcome, 718
  pathophysiology, 718
  prevalence, 718
    increase, 718
  treatment, 718–719
Women, narcolepsy, 728–729
  clinical presentation, 728
Women, nighttime eating disorders, 729
Women, obstructive sleep apnea, 723–725
  anatomic factors, 723
  body mass index/body habitus, 723
  central ventilatory control, 724
  continuous positive airway pressure (CPAP)
    therapy, 725
  hormonal effects, 724
  neuromuscular reflexes, 723
  oral appliance therapy, 725
  physiologic factors, 723–724
  polysomnography, 723
  sleep apnea, 724–725
  sleep arousal, 724
  sleep-disordered breathing, 724
  symptoms, 723
  treatment, 725
  upper airway anatomy, 723
  upper airway compliance, 723
  upper airway surgery, 725
  weight loss, 725
Women, periodic limb movement disorder,
  725–728
  development, familial tendency, 726
  ICSD-2 diagnostic criteria, 727b
  medications, 726
Women, periodic limb movements of sleep, 727
Women, restless legs syndrome, 725–728
  conditions, 726b
  development, familial tendency, 726
  diagnosis, 725–726
  ICSD-2 diagnostic criteria, 725b
  medications, 726
  pathophysiology, 726
  treatment, 727

Women, sleep disorders, 717
Work shift
  schedules, change (management strategies),
    384–385
Work station light unit, 699f
World Association of Sleep Medicine (WASM), 6
World Federation of Sleep Research and Sleep
  Medicine (WFSRSM) Societies, formation,
  6
World Federation of Sleep Research (WFSR)
  Societies, formation, 6
Worry, symptoms, 682–683
Worrying, control, 184
Worry list, creation, 153, 157

X
Xanthine derivatives, chemical structure, 87f

Y
Yi-gan san, usage, 554
Yoga, 134
  safety profile, 134
  side effects, 134

Z
Zaleplon (Sonata)
  impact, 200
  somnambulism, impact, 106
  usage, 460
Ziprasidone, DA D_2/5-HT_2 receptor blockade,
  117–118
Zolpidem (Ambien)
  extended release, usage, 144
  non-nightly use, efficacy, 102
  somnambulism impact, 106
  usage, 460
Z-palatopharyngoplasty (ZPP), 220–221
  goal, 220
  pain/dysphagia, 221
  palatal flaps, outline, 221f
  UPPP modification, 220